A CD-ROM accompanies this book. Please ensure it is enclosed when the book is returned.

Clinical Obstetrics

The Fetus & Mother

Dedication

To Sharon, Kelie, Brynne, and Sharon-Andrea with greatest love and gratitude.

~E. Albert Reece MD, PhD, MBA

To the memory of my father, who was the best role model anyone could have had, and my mother, who always gave me love and support (despite her never quite understanding what I did for a living).

~John C. Hobbins MD

Clinical Obstetrics

The Fetus & Mother

E. Albert Reece MD, PhD, MBA
Vice President for Medical Affairs, University of Maryland, and
John Z. & Akiko K. Bowers Distinguished Professor and
Dean, School of Medicine,
Baltimore, Maryland

John C. Hobbins MD
Professor of Obstetrics and Gynecology
University of Colorado School of Medicine
University of Colorado Health Sciences Center
Denver, Colorado

FOREWORD BY

Norman F. Gant Jr. MD
Professor and Chairman Emeritus
University of Texas Southwestern Medical School
Executive Director, The American Board of Obstetrics and Gynecology
Dallas, Texas

THIRD EDITION

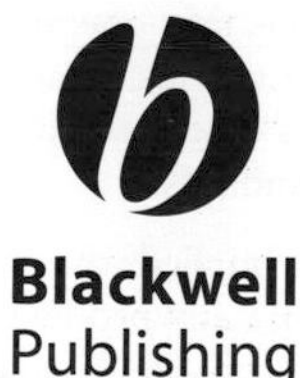

Blackwell
Publishing

Blackwell Publishing, Inc., 350 Main Street, Malden, Massachusetts 02148-5020, USA
Blackwell Publishing Ltd, 9600 Garsington Road, Oxford OX4 2DQ, UK
Blackwell Publishing Asia Pty Ltd, 550 Swanston Street, Carlton, Victoria 3053, Australia

First published 1992 © Lippincott Williams & Wilkins
Second edition 1999 © Lippincott–Raven Publishers
Third edition 2007

1 2007

Library of Congress Cataloging-in-Publication Data

Clinical obstetrics : the fetus & mother / [edited by] E. Albert Reece, John C. Hobbins. – 3rd ed.
p. ; cm.
Rev. ed. of: Medicine of the fetus and mother. 2nd ed. c1999.
Includes bibliographical references and index.
ISBN-13: 978-1-4051-3216-9 (alk. paper)
ISBN-10: 1-4051-3216-7 (alk. paper)
1. Pregnancy. 2. Obstetrics. 3. Pregnancy–Complications. 4. Prenatal diagnosis. 5. Maternal-fetal exchange. I. Reece, E. Albert. II. Hobbins, John C., 1936– . III. Medicine of the fetus and mother.
[DNLM: 1. Fetal Diseases. 2. Embryonic Development. 3. Fetal Development. 4. Maternal-Fetal Exchange. 5. Pregnancy–physiology. 6. Pregnancy Complications. 7. Prenatal Diagnosis.
WQ 211 C641 2006]
RG551.M43 2006
618.3–dc22

A catalogue record for this title is available from the British Library

Set in Sabon 9/12 pt by SNP Best-set Typesetter Ltd., Hong Kong
Printed and bound by Replika Press Pvt. Ltd, India

Commissioning Editor: Stuart Taylor
Development Editor: Rebecca Huxley
Production Controller: Kate Charman
CD production: Meg Barton and Nathan Harris
Production Editor: Karin Skeet

For further information on Blackwell Publishing, visit our website:
http://www.blackwellpublishing.com

The publisher's policy is to use permanent paper from mills that operate a sustainable forestry policy, and which has been manufactured from pulp processed using acid-free and elementary chlorine-free practices. Furthermore, the publisher ensures that the text paper and cover board used have met acceptable environmental accreditation standards.

Contents

Clinical Obstetrics: The Fetus & Mother—Companion CD-ROM
Contents • The complete text • Color versions of over a hundred illustrations from the book • Full text search **Installation** The CD should load automatically on insertion. Alternatively, or to restart after quitting, browse the CD and double-click the file **BMJ_Books_PC** (if using Windows 98 or higher) or **BMJ_Books_MAC** (if using Mac OS 10.2.2 or higher).

Contributors

Kjersti Aagaard-Tillery MD, PhD
MFM Fellow, Division of Maternal–Fetal Medicine, University of Utah, Salt Lake City, UT, USA

Eli Y. Adashi MD
Dean of Medicine and Biological Sciences, Brown Medical School, Providence, RI, USA

Erol Amon
Professor and Director, Department of Obstetrics, Gynecology, and Women's Health, Division of Maternal–Fetal Medicine, St Louis University, St Louis, MI, USA

Janet I. Andrews MD
Associate Maternal–Fetal Medicine, Department of Obstetrics and Gynecology, University of Iowa, Iowa City, IA, USA

Teresita L. Angtuaco MD, FACR, FAIUM, FSRU
Professor of Radiology, Obstetrics, and Gynecology, Director, Division of Imaging and Chief of Ultrasound, Department of Radiology, University of Arkansas for Medical Sciences College of Medicine, Little Rock, AR, USA

R. Lee Archer MD, FAAN
Associate Professor, Department of Neurology, University of Arkansas for Medical Sciences College of Medicine, Little Rock, AR, USA

Masoud Azodi MD
Assistant Professor, Department of Obstetrics and Gynecology, Yale University School of Medicine, New Haven, CT, USA

Ray Bahado-Singh MD
Professor, Department of Obstetrics and Gynecology, Division of Maternal–Fetal Medicine, Wayne State University/Hutzel Women's Hospital, Detroit, MI, USA

Robert H. Ball MD
Associate Professor, Department of Obstetrics, Gynecology, and Reproductive Sciences and Radiology, UCSF Fetal Treatment Center, San Francisco, CA, USA

Frederick C. Battaglia MD
Professor Emeritus, Departments of Pediatrics and Obstetrics–Gynecology, University of Colorado School of Medicine, University of Colorado at Denver and Health Sciences Center, Perinatal Research Center, Aurora, CO, USA

Pamela D. Berens MD
Associate Professor, Department of Obstetrics, Gynecology, and Reproductive Sciences, University of Texas Medical School – Houston, Houston, TX, USA

Matthew J. Bizzarro MD
Assistant Professor, Department of Pediatrics, Yale University School of Medicine, New Haven, CT, USA

D. Ware Branch MD
Professor and H.A. & Edna Benning Presidential Endowed Chair, Department of Obstetrics and Gynecology, University of Utah Health Sciences Center, Salt Lake City, UT, USA

Robert L. Brent MD, PhD, DSc
Distinguished Professor, Departments of Pediatrics, Radiology, and Pathology, Thomas Jefferson University and Alfred I. duPont Hospital for Children, Wilmington, DE, USA

Stephen R. Carr MD
Associate Professor, Department of Obstetrics–Gynecology, Division of Maternal–Fetal Medicine, Brown University, Women and Infants' Hospital, Providence, RI, USA

Véronique Cayol MD
Assistante, Institut de Puériculture et de Périnatalogie, Paris, France

Tim Chard MD, FRCOG
Professor of Obstetrics and Gynaecology, St Bartholomew's Hospital and the Royal London School of Medicine and Dentistry, West Smithfield, London, UK

Frank A. Chervenak MD
Professor and Chairman, Department of Obstetrics and Gynecology, Weill Medical College of Cornell University, New York, NY, USA

Judith L. Chervenak MD, JD
Of Counsel, Heidell, Pittoni, Murphy & Bach, LLP, New York, NY, USA

Edward K.S. Chien MD, FACOG
Assistant Professor, Department of Obstetrics and Gynecology, Women and Infants' Hospital of Rhode Island, Brown University, Providence, RI, USA

Erin A.S. Clark MD
Chief Resident, Department of Obstetrics and Gynecology, University of Utah Hospital, Salt Lake City, UT, USA

Steven L. Clark MD
Director of Perinatal Medicine, Hospital Corporation of America, St. Marks Hospital, Salt Lake City, UT, USA

Richard B. Clark BSM, MD
Professor Emeritus, Departments of Anesthesiology and Obstetrics and Gynecology, University of Arkansas for Medical Sciences College of Medicine, Little Rock, AR, USA

Wayne R. Cohen MD
Chairman, Department of Obstetrics and Gynecology, Jamaica Hospital Medical Center, Professor of Clinical Obstetrics and Gynecology, Weill–Cornell Medical College, Jamaica, NY, USA

Donald R. Coustan MD
Chace/Joukowsky Professor and Chair, Department of Obstetrics and Gynecology, Brown Medical School, Chief Obstetrician and Gynecologist, Women and Infants' Hospital of Rhode Island, Providence, RI, USA

Fernand Daffos MD
Head of the Fetal Medicine Department, Insitut de Puériculture de Paris, CDPMF, Paris, France

Alan H. DeCherney MD
Chief, Reproductive Biology and Medicine Branch, National Institute of Child Health and Human Development, National Institutes of Health, Bethesda, MD, USA

Luis E. De Las Casas MD
Staff Pathologist, Pathology Professional Services, El Paso, TX, USA

Patricia L. Devers MS, CGC
Perinatology Research Branch, National Institute of Child Health and Human Development, National Institutes of Health, Department of Health and Human Services, Wayne State University School of Medicine, Detroit, MI, USA

Gary A. Dildy MD
Associate Professor, Division of Maternal–Fetal Medicine, Department of Obstetrics and Gynecology, University of Utah School of Medicine, UT, USA

Offer Erez MD
Research Associate, Perinatology Research Branch, National Institute of Child Health and Human Development, National Institutes of Health, Department of Health and Human Services, Wayne State University School of Medicine, Detroit, MI, USA

Frederick U. Eruo MD, MPH
Instructor, Department of Obstetrics and Gynecology, University of Cincinnati, Cincinnati, OH, USA

Jimmy Espinoza MSc MD
Assistant Professor, Department of Obstetrics and Gynecology, Wayne State University/Hutzel Women's Hospital, and Perinatology Research Branch, National Institute of Child Health and Human Development, National Institutes of Health, Department of Health and Human Services, Detroit, MI, USA

Mark I. Evans MD
President, Fetal Medicine Foundation of America, Director, Comprehensive Genetics, Professor of Obstetrics and Gynecology, Mt. Sinai School of Medicine, New York, NY, USA

Fred H. Faas MD
Staff Physician, VA Hospital, Professor of Medicine, University of Arkansas for Medical Sciences College of Medicine, Little Rock, AR, USA

Lynda B. Fawcett PhD
Assistant Professor, Department of Pediatrics, Alfred I. duPont Hospital for Children, Wilmington, DE, USA

Helen Feltovich MD, MS
Minnesota Perinatal Physicians, Abbott Northwestern Hospital, Minneapolis, MN, USA

Alan W. Flake MD
Professor, Departments of Surgery and Obstetrics and Gynecology, University of Pennsylvania School of Medicine, Ruth and Tristram C. Colket Jr. Chair of Pediatric Surgery and Director, Children's Institute of Surgical Science, Children's Hospital of Philadelphia, Philadelphia, PA, USA

Alfred D. Fleming MD, FACOG
Professor and Chairman, Department of Obstetrics and Gynecology, Creighton University School of Medicine, Omaha, NE, USA

Jean-Claude Fouron MD, FRCP
Professor, Department of Pediatrics, Université de Montréal, Director of the Fetal Cardiology Unit, Division of Pediatric Cardiology, Hôpital Sainte-Justine, Montréal, QC, Canada

Lara A. Friel MD, PhD
Fellow, Division of Maternal–Fetal Medicine, Department of Obstetrics and Gynecology, Wayne State University/Hutzel Women's Hospital, Detroit, MI, USA

Sandro Gabrielli MD
Attending Physician, Prenatal Medicine, S. Orsola-Malpighi University Hospital, Bologna, Italy

Henry L. Galan MD
Associate Professor, Department of Obstetrics–Gynecology, Division of Maternal–Fetal Medicine, University of Colorado Health Sciences Center, Denver, CO, USA

Norman F. Gant Jr. MD
Professor and Chairman Emeritus, University of Texas Southwestern Medical School, Executive Director, American Board of Obstetrics and Gynecology, Dallas, TX, USA

Ronald S. Gibbs MD
Professor and Chairman, E. Stewart Taylor Chair in Obstetrics and Gynecology, Department of Obstetrics–Gynecology, University of Colorado School of Medicine, Denver, CO, USA

Luís F. Gonçalves MD
Director of Prenatal Diagnosis, Perinatology Research Branch, National Institute of Child Health and Human Development, National Institutes of Health, Department of Health and Human Services, Bethesda, MD, and Detroit, MI, Assistant Professor, Department of Obstetrics and Gynecology, Wayne State University/Hutzel Women's Hospital, Detroit, MI, USA

Ian Gross MD
Professor of Pediatrics, Department of Pediatrics, Yale University School of Medicine, New Haven, CT, USA

Andrée Gruslin MD, FRCS
Associate Professor, Division of Maternal–Fetal Medicine, Department of Obstetrics and Gynecology, University of Ottawa, Ottawa, ON, Canada

James E. Haddow MD
Vice President and Medical Director, Foundation for Blood Research, Scarborough, ME, USA

Zion J. Hagay MD
Professor and Chairman, Department of Obstetrics and Gynecology, Kaplan Medical Center, Rehovot, Israel

Michael R. Harrison MD
Professor of Surgery and Pediatrics, Director, Fetal Treatment Center, Department of Surgery, University of California, San Francisco School of Medicine, San Francisco, CA, USA

Jean C. Hay BSc(Hons), MSc
Associate Professor of Anatomy (retired), Department of Human Anatomy and Cell Science, University of Manitoba, Winnipeg, MB, Canada

Alan Hill MD, PhD
Professor, Department of Pediatrics, University of British Columbia, Consultant Pediatric Neurologist, British Columbia's Children's Hospital, Vancouver, BC, Canada

Washington Clark Hill MD, FACOG
Chairman, Department of Obstetrics and Gynecology, Director, Maternal–Fetal Medicine, Sarasota Memorial Hospital, Sarasota, Clinical Professor, Department of Obstetrics and Gynecology, University of South Florida, College of Medicine, Tampa, Clinical Professor, Department of Clinical Sciences, OB-GYN Clerkship Director-Sarasota, Florida State University College of Medicine, Tallahassee, FL, USA

John C. Hobbins MD
Professor, Department of Obstetrics and Gynecology, University of Colorado School of Medicine, Health Sciences Center, Denver, CO, USA

Calla Holmgren MD
Fellow, Maternal–Fetal Medicine, Department of Obstetrics and Gynecology, University of Utah, Salt Lake City, UT, USA

Carol J. Homko PhD, RN
Assistant Professor, Department of Obstetrics, Gynecology, and Reproductive Sciences, Temple University Hospital, Philadelphia, PA, USA

Judy M. Hopkinson PhD, IBCLC
Associate Professor, Department of Pediatrics, Baylor College of Medicine, Houston, TX, USA

Thomas D. Horn MD, MBA
Chairman, Department of Dermatology, Professor, Departments of Dermatology and Pathology, University of Arkansas for Medical Sciences College of Medicine, Little Rock, AR, USA

Jerri L. Hoskyn MD
Assistant Professor, Department of Dermatology, University of Arkansas for Medical Sciences College of Medicine, Staff Physician, Central Arkansas Veterans' Hospital Administration, Little Rock, AR, USA

Karen A. Hutchinson MD
Director of Medical Education, Bridgeport Hospital, Bridgeport, CT, USA

Philippe Jeanty MD, PhD
Tennessee Women's Care, PC, Nashville, TN, USA

Helen H. Kay MD
Professor and Chair, Department of Obstetrics and Gynecology, University of Arkansas for Medical Sciences College of Medicine, Little Rock, AR, USA

Maureen Keller-Wood PhD
Professor and Chair, Department of Pharmacodynamics, College of Pharmacy, University of Florida, Gainesville, FL, USA

Charles S. Kleinman MD
Professor of Clinical Pediatrics in Obstetrics and Gynecology, Columbia University College of Physicians and Surgeons/Weill Medical College of Cornell University, Chief, Pediatric Cardiac Imaging, New York – Presbyterian Hospital, Division of Pediatric Cardiology, Babies Hospital, New York, NY, USA

Soheila Korourian MD
Associate Professor, Department of Pathology, University of Arkansas for Medical Sciences College of Medicine, Little Rock, AR, USA

Michelle W. Krause MD, MPH
Assistant Professor of Medicine, Division of Nephrology, Department of Internal Medicine, University of Arkansas for Medical Sciences College of Medicine, Little Rock, AR, USA

Juan Pedro Kusanovic MD
Research Associate, Perinatology Research Branch, National Institute of Child Health and Human Development, National Institutes of Health, Department of Health and Human Services, Wayne State University School of Medicine, Detroit, MI, USA

Matthew Laughon MD, MPH
Assistant Professor, Department of Pediatrics, Division of Neonatal/Perinatal Medicine, The University of North Carolina at Chapel Hill, Chapel Hill, NC, USA

Gustavo F. Leguizamón MD
Assistant Professor, Chief, High Risk Pregnancy Unit, Department of Obstetrics and Gynecology, CEMIC University, Buenos Aires, Argentina

Juliana M.B. Leite MD
Nashville, TN, USA

Charles J. Lockwood MD
The Anita O'Keefe Young Professor and Chair, Department of Obstetrics, Gynecology, and Reproductive Sciences, Yale University School of Medicine, New Haven, CT, USA

Curtis L. Lowery MD
Professor and Director, Maternal–Fetal Medicine, Department of Obstetrics and Gynecology, University of Arkansas for Medical Sciences College of Medicine, Little Rock, AR, USA

Barbara Luke ScD, MPH, RN, RD
Professor of Nursing, Obstetrics, and Pediatrics, School of Nursing and Health Studies, University of Miami, Coral Gables, FL, USA

Laurence B. McCullough PhD
Professor of Medicine and Medical Ethics, Center for Medical Ethics and Health Policy, Baylor College of Medicine, Houston, TX, USA

James G. McNamara MD
Chief, Clinical Immunology Branch, Division of Allergy, Immunology, and Transplantation, National Institute of Allergy and Infectious Diseases, National Institutes of Health, Bethesda, MD, USA

Maurice J. Mahoney MD, JD
Professor, Departments of Genetics, Pediatrics, and Obstetrics, Gynecology and Reproductive Sciences, Department of Genetics, Yale University School of Medicine, New Haven, CT, USA

Anita C. Manogura MD
Fellow, Maternal–Fetal Medicine, Department of Obstetrics and Gynecology, University of Maryland, Baltimore, MD, USA

Jennifer L. Melville MD, MPH
Assistant Professor, Department of Obstetrics and Gynecology, University of Washington School of Medicine, Seattle, WA, USA

Aubrey Milunsky MB, BCh, DSc, FRCP, FACMG, DCH
Professor, Departments of Human Genetics, Pediatrics, Pathology, and Obstetrics and Gynecology, Center for Human Genetics, Boston University School of Medicine, Boston, MA, USA

Jeff Milunsky MD, FACMG
Associate Professor, Departments of Pediatrics, Genetics, and Genomics, Boston University School of Medicine, Boston, MA, USA

Howard Minkoff MD
Chairman, Obstetrics and Gynecology, Maimonides Medical Center, Distinguished Professor, Obstetrics and Gynecology, SUNY Downstate, Brooklyn, NY, USA

Fernando R. Moya MD
Director of Neonatology, Coastal AHEC, Wilmington, Professor, Department of Pediatrics, University of North Carolina, Chapel Hill, NC, USA

Thomas D. Myles MD
St. Louis University, Richmond Heights, MO, USA

Jennifer R. Niebyl MD
Professor and Head, Department of Obstetrics and Gynecology, University of Iowa Roy J. and Lucille A. Carver College of Medicine, Iowa City, IA, USA

Jyh Kae Nien MD
Fellow, Perinatology Research Branch, National Institute of Child Health and Human Development, National Institutes of Health, Department of Health and Human Services, Bethesda, MD, and Detroit, MI, USA

The late Carl A. Nimrod MB, BS, FRCS(C)
Formerly Professor and Chair, Department of Obstetrics and Gynecology, University of Ottawa, Ottawa, ON, Canada

Chien Oh MD
Fellow of Maternal–Fetal Medicine, Department of Obstetrics, Gynecology, and Reproductive Sciences, University of Maryland, Baltimore, MD, USA

Lawrence W. Oppenheimer MB, FRCOG, FRCS(UK), FRCS(C)
Associate Professor, Division of Maternal–Fetal Medicine, Department of Obstetrics and Gynecology, University of Ottawa, Ottawa, ON, Canada

Michael J. Paidas MD
Associate Professor, Department of Obstetrics, Gynecology, and Reproductive Sciences, Co-Director, Yale Blood Center for Women and Children, Yale University School of Medicine, New Haven, CT, USA

Glenn E. Palomaki
Director of Biometry, Foundation for Blood Research, Scarborough, MA, USA

Santosh Pandipati MD
Instructor-Fellow, Maternal–Fetal Medicine, University of Colorado Health Sciences Center, Denver, CO, USA

Trivedi Vidhya N. Persaud MD, PhD, DSc, FRCPath(Lond)
Professor Emeritus, Department of Human Anatomy and Cell Science, University of Manitoba, Winnipeg, MB, Canada

Christian M. Pettker MD
Instructor and Clinical Fellow, Division of Maternal–Fetal Medicine, Department of Obstetrics, Gynecology, and Reproductive Sciences, Yale University School of Medicine, New Haven, CT, USA

Gianluigi Pilu MD
Associate Professor, Department of Obstetrics and Gynecology, Prenatal Medicine, S. Orsola-Malpighi University Hospital, Bologna, Italy

Mladen Predanic MSc, MD
Fellow, Division of Maternal–Fetal Medicine, Department of Obstetrics and Gynecology, Weill Medical College of Cornell University, New York, NY, USA

Vivek Raj MB, BS, MD, MRCP(UK)
Associate Professor, Interim Director, Division of Gastroenterology, University of Arkansas for Medical Sciences College of Medicine, Little Rock, AR, USA

E. Albert Reece MD, PhD, MBA
Vice President for Medical Affairs, University of Maryland, and John Z. & Akiko K. Bowers Distinguished Professor and Dean, School of Medicine, and
Professor, Departments of OB/GYN and Reproductive Sciences; Medicine; and Biochemistry and Molecular Biology; Baltimore, MD, USA

Nicola Rizzo MD
Professor of Obstetrics and Gynecology, Prenatal Medicine, S. Orsola-Malpighi University Hospital, Bologna, Italy

Paula K. Roberson PhD
Professor and Chair, Biostatistics, Colleges of Medicine and Public Health, University of Arkansas for Medical Sciences College of Medicine, Little Rock, AR, USA

Roberto Romero MD
Chief, Perinatology Research Branch, Intramural Division, National Institute of Child Health and Human Development, National Institutes of Health, Department of Health and Human Services, Bethesda, MD, and Detroit, MI, USA

Michael G. Ross MD, MPH
Professor and Chairman, Department of Obstetrics and Gynecology, Harbor–UCLA Medical Center, Torrance, CA, USA

Stacy A. Rudnicki MD
Associate Professor of Neurology, University of Arkansas for Medical Sciences College of Medicine, Little Rock, AR, USA

Benjamin P. Sachs MB, BS, DPH, FACOG
Obstetrician-Gynecologist-in-Chief,
Harold H. Rosenfield Professor of Obstetrics, Gynecology, and Reproductive Biology, Harvard Medical School, Department of Obstetrics/Gynecology, Beth Israel Deaconess Medical Center, Boston, MA, USA

Joaquin Santolaya-Forgas MD, PhD
Professor, Wayne State University/Hutzel Women's Hospital, Department of Obstetrics and Gynecology, Perinatology Research Branch, National Institute of Child Health and Human Development, National Institutes of Health, Department of Health and Human Services, Detroit, MI, USA

Peter E. Schwartz MD
John Slade Ely Professor of Gynecology, Yale University School of Medicine, New Haven, CT, USA

Sudhir V. Shah MD, FACP
Professor of Medicine, Division Director of Nephrology, University of Arkansas for Medical Sciences College of Medicine, Little Rock, AR, USA

Eyal Sheiner MD
Attending Physician, Department of Obstetrics–Gynecology, Soroka University Medical Center, Faculty of Health Sciences, Ben-Gurion University, Beer-Sheva, Israel

Bashir S. Shihabuddin MD
Assistant Professor, Department of Neurology, University of Arkansas for Medical Sciences College of Medicine, Little Rock, AR, USA

Baha M. Sibai MD
Professor, Department of Obstetrics and Gynecology, University of Cincinnati College of Medicine, Cincinnati, OH, USA

Robert M. Silver MD
Professor, Department of Obstetrics–Gynecology, Division Chief, Maternal–Fetal Medicine, University of Utah, Salt Lake City, UT, USA

Joe Leigh Simpson MD
Ernst W. Bertner Chairman and Professor, Department of Obstetrics and Gynecology,
Professor, Department of Molecular and Human Genetics, Baylor College of Medicine, Houston, TX, USA

Antonio V. Sison
Chairman, Department of Obstetrics and Gynecology, Robert Wood Johnson University Hospital at Hamilton,
Medical Director, Robert Wood Johnson OB/GYN Group, Hamilton, NJ, USA

Amanda Skoll MD, FRCSC
Associate Professor, Division of Maternal–Fetal Medicine, Department of Obstetrics and Gynecology, University of British Columbia, Vancouver, BC, Canada

Daniel W. Skupski MD
Associate Professor, Obstetrics and Gynecology, Weill Medical College of Cornell University, New York, NY, USA

Michelle Smith-Levitin MD
Director, High Risk Pregnancy Center, North Shore University Hospital, Manhasset, NY, USA

Jessica Spencer MD
Fellow in Reproductive Endocrinology and Infertility, Department of Gynecology and Obstetrics, Emory University, Atlanta, GA, USA

Richard L. Sweet MD
Professor and Vice Chair,
Director, Women's Center for Health, University of California, Davis Medical Center, Sacramento, CA, USA

Kirsten von Sydow PhD
Clinical Psychologist, University of Hamburg, Psychological Institute, Private Psychotherapy Practice, Hamburg, Germany

Brian J. Trudinger MB, BS, MD, FRANZCOG, FRCOG, FRCS(Ed)
Professor of Obstetrics and Gynecology, University of Sydney at Westmead Hospital, Sydney, NSW, Australia

Anthony M. Vintzileos
Professor and Chair, Department of Obstetrics, Gynecology, and Reproductive Sciences, University of Medicine and Dentistry of New Jersey–Robert Wood Johnson Medical School, New Brunswick, NJ, USA

Ronald J. Wapner MD
Professor, Department of Obstetrics and Gynecology, Drexel University College of Medicine, Philadelphia, PA, USA

Josiah F. Wedgwood MD, PhD
Chief, Immunodeficiency and Immunopathology Section, Division of Allergy, Immunology, and Transplantation, National Institute of Allergy and Infectious Diseases, National Institutes of Health, Bethesda, MD, USA

Carl P. Weiner MD, MBA, FACOG
K.E. Krantz Professor and Chair, Department of Obstetrics and Gynecology, University of Kansas School of Medicine, Kansas City, KS, USA

Paul J. Wendel MD
Associate Professor,
Medical Director of Labor and Delivery Division of Maternal–Fetal Medicine, Department of Obstetrics and Gynecology, University of Arkansas for Medical Sciences College of Medicine, Little Rock, AR, USA

Danny Wilkerson MD
Assistant Professor, Departments of Anesthesiology and Obstetrics and Gynecology, University of Arkansas for Medical Sciences College of Medicine, Little Rock, AR, USA

Arnon Wiznitzer MD
Professor and Chairman, Department of Obstetrics and Gynecology, Soroka University Medical Center, Faculty of Health Sciences, Ben-Gurion University, Beer-Sheva, Israel

Kenneth H.H. Wong MD, MBA
Physician, Division of Reproductive Endocrinology and Infertility, Kaiser Permanente, Fontana, CA, USA

Charles E. Wood PhD
Professor and Chair, Department of Physiology and Functional Genomics, University of Florida, Gainesville, FL, USA

Linda L.M. Worley MD
Associate Professor, Departments of Psychiatry and Obstetrics and Gynecology, University of Arkansas for Medical Sciences College of Medicine, Little Rock, AR, USA

Yuval Yaron MD
Director, Prenatal Genetic Diagnosis Unit, Genetic Institute, Tel Aviv Sourasky Medical Center, affiliated to Sackler Faculty of Medicine, Tel Aviv University, Tel Aviv, Israel

Lami Yeo MD
Associate Professor of Obstetrics and Gynecology, Director of Perinatal Ultrasound, Director of Fetal Cardiovascular Unit, Department of Obstetrics, Gynecology, and Reproductive Sciences, Division of Maternal–Fetal Medicine, University of Medicine and Dentistry of New Jersey–Robert Wood Johnson Medical School, New Brunswick, NJ, USA

Edward R. Yeomans MD
Associate Professor, Department of Obstetrics, Gynecology, and Reproductive Sciences, University of Texas-Houston Health Science Center, Lyndon B. Johnson General Hospital, Houston, TX, USA

Foreword

When asked to write the foreword to the third edition of *Clinical Obstetrics—The Fetus & Mother*, I had two immediate thoughts, the first being that I liked the new title better than the former title, *Medicine of the Fetus & Mother*. The second was that those already acquainted with the former title might not recognize the new one. As I had no control over either, I was pleased that I at least could remind readers of the importance of this current work.

When considering a new or forward-thinking idea, concept, or treatise, it is often a good idea to consider where we have been and where we are going. This is especially true when considering clinical obstetrics, which today means both fetus and mother.

Although the fetus could be evaluated prior to the early 1960s, the methods were crude when considered retrospectively. Auscultation and radiography were the primary tools and little could be accomplished to alter fetal outcome other than by delivery. This changed in 1961 with Lily's pioneering work with the use of amniocentesis to manage Rh-isoimmunization.

In less than one professional lifetime, the fetus has become our patient, not just the mother. This rapid evolution has been helped by pioneers in electronic fetal heart rate monitoring, such as Edward Hon, and of course by the use of ultrasound and Doppler evaluations of the fetus. In this last field it is important to acknowledge individuals such as Ian Donald in the United Kingdom. He struggled in the 1960s to develop ultrasound as a useful clinical tool when many of our colleagues in radiology considered such machines to be toys. Certainly, as is obvious in the current textbook, the authors' efforts over the past two decades have proven Dr. Donald right. Many of their own studies have formed the basis for maternal and actual fetal therapy.

It is critically important to recognize in the current textbook that maternal–fetal medicine now encompasses the areas of conception and fetal growth, extending into the neonatal time period. It is now apparent that the basic fundamental biology of conception likely will lead to a better understanding of stem cell biology and basic immunology. Finally, an entire new field of study is developing in understanding how fetal/neonatal illness may result in adult disease(s) many years after birth.

Both the student of obstetrics and the practitioner should read this third edition of what is becoming an essential update of maternal–fetal knowledge. Today's practice is founded upon the principles and practices so clearly presented in this book. This third edition provides the proof that learning can be fun!

Norman F. Gant Jr. MD
2006

Preface

The field of clinical obstetrics and maternal–fetal medicine is undergoing major advances, with rapid strides being made.

The first edition was introduced as the fulfillment of a concept: to combine into one source maternal medicine—an established field focusing primarily on medical complications of pregnancy—and the rapidly evolving field of fetal medicine. The acceptance of this single source book has been overwhelming. The text has been embraced not only by clinical obstetricians but also by maternal–fetal medicine specialists, resident physicians in training, medical students, and others who use the book primarily for its comprehensive obstetrical coverage. The second edition was an updated version of the first edition.

However, this third edition is not only entirely revised, but now has a strong clinical emphasis, while maintaining a scholarly orientation that is expected to be appealing to both clinicians and academicians. The new book title, *Clinical Obstetrics—The Fetus & Mother*, reflects the new orientation of this third edition.

This text is a comprehensive treatise in obstetrics and maternal–fetal medicine. It discusses subjects from the time of conception to delivery, including the normal processes and disease states of the fetus, as well as diagnostic and therapeutic measures that can be used to effect fetal well-being. The fetal medicine section includes prenatal diagnosis and places a strong emphasis on the biology of early pregnancy and the fetal–placental unit, fetal development, and variations in normal embryonic and fetal growth. The influence of teratogens, infections, and fetal diseases on outcome is also discussed. Extensive coverage is given to the prenatal diagnosis of congenital malformations using a variety of modalities, both noninvasive and invasive. The various biophysical and biochemical means of evaluation of fetal well-being are also discussed in great detail. The application of fetal therapy, both surgical and medical, is presented, with limited coverage on the evolving field of gene and cell therapy. In addition, maternal medical complications of pregnancy are thoroughly covered.

Although comprehensive, this book is designed to provide readily accessible information. The overall balance, scope, content, and design fully serve the needs of academic subspecialists, obstetricians, and house staff physicians, as well as other keen students of medicine.

E. Albert Reece MD, PhD, MBA
John C. Hobbins MD
2006

Preface to the first edition

The field of maternal–fetal medicine developed into a recognized subspecialty from the 1950s through the 1970s and subsequently has become the academic arm of obstetrics. With greater sophistication, the field has widened to encompass many other allied areas, including genetics, teratology, diagnostic imaging, fetal and maternal physiology, and endocrinology. In spite of these advances the fetus remained, until recently, inaccessible to the obstetrician/perinatologist. Specialized medical care was provided primarily to the mother with the hope that improving the maternal condition would benefit the fetus. In recent years, the fetus has become accessible through various technologic advances, permitting fetal disease to be diagnosed by various methods including genetics, sonographic or direct *in utero* testing, and treatment administered either medically or surgically.

With the fetus having emerged as a bona fide patient, the field of maternal–fetal medicine has entered a new era. It may no longer be regarded as dealing with medical complications of the mother during pregnancy, but, rather, is to be seen as embodying both normal and diseased processes of both the fetus and the mother. The editors of this textbook believe that physicians in the practice of maternal–fetal medicine need, therefore, to become familiar with the complications of pregnancy that affect the fetus and/or the mother as well as the variety of modalities that are available for diagnosis, evaluation, and treatment.

This textbook is a comprehensive treatise on maternal–fetal medicine. It discusses subjects from the time of conception to delivery, including normal processes and disease states of the fetus, as well as diagnostic and therapeutic measures that can be used. In addition, all maternal medical complications of pregnancy are discussed in detail. A separate volume consisting of a compilation of questions and answers corresponding to each chapter is available for the student of medicine who wishes to test his or her knowledge of the subject.

Although this textbook is comprehensive, it is designed in such a manner that information relating to either the fetus or the mother is readily accessible. The overall balance in scope, content, and design will serve the needs of academic subspecialists, obstetricians, and house staff physicians, as well as other keen students of medicine, very well.

E. Albert Reece MD
John C. Hobbins MD
Maurice J. Mahoney MD
Roy H. Petrie, MD ScD

Acknowledgments

The editors are deeply indebted to all of the contributors, who have invested an enormous amount of time and energy in this project. We count ourselves extremely fortunate to have colleagues and friends who are willing to make this type of investment. The collective efforts have resulted in an entirely revised and most up-to-date book series.

We truly appreciate the invaluable efforts of Ms. Veronika Guttenberger, project specialist in the College of Medicine at the University of Arkansas for Medical Sciences, who assisted in coordinating this entire project. We remain grateful and indebted to her. Carol Homko, PhD, from Temple University School of Medicine made invaluable editorial contributions to this project and we are most appreciative of her assistance.

Finally, we are greatly appreciative of the editors at Blackwell Publishing Ltd., especially Ms. Rebecca Huxley and Dr. Stuart Taylor, for their wise counsel and enduring patience.

The collective efforts of all who contributed to this project are a true testimony of scholarship, commitment, and selflessness. Our lives have been touched by the willingness of everyone to be so generous in sharing their time and talents. Thank you very kindly.

We want to especially acknowledge and thank our good friend and colleague the late Dr. Carl Nimrod, MB, BS, FRCS(C), who contributed so generously to this book series and prior editions. His untimely death saddens us all, but his life and scholarly contributions will brighten our memories.

E. Albert Reece MD, PhD, MBA
John C. Hobbins MD
2006

Abbreviations

17P	17α-hydroxyprogesterone caproate
2,4,5-T	2,4,5-trichlorophenoxyacetic acid
3D	three-dimensional
3DHCT	three-dimensional helical computed tomography
4D	four-dimensional
AA	ascorbic acid
AAP	American Academy of Pediatrics
AC	abdominal circumference
ACA	anticardiolipin antibodies
ACC	agenesis of the corpus callosum
ACE	angiotensin-converting enzyme
ACIP	Advisory Committee on Immunization Practices
ACLA	anticardiolipin antibodies
ACOG	American College of Obstetricians and Gynecologists
ACR	American College of Rheumatology
ACS	acute chest syndrome
ACTH	adrenocorticotropic hormone
ADCC	antibody-dependent cellular cytotoxicity
ADP	adenosine triphosphate
ADPase	adenosine diphosphatase
AED	antiepileptic drug
AF	amniotic fluid
AFE	amniotic fluid embolism
AFI	amniotic fluid index
AFLP	acute fatty liver of pregnancy
AFP	alpha-fetoprotein
AFV	amniotic fluid volume
AGA	appropriate for gestational age
AHA	American Heart Association
AHRQ	Agency for Healthcare Research and Quality
AHT	antihuman globulin
AIDS	acquired immunodeficiency syndrome
AIHA	autoimmune hemolytic anemia
AIT	alloimmune thrombocytopenia
AITP	alloimmune thrombocytopenic purpura
AIUM	American Institute of Ultrasound in Medicine
ALARA	as low as reasonably achievable
ALP	alkaline phosphatase
ALPL	alkaline phosphatase liver gene
ALT	alanine aminotransferase
AMA	advanced maternal age
AMC	arthrogryposis multiplex congenita
ANAs	antinuclear antibodies
AOR	adjusted odds ratio
AP	anteroposterior
APA	antiphospholipid antibodies
APAS	antiphospholipid antibody syndrome
APC	activated protein C
APE	acute pulmonary embolus
APO	adverse pregnancy outcomes
APS	antiphospholipid antibody
aPTT	activated partial thromboplastin time
AR	acrosome reaction
ARDS	acute respiratory distress syndrome
ARF	acute renal failure
ART	assisted reproductive technology
AS	Angelman syndrome
ASB	asymptomatic bacteriuria
ASD	atrial septal defect
ASHA	American Social Health Association
AST	aspartate aminotransferase
ATD	asphyxiating thoracic dystrophy
ATP	adenosine triphosphate
ATPase	adenosine triphosphatase
AV	atrioventricular
AVP	arginine vasopressin
βhCG	β subunit of human chorionic gonadotropic hormone
b.p.m.	beats per minute
BCA	bichloroacetic acid
BCR	B-cell receptor
BEP	bleomycin, etoposide, and platinum
BMI	body mass index
BMT	bone marrow transplantation
BP	blood pressure
BPD	biparietal diameter
BPP	biophysical profile
BR	bilirubin
Btk	Bruton's tyrosine kinase
BUN	blood urea nitrogen
BV	bacterial vaginosis
CAH	congenital adrenal hyperplasia
cAMP	cyclic adenosine monophosphate
CAPS	catastrophic antiphospholipid antibody syndrome

CBC	complete blood count
CBD	common bile duct
CBFA-1	core binding factor A-1
CBT	cognitive behavioral therapy
CCAM	cystic adenomatoid malformation
CCB	calcium channel blockers
CD40L	CD40 ligand
CDC	Centers for Disease Control
CDH	congenital diaphragmatic hernia
CDMP-1	cartilage-derived morphogenetic protein-1
CDs	clusters of differentiation
CEA	carcinoembryonic antigen
CF	cystic fibrosis
cGMP	cyclic guanosine monophosphate
CHB	congenital heart block
CHM	complete hydatidiform mole
CHTN	chronic hypertension
CI	confidence interval
CID	cytomegalic inclusion disease
CKD	chronic kidney disease
CMD	campomelic dysplasia
CMV	cytomegalovirus
CNS	central nervous system
CO	cardiac output
COXIBs	cyclo-oxygenase-2-selective inhibitors
CP	cholestasis of pregnancy
CPD	cephalopelvic disproportion
CPF	chlorpyrifos
CPM	confined placental mosaicism
CREST	calcinosis, Raynaud's phenomenon, esophageal dysmotility, sclerodactyly, and telangiectasia
CRH	corticotropin releasing hormone
CRI	congenital rubella infection
CRL	crown–rump length
CRP	C-reactive protein
CRS	congenital rubella syndrome
CS	Cesarean section
CSE	combined spinal epidural
CSF	cerebrospinal fluid
CSF	colony-stimulating factor
CST	contraction stress test
CT	computed tomography
CVP	central venous pressure
CVS	congenital varicella syndrome
D&C	dilatation and curettage
DAO	diamine oxidase
DC	diamnionic–dichorionic
DES	diethylstilbestrol
DGI	disseminated gonococcal infection
DHA	docosahexanoic acid
DHAS	dehydroepiandrosterone sulfate (Chapter 9)
DHC	dehydrocholesterol
DHEA	dehydroepiandrosterone
DHEAS	dehydroepiandrosterone sulfate (Chapter 5)
DHODH	dihydroorotate dehydrogenase
DHT	dihydroxytestosterone
DIC	disseminated intravascular coagulation
DIF	direct immunofluorescence
DKA	diabetic ketoacidosis
DMARDs	disease-modifying antirheumatic drugs
DMD	Duchenne muscular dystrophy
DNA	deoxyribonucleic acid
DORV	double outlet right ventricle
DS	Down syndrome
DSPC	disaturated phosphatidylcholine
DTDST	diastrophic dysplasia sulfate transporter
DVT	deep vein thrombosis
DZ	dizygotic
E_2	estradiol
E_3	estriol
EBV	Epstein–Barr virus
ECG	electrocardiogram
ECT	electroconvulsive therapy
EDD	estimated delivery date
EDPAF	embryo-derived platelet activating factor
EFM	estimated/electronic/external fetal monitoring
EFW	estimated fetal weight
EGF	epidermal growth factor
EHRF	embryo-derived histamine releasing factor
ELISA	enzyme-linked immunosorbent assay
EMF	electromagnetic fields
EP	ectopic pregnancy
EPA	Environmental Protection Agency
EPCR	endothelial protein C receptor
EPG	early pregnancy factor
ERCP	endoscopic retrograde cholangiopancreatography
ERPF	effective renal plasma flow
ERV	expiratory reserve volume
ESRD	endstage renal disease
ET	essential thrombocytosis
EXIT	*ex utero* intrapartum treatment
FACS	fluorescence-activated cell sorting
FAS	fetal alcohol syndrome
FBM	fetal breathing movements
FBP	fetal biophysical profile
FDA	Food and Drug Administration
FEV	forced expiratory volume
FEV_1	forced expiratory volume in 1 second
FFA	free fatty acid
fFN	fetal fibronectin
FFP	fresh frozen plasma
FGF	fibroblast growth factor
FGFR3	fibroblast growth factor receptor-3 gene
FGR	fetal growth restriction
FHR	fetal heart rate

FIGO	International Federation of Gynecology and Obstetrics
FIGS	fetal intervention guided by sonography
FIL	feedback inhibitor of lactation
F_IO_2	fractional percentage of inspired oxygen
FIRS	fetal inflammatory response syndrome
FISH	fluorescence *in situ* hybridization
FL	femur length
FL/AC	ratio of femur length to abdominal circumference
FM	fetal movements
FMH	fetal–maternal hemorrhage
FNA	fine needle aspiration
FPO	fetal pulse oximetry
FRC	functional residual capacity
FSGS	focal segmental glomerulosclerosis
FSH	follicle-stimulating hormone
FSI	foam stability index
FT	fetal tone
FTA-ABS	fluorescent treponemal antibody absorbed
FVC	forced vital capacity
FVW	flow velocity waveform
G6PD	glucose 6-phosphate dehydrogenase
GALT	galactose-1-phosphate uridyltransferase
GBS	group B *Streptococcus*
GDM	gestational diabetes mellitus
GEE	generalized estimating equations
GFR	glomerular filtration rate
gG	glycoprotein G
GGT	gamma-glutamyltransferase
GH	growth hormone
GH-RH	growth hormone-releasing hormone
GHS	glutathione
GI	gastrointestinal
GIFT	gamete intrafallopian transfer
GM-CSF	granulocyte–macrophage colony-stimulating factor
GMH-IVH	germinal matrix-intraventricular hemorrhage
GnRH	gonadotropin-releasing hormone
GT	gestational thrombocytopenia
GTD	gestational trophoblastic disease
GU	genitourinary
GVHD	graft-versus-host disease
HAART	highly active antiretroviral therapy
HASTE	Half-Fourier Acquisition Single Shot Turbo Spin Echo
HAV	hepatitis A virus
Hb	hemoglobin
HBIG	hepatitis B immune globulin
HBsAg	hepatitis B surface antigen
HBV	hepatitis B virus
HC	head circumference
hCG	human chorionic gonadotropin
HCM	hypertrophic cardiomyopathy
HCQ	hydroxychloroquinone
hCS	human chorionic somatomammotropin
hCT	human chorionic thyrotropin
HCV	hepatitis C virus
HDL	high-density lipopolysaccharide
HE	hereditary elliptocytosis
HELLP	hemolysis, elevated liver enzymes, and low platelets
HEV	hepatitis E virus
Hgb	hemoglobin
HHC	hyperhomocysteinemia
HIT	heparin-induced thrombocytopenia
HIV	human immunodeficiency virus
HLA	human leukocyte antigen
HMO	human milk oligosaccharides
HPA	hypothalamus–pituitary–adrenal (axis)
HPG	hypothalamus–pituitary–gonadal (axis)
HPP	hereditary pyropoikilocytosis
HPT	hypothalamus–pituitary–thyroid (axis)
HPV	human papillomavirus
HS	hereditary spherocytosis
HSC	hematopoietic stem cell
HSD	hydroxysteroid dehydrogenase
HSV	herpes simplex virus
HUAM	home uterine activity monitoring
HUS	hemolytic uremic syndrome
HYN	hypertension
i.m.	intramuscular/intramuscularly
i.v.	intravenous/intravenously
IAT	indirect antiglobulin
ICH	intracranial hemorrhage
ICP	intrahepatic cholestasis of pregnancy
ICSI	intracytoplasmic sperm injection
ICU	intensive care unit
IF	immunosuppressive factor
IFI	isthmic flow index
IFN	interferon
Ig	immunoglobulin
IGF	insulin-like growth factor
IGFBP	insulin-like growth factor binding protein
IgG	immunoglobulin G
IH	impetigo herpetiformis
IHSS	idiopathic hypertrophic subaortic stenosis
IL	interleukin
INH	isoniazid
iNO	inhaled nitric oxide
INR	international normalized ratio
IOM	Institute of Medicine
IPT	intraperitoneal transfusion
IRV	inspiratory reserve volume
ITP	immune thrombocytopenic purpura
IUD	intrauterine contraceptive devices
IUFD	intrauterine fetal demise

IUGR	intrauterine growth restriction
IUT	intrauterine transfusion
IVC	inferior vena cava
IVF	*in vitro* fertilization
IVH	intraventricular hemorrhage
IVIC	Instituto Venezolano de Investigaciones Cientificas
IVIG	intravenous immunoglobulin
IVT	intravascular transfusion
Jak-3	janus kinase 3
kDa	kilodalton
L/S	lecithin–sphingomyelin
LAC	lupus anticoagulant
LARD	lacrimo-auriculo-radial-dental
LBW	low birthweight
LCHAD	long-chain 3-hydroxyl acyl-coenzyme dehydrogenase
LCR	ligase chain reaction
LCSW	licensed clinical social worker
LDA	low-dose aspirin
LDH	lactate dehydrogenase
LET	low energy transfer
LFA	leukocyte function-associated antigen
LGA	large for gestational age
LGSIL	low-grade squamous intraepithelial lesion
LH	luteinizing hormone
LHR	lung–head ratio
LIF	leukemia inhibitory factor
LMA	laryngeal mask airway
LMP	last menstrual period
LMWH	low-molecular-weight heparin
LOR	loss of resistance
LPD	luteal phase defect
LUD	left uterine displacement
LV	left ventricle
LVEDV	left ventricular end-diastolic volume
MA	monoamnionic–monochorionic
MACS	magnetic-activated cell separation
MAOI	monoamine oxidase inhibitors
MAP	mean arterial pressure
MC	diamnionic–monochorionic
MCA	middle cerebral artery
MCHC	mean corpuscular hemoglobin concentration
MCP	metacarpophalangeal
MCV	mean corpuscular volume
MDKD	multicystic dysplastic kidney disease
MDR3	multidrug resistance protein 3
MDR-TB	multidrug-resistant tuberculosis
MED	multiple epiphyseal dysplasia
MFPR	multifetal pregnancy reduction
MG	myasthenia gravis
MHATP	microhemagglutination assay for antibody to *T. pallidum*
MHC	major histocompatibility complex
MIAC	microbial invasion of the amniotic cavity
MIS	mullerian-inhibiting substance
MMA	methylmalonic acidemia
MMC	myelomeningocele
MMI	methimazole
MMP	matrix metalloproteinase
MOA	method of action
MOPP	Mustargen, Oncovin, procarbazine, and prednisone
MPE	maximum permissible exposure
MRI	magnetic resonance imaging
mRNA	messenger RNA
MSAFP	maternal serum alpha fetoprotein
MSD	mean gestational sac diameter
MSH	melanocyte-stimulating hormone
MTCT	mother-to-child transmission
MTHFR	methylene tetrahydrofolate reductase
MTP	metatarsophalangeal
MTR	methionine synthase
MUAC	mid-upper arm circumference
MZ	monozygotic
NE	neutrophil elastase
NEC	necrotizing enterocolitis
NG	*Neisseria gonorrhoea*
NICHD	National Institute of Child Health and Human Development
NICU	neonatal intensive care unit
NIH	National Institutes of Health
NK	natural killer
NLS	neonatal lupus syndrome
NNRTI	non-nucleoside reverse transcriptase inhibitor
NOAEL	no-observed adverse effect level
NPH	neutral protamine Hagedorn
NPO	normal pregnancy outcomes
NPV	negative predictive value
NRFHR	nonreassuring fetal heart rate
NRTI	nucleoside reverse transcriptase inhibitor
NSAIDs	nonsteroidal anti-inflammatory drugs
NSFT	nuchal skinfold thickness
NST	nonstress test
NT	nuchal translucency
NTD	neural tube defect
NVP	nevirapine
OCD	obsessive compulsive disorder
OCT	oxytocin challenge test
OEIS	omphalocele, exstrophy of the bladder, imperforated anus, and spinal defects
OFD	occipitofrontal diameter
OGTT	oral glucose tolerance test

OLEDAID osteopetrosis, lymphedema, ectodermal dysplasia and immunodeficiency
OMIM Online Mendelian Inheritance of Man
OR odds ratio
OSMED otospondylomegaepiphyseal dysplasia
OVD operative vaginal delivery
OVLT organum vasculosum of the lamina terminalis

p.c. post coital
p.o. per os
PAC premature atrial contraction
PACS picture archiving and communication systems
PAF platelet-activating factor
PAI-1 plasminogen activator inhibitor type 1
$P_{a}O_2$ arterial oxygen partial pressure
$P_{A}O_2$ alveolar oxygen partial pressure
PAPP-A pregnancy-associated plasma protein A
PAPSS2 phosphoadenosine-phosphosulfate-synthase 2
PAR protease-activated receptor
PB barometric pressure
PBEF preB-cell colony-enhancing factor
PBMC peripheral blood mononuclear cell
PC phosphatidylcholine
EPCR endothelial protein C receptor
PCA patient-controlled anesthesia
PCB polychlorinated biphenyl
$P\text{CO}_2$ carbon dioxide partial pressure
PCP *Pneumocystis carinii* pneumonia
PCR polymerase chain reaction
PCWP pulmonary capillary wedge pressure
PDA patent ductus arteriosus
PDGF platelet-derived growth factor
PDR *Physicians' Desk Reference*
PEEP positive end-expiratory pressure
PEFR peak expiratory flow rate
PEP polymorphic eruption of pregnancy
PF pruritic folliculitis
PG phosphatidylglycerol (Chapters 6 and 63), pemphigoid gestationis (Chapter 52)
PGE_2 prostaglandin E_2
PHH posthemorrhagic hydrocephalus
PHM partial hydatidiform mole
PHQ patient health questionnaire
PI pulsatility index
PI3 protein inhibitor 3
PID pelvic inflammatory disease
PIH prenancy-induced hypertension
PIOPED Prospective Evaluation of Pulmonary Embolism Diagnosis
PIP proximal interphalangeal
PKU phenylketonuria
PlGF placental growth factor
PMNs polymorphonuclear leukocytes
PNH paroxysmal nocturnal hemoglobinuria
PNM perinatal morbidity
PNMT phenylethanolamine-N-methyltransferase
$P\text{O}_2$ oxygen partial pressure
POMC proopiomelanocortin
PP prurigo of pregnancy
PPD purified protein derivative
p.p.m. parts per million
PPNG penicillin-producing *N. gonorrhoeae*
PPROM preterm premature rupture of membranes
PPV positive predictive value
PRMP pregnancy-related mortality ratio
PROM prelabor rupture of the membranes
PS protein S
PSV peak systolic volume
PT prothrombin time
PTH parathyroid hormone
PTHrp parathyroid hormone-related peptide
PTSD post-traumatic stress disorder
PTT partial thromboplastin time
PTU propylthiouracil
PUBS percutaneous umbilical blood sampling
PVI periventricular hemorrhagic infarction
PVL periventricular leukomalacia
PVN paraventricular nuclei
PWM pokeweed mitogen
PWS Prader–Willi syndrome
PZ protein Z

RAAS renin–angiotensin–aldosterone system
RBC red blood cell
RCT randomized controlled trial
RDA recommended dietary allowance
RFA radiofrequency ablation
RFLP restriction fragment length polymorphism
Rh rhesus
RhIG rhesus immune globulin
rMED recessive multiple epiphyseal dysplasia
RNA ribonucleic acid
ROC receiver–operator curve
ROP retinopathy of prematurity
RPL recurrent pregnancy loss
RPR rapid plasma regain
RPVE re-evaluated pulmonary volume equation
RR relative risk
RT PCR reverse transcription polymerase chain reaction
RV right ventricle (Chapter 7), residual volume (Chapter 40)

SADDAN severe achondroplasia with developmental delay and acanthosis nigricans
SAGES Society of American Gastrointestinal Endoscopic Surgeons
SAH subarachnoid hemorrhage
SAO South-east Asian ovalocytosis
SBE subacute bacterial endocarditis
SCD sickle cell disease

SCID	severe combined immunodeficiency
SCT	sacrococcygeal teratoma
SED-XL	X-linked spondyloepiphyseal dysplasia
SEM	skin, eye, mouth (disease)
SES	socioeconomic status
SGA	small for gestational age
SIADH	syndrome of inappropriate antidiuretic hormone secretion
SIDS	sudden infant death syndrome
SIgA	secretory immunoglobulin A
SLDH	serum lactic dehydrogenase
SLE	systemic lupus erythematosus
SLOS	Smith–Lemli–Opitz syndrome
SLPI	secretory leukocyte protease inhibitor
SM	somatomedin
SNP	single nucleotide polymorphism
SP-A	surfactant protein A
SP-B	surfactant protein B
SP-C	surfactant protein C
SP-D	surfactant protein D
SSFSE	Single Shot Fast Spin Echo
SSRI	selective serotonin reuptake inhibitor
STAN	ST segment automated analysis
STD	sexually transmitted disease
STIC	spatiotemporal image correlation
Sv	sievert
SV	stroke volume
SVR	systemic vascular resistance
SVT	supraventricular paroxysmal tachycardia
SXT	trimethoprim–sulfamethoxazole
T	testosterone
T_3	triiodothyronine
T_4	thyroxine
TAFI	thrombin-activatable fibrinolysis inhibitor
TAR	thrombocytopenia with absent radius (syndrome)
TAS	transabdominal sonography
TAT	thrombin–antithrombin
TBA	total bile acid
TBG	thyroid-binding globulin
TBR	total bilirubin
TCA	tricyclic antidepressants
TCD	transverse cerebellar diameter
TCE	trichloroethylene
TCR	T-cell receptor
Td	tetanus and diphtheria
TEG	thromboelastography
TF	tissue factor
TFPI	tissue factor pathway inhibitor
TGF	transforming growth factor
Th1	type 1 T helper
Th2	type 2 T helper
TIBC	total iron-binding capacity
TIMP	tissue inhibitors of metalloproteinases
TLC	total lung capacity
TMA	transcription-mediated amplification
TNF	tumor necrosis factor
TNSALP	tissue non-specific alkaline phosphatase
TP	thrombophilia
tPA	tissue-type plasminogen activator
TPH	transplacental hemorrhage
TPN	total parenteral nutrition
TPO	thrombopoietin
TRAP	twin reversed arterial perfusion
TRF	thyroid-releasing factor
TRH	thyrotropin-releasing hormone
TRI	trimester
TRNG	tetracycline-resistant *N. gonorrhoeae*
TSH	thyroid-stimulating hormone
TTP	thrombotic thrombocytopenic purpura
TTTS	twin–twin transfusion syndrome
TV	tidal volume (Chapter 40), *Trichomonas vaginalis* (Chapter 63)
TVS	transvaginal sonography
UA	umbilical artery
UC	uterine contractions
UDCA	ursodeoxycholic acid
uPA	urokinase-type plasminogen activator
UPD	uniparental disomy
UPJ	ureteropelvic junction
US	ultrasound
UTI	urinary tract infection
UVB	ultraviolet light
UVpH	umbilical vein pH
V/Q	ventilation–perfusion
VAC	vincristine, actinomycin D, and cyclophosphamide
VACTERL	vertebral, anorectal, cardiac anomalies, tracheo-esophageal fistula, esophageal atresia, renal anomalies, and limb anomalies
VAS	vibroacoustic stimulation
VBAC	vaginal birth after Cesarean section
VDDR1	vitamin D-dependent rickets type 1
VDRL	Venereal Disease Research Laboratory
VE	vacuum extractor
VEE virus	Venezuelan equine encephalitis virus
VEGF	vascular endothelial growth factor
VIP	vasoactive intestinal polypeptide
VLBW	very low birthweight
VLDL	very low-density lipoprotein
VMA	vanylmandelic acid
VPA	valproic acid
VSD	ventricular septal defect
VTE	venous thromboembolism
VTI	velocity time integral
VUR	vesicoureteral reflux
vWD	von Willebrand's disease

vWF von Willebrand's factor
VZIG varicella zoster immune globulin
VZV varicella-zoster virus

WBC white blood cell

ZAM zone of altered morphology
ZDV zidovudine
ZIFT zygote intrafallopian transfer
ZP zona pellucida
ZPI PZ-dependent protease inhibitor

Overview: historical perspectives of fetal medicine

Edward J. Quilligan and Fredrick P. Zuspan

The fetus has never been considered a separate patient but rather an integral part of the pregnancy. It was thoroughly protected from any diagnosis or manipulation; nothing could be done to alter the course or condition of the fetus. It was a passenger, not a patient.

If we can define a patient as someone about whom we can make a diagnosis and treat so as to alter that individual's course, then the fetus became a patient in the period between 1500 and 1600. In 1500, Jacob Nufer, a swine gelder, performed the first recorded successful Cesarean section on his wife. Rousset published a book on Cesarean section in 1588, and in the first Italian book on obstetrics, Mercurio advocated Cesarean section for patients with contracted pelvises.[1] Peter the Elder of the Chamberlen family invented the obstetric forceps.[2] Both of these methods of delivering the fetus, although developed primarily to assist the mother during a difficult delivery, had the potential to alter the fetal environment and thus could be said to treat the fetus, albeit indirectly. The first attempts at fetal diagnosis can be attributed to Marsac, who, in the seventeenth century, first heard the fetal heart beat. In 1818, Mayor, a Swiss surgeon, reported the presence of fetal heart tones; 3 years later, Kergaradec suggested auscultation would be helpful in the diagnosis of twins and the fetal lie and its position.[3] In 1833, Kennedy[4] suggested that the fetal heart rate was indicative of fetal distress. Such distress, if diagnosed late in pregnancy, could be treated using forceps for delivery; however, it was not until relatively recent times that Cesarean section was used to treat fetal distress during the first stage of labor. Douglas and Stromme,[1] in their 1957 text *Operative Obstetrics*, state that "fetal distress was virtually nonexistent as a cause for Cesarean section on our service [New York Hospital] until 10 years ago."

Rh disease

The next major diagnostic step was made by Bevis[5] in 1952. He found a good correlation between amniotic fluid nonheme iron (obtained by amniocentesis) and the severity of fetal anemia. This pioneering work was amplified by Liley,[6] who in 1961 demonstrated that the spectral peak at 450 mU reflected the severity of hemolysis. This gave the obstetrician a method with which to follow the patient with Rh sensitization and, in some cases, deliver the fetus prematurely for fetal salvage. The next major step in the treatment of these Rh-sensitized fetuses was also made by Liley,[7] who in 1964 demonstrated that one could successfully treat these anemic fetuses *in utero* by transfusing blood into the fetal abdomen.

Fetal heart rate monitoring

During this same period, Hon[8] was developing methods for continuous recording of the fetal heart rate and, more important, the factors acting in the fetus that altered the fetal heart rate in response to uterine contractions. He identified three basic patterns: early, late, and variable decelerations, which were due to head compression, uteroplacental insufficiency, and umbilical cord compression, respectively. This permitted the attending obstetrician to assign a cause for the fetal heart rate decelerations that had been described in the 1800s. It also permitted a more individualized therapy for the deceleration: change of position for the variable deceleration and maternal oxygen for the late decelerations. Baseline heart rate change and heart rate variability were also related to specific fetal or maternal conditions.

The association of late decelerations and fetal oxygen deficiency was carried into the antepartum period by Hammacher[9] in 1966. He observed that those infants who had late decelerations of their fetal heart rate in association with spontaneous uterine contractions had lower Apgar scores at birth and a higher stillbirth rate. Pose and Escarcena[10] induced the contractions with oxytocin and found a similar correlation. Ray et al.[11] conducted the first prospective blind trial in the USA and confirmed the results of Hammacher and Pose and Escarcena.

Biochemical monitoring

The fetal heart rate changes are best characterized as biophysical changes. During this same period, fetal biochemical changes related to fetal well-being were being observed. The initial biochemical change associated with fetal health was its ability to make estriol.

Although Spielman et al.[12] and Smith and Smith[13] demonstrated the association between maternal urinary estriol excretion and fetal health in 1933, the test was not used extensively until the 1950s owing to the lack of a reliable and easily performed chemical assay. Brown developed such an assay, and the test was used for many years, finally succumbing to less expensive, more accurate biophysical tests.[14] Another biochemical marker of fetal distress was the acid–base balance of the fetal scalp blood introduced by Saling and Schneider[15] in 1963. This is still a reasonable test to use in selected situations.

Genetic testing

The foregoing discussion of fetal monitoring deals primarily with the oxygenation of the fetus. The development of a method of culturing and examining the chromosomes of the fetal cells residing in the amniotic fluid of the first- and early second-trimester fetus permitted the diagnosis of chromosomal abnormalities when pregnancy could be safely interrupted. In 1949, Barr and Bertram[16] identified the sex chromatin that allowed several investigators[17–20] to use amniotic fluid to determine whether a sex-linked genetic aberration was a possibility in a given pregnancy. Culture of amniotic fluid cells was reported by Jacobson and Barter[21] in 1967. They used available techniques to search for chromosomal abnormalities in 56 pregnancies before 20 weeks of gestation, with a greater than 90% success rate in obtaining adequate chromosomal patterns. Knowledge of chromosomal abnormalities has increased as new techniques such as banding allowed the geneticist a more detailed look at the chromosomal structure; more recently, the development of genetic probes has significantly widened the field of genetic diagnosis. Chromosomal abnormalities were not the only fetal problems that could be determined using amniotic fluid; biochemical determinations allowed the diagnosis of such inheritable diseases as Tay–Sachs disease and many others. Although amniotic sac puncture to obtain fluid had relatively few risks, there were some. This, coupled with the significant work and cost associated with analyzing amniotic fluid for chromosomal abnormalities, has led to restricting the test to those most at risk: older pregnant patients and patients who have a genetic problem in the family or had an abnormal prior pregnancy. The development of maternal blood markers for fetal abnormalities was extremely important because, using the criteria described above, one would miss a significant proportion of fetal problems. For example, although the risk of trisomy 21 is much greater in infants of patients older than age 35 years, screening only these patients failed to detect 75% of the trisomy 21 patients, because these patients were younger than 35 years of age. In 1944, Pederson[22] described a protein found only in the fetus, fetuin. This was the first specific fetal protein. Bergstrand and Czar[23] found another fetal-specific protein, which migrated between the albumen and α globulin fraction. This was named *α-fetoprotein* by Gitlin and Boesman[24] in 1966. In 1972, Brock and Sutcliffe[25] reported elevated levels of α-fetoprotein in the amniotic fluid surrounding fetuses with neural tube defects, and, in 1984, Merkatz and his colleagues[26] noted that pregnant patients with a trisomy 21 fetus had lower than expected maternal levels of α-fetoprotein. This marker allows all pregnant patients to be offered screening for neural tube defects and some trisomics. Placental and fetal cells enter the maternal circulation, albeit in small numbers. Investigators are currently working on methods of harvesting and culturing these cells, which would obviate the need for amniocentesis.

Sonography

In 1955, Ian Donald[27,28] introduced a technical innovation to obstetrics and gynecology that brought the fetus to the obstetrician's fingertips. Ultrasound changed the way obstetrics was practiced because, for the first time, the fetus, placenta, and umbilical cord were visualized with increasing clarity. One could assess fetal position, fetal growth, fetal weight, and fetal structure for anomalies, as well as placental and umbilical cord location and vessel number. As ultrasound improved technically, it became possible to perform fetal echocardiograms and evaluate fetal blood flow through umbilical, uterine, and numerous fetal vessels. This clarity of observation allowed the obstetrician fetal access in terms of placing needles in the umbilical vessels to perform fetal diagnostic studies or therapy such as transfusion.

Although the fetus could be very accurately visualized, and sometimes treated, using ultrasound, there were some conditions, such as diaphragmatic hernia, that required a surgical approach during the second trimester if pulmonary hypoplasia was to be avoided. Although removal of the fetus from the uterus had been tried since 1980, it was not successful owing to premature labor or fetal death *in utero*. In 1990, Harrison and his colleagues[29] reported the successful repair of a diaphragmatic hernia on a midtrimester fetus that was placed back into the uterus. The pregnancy continued into the third trimester, with delivery of a live fetus.

Development of maternal–fetal medicine

The fetus has become a patient the obstetrician can diagnose and treat. This is recognized in a variety of ways. The American Board of Obstetrics and Gynecology developed certification for the specialist in maternal–fetal medicine in 1974. Centers of excellence in care of the fetus have developed throughout the country, receiving referrals for difficult maternal and fetal management problems from the generalist obstetrician–gynecologist. Texts such as this stress fetal diagnostic and therapeutic approaches.

The saying "you've come a long way, baby" has never been

so true from the standpoint of both the fetus and the newborn. This is reflected in the continuing decline in perinatal mortality; however, the statement "you still have a long way to go" is also very true. We still do not know for certain precisely what triggers the onset of premature labor, which is responsible for the greatest number of perinatal deaths. Research needs to continue at an accelerated pace, taking diagnosis and treatment to the molecular level. In addition to providing the known material in this field at a very high level, this text asks the questions that need to be asked.

References

1 Douglas RG, Stromme WB. *Operative obstetrics*. New York: Appleton-Century-Crofts, 1957:413.
2 Da KN. *Obstetric forceps: its history and evolution*. St Louis: Mosby, 1929.
3 Goodlin R. History of fetal monitoring. *Am J Obstet Gynecol* 1979;33:325.
4 Kennedy E. *Observations on obstetric auscultation*. Dublin: Hodges and Smith, 1833.
5 Bevis DCA. The prenatal prediction of antenatal disease of the newborn. *Lancet* 1952;1:395.
6 Liley AW. Liquor amnii analysis in the management of the pregnancy complicated by rhesus sensitization. *Am J Obstet Gynecol* 1961;82:1359.
7 Liley AW. Technique of fetal transfusion in treatment of severe hemolytic disease. *Am J Obstet Gynecol* 1964;89:817.
8 Hon EH. The electronic evaluation of the fetal heart rate (preliminary report). *Am J Obstet Gynecol* 1958;75:1215.
9 Hammacher K. Fruherkennung intrauterineo gefahrenzustande durch electrophonocardiographie und focographie. In: Elert R, Hates KA, eds. *Prophylaxe frunddkindicher hirnschaden*. Stuttgart: Georg Thieme Verlag, 1966:120.
10 Pose SV, Escarcena L. The influence of uterine contractions on the partial pressure of oxygen in the human fetus. In: Calderyo-Barcia R, ed. *Effects of labor on the fetus and newborn*. Oxford, UK: Pergamon Press, 1967:48.
11 Ray M, Freeman RK, Pine S, et al. Clinical experience with the oxytocin challenge test. *Am J Obstet Gynecol* 1972;114:12.
12 Spielman F, Goldberger MA, Frank RT. Hormonal diagnosis of viability of pregnancy. *JAMA* 1933;101:266.
13 Smith GV, Smith OW. Estrogen and progestin metabolism in pregnancy: endocrine imbalance of preeclampsia and eclampsia. Summary of findings to February 1941. *Endocrinology* 1941; 1:470.
14 Brown JB. Chemical method for determination of oestriol, oestrone, and oestradiol in human urine. *Biochem J* 1955;60:185.
15 Saling E, Schneider D. Biochemical supervision of the fetus during labor. *Br J Obstet Gynecol* 1967;74:799.
16 Barr ML, Bertram LF. A morphologic distinction between neurons of the male and the female and the behavior of the nuclear satellite during accelerated nucleoprotein synthesis. *Nature* 1949;163: 676.
17 Fuchs F, Riis P. Antenatal sex determination. *Nature* 1956; 177:330.
18 Serr DM, Sachs L, Danon M. Diagnosis of fetal sex before birth using cells from the amniotic fluid. *Bull Res Council Israel* 1955;E5B:137.
19 Makowski EL, Prem KA, Kaiser IH. Detection of sex of fetuses by the incidence of sex chromatin body in nuclei of cells in amniotic fluid. *Science* 1956;123:542.
20 Shettles LB. Nuclear morphology of cells in human amniotic fluid in relation to sex of the infant. *Am J Obstet Gynecol* 1956;71:834.
21 Jacobson CB, Barter RH. Intrauterine diagnosis and management of genetic defects. *Am J Obstet Gynecol* 1967;99:796.
22 Pedersen K. Fetuin, a new globulin isolated from serum. *Nature* 1944;154:575.
23 Bergstrand CG, Czar B. Demonstration of a new protein fraction in the serum from the human fetus. *Scand J Clin Lab Invest* 1956;8:174.
24 Gitlin D, Boesman M. Serum alpha-fetoprotein albumen and gamma G-globulin in the human conceptus. *J Clin Invest* 1966;45:1826.
25 Brock DJH, Sutcliffe RG. Alpha fetoprotein in the diagnosis of anencephaly and spine bifida. *Lancet* 1972;2:197.
26 Merkatz IR, Nitowsky IJM, Macri JN, Johnson WE. An association between low serum alpha-fetoprotein and fetal chromosomal abnormalities. *Am J Obstet Gynecol* 1984;148:886.
27 Donald I, MacVicar J, Brown TG. Investigation of abdominal masses by pulsed ultrasound. *Lancet* 1958;1:1188.
28 Donald I. On launching a new diagnostic science. *Am J Obstet Gynecol* 1969;103:609.
29 Harrison MR, Odzick NS, Longaker MT, et al. Successful repair in-utero of a fetal diaphragmatic hernia after removal of herniated viscera from the left thorax. *N Engl J Med* 1990;322:1582.

Part
I

Conception and Conceptus Development

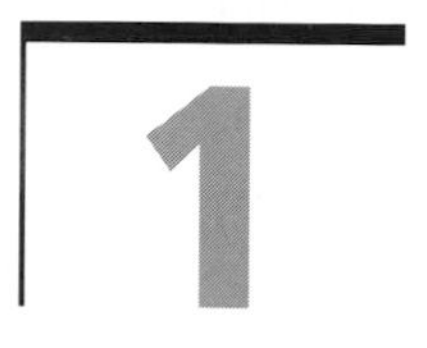

Early conceptus growth and immunobiologic adaptations of pregnancy

Kenneth H.H. Wong and Eli Y. Adashi

Reproduction will only be successful if a multitude of intricate sequences and interactions occur. This reproductive process begins with the formation of individual male and female gametes. Following gamete formation, a mechanism must be provided to ensure that these gametes attain close proximity to each other so fertilization may take place. After successful fertilization, the newly formed embryo must develop correctly and finally implant in a nourishing environment. Recently, there have been many advances in the understanding of these reproductive processes; however, it is beyond the scope of this chapter to provide detailed information on gamete formation, fertilization, and implantation. The interested reader is referred to several excellent texts for more specific information.[1,2] Rather, this chapter summarizes key normal developmental and physiologic events in early conceptus growth and immunobiologic adaptation of a pregnancy.

Gametogenesis

Gametogenesis is the maturational process that produces specialized gametes: the spermatozoon in the male and the oocyte in the female. Both cytoreduction and division prepare gametes for fertilization, which involves the union of male and female gametes. In order to maintain a constant chromosome number, the gametes undergo meiosis, a specialized form of cell division responsible for reducing the diploid number (46) of chromosomes to the haploid number (23).

At approximately 5 weeks of gestation, primitive germ cells migrate, presumably by way of ameboid movement from the yolk sac to the gonadal ridges. Following their migration, the germ cells are surrounded by somatic cells derived from the mesonephros forming the primary sex cords.[3]

In the first meiotic division, homologous chromosomes pair during prophase. In the pachytene stage of prophase, independent assortment and recombination of genetic material occurs among the gametes. Separation of the paired chromosomes occurs in anaphase, whereupon each new daughter cell contains the haploid chromosome number or 23 double-structured chromosomes.

Shortly after the first division, the cell enters the second meiotic division. Each double-structured chromosome divides to form two separate chromosomes containing one chromatid. The resultant products include four daughter cells each containing the haploid number of chromosomes. Thus, one primary oocyte gives rise to four daughter cells, each receiving 22 autosomes and an X chromosome, and the primary spermatocyte gives rise to four daughter cells, each receiving 22 autosomes and either an X or a Y chromosome.

Fertilization

Embryonic development begins with the process of fertilization, the union of individual male and female gametes (Fig. 1.1). The fusion of two haploid cells, each bearing 22 autosomes and one sex chromosome, creates an offspring whose genetic makeup is different from that of both parents. Fertilization consists of a regulated sequence of interactions that will ultimately result in embryo development (Fig. 1.2).

Prior to any sperm–egg interaction, a requisite maturation of spermatozoa, termed capacitation, must occur.[4,5] The spermatozoa gain this ability during the transit through the female reproductive tract. Triggered exocytosis is the final consequence of capacitation.[6] The importance of capacitation has long been recognized, with the initial observation that capacitated sperm can readily penetrate the cumulus.[7] Capacitation is characterized by the acrosome reaction (AR) , the ability to bind to the zona pellucida (ZP), and the acquisition of hypermobility.

Spermatozoa must pass through an investment of cells and matrices, the cumulus, before any sperm–egg interaction may take place. The cumulus is composed of granulosa cells and a matrix consisting primarily of hyaluronic acid and proteins. Sperm capacitation and the hyperactivated motility seem to be important in the sperm's ability to penetrate the cumulus. Investigations have revealed that the sperm protein PH-20 is

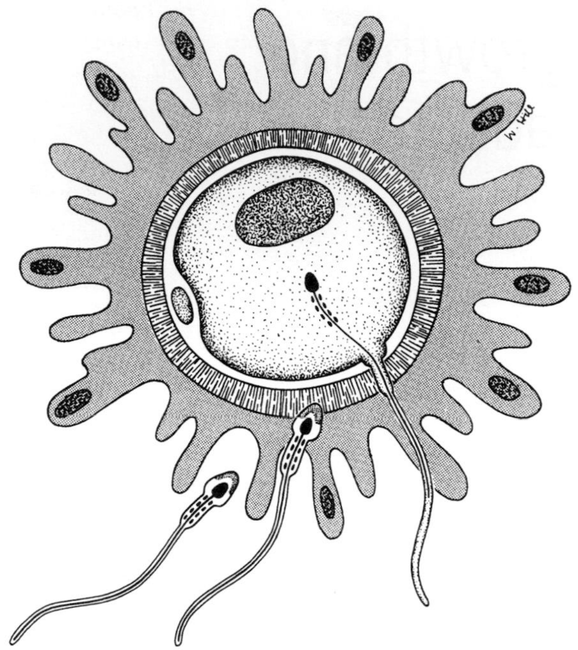

Figure 1.1 Fertilization. A sperm is shown penetrating an oocyte. The spermatozoon must first undergo capacitation. Next, the sperm must penetrate the cumulus (the investment of cells and matrix surrounding the oocyte). After cumulus penetration, the sperm binds to the zona pellucida via specific receptors. The plasma membranes of the sperm and oocyte fuse. The sperm and tail of the sperm enter the oocyte, leaving the sperm's plasma membrane.

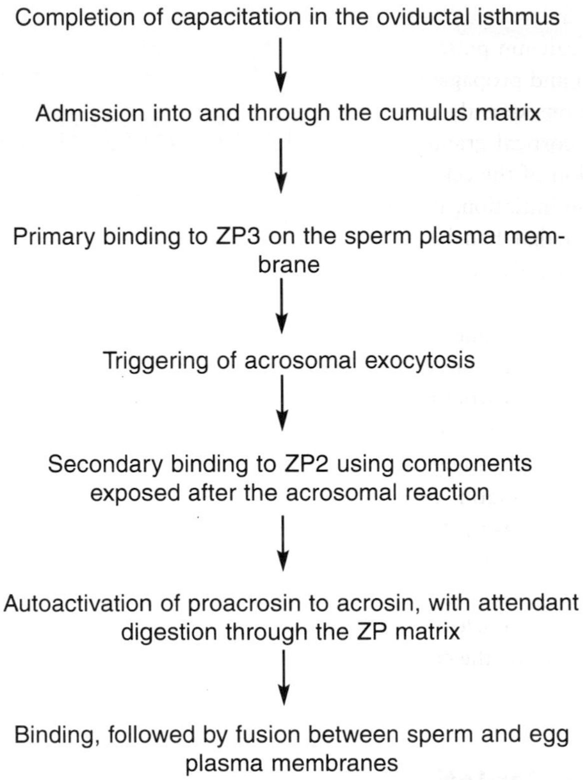

Completion of capacitation in the oviductal isthmus

↓

Admission into and through the cumulus matrix

↓

Primary binding to ZP3 on the sperm plasma membrane

↓

Triggering of acrosomal exocytosis

↓

Secondary binding to ZP2 using components exposed after the acrosomal reaction

↓

Autoactivation of proacrosin to acrosin, with attendant digestion through the ZP matrix

↓

Binding, followed by fusion between sperm and egg plasma membranes

Figure 1.2 Proposed sequence for mammalian gamete interaction. ZP, zona pellucida. (Adapted from ref. 35, with permission.)

also involved with cumulus matrix penetration.[8] Although PH-20 degrades hyaluronic acid and possesses similar protein properties to hyaluronidase, the exact role of this enzyme still remains uncertain.

The ZP is an acellular glycoprotein coat that covers and protects the ovum. The ZP is the last physical barrier that spermatozoa must pass before fertilization with the ovum. The initial interaction between the sperm and the oocyte ZP appears to be a receptor-mediated process. The ZP consists principally of three heavily glycosylated proteins: ZP1, ZP2, and ZP3.[9,10] Extensive studies, especially in the mouse, have revealed ZP2 and ZP3 function in sperm binding, whereas ZP1 serves a structural role.[5,11] Moreover, ZP3 has been demonstrated to be responsible for primary sperm binding (binding prior to the acrosome reaction) and triggers the acrosome reaction, while ZP2 is involved with secondary binding (binding with sperm following the acrosome reaction).[12,13]

The AR involves fusion between the sperm's plasma and acrosomal membrane with exocytosis of the enzyme contents of the acrosome. These enzymes, including hyaluronidase and acrosin, appear to play a role in ZP penetration. Furthermore, the AR changes the sperm head membranes in preparation for the eventual fusion of the inner acrosomal membrane with the oocyte's plasma membrane. Acrosome-intact sperm are unable to fuse with oocytes.[14] Thus, the AR is an absolute prerequisite for sperm fusion with the oocyte membrane.

Once the ZP has been penetrated, the spermatozoon enters the perivitelline space at an angle and crosses quickly. The sperm then binds to the oocyte plasma membrane (oolemma) and soon the entire head enters the cytoplasm of the oocyte (ooplasm). Subsequently, there is fusion of the sperm and egg membranes with specific proteins mediating this process. One such fusion protein is fertilin (formerly called PH-30).[8,15] This sperm membrane protein appears to bind to the oolema via an integrin receptor-mediated mechanism.[8] Following fusion, several morphologic and biochemical events are initiated in the fertilized ovum.

Upon fusion of the egg and sperm membranes, there is a triggering of the cortical and zona reactions. As a result of the release of cortical granules in the oocyte, the oolema becomes impenetrable to spermatozoa. Furthermore, the ZP alters its structure, possibly due to ZP2 and ZP3 protein rearrangement, to prevent further sperm binding.[5] These are the primary blocking mechanisms to polyspermy.

Besides the cortical and zona reactions, a number of biochemical and molecular events are activated in the oocyte after sperm–egg fusion. Initially, there is a transient release of intracellular calcium in a repeated oscillatory fashion.[16,17] These calcium pulses may be initiated by membrane depolarization and propagated through inositol triphosphate production. Consequently, the release of calcium induces exocytosis of the cortical granules. Eventually, these events will lead to initiation of the cell cycle and DNA synthesis.

Upon initiation, the oocyte will resume the second meiotic division that had been arrested at metaphase 2. One of the daughter cells will be extruded as the second polar body, while the other daughter cell, containing a haploid number of chromosomes, becomes the definitive oocyte. Restoration of the diploid number of chromosomes results from the addition of chromosomes from the sperm upon fertilization.

The female pronucleus is formed from the maternal chromosomes remaining in the oocyte. Meanwhile, the sperm head's chromatin decondenses, while enlarging the head in the ooplasm, forming the male pronucleus. The two pronuclei enlarge and migrate toward each other in the center of the fertilized egg. As the pronuclei move into close proximity, the nuclear membranes break down. Syngamy then begins as the chromosomes condense during the first cell division.

Preimplantation embryo

The initial phases of embryonic growth following fertilization are concerned with rapid cell division (Fig. 1.3). This initial increase in cell numbers is critical in establishing a sufficient number of cells in the embryo, which can then initiate differentiation. These cells are known as blastomeres. Beginning with the first division, approximately 24–30 hours after fertilization, the blastomeres become smaller with successive divisions. Until the eight-cell stage, the cells are in a loosely arranged clump; however, following this cleavage stage, blastomeres begin merging into a coherent mass of cells marked by the formation of gap and tight junctions.[18,19] This process of compaction segregates inner cells from outer cells and represents the onset of embryonic differentiation. Approximately 3 days after fertilization, the berry-like mass of cells, termed the morula, enters the uterus.

The next event in embryo development is the formation of a fluid-filled cavity, the blastocele. With blastocyst formation, there is a partitioning of cells between an inner cell mass, the embryoblast, and an outer mass of cells, the trophectoderm. E-cadherin, a molecule involved with cell–cell binding, seems to be important for trophectoderm and blastocyst formation.[20] This polarization of blastomeres permits differentiation to proceed. Differentiation allows for the development of the three primitive tissue layers: the endoderm, mesoderm, and ectoderm. The primitive endoderm arises from a flattened layer of cells, the hypoblast, which lies on the surface of the inner cell mass and faces the blastocoele. Meanwhile, both the mesoderm and the ectoderm develop from the epiblast, the high columnar cell of the inner cell mass.

Until this stage in its growth, the blastocyst is still entirely surrounded by the ZP. The primary function of the ZP appears to be prevention of polyspermy. However, the ZP must be shed prior to embryo implantation to allow for the increasing cell mass and to enable contact between the embryo and the endometrium. This is achieved by hatching, where the embryo wiggles and squeezes out of this investment through a hole. In

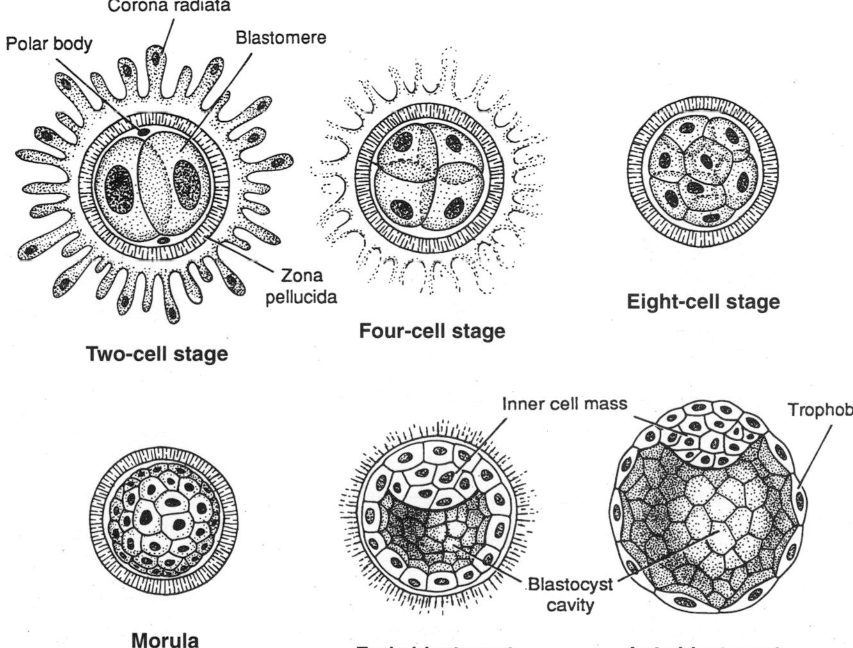

Figure 1.3 Cleavage and blastogenesis. Cleavage occurs in stages and results in the formation of blastomeres. The morula is composed of 12–16 blastomeres. The blastocyst forms when approximately 60 blastomeres are present. Note that the zona pellucida has disappeared by the late blastocyst stage. Until the zona pellucida is shed, the developing embryo essentially does not increase in size.

mice, the initial hole in the ZP is created by the enzyme trypsin.[21] In contrast, the exact mechanism in the human is still unknown, and human hatching has only been seen *in vitro*.[22]

After entering the uterus, the developing blastocyst floats inside the endometrial cavity for about 2–3 days. The embryo begins implantation approximately 6 days after fertilization, while the primitive germ layers develop between days 6 and 8. Following initial implantation, the embryo is completely imbedded within the endometrium by approximately 8–9 days after ovulation.

Intermediary metabolism in the developing embryo

Like all other cells, the developing embryo has nutritional requirements and possesses few nutrient stores, so it must depend on external sources. The metabolic requirements may vary depending on the particular embryonic stage of development. One requirement of particular interest is that pyruvate appears to be the major energy source for early embryo development, while glucose metabolism becomes activated in later cleavage stages. Besides pyruvate and glucose, there are many embryo nutrients and stimulants, including amino acids, intermediaries regulating calcium, and free radical scavengers, to name a few (see Fig. 1.4).

Molecular synthesis in the developing conceptus

The early conceptus exhibits a high level of metabolic activity and is capable of the synthesis and secretion of a number of macromolecules that have diverse effects on the success of implantation, placentation, and maintenance of pregnancy.

Among the earliest substances secreted by the preimplantation embryo is a soluble ether phospholipid, platelet activating factor (PAF). Correlation between the production of embryo-derived (ED)PAF and the pregnancy potential of embryos suggests that it may serve a fundamental role in the establishment of pregnancy.[23] Apparently, human embryos release variable amounts of PAF within 48 hours after fertilization.[24] Conclusive evidence for the essential role of PAF in the establishment of pregnancy was provided by Spinks and O'Neill, who used inhibitors of PAF activity *in vivo* to induce implantation failure in animals.[25]

Human chorionic gonadotropin (hCG) is a glycoprotein composed of one α and one β subunit with amino acid sequences similar to luteinizing hormone. It is produced by the early human trophoblast beginning about the eight-cell stage and is essential for the survival of the conceptus by stimulating progesterone production from the corpus luteum and thus preventing luteolysis and menstruation. In the human, implantation occurs on day 6 after ovulation, and hCG is first measurable on day 9 following ovulation.[26] The hCG production of human blastocysts *in vitro* has been correlated with their morphology and maturity, with the best embryos producing more hCG.[27]

Early pregnancy factor (EPF) has been described based on an alteration in lymphocytic reactivity in the lymphocyte rosette test, which was devised to assess the immunosuppressive characteristics of antilymphocyte serum *in vitro*.[28] Isolation of EPF in embryo growth media has been reported in several species. An immunosuppressive role has been implicated, possibly by modulating the maternal immune system.[29] Recently identified as part of a highly conserved heat shock family of molecules, EPF consists of an amino acid sequence with approximately 70% homology to chaperonin 10 and may be involved in protein binding.[30] EPF becomes positive in maternal serum as early as 24–48 hours after conception and therefore may be useful in the evaluation of early pregnancy failure.[31] Consequently, disorders of menstruation may be distinguished from early spontaneous abortion.

The human zygote produces a factor *in vitro* that is directly immunosuppressive.[32] Unlike the immunosuppressive actions of EPF or EDPAF, the actions of immunosuppressive factor (IF) are direct. The factor obtained from culture media of human embryos after *in vitro* fertilization suppresses mitogen-induced proliferation of peripheral lymphocytes, and those embryos producing the factor alone result in pregnancy. The presence of embryo-associated IFs at various stages of gestation may play a role in suppressing maternal cellular immune responses and prevent maternal rejection of the fetal allograft. Although IF was thought initially to derive from the developing embryo, recent evidence has localized IF to decidual cells.[33]

Although the mechanism has not been elucidated, histamine is thought to play a role in implantation of the blastocyst. Embryo-derived histamine releasing factor (EHRF) has been identified in culture medium used to grow developing embryos.[34] Both calcium and temperature dependent, EHRF induces histamine release from sensitized basal cells. Although the role of this factor remains to be clarified, EHRF could represent a message sent by the embryo to the mother to induce histamine release at the time of implantation.

Cytokines and growth factors regulating implantation

A critical stage in development involves embryonic implantation, a continual synchrony between the embryo itself and a complex series of molecular and cellular events induced in the uterus by estrogen and progesterone. Much of this maternal environment/embryonic "talk" is mediated in an autocrine/paracrine manner by cytokines and growth factors produced by both the embryo and the uterus. Although there exists a myriad of information concerning cytokine and growth factor involvement with implantation, the complete details of this mechanism are still incomplete. For a more comprehensive

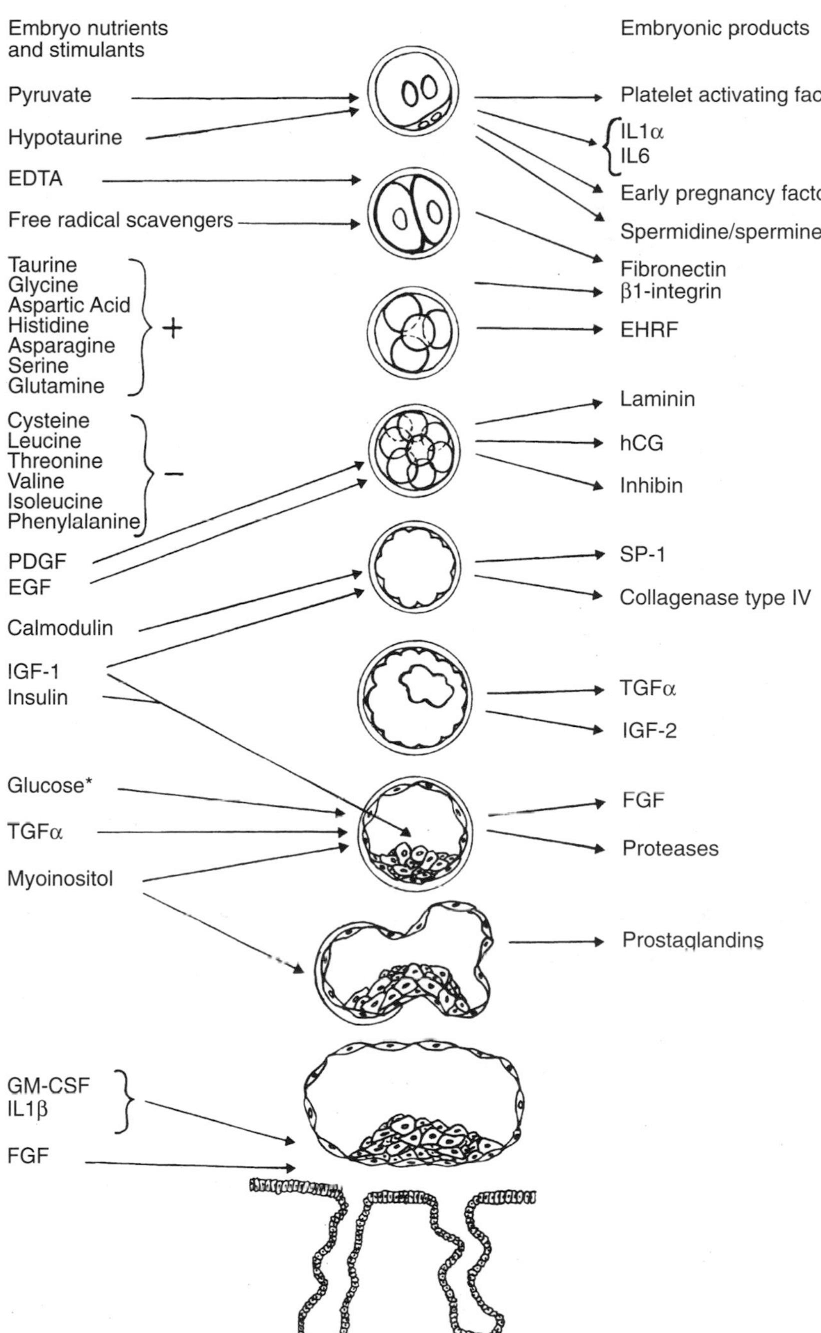

Figure 1.4 Embryonic nutrients and secreted products. EDTA, ethylenediaminetetraacetic acid; EGF, epidermal growth factor; EHRF, embryo-derived histamine-releasing factor; FGF, fibroblast growth factor; GM-CSF, granulocyte-macrophage colony-stimulating factor; hCG, human chorionic gonadotropin; IGF, insulin-like growth factor; IL, interleukin; PDGF, platelet-derived growth factor; TGF, transforming growth factor. (From ref. 55, with permission.)

review, the interested reader is referred to several reviews.[35,36] At least three cytokines, colony-stimulating factor 1 (CSF-1), leukemia inhibitory factor (LIF) and interleukin 1 (IL-1) appear to be involved in implantation.[37]

Apposition and adhesion of the embryo to the endometrium

The blastocyst lies unattached in the uterine endometrial cavity for approximately 2 days before implantation. Implantation begins as the embryo becomes closely apposed to the endometrial epithelium (Fig. 1.5). The initial contact is made via the polar trophectoderm. Apposition seems to allow the complementary binding proteins of the embryo and endometrial epithelium to function effectively during implantation by the interdigitating of epithelial cells and trophoblast with microvilli.

The adherence of the blastocyst to the endometrial epithelium appears to be mediated through ligand–receptor complexes. The expression of specific adhesion molecules, such as integrins, in the embryo and specific substrates and receptors,

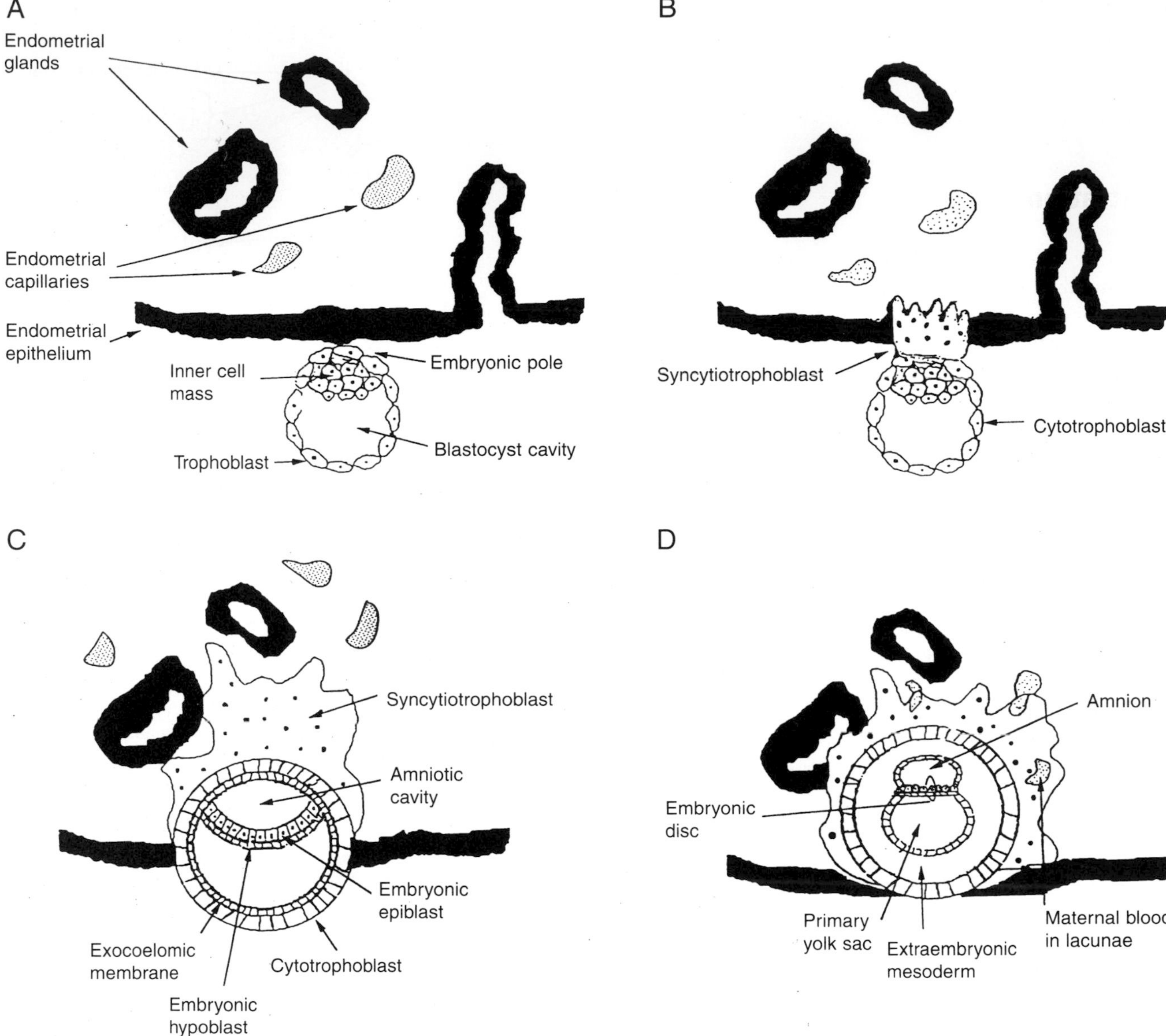

Figure 1.5 Implantation. (A) After floating free for 2 days, the polar trophectoderm of the embryo apposes the endometrial epithelium. (B) Penetration begins with rapid proliferation and differentiation into two cell types, the cytotrophoblast and the syncytiotrophoblast. The syncytiotrophoblast, a multinucleated mass of cells with no cell boundaries, extends through the endometrial epithelium to penetrate the stroma. (C) The inner cell mass differentiates into the epiblast, which gives rise to the mesoderm and ectoderm, and the hypoblast, which gives rise to the endoderm. (D) The embryo becomes completely embedded 7–13 days after ovulation.

such as laminin, fibronectins, and collagen IV, in the uterine epithelium and decidua appears to be involved with these ligand–receptor complexes. After adhering to the uterine epithelium, the blastocyst will begin penetrating through the basement membrane and into the uterine stroma.

Penetration of the epithelium

Immediately following adhesion, the blastocyst begins penetration into the endometrial epithelium and stroma (Fig. 1.5). For trophoblast cells to invade, they have to degrade and remodel the epithelium and stroma. Thus, embryos must produce specific molecules and other enzymes to assist in their penetration. A delicate coordination must exist, however, between the invading embryo and the underlying endometrium to prevent excessive penetration and yet provide adequate invasiveness.

The enzymes and molecules implicated in implantation include the proteases, proteinases, and their inhibitors, which are all involved with degradation of the extracellular matrix. There is a high degree of tissue reorganization that occurs during implantation. At present, the significance of these substances is not fully understood, although their importance in implantation is paramount. Clearly, further studies are needed to elucidate whether one or more of these systems are involved in embryo penetration or if they are redundant systems for "back up" in case one of the systems should become ineffective.

The early human trophoblast

The blastocyst attaches to the endometrial epithelium at the embryonic pole 6 days after fertilization (Fig. 1.5). After the trophoblast has attached to the endometrial epithelium, rapid cellular proliferation occurs, and the trophoblast differentiates into two layers consisting of the inner cytotrophoblast and an outer syncytiotrophoblast, a multinucleated mass without cellular boundaries. Syncytial trophoblast processes extend through the endometrial epithelium to invade the endometrial stroma. Stromal cells surrounding the implantation site become laden with lipids and glycogen, become polyhedral in shape, and are referred to as decidual cells. These decidual cells degenerate in the region of the invading syncytiotrophoblast and provide nutrition to the developing embryo. The blastocyst superficially implants in the stratum compactum of the endometrium by the end of the first week. The trophoblast then invades the surrounding myometrium as the blastocyst becomes completely imbedded in the decidua. Capillary connections are formed as the trophoblast invades, and the blood supply to the developing fetus is established through which it will obtain its support until delivery occurs.

Immunobiologic adaptations of pregnancy

The primary role of the immune system is to protect the body from invasion by foreign organisms and their toxic products. This requires an ability to discriminate between self and nonself antigens, so that immune destruction can be targeted against the invading organism and not against the animal's own tissues. In pregnancy, the antigenically foreign fetus grows in its mother for 9 months, unharmed by her immune system. Clearly, immune adaptations must occur in pregnancy that are central to the survival of the fetus while maintaining the mother's ability to fight infection.

The maternal–fetal interface

Trophoblast

The fetus itself does not come into direct contact with maternal tissue. The trophoblast of the placenta and fetal membranes forms the interface between mother and fetus. Two areas of contact between mother and fetus are established: (1) a large surface area formed by the syncytiotrophoblast of the chorionic villi that is bathed by maternal blood; and (2), within the deciduas, extravillous trophoblast (mostly cytotrophoblast but with some syncytial elements) that mingles directly with maternal tissues.

Fetal–maternal cell traffic

The villous syncytiotrophoblast, adjacent to blood, and the nonvillous cytotrophoblast, in contact with maternal deciduas, are the main areas where maternal lymphocytes might be sensitized to trophoblasts. However, the interface between mother and fetus is extended by the traffic of fetal cells into the maternal circulation, carrying fetal antigens to other parts of the maternal immune system, where priming responses could also occur (Table 1.1).

Trophoblast deportation

It has been known for many years that trophoblast cells enter the maternal circulation.[38] There are two ways in which this might happen. First, trophoblast "buds" (called syncytial sprouts) often form on the syncytiotrophoblast surface and

Table 1.1 Contact between maternal and fetal tissues.

Local	Syncytiotrophoblast lining intervillous space Cytotrophoblast in decidua
Systemic	Fetal red and white cells entering maternal blood Trophoblast deportation

may break free and enter the maternal blood. This disruption of the syncytiotrophoblast could also lead to the underlying villous cytotrophoblast entering the mother's blood. Alternatively, the endovascular cytotrophoblast that lines the spiral arteries may be carried away into the bloodstream. There is evidence for both multinucleate (syncytiotrophoblast) and mononuclear (cytotrophoblast) cells entering the maternal uterine vein,[39] but it is not yet established whether the mononuclear cells are villous or extravillous cytotrophoblasts in origin. It is also a matter of great controversy whether trophoblasts enter the peripheral circulation to a major extent in pregnancy,[40] or whether they become trapped in the lungs.[41]

Traffic of fetal blood cells

Direct contact of fetal (as opposed to placental) cells with maternal cells can come about only by the passage of fetal blood into the maternal circulation. There is now good evidence that fetal nucleated erythrocytes can enter the maternal blood in early pregnancy,[42] and it must be assumed that fetal leukocytes will enter at the same time.[43] Therefore, it appears that more cells traverse the placental barrier as the fetus and the placenta grow.[44] Their presence is presumed to result from fetal–maternal hemorrhage, although the mechanism by which this occurs has yet to be defined.

Maternal immune cells in decidua

The decidua is the tissue in which immune recognition of trophoblasts is most likely to occur. Immunohistologic and flow cytometric studies of the first-trimester pregnancy decidua into which trophoblast invades have shown that it is composed predominantly of immune cells.[45] Approximately 10% of the stromal cells are T lymphocytes (although there are virtually no B cells) and 20% are macrophages;[46] these two cell types are essential for cell-mediated graft rejection responses. However, the main immune cell population is large granular lymphocytes or natural killer (NK) cells, comprising 45% of the decidual cells.[47] Immunohistologic studies show that the extravillous cytotrophoblast is in close contact with these immune cells, which raises the question as to how the trophoblast avoids recognition and rejection.

Maternal immune responses to trophoblast

Expression of major histocompatibility complex (MHC) antigens by trophoblast

The way in which the mother's immune system responds to trophoblast cells will depend on which, if any, MHC antigens they express; therefore, this has been an area of intense study. Studies using monoclonal antibodies that recognized all forms of class I antigens [human leukocyte antigen (HLA)-A, -B, and -C] revealed that, although the syncytiotrophoblast and underlying villous cytotrophoblast were negative for class I, the invasive extravillous cytotrophoblast in the placental bed and the amniochorion strongly expressed this antigen.[48] Subsequent biochemical[49,50] and molecular analyses[51] have shown that the trophoblast class I antigen is in fact HLA-G. HLA-G differs from HLA-A, -B, and -C in that it is nonpolymorphic and has a lower molecular weight. The latter characteristic arises from a termination codon in exon 6, resulting in the transcription of a protein with a truncated cytoplasmic tail.[52]

Table 1.2 MHC expression in human development.

	Class I MHC		Class II MHC
	HLA-G	HLA-A, -B, -C	HLA-DR, -DP, -DQ
Oocyte	–	–	–
Sperm	–	–	–
Blastocyst	+	?	?
Syncytiotrophoblast	–	–	–
Villous cytotrophoblast	–	–	–
Extravillous cytotrophoblast	+	–	–
Fetal tissue	–	+	+

MHC, major histocompatibility complex; –, antigen absent; +, antigen present; ?, not yet known.

Polyclonal antibody studies have confirmed that HLA-G protein is expressed only by extravillous cytotrophoblast[53] (Table 1.2). Neither oocytes[54] nor sperm express surface class I or class II antigens, although sperm are reported to express mRNA for both HLA-B and -G.[55] Similarly, oocytes appear to be negative for both class I and class II antigens. Cleavage-stage embryos and blastocysts were also thought to be negative for class I,[56] but there is no evidence that a proportion of blastocysts express both HLA-G mRNA and protein, which may be associated with more rapid cleavage rates.[57] Thus, expression of HLA-G at this stage could be vital to protect the embryo as it implants into the decidua.

Immunoregulatory role of HLA-G

Soluble class I HLA molecules are known to be shed into the serum of patients with HLA-mismatched organ grafts.[58] These donor-derived, soluble, class I antigens are believed to prolong graft survival by inhibiting the activity of alloreactive cytotoxic lymphocytes.[59] This may occur through their binding to the T-cell receptor or its coreceptor, CD8, which induces apoptosis of the cytotoxic T cell.[60] It has been proposed that soluble HLA-G may likewise be shed from the surface of the trophoblast and may eliminate maternal cytotoxic T cells by a similar mechanism.[61] In support of the hypothesis, evidence for a soluble HLA-G molecule has been obtained at both the

Table 1.3 Properties and functions of HLA-G.

Protein expression restricted to extravillous cytotrophoblast
Exists in both membrane-bound and soluble forms
Heavy chain (40-kDa) has truncated cytoplasmic tail
May have limited polymorphism or is nonpolymorphic
Forms class I complexes with β_2-microglobulin and antigenic peptides
Expression is associated with TAP1
Appears not to stimulate maternal T-cell responses
Downregulates NK cell-mediated cytotoxicity

NK cell, natural killer cell; TAP1, transporter associated with peptide presentation.

molecular[62] and the protein level,[50] and other studies have shown that HLA-G binds to CD8.[63]

HLA-G expression may also serve a protective role for trophoblasts. HLA-G inhibits the proliferation of CD4+ T lymphocytes[64] and decreases decidual cell production of interferon (IFN)-γ and tumor necrosis factor (TNF)-α.[65] Addition of HLA-G to mixed lymphocyte cultures increases the production of IL-10 and decreases IFN-γ and TNF-α production causing a shift from a Th1 to a Th2 phenotype.[66]

Protection against NK cell attack

It might seem that, in evolutionary terms, it would be simpler for the trophoblast not to express class I MHC and thereby avoid immune recognition. However, a major threat to trophoblast invading the decidua is presented by the large granular lymphocytes (NK cells). NK cells preferentially kill target cells that lack class I MHC. The presence of class I antigens on the cell surface is thought to be essential for protection from NK cell-mediated attack. Experiments using cell lines have shown that variants with low levels of class I expression are highly susceptible to NK lysis,[67] but that transfection with both classical class I and HLA-G genes can confer protection.[61,68] The expression of HLA-G may therefore be essential to protect extravillous cytotrophoblast from decidual NK cells.[69,70] Thus, HLA-G may serve a dual role in protecting trophoblast from both cytotoxic T cells and NK cells.

The properties and possible functions of HLA-G are summarized in Table 1.3.

Maternal immune responses to trafficking cells

Fetal leukocytes

In the placenta, class I antigen expression occurs in the mesenchyme of the chorionic villi as early as 2.5 weeks, although it is sporadic and weak. Class II-positive cells are found in the placenta by 14 weeks' gestation.[71] In the fetus itself, class I- and class II-positive cells have been found in the thymic epithelium at 7 weeks' gestation.[72] Thus, if fetal leukocytes enter the maternal circulation, they could potentially stimulate maternal immune responses.

Antibody responses

Antifetal (paternal) HLA alloantibodies can develop during a first pregnancy,[73] and may occur after an abortion,[74] which indicates that immunization is not necessarily the result of events at delivery, but usually develops after 28 weeks, with the incidence increasing with parity.[75] These antibodies do not develop in all pregnancies. The rate is approximately 15% of women in their first pregnancies and never more than approximately 60% among multiparous women.[76] Antibodies may develop against both class I and class II antigens.[77]

None of these antifetal antibodies appears to cause harm to the fetus, probably because they cannot bind to the syncytiotrophoblast, given that it does not express MHC antigens. This would be sufficient protection were it not for the placenta's role in the transfer of immunoglobulins from the maternal to the fetal circulation – a process by which the fetus acquires immunity from infection in the perinatal period. Fc receptors on the surface of the syncytiotrophoblast bind free immunoglobulin G (IgG) molecules and transport them to the villous stroma, where they enter the fetal circulation. Only IgG is transported; antibodies of other classes remain in the maternal blood. However, antibodies to fetal (paternal) HLA appear to be effectively filtered out by binding HLA antigens on cells in the villous stroma. IgG that is aggregated or complexed with antigen is removed by Fc receptor-bearing macrophages.[78] This illustrates the concept of the placental "sponge." Thus, only maternal IgG antibodies to antigens not represented in placental tissues escape the "sponge" and reach the fetal circulation.[79]

Cell-mediated responses

If the mother can develop antibodies to fetal HLA antigens, it would be expected that she can also develop cell-mediated immunity because T- and B-cell sensitization to fetal HLA should occur together. It is therefore surprising that there is only sporadic evidence for T-cell sensitization, as judged by the detection of a secondary maternal–paternal (fetal) mixed lymphocyte reaction or paternal (fetal)-specific cytotoxic T cells.[80]

A search for maternal cytotoxic T cells against paternal and unrelated control target cells at term found clear evidence for their presence in only 2 of 20 pregnant women.[81] In a further series of experiments, no sensitization to paternal HLA was seen in 25 normal first-trimester pregnancies.[82] Even when cytotoxic T cells were found, they did not appear to harm the fetus because these women had normal pregnancies. This implies that cytotoxic T cells cannot cross the placental barrier to gain access to the fetus.

Table 1.4 Maternal immune responses to fetal cells.

	Antibody response	Cell-mediated response
Fetal leukocytes	+	+/–
Trophoblast	+/– (?)	–

+, response; –, no response; (?), conflicting evidence.

Table 1.5 Alterations in maternal cellular immunity during pregnancy.

Component	Alteration in pregnancy	Reference
B-cell numbers	No change	102, 103
T-cell numbers	No change	104, 105, 106
T-cell function	No change	107
	Decreased	108, 109
NK-cell function	Decreased	110, 111

Immunoregulation

From the discussion above, it is clear that there is a paradox in pregnancy in that, although the mother's ability to produce antibodies is apparently normal, her ability to mount cell-mediated immune responses is weakened (Table 1.4). This concept is supported by clinical observations that pregnant women, although not grossly immunocompromised, are more susceptible to diseases that are normally dealt with by cell-mediated immune responses. Certain viral infections, such as hepatitis, herpes simples, and Epstein–Barr virus, are more common in pregnancy.[83] Diseases caused by intracellular pathogens (e.g., leprosy, tuberculosis, malaria, toxoplasmosis, and coccidioidomycosis) appear to be exacerbated by pregnancy. Furthermore, approximately 70% of women with rheumatoid arthritis (caused by cytotoxic T cells in the joints) experience a temporary remission of their symptoms during gestation, whereas systemic lupus erythematosus (caused by autoantibodies) tends to get worse during pregnancy.[84]

Many investigators have attempted to characterize the maternal immune response by determining immune cell subsets and immune cell function during pregnancy. In general, immune function is similar in pregnant and nonpregnant women (Table 1.5). Taken together, there is no clear trend toward either the enhancement or the suppression of immune function during pregnancy.

Immunoregulatory factors

Placental suppressor factors

The placenta itself can release factors that suppress T-cell and NK-cell activity.[85] Microvillous preparations of syncytiotrophoblast and culture supernatants from placental cells and choriocarcinoma cell lines[86,87] nonspecifically suppress mitogen responsiveness and allogenetically stimulated lymphocytes in the mixed lymphocyte reaction along with the cytolytic activity of cytotoxic T cells and NK-cell activity.[88] Suppressive activity may appear very early in gestation, given that animal[89] and human preimplantation embryos have been reported to produce inhibitory factors within 24 hours of fertilization.[90]

Decidual suppressor factors

Suppressive factors released by the placenta into the blood may inhibit lymphocyte responses systematically, but other mechanisms may be involved locally to prevent alloimmune recognition of extravillous cytotrophoblast that invades the decidua. Suppression of cell-mediated responsiveness *in vitro* by cell populations[91] from first-trimester human decidua has also been demonstrated. Decidual cells secrete various proteins that might mediate these suppressive activities. Transforming growth factor β, a cytokine that strongly inhibits proliferation of B cells and T cells and the cytolytic activity of NK cells, has been localized to the large granular lymphocytes in the human decidua.[92]

Cytokines and pregnancy

The strongest candidates for the suppressor factors derived from the placenta and decidua are cytokines. It has been proposed that the maternal immune changes in pregnancy are brought about by a shift in the balance of cytokines that favors antibody production and depresses the potentially harmful cell-mediated immune responses.

Type I and type 2 cytokines and the immune response

It has become apparent that antibody production and cell-mediated responses are controlled through two distinct populations of CD4+ Th cells.[93] Type 1 CD4+ Th cells (Th1) control cell-mediated responses by secreting cytokines such as IL-2, TFN-β, and IFN-γ, which stimulate cytotoxic T cells and NK cells (Th1 response). Type 2 CD4+ Th cells (Th2) produce IL-4, which stimulates IgE and IgG antibody production by B cells (Th2 response) (Fig. 1.6A). These two systems are also interactive in that IFN-γ produced by T1 cells inhibits B-cell development induced by Th2 cells, and Th2 cells in turn produce IL-10, which inhibits cytokine synthesis by Th1 cells (Fig. 1.6B). Thus, Th1 and Th2 cytokines are mutually inhibitory but, in the normal state, they are in balance, allowing both forms of immune response to coexist. However, a deviation in the pattern of cytokine production could lead to one type of response being favored over the other.

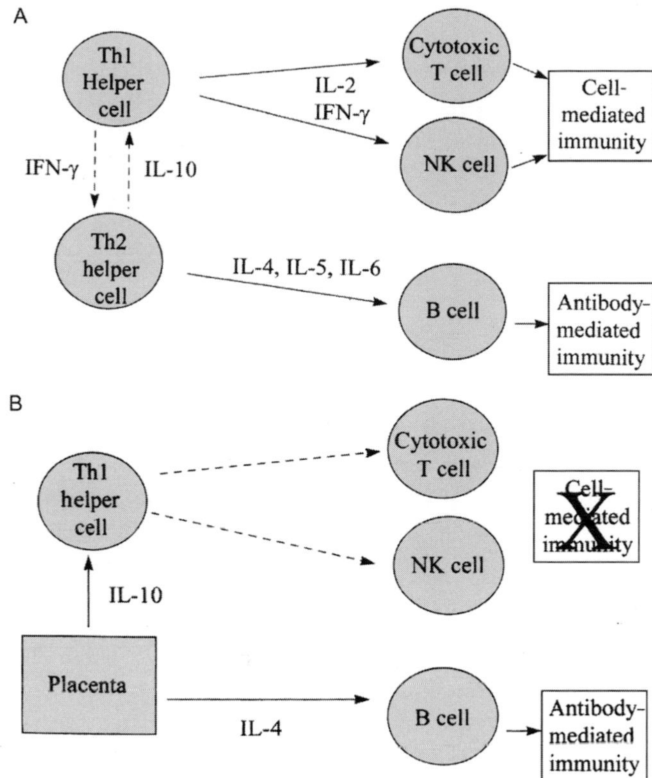

Figure 1.6 (A) Th1 and Th2 cytokines in immune responses. (B) Th1 and Th2 cytokines in pregnancy. IFN, interferon; IL, interleukin; NK, natural killer; Th1, type 1 T helper cells; Th2, type 2 T helper cells.

Type 1 and type 2 cytokines in pregnancy

In pregnancy, it is proposed that there is a shift away from Th1 responses and toward Th2 responses.[94] The cause of this shift is thought to be the production of Th2 cytokines by the placenta (Fig. 1.6B). Thus, excess IL-4 released from the placenta would stimulate maternal antibody responses. At the same time, excess IL-10 production would inhibit Th1 cells, leading to the suppression of cytotoxic T cells and NK-cell activity, which has been observed.

Experimental evidence for this hypothesis is largely confined to the mouse. Several groups have demonstrated that production of Th2 cytokines by tissues at the maternal–fetal interface[95,96] and injection of Th1 cytokines TNF-α, IFN-γ, and IL-2 into pregnant mice can increase fetal resorption rates and inhibit mouse embryo development and implantation *in vitro*.[97] So far, evidence in the human is restricted to localization studies showing that IL-4 is present in the syncytiotrophoblast, the cytotrophoblast of the fetal membranes, and decidual macrophages,[98] and that IL-10 is secreted by HLA-G-positive cytotrophoblast.[99] In contrast, IL-10 knockout mice[100] and IL-10, IL-4 double knockouts[101] have normal pregnancies. Thus, the immunologic relationship between mother and fetus may be more complex than originally thought.

Immune circuit

It is clear form the foregoing discussion that, in normal pregnancy, fetal growth progresses side by side with the development of a number of immune mechanisms that function at several levels. These can be summarized by constructing an immune circuit (Fig. 1.7A). The first stage in this circuit is the exposure of the maternal immune system to both fetal trophoblast and leukocytes. This could potentially lead to immune recognition and the development of cell-mediated and antibody responses to fetal antigens, which in turn would lead to rejection of the fetus (placenta). However, this circuit is broken at several stages (Fig. 1.7B). First, on the basis of current evidence, the maternal immune system does not recognize the trophoblast because it either fails to express HLA or expresses HLA-G. Second, although fetal leukocytes can be recognized by maternal immune cells, only antibody responses occur because the placenta's production of Th2 cytokines downregulates cell-mediated immunity. Finally, the production of antipaternal antibodies is not harmful because the placenta filters out these antibodies before they reach the fetal circulation. Thus, it is the combination of these many immune adaptations of pregnancy that ensure the success of the fetus.

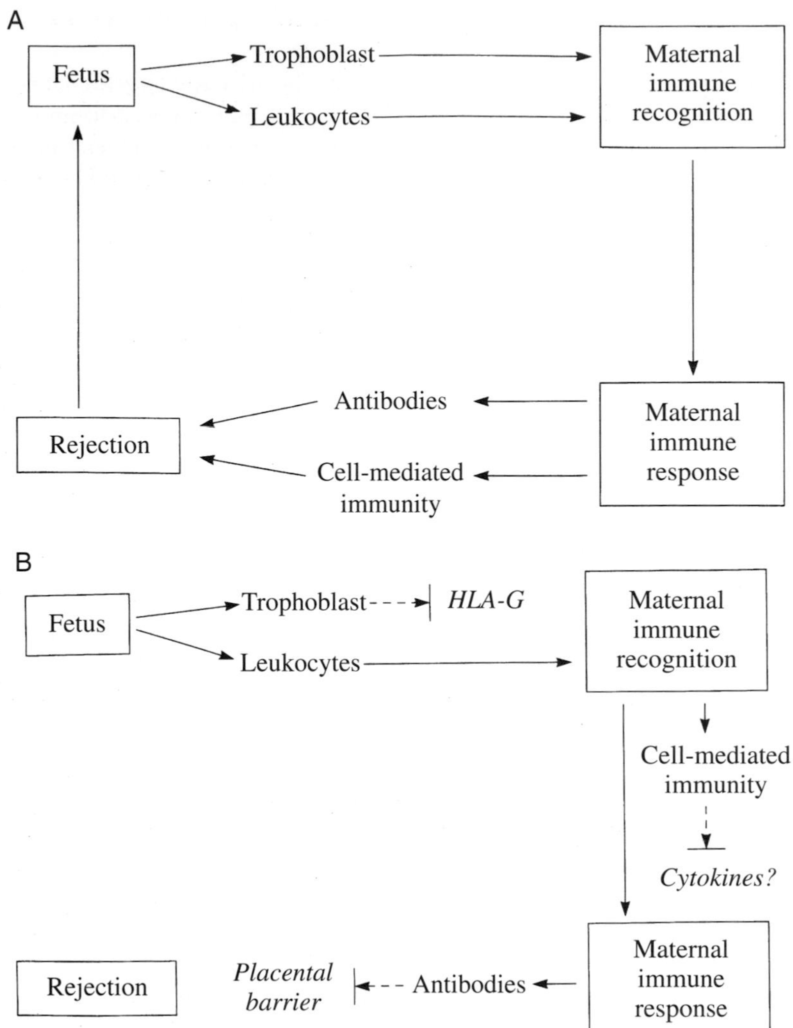

Figure 1.7 (A) Immune responses in pregnancy that could lead to rejection of the fetus. (B) Immunoregulatory mechanisms in pregnancy that prevent the rejection of the fetus.

Key points

1 During meiosis, the primary oocyte gives rise to four daughter cells, each receiving 22 autosomes and an X chromosome. The primary spermatocyte also gives rise to four daughter cells, each receiving 22 autosomes and either an X or a Y chromosome.

2 Prior to sperm–egg interaction, capacitation of the spermatozoa must occur.

3 Capacitation is characterized by the acrosome reaction, fusion between the sperm's plasma and acrosomal membrane with exocytosis of the enzyme contents.

4 The zona pellucida is an acellular glycoprotein coat covering the ovum and consists of three principal proteins: ZP1, ZP2, and ZP3.

5 Upon fusion of the egg and sperm membranes, the cortical and zona reactions are triggered.

6 After egg–sperm fusion, the oocyte will resume the second meiotic division and extrude the second polar body.

7 The morula enters the uterus 3 days after fertilization and floats inside the endometrial cavity for 2–3 days. The embryo begins implantation approximately 6 days after fertilization.

8 Human chorionic gonadotrophin is a glycoprotein produced by the early conceptus and is essential in stimulating the corpus luteum to produce progesterone.

9 Three cytokines appear to be involved in implantation, colony-stimulating factor 1, leukemia inhibitory factor, and interleukin 1.

10 The adherence of the blastocyst to the endometrial epithelium is mediated through ligand–receptor complexes.

11 HLA-G protein is expressed only by extravillous cytotrophoblast.

12 Fetal nucleated erythrocytes and leukocytes can enter the maternal blood in early pregnancy.

13 First-trimester pregnancy decidua is composed predominantly of immune cells. Approximately 10% of the stromal cells are T lymphocytes, 20% are macrophages, and the main immune cell population is large granular lymphocytes or NK cells, comprising 45% of the decidual cells.

14 HLA-G inhibits the proliferation of CD4+ T lymphocytes and decreases decidual cell production of IFN-γ and TNF-α.

15 HLA-G may serve a dual role in protecting trophoblast from both cytotoxic T cells and NK cells.

16 In the placenta, class I antigen expression occurs in the mesenchyme of the chorionic villi as early as 2.5 weeks; class II-positive cells are found in the placenta by 14 weeks' gestation.

17 There is no clear trend toward either the enhancement or the suppression of immune function during pregnancy.

18 The placenta can release factors that suppress T-cell and NK-cell activity.

19 Type 1 CD4+ Th cells (Th1) control cell-mediated responses by secreting cytokines such as IL-2, TFN-β, and IFN-γ, which stimulate cytotoxic T cells and NK cells (Th1 response).

20 Type 2 CD4+ Th cells (Th2) produce IL-4, which stimulates IgE and IgG antibody production by B cells (Th2 response).

References

1 Knobil E, Neill JD, eds. *The physiology of reproduction*, 2nd edn. New York: Raven Press, 1994.

2 Adashi EY, Rock JA, Rosenwaks Z, eds. *Reproductive endocrinology, surgery and technology*. Philadelphia, PA: Lippincott-Raven, 1996.

3 Yoshinaga K, Hess DL, Hendrickx AG, et al. The development of the sexually indifferent gonad in the prosimian, *Galago crassicaudatus crassicaudatus*. *Am J Anat* 1988;181:89–105.

4 Austin CR. The capacitation of the mammalian sperm. *Nature* 1952;190:326.

5 Yanagimachi R. Mammalian fertilization. In: Knobil E, Neill JD, eds. *The physiology of reproduction*. New York: Raven Press; 1994:189–317.

6 Bedford JM. Significance of the need for sperm capacitation before fertilization in eutherian mammals. *Biol Reprod* 1983;28: 108–120.

7 Austin CR. Capacitation and the release of hyaluronidase from spermatozoa. *J Reprod Fertil* 1960;3:310–311.

8 Saling PM. Fertilization: mammalian gamete interactions. In: Adashi EY, Rock JA, Rosenwaks Z, eds. *Reproductive endocrinology, surgery and technology*. Philadelphia, PA: Lippincott-Raven; 1996:404–420.

9 Liang LF, Dean J. Oocyte development: molecular biology of the zona pellucida. *Vitam Horm* 1993;158:35–45.

10 Wassarman PM, Albertini DF. The mammalian ovum. In: Knobil E, Neill J, eds. *The physiology of reproduction*. New York: Raven Press; 1994:69–102.

11 Wassarman PM. Zona pellucida glycoproteins. *Annu Rev Biochem* 1988;57:415–442.

12 Wassarman PM. Gamete interactions during mammalian fertilization. *Theriogenology* 1994;41:31–44.

13 Foltz KR. Sperm-binding proteins. *Int Rev Cytol* 1995;163: 249–303.

14 Yanagimachi R. Sperm–egg fusion. In: Duzgunes N, Bronner F, eds. *Current topics in membranes and transport*. San Diego, CA: Academic Press; 1988:3–43.

15 Green DP. Mammalian fertilization as a biological machine: a working model for adhesion and fusion of sperm and oocyte. *Hum Reprod* 1993;8:91–96.

16 Miyazaki S, Shirakawa H, Nakada K, et al. Essential role of the inositol 1,4,5 triphosphate receptor/Ca2+ release channel in Ca2+ waves and oscillations at fertilization of mammalian eggs. *Dev Biol* 1993;158:62–78.

17 Taylor CT, Lawrence YM, Kingsland CR, et al. Oscillations in intracellular free calcium induced by spermatozoa in human oocytes at fertilization. *Hum Reprod* 1993;8:2174–2179.

18 Dale B, Gualtieri R, Talevi R, et al. Intercellular communication in the early human embryo. *Mol Reprod Dev* 1991;29:22–28.

19 Lo CW. The role of gap junction membrane channels in development. *J Bioenerg Biomembr* 1996;28:379–385.

20 Larue L, Mami O, Hirchenhain J, et al. E cadherin null mutant embryos fail to form a trophectoderm epithelium. *Proc Natl Acad Sci USA* 1994;91:188–195.

21 Perona RM, Wassarman PM. Mouse blastocysts hatch *in vitro* by using a trypsin-like proteinase associated with cells of mural trophectoderm. *Dev Biol* 1986;114:42–52.

22 Sathananthan H. Ultrastructure of preimplantation human embryos co-cultured with human ampullary cells. *Hum Reprod* 1990;5:309–318.

23 Minhas BS, Ripps BA, Zhu YP, et al. Platelet activating factor and conception. *Am J Reprod Immunol* 1996;35:267–271.

24 O'Neill C, Gidley-Baird AA, Pike IL, et al. Maternal blood platelet physiology and luteal phase endocrinology as a means of monitoring pre- and post-implantation embryo viability following *in vitro* fertilization. *J In Vitro Embryo Transfer* 1985;2: 87–93.

25 Spinks NR, O'Neill C. Embryo-derived platelet-activating factor is essential for establishment of pregnancy in the mouse. *Lancet* 1987;1:106–107.

26 Lenton EA. Gonadotrophins of the menstrual cycle and implantation. *Serono Symp Publ* 1990;66:33–48.

27 Dokras A, Sargent IL, Gardner RL, et al. Human trophectoderm biopsy and secretion of chorionic gonadotrophin. *Hum Reprod* 1991;6:1453–1459.

28 Morton H, Rolfe B, Clunie GJA, et al. An early pregnancy factor detected in human serum by the rosette inhibition test. *Lancet* 1977;1:394–397.

29 Bose R, Cheung H, Sabbadini E, et al. Purified human early pregnancy factor from preimplantation embryo possesses immunosuppressive factors. *Am J Obstet Gynecol* 1989;160:954–960.

30 Cavanagh AC, Morton H. The purification of early-pregnancy factor to homogeneity from human platelets and identification as chaperonin 10. *Eur J Biochem* 1994;222:551–560.
31 Straube W, Romer T, Zeeni L, et al. The early pregnancy factor (EPF) as an early marker of disorders in pregnancy. *Zentralbl Gynakol* 1995;117:32–34.
32 Sheth KV, Roca GL, Al Sediary ST, et al. Prediction of successful embryo implantation by measuring interleukin-1α and immunosuppressive factor(s) in preimplantation embryo culture fluid. *Fertil Steril* 1991;55:952–957.
33 Bose R, Lacson AG. Embryo-associated immunosuppressor factor is produced at the maternal–fetal interface in human pregnancy. *Am J Reprod Immunol* 1995;33:373–380.
34 Cocchiara R, Di Trapani G, Azzolina A, et al. Identification of a histamine-releasing factor secreted by human pre-implantation embryos grown *in vitro*. *J Reprod Immunol* 1988;13:41–52.
35 Harvey MB, Leco KJ, Arcellana-Panlilio MY, et al. Roles of growth factors during peri-implantation development. *Hum Reprod* 1995:712–718.
36 Tabibzadeh S, Babaknia A. The signals and molecular pathways involved in implantation, a symbiotic interaction between blastocyst and endometrium involving adhesion and tissue invasion. *Hum Reprod* 1995:1579–1602.
37 Simon C. Potential molecular mechanisms for the contraceptive control of implantation. *Mol Hum Reprod* 1996;2(7):475–479.
38 Thomas L, Douglas GW, Carr MC. The continual migration of syncytial trophoblasts from the fetal placenta into the maternal circulation. *Trans Assoc Am Physiol* 1959;72:140–148.
39 Chua S, Wilkins T, Sargent I, et al. Trophoblast deportation in pre-eclamptic pregnancy. *Br J Obstet Gynaecol* 1991;98(10): 973–979.
40 Mueller UW, Hawes CS, Wright AE, et al. Isolation of fetal trophoblast cells from peripheral blood of pregnant women. *Lancet* 1990;336(8709):197–200.
41 Sargent IL, Johansen M, Chua S, et al. Clinical experience: isolating trophoblasts from maternal blood. *Ann NY Acad Sci* 1994;731:154–161.
42 Bianchi DW, Zickwolf GK, Yih MC, et al. Erythroid-specific antibodies enhance detection of fetal nucleated erythrocytes in maternal blood. *Prenat Diagn* 1993;13(4):293–300.
43 Zilliacus R, De la Chapelle A, Schroder J, et al. Transplacental passage of foetal blood cells. *Scand J Haematol* 1975;15(5): 333–338.
44 Hamada H, Arinami T, Kubo T, et al. Fetal nucleated cells in maternal peripheral blood: frequency and relationship to gestational age. *Hum Genet* 1993;91(5):427–432.
45 Bulmer JN, Sunderland CA. Bone-marrow origin of endometrial granulocytes in the early human placental bed. *J Reprod Immunol* 1983;5(6):383–387.
46 Starkey PM, Sargent IL, Redman CW. Cell populations in human early pregnancy decidua: characterization and isolation of large granular lymphocytes by flow cytometry. *Immunology* 1988; 65(1):129–134.
47 Giacomini P, Tosi S, Murgia C, et al. First-trimester human trophoblast is class II major histocompatibility complex mRNA+/antigen. *Hum Immunol* 1994;39(4):281–289.
48 Sunderland CA, Naiem M, Mason DY, et al. The expression of major histocompatibility antigens by human chorionic villi. *J Reprod Immunol* 1981;3(6):323–331.
49 Ellis SA, Sargent IL, Redman CW, et al. Evidence for a novel HLA antigen found on human extravillous trophoblast and a choriocarcinoma cell line. *Immunology* 1986;59(4):595–601.
50 Kovats S, Main EK, Librach C, et al. A class I antigen, HLA-G, expressed in human trophoblasts. *Science* 1990;248(4952): 220–223.
51 Ellis SA, Palmer MS, McMichael AJ. Human trophoblast and the choriocarcinoma cell line BeWo express a truncated HLA Class I molecule. *J Immunol* 1990;144(2):731–735.
52 Geraghty DE, Koller BH, Orr HT. A human major histocompatibility complex class I gene that encodes a protein with a shortened cytoplasmic segment. *Proc Natl Acad Sci USA* 1987;84(24):9145–9149.
53 Chumbley G, King A, Gardner L, et al. Generation of an antibody to HLA-G in transgenic mice and demonstration of the tissue reactivity of this antibody. *J Reprod Immunol* 1994;27(3):173–186.
54 Dohr G. HLA and TLX antigen expression on the human oocyte, zona pellucida and granulosa cells. *Hum Reprod* 1987;2(8): 657–664.
55 Chiang MH, Steuerwald N, Lambert H, et al. Detection of human leukocyte antigen class I messenger ribonucleic acid transcripts in human spermatozoa via reverse transcription-polymerase chain reaction. *Fertil Steril* 1994;61(2):276–280.
56 Roberts JM, Taylor CT, Melling GC, et al. Expression of the CD46 antigen, and absence of class I MHC antigen, on the human oocyte and preimplantation blastocyst. *Immunology* 1992;75(1):202–205.
57 Jurisicova A, Casper RF, MacLusky NJ, et al. HLA-G expression during preimplantation human embryo development. *Proc Natl Acad Sci USA* 1996;93(1):161–165.
58 Puppo F, Scudeletti M, Indiveri F, et al. Serum HLA class I antigens: markers and modulators of an immune response? *Immunol Today* 1995;16(3):124–127.
59 Hausmann R, Zavazava N, Steinmann J, et al. Interaction of papain-digested HLA class I molecules with human alloreactive cytotoxic T lymphocytes (CTL). *Clin Exp Immunol* 1993;91(1): 183–188.
60 Zavazava N, Kronke M. Soluble HLA class I molecules induce apoptosis in alloreactive cytotoxic T lymphocytes. *Nature Med* 1996;2(9):1005–1010.
61 Kovats S, Librach C, Fisch P, et al. Expression and possible function of the HLA-G a chain in human cytotrophoblasts. In: Chaouat G, Mowbray J, eds. *Cellular and molecular biology of the materno-fetal relationship*. Paris: John Libbey; 1991:21–29.
62 Ishitani A, Geraghty DE. Alternative splicing of HLA-G transcripts yields proteins with primary structures resembling both class I and class II antigens. *Proc Natl Acad Sci USA* 1992;89(9):3947–3951.
63 Sanders SK, Giblin PA, Kavathas P. Cell–cell adhesion mediated by CD8 and human histocompatibility leukocyte antigen G, a nonclassical major histocompatibility complex class 1 molecule on cytotrophoblasts. *J Exp Med* 1991;174(3):737–740.
64 Bainbridge DR, Ellis SA, Sargent IL. HLA-G suppresses proliferation of CD4(+) T-lymphocytes. *J Reprod Immunol* 2000;48(1):17–26.
65 Kanai T, Fujii T, Unno N, et al. Human leukocyte antigen-G-expressing cells differently modulate the release of cytokines from mononuclear cells present in the decidua versus peripheral blood. *Am J Reprod Immunol* 2001;45(2):94–99.
66 Kapasi K, Albert SE, Yie S, et al. HLA-G has a concentration-dependent effect on the generation of an allo-CTL response. *Immunology* 2000;101(2):191–200.
67 Harel-Bellan A, Quillet A, Marchiol C, et al. Natural killer susceptibility of human cells may be regulated by genes in the HLA

region on chromosome 6. *Proc Natl Acad Sci USA* 1986;83(15): 5688–5692.

68 Pazmany L, Mandelboim O, Vales-Gomez M, et al. Protection from natural killer cell-mediated lysis by HLA-G expression on target cells. *Science* 1996;274(5288):792–795.

69 Riteau B, Rouas-Freiss N, Menier C, et al. HLA-G2, -G3, and -G4 isoforms expressed as nonmature cell surface glycoproteins inhibit NK and antigen-specific CTL cytolysis. *J Immunol* 2001;166(8):5018–5026.

70 Rieger L, Hofmeister V, Probe C, et al. Th1- and Th2-like cytokine production by first trimester decidual large granular lymphocytes is influenced by HLA-G and HLA-E. *Mol Hum Reprod* 2002;8(3):255–261.

71 Sutton L, Mason DY, Redman CW. HLA-DR positive cells in the human placenta. *Immunology* 1983;49(1):103–112.

72 Haynes BF, Scearce RM, Lobach DF, et al. Phenotypic characterization and ontogeny of mesodermal-derived and endocrine epithelial components of the human thymic microenvironment. *J Exp Med* 1984;159(4):1149–1168.

73 Van der Werf AJM. Are lymphocytotoxic iso-antibodies produced by the early human trophoblast? *Lancet* 1971(1):95.

74 Nakajima H, Mano Y, Tokunaga E, et al. Influence of previous pregnancy on maternal response to foetal antigens. *Tissue Antigens* 1982;19(1):92–94.

75 Regan L, Braude PR. Is antipaternal cytotoxic antibody a valid marker in the management of recurrent abortion? *Lancet* 1987;2(8570):1280.

76 Van Rood GG, Eernisse G, Van Leuween A. Leukocyte antibodies in sera from pregnant women. *Nature* 1958(181):1735–1736.

77 Borelli I, Amoroso A, Richiardi P, et al. Evaluation of different technical approaches for the research of human anti-Ia alloantisera. *Tissue Antigens* 1982;19(5):380–387.

78 Wood GW, Bjerrum K, Johnson B. Detection of IgG bound within human trophoblast. *J Immunol* 1982;129(4):1479–1484.

79 Tongio MM, Mayer S, Lebec A. Transfer of HL-A antibodies from the mother to the child. Complement of information. *Transplantation* 1975;20(2):163–166.

80 Sargent IL. Maternal and fetal immune responses during pregnancy. *Exp Clin Immunogenet* 1993;10(2):85–102.

81 Sargent IL, Arenas J, Redman CW. Maternal cell-mediated sensitisation to paternal HLA may occur, but is not a regular event in normal human pregnancy. *J Reprod Immunol* 1987;10(2): 111–120.

82 Sargent IL, Wilkins T, Redman CW. Maternal immune responses to the fetus in early pregnancy and recurrent miscarriage. *Lancet* 1988;2(8620):1099–104.

83 Larsen B, Galask RP. Host–parasite interactions during pregnancy. *Obstet Gynecol Surv* 1978;33(5):297–318.

84 Piccinni MP, Romagnani S. Regulation of fetal allograft survival by a hormone-controlled Th1- and Th2-type cytokines. *Immunol Res* 1996;15(2):141–150.

85 Menu E, Kaplan L, Andreu G, et al. Immunoactive products of human placenta. I. An immunoregulatory factor obtained from explant cultures of human placenta inhibits CTL generation and cytotoxic effector activity. *Cell Immunol* 1989;119(2):341–352.

86 Matsuzaki N, Okada T, Kameda T, et al. Trophoblast-derived immunoregulatory factor: demonstration of the biological function and the physicochemical characteristics of the factor derived from choriocarcinoma cell lines. *Am J Reprod Immunol* 1989; 19(4):121–127.

87 Arkwright PD, Rademacher TW, Boutignon F, et al. Suppression of allogeneic reactivity *in vitro* by the syncytiotrophoblast membrane glycocalyx of the human term placenta is carbohydrate dependent. *Glycobiology* 1994;4(1):39–47.

88 Degenne D, Khalfoun B, Bardos P. *In vitro* inhibitory effect of human syncytiotrophoblast plasma membranes on the cytolytic activities of CTL and NK cells. *Am J Reprod Immunol Microbiol* 1986;12(4):106–110.

89 Murray MK, Segerson EC, Hansen PJ, et al. Suppression of lymphocyte activation by a high-molecular-weight glycoprotein released from preimplantation ovine and porcine conceptuses. *Am J Reprod Immunol Microbiol* 1987;14(2):38–44.

90 Clark DA, Lee S, Fishell S, et al. Immunosuppressive activity in human *in vitro* fertilization (IVF) culture supernatants and prediction of the outcome of embryo transfer: a multicenter trial. *J In Vitro Fertil Embryo Transf* 1989;6(1):51–58.

91 Daya S, Clark DA, Devlin C, et al. Suppressor cells in human decidua. *Am J Obstet Gynecol* 1985;151(2):267–270.

92 Clark DA, Vince G, Flanders KC, et al. CD56+ lymphoid cells in human first trimester pregnancy decidua as a source of novel transforming growth factor-beta 2-related immunosuppressive factors. *Hum Reprod* 1994;9(12):2270–2277.

93 Mosmann TR, Coffman RL. TH1 and TH2 cells: different patterns of lymphokine secretion lead to different functional properties. *Annu Rev Immunol* 1989;7:145–173.

94 Wegmann TG, Lin H, Guilbert L, et al. Bidirectional cytokine interactions in the maternal-fetal relationship: is successful pregnancy a TH2 phenomenon? *Immunol Today* 1993;14(7): 353–356.

95 Lin H, Mosmann TR, Guilbert L, et al. Synthesis of T helper 2-type cytokines at the maternal–fetal interface. *J Immunol* 1993;151(9):4562–4573.

96 Delassus S, Coutinho GC, Saucier C, et al. Differential cytokine expression in maternal blood and placenta during murine gestation. *J Immunol* 1994;152(5):2411–2420.

97 Haimovici F, Hill JA, Anderson DJ. The effects of soluble products of activated lymphocytes and macrophages on blastocyst implantation events *in vitro*. *Biol Reprod* 1991;44(1):69–75.

98 de Moraes-Pinto MI, Vince GS, Flanagan BF, et al. Localization of IL-4 and IL-4 receptors in the human term placenta, decidua and amniochorionic membranes. *Immunology* 1997;90(1): 87–94.

99 Roth I, Corry DB, Locksley RM, et al. Human placental cytotrophoblasts produce the immunosuppressive cytokine interleukin 10. *J Exp Med* 1996;184(2):539–548.

100 Kuhn R, Lohler J, Rennick D, et al. Interleukin-10-deficient mice develop chronic enterocolitis. *Cell* 1993;75(2):263–274.

101 Svensson L, Arvola M, Sallstrom MA, et al. The Th2 cytokines IL-4 and IL-10 are not crucial for the completion of allogeneic pregnancy in mice. *J Reprod Immunol* 2001;51(1):3–7.

102 Sridama V, Pacini F, Yang SL, et al. Decreased levels of helper T cells: a possible cause of immunodeficiency in pregnancy. *N Engl J Med* 1982;307(6):352–356.

103 Dodson MG, Kerman RH, Lange CF, et al. T and B cells in pregnancy. *Obstet Gynecol* 1977;49(3):299–302.

104 Siegel I, Gleicher N. Changes in peripheral mononuclear cells in pregnancy. *Am J Reprod Immunol* 1981;1(3):154–155.

105 Moore MP, Carter NP, Redman CW. Lymphocyte subsets in normal and pre-eclamptic pregnancies. *Br J Obstet Gynaecol* 1983;90(4):326–331.

106 Bardeguez AD, McNerney R, Frieri M, et al. Cellular immunity in preeclampsia: alterations in T-lymphocyte subpopulations during early pregnancy. *Obstet Gynecol* 1991;77(6):859–862.

107 Gill TJ, 3rd, Repetti CF. Immunologic and genetic factors influencing reproduction. A review. *Am J Pathol* 1979;95(2): 465–570.
108 Gehrz RC, Christianson WR, Linner KM, et al. A longitudinal analysis of lymphocyte proliferative responses to mitogens and antigens during human pregnancy. *Am J Obstet Gynecol* 1981;140(6):665–670.
109 Petrucco OM, Seamark RF, Holmes K, et al. Changes in lymphocyte function during pregnancy. *Br J Obstet Gynaecol* 1976;83(3):245–250.
110 Toder V, Nebel L, Gleicher N. Studies of natural killer cells in pregnancy. I. Analysis at the single cell level. *J Clin Lab Immunol* 1984;14(3):123–127.
111 Vaquer S, de la Hera A, Jorda J, et al. Diminished natural killer activity in pregnancy: modulation by interleukin 2 and interferon gamma. *Scand J Immunol* 1987;26(6):691–698.

2 Normal embryonic and fetal development

Trivedi Vidhya N. Persaud and Jean C. Hay

This chapter is a synopsis of the main events in normal human development. The reader should consult the references[1–9] for a more detailed discussion of individual topics.

Fertilization normally occurs in the ampulla of the uterine tube and results in the formation of a zygote (Fig. 2.1). The zygote undergoes cleavage to form blastomeres. Contraction of smooth muscle in the wall of the uterine tube propels the dividing zygote toward the uterine cavity. About day 3, the morula, composed of approximately 16 blastomeres, enters the uterine cavity and forms a blastocyst consisting of the outer cell mass or trophoblast, the inner cell mass or embryoblast, and the blastocyst cavity. At about day 6, the blastocyst begins to implant in the endometrium. As the trophoblast penetrates the endometrium, it differentiates into the syncytiotrophoblast and cytotrophoblast. By the end of this week, a layer of cells, the hypoblast, appears on the side of the inner cell mass facing the blastocyst cavity.

The second week is marked by the completion of implantation and the formation of the bilaminar embryonic disk (Fig. 2.2). The amniotic cavity develops between the inner cell mass and the cytotrophoblast. The epithelial roof of this cavity is the amnion. The layer of inner cell mass cells forming the floor of the cavity constitutes the epiblast. The epiblast and hypoblast form the bilaminar embryonic disk. The exocoelomic membrane, continuous with the hypoblast, surrounds a cavity called the primary yolk sac. Cells from the trophoblast form the extraembryonic mesoderm, which surrounds the amnion and primary yolk sac. Fluid-filled spaces in the extraembryonic mesoderm coalesce to form the extraembryonic coelom or chorionic cavity. As the extraembryonic coelom develops, the primary yolk sac is reduced and, as hypoblast cells grow out and line it, the secondary or definitive yolk sac forms. Except for the connecting or body stalk, the extraembryonic coelom splits the extraembryonic mesoderm into two layers: the extraembryonic splanchnic mesoderm covering the yolk sac; and the extraembryonic somatic mesoderm that covers the amnion and lines the trophoblast. The trophoblast and the extraembryonic mesoderm lining it form the chorion. The prechordal plate, a midline circular thickening of the hypoblast, marks the future mouth region and the cranial end of the embryonic disk.

During the third week, the trilaminar embryonic disk is formed, differentiation of the germ layers begins, and a primitive circulatory system is established (Fig. 2.3). A midline thickening of epiblast, the primitive streak, appears in the caudal region of the embryonic disk. Epiblast cells move to the primitive streak and pass laterally and cranially between the epiblast and the hypoblast to form the intraembryonic mesoderm. The epiblast is now called the embryonic ectoderm. Epiblast cells are thought to displace much of the hypoblast to form the embryonic endoderm. Cells from the primitive node pass between the endoderm and the ectoderm in the midline and extend cranially to the prechordal plate, which will give rise to the notochord. At the cranial and caudal ends of the embryonic disk, the endoderm and the overlying ectoderm fuse to form the oropharyngeal membrane and the cloacal membrane respectively. Embryonic mesoderm passes between the ectoderm and the endoderm except at the oropharyngeal and cloacal membranes, and where the notochord extends in the midline. Mesoderm cranial to the oropharyngeal membrane forms the cardiogenic area. Normally, the primitive streak will regress and disappear.

The notochord and adjacent mesoderm induce the overlying ectoderm to form the neural plate. Differential growth gives rise to a neural groove flanked by neural folds. The neural folds fuse to form the neural tube with a central neural canal. Fusion of the neural folds commences in the future cervical region and extends cranially and caudally (the anterior neuropore closes between days 25 and 26 of gestation, followed by the posterior neuropore 2 days later). It has been suggested that there are multiple closure sites involved in the formation of the neural tube. Some neuroectodermal cells are not incorporated into the neural tube and form the neural crests. The neural tube detaches from the ectoderm, and the surface ectoderm mainly forms the epidermis and the structures derived from it.

Differentiation of the mesoderm on each side of the notochord forms the paraxial mesoderm, which becomes

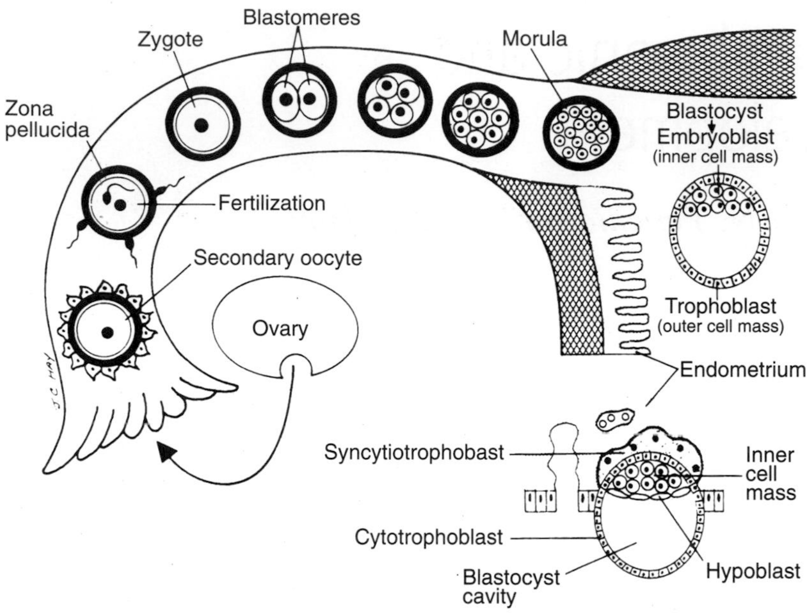

Figure 2.1 Diagram illustrating the first week of development.

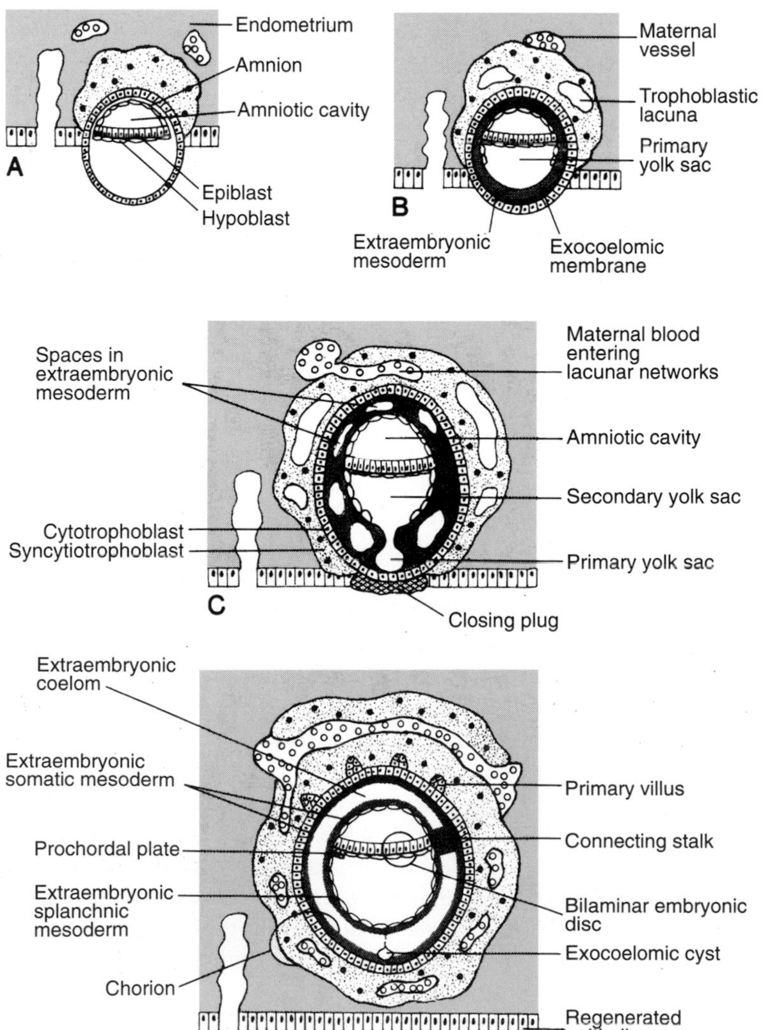

Figure 2.2 Diagrams illustrating the second week of development. Sections of the implanting blastocyst at approximately 8 days (A), 9 days (B), 12 days (C), and 14 days (D).

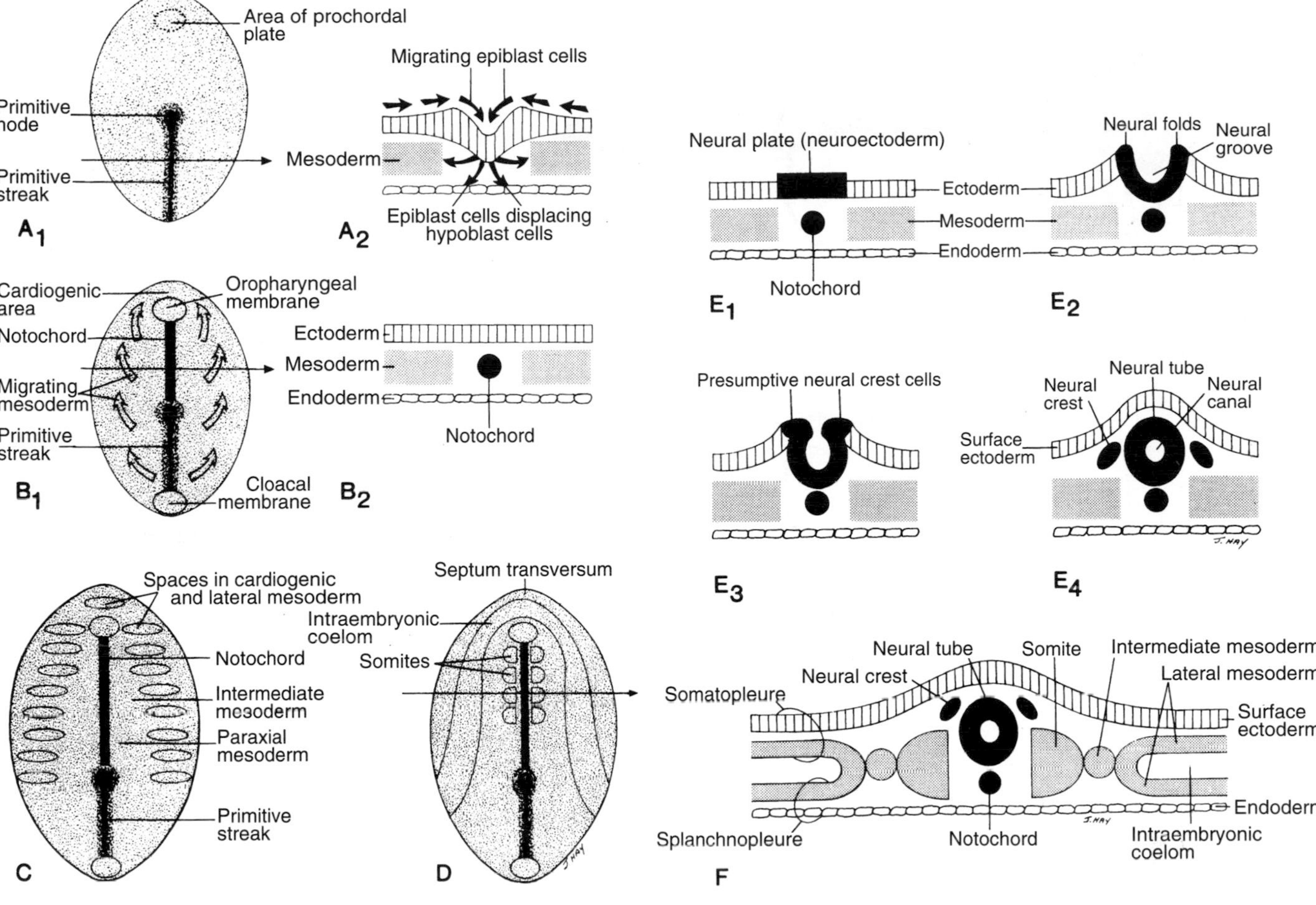

Figure 2.3 Diagrams illustrating some of the developmental events in the third week. (A_1 and B_1) Dorsal views of the embryonic disk. (A_2 and B_2) Transverse sections of the embryonic disk at the levels indicated in (A_1) and (B_1). (C and D) Dorsal views of the embryonic disk showing differentiation of the mesoderm and formation of the intraembryonic coelom (the developing neural tube has been omitted). (E_1 to E_4) Development of the neural tube and neural crests. (F) Transverse section of the embryonic disk at the level indicated in (D).

organized into 42–44 pairs of somites. Each somite is composed of a dermatome, which contributes to the dermis; a myotome, which gives rises to skeletal muscle; and a sclerotome, the cells of which migrate around the neural tube and notochord to form the precursors of the vertebrae and the ribs. It also forms the intermediate mesoderm, a small area of mesoderm lateral to the paraxial mesoderm. This is associated with the development of the urogenital system. Finally, it forms the lateral mesoderm at the margins of the disk. Spaces in this mesoderm coalesce to form the horseshoe-shaped intraembryonic coelom, which will form the pericardial, pleural, and peritoneal cavities. This coelom splits the lateral mesoderm into somatic and splanchnic layers. The somatopleure, the embryonic somatic mesoderm and ectoderm, will form the body walls. The splanchnopleure, the embryonic splanchnic mesoderm and endoderm, will form the primitive gut and the structures derived from it. In the cardiogenic area, mesoderm cranial to the embryonic coelom forms the septum transversum, which will form part of the diaphragm.

Concurrently, chorionic villi, consisting of a core of extraembryonic mesoderm covered with cytotrophoblast and syncytiotrophoblast, develop around the chorionic sac. The allantois, a finger-like extension of endoderm from the caudal wall of the yolk sac, extends into the mesoderm of the connecting stalk.

Blood vessels first appear in the extraembryonic mesoderm (except that covering the amnion) and shortly thereafter in the embryo. Clusters of cells, the blood islands, acquire lumina. The surrounding cells form the endothelium and other layers of the vessel wall. As the vessels develop and sprout, the intra- and extraembryonic vessels are linked. Blood cells develop in association with the vessels of the yolk sac and allantois. Blood cells may arise from cells trapped within the lumen as the vessel forms, or from cells shed into the lumen. Paired endothelial heart tubes develop in the cardiogenic area. These fuse to form a single contractile heart tube and, by the end of the third week, a primitive circulation is established between the embryo and the chorion.

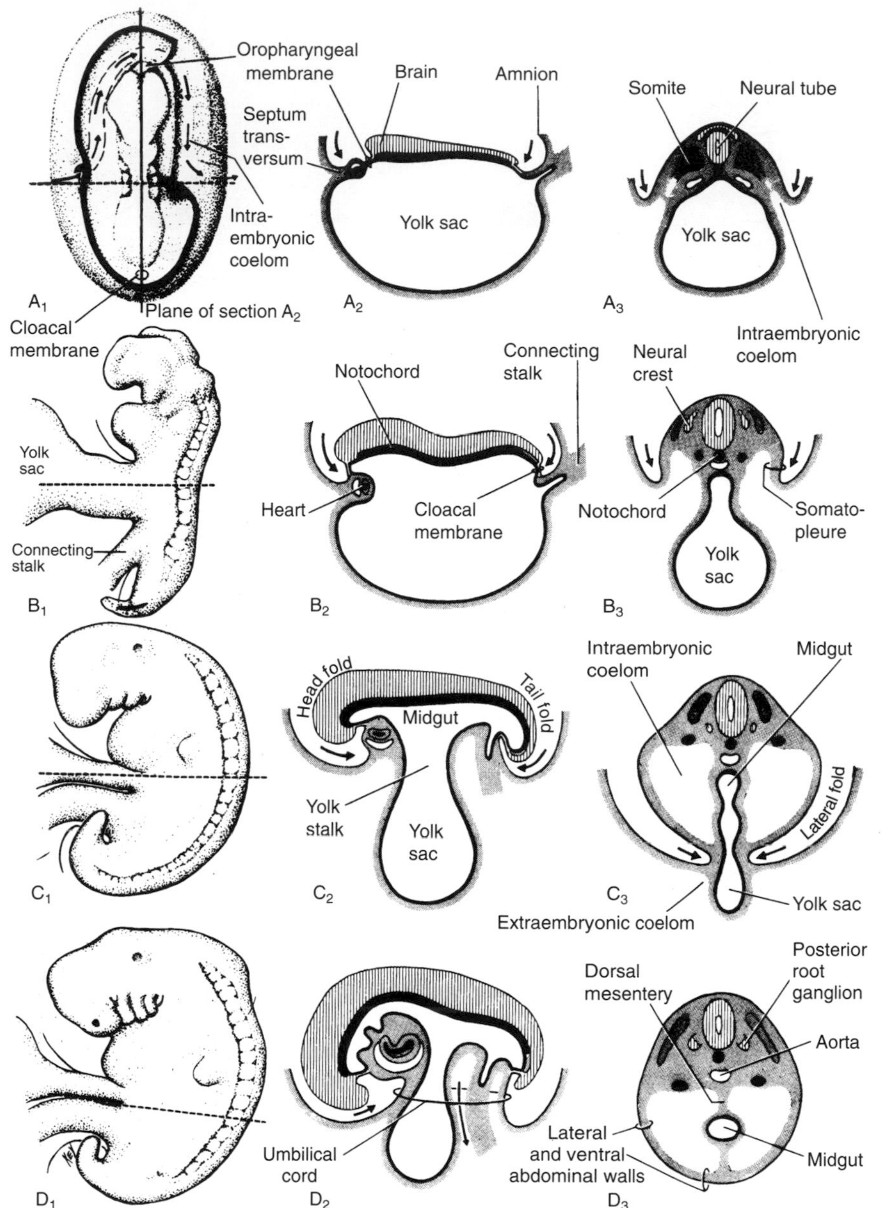

Figure 2.4 Diagrams illustrating folding of the embryonic disk during the fourth week. (A_1) Dorsal view. (B_1 to D_1) Lateral views of the embryo. (A_2 to D_2) Longitudinal sections at the levels shown in (A_3 to D_1). (From Moore KL. *The developing human*, 4th edn. Philadelphia, PA: W.B. Saunders, 1988 with permission.)

The embryonic period

The embryonic period extends from the beginning of the fourth week to the end of the eighth week. During this period, all the major internal and external structures begin their development. By the end of this period, the embryo has acquired characteristic human features. In the fourth week, the embryonic disk undergoes folding (Fig. 2.4). Folding converts the flat embryonic disk into a cylindrical embryo. Folding in the longitudinal axis results in the formation of the head and tail folds. With the head fold, the developing heart and pericardial cavity are swung onto the ventral surface, and the septum transversum then lies caudal to the developing heart. The dorsal part of the yolk sac is incorporated into the embryo to form the foregut. This is separated by the oropharyngeal membrane from the stomodeum or primitive oral cavity. With the tail fold, the body or connecting stalk, the future umbilical cord, is swung onto the ventral surface, and part of the allantois is incorporated into the embryo. The dorsal part of the yolk sac is incorporated into the embryo to form the hindgut. The terminal portion of the hindgut dilates to form the cloaca, which is separated from the amniotic cavity by the cloacal membrane. Folding in the transverse axis results in the somatopleure forming the lateral and ventral body walls. As the dorsal part of the yolk sac is incorporated into the embryo, the splanchnopleure forms the primitive gut. The midgut is connected to the yolk sac by the narrow vitelline duct. The remnant of the yolk sac ultimately degenerates. As the caudal limbs of the intraembryonic coelom are moved ventrally,

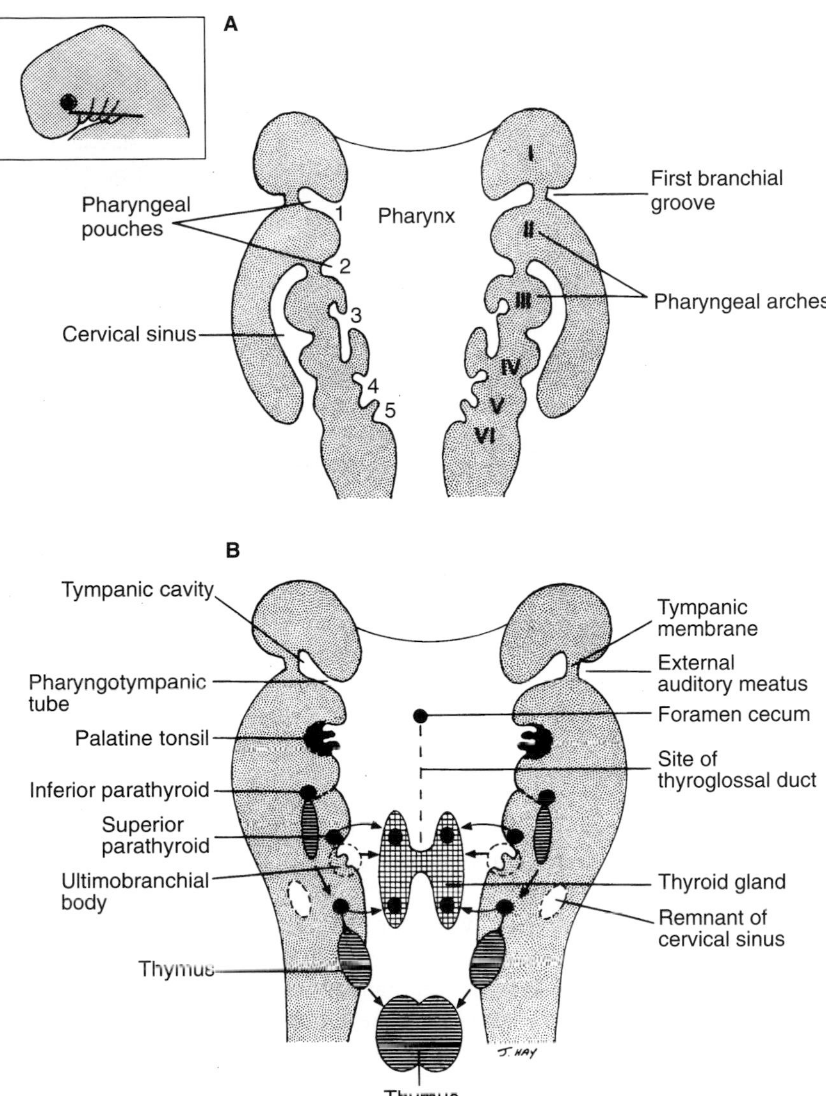

Figure 2.5 Diagrams illustrating the pharyngeal apparatus. Inset indicates the level of the horizontal sections shown in (A) and (B).

they are initially separated by a ventral mesentery. This mesentery disappears, except in the region of the foregut, and a single peritoneal cavity is formed. From the pericardial cavity, the pericardioperitoneal canals or future pleural cavities pass dorsally and caudally to communicate with the peritoneal cavity.

The fetal period

The fetal period extends from the beginning of the ninth week until birth. The main features of this period are the growth and differentiation of those tissues and organs that began their development in the embryonic period. Few new structures (hairs, nails) appear. During this period, fetal movement begins, and the life-sustaining reflexes (sucking, swallowing, etc.) are established.

Pharyngeal apparatus

In the fourth week, ridges and grooves appear in the future neck region (Fig. 2.5). These form part of the pharyngeal apparatus, which consists of the following: six pairs of pharyngeal arches numbered in a craniocaudal sequence (in humans, the fifth pharyngeal arch is absent); the pharyngeal grooves or clefts between the arches; the pharyngeal pouches (lined by endoderm and occurring internally between the arches); and the pharyngeal membranes, formed by the ectoderm and endoderm between the arches. The first or mandibular arch gives rise to the maxillary and mandibular prominences. The second or hyoid arch enlarges and grows caudally, concealing the posterior arches and creating an ectodermal depression, the cervical sinus; this arch ultimately fuses with the upper thoracic wall, giving the neck a smooth

Table 2.1 Major derivatives of the pharyngeal arch components.

Arch	Nerve	Muscles	Cartilages	Arteries
I	Trigeminal (V)	Muscles of mastication	Malleus, incus	Part of maxillary
II	Facial (VII)	Muscles of facial expression	Stapes, styloid process, part of hyoid bone	None
III	Glossopharyngeal (IX)	Stylopharyngeus	Remainder of hyoid bone	Common carotids, part of internal carotids
IV	Vagus (X) superior laryngeal branch			Part of arch of aorta and right subclavian
V		Muscles of palate, pharynx and larynx	Laryngeal cartilages (except epiglottis)	None
VI	Vagus (X) recurrent laryngeal branch			Pulmonary arteries and ductus arteriosus

contour. The first branchial groove, between the first and second arches, persists as the primordium of the external auditory meatus. In the mesodermal core of each arch are a cranial nerve, a skeletal muscle element, an artery, and a rod or bar of hyaline cartilage that is derived from neural crest cells. The ventral portions of the first arch or Meckel's cartilage disappear, and the mandible is derived from intramembranous ossification. The second arch cartilage is also called Reichert's cartilage. The derivatives of the branchial arch components are summarized in Table 2.1.

The first pair of pouches (between the first and second arches) forms the tympanic cavity and pharyngotympanic tube. The first branchial or closing membrane forms the tympanic membrane. The second pair of pouches persists in part to form the tonsillar fossa. This pair is associated with development of the palatine tonsils. The third pair of pouches develops dorsal and ventral portions. The dorsal portions separate, attach to the posterior aspect of the thyroid gland, and form the inferior parathyroid glands. The ventral portions fuse to form the thymus, which descends into the thorax. The fourth pair of pouches also develops dorsal and ventral portions and loses the connection with the pharynx. The dorsal portions separate, attach to the posterior aspect of the thyroid gland, and form the superior parathyroid glands. The small ventral portions of the fourth pouches and the rudimentary fifth pouches form the ultimobranchial bodies, which are incorporated into the thyroid gland to form the parafollicular cells.

In the fourth week, a thickening of endoderm appears in the floor of the pharynx; this grows downward to form the thyroid diverticulum. It grows caudally, becomes bilobed and is connected by the isthmus. The gland reaches its definitive position in the seventh week and is attached to its site of origin by the thyroglossal duct. This duct normally degenerates except for a small pit, the foramen cecum, in the tongue (see Fig. 2.5). In about 50% of individuals, the caudal portion of the duct persists to form a pyramidal lobe that extends upward from the isthmus. The endoderm becomes organized into follicles, and the parafollicular cells are derived from the ultimobranchial bodies. The thyroid gland is functional by the 12th week of gestation.

The primordia of the tongue appear in the floor of the pharynx in the fourth week.

The body or oral part consists of the anterior two-thirds. Proliferation of mesoderm at the ventromedial ends of the first branchial arches forms the median tongue bud (tuberculum impar) just anterior to the foramen cecum. This bud is flanked by the two distal tongue buds (lateral lingual swellings). The median tongue bud is overgrown as the distal tongue buds enlarge and fuse, and the median sulcus indicates the plane of fusion. The root or pharyngeal part consists of the posterior one-third. The copula, just posterior to the foramen cecum, is formed by proliferation of mesoderm at the ventromedial ends of the second branchial arches. Posterior to the copula, the hypobranchial eminence is derived from proliferation of mesoderm at the ventromedial ends of the third and fourth branchial arches. The cranial part of this eminence overgrows the copula; the caudal portion will form the epiglottis. The sulcus terminalis roughly demarcates the junction of the root and the body. The intrinsic muscles of the tongue are derived from myoblasts that migrate from the occipital somites, and this explains why they are innervated by the hypoglossal nerve rather than by the branchial arch nerves.

The face

The primordia of the face appear at the end of the fourth week and are related to the stomodeum or primitive oral cavity as follows: the frontonasal prominence forms the cranial boundary, the maxillary prominences form the lateral boundaries, and the mandibular prominences form the caudal boundary. These prominences, formed by accumulations of mesenchyme, are separated by grooves and furrows. During development, the prominences merge with one another as the grooves are smoothed out by proliferation of the underlying mesenchyme. Much of the mesenchyme in the facial region is considered to be of neural crest origin. Merging occurs mainly during the fifth to eighth weeks. Ectodermal thickenings on the inferolateral aspects of the frontonasal prominence form the nasal placodes. Mesenchyme around the placodes proliferates to form the medial and lateral nasal prominences, and the placodes then lie in depressions, the nasal pits or future nostrils. Expansion of the back of the head moves the eyes forward and contributes to the growth of the facial components toward the midline. The maxillary prominences merge with the medial nasal prominences, and the medial nasal prominences merge with each other to form the intermaxillary segment. The mandibular prominences merge with each other in the midline. The adult derivatives are the frontonasal prominence – the forehead, dorsum, and apex of the nose; the lateral nasal prominences – the alae of the nose; the merged medial nasal prominences (intermaxillary segment) – the columella, philtrum of the upper lip, the maxilla that bears the incisors (the premaxilla), and the primary palate; the maxillary prominences – the lateral portions of the upper lip, the upper cheeks and face, the rest of the maxilla, and the secondary palate; and the mandibular prominences – the lower lip, lower cheeks and face, and the mandible. Myoblasts from the second branchial arch migrate into the facial region to form the muscles of facial expression. Along the nasolacrimal groove between the lateral nasal and maxillary prominences, a cord of cells sinks into the underlying mesenchyme; this canalizes to form the nasolacrimal duct.

The palate

The palate develops from two primordia: the primary palate, a wedge-shaped mass of mesoderm from the innermost aspect of the intermaxillary segment that appears in the fifth week, and the secondary palate, which develops from the lateral palatine processes, shelf-like projections of mesoderm from the medial aspects of the maxillary prominences. These processes appear in the sixth week. As the developing tongue occupies most of the oral cavity, the lateral palatine processes assume a vertical position. As the stomodeum enlarges, the tongue drops down to the floor of the stomodeum, and the lateral palatine processes elevate to a horizontal position; this elevation occurs slightly later in females. Beginning anteriorly and proceeding posteriorly, the lateral palatine processes fuse with the posterior margin of the median palatine process, the inferior border of the nasal septum, and each other. Fusion involves epithelial contact, adhesion, and the replacement of the epithelial seam by mesoderm. Fusion begins in the ninth week and is completed by the 11th week in males and the 12th week in females. Intramembranous ossification spreads into the palate from the maxillary and palatine bones and extends to the posterior border of the nasal septum. Posterior to this, the unossified portion forms the soft palate and uvula. The palatal muscles are derived from the branchial arches.

The respiratory system

The nasal pits deepen to form the nasal sacs. The oronasal membrane separating the oral and nasal cavities ruptures, and the cavities communicate just posteriorly to the primary palate. The nasal septum, a midline downgrowth from the frontonasal prominence, separates the nasal cavities. In the late fetal period, the paranasal sinuses develop as bone is resorbed, and most of their expansion occurs postnatally. The epithelium of the nasal placodes, located in the roof of the nasal cavities, forms the olfactory epithelium. In the fourth week, the laryngotracheal groove appears in the floor of the pharynx; it deepens to form the laryngotracheal diverticulum. As it grows caudally, longitudinal folds of mesenchyme fuse to form the tracheoesophageal septum, which separates the laryngotracheal tube (ventrally) from the esophagus (dorsally). The laryngotracheal tube gives rise to the larynx and trachea. A lung bud develops at the caudal end of the tube, and this soon bifurcates to give two bronchopulmonary or lung buds. The right lung bud develops two secondary buds, and the left lung bud gives rise to one secondary lung bud; these buds demarcate the future lobes of the lung. Dichotomous branching forms the air-conducting passages, the bronchi and bronchioles. Respiratory tissue – the respiratory bronchioles, alveolar ducts and sacs, and the alveoli – develops at the terminal ends of the bronchioles and continues to develop postnatally. As the lungs grow into the medial aspects of the pericardioperitoneal or pleural canals, they acquire a layer of visceral pleura.

The digestive system

The primitive gut forms during the fourth week as the head, tail, and lateral folds incorporate the dorsal part of the yolk sac into the embryo (see Fig. 2.4). The endoderm of the primitive gut gives rise to the epithelium and glands of most of the digestive tract; the epithelium at the cranial and caudal ends of the tract is derived from the ectoderm of the primitive oral cavity (stomodeum) and the anal pit (proctodeum) respectively. The muscular and fibrous elements of the digestive tract and the visceral peritoneum are derived from splanchnic mesenchyme. The primitive gut is divided into three parts: the foregut, midgut, and hindgut. The derivatives of the foregut are the pharynx and its derivatives, the lower respiratory tract, the esophagus, the stomach, the duodenum, proximal to the common bile duct, and the liver, biliary tract, gallbladder, and pancreas. The esophagus develops from the cranial part of the foregut. The striated muscle of the esophagus is derived from the caudal branchial arches, and the smooth muscle of the lower esophagus develops locally from the surrounding splanchnic mesenchyme. The lumen of the esophagus becomes occluded by proliferation of the endodermal cells, but these cells degenerate and the lumen is recanalized. The stomach appears during week 4 as a fusiform dilation of the caudal part of the foregut; this primordium soon expands and broadens dorsoventrally. The dorsal border grows more rapidly than the ventral border and forms the greater curvature. As the stomach enlarges and acquires its adult shape, it rotates 90° in a clockwise direction about its longitudinal axis. Thus, the ventral border (lesser curvature) moves to the right, and the dorsal border (greater curvature) moves to the left. The original left side becomes the ventral surface, and the right side becomes the dorsal surface. The stomach is suspended from the dorsal wall of the abdominal cavity by the dorsal mesentery (dorsal mesogastrium). As the dorsal mesogastrium is carried to the left during rotation of the stomach, the lesser sac forms. Isolated clefts develop in the dorsal mesogastrium and coalesce to form the lesser peritoneal sac, which communicates with the greater peritoneal cavity through the epiploic foramen. The dorsal mesogastrium, the greater omentum, hangs from the greater curvature anterior to the developing intestines. As the embryo lengthens, the caudal part of the septum transversum thins and becomes the ventral mesentery, which attaches the stomach and the duodenum to the ventral wall of the abdominal cavity. The ventral mesentery persists only where it is attached to the caudal part of the foregut. The final shape and position of the stomach are influenced by the development of the liver and the omental bursa. The duodenum develops from the most caudal part of the foregut and the most cranial part of the midgut. These parts grow rapidly and form a C-shaped loop that projects ventrally. The junction of the foregut and the midgut is at the apex of this duodenal loop, and is demarcated by the duodenal papilla.

The liver arises as an endodermal bud from the most caudal part of the foregut; this hepatic diverticulum extends into the septum transversum, enlarges rapidly, and divides into a larger cranial part, the primordium of the liver, and a smaller caudal part, which will form the gallbladder and cystic duct. The stalk connecting the hepatic and cystic ducts to the duodenum becomes the common bile duct. The proliferating endodermal cells give rise to interlacing cords of liver cells and the epithelial lining of the intrahepatic portion of the biliary apparatus. As the liver cords invade the septum transversum, they break up the umbilical and vitelline veins to form the hepatic sinusoids. Hemopoiesis begins in the liver during the sixth week. The lobes of the liver grow extensively and soon fill most of the abdominal cavity. Initially, the lobes are about the same size, but the right lobe becomes much larger; the caudate and quadrate lobes develop as subdivisions of the left lobe. The ventral mesentery gives rise to the lesser omentum (gastrohepatic ligament and duodenohepatic ligament), the falciform ligament (liver to the anterior abdominal wall), and the visceral peritoneum of the liver.

The pancreas develops from dorsal and ventral pancreatic buds. The ventral pancreatic bud forms as an evagination of the hepatic diverticulum, and the dorsal pancreatic bud is derived from the proximal part of the duodenum, opposite the hepatic diverticulum. As the duodenum grows and rotates to the right, the two buds come together and fuse. The ventral pancreatic bud gives rise to the main pancreatic duct, the uncinate process, and the lower part of the head of the pancreas. The rest of the pancreas and the accessory pancreatic duct are formed from the dorsal pancreatic bud. The two pancreatic ducts usually anastomose to form a single pancreatic duct. The spleen is derived from the fusion of mesenchymal nodules located in the dorsal mesogastrium.

The derivatives of the midgut are the small intestines (except for the duodenum from the stomach to the entry of the common bile duct), the cecum and appendix, the ascending colon, and the proximal one-half to two-thirds of the transverse colon.

The dorsal mesentery, which suspends the midgut from the dorsal abdominal wall, elongates rapidly. The midgut elongates during the sixth week, forming a ventral, U-shaped intestinal loop.

The midgut loop has a proximal or cranial limb, and a distal or caudal limb. The communication of the midgut with the yolk sac is reduced to the narrow yolk stalk or vitelline duct, which is attached to the apex of the loop and marks the junction between the two limbs. The midgut loop migrates into the umbilical cord. This "herniation" of the intestines occurs because there is not enough room in the abdomen, mainly because of the relatively large size of the liver and kidneys. The proximal limb grows rapidly and forms intestinal loops, but the caudal limb undergoes very little change except for development of the cecal diverticulum. The midgut loop then rotates within the umbilical cord. During the 10th week, as the intestines return rapidly to the abdomen, they undergo further rotation. The midgut segment undergoes a total counterclockwise rotation of 270°. This "reduction of the midgut hernia" is usually attributed to an increase in the size of the abdominal cavity and a decrease in the relative size of the liver and kidneys. The primordium of the cecum and appendix appears during the sixth week as the cecal bud, a conical pouch of the caudal limb of the midgut loop. The apex of this blind pouch does not grow as rapidly as the rest of the cecum and forms the vermiform appendix. Elongation of the proximal part of the colon results in the cecum and appendix "descending" from the upper to the lower right quadrant of the abdomen. As the intestines assume their final positions, in some places the mesentery fuses with the parietal peritoneum and disappears; those parts of the midgut become retroperitoneal. The proximal part of the duodenum and the ascending colon become retroperitoneal. Other derivatives of the midgut loop retain their mesenteries. The transverse colon is attached to the greater omentum.

The derivatives of the hindgut are the distal one-third to one-half of the transverse colon, the descending colon, the sigmoid colon, the rectum and the upper portion of the anal canal, and part of the urogenital system. The expanded terminal part of the hindgut, the cloaca, is separated from the amniotic cavity by the cloacal membrane. The cloaca receives the allantois ventrally. A mesodermal partition, the urorectal septum, which develops between the allantois and the hindgut, divides the cloaca into the rectum and upper anal canal dorsally and the urogenital sinus ventrally. By the end of the seventh week, the urorectal septum fuses with the cloacal membrane, dividing it into a dorsal anal membrane and a ventral urogenital membrane. Proliferation of mesenchymal tissue around the anal membrane elevates the surface ectoderm and forms the shallow anal pit or proctodeum. The anal membrane at the floor of this pit ruptures by the end of the seventh week, forming the anal canal. The caudal part of the digestive tract is now in communication with the amniotic cavity. The proximal (upper) two-thirds of this canal is derived from the hindgut; the distal (lower) one-third develops from the proctodeum. The pectinate line indicates the approximate former site of the anal membrane and the junction of endoderm and ectoderm. The other layers are mesenchymal in origin.

The urinary system

At the beginning of the fourth week, the intermediate mesoderm on each side detaches from the somites and forms the nephrogenic cords. From the nephrogenic cords, three successive sets of excretory organs develop: the pronephros, the mesonephros, and the metanephros. The pronephros is formed in the cervical region and is a transitory nonfunctional structure. It regresses soon after its formation, leaving the pronephric ducts, which run caudally to enter the cloaca. These ducts will become the mesonephric ducts. The mesonephros also appears during the fourth week, caudal to the degenerating pronephros. Cell clusters in the nephrogenic cords give rise to mesonephric tubules, which drain into the mesonephric duct. The mesonephros serves as a temporary excretory organ and probably functions in urine production, but it degenerates during the latter part of the embryonic period. In the male, the mesonephric ducts form some components of the reproductive system. In the female, the mesonephric ducts degenerate, except for vestigial remnants. The permanent adult kidney, the metanephros, begins to develop early in the fifth week and is functional 2–3 weeks later. The ureteric bud develops as an outgrowth from the mesonephric duct, close to its entry into the cloaca. The ureteric bud grows dorsally and cranially to meet the metanephrogenic blastema (intermediate mesoderm). The ureteric bud forms the ureter, renal pelvis, calyces, and collecting tubules. The nephrons are derived from the metanephric blastema. At birth, the nephrons, approximately one million in each kidney, are formed, but are still short. No new nephrons are formed after birth. During infancy, the nephrons complete their differentiation and increase in size until adulthood. Initially, the metanephros is located in the sacral region of the embryo and receives its blood supply from the dorsal aorta at that level. The metanephros gradually ascends, probably as a result of caudal growth of the embryo. This results in a relative change in the position of these organs, and they receive their blood supply from progressively higher levels. As the kidney ascends, it rotates, and the position of the hilum changes from ventral to medial.

The urinary bladder is derived from the cranial part of the urogenital sinus. It is lined by endoderm; the other layers are derived from the adjacent splanchnic mesenchyme. The mucosa and musculature of the trigone area are mesodermal in origin; possibly this mucosa is later overgrown by endodermal epithelium. The allantois, continuous with the bladder, constricts to form the urachus. The adult derivative of the urachus is the median umbilical ligament, which passes from the apex of the bladder to the umbilicus. In both sexes, the urethra is derived from the caudal part of the urogenital sinus. The epithelium of the entire female urethra is derived from the endoderm of the urogenital sinus. In the male, except for its most distal part, which is derived from ectoderm, the urethral epithelium has a similar origin. In both sexes, the other layers of the urethra are derived from adjacent splanchnic mesenchyme. Rupture of the urogenital membrane brings the urinary system into communication with the amniotic cavity. The suprarenal (adrenal) glands: aggregates of mesenchymal cells, derived from the mesothelium lining the posterior body wall, form the cortex. The medulla is derived from cells of neural crest origin.

The genital system

The genetic sex of the embryo is determined at fertilization by the type of spermatozoon that fertilizes the oocyte. There is no morphological indication of sexual differences until the eighth week, when the gonads begin to acquire sexual characteristics. Initially, all normal human embryos are potentially bisexual; male and female embryos have identical gonads, genital ducts, and external genitalia. This period of early genital development is referred to as the indifferent stage of the reproductive organs. The gonads appear during the fifth week of development, as the intermediate mesoderm on the dorsal body wall forms the gonadal ridges. The coelomic epithelium grows into the underlying mesenchyme and forms the primary sex cords. A week later, the cords become populated by primordial germ cells, precursors of the spermatogonia or oogonia. The Y chromosome has a strong testis-determining effect on the indifferent gonad. Under its influence, the primary sex cords differentiate into seminiferous tubules. Absence of a Y chromosome results in the formation of an ovary. Thus, the type of sex chromosome complex established at fertilization determines the type of gonad that develops from the indifferent gonad. The type of gonad then determines the sexual differentiation of the genital ducts and external genitalia.

Two pairs of genital ducts develop in both sexes: mesonephric (wolffian) ducts and paramesonephric (müllerian) ducts. In the male, the fetal testes produce at least two hormones: one stimulates development of the mesonephric ducts into the male genital tract, and the other suppresses development of the paramesonephric ducts. Some mesonephric tubules near the testis persist and are transformed into efferent ductules or ductuli efferentes, which connect the rete testis to the epididymis. The mesonephric duct becomes the ductus epididymis and the vas deferens. The seminal vesicles develop from paired lateral diverticula from the caudal ends of the mesonephric ducts. The part of the mesonephric duct between the duct of this gland and the urethra becomes the ejaculatory duct. The appendix of the epididymis and the paradidymis are nonfunctional rudiments of the mesonephric duct and mesonephric tubules respectively. In the male, the paramesonephric ducts largely degenerate, except for two vestigial remnants: the appendix of the testis and the prostatic utricle.

In female embryos, the mesonephric ducts regress and the paramesonephric ducts give rise to the female genital tract. The cranial unfused ends of the paramesonephric ducts form the uterine tubes. The caudal portions of the ducts converge and fuse in the midline to form the uterovaginal primordium, which gives rise to the uterus, cervix, and possibly part of the vagina. The development of the vagina is not entirely settled. One theory is that the uterovaginal primordium induces the formation of paired, endodermally derived outgrowths from the urogenital sinus. These fuse to form a solid vaginal plate, which eventually canalizes to become the vagina. Thus, the vaginal epithelium is derived from the endoderm of the urogenital sinus, and the fibromuscular wall of the vagina develops from the mesenchymal cells of the uterovaginal primordium. Another view is that the uterus and upper third of the vagina are formed from the uterovaginal primordium and surrounding mesenchyme, while the lower two-thirds of the vagina is presumed to be derived from the vaginal plate and the surrounding mesenchyme. A few blind mesonephric tubules, the epoophoron, may persist in the mesovarium. Parts of the mesonephric duct may persist as Gartner's duct in the broad ligament along the lateral wall of the uterus, or as a Gartner's cyst in the wall of the vagina.

The external genitalia also pass through an indifferent stage that is not distinguishable as male or female. Early in the fourth week, a genital tubercle develops ventrally to the cloacal membrane; this elongates to form the phallus. By the sixth week, labioscrotal swellings and urogenital folds develop on each side of the future urogenital membrane. In the male, masculinization of the indifferent external genitalia is caused by androgens produced by the testes. The phallus will form the penis. The urogenital folds fuse with each other along the ventral (under) surface of the penis and form the penile urethra. The paired labioscrotal swellings grow toward each other and fuse to form the scrotum. In the female, because of the absence of androgens, feminization of the indifferent external genitalia occurs. The phallus elongates rapidly at first but, as its growth gradually slows, it becomes the relatively small clitoris. The unfused urogenital folds form the paired labia minora, whereas the labioscrotal swellings give rise to the labia majora. The caudal portion of the urogenital sinus gives rise to the vestibule of the vagina.

The cardiovascular system

The development of the heart begins in the third week in the cardiogenic area (see Fig. 2.3). Splanchnic mesoderm ventral to the pericardial cavity aggregates to form a pair of elongated heart cords. By day 17 of gestation, these cords are canalized to form endothelial tubes, called endocardial heart tubes. As the lateral folds develop, the heart tubes fuse to form a single median endocardial heart tube; fusion begins cranially and rapidly extends caudally. A single endocardial tube is formed by day 22. It is surrounded by a myoepicardial mantle and separated from the endothelial lining by cardiac jelly. With the development of the head fold, the cardiac tube comes to lie dorsal to the pericardial cavity and ventral to the foregut (see Fig. 2.4). As the tubular heart elongates, it differentiates into four main regions. From cranial to caudal, these are the bulbus cordis, ventricle, atrium, and the sinus venosus. The bulbus cordis represents the arterial end of the heart and consists of a proximal part, the conus, and a distal part, the truncus arteriosus. The sinus venosus represents the venous end of the heart. It receives the umbilical veins from the placenta, the vitelline veins from the yolk sac, and the common cardinal veins from the embryo. The arterial and venous ends of the heart tube are fixed by the pharyngeal arches and the septum transversum respectively. Because the bulbus cordis and the ventricle grow faster than the other regions, the heart tube bends upon itself, forming a U-shaped bulboventricular loop. It later becomes S-shaped. As the heart tube bends, the atrium and the sinus venosus come to lie dorsal to the bulbus cordis, truncus arteriosus, and ventricle. By this stage, the sinus venosus has developed lateral expansions, called right and left horns. The right horn of the sinus venosus subsequently becomes larger than the left. The developing heart tube now gradually invaginates into the dorsal aspect of the pericardial cavity.

Partitioning of the atrioventricular canal, the atrium, and the ventricle begins about the middle of the fourth week and is essentially complete by the end of the seventh week. At first, the atrioventricular opening is round. In the region of the atrioventricular canal, two thickenings of subendocardial tissue, the endocardial cushions, appear in the dorsal and ventral walls of the heart. During the fifth week, these cushions grow toward each other and fuse, dividing the atrioventricular canal into right and left atrioventricular canals. The primitive atrial chamber communicates posteriorly with the sinus venosus, and inferiorly with the ventricle through the atrioventricular canal. A crescent-shaped membrane, the septum primum, grows down toward the endocardial cushions. A large gap, the foramen primum, exists between its lower free edge and the endocardial cushions. As the septum primum grows toward the endocardial cushions, the foramen primum becomes progressively smaller. Before the foramen primum is obliterated, an opening, the foramen secundum, appears in the upper part of septum primum. Concurrently, the free edge of the septum primum fuses with the left side of the fused endocardial cushions and obliterates the foramen primum. At this stage, the left atrium receives most of its blood from the right atrium via the foramen secundum. Toward the end of the fifth week, a second membrane, the septum secundum, arises from the roof of the atrium on the right side of the septum primum. As this septum grows downward toward the endocardial cushions, it gradually overlaps the foramen secundum. The septum secundum forms an incomplete partition with an oblique opening, the foramen ovale, through which the two atria communicate. The upper part of the septum primum gradually degenerates, while the remaining part of the septum primum persists as the valve of the foramen ovale. Whereas the lower border of the septum secundum (crista dividens) is thick and firm, the edge of the septum primum is thin and mobile, and offers no obstruction to blood flow from the right to the left atrium. The foramen ovale persists throughout fetal life. Initially, the sinus venosus is a separate chamber, opening into the part of the primitive atrium that will become the right atrium. The left horn of the sinus venosus and its tributaries regress, leaving the coronary sinus. After the formation of the interatrial septum, the right horn of the sinus venosus becomes incorporated into the wall of the right atrium, forming the smooth part of its wall. Most of the wall of the left atrium is smooth and is derived from the primitive pulmonary vein. Initially, a single pulmonary vein opens into the primitive left atrium. As the atrium expands, this vein is gradually incorporated into the wall of the left atrium, and the proximal portions of its branches are progressively absorbed. This results in four pulmonary veins, which open separately into the atrium.

The ventricles are derived from the primitive ventricular chamber and the proximal part of the bulbus cordis, the conus. The infundibulum of the right ventricle and the aortic vestibule of the left ventricle arise from the conus. Partitioning of the primitive ventricle into right and left ventricles is first indicated by a muscular ridge, the interventricular septum, which grows upward from the floor of the bulboventricular cavity, and divides it into right and left halves. Initially, most of the growth of the interventricular septum results from dilation of the ventricles on each side of it. Later, there is active growth of septal tissue as the muscular portion of the interventricular septum forms. The gap between the upper free edge of the interventricular septum and the endocardial cushions permits communication between the right and left ventricles until about the end of the seventh week. Proliferation of tissue from several sources forms the membranous portion of the interventricular septum, and it completes the partitioning of the ventricles. During the fifth week, opposing ridges of subendocardial tissue, the bulbar ridges, arise in the wall of the bulbus cordis. Similar ridges also form in the truncus arteriosus and are continuous with those in the bulbus cordis. The spiral orientation of the ridges is possibly caused by the streaming of blood from the ventricles. Fusion of these ridges results in a spiral aorticopulmonary septum. The septum subdivides the bulbus cordis and the truncus arteriosus into two channels, the ascending aorta and the pulmonary trunk. Blood from the aorta now passes into the third and fourth pairs of aortic arch arteries, and blood from the pulmonary trunk flows into the sixth pair of aortic arch arteries. Because of the spiral orientation of the septum, the pulmonary trunk twists around the ascending aorta. Proximally, the pulmonary trunk lies ventral to the aorta but, distally, it lies to the left of the aorta. The bulbus cordis is gradually incorporated into the walls of the ventricles. Closure of the interventricular foramen, at about the end of the seventh week, results from the fusion of subendocardial tissue from the right bulbar ridge, the left bulbar ridge, and the fused endocardial cushions. The membranous part of the interventricular septum is derived from proliferation of tissue from the right side of the fused endocardial cushions. This tissue fuses with the aorticopulmonary septum and the muscular part of the interventricular septum. Following closure of the interventricular foramen, the pulmonary trunk is in communication with the right ventricle and the aorta with the left ventricle. Cardiac valves develop as swellings or ridges of subendocardial tissue that become hollowed out and reshaped.

Six pairs of aortic or branchial arch arteries arise from the aortic sac, a dilated region of the truncus arteriosus, and terminate in the dorsal aorta of the corresponding side. Their derivatives are: first pair, parts of the maxillary arteries; second pair, no adult derivatives; third pair, common carotid arteries and part of internal carotid arteries; fourth pair, left – part of arch of aorta; and right – part of right subclavian artery; fifth pair, no adult derivatives; sixth pair, left – proximal: proximal part of left pulmonary artery; distal: ductus arteriosus (acts as a shunt in prenatal life); and right – proximal: proximal part of right pulmonary artery; distal: degenerates.

Fetal circulation

Well-oxygenated blood returns from the placenta in the umbilical vein. About half the blood passes through the hepatic sinusoids; the remainder bypasses the sinusoids by going through the ductus venosus into the inferior vena cava. This blood flow is regulated by a muscular sphincter in the ductus venosus near the umbilical vein. After a short course in the inferior vena cava, the blood enters the right atrium. Because the inferior vena cava also receives deoxygenated blood from the lower limbs and viscera, the blood entering the right atrium is less oxygenated than that in the umbilical vein. The blood from the inferior vena cava is largely directed by the lower border of the septum secundum (the crista dividens) through the

Table 2.2 Major derivatives of the three primary brain vesicles.

Primary vesicles	Secondary vesicles	Derivatives	Lumen
Prosencephalon	Telencephalon	Cerebral hemispheres consisting of the olfactory system, corpus striatum, cortex, and medullary center	Lateral ventricles and part of the third ventricle
	Diencephalon	Thalamus, epithalamus, hypothalamus, and subthalamus	Major part of the third ventricle
Mesencephalon	Mesencephalon	Midbrain: colliculi and cerebral peduncles	Cerebral aqueduct
Rhombencephalon	Metencephalon	Pons and cerebellum	Fourth ventricle
	Myelencephalon	Medulla oblongata	Fourth ventricle and part of the central canal

foramen ovale into the left atrium. In the left atrium, it mixes with a relatively small amount of deoxygenated blood returning from the lungs via the pulmonary veins. From the left atrium, the blood passes into the left ventricle and leaves via the ascending aorta. Consequently, the vessels to the heart, head and neck, and upper limbs receive rather well-oxygenated blood. A small stream of oxygenated blood from the inferior vena cava is diverted by the crista dividens and remains in the right atrium. This blood mixes with deoxygenated blood from the superior vena cava and coronary sinus and passes into the right ventricle. From the right ventricle, the blood enters the pulmonary trunk. Only a small amount of this blood reaches the lungs. The greater part of the blood is diverted through the ductus arteriosus into the aorta. Some of this blood circulates to the abdominal and pelvic viscera and the lower limbs and is returned to the fetal heart, but much of the blood in the aorta is transported by the umbilical arteries to the placenta.

Changes occur in several fetal blood vessels. Muscle in the walls of the umbilical arteries contracts, occludes the lumen, and thus prevents the loss of fetal blood. When the umbilical vein is occluded and blood flow from the placenta ceases, the pressure in the right atrium is lowered. The ductus venosus also becomes occluded. Occlusion of the ductus arteriosus results in all the blood from the right ventricle going to the lungs for oxygenation. Because this increases the volume of blood returning to the left atrium from the lungs, the pressure in the left atrium is raised. As a result of the difference in pressure between the right and left atria, the valve of the foramen ovale closes. Anatomical closure of the fetal blood vessels by fibrous tissue forms various ligamentous remnants: umbilical arteries, medial umbilical ligaments; left umbilical vein, ligamentum teres of the liver; ductus venosus, ligamentum venosum; ductus arteriosus, ligamentum arteriosum.

The nervous system

The neural tube (see Fig. 2.3) gives rise to the entire central nervous system, with the exception of its blood vessels and certain neuroglial cells. At first, the neural tube consists of a layer of pseudostratified columnar neuroepithelial cells. As a result of continuous cell proliferation, the walls of the neural tube become thickened and develop an inner ventricular (ependymal) layer, an intermediate (mantle) layer, and an outer marginal layer. All nerve and macroglial cells (astrocytes and oligodendrocytes) are derived from the neuroepithelial cells; the microglial cells differentiate from mesenchymal cells that have entered the central nervous system with developing blood vessels. The sulcus limitans separates the dorsal alar plate (sensory) from the ventral basal plate (motor). The cranial part of the neural tube grows rapidly to form the three primary brain vesicles: the forebrain vesicle (prosencephalon), the midbrain vesicle (mesencephalon), and the hindbrain vesicle (rhombencephalon). The lumen of the neural tube mainly forms the ventricles of the brain. The derivatives of the primary brain vesicles are summarized in Table 2.2. The rapid growth of the brain results in the formation of two flexures, the cranial (midbrain) and caudal (cervical) flexures. Later, a third flexure, the pontine flexure, appears between the metencephalon and myelencephalon

The spinal cord develops from the caudal part of the neural tube. From the alar and basal plates, the posterior and anterior horns are derived respectively. These plates contribute to the formation of the lateral horn. The neural canal becomes the central canal of the spinal cord. From the neural crest cells, the following structures differentiate: sensory ganglia of the cranial and spinal nerves, autonomic ganglia, neurilemmal (Schwann) cells, cells of the suprarenal medulla, and melanocytes. Neural crest cells contribute to the development of the connective tissues of the head, the meninges, and the pharyngeal arches.

The pituitary gland (hypophysis) develops from two sources: the neurohypophysis develops as a downgrowth from the floor of the diencephalon, and the adenohypophysis develops from an ectodermal outgrowth (Rathke's pouch) from the roof of the stomodeum.

The musculoskeletal system

By the end of the fourth week, the limb buds appear as paddle-shaped thickenings of the somatic mesoderm at the level of the lower cervical and lumbosacral somites. At the apex of each limb bud, the overlying ectoderm thickens to form the apical ectodermal ridge. The apical ectodermal ridge induces proliferation of the underlying mesenchyme, some of which differentiates into cartilage. The cartilaginous segments of the limbs are sequentially established in a proximodistal order. The flattened hand and foot plates develop five mesenchymal condensations (digital rays), which will give rise to the metacarpals, metatarsals, and phalanges. Programmed cell death or apoptosis is responsible for the degeneration of the loose mesenchyme between the digital rays which separates the fingers and toes (interdigital clefts). By the seventh week, endochondral ossification begins. The limb muscles develop from myogenic precursor cells in the limb buds, which probably originate from the somites. Immediately following their formation, the muscles are penetrated by nerves. The muscle masses separate into extensor (dorsal) and flexor (ventral) compartments. Between the seventh and ninth weeks, the developing limbs rotate longitudinally in opposite directions at the elbow and knee regions. Whereas the arm buds rotate laterally, the limb buds rotate medially. Thus, the anterior (flexor) compartments of the arm and forearm are homologous to the posterior compartments of the thigh and leg.

The skull consists of the neurocranium, which surrounds the brain, and the viscerocranium or facial skeleton. The flat bones surrounding the brain form the membranous part of the

Key points

1 The fertilized oocyte (zygote) undergoes cleavage, forming a morula and, by day 6, it differentiates into a blastocyst, which then implants in the endometrium.

2 Implantation is completed by the end of the second week as a bilaminar embryonic disk of epiblast and hypoblast is formed.

3 Intraembryonic mesoderm forms the somites, which give rise to the dermis and skeletal muscle, and precursors of the vertebrae and the ribs.

4 The intraembryonic coelom, which is formed in the lateral mesoderm, gives rise to the pericardial, pleural, and peritoneal cavities.

5 Blood vessels first appear as clusters of differentiated mesenchymal cells (blood islands) that acquire lumina.

6 The embryonic period extends from the beginning of the fourth week to the end of the eighth week; the fetal period is from the beginning of the ninth week until birth.

7 Folding converts the flat embryonic disk into a cylindrical embryo.

8 The thyroid diverticulum forms in the floor of the pharynx, grows caudally, and becomes functional by the 12th week of gestation.

9 The primordia of the face (the frontonasal prominence, the maxillary prominences, and the mandibular prominences) merge during the fifth to eighth weeks to form the facial structures.

10 The palate develops from two primordia: the primary palate, a wedge-shaped mesodermal mass from the innermost aspect of the intermaxillary segment (fifth week); and the secondary palate from the medial aspects of the maxillary prominences (sixth week).

11 Fusion of the primordia of the palate begins in the ninth week and is completed by the 11th week in males and the 12th week in females.

12 The larynx, trachea, and lung buds develop from the laryngotracheal tube.

13 The foregut derivatives are the pharynx and its derivatives, the lower respiratory tract, the esophagus, the stomach, the duodenum, proximal to the common bile duct, and the liver, biliary tract, gallbladder, and pancreas.

14 Three successive sets of excretory organs develop: transitory, the pronephros; a temporary mesonephros; and the definitive metanephros that will give rise to the kidneys.

15 Two pairs of genital ducts develop in both sexes: mesonephric (wolffian) ducts and paramesonephric (müllerian) ducts, which contribute to the male and female urogenital systems.

16 In female embryos, the mesonephric ducts regress, the paramesonephric ducts give rise to the female genital tract, and the cranial unfused ends of the paramesonephric ducts form the uterine tubes.

17 The caudal portions of the ducts fuse in the midline to form the uterovaginal primordium, which gives rise to the uterus, cervix, and possibly part of the vagina.

18 The development of the heart begins as a single endocardial heart tube, which forms the heart by the end of the embryonic period.

19 The notochord induces the overlying ectoderm to form the neural plate, which gives rise to the neural tube, the primordium of the central nervous system: the forebrain vesicle (prosencephalon), the midbrain vesicle (mesencephalon), and the hindbrain vesicle (rhombencephalon).

neurocranium, and the cartilaginous part gives rise to the bones of the base of the skull. The skull develops from the mesenchyme surrounding the developing brain, with contributions from the first four occipital somites and the first pharyngeal arch. The frontal, parietal, zygomatic, palatine, nasal, and lacrimal bones, the maxilla, and the vomer are formed by intramembranous ossification. Only the ethmoid bone and the inferior nasal conchae are completely formed in cartilage. Bones formed by intramembranous and endochondral ossifications include the occipital, sphenoid, and temporal bones, and the mandible.

References

1 Carlson BM. *Human embryology and developmental biology*, 3rd edn. Philadelphia, PA: Mosby, 2004.

2 Drews V. *Color atlas of embryology*. New York: Thieme Medical Publishers: 1995.

3 England MA. *Color atlas of life before birth*. Chicago, IL: Year Book Medical, 1983.

4 Hinrichsen KV, ed. *Human embryologie*. Berlin: Springer Verlag, 1995.

5 Larsen WJ. *Human embryology*, 3rd edn. New York: Churchill Livingstone, 2001.

6 Moore KL, Persaud TVN. *The developing human. Clinically oriented embryology*, 7th edn. Philadelphia, PA: W.B. Saunders, 2003.

7 Moore KL, Persaud TVN, Shiota K. *Color atlas of clinical embryology*, 2nd edn. Philadelphia, PA: W.B. Saunders, 2000.

8 O'Rahilly R, Müller F. *Human embryology and teratology*, 3rd edn. New York: Wiley-Liss, 2001.

9 Sadler TW. *Langman's medical embryology*, 9th edn. Baltimore, MD: Lippincott Williams & Wilkins, 2004.

Part II

Pregnancy and the Fetoplacental Unit

3 Normal and abnormal placentation

Soheila Korourian and Luis De Las Casas

Anatomy, structure, and function

Proper function and development of the placenta is critical to the survival of the embryo. The placenta is not only responsible for implantation but it is also necessary for the transport of nutrients and redirection of the maternal endocrine, immune, and metabolic functions to support the embryo.

The ovum is fertilized in the fallopian tube and develops rapidly, reaching the endometrial cavity as a blastocyst. A surge of estrogens, secreted by ovarian follicles, triggers and induces implantation. In the absence of this surge, implantation cannot occur.[1–5]

The trophoblasts grow rapidly and circumferentially, invading the endometrium and the wall of the spiral arteries of the endometrium. Table 3.1 shows some of the crucial developmental stages of the conceptus during the first postcoital (p.c.) month. Allantoic vessels establish connectivity with the vessels developing in the villi, resulting in fetoplacental circulation by the fifth week of gestation (Fig. 3.1). Initially, villi surround the entire chorionic cavity, but as the chorion grows into the endometrial cavity, the villi on the implantation aspect continue to proliferate, forming the definitive chorionic plate, while the villi oriented toward the uterine cavity undergo atrophy resulting in formation of the fetal membrane.[6–12]

Between the 14th and 20th weeks of pregnancy, intermediate trophoblasts invade the myometrial segments of the spiral arteries. Continued growth and enlargement of the chorion result in obliteration of the uterine cavity at around 20 weeks' gestation (Fig. 3.2). The Po_2 rises sharply at the start of the second trimester. As the villi mature, the barrier between maternal and fetal circulation is reduced.[13–16]

A term placenta consists of 40–60 functional units. These units receive oxygenated blood from the branches of the maternal spiral arteries, which are present in the stem villi. Each lobular unit depends on its own spiral artery (Fig. 3.3). Thrombosis of the spiral arteries results in infarction of the dependent unit.[17]

Umbilical cord

The umbilical cord is a counterclockwise spiraled cord that usually has three vessels: two arteries, which originate from the internal iliac arteries, and one vein, which drains into the hepatic vein. Usually, 96% of umbilical arteries are either fused or connected via an anastomosis. The umbilical arteries have no internal elastic membrane, whereas the vein has an elastic sublayer.[7,18–20] A single umbilical artery is seen in less than 1% of deliveries. Single artery cords are more common in diabetic mothers and in fetuses with chromosomal abnormalities (Fig. 3.4). Infants with a single umbilical artery have a lower birthweight and higher perinatal mortality rate.[21–23] Closure of the umbilical cord at birth is caused by irregular constrictions of the arteries; this is mediated by serotonin, angiotensin, and oxytocin as well as by prostaglandins.[24,25]

A normal cord is 37.7 ± 7.73 mm in diameter. A diminished size seems to be due to a reduction in Wharton's jelly, and can cause vascular occlusion.[26–28] The length of the umbilical cord is important and can most accurately be measured in the delivery room. Short cords, defined as cords less than 32 cm long, are seen in 0.4–0.9% of pregnancies. They are often seen in conditions restricting fetal mobility, such as oligohydramnios, and crowding (multiple pregnancy) and have been linked to fetal distress. Short cords have also been seen in children with Down syndrome. In the absence of fetal anomalies, short cords have been associated with neonatal hypotonia and an increased need for resuscitation. At the extreme, there may be complete or near complete absence of the cord (acordia), associated with fetal anterior wall defects. This condition is uniformly fatal. Abnormally long cords, defined as cords longer than 80 cm according to some references or 100 cm according to others, are seen in 3.7% and 0.5% of pregnancies respectively.[29–38] Abnormally long cords have been associated with excess knotting, torsion, encirclement around body parts, prolapsed cord, and vascular occlusions.

Table 3.1 Stages of placental development, postcoital days 1–29.

Postcoital days	Stage	Diameter (mm)	Size of embryo	Placental state
1	1 fertilized egg	0.1		
2	2–4 cells	0.1–0.2		
3	4–16 cells	0.1–0.2		
4	16 ± 64 cells	0.2		
5 to early day 6	128 ± 256 cells	0.2–0.3		Blastocyst attaches to endometrium
6 to early day 8	Prelacunar stage	0.3 × 0.3 × 0.15		Blastocyst partially implanted
Late day 8 to day 12	Lacunar or trabecular stage	0.5 × 0.5 × 0.3 to 0.9 × 0.9 × 0.6	0.1 mm	Implantation pole exhibits vacuoles (first lacunae), endometrium 0.5 mm at implantation site
13–14	Villous stage	1.2–2.1	0.2–0.4 mm, yolk sac appears	Development of primary villi
15–18	Secondary villous stage	5–8	<0.9 mm, development of notochordal and neuroenteric canals	Mesenchyme invades the villi, transforming them to secondary villi
19–23	Early tertiary villi	12–15	1.5–3.5 mm, neural tube starts to fuse	First appearance of villous capillaries
23–29	Early tertiary villi	18–21	Crown–rump length 2.5–5 mm, 21–29 closure of caudal somites, neuropore, three visceral arches, appearance of upper limb buds	First appearance of villous stems characterized by fibrous stroma

Adopted and modified from ref. 8.

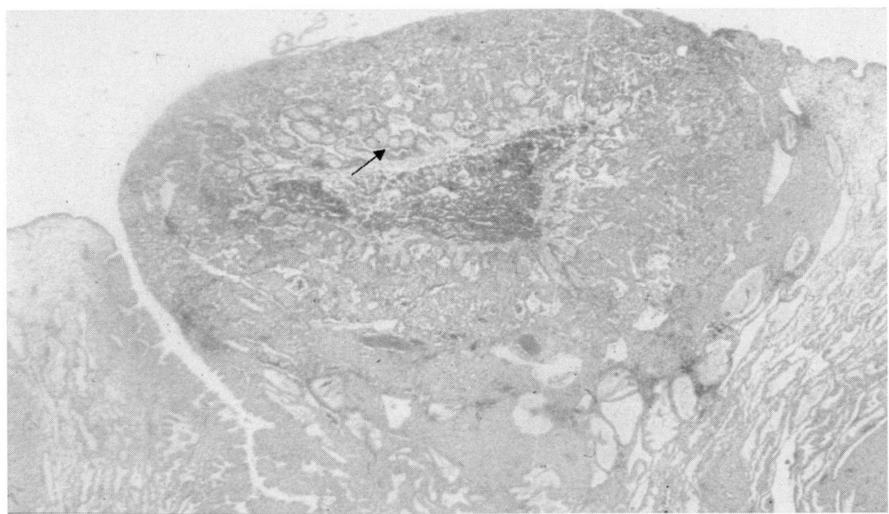

Figure 3.1 Implantation site; arrow marks the tertiary villi seen in the first trimester. Lacunar stage; fetal circulation is established.

Most investigators agree that spiraling of the cord is due to fetal activity. Absence of spiraling is likely due to either disturbances of the central nervous system or the presence of chromosomal abnormalities.

True umbilical knots are reported in 0.35–0.5% of pregnancies (Fig. 3.5). True knots are associated with an overall perinatal mortality rate of 8–11%, and acutely tightened or longstanding knots may be responsible for intrauterine or intrapartum fetal death. False knots are generally of no clinical significance.[39–41]

Hematomas of the umbilical cord cause red–purple swelling at the fetal end (Fig. 3.6); they are usually single but may be multiple. The perinatal mortality rate of cord hematomas is 40–50%.[42,43]

Thrombosis of the umbilical cord is uncommon and may be associated with cord compression, abnormal coiling, knots, torsion, stricture, hematomas, funisitis, anomalous insertion, amniotic band, or entanglements. Fetal morbidity and mortality are very high.[44–46]

Complete cord rupture is rare. Partial rupture with the formation of hemorrhage and hematomas is more common.[47]

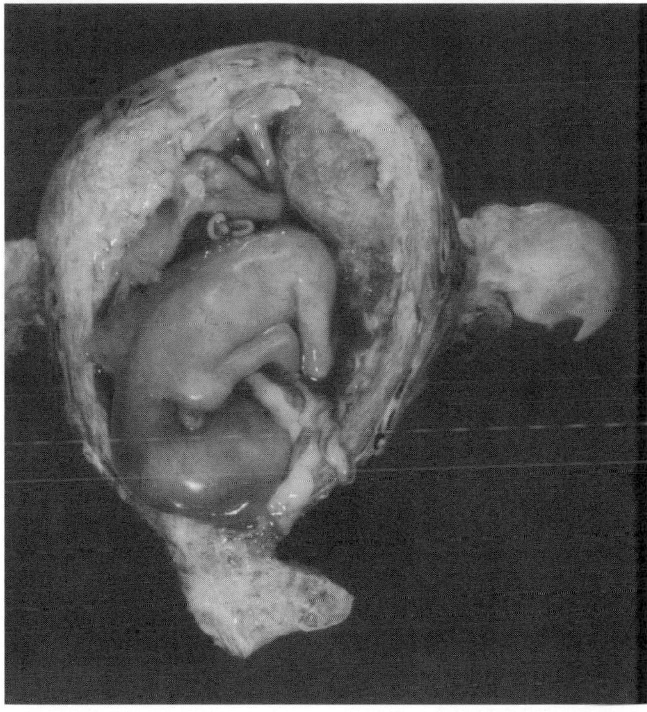

Figure 3.2 Continued growth and enlargement of the chorion results in the obliteration of the uterine cavity at approximately 20 weeks' gestation.

Circulatory disorders

The placenta is a vascular organ with a dual blood supply. The integrity of both maternal and fetal circulation is essential to placental function.

Placental infarct

Placental infarcts occur when the maternal blood flow through spiral arteries is obstructed by thrombi or in the presence of a retroplacental hematoma. Small placental infarcts, usually less than 3 cm in greatest dimension, are found in approximately 25% of placentas from uncomplicated pregnancies. Multiple or large infarcts, and especially centrally located infarcts and infarcts occurring in the first and second trimester, are clinically significant (Fig. 3.7).

Clinically significant infarcts can cause neonatal asphyxia, low birthweight, and fetal death. There is a consistent positive correlation between infarcts and maternal thrombophilia, and with intrauterine growth retardation (IUGR), in both term and preterm infants.

Recurrent pregnancy loss related to acute atherosis is a recognized complication in women with circulating antiphospholipid antibodies (scleroderma and systemic lupus) and in women with coagulation disorders (antithrombin III, protein C or S deficiency).[48–64]

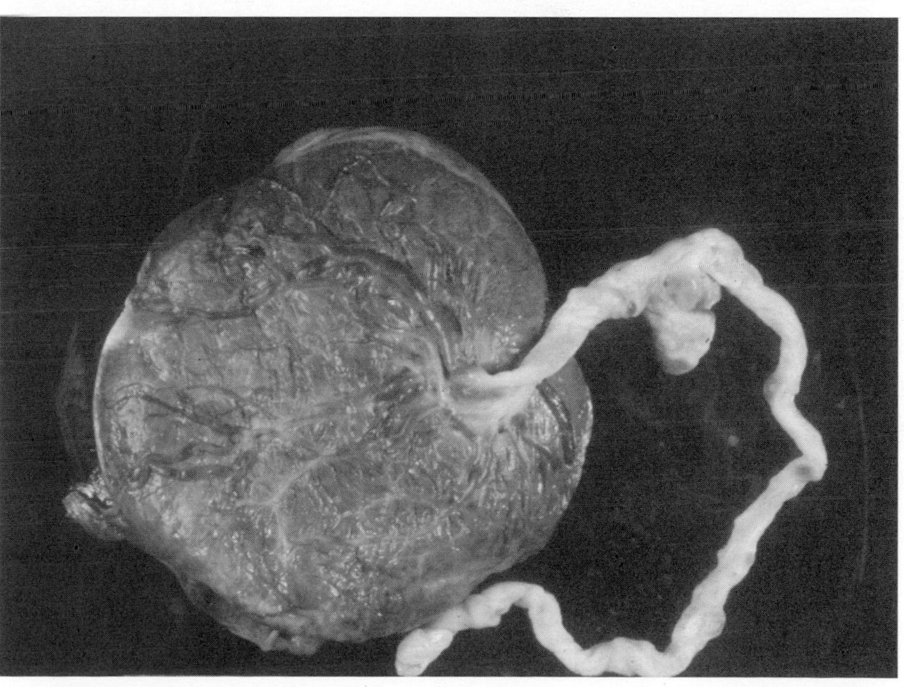

Figure 3.3 Term placenta; fetal surface is steel gray and glistening. Umbilical cord usually inserts slightly off center.

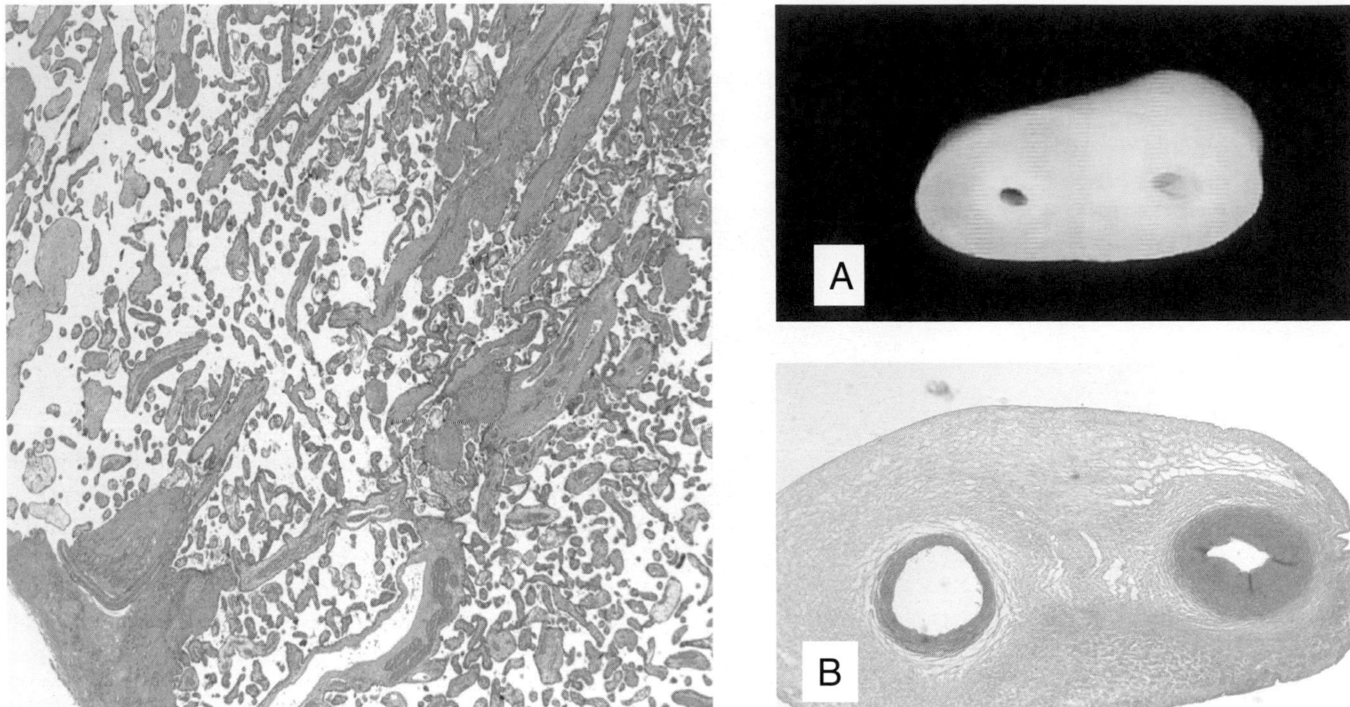

Figure 3.4 Left: underdeveloped placenta weighing 220 g at 40 weeks' gestation, below 5% of placental weight for the gestational age. Right: two-vessel umbilical cord (A, gross picture, from ref. 158, with permission; B, microscopic image).

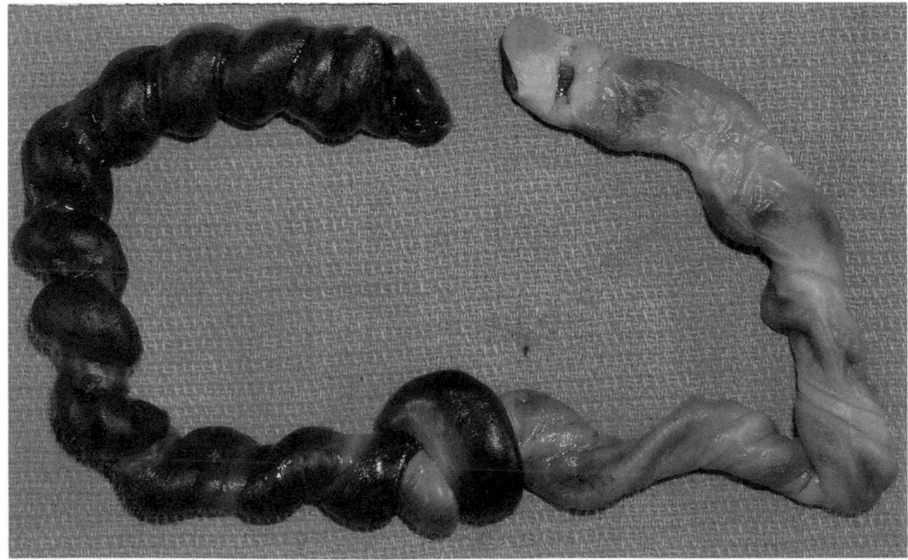

Figure 3.5 Umbilical cord knot with complete torsion and umbilical cord hematoma.

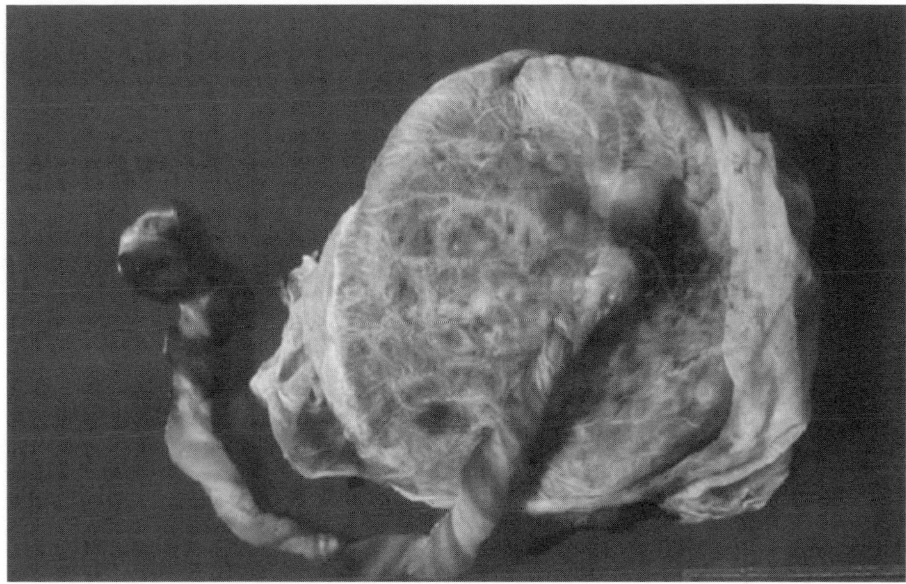

Figure 3.6 Thrombosis of umbilical cord.

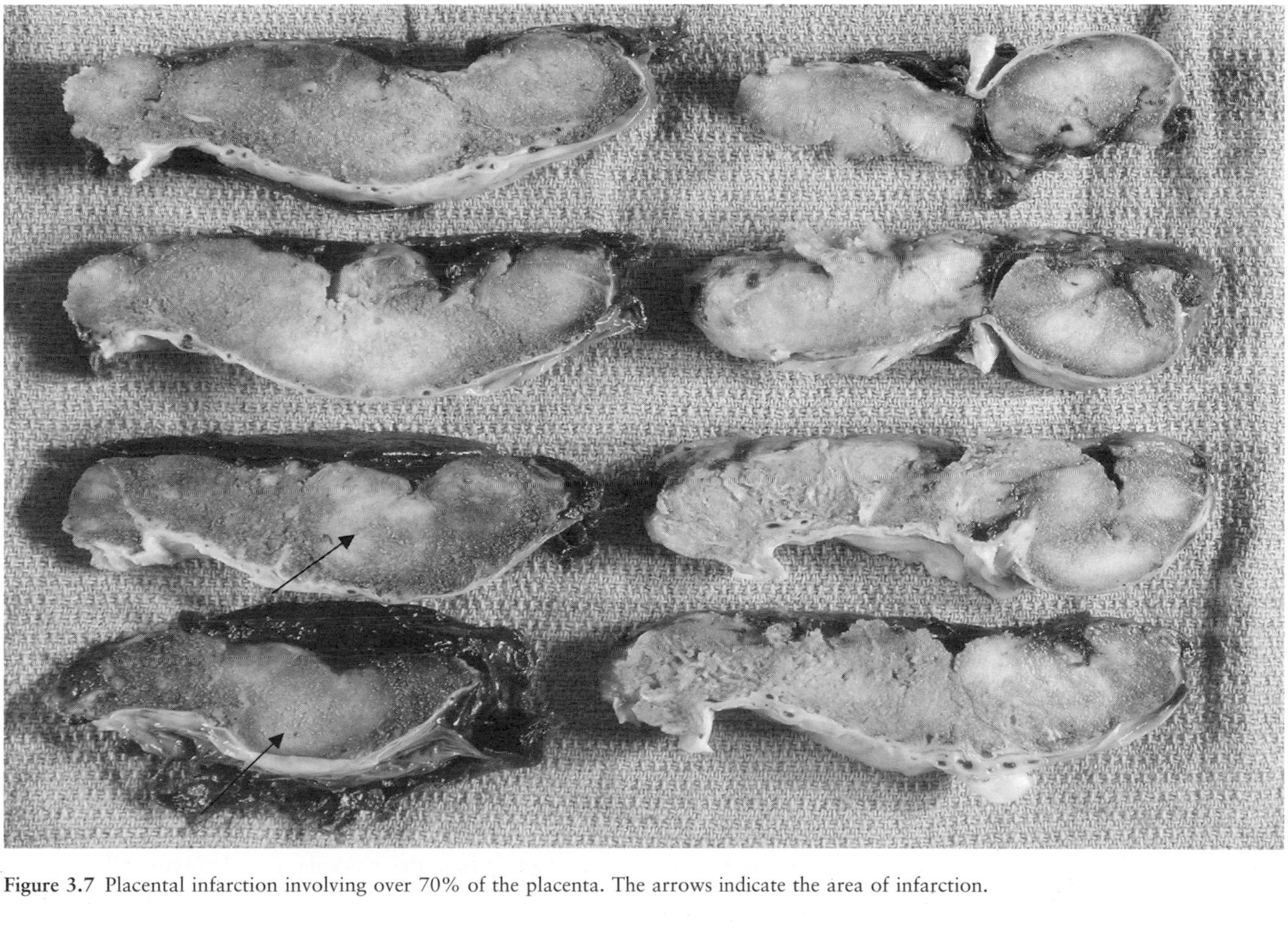

Figure 3.7 Placental infarction involving over 70% of the placenta. The arrows indicate the area of infarction.

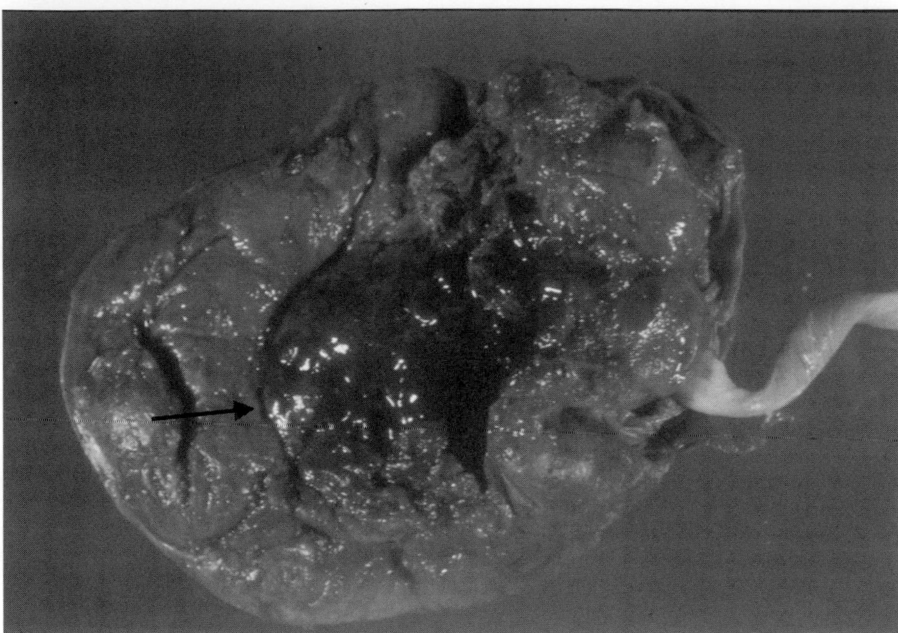

Figure 3.8 Retroplacental hematoma; arrow marks the area of depression secondary to the hematoma.

Maternal floor infarct

Maternal floor infarct is characterized by heavy deposition of fibrin in the region of basal villi adjacent to the decidua basalis. The fibrin extends to the intervillous space. It is reported in 0.09–5% of pregnancies and is associated with a high mortality rate (17–40%) and IUGR. It frequently recurs in successive pregnancies.[65–67]

Retroplacental hematomas and placental abruption

Retroplacental hematomas are clots located in the decidua between the placental floor and the muscular wall of the uterus (Fig. 3.8). They may cause a characteristic depression in the placenta. Acute bleeding from a ruptured decidual artery spreads along the decidua between the placenta and the uterine wall, often resulting in complete detachment of the placenta. In these types of cases, placentas do not show any deformity.

The predisposing factors for retroplacental hematoma and placental abruption are similar. These include pre-eclampsia, trauma, essential hypertension, smoking, and chorioamnionitis. Recent studies also implicate thrombophilic states.

Small hematomas in the decidual layer can occur days or weeks before delivery, sometimes in association with a circumvallate placenta. This condition is frequently referred to as chronic abruption.

Retroplacental hematoma is related to, but not synonymous with, placental abruption. Placental abruption is an acute clinical syndrome characterized by pain, uterine tetany, fetal distress, and sometimes consumption coagulopathy. It occurs in 1.1% of pregnancies and is associated with a 20–40% fetal mortality rate. It accounts for 10% of all stillbirths and 5% of maternal deaths.

In approximately 65% of cases of retroplacental hematomas, placental abruption does not occur.[68–77]

Placental inflammation and intrauterine infections

Placental inflammation is common. Different patterns of inflammation are associated with different routes of infection. Ascending infection, commonly caused by bacteria, induces acute inflammation of the membrane (chorioamnionitis) and umbilical cord (funisitis), and ultimately causes fetal infection. Hematogenous infections, usually caused by viruses, induce inflammation of the villous parenchyma.

Acute chorioamnionitis and funisitis

This is caused by the inflammatory response of membranes to the ascending infection (Fig. 3.9). The infection is usually caused by bacteria, including normal cervicovaginal flora such as group B β-hemolytic streptococci, *Ureaplasma urealyticum*, *Mycoplasma hominis*, *Fusobacterium*, and, rarely, *Candida* species.

In most cases, the placenta is macroscopically normal. Occasionally, the membrane may be opaque, friable, or foul smelling.

The maternal reaction is demonstrated by an accumulation of neutrophils in the decidua that migrate progressively through the chorion, amnion, and into the amniotic fluid. The

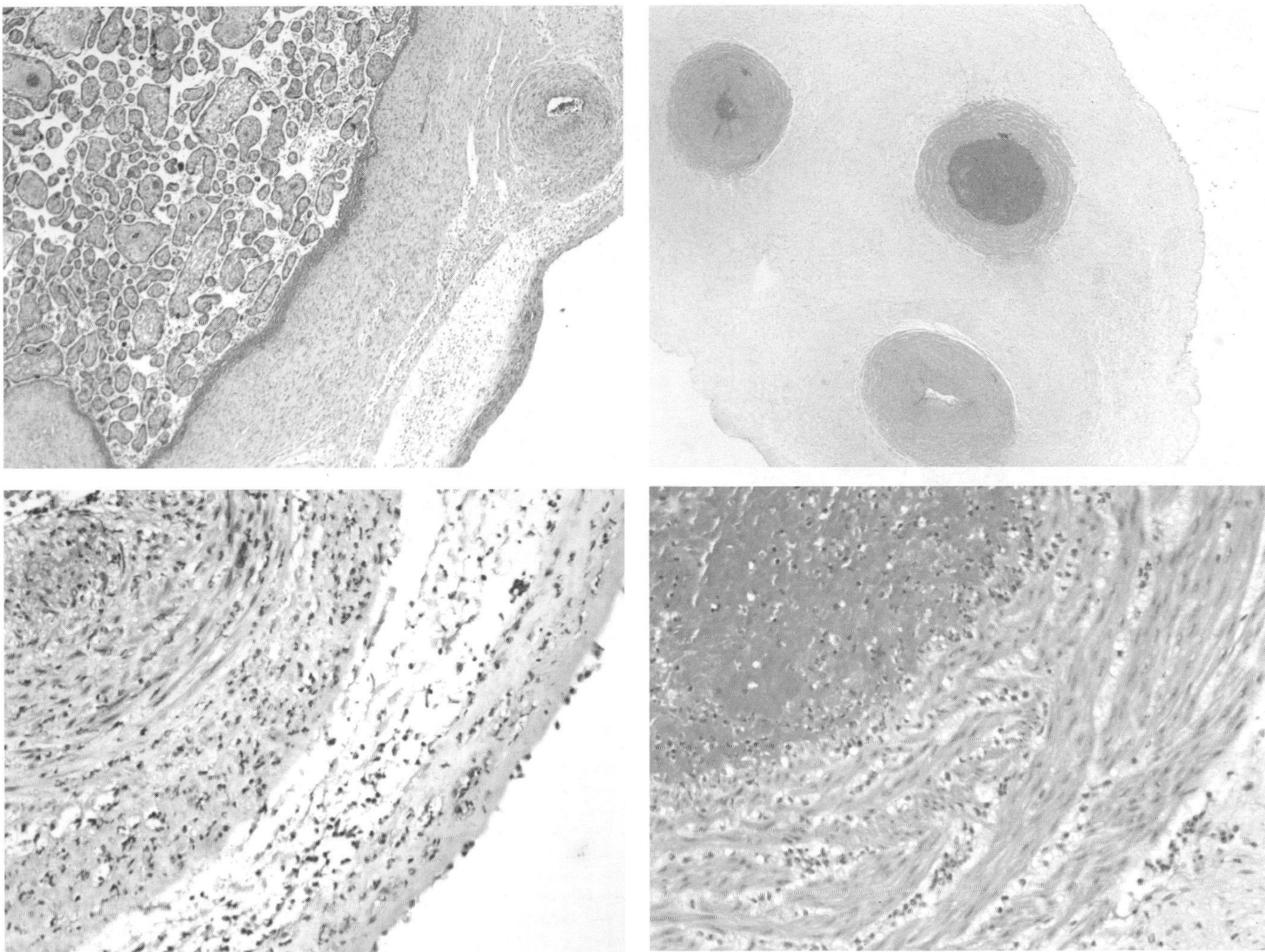

Figure 3.9 Acute chorioamnionitis (left), and funisitis (right).

fetal reaction is manifested by the migration of fetal neutrophils from the umbilical cord and chorionic plate vessels into Wharton's jelly or the chorionic plate.

The clinical significance of this placental inflammation includes preterm labor and neonatal infection. Chorioamnionitis is a major cause of premature labor. Neonatal infection can occur through the skin, eyes, nose, or ear canal or by aspiration or swallowing of infected fluid. It is commonly caused by group B β-hemolytic streptococci, *Escherichia coli*, and *Haemophilus influenzae*, and the neonate may develop bronchopneumonia, gastritis, ileitis, or gastrointestinal perforation with peritonitis and sepsis.[78,79]

Acute and chronic villitis

Hematogenous maternal infection can affect the placenta and cause villitis (Figs 3.10 and 3.11). The inflammatory infiltrate is commonly chronic, composed of lymphocytes, histiocytes, and plasma cells (Fig. 3.10). Granulomatous inflammation, and rarely neutrophils (Fig. 3.10), can be seen. The inflammatory infiltrate may also extend into the surrounding perivillous and intervillous space. The majority of chronic villitis cases (95%) are of unknown etiology. Table 3.2 shows the infectious agents which can cause villitis and their possible clinical manifestations.[80–102]

Hydrops fetalis and placental hydrops

Hydrops fetalis is a state of profound generalized fetal edema, with marked accumulation of fluid in subcutaneous tissue and all body cavities. It represents the end stage of a variety of fetal diseases, including genetic anomalies, hypoproteinemia, and cardiac failure. The placenta and umbilical cord also become edematous. The placenta does not always appear grossly hydropic, but villous edema is usually evident microscopically. A hydropic placenta is often massively enlarged, soft, and friable.

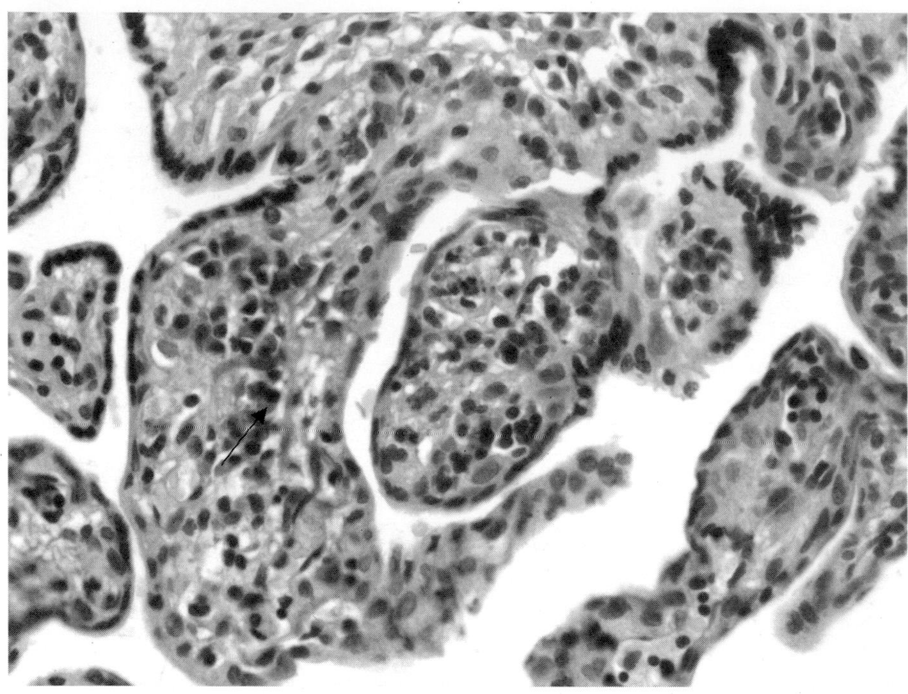

Figure 3.10 Chronic villitis; arrow marks a plasma cell.

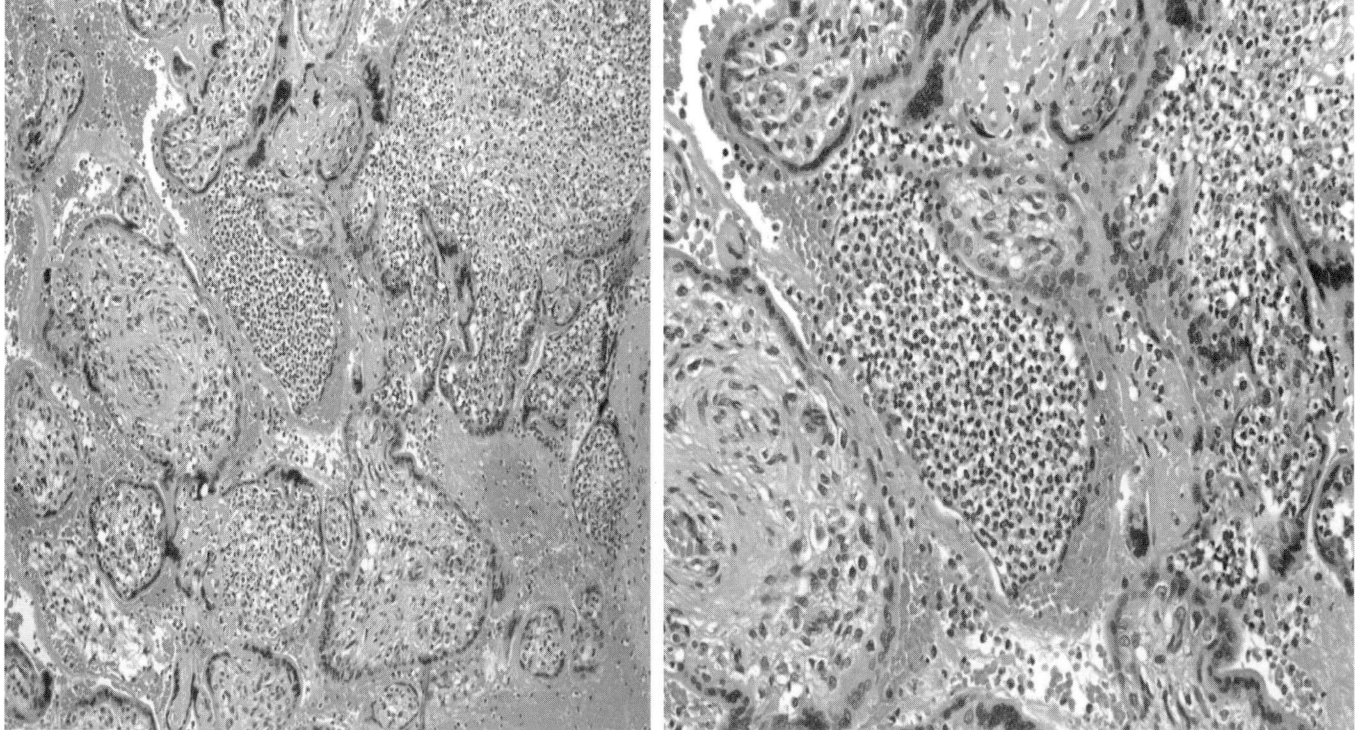

Figure 3.11 Acute villitis.

Table 3.2 Microorganisms associated with acute and chronic villitis and their clinical manifestation.

Infectious agent	Type of inflammatory response	Clinical manifestation
Cytomegalovirus (CMV)	Chronic villitis with CMV inclusion	Hepatosplenomegaly with microencephaly Late complication: mental retardation, chorioretinitis, and seizure
Herpes simplex virus	Villous necrosis, agglutination, lymphocytic villitis, and fibrinoid necrosis of vessels Chronic lymphoplasmacytic chorioamnionitis	Spontaneous abortion Congenital malformation
Varicella zoster	Grossly visible necrotic foci of villous necrosis	Wide range from completely asymptomatic to full-blown embryopathy
Parvovirus B19 (agent of fifth disease)	Large, pale placenta with edematous immature villi Fetal erythrocytes show intranuclear inclusion	Nonimmune hydrops, abortion Malformation similar to rubella
Human immunodeficiency virus (HIV)	No specific finding	Variable
Treponema pallidum	Large and edematous placenta with lymphoplasmacytic villitis and possible microabscesses	Abortion and stillbirth, and congenital syphilis
Listeria monocytogenes	Acute villitis with villous necrosis and abscess formation	Spontaneous abortion Prematurity Neonatal sepsis
Toxoplasmosis gondii (risk of transmission 50% during parasitemia)	Wide range (lymphocytic villitis, placental necrosis, and fibrosis)	Wide range (asymptomatic to severe damage to central nervous system and eyes)
Unknown etiology (severity of villitis correlates with the complications)	Chronic villitis	Asymptomatic to intrauterine growth retardation and increased perinatal mortality rate

Immune hydrops

Immune hydrops, also referred to as erythroblastosis fetalis, was once the most common cause of fetal hydrops. It is caused by severe hemolytic anemia, which results from the transplacental passage of maternal rhesus (Rh) antibodies to the Rh antigen-negative fetus. Hypoalbuminemia, or high output cardiac failure resulting from severe anemia, is the cause for the hydropic changes. Occasionally, other red blood cell antigens (e.g., Kell) show a similar, but usually less severe, effect.[103–105]

Nonimmune hydrops

A heterogeneous group of conditions is responsible for nonimmune hydrops. Most causes can be categorized as cardiac failure, anemia, or hypoproteinemia (Table 3.3). Homozygous α-thalassemia is a common cause of hydrops and should be considered first among ethnic Southeast Asian parents. A fetus with homozygous sickle cell disease or β-thalassemia is protected from hemolysis before birth by the presence of fetal hemoglobin. Parvovirus B19 infection, seen only in fetuses with group p antigen, is responsible for 14–18% of cases of nonimmune placental and fetal hydrops.[105–115]

Disorders of placental development

Abnormal placental development can be caused by multiple factors, including abnormalities of placental gene expression, an abnormal maternal environment, or as a result of disruption of normal development.[116]

Disorders of membrane development

Placental membranacea

This extremely rare condition is characterized by the failure of normal membrane formation, leading to a gestational sac surrounded by chorionic villi. The placenta tends to be abnormally thin and the maternal surface is often disrupted owing to placenta accreta. Clinical features include premature separation and placenta previa, resulting in maternal hemorrhage and life-threatening fetal hemorrhage at the time of membrane rupture.[117,118]

Circumvallation

This is the complete or partial insertion of fetal membrane into the placental disk, away from the peripheral margin, with or without a distinct ridge of degenerating blood clot. The inci-

Table 3.3 Etiology of nonimmune hydrops.

Congenital	Chromosomal aberration	Infection	Other
Hemoglobinopathies, α-thalassemia	Down syndrome	Parvovirus	Fetomaternal hemorrhage
Cardiac anomalies and cardiomyopathies	Turner syndrome	Toxoplasma	Twin–twin transfusion
Adenomatoid malformation of the lung	Trisomy 13	Syphilis	Large tumors, hemangiomas
Urinary tract malformation	Trisomy 18	Rubella	
Lysosomal storage disease			

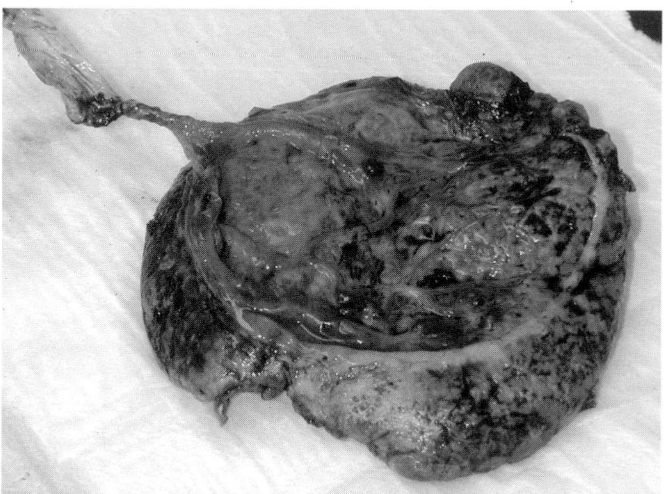

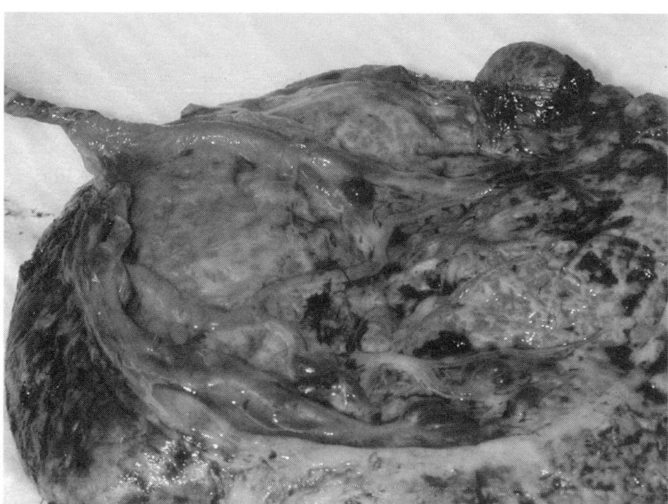

Figure 3.12 Term placenta showing abnormal placentation with circummargination and marginal insertion of the umbilical cord.

dence in normal pregnancies is reported to be 1–7%, and these placentas tend to be smaller. Most investigators have observed that marginal venous hemorrhage is often present, which pushes the membrane inward over the chorionic plate (Fig. 3.12).

Clinical features include recurrent vaginal bleeding in all trimesters. Circumvallation can also cause placental hematomas, marginal hematomas, oligohydramnios, and placental abruption. Clinical sequelae reflect the amount of associated hemorrhage. Term infants with circumvallation or chronic marginal hemorrhage may have mild IUGR and be at increased risk of neurological impairment.[119–124]

Disorders of uterine implantation

Placenta previa

In placenta previa, implantation is in the lower uterine segment with some tissue near or overlying the uterine cervical os. Complete previa occurs when the placenta completely covers the cervical os. Partial previa is when the edge of the placenta is within 2 cm of the os.

Placenta previa occurs in 0.3–0.5% of deliveries. Epithelial alterations, which might have changed the extracellular matrix, may increase the risk for placenta previa. These include previous history of curettage, prior Cesarean section, or multiple vaginal deliveries, as well as abnormalities of the uterine fundus including intrauterine and submucosal leiomyomata and uterine malformations.

Clinically, placenta previa often results in premature separation of the placenta, leading to severe vaginal bleeding and premature labor, or both.[125]

Placenta accreta, increta, and percreta

These conditions are caused by implantation of anchoring villi on uterine smooth muscle without intervening decidua. In placenta accreta, the villi are limited to superficial myometrium; in increta, the villi extend into the myometrium; and in percreta, the villi extend to or through the uterine serosa (Fig. 3.13).

The incidence has apparently increased in recent years and is reported to be as high as 1 in 540 pregnancies. Predisposing conditions include a maternal age greater than 35, previous instrumentation, congenital or acquired uterine defects such as uterine septa, leiomyomata, and ectopic implantation such as placenta previa or cornual pregnancy.[126–128]

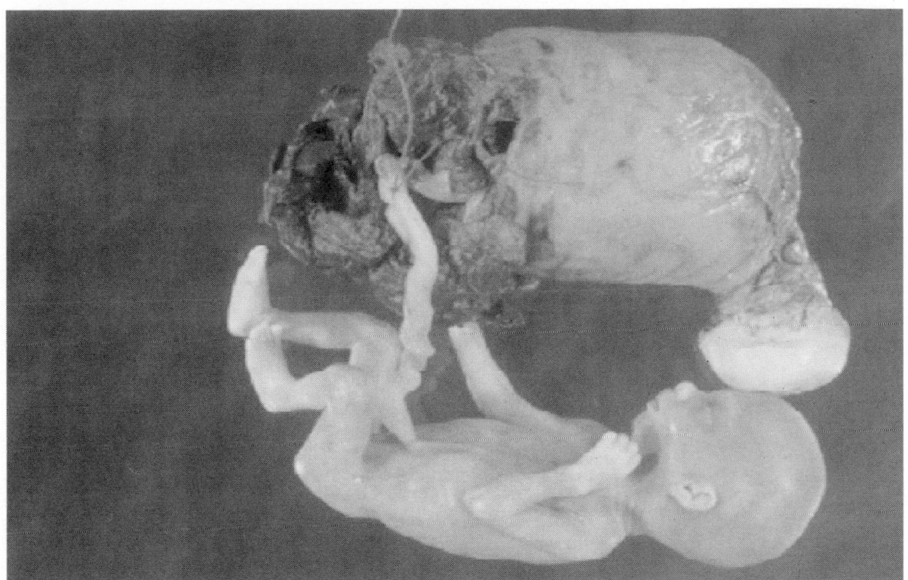

Figure 3.13 Placenta percreta with complete perforation of the uterus.

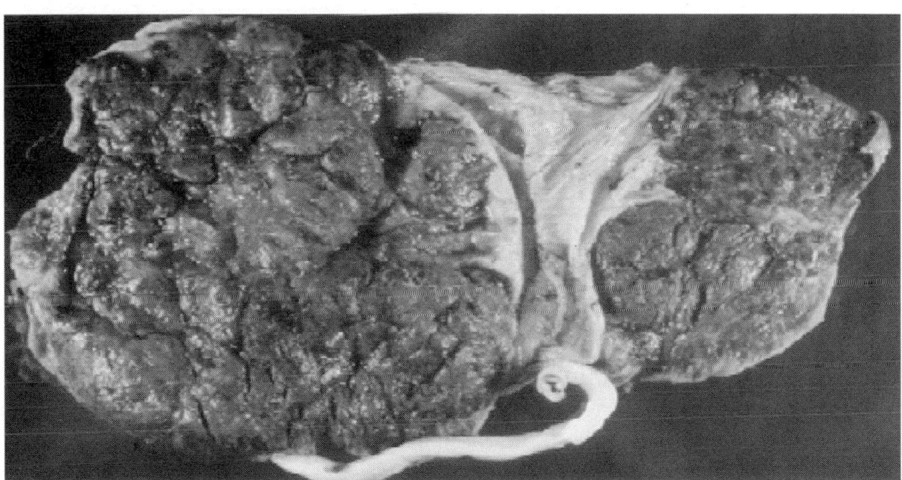

Figure 3.14 Accessory lobe.

Grossly, the maternal surface of the placenta is always disrupted. In most cases, smooth muscle cells are seen in close proximity to the anchoring villi, with fibrin and intermediate trophoblasts intervening.

Clinically, patients often present with recurrent vaginal spotting or overt hemorrhage, and occasionally with uterine rupture. Patients may also present with early or delayed postpartum hemorrhage, necessitating gravid hysterectomy.[129]

Superficial implantation

A deficiency of the interstitial and endovascular intermediate trophoblasts in the decidua basalis and basal plate arteries results in superficial implantation. Superficial implantation is the underlying anatomic abnormality in preeclampsia, which affects 2.6% of all pregnancies. Other related disorders include maternal thrombophilia and placental abruption. Superficially implanted placentas are often small for the gestational age.

Clinically, superficial implantation is related to maternal underperfusion of the intervillous space. It is not clear whether superficial implantation occurs in all cases of preeclampsia.[130]

Disorders of placental migration

Accessory lobe and multilobulation

An accessory lobe and multilobulation occur when a portion of placental parenchyma is completely separated from the main placental disk by the surrounding membrane. It is found in 3–6% of placentas. Shape abnormalities occur in response to a local reduction of uterine perfusion (Fig. 3.14). Shape abnormalities are of little clinical significance except as

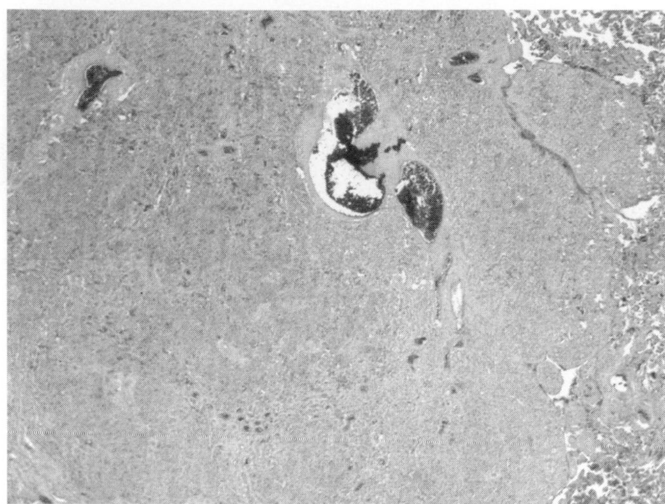
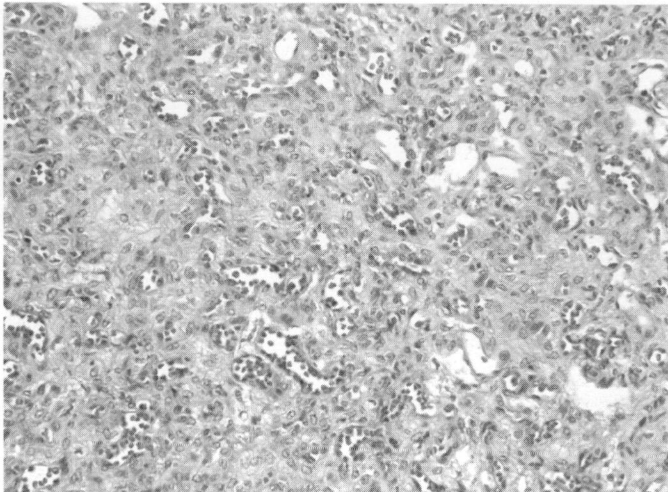

Figure 3.15 Choriangioma: note the well-circumscribed mass surrounded by trophoblasts and composed of tightly packed capillaries separated by fibrous connective tissue.

markers for uterine pathology. Both placenta accreta and previa are commonly associated with abnormal shape.[125]

Peripheral cord insertion

Membranous insertion (velamentous insertion) and marginal insertion

In velamentous insertion, the umbilical cord terminates in the placental membrane rather than in the chorionic disk; this occurs in 1.3–1.6% of pregnancies. In marginal insertion, the cord inserts at the placental margin; this occurs in 6–9% of pregnancies.

Velamentous and marginal cord insertion are thought to occur as a result of asymmetry in the vascular supply in singletons, or competition for uterine vascular supply in twins. Abnormal insertion is more common in twin pregnancies.

Clinically, these conditions are associated with a slightly increased incidence of fetal growth retardation. The major risk is the rupture of membranous vessels at the time of membrane rupture. Twisting of the vessel can lead to progressive variable deceleration and fetal acidosis.[125]

Disorders of fetal vascular development

Chorangioma

Chorangiomas are expansile single or multiple nodular lesions composed of capillary channels and intervening stroma cells surrounded by trophoblasts (Fig. 3.15). Small chorangiomas are usually incidental findings of no clinical significance; intermediate sized chorangiomas are associated with IUGR, and masses larger than 9 cm are associated with shunting of blood and multiple complications. They are thought to be induced by hypoxia.[126,127,131]

Chorangiomatosis

This term is used when excessive capillary growth affects scattered secondary and tertiary stem villi. It is associated with preeclampsia, multiple gestation, and premature delivery. It is also associated with extreme prematurity (<32 weeks), congenital malformations, and IUGR.[131]

The placenta in maternal disorders

There is a great deal of disagreement and direct contradiction about the nature and significance of lesions seen in various maternal disorders.

Preeclampsia (pregnancy-induced hypertension) and eclampsia

No single or specific abnormality is found in the placentas affected by these conditions. In the majority of cases, the placenta shows the effect of low uteroplacental flow.

The placenta is smaller than those from uncomplicated pregnancies. Infarcts are more common and centrally located. The villi may show cytotrophoblastic proliferation, trophoblastic basement membrane thickening, small inconspicuous fetal capillaries, and prominence of villous stroma. The villi show accelerated maturation and are often abnormally small with increased syncytial knots (greater than 30% of the villi). The spiral arteries show a lack of adaptive remodeling features. In these women, the second wave of intravascular trophoblastic migration does not occur. The intramyometrial segment of spiral arteries retains the musculoelastic media and cannot dilate. Spiral arteries show an acute necrotizing arteropathy (see Fig. 3.9: right, upper and lower). This type of arteropathy has also been described in other complications, including other hypertensive placentas, diabetes, systemic lupus erythromatosus, and antiphospholipid syndrome.

A smaller group of preeclamptic patients show large placentas with abundant immature trophoblasts. These patients usually have other underlying causes including diabetes, multiple gestation, or hydatidiform mole.[132–143]

Acquired thrombophilia

Acquired thrombophilia, especially the presence of antiphospholipid antibodies, promotes intraplacental clotting. The most common inherited coagulopathies are mutations in the factor V gene (factor V Leiden), the prothrombin gene, and the methylene tetrahydrofolate reductase gene. Diabetes mellitus is also commonly associated with a hypercoagulable state.

The maternal risk is mainly venous thromboembolism, but arterial thrombosis also occurs. There is also a strong association with maternal preeclampsia. Adverse pregnancy outcomes occur in approximately 54% of women with thrombophilia. The fetus of a mother with thrombophilia is at risk for IUGR and stillbirth.[54–60,138,144–148]

Diabetes mellitus

The gross and microscopic features of diabetic placentas vary considerably. A large study demonstrated that about one-half of the placentas of diabetic mothers had a normal weight and size. However, placentas that are abnormal are larger, thicker, more friable, and heavier than normal placentas of the same gestational age, and the umbilical cord is often notoriously thicker.

The microscopic appearance of the placenta can also be normal, but some abnormalities are distinctive when they are present. Villi commonly appear immature with stromal edema, enlarged villous diameters, and an increase in the prominence of the cytotrophoblastic cells. The decidual arteries are unremarkable except in cases of superimposed hypertension or preeclampsia.

Thrombotic vasculopathy is common. In the presence of maternal vascular disease, renal failure, or preeclampsia, the placenta may be smaller than expected with infarcts and accelerated maturation. There is generally no correlation between the severity and duration of diabetes and the severity of the placental lesions.[59]

Maternal anemia

There are no specific histopathological features associated with maternal anemia. Placentas can be larger or smaller than expected for the gestational age. In maternal sickle cell anemia, placental infarctions are common with the infarcts generally showing sickled erythrocytes. Both placenta and newborn are small for the gestational age and hydropic villi and placental abruption may occur. Uncomplicated sickle cell trait is unlikely to cause placental lesions.

Homozygous α-thalassemia produces severe fetal anemia and, consequently, hydropic changes in the placenta and fetus, as well as intrauterine fetal death or death soon after birth. In contrast, the placenta and fetus in homozygous β-thalassemia are normal at birth, but the infant soon becomes markedly anemic as the protective hemoglobin F declines.[62,63,149]

Toxic damage to the placenta

Some of the most common toxic exposures to the placenta are initiated by smoking and cocaine use. Cigarette smoking causes low birthweight, and the placentas of women who smoke more often show necrotic damage. Women who smoke have a higher incidence of placenta previa, abnormalities of the placenta, and fetal malformations. On the other hand, the prevalence of preeclampsia is significantly lower than in nonsmokers. Both nicotine and cocaine can induce vasoconstriction of uterine vessels, causing restriction in the blood supply to the placenta. Cocaine-induced complications during pregnancy are numerous and multifactorial. These complications include placental bleeding, abruption, premature labor, and malnutrition of the developing fetus.[63,147,149–151]

Metabolic storage disorders

On gross examination, the placenta and the fetus may be hydropic or show no specific gross findings. The accumulated metabolites in these disorders are generally soluble in water; therefore, routinely processed histological slides of the placenta may show only diffuse cytoplasmic vacuolation.[152]

Chromosomal abnormalities

Certain patterns of villous morphology are suggestive of an abnormal karyotype. The incidence of chromosomal abnormalities increases with advanced maternal age. Abnormal karyotype limited to the placenta is seen in 1–3% of all first-trimester chorionic villous sampling. The clinical outcome for chromosomal abnormalities depends on the nature of the abnormality.

Multiple pregnancies

Multiple pregnancies are common, and their rate is increasing owing to assisted reproductive technology (ART). In the USA, ART accounted for 14% of all twin gestations in 2000. Multiple pregnancies are associated with a disproportionate share of complications, including higher rates of morbidity, mortality, malformation, and anomalous development and low birthweight.

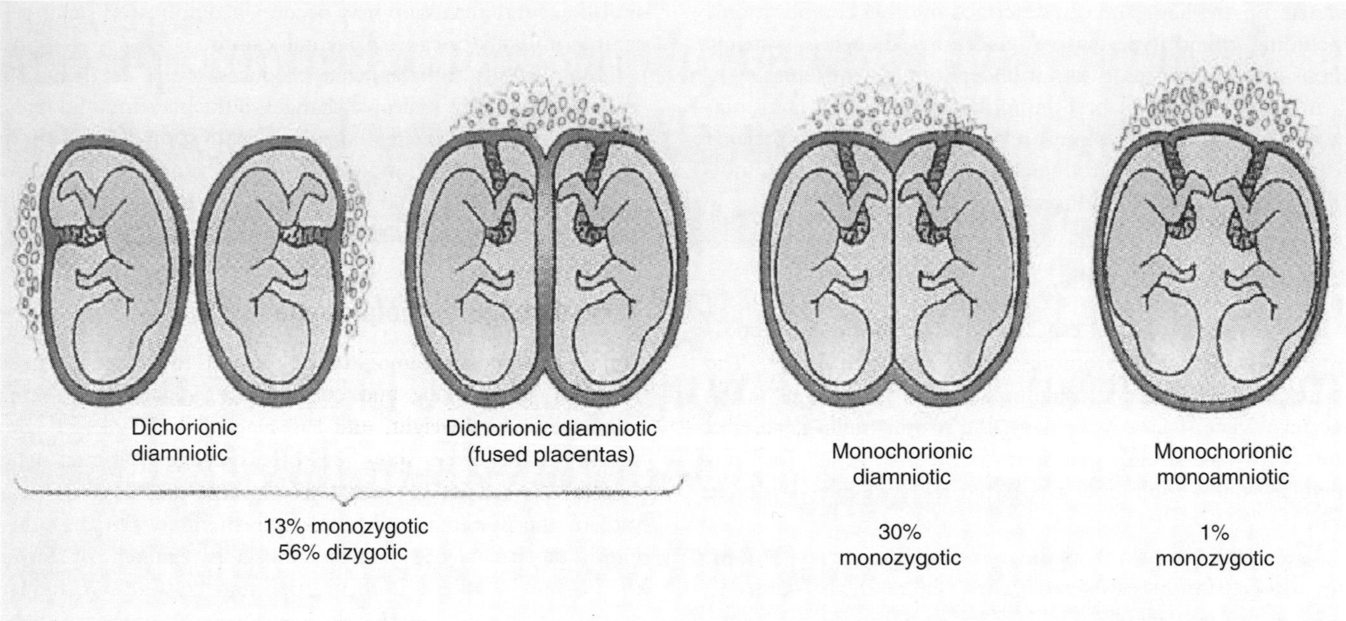

Figure 3.16 Zygosity in twin placentas. Adapted from ref. 158, with permission.

Zygosity

Twins are classified as dizygous (fraternal) or monozygous (identical). Dizygous twins are the result of the fertilization of two separate ova. Monozygous twins are the result of division of a single fertilized ovum (Fig. 3.16). Monozygous twins are genetically and, usually, phenotypically identical.[153–162]

Frequency

The frequency of monozygous twins is relatively constant worldwide (3.5 in 1000 pregnancies). There are marked geographic differences in dizygous twin pregnancies. This reflects a genetic predisposition for high follicle-stimulating hormone (FSH) levels in certain populations which results in polyovulation. The frequency also increases with advancing maternal age (greater than 35), probably as the result of increasing FSH levels with age. Approximately 30% of Caucasian twin pregnancies in the USA are monozygotic.

Placentation

Features unique to multiple gestations include the relationship of the placental disk, fetal membrane, and the pattern and degree of anastomosis of the vessels.

Placentas in twin gestations are either dichorionic or monochorionic. All dizygous twins have dichorionic placentas (dichorionic diamniotic: DiDi).

A monozygous twin gestation can show any type of placentation depending on the time of splitting of the blastocyst. If the single fertilized ovum divides before day 3, the situation is analagous to dizygous twinning. If the split occurs between days 3 and 8 there will be a monochorionic diamniotic placenta (DiMo) (Fig. 3.17). A split after formation of the amnion (days 8–13) results in a monochorionic monoamniotic (MoMo) placenta (Fig. 3.17). The majority of monozygous twins have a monochorionic placenta. Twins with monochorionic placentas have a much higher mortality rate. Monoamniotic placentas have a fetal mortality rate of almost 50%.

Two entirely separate placentas are dichorionic. The septum in a dichorionic fused placenta is relatively thick and variably opaque owing to the presence of chorionic tissue between the two amniotic layers. The septum in monochorionic diamniotic placentas is thin and translucent, composed of only two directly opposed layers of amnion. This type of septum is easily detached from the placental surface. There is an important difference in the distribution of fetal vessels between DiDi fused placentas and DiMo placentas. In a DiDi fused placenta, the fetal chorionic vessels approach, but do not cross, the area of fusion.

Complications of multiple pregnancy

Twin–twin transfusion syndrome

Vascular communications in monochorionic placentas create the potential for blood flow between twins. Large vessel anastomoses are likely bidirectional, and arteriovenous anastomoses are likely unidirectional (Fig. 3.18).

Chronic unidirectional blood flow results in anemia and growth retardation of the donor fetus. Hypervolemia can cause hypertension, high urine output, and polyhydramnios in the recipient. A relatively selective criterion for twin–twin transfusion is a recipient heart weight that is 2–4 times that of the donor.

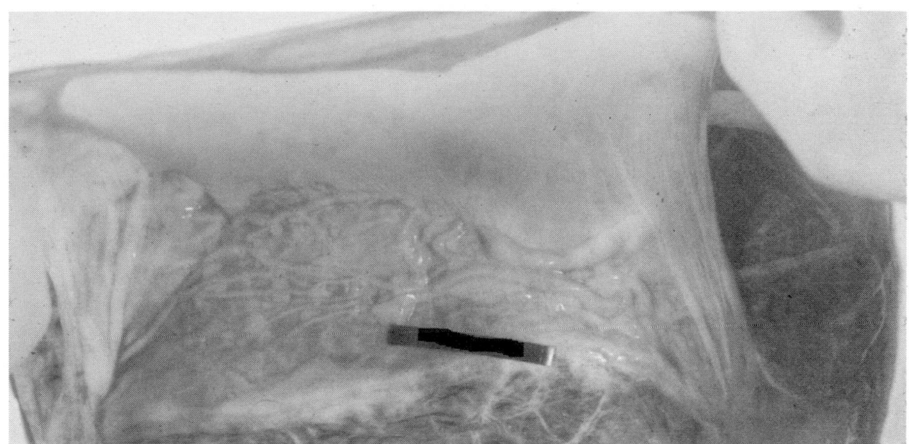

Figure 3.17 Diamniotic monochorionic twin placenta.

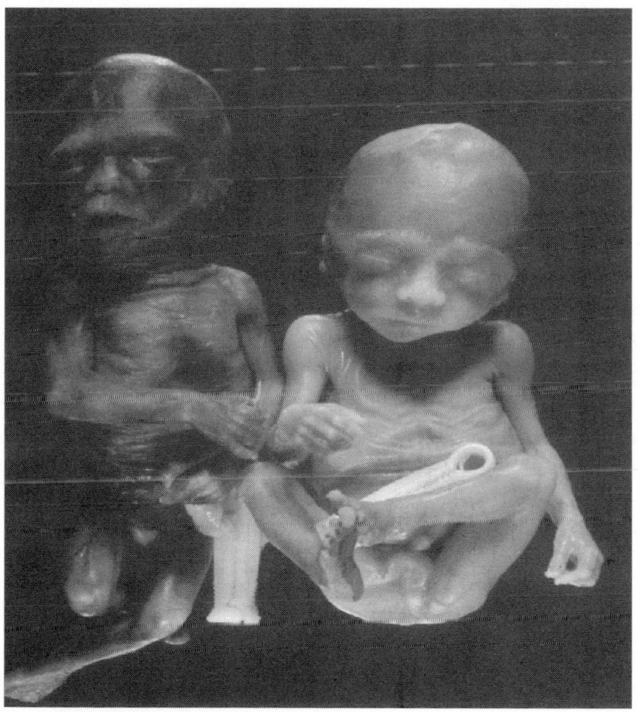

Figure 3.18 Twin–twin transfusion.

Clinically, twin–twin transfusion is manifested in the second trimester with acute hydramnios. The mortality rate is as high as 70–100%. The recipient twin can develop cardiac failure, hemolytic jaundice, kernicterus, and thrombosis. The donor twin may be severely anemic, hypoglycemic, and is at risk for ischemic lesions.

Asymmetric growth

The growth curves of twins approximate those of singletons up to 34 weeks. Thereafter, twins weigh progressively less than singletons. Twin birthweight discordance is associated with preterm labor, perinatal death, and postnatal morbidity.

Duplication abnormalities

Monozygotic twins occasionally show a marked discrepancy in size and configuration, asymmetry, and incomplete duplication. Acardiac twinning is the most common asymmetric duplication, occurring in 1% of monochorionic twins.

Cord anomalies

Anomalies of the umbilical cord are more common in multiple pregnancies. Velamentous cord insertion is nine times higher in multiple pregnancies. Single artery cords are also more common in multiple pregnancies. Monoamnionic twins are at increased risk for cord entanglement (Fig. 3.19).

Higher multiple births

The same principles of placentation and zygosity apply to triplets, quadruplets, and higher multiple births. Combinations of monozygous and polyzygous multiples are common.

Preterm labor, premature rupture of the membranes

Labor, including preterm labor, is induced by prostaglandin release, which mediates the release of cytokines. The most common cause of preterm labor is bacterial infection, with the second most common cause being vascular sequelae.

Neonatal complications include hyaline membrane disease, periventricular leukomalacia, intraventricular hemorrhage, retinopathy, necrotizing enterocolitis, and death.[163]

Post-term pregnancy

Postmaturity is defined as a pregnancy of 42 or more weeks (294 days) following the onset of the last menses. It is important to note that many supposed cases of

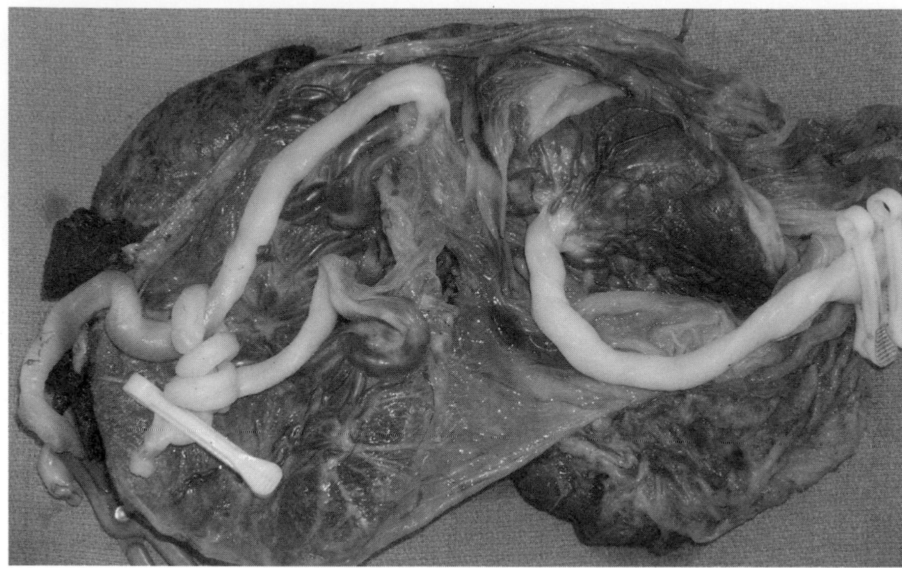

Figure 3.19 Umbilical cord entanglement seen in a monoamniotic monochorionic component of a triplet placenta.

postmaturity result from an incorrect estimation of gestational age.[164]

There is a marked increase in perinatal mortality in pregnancies of more than 43 weeks. The fetus can experience a combination of progressive oligohydramnios and meconium impregnation with cord compression and be at risk of pulmonary failure, possibly due to aspiration of viscous meconium.[163]

Recurrent spontaneous abortion

This diagnosis is usually based on the occurrence of three or more consecutive spontaneous abortions. The probability that a recognizable cause can be demonstrated is small, but the identifiable causes are potentially significant. They include maternal thrombophilias, especially those related to autoimmune antibodies; anatomic problems such as an incompetent cervix or leiomyomata; and poorly controlled diabetes mellitus. Rare placental lesions such as maternal floor infarcts and extensive chronic villitis may cause repeated miscarriage often in the third trimester. Early gestational problems can include massive chronic intervillositis, lymphoplasmacytic deciduitis, and chronic decidual perivasculitis.[165–167]

Intrauterine growth retardation and small for gestational age newborn

A small for gestational age (SGA) infant is a baby who has a birthweight below the 10th percentile for gestational age. Term babies born with a weight below 2500 g are considered to be of low birthweight. Many of these babies are normal and healthy but small because of genetic factors such as parental size or ethnicity. For those below the third percentile, the death rate is nearly 20 times the average population.[168]

In addition to fetal demise, the prevalence of seizures in the first day of life, respiratory insufficiency, sepsis, hypothermia, hypoglycemia, and meconium aspiration is increased. The medical problems of the survivors persist into adulthood and include hypertension, coronary artery disease, and type 2 diabetes mellitus.[169,170]

Maternal factors associated with IUGR are poor nutrition, hypertension, preeclampsia, chronic renal disease, tobacco, and other drug abuse. Fetal factors include chromosomal anomalies, congenital malformations, and multiple gestations.

Placental lesions associated with IUGR include maternal vasculopathy, chronic abruption, fetal thrombotic vasculopathy, large chorangiomas, villitis of unknown etiology, and maternal floor infarction.[171,172]

Meconium staining

The passage of meconium *in utero* is due to bowel peristalsis and relaxation of the anal sphincter; it may indicate fetal distress and can be associated with meconium aspiration. It is seen in 14% of pregnancies. Meconium staining should be differentiated from the deposition of slimy green meconium across the placental surface that can be washed off by gentle rinsing with water, which indicates a normal fetus that has passed meconium shortly before delivery. True meconium staining results from exposure to meconium for several hours. Damage to the fetus increases with length of exposure to meconium. Over time, soluble meconium components diffuse into the placenta and cord, inducing vasoconstriction and resulting in fetal hypoperfusion.

Chorioamnionitis is an especially common association and may play an important role in neonatal morbidity.

Abnormal amniotic fluid volume

The presence of an excess of amniotic fluid is called hydramnios or polyhydramnios. A diminished amount is called oligohydramnios. Amniotic fluid provides the medium for free fetal movements and has a cushioning effect to prevent possible fetal injury. Secretions from amniotic epithelium and fetal urine are the main sources of amniotic fluid. The most common significant anomalies associated with hydramnios are anencephaly, spina bifida, esophageal atresia, nonimmune hydrops, and various abnormal karyotypes. The recipient twin affected by twin–twin transfusion syndrome commonly has polyhydramnios.

The most common cause of oligohydramnios is leakage of the amniotic fluid caused by premature rupture of membranes. Oligohydramnios also occurs in nearly all cases of bilateral renal agenesis and fetal urinary tract obstruction. Other associations include abnormal karyotype, IUGR, post-term pregnancies, preeclampsia, maternal hypertension, and the donor twin in twin–twin transfusion syndrome. The umbilical cord is subject to compression, especially with severe oligohydramnios, and pulmonary hypoplasia occurs secondarily. These fetuses are at risk for amniotic band syndrome.

Gestational trophoblastic disease

There is a heterogeneous group of gestational and neoplastic conditions of trophoblastic origin.[173] The incidence of gestational trophoblastic disease (GTD) varies widely among different populations. It is reported to occur in 8.3 in 1000 pregnancies in some areas of Asia and South America compared with 0.1–0.6 in 1000 pregnancies in the USA. The incidence of this disease is higher in women aged 40 or over and is also increased in those younger than 20. Other risk factors include a diet that is low in vitamin E, low socioeconomic status, and blood group A women who have children with blood group O men.

Complete and partial hydatidiform mole

Complete hydatidiform mole (CHM) results from fertilization of an empty ovum. The majority of CHMs are diploid and show a 46,XX karyotype, whereas the partial hydatidiform mole (PHM) is triploid and shows a 69,XXY karyotype. Up to 50% of gestational choriocarcinomas follow CHM.

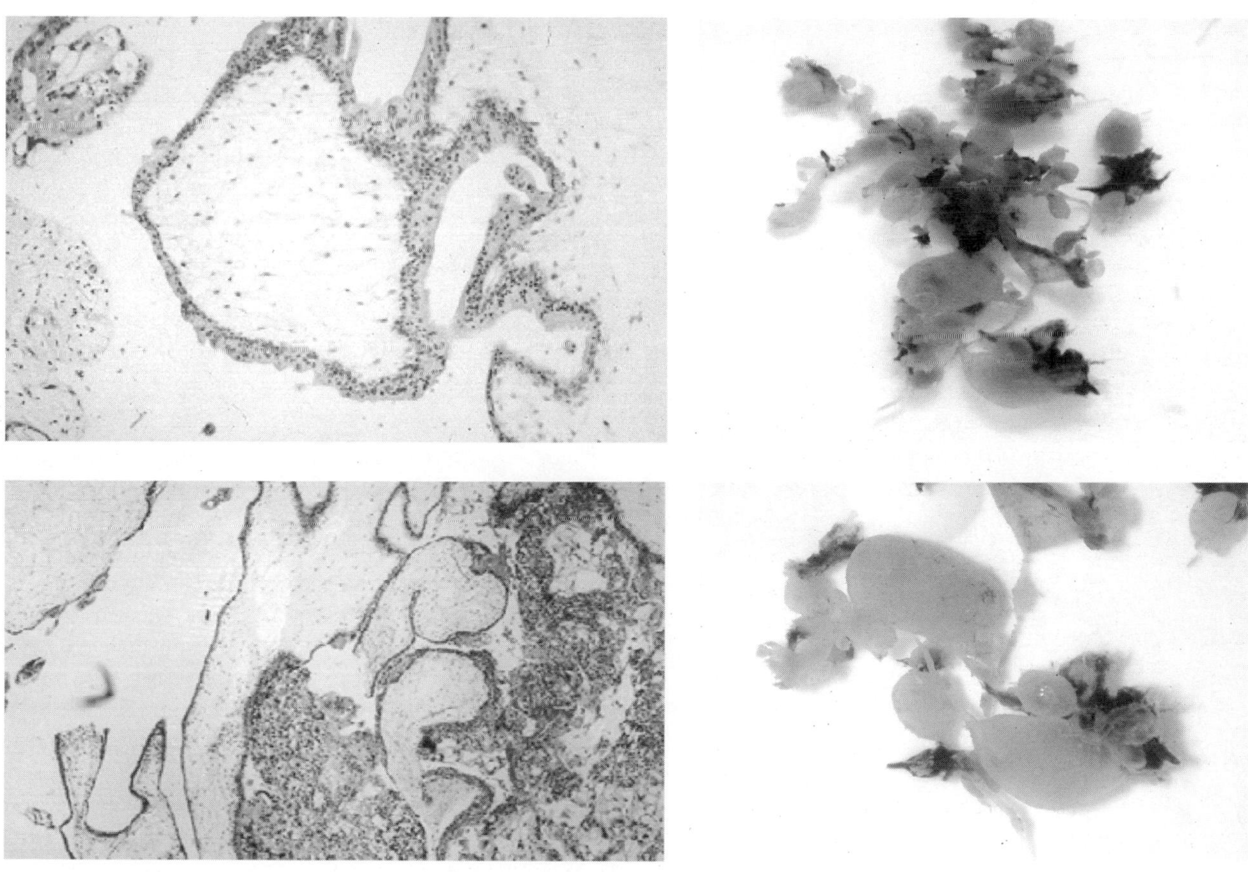

Figure 3.20 Complete hydatidiform mole.

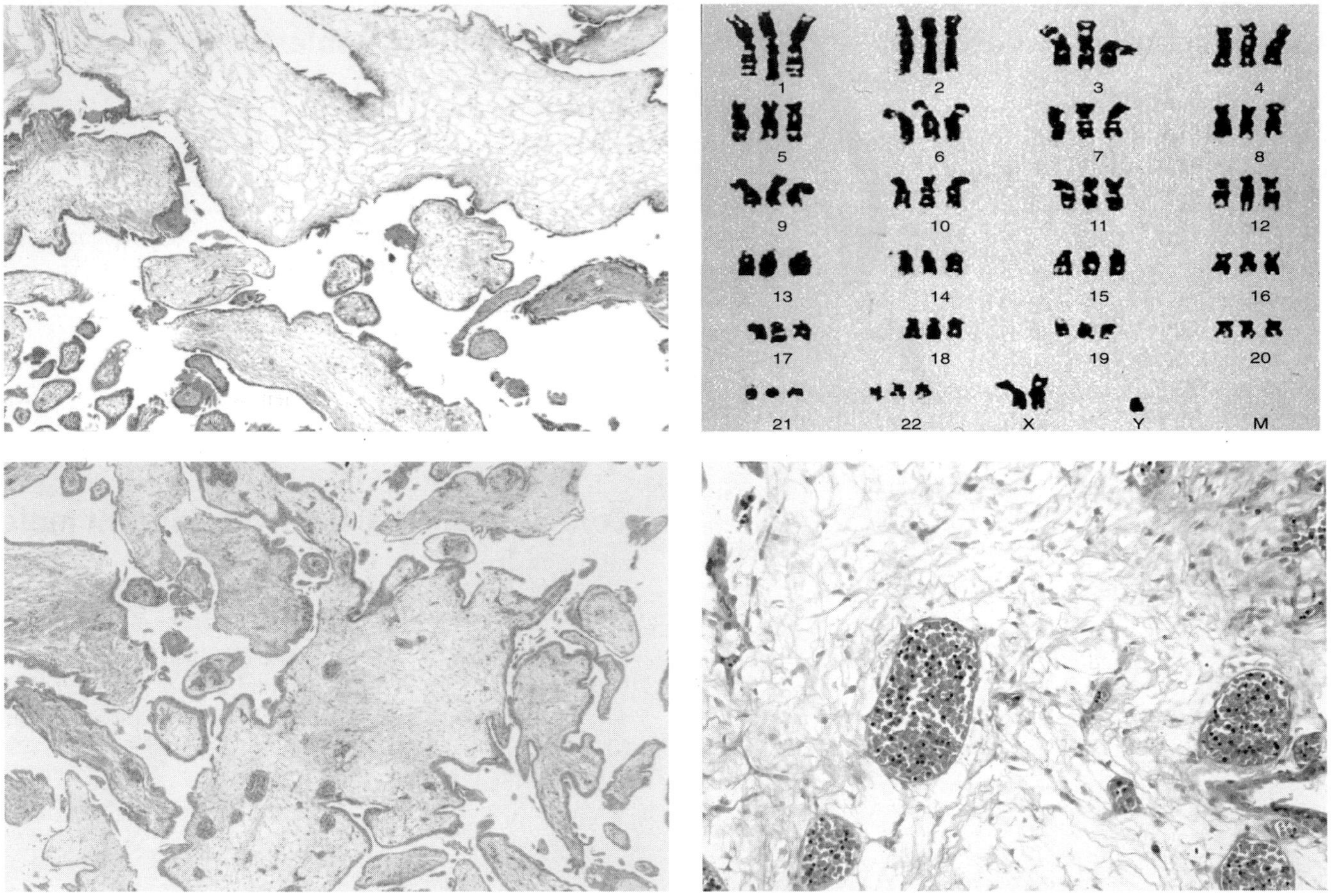

Figure 3.21 Partial mole. Note the presence of nucleated red blood cells indicative of fetal circulation. Partial moles are in general triploid (69,XXY).

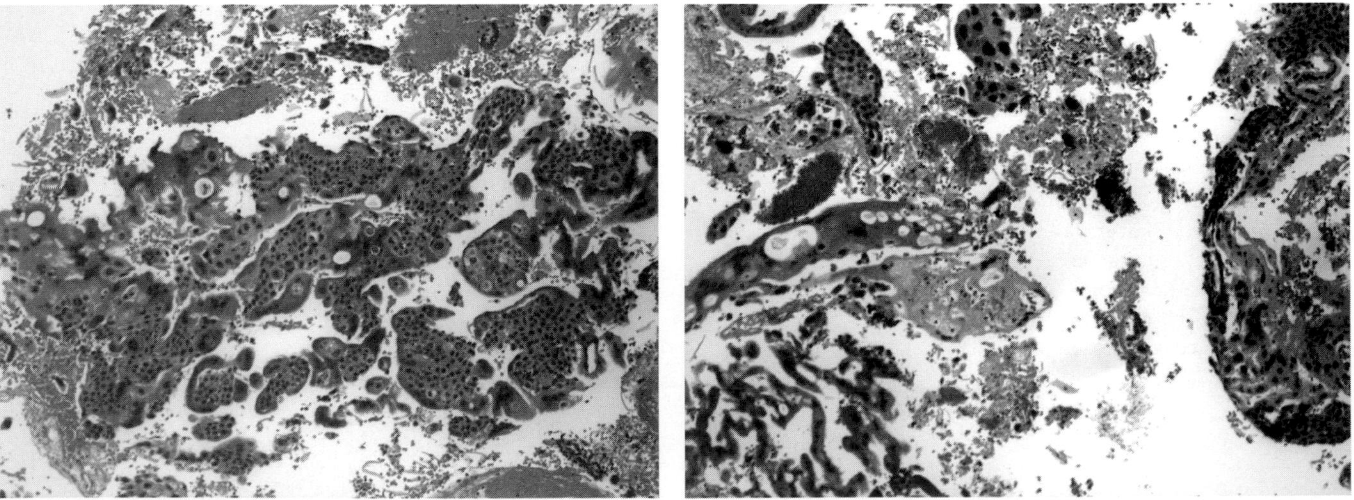

Figure 3.22 Choriocarcinoma.

Key points

1 The fertilized ovum at day 1 (post coital) has a diameter of 0.1 mm. The blastocyst measures approximately 0.3 mm. The embryo grows from 0.1 mm at days 8–12 to 3.5 mm by day 23.

2 Steroid hormones prepare the endometrium for implantation of the blastocyst. A surge of estrogens, secreted by the ovary, triggers and induces implantation.

3 The fetal–placental circulation is developed by the fifth gestational week. Between 14 and 20 weeks, the trophoblast invades the myometrium, resulting in obliteration of the uterine cavity by the 20th week.

4 The term placenta consists of 40–60 functional units that receive oxygenated blood from the branches of the maternal spiral arteries. Each unit depends on its own spiral artery. Thrombosis of the spiral arteries results in infarction of the dependent unit.

5 The mean length of the umbilical cord at term is 32–45 cm. Markedly long cords (greater than 80 cm in length) have been associated with encirclement around the neck, knots, torsion, prolapse, and variable degrees of vascular occlusion. Short cords (less than 32 cm in length) may predispose to intrauterine hypoxia, cord rupture and hemorrhage, retroplacental hematomas and abruption, and uterine inversion.

6 Wharton's jelly acts as a cushion between umbilical cord vessels. A diminished size of cord is related to a decrease in the amount of Wharton's jelly and can cause vascular occlusion.

7 Small placental infarcts (<3 cm) can be found in uncomplicated pregnancies. However, large or multiple infarcts can be associated with neonatal asphyxia, low birthweight, and intrauterine fetal death.

8 Maternal floor infarcts are characterized by heavy deposition of fibrin around basal villi adjacent to the decidua basalis. Infarcts can be associated with perinatal death and intrauterine growth retardation.

9 Retroplacental hematomas are intradecidual clots between the placental floor and the myometrium. They can cause a characteristic area of placental depression. Acute bleeding from a ruptured decidual artery, spreading between the placenta and uterine wall, can cause placental detachment (abruption).

10 Premature rupture of the membranes is very commonly associated with preterm delivery. In the majority of cases, the reason for membranes becoming weak and rupturing is not known. Known reasons for premature rupture of the membranes are subclinical infections, hydramnios, incompetence of the cervix, retroplacental hematomas, and amniocentesis.

11 Acute chorioamnionitis is caused by an inflammatory response of the membranes to an ascending infection caused by bacteria, including normal cervicovaginal flora, such as group B β-hemolytic streptococci, *Ureaplasma urealyticum, Mycoplasma hominis, Fusobacterium*, and, rarely, *Candida* species. Chorioamnionitis can predispose to, and be associated with, preterm labor and neonatal infection.

12 Hematogenous infection of the placenta can occasionally be associated with chronic endometritis, localized maternal infection, or pelvic inflammatory disease.

13 Immune hydrops is caused by severe hemolytic anemia, which is mostly the result of transplacental passage of maternal Rh antibodies to the Rh-negative fetus. Rarely, other blood groups than Rh are responsible for the hemolysis (e.g., Kell). Various different conditions can cause or be associated with nonimmune hydrops fetalis. Some of these conditions are homozygous α-thalassemia, infection with parvovirus B19, and metabolic disorders.

14 The term placenta previa refers to a placenta that is implanted at the lower uterine segment near, or overlying, the cervical os. Placenta previa can cause premature separation of the placenta, resulting in severe bleeding and/or premature labor.

15 In placenta accreta, the villi are implanted into the superficial myometrium. In placenta increta, the villi invade the myometrium. In placenta percreta, the villi penetrate through the entire uterine wall.

16 Chorangiomas are expansile nodules composed of capillaries and stroma surrounded by trophoblasts. Small lesions are of no clinical significance, but larger lesions (>9 cm) are associated with shunting of blood and multiple related complications.

17 Preeclampsia is related to low uteroplacental blood flow and can be associated with other conditions such as diabetes, multiple gestation, and hydatidiform mole.

18 Acquired thrombophilic disorders, especially those associated with antiphospholipid antibodies, promote intraplacental clotting. The maternal risk is mainly venous thromboembolism; however, arterial thrombosis may also occur.

19 Assisted reproductive technology is increasing the rate of multiple pregnancies. Multiple pregnancies are associated with an increased incidence of complications related to prematurity, low birthweight, malformations, and developmental anomalies.

20 Excess of amniotic fluid is called polyhydramnios and is associated with anencephaly, spina bifida, esophageal atresia, nonimmune hydrops, and abnormal karyotypes. A diminished amount is called oligohydramnios. The most common cause of oligohydramnios is premature rupture of membranes. Other important causes include bilateral renal agenesis and fetal urinary tract obstruction.

Clinically, patients with CHM usually present in the first trimester with bleeding, enlarged uteri for expected gestational age, an absence of fetal parts on ultrasound, and markedly elevated β-human chorionic gonadotropin (β-hCG). Other signs include hyperemesis and toxemia during the first or second trimester.

CHM shows a diffusely edematous placenta in which the macroscopically enlarged villi lack blood vessels and have cyst-like fluid-filled cavities. Complete hydatidiform mole can also be seen in a twin gestation; in these cases, the diagnosis is often delayed. The majority of complete moles arise in uterine pregnancy, although occasional molar pregnancies are seen in ectopic pregnancies. As a comparison, PHM is composed of large and small villi, and fetal parts are present (Figs 3.20 and 3.21).

Invasive hydatidiform mole

This condition is characterized by molar villi and trophoblasts infiltrating the uterine wall, and occurs more frequently after CHM. Molar tissue may be transported to distant organs such as the lung, and may result in acute pulmonary hypertension, edema, and even death. In these cases, clinical follow-up and therapy do not differ from patients with CHM confined to the uterus.

Gestational choriocarcinoma

This is a malignant neoplasm composed exclusively of cytotrophoblasts and syncytiotrophoblasts. In the USA, the incidence is 1 in 40 000 pregnancies and correlates with the rate of CHM occurrence (Fig. 3.22). Choriocarcinoma spreads hematogenously; metastatic sites include lung (80%), vagina (30%), pelvis (20%), brain (17%), and liver (10%).

References

1 Cross JC, Werb Z, Fisher SJ. Implantation and the placenta: key pieces of the development puzzle. *Science* 1994;266:1508–1518.

2 Das SK, Wang XN, Paria BC, et al. Neonatal alloimmune thrombocytopenia with HLA alloimmunization: case report with immuno-hematologic and placental findings. *Pediatr Dev Pathol* 2002;5:200–205.

3 Shen MM, Leder P. Leukemia inhibitory factor is expressed by the preimplantation uterus and selectively blocks primitive ectoderm formation in vitro. *Proc Natl Acad Sci USA* 1992;89:8240–8244.

4 Stewart CL, Kaspar P, Brunet LJ, et al. Blastocyst implantation depends on maternal expression of leukemia inhibitory factor. *Nature* 1992;359:76–79.

5 Barash A, Dekel N, Fieldust S, et al. Local injury to the endometrium doubles the incidence of successful pregnancies in patients undergoing in vitro fertilization. *Fertil Steril* 2003;79:1317–1322.

6 Brosenesens I, Robertson WB, Dickson AG. The physiological response to the vessels of the placenta predicts normal pregnancy. *J Pathol Bacteriol* 1967;93:569–579.

7 Boyd JD, Hamilton WJ. The human placenta. Cambridge: Heffer, 1970.

8 Benirschke K, Kaufmann P. Pathology of the human placenta, 3rd edn. New York, NY: Springer; 1995:151–181.

9 Benirschke K, Kaufmann P. Pathology of the human placenta, 4th edn. New York, NY: Springer, 2000.

10 Kaufman P, Castellucci M. Development and anatomy of the placenta. In: Fox H, Wells M, eds. *Haines' and Taylor's textbook of obstetrical and gynecological pathology*, 4th edn. New York: Churchill Livingstone, 1994.

11 Sinha AA. Ultrastructure of human amnion and amniotic plaques of normal pregnancy. *Z Zellforsch Mikrosk Anat* 1971;122:1–14.

12 Jones CJP, Jauniaux E, Campbell S. Development and degeneration of the secondary human yolk sac. *Placenta* 1993;14:A32.

13 Charnock-Jones DS, Burton GJ. Placental vascular morphogenesis. *Best Pract Res Clin Obstet Gynecol* 2000;14:953–968.

14 Jaffe R. First trimester utero-placental circulation. Maternal-fetal interaction. *J Perinat Med* 1998;26:168–174.

15 Carbillon L, Uzan M, Uzan S. Pregnancy, vascular tone, and maternal hemodynamics: a crucial adaptation. *Obstet Gynecol* 2000;55:574–581.

16 Kraus FT, Redline RW, Gersell DJ, et al. AFIP Atlas of non tumor pathology: Placental pathology. Washington DC: American Registry of Pathology, 2004.

17 Rayne SC, Kraus FT. Placental thrombi and other vascular lesions. Classifications, morphology, and clinical correlations. *Pathol Res Pract* 1993;189:2–17.

18 Fletcher S. Chirality in umbilical cord. *Br J Obstet Gynaecol* 1993;100:234–236.

19 Nikolov SD, Schiebler TH. Das fetale gefaesz system der reifen menschlische placenta. *Z Zellforsch Mikrosk Anat* 1973;139:333–350.

20 Las Heras J, Haust D. Ultrastructure of fetal stem arteries of human placenta in normal pregnancy. *Virchows Arch* 1981;393:133–144.

21 Froelich LA, Fujkura T. Significance of a single umbilical artery. Report of collaborative study on cerebral palsy. *Am J Obstet Gynecol* 1976;94:274–279.

22 Lilja M. Infants with single umbilical artery studied in a national registry. 2. Survival and malformation in infants with single umbilical artery. *Pediatr Perinat Epidemiol* 1992;6:416–422.

23 Lacro RV, Jones KL, Benirschke K. The umbilical twist: origin, direction, and relevance. *Am J Obstet Gynecol* 1987;157:833–838.

24 Dyer DCC. Comparison of constricting action produced by serotonin and prostaglandin on isolated sheep umbilical arteries and veins. *Gynecol Invest* 1970;1:204–209.

25 Harold JG, Segal RJ, Fitzgerald GA, et al. Differential prostaglandin production by human umbilical vasculature. *Arch Pathol Lab Med* 1988;112:43–46.

26 Heifetz SA. Pathology of umbilical cords. In: Lewis SH, Perrin E, eds. *Pathology of the placenta*. New York, NY: Churchill Livingstone, 1999.

27 Patel D, Dawson M, Kalyanam P, et al. Umbilical cord circumference at birth. *Am J Dis Child* 1989;143:638–639.

28 Kristoffersen K. The significance of absence of one umbilical artery. *Acta Obstet Gynecol Scand* 1969;48:195–214.

29 Mills JL, Harley EE, Moessinger AC. Standards for measuring umbilical cord length. *Placenta* 1983;4:423–426.

30 Rosen RH. The short umbilical cord. *Am J Obstet Gynecol* 1955;66:1253–1259.

31 Miller ME, Higgin-Bottom M, Smith TW. Short umbilical cord: its origin and relevance. *J Pediatr* 1981;67:618–621.

32 Miller ME, Jones MC, Smith DW. Tension: the basis of umbilical cord growth. *J. Pediatr* 1982;101:844.

33 Moessinger AC, Blanc WA, Marone PA, et al. Umbilical cord length in Down syndrome. *Am J Dis Child* 1986;140: 1276–1277.

34 Burg TG, Raburn WF. Umbilical cord length and acid base balance at delivery. *J Reprod Med* 1995;40:19–22.

35 Naeye RL. Umbilical length: clinical significance. *J Pediatr* 1985;107:278–281.

36 Robinson JN, Abuhamad AZ. Abdominal wall in umbilical cord anomalies. *Clin Perinatol* 2000;27:947–978.

37 Nelson KB, Grether JK. Potentially asphyxiating conditions and spastic cerebral palsy in infants of normal birth weight. *Am J Obstet Gynecol* 1998;179:507–513.

38 Goodland RRC. Fetal dismaturity, "thin cords" and fetal distress. *Am J Obstet Gynecol* 1987;156:1357.

39 Rolschau J. The relationship between some disorders of umbilical cord and intrauterine growth retardation. *Acta Obstet Gynecol Scand* 1978;72(Suppl.):15–21.

40 Fox H. Pathology of the placenta, 2nd edn. Philadelphia, PA: WB Saunders, 1997.

41 McLennan H, Price E, Urbanska M, et al. Umbilical cord knots and encirclements. *Aust NZ J Obstet Gynecol* 1988;28: 116–119.

42 Shen-Schwarz S, Ananth CV, Smulian JC, et al. Umbilical cord twist patterns in twins gestations. *Am J Obstet Gynecol* 1997; 176:154.

43 Machin GA, Ackerman J, Gillbert-Barness E. Abnormal umbilical cord coiling is associated with adverse prenatal outcomes. *Pediatr Dev Pathol* 2000;3:462–471.

44 Ruvinsky ED, Wiley TL, Morrison JC, et al. In utero diagnosis of umbilical cord hematoma by ultrasonography. *Am J Obstet Gynecol* 1981;140:833–834.

45 Kraus FT. Cerebral palsy and thrombi in placental vessels of the fetus. *Hum Pathol* 1997,28:246–248.

46 Rhen K, Kinnunen O. Ante-partum rupture of the umbilical cord: case report. *Acta Obstet Gynecol Scand* 1962;41:86–89.

47 Torry RJ, Schwartz GS, Torry DS. Vascularization of the placenta. In: Tomanek RJ, ed. *Cardiovascular molecular morphogenesis: assembly of the vasculature and its regulation*. New York, NY: Springer, 2002.

48 Torry DS, Hinrichs M, Torry RJ. Determinants of placental vascularity. *Am J Reprod Immunol* 2004;51:257–268.

49 Many A, Schreiber L, Rosner S, et al. Pathologic features of the placenta in women with severe pregnancy complications and thrombophilia. *Obstet Gynecol* 2001;98:1041–1044.

50 Salafia CM, Vintzileos AM, Silberman L, et al. Placental pathology of idiopathic intrauterine growth retardation at term. *Am J Perinatol* 1992;9:179–184.

51 Salafia CM, Minio VK, Pezullo JC, et al. Intrauterine growth restriction in infants of less than thirty-two weeks gestation: associated placental pathologic features. *Am J Obstet Gynecol* 1995;173:1049–1057.

52 Wentworth P. The incidence and significance of intervillous thrombi in the human placenta. *J Obstet Gynaecol Br Commonw* 1964;71:894–898.

53 Fox H. Thrombosis of fetal stem arteries in the human placenta. *J Obstet Gynaecol Br Commonw* 1966;73:961–965.

54 Rand JH, Wu XX, Andree HA, et al. Pregnancy loss in the antiphospholipid–antibody syndrome: a possible thrombogenic mechanism. *N Engl J Med* 1997;337:154–160.

55 Sowers JR, Lester MA. Diabetes and cardiovascular disease. *Diabetes Care* 1999;22(Suppl. 3):14–20.

56 Greer IA. Thrombosis in pregnancy: maternal and fetal issues. *Lancet* 1999;353:1258–1265

57 Seligsohn U, Lubetsky A. A genetic susceptibility to venous thrombosis. *N Engl J Med* 2001;344:1222–1231.

58 Alfirevic Z, Roberts D, Martlew V. How strong is the association between maternal thrombophilia and adverse pregnancy outcome? A systematic review. *Eur J Obstet Gynecol Reprod Biol* 2002;101:6–14.

59 Ogueh O, Chen MF, Spurli G, et al. Outcome of pregnancy in women with hereditary thrombophilia. *Int J Gynecol Obstet* 2001;71:247–253.

60 de Tar MW, Klohe E, Grosset A, et al. Neonatal alloimmune thrombocytopenia with HLA alloimmunization: case report with immuno-hematologic and placental findings. *Pediatr Dev Pathol* 2002;5:200–205.

61 Many A, Elad R, Yaron Y, et al. Third trimester unexplained intrauterine fetal death is associated with inherited thrombophilia. *Obstet Gynecol* 2002;99:684–687.

62 Arias F, Romero R, Joist H, et al. Thrombophilia: a mechanism of disease in women with adverse pregnancy outcome and thrombotic lesions in the placenta. *J Matern Fetal Med* 1998;7: 277–286.

63 Kraus FT, Acheen VI. Fetal thrombotic vasculopathy in the placenta: cerebral thrombi and infarcts, coagulopathies, and cerebral palsy. *Hum Pathol* 1999;30:759–769.

64 Andres RL, Kuyper W, Resnik R. The association of maternal floor infarction of the placenta with adverse perinatal outcome. *Am J Obstet Gynecol* 1990;163:935–938.

65 Clewell WH, Manchester DK. Recurrent maternal floor infarction: a preventable cause of fetal death. *Am J Obstet Gynecol* 1983;147:346–347.

66 Naeye RL. Maternal floor infarction. *Hum Pathol* 1985;16: 823–828.

67 Darby MJ, Caritis SN, Shen-Schwarz S. Placental abruption in the preterm gestation: an association with chorioamnionitis. *Obstet Gynecol* 1989;74:88–92.

68 Cejtin HE, Young SA, Ungaretti J, et al. Effects of cocaine on the placenta. *Pediatr Dev Pathol* 1999;2:143–147.

69 Sherer DM, Schenker JG. Accidental injury during pregnancy. *Obstet Gynecol Surv* 1989;44:330–338.

70 Elliot JP, Gilpin B, Strong TH, Jr, et al. Chronic abruption-oligohydramnios sequence. *J Reprod Med* 1998;43:418–422.

71 Redline RW, Wilson-Costello D. Chronic peripheral separation of the placenta. The significance of diffuse chorionic hemosiderosis. *Am J Clin Pathol* 1999;111:804–810.

72 Gersell DJ, Kraus FT. Diseases of the placenta. In: Kurman RJ, ed. *Blaustein's pathology of the female genital tract*, 5th edn. New York, NY: Springer-Verlag, 2002.

73 Baergen RN, Chacko SA, Edersheim T, et al. The placenta in thrombophilias: a clinicopathologic study. *Mod Pathol* 2001;14: 213A.

74 Kramer MS, Usher RH, Pollack R, et al. Etiologic determinants of abruptio placentae. *Obstet Gynecol* 1997;89:221–226.

75 Shanklin DR, Scott JS, Massive subchorial thrombohaematoma (Breu's mole). *Br J Obstet Gynaecol* 1975;82:476–487.

76 Kirkinen P, Jouppia P. Intrauterine membranous cyst. *Obstet Gynecol* 1986;67:26-30.

77 Blanc WA. Pathology of the placenta and cord in ascending and hematogenous infection. *Ciba Found Symp* 1980;77:17–38.
78 Goldenberg RL, Hauth JC, Andrews WW. Intrauterine infection and preterm delivery. *N Engl J Med* 2000;342:1500–1507.
79 Redline RW, Zaragoza M, Hassold T. Prevalence of developmental and inflammatory lesions in nonmolar first-trimester spontaneous abortions. *Hum Pathol* 1999;30:93–100.
80 Jordan JA. Identification of human parvovirus B-19 infection in idiopathic nonimmune hydrops fetalis. *Am J Obstet Gynecol* 1996;174:37–42.
81 Rogers BB, Mark Y, Over CE. Diagnosis and incidence of fetal parvovirus infection in an autopsy series: I. Histology. *Pediatr Pathol* 1993;13:371–379.
82 Brown KE, Hibbs JR, Gallinella G, et al. Resistance to parvovirus B19 infection due to lack of virus receptor (erythrocyte p antigen). *N Engl J Med* 1994;330:1192–1196.
83 Altshuler G, Hyde S. Fusobacteria. An important cause of chorioamnionitis. *Arch Pathol Lab Med* 1985;109:739–743.
84 Ohyama M, Itani Y, Yamanaka M, et al. Re-evaluation of chorioamnionitis and funisitis with a special reference to subacute chorioamnionitis. *Hum Pathol* 2002;33:183–190.
85 Young SA, Crocker DW. Occult congenital syphilis in macerated stillborn fetuses. *Arch Pathol Lab Med* 1994;118:44–47.
86 Hood IC, Desa DJ, White RK. The inflammatory response in candida chorioamnionitis. *Hum Pathol* 1983;14:984–990.
87 Genest DR, Choi-Hong SR, Tate JE, et al. Diagnosis of congenital syphilis from placental examination: comparison of histopathology, Steiner stain, and polymerase chain reaction for *Treponema pallidum* DNA. *Hum Pathol* 1996;27:366–372.
88 Schwartz DA, Larsen SA, Beck-Sague C, et al. Pathology of the umbilical cord in congenital syphilis: analysis of 25 specimens using histochemistry and immunofluorescent antibody to *Treponema pallidum. Hum Pathol* 1995;26:784–791.
89 Muhlemann K, Miller RK, Metlay L, et al. Cytomegalovirus infection of the human placenta: an immunocytochemical study. *Hum Pathol* 1992;23:1234–1237.
90 Diagne N, Rogier C, Sokhna C, et al. Increased susceptibility to malaria during the early postpartum period. *N Engl J Med* 2000;343:598–603.
91 Ismail MR, Ordi J, Menendez C, et al. Placental pathology in malaria: a histological, immunohistochemical and quantitative study. *Hum Pathol* 2003;31:85–93.
92 MacGregor I. Epidemiology, malaria, and pregnancy. *Am J Trop Med Hyg* 1984;33:517–525.
93 Heifetz SA, Bauman M. Necrotizing funisitis and herpes simplex infection of placental and decidual tissues: study of four cases. *Hum Pathol* 1994;25:715–722.
94 Qureshi F, Jacques SM. Maternal varicella during pregnancy. *Hum Pathol* 1996;27:191–196.
95 Mattern CFT, Murray K, Jensen A, et al. Localization of human immunodeficiency virus core antigen in term placenta. *Pediatrics* 1992;89:207–209.
96 Jauniaux E, Nessmann C, Imbert C, et al. Morphological aspects of placenta in HIV pregnancies. *Placenta* 1988;9:633–642.
97 Doss BJ, Greene MF, Hill J, et al. Massive chronic intervillitis associated with recurrent abortions. *Hum Pathol* 1995;26: 1245–1251.
98 Knox TA, Fox H. Villitis of unknown etiology. *Placenta* 1984;5:395–402.
99 Martin AW, Brady K, Smith SI, et al. Immunohistochemical localization of human immunodeficiency virus p24 antigen in placental tissue. *Hum Pathol* 1992;23:411–414.
100 Redline RW, Abramowsky CR. Clinical and pathologic aspects of recurrent placental villitis. *Hum Pathol* 1985;16:727–731.
101 Boyd TK, Redline RW. Chronic histiocytic intervillositis: a placental lesion associated with recurrent reproductive loss. *Hum Pathol* 2000;31:1389–1396.
102 Cannon M, Pierce R, Taber EB, et al. Fatal hydrops fetalis caused by anti-D in a mother with partial D. *Obstet Gynecol* 2003;102:1143–1145.
103 Denomme GA, Ryan G, Seaward PG, et al. Maternal ABO-mismatched blood for intrauterine transfusion of severe hemolytic disease of the newborn due to anti-Rh17. *Transfusion* 2004;44:1357–1360.
104 Lujan-Zilbermann J, Lacson A, Gilbert-Barness E, et al. Clinicopathologic conference: newborn with hydrops fetalis caused by CMV infection case report. *Pediatr Pathol Mol Med* 2003;22: 481–494.
105 Favre R, Dreux S, Dommergues M, et al. Nonimmune fetal ascites. *Am J Obstet Gynecol* 2004;190:407–412.
106 Kalpatthi R, Lieber E, Rajegowda B, et al. Hydrocephalus in a hydropic fetus with Turner syndrome: a rare association. *J Maternal Fetal Neonatal Med* 2003;14:136–138.
107 Rodriguez MM, Chaves F, Romaguera RL, et al. Value of autopsy in nonimmune hydrops fetalis. *Pediatr Dev Pathol* 2002;5:365–374.
108 Wraith JE. Lysosomal disorders. *Semin Neonatol* 2002;7:75–83.
109 D'Ercole C, Cravello L, Boubli L, et al. Large chorioangioma associated with hydrops fetalis. *Fetal Diagn Ther* 1996;11: 357–360.
110 Parilla BV, Socol ML. Hydrops fetalis with Kell isoimmunization. *Obstet Gynecol* 1996;88:730.
111 Knisely AS. The pathologist and the hydropic placenta, fetus, or infant. *Semin Perinatol* 1995;19:525–531.
112 Arcasoy MO, Gallagher PG. Hematologic disorders and nonimmune hydrops fetalis. *Semin Perinatol* 1995;19:502–515.
113 Barron SD, Pass RF. Infectious causes of hydrops fetalis. *Semin Perinatol* 1995;19:493–501.
114 Knilans TK. Cardiac abnormalities associated with hydrops fetalis. *Semin Perinatol* 1995;19:483–492.
115 Kraus FT, Redline RW, Gersell DJ, et al. AFIP Atlas of non tumor pathology: Placental pathology. Washington DC: American Registry of Pathology; 2004:47–73.
116 Ahmad A, Gilbert Barnes E. Placenta membranacea: a developmental anomaly with diverse clinical presentation. *Pediatr Dev Pathol* 2003;6:201–202.
117 Greenberg JA, Sorem KA, Shifren JL, et al. Placenta membranacea with placenta increta. *Obstet Gynecol* 1991;92:512–514.
118 Fox H. Pathology of the placenta, 2nd edn. *Major problems in pathology*. Philadelphia, PA: WB Saunders; 1997:54–60.
119 Naftolin F, Khudr G, Bernischke K, et al. The syndrome of chronic abruptio placentae, hydrorrhea, and circumvallate placenta. *Am J Obstet Gynecol* 1973;116:347–350.
120 Eriksen G, Wohlert M, Ersbak V, et al. Placental abruption. A case-control investigation. *Br J Obstet Gynaecol* 1991;98: 448–452.
121 Redline RW, O'Riordan MA. Placental lesions associated with cerebral palsy and neurological impairment following term birth. *Arch Pathol Lab Med* 2000;124:1785–1791.
122 Williams MA, Hickok DE, Zingheim RW, et al. Low birth weight and preterm delivery in relation to early-gestation vaginal bleeding and elevated maternal serum alpha-fetoprotein. *Obstet Gynecol* 1992;80;745–749.

123 Cunningham FG, MacDonald P, Gant N, et al. Williams obstetrics, 20th edn. Stamford, CT: Appleton & Lange; 1997:765–767.

124 Han VK, Hunter ES 3rd, Pratt RM, et al. Expression of rat transforming growth factor alpha mRNA during development occurs predominantly in the maternal decidua. *Mol Cell Biol* 1987;7: 2335–2343.

125 Librach CL, Werb Z, Fitzgerald ML, et al. 92-kD type IV collagenase mediates invasion of human cytotrophoblasts. *J Cell Biol* 1991;113:437–449.

126 Bass KE, Morrish D, Roth I, et al. Human cytotrophoblast invasion is up-regulated by epidermal growth factor: evidence that paracrine factors modify this process. *Dev Biol* 1994;164: 550–561.

127 Shimonovitz S, Hurwitz A, Dushnik M, et al. Developmental regulation of the expression of 72 and 92 kd type IV collagenases in human trophoblasts: a possible mechanism for control of trophoblast invasion. *Am J Obstet Gynecol* 1994;171: 832–838.

128 American College of Obstetricians and Gynecologists Committee on Obstetric Practice. Placenta accreta. Committee Opinion, No. 266. *Obstet Gynecol* 2002:99;169–170.

129 Read JA, Cotlon DB, Miller FC. Placenta accreta: changing clinical aspects and outcome. *Obstet Gynecol* 1980;56:31–34.

130 Jacques SM, Qureshi F. The significance of placental basal plate myometrial fibers. *Mod Pathol* 1999;12:118A.

131 Bernischke K, Kaufman P. Pathology of human placenta, 4th edn. New York, NY: Springer; 2000:778–785.

132 Tonkin IL, Setzer ES, Ermocilla R. Placental chorangioma: a rare cause of congestive heart failure and hydrops fetalis in the newborn. *Am J Roentgenol* 1980:134:181–183.

133 Jones CE, Rivers RP, Taghizadeh A. Disseminated intravascular coagulation and fetal hydrops in a newborn infant associated with a chorangioma of placenta. *Pediatrics* 1992;50:901–905.

134 Ogino S, Redline RW. Villous capillary lesions of the placenta: distinctions between chorangioma, chorangiomatosis, and chorangiosis. *Hum Pathol* 2000;31:945–954.

135 Duley L. Pre-eclampsia and hypertension (update). *Clin Evid* 2003;9:1584–1600.

136 Moroni G, Ponticelli C. The risk of pregnancy in patients with lupus nephritis. *J Nephrol* 2003;6:161–167.

137 de Groot CJ, Taylor RN. New insights into the etiology of preeclampsia. *Ann Med* 1993;25:243–249.

138 Friedman SA, Taylor RN, Roberts JM. Pathophysiology of preeclampsia. *Clinics Perinatol* 1991;18:661–682.

139 Lindheimer MD, Katz AI. Preeclampsia: pathophysiology, diagnosis, and management. *Annu Rev Med* 1989;40:233–250.

140 Crocker A. Farrell T. Pregnancy and pre-existing diabetes: key concerns. *Hosp Med (London)* 2004;65:351–354.

141 Kaufmann P, Black S, Huppertz B. Endovascular trophoblast invasion: implications for the pathogenesis of intrauterine growth retardation and preeclampsia. *Biol Reprod* 2003;69:1–7.

142 Redman CW, Sargent IL. Pre-eclampsia, the placenta and the maternal systemic inflammatory response: a review. *Placenta* 2003;24(Suppl. A):21–27.

143 Sibai BM, Caritis S, Hauth J. National Institutes of Child Health and Human Development Maternal–Fetal Medicine Units Network. What we have learned about preeclampsia. *Semin Perinatol* 2003;27:239–246.

144 Goldman-Wohl D, Yagel S. Regulation of trophoblast invasion: from normal implantation to pre-eclampsia. *Mol Cell Endocrinol* 2002;187:233–238.

145 Ness RB, Roberts JM. Heterogeneous causes constituting the single syndrome of preeclampsia: a hypothesis and its implications. *Am J Obstet Gynecol* 1996;175:1365–1370.

146 Paria BC, Ma W, Tan J, et al. Cellular and molecular responses of the uterus to embryo implantation can be elicited by locally applied growth factors. *Proc Natl Acad Sci USA* 2001;98: 1047–1052.

147 Altshuler G. Chorangiosis. An important placental sign of neonatal morbidity and mortality. *Arch Pathol Lab Med* 1984;108: 71–74.

148 Unfried G, Griesmacher A, Weismuller W, et al. The C677T polymorphism of the methylene tetrahydrofolate reductase gene and idiopathic recurrent miscarriage. *Obstet Gynecol* 2002;99: 614–619.

149 Gunther G, Junker R, Strater R, et al. Symptomatic ischemic stroke in full term neonates: role of acquired and genetic prothrombotic risk factors. *Stroke* 2000;31:2437–2441.

150 Haust MD. Maternal diabetes mellitus: effects on the fetus and placenta. In: Naeye RL, Kissane JM, Kaufman N, eds. *Perinatal disease*. Baltimore, MD: Williams &Wilkins; 1981:201–285.

151 Fox H. Thrombosis of foetal stem arteries in the human placenta. *J Obstet Gynaecol Br Commonw* 1966;73:961–965.

152 Botting BJ, Davis IM, MacFarlane AJ. Recent trends in the incidence of multiple births and associated mortality. *Arch Dis Child* 1987;62:941–950.

153 Kovacs BW, Kirschbaum TH, Paul RH. Twin gestations. I. Neonatal care and complications. *Obstet Gynecol* 1989;74: 313–317.

154 Nylander PP. Perinatal mortality in twins. *Acta Genet Med Gemellol* 1979;28:363–368.

155 Gonsoulin W, Copeland KL, Carpenter RJ Jr, et al. Fetal blood sampling demonstrating chimerism in monozygotic twins discaccording for sex and tissue karyotype (46,XY and 45,X). *Prenat Diagn* 1990;10:25–28.

156 Powers WF, Kiely JL. The risks confronting twins: a national prospective. *Am J Obstet Gynecol* 1994;170:456–461.

157 Williams K, Hennessy E, Alberman E. Cerebral palsy: effects of twinning, birth rate, and gestational age. *Arch Dis Child Fetal Neonatal* 1996;75:F178–182.

158 Robboy SJ, Anderson, MC, Russell, P. Pathology of female reproductive tract, 1st edn. London: Churchill Livingstone; 2002: 736–739.

159 Coughtrey H, Jeffery HE, Henderson-Smart DJ, et al. Possible causes linking asphyxia, thick meconium, and respiratory distress. *Aust NZ J Obstet Gynaecol* 1991;31:97–102.

160 Piper JM, Newton ER, Berkus MD, et al. Meconium: a marker for prepartum infection. *Obstet Gynecol* 1998;91:741–745.

161 Romero R, Hanaoka S, Mazor M, et al. Meconium stained amniotic fluid: a risk factor for microbial invasion of the amniotic cavity. *Am J Obstet Gynecol* 1991;164:859–862.

162 Ghidini A, Spong CY. Severe meconium aspiration syndrome is not caused by aspiration of meconium. *Am J Obstet Gynecol* 2001;185:931–938.

163 Ramin KD, Leveno KJ, Kelly MA, et al. Amniotic fluid meconium: a fetal environmental hazard. *Obstet Gynecol* 1996;87: 181–184.

164 Larsen LG, Clausen HV, Anderson B, et al. A stereologic study of postmature placentas fixed by dual perfusion. *Am J Obstet Gynecol* 1995;172:500–507.

165 Damato N, Filly RA, Goldstein RB, et al. Frequency of fetal anomalies in sonographically detected polyhydramnios. *J Ultrasound Med* 1993;12:11–15.
166 Hillier SL, Martius J, Krohn M, et al. A case control study of chorioamnionic infection and histologic chorioamnionitis in prematurity. *N Engl J Med* 1988;319:972–978.
167 Arias F, Victoria A, Cho K, et al. Placental histology and clinical characteristics of patients with preterm premature rupture of membranes. *Obstet Gynecol* 1997;89:265–271.
168 McIntire DD, Bloom SL, Casey BM, et al. Birth weight in relation to morbidity and mortality among newborn infants. *New Engl J Med* 1999;340:1234–1238.
169 Newham J. Consequences of fetal growth restriction. *Curr Opin Obstet Gynecol* 1998;10:145–149.
170 Lin CC, Santolaya-Forgas J. Current concepts of fetal growth restriction: Part 1. Causes, classification, and pathophysiology. *Obstet Gynecol* 1998;92:1044–1055.
171 World Health Organization (WHO). Recommended definitions, terminology and format for statistical tables related to the perinatal period and use of a new certificate for cause of perinatal deaths. *Acta Obstet Gynecol Scand* 1977;56:247–253.
172 Benirschke K, Kaufmann P. Pathology of the human placenta, 4th edn. New York, NY: Springer; 2000:443–454.
173 Shih IM, Mazur MT, Kurman R. Gestational trophoblastic disease and related lesions, In: *Blaustein's pathology of female genital tract*, 5th edn. New York: Springer, 2002.

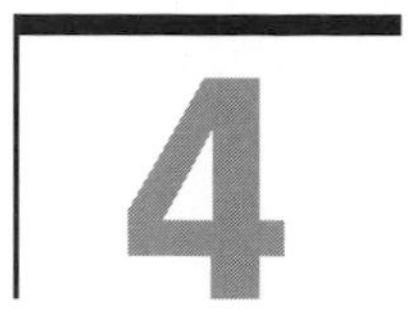

Fetoplacental perfusion and transfer of nutrients

Henry L. Galan and Frederick C. Battaglia

The technical advances in the tools that obstetricians use for the evaluation of a pregnancy have progressed faster than our basic understanding of some of the developmental aspects of fetal and placental physiology. In this chapter, we shall try to bring out those aspects of perinatal physiology that are reasonably well established.

Perfusion and placental transport

A number of concepts relating to placental perfusion and transport, most of which have considerable clinical significance, have become relatively well established. One of these is the absence of autoregulation in the uterine vascular bed. This has been shown in animal studies by the absence of reactive hyperemia after uterine artery occlusion.[1]

The clinical implication of these observations is that the uterine bed in late pregnancy may be regarded as an almost fully dilated bed. Thus, it cannot easily compensate for a sudden decrease in vasodilation. From a clinical perspective, maternal hypotension must be regarded as a direct causal factor in producing a reduction in uterine and placental blood flow. Maternal hypotension should therefore be avoided, particularly in late gestation.

Another characteristic of the uterine vascular bed is the unresponsiveness of the uterine vascular vessels to changes in PO_2 or PCO_2. Again, this has considerable clinical significance because it means that oxygen therapy for the mother does carry with it the risk of increasing fetal hypoxia by vasoconstriction of the uterine bed. It has been well demonstrated in animal studies that oxygen administration to the mother increases fetal oxygenation, lending support to the clinical approach of using maternal oxygen therapy when there are signs of fetal distress during labor and delivery. Unfortunately, as is true with many areas of physiology, we have much less information about the effects of chronic maternal oxygen therapy. Because this is such an important issue in clinical obstetrics, it is worth reviewing in some detail the animal studies that support the use of maternal oxygen therapy for fetal hypoxia. The first study[2] to directly address the question of the impact of maternal oxygen administration upon uterine and umbilical blood flows and fetal oxygenation showed that there was no effect of the increased maternal PO_2 upon uterine or umbilical blood flows and that, as expected, umbilical venous PO_2, representing the most oxygenated blood of the fetus, increased significantly.

Clinically, the first studies demonstrating an effect upon fetal oxygenation by maternal oxygen administration were based upon changes in fetal scalp PO_2 and were carried out by scalp sampling during labor. More recently, maternal oxygen administration has been used in pregnancies complicated by intrauterine growth retardation (IUGR). The beneficial effect is confirmed both by the changes in fetal blood PO_2 and saturation in blood obtained by cordocentesis, and by an apparent improvement in velocity waveform measurements upon the fetal descending aorta, suggesting a reduced placental impedance during maternal oxygen therapy.[3]

The relationship between fetal oxygenation and maternal oxygenation is complex because a number of factors are involved in determining the "normal" umbilical venous PO_2 in any species. These factors include:

1 placental oxygen consumption
2 uterine and umbilical blood flows
3 placental permeability
4 pattern of placental perfusion (i.e., concurrent, cross-current, countercurrent)
5 maternal arterial PO_2 and hemoglobin concentration
6 shape of maternal and fetal oxygen dissociation curves.

For a more complete discussion of the contribution of each of these factors, see references 1 and 4. In man, umbilical venous PO_2 tends to equilibrate with uterine *venous*, not arterial, PO_2, i.e., it simulates a concurrent exchanger. With the advent of techniques to sample umbilical venous blood transabdominally (i.e., cordocentesis), data are now available describing umbilical venous PO_2 through the latter half of gestation. The umbilical venous PO_2 of the human fetus is higher in mid-gestation and decreases as gestation advances.[5,6] However, at any gestational age, it is clear that the human fetal umbilical venous PO_2 is very low by postnatal standards. This highlights the importance of the difference in whole blood oxygen affinity in the fetus versus the adult because the higher affinity of fetal hemoglobin insures that the bulk of the hemoglobin will be oxygenated even at the low PO_2 of fetal umbilical venous blood. The change in fetal PO_2 in late gestation does not imply increasing fetal hypoxia because, associated with this, there is an increasing hemoglobin concentration as gestation progresses. This latter change maintains the oxygen content of umbilical venous blood throughout gestation.[7] For this reason, measurements of fetal oxygen content are particularly useful because they are independent of gestational age. Studies in the mid-gestation fetal lamb have shown a higher PO_2 and oxygen saturation in fetal vessels than in late gestation lambs.[8]

Soothill and coauthors[9] have shown a relationship between fetal lactate concentration and fetal hemoglobin and oxygen concentration in rhesus (Rh)-isoimmunized pregnancies. Similarly, Ferrazzi and coauthors[10] and Soothill and coauthors[3] described lactic acidemia in association with abnormal velocity waveforms in the fetal descending aorta or umbilical artery. Several studies have shown that it is now possible to move beyond velocity measurements alone to measurements of actual blood flow in the umbilical vein.[11,12] These studies have reported a mean umbilical blood flow of 120 mL/min/kg fetal weight in the human fetus during late gestation. The umbilical flow is markedly reduced in IUGR pregnancies.[13]

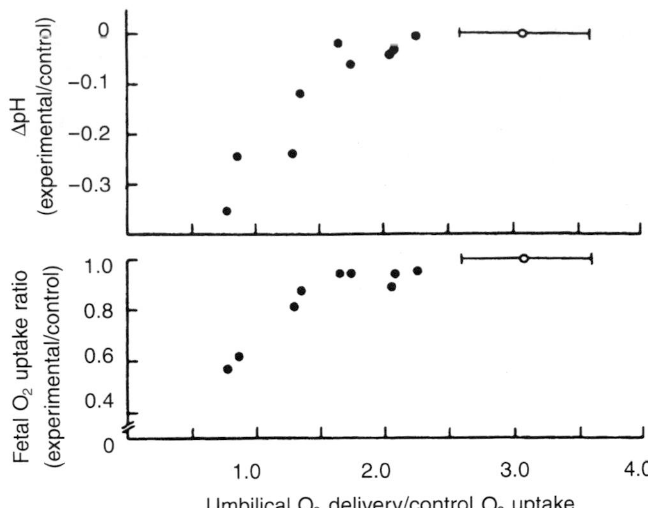

Figure 4.1 Changes in fetal O_2 uptake and fetal arterial blood pH in relation to the ratio of umbilical O_2 delivery to control O_2 uptake. In control periods, the ratio averaged 3.09 (O) and ranged between 2.60 and 3.62. Note that O_2 uptake and pH remained virtually constant for ratios of O_2 delivery to control O_2 uptake >1.6.

Uterine flow and placental transport

Uterine blood flow increases remarkably during late gestation. However, the increase in uterine blood flow does not keep up with the increase in uterine oxygen consumption, which causes the uterine venous PO_2 content to decrease with increasing gestational age. In human pregnancies, it has been shown that a decrease in uterine venous PO_2 leads to a lower umbilical venous PO_2.

In terms of clinical applicability, one of the more important contributions to fetal physiology was made by the studies that described a nonlinear relationship between uterine blood flow and placental transport of oxygen and nutrients to the fetus. Wilkening and Meschia[14] demonstrated that, in pregnant sheep, uterine blood flow can decrease over a fairly wide range without any effect on oxygen transport. A critical point is then reached beyond which any further reduction in uterine blood flow leads to a decrease in oxygen transport. As shown in Fig. 4.1, similar data have been obtained by the same investigators for umbilical blood flow versus placental transport.[15] Although a similar study has not been carried out for other nutrients, the transport of all nutrients should share this common characteristic, namely that there is a margin of safety represented by the range within which uterine blood flow can be reduced without affecting transport. This concept has considerable clinical significance. It would appear that a critical need in obstetrics is to determine whether such relationships exist in high-risk pregnancies, i.e., critical levels of uterine perfusion beyond which reductions in uterine flow profoundly affect fetal oxygenation and fetal nutrition.

There is currently active research from many centers directed at determining the role of specific vasoconstrictors and vasodilators in normal pregnancy and in pathologic pregnancies, particularly in pregnancy-induced hypertension (PIH). However, one common path for the control of vasomotor tone is through nitric oxide production by uterine and placental endothelium. Several studies on human placental tissue by Myatt and co-workers,[16–18] Diiulio and co-workers,[19,20] and others[21,22] have highlighted the importance of this area of research, particularly in terms of endothelial nitric oxide synthase expression in placental tissues. The link between these pathways and other vasodilators and constrictors is likely to remain a major focus of vascular research in perinatal medicine.

Uterine venous drainage

Uterine arterial flow has been relatively well studied in animals; however, uterine venous drainage has not received such careful attention. Maternal position has been considered to be important in clinical obstetrics, principally through the potential to relieve inferior vena caval obstruction by the pregnant uterus and increase right-sided venous return to the heart. Alleviation of signs of fetal distress have been reported

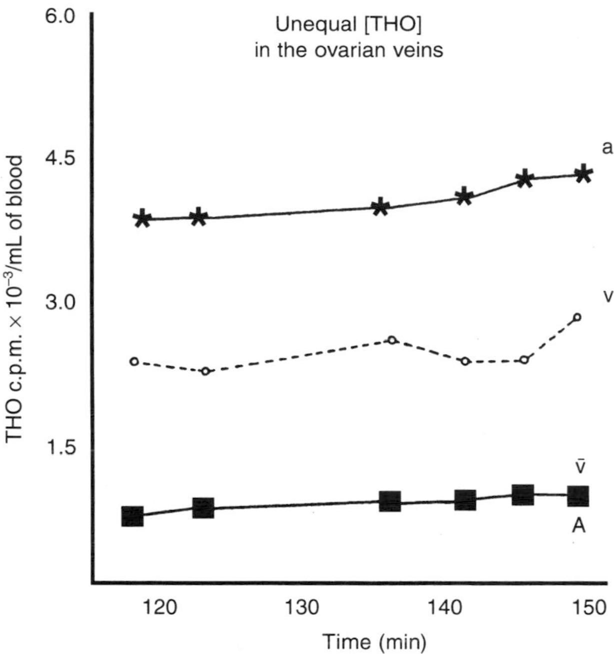

Figure 4.2 Tritiated water concentrations in both arteries and both ovarian veins of a rhesus monkey. It is clear that only one ovarian vein was carrying blood from the placenta whereas the other was draining nonexchange tissues within the uterus; the latter had a ^3H_2O concentration indistinguishable from the maternal artery. It should be stressed that this difference in tissue drainage could not be detected from the gross appearance of the two veins by either color or size of the vessels.[23]

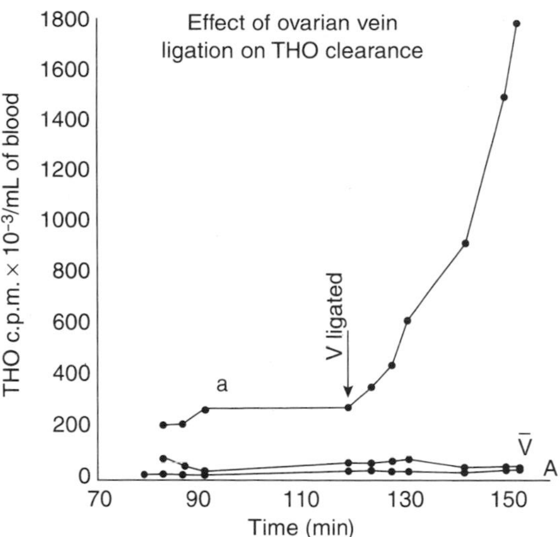

Figure 4.3 Ligation of one ovarian vein produced rapid deterioration of the preparation, as indicated by the rapid rise of ^3H_2O concentration in the fetus and the inability of the system to attain a new steady state. Presumably in this animal, the principal channel for venous drainage of the placenta was the ovarian vein that was ligated.[23]

after positioning the mother from the supine into the left-lateral decubitus position.

Two laboratories have confirmed that, in the rhesus monkey, drainage is not predictable; occasionally, one vein carries essentially all of the placental drainage. This can put the fetus at risk, as shown in Figs 4.2 and 4.3 that were taken from the study of Battaglia and coauthors.[23] Figure 4.2 shows that tritiated water infused into the fetal rhesus monkey as a marker appeared in only one uterine vein. The other vein had a concentration similar to that of maternal arterial blood. Occlusion of this latter vein would have no repercussions upon placental function. However, as shown in Fig. 4.3, obstruction of the vein carrying all of the placental drainage leads to a rapid accumulation of tritiated water in the fetus because placental clearance is virtually zero. Such data are not available in man, but there is sufficient reason to believe that placental drainage in man is not distributed equally to the venous drainage on the two sides of the uterus. One study has shown that, when both uterine veins are sampled across the pregnant uterus during Cesarean section, there is great variability in oxygen saturation and this is independent of the position of the placenta.[5] This suggests that there may be an unequal distribution of placental drainage to one of the other uterine veins. Thus, the question of whether uterine venous obstruction contributes to the maternal positional effects upon fetal well-being is an important one that needs further investigation.

Placental transport and metabolism

The placenta is very active metabolically and has an oxygen consumption and glucose utilization rate similar to brain tissue.[24] One of the characteristics of its metabolism is the production of lactate and ammonia (NH_3) as the end products that are delivered into both the uterine and the umbilical circulations. Because the production of lactate and NH_3 by the pregnant uterus has been a general characteristic among species with very different placental types, it seems reasonable to hypothesize that this reflects the metabolic activity of the trophoblast as this epithelial layer persists in all placental types.

There are several studies that have examined maternal–fetal glucose relationships in human pregnancy utilizing data obtained at cordocentesis. Figure 4.4, taken from Marconi and coauthors,[25] compares fetal and maternal glucose concentrations over a wide gestational age range. The data demonstrate that the maternal–fetal glucose concentration difference increases as gestation advances. The increased transplacental glucose gradient is one means of accommodating the increased glucose requirements of the rapidly growing fetus. In addition, there is probably a substantial increase in placental glucose transport capacity. In fetuses with IUGR, the maternal–fetal glucose gradient is further increased and this appears to correlate with increasing severity, as shown in Figure 4.5. The question of maternal glucose utilization in pregnancy has also

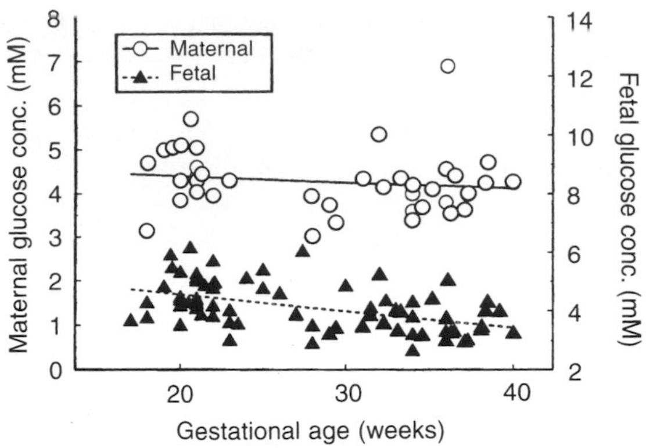

Figure 4.4 Umbilical venous glucose concentrations vs. gestational age for appropriate for gestational age (AGA) pregnancies (▲). Maternal arterial glucose concentration vs. gestational age (○).

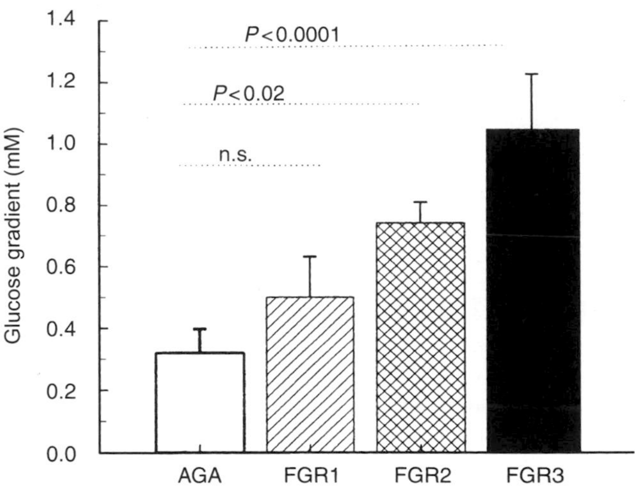

Figure 4.5 Measured mean ± SD values of maternal arterial–umbilical venous glucose concentration (conc.) differences in AGA fetuses and fetal growth restriction (FGR) cases of groups 1, 2, and 3. The *P*-values refer to the significance of the differences for the intercepts of AGA compared with FGR groups (solid lines), and among groups of FGR (dashed lines) for the regression analysis of the maternal–fetal difference vs. gestational age.

been studied from the viewpoint of the increased metabolic demand placed upon the mother by multiple pregnancies. Marconi and coauthors[26] reported that there was a significant correlation between plasma glucose disposal rate and both the maternal glucose concentration and the mass of the conceptus. Thus, maternal glucose disposal rate is a function not only of the glucose concentration but also of the mass of the conceptus (fetus + placenta).

Amino acid transport has been studied under steady-state conditions in sheep *in vivo*[27–30] as well as under a variety of *in vitro* conditions in small mammals and in the human placenta.[31] This is an extensive subject that has been well reviewed recently,[32] but that is not covered in this chapter.

Placental growth

In all mammalian species, placental growth is much more rapid than fetal growth in early gestation. Placental growth then either stops or is at a very low rate during later gestation. Fetal growth, on the other hand, is largely exponential throughout gestation. There is a slower rate of fetal growth in late gestation but this still far exceeds placental growth. The outcome of these differences in growth rate is that the fetal–placental ratio increases markedly as gestation advances. Although the growth rate of the human placenta decreases, its maturation continues. This can be demonstrated by morphometric techniques that bring out the continued exponential increase in surface area of the placenta during late gestation when its weight is no longer increasing.[33] Physiological studies in animals support the morphometric data in that there is a marked increase in the capacity of the placenta to diffuse urea in late gestation, which parallels the changes in surface area.[34]

Fetal growth

Key aspects of fetal growth include not only the rate of change in fetal body weight but also the change in body composition as gestation advances. This is particularly striking for the human fetus, which grows by approximately 1.5% each day. Accompanying this growth there is a reduction in total body water concentration, attributable largely to a decrease in extracellular fluid volume as a fraction of total body water, and large increases in white fat depots. There are a number of clinical implications of these changes in body composition. Water has no caloric density, whereas fat has the highest caloric density of tissues; therefore, the human fetus has a relatively high caloric accretion rate. Also, because fat consists of 78% carbon but is nitrogen free, the human fetus has a relatively low nitrogen accretion rate in late pregnancy but builds up large carbon stores in fat and glycogen.[35]

The accumulation of large white fat depots in the human fetus has important nutritional implications. Fat depots are important storage sites for the fat-soluble vitamins and essential fatty acids, particularly the polyunsaturated, long-chain fatty acids. Intrauterine growth-retarded and very preterm infants are born with depleted fat and glycogen stores and are at risk of developing essential fatty acid deficiency relatively quickly (i.e., within days) compared with term infants (i.e., within weeks).[36,37] Similarly, IUGR and preterm infants are at risk of neonatal hypoglycemia. Fat also helps to insulate the term infant, reducing heat and water loss through the skin – all adaptations that the premature infant does not have.

Fetal metabolism

Fetal metabolism has been fairly intensively studied in the past few years as techniques for the application of tracer methodology have become more available.

Umbilical uptake of nutrients

The net uptake of nutrients into the umbilical circulation from the placenta is an indispensable reference point for understanding fetal metabolism. The reason for this is that the net umbilical uptake represents the dietary supply of nutrients to the fetus. Although it is possible for the fetus to synthesize nutrients such as glucose or nonessential amino acids within the fetal tissues, such interconversions of compounds do not satisfy the absolute requirement for an exogenous (to the fetus) supply of carbon and nitrogen for growth and oxidation.

The main nutrients that the fetus receives include glucose, lactate, and amino acids.[4,38] Glucose and the essential amino acids are derived from the maternal circulation.

The nonessential amino acids are a far more complicated issue. Tracer studies have clearly shown that some amino acids are produced within the placenta in large amounts, with a relatively small component coming from direct transplacental transport. The fetal requirements for some amino acids (glutamate and serine) appear to be met entirely by production within the fetus. Studies of glutamate venous–arterial differences across the human umbilical circulation at the time of Cesarean section have shown a net uptake of glutamate from the fetal circulation into the placenta.[39] Presumably, it is used as a metabolic fuel in the human placenta as it is in the ovine placenta.[40]

Both glucose and lactate have been shown to have fairly high oxidation rates during fetal life. If their transport is increased, their contribution to oxidation will also increase, sparing the utilization of amino acids as metabolic fuels. Conversely, during maternal fasting, placental glucose transport is decreased and amino acid oxidation increased.

Quantitative information about amino acid and nitrogen transport to the human fetus is not as firmly established because it is difficult to obtain reliable data for umbilical venous–arterial differences of amino acids at the time of delivery. Several studies have measured the uptake of amino acids by the umbilical circulation at the time of Cesarean section. Because umbilical blood flow could not be measured reliably, the data were expressed per unit of oxygen uptake. These studies have shown a large uptake of most amino acids (with the exception of glutamate, which is taken up by the placenta). Amino acids are provided to the human fetus in amounts that exceed their net rates of accretion. The data supporting this interpretation come from the observation of a relatively large placental urea gradient, with fetal concentrations being higher than maternal concentrations.[41] Given the large urea clearance in the primate placenta, the urea concentration difference across the placenta implies a fairly high urea production rate during fetal life.

In addition to serving as fuels for the fetus, amino acids are used for protein synthesis. There are a number of conceptual problems in attempting to estimate the rate of protein synthesis during fetal life. However, it is clear that the rate of protein synthesis expressed per gram of fetus is higher in early gestation and decreases towards term, roughly in parallel with the changes in metabolic rate.[42] The rate of protein synthesis exceeds the rate of net protein accretion from growth, reflecting a relatively high rate of protein turnover during normal fetal development.

Fatty acids and ketone bodies cross the placenta in man and in several other species, maintaining relatively small transplacental concentration gradients. Their fate upon entering the fetal circulation has not been well studied, although it is clear that fatty acids are used largely for carbon accretion in white fat depots and are not oxidized extensively during fetal life.[43] Because of their importance for brain growth, there are more studies directed at placental transport of polyunsaturated, long-chain fatty acids.

As alluded to earlier, the limitation in understanding fetal growth has been the inability to measure umbilical volume blood flow accurately. For example, endpoints of many nutritionally based studies, such as those evaluating amino acids, fatty acids, or glucose transport, have required that values be expressed by units other than rate (i.e., mL/min or mL/min/kg). Recent advances in ultrasound technology that include improved imaging and flow velocity data acquisition have given investigators the tools to accurately assess *volume* flow. Although Doppler velocimetry has been a very useful tool in assessing and managing the fetus with IUGR by obtaining information on blood flow resistance,[44–46] determination of oxygenation and nutrient delivery is dictated by *volume* blood flow and not velocimetry. A study in 1999 demonstrated that umbilical venous flow measurements (mL/min) can be obtained in human fetuses with accuracy and precision, and that the examination can be completed on average in less than 5 min.[47] This technique involves the combined use of real-time ultrasound, color Doppler, and pulsed-wave Doppler velocimetry to obtain the necessary measurements for calculation of umbilical vein flow from the following formula:

$$\text{Umbilical vein flow (mL/min)} = \text{vessel cross-sectional area } (\pi r^2) \times \text{mean velocity (cm/s)} \times 60\,\text{s} \quad (4.1)$$

Figures 4.6 and 4.7 show the images required for accurately calculating the umbilical vein flow. Important technical aspects include maximal magnification of the vessel for diameter measurement and vertical orientation of the vessel for acquisition of the Doppler flow velocity waveform. This method of calculating blood flow has been validated in a sheep model in which a well-established technique of measuring flow (steady-state diffusion technique) confirmed the accuracy of

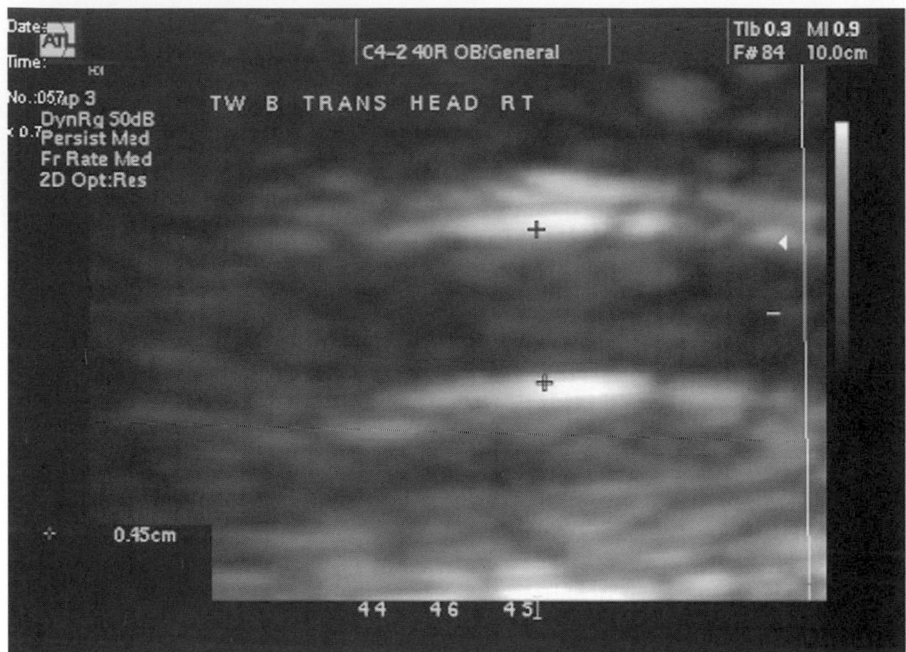

Figure 4.6 Magnified longitudinal image of the umbilical vein for accurate placement of calipers to measure the diameter of the vein from which the radius can be obtained.

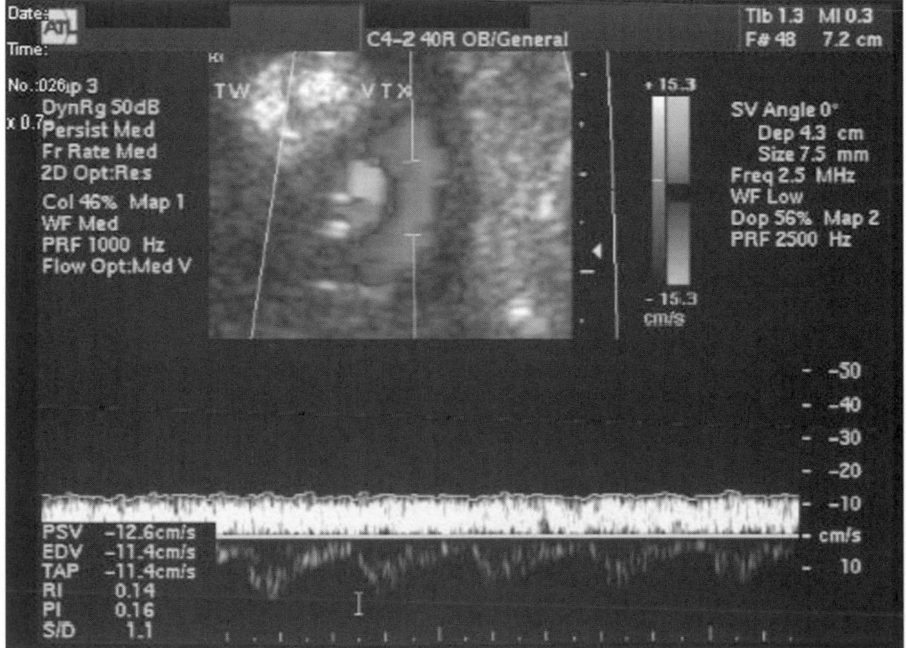

Figure 4.7 Ultrasound and Doppler images depicting the vertically oriented umbilical vein image with color Doppler, and the 0° angle of insonation of the Doppler sample volume for obtaining the Doppler flow velocity waveform.

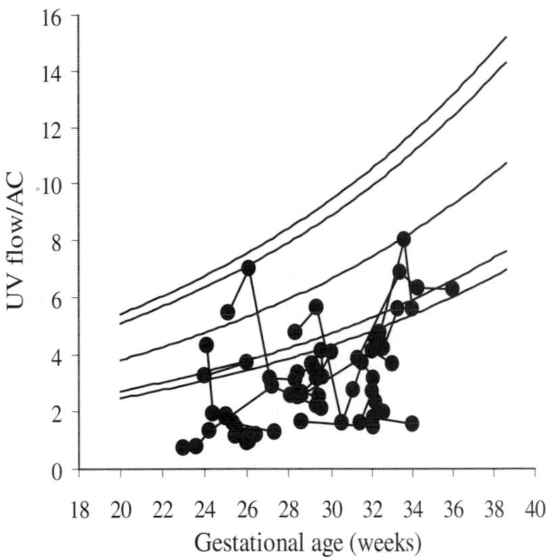

Figure 4.8 Graph showing the reduction of umbilical vein flow in growth-restricted fetuses compared with control subjects across gestation.[13]

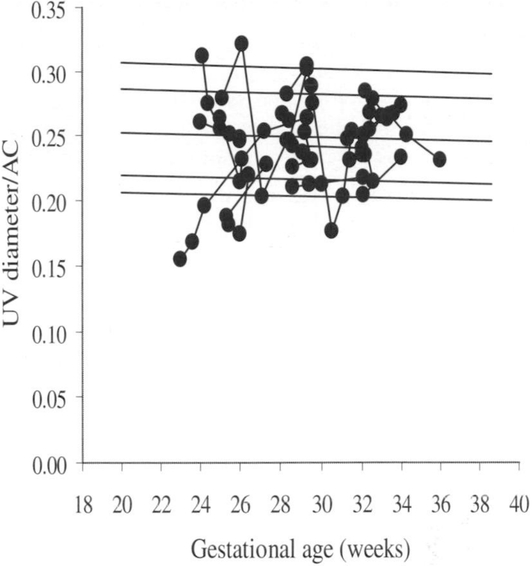

Figure 4.9 Graph demonstrating that there was no difference in umbilical vein diameter adjusted for fetal weight among fetuses with IUGR compared with control subjects.[13]

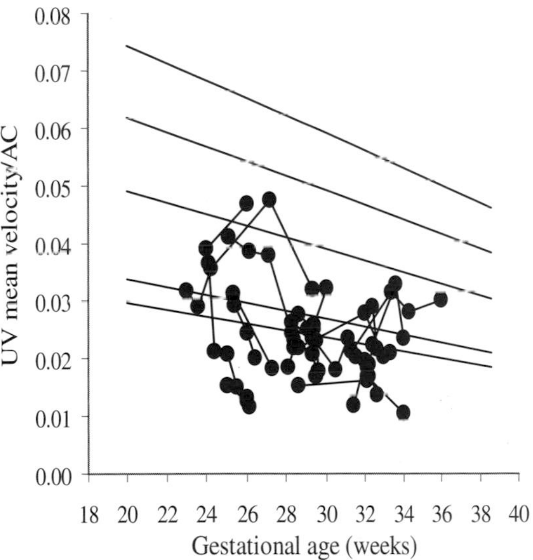

Figure 4.10 Graph demonstrating a reduction in umbilical vein blood velocity adjusted for fetal weight among fetuses with IUGR compared with control subjects.[13]

measuring blood flow with ultrasound.[48] Using this ultrasound technique, absolute umbilical vein volume flow has been shown to be reduced in fetuses with IUGR compared with those growing normally (Fig. 4.8).[13] Furthermore, when adjusted for estimated fetal weight, the reduction in blood flow volume was found to be secondary to a reduction in the velocity of blood and not to a reduction in the diameter of the umbilical vein (Figs 4.9 and 4.10). This study also showed that volume blood flow was reduced by mid-gestation in these fetuses with IUGR. This finding is important from a developmental point of view because if blood flow on a per kilogram basis is reduced by mid-gestation then this suggests that there are factors affecting normal uteroplacental vascularization and angiogenesis (branching). Thus, abnormal placental development and reduction in circulating blood volume at some point in gestation will result in insufficient nutrient delivery and aberrant fetal growth. The ability to calculate volume blood flow will provide the opportunity to better understand nutrient flux across the human placenta. It is anticipated that, with the knowledge accumulated from these types of studies, fetuses with IUGR could potentially be treated in the antepartum period and at the appropriate time.

Key points

1 The oxygen exchange across the human placenta is characterized by the umbilical vein Po_2 following the uterine venous Po_2 but at a somewhat lower level.

2 The transport of oxygen to the fetus is a function of both uterine and umbilical blood flow as well as placental permeability to oxygen.

3 Uterine blood flow can decrease significantly before a critical flow is reached at which oxygen delivery to the baby decreases.

4 Metabolism by the placenta takes place at a very high rate, as indicated by its high oxygen and glucose consumption.

5 There is a persistent maternal–fetal glucose concentration difference that is maintained over a very wide range of maternal glucose concentrations.

6 This gradient is increased in cases of fetuses with intrauterine growth retardation (IUGR).

7 Fetal growth in the human is characterized by a very long gestation period and by the accretion of a large mass of white fat, which accumulates in the last third of gestation.

8 The net umbilical uptake of nutrients represents the dietary supply to the fetus.

9 There is extensive interconversion of nutrients within the placenta; glucose, lactate, and amino acids represent the major sources of carbon and nitrogen for the fetal diet.

10 There is a net umbilical uptake of all of the essential amino acids from the maternal circulation into the fetal circulation.

11 The nonessential amino acids do not all show a significant transport from the maternal circulation to the fetus. There are some nonessential amino acids, e.g., glutamate and aspartate, which are taken up from the fetal circulation into the placenta.

12 It is important to understand the differences between measuring velocity profiles and measuring the actual blood flow, which can now be undertaken for the umbilical circulation and the uterine circulation. In normal pregnancy, umbilical blood flow, expressed per kilogram of fetal weight, decreases as pregnancy advances.

13 Umbilical blood flow per kilogram, as well as absolute flow in millimeters per minute, are both significantly reduced in fetuses with IUGR compared with normal fetuses.

14 Placental growth is characterized by a much more rapid growth rate than fetal growth in early pregnancy.

15 In late pregnancy, the growth rate of the human placenta slows markedly but its maturation continues.

16 There continues to be an exponential increase in surface area of the placenta during late gestation.

17 The uptake of oxygen, glucose, and amino acids in the fetal circulation has been shown to be increased when maternal concentration is increased.

18 Fetal lactic acid concentrations are increased in association with velocimetry changes in fetuses with IUGR.

19 Uterine venous Po_2 is an important determinant of umbilical venous Po_2.

20 Both the maternal–fetal Po_2 gradient and the glucose gradient are increased in IUGR pregnancies.

References

1 Wilkening RB, Meschia G. Current topic: comparative physiology of placental oxygen transport. *Placenta* 1992;13:1–15.

2 Battaglia FC, Meschia G, Makowski EL, et al. The effect of maternal oxygen inhalation upon fetal oxygenation. *J Clin Invest* 1968;47:548–555.

3 Soothill PW, Nicolaides KH, Bilardo CM, et al. Relation of fetal hypoxia in growth retardation to mean blood velocity in the fetal aorta. *Lancet* 1986;2:1118–1120.

4 Battaglia FC, Meschia G. An introduction to fetal physiology. Orlando, FL: Academic Press Inc., 1986.

5 Pardi G, Cetin I, Marconi AM, et al. The venous drainage of the human uterus: respiratory gas studies in normal and fetal growth retarded pregnancies. *Am J Obstet Gynecol* 1992;166: 699–706.

6 Soothill PW, Nicolaides KH, Rodeck CH, et al. Blood gases and acid-base status of the human second-trimester fetus. *Obstet Gynecol* 1986;68:173–176.

7 Bozzetti P, Buscaglia M, Cetin I, et al. Respiratory gases, acid-base balance and lactate concentrations in the mid-term human fetus. *Biol Neonate* 1987;51:188–197.

8 Bell AW, Kennaugh JM, Battaglia FC, et al. Metabolic and circulatory studies of fetal lamb at mid gestation. *Am J Physiol* 1986;250:E538–E544.

9 Soothill PW, Nicolaides KH, Rodeck CH, et al. Relationship of fetal hemoglobin and oxygen content to lactate concentration in Rh isoimmunized pregnancies. *Obstet Gynecol* 1987;69:268–270.

10 Ferrazzi E, Pardi G, Buscaglia M, et al. The correlation of biochemical monitoring versus umbilical flow velocity measurements of the human fetus. *Am J Obstet Gynecol* 1988;159:1081–1097.

11 Gill RW, Kossoff G, Warren PS, et al. Umbilical venous flow in normal and complicated pregnancy. *Ultrasound Med Biol* 1984; 10:349–363.

12 Jouppila P, Kirkinem P. Umbilical vein blood flow in the human fetus in cases of maternal and fetal anemia and uterine bleeding. *Ultrasound Med Biol* 1984;10:365–370.

13 Rigano S, Bozzo M, Ferrazzi E, et al. Early and persistent reduction in umbilical vein blood flow in the growth-restricted

fetus: a longitudinal study. *Am J Obstet Gynecol* 2001;185: 834–838.

14 Wilkening RB, Meschia G. Fetal oxygen uptake, oxygenation, and acid-base balance as a function of uterine blood flow. *Am J Physiol* 1983;244:H749–H755.

15 Wilkening RB, Meschia G. Effect of umbilical blood flow on transplacental diffusion of ethanol and oxygen. *Am J Physiol* 1989;256:H813–H820.

16 Myatt L, Eis ALW, Brockman DE, et al. Endothelial nitric oxide synthase in placental villous tissue from normal, pre-eclamptic and intrauterine growth restricted pregnancies. *Hum Reprod* 1997; 12:167–172.

17 Myatt L, Rosenfield RB, Eis ALW, et al. Nitrotyrosine residues in placenta – evidence of peroxynitrite formation and action. *Hypertension* 1996;28:488–493.

18 Lyall F, Greer IA, Young A, et al. Nitric oxide concentrations are increased in the feto-placental circulation in intrauterine growth restriction. *Placenta* 1996;17:165–168.

19 Diiulio JL, Gude NM, King RG, et al. Human placental and fetal membrane nitric oxide synthase activity before, during and after labour at term. *Reprod Fertil Dev* 1996;7:1505–1508.

20 King RG, Gude NM, Diiulio JL, et al. Regulation of human placental fetal vessel tone – role of nitric oxide. *Reprod Fertil Dev* 1996;7:1407–1411.

21 Boccardo P, Soregaroli M, Aiello S, et al. Systemic and fetal–maternal nitric oxide synthesis in normal pregnancy and pre-eclampsia. *Br J Obstet Gynaecol* 1996;103:879–886.

22 Schonfelder G, John M, Hopp H, et al. Expression of inducible nitric oxide synthase in placenta of women with gestational diabetes. *FASEB J* 1996;10:777–784.

23 Battaglia FC, Makowski EL, Meschia G. Physiologic study of the uterine venous drainage of the pregnant rhesus monkey. *Yale J Biol Med* 1970;42:218–228.

24 Meschia G, Battaglia FC, Hay WW, et al. Utilization of substrates by the ovine placenta in vivo. *Fed Proc* 1980;39:245–249.

25 Marconi AM, Paolini C, Cetin I, et al. The impact of gestational age and of intrauterine growth upon the maternal–fetal glucose concentrations difference. *Obstet Gynecol* 1996;87:937–942.

26 Marconi AM, Davoli E, Cetin I, et al. The impact of conceptus mass upon glucose disposal rate in pregnant women. *Am J Physiol* 1993;27:E514–E518.

27 Marconi A, Battaglia FC, Meschia G, et al. A comparison of amino acid arteriovenous differences across the placenta and liver in the fetal lamb. *Am J Physiol* 1989;257:E909–E915.

28 Lemons JA, Adcock EW, III, Jones MD, Jr, et al. Umbilical uptake of amino acids in the unstressed fetal lamb. *J Clin Invest* 1976; 58:1428–1434.

29 Lemons JA, Schreiner RL. Metabolic balance of the ovine fetus during the fed and fasted states. *Ann Nutr Metab* 1984;28: 268–280.

30 Lemons JA, Schreiner RL. Amino acid metabolism in the ovine fetus. *Am J Physiol* 1983;244:E459–E466.

31 Yudilevich DL, Sweiry JH. Transport of amino acids in the placenta. *Biochim Biophys Acta* 1985;822:169–201.

32 Regnault TRH, de Vrijer B, Battaglia FC. Transport and metabolism of amino acids in placenta. *Endocrine* 2002;19:23–41.

33 Baur R. Morphometry of the placental exchange area. Advances in anatomy, embryology and cell biology. Berlin: Springer-Verlag, 1977.

34 Kulhanek JF, Meschia G, Makowski EL, et al. Changes in DNA content and urea permeability of the sheep placenta. *Am J Physiol* 1974;226:1257–1263.

35 Sparks JW, Girard J, Battaglia FC. An estimate of the caloric requirements of the human fetus. *Biol Neonate* 1980;38:113–119.

36 Clandinin MT, Chappell JE, Heim T, et al. Fatty acid utilization in perinatal de novo synthesis of tissues. *Early Hum Dev* 1981; 5:355–366.

37 Clandinin MT, Chappell JE, Heim T, et al. Fatty acid accretion in fetal and neonatal liver: implications for fatty acid requirements. *Early Hum Dev* 1981;5:7–14.

38 Battaglia FC, Meschia G. Fetal nutrition. *Annu Rev Nutr* 1988;8:43–61.

39 Hayashi S, Sanada K, Sagama N, et al. Umbilical vein–artery differences of plasma amino acids in the last trimester of human pregnancy. *Biol Neonate* 1978;34:11–18.

40 Moores RR, Jr, Vaughn PR, Battaglia FC, et al. Glutamate metabolism in the fetus and placenta of late gestation sheep. *Am J Physiol* 1994;267:R89–R96.

41 Gresham EL, Simons PS, Battaglia FC. Maternal–fetal urea concentration difference in man: metabolic significance. *J Pediatr* 1971;79:809–811.

42 Kennaugh JM, Bell AW, Meschia G, et al. Ontogenetic changes in protein synthesis rate and leucine oxidation rate during fetal life. *Pediatr Res* 1987;22:688–692.

43 Warshaw JB. Fatty acid metabolism during development. *Semin Perinatol* 1979;3:131–139.

44 Karlesdrop VHM, van Vugt JMG, van Geijn HP, et al. Clinical significance of absent or reversed end diastolic velocity waveforms in umbilical artery. *Lancet* 1994;344:1664–1668.

45 Pardi G, Cetin I, Marconi AM, et al. Diagnostic value of blood sampling in fetuses with growth retardation. *N Engl J Med* 1993;328:692–696.

46 Ferrazzi E, Bozzo M, Rigano S, et al. Temporal sequence of abnormal Doppler changes in the peripheral and central circulatory systems of the severely growth restricted fetuses. *Ultrasound Obstet Gynecol* 2002;19:140–146.

47 Barbera A, Galan HL, Ferrazzi E et al. Relationship of umbilical vein blood flow to growth parameters in the human fetus. *Am J Obstet Gynecol* 1999;181:174–179.

48 Galan HL, Jozwik M, Rigano S, et al. Umbilical vein blood flow determination in the ovine fetus: Comparison of Doppler ultrasonographic and steady-state diffusion techniques. *Am J Obstet Gynecol* 1999;181:1149–1153.

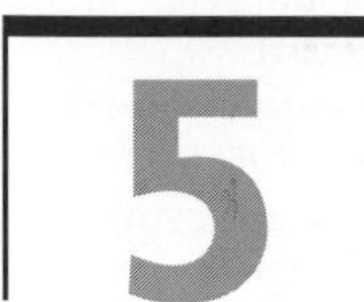

Endocrinology of pregnancy and the placenta

Alan DeCherney, Jessica Spencer, Tim Chard, and Karen A. Hutchinson

The synthesis and role of hormones in pregnancy is a unique interplay between the three major compartments of pregnancy: the fetus, the placenta, and the mother. Some hormones are produced in the nonpregnant state and upregulated in pregnancy (quantitative hormones), whereas others are largely unique to the pregnant state (qualitative hormones). This chapter will review each of these compartments and their respective hormone products by axis, emphasizing their function and the consequences of pathological change.

The corpus luteum

The corpus luteum forms from the ovulated follicle and, in the absence of pregnancy, undergoes luteolysis at the onset of menses. Maximal activity is achieved 1 week after the luteinizing hormone (LH) surge and the normal lifespan is 14 days. The corpus luteum in early pregnancy synthesizes crucial hormones until the fetoplacental unit can take over. These include progesterone, estradiol, inhibin A, relaxin, and vascular endothelial growth factor (VEGF), all of which promote the growth and development of the embryo, inhibit spontaneous uterine activity, and suppress further folliculogenesis. The corpus luteum can also produce metalloproteases and other cytolytic enzymes that initiate luteolysis. Human chorionic gonadotropin (hCG), which is secreted by the trophoblast, inhibits this cascade and is therefore essential for rescuing the corpus luteum. This is discussed in more detail at the end of the chapter.

Estrone, estradiol, and estriol

These estrogen molecules share the same basic 18-carbon estrone nucleus and differ only in the number and arrangement of hydroxyl groups as depicted in Figure 5.1. All three estrogens increase dramatically in pregnancy. Estrone (E_1) is a precursor to estradiol (E_2) and is the predominant estrogen in menopause.

E_2 is the predominant estrogen secreted by the ovary. The endometrium contains receptors for both E_2 and progesterone,[1] creating a secretory environment that permits embryonic implantation and development.[2]

Estriol (E_3) is almost exclusively produced in pregnancy by the placenta, with its precursor dehydroepiandrosterone sulfate (DHEAS), produced in the fetal and maternal adrenal glands. It is believed to be the primary estrogen responsible for increased uterine blood flow during pregnancy.[3] It is excreted rapidly and may provide an important route of elimination for the estrogen precursors of pregnancy. The maternal system tolerates higher levels of E_3 than more potent compounds.

Progesterone

Progestins differ in the number and arrangement of their hydroxyl groups as shown in Figure 5.2. Progesterone is clearly the more biologically active progestin.

The effects of progesterone begin early in pregnancy. The pre-implantation corona cells of the conceptus secrete progesterone and E_2 before implantation.[4,5] En route to the uterus, the conceptus secretes progesterone, which is believed to relax uterotubal musculature. The site where ova and sperm meet, in the distal one-third of the fallopian tube, contains many progesterone receptors. It is possible that E_2 secreted by the conceptus may balance the effects of progesterone to maintain an optimal level of tubal motility and tone.[5,6]

At the time of implantation, progesterone inhibits T lymphocyte-mediated tissue rejection. Human chorionic gonadotropin and decidual cortisol are also involved in this process.[7] This inhibition of rejection may well offer immunological protection to the implanted conceptus and evolving placenta. In addition, progesterone decreases uterine blood flow. Progesterone and estrogens thus appear to balance one another in the maintenance of optimal blood flow to the implantation site.[8,9]

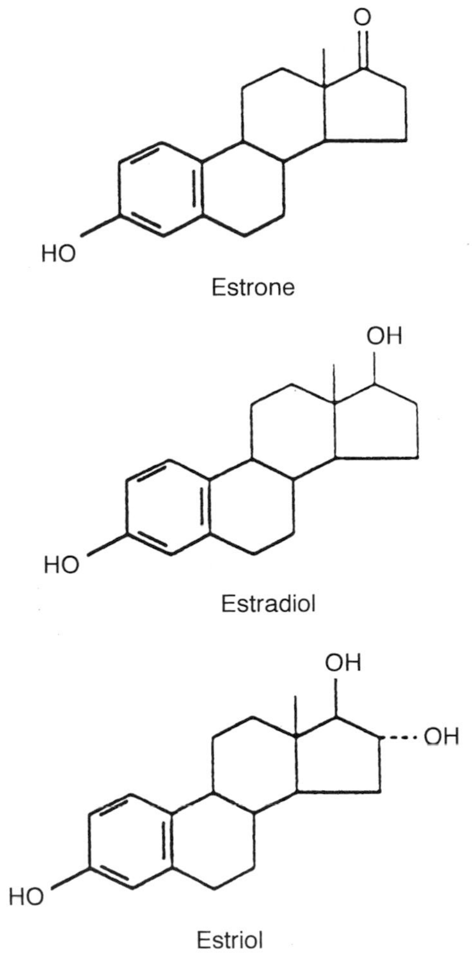

Estrone

Estradiol

Estriol

Figure 5.1 Molecular structures of estrogens. The basic 18-carbon estrane nucleus is shared by estrone, estradiol, and estriol. Each estrogen is different as a result of the arrangement of hydroxyl groups.

The fetal allograft and maternal immune tolerance

Several changes occur in the maternal immune system and the decidual immunological environment to allow the conceptus to coexist with the mother. Normal pregnancy is characterized by a type 1 to type 2 T helper (Th1 to Th2) cytokine deviation in the mother. Pathologically, this change is not seen in preeclampsia.[10] Recurrent abortion and endometriosis, both major causes of infertility, have also been linked to a Th1 cytokine deviation (tumor necrosis factor alpha, TNF-α, being the main factor).[11] Several studies have also demonstrated significant changes in the levels of peripheral maternal $CD4^+$ and $CD8^+$ cells during pregnancy. Deletion of alloreactive B cells, which are detectable in early pregnancy and which rise with each subsequent gestation, may also occur.[12]

The physical barrier which develops after implantation is composed of the outer syncytiotrophoblast layer (which is in direct contact with maternal blood) and an inner cytotrophoblast layer. This barrier is not impermeable; fetal DNA has been isolated from maternal blood[13] and has even been detected in women 27 years after giving birth.[14] On the fetal side of the barrier, major histocompatibility complex I (MHC-

Progesterone

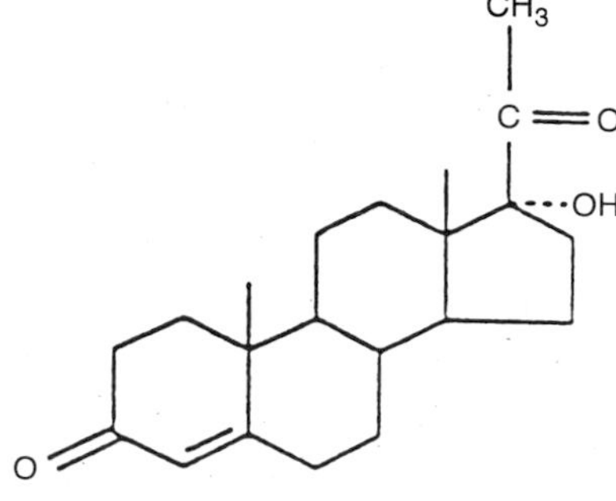

Figure 5.2 Molecular structure of progestogens. The basic 21-carbon pregnene structure is shared by progesterone and 17α-hydroxyprogesterone. These compounds differ in the number and arrangements of the hydroxyl groups.

I) is replaced by human leukocyte antigen (HLA)-G and -E, which are much less polymorphic, allowing the fetal cells to "hide" from maternal cytotoxic T lymphocytes. Interestingly, maternal serum and placental HLA-G expression appears to be reduced in preeclampsia according to one small study.[15]

Several studies have also implicated the Fas–FasL pathway, critical in apoptosis, as playing an integral role in deleting alloreactive T cells. Fetal cells and decidua express high levels of Fas ligand, which prevents the infiltration of cytotoxic T lymphocytes.[12]

Additionally, complement regulation at the maternal–fetal interface helps prevent complement-mediated cellular lysis. When antibodies exist in very high levels, however, such as in antiphospholipid antibody syndrome, fetal loss may occur.

The recently implicated uterine natural killer (NK) cells appear to be the dominant lymphocyte in the decidua and are concentrated most highly around the invading trophoblast. Natural killer cells seem to play a pivotal role in the acceptance of trophoblast invasion.[16] Indeed, mice with deficient NK cells have been shown to have higher levels of fetal loss than their wild-type equivalent. Furthermore, rescuing their NK population with a bone marrow transplantation decreases the frequency of fetal loss.[17]

All of these mechanisms represent a delicate balance in cytokines, lymphocyte proliferation and apoptosis, and receptor expression, which ultimately allows the immunotolerance of the fetal allograft.

Maternal cardiovascular adaptation to pregnancy

The average blood volume in pregnant women increases by approximately 40%, peaking at 32 weeks. In contrast, the absolute red blood cell count increases by only 33%, creating a physiological anemia. This cardiovascular metamorphosis provides enough blood for the rapidly enlarging uterus, placenta, and fetus. It also safeguards the mother from blood loss in delivery, which averages 500 mL.

Angiotensin II resistance occurs in normal pregnancy causing a mild hyponatremia with a lower plasma osmolality. Several mediators including progesterone, prostaglandins, and nitric oxide also cause vasodilation. This increase in volume brings about a decrease in peripheral vascular resistance and maternal blood pressure lowers by approximately 10–20 mmHg. In contrast, maternal heart rate will increase by approximately 25%.

This characteristic volume expansion and vasodilation is pathologic in preeclampsia, when arteriolar constriction is a key feature. Leaking capillaries lead to a depletion of intravascular volume and fluid collection in interstitial spaces (e.g., liver and brain edema). Furthermore, endothelial dysfunction is characterized by higher levels of thromboxane A_2, which increases platelet activation. Corticotropin-releasing factor and neurokinin B are additional endocrine factors that may perpetuate platelet dysfunction.[18,19]

Nutrition and the fetus

Glucose is the primary fuel of fetal growth and its turnover in a neonate is twice that of a normal adult. The fetal glucose level is usually 10–20 mg/mL lower than in its mother, because glucose crosses the placenta by carrier-mediated facilitated diffusion. Once inside the fetus, glucose serves as a precursor for fat and glycogen. In contrast, maternal insulin and glucagon are unable to cross the placenta and are instead produced by the fetus itself. Amino acids are also actively transported by the placenta and can stimulate fetal insulin secretion. Additionally, free fatty acids cross the placenta and are esterified in the fetal liver into very low-density lipoprotein (VLDL).

This enormous maternal glucose drain favors an insulin-resistant environment that has been attributed previously to the increase in human placental lactogen (hPL) and growth hormone, progesterone, cortisol, and prolactin. Newer studies, however, have implicated TNF-α and leptin and, most recently, the so-called resistin protein, which may be the missing link between obesity and insulin resistance. Its role in pregnancy, however, has yet to be established.[20]

Obesity is now a problem that affects over 40% of women of childbearing age. Besides its known detrimental effect on fertility (via anovulation) and the increase in miscarriage rates, obesity significantly increases a pregnant woman's chances of developing gestational diabetes and hypertensive disorders such as preeclampsia. This, in turn, increases Cesarean section rates and overall morbidity in obese women.[21]

Hypothalamic and pituitary development in the fetus

The earliest embryonic development of the brain can be identified by day 22 after conception, and the primitive diencephalon by day 35. Within the ventral portion of the diencephalon (which later develops into the hypothalamus), primitive fiber tracts and neuroblasts can be observed. By gestational day 42, the hypothalamus has coalesced beneath the third ventricle and already contains thyroid releasing factor (TRF).

Much of what we know about the development of the fetal endocrine system comes from a review by Kaplan and coauthors.[22] All of the hypothalamic nuclei are differentiated by 14 weeks' gestation and the continuity of the primary and secondary plexus of the portal system is finally completed by gestational weeks 19–21.

The pituitary gland is formed at about this time and develops from the outpocketing of oral ectoderm from the floor of the diencephalon (Rathke's pouch), which gives rise to the adenohypophysis anteriorly, and neuroectoderm from the ventral diencephalon posteriorly. Capillaries appear within the mesenchymal tissue adjoining Rathke's pouch and the diencephalon by 9 weeks' gestation. Rapid vascularization begins with the development of the primary plexus of the portal system at approximately 100 days. The anterior portion of the pituitary will differentiate into five cellular subtypes: thyrotrophs, corticotrophs, somatotrophs, gonadotrophs, and lactotrophs. The posterior pituitary will eventually produce oxytocin (Chapter 66) and vasopressin (Chapter 35), which is not discussed in this chapter. Many of the specific genes responsible for cellular differentiation in the pituitary have been elucidated and seem to be controlled by local signals that are derived from adjacent tissues.[23]

Pituitary and hypothalamic-like peptides in the placenta

Pituitary-like hormones [adrenocorticotropic hormone (ACTH), hCG, human chorionic somatomammotropin (hCS), and human chorionic thyrotropin (hCT)] have been histochemically localized to the syncytiotrophoblast.[24–26] Hypothalamic-like hormones [corticotropin-releasing hormone (CRH), gonadotropin-releasing hormone (GnRH), somatotropin-release inhibiting factor, and thyrotropin-releasing hormone (TRH)] have been similarly localized to the cytotrophoblastic layer.[27–30] It would appear that there is a paracrine analog within these tissues that is similar to the hypothalamic–pituitary axis. The end organ feedback within this system is not exclusively inhibitory (see below). Indeed, selective placental proteins may well have a positive feedback relationship with fetal steroids.

The endocrine axes of the fetus and placenta

GnRH, FSH and LH, and the gonads

Immunoreactive GnRH is present in the fetal hypothalamus by 10 weeks. Follicle-stimulating hormone (FSH) and LH secretion first begin at 9–10 weeks' gestation and peak at about 20–22 weeks. Unlike GnRH, which is secreted in equal concentration in the male and female fetus, the female pituitary appears to contain more FSH and LH than the male gland.[22] Gonadotrope activity then gradually declines during late gestation, remaining dormant until puberty. As demonstrated in fetal sheep, this is likely due to decreased secretion of GnRH from the fetal hypothalamus as the gonadaotropes are unstimulated, not inactive.[31]

At approximately 6 weeks' gestation, the structure of the fetal testes can be recognized including prominent interstitial (Leydig) cells. These cells produce testosterone, which is critical for male internal secondary sexual development. In contrast, dihydroxytestosterone (DHT), a reduced metabolite of testosterone formed in certain androgen target tissues by 5α-reductase, is the trophic hormone for the external genitalia. Testosterone also stimulates the production of two proteins within the adjacent Sertoli cells of the testes: müllerian-inhibiting substance (MIS) and androgen-binding protein. The former causes inhibition of müllerian duct development; the latter binds testosterone and possibly DHT within the wolffian duct system and may be involved in the transduction of androgens into their target tissues. Maximal hCG production by the placenta coincides with the time of greatest biosynthetic activity by the interstitial cells, suggesting that these events are interrelated.[32–34]

The fetal ovary can be histologically recognized by gestational week 10. The female gonad lacks the impressive biosynthetic capacity of the testis at this point *in utero*. *In vitro* studies have demonstrated that fetal ovarian tissue has the capacity to cleave pregnenolone sulfate and further metabolize pregnenolone to the C-19 steroids dehydroepiandrosterone and androstenedione. However, ovarian production of free progesterone, testosterone, or estrogens has not been documented.[35]

Placental GnRH, hCG, and inhibin

Placental GnRH is similar in structure to the hypothalamic decapeptide of the same name. Its activity has been localized to the cytotrophoblastic cells along the outer surface layer of the syncytiotrophoblast.[36] The structure and additional functions of hCG are described below (see section on human chorionic gonadotropin). Inhibin is a heterodimeric glycoprotein with α- and β-subunits and its immunoreactivity has been localized to the cytotrophoblast layer.

Syncytiotrophoblastic GnRH activity peaks at approximately 8 weeks' gestation and decreases with advancing fetal age. These changes in GnRH activity parallel those seen in placental hCG.[36] Information regarding inhibin variation during pregnancy is not available.

It is clear that placental GnRH stimulates the release of hCG through a dose-dependent paracrine mechanism.[37] *In vitro* work with first-trimester placentas has shown that GnRH has little stimulatory effect on hCG production when the latter is close to maximum.[36] However, in midtrimester, GnRH markedly increases hCG release. Not surprisingly, this effect diminishes in the term placenta. A complete intraplacental regulatory system can be hypothesized whereby cytotrophoblastic GnRH stimulates the production of syncytiotrophoblastic hCG, which, in turn, influences steroidogenesis. It has been postulated that placental inhibin functions also go through a paracrine mechanism to inhibit GnRH release and thereby hCG release.

TRH, TSH, and the thyroid

Immunoreactive TRH has been detected in significant levels in the fetal hypothalamus by 10 weeks. As noted with GnRH, there is not an appreciable correlation between gestational age or sex. Secretion of thyroid-stimulating hormone (TSH) *in utero* is regulated by both hypothalamic TRH and the intact pituitary–thyroid feedback system (mature by mid-gestation).

The thyroid gland first appears at 16–17 days of gestation and the capacity of the developing follicular cells to produce thyroglobulin is established by day 29. However, the development necessary to concentrate iodide into synthesized thyroxine (T_4) is not operational until the 11th week.[38] Furthermore, pituitary thyrotropes are not detectable until approximately 13 weeks' gestation. Once the thyrotropes mature, iodine uptake and the synthesis of iodothyronines in the thyroid commences.

Interestingly, fetal thyroid function is not affected to any significant degree by the limited transplacental passage of TSH and iodothyronines. Indeed, the human placenta appears to contain a highly active 5-monodeiodinase that converts T_4 to the inert iodothyronine, reverse triiodothyronine (reverse T_3).[39]

The metabolism of T_4 *in utero* differs dramatically from the situation found in adults. Not only are production and degradation rates greater in the fetus (on the basis of unit body mass), but also the specific enzymatic pathway by which T_4 is metabolized favors the formation of the inert, reverse T_3, at the expense of the metabolically active product generally found in adults, T_3.

Thyroxine-binding globulin (TBG) can be detected in serum by the 10th gestational week, progressively increasing in concentration to term. The second- and third-trimester increase in serum T_4 concentration reflects not only this increase in TBG, but also the greater secretory capacity of the fetal thyroid gland under the influence of the maturing hypothalamic–hypophyseal portal system (Fig. 5.3).[40]

Somatic development *in utero* is not a phenomenon that is dependent on thyroid hormones. However, thyroid hormones do appear to be necessary for late-phase skeletal maturation and late prenatal pulmonary development, as well as the normal development of the brain and intellectual function.[38]

Human chorionic thyrotropin

TRH has been detected in the cytotrophoblast layer of the placenta and is then called human chorionic thyrotropin (hCT). However, this molecule appears to be chromatographically different from synthetic TRH, which is a tripeptide.[41] The structure of hCT is similar to pituitary TSH α-subunits, but it has negligible thyrotrophic activity[32] and its role is unclear.

The excessive amount of thyroid-stimulating activity found in neoplastic trophoblast tissue is not secondary to an hCT effect. Indeed, studies in molar pregnancy have failed to identify hCT.[32] The hyperstimulation of thyroid tissue that occurs in some women with molar pregnancy is attributed to the high circulating concentration of hCG which has 1/4000th of the activity of TSH.[42]

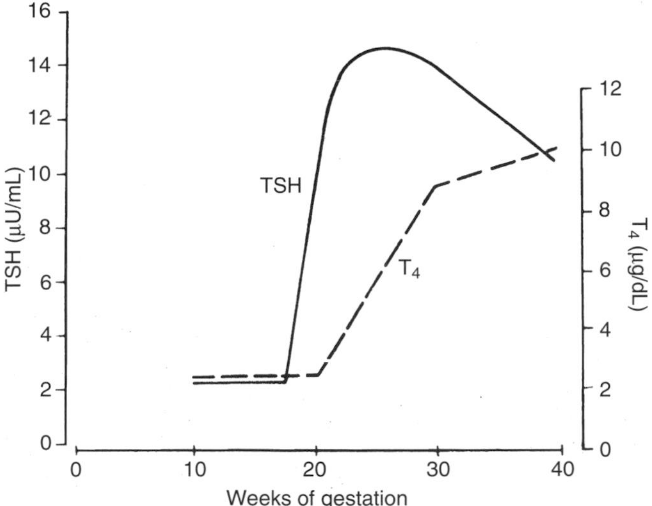

Figure 5.3 Patterns of maturation of serum thyroid-stimulating hormone (*TSH*) and thyroxin (*T_4*) concentrations in the human fetus. (From Fisher DA, Klein AH. Thyroid development and disorders of thyroid function in the newborn. *N Engl J Med* 1981;304:702, with permission.)

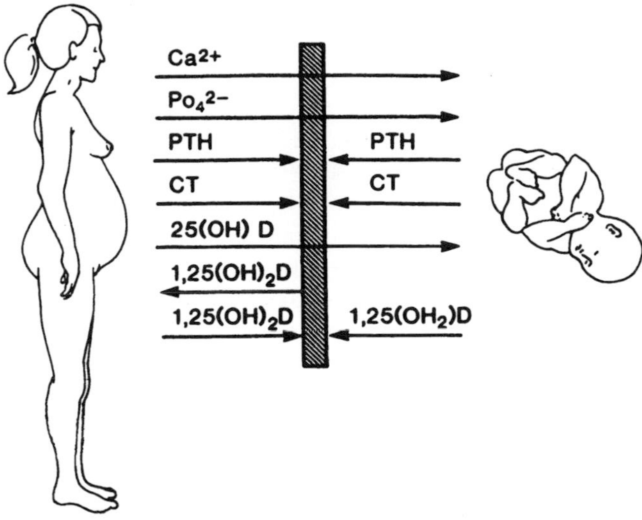

Figure 5.4 Schematic representation of transplacental transport of calcium (*Ca^{2+}*), phosphorus (*PO_4^{-1}*), parathyroid hormone (*PTH*), calcitonin (*CT*), and mono- and dihydroxyvitamin D (*25(OH)D* and *$1,25(OH)_2D$* respectively). (From Fuchs F, Klopper A, eds. *Endocrinology of pregnancy*. Philadelphia: Harper & Row, 1983:186, with permission.)

The parathyroid and calcium homeostasis

Fetal parathyroid hormone (PTH) is detected between the tenth and thirteenth gestational weeks (Fig. 5.4). Parathyroid function, however, remains suppressed throughout most of pregnancy owing to the relatively hypercalcemic state of the fetus (secondary to the considerable placental transport of calcium, critical for bone formation). Calcitonin levels are elevated, which enhances bone development.

At term, fetal 1,25-dihydroxyvitamin D levels are considerably below maternal levels, supporting the concept that 1,25-dihydroxyvitamin D does not cross the placenta, although 25-hydroxyvitamin D probably does cross. Direct comparisons of serum concentrations of vitamin D in mother and fetus are complicated by the fact that there are estrogen-induced changes in vitamin D-binding protein. The fetal kidney can hydroxylate 25-hydroxyvitamin D although the placenta can synthesize 1,25-dihydroxyvitamin D directly. Excellent reviews of vitamin D and its metabolism have been published.[43–45]

Prolactin

Immunoreactive prolactin is present in the pituitary gland in small but measurable amounts early in gestation. However, in both males and females, the concentration increases rapidly between 20 and 30 weeks' gestation and term. Several authors have proposed that the major modulating force behind the late-trimester increase in fetal prolactin is placenta-derived estrogens. It is also possible that, developmentally, the pituitary is functionally able to respond to tropic agents including TRF after 20 weeks' gestation.

Fetal prolactin may play a role in the regulation of normal fetal osmolality.[46] Prolactin receptors are expressed in a range of fetal tissues as early as the seventh gestational week and may play a role in bone, adrenal gland, lung, brain, and pancreatic β-cell development and function.[47] In fact, cord blood from preterm infants who develop respiratory distress syndrome has been shown to have lower mean prolactin levels.[48,49]

GH-RH, GH, and somatostatin

The presence of growth hormone-releasing hormone (GH-RH) late in gestation is suggested by the elevated levels of plasma growth hormone (GH) in premature neonates.[22] However, this peptide has yet to be identified in fetal tissues.

By 7–9 weeks' gestation, GH is present in the fetal pituitary. "Little" or monomeric GH predominates in the fetal pituitary with only a small amount of "big" GH present. This pattern is similar to that observed in adults.[22] Because GH does not cross the placenta, circulating GH is entirely of pituitary origin. Peak concentrations of immunoreactive GH occur between 25 and 30 weeks' gestation, followed by a decrease in the third trimester. This coincides with maturation of hypothalamic neuroregulation (Fig. 5.5). The reader is referred to an excellent review by Gluckman and coauthors.[46]

The exact role of GH in development is unknown; however, many fetal tissues express GH receptors and GH stimulates the synthesis of insulin-like growth factors (IGF-1 and -2). Fetal IGF-1 and its binding protein seem to be altered in chronic hypoxemia and malnutrition, and IGF-2 may be closely related to steroid hormone biosynthesis.[50]

Growth hormone release-inhibiting hormone (also known as somatostatin) more than triples from 10 to 20 weeks' gestation.[22] Studies have identified somatostatin receptors as early as 16 weeks' gestation in the hypothalamus, pituitary, and central nervous system.[51] It has been suggested that the pattern of GH secretion in the fetus reflects maturational changes in the secretion of GH-RH and somatostatin.[46]

Somatomedin

Somatomedin activity in umbilical cord blood increases during gestation from 24 weeks to term, although somatomedin activity can be detected in fetal sera by 14 weeks.[46] A growth-promoting function for somatomedin in the fetus is supported indirectly by the observations that cord somatomedin concentrations correlate directly with body weight,[52,53] and infants with intrauterine growth retardation (IUGR) have lower somatomedin levels than normal newborns of a similar gestational age.[52,54–56] Moreover, fetal chondrocytes are responsive to the growth-promoting effects of this peptide.

In the human fetus, somatomedin secretion is not GH dependent. Because a transient increase in neonatal

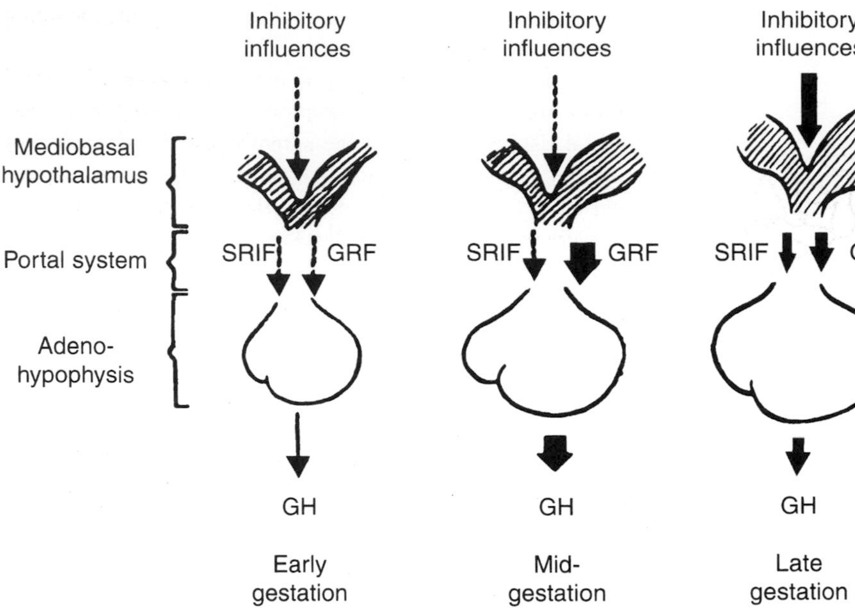

Figure 5.5 Schematic illustration of the proposed ontogenesis of hypothalamic neurohormonal control of fetal growth hormone (*GH*) secretion. GRF, growth-hormone-releasing factor; SRIF, somatotropin release-inhibiting factor. (From Gluckman PD, Grumbach MM, Kaplan SL. The neuroendocrine regulation and function of growth hormone and prolactin in the mammalian fetus. *Endocrine Rev* 1981;2:363, with permission.)

somatomedin has been observed during the first month of life when estrogen levels are declining, it has been suggested that estrogens may serve some suppressive regulatory function *in utero*.

CRH, ACTH, and the adrenal gland

After the seventh week of gestation, the corpus luteum ceases to be the dominant steroid-producing organ and the fetoplacental unit takes over. The interdependence of the fetal adrenal cortex and the placenta reflects their incomplete, but complementary steroidogenic, enzyme systems. The characteristic steroid profile of pregnancy results from their constant exchange of steroid precursors. However, there appears to be little maternal contribution to the fetal pool of ACTH.

Bioassayable ACTH can be detected in the fetal pituitary by 8–10 weeks' gestation, peaks between 12 and 19 weeks, and then declines slowly throughout the third trimester. At midgestation it appears to play a critical tropic role in the developing fetal zone of the adrenal gland. However, pituitary ACTH may not provide the only stimulus for adrenal growth: placental-derived proopiomelanocortin (POMC, the precursor of ACTH and β-lipotropin) may also share this activity.

Placental CRH is structurally similar to hypothalamic CRH.[57] Both are products of the same gene located on the long arm of chromosome 8.[58] Likewise, placental ACTH appears to be structurally similar to the pituitary ACTH 1–39 peptide.[59] The activity of CRH is highest during the first trimester and diminishes as term approaches. Of note, pro-CRH mRNA has been found in the cytotrophoblast[58], and placental ACTH activity has been localized to the syncytiotrophoblast.[24]

Similarly to their hypothalamic pituitary counterparts, there is a dose-dependent stimulation of placental ACTH by placental CRH.[60] However, a paradoxical relationship is observed between the endorgan product, cortisol, and these placental peptides (Fig. 5.6). Glucocorticoids increase placental CRH and ACTH secretion.[60] Placental CRH, once released into the maternal and fetal circulations, stimulates the respective pituitary glands and the placenta to secrete ACTH. In turn, ACTH from the maternal and fetal adrenal cortex, as well as from the placenta, stimulates more glucocorticoid secretion (see Fig. 5.6). This positive feedback mechanism may allow an increase in glucocorticoid secretion during times of stress, beyond the amount available if the woman were not pregnant.

Placental CRH and ACTH probably participate with the fetal hypothalamus and pituitary in the observed surge of fetal glucocorticoids associated with the late third trimester.[61]

The fetal adrenal gland

At term, the fetal adrenal glands are as large as those of adults, weighing 10g or more. What ultimately develops into the adult adrenal cortex, the outer or definitive zone, accounts for only 15% of the fetal gland (Fig. 5.7). The unique inner or fetal zone constitutes 85% of the volume of the adrenal gland *in utero* but involutes after delivery and completely disappears by the first year of life. Work in nonhuman primates suggests that the fasciculata zone of the adult adrenal gland may stem from the fetal zone.[62]

In late gestation, the fetal zone appears to be dependent on the fetal pituitary. This is indirectly supported by observations of fetal zone atrophy in anencephalic and apituitary fetuses, and gland atrophy and reduced DHEAS secretion subsequent to glucocorticoid treatment.[63–65] However, before midgestation, the endocrine support of the pituitary appears unnecessary because anencephalic fetuses demonstrate normal adrenal growth and development up to week 20.[66] Peptides,

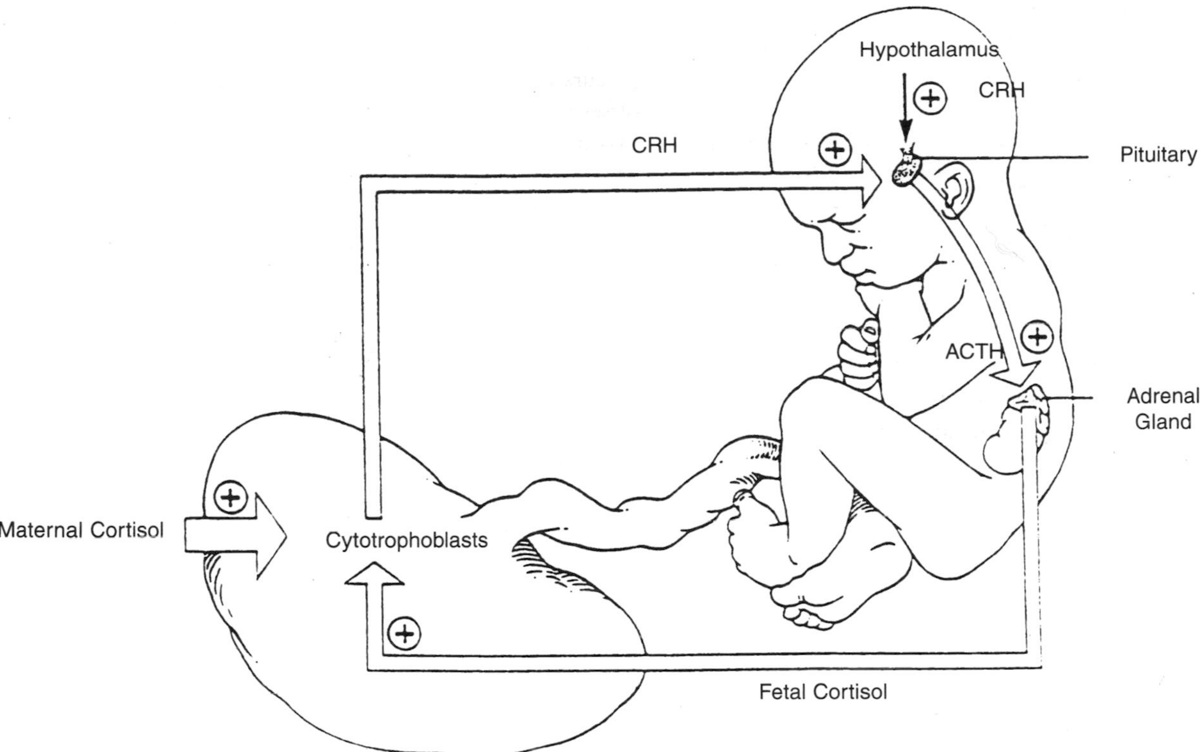

Figure 5.6 The fetoplacental corticotropin-releasing hormone (*CRH*)–glucocorticoid positive feedback hypothesis. CRH, secreted by the placental trophoblast, enters the fetal circulation via the umbilical vein and stimulates (+) fetal adrenocorticotropic hormone (*ACTH*) release from the fetal pituitary. Fetal ACTH stimulates secretion of fetal adrenal cortisol, which enters the placental circulation via the umbilical artery. Cortisol further stimulates placental CRH secretion, thereby completing the positive feedback loop. Fetal CRH, secreted from the fetal hypothalamus, may independently stimulate fetal ACTH release, and placental and fetal hypothalamic CRH may be directly stimulated by environmental stresses. In addition, placental ACTH may stimulate the fetal adrenal directly. (From Buster JE, Carson SA. Placental endocrinology and diagnosis of pregnancy. In: Gabbe SG, Niebyl JR, Simpson JL, eds. *Obstetrics: normal and problem pregnancies*. New York: Churchill Livingstone, 1991:59, with permission.)

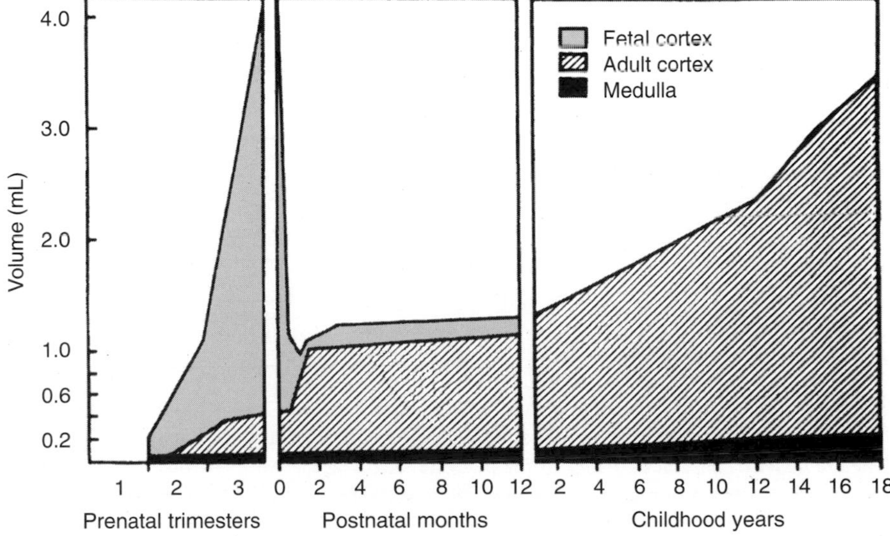

Figure 5.7 Size of adrenal gland and its component parts *in utero*, during infancy, and during childhood. (From Bethune JE. *The adrenal cortex. A Scope Monograph*. Kalamazoo, MI: Upjohn, 1974:11, with permission.)

including hCG, prolactin, hPL, GH, and α-melanocyte-stimulating hormone (α-MSH), as well as epidermal and fibroblast growth factors, have all been proposed to play a tropic role in adrenal development.[32,67,68]

Catecholamine production occurs in the fetal adrenal medulla, which is derived from sympathetic cell precursors from the neurocrest and neurotube. These subsequently differentiate into neuroblasts, then sympathetic ganglion cells, and eventually pheochromoblasts which invade the developing adrenal cortex by the seventh gestational week and become pheochromocytes or mature chromaffin cells. The adrenal medulla, however, is not fully developed until 3 years of age.[69,70] Catecholamines are critical for optimal regulation of the central nervous, cardiovascular, and metabolic systems. Catecholamine release is predominantly regulated by sympathetic nerves that secrete acetylcholine.[71]

DHEAS

The fetal adrenal cortex is functionally deficient in the enzyme 3β-hydroxysteroid dehydrogenase, which converts pregnenolone and dehydroepiandrosterone (DHEA) to progesterone and androstenedione, respectively,[72,73] the immediate precursors of the sex steroids. These enzyme deficiencies are offset by the enzyme activities of the placenta, allowing these two organs to work together to produce a range of steroids not otherwise possible (Fig. 5.8). The fetal adrenal cortex extracts LDL from the fetal circulation and converts it to pregnenolone sulfate and DHEAS.[73,74] Pregnenolone sulfate is delivered to the placenta through the umbilical artery. The placenta, which has an abundance of 3β-hydroxysteroid dehydrogenase, converts pregnenolone to progesterone and this is then returned to the fetus for mineralocorticoid and glucocorticoid synthesis. Of note, the placenta also has the enzymatic capacity to extract LDL cholesterol and convert it to progesterone.

The fetal zone produces DHEAS in large concentrations. This reflects the restricted availability of Δ3β-hydroxysteroid dehydrogenase and Δ4,5 isomerase activity necessary for the biosynthesis of progesterone, cortisol, and testosterone. The high circulating levels of progesterone and estradiol found

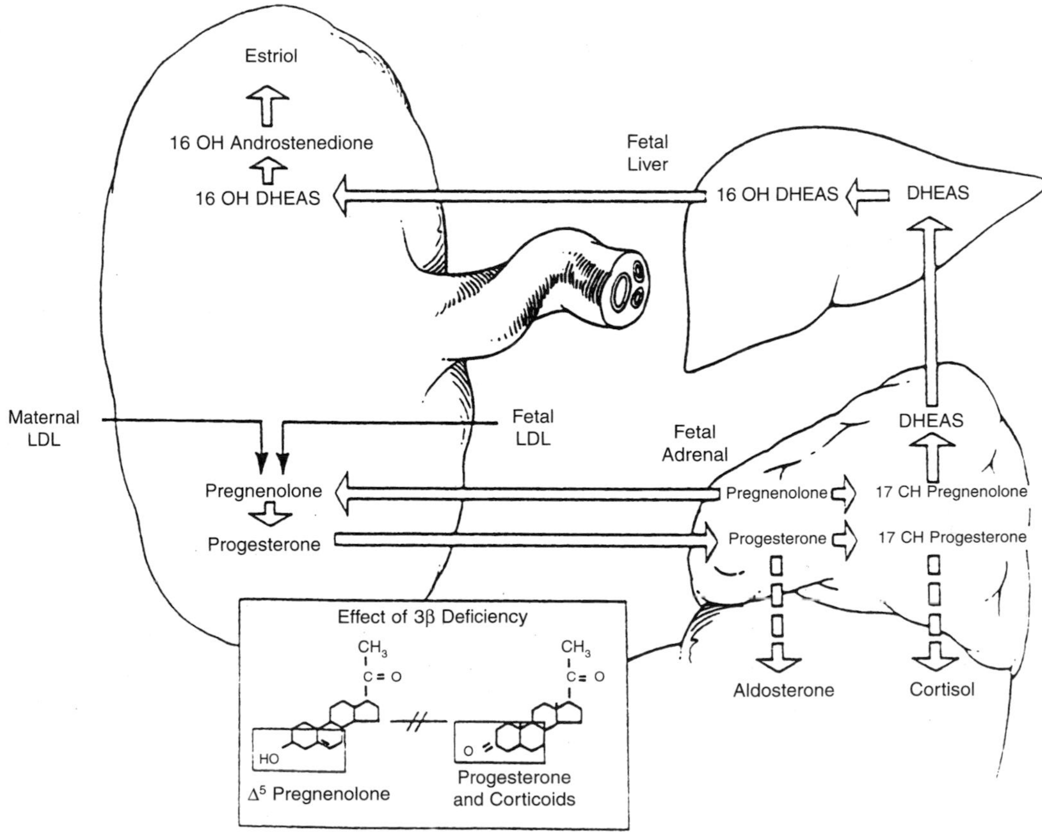

Figure 5.8 Exchange of circulating steroid intermediates between the adrenal fetal zone and placenta. Enzyme deficiencies of the fetal zone are offset by enzyme activities of the placenta, enabling the two organs to work as a mutual cooperative to produce an extensive profile of steroids not otherwise possible. The fetal adrenal cortex is functionally deficient in 3β-hydroxysteroid dehydrogenase, the enzyme that converts pregnenolone to progesterone and dehydroepiandrosterone sulfate (*DHEAS*) to androstenedione. The placenta contains 3β-hydroxysteroid dehydrogenase in abundance and can make this conversion. The placenta is deficient, however, in 17α-hydroxylase and cannot make corticoids. LDL, low-density lipoprotein. (From Buster JE, Carson SA. Placental endocrinology and diagnosis of pregnancy. In: Gabbe SG, Niebyl JR, Simpson JL, eds. *Obstetrics: normal and problem pregnancies*. New York: Churchill Livingstone, 1991:59, with permission.)

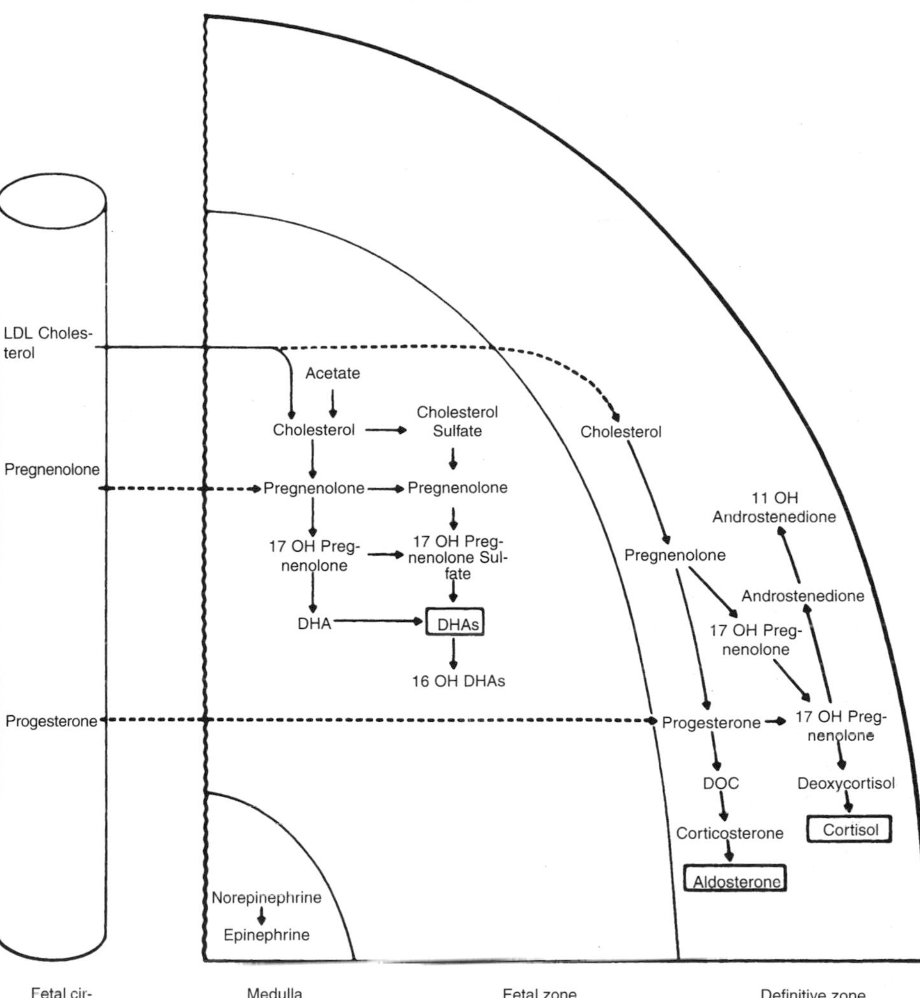

Figure 5.9 Schematic illustration of generalized pathways of hormone formation in the human fetal adrenal gland. DHA, dehydroepiandrosterone; DHAS, dehydroepiandrosterone sulfate; LDL, low-density lipoprotein. (From Seron-Ferre M, Jaffe RB. The fetal adrenal gland. *Annu Rev Physiol* 1981;43:141, with permission.)

during pregnancy inhibit this enzyme complex and thereby indirectly promote DHEAS production. Maternal LDL cholesterol appears to be the major precursor of fetal adrenal DHEAS. Other steroid sulfates can also be converted to DHEAS without loss of the sulfate sidechain. DHEAS is delivered to the fetal liver, where it is converted to 16α-hydroxyandrostenedione and then further aromatized into estriol.[73] Estrogens are subsequently secreted into the fetal and maternal circulations.[73] Jaffe and Payne[75] have demonstrated that the human fetal testis has the capacity to use DHEAS *in vitro* to form active steroids.

Cortisol

Together with aldosterone, cortisol is the major steroid produced by the definitive zone (Fig. 5.9). The adrenocorticoids share the same 21-carbon pregnane structure with progesterone. However, these compounds differ markedly in their biological activity because of the additional hydroxyl and ketone groups as shown in Fig. 5.10. Low-density lipoprotein cholesterol is used as a substrate for the synthesis of cortisol via the pathways of 17α-, 21-, and 11β-hydroxylation. Progesterone derived from the placental circulation can also be used within the definitive zone for the production of cortisol, deoxycorticosterone, corticosterone, and aldosterone.[66] As described below, cortisol has many roles in fetal development.

Cortisol stimulates pulmonary surfactant production by type 2 pneumocytes.[76] At approximately 34–36 weeks' gestation, cortisol, together with thyroxin, prolactin, and estrogens, stimulates choline phosphotransferase to produce dipalmitoyl lecithin, the principal surface-active phospholipid.[77,78] This increases the lecithin–sphingomyelin ratio, characteristic of fetal lung maturity.

Corticosteroids induce the development and maturation of a number of hepatic enzyme systems necessary for carbohydrate, protein, and fat metabolism. The concentration of liver glycogen increases with advancing gestational age, and glycogen deposition appears to be controlled by cortisol.[79] This role of cortisol is critical considering the fact that glycogen availability in the newborn is necessary for its extrauterine adaptation. Indeed, during the first 24 h of life, continuous blood glucose delivery to the neonatal brain is dependent on liver glycogen stores.[77]

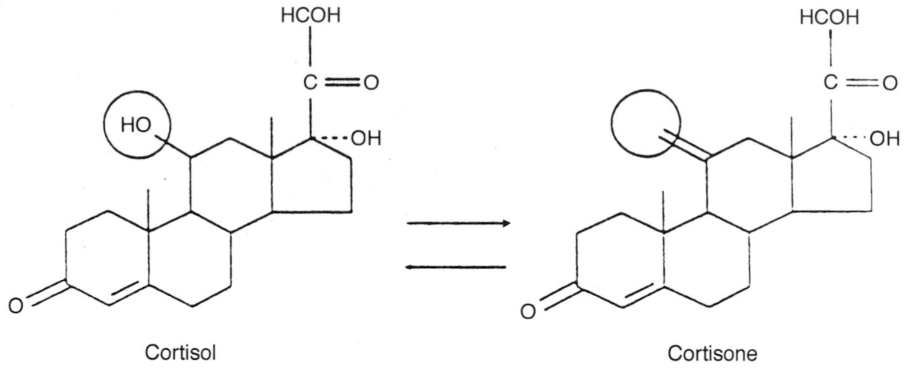

Figure 5.10 Molecular structure of the corticoids. Cortisol and cortisone differ from progesterone in the number and arrangements of hydroxyl groups.

In nonhuman models, cortisol has also been shown to participate in the maturation of the hypothalamic–pituitary–adrenal (HPA) axis, in central nervous system growth, and the establishment of hypothalamic rhythmicity.[77] Intrauterine stressors may set this axis at an early age to favor short-term benefits such as restricting growth and increasing fuel availability, but this may have long-term adult consequences such as coronary heart disease.[80]

Maternal free and bound cortisol levels increase in pregnancy, peaking in the early third trimester and then declining again. In parturition, a transient increase in cortisol is again observed. Placental CRH production has been hypothesized to initiate labor and even preterm labor. In sheep, fetal cortisol production is responsible for the initiation of labor but this has not been demonstrated in humans. However, concentrations are slightly higher in spontaneous labor than in induced labor.[81]

Cortisol may also play a role in the transfer from fetal- to adult-type hemoglobin. However, most of the work on the function of cortisol in the fetus has been carried out in animal models and human data are lacking.

Renin–angiotensin system

Renin secretion clearly doubles as early as the eighth week of gestation, and then increases to 32 weeks, after which no further significant changes occur. Plasma renin substrate, however, doubles by the eighth week of pregnancy, plateaus by the 20th week, and remains steady thereafter.[82] This concurrent stimulation of enzyme and substrate levels results in a dramatic increase in plasma renin activity. The large size of renin (molecular weight 43 kDa) makes it unlikely that this molecule crosses the placenta. Not surprisingly, anephric infants have been found to have undetectable renin levels.

The circulating concentration of the octapeptide, angiotensin II, in the fetus is similar to or greater than the maternal level, and both are higher than those observed in the nongravid state. Placental metabolism of angiotensin I into angiotensin II, or production of angiotensin II by the placenta, is suggested by the observation that venous blood from the umbilical cord has higher levels of angiotensin II than arterial cord blood. It has been suggested that these findings support a significant role of the renin–angiotensin system in the regulation of fetoplacental blood pressure.

The pattern of aldosterone secretion, as well as plasma aldosterone levels, may diverge from that of plasma renin activity in pregnancy. Although changes in plasma renin activity begin to plateau as early as 20–32 weeks, plasma and urine aldosterone continue to increase progressively throughout pregnancy. This pattern appears to closely parallel the profile of other steroid hormones, such as progesterone, E_3, and E_2.[83]

Fetoplacental peptides

Considering the totipotential nature of the trophoblast, it is not surprising that this tissue secretes a variety of substances, including several proteins that are produced early in human pregnancy. The following discussion considers the most prominent of these and their role in gestation.

Human chorionic gonadotropin

Human chorionic gonadotropin (hCG) has a molecular weight of 36–40 kDa and is a glycoprotein that is biologically and immunologically similar to LH but with a longer half-life.[84–86] All of the glycoprotein hormones (hCG, LH, FSH, and TSH) have a similar biological activity which is characteristic of the β-subunit component. It is because of this that hCG seems to have a stimulatory effect on the maternal thyroid in early pregnancy when hCG levels are highest. The α-subunit and carbohydrate component are required for expression of the biological activity unique to the β-subunit. The 28–30 amino acids on the carboxy-terminal end of the β-subunit of hCG are unique compared with LH. The specific immunoreactive properties of the hCG β-subunit allow the diagnosis of pregnancy or extrapregnancy sources of hCG (i.e., gonadal tumors) with great accuracy. Even in the presence of LH, hCG is produced by the syncytiotrophoblast during pregnancy. It is also produced by all other types of trophoblastic tissue, including that derived from choriocarcinoma and hydatidiform mole.[32]

The physiological role of hCG in human pregnancy has yet to be fully elucidated. As described earlier, it is known to play a luteotropic role early in pregnancy. Late in pregnancy, hCG assumes a gonadotropic role by inducing the secretion of testosterone from the fetal testes prior to the availability of LH secretion from the fetal pituitary. It may also regulate DHEAS production by the fetal zone of the adrenal gland[69] and play a critical immunosuppressive role *in vivo* by preventing the rejection of the fetal allograft by its maternal host.[87] However, data from recent studies are mixed, and the relative contributions of progesterone, hCG, and cortisol to DHEAS production and immunosuppression continue to be the subject of investigation.

In spontaneous pregnancy, hCG can be detected by the ninth day after the LH surge.[84] This initial detection in maternal blood has been found to correlate with the implantation of the blastocyst and, specifically, with the moment that lacunae receive maternal blood.[88,89] The concentration of intact hCG peaks by 60–90 days' gestation and then decreases to a plateau that is maintained throughout the duration of the pregnancy. The production of the β-subunit by the trophoblast parallels that of intact hCG throughout the first trimester.[90] During this period, free α-subunit levels are low or absent. Thereafter, the relative production of α- and β-subunits reverses and levels of the α-subunit increase until term.

Key points

1. The corpus luteum synthesizes crucial hormones that maintain pregnancy until the placenta can take over. These include progesterone, estradiol (E_2), inhibin A, relaxin, and vascular endothelial growth factor (VEGF) which maintain the endometrial lining, prevent contractions, and promote the growth of the embryo.
2. All three estrogens share the same 18 carbon nucleus. Estrone (E_1) predominates in menopause, E_2 is the major estrogen secreted by the ovary during the reproductive years, and estriol (E_3) is produced almost exclusively in pregnancy.
3. Physiological changes of pregnancy include:
   - physiologic anemia;
   - angiotensin II resistance and a decrease in blood pressure;
   - propensity toward insulin resistance.
4. The pituitary is composed of two distinctly derived parts: the anterior pituitary is derived from Rathke's pouch and secretes thyroid-stimulating hormone (TSH), adrenocorticotropic hormone (ACTH), growth hormone (GH), prolactin, follicle-stimulating hormone (FSH), and luteinizing hormone (LH), whereas the posterior pituitary is derived from neuroectoderm and produces oxytocin and vasopressin.
5. The α-subunits of TSH, FSH, LH, and human chorionic gonadotropin (hCG) are homologous. It is the β-subunit that confers each hormone's specificity.
6. β-hCG has partial thyrotropic activity and its high levels probably cause the suppression of TSH in early pregnancy and the potential hyperthyroid state sometimes observed in molar pregnancies.
7. Each endocrine axis of the fetus is intricately tied to the endocrine function of the placenta and the mother.
8. Gonadotropin-releasing hormone (GnRH) activity peaks at 20 weeks' gestation during gonadal development and then gradually becomes dormant until puberty.
9. Testosterone is converted by 5α-reductase to its more active form, dihydroxytestosterone (DHT). DHT is responsible for virilization of external genitalia.
10. The fetal adrenal cortex is mostly composed of an inner fetal zone that involutes after birth, and a smaller outer definitive zone that ultimately becomes the adult adrenal cortex.
11. The fetal cortex produces dehydroepiandrosterone sulfate (DHEAS) from maternal low-density lipoprotein (LDL). DHEAS serves as a precursor to multiple hormones including estrogens, testosterone, and androstenedione.
12. Cortisol stimulates the production of surfactant in developing fetal lungs, matures fetal liver enzymes, and may be involved in the initiation of labor.
13. β-hCG is produced by the syncytiotrophoblast of the placenta and maintains the corpus luteum, stimulates the testes to produce testosterone (in place of LH), and regulates DHEAS production.
14. β-hCG is detectable 9 days after the LH surge at the time of implantation. The level of β-hCG peaks at 2–3 months' gestation.
15. Human chorionic somatomammotropin (hCS, also known as human placental lactogen, hPL) shares 96% identity with GH and serves as a key stimulatory hormone for fetal growth.

Human chorionic somatomammotropin (human placental lactogen)

Human chorionic somatomammotropin (hCS), also known as hPL, is a single-chain polypeptide of 190 amino acids with two disulfide bridges. It has a short half-life and is produced in massive daily quantities by the syncytiotrophoblast layer of the placenta. Circulating levels increase 10-fold from the first trimester and plateau in the third trimester. It shares 96% identity with GH and its levels have been shown to relate to fetal and placental weight. Despite this, hCS has only 3% of the somatotrophic activity of GH. In animal studies it has been found to display 50% of the lactogenic activity of prolactin.

hCS can be detected in the urine and serum in normal and molar pregnancies, as well as in the urine of patients with trophoblastic tumors and in men with choriocarcinoma of the testes.

The major metabolic role of hCS during pregnancy is to ensure the nutritional needs of the fetus. Hypoglycemia stimulates hCS secretion. As the supply of glucose decreases during the fasting state, hCS levels rise, stimulating lipolysis over carbohydrate metabolism. The increased ketones induced by metabolism of free fatty acids are an important energy source for the fetus. During the fed state, and in response to rising glucose levels, insulin secretion increases and hCS secretion decreases, leading to glucose use and lipogenesis. Because of increasing substrate requirements by the fetus as pregnancy progresses, the functional role of hCS assumes great significance in the second and third trimesters.[91]

Conclusion

Endocrine influences on fetal growth and development are complex. Although there are significant gaps in our knowledge, tremendous progress has been made. The fetoplacental–maternal unit stands as a wondrous example in human biology of interrelated systems that allow for the concurrent processes of fetal progression and maternal adaptation.

References

1 Kreitmann-Gimbal B, Bayad F, Nixon WE, et al. Patterns of estrogen and progesterone receptors in monkey endometrium during the normal menstrual cycle. *Steroid* 1980;35:47.

2 Johnannisson E, Parker RA, Landgren BM, et al. Morphometric analysis of the human endometrium in relation to peripheral hormone levels. *Fertil Steril* 1982;38:564.

3 Resnik R, Killam AP, Battaglia FC, et al. The stimulation of uterine blood flow by various estrogens. *Endocrinology* 1974;94:1192.

4 Shutt TA, Lopata A. The secretion of hormones during the culture of human preimplantation embryos with corona cells. *Fertil Steril* 1981;35:413.

5 Laufer N, Decherney AH, Haseltine FP, et al. Steroid secretion by the human egg–corona cumulus complex in culture. *J Clin Endocrinol Metab* 1984;58:1153.

6 Punnonen R, Lukola A. Binding of estrogen and progestin in the human fallopian tube. *Fertil Steril* 1981;37:610.

7 Siiteri PK, Febres F, Clemens LE, et al. Progesterone and maintenance of pregnancy: is progesterone nature's immunosuppressant? *Ann NY Acad Sci* 1977:286:3384.

8 Resnik R, Brink GW, Plumer MH. The effect of progesterone on estrogen-induced uterine blood flow. *Am J Obstet Gynecol* 1977:128:251.

9 Hsueh AJW, Peck EJ, Clark JH. Progesterone antagonism of the estrogen receptor and estrogen-induced uterine blood flow. *Am J Obstet Gynecol* 1977;128:251.

10 Darmochwal-Kolarz D, Leszczynska-Gorzelak B, Rolinski J, et al. Th1 and Th2 type cytokine imbalance in women with preeclampsia. *J Obstet Gynecol Reprod Biol* 1999;86:165.

11 Clark, D. Is there any evidence for immunologically mediated or immunologically modifiable early pregnancy failure? *J Assisted Reprod Gen* 2003;20:63.

12 Koch C, Platt J. Natural mechanisms for evading graft rejection: the fetus as an allograft. *Springer Semin Immunopathol* 2003; 25:95.

13 Lo YM, Lo ES, Watson N, et al. Two way cell traffic between mother and fetus: biologic and clinical implications. *Blood* 1996;88:4390.

14 Bianchi DW, Zickwolf GK, Weil GJ, et al. Male fetal progenitor cells persist in maternal blood for as long as 27 years postpartum. *Proc Natl Acad Sci USA* 1996;93:705.

15 Yie SM, Li LH, Li YM, et al. HLA-G protein concentrations in maternal serum and placental tissue are decreased in preeclampsia. *Am J Obstet Gynecol* 2004;191:525.

16 Trundley A, Moffett A. Human uterine leukocytes and pregnancy. *Tissue Antigens* 2004;63:1.

17 Guimond M-J, Wang B, Croy BA, et al. Engraftment of bone marrow from SCID mice reverses the reproductive deficits in NK cell deficient tg epsilon 26 mice. *J Exp Med* 1998;187:217.

18 Graham GJ, Stevens JM, Page NM, et al. Tachykinins regulate the function of platelets. *Blood* 2004;104:1058.

19 Pridjian G, Puschett J. Preeclampsia. Part 1: clinical and pathophysiologic considerations. *Obstet Gynecol Surv* 2002;57: 598.

20 Page NM. The endocrinology of pre-eclampsia. *Clin Endocrinol* 2002;57:413.

21 Ryan E. Hormones and insulin resistance in pregnancy. *Lancet* 2003;362:1777.

21 Linné Y. Effects of obesity on women's reproduction and complications during pregnancy. *Obes Rev* 2004;5:137.

22 Kaplan SL, Grumbach MM, Aubert ML. The ontogenesis of pituitary hormones and hypothalamic factors in the human fetus: maturation of central nervous system regulation of anterior pituitary function. *Recent Prog Horm Res* 1976;32:161.

23 Sheng H, Westphal H. Early steps in pituitary organogenesis. *Trends Genet* 1999;15:236.

24 Al-Timim A, Fox H. Immunohistochemical localization of follicle-stimulating hormone, luteinizing hormone, growth hormone, adrenocorticotropic hormone and prolactin in the human placenta. *Placenta* 1986;7:163.

25 Hay DL. Placental histology and the production of human chorionogonadotropin and its subunits in pregnancy. *Br Obstet Gynaecol* 1988;95:1268.

26 Harada A, Hershman JM. Extraction of human chorionic thyrotropin (hCT) from term placentas: failure to recover thyrotropic activity. *J Clin Endocrinol Metab* 1978;47:681.

27 Khodr GS, Siler-Khodr TM. Placental luteinizing hormone-releasing factor and its synthesis. *Science* 1980;207:315.

28 Hoshina M, Hussa R, Pattillo R, et al. The role of trophoblast differentiation in the control of the hCG and hPL genes. *Adv Exp Med Biol* 1984;176:299.

29 Hosina M, Boime I, Mochizuki. Cytological localization of hPL, hCG, and mRNA in chorionic tissue using in situ hybridization. *Acta Obstet Gynaecol Jpn* 1984;36:397.

30 Kurman RJ, Young RH, Norris JH, et al. Immunocytochemical localization of placental lactogen and chorionic gonadotropin in the normal placenta and trophoblastic tumors, with emphasis on intermediate trophoblast and the placental site trophoblastic tumor. *Int J Gynecol Pathol* 1984;3:101.

31 Thomas GB, Brooks AN. Pituitary and gonadal responses to the long-term pulsatile administration of gonadotrophin-releasing hormone in fetal sheep. *J Endocrinol* 1997;153:385.

32 Jaffe RB. Endocrine physiology of the fetus and fetoplacental unit. In: Yen SSC, Jaffe RB, eds. *Reproductive endocrinology: physiology, pathophysiology and clinical management.* Philidelphia, PA: WB Saunders; 1986:737.

33 Siiteri PK, Wolfson JD. Testosterone formation and metabolism during male sexual differentiation in the human embryo. *J Clin Endocrinol Metab* 1974;38:113.

34 Jaffe RB. Fetoplacental endocrine and metabolic physiology. *Perinat Endocrinol* 1983;10:669.

35 Payne AH, Jaffe RB. Androgen formation from pregnenolone sulfate by the human fetal ovary. *J Clin Endocrinol Metab* 1974:39:300.

36 Siler-Khodr TM, Khodr GS, Valenzuela G. Gonadotropin-releasing hormone effects on placental hormones during gestation. I: alpha-human chorionic gonadotropin, human chorionic gonadotropin and human chorionic somatomammotropin. *Biol Reprod* 1986;34:245.

37 Barnea ER, Kaplan M. Spontaneous, gonadotropin-releasing hormone-induced, and progesterone-inhibited pulsatile secretion of human chorionic gonadotropin in the first trimester placenta in vitro. *J Clin Endocrinol Metab* 1989;69:215.

38 Ingbar SH. The thyroid gland. In: Wilson JD, Foster DW, eds. *Williams textbook of endocrinology*, 7th edn. Philidelphia, PA: WB Saunders; 1985:682.

39 Roti E, Gnudi A, Braverman LE, et al. Human cord blood concentrations of thyrotropin, thyroglobulin and iodothyronines after maternal administration of thyrotropin-releasing hormone. *J Clin Endocrinol Metab* 1981;53:813.

40 Fisher DA, Klein AH. Thyroid development and disorders of thyroid function in the newborn. *N Engl J Med* 1981;304: 702.

41 Youngblood WW, Humm J, Kizer S. Thyrotropin-releasing hormone-like bioactivity in placenta: evidence for the existence of substances other than pyro-Glu-His-Pro-NH_2 (TRH) capable of stimulating pituitary thyrotropin release. *Endocrinology* 1980; 106:541.

42 Kenimer JG, Herschman JN, Higgins HP. The thyrotropin in hydatidiform moles is human chorionic gonadotropin. *J Clin Endocrinol Metab* 1975;40:482.

43 Gray TK, Lame W, Lester GE. Vitamin D and pregnancy: the maternal fetal metabolism of vitamin D. *Endocrine Rev* 1981; 2:264.

44 Lester GE, Gray TK, Lorenc RS. Evidence for maternal and fetal differences in vitamin D metabolism. *Proc Soc Exp Biol Med* 1978;159:303.

45 Reddy GS, Normon AW, Willis DM, et al. Regulation of vitamin D metabolism in normal human pregnancy. *J Clin Endocrinol Metab* 1983;56:363.

46 Gluckman PD, Grumbach MM, Kaplan SL. The neuroendocrine regulation and function of growth hormone and prolactin in the mammalian fetus. *Endocrine Rev* 1981;2:363.

47 Freemark M, Driscoll P, Maaskant R, et al. Ontogenesis of prolactin receptors in the human fetus: roles in fetal development. *J Clin Invest* 1997;99:1107.

48 Hauth JC, Parker CR, McDonald PC, et al. A role of fetal prolactin in lung maturation. *Obstet Gynecol* 1978;51:81.

49 Gluckman PD, Ballard PL, Kaplan SL, et al. Prolactin in umbilical cord blood and the respiratory distress syndrome. *J Pediatr* 1978;93:1011.

50 Han VK. The ontogeny of growth hormone, insulin-like growth factors and sex steroids: molecular aspects. *Horm Res* 1996;45:61.

51 Goodyer CG, Grigorakis SI, Patel YC, et al. Developmental changes in the expression of somatostatin receptors (1–5) in the brain, hypothalamus, pituitary and spinal cord of the human fetus. *Neuroscience* 2004;125:441.

52 Gluckman PD, Brinsmead MW. Somatomedin in cord blood: relationship to gestational age and birth size. *J Clin Endocrinol Metab* 1976;43:1378.

53 Kastrup KW, Anderson HT, Lebech P. Somatomedin in newborns and the relationship to human chorionic somatotropin and fetal growth. *Acta Pediatr Scand* 1978;67:757.

54 Ashton IK, Vesey J. Somatomedin activity in human cord plasma and relationship to birth size, insulin, growth hormone and prolactin. *Early Hum Dev* 1978;2:115.

55 Heinrick UE, Schlach DS, Jawadi MH, et al. NSILA and fetal growth. *Acta Endocrinol (Copenh)* 1979;90:534.

56 Foley TP, DeFilip R, Pericelli A, et al. Low somatomedin activity in cord serum from infants with intrauterine growth retardation. *J Pediatr* 1980;96:605.

57 Stalla GK, Hartwimmer J, von-Werder K, et al. Immunocytochemical localization of placental lactogen and chorionic gonadotropin in the normal placenta and trophoblastic tumors, with emphasis on intermediate trophoblast and the placental site trophoblastic tumor. *Int J Gynecol Pathol* 1984;3:101.

58 Shibahara S, Morimoto Y, Furutani Y, et al. Isolation and sequence analysis of the human corticotropin-releasing factor precursor gene. *EMBO J* 1983;2:775.

59 Chrousos GP, Calabrese JR, Avgerinos P, et al. Corticotropin releasing factor: basic studies and clinical applications. *Prog Neuropsychopharmacol Biol Psychiatry* 1985;9:349.

60 Robinson BC, Emanuel RL, Frim DN, et al. Glucocorticoid stimulates expression of corticotropin-releasing hormone gene in human placenta. *Proc Natl Acad Sci USA* 1988;85:5244.

61 Buster JE, Carson SA. Placental endocrinology and diagnosis of pregnancy. In: Gabbe SG, Niebyl JR, Simpson JL, eds. *Obstetrics: normal and problem pregnancies.* New York: Churchill Livingstone; 1991:59.

62 McNulty WP, Novy MJ, Walsh SW. Fetal and postnatal development of the adrenal glands in *Macaca mulatta. Biol Reprod* 1981;25:1079.

63 Benirschke K. Adrenals in anencephaly and hydrocephaly. *Obstet Gynecol* 1956;8:412.

64 Ballard PL, Gluckman PD, Liggins GC, et al. Steroid and growth hormone levels in premature infants after perinatal betamethasone therapy to prevent respiratory distress syndrome. *Pediatr Res* 1980:14:112.

65 Simmer HH, Tulchinsky D, Gold EM, et al. On the regulation of estrogen production by cortisol and ACTH in human pregnancy at term. *Am J Obstet Gynecol* 1974;119:283.

66 Heinrichs WL, Gibbons WE. Endocrinology of pregnancy. In: Brody SA, Ueland K, eds. *Endocrine disorders in pregnancy.* Norwalk, CT: Appleton & Lange; 1989:65.

67 Jaffe RB, Seron-Ferre M, Crickard K, et al. Regulation and function of the primate fetal adrenal gland and gonad. *Recent Prog Horm Res* 1981:37:41.
68 Crickard K, Ill CR, Jaffe RB. Control of proliferation of human fetal adrenal cells in vitro. *J Clin Endocrinol Metab* 1981;53:790.
69 Seron-Ferre M, Jaffe RB. The fetal adrenal gland. *Annu Rev Physiol* 1981;43:141.
70 Wurtman RJ. Controlled epinephrine synthesis in the adrenal medulla by the adrenal cortex: hormonal specificity and dose response characteristics. *Endocrinology* 1966;79:608.
71 Healey DL, Herrington AC, O'Herlihy C. Chronic polyhydramnios is a syndrome with a lactogen receptor defect in the chorion laeve. *Br J Obstet Gynaecol* 1985;92:461.
72 Buster J. Fetal adrenal cortex. *Clin Obstet Gynecol* 1980;23:804.
73 Diczfalusy E. Steroid metabolism in the feto-placental unit. In: Pecile A, Finzi C, eds. *The feto–placental unit.* Amsterdam: Excerpta Medica; 1969.
74 Simpson ER, Carr BR, Parker CR, et al. The role of serum lipoproteins in steroidogenesis by the human fetal adrenal cortex. *J Clin Endocrinol Metab* 1979;49:146.
75 Jaffe RB, Payne AH. Gonadal steroid sulfates and sulfatase. IV: comparative studies on the steroid sulfokinase in the human fetal testes and adrenal. *J Clin Endocrinol Metab* 1971;33:592.
76 Kittermann JA, Liggins CT, Campos GA, et al. Prepartum maturation of the lung in fetal sheep: relation to cortisol. *J Appl Physiol* 1981;51:384.
77 Liggins GC. Endocrinology of the feto-maternal unit. In: Shearman RP, ed. *Human reproductive physiology*. Oxford: Blackwell Science; 1972:138.
78 Colacicco G, Ray AK, Basu MK, et al. Cultured lung cells: interplay effects of beta-mimetics, prostaglandins and corticosteroids in the biosynthesis of dipalmitoyl lecithin. *J Biosci* 1979;34:101.
79 Fowden AL, Comline RS, Silver M. The effects of cortisol on the concentration of glycogen in different tissues in the chronically catheterized fetal pig. *J Exp Physiol* 1985;70:23.
80 Phillips DI. Fetal growth and programming of the hypothalamic-pituitary-adrenal axis. *Clin Exp Pharm Phys* 2001;28:967.
81 Goldkrand JW, Schulte RL, Messer RH. Maternal and fetal plasma cortisol levels at parturition. *Obstet Gynecol* 1976;47:41.
82 Wilson M, Morganti AG, Zervoudakis I, et al. Blood pressure, the renin aldosterone system and sex steroids throughout normal pregnancy. *Am J Med* 1980;68:97.
83 Resnik LM, Laragh JH. The renin-angiotensin-aldosterone system in pregnancy. In: Fuchs F, Klopper A, eds. *Endocrinology of pregnancy*. Philadelphia, PA: Harper & Row; 1983:191.
84 Jaffe RB, Lee PA, Midgley AR, Jr. Serum gonadotropin before, at the inception of, and following human pregnancy. *J Clin Endocrinol Metab* 1969;29:1281.
85 Midgley AR, Pierce GB. Immunohistochemical localization of human chorionic gonadotropin. *J Exp Med* 1962;111:289.
86 Jaffe RB. Protein hormones of the placenta, deciduas and fetal membranes. In: Yen SSC, Jaffe RB, eds. *Reproductive endocrinology*. Philadelphia, PA: WB Saunders; 1988:758.
87 Teasdale F, Adcock EA, III, August CS, et al. Human chorionic gonadotropin: inhibitory effect on mixed lymphocyte cultures. *Gynecol Invest* 1973;4:263–269.
88 Khodr GS, Siler-Khodr TM. Localization of leutinizing hormone-releasing factor in the human placenta. *Fertil Steril* 1978;29:523.
89 Khodr GS, Siler-Khodr TM. The effect of leutinizing hormone-releasing factor on human chorionic gonadotropin secretion. *Fertil Steril* 1978;30:301.
90 Cole LA, Kroll TG, Ruddon RW, et al. Differential occurrence of free β and free α subunit of human chorionic gonadotropin in pregnancy sera. *J Clin Endocrinol Metab* 1984;48:1200.
91 Kaplan S. The endocrine mileu of pregnancy. In: Jaffe RB, ed. *Puerperium and childhood*. Report of the Third Roth Conference on Obstetric Research. Columbus, OH: Roth Laboratories; 1974:77.

Part III

Fetal Developmental Biology

Fetal lung development and amniotic fluid analysis

Ian Gross and Matthew J. Bizzarro

Respiratory distress syndrome (RDS) is a developmental disorder of prematurely born infants, characterized by progressive atelectasis and respiratory insufficiency. RDS occurs as a result of the structural and functional immaturity of the lung. The primary biochemical deficiency is immaturity of the surfactant system, which results in increased surface tension at the air–alveolar interface and a tendency for alveolar collapse and generalized atelectasis.

Composition and function of surfactant

Pulmonary surfactant is a complex mixture of phospholipids and proteins that is synthesized in type 2 alveolar cells. The major phospholipids in surfactant are phosphatidylcholine (PC, also called lecithin), which accounts for 80–85% of total phospholipid, and phosphatidylglycerol (PG), which accounts for 8–11%. Approximately one-half of the phosphatidylcholine is in the disaturated form (DSPC).[1] At 80–90% gestation, a marked increase in total lung phospholipid occurs, with a large increase in PC accounting for most of the change.[2] An increase in the surface activity of lung extracts and in lung distensibility and stability also occurs at this time.

In addition to the phospholipid components of surfactant, four surfactant-related proteins have been described and characterized. Surfactant protein A (SP-A) is a highly glycosylated protein with a molecular weight of 28–36 kDa. SP-A is a component of the innate immune system of the lung and recent studies indicate that mice deficient in SP-A are more likely to develop pulmonary and systemic infections when challenged with an intratracheal administration of bacteria, including group B streptococcus.[3] Two smaller hydrophobic proteins, SP-B and SP-C, with molecular weights of 4 and 8 kDa, respectively, are important for the surface-active properties of surfactant and are present in clinically effective surfactant preparations. SP-D is a lectin-like protein and, similar to SP-A, is important for defense against infection.[4]

Regulation of lung maturation

Clinical observations

A variety of physical, chemical, and hormonal stimuli can alter lung development and phospholipid synthesis and secretion. The incidence of RDS is lower in infants who are delivered after labor, whether by vaginal delivery or Cesarean section, than in those delivered without labor at the same gestational age.[5] Gender appears to play a role in lung maturation; at the same gestational age, males are more likely than females to develop RDS. Differences in amniotic fluid phospholipids indicate that the biochemical maturity of the female lung precedes that of the male by approximately 1 week.[6] Maternal diabetes also influences lung maturity; there is a higher incidence of RDS in infants born prematurely to mothers with class A–C diabetes in whom there is no strict control of blood glucose. This delay in lung maturation could be due to hyperglycemia, hyperinsulinemia, excess butyric acid derivatives, or a combination of all three factors.[7] Acute asphyxia with hypoxia and acidosis also appears to inhibit surfactant production. The incidence of RDS is higher in the second of twins, as are a variety of other problems; it is not clear whether this is related to asphyxia. Finally, there appears to be a familial tendency to develop RDS, and a history of a previous infant with RDS places a subsequent premature infant at a higher risk.

Conversely, some clinical conditions appear to accelerate lung maturation and decrease the incidence of RDS. These include long-term maternal stress, e.g., toxemia and hypertension, intrauterine growth retardation, maternal infection, class F and R diabetes, and maternal heroin exposure. Chronic low-grade maternal stress, as opposed to acute asphyxia, accelerates lung maturation by a mechanism that may involve hormones such as glucocorticoids and catecholamines.

The pharmacological acceleration of lung maturation by antenatal hormone administration will be discussed in more detail below.

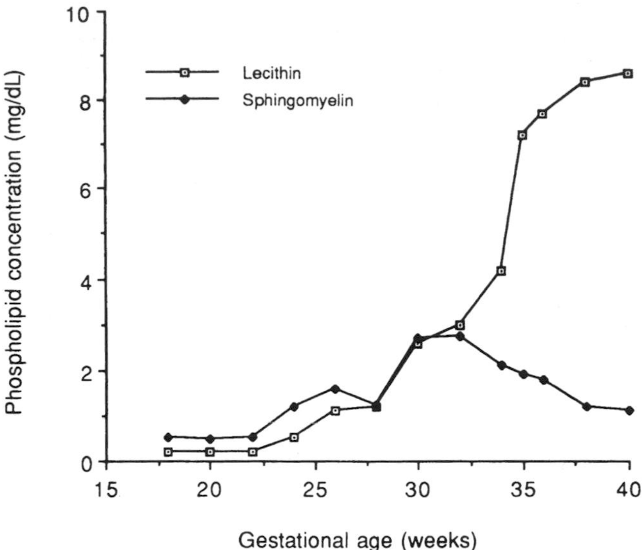

Figure 6.1 Amniotic fluid phospholipid concentration vs. gestational age.

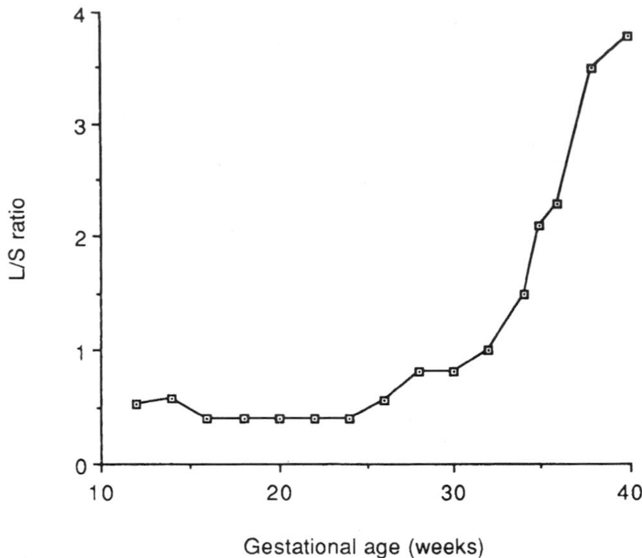

Figure 6.2 Lecithin–sphingomyelin (L/S) ratio vs. gestational age.

Experimental findings

Surfactant synthesis is stimulated by a variety of hormones, growth factors, and transcription factors including glucocorticoids, thyroid hormones, thyrotropin-releasing hormone (TRH), prolactin, cyclic adenosine monophosphate (cAMP), retinoic acid, epidermal growth factor, and thyroid transcription factor. Of these, glucocorticoids have been most extensively studied.[7,8] The administration of glucocorticoids to a fetus results in morphological changes indicative of accelerated lung maturity including larger alveoli, thinner interalveolar septae, increased number of type 2 cells, and increased lamellar bodies within the type 2 cells. In addition, glucocorticoids enhance the biosynthesis of both lung phospholipids and surfactant proteins. Secretion of surfactant is also stimulated by a number of agents, including β-adrenergic agonists, such as terbutaline, and purinoceptor agonists, such as adenosine.

Evaluation of fetal lung maturity

The assessment of fetal lung maturity by the analysis of phospholipids in amniotic fluid began in 1971, when Gluck and coauthors[9] reported on gestational changes in amniotic fluid phospholipid concentrations. In an analysis of amniocenteses from both normal and abnormal pregnancies, from 12 weeks to term, they showed that total phospholipids in amniotic fluid increased throughout gestation, but that there was a sharp increase at 35 weeks. Both lecithin (PC), which originates in the fetal lung, and sphingomyelin were measured. The concentrations of lecithin and sphingomyelin were nearly equal until approximately 32 weeks, after which lecithin concentration increased while sphingomyelin declined (Fig. 6.1). The concept of the lecithin–sphingomyelin (L/S) ratio emerged from this report. The ratio between the two phospholipids was used to correct for changes in amniotic fluid volume.

This report was followed by a number of studies on the clinical utility of the L/S ratio for predicting lung maturity. In an early report, Hobbins and coauthors[10] used a lecithin concentration greater than the sphingomyelin concentration as a definition of maturity and found that, regardless of birthweight, infants did not develop RDS if the amniotic fluid phospholipids indicated maturity.

An L/S ratio of 2 : 1 occurs at approximately 35 weeks' gestation (Fig. 6.2) and, in subsequent clinical studies,[11,12] RDS was reported in only 2–3% of infants with a ratio of 2 : 1 or greater. Most of these cases of RDS occurred in infants born to women with diabetes. However, a L/S ratio of less than 2 : 1 was found to have a low predictive value for RDS as almost one-half of the infants with a low L/S ratio failed to develop RDS. In an effort to improve the accuracy of amniotic fluid phospholipid analysis at predicting RDS, other phospholipids such as PG were studied in normal and complicated pregnancies.[12,13] PG was first detected at 34–35 weeks' gestation and the concentration then increased with gestational age. The presence of PG as 3% or more of total phospholipids was found to predict lung maturity. Combining the L/S ratio and PG measurements improved both the positive and the negative predictive accuracy of amniotic fluid phospholipid analysis. This was particularly important in diabetic pregnancies. Class A–C diabetics showed a delayed appearance of PG until 37–39 weeks, whereas class D, F, and R diabetics had a normal or early appearance of PG.

The L/S ratio and PG measurements (L/S–PG) have become a standard means of determining fetal lung maturity. A mature L/S with a positive PG has a negative predictive value (a mature test = clinical maturity) of close to 100%. However, the positive predictive value (an immature test = clinical immaturity) is only around 70%. The L/S–PG test has other drawbacks as well. The test is done by the time-consuming method of thin-layer chromatography. Blood and meconium in the amniotic fluid can greatly reduce the accuracy of the L/S ratio. As a result of these limitations, other methods of determining fetal lung maturity have been evaluated. The ideal method would be reproducible, technically simple, and have a short turnaround time, and it would have both positive and negative predictive accuracy. However, to date, no ideal method has been developed.

In 1972, Clements and coauthors[14] reported a rapid test for surfactant in amniotic fluid called the foam stability or shake test. This was based on the ability of surfactant to produce a stable foam in the presence of ethanol. The technique is fairly simple, requires no special equipment, and results are available rapidly: a "mature" test is indicated by the presence of foam at a 1:2 dilution of amniotic fluid; an "immature" test is indicated by the absence of foam at a 1:1 dilution. The shake test is as good at predicting maturity as the L/S ratio; however, it has a higher false immature rate.[15] As with the L/S ratio, the shake test is not accurate in the presence of blood or meconium. Although it is more easily and rapidly performed than the L/S ratio, the shake test has only been used as a screen and an immature result should be confirmed with an L/S–PG test.

The concentration of lamellar bodies in amniotic fluid is directly related to its absorbance at 650 nm,[16] and this absorbance has been used as a rapid test for fetal lung maturity. However, this test is limited by a very high, false immaturity rate.

Amniotic fluid microviscosity, as determined by fluorescence polarization, has also been used as a fairly rapid method of evaluating lung maturity. Amniotic fluid has a high, constant viscosity until approximately 30–32 weeks' gestation when there is an abrupt decrease followed by a steady decline to term. As with other tests, determination of microviscosity accurately predicts maturity but overestimates immaturity.[17] A refinement of fluorescence polarization uses a ratio of surfactant to albumin rather than microviscosity.[18] As an automated test it is simple to perform and can be carried out quickly, although it does require special instrumentation. A "mature" test correlates well with clinical maturity, but an immature test is not as good a predictor of who will actually develop RDS.

Surfactant proteins in the amniotic fluid have been examined as a way of predicting lung maturity more accurately. King and coauthors[19] assayed amniotic fluid from 12 weeks to term for "surfactant-associated protein," now known to be SP-A. Between 12 and 32 weeks of gestation essentially no protein was found; the protein titers increased from 32 to 37 weeks and then plateaued. This pattern parallels the gestational age-related increase in phospholipids. A more specific monoclonal antibody assay for SP-A was subsequently used to determine the predictive accuracy of protein assay of amniotic fluid.[20] Little protein was found before 32 weeks, there was a slow increase at between 32 and 37 weeks, and a sharp increase after 37 weeks. An SP-A concentration of 3 µg/mL or greater accurately predicted clinical lung maturity but the test was much less accurate in predicting immaturity with a large false-positive rate. When surfactant protein determination was combined with an L/S–PG, the ability to correctly predict immaturity increased. Studies have also indicated that SP-A levels are decreased in amniotic fluid in diabetic pregnancies,[21,22] but a clear clinical role for surfactant protein determination in diabetic pregnancies has not yet been established.

Table 6.1 Predictive value of prenatal tests for lung maturity.

Test	Positive accuracy	Negative accuracy	References
L/S	0.54	0.98	11, 12, 15–18, 20
L/S–PG	0.47	0.99	20, 22
Shake test	0.12	1.0	15
A_{650}	0.13	0.99	16
SP-A	0.32	1.0	20
L/S–PG + 35 kDa	0.71	1.0	20
FELMA	0.33	1.0	17
TDx-FLM	0.31	0.97	18

FELMA, microviscosity by fluorescence polarization; L/S, lecithin–sphingomyelin ratio; PG, phosphatidylglycerol; TDx-FLM, fluorescence polarization, Abbot Laboratories.
Negative test, maturity; *positive test*, immaturity; *negative predictive accuracy*, accuracy with which a mature test predicts no RDS; *positive predictive accuracy*, the accuracy with which an immature test predicts RDS.
The values above were calculated using data from the references cited. (Definitions from Feinstein AR. On the sensitivity, specificity, and discrimination of diagnostic tests. In: Feinstein AR, ed. *Clinical biostatistics*. St. Louis, MO: CV Mosby; 1997.)

Table 6.1 summarizes the predictive accuracy of each of the methods discussed. The values in this table were calculated from the data in the references cited. All of the tests accurately predict lung maturity with a very low false-negative rate. This means that an infant with a mature test has a very low risk of developing RDS, which is of great value in determining the timing of delivery of a complicated pregnancy. Conversely, an infant with an immature L/S ratio has about a 50% chance of developing RDS. Using the presence of PG or surfactant protein analysis together with the L/S ratio reduces the chance of a false mature test.

Acceleration of lung development by antenatal hormone administration

Glucocorticoids

The seminal observation by Liggins that antenatal glucocorticoid administration accelerated lung maturity and improved

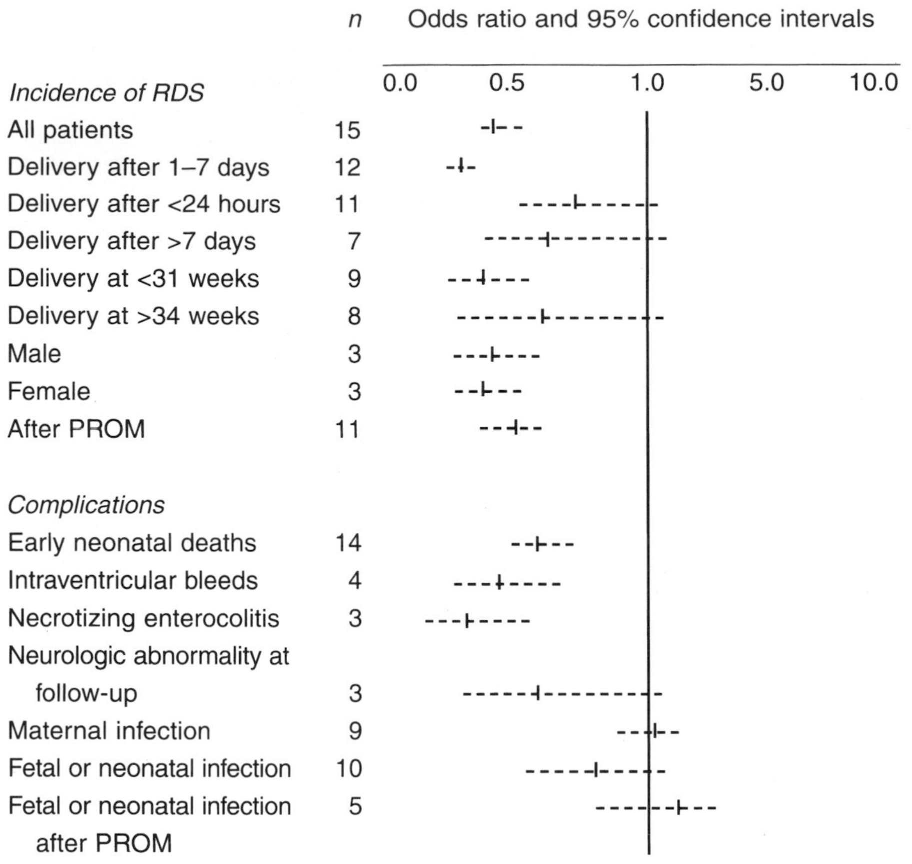

	n	Odds ratio and 95% confidence intervals
		0.0 0.5 1.0 5.0 10.0
Incidence of RDS		
All patients	15	
Delivery after 1–7 days	12	
Delivery after <24 hours	11	
Delivery after >7 days	7	
Delivery at <31 weeks	9	
Delivery at >34 weeks	8	
Male	3	
Female	3	
After PROM	11	
Complications		
Early neonatal deaths	14	
Intraventricular bleeds	4	
Necrotizing enterocolitis	3	
Neurologic abnormality at follow-up	3	
Maternal infection	9	
Fetal or neonatal infection	10	
Fetal or neonatal infection after PROM	5	

Figure 6.3 The effects of antenatal glucocorticoids. Modified from ref. 44. Original data from ref. 24.

viability in prematurely born lamb fetuses led to clinical trials of antenatal steroids and other agents, including TRH. In 1994, the National Institutes of Health (NIH) convened a Consensus Conference to study the impact of glucocorticoid therapy on fetal maturation and perinatal outcome.[23] The conferees relied to a large extent on Crowley's[24] meta-analysis of published randomized trials of antenatal glucocorticoid therapy and on the data from several "observational databases." The latter consisted of treatment and outcome information collected from five sources and involving more than 30 000 infants.

Effect on the incidence of RDS

The meta-analysis[24] (Fig. 6.3) revealed that antenatal glucocorticoid therapy significantly reduced the overall incidence of RDS by approximately 50%. Whereas the effect was statistically significant only in those infants who delivered from 1 to 7 days after the initiation of maternal treatment, there was a trend toward decreased RDS in infants born less than 24 h or more than 7 days after the initiation of steroid treatment. Also, treatment was effective in boys and girls.

Taken as a group, there was a significant reduction in the incidence of RDS in babies born before 31 weeks, but the effectiveness of glucocorticoids in infants born before 28 weeks of gestation was not resolved by these studies. Although it is not clear whether the incidence of RDS was decreased, there was a benefit in terms of diminished severity of RDS, decreased mortality, and a lower incidence of intraventricular hemorrhage (IVH).

Effect on complications of prematurity

The use of antenatal steroid therapy reduces early neonatal mortality as well as two major complications of prematurity, IVH and necrotizing enterocolitis (NEC).

It is reassuring that long-term follow-up of infants exposed to antenatal glucocorticoids revealed no adverse effects on developmental outcome. Studies conducted at 12 years of age found no deficits in motor skills, cognition, or scholastic achievement despite the greater survival rate of premature infants after steroid therapy.[25,26] The meta-analysis actually revealed a trend toward decreased neurological abnormalities at follow-up.

Effects on neonatal and maternal infection

Glucocorticoid therapy does not have a significant effect on the overall incidence of maternal or fetal infection. When steroids were administered in the presence of premature rupture of the membranes (PROM), there was a trend toward an increase in fetal and neonatal infection, but this effect was not statistically significant. The meta-analysis also indicated that steroids decreased the incidence of RDS in the presence of PROM. Furthermore, the observational database revealed that when steroids are administered to women with PROM, there is a decrease in neonatal IVH and mortality. The advantages of using steroids in the presence of PROM appear to outweigh the disadvantages.

Complicated pregnancies

An early report[27] that there was increased fetal mortality when women with hypertension and proteinuria received antenatal steroid therapy has not been confirmed.[28,29] Glucocorticoid administration, however, may adversely affect pregnant women with diabetes and the use of steroids in this situation is a matter of judgment.

Information on the use of glucocorticoids in pregnancies complicated by multiple gestation, intrauterine growth retardation, or hydrops fetalis is, at present, inadequate. Until more information is available, glucocorticoid therapy should probably be used in these situations.

Repeat courses of antenatal glucocorticoids

The incidence of RDS is not significantly decreased in newborns delivered more than 7 days after maternal glucocorticoid treatment.[30] As a result, some obstetricians administer repeated courses of antenatal glucocorticoids during pregnancies threatened by preterm delivery. This practice has raised major concerns. In 2000, a NIH Consensus Development Conference[31] recommended that "because of insufficient data from randomized clinical trials regarding efficacy and safety, repeat courses of corticosteroids should not be used routinely." The American College of Obstetricians and Gynecologists (ACOG)[32] supported this recommendation in 2002. Three trials addressing this issue have now been completed[33–35] and their data have been summarized in a systematic review.[36] These trials found that there is a reduction in the severity of lung disease or decreased need for surfactant therapy in patients who receive repeated doses of glucocorticoids. However, there was no statistically significant difference between groups with regard to the incidence of RDS, chronic lung disease, IVH, periventricular leukomalacia (PVL), and fetal, neonatal, or infant death.[36] Concern over the safety of repetitive courses of antenatal glucocorticoids stems from animal studies that have reported adverse long-term outcomes such as growth retardation,[37] suppression of brain growth,[38] and neuronal myelination,[39] and clinical trials that have reported suppression of adrenal function,[40] increased risk of destructive and hyperactive behavior in children,[41] and increased mortality.[40] Sufficient concern has been raised by these observations to support limiting the number of courses of antenatal corticosteroids to one, as recommended by ACOG (or perhaps at most two, with the second course being administered if the patient again demonstrates threatened preterm labor, weeks after the initial course of glucocorticoid).

Betamethasone versus dexamethasone

Dexamethasone and betamethasone are structurally similar glucocorticoids that differ only in the configuration of a single methyl group, and that have equal ability to cross the placenta and influence fetal function.[42] However, there is a growing body of evidence suggesting that dexamethasone may have more significant side-effects than betamethasone. In addition, Crowley's systematic review indicated that there was a significant reduction in neonatal mortality in the patients treated with betamethasone compared with those treated with dexamethasone.[24]

In 1999, Baud and coauthors[42] retrospectively examined the effects of antenatal betamethasone, dexamethasone, or no glucocorticoid treatment on neonates of 24–31 weeks' gestation. After adjusting for differences in gestational age, number of courses of glucocorticoids, and other possible confounding variables, they found no significant differences between the two glucocorticoids with respect to the incidence of RDS, bronchopulmonary dysplasia, IVH, or necrotizing enterocolitis. However, there was a significant reduction in the risk of cystic PVL in the group treated with betamethasone compared with the no-treatment group, whereas those neonates whose mothers had received antenatal dexamethasone had an increased risk of cystic PVL compared with the no-treatment group.

A number of theories have been put forward to account for the increased toxicity of dexamethasone. One suggestion is that it relates to sulfite preservatives which are used in dexamethasone preparations.[43] An *in vivo* and *in vitro* study found that there is increased neuronal death after exposure to pharmacological preparations of dexamethasone-containing sulfites or to isolated sulfites. The dose of glucocorticoid used in this study was approximately 10 times that recommended for antenatal administration. An alternative, and probably more likely, explanation is that when dexamethasone is administered intravenously or intramuscularly, it reaches higher peak blood levels than the slowly released intramuscular (i.m.) betamethasone. These high circulating levels of dexamethasone may cause the observed neuronal damage.[44] At this stage, betamethasone should be regarded as the glucocorticoid of choice.

Synergism between antenatal glucocorticoid and postnatal surfactant therapies

Animal and clinical data indicate that there is a positive interaction between antenatal glucocorticoid administration and postnatal surfactant therapy. In a clinical trial, infants who were treated with antenatal steroids and received surfactant, if indicated, had significantly less respiratory disease as well as a lower incidence of IVH or periventricular leukomalacia than infants who did not receive antenatal steroids.[45]

Conclusions

The recommendations of the NIH Consensus Conference[23] are summarized in Table 6.2. It is clear that there are few situations when steroids should not be used in women with threatened preterm labor. Repeated courses of glucocorticoid, however, should not be routinely administered during pregnancy. Betamethasone is the glucocorticoid of choice.

At present, optimal management of premature infants includes assessment of fetal lung maturation, antenatal glucocorticoid administration, and postnatal surfactant therapy. This approach has been shown to be highly beneficial for the prevention and treatment of RDS and other major complications of prematurity.

Table 6.2 NIH Consensus Development Conference. Recommendations for use of antenatal glucocorticoids.

The benefits of antenatal corticosteroids "vastly" outweigh the risks
All fetuses at risk for preterm delivery between 24 and 34 weeks of gestation are candidates for treatment
This decision should not be altered by race, gender, or availability of surfactant therapy
Patients who are eligible for tocolytic therapy are also eligible for steroid therapy
Treatment should be given unless immediate delivery is expected; treatment for less than 24 h is associated with decreased mortality, RDS, and intraventricular hemorrhage
In cases of PROM at less than 30–32 weeks of gestation, treatment is recommended in the absence of clinical chorioamnionitis
In complicated pregnancies in which delivery before 34 weeks is expected, treatment is recommended unless there is evidence that it will have an adverse effect on the mother
Dosing: betamethasone, 12 mg i.m. q24 h × 2 (or dexamethasone, 6 mg i.m. q12 h × 4)

Key points

1 The major phospholipids in surfactant are phosphatidylcholine (PC, also called lecithin), which accounts for 80–85% of total phospholipid, and phosphatidylglycerol (PG), which accounts for 8–11%.

2 Surfactant protein A (SP-A) is a component of the innate immune system of the lung; mice deficient in SP-A are more likely to develop pulmonary and systemic infections.

3 Two smaller proteins, SP-B and SP-C, are important for the surface-active properties of surfactant and are present in clinically effective surfactant preparations.

4 At the same gestational age, males are more likely than females to develop RDS. Amniotic fluid phospholipid analysis indicates that the biochemical maturity of the female lung precedes that of males by around 1 week.

5 An L/S ratio of 2 : 1 occurs at approximately 35 weeks of gestation. RDS was reported in only 2–3% of infants with a ratio of 2 : 1 or greater.

6 Combining L/S ratio and PG measurements improves both the positive and the negative predictive accuracy of amniotic fluid phospholipid analysis. This is particularly important in diabetic pregnancies.

7 Some clinical conditions appear to accelerate lung maturation and decrease the incidence of RDS. These include long-term maternal stress, e.g., toxemia and hypertension, intrauterine growth retardation, maternal infection, and maternal heroin exposure.

8 The benefits of antenatal corticosteroids vastly outweigh the risks.

9 All fetuses at risk for preterm delivery between 24 and 34 weeks of gestation are candidates for antenatal glucocorticoid treatment.

10 Glucocorticoid therapy significantly reduces the overall incidence of RDS by approximately 50%.

11 The effect of glucocorticoid therapy on RDS is statistically significant in infants who deliver from 1 to 7 days after the initiation of maternal treatment. There is a trend toward decreased RDS in babies born less than 24 h or more than 7 days after the initiation of steroid treatment.

12 Although it is not clear whether glucocorticoids decrease the incidence of RDS in infants below 28 weeks' gestation, there is a benefit in terms of diminished severity of RDS, and reduced incidence of intraventricular hemorrhage (IVH) and necrotizing enterocolitis (NEC) as well as decreased neonatal mortality.

13 Glucocorticoid therapy does not have a significant effect on the overall incidence of maternal or fetal infection.

14 In cases of prolonged rupture of the membranes (PROM) at less than 30–32 weeks of gestation, treatment is recommended in the absence of clinical chorioamnionitis.

15 A National Institutes of Health (NIH) Consensus Development Conference and the American College of Obstetricians and Gynecologists (ACOG) recommend that repeat courses of corticosteroids should not be used routinely during pregnancy.

16 Administration of antenatal betamethasone has been reported to result in a significant reduction in the risk of cystic periventricular leukomalacia (PVL), whereas neonates whose mothers receive antenatal dexamethasone have an increased risk of cystic PVL.

17 Betamethasone is the glucocorticoid of choice for antenatal steroid therapy.

18 Antenatal betamethasone, if indicated, should be given unless immediate delivery is expected. Treatment for less than 24 h is associated with decreased mortality and IVH, and a trend to reduced severity of RDS.

19 The recommended dose of betamethasone is 12 mg i.m. q24 h × 2. If dexamethasone is used, the dose is 6 mg i.m. q12 h × 4.

20 Infants whose mothers were treated with antenatal steroids and who then received postnatal surfactant, if indicated, showed a significant reduction in respiratory disease as well as a lower incidence of IVH or PVL than infants whose mothers did not receive antenatal steroids.

References

1 Rooney SA. The surfactant system and lung phospholipid biochemistry. *Am Rev Resp Dis* 1985;131:439–460.

2 Rooney SA, Wai Lee TS, Gobran L, et al. Phospholipid content, composition and biosynthesis during fetal lung development in the rabbit. *Biochim Biophys Acta* 1976;431:447–458.

3 LeVine AM, Kurak KE, Wright JR, et al. Surfactant protein-A binds group B streptococcus enhancing phagocytosis and clearance from lungs of surfactant protein-A-deficient mice. *Am J Respir Cell Mol Biol* 1999;20:279–286.

4 LeVine AM, Elliott J, Whitsett JA, et al. Surfactant protein-d enhances phagocytosis and pulmonary clearance of respiratory syncytial virus. *Am J Respir Cell Mol Biol* 2004;31:193–199.

5 Olver RE. Of labor and the lungs. *Arch Dis Child* 1981;56:659–662.

6 Torday JS, Nielson HC, Fencl MDM, et al. Sex differences in fetal lung maturation. *Am Rev Resp Dis* 1981;123:205–208.

7 Gross I. Regulation of fetal lung maturation. *Am J Physiol (Lung Cell Mol Physiol)* 1990;259:L337–L344.

8 Ballard PL, Ballard RA. Scientific basis and therapeutic regimens for use of antenatal glucocorticoids. *Am J Obstet Gynecol* 1995;173:254–262.

9 Gluck L, Kulovich MV, Borer RC, et al. Diagnosis of the respiratory distress syndrome by amniocentesis. *Am J Obstet Gynecol* 1971;109:440–445.

10 Hobbins JC, Brock W, Speroff L, et al. L/S ratio in predicting pulmonary maturity *in utero*. *Obstet Gynecol* 1972;39:660–664.

11 Donald IR, Freeman RK, Goebelsmann U, et al. Clinical experience with the amniotic fluid lecithin/sphingomyelin ratio. I: antenatal prediction of pulmonary maturity. *Am J Obstet Gynecol* 1973;115:547–552.

12 Kulovich M, Hallman M, Gluck L. The lung profile. I: normal pregnancy. *Am J Obstet Gynecol* 1979;135:57–63.

13 Kulovich M, Gluck L. The lung profile. II: complicated pregnancy. *Am J Obstet Gynecol* 1979;135:64–70.

14 Clements JA, Platzker ACG, Tierney DF, et al. Assessment of the risk of the respiratory distress syndrome by a rapid test for surfactant in amniotic fluid. *N Engl J Med* 1972;286:1077–1081.

15 Goldstein AS, Fukunaga K, Malachowski N, et al. A comparison of the lecithin/sphingomyelin ratio and shake test for estimating fetal pulmonary maturity. *Am J Obstet Gynecol* 1972;118: 1132–1135.

16 Copeland W. Rapid assessment of fetal pulmonary maturity. *Am J Obstet Gynecol* 1979;135:1048–1050.

17 Golde SH, Mosley GH. A blind comparison study of the lung phospholipid profile, fluorescence microviscosimetry and the lecithin/sphingomyelin ratio. *Am J Obstet Gynecol* 1980;136. 222–227.

18 Russell JC, Cooper CM, Ketchum CH, et al. Multicenter evaluation of TD_x test for assessing fetal lung maturity. *Clin Chem* 1989;35:1005–1010.

19 King RJ, Ruch J, Gikas EG, et al. Appearance of apoproteins of pulmonary surfactant in human amniotic fluid. *J Appl Physiol* 1975;39:735–741.

20 Hallman M, Arjomaa P, Mizumoto M, et al. Surfactant proteins in the diagnosis of fetal lung maturity. I: predictive accuracy of the 35 kd protein, the lecithin/sphingomyelin ratio, and phosphatidylglycerol. *Am J Obstet Gynecol* 1988;158:5315.

21 Snyder JM, Kwun JE, O'Brien JA, et al. The concentration of the 35-kDa surfactant apoprotein in amniotic fluid from normal and diabetic pregnancies. *Pediatr Res* 1988;24:728–734.

22 Katyal SL, Amenta JS, Singh AG, et al. Deficient lung surfactant apoproteins in amniotic fluid with mature phospholipid profile from diabetic pregnancies. *Am J Obstet Gynecol* 1984;148:48–53.

23 National Insitutes of Health Consensus Development Panel. Effect of corticosteroids for fetal maturation on perinatal outcomes. *JAMA* 1995;273:413–418.

24 Crowley P. Antenatal corticosteroid therapy: a meta-analysis of the randomized trials, 1972 to 1994. *Am J Obstet Gynecol* 1995;173:322–335.

25 Smolders-de Haas H, Neuvel J, Schmand B, et al. Physical development and medical history of children who were treated antenatally with corticosteroids to prevent respiratory distress syndrome: a 10 to 12 year follow-up. *Pediatrics* 1989;86:65–70.

26 Schmand B, Neuvel J, Smolders-de Haas H, et al. Psychological development of children who were treated antenatally with corticosteroids to prevent respiratory distress syndrome. *Pediatrics* 1990;86:58–64.

27 Liggins GC, Howie RN. A controlled trial of antepartum glucocorticoid treatment for prevention of the respiratory distress syndrome in premature infants. *Pediatrics* 1972;50:515–525.

28 Collaborative Group on Antenatal Steroid Therapy. Effects of antenatal dexamethasone administration on the prevention of respiratory distress syndrome. *Am J Obstet Gynecol* 1981;141: 276–287.

29 Gamsu HR. Antenatal administration of betamethasone to prevent respiratory distress syndrome in preterm infants: report of a UK multicentre trial. *Br J Obstet Gynaecol* 1989;96:401–410.
30 Crowley P. Prophylactic corticosteroids for preterm birth. *Cochrane Database Syst Rev* 2004;2.
31 National Institutes of Health Consensus Development Conference Statement. *Antenatal corticosteroids revisited: repeat courses*. NIH Consensus Statement. August 17–18, 2000;17:1–10.
32 American College of Obstetricians and Gynecologists. *Antenatal corticosteroid therapy for fetal maturation*. Committee Opinions 2002;273:9–11.
33 Aghajafari F, Murphy K, Ohlsson A, et al. Multiple versus single courses of antenatal corticosteroids for preterm birth: a pilot study. *J Obstet Gynaecol Canada* 2002;24:321–329.
34 Guinn D, Atkinson M, Sullivan L, et al. Single versus weekly courses of antenatal corticosteroids for women at risk of preterm delivery. *JAMA* 2001;286:1581–1587.
35 McEvoy C, Bowling S, Williamson R, et al. The effect of a single remote course versus weekly courses of antenatal corticosteroids on functional residual capacity in preterm infants: a randomized trial. *Pediatrics* 2002;110:280–284.
36 Crowther CA, Harding J. Repeat doses of prenatal corticosteroids for women at risk of preterm birth for preventing neonatal respiratory disease. *Cochrane Database Syst Rev* 2004;2.
37 Ikegami M, Jobe AH, Newnham J, et al. Repetitive prenatal corticosteroids improve lung function and decrease growth in preterm lambs. *Am J Respir Crit Care Med* 1997;156;178–184.
38 Modi N, Lewis H, Al-Naqeeb N, et al. The effects of repeated antenatal glucocorticoid therapy on the developing brain. *Pediatr Res* 2001;50:581–585.
39 Dunlop SA, Archer MA, Quinlivan JA, et al. Repeated prenatal corticosteroids delay myelination in the ovine central nervous system. *J Matern Fet Med* 1997;6:309–313.
40 Banks BA, Cnaan A, Morgan MA, et al. Multiple courses of antenatal corticosteroids and outcome of premature neonates. North American thyrotropin-releasing hormone study group. *Am J Obstet Gynecol* 1999;181:709–717.
41 French NP, Hagan R, Evans SF, et al. Repeated antenatal corticosteroids: effects on cerebral palsy and childhood behavior. *Am J Obstet Gynecol* 2004;190:588–595.
42 Baud O, Foix-L'Helias L, Kaminski M, et al. Antenatal glucocorticoid treatment and cystic periventricular leukomalacia in very premature infants. *N Engl J Med* 1999;341:1190–1196.
43 Baud O, Laudenbach V, Laudenbach E, et al. Neurotoxic effects of fluorinated glucocorticoid preparations on the developing mouse brain: role of preservatives. *Pediatr Res* 2001;50:706–711.
44 Gross I, Ballard PL. Hormonal therapy for prevention of respiratory distress syndrome. In: Polin RA, Fox WW, Abman SH, eds. *Fetal and neonatal physiology*, 3rd edn. Philadelphia, PA: Elsevier; 2003:1069–1074.
45 Kari MA, Hallman M, Eronen M, et al. Prenatal dexamethasone treatment in conjunction with rescue therapy of human surfactant: a randomized placebo-controlled multicenter study. *Pediatrics* 1994;93:730–736.

7 Fetal cardiovascular physiology and response to stress conditions

Jean-Claude Fouron and Amanda Skoll

Fetal cardiovascular physiology

Functional characteristics of the fetal heart

Functional maturational processes

Significant maturational changes are observed in the structure of the myocardium prior to birth.[1] In more immature myocardial cells, the myofibrils are chaotically organized and often not oriented along the long axis of the cell. These cells are also characterized by a proportionally greater amount of noncontractile proteins than in adult cells. A maturational increase in the myofilament content of myocytes is observed progressively along with a rearrangement of these filaments into an orientation along the long axis of the cells. The nuclei and mitochondria, which were localized at the centre of the cell, are ultimately distributed in an ordered arrangement along the myofilaments. Primitive mesodermal cells lose their ability to differentiate into cardiomyocytes at approximately the time of birth; consequently, fetal cardiomyocytes may divide and increase in number, whereas mature adult cardiomyocytes can only increase in size.

The sarcoplasmic reticulum is also the site of developmental changes.[2,3] In the mature myocardium, the sarcoplasmic reticulum serves as the site of calcium release and removal, which activates the contractile process. The process of calcium removal from troponin C, responsible for myocardial relaxation, has also been shown to be less rapid in the fetus[4] compared with the adult myocardium. Many elements suggest that the effectiveness of the sarcoplasmic reticulum in storing and releasing calcium is quantitatively enhanced with maturation. Thus, more immature cells rely mainly on trans-sarcolemmal movement of calcium to modulate their cytosolic concentration.

In addition to these structural modifications, there are biochemical differences in fetal and adult forms of the myocardial contractile proteins myosin, actin, and the troponins, as well as in their sensitivity to cytosolic calcium concentration.[5,6] As far as we know, cardiac myosin is made up of two heavy chains, alpha and beta. There are three known myosin isozymes based on the distribution of these two chains. The V1 isozyme contains two alpha chains, V2 contains an alpha and a beta chain, and V3 has two beta chains. The slower V3 myosin is the predominant adult form in larger animals, including humans. Ventricles with different proportions of myosin V1 and V3 may perform similar amounts of work. However, the myocardium, with a higher proportion of V3, consumes a relatively smaller amount of oxygen and adenosine triphosphate (ATP) and, therefore, demonstrates greater efficiency. Lactate is the primary agent metabolized in the immature heart, whereas the adult myocardium preferentially consumes long-chain fatty acids.[7] A fetal deficiency in carnitine palmitoyl transferase hampers the transport of long-chain fatty acids into the mitochondria.

Another contractile protein, titin, also known as connectin, has been shown to play a major role in myocardial mechanics.[8] Titin is likely to be a factor in setting the lower sarcomere length limit during systole and in the elastic recoil responsible for early diastolic filling. A recent report, showing that fetal cardiac titin contains additional spring elements not found in adults, suggests that regulation of titin's spring composition may allow adjustment of diastolic filling behavior during the development of the heart.[9]

Fetal myocardial contractility

When isolated fetal muscle strips are studied, there is a significant reduction in the active tension that can be generated compared with adult samples, at all muscle lengths along the length–tension curve.[10] Resting tension is, however, higher in fetal tissue. These contractile characteristics of fetal myocytes have been related to their significantly greater proportion of noncontractile protein (60% in the fetal myocardium compared with 30% in adults)[10] and also to the differences in the activity of ATPase of fetal and adult myosin isoforms.[6]

Effect of changes in preload

The concept that the fetus has a stiff heart was the basis of a controversy concerning its ability to respond to the Frank–Starling mechanism. For some time, it had been accepted that

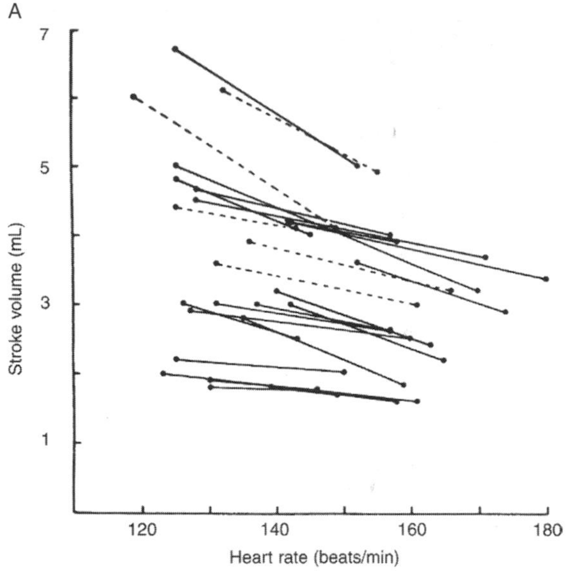

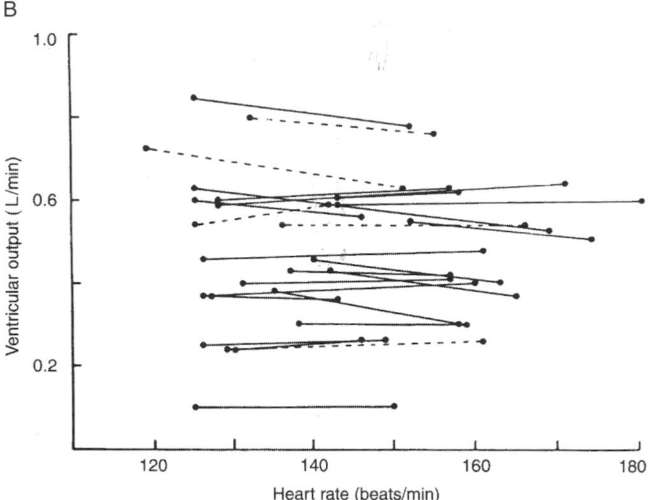

Figure 7.1 (A) Demonstration of the capacity of fetal ventricles to increase their stroke volume with a decrease in heart rate. (B) Consequently, no change is observed in ventricular outputs with bradycardia. Solid line, left ventricle; dotted line, right ventricle (reprinted with permission from ref. 14).

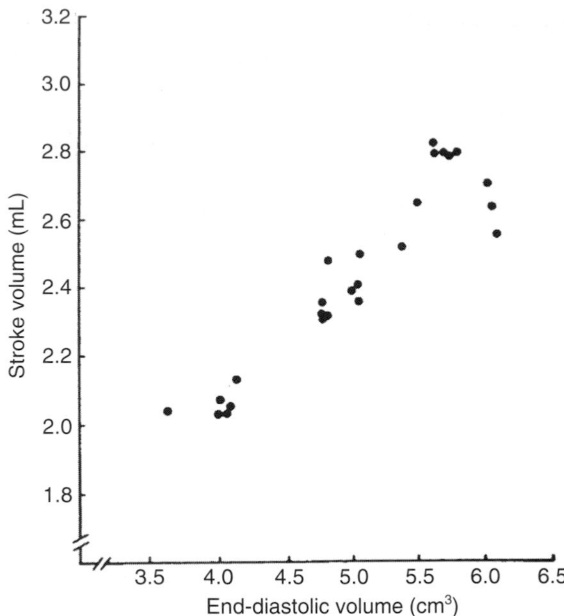

Figure 7.2 Relationship between end-diastolic volume (LVEDV) and stroke volume (SV) of the left ventricle in the fetal lamb (reprinted with permission from ref. 1).

variation in fetal cardiac output was essentially linked to changes in heart rate.[11] This position was apparently strengthened by observations that volume infusion in fetal lambs did not result in any significant increase in either right or left ventricular output.[12,13] However, because of great compliance of the umbilical placental circulation, volume infusion in the fetal circulation requires a relatively greater amount of fluid to achieve a significant change in venous return.

More recent investigations based on Doppler echocardiography have revealed that changes in fetal heart rate are not necessarily associated with alterations in cardiac output[14] (Fig. 7.1). Furthermore, the Frank–Starling relationship has been shown to be present in the isolated fetal myocardium.[10] As would be anticipated, when the relationship is plotted between muscle tension and the extent or velocity of shortening, the fetal value always falls below that of the adult myocardium. Other evidence of a functional Frank–Starling mechanism was demonstrated when the maximum rate of rise of left ventricular pressure (dp/dt max) was used to assess the effect of changes in end-diastolic volume in fetal lambs.[1] In addition, because of its relative stiffness,[15] end-diastolic pressure is not a reliable index for evaluation of the Frank–Starling relationship in the fetal heart. A large change in diastolic pressure may produce relatively little change in end-diastolic volume. In fact, when ventricular dimensions are used to assess the effect of preload on fetal ventricular stroke volume, a significant positive relationship between end-diastolic volume and stroke volume is found in the fetal heart[1] (Fig. 7.2). Echocardiography permits the documentation of two clinical examples of the capacity of the fetal heart to respond to myocardial fiber stretching: first, fetuses with congenital atrioventricular block with heart rates around 60 b.p.m. show an increase in end-diastolic diameters of both ventricles without cardiac failure and, secondly, there is evidence of a postectopic increase in stroke volume in fetuses with arrhythmia. Finally, it must be remembered that, in the fetal heart, manifestations of the Frank–Starling mechanism can be hampered by diastolic–ventricular interaction. Indeed, because of the widely patent foramen ovale, any increase in right ventricular end-diastolic pressure should be transmitted to the left ventricle. The simultaneous increase in diastolic pressures on both sides of the ventricular septum should limit the possibility of volume expansion of one ventricle and, by the same token, should impose limitations on the Frank–Starling mechanism. Similarly, extrinsic compression of the fetal heart by the chest wall, pleural pressure, and fluid-filled lungs and pericardium have also been proposed as factors constraining fetal stroke volume.[16]

Thus, the fetal myocardium has the ability, albeit limited, to respond to the Frank–Starling mechanism. The various components of fetal ventricular preload must be clarified, however, as they are quite different from those of extrauterine life. *In utero*, each ventricle must be considered separately. In a normal fetus, left ventricular preload will be greatly influenced not only by the size of the foramen ovale but also by approximately 30–40% of the volume flow coming from the inferior vena cava, by pulmonary venous return, and by the diastolic filling characteristics of the right side. Based on data gathered from experimental lamb preparations, it had been widely accepted that no more than 7–10% of combined cardiac output goes to the lungs, a phenomenon explained by elevated pulmonary vascular resistance during fetal life.[17,18] More recent reports using the Doppler technique on normal human fetuses showed that pulmonary blood flow increased by almost fourfold over the period of gestation studied and amounted to a mean of 22–25% of combined ventricular output. Thus, pulmonary venous return becomes a significant component of left ventricular preload, at least during the third trimester of gestation.[19,20] Diastolic function of the right ventricle should also influence left ventricular preload during fetal life via the widely patent foramen ovale, which allows the transmission of flow and pressure from the right to the left atrium.

On the other hand, right ventricular volume load during fetal life is normally made up of the entire volume flow coming from the superior vena cava (21% of total venous return)[18] and the fraction of inferior vena cava return that does not go through the foramen ovale. Consequently, factors that will influence right to left shunting through the foramen will also modify right ventricular preload. For example, although an increase in left atrial pressure, such as that observed in left ventricular diastolic dysfunction, will have little repercussion on right atrial pressure because of secondary sealing of the foramen ovale by the septum primum, this will nevertheless cause significant volume overload of the right ventricle by rerouting the entire inferior vena cava blood toward the right ventricle.

Effect of changes in afterload

In all cardiac preparations, including those using fetal tissue, the shortening ability of the myocardium is decreased as afterload is increased.[10] When the relationship between shortening velocity and afterload of the fetal myocardium is compared with that of the adult, the fetal myocardium shortens more slowly against the same relative load than does the adult myocardium. Interestingly, studies on fetal lambs have shown that, for a similar increase in afterload, a significantly greater reduction in right compared with left ventricular stroke volume was observed.[21,22]

Approximately 65% of the blood ejected by the left ventricle perfuses the upper body.[18] Therefore, any changes in resistance or pressure of the vascular beds in this region will specifically influence afterload of the fetal left heart. On the other hand, the right ventricular outlet during intrauterine life consists of a large main pulmonary artery from which smaller left and right arteries branch off at very sharp angles. The widely patent ductus arteriosus forms a natural prolongation of the main pulmonary artery toward the descending thoracic aorta. Somewhere between 80% and 90% of blood ejected by the right ventricle flows with minimal resistance through the ductus arteriosus into the descending thoracic aorta. Because of this arrangement, fetal right ventricular afterload is essentially dictated by resistances of the various vascular beds perfused by the descending aorta. Among these vascular networks, the placenta plays a key role in establishing the level of right ventricular afterload because of its significantly lower resistance and higher volume flow.

Fetal systolic and diastolic ventricular performances

When combined right and left ventricular output/min normalized to unit fetal body weight is used to examine the ability of the developing heart to eject blood, very little difference is noted from 18 weeks of gestation to term in the human fetus, similar to that in the fetal lamb. At term, combined ventricular output of the human fetus, calculated by Doppler echocardiography, is approximately 450 mL/kg/min.[23,24] The same value has also been found in fetal lambs by radioactive microsphere techniques.[18] Likewise, right ventricular preponderance has been found in the human fetus, as described previously in sheep, and is expressed by right ventricular stroke volume approximately 20% greater than that of the left ventricle. Pressure development in the fetal left ventricle appears to be similar to that in the adult. For example, the peak first derivative of left ventricular pressure (dp/dt max) has the same range in fetal lambs as it has in adult sheep (1500–3000 mmHg/s).[1] This range is the same as that observed in the human child and adult. Likewise, the mean value of 0.36 ± 0.06 found in normal human fetuses for the myocardial performance index,[25] a global index of cardiac function, is similar to values for the same index in normal adults (0.39 ± 0.05) .[26] Peak velocity and acceleration time in the ascending aorta have also been used as a Doppler index of myocardial performance. Unlike adults, in normal fetuses, acceleration time or time to peak velocity is known to be shorter in the fetal pulmonary artery than in the aorta.[27] This finding has been explained by the higher resistance of the fetal pulmonary vascular system. However, as mentioned previously, the right ventricle is ejecting blood toward the placenta through the widely patent ductus arteriosus. The possibility deserves investigation that, in normal fetuses, the shorter acceleration time is due to better right ventricular

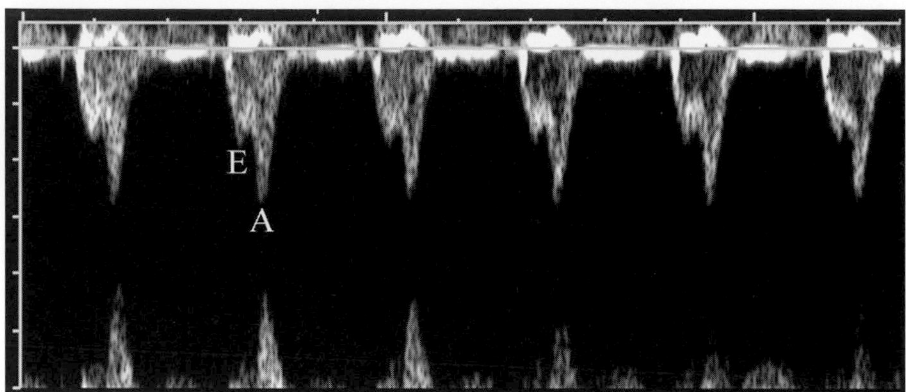

Figure 7.3 Example of Doppler flow velocity waveforms through the tricuspid valve of a fetus at 22 weeks of gestation. The A waves are predominant.

performance with a higher stroke volume and a lower afterload.

In summary, the systolic performance of the fetal heart does not seem to be affected by the maturational changes observed in sarcomeres throughout gestation. In contrast, the limitations are more apparent during diastole. With the advent of Doppler ultrasound technology, it has been possible to study blood flow velocity patterns through the fetal atrioventricular valves; they are quite different from those seen during postnatal life. In extrauterine life, there is a predominance of the E wave, reflecting the major contribution of the early relaxation process causing rapid filling of the ventricles during the first part of diastole. In contrast, the fetal profile is characterized by a higher peak A than E wave[28] (Fig. 7.3). Throughout pregnancy, the peak velocity of the A wave does not change significantly, whereas that of the E wave rises steadily and is entirely responsible for the increase in the E/A ratio[29] (Fig. 7.4). This observation would support the concept of a progressive maturational change predominantly involving the active process of ventricular relaxation.

Fetal circulatory dynamics

Four basic elements characterize the dynamics of the fetal circulation: parallel arrangement of the ventricles; high resistance of the pulmonary circulation; the placental vascular system with its low resistance and relatively high flow; and the presence of shunts.

Parallel arrangement of the ventricles

In the fetus, both ventricular pumps are perfusing the same systemic circulation, the left via the ascending aorta, the right via the pulmonary trunk and the ductus arteriosus. Figure 7.5 is a schematic representation of this feature. The hemodynamic implications of this arrangement are presented in Table 7.1. In this situation, the individual ventricular outputs are not necessarily equal, and fetal cardiac output is logically expressed as combined ventricular output. Another consequence of this arrangement is that both ventricles share the same systolic ejection pressure of approximately 70–80 mmHg. Close to term, a slight increase in pressure has been reported in the pulmonary trunk compared with systemic pressure. This could be due to either greater flow through the right ventricle and/or active constriction of the ductus arteriosus. As a third consequence, there is the reciprocal influence of diastolic function of the two ventricles through a widely patent foramen ovale. The parallel arrangement of the two ventricles is also a key element in the intrauterine survival of fetuses with complex malformations; in cases of hypoplasia of one ventricle, for example, blood can be diverted toward the contralateral ventricle without significant impairment of peripheral perfusion.

Table 7.1 Hemodynamic implications of the parallel arrangement of the two ventricles.

Inequality of ventricular outputs
Similarity of systolic pressures
Reciprocal influence of ventricular diastolic functions
Possibility of adequate perfusion by a single ventricle
Special status of the aortic isthmus

Finally, the parallel arrangement of the two ventricles confers special status to the aortic isthmus. This vascular segment, localized between the origin of the left subclavian artery and the aortic end of the ductus arteriosus, establishes communication between the two parallel systems. The direction of blood flow through the fetal aortic isthmus should reflect the balance between both left and right ventricular outputs, and the vascular resistances, of the upper body on one side and the subdiaphragmatic circulation on the other side. This specific aspect will be discussed later in the chapter.

The pulmonary circulation

The fetal pulmonary arteries, offering high resistance to flow, are responsible for relatively minor pulmonary flow. This proportion, however, increases with advancing gestation. As mentioned previously, recent reports using Doppler technology found that, in term human fetuses, as much as 25% of combined ventricular output goes through the lungs.[14,15] This

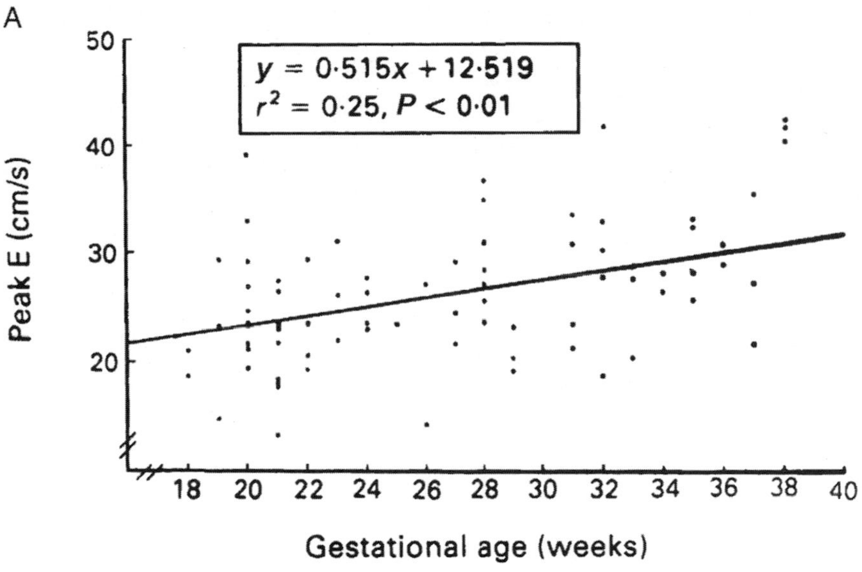

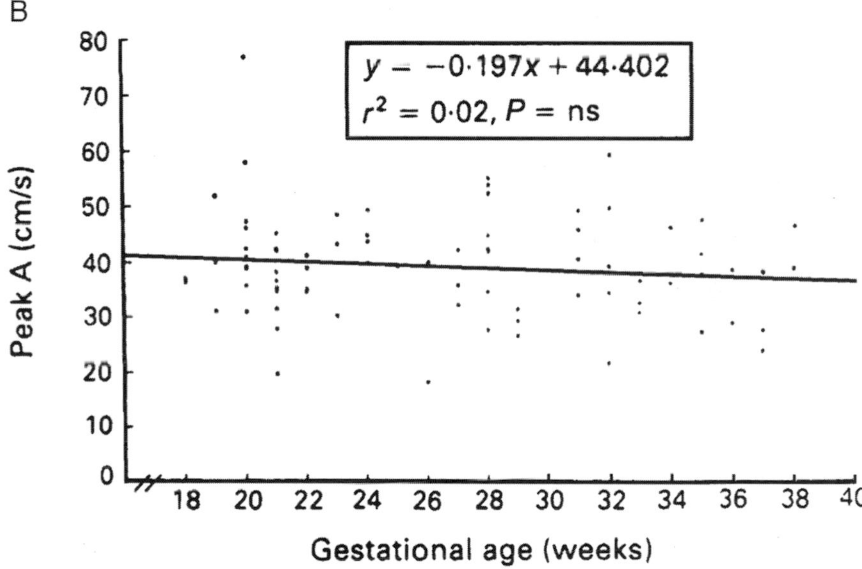

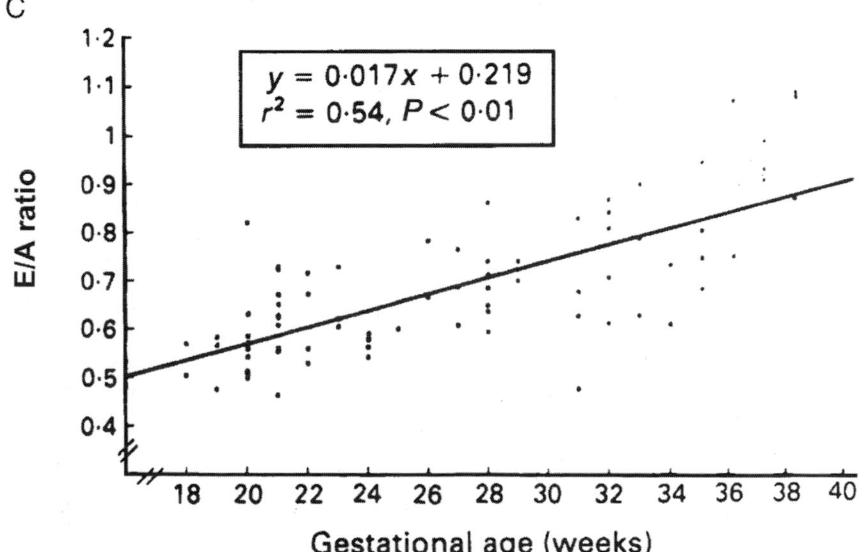

Figure 7.4 (A) With advancing gestation, the early peak velocity (E wave) of the fetal atrioventricular valves increases, while (B) the second peak (A wave) remains unchanged, resulting in (C) a progressive increase in the E/A ratio (adapted with permission from ref. 29).

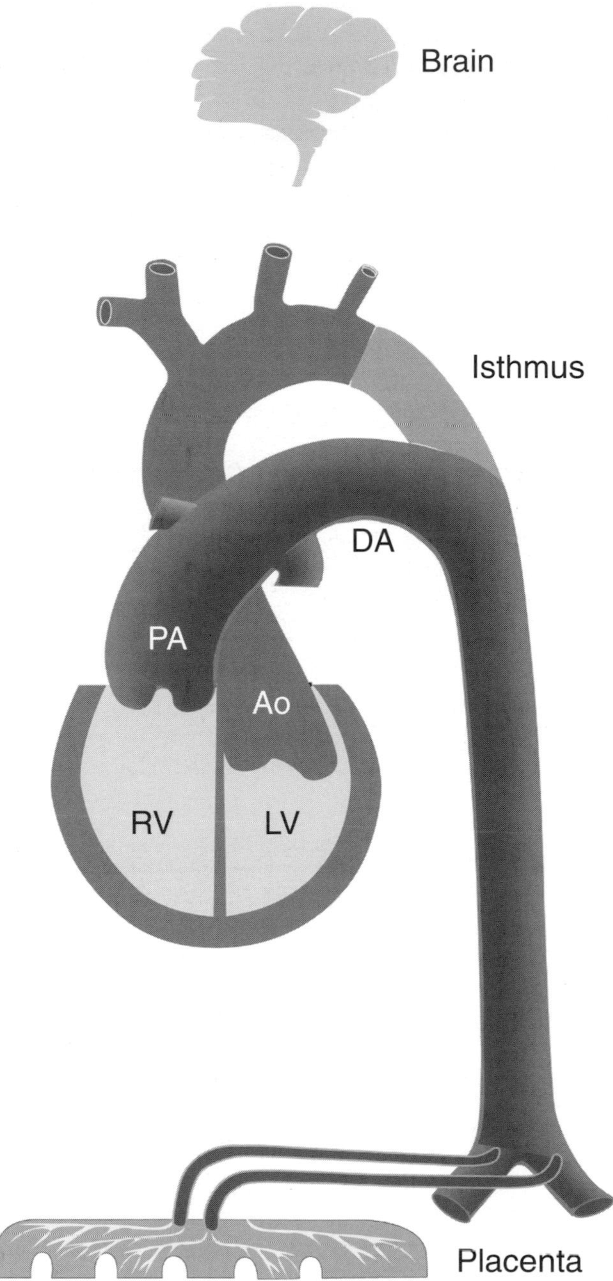

Figure 7.5 Schematic representation of the fetal circulatory dynamics. The right (RV) and left (LV) ventricles are perfusing the systemic circulation in parallel. The upper part of the body receives blood exclusively from the LV. In addition to the lungs, RV perfuses the subdiaphragmatic part of the circulation via the ductus arteriosus (DA). The parallel disposition of the pulmonary (PA) and the aortic (Ao) arches is well illustrated. The isthmus represents a vascular segment connecting these two parallel systems.

unique feature of intrauterine life is related to both morphological and dynamic factors. Major developmental changes occur in the pulmonary circulation throughout pregnancy, and these changes continue after birth.[30,31] In humans, the preacinar branching pattern of the pulmonary arteries is complete by 20 weeks of gestation; subsequently, extensive ramification of small pulmonary arteries is observed, with these arteries increasing in number until term. Some intra-acinar arteriolar growth occurs late in gestation, but this developmental process is mainly associated with alveolar growth in the first years of life. The progressive morphological changes are responsible for a low total cross-sectional pulmonary vascular area in the first half of gestation and, at least in part, for the high vascular resistance observed *in utero*. However, a 20-fold increase in the cross-sectional area of the pulmonary vascular bed has been documented during the latter half of gestation. This growth would cause a significant drop in vascular resistance if it was not for the concomitant development of a thick muscular layer in the walls of the pulmonary arteries to the level of the terminal bronchioles. This muscular layer is the site of reactivity of fetal intrapulmonary arterial branches.

One of the main determinants of pulmonary vascular tone during fetal and extrauterine life is oxygen. Reduced pulmonary (mixed venous) and systemic arterial blood oxygen tension has been demonstrated to cause pulmonary vasoconstriction in fetal sheep.[32,33] Normally low fetal mixed venous PO_2 (16–18 mmHg) therefore plays a major role in maintaining elevated pulmonary vascular resistance during intrauterine life. The mechanisms by which oxygen influences pulmonary vascular tone and the role played by other elements have been the subjects of extensive investigation.[34-37] From these studies, it appears that the pulmonary circulation can be influenced not only by local changes in O_2, but also by many other factors, acting either directly or as mediators or messengers. Among them, neurochemicals, such as alpha-adrenergic agonists and beta-antagonists, constrict whereas alpha-adrenergic antagonists and beta-agonists dilate the pulmonary circulation before and after birth. Vasoconstrictors, such as endothelin, have also been shown to be involved in the modulation of high basal pulmonary vascular resistance in normal lamb fetuses.[38] Another important determinant of pulmonary vascular tone is the blood pH level. Acidosis, either metabolic or respiratory, has been demonstrated to cause pulmonary vasoconstriction, and alkalosis elicits vasodilation at all stages of development.[39,40]

The influence of the central nervous system on pulmonary vasomotor tone has been documented experimentally. In dogs, hypothalamic stimulation alters the distensibility of large pulmonary arteries, and this influence is mediated by the sympathetic nervous system.[41] Electrical stimulation of the brainstem vasomotor center of the newborn piglet has been shown to cause significant increases in pulmonary artery pressure without changing pulmonary flow, indicating pulmonary vasoconstriction.[42] The effects of eicosanoids derived from arachidonic acid (prostaglandins, thromboxane, and leukotrienes) on the fetal and perinatal pulmonary circulation have also been studied extensively. Thromboxane, leukotrienes, and prostaglandin $F_{2\alpha}$ are pulmonary vasoconstrictors.[42–45] All the other products of cyclo-oxygenase have been found to be pulmonary vasodilators, among which prostacyclin is one of the most

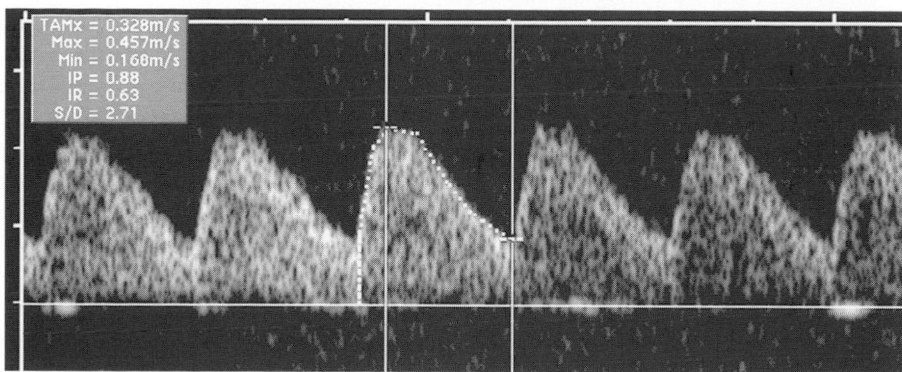

Figure 7.6 Pulsed Doppler recording in the umbilical artery of a 24-week fetus. Systolodiastolic forward velocities confirm the low vascular placental resistance.

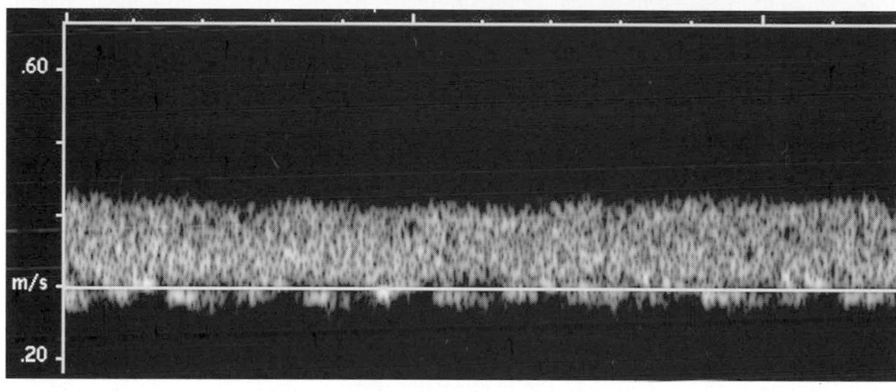

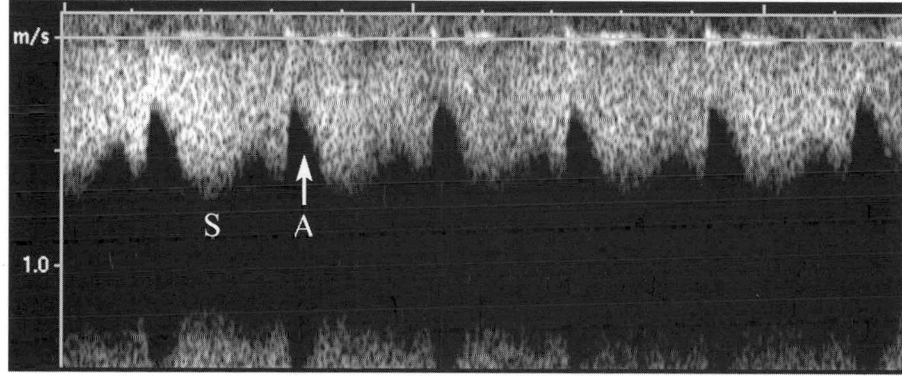

Figure 7.7 (A) Pulsed Doppler recording in the intra-abdominal portion of the umbilical vein, showing continuous low velocities. (B) In the ductus venosus, peak velocities reach 0.7 m/s. Two forward waves are seen: one during ventricular systole (S) and the other during the early part of diastole. A deceleration wave is recorded during atrial (A) contractions.

potent.[46,47] The purine nucleotides adenosine and ATP also have significant pulmonary vasodilatory effects in fetal lambs.[48]

The placental circulation

Unlike fetal lungs, the normal placenta is a vascular bed with very low resistance to flow. Consequently, approximately 50% of the combined cardiac output of lamb fetuses flows into the umbilical circulation.[18] This unique feature of the fetal circulation is well illustrated by the Doppler velocimetric assessment of blood flow through the umbilical artery (Fig. 7.6); fetuses with a normal placental vasculature show Doppler flow velocity waveforms with significant diastolic forward flow, increasing as gestation progresses.[49]

Many investigators have studied the mechanisms regulating placental blood flow. The absence of innervation in either the umbilical cord or the placenta makes it very unlikely that neural control plays any physiological role.[50] Similarly, despite experimental evidence of placental vascular reactivity to some vasoactive hormones, such as angiotensin II[51] and norepinephrine,[52] administration of their respective blockers has no effect on placental vascular resistance.[52] Prostaglandins have also been proposed as local vasoactive agents.[53] Intriguing evidence of maternal and fetal placental blood flow matching[54] strongly suggests some form of intrinsic regulation. For the time being, however, the mediator(s) of this physiological and important mechanism has(ve) not yet been clearly identified.

The umbilical vein drains oxygenated blood coming from the placenta into the left branch of the portal vein. Umbilical venous flow has a continuous low velocity (mean 15 cm/s) (Fig. 7.7A). Placental flow depends on the umbilical arteriovenous gradient. The venous component of this relationship is influenced by resistance in the ductus venosus, in the liver parenchyma, and also by right atrial filling pressure.

The shunts

Three shunts are classically described within the fetal circulation. The first occurs at the level of the ductus venosus. This short venous segment links the umbilical and portal veins to the inferior vena cava, allowing a portion of blood coming from the umbilical vein to bypass the hepatic circulation and directly enter the inferior vena cava. From Doppler investigations in normal human fetuses, this shunt amounts to approximately 30% of umbilical venous return.[55] Because of its trumpet-shaped appearance, the ductus venosus functions as an important regulator of the placental circulation, protecting the fetal heart from excessive blood flow to the placenta. The continuous low velocity of umbilical venous blood is transformed within the ductus venosus into a pulsatile high-velocity jet with peak flows up to 75 cm/s, suggesting a gradient between the umbilical vein and the central venous system. The gradient has been estimated to reach a peak of 3 mmHg during atrial and early ventricular filling.[56] This flow acceleration is responsible for the preferential streaming of highly oxygenated blood across the foramen ovale into the left heart.[18] Flow in the ductus venosus is normally phasic, characterized by two forward waves, one during ventricular systole, the other early in diastole. Atrial contraction causes the deceleration of blood velocities, which normally never results in complete absence of anterograde flow toward the heart (Fig. 7.7B).

A second shunt takes place at the level of the foramen ovale, which corresponds to an opening in the septum secundum between the two atria, associated with a flap valve formed by the septum primum. This valve allows blood to pass only from the right to the left atrium. Recent Doppler investigations of human fetuses estimated the shunt through the foramen ovale to drop from 34% to 18% of combined ventricular output during the period from 20 to 30 weeks of gestation.[20]

Finally, the ductus arteriosus, which is a prolongation of the main pulmonary artery toward the descending aorta, is also usually considered as a shunt, allowing much of the blood ejected by the right ventricle to bypass the lungs. Convincing data now demonstrate that, during fetal life, the patency of the ductus arteriosus is regulated by both contractile and dilatory factors. Oxygen was the first constrictor of the ductus arteriosus to be recognized.[57] The sensitivity of the ductus arteriosus to O_2 increases during the last trimester of gestation.[58] The oxygen-constrictive effect appears to be linked to accelerated endothelin-1 production.[59] Although circulating adenosine has been suggested to be a dilator of the ductus,[60] numerous reports favor the prostaglandins (E_1 and particularly E_2) as major elements maintaining ductal patency.[61–63]

The idea of considering the ductus arteriosus as the site of a vascular shunt is certainly valid in extrauterine life where the two ventricles are disposed in series. In this situation, the ductus arteriosus is obviously diverting blood from the pulmonary or the systemic circulations, depending on the balance between downstream resistances of the two circulations. During fetal life, however, classification of the ductus arteriosus as a shunt must be questioned, as it is incompatible with the concept of parallel arrangement of the prenatal circulation. Indeed, because of its parallel disposition, the fetal ductus arteriosus is a segment of the pulmonary arch and does not actually divert any blood, but rather participates in combined output by channeling right ventricular output toward the systemic circulation. This is well illustrated in Figure 7.5. The concept of parallel disposition of the two ventricles implies, as a rational conclusion, that, in fetal life, the only arterial segment corresponding to the definition of a shunt would be the aortic isthmus.[64] Indeed, this vascular segment normally transfers blood from the upper body toward the lower body by connecting the two parallel systems (Fig. 7.5). Approximately 65% of the blood ejected by the left ventricle perfuses the upper body, the rest going through the aortic isthmus toward the subdiaphragmatic circulation.[18] The factors influencing the direction of blood flow through the isthmus are illustrated in Figs 7.8 and 7.9. In systole, the direction of blood flow is dictated by both individual performances of the ventricles and downstream resistance of the upper and lower body vascular networks. The ventricles have opposite influences on the direction of flow: the left ventricle causes forward flow through the isthmus (Fig. 7.8A), while blood ejected by the right ventricle has a retrograde influence (Fig. 7.8B). In normal conditions, the presence of the placenta with its low vascular impedance explains the forward systolic flow observed in the isthmus.[65] With advancing gestation, however, two physiological events alter flow patterns through the isthmus: first, the fall in cerebral vascular impedance causes a reduction in the diastolic component of the waveform; secondly, the progressive preponderance of right ventricular output evokes a brief end-systolic reversal of isthmic flow; this process starts at about 30 weeks and increases progressively up to the end of gestation (Fig. 7.10). To facilitate the objective monitoring of flow patterns through the fetal aortic isthmus, an isthmic flow index (IFI) has been developed. The proposed index was obtained by dividing the sum of systolic (S) and diastolic (D) Doppler flow velocity integrals by systolic flow integrals: $IFI = S + D/S$. Positive and negative signs are assigned to antegrade and retrograde velocity values respectively. The normal reference ranges of the IFI have been published recently.[66] In cases of severe fetal left ventricular dysfunction, reverse flow is recorded even during systole through the isthmus because of the isolated influence of the right ventricle. In diastole, the two semilunar valves being closed, the direction of blood in the isthmus will be essentially influenced by downstream vascular resistance (Fig. 7.9); any significant fall in upper body vascular resistance (cerebral arteriovenous fistula[67]) or increase in lower body vascular resistance (placental vascular impairment[68]) should cause a reversal

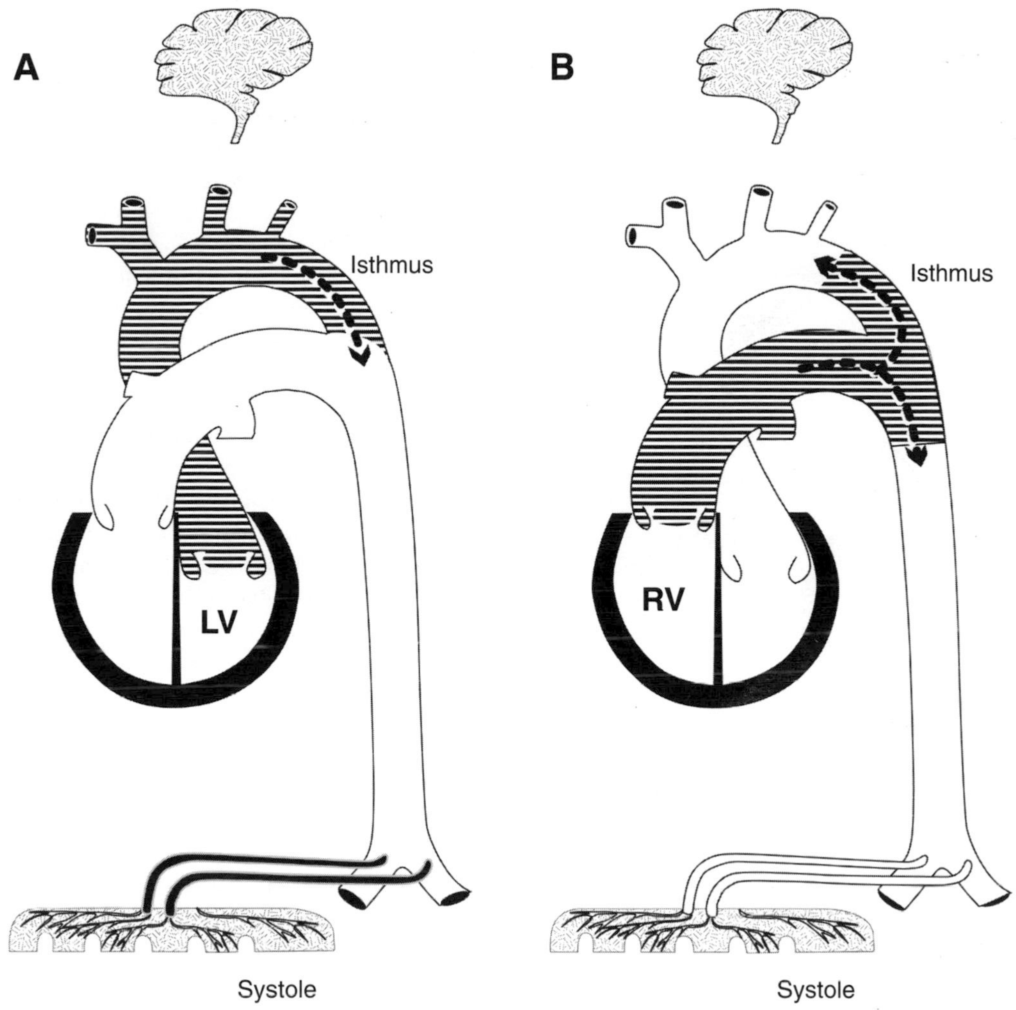

Figure 7.8 Influences of individual ventricular ejection on the direction of blood flow through the aortic isthmus during systole. (A) The left ventricle (LV) causes a forward flow, while (B) blood ejected by the right ventricle (RV) has a retrograde influence.

of the diastolic component of flow velocity waveforms in the isthmus.

Fetal cardiocirculatory adjustments to stress

Abnormal loading conditions

Abnormal loading conditions of the fetal circulation can be observed in a variety of disorders, such as arteriovenous malformation, anemia or the twin–twin transfusion syndrome (TTTS). Each of these conditions represents situations in which cardiac preload is increased but afterload varies. Furthermore, in each case, the etiology of the loading disturbance is different. The specific cardiocirculatory adjustments will, therefore, be underlined for each condition, considering separately the impact on the heart and on the peripheral circulation.

Arteriovenous malformations

A large arteriovenous shunt in the fetal circulation may occur in tumors such as sacrococcygeal teratomas, placental

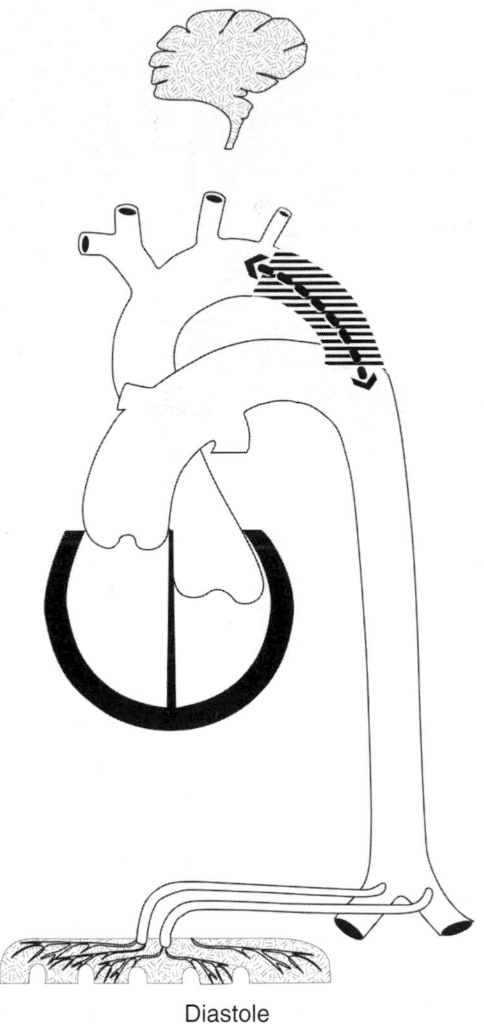

Figure 7.9 In diastole, the direction of flow in the isthmus is simultaneously influenced by the downstream vascular resistances of the two parallel systems.

chorioangiomas or in the presence of cerebral vascular malformation associated with an aneurysm of the vein of Galen.

Cardiac impact

All these conditions are characterized by both elevated preload, because of increased venous return from the shunts, and reduced afterload due to arteriovenous runoff. Dramatic rises in combined cardiac output have been documented in these cases, reaching twice the estimated normal range.[69] In fetuses with cerebral arteriovenous malformations, close to 70% of the combined cardiac output comes from the right ventricle because of the increment in blood flow through the superior vena cava going directly through the right ventricle.[70] As cardiac output increases, the fetal heart compensates by a linear augmentation in size.[71] With progression of the disease, cardiac failure may develop with worsening of the degree of atrioventricular valve regurgitation and the appearance of fetal hydrops.

The peripheral circulation

During fetal life, changes in the peripheral circulation caused by localized declines in vascular impedance will be very much influenced by the parallel disposition of the two ventricles and their arterial outlets. In fetuses with arteriovenous malformations in the upper part of the body (cerebral arteriovenous fistula), retrograde diastolic flow is observed in the aortic isthmus while the flow pattern in the descending aorta remains normal.[70] The right ventricle then perfuses both the lower and the upper body. In contrast, when the arteriovenous malformation is in the lower body, both ventricles share the volume load. Antegrade flow through the aortic isthmus is then increased. Reversal of diastolic flow in the umbilical artery has also been reported, suggesting a "steal" phenomenon from the placental circulation.[71]

Anemia

Cardiac impact

In fetal anemia resulting from isoimmunization, left and right ventricular outputs are significantly elevated, and right cardiac output over the left ventricular output ratio is normal.[72,73] Oxygen delivery can thus be preserved. This rise in cardiac output is related to both higher preload (decreased blood viscosity leading to increased venous return) and lower afterload (diminished blood viscosity and peripheral vasodilatation due to reduced O_2 content). Peak velocities are augmented through both semilunar valves.

The peripheral circulation

Peripheral adjustments to the stress of anemia reflect the hyperdynamic state of these fetuses. Peak velocities tend to increase in both parallel circulatory systems. An inverse correlation has been found between the rise in peak velocity in the middle cerebral artery and the level of hematocrit.[74] Venous flows are also affected, and peak velocities are elevated in the ductus venosus, which also shows less pulsatility than normal.[73–75]

Twin–twin transfusion syndrome (TTTS)

This condition occurs in about 15% of monochorionic–diamniotic twin gestations. Vascular connections deep within the placenta cause a shift in blood volume from the donor to the recipient twin.[76] However, this classic pathophysiological background does not explain some intriguing cardiocirculatory perturbations found in TTTS.

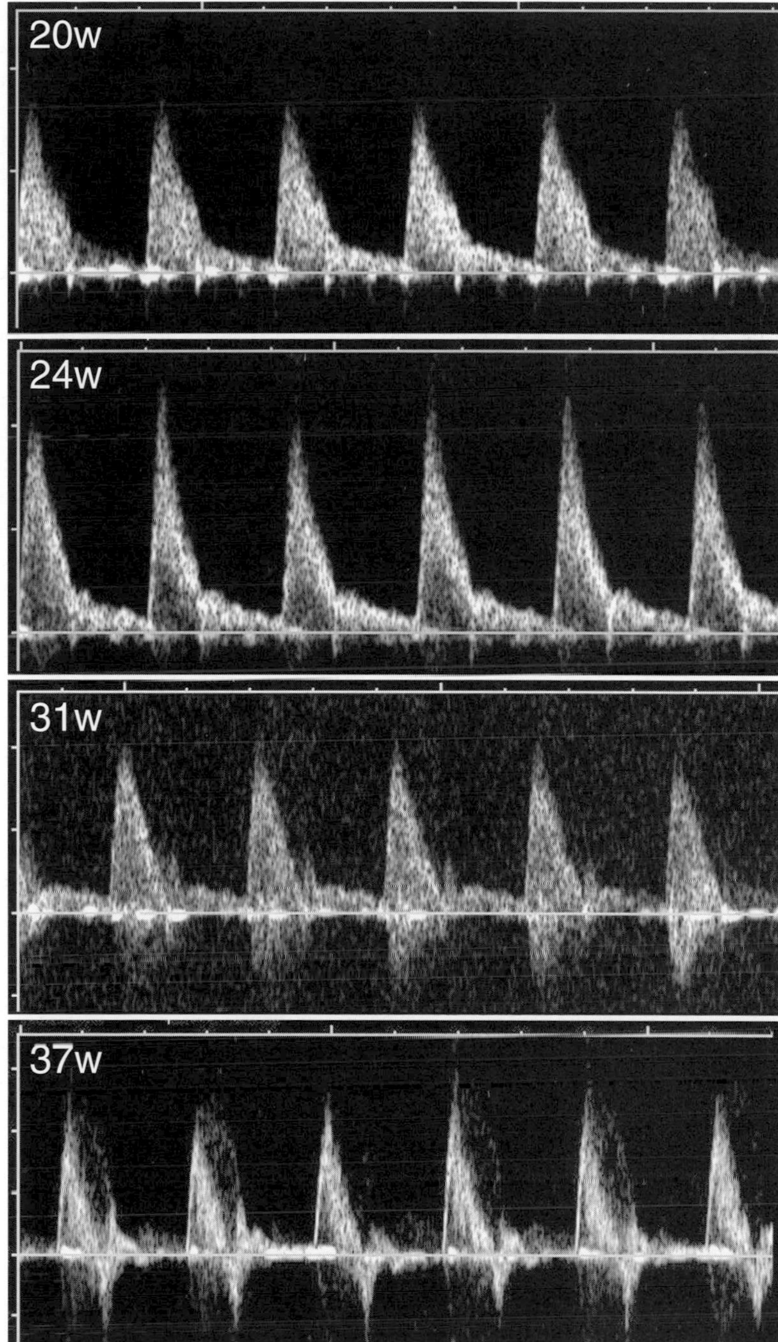

Figure 7.10 Doppler flow velocity waveforms in the aortic isthmus. At 20 weeks of gestation, forward systolic and diastolic waves are observed. An end-systolic incisura appears at about 25 weeks and increases thereafter; late in gestation, a brief reversal of flow is observed at the end of systole. Note on the tracing recorded at 37 weeks (bottom), the superimposed velocity Doppler signals from the ductus arteriosus, demarcating the end of systole.

Cardiac impact

Although the donor twin becomes anemic, his/her hemodynamic picture is mainly marked by the consequences of his/her volume depletion. Reports of elevated blood levels of endothelin[77] and evidence of renin–angiotensin system stimulation[78] are convincing elements in favor of chronic hypotension and peripheral hypoperfusion in these fetuses. Ventricular function is usually preserved. Increased arterial pulsed wave velocity has been found in surviving postnatal donor twins, suggesting intrauterine vascular remodeling with lifelong consequences.[79]

In contrast, hypertrophic cardiomyopathy is typically described in the recipient twin.[80] The progressive nature of the process and the fact that marked ventricular hypertrophy can be observed with little or no evidence of dilation strongly favor the renin–angiotensin pathophysiologic hypothesis to the detriment of a simple volume shift. Subclinical cardiomyopathy, essentially manifested by early signs of diastolic dysfunction, has also been documented and goes along well with the renin–angiotensin hypothesis.[81] According to this concept, the hypervolemic recipient twin is exposed to mediators (renin, angiotensin) released by the hypovolemic donor twin, mediators responsible for vasoconstriction and ventricular hypertrophy. In severe cases, this process can lead to ventricular dysfunction with hydrops and fetal demise. Right ventricular hypertrophy rarely evolves to pulmonary infundibular stenosis and even pulmonary atresia.[82]

The peripheral circulation
Serial Doppler recordings in the donor twin do not reveal any significant change until the appearance of fetal distress;[83] at this last stage, the donor presents signs consistent with anemia (increased peak velocities), indicating a massive shift in blood volume. In the recipient twin, diastolic myocardial dysfunction causes heightened pulsatility in the ductus venosus (deep "a" waves) with umbilical vein pulsations.

Hypoxic stress

The stress encountered most frequently during fetal life is lack of oxygen. For obvious reasons, most of our information on this subject comes from experimental studies, assuming that findings in laboratories reflect what is actually occurring in the human fetus. Another problem arises from the fact that the bulk of experimental protocols are designed to provide relatively short exposure to hypoxemia; here again, assumptions have to be made about the outcome in human fetuses in whom hypoxemia is sustained for days or weeks. A third drawback is the lack of homogeneity in protocols of the experimental studies. As shown in Tables 7.2 and 7.3, the designs of studies cited as references in this chapter vary not only in terms of the duration of the hypoxemia, but also in the way hypoxemia was created experimentally.

The advent of Doppler ultrasonography has undoubtedly opened new horizons in investigations of the human fetal cardiovascular system. This technology has been instrumental in introducing into clinical practice a fundamental notion already demonstrated in acute experiments, that is the importance of placental vascular resistance. Indeed, as the placenta offers the lowest resistances within the entire fetal vascular system, any increase in those resistances should have repercussions on both flows and pressures, which are not necessarily related to the secondary hypoxemia. The assessment of circulatory responses to fetal hypoxemia can no longer be made without first establishing the state of the placental vascular system. The two situations will, therefore, be discussed separately. Adaptive mechanisms in the presence of hypoxemia, such as increased O_2 extraction from erythrocytes[84] or reduction of fetal O_2 consumption,[85] which are not directly related to the circulatory system, will not be discussed here, despite their potential importance *in vivo*.

Hypoxemia with normal placental vascular resistances

Blood gases
In humans, this condition is usually observed in mothers suffering from chronic pulmonary or cardiac disorders or living at high altitudes, or in fetuses with acute or chronic anemia. Placental vascular resistance is usually normal in these cases. Most of our knowledge concerning this type of fetal

Table 7.2 Examples of studies of fetal hypoxic hypoxemia.

Experimental technique	First author	Duration
Low maternal FiO_2	Assali et al. (1962)[86]	15 min
	Cohn et al. (1974)[87]	4–44 min
	Peeters et al. (1979)[88]	1 h
	Sheldon et al. (1979)[89]	7 days
	Alonso et al. (1989)[90]	2 weeks
	Kitanaka et al. (1989)[91]	28 days
	Morrow et al. (1990)[92]	1 h
	Fouron et al. (1990)[93]	3 h
	Piacquadio et al. (1990)[94]	30 min
	Rurak et al. (1990)[95]	8 h
	Itskovitz et al. (1991)[96]	20 min
	Paulick et al. (1991)[97]	± 30 min
	Kamitomo et al. (1992)[98]	105 days
Uterine blood flow restriction	Creasy et al. (1973)[99]	21–28 days
	Moutquin (1981)[100]	30 min
	Abitbol (1982)[101]	1 min
	Yaffe et al. (1987)[102]	15 min
	Bocking et al. (1988)[103]	48 h
	van Huisseling et al. (1989)[104]	90 s
	Reid et al. (1991)[105]	19 ± 3 min
Reduction in fetal hematocrit	Fumia et al. (1984)[106]	–

Table 7.3 Examples of studies of hypoxemia due to placental circulatory insufficiency.

Experimental technique	First author	Duration
Umbilical cord constriction	Lewis et al. (1984)[118]	5–10 min × 5 for 1 h
	Itskowitz et al. (1987)[119]	4–5 min
	Richardson et al. (1996)[120]	1 min every 5 min for 1 h
	De Haan et al. (1997)[121]	1–2 min every 5 min
	Ley et al. (2004)[122]	
Placental embolization	Trudinger et al. (1987)[123]	9 days
	Morrow et al. (1989)[124]	2.5 h
	Lewinsky et al. (1993)[125]	Every 15 min × 5
	Gagnon et al. (1995)[126]	10 days
	Murotsuki et al. (1997)[127]	21 days
Umbilical vein constriction	Fouron et al. (1991)[130]	3 h

hypoxemia is derived from instrumented fetal lambs under hypoxemic stress created either by decreasing the O_2 concentration of the gas mixture inspired by the ewe[86–98] or by uterine blood flow restriction[99–105] (Table 7.2). Less frequently, hypoxia has been achieved by changing the hematocrit level by isovolemic exchange transfusion.[106] Except for this last condition, where the fall in blood O_2 content is related to a lack of O_2 carriers, the oxymetric feature that characterizes all the other fetuses in this group is the low PO_2 of the umbilical venous return, explaining the term "hypoxic hypoxemia" frequently assigned to the group. In these circumstances, fetal blood gases will be dependent on maternal blood gas status. As placental exchange is preserved, relatively low levels of PO_2 can be reached without significant buildup of acid metabolites in the fetus. The level of fetal PCO_2 will also depend on maternal PCO_2, which may be perfectly normal. A resultant gradual increase in fetal hematocrit serves as a compensatory mechanism to cause an elevation in arterial O_2 content.

Cardiocirculatory responses

During acute hypoxic hypoxemia, blood pressure rises and heart rate decreases, with a redistribution of cardiac output.[87,89] Hypoxia stimulates catecholamine secretion from the adrenal medulla either directly[107] or, in more mature fetuses, by a reflex effect through the splanchnic nerves. The consequences of adrenal norepinephrine secretion during fetal hypoxemia can be blocked by alpha-adrenergic blockers, resulting in a return of vascular resistance and blood pressure to normal values.[97,108] An increase in vasopressin has also been documented during fetal hypoxemia, and could be another factor contributing to the rise in vascular resistance.[94,108] Bradycardia as well as peripheral vasoconstriction has been related to neural reflexes via both baro- and chemoreceptors in the aortic and carotid bodies.[96,110] Animal studies have consistently shown blood flow redistribution to the brain, heart, and adrenals when hypoxic hypoxemia is induced experimentally[87–89,102,105] (Fig. 7.11). This redistribution, mediated via humoral and reflex mechanisms, is caused by local vasodilatation in these three organs concomitant with vasoconstriction in the lungs, digestive tract, spleen, pancreas, kidneys, carcass, skin, etc. In acute experiments, absolute flow and the proportion of cardiac output going to the brain increase.[86,88,89] Meanwhile, placental blood flow and combined cardiac output do not change significantly. In severe hypoxia, however, the deleterious effect of acidosis on fetal heart rate and myocardial contractility will be responsible for a fall in combined ventricular output.[87,93]

A few experimental protocols have studied chronic hypoxic hypoxemia. In these experiments, blood flow increased to the brain, myocardium, and adrenals, and remained elevated after at least 8[95] to 48 h[103] of fetal hypoxic hypoxemia. Elevated concentrations of plasma epinephrine have been found in lambs and fetuses after 28 days of hypoxemia.[91] In contrast, a longer period of hypoxemia maintained by exposure of pregnant ewes to high altitude did not cause any increase in fetal cerebral blood flow[111] or changes in left ventricular function.[98] Likewise, in fetal lambs exposed to hypoxic hypoxemia for 2 weeks, right ventricular output and stroke volume fell to 30% on the third day of the experiments, but recovered to normal values in the following days.[90] One important finding documented in all studies is that the umbilical circulation is not significantly affected until severe acidemia causes a fall in combined cardiac output.

Because of the parallel arrangement of the two ventricles and the dynamic nature of vascular shunts, the fetus has the capacity to selectively adjust its arterial O_2 content. This mechanism is unique to intrauterine life, and is not available after birth. Indeed, *in utero*, arterial O_2 content is closely dependent on the redistribution of placental venous return. In normoxemic conditions, approximately 30% of the umbilical venous return bypasses the hepatic microcirculation and directly enters the inferior vena cava through the ductus venosus.[55] It has been demonstrated in both fetal sheep[18] and primates[112] that this highly oxygenated stream of blood preferentially enters the left atrium via the foramen ovale, and is thus distributed to the upper body. In normoxemic conditions, this preferential streaming is responsible for the slightly higher arterial Po_2 of blood in the ascending aorta (~20 mmHg) compared with postductal blood in the descending aorta (~17 mmHg). During hypoxemia, an increase in the proportion of blood that bypasses the liver and goes directly to the inferior vena cava through the ductus venosus has been demonstrated repeatedly.[112–114] This shunting pattern should reduce transit time from the placenta to the heart, favoring rapid filling of the right atrium by better oxygenated blood. What happens to the transfer of this blood through the foramen ovale is less clear. It is generally accepted that preferential shunting of ductus venosus blood across the foramen ovale does not increase during hypoxemia.[112]

In most cases of hypoxic hypoxemia, the O_2 content of the umbilical vein is low, but this should be compensated by the preservation of umbilical blood flow and increased cerebral perfusion. This last element, however, causes a rise in the volume of poorly oxygenated blood that returns to the right atrium through the superior vena cava. The effect of this rise in superior vena cava blood flowing into the right atrium on the shunting pattern through the foramen ovale has not been clearly established.

Doppler findings

Doppler echocardiography, which allows the indirect assessment of peripheral vascular impedance and the early recognition of circulatory adjustments, is widely integrated in contemporary fetal monitoring. Many studies have confirmed that hypoxic hypoxemia does not alter Doppler flow velocimetry waveforms in the umbilical artery[92,115,116] or, if it does, it is only secondary to the changes in heart rate.[116] This is in all likelihood related to the fact that placental resistance does not change significantly in this condition. In one report, 1 min of maternal abdominal aortic compression caused a 10% increase in the Doppler-derived umbilical resistance index, and a 10% fall in umbilical blood flow associated with a 20% reduction in the cerebral resistance index[117]; fetal heart rate decelerations were, however, observed during the same period. In another study in which abdominal aortic compression was also created, parasympathetic blockade with atropine prevented both fetal heart rate deceleration and Doppler velocimetric changes in the umbilical artery.[104]

Hypoxemia with elevated placental vascular resistance

Blood gases

Uteroplacental insufficiency with secondary fetal growth restriction affects 3–7% of all deliveries and is a major cause of perinatal morbidity and mortality. Maternal blood gases are usually normal in this condition. In contrast to fetal hypoxic hypoxemia, hypoxemia due to placental insufficiency is characterized by an increase in placental vascular impedance and a secondary fall in umbilical blood flow. As a consequence of the decrease in umbilical venous return, the proportion of poorly oxygenated blood coming from the distal inferior vena cava that reaches the right atrium increases, lowering the O_2 available to the fetus. Contrary to what was observed in the previous setting, pCO_2 tends to rise very early because of the primary disorder in placental exchange. Similarly, acid metabolites have less chance of crossing the placental barrier and, therefore, tend to accumulate in the fetus. Consequently, for the same level of hypoxemia, respiratory and metabolic acidemia should develop early, compared with the group with normal placental vascular resistance and flow. This point is important in view of the deleterious effect of acidemia on tissue O_2 extraction and myocardial contractility.

Cardiocirculatory responses

In an attempt to reproduce, at least in part, the conditions created by an increase in placental vascular resistance, various techniques have been used in fetal lambs, such as umbilical cord compression[118–122] or embolization of the placental vascular network[123–127] (Table 7.3). The hemodynamic characteristics created by compression of the whole cord differ somewhat from the human situation as both arterial and venous umbilical flows are impaired. Doppler investigations have shown that the pattern of umbilical Doppler flow velocities in fetuses exhibiting growth restriction due to placental insufficiency cannot be reproduced by compression of the umbilical arteries.[128] Nevertheless, in all these experiments, a drop in combined cardiac output is observed and, more importantly, cardiac output decreases linearly with umbilical blood flow.[119,129] In experiments in which resistance to placental flow

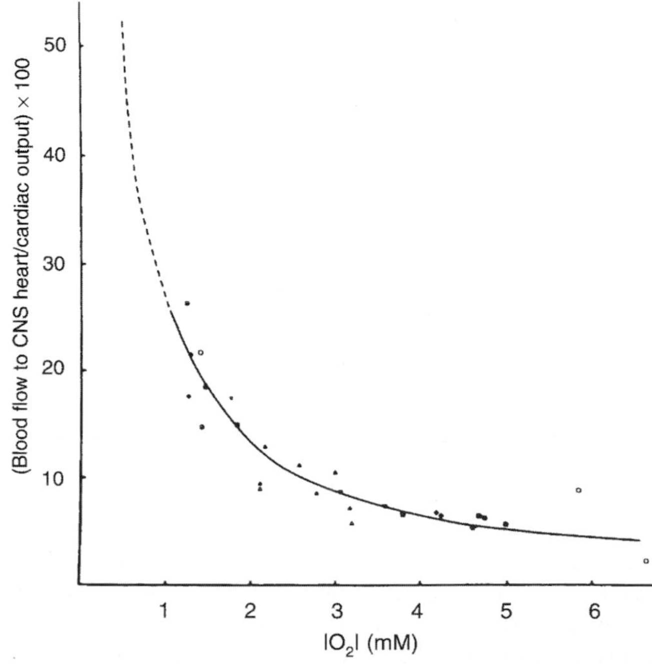

Figure 7.11 Variation in the proportion of the combined ventricular output flowing to the heart and brain of fetal lambs according to arterial O_2 content. This proportion increases by 25% with a reduction from 6 to 1 mM (reprinted with permission from ref. 89).

was increased by selective umbilical vein compression, not only could the Doppler velocimetric pattern usually seen in growth-restricted fetuses be reproduced, but a significant drop in combined cardiac output could also be documented.[130–132]

Available reports on fetal lambs demonstrate that most of the other peripheral vascular reactions described in hypoxic hypoxemia are also present with hypoxemia caused by an increase in placental vascular resistance. Mesenteric vasoconstriction is observed as well as a decrease in flow to the skeletal muscles. Blood flow to the myocardium, adrenal glands and, particularly, the brain has been found to be augmented. This last phenomenon, documented in human fetuses with growth restriction and placental insufficiency, has been called the "brain-sparing effect."

In the presence of hypoxemia related to changes in placental vascular impedance, arterial blood pressure is influenced by two elements acting in opposite directions. On the one hand, the increase in placental vascular resistance and hypoxemia-induced catecholamine release would tend to heighten blood pressure; on the other hand, the concomitant fall in cardiac output would tend to lower it. As a final result, blood pressure tends either to increase moderately[127] or to remain within normal limits in these cases. Heart rate is also quite variable, depending on the influence of catecholamines, baroreceptors, and direct local effects. Bradycardia is noted in the presence of severe hypoxemia with acidemia.

Myocardial function during increases in placental vascular resistance is influenced by factors that could also have opposite effects. In theory, cardiac function should be depressed both by the fall in preload (low venous return) and by the significant rise in afterload (increase in placental resistance). On the other hand, myocardial contractility should be improved by catecholamine release. Evidence of right ventricular dysfunction has been found in this group of fetuses.[127,133] Loss of end-systolic elastance of the left ventricle has been reported in fetal sheep after repeated placental embolization.[125] Others, using the same method to create chronic fetal hypoxemia, have noted a reduction in the myocardial deoxyribonucleic acid synthesis rate that could be a contributing factor in the deterioration of fetal myocardial function associated with increased placental vascular resistance.[126] In human fetuses with severe growth restriction associated with hypoxia and acidosis, changes in ventricular diastolic filling patterns have been documented, indicating impaired diastolic function.[134–136]

Doppler findings

Doppler investigations have detected various degrees of alteration in blood flow velocity waveforms of the umbilical artery in human fetuses with increased placental vascular impedance. Normal forward diastolic flow decreases with the rise in placental vascular resistance, and may completely disappear. In severe cases, reverse diastolic flow can be recorded.[137] The relationship between changes in Doppler velocimetry and the fall in umbilical blood flow has been shown, however, to be nonlinear,[138] as close to a 50% decline in umbilical blood flow must be achieved in the fetal lamb before any significant change in Doppler velocimetric indices can be seen.

Arterial redistribution and blood centralization to vital organs have been confirmed by recent Doppler investigations involving not only the cerebral arteries but also renal,[139] splenic,[140] brachial,[141] coronary,[142] adrenal,[143] and peripheral pulmonary arteries.[144] With such arterial blood redistribution, the fetus can still maintain adequate cerebral oxygenation. This corresponds to the "compensation phase" which, in the clinical setting, justifies an expectant approach and the prolongation of pregnancy. In severe cases, however, the defense system is overwhelmed, resulting in metabolic acidemia with cerebral hypoxia, and reflecting the "decompensation phase." As mentioned previously, because of the unique position of the aortic isthmus, this vascular segment should be the best site in the entire fetal circulatory system at which even subtle changes could be detected in the balance between downstream resistances of the upper body and the subdiaphragmatic circulation. Experimental studies have shown that, when placental resistance to flow in fetal lambs is increased progressively, isthmic diastolic flow disappears quickly and becomes progressively retrograde.[132] In these experiments, a strong correlation has been found between blood flow in the aortic isthmus and flow through the umbilical circulation (Fig. 7.12). As O_2 delivery

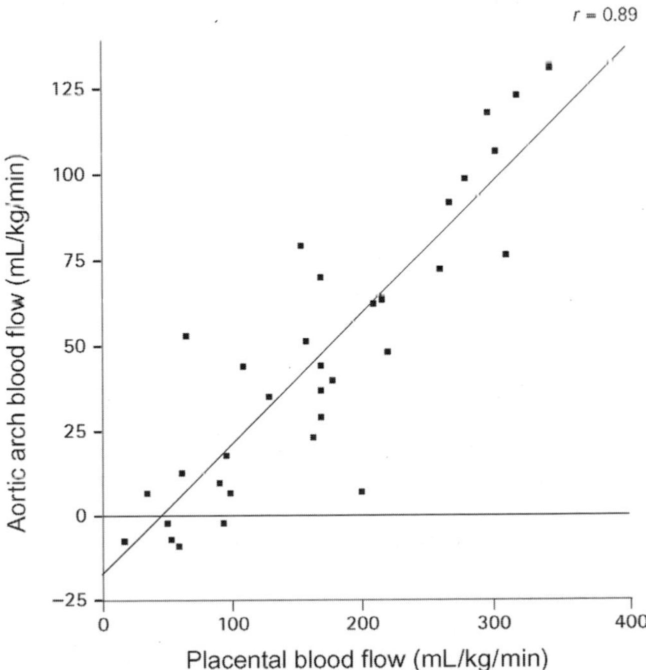

Figure 7.12 Relationship between aortic arch and placental flows in fetal lambs whose resistance to placental perfusion is increased by stepwise compression of the umbilical veins. A strong linear correlation is observed. (In the ovine, the aortic arch is the equivalent of the aortic isthmus in the human.) (Adapted from ref. 132.)

to the fetus is closely related to umbilical blood flow, one can extrapolate and consider that, in these circumstances, fetal O_2 delivery is also intimately linked to aortic isthmus blood flow. An inverse correlation between the isthmic blood flow velocity index and postnatal neurodevelopmental outcome has been reported recently: as the isthmic flow index diminishes, the probability of a nonoptimal neurodevelopmental outcome increases.[145]

Acknowledgments

The authors are grateful to Mrs Nathalie Ishmael for her precious secretarial contribution.

Key points

1 The fetal heart is functionally immature because of differences in myofibril arrangement and a greater proportion of noncontractile proteins. Also, the fetal sarcoplasmic reticulum is less efficient at releasing calcium.

2 Isolated fetal cardiac muscle strips generate reduced active tension compared with the adult muscle, although they exhibit higher resting tension.

3 The fetal heart *does* respond to the Frank–Starling mechanism, although fetal muscle shortening is less than that of adult muscle for the same tension.

4 Fetal left ventricular (LV) preload is influenced by: the size of the foramen ovale; 30–40% of inferior vena cava (IVC) flow; pulmonary venous return; and diastolic filling characteristics of the right ventricle (RV).

5 Fetal RV preload consists of: all venous return from the superior vena cava and blood from the IVC, which does not cross the foramen ovale and the gradient between the right and left atria.

6 LV afterload is primarily determined by vascular resistance in the upper body. RV output – through the widely patent ductus arteriosus – is primarily directed to the placenta. Thus, RV afterload is determined by resistance at the placental level.

7 Combined ventricular output is fairly stable from 18 weeks of gestation at 450 mL/kg/min, with an increasing preponderance of RV stroke volume. Pressure development is similar to that of the adult heart.

8 It is primarily the diastolic function of the fetal heart that reflects maturational changes. Doppler flow through the atrioventricular (AV) valves demonstrates this, with a gradual increase in the E wave (resulting from active ventricular relaxation) as gestation progresses.

9 The fetal ventricles are arranged in parallel. However, individual ventricular outputs are not equal. Flow in the aortic isthmus represents a reflection of the relative ventricular outputs and relative resistance in vascular beds perfused by the two ventricles.

10 The pulmonary circulation is a relatively high-resistance, low-flow vascular bed. However, the proportion of blood flowing through this bed increases to as much as 25% of cardiac output at term.

11 The placental circulation is a very low-resistance, high-flow vascular bed, receiving approximately 50% of combined cardiac output.

12 Vascular shunts traditionally described in the fetal circulation include: the ductus venosus, which allows some of the umbilical venous flow to enter the IVC directly; the foramen ovale, which permits flow from the right atrium to the left atrium; and the ductus arteriosus. The last vascular segment actually channels RV outflow toward the systemic circulation.

13 The aortic isthmus, located between the origin of the left subclavian artery and the aortic end of the ductus arteriosus, is a shunt between the two parallel circulations of the LV and the RV.

14 The direction of flow in the isthmus is determined by the relative influences of the two ventricles and the resistance of their respective downstream vascular beds.

15 Arteriovenous malformations lead to increased preload and decreased afterload. There is a marked elevation in cardiac output, and then progressively in cardiac size. Failure may occur from AV valve regurgitation. Peripheral circulatory changes vary, depending on the location of the malformation (upper versus lower body).

16 Fetal anemia also results in increased preload and decreased afterload. Cardiac output rises, and peripheral blood velocities tend to climb.

17 The twin–twin transfusion syndrome is characterized by chronic hypotension and hypoperfusion in the donor twin, while the recipient develops hypertrophic cardiomyopathy potentially leading to ventricular dysfunction and hydrops.

18 Fetal hypoxic hypoxemia causes elevated blood pressure and decreased heart rate, with redistribution of cardiac output to the brain, heart, and adrenals. Placental blood is maintained until the progression to

severe acidemia with a fall in cardiac output. Highly oxygenated umbilical venous blood is increasingly shunted through the ductus venosus to the IVC.

19 Hypoxemia resulting from placental insufficiency involves heightened placental vascular impedance and decreased umbilical blood flow. pCO_2 increases more quickly, and acidemia develops earlier than in the setting of normal placental resistance. Blood flow is markedly redistributed to the brain, heart, and adrenal glands. Ventricular dysfunction may develop in the face of hypoxia and acidosis.

20 With increased placental resistance, diastolic flow velocity in the umbilical artery (UA) decreases and may eventually become retrograde. Doppler flows in the aortic isthmus predate the changes in the UA. There is an inverse correlation between the isthmic blood flow velocity index and postnatal neurodevelopmental outcome.

References

1 Anderson PAW. Myocardial development. In: Long W, ed. *Fetal and neonatal cardiology.* Philadelphia, PA: W.B. Saunders Co.; 1990:17–38.

2 Nayler WG, Fassold E. Calcium accumulating and ATPase activity of cardiac sarcoplasmic reticulum before and after birth. *Cardiovasc Res* 1977;11:231–237.

3 Nakanishi T, Jarmakani JM. Developmental changes in myocardial mechanical function and subcellular organelles. *Am J Physiol* 1984;246:H615–625.

4 Mahoney L. Calcium homeostasis and control of contractility in the developing heart. *Semin Perinatol* 1996;20:510–519.

5 Lompre AM, Mercadier JJ, Wisnewsky C, et al. Species and age-dependent changes in the relative amounts of cardiac myosin isoenzymes in mammals. *Dev Biol* 1981;84:286–290.

6 Sweeney LJ, Nag AC, Eisenberg B, et al. Developmental aspects of cardiac contractile protein. *Basic Res Cardiol* 1985;80(Suppl. 2):123–127.

7 Fisher DJ, Heymann MA, Rudolph AM. Myocardial consumption of oxygen and carbohydrates in newborn sheep. *Pediatr Res* 1981;15:843–846.

8 Granzier HL, Labeit S. The giant protein titin. A major player in myocardial mechanics, signaling, and disease. *Circ Res* 2004; 94:284.

9 Lahmers S, Wu Y, Call DR, et al. Development control of titin isoform expression and passive stiffness in fetal and neonatal myocardium. *Circ Res* 2004;10:1161/01.

10 Friedman WF. The intrinsic physiologic properties of the developing heart. *Prog Cardiovasc Dis* 1972;15:87–111.

11 Rudolph AM, Heymann MA. Cardiac output in the fetal lamb: the effects of spontaneous and induced changes of heart rate on right and left ventricular output. *Am J Obstet Gynecol* 1976; 124(2):183–192.

12 Gilbert RD. Control of fetal cardiac output during changes in blood volume. *Am J Physiol* 1980;238:H80–86.

13 Thornburg KL, Morton MJ. Filling and arterial pressures as determinants of RV stroke volume in the sheep fetus. *Am J Physiol* 1983;244:H656–663.

14 Kenny J, Plappert T, Doubilet P, et al. Effects of heart rate on ventricular size, stroke volume and output in the normal human fetus: a prospective Doppler echocardiographic study. *Circulation* 1987;76:52–58.

15 Romero T, Covell J, Friedman WF. A comparison of pressure–volume relations of the fetal, newborn, and adult heart. *Am J Physiol* 1972;222(5):1285–1290.

16 Grant DA. Ventricular constraint in the fetus and newborn. *Can J Cardiol* 1999;15:95–104.

17 Dawes GS. The fetal circulation. In: Dawes GS, ed. *Fetal and neonatal physiology*. Chicago, IL: Year Book Medical Publishers; 1968;91–105.

18 Rudolph AM. Distribution and regulation of blood flow in the fetal and neonatal lamb. *Circ Res* 1985;57:811–820.

19 St John Sutton M, Groves A, MacNeil A, et al. Assessment of changes in blood flow through the lungs and foramen ovale in the normal human fetus with gestational age: a prospective Doppler echocardiographic study. *Br Heart J* 1994;71:232–237.

20 Rasanen J, Wood DC, Weiner S, et al. Role of the pulmonary circulation in the distribution of human fetal cardiac output during the second half of pregnancy. *Circulation* 1996;94:1068–1073.

21 Reller MD, Morton MJ, Reid DL, Thornburg KL. Fetal lamb ventricles respond differently to filling and arterial pressures and to in utero ventilation. *Pediatr Res* 1987;22:621–626.

22 Fouron JC, Drblik SP. Fetal cardiovascular dynamics in intrauterine growth retardation. In: Copel JA, Reed KL, eds. *Doppler ultrasound in obstetrics and gynecology.* New York: Raven Press; 1995:281–290.

23 Kenny JF, Plappert E, Doubilet P, et al. Changes in intracardiac blood flow velocities and right and left ventricular stroke volumes with gestational age in the normal human fetus: A prospective Doppler echocardiographic study. *Circulation* 1986; 74:1208–1216.

24 St-John Sutton MG, Gewitz MH, et al. Quantitative assessment of growth and function of the cardiac chamber in the normal human fetus: a prospective longitudinal study. *Circulation* 1984;69(4):645–654.

25 Tei C, Ling LH, Hodge DO, et al. New index of combined systolic and diastolic myocardial performance: A simple and reproducible measure of cardiac function – A study in normals and dilated cardiomyopathy. *J Cardiol* 1995;26:357–366.

26 Eidem BW, Edwards JM, Cetta F. Quantitative assessment of fetal ventricular function: establishing normal values of the myocardial performance index in the fetus. *Echocardiography* 2001;18:9–13.

27 Machado MVL, Chita SC, Allan LD. Acceleration time in the aorta and pulmonary artery measured by Doppler echocardiography in the midtrimester normal human fetus. *Br Heart J* 1987;58:15–18.

28 Reed KL, Sahn DJ, Scagnelli S, et al. Doppler echocardiographic studies of diastolic function in the human fetal heart: Changes during gestation. *J Am Coll Cardiol* 1986;8:391–395.
29 Carceller-Blanchard AM, Fouron JC. Determinants of the Doppler flow velocity profile through the mitral valve of the human fetus. *Br Heart J* 1993;70:457–460.
30 Hislop A, Reid L. Intrapulmonary arterial development during fetal life – branching pattern and structure. *J Anat* 1972;113: 35–48.
31 Hislop A, Reid L. Pulmonary arterial development during childhood: Branching pattern and structure. *Thorax* 1973;28: 129–135.
32 Cook CD, Drinker PA, Jacobson HN, et al. Control of pulmonary blood flow in the fetal and newly born lamb. *J Physiol* 1963;169:10–29.
33 Campbell AGM, Cockburn F, Dawes GS, Miligan JE. Pulmonary vasoconstriction in asphyxia during cross-circulation between twin foetal lambs. *J Physiol (Lond)* 1967;192:111–121.
34 Fishman AP. Hypoxia on the pulmonary circulation: how and where it acts. *Circ Res* 1986;38:221–231.
35 Goetzman BW, Milstein JM. Pulmonary vasodilator action of tolazoline. *Pediatr Res* 1979;13:942–944.
36 Goldring RM, Turino GM, Cohen G, et al. The catecholamines in the pulmonary arterial pressor response to acute hypoxia. *J Clin Invest* 1962;41:1211–1212.
37 Locke JE, Olley PM, Coceani F. Enhanced beta-adrenergic function in fetal sheep. *Am J Obstet Gynecol* 1981;112: 1114–1121.
38 Ivy DD, Kinsella JP, Abman SH. Physiologic characterization of endothelin A and B receptor activity in the ovine fetal pulmonary circulation. *J Clin Invest* 1994;93:2141–2148.
39 Rudolph AM, Yvan A. Response of the pulmonary vasculature to hypoxia and H^+ ion concentration changes. *J Clin Invest* 1966;45:399–411.
40 Morin FC III. Hyperventilation, alkalosis, prostaglandin and pulmonary circulation of the newborn. *J Appl Physiol* 1986;61: 2088–2094.
41 Szidon JP, Fishman AP. Autonomic control of the pulmonary circulation. In: Fishman HP, Hecht HH, eds. *The pulmonary circulation and interstitial space*. Chicago, IL: The University of Chicago Press; 1969:239–268.
42 Long WA. Developmental pulmonary circulatory physiology. In: Long WA, ed. *Fetal and neonatal cardiology*. Philadelphia, PA: W.B. Saunders Co.; 1990:76–96.
43 Noonan TC, Malik AB. Pulmonary vascular responses to leukotriene D4 in unanesthetized sheep: role of thromboxane. *J Appl Physiol* 1986;60:765–769.
44 Adowitz PJ, Hyman AL. Analysis of responses to leukotriene D4 in the pulmonary vascular bed. *Circ Res* 1984;55:707–717.
45 Prague RS, Stephenson AH, Heitmann LJ, Lonigro AJ. Differential response of the pulmonary circulation to prostaglandin E_2 and $F_{2\alpha}$ in the presence of unilateral alveolar hypoxia. *J Pharmacol Exp Ther* 1984;229:38–43.
46 Cassin S, Winikor I, Tod M, et al. Effects of prostacyclin on the fetal pulmonary circulation. *Pediatr Pharmacol* 1981;1:197–207.
47 Sideris EB, Yokochi K, Van Helder T, et al. Effects of indomethacin, and prostaglandins E_2, I_2, and D_2 on the fetal circulation. *Adv Prostaglandin Thromboxane Leukotriene Res* 1983;12:477–482.
48 Konduri GG, Theodorou AA, Mukhopadhyay A, Deshmukh DR. Adenosine triphosphate and adenosine increase the pulmonary blood flow to postnatal levels in fetal lambs. *Pediatr Res* 1992;31:451–457.
49 Sonesson SE, Fouron JC, Tawile C, et al. Reference values for Doppler velocimetric indices from the fetal and placental ends of the umbilical artery during normal pregnancy. *J Clin Ultrasound* 1993;21:317–324.
50 Reilly FD, Russell PT. Neurohistochemical evidence supporting an absence of adrenergic and cholinergic innervation in the human placenta and umbilical cord. *Anat Rec* 1977;188:277.
51 Iwamoto HS, Rudolph AM. Effects of angiotensin II on the blood flow and its distribution in fetal lambs. *Circ Res* 1981;48: 183–189.
52 Rankin JHG, Phernetton TM. Alpha and angiotensin receptor tone in the near-term sheep fetus. *Proc Soc Exp Biol Med* 1978;158:166.
53 Rankin JHG. A role for prostaglandins in the regulation of the placental blood flows. *Prostaglandins* 1976;11:343.
54 Stock MK, Anderson DF, Phernetton TM, et al. Vascular response of the fetal placenta to local occlusion of the maternal placental vasculature. *J Dev Physiol* 1980;2:339–346.
55 Kiserud T, Rasmussen S, Skulstad S. Blood flow and the degree of shunting through the ductus venosus in the human fetus. *Am J Obstet Gynecol* 2000;182:147–153.
56 Kiserud T, Hellevik LR, Eik-Nes SH, et al. Estimation of the pressure gradient across the fetal ductus venosus based on Doppler velocimetry. *Ultrasound Med Biol* 1994;20(3):225–232.
57 Kennedy JA, Clark SL. Observations on the physiological reactions of the ductus arteriosus. *Am J Physiol* 1942;136: 140–147.
58 McMurphy DM, Heymann MA, Rudolph AM, Melmon KL. Developmental changes in constriction of the ductus arteriosus: Responses to oxygen and vasoactive substances in the isolated ductus arteriosus of the fetal lamb. *Pediatr Res* 1972;6:231–238.
59 Coceani F, Liu Y, Seidlitz E, Kelsey L, et al. Endothelin A receptor is necessary for O_2 constriction but not closure of ductus arteriosus. *Am J Physiol* 1999;227:H1521–H1531.
60 Mentzer RM, Ely SW, Lasley RD, et al. Hormonal role of adenosine in maintaining patency of the ductus arteriosus in fetal lambs. *Ann Surg* 1985;202:223–230.
61 Coceani F, Olley PM. The response of the ductus arteriosus to prostaglandins. *Can J Physiol Pharmacol* 1973;51:220–225.
62 Sharpe GL, Thalme B, Larsson KS. Studies on closure of the ductus arteriosus. XI. Ductal closure in utero by a prostaglandin synthetase inhibitor. *Prostaglandins* 1874;8:363–368.
63 Clyman RI, Mauray F, Koerper MA, et al. Formation of prostacyclin (PGI_2) by the ductus arteriosus of fetal lambs at different stages of gestation. *Prostaglandins* 1978;16:633–642.
64 Fouron JC. The unrecognized physiological and clinical significance of the fetal aortic isthmus. *Ultrasound Obstet Gynecol* 2003;22:441–447.
65 Fouron JC, Zarelli M, Drblik SP, Lessard M. Normal flow velocity profile of the fetal aortic isthmus through normal gestation. *Am J Cardiol* 1994;74:483–486.
66 Ruskamp J, Fouron JC, Gosselin J, et al. Reference values for an index of fetal aortic isthmus blood flow during the second half of pregnancy. *Ultrasound Obstet Gynecol* 2003;21:441–444.
67 Patton DJ, Fouron JC. Cerebral arteriovenous malformations: comparison of pre- and postnatal central blood flow dynamics. *Pediatr Cardiol* 1995;16:141–144.
68 Fouron JC, Teyssier G, Bonnin P, et al. Blood flow velocity profile in the fetal aortic isthmus. A sensitive indicator of changes in systemic peripheral resistance II: Clinical observations. *J Matern Fetal Invest* 1993;3:219–224.

69 Schmidt KG, Silverman NH, Harrison MR, Callen PW. High output cardiac failure in fetuses with large sacrococcygeal teratoma: diagnosis by echocardiography and Doppler ultrasound. *J Pediatr* 1989;114:1023–1028.

70 Patton DJ, Fouron JC. Cerebral arteriovenous malformation: prenatal and postnatal central blood flow dynamics. *Pediatr Cardiol* 1995;16:141–144.

71 Rychik J. Fetal cardiovascular physiology. *Pediatr Cardiol* 2004;25:201–209.

72 Fumia FD, Edelstone DI, Holzman IR. Blood flow and oxygen delivery as functions of fetal hematocrit. *Am J Obstet Gynecol* 1984;150:274–282.

73 Oepkes D, Vandenbussche FP, Van Bel F, Kanhai HHH. Fetal ductus venosus blood flow velocities before and after transfusion in red-cell alloimmunized pregnancies. *Obstet Gynecol* 1993; 82:237–241.

74 Mari G, Adrignolo A, Abuhamad AZ, et al. Diagnosis of fetal anaemia with Doppler ultrasound in the pregnancy complicated by maternal blood group immunization. *Ultrasound Obstet Gynecol* 1995;5:400–405.

75 Hecker K, Snijders R, Campbell S, Nicolaides K. Fetal venous, arterial and intracardiac blood flows in red blood cell isoimmunization. *Obstet Gynecol* 1995;85:122–128.

76 Bajoria R, Wigglesworth J, Fisk NM. Angioarchitecture of monochorionic placentas in relation to the twin–twin transfusion syndrome. *Am J Obstet Gynecol* 1995;172:856–863.

77 Bajoria R, Sullivan M, Fisk NM. Endothelin concentrations in monochorionic twins with severe twin–twin transfusion syndrome. *Hum Reprod* 1999;14:1614–1618.

78 Mahieu-Caputo D, Muller F, Joly D, et al. Pathogenesis of twin–twin transfusion syndrome: the renin–angiotensin system hypothesis. *Fetal Diagn Ther* 2001;16:241–244.

79 Cheung YF, Taylor MJ, Fisk NM, et al. Fetal origins of reduced arterial distensibility in the donor twin in twin–twin transfusion syndrome. *Lancet* 2000;355:1157–1158.

80 Fesslova V, Villa L, Nava S, et al. Fetal and neonatal echocardiographic findings in twin–twin transfusion syndrome. *Am J Obstet Gynecol* 1998;179:1056–1062.

81 Raboisson MJ, Fouron JC, Lamoureux J, et al. Early in-tertwin differences in myocardial performance during the twin-to-twin transfusion syndrome. *Circulation* 2004;110:3043–3048.

82 Lougheed J, Sinclair BG, Fung KFK, et al. Acquired right ventricular outflow tract obstruction in the recipient twin in twin–twin transfusion syndrome. *J Am Coll Cardiol* 2001;38: 1533–1538.

83 Rizzo G, Arduini D, Romanini C. Cardiac and extra-cardiac flows in discordant twins. *Am J Obstet Gynecol* 1994;170:1321–1327.

84 Jones MD, Rosenberg AA, Simmons MA, et al. Oxygen delivery to the brain before and after birth. *Science* 1982;216:324–325.

85 Sidi D, Kuipers JRG, Teitel D, et al. Developmental changes in oxygenation and circulatory responses to hypoxemia in lambs. *Am J Physiol* 1983;245:H674–682.

86 Assali NS, Holm LW, Sehgal N. Hemodynamic changes in fetal lamb in utero in response to asphyxia, hypoxia, and hypercapnia. *Circ Res* 1962;11:423–430.

87 Cohn HE, Sacks EJ, Heymann MA, Rudolph AM. Cardiovascular responses to hypoxemia and acidemia in fetal lambs. *Am J Obstet Gynecol* 1974;120:817–824.

88 Peeters LL, Sheldon RE, Jones MD, et al. Blood flow to fetal organs as a function of arterial oxygen content. *Am J Obstet Gynecol* 1979;135:637–646.

89 Sheldon RE, Peeters LLH, Jones Jr MD, et al. Redistribution of cardiac output and oxygen delivery in the hypoxemic fetal lamb. *Am J Obstet Gynecol* 1979;135:1071–1078.

90 Alonso JG, Okai T, Longo LD, Gilbert RD. Cardiac function during long-term hypoxemia in fetal sheep. *Am J Physiol* 1989;257:H581–589.

91 Kitanaka T, Alonso JG, Gilbert RD, et al. Fetal responses to long-term hypoxemia in sheep. *Am J Physiol* 1989;256:R1348–1354.

92 Morrow RJ, Adamson SL, Bull SB, Knox Ritchie JW. Acute hypoxemia does not affect the umbilical artery flow velocity waveform in fetal sheep. *Obstet Gynecol* 1990;75:590–593.

93 Fouron JC, Lafond J, Bard H. Effects of hypoxemia with and without acidemia on the isometric contraction time and the electromechanical delay of the fetal myocardium: an experimental study on the ovine fetus. *Am J Obstet Gynecol* 1990;162: 262–266.

94 Piacquadio KM, Brace RA, Cheung CY. Role of vasopressin in medication of fetal cardiovascular responses to acute hypoxia. *Am J Obstet Gynecol* 1990;163:1294–1300.

95 Rurak DW, Richandson BS, Patrick JE, et al. Blood flow and oxygen delivery to fetal organs and tissues during sustained hypoxemia. *Am J Physiol* 1990;258:R1116–1122.

96 Itskovitz J, LaGamma EF, Bristow J, Rudolph AM. Cardiovascular responses to hypoxemia in sinoaortic-denervated fetal sheep. *Pediatr Res* 1991;30:381–385.

97 Paulick RP, Meyers RL, Rudolph CD, Rudolph AM. Hemodynamic responses to alpha-adrenergic blockade during hypoxemia in fetal lamb. *J Dev Physiol* 1991;16:63–69.

98 Kamitomo M, Longo LD, Gilbert RD. Right and left ventricular function in fetal sheep exposed to long-term high altitude hypoxemia. *Am J Physiol* 1992;262:H399–405.

99 Creasy RK, Barrett CT, Swiet M de, et al. Experimental intrauterine growth retardation in the sheep. *Am J Obstet Gynecol* 1972;112:566–573.

100 Moutquin JM, Liggins GC. Effects of partial lower aortic obstruction in the pregnant ewe on fetal arterial pressure, heart rate, plasma renin activity and prostaglandin E concentration. *J Dev Physiol* 1981;3:75–84.

101 Abitbol MM. Fetal heart rate and tissue pH changes associated with repetitive aortic occlusion in the pregnant ewe dog. *Am J Obstet Gynecol* 1982;143:430–439.

102 Yaffe H, Parer JT, Block BS, Leanos AJ. Cardiorespiratory responses to graded reductions of uterine blood flow in the sheep fetus. *J Dev Physiol* 1987;9:325–336.

103 Bocking AD, Gagnon R, White SE, et al. Circulatory responses to prolonged hypoxemia in fetal sheep. *Am J Obstet Gynecol* 1988;159:1418–1424.

104 van Huisseling H, Hasaart TH, Ruissen CJ, et al. Umbilical artery flow velocity waveforms during acute hypoxemia and the relationship with hemodynamic changes in the fetal lamb. *Am J Obstet Gynecol* 1989;161:1061–1064.

105 Reid DL, Parer JT, Williams K, et al. Effects of severe reduction in Develop Physiol maternal placental blood flow on blood flow distribution in the sheep fetus. *J Dev Physiol* 1991;15:183–188.

106 Fumia FD, Edelstone DI, Holzman IR. Blood flow and oxygen delivery to fetal organs as functions of fetal hematocrit. *Am J Obstet Gynecol* 1984;150:274–282.

107 Comline RS, Silver M. Development of activity in the adrenal medulla of the fetus and newborn animal. *Br Med Bull* 1966;22:16–20.

108 Reuss ML, Parer JT, Harris JL, Krueger TR. Hemodynamic effects of alpha-adrenergic blockade during hypoxia in fetal sheep. *Am J Obstet Gynecol* 1982;142:410–415.

109 Rurak DW. Plasma vasopressin levels during hypoxemia and the cardiovascular effects of exogenous vasopressin in foetal and adult sheep. *J Physiol (Lond)* 1978;277:341–357.

110 Dawes GS, Lewis BV, Nilligan JE, et al. Vasomotor responses in the hind limbs of foetal and newborn lambs to asphyxia and aortic chemoreceptor stimulation. *J Physiol* 1968;195:55–81.

111 Gilbert RD, Pearce WJ, Ashwal S, Longo LD. Effects of hypoxia on contractility of isolated fetal lamb cerebral arteries. *J Dev Physiol* 1990;13:199–203.

112 Behrman RE, Lees MH, Peterson EN, et al. Distribution of the circulation in the normal and asphyxiated fetal primate. *Am J Obstet Gynecol* 1970;108:956–969.

113 Reuss ML, Rudolph AM. Distribution and recirculation of umbilical and systemic venous blood flow in fetal lambs during hypoxia. *J Dev Physiol* 1980;2:71.

114 Edelstone DI. Regulation of blood flow through the ductus venosus. *J Dev Physiol* 1980;2:219–238.

115 Muijsers GJJM, Hasaart THM, van Huisseling H, de Haan J. The response of the umbilical artery pulsatility index in fetal sheep to acute and prolonged hypoxaemia and acidaemia induced by embolization of the uterine microcirculation. *J Dev Physiol* 1990;13:231–236.

116 Downing GJ, Yarlagadda P, Maulik D. Effects of acute hypoxemia on umbilical arterial Doppler indices in a fetal ovine model. *Early Human Dev* 1991;25:1–10.

117 Arbeille P, Maulik D, Fignon A, et al. Assessment of the fetal PO_2 changes by cerebral and umbilical Doppler on lamb fetuses during acute hypoxia. *Ultrasound Med Biol* 1995;21:861–870.

118 Lewis AB, Wolf WS, Sischo W. Cardiovascular and catecholamine responses to successive episodes of hypoxemia in the fetus. *Biol Neonate* 1984;45:105–111.

119 Itskowitz J, LaGamma EF, Rudolph AM. Effects of cord compression on fetal blood flow distribution and O_2 delivery. *Am J Physiol* 1987;252:H100–109.

120 Richardson BS, Carmichael L, Homan J, et al. Fetal cerebral circulatory and metabolic responses during heart rate decelerations with umbilical cord compression. *Am J Obstet Gynecol* 1996; 175:929–936.

121 De Haan HH, Gunn AJ, Williams CE, Cluckman PD. Brief repeated umbilical cord occlusions cause sustained cytotoxic cerebral edema and focal infants in near-term fetal lambs. *Pediatr Res* 1997;41:96–104.

122 Ley D, Oskarsson G, Bellander M, Hernandez-Andrade E, et al. Different responses of myocardial and cerebral blood flow to cord occlusion in exteriorized fetal sheep. *Pediatr Res* 2004;55:568–575.

123 Trudinger BJ, Stevens D, Connely A. Umbilical artery flow velocity waveforms and placental resistance: The effects of embolization of the umbilical circulation. *Am J Obstet Gynecol* 1987;157:1443–1448.

124 Morrow RJ, Adamson SL, Bull SB, Ritchie JWK. Effect of placental embolization on the umbilical arterial velocity waveform in fetal sheep. *Am J Obstet Gynecol* 1989;161:1055–1060.

125 Lewinsky RM, Szwarc RS, Benson LN, Ritchie JW. The effects of hypoxic acidemia on left ventricular end-systolic elastance in fetal sheep. *Pediatr Res* 1993;34:38–43.

126 Gagnon R, Rundle H, Johnston L, Han VK. Alterations in fetal and placental deoxyribonucleic acid synthesis rates after chronic fetal placental embolization. *Am J Obstet Gynecol* 1995; 172:1451–1458.

127 Murotsuki J, Challis JRG, Han VKM, et al. Chronic fetal placental embolization and hypoxemia cause hypertension and myocardial hypertrophy in fetal sheep. *Am J Physiol* 1997;41: R201–207.

128 Adamson SL, Morrow RJ, Langille BL, et al. Site-dependent effects of increases in placental vascular resistance on the umbilical arterial velocity waveform in fetal sheep. *Ultrasound Med Biol* 1990;16:19–27.

129 Iwamoto HS, Stucky E, Roman CM. Effect of graded umbilical cord compression in fetal sheep at 0.6–0.7 gestation. *Am J Physiol* 1991;261:H1268–1274.

130 Fouron JC, Teyssier G, Maroto E, et al. Diastolic circulatory dynamics in the presence of elevated retrograde diastolic flow in the umbilical artery: a Doppler echocardiographic study in lambs. *Am J Obstet Gynecol* 1991;164:195–203.

131 Sonesson SE, Fouron JC, Teyssier G, Bonnin P. Effects of increased resistance to umbilical blood flow on fetal hemodynamic changes induced by maternal oxygen administration: a Doppler velocimetric study on the sheep. *Pediatr Res* 1993;34: 796–800.

132 Bonnin P, Fouron JC, Teyssier G, et al. Quantitative assessment of circulatory changes in the fetal aortic isthmus during progressive increase of resistance to umbilical blood flow. *Circulation* 1993;88:216–222.

133 Rasanen J, Kirkinen P, Jouppila P. Right ventricular dysfunction in human fetal compromise. *Am J Obstet Gynecol* 1989;161: 136–140.

134 Reed KL, Anderson CF, Shenker L. Changes in intracardiac Doppler blood flow velocities in fetuses with absent umbilical artery diastolic flow. *Am J Obstet Gynecol* 1987;157:774–779.

135 Rizzo C, Arduini D, Romanini C, Mancuson S. Doppler echocardiographic assessment of atrioventricular velocity waveforms in normal and small-for-gestational-age fetuses. *Br J Obstet Gynaecol* 1988;95:65–69.

136 Kiserud T, Eik-Nes SH, Blaas HG, et al. Ductus venosus blood velocity and the umbilical circulation in the seriously growth-retarded fetus. *Ultrasound Obstet Gynecol* 1994;4: 109.

137 Farine D, Kelly EN, Ryan G, et al. Absent and reversed umbilical artery end-diastolic velocity. In: Copel JA, Reed KL, eds. *Doppler ultrasound in obstetrics and gynecology.* New York: Raven Press; 1995:187–197.

138 Schmidt KG, Di Tommaso M, Silverman NH, Rudolph AM. Evaluation of changes in umbilical blood flow in the fetal lamb by Doppler waveform analysis. *Am J Obstet Gynecol* 1991; 164:1118–1126.

139 Vyas S, Nicolaides KH, Campbell S. Renal flow-velocity waveforms in normal and hypoxemic fetuses. *Am J Obstet Gynecol* 1989;16:1168–1172.

140 Mari G, Abuhamad AZ, Verpairojkit B, et al. Blood flow velocity waveforms of the abdominal arteries in appropriate and small for gestational age fetuses. *Ultrasound Obstet Gynecol* 1995; 6:15–18.

141 Sepulveda W, Bower S, Nicolaides P, et al. Discordant blood flow velocity waveforms in left and right brachial arteries in growth-retarded fetuses. *Obstet Gynecol* 1995; 86:734–738.

142 Gembruck U, Baschat AA. Demonstration of fetal coronary blood flow by color-coded and pulsed wave Doppler sonography: a possible indicator of severe compromise and impending demise in intrauterine growth retardation. *Ultrasound Obstet Gynecol* 1996;7:10–16.

143 Mari G, Verpairojkit B, Abuhamad AZ, Copel JA. Adrenal artery

velocity waveforms in the appropriate and small for gestational age fetus. *Ultrasound Obstet Gynecol* 1996;8:82–86.

144 Rizzo G, Capponi A, Choui R, et al. Blood flow velocity waveforms from peripheral pulmonary arteries in normally grown and growth retarded fetuses. *Ultrasound Obstet Gynecol* 1996;8: 87–92.

145 Fouron JC, Gosselin J, Raboisson MJ, et al. The relationship between an aortic isthmus blood flow velocity index and the postnatal neurodevelopment status of fetuses with placental circulatory insufficiency. *Am J Obstet Gynecol* 2005;192:497–503.

8 Immunology of the fetus

Josiah F. Wedgwood and James G. McNamara

This chapter provides an overview of the developing fetal immune system from molecular, cellular, and functional perspectives. Many questions and issues remain unresolved, but the framework reveals a tightly regulated process of development and provides a basis for understanding future insights into the ontogeny of the immune system.

The purpose of the developing immune system is to recognize virtually all foreign pathogens (i.e., to have a very broad repertoire of responses) and yet not respond to normal host products (i.e., not react to self). This is accomplished through the innate and adaptive immune systems and the interactions between them. The generation of B- and T-cell receptor (BCR and TCR) diversity, which is critical to the adaptive immune system, has been the subject of intense investigation and has provided a number of useful models of how the developing fetus acquires functional competence. The role of changes (or lack of changes) in the innate immune system during fetal development is much less well understood. Before going further, a summary of some general concepts will allow us to consider developmental immunology issues from a common framework.

Relevant concepts in immunology

The innate immune system consists of receptors and other proteins that respond to foreign pathogens but do not change over time.[1] Table 8.1 lists the components of the innate immune system; this list will undoubtedly grow as our understanding of the innate immune system increases. In contrast with the innate immune system, the adaptive immune system uses receptors that can become more refined over time.[2] The two systems can cooperate in a number of ways.

All of the cells of the immune system originate from hematopoietic stem cells located in the bone marrow of adults.[3] These pluripotent cells initially generate the myeloid progenitors (the precursor of granulocytes, macrophages, dendritic cells, and mast cells) and the common lymphoid progenitors [the precursor of lymphocytes and natural killer (NK) cells]. Cells of the myeloid lineage mature in the bone marrow or after taking up residence in the tissues. The lymphocytes mature in the bone marrow (B cells) or thymus (T cells). After maturation, the lymphocytes circulate through the bloodstream to the peripheral lymphoid organs, where they can become exposed to antigens on dendritic cells. From the peripheral lymphoid organs, the lymphocytes enter the lymph ducts and are returned to the bloodstream. This allows the formation of immunologic memory and refinement of the receptors of the adaptive immune system.

Immunologic nomenclature

The nomenclature used in immunology can be very cumbersome and confusing. The term "clusters of differentiation" (CD) is used to describe antigens expressed by groups or subsets of cells of the hematopoietic system. More than 300 CDs have been defined.[4] This designation is used for all species in which homologous structures have been identified. Antibodies to specific CDs are often used to enumerate important types of leukocytes by flow cytometry. Table 8.2 lists the commonly encountered leukocyte groups.

Chemokines are small secreted proteins that act as chemoattractants for leukocytes and some other cells during inflammation.[5] Chemokines interact with specific chemokine receptors. Table 8.3 lists the chemokines, chemokine receptors, and target cells.

Cytokines are also secreted proteins that affect the behavior of other cells.[6] Cytokines interact with specific cytokine receptors. Cytokines made by lymphocytes are sometimes referred to as lymphokines or interleukins. Table 8.4 lists the cytokines, cytokine receptors, producer cells, and cytokine actions.

Pathogen recognition in the innate immune system

The innate immune system recognizes pathogens through invariant receptors that take advantage of molecular structures that are unique to pathogens.[7] The system is static, although changes in the number of receptors present can occur. For example, the collectins, which include mannose-binding protein (MBP), surfactant protein A (SpA) and surfactant protein D (SpD), bind to repeating carbohydrates in particular spatial arrangements that are present only on pathogens.[8] Binding of SpA to the respiratory syncytial virus fusion protein neutralizes this virus, and thus can prevent infection or spread of virus.[9]

Toll-like receptors (TLRs) were originally described in the fruit fly, in which they were found to confer protection from some fungal infections.[10] In humans, TLRs respond to various microbial products, including peptidoglycan, flagellin, and unmethylated CpG DNA.[11] Lipopolysaccharide (LPS) bound to CD14 is recognized by TLR-4. TLR-3 recognizes double-stranded RNA, which is sometimes expressed during viral infections and is not normally found in mammalian cells. Unmethylated CpG DNA is typically found in bacteria and is recognized by TLR-9. Single-stranded RNA, which is typical of many viruses, is recognized by TLR-7 and TLR-9. The activation of TLRs triggers the production of proinflammatory cytokines [IL (interleukin)-1, IL-6, IL-12, tumor necrosis factor

Table 8.1 Components of the innate immune system.

Type of system	Examples
Physical barriers	Skin, gut, and respiratory epithelium, hairs, cilia, mucin, normal flora
Host cells	Macrophages/dendritic cells, neutrophils, NK cells, mast cells, γ/δ T cells, CD5+ B lymphocytes
Antimicrobial agents	Defensins, lactoferrin, transferrin, lysozyme, myeloperoxidase, serprocidins, bacterial permeability-increasing protein
Opsonins	Complement, fibronectin
Reactive oxygen and nitrogen species	Superoxide, hydrogen peroxide, hydroxyl radical, hypochlorite ion, nitric oxide
Receptors	Collectins, conglutinin, selectins, CD14, TLR
Cytokines	IL-1, TNF-α, IL-6, IL-8, MIP, MCP, IFN-γ, IL-12, IL-15, IL-18, GM-CSF, G-CSF, M-CSF

Table 8.2 CD antigens used to define important leukocyte groups.

Leukocyte group	Description
Lymphocyte subgroups	
CD3+	T cells
CD4+/CD3+	Helper T cells
CD8+/CD3+	Cytotoxic T cells
CD25+/CD4+/CD3+	Regulatory T cells
CD45RA+/CD3+	Naive T cells
CD45RO+/CD3+	Memory T cells
CD19+	B cells
CD20+	B cells
IgM+/IgD–/CD19+	Immature B cells
IgM+/IgD+/CD19+	Mature naive B cells
IgM–/IgD–/CD19+	Memory B cells
Other cell types	
CD56+	NK cells
CD14+	Monocytes/neutrophils (myelomonocytic lineage)

Table 8.3 Chemokines.

Family*	Chemokines	Examples of other names	Human chromosome	Target cell	Specific receptor
CXCL (ELR+: chemotactic for neutrophils)	CXCL1, CXCL2, CXCL3, CXCL5, CXCL6, CXCL7, CXCL8, CXCL14, CXCL15	GROα, GROβ, GROγ, IL-8	4, occasionally 5	Predominantly neutrophils	CXCR1, CXCR2, some unknown
CXCL (ELR–: chemotactic for lymphocytes)	CXCL4, CXCL9, CXCL10, CXCL11, CXCL12, CXCL13, CXCL16	PF4, Mig, IP-10, I-TAC, SDF-1	4, occasionally 10 or 17	Predominantly activated T cells	CXCR3, CXCR4, CXCR5, CXCR6
CCL	CCL1–28 (some only in mouse)	MCP-1, MIP-1α, MIP-1β, RANTES	17, occasionally 2, 5, 7, 9, or 16	Predominantly monocytes/macrophages, also dendritic cells, T cells, eosinophils, basophils	CCR1–10, some unknown
C and CX3C	XCL1, XCL2, CX3CL1	Lymphotactin, SCM-1β, fractalkine	1 or 16	Predominantly T cells and NK cells	XCR1, XCR2, CXCR1

*Chemokine families are characterized by the amino acid sequence surrounding the critical cysteine(s).

Table 8.4 Representative cytokines.

	Cytokine	Receptor	Producer cells	Action
Hematopoietins	Epo (erythropoietin)	EpoR	Kidney cells, hepatocytes	Stimulation of erythroid progenitors
	IL-2 (T-cell growth factor)	IL-2R (CD25 α-chain, CD122 β-chain, CD132 common γ-chain)	T cells	T-cell proliferation
	IL-4 (BCGF-1, BSF-1)	IL-4R (CD124 α-chain, CD132 common γ-chain)	T cells, mast cells	B-cell activation, IgE switch, differentiation into Th2
	G-CSF	G-CSFR	Fibroblasts and monocytes	Neutrophil development and differentiation
	GM-CSF	GM-CSFR (CD116 α-chain, CDw131 common β-chain)	Macrophages, T cells	Growth and differentiation of myelomonocytic lineage, particularly dendritic cells
Interferons	IFN-α	CD118 (IFNAR2)	Leukocytes, dendritic cells	Antiviral, increased MHC class I expression
	IFN-β	CD118 (IFNAR2)	Fibroblasts	Antiviral, increased MHC class I expression
	IFN-γ	CD119 (IFNGR2)	T cells, NK cells	Macrophage activation, increased MHC/antigen expression, Ig class switch, suppression of Th2
TNF family	TNF-α (cachectin)	CD120a, CD120b	Macrophage, NK cells, T cells	Local inflammation, endothelial activation
	TNF-β (lymphotoxin)	CD120a, CD120b	T cells, B cells	Killing, endothelial activation
	CD40 ligand (CD40L, CD154)	CD40	T cells, mast cells	B-cell activation, Ig class switch
	Fas ligand	CD95 (Fas)	T cells	Apoptosis, Ca^{2+}- independent cytotoxicity
IL-10 family	IL-10	IL-10R	T cells, macrophages	Potent suppressant of macrophage functions
IL-12 family	IL-12	IL-12R	Macrophages, dendritic cells	Activation of NK cells, induction of CD4+ T- cell differentiation into Th1-like cells
Unassigned	TGF-β	TGF-βR	Chondrocytes, monocytes, T cells	Inhibition of cell growth, anti-inflammatory, induction of IgA switch
	IL-1α	CD121a, CD121b	Macrophages, epithelial cells	Fever, T-cell activation, macrophage activation
	IL-1β	CD121a, CD121b	Macrophages, epithelial cells	Fever, T-cell activation, macrophage activation

(TNF)-α] and chemokines (CXCL8 or IL-8) and the expression of co-stimulatory molecules.

TLRs are not the only pattern recognition receptors (PRRs) of the innate immune system. The nucleotide-binding oligomerization domain (NOD) proteins, which recognize muroproteins from the bacterial cell wall, and RNA helicases, which respond to double-stranded RNA from viral infections, have recently been described,[12] and the discovery of other PRRs can be expected.[7]

Killer cell immunoglobulin-like receptors (KIRs) represent a recently described and complex series of receptors that are present on subsets of NK cells, γ/δ TCR+ T cells, and some memory/effector α/β TCR+ T cells.[13] In humans, the *KIR* gene family contains up to 15 genes and two pseudogenes that are closely linked on chromosome 19. The selection of varying numbers of *KIR* genes for expression appears to be a random event. The subset of expressed *KIR* genes becomes fixed by methylation of the unexpressed *KIR* genes. The KIR ligands are major histocompatibility complex (MHC) class I molecules including human leukocyte antigen (HLA)-A, HLA-B, and HLA-C proteins. Binding of KIR to these molecules is usually inhibitory, leading to suppression of cytotoxicity and cytokine secretion. The interaction of KIR with HLA-G and HLA-E may help in the maintenance of pregnancy.[14] Because

NK cells are involved in vascular remodeling of the placenta, preeclampsia and spontaneous abortion may result from abnormal KIR–ligand interactions.[15]

The various components of the innate immune system are able to: (1) prevent infection or slow the spread of infection; (2) kill cells harboring or replicating the pathogen; and (3) recruit other components of the innate and adaptive immune systems to the site of infection.

Pathogen recognition in the adaptive immune system

By definition, mature B cells or T cells express cell-surface receptors that they use to recognize foreign antigens. The BCR is made up of a membrane-anchored immunoglobulin (two heavy chains and two light chains), together with associated signaling molecules.[16] The BCR is able to recognize both membrane-associated and soluble antigens. The TCR is composed of two glycoprotein chains (α/β or γ/δ heterodimers) that are able to recognize antigens in association with MHC class I or class II molecules.[17] TCRs are also associated with nonpolymorphic proteins that are involved in signal transduction.

The generation of functional BCRs and TCRs is the result of ordered rearrangements and expression of families of genes. The immunoglobulin family of genes that generate BCRs was the first to be described and became the prototype for the study of TCR genes.[18] Immunoglobulin genes have coding sequences (exons) for constant regions (C), variable regions (V), joining regions (J), and, in heavy chains, diversity regions (D), which are encoded in a nonrearranged form (germline configuration) on different chromosomes: chromosome 14 for immunoglobulin heavy chains, chromosome 2 for κ light chains, and chromosome 22 for λ light chains.

The cascade of events leading up to a productively rearranged IgM heavy chain can be summarized as follows. First, a D-gene exon is transposed next to a J-chain exon, with the intervening genes being deleted as a result of the rearrangement. Then a V-gene exon is similarly transposed to form a V/D/J recombinant. This recombination alters nuclear regulatory genes and allows the transcription of the V/D/J complex as well as the downstream C exon. Subsequently, the transcribed RNA is spliced to remove the intervening sequences to produce mature messenger RNA (mRNA); this is translated to produce a functional IgM heavy chain with a hydrophobic tail, which anchors the BCR in the cell membrane. Similar events lead to the production of light chains except that no D gene is involved.

Immunologic diversity is generated through four mechanisms.[19] First, a large combinatorial contribution comes from the number of different V, D, and J exons that are available to produce the heavy chain, or the different V and J exons that are available to produce the light chain. Second, junctional diversity is introduced as a result of the addition or deletion of base pairs at the time of recombination. Third, additional combinatorial diversity results from the different possible combinations of heavy and light chains. Finally, in a process that is unique to B cells, somatic mutations, or the mutational events that occur within genes after rearrangement, occur with activation. By the process known as allelic exclusion, only one chromosomal allele at a time can be productively rearranged for each heavy- or light-chain immunoglobulin gene. Significantly, the entire process of gene rearrangements to form immunoglobulins in immature B cells occurs as an antigen-independent event. The signals that drive the initiation of this cascade, which culminates with the production of a highly sophisticated mechanism of protection, are not known.

TCRs are composed of heterodimers of α/β chains or the numerically much less common γ/δ chains (< 5% of peripheral blood T cells).[20] TCR diversity is generated in the same way as BCR diversity: V/D/J recombinations generate the variable region of the TCR δ-chain or γ-chain and V/J recombinations generate the variable region of the TCR β-chain or δ-chain. Similarly, the diversity of TCR antigen specificities is generated through combinatorial and junctional mechanisms; however, somatic mutation is responsible for much less receptor diversity than in immunoglobulins. As with BCR, the TCR gene rearrangement is not driven by antigen-dependent mechanisms. Generation of the TCR results in formation of a TCR excision circle (TREC) that persists until the cell undergoes mitosis.[21] Thymic output of T cells can be assessed by determining the fraction of TREC+ T cells.

The BCR is unique in its ability to switch isotypes by recombination between the V/D/J cluster and sequences for switch sites further downstream; this brings the complex to regions encoding other heavy-chain exons, which again undergo RNA splicing to generate the final mRNA product. This process is termed "isotype switching."[22]

Clonal selection hypothesis

The random generation of BCRs and TCRs described above will lead to the generation of cells that can be expected to respond to self (auto)-antigens. Burnet's clonal selection hypothesis includes a postulate that explains why these clones are not observed;[23] they are deleted at an early stage in lymphoid cell development. Experimental evidence has demonstrated that this hypothesis is correct.

T-cell clonal deletion in the thymus and peripheral lymphoid tissues

The development of the thymus is essential to the normal evolution of a functional immune system. Patients with the complete DiGeorge's anomaly (triad of cardiac abnormalities, hypoparathyroidism, and absent thymus) fail to develop T-cell lymphocytes and have a severe combined immunodeficiency.[24]

The thymus consists of numerous lobules, each of which has an outer cortical region and an inner medulla. The cortical region consists of a network of epithelial cells that provide signals to lymphoid progenitors to differentiate into T cells through the Notch1 receptor, in addition to providing other critical cytokines which allow T-cell development.[25] One of the signals that is necessary for a T cell to survive is the ability of the TCR to bind to MHC self-molecules in the absence of antigen. At the time of this positive selection, the developing T cell expresses both CD4 and CD8. The selection results in CD4+ T cells, which recognize MHC class II molecules, and CD8+ T cells, which recognize MHC class I molecules. Negative selection occurs when these cells bind tightly to cortical epithelial cells expressing self-antigens that are bound to MHC molecules. A second round of negative selection occurs when developing T cells are exposed to self-antigens on dendritic cells at the corticomedullary junction. A substantial fraction of T-cell clones are removed through this selection process.[26]

In addition to selection in the thymus, T cells are actively selected in peripheral lymphoid tissue. Repeated contact with MHC–self-peptide complexes is necessary for the continued survival of naive T cells. Negative selection of autoreactive T-cell clones also occurs in the periphery.[27]

B-cell clonal deletion in the bone marrow and peripheral lymphoid tissues

In the bone marrow, developing B cells, which are cross-linked to BCRs by multivalent self-molecules, are either deleted or undergo additional receptor editing.[28] B cells that encounter soluble self-molecules in the bone marrow downregulate the μ-chain of the BCR and become anergic (unresponsive) to further exposure to antigen. Naive B cells must enter the follicular region of peripheral lymphoid tissue to receive signals to prevent cell death. Naive B cells that encounter a strongly cross-linking self-antigen also undergo clonal deletion. Again, a substantial fraction of clones are deleted through this selection process.

Immunologic memory

B cells or T cells that have not been exposed to antigen are called naive. Exposure of B cells to antigen (first signal) together with signals from activated T cells or antigen-presenting cells (APC) result in activation of the B cell, cellular proliferation, and generation of scattered somatic mutations throughout the antibody variable regions.[29] Somatic mutations that improve antigen binding are able to undergo additional expansion whereas mutations with diminished binding undergo apoptosis. In addition, some B cells may also undergo an isotype switch, which is regulated by T-cell-derived signals.[30] The resulting B cells are termed memory B cells, and are responsible for the robust secondary antibody response seen on re-exposure to an antigen. Finally, some of the B cells will mature into plasma cells and produce secreted antibody.[31]

T cells respond to antigen which has been processed by APC. Small peptides derived from the antigen are bound to class I MHC or class II MHC molecules transferred to the cell membrane.[32,33] A second signal, usually the result of activation of the APC, is required for T-cell proliferation and maturation.[34] Immediately after exposure to antigen, the number of reactive T cells increases as effector T cells are produced. Some of these cells persist and are called memory T cells.

Ontogeny of the innate immune system

The ontogeny of some components of the innate immune system has been investigated; however, further information is still required in many areas.

Physical barriers

The incomplete keratinization of the skin of premature infants is well known.[35] After premature delivery, accelerated maturation occurs. Studies of skin treatments to reduce infections have yielded inconsistent results.[36] What is clear is that there is a markedly increased absorption of topically applied compounds through the skin of newborns, which can result in toxicity (e.g., hexachlorophene, povidone–iodine).[37] Proponents of probiotics argue that establishing an appropriate gut flora reduces the risk of infection and necrotizing enterocolitis.[38,39] One recent report has suggested that erythema toxicum neonatorum may be the result of the innate immune response to commensal bacteria penetrating the skin of the newborn around the hair follicle.[40]

Host cells

The numbers of macrophages/dendritic cells, neutrophils, NK cells, mast cells, γ/δ T cells, and B1 lymphocytes appear normal at birth. Neonatal dendritic cellular function is impaired and may contribute to the impaired specific immune response observed in this group.[41] Newborn neutrophil chemotaxis in response to chemokines is decreased when compared with adults.[42] NK cells from newborns function poorly against herpes simplex virus (HSV)-infected target cells, which may explain the unusual susceptibility of this group to *Herpes simplex* infections.[43]

Antimicrobial agents

Antimicrobial proteins such as defensins, bacterial permeability-increasing protein (BPI), and lysozyme are developmentally regulated and expressed in lower levels in premature infants than in term infants.[44–46] These proteins contribute to the antimicrobial properties of amniotic fluid and vernix.[47]

Opsonins

Most complement components, including C3, are decreased in newborns. Diminished C3 levels may result in an increased risk of infection as well as a diminished response to vaccination. Serum fibronectin levels are related to gestational age at birth. This may have clinical implications because fibronectin serves as an opsonin for staphylococci and group B streptococci.

Reactive oxygen and nitrogen species

Functional comparisons of adult and newborn neutrophils give conflicting results.[48] Oxidative metabolism (H_2O_2 and O^{2-} production) is normal or increased in newborn neutrophils, but chemiluminescence (·OH production) is diminished for many stimuli; this may be the result of decreased lactoferrin content. LPS dramatically increases oxidative metabolism and chemiluminescence in adult neutrophils but has little effect in newborns as expression of CD14, an LPS receptor, is decreased.[49] *In vivo*, the relative inability of newborn neutrophils to generate reactive oxygen and nitrogen species and hence kill bacteria is accentuated by defects in adherence to activated endothelial cells and chemotaxis,[50] defects in phagocytosis resulting from poor serum opsonization,[51] and a smaller neutrophil storage pool.[52]

Innate receptors

Many of the TLR responses of newborn cells are diminished for reasons that are not completely understood. For example, the response of cord blood monocytes to LPS exposure is diminished.[53] Some have argued that this is the result of decreased expression of TLR-4 on fetal and newborn monocytes, but others have noted decreased intracellular levels of MyD88, a TLR-adaptor protein.[54] Other relative defects in the TLR signaling pathway have also been described.[55] Whatever the mechanism, activation of TLRs in the newborn results in smaller amounts of proinflammatory cytokines and chemokines as well as diminished expression of co-stimulatory molecules. The predicted result of this decreased TLR function is an increased susceptibility to infection and a decreased ability to develop a robust adaptive immune response. Negative regulators of TLRs have been described but have not been studied in newborns.[56]

Inflammatory cytokines

Newborn mononuclear cells produce decreased amounts of CCL3 (MIP-1α) compared with adult cells.[57] In contrast, production of IL-8 by newborn neutrophils is increased.[58] Few studies have been conducted to evaluate other cytokines. The implications of reported differences in cytokine production for clinical practice are unclear.

Ontogeny of the adaptive immune system

Serum immunoglobulin

Term newborns have total serum IgG levels that are slightly higher than their mothers. This IgG is produced by the mother's immune system and is actively transported across the placenta starting in the second half of the second trimester. Transport is mediated by neonatal Fc receptors in the syncytiotrophoblast, which are able to bind IgG at the acidic pH present in the vacuoles containing pinocytosed maternal serum.[59] IgG1 is transported more efficiently than the other IgG subclasses. IgM, IgA, and IgE do not bind to the neonatal Fc receptor involved in this transport process and are virtually absent from newborn serum unless the fetal immune system has been stimulated (e.g., by a congenital infection; Table 8.5).

Table 8.5 Serum immunoglobulin levels (mgdL) in fetuses and newborns.

Group	IgG1	IgG2	IgG3	IgG4	IgA	IgM
17–22 weeks	0.93	0.31	0.05	0.04	0.001	–
28–32 weeks	3.7	0.93	0.19	0.21	0.002	–
Term	10.43	1.56	0.41	0.47	0.004	< 0.2
Adult	10	4	1	0.5	2.5	2

The presence of maternal antibodies protects the newborn (passive immunity) from some infections for several months. However, the presence of maternal antibodies also interferes with the antibody response generated by immunization.[60] Interestingly, T cells are usually primed in a normal fashion to immunogens.[61] These maternal antibodies can also prevent the early replication of live viral vaccines, leading to vaccine failure.

Preterm infants have immunoglobulin levels that are similar to those seen in congenital immunodeficiency diseases involving antibody formation, which are associated with an increased risk of infections.[62] Immunoglobulin replacement therapy in preterm infants has not been associated with decreased numbers of infections.[63] This may reflect alterations in complement levels, neutrophil function, and phagocytic capability, which are also present in newborns, as well as the fact that the most frequent cause of newborn sepsis is *Staphylococcus epidermidis*.

T-cell development

Pre-T cells can be identified in the fetal liver as early as 7 weeks of gestation; these cells seed the thymus at 8–9 weeks, and T cells (TCR+) appear shortly thereafter. By 18 weeks, CD4+ T cells and CD8+ T cells are present in the blood. At term, the numbers of CD4+ T cells and CD8+ T cells in blood are approximately the same as those seen in adults. However, there are some significant differences. Almost all of the peripheral blood T cells in the fetus are naive compared with 40% of the adult T cells. A much larger percentage of newborn T cells are recent emigrants from the thymus and have the DNA excision circles that are formed during the TCR recombination process. Finally, the newborn T cells have a random distribution of TCRs, whereas adult T cells have evidence of clonal expansion.[64] CD25+/CD4+ regulatory T cells are observed early in the second trimester.[65]

B-cell development

In the human fetus, pre-B cells can be identified in fetal liver samples as early as 7–8 weeks' gestation.[66] B cells bearing surface IgM are first detected in fetal liver at 9–10 weeks' gestation. Shortly after this time, B cells that also express surface IgG or surface IgA can be found in small numbers, and, by weeks 12–13, surface IgD cells can also be found. Although B cells are first observed in fetal liver, they are rapidly observed subsequently in fetal bone marrow, spleen, and blood. The number of circulating B cells found in fetal blood reaches the level seen in adults by approximately 15 weeks' gestation. By the end of the first trimester, the generation of new B cells switches from the fetal liver to the bone marrow. Primary nodules develop around the follicular dendritic cells of the lymph nodes at about 17 weeks of gestation, but do not develop in the spleen until about 24 weeks.[67] Germinal centers are generally absent until after birth, probably from lack of response to antigens.

CD5+ B cells are largely T-independent and produce polyreactive antibodies that may be important in the primary immune response.[68] The percentage of CD5+ B cells is significantly elevated in the fetus and declines during gestation. At birth, most B cells are CD5+, whereas CD5+ cells represent a small fraction of the B cells found in adults. CD5+ B cells may be a distinct lineage of B cells, not a precursor of CD5– B cells.

Plasma cells secreting IgM can first be detected at 15 weeks' gestation, followed by IgG- and IgA-secreting plasma cells at approximately 20 and 30 weeks' gestation respectively.[69] As noted in the discussion above, the amount of immunoglobulin produced by these cells is very small compared with that transferred from the mother.

Functional adaptive immunity

Although the number of B cells and T cells in the fetus and newborn are similar to those observed in adults, the function of the cells is abnormal. Neonatal T cells spontaneously proliferate *in vitro*, to a small extent, and respond well to IL-7, the interleukin responsible for regulating the size of the lymphocyte pool. However, neonatal T cells do not proliferate well in response to activation through the TCR.

The fetus is able to develop memory CD4+ T cells to transplacental antigen exposure such as tetanus toxoid, cat dander, and dust mites;[70] generally, the response is weak. Newborns are also able to respond to immunization with bacille Calmette–Guérin (BCG) and can develop a strong antiviral response after infection.[71] Still, the amount of cytokines (IL-2, IL-4, IFN-γ) secreted is lower than that seen in adults and the expression of the activation marker CD154 (CD40L), which is a second signal for B cells, is diminished.[72] This means that fetal and newborn T cells are not as effective in helping B cells as adult T cells. The CD25+/CD4+ regulatory T cells observed in the newborn are able to suppress other T-cell functions. The functional capabilities of newborn CD8+ cytotoxic T cells have not been well studied.

Newborn B cells are able to respond to activation through the BCR and CD154 (CD40L).[73] Newborn B cells require higher levels of IL-4 to undergo class switch in culture.[74] The absence of germinal centers in the lymph nodes and spleen of the newborn may also play a role in the poor antibody response observed after infection or immunization.

Conclusion

The immune system develops in a highly orchestrated and integrated fashion. B- and T-lymphocyte development begins midway through the first trimester and, in many ways, achieves significant maturity (equal to that seen in the term neonate) during the second trimester of pregnancy. The early stages of lymphocyte maturation occur as the result of mechanisms that do not depend on antigenic stimulation, providing humans with an immunologic repertoire that is capable of responding to virtually any antigenic challenge. Further maturation of the immune system, such as the development of specific immunologic memory and more potent humoral and cellular effector mechanisms, occurs after exposure to the myriad environmental challenges that occur in postnatal life. Thus, the immune system is a highly responsive organ system that has its origins early in gestation, reaches maturity during the first decade of life, but continues to evolve and respond to pathogenic insults throughout life until immunologic senescence occurs.

Key points

1 Components of the innate immune system do not change with exposure.

2 The innate immune system includes pattern recognition receptors such as the toll-like receptors (TLRs).

3 The innate immune response can recruit other components of the innate and adaptive immune system to the site of infection.

4 T-cell receptor (TCR) and B-cell receptor (BCR) diversity results from recombination of multiple exons, junctional diversity, and random combinations of the two chains present in each receptor.

5 Self-reaction T cells are deleted primarily in the thymus.

6 T cells recognize small peptides bound to class I or class II major histocompatibility complex (MHC) molecules.

7 Repeated exposure of B cells to antigen results in somatic mutations of the antibody variable region and selection of B cells with improved antigen binding. Somatic mutation does not occur in T cells.

8 T-cell memory is a result of clonal expansion.

9 The following defects of the innate immune system are observed in newborns: incomplete keratinization of the skin; decreased neutrophil chemotaxis; decreased natural killer (NK) cell function against herpes simplex virus (HSV)-infected cells; decreased antimicrobial proteins; decreased complement C3 and fibronectin; decreased response of neutrophil oxidative metabolism to lipopolysaccharide (LPS) exposure; and a decreased neutrophil storage pool.

10 Many components of the innate immune system have not been studied in the fetus or newborn.

11 Defects in the innate immune system contribute to the susceptibility of the fetus and newborn to infection.

12 Maternal IgG is actively transported to the fetus during the third trimester. IgG1 is more efficiently transported than IgG2, IgG3, or IgG4. Maternal IgM, IgA, and IgE are not transported and are typically present in very small amounts.

13 Maternal IgG interferes with the newborn's ability to generate an antibody response to vaccination, but not a T-cell response to vaccination.

14 Immunoglobulin replacement therapy in preterm infants has not been associated with decreased numbers of infections.

15 Fetal T cells appear in the first trimester.

16 At birth, neonatal T cells have not undergone clonal expansion. Almost all neonatal T cells are naive.

17 The fetus is able to generate T-cell responses to transplacental antigen exposure.

18 Fetal B cells appear in the first trimester.

19 The fetus is able to make IgM, IgG, and IgA by the second trimester, but very little immunoglobulin is produced.

20 Fetal and newborn T cells have diminished expression of CD154 (CD40L), which is required to generate an appropriate antibody response.

References

1 Hill HR, Bohnsack JF, La Pine TR. The natural (innate) defense system. In: Stiehm ER, Ochs HD, Winkelstein JA, eds. *Immunologic disorders in infants and children*, 5th edn. Philadelphia, PA: Elsevier; 2004:245–272.

2 Janeway CA, Jr, Travers P, Walport W, Shlomchik MJ. *Immunobiology*, 6th edn. New York: Garland Science Publishing, 2005.

3 Adams GB, Scadden DT. The hematopoietic stem cell in its place. *Nat Immunol* 2006;7:333–337.

4 Swart B, Salganik MP, Wand MP, et al. The HLDA8 blind panel: findings and conclusions. *J Immunol Methods* 2005;305: 75–83.

5 Charo IF, Ransohoff RM. The many roles of chemokines and chemokine receptors in inflammation. *N Engl J Med* 2006;354: 610–621.

6 Park JS, Park CW, Lockwood CJ, Norwitz ER. Role of cytokines in preterm labor and birth. *Minerva Ginecol* 2005;57:349–366.

7 Akira S, Uematsu S, Takeuchi O. Pathogen recognition and innate immunity. *Cell* 2006;124:783–801.

8 Davies J, Turner M, Klein N. The role of the collectin system in pulmonary defence. *Paediatr Respir Rev* 2001;2:70–75.

9 Ghildyal R, Hartley C, Varrasso A, et al. Surfactant protein A binds to the fusion glycoprotein of respiratory syncytial virus and neutralizes virion infectivity. *J Infect Dis* 1999;180:2009–2013.

10 Lemaitre B, Nicolas E, Michaut L, et al. The dorsoventral regulatory gene cassette spatzle/Toll/cactus controls the potent antifungal response in *Drosophila* adults. *Cell* 1996;86:973–983.

11 Takeda K, Akira S. Toll-like receptors in innate immunity. *Int Immunol* 2005;17:1–14.

12 Strober W, Murray PJ, Kitani A, Watanabe T. Signalling pathways and molecular interactions of NOD1 and NOD2. *Nat Rev Immunol* 2006;6:9–20.

13 Parham P. MHC class I molecules and KIRs in human history, health and survival. *Nat Rev Immunol* 2005;5:201–214.

14 Varla-Leftherioti M. The significance of the women's repertoire of natural killer cell receptors in the maintenance of pregnancy. *Chem Immunol Allergy* 2005;89:84–95.

15 Redman CW, Sargent IL. Latest advances in understanding preeclampsia. *Science* 2005;308:1592–1594.

16 Ulivieri C, Baldari CT. The BCR signalosome: where cell fate is decided. *J Biol Regul Homeost Agents* 2005;19:1–16.
17 Rudolph MG, Stanfield RL, Wilson IA. How TCRs bind MHCs, peptides, and coreceptors. *Annu Rev Immunol* 2006;24:419–466.
18 Jung D, Giallourakis C, Mostoslavsky R, Alt FW. Mechanism and control of V(D)J recombination at the immunoglobulin heavy chain locus. *Annu Rev Immunol* 2006;24:541–570.
19 Zemlin M, Schelonka RL, Bauer K, Schroeder HW, Jr. Regulation and change in the ontogeny of B and T cell antigen receptor repertoires. *Immunol Res* 2002;26: 265–278.
20 Girardi M. Immunosurveillance and immunoregulation by gammadelta T cells. *J Invest Dermatol* 2006;126:25–31.
21 Hazenberg MD, Verschuren MC, Hamann D, et al. T cell receptor excision circles as markers for recent thymic emigrants: basic aspects, technical approach, and guidelines for interpretation. *J Mol Med* 2001;79:631–640.
22 Notarangelo LD, Lanzi G, Peron S, Durandy A. Defects of class-switch recombination. *J Allergy Clin Immunol* 2006;117: 855–864.
23 Silverstein AM. The clonal selection theory: what it really is and why modern challenges are misplaced. *Nat Immunol* 2002;3: 793–796.
24 Sullivan KE. The clinical, immunological, and molecular spectrum of chromosome 22q11.2 deletion syndrome and DiGeorge syndrome. *Curr Opin Allergy Clin Immunol* 2004;4:505–512.
25 Minato Y, Yasutomo K. Regulation of acquired immune system by notch signaling. *Int J Hematol* 2005;82:302–306.
26 Siggs OM, Makaroff LE, Liston A. The why and how of thymocyte negative selection. *Curr Opin Immunol* 2006;18: 175–183.
27 Stefanova I, Dorfman JR, Tsukamoto M, Germain RN. On the role of self-recognition in T cell responses to foreign antigen. *Immunol Rev* 2003;191:97–106.
28 Edry E, Melamed D. Receptor editing in positive and negative selection of B lymphopoiesis. *J Immunol* 2004;173:4265–4271.
29 Lawton AR, Crowe JE, Jr. Ontogeny of immunity. In: Stiehm ER, Ochs HD, Winkelstein JA, eds. *Immunologic disorders in infants and children*, 5th edn. Philadelphia, PA: Elsevier; 2004:3–19.
30 Zhang K. Accessibility control and machinery of immunoglobulin class switch recombination. *J Leukoc Biol* 2003;73:323–332.
31 Shapiro-Shelef M, Calame K. Regulation of plasma-cell development. *Nat Rev Immunol* 2005;5:230–242.
32 Groothuis T, Neefjes J. The ins and outs of intracellular peptides and antigen presentation by MHC class I molecules. *Curr Top Microbiol Immunol* 2005;300:127–148.
33 Busch R, Rinderknecht CH, Roh S, et al. Achieving stability through editing and chaperoning: regulation of MHC class II peptide binding and expression. *Immunol Rev* 2005;207:242–260.
34 Subudhi SK, Alegre ML, Fu YX. The balance of immune responses: costimulation versus coinhibition. *J Mol Med* 2005;83:193–202.
35 Shwayder T, Akland T. Neonatal skin barrier: structure, function, and disorders. *Dermatol Ther* 2005;18:87–103.
36 Conner JM, Soll RF, Edwards WH. Topical ointment for preventing infection in preterm infants. *Cochrane Database Syst Rev* 2004;1: CD001150.
37 Mancini AJ. Skin. *Pediatrics* 2004;113(Suppl.):1114–1119.
38 Caicedo RA, Schanler RJ, Li N, Neu J. The developing intestinal ecosystem: implications for the neonate. *Pediatr Res* 2005;58: 625–628.
39 Zhang L, Li N, Neu J. Probiotics for preterm infants. *NeoReviews* 2005;6:227–232.
40 Marchini G, Nelson A, Edner J, et al. Erythema toxicum neonatorum is an innate immune response to commensal microbes penetrated into the skin of the newborn infant. *Pediatr Res* 2005;58: 613–616.
41 Vanden Eijnden S, Goriely S, De Wit D, et al. Preferential production of the IL-12(p40)/IL-23(p19) heterodimer by dendritic cells from human newborns. *Eur J Immunol* 2006;36:21–26.
42 Carr R. Neutrophil production and function in newborn infants. *Br J Haematol* 2000;110:18–28.
43 Leibson PJ, Hunter-Laszlo M, Douvas GS, Hayward AR. Impaired neonatal natural killer-cell activity to herpes simplex virus: decreased inhibition of viral replication and altered response to lymphokines. *J Clin Immunol* 1986;6:216–224.
44 Starner TD, Agerberth B, Gudmundsson GH, McCray Jr, PB. Expression and activity of beta-defensins and LL-37 in the developing human lung. *J Immunol* 2005;174:1608–1615.
45 Levy O. Impaired innate immunity at birth: deficiency of bactericidal/permeability-increasing protein in the neutrophils of newborns. *Pediatr Res* 2002;51:667–669.
46 Nupponen I, Venge P, Pohjavuori M, et al. Phagocyte activation in preterm infants following premature rupture of the membranes or chorioamnionitis. *Acta Paediatr* 2000;89:1207–1212.
47 Marchini G, Lindow S, Brismar H, et al. The newborn infant is protected by an innate antimicrobial barrier: peptide antibiotics are present in the skin and vernix caseosa. *Br J Dermatol* 2002;147:1127–1134.
48 Urlichs F, Speer CP. Neutrophil function in preterm and term infants. *Neo Rev* 2004;5:417–429.
49 Qing G, Rajaraman K, Bortolussi R. Diminished priming of neonatal polymorphonuclear leukocytes by lipopolysaccharide is associated with reduced CD14 expression. *Infect Immun* 1995;63:248–252.
50 Kim SK, Keeney SE, Alpard SK, Schmalstieg FC. Comparison of L-selectin and CD11b on neutrophils of adults and neonates during the first month of life. *Pediatr Res* 2003;53:132–136.
51 Koenig JM, Yoder MC. Neonatal neutrophils: the good, the bad, and the ugly. *Clin Perinatol* 2004;31:39–51.
52 Bracho F, Goldman S, Cairo MS. Potential use of granulocyte colon-stimulating factor and granulocyte-macrophage colony-stimulating factor in neonates. *Curr Opin Hematol* 1998;5:215–220.
53 Levy O. Innate immunity of the human newborn: distinct cytokine response to LPS and other toll-like receptor agonists. *J Endotoxin Res* 2005;11:113–166.
54 Forster-Waldl E, Sadeghi K, Tamandl D, et al. Monocyte toll-like receptor 4 expression and LPS-induced cytokine production increase during gestational aging. *Pediatr Res* 2005;58:121–124.
55 Marodi L. Innate cellular immune responses in newborns. *Clin Immunol* 2006;118:137–144.
56 Liew FY, Xu D, Brint EK, O'Neill LAJ. Negative regulation of toll-like receptor-mediated immune responses. *Nat Rev Immunol* 2005;5:446–458.
57 Vigano A, Esposito S, Arienti D, et al. Differential development of type 1 and type 2 cytokines and beta-chemokines in the ontogeny of healthy newborns. *Biol Neonate* 1999;75:1–8.
58 Fox SE, Lu W, Maheshwari A, et al. The effects and comparative differences of neutrophil specific chemokines on neutrophil chemotaxis of the neonate. *Cytokine* 2005;29:135–140.
59 Simister NE. Placental transport of immunoglobulin G. *Vaccine* 2003;21:3365–3369.
60 Glezen WP. Effect of maternal antibodies on the infant immune response. *Vaccine* 2003;21:3389–3392.

61 Siegrist CA. Neonatal and early life vaccinology. *Vaccine* 2001;19:3331–3346.
62 Sasidharan P. Postnatal IgG levels in very-low-birth-weight infants. Preliminary observations. *Clin Pediatr* 1988;27:271–274.
63 Ohlsson A, Lacy JB. Intravenous immunoglobulin for preventing infection in preterm and/or low-birth-weight infants. *Cochrane Database Syst Rev* 2004;1. CD001239.
64 Schonland SO, Zimmer JK, Lopez-Benitez CM, et al. Homeostatic control of T-cell generation in neonates. *Blood* 2003;102: 1428–1434.
65 Michaelsson J, Mold JE, McCune JM, Nixon DF. Regulation of T cell responses in the developing human fetus. *J Immunol* 2006;176:5741–5748.
66 Cooper MD. Pre-B cells; normal and abnormal development. *J Clin Immunol* 1981;1:81–89.
67 Asano S, Akaike Y, Muramatsu T, et al. Immunohistologic detection of the primary follicle (PF) in human fetal and newborn lymph node anlages. *Pathol Res Pract* 1993;189:921–927.
68 Dono M, Cerruti G, Zupo S. The CD5+ B-cell. *Int J Biochem Cell Biol* 2004;36:2105–2111.
69 Gathings WE, Kubagawa H, Cooper MD. A distinctive pattern of B cell immaturity in perinatal humans. *Immunol Rev* 1981;57: 107–126.
70 Prescott SL, Macaubas C, Smallacombe T, et al. Development of allergen-specific T-cell memory in atopic and normal children. *Lancet* 1999;353:196–200.
71 Davids V, Hanekom WA, Mansoor N, et al. The effect of bacille Calmette-Guérin vaccine strain and route of administration on induced immune responses in vaccinated infants. *J Infect Dis* 2006;193:531–536.
72 Han P, McDonald T, Hodge G. Potential immaturity of the T-cell and antigen-presenting cell interaction in cord blood with particular emphasis on the CD40–CD40 ligand costimulatory pathway. *Immunology* 2004;113:26–34.
73 Durandy A, De Saint Basile G, Lisowska-Grospierre B, et al. Undetectable CD40 ligand expression on T cells and low B cell responses to CD40 binding agonists in human newborns. *J Immunol* 1995;154:1560–1568.
74 Nagumo H, Agematsu K, Kobayashi N, et al. The different process of class switching and somatic hypermutation; a novel analysis by CD27(–) naive B cells. *Blood* 2002;99:567–575.

9 Fetal endocrinology

Charles E. Wood and Maureen Keller-Wood

The endocrine systems of the fetus are modulators of the classical physiological organ systems. For example, the basic components of the cardiovascular system work together to transport nutrients and waste products and to perfuse the tissues with blood. However, the blood volume and osmolality is controlled via the actions of endocrine feedback mechanisms, and the distribution of combined ventricular output is affected by several hormones that are released after fetal stress. The fetal lung makes lung liquid prior to birth and serves as an organ of gas exchange after birth. However, the reabsorption of lung liquid is likely to be coordinated by several hormones that are secreted at birth. This chapter will focus on the endocrinology of the developing fetus. Because of the inherent difficulty in studying developing human fetuses, much of what we know about the developing human has its origins in the study of animal models, mostly fetal sheep; although more pertinent to the human being, less information has been obtained from primate models of fetal development. Rodents are altricial species (relatively immature at birth); however, useful information about endocrine development (especially relating to first- and second-trimester fetuses) has been obtained from developing rats and mice. There are notable exceptions, however, for example the biosynthesis of estrogens in humans and primates involves a "fetoplacental unit," while the biosynthesis of estrogens in sheep is more straightforward. It is, perhaps, the differences among species that allow us to identify the truly basic principles of endocrine control in fetuses. This chapter is intended to be an overview of the current knowledge of several aspects of this large field, not a comprehensive review of the literature. The focus of this chapter will be the major endocrine axes of the fetus including estrogen biosynthesis, and hypothalamic and pituitary control of adrenal, gonad, and thyroid function, with special emphasis on the roles that these endocrine axes play in the development of the fetus and its adaptation to extrauterine life. We will address each of these major endocrine systems separately.

Hypothalamus–pituitary–gonadal axis

Gonadotropin-releasing hormone (GnRH) is secreted into the hypophyseal–portal blood at the median eminence, and stimulates the release of both luteinizing hormone (LH) and follicle-stimulating hormone (FSH) from gonadotropes in the anterior pituitary. At mid-gestation or before, in the sheep fetus, LH and FSH are present in gonadotropes and GnRH is present in the hypothalamus at both the mRNA and the protein level. (Prior to the maturation of the fetal pituitary, chorionic gonadotropin (CG) from the placenta stimulates fetal gonadal growth, differentiation, and secretory activity.) The levels of LH and FSH appear to be greater in female fetuses than in male fetuses and pulsatile secretion of these hormones becomes established during the fetal period. The overall activity of the hypothalamus–pituitary–gonadal (HPG) axis reaches a peak at approximately 30–40% gestation in the sheep fetus, decreasing until birth (Fig. 9.1).[1] In the rat fetus, a species that is relatively immature at birth, the protein and mRNA tissue concentrations of GnRH, LH, and FSH increase continuously until birth. GnRH neurons have been identified in the region of the organum vasculosum of the lamina terminalis (OVLT), in the medial preoptic nucleus, and in the nucleus of the diagonal band of Broca.

In the sheep fetus, testosterone secretion from the fetal gonads peaks at about the same time as the peak in plasma concentrations of gonadotropins, at approximately 30–40% gestation (Fig. 9.1). The mid-gestational peak in gonadal steroid hormone secretion appears to stimulate gonadal growth and differentiation. However, later in gestation, the placenta synthesizes increasing quantities of both estrogens and androgens, which is controlled by the fetal hypothalamus–pituitary–adrenal (HPA) axis.[2]

Fetal estrogen and androgen biosynthesis

The major source of androgens and estrogens in the late-gestation fetus is the placenta.[3] In primate species, including humans, the biosynthesis of estrogens and androgens depends upon an intact fetoplacental unit. The placenta lacks cytochrome $P450_{c17\alpha}$ (CYP17), and therefore, 17α-hydroxylase and 17,20-lyase activities (Fig. 9.2). Nevertheless, the placenta is able to synthesize large amounts of estrogen as it receives a supply of estrogen biosynthetic precursor from the fetal adrenal cortex. The *adult zone* or *definitive zone* of the fetal adrenal cortex lacks the enzyme 3β-hydroxysteroid dehydrogenase (Fig. 9.2) and cannot, therefore, convert either pregnenolone to progesterone or 17α-hydroxypregnenolone to 17α-hydroxyprogesterone. However, the *fetal* zone of the fetal adrenal cortex secretes dehydroepiandrosterone (DHEA) and dehydroepiandrosterone sulfate (DHAS) in response to adrenocorticotropic hormone (ACTH), and these steroidogenic intermediates are taken up by the placenta and used in the biosynthesis of estrogens, bypassing the lack of CYP17 (Figs 9.2 and 9.3). Alterations in fetal HPA axis activity are reflected in changes in circulating concentrations of estrogens in maternal plasma. For example, fetal death dramatically reduces maternal plasma concentrations of estriol. In rhesus monkeys, infusion of ACTH into the fetal blood has been shown to increase the circulating concentrations of estrogens in maternal plasma, and negative feedback inhibition of fetal ACTH secretion by infusion of glucocorticoids reduces maternal plasma estrogen concentrations.[4] Estrogen biosynthesis and release into the fetal bloodstream creates an endocrine environment that allows fetal growth and development. For example, uterine blood flow during pregnancy is critically influenced by placental estrogen biosynthesis. The estrogen environment *in utero* is also important, however, at the final stages of pregnancy; increases in estrogen biosynthesis at the end of gestation are thought to be a central feature of the events that increase myometrial contractility and initiate labor.

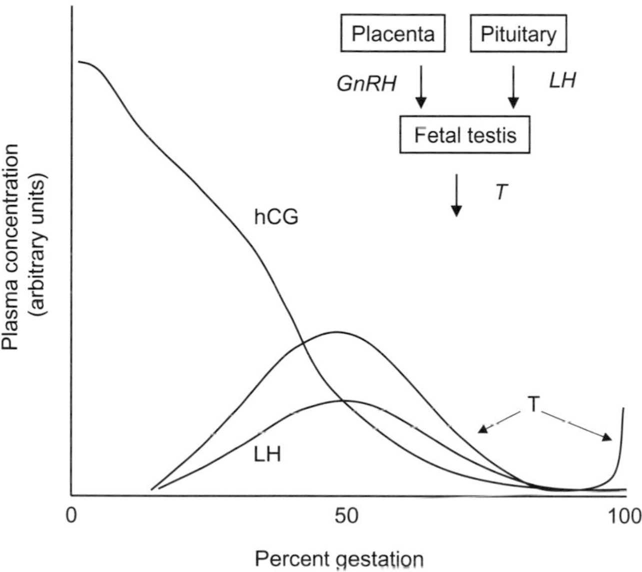

Figure 9.1 Schematic representation of the ontogeny of hCG, LH, and testosterone (T) in the plasma of a male fetus. The relationship of GnRH, FSH, LH, and T is represented in the upper right corner of the figure.

Hypothalamus–pituitary–adrenal axis

The endocrine hierarchy within the fetal HPA axis[5] is similar to that of the adult (Fig. 9.2). ACTH is synthesized and

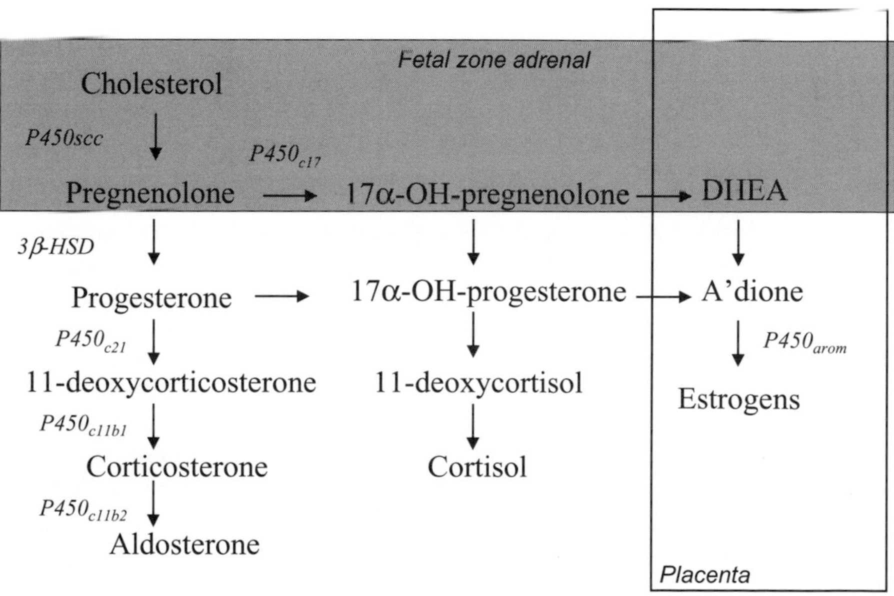

Figure 9.2 Steroid biosynthesis in the developing primate fetus. Steroidogenic enzymes are represented by the following abbreviations: $P450_{c17}$ (17α-hydroxylase and 17,20-lyase activities); 3β-HSD (3β-hydroxysteroid dehydrogenase activity); $P450_{c11b1}$ (11α-hydroxylase activity); $P450_{c11b2}$ (aldosterone synthase activity); $P450_{arom}$ (aromatase activity). The fetal zone of the fetal adrenal cortex is capable of performing the reactions in the shaded area. The overlapping box (right) represents estrogen biosynthesis by the placenta. A'dione, androstenedione.

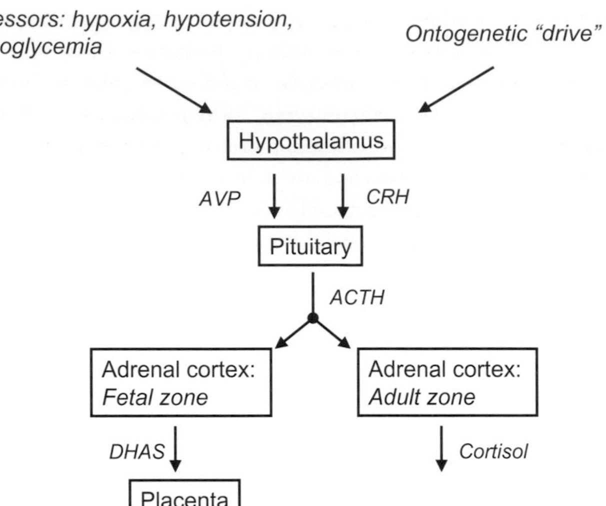

Figure 9.3 Relationship between hypothalamus, pituitary, and fetal and definitive zones of the fetal adrenal. Both zones of the fetal adrenal cortex are stimulated by ACTH secreted by the fetal anterior pituitary. The secretion of ACTH is stimulated acutely in response to stressors *in utero*, and chronically in a pattern that produces increased activity of the fetal hypothalamus–pituitary–adrenal axis independent of stressors at the end of gestation.

secreted by the corticotropes of the anterior pituitary in response to two hypothalamic releasing factors: arginine vasopressin (AVP) and corticotropin-releasing hormone (CRH). The two releasing hormones work in concert: each increases the sensitivity of the corticotrope to the other. The fetal HPA axis appears to be controlled by the paraventricular nuclei (PVN); in sheep fetuses, destruction of the PVN or implantation of dexamethasone crystals near the PVN disrupts the function of the axis.[6]

ACTH stimulates the release of glucocorticoid hormones (i.e., cortisol in the human, primate, and sheep, and corticosterone in rodents) from the *definitive zone*. This zone contains the full complement of steroidogenic enzymes that are found in the adult adrenal cortex (Fig. 9.2) and it responds to ACTH with an increase in cortisol secretion, and to angiotensin II and K^+ with an increase in aldosterone secretion. In the *fetal zone*, ACTH stimulates the release of the estrogen precursors, DHEA and DHAS. The overall size of the fetal zone increases in late gestation, reaching a peak at the time of birth and regressing thereafter.

The fetal HPA axis is activated progressively throughout the latter part of gestation as a normal consequence of ontogenetic development. This has been well documented in fetal sheep and there is good evidence that this is also true in primate fetuses. The activation of the fetal HPA axis can be seen as a semilogarithmic increase in circulating concentrations of ACTH and cortisol in nonhuman fetal blood, and DHEA, DHAS, and estrogens in human fetal blood (Fig. 9.4). In sheep fetuses, the increase in fetal HPA axis activity includes increased biosynthesis of CRH and AVP in the hypothalamus, and proopiomelanocortin (POMC) in the fetal pituitary, as well as increased abundance of steroidogenic enzymes in the adrenal cortex. The molecular processing of POMC to ACTH is also increased in the latter stages of development (Fig. 9.5); this increased processing is in part the result of stimulation by estrogens from the placenta. Prior to term, as in the adult animal, there is an effective negative feedback mechanism by which cortisol inhibits fetal ACTH secretion. In the final few days of fetal life, however, the negative feedback mechanism is interrupted, allowing both ACTH and cortisol to increase simultaneously (Fig. 9.6); this may allow for the large increases in secretion of both hormones that occurs prior to birth.

Throughout the third trimester, the adrenal cortex increases in size and there is an increase in the sensitivity of the steroidogenic tissue to ACTH; this is a function of adrenal mass, as well as several endocrine and neural influences. For example, POMC and 22-kDa "pro-ACTH" reduce adrenal sensitivity to ACTH (Fig. 9.5), whereas splanchnic nerve stimulation increases adrenal responsiveness to ACTH. In sheep, the increases in adrenal cortisol secretion are accompanied by an increase in the binding capacity for cortisol. This effectively exaggerates the increase in fetal plasma cortisol concentration and provides an increased supply of bound cortisol in plasma.

The ontogenetic increase in fetal HPA axis activity at the end of gestation is a critical part of the process by which fetal visceral and pulmonary maturation are accelerated in preparation for extrauterine life. In sheep, the fetal HPA axis plays a critical role in the triggering of parturition.[7] It is likely that the role is essentially similar in the human fetus because placental estrogen biosynthesis is controlled by fetal ACTH secretion in both species. There is a clear functional relationship between the fetal HPA axis and placental estrogen biosynthesis. In sheep, and likely in human fetuses, placental estrogen potently stimulates fetal HPA axis activity. At the end of gestation, the interplay between the placenta and the fetal

HPA axis functions as a positive feedback cycle, progressively increasing fetal HPA activity, thus preparing the fetus for birth.

The placenta expresses 11β-hydroxysteroid dehydrogenase (HSD), the enzyme that interconverts cortisol and cortisone (biologically inactive at the corticosteroid receptor). Placental 11β-HSD-2, which predominantly converts cortisol to cortisone, partially isolates the fetus from the cortisol in the maternal circulation. As the fetus matures, the activity of 11β-HSD is increased, perhaps itself the result of increased estrogen biosynthesis by the placenta.[8]

Primate placenta contains significant amounts of immunoreactive ACTH and CRH.[9] It has been proposed that the release of ACTH and/or CRH into the fetal blood might be a physiologically important mechanism by which the placenta affects the timing of parturition in these species. The concentration of CRH is substantial in both fetal and maternal plasma in primates. However, CRH is partially protein bound in fetal plasma by a CRH-binding protein that is synthesized and secreted by the placental tissue. The function of the binding protein is not known; its presence in plasma suggests that the high circulating concentrations of CRH in plasma might represent spillover from sites of production and (paracrine or autocrine) action in the placenta and other sites within the peripheral circulation. In the human placenta, CRH causes the release of ACTH locally, followed by an alteration in placental steroidogenesis. It has also been proposed that the release of CRH from the human placenta into the fetal umbilical venous blood stimulates the activity of the fetal HPA axis at the end of gestation, which ultimately might initiate parturition.

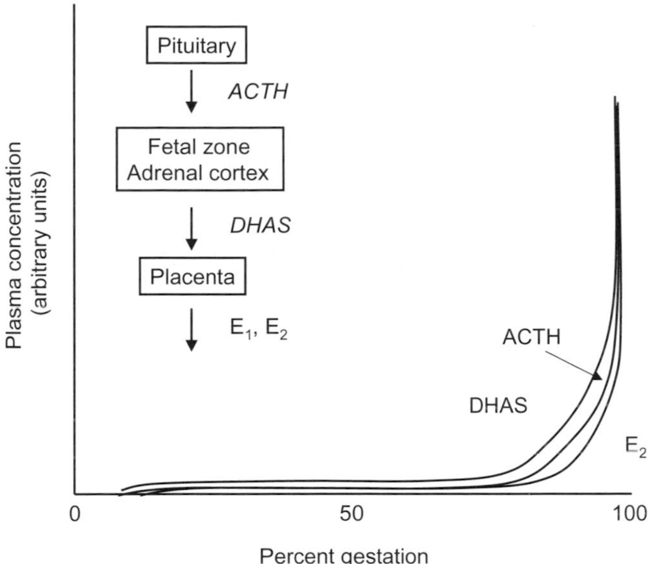

Figure 9.4 Ontogeny of fetal ACTH, DHAS, and estrone (E_1), estradiol (E_2), and estriol (E_3) in the primate fetus. The relationship of these hormones is represented in the upper right corner of the figure.

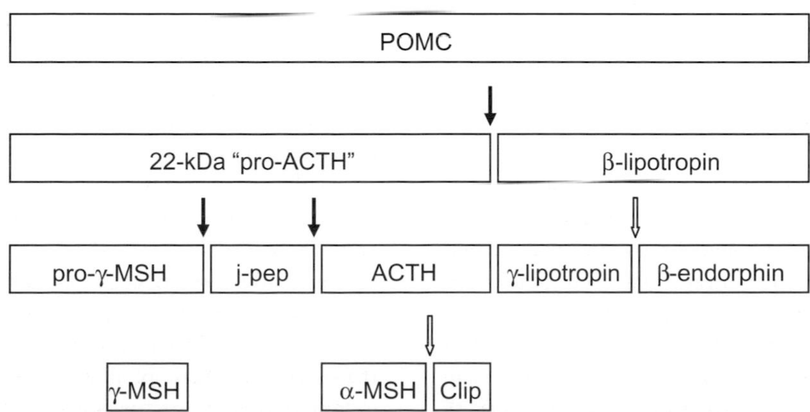

Figure 9.5 Post-translational processing of POMC. POMC is cleaved to β-lipotropin and 22-kDa "pro-ACTH" by the prohormone convertase 1/3 (PC1/3, solid arrows). β-Lipotropin is further processed to lipotropin and endorphin by prohormone convertase 2 (PC2, hollow arrow). Pro-ACTH is cleaved to ACTH, pro-γ-MSH, and joining peptide (j-pep) by PC1/3. ACTH is cleaved to α-MSH and corticotropin-like immunoreactive peptide (CLIP) by PC2. The specific peptide products of POMC are cell specific. For example, corticotropes synthesize ACTH, whereas the neurointermediate lobe synthesizes α-MSH predominantly.

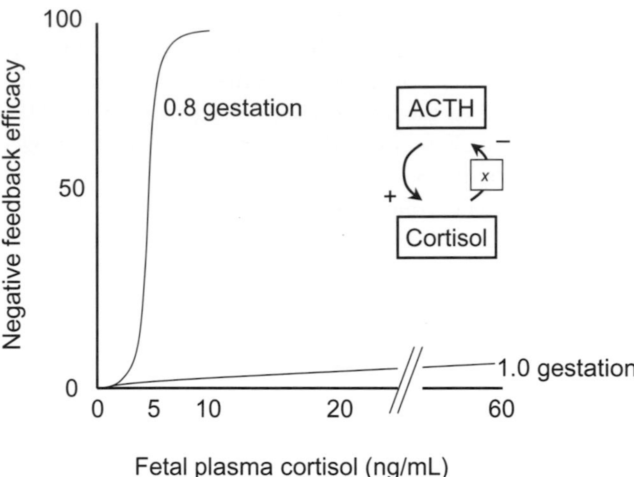

Figure 9.6 Graphical representation of the efficacy of negative feedback inhibition of stimulated ACTH secretion by cortisol in fetal plasma. Negative feedback inhibition of ACTH secretion is apparent at 80% gestation, but not in the last several days of fetal life (100% gestation). The relationship between cortisol and ACTH in the fetus is represented by the inset (upper right).

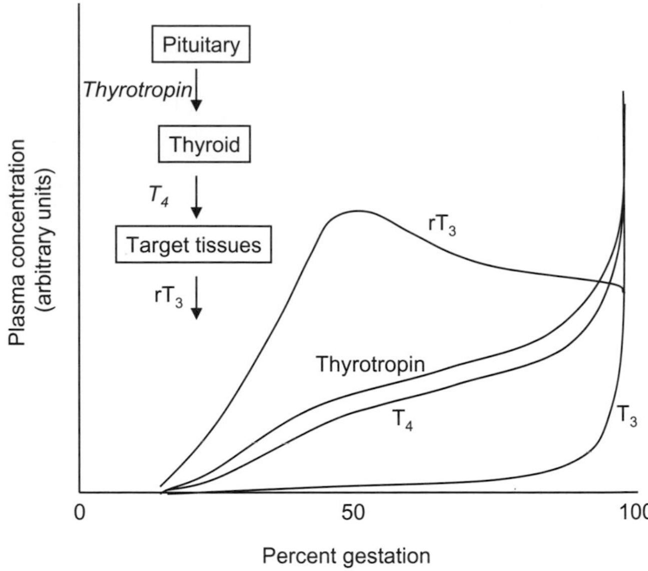

Figure 9.7 The ontogeny of thyrotropin, T_4, T_3, and rT_3 in fetal plasma. The relationship of thyrotropin, T_4, T_3, and rT_3 is represented in the upper left corner of the figure.

Neurointermediate lobe of the pituitary

The cells of the neurointermediate lobe synthesize POMC. The major processing products of the POMC-synthesizing cells are α-melanocyte-stimulating hormone (α-MSH) and γ-MSH. One report[10] suggested that neurointermediate lobe cells from fetal sheep respond to CRH and/or AVP with increased secretion of immunoreactive ACTH, whereas neurointermediate lobe cells from neonatal sheep did not respond to CRH and/or AVP. The responsiveness of the cells to CRH and/or AVP was altered by prior adrenalectomy. The authors suggested that neurointermediate lobe cells mature in late gestation, perhaps in response to cortisol in fetal plasma.

Adrenal medulla

The adrenal medulla becomes innervated by sympathetic preganglionic nerves at approximately 80% gestation (in sheep), and secretes the catecholamines, epinephrine and norepinephrine,[11] whereas prior to innervation, the fetal adrenal is directly responsive to hypoxia. The adrenal medullary biosynthesis of epinephrine is dependent upon the expression of phenylethanolamine-N-methyltransferase (PNMT), which is, in turn, induced by cortisol. For this reason, the secretory capacity of the adrenal medulla for epinephrine increases late in gestation.

The adrenal medulla responds to various stresses such as hypoxia and hypotension with increased secretion of catecholamines. The increase in response to hypoxia is important for redistributing fetal combined ventricular output away from somatic tissues and towards the umbilical–placental circulation. The adrenal medulla also plays an important role in fetal glucose homeostasis; an increase in fetal epinephrine secretion elevates the fetal plasma glucose level, which is seen, for example, following periods of fetal distress.

Hypothalamus–pituitary–thyroid axis[12,13]

In humans, the fetal thyroid is sufficiently developed to support thyroglobulin biosynthesis by approximately 25% gestation (Fig. 9.7). Thyrotropin is present in the fetal pituitary and in fetal plasma at the beginning of the second trimester, at approximately the time of hypothalamo–hypophyseal portal system development. Thyrotropin and thyroxine (T_4) circulate in fetal plasma in increasing concentrations, starting early in the second trimester. Type 3 deiodinase (D3), which converts T_4 to reverse 3,5,5′ triiodothyronine (rT_3), is expressed leading to an abundance of rT_3 circulating in fetal plasma throughout the second and third trimesters (Fig. 9.8). Circulating concentrations of 3,5,3′ triiodothyronine (T_3), however, increase only in the final stages of fetal development, suggesting late development of types 1 and 2 deiodinases (D1 and D2 respectively) in liver and other tissues (Fig. 9.7). In the first trimester of human pregnancy, the abundance of TRH in extrahypothalamic tissue is greater than in the fetal hypothalamus, suggesting a role for extrahypothalamic TRH in the stimulation of thyrotropin secretion from the developing anterior pituitary. In the sheep fetus, the development of the thyrotrope starts at approximately 30% gestation, followed by the development of the thyroid gland at approximately 40%

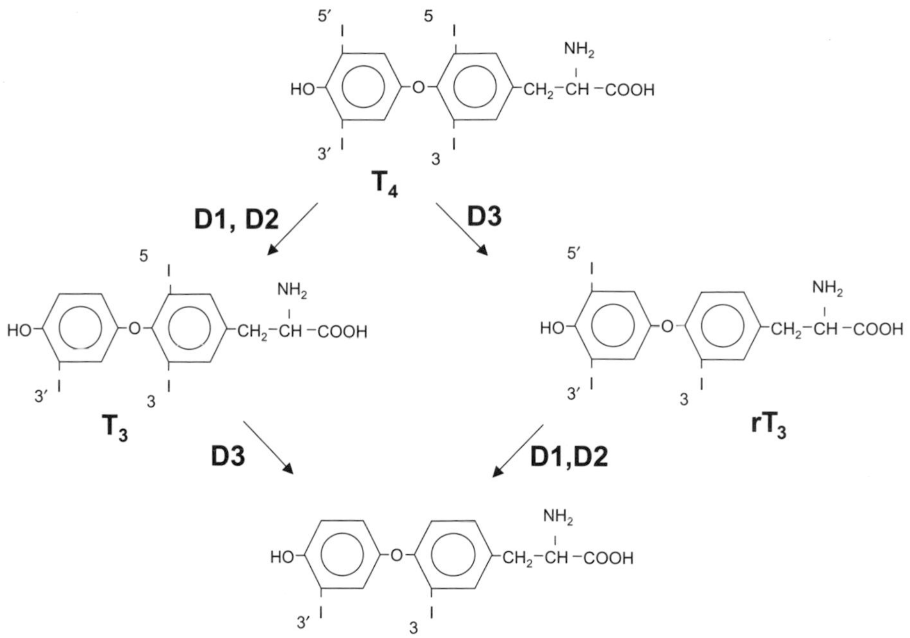

Figure 9.8 The metabolism of thyroid hormones by types 1 and 2 (D1 and D2) deiodinases, and type 3 (D3) deiodinase. Thyroxine, triiodothyronine, and reverse triiodothyronine are represented as previously defined (T_4, T_3, and rT_3 respectively).

gestation, and the development of hypothalamic TRH at around 50% gestation. Plasma concentrations of thyrotropin in the sheep fetus increase from approximately 30% gestation, leading investigators to speculate that extrahypothalamic TRH synthesis and release might be relevant for control of pituitary thyrotropes. True neuroendocrine control of the hypothalamus–pituitary–thyroid (HPT) axis develops near the end of human and ovine pregnancies.

The maternal and fetal HPT axes operate somewhat independently. The placenta is relatively impermeable to T_4 and T_3 because of the presence of the deiodinase that converts T_4 to rT_3. The placenta is also impermeable to the relatively large thyrotropin and thyroid-binding globulins. On the other hand, the human placenta is relatively impermeable to TRH, a fairly small molecule (the ovine placenta is also impermeable to TRH). For this reason, there is usually a gradient of both T_4 and T_3 from maternal to fetal plasma.

Development of the HPT axis of the fetus is critically important for differentiation of the nervous system. Congenital hypothyroidism causes mental retardation in human infants. Although the infant can be treated with some success after birth, it will tend to be less responsive if the mother also suffered from hypothyroidism during pregnancy. The HPT axis also plays a role in the adaptation to extrauterine life. This has been illustrated in sheep; thyroidectomy, days before birth, causes severe neonatal hypothermia, in part because of a failure of thermogenesis in the brown adipose tissue. The effect of thyroid hormones in this process is to accelerate development of the brown adipose tissue in the last few days of gestation.

Posterior pituitary

Both AVP and oxytocin are synthesized by magnocellular neurons in the supraoptic and paraventricular nuclei. Axons from these neurons terminate in the posterior pituitary. AVP is a hormone with at least three biological activities (Fig. 9.9). The vasopressor action of this hormone is mediated by V_{1a} vasopressin receptors on vascular smooth muscle cells in the peripheral vasculature. Corticotropin-releasing activity is mediated by the V_{1b} vasopressin receptor (AVP acting as a corticotropin-releasing factor is derived from parvocellular neurons and released into the hypothalamo–hypophyseal portal blood at the median eminence). The antidiuretic activity is mediated by the V_2 vasopressin receptor. The potency of vasopressin action in the fetal kidney appears to be somewhat less than in the adult. The fetal sheep excretes a relatively large volume of dilute urine. The renal concentrating mechanisms are immature, therefore the increase in urine osmolality after exposure to vasopressin is not as dramatic as in the adult.

AVP is an important cardiovascular hormone in the fetus.[14] Hemorrhage greatly increases its concentration in plasma, and pharmacologic blockade of V_{1a} receptors impairs blood pressure regulation during hypovolemia. Increases in plasma vasopressin concentration redistribute fetal combined ventricular output toward the umbilical–placental circulation, maximizing transfer of gases between the maternal and fetal circulations.

Oxytocin circulates in fetal plasma in relatively high concentrations, which increase during active labor. Immuno-

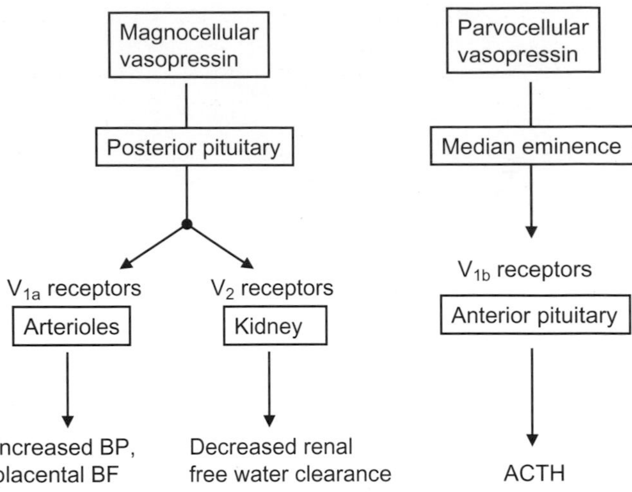

Figure 9.9 The synthesis, release, and action of AVP in the fetus. Magnocellular neurons in the paraventricular nucleus synthesize vasopressin, releasing the peptide into the bloodstream at the posterior pituitary. Parvocellular neurons in the hypothalamic nucleus synthesize vasopressin, which is released into the hypothalamo–hypophyseal portal blood at the median eminence. Portal blood vasopressin acts as a corticotropin-releasing factor at the corticotrope of the anterior pituitary.

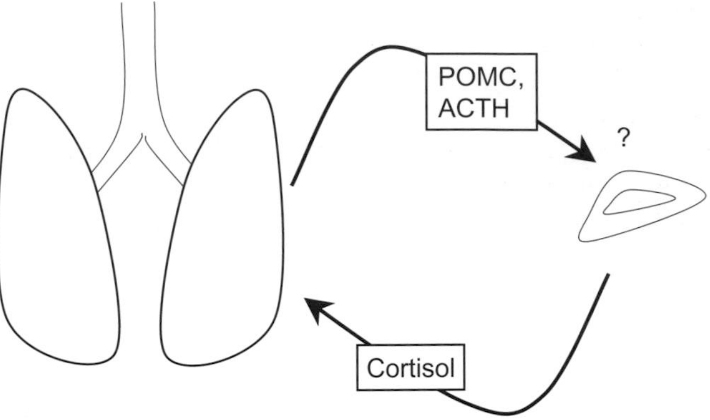

Figure 9.10 The fetal lung synthesizes and secretes POMC into the fetal bloodstream. This peptide is known to alter adrenal sensitivity to ACTH. It has been proposed that there is an interplay among the lung, pituitary, and adrenal that modulates fetal adrenal responsiveness to stress and the timing of parturition as the lung matures.

reactive oxytocin in fetal plasma is present as a mixture of processed and unprocessed forms. As the fetus matures, the proportion of processed oxytocin in fetal plasma increases. The function of oxytocin in the fetus is not clear, although the placental barrier prevents fetal oxytocin from reaching the myometrium. It is possible that oxytocin stimulates the release of ACTH via an interaction with the V_{1b} receptor.

Ectopic hormones

In addition to the placenta, "pituitary" hormones are synthesized and released from other tissue in the fetal body (Fig. 9.10). One example of this phenomenon is the synthesis and release of POMC and POMC-related peptides by the neuroendocrine cells of the fetal lung. It has been proposed that POMC secreted by the lung might play a role in stress responsiveness, or in the timing of parturition, by altering

Key points

1 The fetal hypothalamus–pituitary–adrenal axis controls estrogen biosynthesis by the placenta in late gestation.
2 The fetal hypothalamus–pituitary–gonadal axis is a more effective controller of circulating sex steroids at mid-gestation than in late gestation.
3 Various hormones in fetal blood, including glucocorticoids and thyroid hormones, are either activated or inactivated at the target tissue.
4 The placenta synthesizes and secretes various hormones that have been proposed to modulate the activity of fetal endocrine axes.
5 The adrenal medulla actively secretes catecholamines and plays an important role in the fetal response to stress; however, innervation by sympathetic preganglionic nerves does not occur until late in gestation.
6 The posterior pituitary of the fetus actively secretes both vasopressin and oxytocin. Vasopressin plays an important role in fluid balance and blood pressure control prenatally.
7 Ectopic hormones, secreted by the lung and other visceral tissues, may play important roles in parturition and in other integrated physiologic processes.

adrenal sensitivity to circulating ACTH (Fig. 9.10). It is interesting that these cells, after transformation, form the basis of small cell carcinoma of the lung, a disease in which significant secretions of POMC and ACTH can produce symptoms of hyperadrenocorticism in the adult. The neuroendocrine cells of the lung synthesize many hormones in addition to POMC, such as vasoactive intestinal polypeptide (VIP) and serotonin.

References

1 Sklar CA, Mueller PL, Gluckman PD, et al. Hormone ontogeny in the ovine fetus VII: circulating luteinizing hormone and follicle stimulating hormone in mid- and late-gestation. *Endocrinology* 1981;108:874–880.

2 Pepe GJ, Albrecht ED. Regulation of the primate adrenal cortex. *Endocrine Rev* 1990;11:151–176.

3 Diczfalusy E. Endocrine functions of the human fetoplacental unit. *Fed Proc* 1964;23:791–798.

4 Walsh SW, Norman RI, Novy MJ. *In utero* regulation of rhesus monkey fetal adrenals: effects of dexamethasone, adrenocorticotropin, thyroid-releasing hormone, prolactin, human chorionic gonadotropin, and alpha-melanocyte-stimulating hormone on fetal and maternal plasma steroids. *Endocrinology* 1979;104: 1805–1813.

5 Wood CE. Estrogen/hypothalamus-pituitary-adrenal axis interactions in the fetus: the interplay between placenta and fetal brain. *J Soc Gynecol Invest* 2005;12:67–76.

6 Myers DA, McDonald TJ, Nathanielsz PW. Effect of bilateral lesions of the ovine fetal hypothalamic paraventricular nuclei at 118–122 days of gestation on subsequent adrenocortical steroidogenic enzyme gene expression. *Endocrinology* 1992;131:305–310.

7 Liggins GC, Fairclough RJ, Grieves SA, et al. The mechanism of initiation of parturition in the ewe. *Rec Prog Horm Res* 1973; 29:111–159.

8 Pepe GJ, Albrecht ED. Central integrative role of oestrogen in the regulation of placental steroidogenic maturation and the development of the fetal pituitary–adrenocortical axis in the baboon. *Hum Reprod Update* 1998;4:406–419.

9 McLean M, Smith R. Corticotrophin-releasing hormone and human parturition. *Reproduction* 2001;121:493–501.

10 Fora MA, Butler TG, Rose JC, Schwartz J. Adrenocorticotropin secretion by fetal sheep anterior and intermediate lobe pituitary cells in vitro: effects of gestation and adrenalectomy. *Endocrinology* 1996;137:3394–3400.

11 Comline RS, Silver M. Development of activity in the adrenal medulla of the foetus and new-born animal. *Br Med Bull* 1966;22:16–20.

12 Darras VM, Hume R, Visser TJ. Regulation of thyroid hormone metabolism during fetal development. *Mol Cell Endocrinol* 1999;151:37–47.

13 Polk DH. Thyroid hormone metabolism during development. *Reprod Fertil Dev* 1995;7:469–477.

14 Wood CE, Tong H. Central nervous system regulation of reflex responses to hypotension during fetal life. *Am J Physiol* 1999;277:R1541–R1552.

10 Fetal hematology

Véronique Cayol and Fernand Daffos

Fetal hematopoiesis

Details of hematopoiesis in the newborn are well known but, because of the difficulties encountered in sampling, such is not the case with the fetus.

Blood cells are of mesenchymal origin. The mesenchyme, which stems from the cytotrophoblast surrounding the egg, forms the inner layers of the chorion and surrounds the unit created by the amniotic cavity, the embryonic button, and the yolk sac. The reunion of these two mesenchymal blades forms an embryonic film. When the first vascular elements appear, the conceptus is wholly embedded in the inner mucosa (Fig. 10.1).

First stage: mesoblastic hematopoiesis of the yolk sac

On day 19 of pregnancy, the first blood cells outside the embryo become apparent in the many vascular islets that appear in the mesenchymal wall of the yolk sac. These islets appear as dark lumps of cells. Two systems – the vascular and the hematopoietic – originate from the islets: the peripheral cells of these lumps constitute the original endothelium of the developing vascular system. Some central cells of these islets leave the vascular walls, become free in the lumen, and form the primitive blood cells, or hematocytoblasts. These cells remain nucleated throughout their functional lives. The primitive erythroblasts, or pronormoblasts, stem directly from the hematocytoblasts. The separate islets gradually connect to each other to form an irregular network enveloping the yolk sac, which will give rise to the vitelline vessels.

Toward day 22 of pregnancy, similar vascular islets begin to appear in the mesenchyme of the chorion and all along the allantoic pedicle. These vascular islets create an extraembryonic network, the chorioallantoic network, which constitutes the future umbilical vessels. In both cases, hematopoiesis is intravascular; the two vascular networks connect to the vessels formed in the embryo at a later stage. Between 6 and 8 weeks' gestation, the vascular islets begin to regress, as does the intravascular hematopoiesis, with its large, nucleated megaloblasts. The first-generation erythropoietic cells disappear completely from the embryoplacental circulation at between 12 and 15 weeks' gestation.

The role of the yolk sac seems to be primary. Although the chorion's mesenchyme proves to be quantitatively greater than that of the yolk sac (which means, in theory, a greater participation in hematopoiesis), the cells of the vascular islets in the wall of the yolk sac remain undifferentiated until the fourth week. In contrast, everywhere else, the primitive vessels already contain erythroblasts.

Second stage: visceral hematopoiesis

Visceral hematopoiesis begins in the liver around 5–6 weeks' gestation and appears to reach an adequate development around 9 weeks. Nests of hematopoiesis appear in the liver sinusoids and increase rapidly. Hematopoiesis becomes extravascular. Clear morphologic differences exist between the cells formed in the liver and the earlier lineages of the yolk sac. The cells originating in the liver are smaller, and their nuclear structure is nearer the normoblast lineage of erythrocytic precursors. These are few in number when they appear in the blood around 5 weeks, becoming predominant between 8 and 9 weeks' gestation (Fig. 10.2).

Although granulocytes and platelets are found in the circulation, the fetal liver seems to be the seat of an almost pure hematopoiesis. From the third to the fifth months of pregnancy, the erythrocytic precursors represent approximately 50% of the liver's nucleated cells.

From 9 to 12 weeks, some hematopoietic activity also can be observed in the thymus, the lymph nodes, and the kidneys. Nucleated red corpuscles are also observed in the spleen.

Their presence has been interpreted in different ways. Some people think that it corresponds to local production as well as sequestration and destruction; others think it is nothing but sequestration at different stages of degeneration. In any case, the role of splenic nucleated red corpuscles is only accessory in the human fetus. As for the yolk sac, it appears to be entirely fibrous at 11 weeks of pregnancy.

We have not been able to detect any erythrocytic activity elsewhere. Visceral, mainly hepatic, hematopoiesis reaches its highest level of production around the fifth and sixth months, gradually regressing until delivery. Visceral hematopoiesis can still be observed during the first week of postnatal life in the liver and occasionally even in the spleen.

Although it disappears almost entirely under normal conditions, extramedullary hematopoiesis is apt to increase noticeably in a large variety of diseases and infections in the fetus as well as in the newborn.

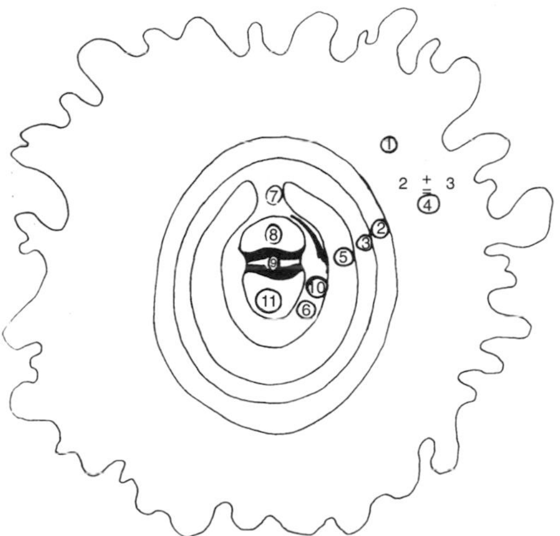

Figure 10.1 Schematic picture of the structures of the egg. (1) Undivided mass of the syncytiotrophoblast; (2) cytotrophoblast; (3) mesenchyme; (4) chorion; (5) extraembryonic coelom; (6) mesenchyme of the wall of the yolk sac; (7) mesenchyme of the embryonic pedicle; (8) amniotic cavity; (9) tridermal embryonic button: ectoblast, mesoblast, endoblast; (10) allantoic pedicle generated by the endoblast; (11) yolk sac.

Third stage: medullary hematopoiesis

Medullary hematopoiesis begins at about the fourth month. Medullary spaces develop in cartilaginous portions of the long bones by a resorptive process. Toward the fifth month, medullary cellularity is still poor and predominantly leukopoietic. The erythropoietic tissues multiply rapidly, and the marrow reaches its maximal cellularity toward 30 weeks' gestation, with each lineage being adequately represented. However, the volume of marrow occupied by the hematopoietic tissue continues to rise until full term. During the last 3 months of pregnancy, the marrow is the privileged seat of blood cell formation, the whole expanding medullary space being occupied by active hematopoietic tissues. The marrow's relative volume in the fetus and the newborn, however, is smaller than that in the grown child or the adult because a large part of the fetal skeleton is cartilaginous and the bones are comparatively small.

Nonerythroid lineage

Leukocytes first develop in the wall of the yolk sac, then in the embryo. Very few circulating granulocytes are found during the first weeks of fetal life. At 8 weeks of pregnancy, some myelocytes are observed, but mature polymorphonuclear leukocytes do not appear until around 12 weeks. The circulating rate remains at less than 1000 elements/μL during the whole of the earlier part of pregnancy and does not increase significantly until the myeloid stage of hematopoiesis; it then increases rapidly until 28 weeks.

Lymphopoiesis begins in the lymphoid plexuses toward the eighth week and spreads first to the thymus, in the ninth week, and then to the lymph nodes from the third month on. After

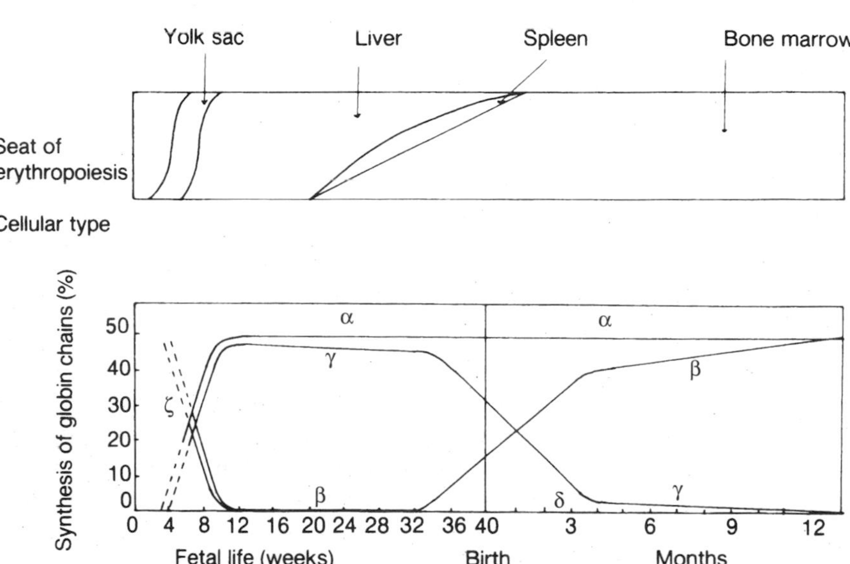

Figure 10.2 Ontogenesis of the chains of hemoglobins and erythropoiesis.

they have begun to appear, the circulating lymphocytes increase rapidly, reaching a peak of 10 000 elements/μL at 20 weeks. The level then decreases gradually to 3000 elements/μL at birth. The megakaryocytes can be found in the wall of the yolk sac between 5 and 6 weeks and then in the liver after the visceral stage of hematopoiesis has begun. They persist there until the end of pregnancy and can be found in significant quantities in the marrow after the third month. Platelets are found in the blood from 11 weeks' gestation and, after 18 weeks, they exist in numbers equal to those in adult blood.

Origin and differentiation of the hematopoietic cells

For years, a controversy raged between the supporters of a unitary thesis and those of a pluricellular origin of the different hematopoietic lineages. The current opinion – based on experiments in animals, on clinical data in human pathology and, more recently, on the culture of hematopoietic cells from healthy subjects – is that there exists a pluripotent stem cell, the colony-forming unit, from which the various lineages stem. This pluripotent stem cell, which cannot be morphologically identified by maturation criteria, is capable of differentiation and self-renewal. It is the precursor of the erythroid, myeloid, and lymphoid lineages, and its existence was confirmed through the technique of splenic lineages described by Iscove et al.[1] We now distinguish a second generation of stem cells with a restricted differentiation potential in either the lymphoid lineage or the myeloid lineage, but their capacity for self-renewal persists. The stem cells are present in the marrow and the blood.

Kelemen et al., in their *Atlas of human haemopoietic development*,[2] suggest the following pattern. Everything stems from a pool of stem cells appearing on the mesenchymal wall of the yolk sac. It is the function of these first-generation intravascular stem cells, after the vascular intra- and extraembryonic networks are linked, to migrate into the embryo and multiply there. Moore and Metcalf[3] demonstrated the necessity of this first migration. No hematopoiesis occurs in an embryo that has been prematurely separated from its yolk sac. The seeding of the liver gives birth to a stem cell, called a *second-generation stem cell*, which is smaller than the first and nearer to the normoblastic lineage. These pluripotent cells proliferate in the liver, becoming half as numerous as the liver's nucleated cells. Then, they migrate toward and seed other areas of the embryo (marrow, spleen, lymph nodes, and thymus) as well as the extraembryonic areas. Some vascular islets of the yolk sac especially are colonized by second-generation stem cells (the first-generation cells are short-lived, with a half-life of approximately 8–12 weeks). A third generation of pluripotent cells gives rise to all the blood cells made during pre- and postnatal life. Given what we know at present, it is difficult to speak of well-defined stages, and modification in the population of stem cells is not proved, particularly as concerns the passage from primitive to fetal erythropoiesis. The current theory is that the passage from fetal to adult erythropoiesis represents a gradual modification of the stem cells rather than a change of population.

Purity of fetal blood samples

Fetal blood sampling under ultrasound guidance is a safe procedure that has enabled us to study fetal biology and to obtain prenatal diagnoses of an increasing variety of disorders.[4] The first step in establishing reference values and ensuring the accuracy or diagnosis is to be sure that the fetal blood sample is not contaminated.[5]

In our samples of fetal blood, contamination can be caused by maternal blood, amniotic fluid, or sodium citrate solution. The overall incidence of contamination in our study was small (1.8%), but it must be viewed in relation to both the disorder under investigation and the type of contamination.

Each type of contamination has differing consequences, depending on the disorder under investigation. During diagnosis of fetal infection in the presence of maternal infection, contamination with maternal blood causes a false-positive result. The presence of amniotic fluid, which is often collected for culture at the same time, does not affect the results, but the hematologic parameters and specific immunoglobulin M must be evaluated with caution. Similarly, the presence of maternal blood cells in a specimen for investigation of fetal karyotype makes the specimen useless, but amniotic fluid or sodium citrate has negligible effects.

Investigation of disorders of hemostasis (platelets or coagulation factors) is severely affected by amniotic fluid contamination because amniotic fluid activates some coagulation factors and can cause platelet aggregation.

We evaluated the sensitivity of each method and measured dilutions of maternal blood, amniotic fluid, and sodium citrate. We believe that each test must be done in all cases because results differ under various conditions.

Depending on the gestational age and the indication for fetal blood sampling, we collect 2–3 mL of blood. This is divided into 500 μl anticoagulated in lyophilized ethylene-diamine tetraacetic acid [EDTAJ K_2 (Sarstedt reference 32332)], 400 μL collected in 0.129 mol/L sodium citrate solution (ratio 9 : n) and, if karyotype is required, 500 μL drawn into a lithium heparin dry mixture. The remaining blood is not anticoagulated.

Hematologic indexes are determined with a Coulter Counter MD II. Leukocytes, erythrocytes, platelets, hemoglobin, hematocrit, and mean corpuscular volume are measured immediately after sampling. The distributions of the volumes of leukocytes, erythrocytes, and platelets are shown in Figs 10.3 and 10.4.

Smears are obtained after leukoconcentration and stained with the May–Grünwald–Giemsa stain for the differential count. The Kleihauer–Betke test to differentiate fetal from adult red cells is performed with the Boehring kit.

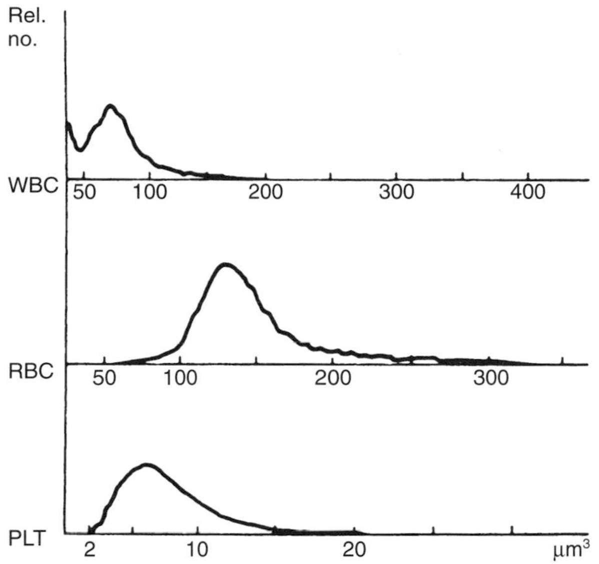

Figure 10.3 Histograms of fetal white blood cell (WBC), red blood cell (RBC), and platelet (PLT) distribution curves.

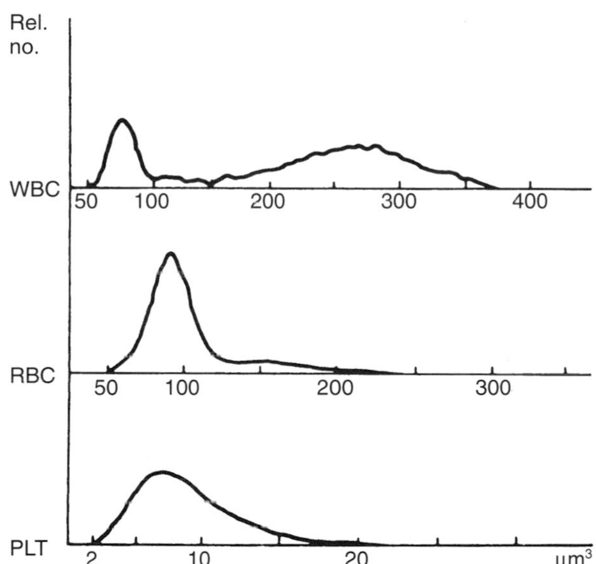

Figure 10.4 Histograms of maternal white blood cell (WBC), red blood cell (RBC), and platelet (PLT) distribution curves.

Anti-I and anti-i cold agglutinins (against erythrocyte antigens), which are active at room temperature, are used in appropriate dilution.

The levels of β-subunit of human chorionic gonadotropic hormone (βhCG) in maternal and fetal serum are determined with the enzyme-linked immunosorbent assay method using an anti-J3-hCG monoclonal antibody (Tandem Biotrol, France).

Coagulation factors IX and VIIIC arc measured by a single-stage method, as described by Mibashan and colleagues[6] adapted for automated coagulation testing (KC 10 from

Table 10.1 Fetal hemostasis expressed as a percentage (mean ± SD) of normal adult value.

Coagulation factor	%	Inhibitor	%
VIIIC	40 ± 12	Fibronectin	40 ± 10
VIIIRAg	60 ± 13	Protein C	11 ± 3
VII	28 ± 5	α_2-Macroglobulin	18 ± 4
IX	9 ± 3	α_2-Antitrypsin	40 ± 4
V	47 ± 10	AT III	30 ± 3
II	12 ± 3	α_2-Antiplasmin	61 ± 6
XII	22 ± 3		
Prekallikrein	19 ± 2		
Fibrin-stabilizing factor	30 ± 5		
Fibrinogen	40 ± 15		
Plasminogen	24 ± 15		

Data from fetuses of 19–27 weeks' gestation.

DADE AHS, Miami, FL, USA). Factor VIII activity is tested against the World Health Organization reference plasma 80/511. Factors II and V are measured by one-stage assay by means of thromboplastin, calcium, and substrate-deficient plasma for both factors II and V. Reference levels are shown in Table 10.1.

The percentage of contamination detectable by each method is determined with fetal blood specimens by means of measured amounts of maternal blood, amniotic fluid, and sodium citrate until minimum detectable contamination is determined.

Each test is performed on all samples. Hematologic indexes are undertaken immediately as an initial screening test before the patient leaves the hospital. It is possible, depending on the clinical circumstances, to repeat the fetal blood sampling, if necessary. No individual test is infallible under all circumstances, and the reliability of each test depends on the clinical situation and the type of contamination. The percentages of contamination detectable by each method are summarized in Table 10.2.

Typical cell size distribution curves for maternal and fetal hematologic indexes are shown in Figs 10.3 and 10.4. Three major differences distinguish maternal from fetal blood. There is only one peak of leukocytes in the fetus (corresponding to lymphocytes and nucleated erythrocytes), the average erythrocyte volume is much higher in the fetus, and red cell distribution width is broader in the fetus.

In leukocytes, there are mainly lymphocytes; granulocytes appear later in pregnancy. Platelet volume is similar in mother and fetus.

In cases of maternal blood contamination, a second peak of leukocytes is usually seen with a larger volume; this peak is the granulocyte peak. The gestational age at the time of sampling must be taken into account because of the change in granulocytes toward term. Contamination of 10% or more by either amniotic fluid or sodium citrate causes a decrease in the

Table 10.2 Percentage of contamination detectable by each method.

Method	Amniotic fluid (%)	Maternal blood (%)	Sodium citrate (%)
Hematologic indexes	20	>5	20
Smear (Giemsa)	10	10	NC
Erythrocyte antigens	NC	15	NC
βhCG	>0.1	0.2	NC
Coagulation factors V or VII, IX, or II	NC	30	10–50
Kleihauer–Betke test		5*	NC

βhCG, β-subunit of human chorionic gonadotropin; NC, noncontributory.
*Depending on the gestational age.

same ratio compared with the normal range of erythrocytes, leukocytes, and platelets.

The Kleihauer–Betke test relies on detecting differences in hemoglobins present in adult and fetal red cells. In theory, this test should be able to detect a maternal blood contamination of as little as 0.5%. In practice, although the test is rapid and simple to perform, absolutely accurate results are not possible because of the gradual appearance of hemoglobin A in fetal erythrocytes. After staining, erythrocytes containing only hemoglobin A appear as empty "cell ghosts." Those containing mainly or exclusively hemoglobin F stain darkly, and those with both hemoglobin A and F have an intermediate level of staining. This causes difficulties and technical errors in the differentiation of immature fetal cells from maternal erythrocytes. We have never demonstrated maternal blood contamination by this method after 30 weeks.

Blood smears stained for differential count clearly show amniotic fluid squames if contamination with amniotic fluid has occurred. The presence of the squames depends on both the gestational age at the time of sampling and the percentage of contamination.

Erythrocyte antigen expression differs from fetus to adult. I antigen is present only on adult erythrocytes; i antigen is present only on fetal erythrocytes. Monoclonal antibody agglutination (anti-I and anti-i) is simple to perform and can detect a maternal blood contamination of 5%.

The βhCG is of maternal origin, has a steep gradient across the placenta, and is found in only minute quantities in fetal blood, although higher levels are found in amniotic fluid. The ratio is approximately 1:100:400 (fetal blood to amniotic fluid to maternal blood). It is probably the most sensitive method for determining whether the sample is contaminated, allowing detection of as little as 0.2% maternal blood or 1% amniotic fluid contamination. In practice, if we detect βhCG in fetal serum, the specimen is regarded as contaminated. A markedly elevated level suggests contamination by maternal blood rather than amniotic fluid, but βhCG levels do not allow differentiation between the types of contamination, so other tests must be used for clarification.

Coagulation factors V and VIII detect both amniotic fluid and sodium citrate contamination, but must be interpreted with caution. Less than 1% contamination with amniotic fluid activates coagulation and falsely increases the activities of factors V and VIII when tested against adult reference plasma. These values need to be compared with vitamin K-dependent factors, such as IX or II, which are not activated by amniotic fluid. In contrast, a large amniotic fluid contamination (greater than 10% and detectable on blood smears) causes lower levels by dilution.

Fetal hematology

Starting from ultrasonically guided fetal blood samplings carried out between 18 and 29 weeks' gestation for various prenatal diagnoses (usually toxoplasmosis), we have been able to determine the reference values of some hematologic parameters in 2860 fetuses.[7] The subjects' prenatal diagnosis tests were normal, and they were confirmed to be healthy at birth.

Fetal blood was sampled into EDTA tubes, and we worked with a Coulter Counter S Plus II on prediluted samples.

Table 10.3 shows the main hematologic results obtained from 2860 normal fetuses between 18 and 36 weeks of pregnancy. There is no significant increase in the number of platelets (which stays at approximately $250 \times 10^3/\mu l$). On the contrary, the red blood cell count gradually increases from 2.85 to $3.82 \times 10^6/\mu l$, and the white blood cell count increases from 4.7 to $7.7 \times 10^3/\mu l$. The concentration of hemoglobin also increases significantly during the second trimester of pregnancy. Conversely, the mean corpuscular volume decreases significantly from 131.5 to 114 fL.

Fetal cytology

The evolution of the fetal leukocyte differential according to the stage of pregnancy is shown in Table 10.4. Also shown are the distribution of polymorphonuclear leukocytes (neutrophils, eosinophils), monocytes, lymphocytes, and erythroblasts. Two reasons led us to include the erythroblasts in the leukocyte differential, even though they belong to the red cell lineage and not to the white cells: (1) erythroblasts are a normal component of fetal blood; and (2) the nuclei of these

Table 10.3 Evolution of hematologic values of 2860 normal fetuses during pregnancy (mean ± SD).[8]

Weeks of gestation	WBC ($\times 10^3/\mu L$)	Platelets ($\times 10^3/\mu L$)	RBC ($\times 10^6/\mu L$)	Hb (g/100 mL)	Ht (%)	MCV (fL)
10–17	1.87 ± 3.42	159 ± 68	1.81 ± 0.78	9.92 ± 2.24	27.4 ± 7.4	154.9 ± 26.8
18–21 (*n* = 760)	4.68 ± 2.96	234 ± 57	2.85 ± 0.36	11.69 ± 1.27	37.3 ± 4.32	131.11 ± 10.97
22–25 (*n* = 1200)	4.72 ± 2.82	247 ± 59	3.09 ± 0.34	12.2 ± 1.6	38.59 ± 3.94	125.1 ± 7.84
26–29 (*n* = 460)	5.16 ± 2.53	242 ± 69	3.46 ± 0.41	12.91 ± 1.38	40.88 ± 4.4	118.5 ± 7.96
>30 (*n* = 440)	7.71 ± 4.99	232 ± 87	3.82 ± 0.64	13.64 ± 2.21	43.55 ± 7.2	114.38 ± 9.34

SD, standard deviation; Hb, hemoglobin concentration; Ht, hematocrit; MCV, mean corpuscular volume; RBC, red blood cell count; WBC, white blood cell count.

Table 10.4 Fetal differential count of 732 normal fetuses according to the stage of gestation.

Weeks of gestation	Lymphocytes (%)	Neutrophils (%)	Eosinophils (%)	Basophils (%)	Monocytes (%)	Erythroblasts (% white blood cells)
18–21 (*n* = 186)	88 ± 7	6 ± 4	2 ± 3	0.5 ± 1	3.5 ± 2	45 ± 86
22–25 (*n* = 230)	87 ± 6	6.5 ± 35	3 ± 3	0.5 ± 1	3 ± 2.5	21 ± 23
26–29 (*n* = 144)	84 ± 6	8.5 ± 4	4 ± 3	0.5 ± 1	3 ± 2.5	21 ± 67
>30 (*n* = 172)	685 ± 15	23 ± 15	5 ± 3	0.5 ± 1	3 ± 2	17 ± 40

erythroblasts are counted as white blood cells by the Coulter Counter.

First, we found few or no basophils in the fetus. Second, a very high lymphocytosis was present from 18 weeks' gestation, along with erythroblastosis. The percentage of lymphocytes decreases from 88% at 18 weeks to 68.5% by 30 weeks, and the erythroblast percentage gradually decreases from 45% at 18 weeks to 17% at 30 weeks. This reduction in the number of erythroblasts is made up for by a gradual increase in neutrophils as fetal life advances, from 6% at 18 weeks to 23% at 30 weeks.

The importance of this evolution of the fetal differential is threefold. First, we have been able retrospectively to establish reference values related to different stages of pregnancy. Second, the blood differential is an extremely useful tool to check the purity of fetal blood. For instance, blood that contains no erythroblasts at 18 weeks, or 40% neutrophils at 20 weeks, could have been contaminated by maternal blood or by blood of placental origin. Third, we have noticed that the fetal differential varies greatly in cases of parasitic (toxoplasmosis) or viral (rubella) infections.

Fetal red blood cell antigens

We compared 72 samples of fetal blood ranging from 20 to 25 weeks of pregnancy with samples of full-term neonates (cord blood) and adults. We tested 38 red blood cell antigens, using specific antibodies:

- Polymorphic antigens: A, A_1, B, D, C, C^w, c, E, e, K, k, Kp^a, Fy^a, Fy^b, JK^a JK^b, M, N, S, s, Lu^a, Lu^b, Le^a, Le^b, P_1, Xg^a.
- Monomorphic antigens: H, Rh17, Kp^b, Js^b, Fy^3, Jk^3, P, I, i, Ve^a, Ge^a, Emma.

Among these 38 antigens, identical reactions were observed in fetus, newborn, and adult, except for A, A_1, B, H, Le^a, Le^b, Lu^a, Lu^b, P^1, P, I, and i.

Table 10.5 shows that some antigens are not expressed or have hardly developed in fetuses. Test results on newborns show an intermediate expression between the fetal and adult periods.

Fetal platelet antigens

From 18 to 29 weeks, the number of platelets remains stable at around 250 × $10^3/\mu L$. On stained blood smears (with May–Grünwald–Giemsa), fetal platelets present no particular cytologic differences from adult platelets. Fetal platelets aggregate with adenosine triphosphate (ADP), thrombin, ristocetine, collagen, arachidonic acid, but not with epinephrine.

The study of the glycoproteins of platelet membranes has made it possible to identify glycoproteins Ib, IIa/b, IIIa/b, with molecular weights of 160, 134, and 90 Da. The PLA_1 antigen is present, which explains the risk of fetal anti-PLA alloimmunization as early as the first trimester of pregnancy.

Working in cooperation with Y. Gruel, we have been able to quantify HPA-1a (PLA1a) and HPA-3a (LeKa or Bak a) antigens, as well as the membrane glycoproteins, from 16 weeks (Table 10.6).[8]

Quantification of glycoproteins GPIIb/IIIa is similar in fetus and adult; antibody anti-GPIb (AN51) and anti-GPIb (6D1) fixed more easily in fetal platelets than in adult platelets.

Table 10.5 Percentage of reactivity of some red blood cell antigens in adult, neonate (cord), and fetus.

Antigens (%)	A	A_1	B	H	Le^a	Le^b	Lu^a	Lu^b	P_1	P	I	i
Adult	45	35	9	100	20	70	7	100	75	100	100	0
Birth	45	37	12	90	0	4	3	100	38	100	12	100
Fetus	36	0	11	64	0	2	1	99	17	88	0	100

Table 10.6 Platelet antigens in fetus (>16 weeks) and adult expressed as mean fluorescence values (± SEM).

Platelets	Immunofluorescence intensity	
	Fetus (mean ± SD)	Adults (mean ± SD)
Antigens		
HPA-1a	433.0 ± 30.0	427 ± 13.5
HPA-3a	441.5 ± 25.0	459 ± 15.0
Glycoproteins		
GPIIb IIIa, IgG	427.0 ± 23.0	420.0 ± 30.0
GPIIb IIIa, AP-2	459.5 ± 23.0	498.0 ± 11.0
GPIIIa, AP-3	536.0 ± 14.0	515.0 ± 13.0
GPIb, AN-51	491.5 ± 14.0	426.5 ± 9.0
GPIb, 6D1	479.0 ± 15.0	443.0 ± 8.7

SD, standard deviation; SEM, standard error of the mean.

Prenatal diagnostic of Glanzmann thrombasthenia (GPIIb/IIIa) or Bernard–Soulier syndrome (GPIb) is now available early in pregnancy.

Lymphocyte subpopulation

Lymphocyte count

Leukocytes are numbered while the Coulter S Plus II monitors the purity of fetal blood. The absolute number of lymphocytes is observed from the leukocyte differential performed on a blood smear stained by May–Grünwald–Giemsa stain.

Separation of the mononucleated cells

Separation of the mononucleated cells is carried out by differential centrifugation in a density gradient.

Lymphocyte phenotype

The development of hybridization techniques now permits the production of commercialized monoclonal antibodies and provides the means of investigating lymphocyte subpopulations.

The main markers of lymphocyte differentiation, as currently defined, have been characterized using Coulter monoclonal antibodies labeled with fluorescein isothiocyanate. Detection was carried out by direct or indirect immunofluorescence. It proved necessary to implement a micromethod, considering the reduced volume of fetal blood.

The following monoclonal antibodies were used:

- Coulter Clone T11 – specific for the receptor of T lymphocytes for the sheep erythrocytes and associated with an antigen that is 50 000 Da in molecular mass.
- Coulter Clone T_3 – specific for an antigen T3 (30 000 Da in molecular mass). This antigen is present in the mature T lymphocytes of peripheral blood and on 20–30% of thymocytes.
- Coulter Clone T4 – specific for an antigen of 64 000 Da molecular mass, present on 80% of thymocytes and 60% of circulating T lymphocytes. It is associated with T lymphocytes whose target is an antigen belonging to the major system of class II histocompatibility. This antigen is stable and is not lost during T-cell activation.
- Coulter Clone T8 – specific for an antigen present in the suppressive and cytotoxic T subpopulations; it is 33 000 Da in molecular mass in its reduced state, 76 000 Da in its nonreduced state. This antigen can be found on 80% of human thymocytes and on approximately 35% of the T lymphocytes of peripheral blood.
- Coulter Clone B1 – specific for an antigen of human B lymphocytes, 35 000 Da in molecular mass. This antigen is found in the B cells of peripheral blood, of the lymphoid organs, and of bone marrow.
- Coulter Clone B_4 – specific for an antigen that is bimolecular in structure, 40 000 and 80 000 Da in molecular mass. It is expressed by the normal B lymphocytes and is present in all isolated B cells. Antigen B4 seems to be the first antigen associated with B cells that can be detected in fetal tissues.
- E 135 – monomorphic anti-DR, kindly provided by Professor Charron (Pitié-Salpêtrière).
- Leu_7, Leu11 (Becton) – antibodies that recognize the natural. killer (NK) cytotoxic cells of peripheral blood and some granulocytes. Antibody NKH!A recognizes all the cells with NK activity; anti-NKH_2 determines a population of large-grained lymphocytes with poor cytotoxic activity.
- Coulter Clone My 4 – recognizes macrophages and some granulocytes.

Results

The following is an outline of the results:

1 Lymphocyte count:
   - Fetal blood (20–26 weeks of amenorrhea): $3.8 \pm 0.9 \times 10^3/\mu L$.
   - Cord blood at birth: $7.1 \pm 2.3 \times 10^3/\mu L$.
   - Adult blood: $2.5 \pm 0.95 \times 10^3/\mu L$.

2 Phenotyping of lymphocyte subpopulations: T-lymphocyte phenotyping is presented in Table 10.7; B-lymphocyte phenotyping is presented in Table 10.8.

The percentages of circulating mononucleated cells recognized by the Leu_{11}, NKH_1A, NKH_2 antibodies are, respectively, 21% ± 7%, 5.8% ± 2.3%, 2.5% ± 1.5% in the fetus between 20 and 26 weeks of gestation and 13% ± 5%, 12% ± 3%, 5% ± 1.5% in the adult. Of fetal circulating nucleated cells, 10% ± 3% react with Coulter Clone MY4.

The study of lymphocytes subpopulations is interesting in cases of maternofetal infection. T4/T8 is decreased in infected fetuses (toxoplasmosis or cytomegalovirus), and CD3 lymphocytes count is increased in mothers and fetus when infection is certain.

Table 10.7 Evolution of T-lymphocyte subpopulations in fetal blood, cord blood at birth, and adult, expressed as a percentage of the absolute number of lymphocytes (mean ± SD).

	T11	T3	T4	T8	T4/T8
Fetus					
19–23 weeks	44 ± 14	54.7 ± 9.6	39.9 ± 6.7	12.7 ± 3.7	3.5 ± 0.5
24–28 weeks		61.9 ± 10.5	43.1 ± 9.3	14.4 ± 4.5	3.3 ± 1.4
29–32 weeks		67.7 ± 7	45.5 ± 8.3	16.8 ± 6.1	3.1 ± 1.5
Neonate	71.4 ± 3.9		52.2 ± 10		
Adult	78.3 ± 12.1	74.2 ± 6.9	46.2 ± 13.3	15.6 ± 4.1	3.1 ± 1.1

SD, standard deviation.

Table 10.8 B-lymphocyte markers in fetus and adult as a percentage of absolute numbers of lymphocytes.

	B_1	B_4	E_{135}
Fetus (20–26 weeks)	4.4 ± 1.7	5 ± 3.8	28.6 ± 8.5
Adult	2.7 ± 2.3	3.2 ± 1.3	12.3 ± 1.5

Key points

1 Mesoblastic hematopoiesis of the yolk sac is the first stage of embryonic hematopoiesis and appears on day 19 of pregnancy.

2 Visceral hematopoiesis is the second stage of embryonic hematopoiesis, begins in the liver sinusoids around 5–6 weeks' gestation, and increases rapidly.

3 Although granulocytes and platelets are found in the circulation, the fetal liver seems to be the seat of an almost pure hematopoiesis. From the third to the fifth months of pregnancy, the erythrocytic precursors represent approximately 50% of the liver's nucleated cells.

4 From 9 to 12 weeks, some hematopoietic activity can also be observed in the thymus, the lymph nodes, the kidneys, and even in the spleen.

5 Visceral, mainly hepatic, hematopoiesis reaches its highest level of production around the fifth and sixth months, gradually regressing until delivery. Visceral hematopoiesis can still be observed during the first week of postnatal life in the liver and occasionally even in the spleen.

6 Medullary hematopoiesis begins about the fourth month and is initially predominantly leukopoietic. The erythropoietic tissues multiply rapidly, and the marrow reaches its maximal cellularity toward 30 weeks' gestation, with each lineage being adequately represented.

7 Leukocytes first develop in the wall of the yolk sac, then in the embryo. Very few circulating granulocytes are found during the first weeks of fetal life.

8 Platelets are found in the blood from 11 weeks' gestation, and, after 18 weeks, they exist in numbers equal to those in adult blood.

9 The current opinion is that there exists a pluripotent stem cell, the colony-forming unit, from which the various lineages stem. This pluripotent stem cell, which cannot be morphologically identified by maturation criteria, is capable of differentiation and self-renewal.

10 Investigation of disorders of hemostasis in fetal blood samplings (platelets or coagulation factors) is severely affected by amniotic fluid contamination because

amniotic fluid activates some coagulation factors and can cause platelet aggregation.

11 Three major differences distinguish maternal from fetal blood. There is only one peak of leukocytes in the fetus (corresponding to lymphocytes and nucleated erythrocytes), the average erythrocyte volume is much higher in the fetus, and red cell distribution width is broader in the fetus.

12 In leukocytes, there are mainly lymphocytes; granulocytes appear later in pregnancy. In cases of maternal blood contamination. a second peak of leukocytes is usually seen with a larger volume; this peak is the granulocyte peak.

13 Fetal blood sampling under ultrasound guidance is a safe procedure to study fetal biology and to obtain prenatal diagnoses of an increasing variety of disorders. The first step in establishing reference values and ensuring the accuracy of diagnosis is to be sure that the fetal blood sample is not contaminated, by detection of βhCG in fetal serum or erythrocyte antigen expression that differs from fetus to adult.

14 Fetal blood sampling contamination can be caused by maternal blood, amniotic fluid, or sodium citrate solution.

15 The red blood cell count gradually increases from 2.85 to 3.82 × 10.6/μL. The concentration of hemoglobin also increases significantly during the second trimester of pregnancy. Conversely, the mean corpuscular volume decreases significantly from 131.5 to 114 fL.

16 The evolution of the fetal leukocyte differential according to the stage of pregnancy shows that there are few or no basophils in the fetus. A very high lymphocytosis is present from 18 weeks' gestation along with erythroblastosis, decreasing to 30 weeks.

17 Quantification of platelet glycoproteins GPIIb/IIIa is similar in fetus and adult; antibody anti-GPIa AN51) and anti GP-Ib (6D1) fix more easily in fetal platelets than in adult platelets.

18 The study of lymphocyte subpopulations is interesting in cases of maternofetal infection. T4/T8 is decreased in infected fetuses (toxoplasmosis or cytomegalovirus), and CD3 lymphocyte count is increased in mothers and fetus when infection is certain.

References

1 Iscove NN, Till JE, McCulloch EA. The proliferative states of mouse granulopoietic progenitor cells. *Proc Soc Exp Biol Med* 1970;134(1):33–36.

2 Kelemen E, Calvo W, Fliedner TM. *Atlas of human haemopoietic development*. Berlin: Springer-Verlag; 1979:1.

3 Moore MAS, Metcalf D. Ontogeny of the hematopoietic system. Yolk sac origin of *in vivo* and *in vitro* colony forming cells in the developing mouse embryo. *Br J Haemotol* 1970;18(3):279–296.

4 Daffos F, Forestier F (eds). Biologie du sang foetal. In: *Medecine et biologie du foetus humain*. Paris: Maloine; 1988:81–116.

5 Forestier F, Cox W, Daffos F, et al. The assessment of fetal blood samples. *Am J Obstet Gynecol* 1988;158:1184.

6 Mibashan RS, Peake IR, Rodeck CH, et al. Dual diagnosis of prenatal hemophilia A by measurement of fetal factor VIIIC and VIIIC antigen (VIIICAg). *Lancet* 1980;ii:994.

7 Forestier F, Daffos F, Catherine N, et al. Developmental hematopoiesis in normal human fetal blood. *Blood* 1991; 77(11):2360–2363.

8 Jacquemard F, Daffos F. *Medecine prénatale; grossesses pathologiques pour raisons foetales*. Paris: Elsevier, 2003.

9 Gruel Y, Boizard B, Daffos P, et al. Determination of platelet antigens and glycoproteins in the human fetus. *Blood* 1986;68(2): 488–492.

Part IV

Variations in Embryonal and Fetal Growth and Development

11 Sporadic and recurrent pregnancy loss

Robert M. Silver and D. Ware Branch

Pregnancy loss is one of the most common medical problems in reproductive-aged couples, with as many as 25% of all women attempting pregnancy experiencing at least one spontaneous abortion. A miscarriage is an emotional event for most individuals, and physicians are often called on to provide insight and counseling. An estimated 0.5–1.0% of couples attempting pregnancy suffer three or more consecutive losses, and an even higher proportion have two or more consecutive losses. These couples with recurrent pregnancy loss (RPL) are often distraught and sometimes desperate, especially when childbearing has been put off until later in life. Despite the anguish associated with RPL, modern medical science has made surprisingly little progress in identifying causes or devising rational treatments. Some physicians believe there are few cost-effective evaluations and few effective treatments. At the other extreme, "pregnancy loss centers" now exist in many larger metropolitan areas, with personnel claiming special insight into the causes of RPL and offering therapies not universally accepted by mainstream medicine. The truth about RPL may lie somewhere between these two contrasting views. The purpose of this chapter is to review the known and suspected causes and management of sporadic pregnancy loss and RPL.

Terminology and frequency of pregnancy loss in humans

Traditionally, physicians have termed all pregnancy losses before 20 weeks' gestation, *abortions*, and death *in utero* thereafter, as a *stillbirth* or *fetal death*. Advances in reproductive biology indicate that this classification is arbitrary, inconsistent with embryonic and fetal development, and not clinically useful. A more worthwhile approach is to classify pregnancy loss in terms of developmental stages of gestation. The *pre-embryonic* period lasts from conception to approximately 5 weeks after the first day of the last menstrual period. The *embryonic* period begins at 6 weeks and continues through 9 weeks' gestation. The *fetal* period begins at 10 weeks' gestation, or 70 days from the last menstrual period, and extends through pregnancy until delivery. Thus, from the perspective of a developmental biologist, pregnancy loss may be categorized as *pre-embryonic (anembryonic)*, *embryonic*, or *fetal*.

Fifty percent or more of human pregnancies are lost before term.[1] The majority are unrecognized pregnancy losses occurring before or with the expected next menses.[2] Approximately 10–12% of all clinically recognized pregnancies are lost as first-trimester or early second-trimester spontaneous abortions. The rate of fetal death after 14 weeks' gestation is much lower than the rate of pre-embryonic and embryonic loss. If neonatal deaths due to prematurity or malformations are excluded, less than 5% of all pregnancies are lost between early second trimester and term.[3–6] The rate of pregnancy loss is greatly influenced by a patient's past obstetric history.[7] Both spontaneous abortion and fetal death are more likely to occur among women with previous pregnancy losses, and less likely to occur in those with prior live births.

The vast majority of pregnancy losses are *sporadic* in nature (i.e., they occur as an isolated event in a woman whose other pregnancies are successful). *Recurrent* miscarriage, traditionally defined as the loss of three or more consecutive pregnancies, occurs in an estimated 0.5–1.0% of women. Women with two successive early spontaneous abortions have a recurrence risk similar to that of women with three previous losses.[7–9] Thus, depending on the patient's age and attitude, investigations into the cause of the recurrent losses may be indicated after two or three successive miscarriages. Some investigators have found that the risk of spontaneous abortion in the subsequent pregnancy increases after four or more successive abortions.[10] The risk of RPL is also increased in couples with prior fetal death as opposed to early pregnancy loss.[11]

Sporadic pregnancy loss

Sporadic pregnancy loss is perhaps the most common adverse outcome in human reproduction. In the vast majority of sporadic spontaneous abortions, an etiology is neither readily apparent nor sought. Nonetheless, most couples who suffer a spontaneous abortion feel a sense of loss and seek an explanation.

Causes of sporadic pregnancy loss

Morphological abnormalities

Abnormalities of growth and development are the immediate cause of most pre-embryonic pregnancy losses (Table 11.1). One-half of pre-implantation conceptuses and one-third of implanted conceptuses are morphologically abnormal.[12] Many of these conceptuses are cytogenetically abnormal and are presumably destined to be miscarried around the time of the expected next menses.

Abnormalities of growth and development are also the immediate cause of most recognized pregnancy losses. Nearly one-fifth of specimens from losses occurring in the first half of pregnancy, and one-third of those occurring at 8 weeks' gestation or earlier, are anembryonic (i.e., the abortus specimen consists of an intact or ruptured gestational sac with no apparent embryo, yolk sac, or umbilical cord).[12] Approximately 35% of women presenting with symptoms of spontaneous abortion have an empty gestational sac or a gestational sac with only a yolk sac present.[13] It is likely that such cases of "blighted ovum" or "anembryonic pregnancy" failed during the pre-embryonic or early embryonic period.

Identifiable embryos or fetuses are found in 50–60% of first-trimester or early second-trimester abortus specimens, but only one-half of these are morphologically normal.[12] The remainder exhibit disorganized growth (25%), are growth impaired (15%), or are too macerated for examination. Ultrasonographic data are consistent with these morphological observations. Fifty percent of women presenting with symptoms of spontaneous abortion who undergo ultrasonographic examination have a dead embryo.[13] Because failure of growth and death of the conceptus commonly precedes physically evident spontaneous abortion by one or more weeks, the gestational age at which the abortion is recognized does not necessarily indicate when pregnancy failure occurred.

Table 11.1 Potential causes of sporadic pregnancy loss.

Morphologic abnormalities/birth defects
Genetic abnormalities
Medical and hormonal disorders
Diabetes mellitus
Thyroid disease
Luteal phase defect
Infections
Treponema pallidum
Borrelia burgdorferi
Listeria monocytogenes
Ureaplasma urealyticum
Viral infections (e.g., parvovirus; herpes simplex)
Bacterial infections (e.g., group B streptococcus)
Other causes
Tobacco
Drugs and chemicals
Ethanol

Interestingly, spontaneous pregnancy loss appears to be biphasic in distribution. Using transvaginal ultrasound, Goldstein[6] found that 13.4% of 232 women with apparently normal early pregnancies had a pregnancy loss. A total of 87% of the losses (12% of all pregnancies) occurred before 10 weeks' gestation, and all embryos that were alive at 8.5 weeks' gestation survived beyond 14 weeks. Thirteen percent of the losses (1–2% of all pregnancies) occurred from 14 to 20 weeks' gestation. Similarly, Simpson and colleagues[14] reported in 1987 that only 3.2% of normal women with a live embryo seen at 8 weeks' gestation eventually suffered a pregnancy loss, and all losses occurred in the period between 10.5 and 16 weeks' gestation. Thus, embryos surviving to 8 weeks' gestation have a very low mortality rate during the next few weeks. The overall rate of pregnancy loss rises again in the early fetal period. The subsequent pregnancy loss rate is only 1% if a live fetus is seen at 14–16 weeks' gestation.[14]

Cytogenetic abnormalities

Overall, approximately 50% of sporadic spontaneous abortions are cytogenetically abnormal.[15,16] Chromosome abnormalities are present in more than 90% of anembryonic abortus tissues,[12] two-thirds of malformed or growth-disorganized embryos, and one-third of malformed fetuses.[17] Approximately 60% of karyotypic abnormalities in early pregnancy losses are autosomal trisomies, 20% are polyploid, and 20% are monosomy X (Table 11.2).

The autosomal trisomies found in spontaneous abortions arise *de novo* as a result of meiotic nondisjunction during gametogenesis in parents with normal karyotypes. Except for trisomy 1, all chromosomal trisomies have been reported in abortus material. The single most common trisomy seen in spontaneous abortion is trisomy 16, accounting for 20–30% of all abortus trisomies. Some autosomal trisomies are seen only in spontaneous abortions (e.g., trisomies 2, 15, 16, and 22) or very early induced abortions, whereas trisomies 13, 18, and 21 are found in spontaneous abortions and also occur in live births. The rate of chromosomally abnormal abortions increases with increasing maternal age because of an increase in the rate of trisomy abortuses.[18] However, the rate of abortions with polyploidy or monosomy X decreases with increasing maternal age.

The proportion of karyotypically abnormal abortuses drops from a high of approximately 50% at 8–11 weeks' gestation to approximately 30% at 16–19 weeks' gestation according to some reports.[16] However, one group of investigators noted that very early first-trimester losses (less than 8 weeks' gesta-

Table 11.2 Chromosomal complements in spontaneous abortions that are recognized clinically in the first trimester.

Complement	Percentage
Normal	54.1
46,XX or 46,XY	
Triploidy	7.7
69,XXX	(2.7)
69,XYX	(0.2)
69,XXY	(4.0)
Other	(0.8)
Tetraploidy	2.6
92,XXX	(1.5)
92,XXYY	(0.55)
Not stated	(0.55)
Monosomy X	8.6
Structural abnormalities	1.5
Sex chromosomal polysomy	0.2
47,XXX (0.05)	
47,XXY (0.15)	
Autosomal monosomy (G)	0.1
Autosomal trisomy	22.3
Chromosome	
No. 1	(0)
No. 2	(1.11)
No. 3	(0.25)
No. 4	(0.64)
No. 5	(0.04)
No. 6	(0.14)
No. 7	(0.89)
No. 8	(0.79)
No. 9	(0.72)
No. 10	(0.36)
No. 11	(0.04)
No. 12	(0.18)
No. 13	(1.07)
No. 14	(0.82)
No. 15	(1.68)
No. 16	(7.27)
No. 17	(0.18)
No. 18	(1.15)
No. 19	(0.01)
No. 20	(0.61)
No. 21	(2.11)
No. 22	(2.26)
Double trisomy	0.7
Mosaic trisomy	1.3
Other abnormalities or not specified	0.9

From Simpson JL, Bombard, AT. Chromosomal abnormalities in spontaneous abortion: frequency, pathology, and genetic counseling. In: Edmonds K, Bennett MJ, eds. *Spontaneous abortion.* London: Blackwell; 1987:51, with permission.

tion) were less likely to be karyotypically abnormal than abortuses from more advanced gestations.[15] The discrepancy in these findings may be due to selection bias.

Traditional cytogenetic analysis involves metaphase analysis of successfully cultured cells. However, culture failure is common with cells obtained from products of conception, occurring in up to 40% of cases.[19] This problem can be circumvented with the use of comparative genomic hybridization (CGH), a molecular genetic technique that allows for the identification of differences in copy number among chromosome regions. Indeed, CGH has been successfully used to determine karyotype in several cases of culture failure after pregnancy loss.[20,21] The technique can even be used in cells obtained from macerated tissues or stored tissue blocks.

Medical and hormonal disorders

Diabetes and thyroid abnormalities have been associated with sporadic pregnancy loss. However, only poorly controlled diabetes, as indicated by an elevated glycosylated hemoglobin, is associated with first-trimester or early second-trimester pregnancy loss.[22] Several groups of investigators have shown that women with antithyroid antibodies detected early in pregnancy have increased rates of first- or early second-trimester loss.[23,24] Most of the affected women do not have biochemical evidence of thyroid disease, and virtually none has clinically apparent disease. It is uncertain whether or not the presence of antithyroid antibodies is specific for pregnancy loss or is simply a marker for an underlying autoimmune disorder also linked to pregnancy loss. Regardless, assessment of thyroid function or antithyroid antibodies is *not recommended* for sporadic pregnancy loss.

Infections

Case reports indicate that infections are a rare cause of some first- or early second-trimester pregnancy losses. Infectious agents such as *Treponema pallidum*,[25] *Borrelia burgdorferi*,[26] and *Listeria monocytogenes*[27] have been identified in first- or early second-trimester miscarriage specimens. *Chlamydia trachomatis* does not appear to be a cause of sporadic abortion.[28,29] Although some data suggest that mycoplasmas and ureaplasmas may be associated with spontaneous abortion,[30,31] these organisms are present in up to 70% of healthy women. Thus, screening for these organisms in women with sporadic abortion is not advised. Other organisms such as group B streptococcus, bacterial vaginosis, parvovirus, herpes simplex virus, *Toxoplasma gondii*, etc. have been linked to second- and third-trimester pregnancy loss.[32] However, they are rarely associated with early losses and routine assessment is not recommended.

Other causes of sporadic early pregnancy loss

Certain drugs and chemical agents, ethanol, coffee, and cigarette smoking have been proposed as causes of sporadic early pregnancy loss. Drugs and chemicals that may cause early pregnancy loss include anesthetic gases, chloroquine, oral hypoglycemic agents, arsenic, heavy metals, and some industrial organic chemicals. It is questionable, however, as to whether any of these is an abortifacient at typical levels of exposure. Antineoplastic agents, such as aminopterin and methotrexate, may cause miscarriage at therapeutic doses. The contention that exposure to video display terminals for more than 20h per week is related to miscarriage has been refuted.[33, 34]

Effect of maternal age, parity, and prior pregnancy outcomes

Sporadic spontaneous abortion is influenced by maternal age and parity. In a cross-sectional study of women in a large healthcare plan,[35] investigators found that the ratio of observed versus expected cases of first-trimester abortion was higher in women younger than 18, lower in women aged 20–35, and rose sharply after age 35. Stein and coauthors[36] found that the overall spontaneous abortion rate was constant until women were in their mid-30s, when it started to rise. The rate of rise increased dramatically at about age 35. Significantly, most of the increase in the rate of spontaneous abortion in older women is not due to an increase in the rate of chromosomally abnormal conceptions.[36] The rate of second-trimester (fetal) loss follows a pattern similar to that of early pregnancy loss, but the increased rate seen in older gravidas begins at age 30.[35] Fretts and Usher[37] showed that approximately 1 in 440 births among women age 35 or older end in unexplained fetal death, a rate more than double that of younger women.

Several investigators have found a direct relationship between gravidity and crude abortion rates, with a noticeable increase after the second pregnancy.[7,8,38,39] These findings are widely considered to be influenced by two factors. First, in modern Western society the third pregnancy and beyond are likely to occur in older women, allowing maternal age to influence the abortion rate. Second, because the average number of desired children in most Western countries is two, many women undertaking a third pregnancy will have experienced pregnancy loss in their prior pregnancies. These women are more likely to have another pregnancy loss than women who have never lost a pregnancy.

Women with one or two previously unsuccessful pregnancies are more likely to suffer a spontaneous loss in their next pregnancy than women undertaking a first pregnancy, or women with one or two previous live births and no abortions. The best data are from Regan's Cambridge Early Pregnancy Loss study.[7] Women with one previous abortion had a recognized abortion rate of 11.5% in their second pregnancy, and women with two previous abortions had an abortion rate of 29.4% in their third pregnancy. By comparison, primigravidas volunteering for the study had a pregnancy loss rate of 5.6%, and women with only live births in the past had an abortion rate of 2.2% in their next pregnancy.

Table 11.3 Recommended evaluation of fetal death.

Generally accepted evaluation
Review of the medical history
Ultrasonography
Indirect Coombs' test
Karyotype
Kleihauer–Betke test
Serological test for syphilis
Toxicology screen
Autopsy
Additional evaluation
Antiphospholipid antibodies
TORCH titers (questionable utility)
Parvovirus serology
Thyroid function tests
Glucose tolerance testing
Testing for heritable thrombophilias

TORCH: toxoplasmosis, and other agents, rubella, cytomegalovirus, herpes simplex.

Fetal death

Clinicians should recognize that the etiologies of late pregnancy loss differ from first-trimester abortions. Potential causes of fetal death include chromosomal abnormalities, fetal malformations, fetal anemia secondary to alloimmunization or fetal–maternal hemorrhage, cord accidents, fetal infections (e.g., syphilis), antiphospholipid syndrome (APS), and heritable thrombophilias. Obstetric disorders such as preeclampsia, abruption, and fetal growth retardation can also lead to fetal death. At present, there is no generally accepted standard evaluation for fetal death. Studies conducted by the Multicenter Stillbirth Collaborative Research Network sponsored by the National Institute of Child Health and Human Development (NICHD) should help to clarify the issue. Meanwhile, Table 11.3 lists our suggested evaluation of patients with fetal death. Amniocentesis should be considered soon after the diagnosis of fetal demise because viable fetal cells can be difficult to obtain from macerated tissues. As CGH becomes more widely available, it will be another option for genetic analysis in cases when culture of live cells is not possible.

Evaluation and management of sporadic pregnancy loss

No specific evaluation of the mother or abortus tissue is indicated in the case of a single pre-embryonic or embryonic loss occurring in an otherwise healthy woman. It may be reassuring to tactfully inform the patient that most sporadic early pregnancy losses are the inevitable consequence of morphological or cytogenetic abnormalities of the conceptus. The clinician should also inform the patient of the high pregnancy success rate after a single spontaneous abortion, taking the maternal age and past obstetric history into account. Recall that several studies have demonstrated that approximately 80–90% of women experiencing a single early spontaneous abortion deliver a viable live infant in the next pregnancy.[7,40,41]

Ultrasound in the management of spontaneous abortion

Endovaginal ultrasonography can play an important role in the management of threatened abortion (Table 11.4). Traditional medical thinking holds that a patient with bleeding in the first 10 weeks of pregnancy has an approximately 50% chance of miscarriage. Ultrasonographic studies have shown, however, that the embryo is usually absent or dead at the time of presentation in patients who are destined to miscarry. In contrast, fewer than one-third of live embryos found in women with uterine bleeding before 10 weeks' gestation will abort.

Precise knowledge of gestational age can facilitate the interpretation of ultrasonographic findings in women with threatened abortion. Ultrasound findings are unreliable at 3–4 weeks' gestation as the uterus usually appears to be empty. At 5–6 weeks, the diagnosis of pregnancy loss is based on yolk sac and gestational sac findings. At 7–8 weeks, gestational sac and embryo findings are germane.

Table 11.4 Sonographic criteria for pregnancy loss.

Criteria diagnostic of pregnancy loss
MSD ≥ 8 mm without yolk sac*
MSD ≥ 16 mm without an embryo*
Embryo without cardiac activity
Findings associated with poor prognosis
MSD minus CRL ≤ 5 mm before 9 weeks' gestation
Yolk sac diameter ≥ 6 mm
Embryonic heart rate ≤ 80 b.p.m.
Subchorionic hemorrhage ≥40% sac volume

B.p.m., beats per min; CRL, crown–rump length; MSD, mean gestational sac diameter.
*High-resolution endovaginal ultrasound (6.25 MHz or greater probe).

The most reliable gestational sac indicator of impending abortion is abnormal sac size relative to other gestational tissue features. For example, one group of investigators have found that when the mean gestational sac diameter (MSD) minus the embryo crown–rump length (CRL) equals 5 mm or less before 9 weeks' gestation (MSD − CRL ≤ 5), the likelihood of miscarriage is greater than 80%.[42] Virtually definitive proof of impending pregnancy loss can be reached with high-resolution (6.25 MHz or greater probe) endovaginal scanning when one sees (1) an MSD of 8 mm or more without a demonstrable yolk sac or (2) an MSD of 16 mm or more without a demonstrable embryo (Fig. 11.1).[43–45] The use of lower resolution equipment requires modification of these criteria.

Abnormally large yolk sac diameter is also associated with pregnancy loss, although it would be unwise to use this feature alone to diagnose pregnancy loss. As a general rule, large yolk sac diameters (6 mm or greater) are associated with abnormal pregnancies destined to miscarry (Fig. 11.2).[46]

A dead embryo (i.e., without cardiac activity) is definitive for pregnancy failure. As a general rule, the presence of a normal cardiac rate in an embryo is encouraging, but there are three important caveats regarding embryonic cardiac activity. First, normal embryos with a CRL of less than 5 mm may have no ultrasonographically apparent cardiac activity. A diagnosis of embryonic death should not be made in this setting. Second, the earlier in pregnancy that embryonic cardiac activity is detected, the less likely it is to predict a successful pregnancy. Among women presenting with uterine bleeding and found to have a live embryo with a CRL of less than 5 mm, the rate of abortion is approximately 30%. After 7 weeks' gestation (CRL approx-

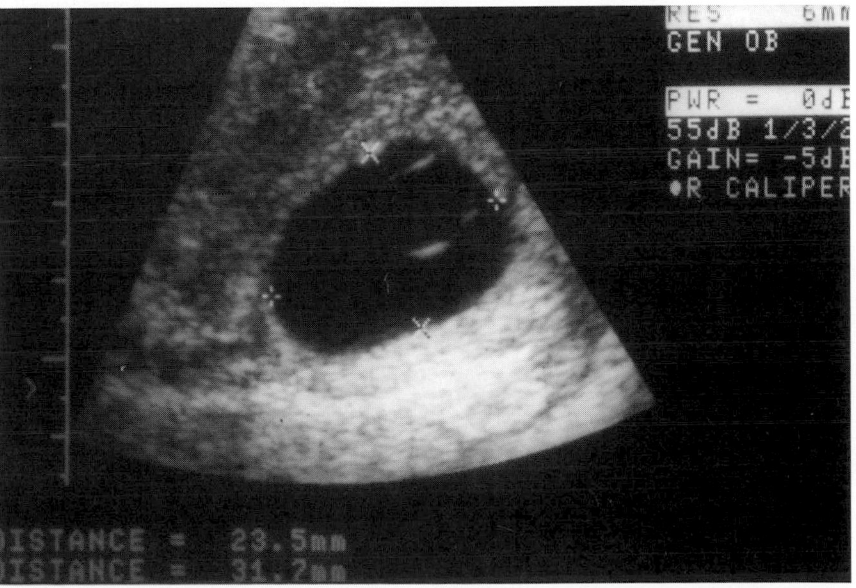

Figure 11.1 Anembryonic pregnancy loss with mean sac diameter of ≥16 mm without a demonstrable embryo.

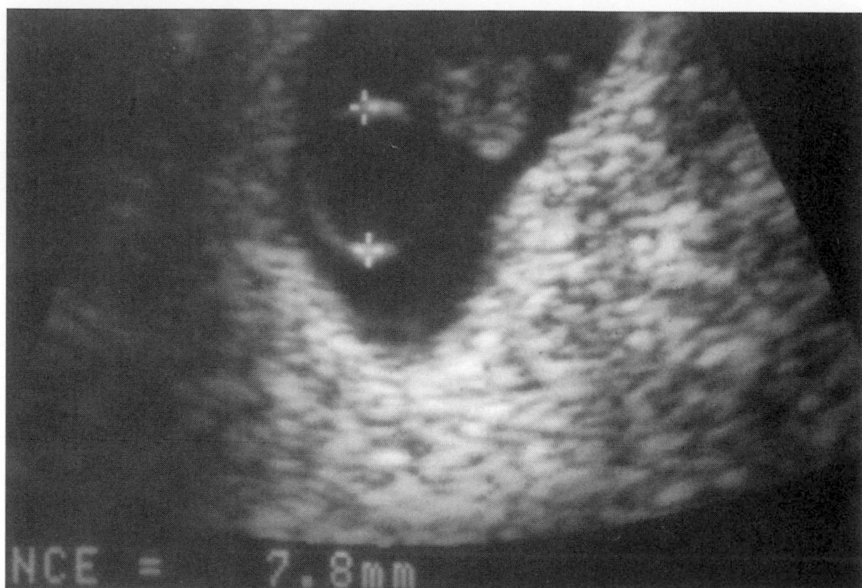

Figure 11.2 Embryonic demise with a large (≥6 mm) yolk sac.

imately 9.5 mm), the finding of a live embryo in the setting of vaginal bleeding is associated with a 10% miscarriage rate. At 9–11 weeks' gestation (CRL approximately 23 mm), the finding of a live embryo or fetus is associated with a 3–4% miscarriage rate. Finally, the cardiac rate provides some predictive value as to the likelihood of miscarriage.[47] At any gestational age, an embryonic heart rate of less than 80 beats per min carries a very poor prognosis. With CRLs of less than 5 mm, cardiac rates of 80–90 beats per min are associated with pregnancy loss in two-thirds of cases, and rates of 90–100 beats per min are associated with losses in one-third of cases. In embryos with a CRL of 5–9 mm, heart rates of less than 100 beats per min are ominous.

Recurrent pregnancy loss

Up to 1% of couples experience three consecutive pregnancy losses, a figure at least two or three times higher than expected based on the observed pregnancy loss rate per pregnancy in the general population. RPL is a particularly difficult clinical problem because no definite etiology is discovered in a substantial proportion of cases. In the face of this emotional and frustrating situation, both physicians and patients may feel the need to perform evaluations for uncertain or unproven "causes" and to try experimental treatments. Table 11.5 presents causes of RPL.

Table 11.5 Proposed causes of recurrent pregnancy loss.

Genetic abnormalities
Parental structural chromosome abnormalities
Numerical chromosome abnormalities of the conceptus
Molecular genetic abnormalities of the conceptus or placenta
Hormonal and metabolic disorders
Luteal phase defects
Diabetes
Thyroid disease
Uterine anatomical abnormalities
Congenital uterine malformations
Uterine synechiae
Uterine fibroids
Autoimmune causes
Antiphospholipid syndrome
Infections
Thrombophilia
Factor V resistance to activated protein C (factor V Leiden)
Prothrombin gene G20210A mutation
Deficiencies of antithrombin III, protein C, or protein S

Causes of recurrent pregnancy loss

Genetic abnormalities

Parental structural chromosome abnormalities

In approximately 3–5% of couples with two or more spontaneous losses, one of the partners has a genetically balanced structural chromosome rearrangement.[48,49] Balanced translocations account for the largest proportion of these karyotypic abnormalities and occur as either reciprocal or robertsonian translocations. In reciprocal translocations, segments are exchanged between two nonhomologous chromosomes. In robertsonian translocations, two acrocentric chromosomes (chromosomes 13 to 15 and 21 to 22) fuse at the centromeric region and lose their short arms. Although the carrier of a balanced translocation is usually phenotypically normal, balanced translocations may cause pregnancy loss because segregation during meiosis results in gametes with duplication or deficiency of chromosome segments. A chromosome inversion occurs when a segment of the chromosome is reinserted in the reverse order after the chromosome breaks. Inversions may result in pregnancy loss because crossovers between abnormally paired chromatids during meiosis I result in duplications or deficiencies of genetic material.

Phenotypically normal offspring do not exclude the possibility of a balanced chromosome abnormality in a couple with RPL. The recurrence risk for spontaneous abortion in a couple with a parental structural chromosome abnormality is related to many variables, the most important of which is the specific type of abnormality. Some couples may wish to consider a preimplantation genetic diagnosis and all should be offered genetic counseling. Couples with one partner who has a balanced translocation or inversion should be offered prenatal genetic diagnosis because of the increased risk of a karyotypic abnormality.

Numerical chromosome abnormalities of the conceptus

Karyotypes in consecutive abortions suggest that recurrent aneuploidy in the conceptus may be a cause of RPL. In one set of data, the karyotype of the second successive spontaneous abortion was abnormal in nearly 70% of cases in which aneuploidy was found in the first abortus, but in only 20% of cases in which the first abortus was chromosomally normal.[50] However, this observation may have been due to the age of the mothers rather than to a nonrandom event in predisposed couples.[51]

Molecular genetic abnormalities of the conceptus

Since the 1980s, the importance of single gene mutations as a cause of numerous human diseases has been brought to light by the development of techniques for DNA analysis. The question of whether mutations may cause RPL is now pertinent, and the potential mechanisms for such a defect to result in pregnancy loss are innumerable. For example, a mutation in genes critical for trophoblast growth and development, or blood vessel formation, could preclude successful implantation or development. There are many examples of embryonic-lethal mutations in mice but, as yet, none has been found in the human.

Hormonal and metabolic disorders

Luteal phase defect

Removal of progesterone production in early pregnancy (via resection of the corpus luteum) results in spontaneous abortion, and progesterone replacement after removal of the corpus luteum allows the pregnancy to continue. Antiprogestins, such as RU486, reliably cause pregnancy loss when administered before 7 weeks after the last menstrual period, confirming the necessity of progesterone (and adequate progesterone response) for the maintenance of early pregnancy. Thus, it is no surprise that investigators hypothesized a role for inadequate progesterone production or effect as a cause of pregnancy loss. Some investigators consider this condition, often referred to as luteal phase defect (LPD), to be a rather common cause of RPL, accounting for approximately 25–40% of cases.[17,52] Nonetheless, properly controlled trials to prove that LPD is a cause of RPL are lacking.

Many authorities believe that a timed, late-luteal phase, endometrial biopsy taken from the fundal portion of the uterus is the gold standard for diagnosing LPD. The timing of the endometrial biopsy is important; it should be obtained within 3 days of the expected menstrual period. Histological interpretation is compared with the luteal phase day as established by the onset of the next menses (assuming 14 days in a normal luteal phase). The endometrium is considered to be out of phase when the histological dating lags behind the menstrual dating by two or more days. Out-of-phase endometrial histology in a single biopsy is relatively common in normal women.[53] For this reason, it is prudent to require that two consecutive endometrial biopsies be out of phase before a diagnosis of LPD is made. Detractors of the endometrial biopsy as a method of diagnosis point out that as many as 50% of normal women have a single endometrial histology suggestive of LPD, and 25% have abnormal biopsy findings in sequential luteal phases.[53] Interobserver variation in dating endometrial biopsies further limits the usefulness of the assay. In one series, more than 20% of women would have received different therapy depending on the individual interpreting the results of their endometrial biopsies.[54] Morphometric analysis of the endometrial biopsy may offer an improvement over histological analysis in the diagnosis of LPD. Using a standardized examination with morphometry, Serle and coauthors[55] identified a delay in endometrial maturation of more than 2 days in 60% of women with RPL, compared with no delay in any of the control subjects.

It would seem that measuring circulating levels of progesterone or its metabolites would be a reasonable alternative to the endometrial biopsy in the diagnosis of LPD. However, the pulsatile nature of progesterone secretion in the second half of the menstrual cycle results in wide fluctuations in circulating levels and leaves the interpretation of a single progesterone level uncertain. Many investigators use serial (daily) progesterone determinations to diagnose or exclude LPD, and the method has gained wide acceptance among infertility specialists.[56] In one well-carried out study, progesterone levels on days 1–4 of the luteal phase were compared in women with unexplained infertility and in normal fertile control subjects, and a significantly different pattern of progesterone levels was found in the infertile group.[57] Similar studies have not been carried out in women with RPL. Given the relative inaccuracies of each method, it is difficult to say whether one is superior to the other.

Notwithstanding the uncertainty as to the relationship between LPD and RPL, various treatments have been used in patients with RPL and LPD. Because most patients with RPL ovulate, it is assumed that inadequate progesterone synthesis in the luteal phase is the cause. A few patients may actually have a progesterone-resistant endometrium. Although uncontrolled studies suggest that progesterone therapy is beneficial in achieving a successful pregnancy,[58] several controlled, randomized trials of limited numbers of patients have not confirmed this.[59] The usual treatment regimen is 25 mg of progesterone, twice a day, beginning on the third day after ovulation and administered by vaginal suppository. A reasonable alternative is 200–400 mg per day of oral micronized progesterone, taken in divided doses. Treatment is often empirical although efficacy is unproven.

Other endocrinological and metabolic disorders

Poorly controlled diabetes mellitus is a recognized cause of sporadic pregnancy loss as well as severe hypothyroidism or severe hyperthyroidism. Case reports suggest that homocystinuria and Wilson's disease are associated with pregnancy loss. However, none of these conditions is likely to present primarily because of RPL and, if they did, they would easily be detected by clinical evaluation. There is no convincing evidence that asymptomatic systemic endocrinological or metabolic disorders are a cause of RPL.[58,60,61]

Uterine anatomic abnormalities

In total, 10–15% of women with recurrent first-trimester abortions have congenital uterine abnormalities.[58,60,61] The rate of uterine abnormalities is higher in women with fetal deaths and deliveries of premature infants.[62] The most common malformations associated with pregnancy loss are variations of the double uterus (bicornuate, septate, didelphys). Severe uterine synechiae (Asherman syndrome) and uterine abnormalities associated with *in utero* exposure to diethylstilbestrol (DES) may also be associated with miscarriage. An association between submucosal leiomyomata and RPL is controversial. Although not proven, pregnancy loss in patients with uterine abnormalities may be due to space constraints or poorly vascularized uterine tissues, which results in inadequate placentation.

Accurate information concerning the risks of uterine abnormalities and pregnancy loss is lacking because reported series do not include a realistic denominator. Only patients presenting for pregnancy loss or infertility are reported. Many women with uterine abnormalities have acceptable reproductive outcomes and would not be included in case series. For example, the overall reproductive performance of women with bicornuate uterus is reasonably good.[63] Even in highly selected series, less than one-half of prior pregnancies in women with bicornuate uterus end in abortion or premature delivery.[64] Indeed, one prospective study of three-dimensional pelvic ultrasound in relatively unselected patients demonstrated much better outcomes in women with uterine abnormalities than had been reported in retrospective cohorts.[65] Thus, a cautious, circumspect approach is warranted in ascribing pregnancy loss to uterine abnormalities and other causes must be excluded.

Uterine anatomical abnormalities are diagnosed by a variety of imaging techniques. Excellent screening techniques include hysterosalpingogram or sonohysterogram. For the hysterosalpingogram, the uterus should be deflexed using cervical traction so that an *en face* radiograph of the uterus can be obtained. Initially, only a small amount of radiopaque dye should be injected so that subtle defects are not overlooked. Pelvic magnetic resonance imaging (MRI) or hysteroscopy may provide more definitive diagnoses.

The most common congenital abnormalities among women complaining of pregnancy loss or immature delivery are septate uterus and bicornuate uterus (Fig. 11.3), which together account for at least 50% of uterine abnormalities in women with RPL. Women with septate uterus are reported to have previous pregnancy loss rates that vary widely, from approximately 25% to more than 90%.[64,66,67] Previous pregnancy outcomes in women with septate uterus are generally worse than for women with bicornuate uterus.[68] The cause of pregnancy loss in women with septate uterus is uncertain, but diminished blood supply to the septum is often cited as a primary problem.

Surgical repair of uterine abnormalities has never been proven to improve outcome in women with RPL in properly designed studies. Nonetheless, dramatically improved outcomes have been reported in case series in women with RPL and septate uteruses undergoing hysteroscopic resection of the septum.[69,70] Given its low morbidity and cost, we believe hysteroscopic resection of uterine septa should be considered in women with a history of RPL, a single fetal death, or marked preterm delivery. In contrast, the metroplasty required to correct abnormalities such as bicornuate uterus and uterus didelphys is considerably more morbid and expensive. Also, the link between these conditions and RPL is less convincing than for uterine septum. Today, metroplasty is rarely performed as a treatment for RPL and should be reserved for unusual and refractory cases. Treatment of Asherman syndrome or submucosal fibroids is of theoretical benefit in some women with RPL but proof of efficacy is lacking.

Cervical insufficiency (cervical incompetence) is a generally accepted cause of second-trimester loss. Diagnosis is made on clinical grounds (painless dilation of the cervix with passage of the fetus) or via sonogram. The reader is referred to chapter 62 of this book for further discussion.

Infectious causes

It remains controversial as to whether an infectious agent may cause RPL. For an infectious agent to cause multiple pregnancy losses, it would have to establish a chronic infection or colonization that could infect, or at least affect, the gestational tissues in successive pregnancies. No infectious agent has been proven to cause recurrent early pregnancy loss, although case reports and circumstantial evidence raise the possibility. In the absence of additional data, evaluation for infectious causes of RPL is ill advised.

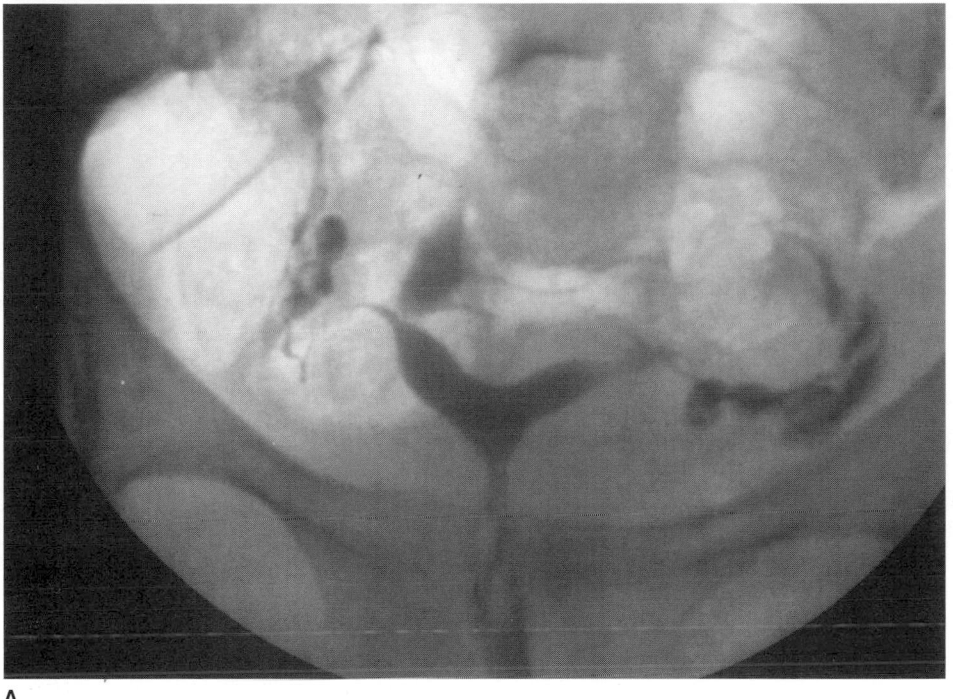

A

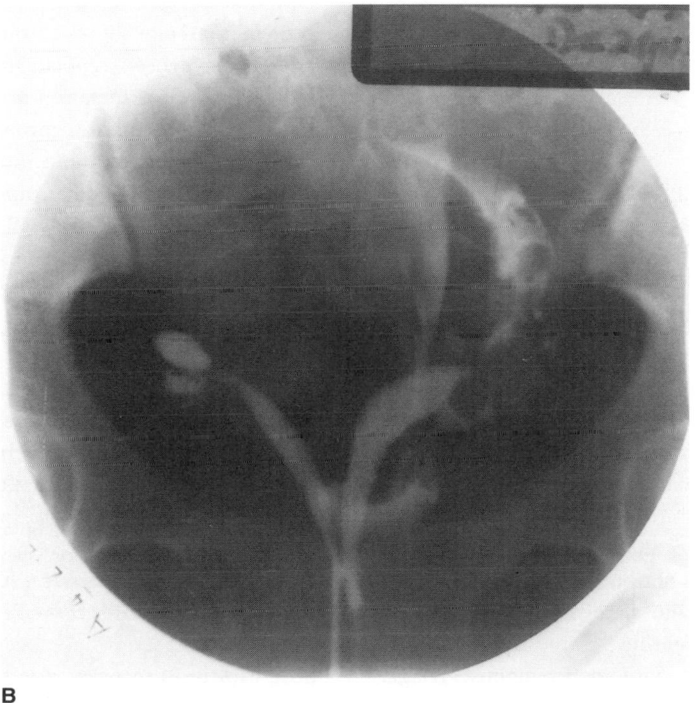

B

Figure 11.3 Septate uterus (A) and bicornuate uterus (B) in women with recurrent pregnancy loss.

Table 11.6 International consensus statement on preliminary criteria for the classification of antiphospholipid syndrome.*

Clinical criteria:

Pregnancy complications

Three or more unexplained early spontaneous abortions
Premature birth before 34 weeks' gestation (placental insufficiency)
Unexplained fetal death

Vascular thrombosis

Venous thrombosis
Arterial thrombosis
Small vessel thrombosis

Laboratory criteria

Lupus anticoagulant
Anticardiolipin antibodies (IgG or IgM)
Medium–high levels (antibodies must be present on two or more occasions at least 6 weeks apart)

From Wilson WA, Gharavi AE, Koike T, et al. International consensus statement on preliminary classification criteria for definite antiphospholipid syndrome: report of an international workshop. *Arthritis Rheum* 1999;42:1309.

*A diagnosis of definite antiphospholipid syndrome requires the presence of at least one of the clinical criteria and one of the laboratory criteria. No limits are placed on the interval between the clinical event and the positive laboratory findings.

Table 11.7 Indications for antiphospholipid antibody testing.

Recurrent spontaneous abortion*
Unexplained second- or third-trimester fetal death
Severe preeclampsia before 34 weeks' gestation
Unexplained venous thrombosis
Unexplained arterial thrombosis
Unexplained stroke
Unexplained transient ischemic attack or amaurosis fugax
Systemic lupus erythematosus or other connective tissue disease
Autoimmune thrombocytopenia
Autoimmune hemolytic anemia
Livedo reticularis
Chorea gravidarum
False-positive serological test for syphilis
Unexplained prolongation in clotting assay
Unexplained severe intrauterine growth retardation

*Three or more spontaneous abortions with no more than one live birth.

Autoimmune causes

Antiphospholipid syndrome (APS) is an autoimmune disorder characterized by the presence of significant levels of antiphospholipid antibodies and one or more clinical features, including pregnancy loss, thrombosis, or autoimmune thrombocytopenia (Table 11.6). This disorder may occur as a secondary condition in patients with underlying autoimmune disease (e.g., systemic lupus erythematosus) or as a primary condition in women with no other recognizable autoimmune disease. Second-trimester fetal death is the most specific type of pregnancy loss associated with APS, but some patients present with recurrent late first-trimester or early second-trimester fetal loss.[71,72] Overall, 5–20% of women with RPL have detectable antiphospholipid antibodies,[71–74] but these low levels of antibodies can be found in 5–10% of otherwise normal women. Thus, APS is identified as the cause of pregnancy loss in 5–10% of women with recurrent miscarriage. Women with a previous fetal death[75–77] and high levels of anticardiolipin IgG antibodies[77] are at greatest risk of fetal loss in subsequent pregnancies.

The two most well-characterized antiphospholipid antibodies are lupus anticoagulant and anticardiolipin. Lupus anticoagulant (a double misnomer and an unconventional name for an antibody) is reported as present or absent. Anticardiolipin antibody results are reported in semiquantitative terms (negative or low/medium/high positive). Low-positive results are of questionable significance:[78] patients with APS virtually always have medium- or high-positive results. Several other antiphospholipid antibodies (e.g., antiphosphatidylserine) and antibodies against β-2-glycoprotein-I (an anticoagulant protein that may be the epitope for antiphospholipid antibodies) have been reported to be associated with APS.[79,80] However, their association with pregnancy loss remains controversial.[81] Thus, we recommend testing for lupus anticoagulant and anticardiolipin antibodies when confirming the diagnosis of APS. Indications for antiphospholipid antibody testing are shown in Table 11.7.

Glucocorticoids, heparin, low-dose aspirin, and intravenous immunoglobulin (IVIG), or combinations of these medications, have been used to treat pregnant women in an attempt to improve pregnancy outcomes among women with APS and pregnancy loss. Direct comparison of these studies is virtually impossible due to differences in patient selection and treatments.[75] The two most widely used treatment regimens have been (1) a combination of prednisone and low-dose aspirin and (2) heparin, with or without low-dose aspirin. Successful pregnancy outcomes have been reported in approximately 55–85% of treated cases. Although none of these studies included appropriate control subjects and efficacy is uncertain, results of case series have been impressive. Heparin and low-dose aspirin is recommended as first-line therapy because it causes fewer side-effects than prednisone[82] and may reduce the risk of thrombosis in women with APS. Thromboprophylactic doses appear to be as effective as anticoagulant doses and have fewer side-effects; thus, they are recommended (e.g., 7500 units twice daily). Low-molecular-weight heparins may safely be used instead of unfractionated heparin. Treatment with IVIG has generated considerable enthusiasm because obstetric outcome has been excellent in a handful of treated pregnancies in women with APS who had previously "failed" treatment with heparin or prednisone.[83,84] However, in a small

Table 11.8 Thrombophilic disorders and risk of pregnancy loss.

Thrombophilic disorder	Prevalence in women with pregnancy loss (%)*	Prevalence in control subjects (%)	Risk of pregnancy loss (OR)
Factor V Leiden	8–32	1–10	2–5
Acquired APC resistance (without factor V Leiden)	9–38	0–3	3–4
Prothrombin gene mutation	4–13	1–3	2–9
Antithrombin deficiency	0–2	0–1.4	2–5
Protein C deficiency	6	0–2.5	2–3
Protein S deficiency	5–8	0–0.2	3–40
Hyperhomocysteinemia	17–27	5–16	3–7
Homozygous MTHFR C677T†	5–21	4–20	0.4–3‡
Combined thrombophilia	8–25	1–5	5–14

From ref. 100, with permission.
*Variably defined as first or recurrent early and/or late pregnancy loss.
†5,10-methylenetetrahydrofolate reductase (MTHFR).
‡No significant difference in prevalence or risk in the majority of studies.

randomized trial,[85] the use of IVIG and heparin was not better than heparin alone, and cannot be recommended as primary therapy in the absence of further study because of its extremely high cost.

Some women with antiphospholipid antibodies have had successful pregnancies without specific medical treatment, but there is no way to identify these patients prospectively. At present, women with APS and a history of second-trimester fetal death or thrombosis should be considered for heparin or heparin and low-dose aspirin treatment,[76] but the empirical nature of the treatment should be discussed with the patient. The treatment of women with recurrent first-trimester miscarriage and antiphospholipid antibodies, but no history of fetal death or thrombosis, is controversial. Results of well-designed clinical trials are mixed.[86–88]

Regardless of treatment, one-half of women with APS in one series developed preeclampsia, with more than one-fourth having severe preeclampsia.[76] Fetal distress requiring delivery developed in more than one-half of cases, and nearly one-third of liveborn infants were small for gestational age. More than one-third of surviving infants were born at, or after, 32 weeks' gestation. Finally, 5% of pregnancies were complicated by maternal thrombosis, including one case of stroke. These high-risk pregnancies demand close maternal and fetal surveillance.

Some investigators have proposed that a subclinical autoimmune condition or conditions might be associated with RPL, and several have found that some women with RPL have detectable antinuclear antibodies (ANAs). However, the proportion of recurrent unexplained miscarriage patients with positive ANAs is not statistically different from that of appropriate control subjects.[89,90] One group found that ANAs having a titer greater than or equal to 1:80 were more frequent in women with RPL than in normal nonpregnant or pregnant women.[91] Subsequent, untreated pregnancy outcomes were no different in this subset than in other women with recurrent miscarriage. Other autoantibodies have also been associated with miscarriage (including anti-SS-A, thyroid autoantibodies) and positive results in autoantibody "profiles." However, these studies were not convincing, or they require confirmation of their significance in women with recurrent miscarriage. Taken together, the data available at present do not support testing women with RPL for ANAs or autoantibodies other than antiphospholipid antibodies.

Thrombophilia

The histological findings of placental infarction, necrosis, and vascular thrombosis (Fig. 11.4) in some cases of pregnancy loss associated with antiphospholipid antibodies have led to the hypothesis that thrombosis in the uteroplacental circulation may lead to placental infarction and fetal death. In turn, these observations have raised the question as to whether other thrombophilic defects (Table 11.8) predispose to fetal loss. Several case series and retrospective studies reported an association between miscarriage,[92] second-trimester pregnancy loss,[93] and stillbirth and deficiencies of the anticoagulant proteins antithrombin III, protein C, and protein S (Fig. 11.5).[94] Placental infarction was noted in many of these cases. Recurrent pregnancy loss has also been linked to the hypercoagulable state, hyperhomocysteinemia,[95] and deficiencies in levels of activated factor XII (Hageman factor).[96]

Abnormal factor V resistance to the anticoagulant effects of activated protein C (APC resistance) has been recognized as the predominant cause of venous thrombosis and familial thrombophilia.[97] It is usually associated with the factor V Leiden mutation in the factor V gene, which is present in approximately 2–8% of the general population in the USA.[98] The second most common thrombophilia is the G20210A mutation in the prothrombin gene, occurring in 2–3% of the general population.[99] Numerous case series and retrospective cohort–control studies have linked both the factor V Leiden

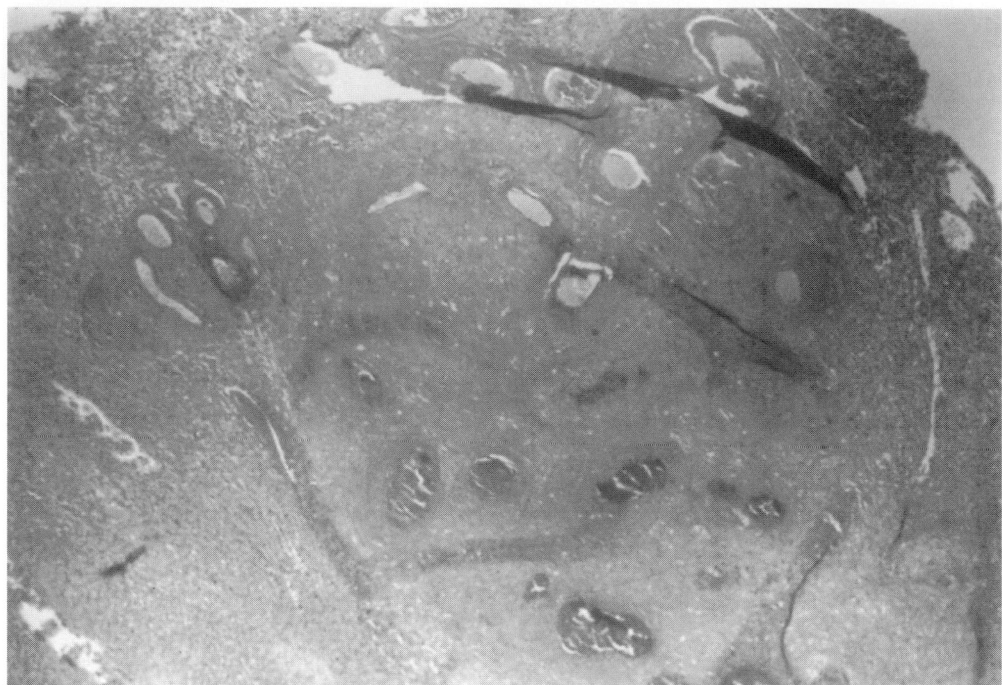

Figure 11.4 Placenta demonstrating extensive infarction and vascular thrombosis taken from a pregnancy resulting in second-trimester fetal death in a patient with antiphospholipid syndrome.

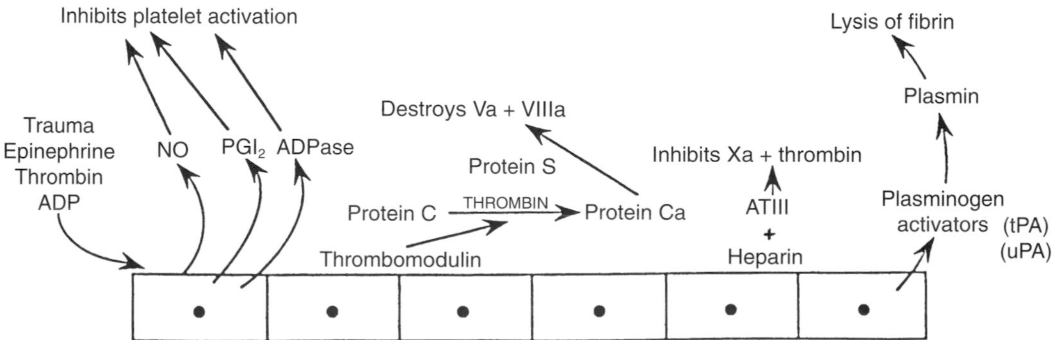

Figure 11.5 Overview of hemostasis. Antithrombin III (*ATIII*) inhibits thrombin and factor Xa, whereas protein C (with protein S as a cofactor) inactivates factor Va and VIIIa. These proteins all inhibit thrombus formation and contribute to the maintenance of vascular patency. ADP, adenosine diphosphate; ADPase, adenosine diphosphatase; NO, nitric oxide; PGI, prostacyclin. (From Colman RW, Marder VJ, Salzman EW, Hirsh J. Plasma coagulation factors. Chapter 1. In: Colman RW et al., eds. *Hemostasis and thrombosis: basic principles and clinical practice*, 3rd edn. Philadelphia: Lippincott, 1994, with permission.)

and G120210A prothrombin gene mutations to pregnancy loss.[100,101] In most studies, thrombophilias were more strongly associated with losses after 10 weeks' gestation as opposed to anembryonic or embryonic losses. A recent meta-analysis indicated an odds ratio of 2 for "early" and 7.8 for "late" RPL for women with the factor V Leiden mutation, and an odds ratio of 2.6 for "early" recurrent fetal loss in those with the prothrombin gene mutation.[101] Protein S deficiency, but not the methylenetetrahydrofolate mutation associated with hyperhomocysteinemia, protein C deficiency, or antithrombin III deficiency were associated with pregnancy loss in the meta-analysis.[101]

It is noteworthy that many heritable thrombophilias are common in normal individuals without a history of thrombosis or pregnancy loss.[100] Thus, although retrospective studies (and one prospective cohort)[102] link thrombophilias to pregnancy loss, most individuals with thrombophilias have uncomplicated pregnancies. Indeed, two large prospective cohort studies indicated no association between the factor V Leiden mutation and heritable thrombophilias, and either pregnancy loss or obstetric complications characterized by placental insufficiency.[103,104] It is clear that thrombophilia alone is insufficient to cause pregnancy loss and such individuals without prior obstetric complications should be reassured.

The association between thrombophilias and pregnancy loss raises the question as to whether thromboprophylaxis may improve outcome in subsequent pregnancies. Several uncontrolled studies report improved outcome in subsequent pregnancies in women with thrombophilias taking thromboprophylactic doses of low-molecular-weight heparin.[100] A recent prospective randomized controlled trial also supports the efficacy of low-molecular-weight heparin in women with thrombophilia and prior pregnancy loss.[105] Out of 80 women taking 40 mg per day of enoxaparin, 69 (86%) had live births compared with 23 out of 80 (29%) taking low-dose aspirin.[105] These data are compelling, but caution is advised regarding the evaluation and treatment of thrombophilias in the setting of RPL. The frequency of thrombophilias in healthy people, the excellent outcome in most women with thrombophilias, and the side-effects and cost of testing and thromboprophylaxis weigh against mass screening and treatment in the absence of additional data from properly designed studies.

Alloimmune causes

The term *alloimmune* refers to immunological differences between individuals of the same species. Allogeneic factors have been proposed as the cause of otherwise unexplained RPL, similar to allograft rejection in organ transplantation. However, there is no direct scientific evidence that alloimmune factors play a role in human pregnancy loss. This concept led to the use of immunological treatments for unexplained RPL, including leukocyte immunization (typically with paternal leukocytes) and IVIG. Although both treatments are still in use, randomized controlled trials failed to demonstrate efficacy.[106,107] These treatments are expensive, have significant adverse effects, and are not recommended at present.

Psychotherapy

Several authorities have proposed that psychotherapy or a program of emotional support and reassurance can improve pregnancy outcome in women with RPL.[108–110] Two studies reported successful pregnancies in approximately 85% of women undergoing "tender loving care" compared with only one-third of control subjects.[109,110] Unfortunately, none of these studies was randomized controlled trials. Nonetheless, couples are likely to benefit emotionally from additional psychological support, as well as medical and ultrasound examinations.

Unexplained recurrent early pregnancy loss

In as many as 55% of couples with RPL, an evaluation that includes parental karyotypes, hysterosalpingography or hysteroscopy, endometrial biopsy, and antiphospholipid antibody testing is negative (Fig. 11.6). Given that an alleged alloimmune cause for RPL is controversial, a substantial majority (approximately 50–75%) of couples with RPL have no diagnosis. Informative and sympathetic counseling appears to serve an important role in this frustrating situation. Livebirth rates ranging from 35% to 85% are commonly reported in couples with unexplained RPL who undertake an untreated subsequent pregnancy,[108,109,111,112] figures that many couples view as optimistic. Good pregnancy outcomes may be achieved using a sympathetic, "tender loving care" approach in early pregnancy.[108–110] Other couples may want to consider the experimental therapies outlined above.

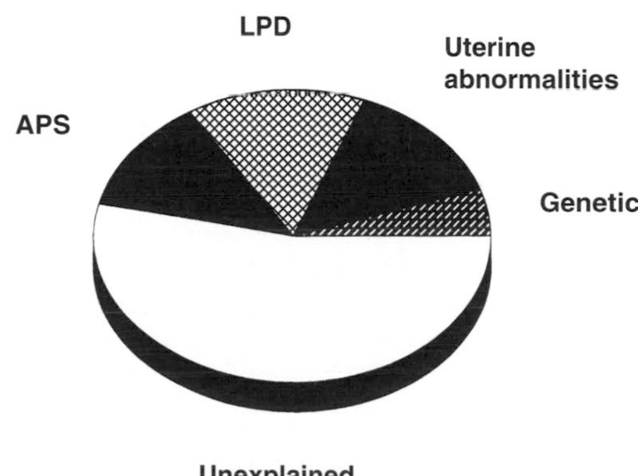

Figure 11.6 Causes of recurrent pregnancy loss in 310 women evaluated at the University of Utah. Luteal phase defect (*LPD*) caused 16% of losses, uterine abnormalities caused 15%, genetic abnormalities caused 5.5%, antiphospholipid syndrome (*APS*) caused 13%, and 57.5% were unexplained. Seven percent of women with "explained" recurrent pregnancy loss had more than one diagnosis.

Conclusions and recommendations

Recurrent pregnancy loss is often a frustrating clinical problem for patients and physicians. Of the known or suspected causes, only parental karyotype abnormalities, APS, uterine malformations, and cervical incompetence are widely accepted. Except for the use of heparin and low-dose aspirin for the treatment of APS, none of the treatments for RPL has been established as efficacious by properly designed studies. A suggested routine for the evaluation of recurrent early pregnancy loss is shown in Table 11.9.

Table 11.9 Suggested routine evaluation for recurrent early pregnancy loss.

History
Pattern and trimester of pregnancy losses and whether a live embryo or fetus was present
Exposure to environmental toxins or drugs
Known gynecologic or obstetric infections
Clinical features associated with antiphospholipid syndrome
Genetic relationship between reproductive partners (consanguinity)
Family history of recurrent miscarriage or syndrome associated with embryonic or fetal loss
Previous diagnostic tests and treatments

Physical
General physical examination
Examination of vagina, cervix, and uterus

Tests
Hysterosalpingogram or sonohysterogram
Luteal phase endometrial biopsy; repeat in the next cycle if abnormal
Parental karyotypes
Lupus anticoagulant and anticardiolipin antibodies
Factor V Leiden mutation
Prothrombin G20210A mutation
Other laboratory tests suggested by history and physical examination

Key points

1 Pregnancy loss is the most common obstetric complication, affecting up to 25% of women attempting pregnancy.

2 In total, 10–14% of clinically recognized pregnancies result in losses.

3 Losses before 20 weeks' gestation are referred to as abortions.

4 *In utero* death after 20 weeks' gestation is referred to as stillbirth.

5 Pre-embryonic losses occur before 6 weeks' gestation. There is an "empty sac" without a discernible embryo. This has previously been referred to as a "blighted ovum."

6 Embryonic losses occur between 6 and 10 weeks' gestation. An embryo without cardiac activity is noted on a sonogram.

7 Spontaneous pregnancy loss is biphasic in distribution. Most occur before 10 weeks' gestation. The second most common time for pregnancy loss is between 14 and 20 weeks' gestation.

8 Approximately 50% of sporadic spontaneous abortions have abnormal karyotypes.

9 The most common abnormal karyotypes in abortus specimens are autosomal trisomies.

10 The most common trisomy in abortus specimens is trisomy 16.

11 Abnormal karyotypes are more common in pregnancy losses occurring early in gestation.

12 Diabetes and thyroid disease may cause pregnancy loss but it is almost always in women with clinically apparent disease. Routine evaluation for diabetes and thyroid disease is not advised.

13 A variety of infections are rare causes of pregnancy loss. Routine evaluation for infection is not advised.

14 The risk of pregnancy loss is increased in women over 35 years of age and in those with two or more previous losses.

15 The causes of fetal death differ from those of spontaneous abortion.

16 Most cases of spontaneous abortion do not require evaluation.

17 Evaluation for possible etiologies should be offered to all women with fetal death.

18 Obstetric sonogram is the best way to diagnose pregnancy loss.
19 A total of 0.5–1.0% of couples suffer three or more losses, termed recurrent pregnancy loss (RPL).
20 Recommended evaluation for couples with RPL includes parental karyotype, assessment of uterine anatomy, exclusion of luteal phase defect, and testing for antiphospholipid syndrome.
21 Of couples with recurrent pregnancy loss, 3–5% will have one partner with a genetically balanced structural chromosome rearrangement.
22 Luteal phase defect (LPD) is diagnosed with endometrial biopsy or serum progesterone determination.
23 LPD is present in 25–40% of women with RPL. However, it is present in many women with normal obstetric outcomes, and it may vary from month to month in the same woman.
24 Typical treatment of LPD consists of progesterone supplementation in the luteal phase, for example 25 mg of progesterone administered by vaginal suppository twice daily, beginning on the third day after ovulation through either the onset of menses or 10 weeks' gestation. Treatment is of unproven efficacy.
25 In total, 10–15% of women with RPL have uterine abnormalities.
26 Most women with uterine abnormalities have normal obstetric outcomes.
27 Uterine septum is the abnormality most strongly associated with pregnancy loss. Hysteroscopic resection of uterine septa may improve outcome in women with RPL.
28 Antiphospholipid syndrome (APS) is an autoimmune disorder characterized by the presence of specified levels of antiphospholipid antibodies and one or more clinical features, including pregnancy loss, thrombosis, or autoimmune thrombocytopenia.
29 The two best-characterized antiphospholipid antibodies are lupus anticoagulant and anticardiolipin antibodies.
30 APS is identified as the cause of pregnancy loss in 5–10% of women with recurrent miscarriage.
31 Treatment with thromboprophylactic doses of heparin (7500 units twice daily) and low-dose aspirin improves obstetric outcome in women with APS.
32 Heritable thrombophilias have also been associated with recurrent pregnancy loss. The association is stronger for fetal death as opposed to early miscarriage.
33 It is noteworthy that many heritable thrombophilias are common in normal individuals without a history of thrombosis or pregnancy loss, and most women with thrombophilias have normal obstetric outcomes.
34 Although of unproven efficacy, improved outcome has been reported in subsequent pregnancies in women with thrombophilias taking thromboprophylactic doses of low-molecular-weight heparin.
35 Treatments such as leukocyte immunization and IVIG are not proven to be efficacious in the treatment of unexplained pregnancy loss.

References

1 Boklage CE. Survival probability of human conceptions from fertilization to term. *Int J Fertil* 1990;35:75–93.
2 Wilcox AI, Weinberg CR, O'Connor JF, et al. Incidence of early loss of pregnancy. *N Engl J Med* 1988;319:189–194.
3 Miller JF, Williamson E, Glue J, et al. Fetal loss after implantation: a prospective study. *Lancet* 1980;2:554–556.
4 Edmonds DK, Lindsay KS, Miller JF, et al. Early embryonic mortality in women. *Fertil Steril* 1982;38:447–453.
5 Whitaker PO, Taylor A, Lind T. Unsuspected pregnancy loss in healthy women. *Lancet* 1983;1:1126–1127.
6 Goldstein SR. Embryonic death in early pregnancy: a new look at the first trimester. *Obstet Gynecol* 1994;84:294–297.
7 Regan L. A prospective study of spontaneous abortion. In: Beard RW, Sharp F, eds. *Early pregnancy loss.* London: Springer-Verlag; 1988:23–37.
8 Warburton D, Fraser FC. Spontaneous abortion risks in man: data from reproductive histories collected in a medical genetics unit. *Am J Hum Genet* 1964;16:1–25.
9 Fitzsimmons J, Jackson D, Wapner R, Jackson L. Subsequent reproductive outcome in couples with repeated pregnancy loss. *Am J Med Genet* 1983;16:583–587.
10 Stirrat GM. Recurrent miscarriage. 1: definition and epidemiology. *Lancet* 1990;336:673–675.
11 Frias AE, Jr, Luikenaar RA, Sullivan AE, et al. Poor obstetric outcome in subsequent pregnancies in women with prior fetal death. *Obstet Gynecol* 2004;104:521–526.
12 Fantel AG, Shepard TH. Morphological analysis of spontaneous abortuses. In: Bennett MI, Edmunds DK, eds. *Spontaneous and recurrent abortion.* Oxford, UK: Blackwell Scientific Publications; 1987:8–28.
13 Mantoni M. Ultrasound signs in threatened abortion and their prognostic significance. *Obstet Gynecol* 1985;65:471–475.
14 Simpson JL, Gray RH, Queenan IT, et al. Low fetal loss rates after demonstration of a live fetus in the first trimester. *JAMA* 1987;258:2555–2557.
15 Kline J, Stein Z. Epidemiology of chromosomal anomalies in spontaneous abortion: prevalence, manifestation and determinants. In: Bennett MI, Edmonds DK, eds. *Spontaneous and recurrent abortion.* Oxford, UK: Blackwell Scientific Publications; 1987:29–50.
16 Geraedts JPM. Chromosomal anomalies and recurrent miscarriage. *Infertil Reprod Med Clin North Am* 1996;7:677–688.
17 Byrne J, Warburton D, Kline J, et al. Morphology of early fetal deaths and their chromosomal characteristics. *Teratology* 1985;32:297–315.

18 Eiben B, Bartels I, Bahr-Porsch S, et al. Cytogenetic analysis of 750 spontaneous abortions with the direct-preparation method of chorionic villi and its implications for studying genetic causes of pregnancy wastage. *Am J Hum Genet* 1990;47:656–663.
19 Lomax B, Tang S, Separovic E, et al. Comparative genomic hybridization in combination with flow cytometry improves results of cytogenetic analysis of spontaneous abortions. *Am J Hum Genet* 2000;66:1516–1521.
20 Christiaens GC, Vissers J, Poddighe PJ, de Pater JM. Comparative genomic hybridization for cytogenetic evaluation of stillbirth. *Obstet Gynecol* 2000;96:281–286.
21 Fritz B, Hallerman C, Olert J, et al. Cytogenetic analyses of culture failures by comparative genomic hybridization (CGH). Re-evaluation of chromosome aberration rates in early spontaneous abortions. *Eur J Hum Genet* 2001;9:539–547.
22 Mills JL, Simpson JL, Driscoll SO, et al. Incidence of spontaneous abortion among normal women and insulin-dependent diabetic women whose pregnancies were identified within 21 days of conception. *N Engl J Med* 1988;319:1617–1623.
23 Stagnaro-Green A, Roman SH, Cobin RH, et al. Detection of at-risk pregnancy by means of highly sensitive assays for thyroid autoantibodies. *JAMA* 1990;264:1422–1425.
24 Lejeune B, Grun JP, Nayer P, et al. Antithyroid antibodies underlying thyroid abnormalities and miscarriage or pregnancy-induced hypertension. *Br J Obstet Gynaecol* 1993;100:669–672.
25 Wendel GD. Gestational and congenital syphilis. *Clin Perinatol* 1988;15:287–303.
26 MacDonald AB. Gestational Lyme borreliosis: implications for the fetus. *Rheum Dis Clin North Am* 1989;15:657–677.
27 Vawter GF. Perinatal listeriosis. *Perspect Pediatr Pathol* 1981;6: 153–166.
28 Gronroos M, Honkonen E, Terho P, Punnonen R. Cervical and serum IgA and serum IgG antibodies to *Chlamydia trachomatis* and herpes simplex virus in threatening abortion: a prospective study. *Br J Obstet Gynaecol* 1983:90:167–170.
29 Munday PE, Porter R, Falder PF, et al. Spontaneous abortion – an infectious aetiology? *Br J Obstet Gynaecol* 1984;91:1177–1180.
30 Capsi E, Salomon F, Sompolinsky D. Early abortion and mycoplasma infection. *Isr J Med Sci* 1972;8:122–127.
31 Kundsin RB, Driscoll SG, Ming PL. Strain of mycoplasma associated with human reproductive failure. *Science* 1967;157: 1573–1574.
32 Goldenberg RL, Thompson C. The infectious origins of stillbirth. *Am J Obstet Gynecol* 2003;89:861–873.
33 Blackwell R, Chang A. Video display terminals and pregnancy: a review. *Br J Obstet Gynaecol* 1988;95:446–453.
34 Schnoor TM, Grajewski BA, Hornung RW, et al. Video display terminals and the risk of spontaneous abortion. *N Engl J Med* 1991;324:727–733.
35 Harlap S, Shiono PH, Ramcharan S. A life table of spontaneous abortions and the effects of age, parity, and other variables. In: Porter IH, Hook EB, eds. *Human embryonic and fetal death.* New York: Academic Press; 1980:145.
36 Stein Z, Kline J, Susser E, et al. Maternal age and spontaneous abortion. In: Porter IH, Hook EB, eds. *Human embryonic and fetal death.* New York: Academic Press; 1980:107.
37 Fretts RC, Usher RH. Causes of fetal death in women of advanced maternal age. *Obstet Gynecol* 1997;89:40–45.
38 Roman EA, Alberman E, Pharoah POD. Pregnancy order and reproductive loss. *Br Med J* 1980;280:715.
39 Naylor AF, Warburton D. Sequential analysis of spontaneous abortion. II. Collaborative study data show that gravidity determines a very substantial increase in risk. *Fertil Steril* 1979;31: 282–286.
40 Boue J, Boue A, Lazar P. Retrospective and prospective epidemiological studies of 1500 karyotyped spontaneous human abortions. *Teratology* 1975;12:11–26.
41 Lauritsen JG. Aetiology of spontaneous abortion. A cytogenetic and epidemiological study of 288 abortuses and their parents. *Acta Obstet Gynecol Scand* 1976;52:1–29.
42 Bromley B, Harlow BL, Laboda LA, Benacereff BR. Small sac size in the first trimester: a predictor of poor fetal outcome. *Radiology* 1991;178:375–377.
43 Levi CS, Lyons EA, Lindsay DJ. Early diagnosis of non-viable pregnancy with endovaginal ultrasound. *Radiology* 1988;167: 383–385.
44 Bree RL, Edwards M, Bohm-Velez M, et al. Transvaginal sonography in the evaluation of normal early pregnancy: correlation with hCG levels. *Am J Roentgenol* 1989;153:75–79.
45 Jain KA, Hamper UM, Sanders RC. Comparison of transvaginal and transabdominal sonography in detection of early pregnancy and its complications. *Am J Roentgenol* 1988;151:1139–1143.
46 Lindsay DJ, Lovett IS, Lyons EA, et al. Yolk sac diameter and shape at endovaginal US: predictors of pregnancy outcome in first trimester. *Radiology* 1992;183:115–118.
47 Doubilet PM, Benson CB. Embryonic heart rate in the early first trimester: what rate is normal? *J Ultrasound Med* 1995;14: 431–434.
48 DeBrackeller M, Dao TN. Cytogenetic studies in couples experiencing repeated pregnancy losses. *Hum Reprod* 1990;5: 519–528.
49 Clifford K, Rai RS, Watson H, Regan L. An informative protocol for the investigation of recurrent miscarriage: preliminary experience of 500 consecutive cases. *Hum Reprod* 1994;9: 1328–1332.
50 Hassold T. A cytogenetic study of repeated spontaneous abortions. *Am J Hum Genet* 1980;32:723–730.
51 Warburton D, Kline J, Stein Z, et al. Does the karyotype of a spontaneous abortion predict the karyotype of a subsequent abortion? Evidence from 273 women with two karyotyped spontaneous abortions. *Am J Hum Genet* 1987;41:465–483.
52 Daya S, Ward S, Burrows E. Progesterone profiles in luteal phase defect cycles and outcome of progesterone treatment in patients with recurrent spontaneous abortion. *Am J Obstet Gynecol* 1988;158:225–232.
53 Davis OK, Berkeley AS, Naus GJ, et al. The incidence of luteal phase defect in normal, fertile women determined by serial endometrial biopsies. *Fertil Steril* 1989;51:582–586.
54 Scott RT, Snyder RR, Strickland DM, et al. The effect of interobserver variation in dating endometrial histology on the diagnosis of luteal phase defects. *Fertil Steril* 1988;50:888–892.
55 Serle E, Aplin JD, Li TC, et al. Endometrial differentiation in the peri-implantation phase of women with recurrent miscarriage: a morphological and immunohistochemical study. *Fertil Steril* 1994;62:989–996.
56 Olive DL. The prevalence and epidemiology of luteal-phase deficiency in normal and infertile women. *Clin Obstet Gynecol* 1991;34:157–179.
57 Lenton EA, Adams M, Cooke ID. Plasma steroid and gonadotropin profiles in ovulatory but infertile women. *Clin Endocrinol* 1978;8:241–255.
58 Tho PT, Byrd JR, McDonough PG. Etiologies and subsequent reproductive performance of 100 couples with recurrent abortion. *Fertil Steril* 1979;32:389–395.

59 Goldstein P, Berrier J, Rosen S, et al. A meta-analysis of randomized control trials of progestational agents in pregnancy. *Br J Obstet Gynaecol* 1989;96:265–274.
60 Harger JH, Archer DF, Marchese SO, et al. Etiology of recurrent pregnancy loss and outcome of subsequent pregnancies. *Obstet Gynecol* 1983;62:574–581.
61 Stray-Pedersen B, Stray-Pedersen S. Etiologic factors and subsequent reproductive performance in 195 couples with a prior history of habitual abortion. *Am J Obstet Gynecol* 1984;148: 140–146.
62 Acien P. Uterine anomalies and recurrent miscarriage. *Infertil Reprod Med Clin North Am* 1996;7:689–719.
63 Rock JA, Jones HW. The clinical management of the double uterus. *Fertil Steril* 1977;28:798–806.
64 Heinonen PK, Saarikoski S, Pystyrien P. Reproductive performance of women with uterine anomalies. *Acta Obstet Gynaecol Scand* 1982;61:157–162.
65 Woelfer B, Salim R, Banerjee S, et al. Reproductive outcomes in women with congenital uterine anomalies detected by three-dimensional ultrasound screening. *Obstet Gynecol* 2000;98: 1099–1103.
66 Musich JR, Behrman SJ. Obstetric outcome before and after metroplasty in women with uterine anomalies. *Obstet Gynecol* 1978;52:63–66.
67 Gray SE, Roberts DK, Franklin RR. Fertility after metroplasty of the septate uterus. *J Reprod Med* 1984;29:185–188.
68 Buttram VC, Gibbons WE. Mullerian anomalies: a proposed classification (an analysis of 144 cases). *Fertil Steril* 1979;32: 40–46.
69 Daly DC, Witten CA, Soto-Albors CE, Riddick DH. Hysteroscopic metroplasty: surgical technique and obstetric outcome. *Fertil Steril* 1983;39:623–628.
70 March CM, Israel R. Hysteroscopic management of recurrent abortion caused by septate uterus. *Am J Obstet Gynecol* 1987;156:834–839.
71 Branch DW, Scott JR. Clinical implication of anti-phospholipid antibodies: the Utah experience. In: Harris EN, Exner T, Hughes GRV, Asherson RA, eds. *Phospholipid-binding antibodies*. Boca Raton, FL: CRC Press; 1991:335–346.
72 Out HJ, Bruinse HW, Christiaens GCML, et al. Prevalence of antiphospholipid antibodies in patients with fetal loss. *Ann Rheum Dis* 1991;50:553–557.
73 Parrazzini F, Acaia B, Faden D, et al. Antiphospholipid antibodies and recurrent abortion. *Obstet Gynecol* 1991;77:854–858.
74 Parke AL, Wilson D, Maier D. The prevalence of antiphospholipid antibodies in women with recurrent spontaneous abortion, women with successful pregnancies, and women who have never been pregnant. *Arthritis Rheum* 1991;34:1231–1235.
75 Branch DW. Immunologic aspects of pregnancy loss: alloimmune and autoimmune considerations. In: Reece EA, Hobbins JC, Mahoney MJ, Petrie RH, eds. *Medicine of the fetus and mother.* Philadelphia: JB Lippincott Company; 1992:217–233.
76 Branch DW, Silver RM, Blackwell JL, et al. Outcome of treated pregnancies in women with antiphospholipid syndrome: an update of the Utah experience. *Obstet Gynecol* 1992;80: 614–620.
77 Lockshin MD, Druzin ML, Qamar T. Prednisone does not prevent fetal death in women with antiphospholipid antibody. *Am J Obstet Gynecol* 1989;160:439–443.
78 Silver RM, Porter TF, van Leeuwen I, et al. Anticardiolipin antibodies: clinical consequences of "low titers." *Obstet Gynecol* 1996;87:494–500.
79 Cabiedes J, Cabral AR, Alarcon-Segovia D. Clinical manifestations of the antiphospholipid syndrome in patients with systemic lupus erythematosus associate more strongly with anti-beta2-glycoprotein-I than with antiphospholipid antibodies. *J Rheumatol* 1995;22:1899–1906.
80 Tsutsumi A, Matsuura E, Ichikawa K, et al. Antibodies to beta2-glycoprotein I and clinical manifestations in patients with systemic lupus erythematosus. *Arthritis Rheum* 1996;39:1466–1474.
81 Branch DW, Silver RM, Pierangelli SS, et al. Antiphospholipid antibodies other than lupus anticoagulant and anticardiolipin antibodies in women with recurrent pregnancy loss, fertile controls, and antiphospholipid syndrome. *Obstet Gynecol* 1997;89: 549–555.
82 Cowchock FS, Reece EA, Balaban D, et al. Repeated fetal losses associated with antiphospholipid antibodies: a collaborative randomized trial comparing prednisone to low-dose heparin treatment. *Am J Obstet Gynecol* 1992;166:1318–1327.
83 Scott JR, Branch DW, Kochenour NK, Ward K. Intravenous immunoglobulin treatment of pregnant patients with recurrent pregnancy loss caused by antiphospholipid antibodies and Rh immunization. *Am J Obstet Gynecol* 1988;159:1055–1056.
84 Spinnato JA, Clark AL, Pierangeli SS, et al. The antiphospholipid syndrome in pregnancy: immunoglobulin therapy. *Am J Obstet Gynecol* 1994;170:334.
85 Branch DW, Peaceman AM, Druzin M, et al. A multicenter, placebo-controlled pilot study of intravenous immune globulin treatment of antiphospholipid syndrome during pregnancy, The Pregnancy Loss Study Group. *Am J Obstet Gynecol* 2000;182: 122–127.
86 Kutteh WH. Antiphospholipid antibody associated recurrent pregnancy loss: treatment with heparin and low-dose aspirin is superior to low-dose aspirin alone. *Am J Obstet Gynecol* 1996;174:1584–1589.
87 Rai RS, Cohen H, Dave M, Regan L. Randomized controlled trial of aspirin and aspirin plus heparin in pregnant women with recurrent miscarriage associated with phospholipid antibodies (or antiphospholipid antibodies). *Br Med J* 1997;314:253–257.
88 Farquharson RG, Quenby S, Greaves M. Antiphospholipid syndrome in pregnancy: a randomized, controlled trial of treatment. *Obstet Gynecol* 2002;100:408–413.
89 Cowchock S, Smith JB, Gocial B. Antibodies to phospholipids and nuclear antigens in patients with repeated abortions. *Am J Obstet Gynecol* 1986;155:1002–1010.
90 Maier DB, Parke A. Subclinical autoimmunity in recurrent aborters. *Fertil Steril* 1989;51:280-285.
91 Harger JH, Rabin BS, Marchese SO. The prognostic value of antinuclear antibodies in women with recurrent pregnancy losses: a prospective controlled study. *Obstet Gynecol* 1989;73: 419–424.
92 Zanardi S, Sanson B, Gavasso S, et al. The incidence of venous thromboembolism during pregnancy and childbirth and the incidence of miscarriages in ATIII-, protein S-, and protein C-deficient women (Abstract). *Thromb Haemost* 1995;73:1263.
93 Bertault D, Mandelbrot L, Tchobroutsky C, et al. Unfavorable pregnancy outcome associated with congenital protein C deficiency: case reports. *Br J Obstet Gynaecol* 1991;98:934–936.
94 Tharakan T, Baxi LV, Diuguid D. Protein S deficiency in pregnancy: a case report. *Am J Obstet Gynecol* 1993;168:141–142.
95 Wouters MG, Boers GH, Blom HJ, et al. Hyperhomocysteinemia: a risk factor in women with unexplained recurrent early pregnancy loss. *Fertil Steril* 1993;60:820-825.

96 Schved JF, Gris IC, Neveu S, et al. Factor Xli congenital deficiency and early spontaneous abortion. *Fertil Steril* 1989;52: 335–336.
97 Svensson PI, Dahlback B. Resistance to activated protein C as a basis for venous thrombosis. *N Engl J Med* 1994;330:517–522.
98 Bertina RM, Koeleman BP, Koster T, et al. Mutation in blood coagulation factor V associated with resistance to activated protein C. *Nature* 1994;369:64–67.
99 Seligsohn U, Lubetsky A. Genetic susceptibility to venous thrombosis. *N Engl J Med* 2001;344:1222–1231.
100 Kujovich JL. Thrombophilia and pregnancy complications. *Am J Obstet Gynecol* 2004;191:412–424.
101 Rey E, Kahn SR, David M, et al. Thromphilic disorders and fetal loss: a meta-analysis. *Lancet* 2003;361:901–908.
102 Preston FE, Rosendaal FR, Walker ID, et al. Increased fetal loss in women with heritable thrombophilia. *Lancet* 1996;348: 913–916.
103 Lindqvist PG, Svensson PJ, Marsaal K, et al. Activated protein C resistance (FV:Q506) and pregnancy. *Thromb Haemost* 1999;81:532–537.
104 Dizon-Townson, D. The factor V leiden mutation does not increase risk of pregnancy-related venous thromboembolism. *Am J Obstet Gynecol SMFM Abstracts* 2003;187(Suppl.159):363.
105 Gris JC, Mercier E, Quere I, et al. Low-molecular-weight heparin versus low-dose aspirin in women with one fetal loss and a constitutional thrombophilic disorder. *Blood* 2004;103:3695–3699.
106 Ober C, Karrison T, Odem RR, et al. Mononuclear-cell immunization in prevention of recurrent miscarriages: a randomized trial. *Lancet* 1999;354:365–369.
107 Scott JR. Immunotherapy for recurrent miscarriage. *Cochrane Database Syst Rev* 2003;1. CD000112. DOI: 10.1002/14651858.
108 Tupper C, Weil RI. The problem of spontaneous abortion. *Am J Obstet Gynecol* 1962;83:421–429.
109 Stray-Pedersen B, Stray-Pedersen S. Recurrent abortion: the role of psychotherapy. In: Beard RW, Sharp P, eds. *Early pregnancy loss*. London: Springer-Verlag; 1988:433–440.
110 Liddell HS, Pattison NS, Zanderigo A. Recurrent miscarriage: outcome after supportive care in early pregnancy. *Aust NZ J Obstet Gynecol* 1991;31:320–322.
111 Mowbray SF, Gibbons C, Liddell H, et al. Controlled trial of treatment of recurrent spontaneous abortion by immunization with paternal cells. *Lancet* 1985;1:941–943.
112 Ho HN, Gill TH, Hsieh HI, et al. Immunotherapy for recurrent spontaneous abortions in a Chinese population. *Am J Reprod Immunol* 1991;25:10–15.

12 Ectopic and heterotopic pregnancies

Arnon Wiznitzer and Eyal Sheiner

Incidence

Ectopic pregnancy, i.e., implantation of a fertilized ovum outside the uterus (Fig. 12.1), is a major health problem for women of reproductive age and is the leading cause of pregnancy-related death during the first 20 weeks of pregnancy.[1] Accurate diagnosis and treatment of ectopic pregnancy decreases the risk of death and optimizes subsequent fertility. A significant increase in the number of cases of ectopic pregnancy has occurred in the USA during the past two decades.[2] In 1970, the rate was 4.5 per 1000 reported pregnancies, whereas in 1992, it was approximately 20 per 1000 pregnancies.[2] Importantly, ectopic pregnancy accounted for around 9% of all pregnancy-related deaths. The incidence of ectopic pregnancy is higher for nonwhite women and this discrepancy increases with age. Available data do not include pregnancies managed in outpatient settings and therefore its true incidence is most likely underestimated.

Etiology

The most common denominator is tubal obstruction and injury. Previous pelvic inflammatory disease, especially when caused by *Chlamydia trachomatis*, is a major risk factor for ectopic pregnancy.[3] The adjusted odds ratio (OR) for previous pelvic infectious disease was recently found to be 3.4 (95% confidence interval, CI: 2.4–5.0).[4] Other factors associated with an increased risk of ectopic pregnancy include prior ectopic pregnancy (which increases the risk for subsequent ectopic pregnancy 10-fold), a history of infertility (and specifically *in vitro* fertilization), cigarette smoking (causing alterations in tubal motility and ciliary activity), prior tubal surgery, diethylstilbestrol exposure (which alters fallopian tube morphology), and advanced maternal age.

Controversy exists regarding the association between ectopic pregnancy and medical abortions. Whereas Bouyer and coauthors[4] found previous, medically induced abortions to be associated with an increased risk of ectopic pregnancy (adjusted OR = 2.8, 95% CI: 1.1–7.2), no such association was observed by Shannon and coauthors[5] who searched MEDLINE for articles on medical abortion regimens.

Intrauterine contraceptive devices (IUDs), progesterone-only contraceptives, and sterilization protect women against developing an ectopic pregnancy.[6–8] Nevertheless, if a woman who has been sterilized or who is a current user of an IUD or progesterone-only contraceptive becomes pregnant, her risk for an ectopic pregnancy is increased six- to 10-fold, as these methods of contraception provide greater protection against intrauterine pregnancy than against ectopic pregnancy.[6–8] The first 2 years after sterilization carry the greatest risk of pregnancy in general and ectopic pregnancy in particular.[9] Sterilization reversal also increases the risk of ectopic pregnancy owing to possible obstruction and abnormal tube anatomy.

The risk of ectopic pregnancy is increased among women who are undergoing assisted reproductive technology and, specifically, *in vitro* fertilization (IVF). The risk is particularly high for women with underlying tubal disease. Hormonal alterations during ovulation induction can cause alterations in tubal function and peristalsis.[10] Other possible explanations include placement of the embryo in embryo transfer high in the uterine cavity (deep fundal transfer), and fluid reflux into the tubes.[11]

Other less common causes of ectopic pregnancy include salpingitis isthmica nodosa (anatomic thickening of the fallopian tube with epithelium leading to multiple lumen diverticula), and possibly vaginal douching and multiple sexual partners (both leading to a higher risk of pelvic infections).[12,13]

Signs and symptoms

Clinical manifestations of ectopic pregnancy are varied and depend on whether rupture has occurred. The classic symptom triad of ectopic pregnancy includes amenorrhea, irregular bleeding, and lower abdominal pain. However, it is present in

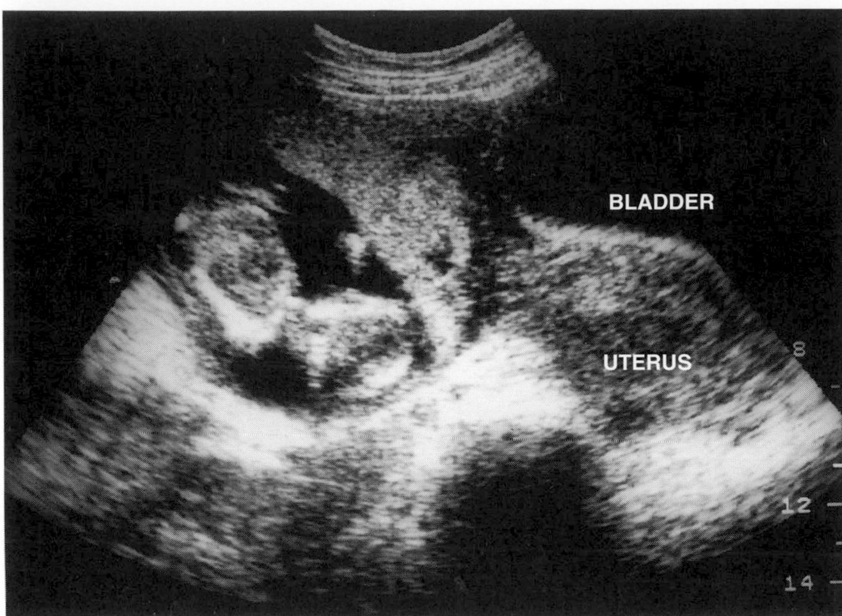

Figure 12.1 Ultrasound image of a well-defined ectopic pregnancy (cornual pregnancy of 15 weeks' gestation).

only one-half of patients and most commonly when rupture has occurred.[14] The most common complaint is sudden severe abdominal pain, which is present in more than 90% of patients.

Any physical examination should include measurements of vital signs. Abdominal and pelvic tenderness, especially cervical motion tenderness, is common when rupture has occurred (and present in approximately 75% of patients). However, pelvic examination before rupture is usually nonspecific, and a palpable pelvic mass on bimanual examination is established in less than one-half of cases.[14] The accuracy of the initial clinical evaluation before rupture is less than 50%, and additional tests are required in order to differentiate ectopic pregnancy from early intrauterine pregnancy (Fig. 12.2).

Laboratory assessment

β-Human chorionic gonadotropin measurements

The first stage in the evaluation of women with a suspected ectopic pregnancy is to determine if the patient is pregnant. The β-human chorionic gonadotropin (β-hCG) enzyme immunoassay, with a sensitivity of 25 mIU/mL, is an accurate screening test and is positive in virtually all cases of ectopic pregnancy.[15]

The levels of β-hCG increase during gestation and reach a peak of approximately 100 000 mIU/mL at 6–10 weeks; they then decrease and remain stable at approximately 20 000 mIU/mL.[16] Many studies have evaluated the increase of β-hCG in normal and abnormal pregnancies. The level of β-hCG in normal pregnancies doubles every 2 days (48 h), and thus, at present, clinicians rely on a normal "doubling time" to characterize a viable gestation. A 66% rise in the β-hCG level over 48 h represents the lower limit of normal values for a viable intrauterine pregnancy.[15] Indeed, there is a consensus that the predictable rise in serial β-hCG values in a viable pregnancy is different from the slow rise or plateau of an ectopic pregnancy.[15–20] However, Barnhart and coauthors[16] recently showed a slower rise in serial β-hCG values for women with viable intrauterine pregnancies. The slowest rise for a normal viable intrauterine pregnancy was 24% at 1 day and 53% at 2 days. Approximately 15% of normal pregnancies are associated with a less than 66% increase in β-hCG, and 17% of ectopic pregnancies have normal doubling times.[15] Thus, limitations of serial β-hCG testing include its inability to distinguish a failing intrauterine pregnancy from an ectopic pregnancy and the inherent 48-h delay. As there is no definitive laboratory level of β-hCG permitting distinction between an ectopic pregnancy and an intrauterine pregnancy, a more conservative approach toward interventions in abnormal pregnancies is mandatory.[16]

Serial β-hCG levels are usually required when the initial ultrasound performed fails to demonstrate either intra- or extrauterine pregnancy. At β-hCG levels of approximately 2000 mIU/mL, a viable intrauterine pregnancy should be seen by vaginal ultrasound.[21] If the β-hCG values fail to decline by 15% after uterine curettage for suspected nonviable intrauterine pregnancy, the possibility of ectopic pregnancy should be kept in mind and treatment may be indicated.[22]

Serum progesterone

Measurement of serum progesterone levels has been shown to be useful in evaluating the chances of early pregnancy failure.[23–25] Serum progesterone levels increase during pregnancy.[26] A baseline serum progesterone level of <20 nmol/L

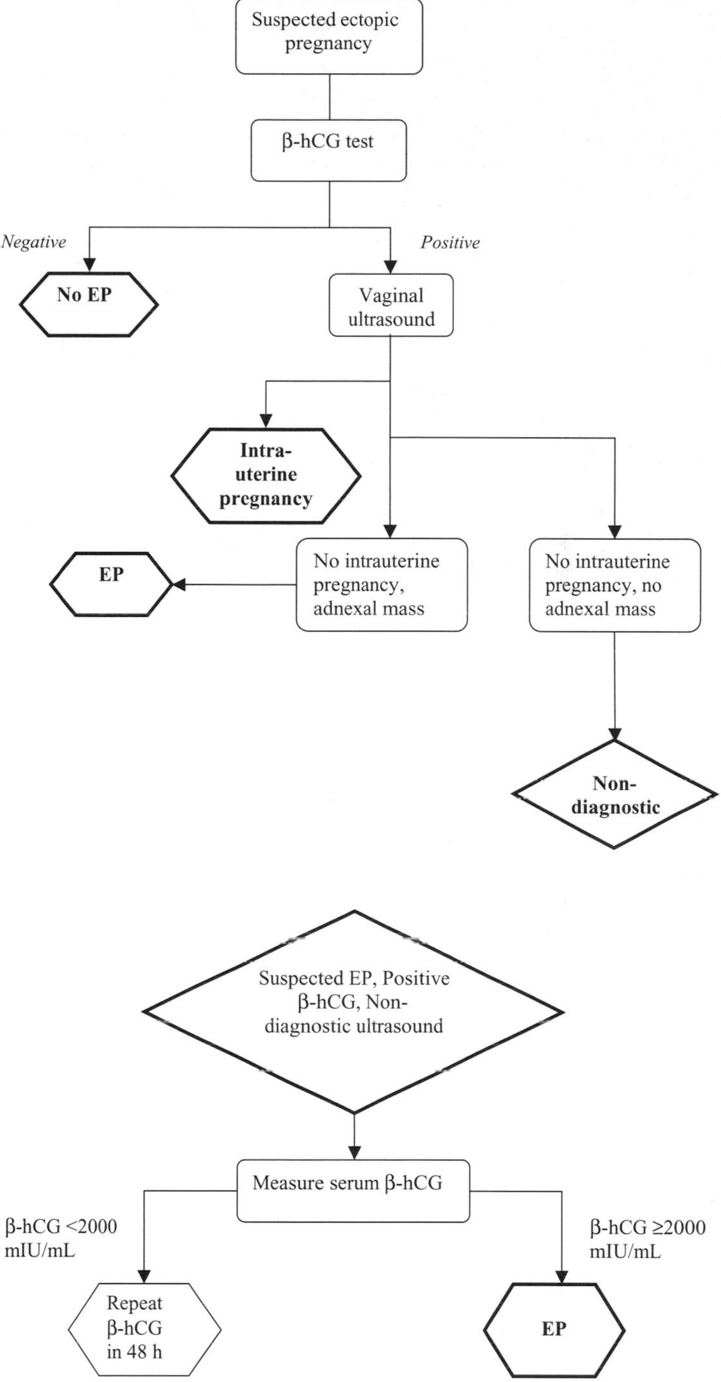

Figure 12.2 Diagnostic management of ectopic pregnancy.

can be used to identify abnormal pregnancy (either intra- or extrauterine) with a positive predictive value (PPV) of ≥95%.[24] Of pregnant patients with serum progesterone values of < 5 nmol/L, 85% have spontaneous abortions, 0.16% have viable intrauterine pregnancies, and 14% have ectopic pregnancies.[27] Most ectopic pregnancies are associated with serum progesterone levels that are lower than 20 nmol/L.[28] On the contrary, the chances of an ectopic pregnancy in patients with serum progesterone levels of 20 nmol/L and above are less than 5%.

However, serum progesterone levels cannot distinguish ectopic pregnancy from spontaneous abortion.[25] Thus, progesterone levels at defined times can be used to predict the immediate viability of a pregnancy, but cannot be used reliably to predict its location.[23]

Ultrasonography

The best diagnosis of ectopic pregnancy is based on the positive visualization of an extrauterine pregnancy (Fig. 12.1) but it is not seen in all cases. Approximately 90% of ectopic pregnancy may be visualized using transvaginal sonography within 5 weeks of the last menstrual period.[29–31]

A viable intrauterine pregnancy should be seen by transvaginal ultrasound[21,32] at β-hCG levels of between 1000 and 2000 mIU/mL or at 5.5 weeks' gestation, as the sensitivity of ultrasound to detect a normally developing intrauterine pregnancy approaches almost 100%.[21,32–34] When the β-hCG level exceeds the transvaginal discriminatory zone (1000–2000 mIU/mL of β-hCG), the absence of an intrauterine gestational sac is suggestive of ectopic pregnancy, but the differential diagnosis includes failed intrauterine pregnancy. The reported sensitivity of transvaginal ultrasonography for identifying ectopic pregnancy ranges from 20.1% to 84% with a specificity of 98.9–100%.[35] The combination of positive β-hCG and transvaginal ultrasound has a PPV of 95% for an ectopic pregnancy.[36]

If an intrauterine pregnancy is detected, this is taken to exclude a diagnosis of ectopic pregnancy because coexistent intra- and extrauterine pregnancies (heterotopic) following spontaneous cycles are rare, with an estimated incidence of 1 in 30 000 normal pregnancies.[1] However, the incidence of heterotopic pregnancy is increased by the use of assisted reproductive technology, with an incidence of up to 1 in 100 normal pregnancies.[37]

The early sonographic appearance of a normal gestational sac is characterized by the double decidual sac sign, i.e., two concentric echogenic rings separated by a hypoechogenic space. The double sac is believed to be the decidua capsularis and decidua parietalis. The double decidual sign is useful to the physician for early diagnosis of intrauterine pregnancy and for the exclusion of ectopic pregnancy. Chiang and coauthors[38] found recently that the sensitivity of the diagnosis of intrauterine pregnancy based on the decidual sign increased when β-hCG levels were equal to or greater than 2000 mIU/mL or the mean sac diameter was equal to or greater than 3 mm. However, the appearance of an intrauterine sac can be seen in some cases of ectopic pregnancy owing to intrauterine fluid or blood collection, i.e., a pseudosac. A pseudosac is a uterine sac without a double decidual ring or a yolk sac. Indeed, the report of a pseudosac is significantly associated with a false-positive diagnosis of ectopic pregnancy.[39] Ahmed and coauthors[39] concluded that a diagnosis of pseudosac should not be interpreted as indicative of an ectopic pregnancy as radiological differentiation between an early intrauterine pregnancy failure and an ectopic pregnancy is not possible. Color flow Doppler may aid in the differentiation between a pseudosac and a normal intrauterine sac; however, it requires advanced technical skills.[40–42]

Dilation and curettage

When serial β-hCG levels do not rise or fall appropriately, an abnormal gestation exists. When the pregnancy has been confirmed to be nonviable and when ultrasound is not sufficient, a uterine dilation and curettage can be performed to distinguish between an ectopic pregnancy and a miscarriage.[22,43–45] Once tissue is obtained by curettage, it can be added to saline in order to investigate if it floats. Because floating of the material is not 100% accurate, histological verification (frozen section is possible) or serial β-hCG measurements are needed. Visualization of villi in the tissue obtained indicates the occurrence of spontaneous intrauterine abortion. The absence of chorionic villi in the curettage specimen indicates the possibility of an ectopic pregnancy. However, a decrease in β-hCG levels of 15% or more, 12 h after the curettage, indicates a complete abortion. A plateau or a rise in the β-hCG levels is diagnostic for ectopic pregnancy. Once the possibility of an abortion is excluded, medical or surgical treatment for ectopic pregnancy is pursued.[22,43–46]

Culdocentesis

Culdocentesis was used as a diagnostic technique for ectopic pregnancy before the widespread availability of the vaginal ultrasound and β-hCG assay. Culdocentesis is positive in around 80% of women with ectopic pregnancy who have hemoperitoneum. In the remaining 20% of cases, the results are nondiagnostic. A nondiagnostic finding cannot be used to exclude ectopic pregnancy, and the test alters management only when it is positive. Thus, it is rarely indicated and is performed only in places where facilities for pregnancy testing and ultrasound are limited.[47]

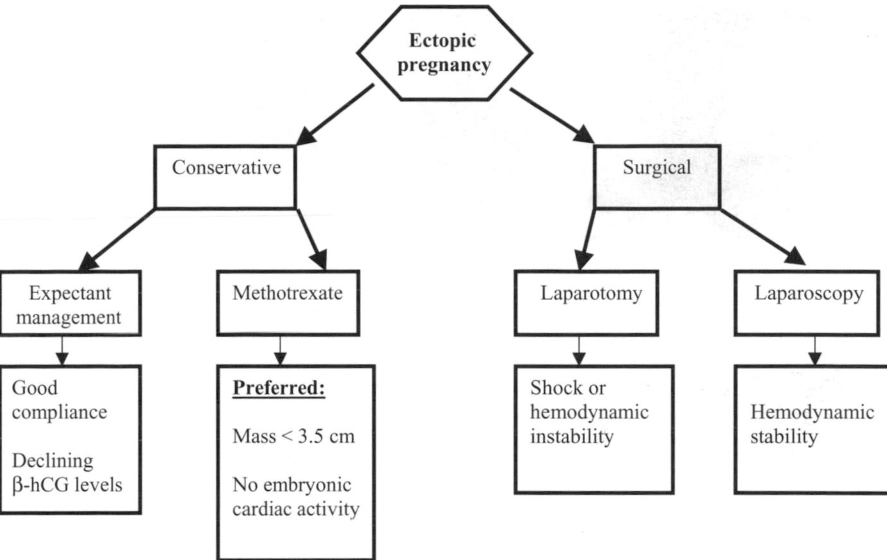

Figure 12.3 Treatment of ectopic pregnancy.

Treatment of ectopic pregnancy

The minority of patients with ectopic pregnancy (less than 10%) present with a surgical abdomen and signs of hypovolemia and shock.[48] They present no diagnostic problem and require no specific intervention besides fluid and blood resuscitation, and immediate operation. Delayed hospital admission and treatment leads to maternal mortality. Indeed, in developing countries, maternal mortality was almost 1% during the year 2000,[49] approximately 100 times higher than that reported in industrialized countries.[50,51] Cases of ectopic pregnancy can be treated by medical (methotrexate), surgical (laparoscopy or laparotomy), or even expectant management alone (Fig 12.3). The choice depends on the medical condition, available resources, and the site of ectopic pregnancy involved.

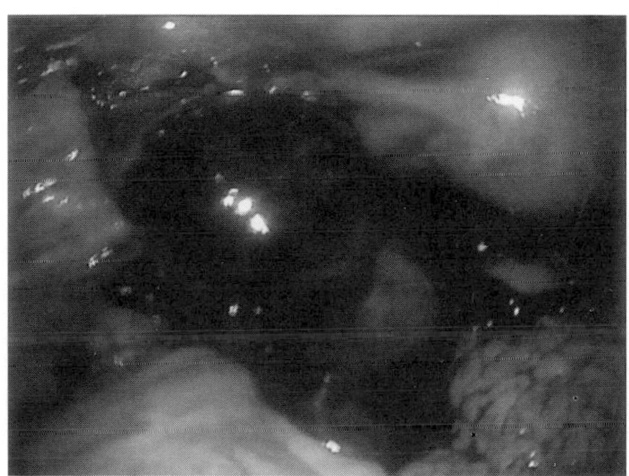

Figure 12.4 Laparoscopy picture of tubal ectopic pregnancy.

Surgical treatment

Laparoscopy versus laparotomy

The standard operative procedure for the treatment of ectopic pregnancy in the developed world is laparoscopy (Fig. 12.4). Almost all tubal pregnancies in hemodynamically stable women can be removed laparoscopically, without the need for laparotomy. The excellent benefits of laparoscopic treatment include less blood loss, less analgesia, less postoperative pain, shorter recovery period, and decreased hospital costs.[52–55]

The laparoscopic treatment of ectopic pregnancy and mainly tubal pregnancies has proven to be safe, but not entirely complication free.[56–60] In a recent meta-analysis, the average laparoscopy resolution rate was above 90%, with an average rate of 2% for intraoperative complications and 9% for postoperative complications.[61]

Because of lower peri- and postoperative morbidity, lower cost, and equivalent efficacy, laparoscopy is preferred to laparotomy for the treatment of ectopic pregnancy. The only absolute contraindication for laparoscopy is shock or hemodynamic instability.[48,52,55]

Salpingectomy, salpingotomy, salpingostomy, and milking

The most commonly performed procedures (by either laparoscopy or laparotomy) are radical salpingectomy (removal of the affected tube – Fig. 12.5), or salpingotomy (tubotomy that is closed) and salpingostomy (tubotomy that is left open) that preserve the tube. Salpingectomy is preferred in cases of ruptured ectopic pregnancy with uncontrolled bleeding, extensive tubal damage, recurrent ectopic pregnancy in the same tube, and sterilization.[62] Higher rates of intrauterine pregnancy have been reported following conservative surgery than with radical surgery.[63] Thus, salpingectomy for

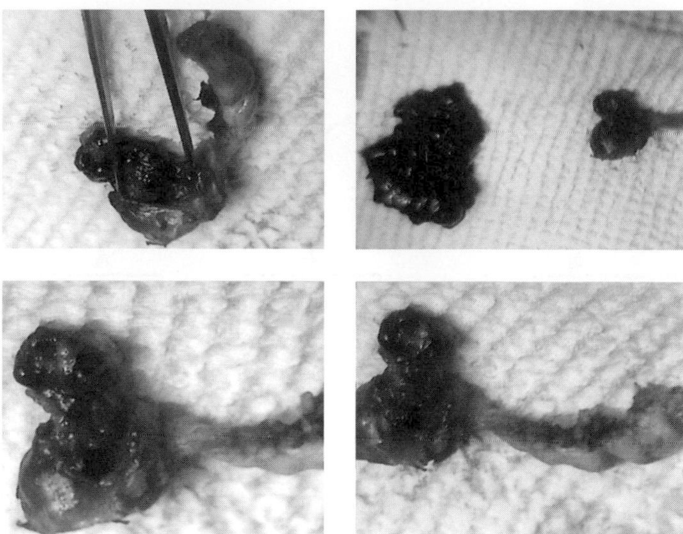

Figure 12.5 Radical salpingectomy (removal of the affected tube) for ruptured ectopic pregnancy.

an unruptured ectopic pregnancy is rarely performed and linear salpingostomy is the procedure of choice. Moreover, linear salpingostomy was found to be as effective as segmental resection with reanastomosis, and is technically easier with a shorter operative time. The ectopic pregnancy is removed through a linear incision of 10–15 mm made into the tube on its antimesenteric border. The products will extrude from the incision and can be flushed out and evacuated. Both livebirth rates and recurrent ectopic pregnancy rates after a tubotomy were similar, regardless of whether the incision was closed (salpingotomy) or left open to heal by secondary intension (salpingostomy).[55,64] Because no differences in prognosis with or without suturing were found, laparoscopic salpingostomy is the preferred surgical procedure for an unruptured ectopic pregnancy.[55]

Manual expression or milking of the tube in order to effect a tubal abortion is possible only in cases of fimbrial pregnancy. The present consensus among tubal surgeons is that milking should be abandoned as it is associated with an inordinately high recurrent rate of ectopic pregnancies, regardless of whether the procedure is performed by laparoscopy or laparotomy.[65]

Medical treatment with methotrexate

Methotrexate is a folinic acid antagonist that inactivates dihydrofolate reductase resulting in the depletion of tetrahydrofolate, a cofactor essential for deoxyribonucleic acid and ribonucleic acid synthesis. It thus interferes with DNA synthesis, repair, and cellular replication.[66] Actively proliferating tissue, such as trophoblast cells of an ectopic pregnancy, is generally more sensitive to these effects of methotrexate.[66] In a meta-analysis study,[61] methotrexate was proven to be a cost-saving treatment for ectopic pregnancy, which is nonsurgical and spares the fallopian tube. Moreover, receiving methotrexate treatment does not subject patients to surgical intervention and the possible associated complications. Thus, at present, methotrexate is considered to be the treatment of choice for ectopic pregnancy.[1]

Table 12.1 Relative and absolute contraindications for methotrexate treatment.

Absolute contraindications	Relative contraindications
Shock, hemodynamic instability	Embryonic cardiac activity
Known sensitivity to methotrexate	Gestational sac of 3.5 cm or more
Breastfeeding	
Immunodeficiency	
Alcoholism	
Hepatic, pulmonary, renal, or hematological dysfunction	
Blood dyscrasias	
Peptic ulcer disease	

Candidates for medical therapy

Hemodynamically stable patients without active bleeding or signs of hemoperitoneum are candidates for medical therapy[1,67] and they should comply with follow-up care. Contraindications for methotrexate treatments are summarized in Table 12.1. Absolute contraindications to medical therapy include breastfeeding, immunodeficiency, alcoholism, hepatic/pulmonary/renal/hematological dysfunction, known sensitivity to methotrexate, blood dyscrasias, or peptic ulcer disease.[1] Relative contraindications for methotrexate treatments include embryonic cardiac activity and a gestational sac of 3.5 cm or more.[1]

Because of its potential toxicity, patients receiving methotrexate should be followed up carefully. Patients using this drug should be aware of the potential side-effects and signs of toxicity. During treatment, patients should be counseled to promptly report any signs and symptoms associated with tubal rupture such as abdominal pain, dizziness, weakness, and syncope. Sexual intercourse, alcohol use, and nonsteroidal anti-inflammatory drugs, as well as folic acid supplements and prenatal vitamins, are prohibited until serum β-hCG is undetectable.[1]

It is clear that the main factor in successful medical treatment is rigorous patient selection. Several parameters aimed at the suitable choice of patients have already been assessed, such as the presence of fetal cardiac activity, size of the ectopic pregnancy, initial levels of β-hCG, and endometrial thickness.[68–70] Interestingly, a history of previous ectopic pregnancy was found to be another independent risk factor for methotrexate failure.[71,72]

Treatment protocols

Presently, there are two commonly used protocols for the administration of methotrexate in the treatment of an ectopic pregnancy. Most commonly, methotrexate can be administered using a single-dose method, based on 50 mg/m^2 of body surface area, without the need for leucovorin rescue. Otherwise, methotrexate can be given using a multidose regimen of 1 mg/kg intramuscularly, alternating with 0.1 mg/kg of leucovorin intramuscularly, for up to four daily doses of each drug.[67,73] Both protocols have been demonstrated to have good success rates in the treatment of ectopic pregnancy.[73–80] The single-dose protocol is easier to administer and monitor, and results in fewer side-effects.[81] However, a recent systematic meta-analysis of the published literature comparing the two regimens found that the single protocol was associated with a higher failure rate. The crude OR was 1.7 (95% CI: 1.04–2.82), and the OR adjusted for β-hCG values and for the presence of embryonic cardiac activity was 4.7 (95% CI: 1.77–12.62).[81]

Direct injection of methotrexate has lower efficacy than systemic administration, and is not considered as a therapeutic alternative for ectopic pregnancy.[82]

Monitoring efficacy of therapy

The overall success rate of methotrexate treatments is almost 90%.[61,73,81] Before treatment with methotrexate, blood analysis is required to establish baseline laboratory values for β-hCG and for renal, liver, and bone marrow function. Blood type should be determined because all patients with ectopic pregnancy who are Rh negative require 50 μg of Rh(D) immunoglobulin.

During treatment, outpatient observation is preferred for its cost-effectiveness and for patients' convenience. However, if there is any question of safety, hospitalization is mandatory. Patient monitoring continues until β-hCG levels are nondetectable. It usually takes a month or longer until β-hCG levels disappear from plasma.[73,83–87] With the single-dose treatment, levels of β-hCG generally increase during the first week after treatment and peak 4 days following injection.[1] Levels should decline 1 week after injection.[73] If a response is observed and the fall in β-hCG levels is greater than 15%, weekly serum β-hCG determinations should be measured until undetectable β-hCG levels are documented. Failure of the β-hCG level to decline requires a second dose of methotrexate.[73,83,88] An additional dose of methotrexate may also be given if β-hCG levels plateau or increase in 1 week.[73,85,86] Ultrasound examination may be repeated to evaluate significant changes in clinical status, such as increased pelvic pain, bleeding, or inadequate decline of β-hCG levels.[73,84–87] Persistent ectopic mass or hemoperitoneum may lead to surgery.

Side-effects

Methotrexate has the potential for serious toxicity and, indeed, high doses can cause bone marrow suppression, hepatotoxicity, stomatitis, pulmonary fibrosis, alopecia, and photosensitivity.[89,90] Toxic effects are usually related to the amount and duration of therapy. Nevertheless, most side-effects during regular treatment for ectopic pregnancy are minor and self-limited, and generally limited to an increase in hepatic transaminases, mild stomatitis, and gastrointestinal disturbances.[81,83–87] This is probably due to the lower dosage and shortened duration of treatment compared with dosages used in treating malignancies. Undoubtedly, the use of the single-dose protocol is associated with fewer side-effects than the multidose regimen.[81]

One of the known problematic side-effects of methotrexate treatment is acute abdominal pain which can be difficult to distinguish from the intra-abdominal hemorrhage of a tubal rupture.[81,84,85] Thus, patients should be counseled regarding this possible side-effect and the continuing risk of tubal rupture during treatment. In such cases, hospitalization is frequently needed for careful surveillance. Interestingly, the presence of side-effects was recently found to be associated with higher rates of resolution of the ectopic pregnancy without surgical intervention.[81]

Reproductive outcome after methotrexate treatment

Recently, Gervaise and coauthors[91] found that within 1 year of seeking to become pregnant, 57.5% of women previously treated with methotrexate for ectopic pregnancy conceived and had ongoing pregnancies. The cumulative intrauterine pregnancy rate was 66.9% after 2 years. The cumulative ectopic pregnancy rate was 15.4% after 1 year and 23.7% after 2 years.[91] Higher conception rates of 79.6%, with a mean time to conception of 3.2 months, were also documented,[10] with 12.8% of the conceptions being recurrent ectopic pregnancies. Similarly, when investigating reproductive outcome following laparoscopic treatment, the intrauterine pregnancy rate was 54% with a recurrent ectopic pregnancy rate of 13%.[92] It seems that fertility depends more on the patients' previous medical history (i.e., a history of infertility) than on her treatment for ectopic pregnancy.[91]

Expectant management

For years, gynecologists have stressed the need for early diagnosis and treatment of ectopic pregnancy in order to reduce morbidity and mortality. However, some patients experience spontaneous resolution of their ectopic pregnancy and in such patients, an expectant management is optional in order to avoid unnecessary treatment. After clear demonstrations that select cases of ectopic pregnancy resolve without therapy, several studies of patients with ectopic pregnancy have been conducted with consistent, reassuring results.[93–95] Candidates for successful expectant management must be asymptomatic with a clear indication of resolution (generally manifested by declining levels of β-hCG). In addition, they should be willing to accept the potential risks of tubal rupture and hemorrhage.[1] Certainly, fetal cardiac activity, adnexal mass of greater than 4cm, and β-hCG levels greater than 2000mIU/mL are considered to be contraindications for expectant management. Patients with early, small tubal gestations with lower (β-hCG < 200mIU/mL) and falling β-hCG levels are the best candidates for expectant management.[1]

A serum β-hCG of less than 1000mIU/mL, accompanied by a small adnexal mass (<4cm), predicts spontaneous resolution in 75% of cases, whereas falling levels of β-hCG predict resolution in around 90% of ectopic pregnancies.[93,94] However, failure of β-hCG levels to decline and suspected tubal rupture due to abdominal pain warrant immediate intervention and abandonment of the expectant management.

Recently, Elson and coauthors[96] have conducted a prospective observational study in which clinically stable women with nonviable pregnancies and no signs of hematoperitoneum were managed expectantly, on an outpatient basis, until their serum β-hCG declined to <20mIU/mL. Women who developed pelvic pain and those with nondeclining serum β-hCG levels were offered surgery. A total of 107 out of 179 (59.8%) tubal ectopic pregnancies were considered to be suitable for expectant management. Ectopic pregnancy resolved spontaneously in 75 out of 107 (70%) women. Initial serum β-hCG level was the best predictor for the successful outcome of expectant management.[96]

Persistent ectopic pregnancy

Incomplete removal of trophoblastic tissue after conservative surgery leads to persistent ectopic pregnancy. Several studies have reported a higher incidence of persistent ectopic pregnancy after laparoscopic surgery than after laparotomy.[97–101] The reported frequency of persistant ectopic pregnancy following conservative laparoscopic surgery varied between 5% and 15% of cases.[102–105]

Management includes methotrexate treatment or sometimes further surgery. Hoppe and coauthors[102] successfully treated all patients with persistent ectopic pregnancy with a single-dose systemic administration of methotrexate. In an attempt to define patients at increased risk of having persistent ectopic pregnancy, β-hCG levels as well as the size of the ectopic pregnancy have been suggested as possible markers. Interestingly, women with a small ectopic pregnancy size (of 8 mm or less), detected by preoperative ultrasound, were at an increased risk for residual tissue.[106,107]

Heterotopic pregnancy

Incidence

Coexistent intrauterine and extrauterine pregnancies are referred to as a heterotopic pregnancy.[108] The occurrence of a heterotopic pregnancy following spontaneous cycles is rare, with an estimated incidence of 1 in 30000 normal pregnancies.[1] It was calculated by multiplying the rate of ectopic pregnancy (0.37%) by that of dizygous twinning (0.8%), thus producing a hypothetical approximation. However, the incidence is increased to around 1% by the use of assisted reproductive technology.[37] It is particularly high among women who are undergoing ovulation induction with gonadotropins, and among women undergoing *in vitro* fertilization, as it has become standard practice to transfer at least two embryos.[109]

Clinical features

Heterotopic pregnancy poses a diagnostic dilemma. Serial β-hCG levels are not helpful because of the intrauterine pregnancy. Routine ultrasound detects only one-half of cases; in cases of viable intrauterine pregnancy, it is more likely that the intrauterine pregnancy will be detected in the course of workup and the ectopic pregnancy dismissed. In cases of nonviable intrauterine pregnancy, the presence of chorionic villi in the curettage specimen serves consistently to delay the correct diagnosis. Indeed, 50% of patients suffer from late diagnosis and arrive at hospital after rupture.[110] There are no specific features to guide the physician to make an accurate, early diagnosis of heterotopic pregnancy other than a general awareness of such a possibility. This is particularly important in cases of abdominal pain and tenderness accompanying normal intrauterine pregnancy, or following uterine curettage for a nonviable intrauterine pregnancy among patients who conceived following assisted reproductive technology. Also, in cases of persistent or rising β-hCG levels following uterine curettage for a nonviable intrauterine pregnancy, the possibility of heterotopic pregnancy should be considered.

Reece and associates[108] performed a review on combined intrauterine and extrauterine pregnancies, which included 589 cases. Approximately 94% were tubal and the rest were ovarian pregnancies. However, combined intrauterine and cervical pregnancies from *in vitro* fertilization and embryo

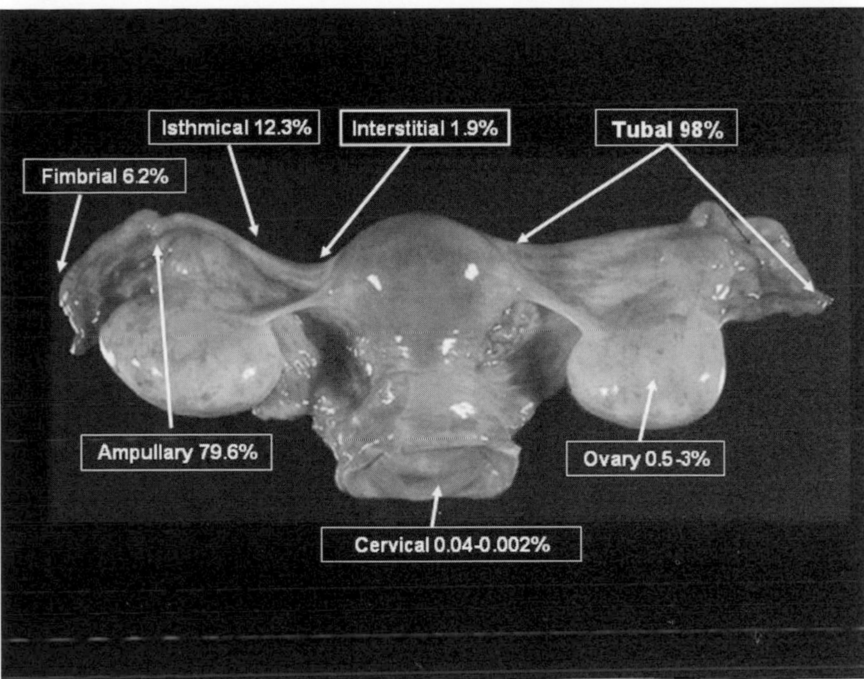

Figure 12.6 Sites of ectopic pregnancy.

transfer were also reported.[111,112] Abdominal pain was found to be the most frequent presenting symptom occurring in more than 80% of patients.[108] A combination of symptoms including abdominal pain, adnexal mass, peritoneal irritation, and an enlarged uterus was the most significant finding in support of a diagnosis of heterotopic pregnancy.

Treatment of heterotopic pregnancy

Treatment consists of removal of the ectopic pregnancy by surgery, and avoidance of intrauterine instrumentation and systemic methotrexate treatment in cases when the pregnancy is desirable (especially following assisted reproductive technology). In hemodynamically unstable patients, an explorative laparotomy is necessary. Expectant management is problematic as β-hCG levels cannot be monitored effectively owing to the intrauterine pregnancy. The prognosis for the intrauterine pregnancy is excellent, and the majority are carried to term.[113]

Treatment is complex in cases of heterotopic cervical pregnancy accompanied by a desirable intrauterine pregnancy. In such cases, hysteroscopic resection of the cervical gestation sac has been tried and the intrauterine pregnancy continued uneventfully until term.[114] The use of cervical Shirodker cerclage as an elective procedure for the management of a heterotopic cervical pregnancy with intrauterine pregnancy has also been described.[115] It resulted in a normal, uneventful term vaginal delivery. Local injection of KCl has been considered as an alternative to methotrexate to avoid exposure of the coexisting intrauterine pregnancy to chemotherapeutic agents. In most reported cases, the intrauterine pregnancy was preserved leading to delivery of liveborn infants.[116–118]

Nontubal ectopic pregnancy

The most common site of ectopic pregnancy implantation is the fallopian tubes, accounting for around 98% of all ectopic pregnancies. The majority of ectopic pregnancies are in the ampullary part of the fallopian tube (79.6%), with 12.3% in the isthmus, 6.2% in the fimbria, and 1.9% in the interstitial part. However, in rare cases implantation can occur in other ectopic sites, including the ovary, uterine cervix, and abdomen (Fig. 12.6).

Interstitial (cornual) pregnancy

The interstitial part of the fallopian tube is the proximal portion that lies within the muscular wall of the uterus. Interstitial implantation of the blastocyst is the rarest form (1.9%) of tubal ectopic pregnancy.[119] Late diagnosis and treatment are the main contributing factors to the poor outcome traditionally linked to these ectopic pregnancies.[120,121] The mortality rate of interstitial pregnancy is about twice that of other ectopic pregnancies.

There are some unique signs in a sonogram that characterize an interstitial ectopic pregnancy. They include the following: an empty uterine cavity with an eccentrically located or a lateral gestational sac, the presence of myometrium between the sac and the uterine cavity, the gestational sac covered with

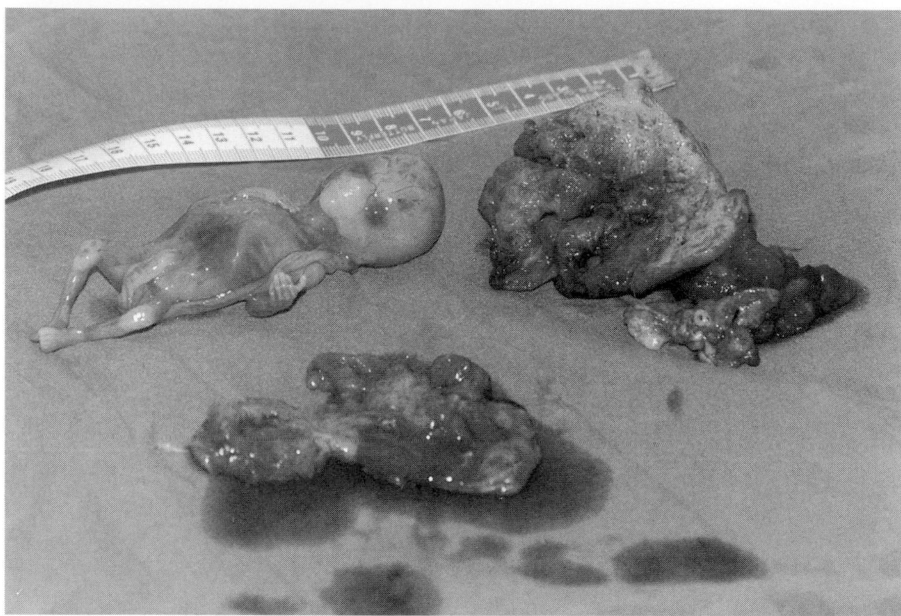

Figure 12.7 Cornual pregnancy of 15 weeks' gestation, after corneal resection.

thin myometrial fold, and no visible sac above the level of the internal os.[122] Recently, Tulandi and Al-Jaroudi[123] summarized 32 cases of interstitial pregnancies reported to the registry of the Society of Reproductive Surgeons and found ultrasound diagnosis of interstitial pregnancy to be accurate in 71.4% of cases, thus allowing conservative treatment.

Important risk factors for interstitial pregnancy include previous ectopic pregnancy (40.6%), ipsilateral salpingectomy (37.5%), *in vitro* fertilization (34.4%), sexually transmitted disease (25.0%), and ovulation induction (3.1%).[123]

The traditional treatment of interstitial pregnancy was hysterectomy or cornual resection by laparotomy.[120] These patients tend to present later in gestation than other tubal pregnancies mainly because the myometrium (cornual part) is more distensible than the fallopian tube (Figs 12.1 and 12.7). However, the progress in diagnostic techniques has led towards conservative management with methotrexate, laparoscopic treatment including cornual resection, cornuostomy, salpingostomy or salpingectomy, and even hysteroscopic removal.[123–127] However, if uncontrolled hemorrhage occurs, hysterectomy might be the preferred treatment.[120]

Abdominal ectopic pregnancy

Abdominal pregnancy occurs in approximately 1 in 8000 normal births and represents 1.4% of ectopic pregnancies.[110] The prognosis is generally poor, with an estimated maternal mortality of 5.1 per 1000 cases (7.7 times higher than other ectopic pregnancies).[128]

Abdominal pregnancies are classified as primary (primary peritoneal implantation) or secondary reimplantation. The latter are more common, resulting from tubal abortion or rupture. Distinction between the two is problematic but treatment is given according to the clinical presentation. Diagnosis is best made by ultrasound.

The incidence of abdominal pregnancy is increased following *in vitro* fertilization, induced abortions, recurrent pelvic infections, previous ectopic pregnancy, and endometriosis.[129,130] There are several reports on abdominal pregnancies reaching near term and their viability. In such cases the survival of the newborns is above 60%, although these pregnancies are associated with a high rate of congenital anomalies (20–40%).[131] Such anomalies, attributed to oligohydramnios, include bone and joint deformities, and central nervous system and skull anomalies,.

Laparotomy was considered to be the treatment of choice with removal of the pregnancy, with or without (if impossible) the placenta.[132,133] The placenta can be detached if its vascular supply can be recognized and ligated. If the vascular supply cannot be identified, the cord is ligated and the placenta is left. In cases where the placenta was left in place, complications such as sepsis, abscess formation, hemorrhage, and intestinal obstruction were noted.[131] However, although removal of the placenta may reduce morbidity, it is associated with a high risk of hemorrhage and subsequent visceral damage.[132] Thus, alternative regimens, including the use of methotrexate or selective embolization of the vessels feeding the placenta prior to definitive surgery, have been successfully tried.[134–137] Laparoscopic management of an early primary abdominal pregnancy has also been reported.[138]

Ovarian pregnancy

Ovarian pregnancy is an infrequent variant of ectopic pregnancy with an incidence of 0.5–3% of all ectopic pregnancies.[139–143] It is likely, however, that the frequency is underestimated as some of the suspected tubal pregnancies that were treated conservatively with methotrexate were in fact early ovarian pregnancies. Also, several cases were only retrospectively confirmed by the pathologist as they had been mistakenly considered as ruptured corpus luteum. Recent improvements in ultrasonography and operative laparoscopy should lead to an earlier and a more accurate diagnosis of these pregnancies.[139]

Risk factors for ovarian pregnancies include multiparity and the use of an IUD.[139,142–144] Interestingly, in two large series, 68–90% of the women with ovarian pregnancies had used this form of contraceptive device.[139,143]

Clinical findings are similar to those encountered in tubal pregnancy. The major presenting symptom (present in almost all patients) is abdominal pain.[139] Other findings include vaginal bleeding and amenorrhea.[142,143] Owing to the increased vascularity of the ovarian tissue, hemodynamic instability and rupture occurs in around 30% of patients.[143]

Historically, oophorectomy was considered as the treatment of choice for ovarian pregnancies. However, improvements in operative laparoscopic skills and instrumentation have led to a more conservative approach, so that laparoscopic wedge resection (Fig. 12.8) and ovarian cystectomy have become the preferred treatment. Successful treatment with methotrexate has also been reported.[145,146] In patients with circulatory collapse, however, immediate laparotomy is mandatory.

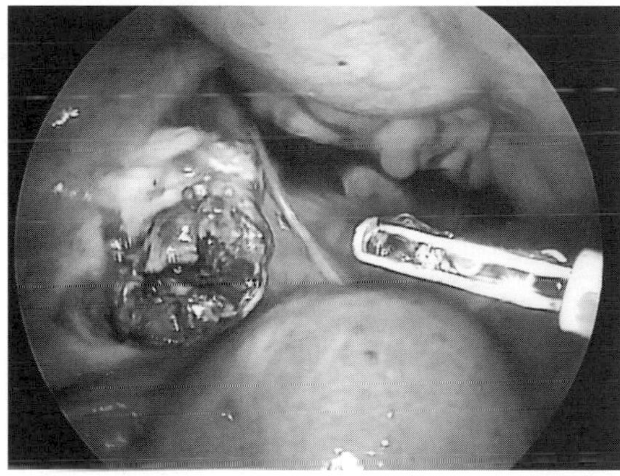

Figure 12.8 Laparoscopic wedge resection for ovarian ectopic pregnancy.

Cervical pregnancy

Cervical pregnancy, which results from implantation of the blastocyst within the cervical canal, is a rare complication of pregnancy. Its incidence varies from 1 in 2400 to 1 in 50 000 normal pregnancies.[147] Appropriate early diagnosis and treatment has led to the remarkable reduction of maternal mortality from 50% in 1911[148] to under 5% in 1983.[147]

A close relationship was found between therapeutic abortions with sharp curettage (dilation and curettage), previous Cesarean sections, *in vitro* fertilization, and cervical pregnancy.[148–150]

Presenting symptoms include painless vaginal bleeding which may be accompanied by abdominal pain and urinary problems.[150] On physical examination, the cervix is usually enlarged, global (barrel shaped), and distended. Occasionally, the external os is dilated.

Accurate diagnosis can be performed by vaginal ultrasound and magnetic resonance imaging, demonstrating an intracervical ectopic sac below a closed internal cervical os (Fig. 12.9). Transvaginal demonstration of an intact part of the cervical

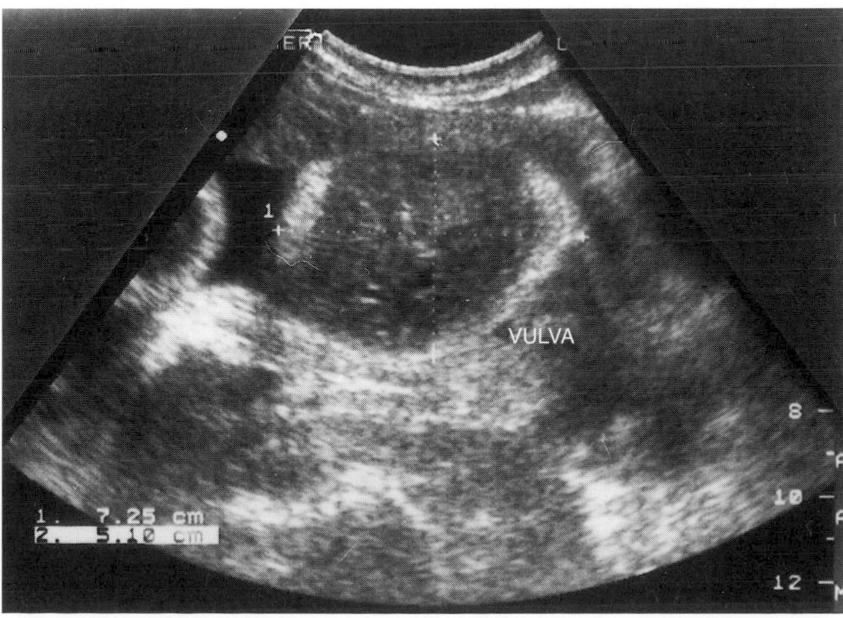

Figure 12.9 Sonographic image of ectopic mass (extrauterine pregnancy) in the cervix area.

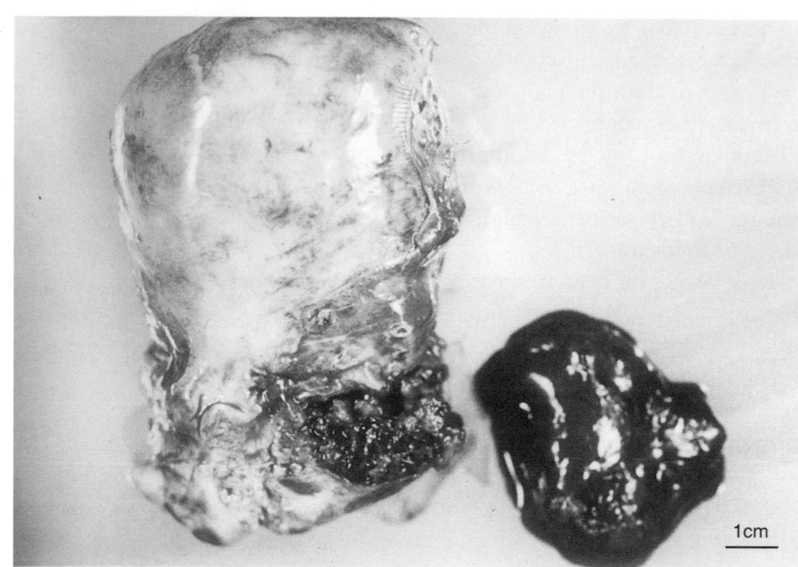

Figure 12.10 Cervical ectopic pregnancy: ruptured in the cervical area with hemorrhagic placental tissue.

Key points

1 Ectopic pregnancy (EP) accounts for approximately 9% of all pregnancy-related deaths.

2 The most common denominator is tubal obstruction and injury.

3 The β-hCG levels in normal pregnancy double every 2 days (48 h), and thus, at present, clinicians rely on a normal "doubling time" to characterize a viable gestation.

4 The accuracy of the initial clinical evaluation before rupture is less than 50%, and additional tests are required in order to differentiate ectopic pregnancy from early intrauterine pregnancy.

5 The risk of EP is increased among women undergoing assisted reproductive technology and specifically *in vitro* fertilization.

6 The most common complaint in EP is sudden severe abdominal pain.

7 Pelvic examination before rupture is usually nonspecific, and a palpable pelvic mass on bimanual examination is established in less than half of the cases.

8 A baseline serum progesterone level of <20 nmol/L can be used to identify abnormal pregnancy (either intra- or extrauterine) with a positive predictive value of ≥95%. However, serum progesterone levels cannot distinguish ectopic pregnancy from spontaneous abortion.

9 The best diagnosis of ectopic pregnancy is based on the positive visualization of an extrauterine pregnancy outside the uterus.

10 At hCG levels between 1000 and 2000 mIU/m, or at 5.5 weeks' gestation, a viable intrauterine pregnancy should be seen by transvaginal ultrasound.

11 Coexistent intra- and extrauterine pregnancies (heterotopic) following spontaneous cycles are rare, with estimated incidence of 1 in 30 000 normal pregnancies.

12 Methotrexate is a cost-saving, nonsurgical fallopian tube-sparing treatment for EP.

13 Absolute contraindications to methotrexate include breastfeeding, immunodeficiency, alcoholism, hepatic, pulmonary, renal, or hematologic dysfunction, known sensitivity to methotrexate, blood dyscrasias, or peptic ulcer disease.

14 The overall success rate of methotrexate treatments is almost 90%.

15 Candidates for successful expectant management must be asymptomatic with an objective evidence of resolution (generally manifested by declining levels of hCG).

canal between the endometrium and gestational sac is suggestive of cervical pregnancy.

Conservative medical management (with systemic methotrexate) has been reported to be successful, obviating the need for surgical treatment, which entails a risk of hysterectomy. Dilation and evacuation, followed by cervical tamponade, was successfully applied using Foley catheter tamponade.[150] Methotrexate is the most commonly used chemotherapy for cervical pregnancies, with a success rate of around 80%.[150–154] Other treatment regimens include arterial embolization and even Shirodkar cerclage placement in order to reduce bleeding. However, in cases of massive and uncontrolled vaginal bleeding, abdominal hysterectomy is necessary (Fig. 12.10).[147]

References

1 ACOG Practice Bulletin. Clinical management guidelines for obstetrician-gynecologists: medical management of tubal pregnancy, no. 3, December 1998.

2 Centers for Disease Control and Prevention. Ectopic pregnancy: United States, 1990–1992. *Morb Mortal Wkly Rep* 1995;44: 46–48.

3 Chow WH, Daling JR, Cates W, Jr, Greenberg RS. Epidemiology of ectopic pregnancy. *Epidemiol Rev* 1987;9:70–94.

4 Bouyer J, Coste J, Shojaei T, et al. Risk factors for ectopic pregnancy: a comprehensive analysis based on a large case-control, population-based study in France. *Am J Epidemiol* 2003;157: 185–194.

5 Shannon C, Brothers PL, Philip NM, et al. Ectopic pregnancy and medical abortion. *Obstet Gynecol* 2004;104:161–167.

6 Ory HM. The women's health study. Ectopic pregnancy and intrauterine contraceptive devices: new perspectives. *Obstet Gynecol* 1981;57:137–144.

7 Westrom L, Bengtsson LP, Mardh PA. Incidence, trends and risks of ectopic pregnancy in a population of women. *Br Med J (Clin Res Ed)* 1981;282:15–18.

8 World Health Organization. Task force on intrauterine devices for fertility regulation. A multinational case-control study of ectopic pregnancy. *Clin Reprod Fertil* 1985;3:131–143.

9 Cheng MC, Wong YM, Rochat RW, et al. Sterilization failure in Singapore: an examination of ligation techniques and failure rates. *Stud Fam Plann* 1977;8:109–115.

10 Karande VC, Flood JT, Heard N, et al. Analysis of ectopic pregnancies resulting from in vitro fertilization and embryo transfer. *Hum Reprod* 1991;6:446–449.

11 Nazari A, Askari HA, Check JH, O'Shaughnessy AO. Embryo transfer techniques as a cause for ectopic pregnancy in in-vitro fertilization. *Fertil Steril* 1993;60:919–921.

12 Homm RJ, Holtz G, Garvin AJ. Isthmic ectopic pregnancy and salpingitis isthmica nodosa. *Fertil Steril* 1987;48:756–760.

13 Ankum WM, Mol BWJ, Van der Veen F, Bossuyt PM. Risk factors for ectopic pregnancy: a meta-analysis. *JAMA* 1996;65: 1093–1099.

14 Weckstein LN, Boucher AR, Tucker H, et al. Accurate diagnosis of early ectopic pregnancy. *Obstet Gynecol* 1985;65:393–397.

15 Kadar N, Caldwell BV, Romero R. A method of screening for ectopic pregnancy and its indications. *Obstet Gynecol* 1981;58: 162–166.

16 Barnhart KT, Sammel MD, Rinaudo PF, et al. Symptomatic patients with an early viable intrauterine pregnancy: hCG curves redefined. *Obstet Gynecol* 2004;104:50–55.

17 Kadar N, Romero R. Observations on the log human chorionic gonadotropin-time relationship in early pregnancy and its practical implication. *Am J Obstet Gynecol* 1987;157:73–78.

18 Kadar N, Freedman M, Zacher M. Further observation on the doubling time of human chorionic gonadotropin in early asymptomatic pregnancy. *Fertil Steril* 1990;54:783–787.

19 Romero R, Kadar N, Copel JA, et al. The value of serial human chorionic gonadotropin testing as a diagnostic tool in ectopic pregnancy. *Am J Obstet Gynecol* 1986;155:392–394.

20 Shepherd RW, Patton PE, Novy MJ, Burry KA. Serial beta-hCG measurements in the early detection of ectopic pregnancy. *Obstet Gynecol* 1990;75:417–420.

21 Fossum GT, Davajam V, Kletzky OA. Early detection of pregnancy with transvaginal ultrasound. *Fertil Steril* 1988;49: 788–791.

22 Carson SA, Buster JE. Ectopic pregnancy. *N Engl J Med* 1993;329:1174–1181.

23 Condous G, Lu C, Van Huffel SV, Bourne T. Human chorionic gonadotrophin and progesterone levels in pregnancies of unknown location. *Int J Gynaecol Obstet* 2004;86:351–357.

24 Banerjee S, Aslam N, Woelfer B, et al. Expectant management of early pregnancies of unknown location: a prospective evaluation of methods to predict spontaneous resolution of pregnancy. *Br J Obstet Gynaecol* 2001;108:158–163.

25 Stovall TG, Ling FW, Carson SA, Buster JE. Serum progesterone and uterine curettage in differential diagnosis of ectopic pregnancy. *Fertil Steril* 1992;57:456–457.

26 Stern JJ, Voss F, Coulam CB. Early diagnosis of ectopic pregnancy using receiver-operator characteristic curves of serum progesterone concentrations. *Hum Reprod* 1993;8:775–779.

27 McCord ML, Muram D, Buster JE, et al. Single serum progesterone as a screen for ectopic pregnancy: exchanging specificity and sensitivity to obtain optimal test performance. *Fertil Steril* 1996;66:513–516.

28 Gelder MS, Boots LR, Younger JB. Use of a single random serum progesterone value as a diagnostic aid for ectopic pregnancy. *Fertil Steril* 1991;55:497–500.

29 Shalev E, Yarom I, Bustan M, et al. Transvaginal sonography as the ultimate diagnostic tool for the management of ectopic pregnancy: experience with 840 cases. *Fertil Steril* 1998;69:62–65.

30 Cacciatore B, Stenman UH, Ylostalo P. Diagnosis of ectopic pregnancy by vaginal ultrasonography in combination with a discriminatory serum hCG level of 1000 IU/l (IRP). *Br J Obstet Gynaecol* 1990;97:904–908.

31 Condous G, Okaro E, Khalid A, et al. The accuracy of transvaginal ultrasonography for the diagnosis of ectopic pregnancy prior to surgery. *Hum Reprod* 2005;20:1404–1409.

32 Goldstein SR, Snyder JR, Watson C, Danon M. Very early pregnancy detection with endovaginal ultrasound. *Obstet Gynecol* 1988;72:200–204.

33 Timor-Tritsch IE, Yeh MN, Peisner DB, et al. The use of transvaginal ultrasound in the diagnosis of ectopic pregnancy. *Am J Obstet Gynecol* 1988;161:157–161.

34 Barnhart KT, Kamelle SA, Simhan H. Diagnostic accuracy of ultrasound, above and below the beta-hCG discriminatory zone. *Obstet Gynecol* 1999;94:583–587.

35 Brown DL, Doubilet PM. Transvaginal sonography for diagnosing ectopic pregnancy: positivity criteria and performance characteristics. *J Ultrasound Med* 1994;13:259–266.

36 Ankum WM, Hajenius PJ, Schrevel LS, Van der Veen F. Management of suspected ectopic pregnancy. *J Reprod Med* 1996;41:724–728.

37 Svare J, Norup P, Grove Thomsen S, et al. Heterotopic pregnancies after in-vitro fertilization and embryo transfer: a Danish survey. *Hum Reprod* 1993;8:116–118.

38 Chiang G, Levine D, Swire M, et al. The intradecidual sign: is it reliable for diagnosis of early intrauterine pregnancy? *Am J Roentgenol* 2004;183:725–731.

39 Ahmed AA, Tom BD, Calabrese P. Ectopic pregnancy diagnosis and the pseudo-sac. *Fertil Steril* 2004;81:1225–1228.

40 Dillon EH, Feyock AL, Taylor KJW. Pseudogestational sacs: Doppler US differentiation from normal or abnormal intrauterine pregnancies. *Radiology* 1990;176:359–364.

41 Kirchler HC, Seebacher S, Alge AA, et al. Early diagnosis of tubal pregnancy: changes in tubal blood flow evaluated by endovaginal color Doppler sonography. *Obstet Gynecol* 1993;82: 561–565.

42 Pellerito JS, Troiano RN, Quedens-Case C, Taylor KJ. Common pitfalls of endovaginal color Doppler flow imaging. *Radiographics* 1995;15:37–47.
43 Barnhart K, Mennuti MT, Benjamin I, et al. Prompt diagnosis of ectopic pregnancy in an emergency department setting. *Obstet Gynecol* 1994;84:1010–1015.
44 Kaplan BC, Dart RG, Moskos M, et al. Ectopic pregnancy: prospective study with improved diagnostic accuracy. *Ann Emerg Med* 1996;28:10–17.
45 Gracia CR, Barnhart KT. Diagnosing ectopic pregnancy in the emergency room setting: a decision analysis comparing six diagnostic strategies. *Obstet Gynecol* 2001;97:464–470.
46 Barnhart KT, Katz I, Hummel A, Gracia CR. Presumed diagnosis of ectopic pregnancy. *Obstet Gynecol* 2002;100:505–510.
47 Vermesh M, Graczykowski JW, Sauer MV. Reevaluation of the role of Culdocentesis in the management of ectopic pregnancy. *Am J Obstet Gynecol* 1990;162:411–413.
48 Maruri F, Azziz R. Laparoscopic surgery for ectopic pregnancies: technology assessment and public health implications. *Fertil Steril* 1993;59:487–498.
49 Leke RJ, Goyaux N, Matsuda T, et al. Ectopic pregnancy in Africa: a population-based study. *Obstet Gynecol* 2004;103:692–697.
50 Dorfman SF. Maternal mortality in New York City, 1981–1983. *Obstet Gynecol* 1990;76:317–323.
51 de Swiet M. Maternal mortality: confidential enquiries into maternal deaths in the United Kingdom. *Am J Obstet Gynecol* 2000;182:760–766.
52 Brumsted J, Kessler C, Gibson C, et al. A comparison of laparoscopy and laparotomy for the treatment of ectopic pregnancy. *Obstet Gynecol* 1988;71:889–892.
53 Tintara H, Choobun T. Laparoscopic adnexectomy for benign tubo-ovarian disease using abdominal wall lift: a comparison to laparotomy. *Int J Gynaecol Obstet* 2004;84:147–155.
54 Vilos GA, Alshimmiri MM. Cost-benefit analysis of laparoscopic versus laparotomy salpingo-oophorectomy for benign tubo-ovarian disease. *J Am Assoc Gynecol Laparosc* 1995;2:299–303.
55 Tulandi T, Saleh A. Surgical management of ectopic pregnancy. *Clin Obstet Gynecol* 1999;42:31–38.
56 Hajenius P, Engelsbel S, Mol B, et al. Randomised trial of systemic methotrexate versus laparoscopic salpingostomy in tubal pregnancy. *Lancet* 1997;350:774–779.
57 Tan H, Tay S. Laparoscopic treatment of ectopic pregnancies: a study of 100 cases. *Ann Acad Med Singapore* 1996;25:665–667.
58 DeCherney AH, Diamond MP. Laparoscopic salpingostomy for ectopic pregnancy. *Obstet Gynecol* 1987;70:948–950.
59 Pouly JL, Mahnes H, Mage G, et al. Conservative laparoscopic treatment of 321 ectopic pregnancies. *Fertil Steril* 1986;46:1093–1097.
60 Bruhat MA, Manhes H, Mage G, Pouly JL. Treatment of ectopic pregnancy by means of laparoscopy. *Fertil Steril* 1980;33:411–414.
61 Morlock RJ, Lafata JE, Eisenstein D. Cost-effectiveness of single-dose methotrexate compared with laparoscopic treatment of ectopic pregnancy. *Obstet Gynecol* 2000;95:407–412.
62 Brezinski A, Schenker JG. Current status of endoscopic surgical management of tubal pregnancy. *Eur J Obstet Gynecol Reprod Biol* 1994;54:43–53.
63 Yao M, Tulandi T. Current status of surgical and nonsurgical management of ectopic pregnancy. *Fertil Steril* 1997;67:421–433.
64 Tulandi T, Guralnick M. Treatment of tubal ectopic pregnancy by salpingotomy with or without tubal suturing and salpingectomy. *Fertil Steril* 1991;55:53–55.
65 Oelsner G, Morad J, Carp H, et al. Reproductive performance following conservative microsurgical management of tubal surgery. *Br J Obstet Gynaecol* 1987;94:1078–1083.
66 Hertz R. Folic acid antagonists: effects on the cell and the patient. Clinical staff conference at NIH. *Ann Intern Med* 1963;59:931–956.
67 Stovall TG, Ling FW, Gray LA, et al. Methotrexate treatment of unruptured ectopic pregnancy: a report of 100 cases. *Obstet Gynecol* 1991;77:749–753.
68 Costa Soares R, Elito J, Han KK, et al. Endometrial thickness as an orienting factor for the medical treatment of unruptured tubal pregnancy. *Acta Obstet Gynecol Scand* 2004;83:289–292.
69 Elito J, Jr, Reichmann AP, Uchiyama MN, Camano L. Predictive score for the systemic treatment of unruptured ectopic pregnancy with a single dose of methotrexate. *Int J Gynecol Obstet* 1999;67:75–79.
70 Lipscomb G, McCord M, Stovall T, et al. Predictors of success of methotrexate treatment in women with tubal ectopic pregnancies. *N Engl J Med* 1999;341:1974–1978.
71 Laibl V, Takacs P, Kang J. Previous ectopic pregnancy as a predictor of methotrexate failure. *Int J Gynecol Obstet* 2004;85:177–178.
72 Lipscomb GH, Givens VA, Meyer NL, Bran D. Previous ectopic pregnancy as a predictor of failure of systemic methotrexate therapy. *Fertil Steril* 2004;81:1221–1224.
73 Stovall TG, Ling FW. Single-dose methotrexate: an expanded clinical trial. *Am J Obstet Gynecol* 1993;168:1759–1765.
74 Saraj AJ, Wilcox JG, Najmabadi S, et al. Resolution of hormonal markers of ectopic gestation: a randomized trial comparing single-dose intra-muscular methotrexate with salpingostomy. *Obstet Gynecol* 1998;92:989–994.
75 Thoen LD, Creinin MD. Medical treatment of ectopic pregnancy with methotrexate. *Fertil Steril* 1997;68:727–730.
76 Jimenez-Caraballo A, Rodriguez-Donoso G. A 6-year clinical trial of methotrexate therapy in the treatment of ectopic pregnancy. *Eur J Obstet Gynecol Reprod Biol* 1998;79:167–171.
77 Lecuru F, Robin F, Bernard JP, et al. Single-dose methotrexate for unruptured ectopic pregnancy. *Int J Gynaecol Obstet* 1998;61:253–259.
78 Lipscomb GH, Bran D, McCord ML, et al. Analysis of three hundred fifteen ectopic pregnancies treated with single-dose methotrexate. *Am J Obstet Gynecol* 1998;178:1354–1358.
79 Sauer MV, Gorrill MJ, Rodi IA, et al. Nonsurgical management of unruptured tubal pregnancy: An extended clinical trial. *Fertil Steril* 1987;48:752–755.
80 Fernandez H, Bourget P, Ville Y, et al. Treatment of unruptured tubal pregnancy with methotrexate: Pharmacokinetic analysis of local versus intra-muscular administration. *Fertil Steril* 1994;62:943–947.
81 Barnhart KT, Gosman G, Ashby R, et al. The medical management of ectopic pregnancy: a meta-analysis comparing "single dose" and "multidose" regimens. *Obstet Gynecol* 2003;101:778–784.
82 Natofsky JG, Lense J, Mayer JC, et al. Ultrasound guided injection of ectopic pregnancy. *Clin Obstet Gynecol* 1999;42:39–47.
83 Corsan GH, Karacan M, Qasim S, et al. Identification of hormonal parameters for successful systemic single-dose methotrexate therapy in ectopic pregnancy. *Hum Reprod* 1995;10:2719–2722.

84 Glock JL, Johnson JV, Brumsted JR. Efficacy and safety of single-dose systemic methotrexate in the treatment of ectopic pregnancy. *Fertil Steril* 1994;62:716–721.
85 Gross Z, Rodriguez JJ, Stalnaker BL. Ectopic pregnancy: nonsurgical, outpatient evaluation and single-dose methotrexate treatment. *J Reprod Med* 1995;40:371–374.
86 Stika CS, Anderson L, Frederiksen MC. Single-dose methotrexate for the treatment of ectopic pregnancy: Northwestern Memorial Hospital three-year experience. *Am J Obstet Gynecol* 1996;174:1840–1846 (discussion 1846–1848).
87 Yao M, Tulandi T, Falcone T. Treatment of ectopic pregnancy by systemic methotrexate, transvaginal methotrexate, and operative laparoscopy. *Int J Fertil* 1996;41:470–475.
88 Wolf GC, Nickisch SA, George KE, et al. Completely nonsurgical management of ectopic pregnancies. *Gynecol Obstet Invest* 1994;37:232–235.
89 Schoenfeld A, Mashiach R, Vardy M, et al. Methotrexate pneumonitis in nonsurgical treatment of ectopic pregnancy. *Obstet Gynecol* 1992;80:520–521.
90 Isaacs JD, Mcgehee RP, Cowan BD. Life threatening neutropenia following methotrexate treatment of ectopic pregnancy: a report of two cases. *Obstet Gynecol* 1996;88:694–696.
91 Gervaise A, Masson L, de Tayrac R, et al. Reproductive outcome after methotrexate treatment of tubal pregnancies. *Fertil Steril* 2004;82:304–308.
92 Vermesh M. Conservative management of ectopic gestation. *Fertil Steril* 1990;53:382–387.
93 Trio D, Strobelt N, Picciolo C, et al. Prognostic factors for successful expectant management. *Fertil Steril* 1995;63:469–472.
94 Shalev E, Peleg D, Tsabari A, et al. Spontaneous resolution of ectopic tubal pregnancy: natural history. *Fertil Steril* 1995;63:15–19.
95 Korhonen J, Stenman UH, Ylöstalo P. Serum human chorionic gonadotropin dynamics during spontaneous resolution of ectopic pregnancy. *Fertil Steril* 1994;61:632–636.
96 Elson J, Tailor A, Banerjee S, et al. Expectant management of tubal ectopic pregnancy: prediction of successful outcome using decision tree analysis. *Ultrasound Obstet Gynecol* 2004;23: 552–556.
97 Vermesh M, Silva PD, Sauer MV, et al. Persistent tubal ectopic gestation: patterns of circulating beta-human chorionic gonadotropin and progesterone, and management options. *Fertil Steril* 1988;50:584–588.
98 Popp LW, Colditz A, Gaetje R. Management of early ectopic pregnancy. *Int J Gynaecol Obstet* 1994;44:239–244.
99 Seifer DB, Gutmann JN, Grant WD, et al. Comparison of persistent ectopic pregnancy after laparoscopic salpingostomy versus salpingostomy and laparotomy for ectopic pregnancy. *Obstet Gynecol* 1993;81:378–382.
100 Vermesh M, Silva PD, Rosen GF, et al. Management of unruptured ectopic gestation by linear salpingostomy: a prospective, randomized clinical trial of laparoscopy versus laparotomy. *Obstet Gynecol* 1989;73:400–404.
101 Hajenius PJ, Mol BW, Ankum WM, et al. Clearance curves of serum human chorionic gonadotrophin for the diagnosis of persistent trophoblast. *Hum Reprod* 1995;10:683–687.
102 Hoppe DE, Bekkar BE, Nager CW. Single-dose systemic methotrexate for the treatment of persistent ectopic pregnancy after conservative surgery. *Obstet Gynecol* 1994;83:51–54.
103 Bengtsson G, Bryman I, Thorburn J, et al. Low-dose oral methotrexate as second-line therapy for persistent trophoblast after conservative treatment of ectopic pregnancy. *Obstet Gynecol* 1992;79:589–591.
104 Pouly JL, Mahnes H, Mage G, et al. Conservative laparoscopic treatment of 321 ectopic pregnancies. *Fertil Steril* 1986;46: 1093–1097.
105 Lundorff P, Hahlin M, Sjoblom P, et al. Persistent trophoblast after conservative treatment of tubal pregnancy: prediction and detection. *Obstet Gynecol* 1991;77:129–133.
106 Nathorst-Böös J, Hamad RR. Risk factors for persistent trophoblastic activity after surgery for ectopic pregnancy. *Acta Obstet Gynecol Scand* 2004;83:471–475.
107 Seifer DB, Gutmann JN, Doyle MB, et al. Persistent ectopic pregnancy following laparoscopic linear salpingostomy. *Obstet Gynecol* 1990;76:1121–1125.
108 Reece EA, Petrie RH, Sirmans MF, et al. Combined intrauterine and extrauterine gestations: a review. *Am J Obstet Gynecol* 1983;146:323–330.
109 Laband SJ, Cherny WB, Finberg HJ. Heterotopic pregnancy: report of four cases. *Am J Obstet Gynecol* 1988;158:437–438.
110 Rojansky N, Schenker JG. Heterotopic pregnancy and assisted reproduction: an update. *J Assist Reprod Genet* 1996;13: 594–601.
111 Bayati J, Garcia JE, Dorsey JH, et al. Combined intrauterine and cervical pregnancy from in vitro fertilization and embryo transfer. *Fertil Steril* 1989;51:725–727.
112 Davies DW, Masson GM, McNeal AD, et al. Simultaneous intrauterine and cervical pregnancies after in-vitro fertilization and embryo transfer in a patient with a history of a previous cervical pregnancy: case report. *Br J Obstet Gynaecol* 1990;97: 634–637.
113 Beckmann CR, Tomasi AM, Thomason JL. Combined interstitial and intrauterine pregnancy: corneal resection in early pregnancy and cesarean delivery at term. *Am J Obstet Gynecol* 1984;149:83–85.
114 Jozwaik EA, Ulug U, Akman MA, et al. Successful resection of a heterotopic cervical pregnancy resulting from intracytoplasmic sperm injection. *Fertil Steril* 2003;79:428–430.
115 Mashiach S, Adom D, Oelsner G, et al. Cervical Shirodker cerclage may be the treatment modality of choice for cervical pregnancy. *Hum Reprod* 2002;17:493–496.
116 Kumar S, Vimala N, Dadhwal V, et al. Heterotopic cervical and intrauterine pregnancy in a spontaneous cycle. *Eur J Obstet Gynecol Reprod Biol* 2004;112:217–220.
117 Monteagudo A, Tarricone NJ, Timor-Tritsch TE, et al. Successful transvaginal ultrasound guided puncture and injection of a cervical pregnancy in a patient with simultaneous intrauterine pregnancy and a history of a previous cervical pregnancy. *Ultrasound Obstet Gynecol* 1996;8:381–386.
118 Carreno CA, King M, Johnson MP, et al. Treatment of heterotopic cervical and intrauterine pregnancy. *Fetal Diagn Ther* 2000;15:1–3.
119 Breen JL. A 21-year survey of 654 ectopic pregnancies. *Am J Obstet Gynecol* 1970;106:1004–1019.
120 Felmus LB, Pedowitz P. Interstitial pregnancy: a survey of 45 cases. *Am J Obstet Gynecol* 1953;66:1271–1279.
121 Sheiner E, Goldstein D, Hershkovitz R, et al. Cornual pregnancy of 15 weeks gestation: case report and current review of management options. *Isr J Obstet Gynecol* 2001;11:121–123.
122 Crvenkovic G, Katz RF, Platt LD. Diagnosis: right side interstitial (cornual) pregnancy. *J Ultrasound Med* 1995;14:325–336.

123 Tulandi T, Al-Jaroudi D. Interstitial pregnancy: results generated from the society of reproductive surgeons registry. *Obstet Gynecol* 2004;103:47–50.
124 Lau S, Tulandi T. Conservative medical and surgical management of interstitial ectopic pregnancy. *Fertil Steril* 1999;72:207–215.
125 Tanaka T, Hayashi H, Kutsuzawa T, et al. Treatment of interstitial ectopic pregnancy with methotrexate: report of a successful case. *Fertil Steril* 1982;37:851–852.
126 Meyer W, Mitchell D. Hysteroscopic removal of an interstitial ectopic gestation. A case report. *J Reprod Med* 1989;34: 928–929.
127 Goldenberg M, Bider D, Oelsner G, et al. Treatment of interstitial pregnancy with methotrexate via hysteroscopy. *Fertil Steril* 1992;58:1234–1236.
128 Atrash HK, Friede A, Hogue CJ. Abdominal pregnancy in the United States: frequency and maternal mortality. *Obstet Gynecol* 1987;69:333–337.
129 Pisarska MD, Carson SA. Incidence and risk factors for ectopic pregnancy. *Clin Obstet Gynecol* 1999;42:2–8.
130 Attapattu JAF, Menson S. Abdominal pregnancy. *Int J Gynaecol Obstet* 1993;43:51–55.
131 Rahman MS, Al-Suleiman SA, Rahman J, et al. Advanced abdominal pregnancy – observations in 10 cases. *Obstet Gynecol* 1982;59:366–372.
132 Martin JN, Jr, McCaul JFT. Emergent management of abdominal pregnancy. *Clin Obstet Gynecol* 1990;33:438–447.
133 Mekki Y, Gilles JM, Mendez L, et al. Abdominal pregnancy: to remove or not to remove the placenta. *Prim Care Update Obstet Gynecol* 1998;5:192.
134 Veerareddy S, Sriemevan A, Cockburn JF, et al. Non-surgical management of a mid-trimester abdominal pregnancy. *Br J Obstet Gynaecol* 2004;111:281–283.
135 Ghezzi F, Lagana D, Franchi M, et al. Conservative treatment by chemotherapy and uterine arteries embolization of a cesarean scar pregnancy. *Eur J Obstet Gynecol Reprod Biol* 2002;103: 88–91.
136 Martin JN, Jr, Ridgway LE, III, Connors JJ, et al. Angiographic arterial embolization and computed tomography-directed drainage for the management of hemorrhage and infection with abdominal pregnancy. *Obstet Gynecol* 1990;76:941–945.
137 Nappi C, D'Elia A, Di Carlo C, et al. Conservative treatment by angiographic uterine artery embolization of a 12 week cervical ectopic pregnancy. *Hum Reprod* 1999;14:1118–1121.
138 Tsudo T, Harada T, Yoshimoka H, et al. Laparoscopic management of early primary abdominal pregnancy. *Obstet Gynecol* 1997;90:687–688.
139 Raziel A, Schachter M, Mordechai E, et al. Ovarian pregnancy: a 12-year experience of 19 cases in one institution. *Eur J Obstet Gynecol Reprod Biol* 2004;114:92–96.
140 Seinera P, Di Gregorio A, Arisio R, et al. Ovarian pregnancy and operative laparoscopy: report of eight cases. *Hum Reprod* 1997;12:608–610.
141 Grimes HG, Nosal RA, Gallagher JC. Ovarian pregnancy: a series of 24 cases. *Obstet Gynecol* 1983;61:174–178.
142 Hallat JG. Primary ovarian pregnancy: a report of 25 cases. *Am J Obstet Gynecol* 1982;143:55–60.
143 Raziel A, Golan A, Pansky M, et al. Ovarian pregnancy: a report of 20 cases in one institution. *Am J Obstet Gynecol* 1990;163:1182–1185.
144 Xie PZ, Feng YZ, Zhao BH. Primary ovarian pregnancy. Report of 15 cases. *Chin Med J* 1991;104:217–220.
145 Chelmow D, Gates E, Penzias AS. Laparoscopic diagnosis and methotrexate treatment of an ovarian pregnancy: a case report. *Fertil Steril* 1994;62:879–881.
146 Raziel A, Golan A. Primary ovarian pregnancy successfully treated with methotrexate. *Am J Obstet Gynecol* 1993;169: 1362–1363.
147 Parente JT, Ou CS, Levy J, et al. Cervical pregnancy analysis. A review and report of five cases. *Obstet Gynecol* 1983;62:79–82.
148 Rubin JC. Cervical pregnancy. *Surg Gynecol Obstet* 1911;13: 625–629.
149 Sheiner E, Yohai D, Katz M. Cervical pregnancy with placenta accreta. *Int J Gynecol Obstet* 1999;65:211–212.
150 Ushakov FB, Elchalal U, Aceman PJ, et al. Cervical pregnancy: past and future. *Obstet Gynecol Surv* 1997;52:45–59.
151 Gun M, Mavrogiorgis M. Cervical ectopic pregnancy: a case report and literature review. *Ultrasound Obstet Gynecol* 2002;19:297–301.
152 Hidalgo LA, Penafiel J, Chedraui PA. Management of cervical pregnancy: risk factors for failed systemic methotrexate. *J Perinat Med* 2004;32:184–186.
153 Kim TJ, Seong SJ, Lee KJ, et al. Clinical outcomes of patients treated for cervical pregnancy with or without methotrexate. *J Korean Med Sci* 2004;19:848–852.
154 Kirk E, Condous G, Haider Z, et al. The conservative management of cervical ectopic pregnancies. *Ultrasound Obstet Gynecol* 2006;27:430–437.

13 Multifetal pregnancies: epidemiology, clinical characteristics, and management

Michelle Smith-Levitin, Daniel W. Skupski, and Frank A. Chervenak

Background

Incidence and epidemiology

In the past, the overall incidence of twins worldwide was about 1 in 80 pregnancies (1.13%), and high-order multiples were rare. During the last 30 years, the incidence of multiple births has been steadily increasing. In the USA, the number of twin births has increased by over 60% since 1980, giving a twin birth rate of 31.1 per 1000 live births. Higher order births increased by 500% for a higher order birth rate of 1.84 per 1000 live births.[1] More than 90% of the increase is estimated to result from the more widespread use of assisted reproductive technologies (ART).[2,3] Patients who conceive after treatment with ovulation-inducing agents or *in vitro* fertilization procedures do so with a multiple gestation 7–50% of the time.[3,4] Recent trends toward delayed childrearing in developed countries have probably contributed to the increase in multiple births as well, as there is a naturally occurring greater incidence of twins among older women.[1,3–5]

Prior to the introduction of ART, the frequency of monozygotic (MZ) twins was relatively constant throughout the world. The incidence was 4 per 1000 births with a 2:1 ratio of DZ:MZ pairs.[6,7] In contrast, the incidence of naturally occurring dizygotic (DZ) twins varies and is affected by maternal race, parity, age, nutritional status, and family history.[6,8] This may be related to higher baseline levels of gonadotropins in certain groups of women.[6,8] For example, the highest incidence of DZ twinning has been found in black women, who have been shown to have larger pituitary glands and higher serum hormone content than other women.[6,8]

Pathogenesis/embryology

Multiple gestations can be either monozygotic (arising form the fertilization of one ovum by one sperm leading to fetuses with an identical genotype) or multizygotic (arising from the fertilization of two or more ova each with one sperm leading to genotypically unique fetuses that happen to share the uterus at the same time). In describing them, one should avoid the terms "identical" and "fraternal", which refer only to phenotypic likeness. Nonetheless, identical generally implies monozygosity, and fraternal generally implies dizygosity.

Monozygous gestations can be diamnionic–dichorionic (DC), diamnionic–monochorionic (MC), or monoamnionic–monochorionic (MA) depending on when the zygote splits (Fig. 13.1).[6,8,9] The zygote splits soon after fertilization resulting in DC placentation in about 30% of MZ twins.[6,8,9] Remnants of blood vessels, ghost villi, and decidual debris can be seen between the four layers of membranes (two amnions and two chorions). The chorions are almost always fused, as seen by a characteristic ridge at the center of the placental mass. If the zygote splits between the third and the eighth days, the resulting single placenta will be MC, which occurs in 70% of MZ twins.[6,8,9] The dividing membranes (two amnions and one chorion) are thin and translucent. Rarely (less than 1%), MZ twins will be MA if the zygote splits after the amnion has formed at about days 9–12.[6,8,9] If the twinning process occurs even later, after the yolk sac has formed, the MZ pair will be conjoined.[6,9] Beyond the 17th day, a singleton gestation will develop.

Interestingly, the rate of zygotic splitting and, therefore, of monozygotic twins appears to be higher following all ART procedures.[3,7,10,11] There is some evidence that it may be related to biochemical or mechanical trauma to the zona pellucida.[10,11] If the timing of events outlined in Fig. 13.1 is correct, one would expect to see only DC multiples in this setting as ART procedures involve manipulation of the zygote within 2 days after ovulation. This has not been the experience.

Multizygotic gestations are generally assumed to be the result of multiple ovulation, as evidenced by their high rate after ovulation induction with sonographically and biochemically confirmed ovulation of multiple ova. All DZ twins have separate DC placentas. Higher order multiple gestations can contain any combination of monozygotic (DC, MC, and MA) and multizygotic (DC) fetuses.

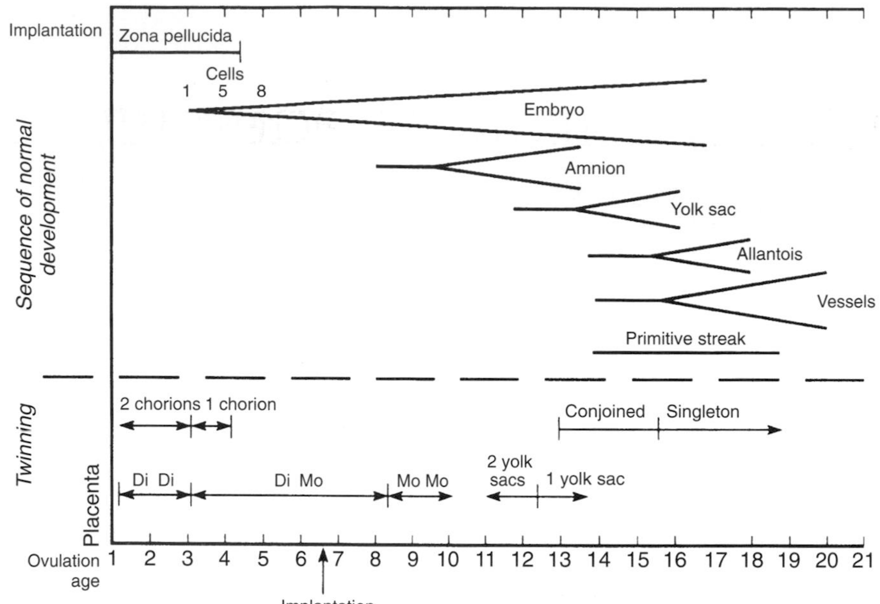

Figure 13.1 The embryology of monozygotic twinning. From Benirschke K, Kim CK. Multiple pregnancy. *N Engl J Med* 1973;288:1276.

Diagnosis

Ultrasound has become indispensable for the identification, assessment, and management of multiple gestations (Table 13.1).[12] An awareness of the risk factors for multiple gestation and the clinical indicators is still important, however, as ultrasound is not routine worldwide.

Risk factors/clinical indicators of multiple gestations

Risk factors for conceiving a multiple gestation include a family or personal history of spontaneous twins and the use of ovulation induction or gamete or zygote transfer procedures. The most common clinical signs or symptoms suggestive of twins include uterine size that is greater than expected for dates, hyperemesis gravidarum, auscultation of two or more fetal heart rates, and accelerated maternal weight gain. Higher levels of biochemical pregnancy markers such as β-human chorionic gonadotropin (βhCG), progesterone, estriol, estradiol, and maternal serum alpha fetoprotein (MSAFP) can also be suggestive of a multiple gestation, although none is specific enough to make the diagnosis of more than one fetus without an ultrasound examination.[6,13]

Ultrasound

At a minimum, patients with the above risks should have a diagnostic ultrasound because outcomes are much better for multiple gestations that are diagnosed early. Although multiple sacs can be seen as early as 4–5 weeks using a transvaginal probe, it is prudent to reserve the diagnosis of twins (or more) until several weeks later when fetal poles with cardiac

Table 13.1 The use of ultrasound in multiple gestations.

First trimester
Diagnosis of multifetal pregnancy
Determination of chorionicity and amnionicity
Accurate pregnancy dating (crown–rump length)
Screening for some anomalies (nuchal translucencies)
Guidance for chorionic villus sampling and multifetal pregnancy reduction
Second trimester
Screening for fetal anomalies
Guidance for amniocentesis
Determination of chorionicity and amnionicity
Determination of placental cord insertion
Biometry to screen for early fetal growth restriction or discordance
Assessment of cervical length
Third trimester
Biometry to screen for fetal growth restriction or discordance
Assessment of cervical length
Fetal status assessment
Amniotic fluid volume
Biophysical profile
Doppler flow studies
Fetal presentation
Intrapartum
Fetal presentation
Guidance for external cephalic version of the second twin

activity are seen, because there is a high frequency of embryonic "disappearance" in patients with a presumed multiple gestation who are scanned in early pregnancy.[14] The prevalence of this "vanishing twin" phenomenon has been reported to range between 22% and 54% of patients with twins or more scanned in the first trimester.[14] Furthermore, a diagnosis of a multiple gestation should not be made simply on the basis of visualization of more than one fluid-filled cavity as a subchorionic hematoma, excessive transducer pressure, or a septate uterus can all mimic a multiple gestation.[12,15]

Determination of chorionicity

There are several ways to determine the placentation in multiple gestations, but the most accurate is assessment in the late first or early second trimester. The visualization of a dividing membrane at any time excludes a diagnosis of a MA pair. Lack of visualization, however, is not necessarily diagnostic of a MA pair as the dividing membrane may be difficult to see until 10–12 weeks in MC multiples (Fig. 13.2). If two fetal poles but only one yolk sac is present, the pregnancy is most likely MA.[16] After the first trimester, the membrane may be completely apposed to a twin with severe oligohydramnios. In this situation, the fetus is trapped or "stuck" against the uterine wall and will not move over time or with maternal position change.[6] A truly MA pair will move away from the uterine wall, and cords will often be visibly entangled.

If the ultrasound reveals separate placental discs, particularly if on opposite uterine surfaces, or fetuses of opposite gender, the pregnancy is DC. If the placentas are close together, attention should be turned to the dividing membranes. A MC membrane will be thin and wispy (Fig. 13.3B), whereas a DC membrane will be thick and more easily visualized (Fig. 13.3A). MC membranes have two layers, and DC membranes have four visible layers. In DC placentas, the "twin peak" sign is a triangular projection of placental tissue from the chorionic plate into a cleft between the layers of the intertwin membrane (Fig. 13.3A).[17] In contrast, a T-shaped junction will be present in an MC placenta (Fig. 13.3B).[18] Assessment of the Y-shaped ipsilon zone can aid in the determination of chorionicity in triplet gestations (Fig. 13.3C).[19] These methods correctly identify chorionicity in the majority of patients who are scanned in early pregnancy.[19,20]

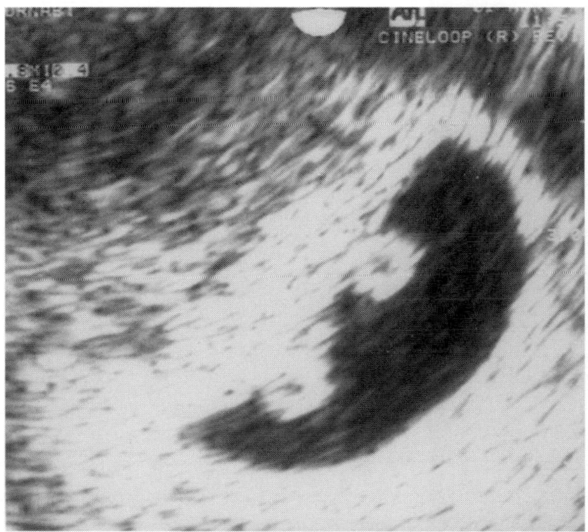

Figure 13.2 Early first-trimester sonogram of diamnionic–monochorionic twins. It is too early to visualize the dividing membrane, but the presence of two yolk sacs suggests diamnionicity. Image courtesy of Birgit Arabin, MD.

The early determination of chorionicity does not always establish the zygosity of multiple gestations as an MZ set can have an MC or DC placenta. More sophisticated methods of zygosity determination can be performed, such as DNA fingerprinting from amniocytes, when the information is needed for antenatal management.[21] It is important to confirm chorionicity and zygosity after birth for the parents and for the future medical care of the children. For example, an MZ twin has a higher chance of developing some medical conditions if the co-twin is affected, and an MZ twin can accept tissue from the co-twin as an isograft. Examination of the placenta after birth, blood grouping, and DNA mapping techniques are methods that are used to determine the zygosity.[6]

Fetal complications

Perinatal morbidity and mortality

Multiple gestations contribute significantly to perinatal morbidity and mortality, although they still account for a relatively small percentage of live births.[4,6,22,23] Twins alone account for 12.6% of the perinatal mortality, although they account for only 3% of live births.[1,22] The overall perinatal mortality rate for twins in developed countries is approximately 50 per 1000 births.[5,15,22] The risk of perinatal death is three- to 10-fold higher for a twin than for a singleton,[15,22] and the risk of cerebral palsy is four times greater.[7] The corrected perinatal mortality rates for triplets and higher order gestations are more striking. The crude perinatal mortality rate for triplets is 121 per 1000 births.[24] Twenty percent of triplets have a major handicap and a triplet is 17 times more likely to have cerebral palsy than a singleton.[7]

Prematurity

The relatively high incidence of perinatal mortality and morbidity is largely due to complications of prematurity. Fifty-eight percent of twins and 92% of triplets are born prior to 37 weeks, because of preterm labor, preterm premature rupture of membranes, or fetal or maternal complications, compared with 10% of singletons.[1] The average length of gestation decreases inversely with the number of fetuses present (Table 13.2). Twelve percent of twins, 36% of triplets,

A

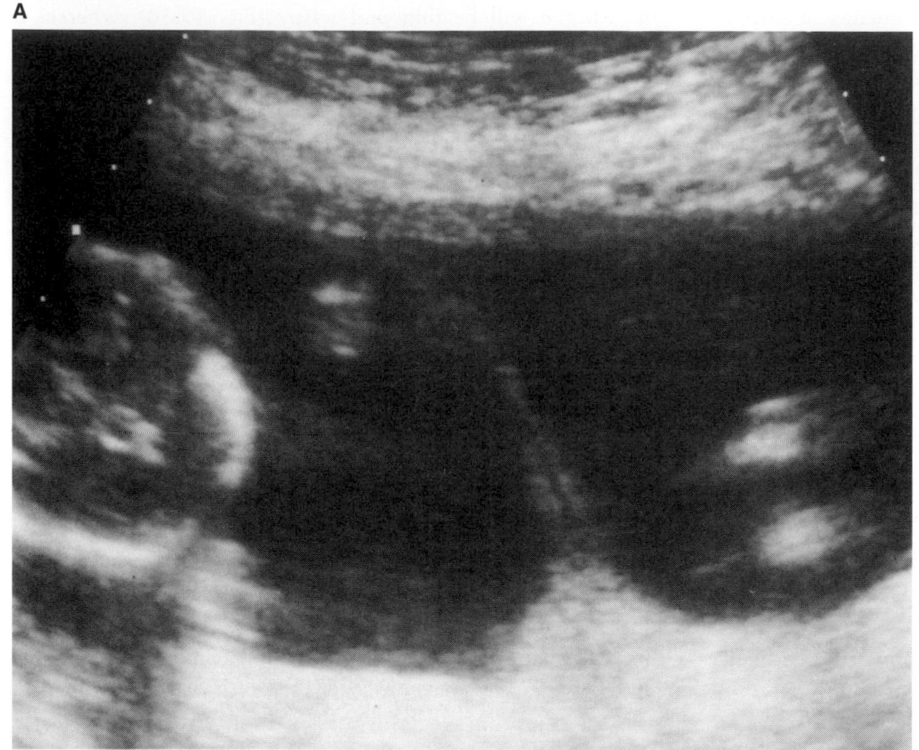

B

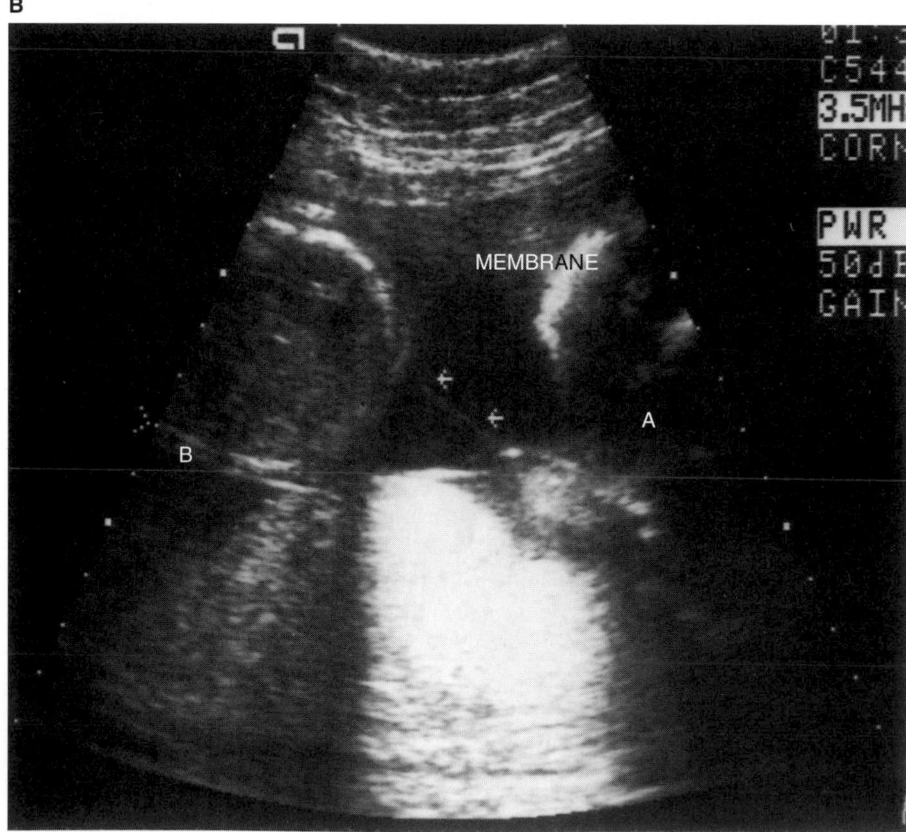

Figure 13.3 (A) The twin peak sign and a thick dichorionic membrane. (B) The T-shaped junction of a monochorionic placenta. (C) The Y-shaped ipsilon zone of a trichorionic triplet gestation.

C

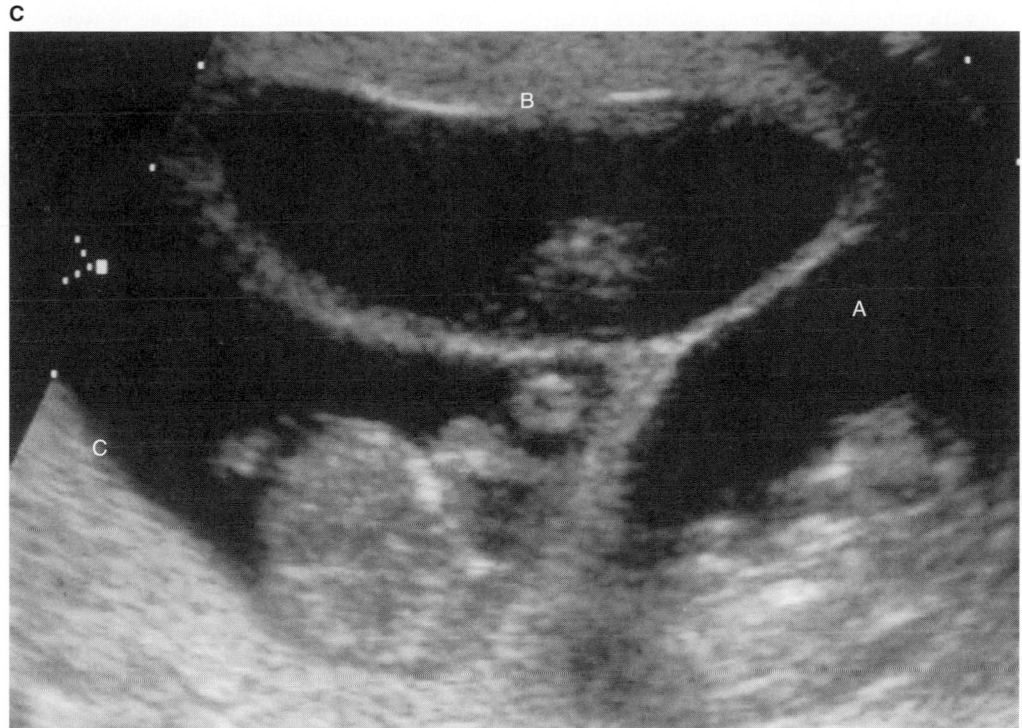

Figure 13.3 *Continued.*

Table 13.2 Gestational age and birthweight in multiple gestations.

	Twins	Triplets	Quadruplets
Average gestational age (weeks)	35.3	32.2	29.9
Average birthweight (g)	2347	1687	1309

Adapted from ref. 1.

and 60% of quadruplets are born prior to 32 weeks, and a significant percentage deliver prior to 28 weeks.[7,25] Furthermore, prematurity results in babies being born at low birthweight, and birthweight has been shown to be the most important factor for predicting morbidity and mortality in twins.[7,23,26] The risk of being born at a low birthweight (< 2500 g) is ninefold higher for a twin than for a singleton and 15-fold higher for a triplet.[1,22,27] The risk of being born at a very low birthweight (< 1500 g) is also 10-fold higher for a twin than for a singleton and is 31-fold higher for a triplet.[1,22,27] Twenty-five percent of twins, 75% of triplets, and all quadruplets are admitted to the neonatal intensive care unit.[7,24,28–30]

Fetal growth

The biometrical parameters that are used to assess fetal growth in singletons have been shown to be accurate in multiple gestations as well. Although femur length measurements between singletons and twins tend to be similar throughout gestation, abdominal circumferences and biparietal diameters tend to be smaller.[31,35] Estimated fetal weights in twins should be determined using formulas that incorporate at least femur length and abdominal circumference.[32–33]

Multiple gestations are at increased risk of being small for gestational age, which also leads to perinatal morbidity and mortality.[6,7,15,23,26] Twins who are born at the same gestational age but who weigh less than 2000 g have a 10-fold greater risk of an adverse outcome compared with twins weighing more than 2000 g, and the risk decreases by 40% for every 250-g increase in birthweight.[23] Fetal growth restriction (FGR) complicates as many as 60% of multiple gestations.[6,7,31,34,35] The degree of FGR tends to increase with increasing numbers of fetuses.[36] The factors that influence growth in multiples are unclear. Theories range from phenomenon that occur early, such as limited vascular supply after the implantation of more than one embryo, to uterine conditions occurring later, such as fetal crowding or limited decidual area for placental growth. Experience with patients undergoing multifetal pregnancy reduction, which reveals correlation between rates of FGR and the starting number of viable embryos, indicates that first-trimester events may play a role.[35,37] However, the fact that fetal growth in the majority of pregnancies, regardless of fetal number, follows the same trajectory until approximately 28–32 weeks when multiple gestations begin to fall behind singletons, and the fact that rates of FGR among multiples increases exponentially with increasing gestational age, suggests that the third-trimester environment is also significant (Fig. 13.4).[6,12,15,31,36,40,41]

The definition of FGR in the setting of multiple gestations is problematic. Some believe that it should be defined as an estimated fetal weight below the 10th percentile at a given gestational age based on specific growth curves for twins or triplets.[31,33,36] Others believe that the use of singleton nomograms is valid and should, in fact, be used, as multiple gestations, at least multizygotic sets, have the same genetic growth potential as singletons.[35,39,40,41] As the validity and accuracy of published twin and triplet growth curves have not been established, singleton curves continue to be used as the gold standard.

Another growth problem seen in multiple gestations is discordance between the fetuses, which complicates at least 15% of twins and up to 54% of triplets.[34] This is associated with even higher morbidity and mortality compared with concordantly grown pairs, especially for the smaller twin or triplet.[7,12,13,42–45] Although discordant growth is not always the result of a pathologic process, it is often due to placental insufficiency or abnormal placentation of one twin, twin–twin transfusion syndrome, or a congenital anomaly of one twin.[12,23,36,46] A combination of some or all of the ultrasonographically detectable indices listed in Table 13.3 identify discordant sets.[12,31,32,47] As with FGR, measurement of abdominal circumference seems to be the most sensitive marker for significant growth discordance.[47]

Congenital anomalies

The incidence of congenital anomalies in multiple gestations is one and a half to three times higher than in singletons.[5,6,28] There is a higher incidence of structural defects seen in MZ twins, some of which are unique to twins and may be due to the twinning process itself.[48] There is also a higher incidence of chromosomal abnormalities, which is related to the older age, in general, of woman conceiving multiples and to the increased probability that a woman carrying more than one fetus will have at least one that is aneuploid at a younger maternal age than if she were carrying a singleton.[7,49–51]

Table 13.3 Sonographic criteria for discordance.

Parameter	
Biparietal diameter	≥ 6 mm
Abdominal circumference	> 20 mm
Femur length	≥ 5 mm
Estimated fetal weight	> 20–25% (expressed as a percentage of the larger fetal weight)
Doppler of the umbilical artery (systolic/diastolic ratio)	> 15% (or > 0.4)

Conjoined twins

Schinzel et al. describe three helpful categories to organize the anomalies encountered in multifetal pregnancies.[48] The first are midline structural defects that are felt to be a consequence of the "teratogenic" event of twinning such as sirenomelia, holoprosencephaly, exstrophy of the cloaca, and neural tube defects.[48,52] Conjoined twins, which are specific to multiple gestations, also fall into this category. The incidence of conjoined twins is 0.2–0.6 per 10 000 births or 40 per 10 000 twin births.[53,54] They can also occur in the setting of a higher order multiple gestation.[12] The twins may be joined by minor, superficial attachments, attachments of major body parts including internal organs, or in the most severe forms (duplicata incompleta), there may be complete union except for duplication of just one body part. Conjoined twins are classified by the most prominent site of union (Table 13.4).[53,54] They can now be diagnosed relatively early in gestation with ultrasound and adjuvant use of three-dimensional ultrasound.[53–55] The signs include lack of a dividing membrane, a fixed position relative one to the other that does not change over time, a bifid appearance to the first-trimester fetal pole, inability to distinguish two complete fetal borders, the appearance of more than three vessels in the umbilical cord, and detection of other anomalies.[13,53–55]

Acardia

The second category of anomalies results from vascular interchanges that occur in most monochorionic placentas.[46,56] Such vascular anastomoses can often be demonstrated by perfusing the placentas after delivery with colored water or milk (Fig. 13.5).[6,46,56,57] The most severe form, acardia or twin reversed arterial perfusion (TRAP), is believed to arise when arterial–arterial and venous–venous anastomoses exist without any arterial–venous connections.[8,9,58,59] As a result, there is uncompensated reversed flow, which is thought to impair development of the heart and often the head (Fig. 13.6). The "pump" twin becomes hydropic, and the "recipient" twin has multiple anomalies, often appearing only as an amorphous mass of tissue.[6,13,58] This anomaly only affects approximately 1 in 35 000 infants or 1 in 100 monozygotic twin pregnancies.[58]

Twin–twin transfusion syndrome

A less severe, but much more common, form of vascular interchange between fetuses leads to the twin–twin transfusion

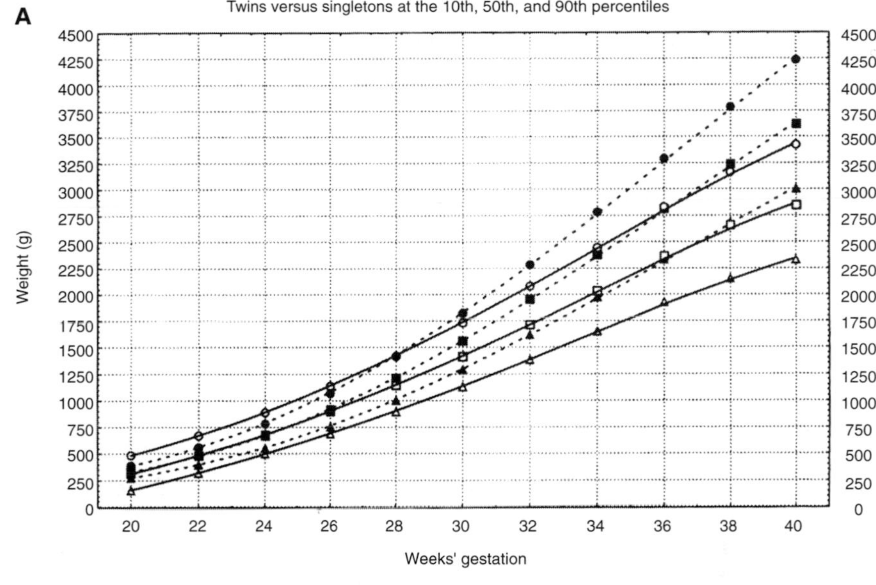

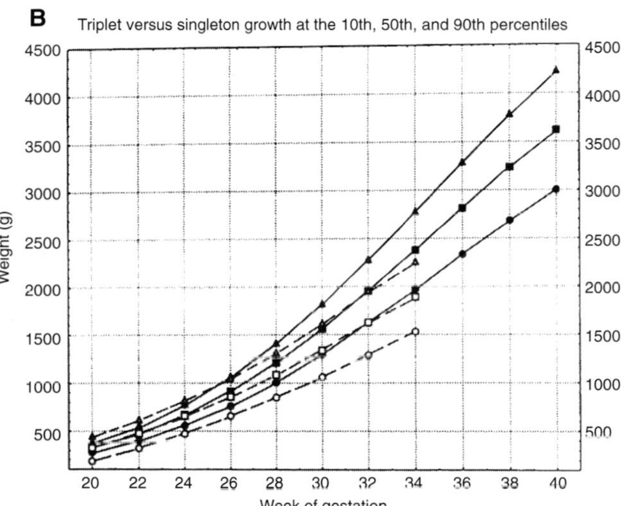

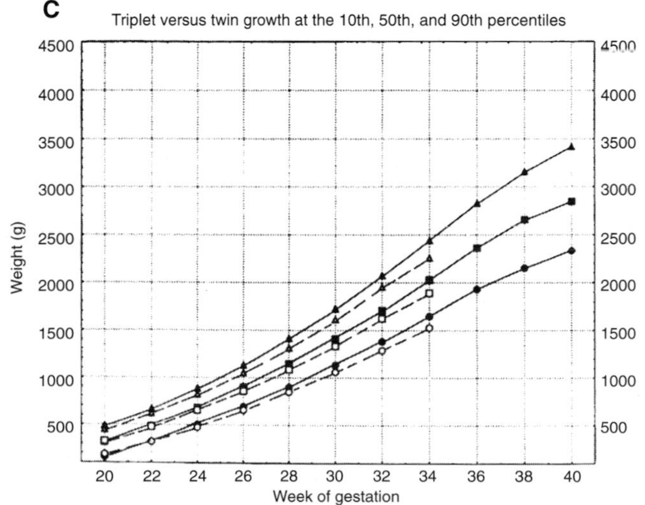

Figure 13.4 (A) Growth rates in twins versus singletons. Twins are represented by open symbols and solid lines. Singletons are represented by solid symbols and dashed lines. Triangles represent the 10th percentiles, squares represent the 50th percentiles, and circles represent the 90th percentiles. From ref 40. (B and C) Growth rates in triplets compared with singletons and twins. Singletons and twins are represented by closed symbols and solid lines, respectively, and triplets are represented by open symbols and dashed lines. Circles represent 10th percentile, squares represent the 50th percentile, and triangles represent the 90th percentile. From ref. 41.

Table 13.4 Classification of conjoined twins.

Type*	Organs commonly shared	Frequency (%)
Thoracopagus (thorax)	Heart, liver, GI tract	29–40
Omphalopagus (abdomen)	Liver, GI tract	25–34
Pypopagus (sacrum)	Spine, GU system, lower GI tract	10–18
Ischiopagus (pelvis)	Pelvis, GU system, GI tract, liver	6–20
Craniopagus (skull)	Brain	2–16

*Extensive areas of union are classified by placing the prefix "di" before the part of the body that is not fused (i.e., dicephalus refers to a conjoined twin with one body but two heads).

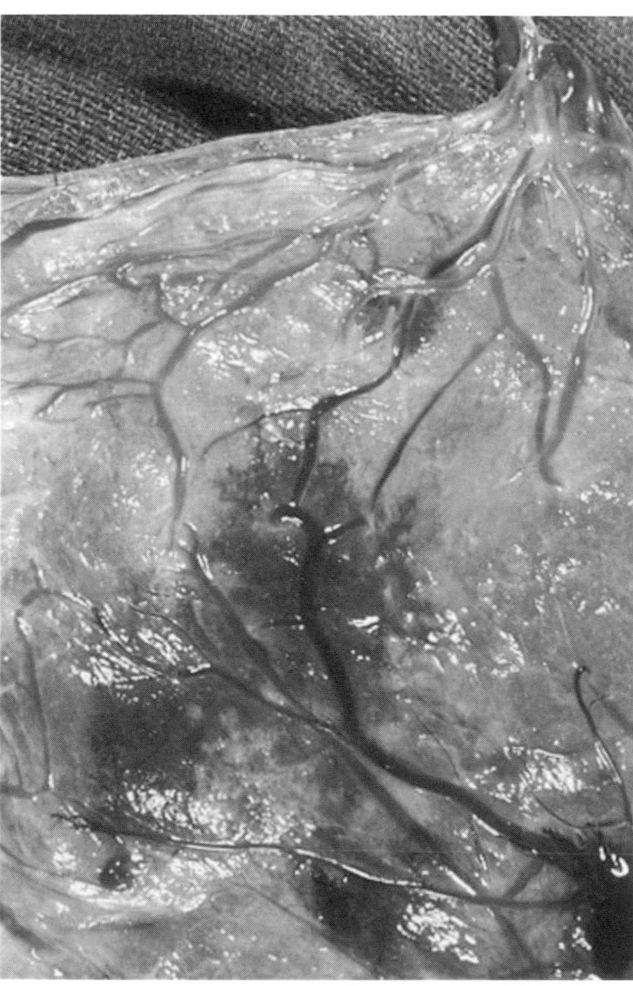

Figure 13.5 Monochorionic placenta perfused with dye demonstrating vascular anastomoses.

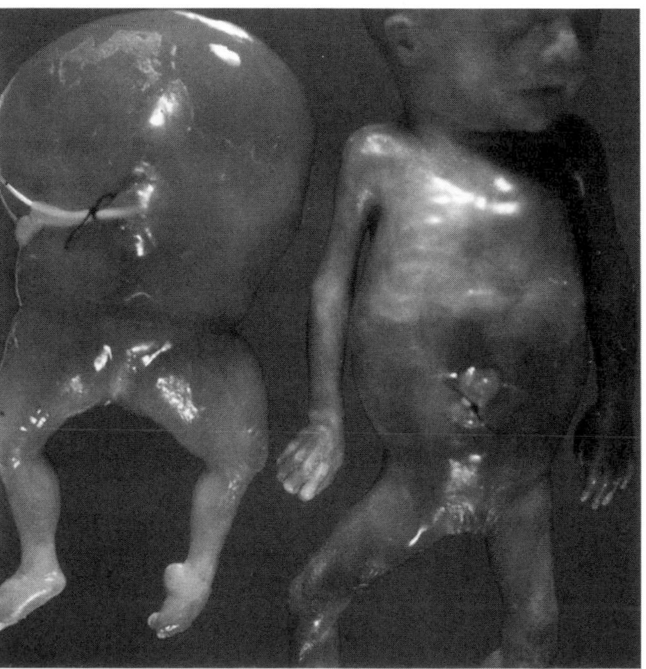

Figure 13.6 Example of twin reversed arterial perfusion (TRAP). The fetus on the left has no head or upper limbs (acardiac), while the fetus on the right is structurally normal. From Ref. 46.

syndrome (TTTS) or polyhydramnios–oligohydramnios sequence. It is thought to occur when deep arterial–venous connections are uncompensated, leading to a one-way shunt between the fetuses (Fig. 13.7).[8,12,46,56,57,60] The exact incidence is unknown as severe forms may present as a "vanished twin" in the first trimester or as the full syndrome later in gestation, and milder forms may be evident only at birth or not at all.[58] Although it has been reported in fused dichorionic placentas, it is largely a complication of monochorionic placentation, probably occurring in 5–15% of such pregnancies.[58,60] The recipient twin becomes hypervolemic and polycythemic, which eventually leads to polyhydramnios, congestive heart failure, and hydrops, while the donor becomes hypovolemic and anemic, which leads to decreased renal perfusion, oligohydramnios, and FGR, and can also eventually lead to heart failure.[12,58,61] An antepartum diagnosis can be made with reasonable certainty using ultrasound. The criteria include a strong suspicion of monochorionicity, oligohydramnios (maximum vertical pocket less than 2 cm) around the smaller twin (often severe enough to make it appear "stuck") with a small or absent urinary bladder on serial scans and polyhydramnios (maximum vertical pocket > 8 cm) around the larger

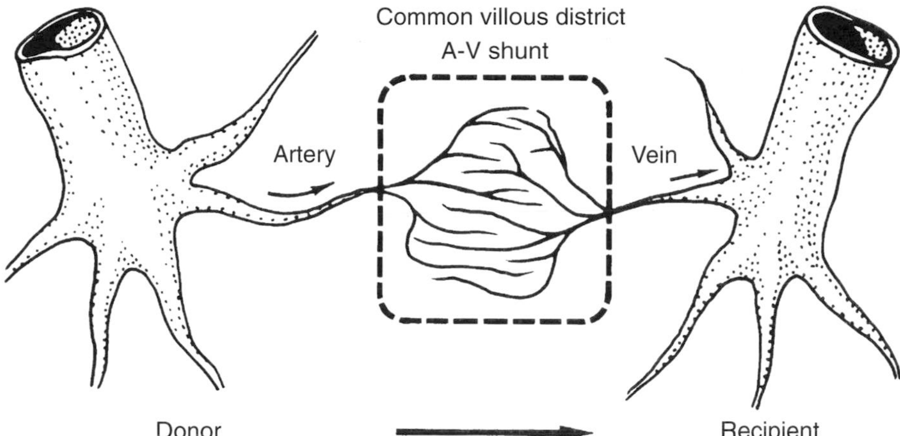

Figure 13.7 The pathologic arteriovenous connection in the twin transfusion syndrome. Redrawn from Benirschke K. Twin gestation: incidence, etiology and inheritance. In: Creasy RK, Resnik R, eds. *Maternal–fetal medicine: principles and practice*, 2nd edn. Philadelphia, PA: W.B. Saunders; 1989:582.

twin (sometimes with evidence of high-output heart failure), with a distended urinary bladder on serial scans.[12,13,58]

In addition to the vascular connections that can occur in the placentas of multiple gestations, other abnormalities of the placenta, membranes, and umbilical cords that can cause fetal complications occur. MA gestations, although rare, are associated with a high perinatal mortality, which often results from entanglement of the two umbilical cords.[46,58,62,63] Bivascular cords (single artery)[8,46] and velamentous cord insertions are also much more common in twin and higher order placentas.[46] The portion of cord that is unprotected is susceptible to thrombosis, compression, or rupture, particularly if it is a vasa previa.[8]

The third group of anomalies that Schnizel et al. described are those resulting from intrauterine crowding. Examples are minor foot deformities, skull asymmetry, and dislocation of the hip.[15,48]

Intrauterine fetal demise

As discussed previously, a vanishing twin early in pregnancy may be a common event that does not usually lead to further problems.[58,64,65] However, death of one fetus later in a multiple gestation, which complicates 4–8% of twins[58,65] and 11–17% of triplets,[58,66] is associated with an increased risk of preterm delivery, FGR, and perinatal mortality in the survivors.[58,64] The risk of fetal demise is at least twice as high in MC as in DC pregnancies,[58,64,65] and there is a 20% risk of organ damage such as microcephaly, hydranencephaly, multicystic encephalomalacia, intestinal atresia, aplasia cutis, or limb amputation in the survivor.[13,48,58,64,67] There is at least a 12% risk of severe neurologic handicap in children who survive the death of a MC co-twin even as early as 18 weeks.[13,58,67] The pathogenesis of such damage is not fully understood, but the most likely theory is hypotension along with hypoxemia and anemia occurring in the survivor due to exsanguination of the survivor into the dead twin's relaxed vascular bed.[8,13,58]

Maternal medical complications

Women carrying multiple fetuses are at greater risk of medical and obstetrical complications than women carrying a singleton because of the increased average maternal age and the increased physiologic demands of multiple fetuses and greater placental mass (Table 13.5). Some of the problems that seem to be more common with multiple gestations are discussed below.

Gastrointestinal

Hyperemesis gravidarum

Nausea and vomiting early in pregnancy complicate almost 50% of multiple gestations.[28] This is probably due to the higher levels of βhCG and steroid hormones. Although there is likely a higher incidence of hyperemesis gravidarum, as well, the exact incidence in multiple gestations has not been quantified.

Cholestasis of pregnancy

There is a higher incidence of intrahepatic cholestasis of pregnancy in multiple gestations, particularly in genetically susceptible populations, in which it occurs in 21% of twins compared with 10% of singletons.[68] As in singletons, intrahepatic cholestasis of pregnancy in multiples usually presents with generalized pruritis and mild jaundice in the third trimester. The recurrence rate is reported to be as high as 70.5%.[68] The differential diagnosis includes viral hepatitis, acute fatty liver of pregnancy, and cholelithiasis. The bile acids (cholic acid, deoxycholic acid, and chenodeoxycholic acid) are increased 10–100 times over normal levels, and should be at least three times normal levels to confirm the diagnosis. The management of intrahepatic cholestasis of pregnancy in a multiple gestation is the same as in a singleton, which must include careful antepartum fetal monitoring and probable early delivery as the condition is associated with adverse perinatal outcome.

Table 13.5 Maternal complications of multiple gestation.

Gastrointestinal
Hyperemesis gravidarum
Cholestasis of pregnancy
Acute fatty liver of pregnancy
Hematologic
Anemia
Thromboembolism
Dermatologic
Pruritic urticaric papules of pregnancy
Metabolic
Gestational diabetes
Infectious
Urinary tract infections
Puerperal infections
Cardiovascular
Pregnancy-induced hypertension
Preeclampsia
Increased susceptibility to pulmonary edema
Complications of tocolysis
Economic
Psychologic morbidity
Obstetric
Preterm labor
Preterm premature rupture of membranes
Antepartum hemorrhage
Abruptio placentae
Postpartum hemorrhage
Increased incidence of Cesarean delivery and subsequent complications
Increased hospitalization

Acute fatty liver of pregnancy

Acute fatty liver of pregnancy (AFLP) is a very rare condition; yet, 16.7% of the cases occur in twin pregnancies.[69] AFLP is a fulminant disease that causes jaundice, nausea, and vomiting in the third trimester. It has historically been associated with poor maternal and perinatal outcome and, if undiagnosed or untreated, may result in somnolence, coma, liver rupture, liver failure, hypoglycemia, disseminated intravascular coagulation (DIC), oliguria, renal failure, metabolic acidosis, multisystem organ failure, maternal death, fetal distress, and fetal demise. Although earlier recognition and treatment of AFLP have decreased maternal mortality, it is still up to 20%.[70] Therefore, the diagnosis must be considered and serum chemistries obtained in symptomatic patients. Important tests include liver transaminases, complete blood count, serum ammonia (all increased), and serum glucose (markedly decreased). Management of AFLP in a multiple gestation is the same as for a singleton.[7,69,70]

Hematologic

The increased demands of a multiple gestation often lead to iron and folate deficiency, and there is more "dilutional" anemia due to the exaggerated increase in plasma volume.[6] Anemia (hemoglobin <10 g/dL or hematocrit <30%) has been reported twice as often in mothers with twins compared with those with singletons,[5,71] It has also been found in 20–70% of triplets and higher order mulitples.[13,25,38] Severe anemia can be defined as a hematocrit <22%, an anemia that requires blood transfusion, or an anemia associated with cardiorespiratory symptoms or decompensation. It is suspected, but has not been shown, that severe anemia is also increased in multiple pregnancy. Thromboembolism is also more common in women carrying a multiple gestation.[72]

Gestational diabetes

It is unclear whether carbohydrate metabolism is affected significantly by the added demands of a multiple gestation.[5] However, it is logical that gestational diabetes (GDM) would be increased in multiples because of the increased human placental lactogen and circulating steroid hormones that are seen in these pregnancies.[38,73,74] The higher incidence observed in triplets (~25%) compared with twins (~5%) supports this logic.[7,74,75] Diabetes education, particularly as it relates to diet, must take into account the increased baseline caloric requirement for women with a multiple gestation and GDM.

Urinary tract infections

Ureteral changes in women carrying a multiple gestation are likely to be exaggerated. Decreased peristalsis from the high progesterone levels or compression at the pelvic brim from the overdistended uterus may lead to increased stasis and more urinary tract infections. Urinary tract infections have been found more commonly in twins than in singletons,[5,71] and in triplets than in twins.[28] However, it is not clear whether the incidence of frank pyelonephritis is increased among multiple gestations.[5]

Cardiovascular complications

The expected physiologic changes in the cardiovascular system are exaggerated in women pregnant with a multiple gestation.[713,76–78] There is an even greater drop in diastolic blood pressure in the second trimester, followed by a greater rise before delivery.[6,13,78] There is a 10–20% greater increase in plasma volume (approximately 500 mL extra) compared with singletons.[6,13,78] As a result, total concentrations of serum proteins and electrolytes are reduced more than expected for singletons. Total intravascular protein mass, however, is unchanged, as are serum sodium, potassium, chloride, and osmolality. Greater increases in stroke volume and heart rate lead to greater increases in cardiac output than singleton pregnancies.[77,78] Most healthy women can adapt to these changes, but women with underlying medical problems and a multiple gestation may be at increased risk of serious consequences.

Preeclampsia/eclampsia

The incidence of gestational hypertension and preeclampsia is significantly increased in women carrying a multiple gestation compared with women carrying a singleton.[5,71,79,80] The average incidence in twins across studies performed from 1982 to 2003 is 16.7% (8.9–37%).[5,15,28,34,70,71,79,80–82] Women carrying triplets have greater placental mass and even higher rates of hypertensive complications, averaging 24.6%.[25,34,38,70,81,83–86] The reported incidence of preeclampsia among patients carrying more than one fetus would undoubtedly be even higher if more of these patients delivered closer to term.[70,80] The onset of preeclampsia is often earlier and the severity and complications are greater in women carrying a multiple gestation compared with a singleton.[15,25,70,80,81,83–85,87] For example, Lynch and colleagues found severe disease in 26% of their cohort of twins presenting with preeclampsia at an average gestational age of 34 weeks.[87] In a series of 100 triplets, 73% of the patients with preeclampsia had severe disease at a mean gestational age of 32.8 weeks.[25] Life-threatening complications such as eclampsia, hemolysis, elevated liver function, and low platelets (HELLP) syndrome, and AFLP occur more often among twins and triplets.[25,28,70,71,79,80,87] For this reason, we recommend obtaining uric acid, transaminases, serum creatinine, and complete blood count with platelets early in pregnancy and again early in the third trimester. Patients with borderline blood pressures or a low platelet count and a multiple gestation are assumed to have a potentially serious hypertensive complication and are evaluated frequently in order to avoid maternal and neonatal morbidity and mortality from missed or delayed diagnosis.[70] A woman with a multiple gestation and preeclampsia is more susceptible to volume overload and pulmonary edema because of the combination of increased afterload (caused by the vasospasm seen in preeclampsia), increased preload (caused by the baseline increase in plasma volume), and decreased baseline colloid oncotic pressure.[88] Therefore, management of preeclampsia in multiple gestations, although similar to management in singletons, must include extra precautions to control blood pressure and to avoid excessive intravenous fluid administration as well as closer monitoring for evidence of life-threatening complications.[70,79,83] There may be a role for expectant management of HELLP syndrome in multiple gestations to avoid a significantly preterm delivery of multiple fetuses using high-dose dexamethasone to improve platelet counts and suppress liver function abnormalities.[70,89]

Psychologic

The psychosocial effects of a multifetal pregnancy and birth can also be significant.[29,85,90–93] Families experience a great deal of stress including feelings of isolation, depression, frustration, and marital difficulties when caring for even healthy, full-term multiples. These feelings are compounded when the infants are preterm, often with handicaps or special needs.[90,91,94]

The complex ethical and bereavement issues that often arise in a multiple gestation (Table 13.6) require a particularly knowledgeable and sensitive approach. Couples often mourn not only for the lost fetus (or baby) or fetuses (or babies) but also for the unique celebrity status that being a parent of multiples confers. With subtotal loss, conflicting feelings of grief and joy can interfere with normal bonding to survivors, a fact that is commonly overlooked by healthcare providers and social supports.[92] In some situations, such as with multifetal pregnancy reduction (MFPR), couples experience grief reactions even when they are comfortable with their decision and do not regret it.[95,96] A detailed discussion of the reactions and responses to loss in the setting of multiple gestations is beyond the scope of this text, but a few pearls for healthcare providers are listed in Table 13.7.

Table 13.6 Loss scenarios in multiple gestations.

First- and second-trimester miscarriage of all fetuses
First-trimester loss of some fetuses (vanishing twin/triplet)
Multifetal pregnancy reduction (MFPR)
Later intrauterine demise of some or all fetuses
Selective or complete termination for anomalies
Expectant management with one or more anomalous fetuses
Complications of monochorionic twins
Intrapartum demise
Delivery at limits of viability
Sudden infant death syndrome (SIDS) (twice as common in twins as in singletons)
Accidental death (more common in multiples)

Adapted from ref. 92.

Table 13.7 A few management pearls for perinatal bereavement after multiple pregnancy loss.

Offer private experiences such as viewing, holding, bathing, and dressing with multiples individually and together (including deceased with survivors)
Offer prenatal mementos (i.e., ultrasound pictures) and matching mementos for each neonate
Offer photos of multiples alone, together, and with parents or other family members: color, black-and-white, digital, or 35 mm
Suggest computer-manipulated photos (Fig. 13.13), sketches, or pastels
Clarify parent preferences for the survivor's crib label (i.e., "twin A" or just "baby Jones")
Clarify parent desires to refer to survivors by the original or the remaining number of babies
Offer multiple-specific grief information and support resources (i.e., Center for Loss in Multiple Birth – www.climb support.org)

Adapted from ref. 92.

Economic

The cost of giving birth to multiple babies is significant for the healthcare system and for the families.[7,30,66,97,98] The expense does not increase linearly with the number of fetuses.[97,98] One study in the USA found the total charges for a triplet delivery to be almost threefold higher than for a twin delivery and 11-fold higher than for a singleton delivery.[30] The lifetime costs of feeding, clothing, and educating multiple children of the same age have not been quantified. Families often lose valuable income when the woman, pregnant with a multiple gestation, is forced to give up her job due to pregnancy complications or to the demands of caring for the children.

Obstetrical complications

Preterm labor

Preterm labor is markedly increased in multiple gestations, with an incidence ranging from 20% to 90%, depending on the study, the definitions used, and the number of fetuses.[7,28,66,71,85,97] The standard treatments for preterm labor have decreased margins of safety in multiple gestations because of the physiologic changes in the cardiovascular system of these women.[7,13,71,78] For example, the combination of pregnancy, multiple gestation, labor, and the administration of tocolytic agents can more than triple cardiac output compared with nonpregnant levels. Intravenous tocolysis, particularly with beta-mimetic agents, but also with magnesium sulfate, is associated with a host of serious cardiovascular and metabolic side-effects that are exaggerated in patients carrying a multiple gestation.[6,7,78,88,99] Volume overload is commonly a precipitating factor in the development of pulmonary edema in patients receiving tocolytics as well as hydration for treatment of preterm labor and, as mentioned previously, patients with a multiple gestation are at higher risk on account of their increased plasma volume.[78] Indeed, multiple gestation appears to have been a predisposing factor in over 19% of the reported cases of pulmonary edema occurring after the use of beta-sympathomimetic agents.[78] In addition, patients with a multiple gestation may be at higher risk for myocardial ischemia and arrhythmias while receiving intravenous beta-sympathomimetics. Maternal death, in this setting, has been reported to have occurred in at least three patients with a multiple gestation.[100]

Preterm premature rupture of membranes

Preterm premature rupture of membranes (PPROM) complicates approximately 14% of twin pregnancies[28,34] and 20% of triplet pregnancies.[25,28,34] The treatment for PPROM, which usually involves prolonged strict bedrest in the hospital, puts the mother at risk of infection, deep venous thromboses, and deconditioning, and is costly.

Hemorrhage

An increased rate of both antepartum and postpartum hemorrhage has been reported for multiple gestations.[28,71] Abruptio placentae, which occurs three times more often in twins than in singletons, is the major reason for the increased risk of antepartum hemorrhage.[13] Placenta previa, other than vasa previa, has not been shown to occur at higher rates in twins.[5] The risk of postpartum hemorrhage is twofold higher for women giving birth to twins,[71] and it occurs in up to 15% of women delivering triplets.[13,25] The average blood loss for a twin vaginal delivery is 500 mL higher than for a singleton.[6] Uterine atony due to overdistention from the multiple gestation is the major etiology. Therefore, patients need to be watched closely for the first 24–48 hours, and treatment, which is the same as in singletons, should be instituted promptly.

Cesarean delivery

More than 50% of twins, 75% of triplets, and almost all higher order multiple gestations are delivered by Cesarean section, often with a classical incision, primarily because of malpresentation.[6,28,66,71,101] There are numerous maternal complications that are increased in incidence in patients undergoing Cesarean delivery compared with patients having vaginal delivery. These include, but are not limited to: puerperal infection (endometritis, pelvic abscess, wound infection, and septic pelvic thrombophlebitis), wound dehiscence and evisceration, deep venous thrombosis, ileus, bowel obstruction, bladder catheter drainage, intraperitoneal or retroperitoneal hemorrhage, and increased need for transfusion of blood products. In a controlled study comparing twin with singleton pregnancies undergoing Cesarean delivery, endometritis was increased nearly threefold (13.1% versus 4.7%) and abdominal wound infections nearly twofold (5.6% versus 3.0%).[102]

Uterine rupture

One retrospective study found a 0% incidence of uterine rupture in patients with twins undergoing a trial of labor after a previous Cesarean section (vaginal birth after Cesarean section; VBAC).[101] A newer, multicenter, retrospective study confirmed the overall safety of attempted VBAC in twins with uterine rupture rates that are comparable to singletons.[103] Until a larger, prospective study is completed, a trial of labor is justifiable for patients with twins as long as they are monitored closely during the antepartum and intrapartum periods, and signs or symptoms of uterine rupture, such as repetitive severe variables or prolonged decelerations, are taken seriously.

Antepartum management

Multifetal pregnancy reduction

Multifetal pregnancy reduction (MFPR), which was introduced in the late 1980s, has proven to be a safe and effective procedure to reduce the maternal and perinatal morbidity and mortality associated with high-order multiple gestations.[34,37,50] It is most commonly performed by transabdominal or transvaginal injection of potassium chloride into the fetal thorax under ultrasound guidance late in the first trimester. The uppermost or technically easiest embryo is chosen for reduction unless one has a smaller crown–rump length or increased nuchal translucency, which can be an early indicator of an anomaly.[104,105] The overall pregnancy loss rates after the procedure are reported to be approximately 3.3–11.7%, depending on the starting and finishing number.[37,50] This must be compared with the background loss rates for high-order multiple gestations prior to viability, which range from 8% to 20%.[13,28] Although there is clear improvement in both maternal and fetal outcome for women with four or more fetuses who undergo the procedure, the medical benefit, although present, is less striking for women pregnant with triplets.[34,74] However, because there is clearly some improvement in outcome for triplets that undergo MFPR to twins, and some women may have compelling economic or psychological reasons for desiring the procedure, we believe that all mothers discovered to have more than two fetuses should be offered the procedure with appropriate counseling.[13,34] The final number of fetuses can safely be left at two or one depending on the woman's medical and emotional background.[37,50] There also appears to be some residual effect of the starting number of fetuses, as the overall pregnancy loss rates and incidence of complications, such as subsequent preterm labor and delivery, and fetal growth restriction, seem to increase in proportion to the starting number.[35,37] MFPR now gives women who find themselves pregnant with a high-order multiple gestation, often after years of emotionally, financially, and physically exhaustive infertility treatments, a chance of a good pregnancy outcome, but the availability of the procedure is not a substitute for judicious monitoring of ovulation induction and the use of advanced reproductive technologies. Patients need to be thoroughly counseled about the likelihood of conceiving multiple fetuses and the risks involved in carrying such a pregnancy before embarking on infertility therapies.

Prenatal diagnosis

Women with multiple gestations frequently have indications for prenatal diagnosis due to the higher incidence of congenital anomalies, the frequency of advanced maternal age, and the increased risk of aneuploidy in at least one fetus at younger ages.[7,13,50,51] The modalities that are available in multiple gestations are similar to those for singletons, although prenatal diagnosis in multiples has some unique problems.[7,50] The noninvasive modalities are ultrasound and biochemical marker screening. The ultrasound markers in twins are similar to those in singletons. As many multiple gestations are scanned early, there is an opportunity to diagnose some anomalies such as anencephaly even in the first trimester. A nuchal translucency thickness greater than 2.5 mm in the first trimester has been shown to be present in a large number of trisomic twin fetuses, as in singletons.[105] It has value, especially when combined with maternal age, as a noninvasive screen for Down syndrome.[13,105] A comprehensive fetal survey should be performed on each fetus at 18–20 weeks to rule out structural anomalies that are not detectable in the first trimester. Biochemical markers, as a screen for aneuploidy, have unproven validity in the setting of multiple gestations, particularly in those of high order, as the normal distributions for both first- and second-trimester proteins have not been established.[13,49] For example, a MSAFP of greater than 2.5 MoM, which is considered abnormal in singletons, occurs in 20–30% of patients with twins.[106] Elevations greater than 4 MoM in a twin gestation, however, are indications for further evaluation.[49] Thus, MSAFP screening alone does have some use in detecting open neural tube and abdominal wall defects in twins that are not the result of MFPR, where the levels are elevated due to the remains of one or more fetuses.

The three invasive methods available for prenatal diagnosis in singletons, chorionic villus sampling (CVS), amniocentesis, and percutaneous umbilical blood sampling (PUBS), are also available for multiple gestations, even those of high order. CVS has been shown to be safe and effective in multiples with loss rates (2–3%) that are similar to those with amniocentesis.[50] The potential problems include inadvertent sampling of the same fetus twice, contamination of one sample with villi from another, and inability to identify the fetus with an abnormal karyotype at a later date.[7,49,50] Some of these problems can be solved by using a combined transcervical and transabdominal route to sample different placentas and by careful ultrasound guidance.[49] The advantages, such as earlier diagnosis, and the disadvantages, such as forgoing amniotic fluid AFP analysis, are the same as for CVS in singletons. An additional use for CVS in high-order multiples is prior to MFPR procedures where it has been used without increasing loss rates from the procedure.[49,50] This saves couples the potential tragedy of finding out later that one of their remaining fetuses has a karyotypic abnormality when embryos that may have been normal were the ones chosen for reduction.

Standard amniocentesis for analysis of karyotype and AFP can be done in multiple gestations at 15–18 weeks with reported loss rates prior to 28 weeks of 2.8%, which are not significantly different from the background loss rates for twins.[49,107,108] Each fetus should be sampled as a separate procedure. To insure that the same fetus is not sampled twice, 1–3 mL of dilute indigo carmine can be injected into the first sac after the fluid is withdrawn.[49] If the second tap produces blue fluid, the same sac has been entered. It is not recommended that methylene blue or other agents be used because of some reports of fetal damage after their use.[49]

PUBS can be performed in twin gestations for the same indications as in singletons. The procedure can be technically difficult, and the cord of one fetus may not be accessible without traversing the sac of another. Although the exact risks of the procedure are not well defined in multiple gestations, the procedure has been performed safely, and there is experience in using it successfully for *in utero* fetal therapy in twins, such as for management of isoimmunization. Whichever method of prenatal diagnosis is chosen by the patient, it is imperative that fetal positions are clearly mapped, preferably by a drawn diagram that identifies the locations of the sacs, placentas, and fetuses, at the time of the procedure, and that the specimens are labeled accordingly. This will decrease the risk that the 'wrong' fetus will be chosen for termination if the parents elect such a procedure at a later date.

Selective termination

Once a fetal abnormality is diagnosed, management options will depend on the severity of the anomaly, the gestational age at the time, and the chorionicity. In the past, patients could either terminate the entire pregnancy, sacrificing the other normal fetus or fetuses, or expectantly manage the pregnancy. Currently, patients have the additional option of selective termination of the abnormal fetus only.[109,110] The procedure is similar to MFPR in which potassium chloride or another cardiotoxic agent is injected directly into the affected fetus's heart under direct ultrasound guidance. Loss of the entire pregnancy occurs in 5–6% of cases if the procedure is done in twins prior to 13 weeks and in 7–9% if the procedure is performed after 13 weeks.[109] Loss rates are slightly higher when the procedure is performed in triplets (12.5%).[109,110] Ongoing pregnancies generally have good outcomes for the remaining fetus or fetuses.[109] It is essential that the abnormal fetus be properly identified prior to the procedure, and a specimen of amniotic fluid or fetal blood should be sent for confirmation in cases of karyotype abnormalities. This injection procedure is not safe in MC gestations discordant for an anomaly because of morbidity and mortality in the survivors similar to that seen with spontaneous death of a monochorionic twin *in utero* (see discussion above). However, a selective termination can still be performed if the ultimate vascular connection between the two fetuses is interrupted by an umbilical cord ligation.[13,111] This can be accomplished using a percutaneous endoscopic technique and is most commonly done using bipolar coagulation.[112–114]

Antenatal care

Specialized clinics

The antepartum care of women carrying more than one fetus requires knowledge of all the maternal and fetal complications that can occur in these pregnancies. In addition, special attention to nutrition, preterm birth prevention, and fetal surveillance has been shown to decrease the perinatal morbidity and mortality that is seen with multifetal pregnancies.[115] In order to provide the most effective care, some have advocated the use of specialized multidisciplinary twin clinics or at least applications of vigilant management protocols.[15,116] The following discussion outlines the interventions that have been recommended to improve outcomes for multiple gestations.

Weight gain/nutrition

Patients pregnant with twins or more have extra nutritional demands.[117,118] It is recommended that supplemental iron (60–80 mg/day) and folate (1 mg/day) be given from the time of diagnosis in addition to standard prenatal vitamins.[15,118] Patients will also need additional calcium, especially in the third trimester, to support the developing skeletons of more than one fetus.[29,99,117] We advocate liberal use of calcium supplements as most patients have difficulty meeting the 1500–2000 mg/day requirement with diet alone. Zinc and magnesium supplementation may be beneficial as well. Increased fluid intake (at least 2 L/day) is necessary to support the expanded plasma volume, amniotic fluid volume, and metabolic demands of multiple gestation. Patients need a diet that is rich in protein (300–400 g/day) and calories (at least 1000 kcal/day) over the requirements for a singleton. Adequate maternal weight gain, especially in the first and second trimesters, has been associated with higher birthweights and better outcomes in multiple gestations.[15,116,118,119] It is currently recommended that women with twins gain 35–45 pounds (16–20 kg), or more if underweight or carrying more than two fetuses.[116–119] Counseling by a certified nutritionist, early in the first trimester, can help patients meet their body mass index (BMI)-based weight gain goals. Screening for gestational diabetes should be performed at 24–26 weeks. Strong consideration should be given to repeating a normal screen at 32 weeks in women with a multiple gestation.

Prevention of prematurity

Prevention, diagnosis, and treatment of preterm labor must be a major focus in the antepartum care of women carrying a multiple gestation as preterm birth is the leading cause of morbidity and mortality in this group. Education and interventions must begin early because most of the mortality (50–80%) occurs before 32 weeks, and the critical period of gestation appears to be between 26 and 29 weeks and between 600 and 900 g. Many methods of preventing premature birth have been explored, with varying levels of success, but little progress has been made. For example, the average gestational age of delivery for triplets (~33 weeks) has not improved since the 1940s.[1] Outcomes have vastly improved, but this is likely due to improvements in neonatal management. It becomes clear as we review current methods that are used to combat prematurity that further clinical investigation is needed.

Identification of patients at risk

The first step in preventing preterm birth is to identify those patients at greatest risk so that they can be targeted for intervention. This process should start with intensive education of the patient regarding the dangers of prematurity, the signs and symptoms of preterm labor, and easy access to a healthcare provider at all times. A cervical length of <25 mm at 24 weeks in twins is strongly predictive of preterm delivery.[15,120–122] A midtrimester short cervix has also been shown to be an increased risk for preterm delivery in triplets.[123] Therefore, the next steps in identifying patients with a multiple gestation who are even more likely to deliver prematurely are a knowledgeable risk assessment combined with serial cervical examinations, both manually and with transvaginal ultrasound.[123] Cervical lengths of at least 3.5 cm at 24 weeks in twins are associated with less than a 5% risk of delivery at less than 34 weeks.[124] Assessments should be made at least every 2 weeks starting in the second trimester in order to be effective. A suspicion of shortening or funneling on a transabdominal sonogram or a digital examination should be followed immediately by a transvaginal sonogram.

Many practitioners use costly home uterine activity monitoring (HUAM) in attempts to identify patients at risk for premature labor. This noninvasive modality is based on the knowledge that baseline uterine activity is increased in twin pregnancies, that there is an increase in the frequency of contractions as early as several weeks before the development of preterm labor, with an even greater rise 24 hours before,[125] and that women with twins are less likely to perceive their contractions.[15] However, the data showing the efficacy of HUAM are limited, even in multiple gestations, and some of the apparent benefit may be from the frequent nursing education and contact that accompanies the programs and not from the use of the monitor *per se*.[15,126]

The detection of fetal fibronectin (fFN) on a simple culture swab from the cervicovaginal secretions, which is commercially available, is a modality that identifies patients at risk for delivering in the near future. The best positive predictor is in twins with serially positive fFN and a short cervix.[120] The high negative predictive value of the test has been confirmed in multiple gestations.[120,127] Unnecessary interventions may be avoided in a patient with increased uterine activity but no cervical change and a negative fFN.[124]

Preventative measures

Cerclage

The placement of a purely prophylactic cerclage in all patients with a multiple gestation is not currently recommended. No benefit from the procedure has been demonstrated in twins without evidence of cervical incompetence.[6,13,121,128] Even in twins with a sonographically short cervix (≤2.5 cm), rescue cerclage placement does not clearly improve outcomes.[121] There is potentially more value to prophylactic cerclage in high-order multifetal pregnancies where the increased weight of the uterine contents may lead to cervical incompetence in patients who have no other risk factors for the condition. Although there are some data that support its use in the management of triplets and quadruplets,[129] there are no randomized clinical trials, and substantial data exist that show no benefit.[29,38,85] Prophylactic cerclage is not an intervention with proven benefit in patients pregnant with more than two fetuses and no history of incompetent cervix.[13]

Bedrest

Bedrest is one of the most commonly prescribed interventions to prevent prematurity in multiple gestations; yet, its efficacy is uncertain. For twins, in fact, prophylactic hospitalized bedrest appears to have no benefit, and it is costly and disruptive to families.[15,28,130,131] There are no randomized trials in higher order pregnancies, but modern management in the USA has essentially abandoned routine hospitalization for these pregnancies as well.[15,29,86,97] The value of prophylactic bedrest at home has not been formally studied, but it is part of the management in most studies of high order multiple gestations.[28,29,86,97] Modification of normal activity and increased rest periods throughout the day may prolong gestation and decrease the incidence of other complications such as hypertension and FGR, even in twins.[15,86] It is the author's opinion that recommendations to women carrying multiple fetuses regarding lifestyle modifications must be individualized depending on additional risk factors for pregnancy complications and the patient's home and work environment, and that strict bedrest and hospitalization be prescribed only when complications occur that warrant it.

Prophylactic tocolytic therapy

The use of currently available tocolytic agents as a prophylactic means to prevent preterm labor in multiple gestations is not supported by the literature.[15,7,132] Furthermore, there is significant risk associated with their use, which is exaggerated in multiple gestations, as discussed above.

Treatment of preterm labor

Tocolytics

Once preterm labor has been diagnosed, however, tocolysis is indicated. The medications, routes of administration, and contraindications are the same as in singleton pregnancies. Unfortunately, multiple gestation is frequently an exclusion criteria in studies that have evaluated the efficacy of tocolysis. Despite the paucity of scientific evidence in multiple gestations, experience has shown that tocolytic agents decrease uterine activity and prolong gestation by at least 24–48 hours in these pregnancies[15,133] and, thus, we believe they should be used to halt (or slow down) labor occurring prior to 34 weeks' gestation. Of course, these agents must be used with extra caution and monitoring in women with multiple gestations because of the increased risk of complications detailed above.[6,78,88]

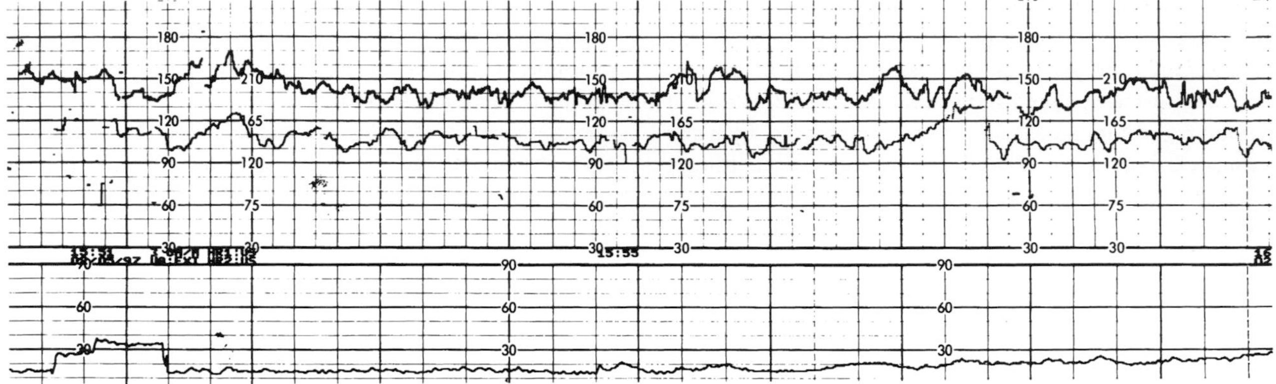

Figure 13.8 A simultaneously reactive twin nonstress test.

Steroids

The administration of betamethasone or dexamethasone within several hours to 7 days of birth between 24 and 34 weeks' gestation clearly decreases the incidence of respiratory distress syndrome, intraventricular hemorrhage, and necrotizing enterocolitis in singleton gestations.[134] The benefit in multifetal pregnancies has not been studied extensively, and there is some question as to whether the currently recommended doses are adequate, given the altered pharmacokinetics in these women.[134,135] However, no harm has been demonstrated, and it is therefore recommended that they be used liberally in multifetal pregnancies for the same indications as in singletons.[134] The efficacy and safety of weekly, prophylactic administration of antenatal steroids has not been demonstrated and is not currently recommended.[134]

Fetal surveillance

Ultrasound

The important uses of ultrasound in multiple gestations are outlined in Table 13.1. As discussed previously, an early sonogram is necessary to confirm the diagnosis, assess chorionicity, and establish good dating.[12] Another sonogram should be performed at 18–20 weeks to screen for anomalies, confirm the chorionicity, and assess the cervix. Frequent sonograms should be performed thereafter (every 3–4 weeks in an uncomplicated multiple gestation) to assess fetal growth, amniotic fluid volume, and cervical length.[15,136] If complications arise, or in particularly high-risk multiple pregnancies, sonograms should be performed more frequently and be done by sonologists experienced in the management of such complications.

Nonstress test

All multiple gestations are at some increased risk for unexplained demise and uteroplacental insufficiency, and they should therefore undergo antepartum fetal testing.[7,137] However, the gestational age at which tests of fetal well-being should be initiated, the frequency of testing, and the modality or combination of modalities that should be used varies depending on the presence of additional maternal or fetal risk factors.[7,15,136] At most centers, the nonstress test (NST) is the primary method, and it is performed at a minimum of weekly from 36 weeks in uncomplicated dichorionic multiples.[15,136] It has been proven to have the same validity in multiple gestations as in singletons and has some of the same problems, such as a high false-positive rate.[15,138] Monitors are available that allow simultaneous testing of multiple fetuses, which shortens testing time and allows for study of the *in utero* behavioral interactions between twins (Fig. 13.8).[136,139] The general principle that an abnormal screening test should be followed immediately by a more sensitive and specific test, such as vibroacoustic stimulation or biophysical profile, applies to multiples as well, but the interpretation and management of nonreassuring testing in a multiple gestation can be much more complex than in a singleton, particularly when the fetuses have discordant test results. Management recommendations must take into account the impact of immediate, often preterm, delivery on the healthy fetus, and the prognosis, which may be poor even with immediate delivery, of the fetus with concerning testing.

Contraction stress test

Although a contraction stress test (CST) may be performed safely in some cases of multiple gestation, this form of fetal surveillance is rarely used. Often, multiple pregnancies are complicated by conditions for which the CST is contraindicated, such as premature labor, abnormal placentation, or abnormal bleeding. If a spontaneous CST arises during a period of antepartum fetal heart rate testing, its interpretation may be of value.[136]

Biophysical profile

The fetal biophysical profile (BPP) is also a reliable method of fetal surveillance in multiples, even in those of high order, with comparable sensitivity and specificity to testing in singletons.[15,136,139] An advantage of using the BPP as an adjunct to the NST in multiple gestations is the ability to assess amniotic fluid volume which, if increased or decreased, may be the first sign of a problem, such as FGR or a twin–twin transfusion. Monochorionic multiple gestations, women with additional risk factors for uteroplacental insufficiency, and fetuses who are already known, from ultrasound, to have a growth problem should have at least an amniotic fluid volume assessment weekly.

Doppler ultrasound

The umbilical artery systolic/diastolic (S/D) ratio in twins is the same as the value in singletons throughout gestation.[12,13] Similar controversies exist regarding the use of umbilical artery Doppler velocimetry as a screening modality for fetal well-being in twins as in singletons. Some have shown that abnormal or discordant values can be detected 4–8 weeks earlier than other evidence of growth problems,[12,13,136,140] and that they are good predictors of poor perinatal outcome.[136,141] It has also been shown to be of use in the surveillance of the twin–twin transfusion syndrome.[12,136,141] However, the utility of Doppler velocimetry in concordant multiples has not been proven, and we feel that its use should be limited to those pregnancies at highest risk. Abnormal results may indicate more frequent surveillance, but other interventions should only be undertaken if a combination of all available test results warrants it.

Timing of delivery

Much controversy exists regarding the timing of delivery in multiple gestations. There is no evidence that fetuses "mature" faster just because they are sharing the same womb. For this reason, uncomplicated twins should not be electively delivered prior to 38 weeks, and there is no contraindication to expectant management until close to the due date as long as there is reassuring testing.[7,15] There is some evidence that twins have higher stillbirth rates and higher than expected rates of FGR after 38–39 weeks.[6,137] The elective delivery of higher order pregnancies, which is almost always by Cesarean section, can be justified slightly earlier, at 36–37 weeks. Many multiple gestations, however, are at higher risk as gestation progresses. Consideration should be given to earlier delivery in these situations, only after confirmation of fetal lung maturity, unless there is an absolute fetal or maternal indication for delivery. As in singletons, the presence of phosphatidylglycerol or a lecithin–sphingomyelin ratio ≥ 2.5 in amniotic fluid is indicative of fetal lung maturity. In at least 50% of twins, there is intersac discordance in lung maturity, so both sacs should be sampled if possible.[6,13,15,142]

Antepartum management of fetal complications

Monoamnionic gestations

Monoamnionic twins were traditionally associated with a mortality rate of 50%, which is predominantly the result of cord entanglement.[13,58,62,63] This occurs in at least 70% of cases and can happen at any time.[58] Contemporary management protocols that involve early diagnosis, ultrasound looking for evidence of cord compression and to evaluate fetal growth, frequent antepartum fetal testing with nonstress tests and continuous fetal monitoring for frequent variable decelerations, and delivery by Cesarean section for nonreassuring testing have decreased the mortality to 20%.[13,58,62,63] Most advocate delivery, usually by Cesarean section, as soon as fetal lung maturity is documented, usually around 34 weeks when mortality is low.[13,58,53] There is some justification for planned Cesarean delivery at 32 weeks.[143]

Conjoined twins

If the diagnosis of a conjoined twin is made early, the option of pregnancy termination should be offered. If the patient declines or if the diagnosis is made later, serial ultrasound and further evaluations such as echocardiography and magnetic resonance imaging (MRI) should be performed to help determine whether extrauterine life is possible, and if there is any chance of successful separation after birth. Management will depend on such assessments.[53,54] If conjoined twins have a possibility of survival, the best perinatal outcome will be achieved with Cesarean delivery, close to term, at a specialized tertiary care center.[54] Abdominal delivery is sometimes necessary, even for nonviable or demised conjoined twins, to avoid maternal trauma. Postnatal prognosis will depend on the site and degree of union, the presence or absence of any other major anomalies, and the degree of prematurity.[54]

Acardiac twins

The mortality for the pump twin in cases of acardia is greater than 50% and is universally lethal for the recipient.[13,59] The *in utero* treatment modalities that have been attempted include medical therapies, selective delivery, and umbilical cord blockade.[13,58,111] The most promising seems to be fetoscopic umbilical cord ligation, which has a relatively low failure rate but a high risk of preterm delivery due to rupture of membranes and preterm labor.[13,111] There is also a role for expectant management when the weight of the acardiac twin $[-1.66(\text{length}) + 1.21(\text{length}^2)]$ divided by the weight of the normal twin (using standard biometry), the twin-weight ratio (TWR), is more than 70%.[58,59] The pump twin needs close surveillance for evidence of cardiac failure and most likely will require early delivery.

Twin–twin transfusion syndrome

When a "stuck twin" is visualized on ultrasound, a fetal anomaly of that twin or a severe growth abnormality with placental insufficiency must be considered. Similarly, if isolated polyhydramnios is seen around one twin, an anomaly or infection may be the etiology. A diagnosis of TTTS should be reserved for those cases that demonstrate the multiple criteria discussed earlier. Once the syndrome is diagnosed with reasonable certainty, prognosis depends on the gestational age and the severity, but the mortality is generally well above 50%

without treatment.[58] A staging system based on the appearance of the bladder in the donor, Doppler values, and the presence of hydrops has some value in patient counseling and comparison of treatment protocols.[144] Four treatment options have been investigated. The first is decompression amniocentesis, whereby large quantities of amniotic fluid are serially removed from the recipient's sac.[145] This serves to decrease maternal respiratory embarrassment and preterm labor from the often massive polyhydramnios, and may reduce compressive forces on the umbilical cord leading to reversal of the shunt. Although some have reported improved outcomes with the procedure (78% survival), there is a question of abnormal neurologic outcome in a significant percentage of the survivors.[145] Another option is amniotic septostomy, which has outcomes similar to serial amniocentesis. There is the possibility of enlargement of the hole in the septum, resulting in an iatrogenic MA pair with its associated risks.[146] A more invasive modality is fetoscopic laser ablation of the anastomotic placental vessels, which has been reported to achieve a 60% survival rate with low neurologic morbidity in the survivors.[60,147–149] By ablating the vascular connections between the fetuses, the now functionally DC pair is probably less susceptible to neurologic injuries that can occur as a result of hypotension or other vascular alterations in a co-twin.[13] Two randomized trials have been performed, one demonstrating no difference in survival between serial amniocentesis and amniotic septostomy,[150] and one showing a significant benefit to laser therapy over serial amniocentesis.[148] The prognosis, including the potential for damage to the survivor in the event of a demise, should be discussed with the patient after the diagnosis is made when deciding between various management options. After therapy, weekly ultrasound and intensive fetal surveillance will be needed. The option of termination of pregnancy needs to be discussed due to the poor prognosis, even with therapy. Delivery should be undertaken as soon as fetal maturity is confirmed or for nonreassuring fetal testing.

Fetal growth restriction of one or more fetuses

When FGR afflicts one or more fetuses, management is similar to that of FGR in a singleton. If it is detected early in pregnancy, an anomaly should be ruled out by careful sonography and karyotype analysis. If it is secondary to uteroplacental insufficiency, the risks of prematurity must be weighed against the risks of continued stress *in utero*. Close fetal surveillance should ensue, with ultrasound examinations every 2 weeks to assess fetal growth, frequent nonstress and biophysical profile testing, and Doppler velocimetry. Delivery of the growth-retarded fetus should await fetal lung maturity of all the fetuses unless the testing is nonreassuring or the affected fetus fails to demonstrate any growth over time.

Growth discordance

The finding of discordant growth among fetuses in a multiple pregnancy is not necessarily pathologic or associated with poor outcome.[36,23,36,42–44] However, severe growth discordance (25–30%), particularly when there is evidence of FGR, is associated with increased morbidity and mortality.[36,42–44] Once etiologies for the discordance, such as TTTS or anomalies of one twin, are dismissed, it is difficult to predict which pairs are truly at risk. For this reason, multiples that are found to be discordant on ultrasound should be followed more frequently for fetal growth and undergo more frequent and earlier fetal testing.[17,13,42,151] As long as each fetus follows its own growth curve and testing is reassuring, there is no indication for early delivery.[6,13,43,151] Early intervention should be undertaken, however, even if premature, if there is progressive growth discordance or signs suggestive of immediate fetal danger.

Single fetal death *in utero*

The management of multiple gestation complicated by the death of one fetus depends on the gestational age at which the loss occurs, the potential cause of the demise, and the chorionicity. If the demise is caused by a pregnancy complication that is likely to affect the survivor, such as uncontrolled diabetes, maternal hypertension, or other medical problems, delivery should be strongly considered even if the fetus will be premature.[152] If the demise is caused by a problem that is unlikely to affect the survivor, such as a known fetal anomaly, expectant management with close surveillance is warranted.[57,58,152] With monochorionic gestations, there is a significant risk to the survivor, as discussed previously.[7,58,64,67] Even immediate delivery may not prevent neurologic deficits. If demise occurs prior to 32 weeks, intensive fetal surveillance should be performed with counseling regarding the substantial risk of morbidity in the survivor that may or may not be detectable on ultrasound or heart rate monitoring.[13,58] Ideally, delivery should be undertaken, even in the face of prematurity, if a complicated MC twin is likely to die shortly.[13] Maternal coagulation profiles should be followed periodically after a single fetal demise, although the risk of maternal DIC is low.[6,7,58,65]

Intrapartum management

Asynchronous birth

Most deliveries of multiple fetuses occur in close proximity to each other. There is a role, however, for delaying delivery of some fetuses after a very premature delivery of one. The criteria for attempting expectant management of the remaining fetuses include reasonable evidence of fetal well-being by heart rate monitoring and ultrasound, absence of signs of abruption or chorioamnionitis, and dichorionic placentation.[153] Although some have had success with the liberal use of antibiotics, tocolysis, and cerclage placement shortly after delivery,[153,154] these interventions are controversial.[155] Indocin, for 48–72 hours after delivery, does appear to work well as a tocolytic in this setting.[153,154] There is a reasonable chance (~50%) of achieving the delivery of a surviving infant or infants weeks after the loss of one in carefully selected patients who have been counseled about the potential risks.[153–155]

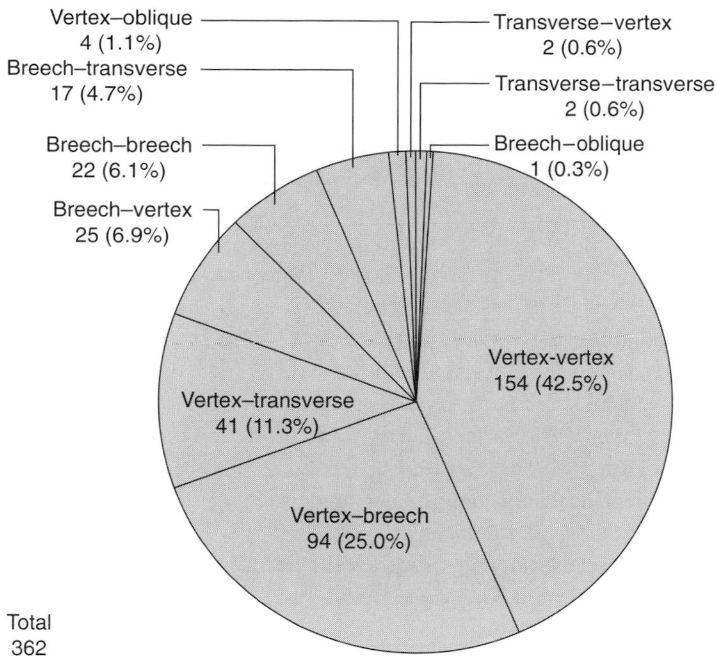

Figure 13.9 The relative occurrence rates of the possible combinations of twin presentations. From ref. 156.

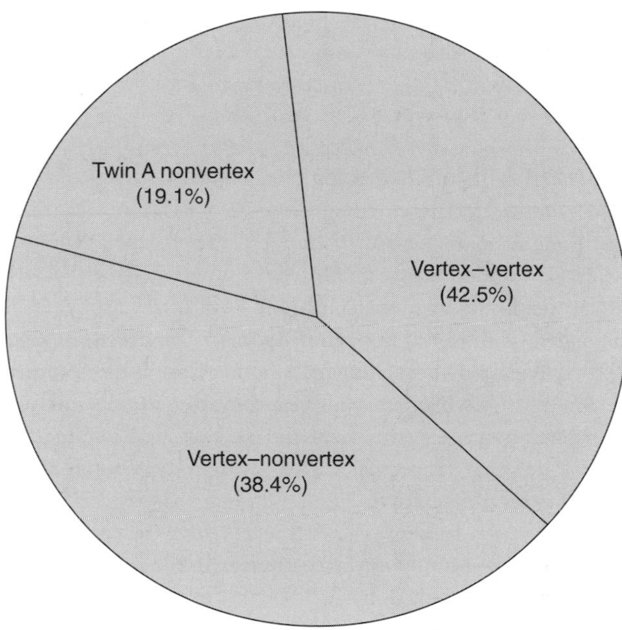

Figure 13.10 The relative occurrence rates of the three broad categories of twin presentations: vertex–vertex, vertex–nonvertex, and twin A nonvertex.

Mode of delivery

The delivery of all multifetal pregnancies, even the seemingly most uncomplicated, has the potential for serious complications including unanticipated malpresentations, cord accidents, abruptions, and postpartum hemorrhage. For this reason, women with more than one fetus should be delivered in centers with capabilities for intrapartum fetal monitoring both electronically and by real-time ultrasound, for immediate Cesarean delivery, and for neonatal resuscitation. Any meaningful discussion of the intrapartum management of twins should consider the relative presentations of twin A and twin B (Fig. 13.9).[156] The possible combinations are varied, but three broad categories provide a working classification: vertex–vertex, vertex–nonvertex, and nonvertex twin A (Fig. 13.10). The authors' management plan is illustrated in Figure 13.11.

Twin A vertex, twin B vertex

There is widespread agreement that vaginal delivery of vertex–vertex twins is appropriate.[13,155–157] Throughout labor, twin A can be monitored with a scalp electrode, once membranes have been ruptured, and twin B can be monitored with an external cardiotocograph. After delivery of twin A, electronic or sonographic monitoring of the fetal heart rate of twin B is carried out until its delivery. Further labor should bring the vertex of twin B into the pelvis, whereupon amniotomy is performed and vaginal delivery is accomplished. If labor has not resumed within 10 min after the delivery of twin A, careful oxytocin augmentation should be used.[158] Although the time interval between delivery of twins is not a critical factor in obtaining a successful outcome, as long as the well-being of the second twin is continuously assessed, there is a higher incidence of an umbilical cord pH less than 7.00 with longer intervals.[156–158] Cesarean delivery of either or both twins should be undertaken for the same indications as in singletons. The safety of internal podalic version with total breech extraction for a second vertex twin who is in distress has not been demonstrated and, therefore, cannot be recommended.[155]

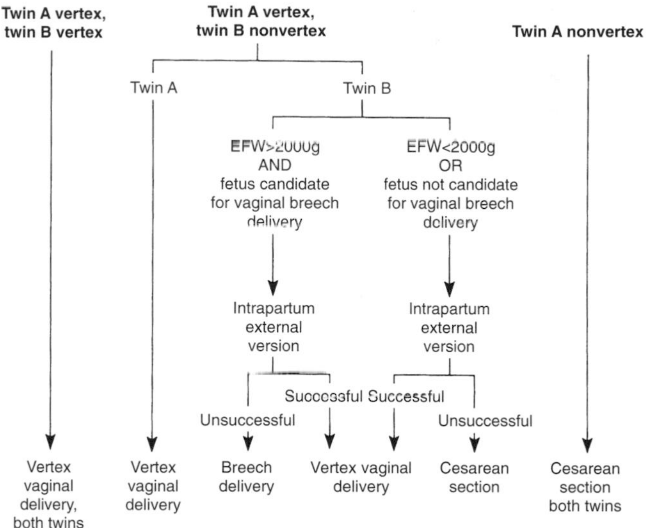

Figure 13.11 Outline of proposed intrapartum management of twin gestation. From ref. 156.

There is some controversy regarding the mode of delivery for very low birthweight infants, even if they are vertex–vertex.[155] However, there is an absence of data demonstrating that Cesarean section is beneficial.[13,156,157]

Twin A vertex, twin B nonvertex

There is no definitive conclusion at this time regarding the optimum management of the vertex–nonvertex twin gestation. One option is that of elective Cesarean delivery because of the possibility of birth trauma and birth asphyxia to the vaginally delivered nonvertex twin.[157] The preponderance of evidence, however, indicates that this is not necessary.[6,155,159–162] Two other options exist after vaginal delivery of the first twin: external cephalic version with subsequent vaginal delivery from the vertex presentation or total or assisted breech extraction.

Several series report a 70% success of external cephalic version for the second twin with good maternal and fetal outcomes.[155,156,160] When considering this option, sonographic assessment of the size of both fetuses should be made and, if twin B is much larger than twin A, the option of elective Cesarean section should be considered. If the patient is a candidate for labor, she should be strongly encouraged to have epidural anesthesia as abdominal wall relaxation will greatly aid attempts at version or breech delivery. The specific maneuver is shown in Figure 13.12. As the first twin is being delivered, the presentation and heart rate of the second twin should be evaluated with real-time ultrasound. Gentle pressure, either with the transducer or with one's hands, is used to guide the vertex toward the pelvis. The shortest arc between the vertex and the pelvic inlet should be followed initially. The version can be accomplished as either a forward or a backward roll, but undue force must be avoided in all patients. When the vertex is brought to the pelvic inlet, the membranes are ruptured and delivery is accomplished, with oxytocin augmentation as needed. If the version is unsuccessful, vaginal breech delivery or Cesarean section is performed depending on whether the fetus is a candidate for breech delivery (see below) and whether the status is reassuring.

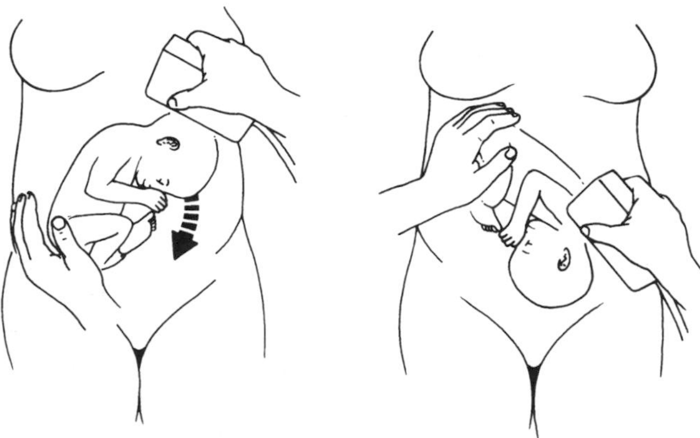

Figure 13.12 The maneuver of external version. From Chervenak FA, Johnson RE, Berkowitz RL, et al. Intrapartum external version of the second twin. *Obstet Gynecol* 1983;62:160.

Vaginal breech delivery of the second twin is the other option to avoid routine abdominal delivery of vertex–nonvertex twins.[155,156,159,162] For twins weighing more than 1500 g, several studies have had up to 95% success rates without any differences in outcome compared with second breech twins delivered by Cesarean section or second vertex twins delivered vaginally.[155,156,] In fact, one study showed improved outcomes and lower hospital charges for the breech extraction group.[162] Even in second breech twins weighing less than 1500 g, there is no evidence that Cesarean section is beneficial.[161,163] We recommend that vaginal breech delivery be performed for the second twin, after a failed version attempt, if the standard criteria for a vaginal breech are met. These include an adequate maternal pelvis, a flexed fetal head, and an estimated fetal weight of 1500–3500 g, and size that is not significantly larger than twin A.[113,155,159,163] If these criteria are not met, or if there is evidence of fetal distress, immediate Cesarean delivery should be performed.

Twin A nonvertex

Cesarean delivery is usually recommended for twins when the first is not vertex because the safety of vaginal delivery in this setting has not been established, and there is the potential complication of interlocking fetal heads.[155] Some have shown, however, that, if the criteria are met for vaginal delivery of a breech singleton, vaginal delivery of a breech first twin may be just as safe as abdominal delivery for the pair.[164]

Higher order births

There are some studies, albeit with small sample sizes, that report good outcomes for triplets that were allowed to deliver vaginally.[165,166] These studies clearly do not provide sufficient evidence to suggest that this is safe, especially given the skill that is required to perform such a delivery, and the increased perinatal mortality inherent with triplet and higher order gestations. Most still recommend Cesarean delivery for all high-order multiple gestations,[7,13,29,155] but the option should be available for motivated patients without other indications for elective Cesarean delivery.

Conclusion

The complexity of both maternal and fetal problems seen with multiple gestation argues for management of the antepartum and intrapartum periods by a multidisciplinary team of experienced personnel, including those skilled in prenatal diagnosis, obstetrical ultrasound, nutrition, prematurity assessment and prevention, and delivery (spontaneous, operative vaginal, and Cesarean deliveries). If complications arise at any time, it is particularly important to have physicians available who are experienced in the management of complications of multiple gestations to optimize successful outcomes and minimize morbidity and mortality.

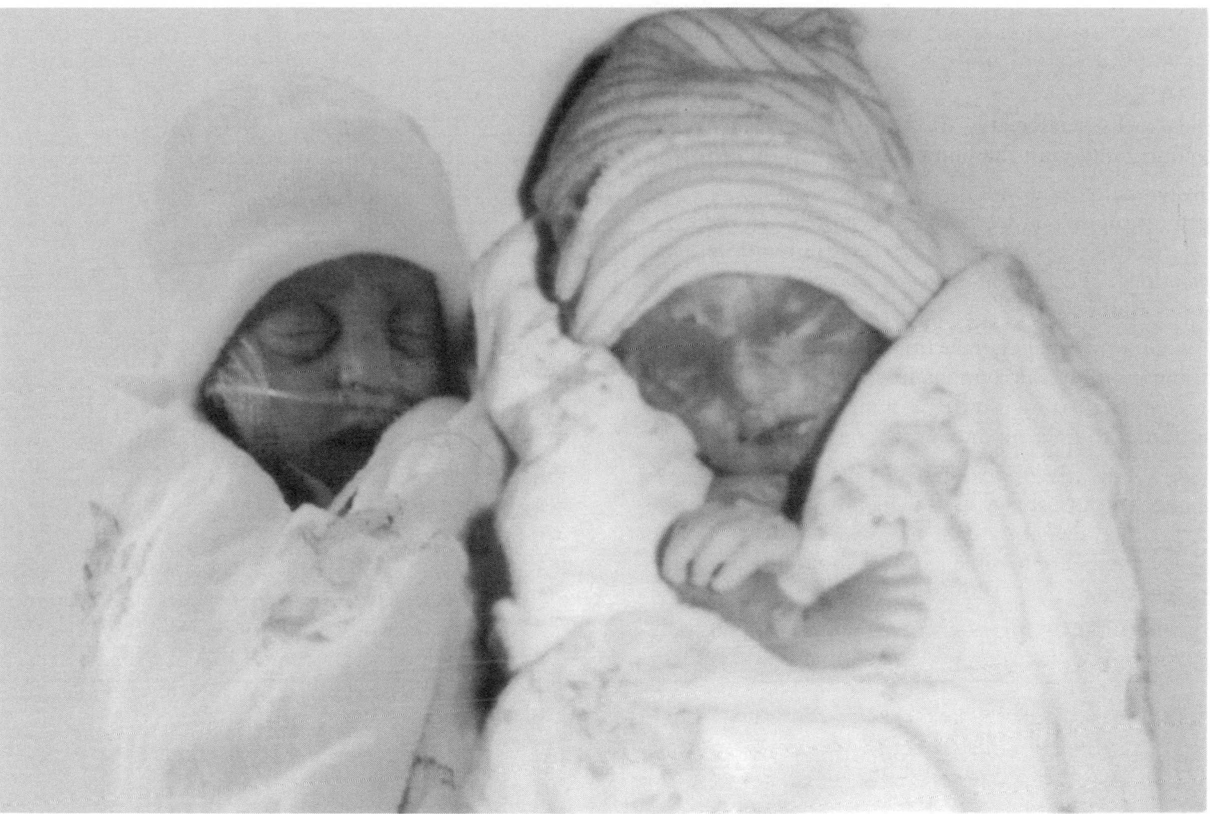

Figure 13.13 Example of twins together created by computerized manipulation of two individual photographs. Twin A (left) is the survivor of TTTS, and twin B (right) was stillborn. Image courtesy of Pam Schachter, with permission.

Key points

1 Widespread use of assisted reproductive technologies has led to dramatic increases in the incidence of twins and higher order multiple births.

2 Multiple gestations can be dizygotic (all diamnionic–dichorionic) or monozygotic (30% diamnionic–dichorionic, 70% diamnionic–monochorionic, or < 1% monoamnionic–monochorionic), or any combination.

3 Ultrasound is indispensable for the identification, assessment including determination of chorionicity, and management of multiple gestations.

4 Multiple gestations contribute significantly to perinatal morbidity and mortality.

5 The majority of twins and most higher order multiple gestations are born prematurely as a result of premature labor, preterm rupture of membranes, or fetal or maternal complications.

6 The risk of being born at a low and very low birthweight is much higher for a multiple because of both prematurity and fetal growth restriction, both of which contribute to morbidity and mortality.

7 Fetal complications such as growth restriction, intrauterine fetal demise, and congenital anomalies and complications unique to multiples, such as discordant growth and twin–twin transfusion syndrome, also lead to significant morbidity and mortality.

8 Maternal medical complications are exaggerated when carrying a multiple gestation.

9 Hyperemesis gravidarum, cholestasis, acute fatty liver of pregnancy, anemia, gestational diabetes, urinary tract infections, and cardiovascular complications occur more frequently and more severely in women carrying a multiple gestation.

10 The incidence of gestational hypertension and preeclampsia is several fold higher in women pregnant with a multiple gestation, and life-threatening complications occur more frequently and at earlier gestational ages.

11 Complex ethical and bereavement issues often arise in a multiple gestation, and psychological stress can be overwhelming.

12 The expenses associated with multiple birth increase exponentially with the number of fetuses.

13 Obstetrical complications such as preterm labor, preterm rupture of membranes, hemorrhage, and Cesarean delivery occur at high rates in multiple gestations, and their management poses additional risks to the mother.

14 Multifetal pregnancy reduction and selective termination are safe options for women who are pregnant with a high-order multiple gestation or who are found to have an anomaly in one fetus.

15 Both noninvasive modalities for prenatal screening such as nuchal translucency as well as invasive modalities for prenatal diagnosis such as CVS, amniocentesis, and cordocentesis are feasible and safe in multifetal pregnancies.

16 Antepartum care for women pregnant with a multiple gestation must focus on good nutrition with adequate supplementation, weight gain, and fluid intake as well as on preterm birth prevention with close surveillance for cervical change and fetal and maternal complications.

17 Antepartum fetal surveillance for multiple gestations must include serial sonograms for fetal growth and cervical length and tests of fetal well-being such as nonstress tests and biophysical profiles.

18 Multiple gestations should not be delivered "early" without documentation of fetal lung maturity unless specific maternal or fetal complications warrant it.

19 Therapeutic interventions such as laser ablation of anastomotic vessels and umbilical cord ligation in complicated monochorionic twins can improve outcomes.

20 Most twins presenting with A vertex can safely be delivered vaginally utilizing external cephalic version or total breech extraction when the second is nonvertex; however, the safest route of delivery for most higher order multiple gestations is by Cesarean section.

References

1 Martin JA, Hamilton BE, Suttton PD, et al. Births: final data for 2002. *Natl Vital Stat Rep* 2003;52(10):1–102.

2 Wilcox LS, Kiley JL, Melvin CL, et al. Assisted reproductive technologies: estimates of their contribution to multiple births and newborn hospital days in the United States. *Fertil Steril* 1996;65:361–366.

3 Markovitz J, Hershlag A. Multiple births resulting from assisted reproductive technologies in the United States, 1997–2001. In Blickstein I, Keith L, eds. *Multiple pregnancy: epidemiology, gestation, and perinatal outcome.* Abingdon: Taylor and Francis; 2005:58–67.

4 Jewell SE, Yip R. Increasing trends in plural births in the United States. *Obstet Gynecol* 1995;85:229–232.

5 Spellacy WN, Handler A, Ferre CD. A case control study of 1253 twin pregnancies from a 1982–1987 perinatal data base. *Obstet Gynecol* 1990;75:168–171.

6 Cunningham FG, Gant NF, Leveno KJ, et al., eds. Multifetal pregnancy. In: *Williams obstetrics,* 21st edn. New York: McGraw-Hill; 2001:chap. 30, pp. 765–810.

7 ACOG. Multiple gestation: complicated twin, triplet, and high-order multifetal pregnancy. *ACOG Pract Bull* 2004;56:869–883.

8 Benirschke K. The biology of the twinning process: how placentation influences outcome. *Semin Perinatol* 1995;19(5):342–350.

9 Benirschke K. Multiple gestation. Incidence, etiology, and inheritance. In: Creasy RK, Resnik R, eds. *Maternal–fetal medicine: principles and practice*, 3rd edn. Philadelphia, PA: W.B. Saunders; 1994:575–588.

10 Blickstein I, Jones C, Keith LG. Zygotic splitting rates after single-embryo transfers in in-vitro fertilization. *N Engl J Med* 2003;348:2366–2367.

11 Milki AA, Jun SH, Hinkley MD, et al. Incidence of monozygotic twinning with blastocyst transfer compared to cleavage-stage transfer. *Fertil Steril* 2003;79:503–506.

12 Divon MY, Weiner Z. Ultrasound in twin pregnancy. *Semin Perinatol* 1995;19(5):404–412.

13 Malone FD, D'Alton ME. Multiple gestation. Clinical characteristics and management. In: Creasy RK, Resnik, R eds. *Maternal–fetal medicine: principles and practice.* Philadelphia, PA: Elsevier; 2004:513–536.

14 Landy HJ, Keith LG. The vanishing twin: a review. *Hum Reprod Update* 1998;14:177–188.

15 Newman RB, Ellings JM. Antepartum management of the multiple gestation: the case for specialized care. *Semin Perinatol* 1995;19(5):387–403.

16 Bromley B, Bernacerraf B. Using the number of yolk sacs to determine amnionicity in early first trimester monochorionic twins. *J Ultrasound Med* 1995;14:415–419.

17 Finberg HJ. The "twin peak" sign. *J Ultrasound Med* 1992;11: 571–577.

18 Monteagudo A, Timor-Tritsch IE, Sharma S. Early and simple determination of chorionic and amniotic type in multifetal gestation in the first fourteen weeks by high-frequency transvaginal ultrasonography. *Am J Obstet Gynecol* 1994;170:824–829.

19 Sepulveda W, Sebire NJ, Odibo A, et al. Prenatal determination of chorionicity in triplet pregnancy by ultrasonographic examination of the ipsilon zone. *Obstet Gynecol* 1996;88:855–858.

20 Scardo JA, Ellings JM, Newman RB. Prospective determination of chorionicity, amnionicity, and zygosity in twin gestations. *Am J Obstet Gynecol* 1995;173:1376–1380.

21 Appleman Z, Manor M, Magal N, et al. Prenatal diagnosis of twin zygosity by DNA fingerprint analysis. *Prenat Diag* 1994; 14:307–309.

22 Powers WF, Kiely L. The risks confronting twins: a national perspective. *Obstet Gynecol* 1994;170:456–461.
23 Fraser D, Picard R, Picard E, et al. Birth weight discordance, intrauterine growth retardation and perinatal outcomes in twins. *J Reprod Med* 1994;39:504–508.
24 Kaufman GE, Malone FD, Harvey-Wilkes KB, et al. Neonatal morbidity and mortality associated with triplet pregnancy. *Obstet Gynecol* 1998;91:342–348.
25 Devine P, Malone F, Athanassiou A, et al. Maternal and neonatal outcome of 100 consecutive triplet pregnancies. *Am J Perinatol* 2001;18:225–235.
26 Kilpatrick SJ, Jackson R, Croughan-Minihane MS. Perinatal mortality in twins and singletons matched for gestational age at delivery at > or = 30 weeks. *Am J Obstet Gynecol* 1996;174: 66–71.
27 Alexander GR, Kogan M, Martin J, et al. What are the fetal growth patterns of singletons, twins, and triplets in the United States? *Clin Obstet Gynecol* 1998;41:114–125.
28 Seoud MAF, Toner JP, Kruithoff C, et al. Outcome of twin, triplet, and quadruplet *in vitro* pregnancies: the Norfolk experience. *Fertil Steril* 1992;57(4):825–834.
29 Elliott JP, Radin TG. Quadruplet pregnancy: contemporary management and outcome. *Obstet Gynecol* 1992:80:421–424.
30 Callahan TL, Hall JE, Ettner SI, et al. The economic impact of multiple gestation pregnancies and the contribution of assisted reproduction techniques to their incidence. *N Engl J Med* 1994;334:244–249.
31 Grumbach K, Coleman BG, Arger PH, et al. Twin and singleton growth patterns compared using ultrasound. *Radiology* 1986; 158:237–241.
32 D'Alton ME, Dudley DKL. Ultrasound in the antepartum management of twin gestation. *Semin Perinatol* 1986;10:30–38.
33 Rodis JF, Vintzilcos AM, Campbell WA, et al. Intrauterine fetal growth in concordant twin gestations. *Am J Obstet Gynecol* 1990;162:1025–1029.
34 Smith-Levitin M, Kowalik A, Birnholz J, et al. Selective reduction of multifetal pregnancies to twins improves outcome over nonreduced triplet gestations. *Am J Obstet Gynecol* 1996;175: 878–882.
35 Depp R, Macones GA, Rosenn MF, et al. Multifetal pregnancy reduction: evaluation of fetal growth in the remaining twins. *Am J Obstet Gynecol* 1996;174:1233–1240.
36 Blickstein I. Intrauterine growth. In: Blickstein I, Keith LG, eds. *Multiple pregnancy: epidemiology, gestation and perinatal outcome.* Abingdon: Taylor and Francis; 2005:505–513.
37 Evans MI, Berkowitz RL, Wapner RJ, et al. Improvements in outcomes of multifetal pregnancy reduction with increased experience. *Am J Obstet Gynecol* 2001;184:97–103.
38 Francois K, Sears C, Wilson R, et al. Twelve year experience of quadruplets at a single institution. *Am J Obstet Gynecol* 2001;S184:113.
39 Rodis JF, Arky L, Egan JF, et al. Comprehensive fetal ultrasonographic growth measurements in triplet gestations. *Am J Obstet Gynecol* 1999;181:1128–1132.
40 Min SJ, Luke B, Gillespie B, Min L, et al. Birth weight references for twins. *Am J Obstet Gynecol* 2000;182:1250–1257.
41 Min SJ, Luke B, Min L, et al. Birth weight references for triplets. *Am J Obstet Gynecol* 2004;191:809–814.
42 Vergani P, Locatelli A, Ratti M, et al. Preterm twins: what threshold of birthweight discordance heralds major adverse outcome: *Am J Obstet Gynecol* 2004;191:1441–1445.
43 Blickstein I, Keith LG. Neonatal mortality rates among growth-discordant twins, classified according to the birthweight of the smaller twin. *Am J Obstet Gynecol* 2004;190:170–174.
44 Hollier LM, McIntire DD, Leveno KJ. Outcome of twin pregnancies according to intrapair birthweight differences. *Obstet Gynecol* 1999;96(6):1006–1010.
45 Jacobs AR, Demissie K, Jain NJ, et al. Birthweight discordance and adverse fetal and neonatal outcomes among triplets in the United States. *Obstet Gynecol* 2003;101:909–914.
46 Machin GA. Advanced placental examination of twins and higher-order multiple pregnancies. In: Blickstein I, Keith LG, eds. *Multiple pregnancies: epidemiology, gestation, and perinatal outcome.* Abingdon: Taylor and Francis; 2005:179–192.
47 Hill LM, Guzick D, Chenevey P, et al. The sonographic assessment of twin growth discordancy. *Obstet Gynecol* 1994;84: 501–504.
48 Schinzel AA, Smith DW, Miller JR. Monozygotic twins and structural defects. *J Pediatr* 1979;95:921.
49 Wapner RJ. Genetic diagnosis in multiple gestations. *Semin Perinatol* 1995;19(5):351–362.
50 Brambati B, Tului L, Camurri L, et al. First trimester fetal reduction to a singleton infant or twins: outcome in relation to final number and karyotyping before reduction by transabdominal chorionic villus sampling. *Am J Obstet Gynecol* 2004;91(16): 2035–2040.
51 Meyers C, Adam R, Dungan J, et al. Aneuploidy in twin gestations: when is maternal age advanced? *Obstet Gynecol* 1997; 89:248–251.
52 Nance WE. Malformations unique to the twinning process. *Prog Clin Biol Res* 1981;69:123.
53 Oleszcuk JJ, Oleszcuk AK. Conjoined twins. In: Blickstein I, Keith LG, eds. *Multiple pregnancy: epidemiology, gestation, and perinatal outcome.* Abingdon: Taylor and Francis; 2005:58–67.
54 Mackenzie TC, Cromblehome TM, Johnson MP et al. The natural history of prenatally diagnosed conjoined twins. *J Pediatr Surg* 2002;37:303.
55 Sepulveda W, Munoz H, Alcalde JL. Conjoined twins in a triplet pregnancy: early diagnosis with three-dimensional ultrasound and review of the literature. *Ultrasound Obstet Gynecol* 2003;22:199–204.
56 Denbow ML, Cox P, Taylor M, et al. Placental angioarchitecture in monochorionic twin pregnancies: relationship to fetal growth, fetofetal transfusion syndrome, and pregnancy outcome. *Am J Obstet Gynecol* 2000;182:417–426
57 Bajoria R, Wigglesworth J, Fisk NM. Angioarchitecture of monochorionic placentas in relation to the twin-twin transfusion syndrome. *Am J Obstet Gynecol* 1995;172:856–863.
58 D'Alton ME, Simpson LL. Syndromes in twins. *Semin Perinatol* 1995;19(5):375–386.
59 Moore TR, Gale S, Benirschke K. Perinatal outcome of forty-nine pregnancies complicated by acardiac twinning. *Am J Obstet Gynecol* 1990;163:907–912.
60 De Lia J, Fisk N, Hecher K, et al. Twin-to-twin transfusion syndrome – debates on the etiology, natural history and management. *Ultrasound Obstet Gynecol* 2000;16:210–213.
61 Hecher K, Ville Y, Snijders R, et al. Doppler studies of the fetal circulation in twin-twin transfusion syndrome. *Ultrasound Obstet Gynecol* 1995;5:318–324.
62 Allen VM, Windrim R, Barrett J, et al. Management of monoamniotic twin pregnancies: a case series and systematic review of the literature. *Br J Obstet Gynaecol* 2001;108:931–936.

63 Shvecky D, Ezra Y, Schenker J, et al. Monoamniotic twins: an update on antenatal diagnosis and treatment. *J Matern Fetal Neonatal Med* 2004;16:180–186.

64 Nicolini U, Poblete A. Single intrauterine death in monochorionic twin pregnancies. *Ultrasound Obstet Gynecol* 1999;14: 297–301.

65 Santema JG, Swaak AM, Wallenburg HCS. Expectant management of twin pregnancy with single fetal death. *Br J Obstet Gynaecol* 1995;102:26–30.

66 Gonen Y, Blankier J, Casper RF. The outcome of triplet, quadruplet and quintuplet pregnancies managed in a perinatal unit: obstetric, neonatal, and follow-up data. *Am J Obstet Gynecol* 1990;162:454–459.

67 Pharoah PO, Adi Y. Consequences of in-utero death in twin pregnancy. *Lancet* 2000;335:1597–1602.

68 Gonzalez MC, Reyes H, Arrese M, et al. Intrahepatic cholestasis of pregnancy in twin pregnancies. *J Hepatol* 1989;9:84–90.

69 Duff P. Acute fatty liver of pregnancy. In: Clark SL, Cotton DB, Hankins GDV, et al., eds. *Critical care obstetrics*, 2nd edn. Cambridge, MA: Blackwell Scientific Publications; 1991;484–497.

70 Smith-Levitin M, Vohra N. Hypertensive disorders during multiple gestations. In: Blickstein I, Keith LG, eds. *Multiple pregnancy: epidemiology, gestation, and perinatal outcome.* Abingdon: Taylor and Francis; 2005:444–450.

71 Conde-Agudelo A, Belizan JM, Lindmark G. Maternal morbidity and mortality associated with multiple gestations. *Obstet Gynecol* 2000;95:899–904.

72 Simpson EL, Lawrenson RA, Nightingale AL, et al. Venous thromboembolism in pregnancy and the puerperium: incidence and additional risk factors from a London perinatal database. *Br J Obstet Gynaecol* 2001;108:56–60.

73 Spellacy WN, Buhi WC, Birk SA. Human placental lactogen levels in multiple pregnancies. *Obstet Gynecol* 1978;52: 210–212.

74 Sivan E, Maman E, Homko CJ, et al. Impact of fetal reduction on the incidence of gestational diabetes. *Obstet Gynecol* 2002; 99:91–94.

75 Schwartz DB, Daoud Y, Zazula P, et al. Gestational diabetes mellitus: metabolic and blood glucose parameters in singleton versus twin pregnancies. *Am J Obstet Gynecol* 1999;181:912–914.

76 Rovinsky JJ, Jaffin H. Cardiac output and left ventricular work in multiple pregnancy. *Am J Obstet Gynecol* 1966;95: 781.

77 Veille JC, Morton MJ, Burry KJ. Maternal cardiovascular adaptations to twin pregnancy. *Am J Obstet Gynecol* 1985;153:261.

78 Nizard J, Arabihn B. Maternal cardiovascular adaptation. In: Blickstein I, Keith LG, eds. *Multiple pregnancies: epidemiology, gestation, and perinatal outcome.* Abingdon: Taylor and Francis; 2005:436–443.

79 Coonrod DV, Hickok DE, Zhu K, et al. Risk factors for preeclampsia in twin pregnancies: a population based cohort study. *Obstet Gynecol* 1995;85:645–650.

80 Sibai BM, Hauth J, Caritis S, et al. Hypertensive disorders in twin versus singleton gestations. National Institute of Child Health and Human Development Network of Maternal–Fetal Medicine Units. *Am J Obstet Gynecol* 2000;182:938–942.

81 Mastrobattista JM, Skupski DW, Monga M, et al. The rate of severe preeclampsia is increased in triplet as compared to twin gestations. *Am J Perinatol* 1997;14:263–265.

82 Fitzsimmons BP, Bebbington MW, Fluker MR. Perinatal and neonatal outcomes in multiple gestations: assisted reproduction versus spontaneous conception. *Am J Obstet Gynecol* 1998; 79:1162–7.

83 Hardardottir H, Kelly K, Bork MD, et al. Atypical presentation of preeclampsia in high-order multifetal gestations. *Obstet Gynecol* 1996;87:370–374.

84 Skupski DW, Nelson SW, Kowalik A, et al. Multiple gestations from *in vitro* fertilization: successful implantation alone is not associated with subsequent preeclampsia. *Am J Obstet Gynecol* 1996;175:1029–1032.

85 Lipitz S, Reichman B, Paret G, et al. The improving outcome of triplet pregnancy. *Am J Obstet Gynecol* 1989;161:1279–1284.

86 Adams DM, Sholl JS, Haney EL, et al. Perinatal outcome associated with outpatient management of triplet pregnancy. *Am J Obstet Gynecol* 1998;178:843–847.

87 Lynch A, McDuffie R, Murphy J, et al. Preeclampsia in multiple gestation: the role of assisted reproductive technologies. *Obstet Gynecol* 2002;99:445–451.

88 Poggi SH, Barr S, Cannum R, et al. Risk factors for pulmonary edema in triplet pregnancies. *J Perinatol* 2003;23:462–465.

89 Heller CS, Elliot JP. High-order multiple pregnancies complicated by HELLP syndrome. *J Reprod Med* 1997;42:743–746.

90 Bryan EM. The consequences to the family of triplets or more. *J Perinat Med* 1991;19:24–28.

91 Garel M, Salobir C, Blondel B. Psychological consequences of having triplets: a four year follow-up study. *Fertil Steril* 1997; 67:1162–1165.

92 Pector EA, Smith-Levitin M. Bereavement: grief and psychological aspects of multiple birth loss. In: Blickstein I, Keith L, eds. *Multiple pregnancy: epidemiology, gestation and perinatal outcome.* Abingdon: Taylor and Francis; 2005:862–873.

93 Spillman JA. Antenatal and postnatal influences on family relationships. In: Sandband AC, ed. *Twin and triplet psychology: a professional guide to working with multiples.* New York: Routledge; 1999:19–35.

94 Kollantai JA. Coping with the impacts of death in multiple birth In: Blickstein I, Keith LG, eds. *Multiple pregnancy: epidemiology, gestation and perinatal outcome.* Abingdon: Taylor and Francis; 2005:874–876.

95 Schreiner-Engel P, Walther VN, Mindes J, et al. First-trimester multifetal pregnancy reduction: acute and persistent psychologic reactions. *Am J Obstet Gynecol* 1995;172:541–547.

96 Bryan E. Loss in higher multiple pregnancy and multifetal pregnancy reduction. *Twin Res* 2002;5:169–174.

97 Newman RB, Hamer C, Miller C. Outpatient triplet management: a contemporary review. *Am J Obstet Gynecol* 1989;161: 547–555.

98 Chelmow D, Penzias AS, Kaufman G, et al. Costs of triplet pregnancy. *Am J Obstet Gynecol* 1995;172:677–682.

99 Levav AL, Chan L, Wapner RJ. Long-term magnesium sulfate tocolysis and maternal osteoporosis in a triplet pregnancy: a case report. *Am J Perinatol* 1998;15:43–46.

100 Hudgens DR, Conradi SE. Sudden death associated with terbutaline sulfate administration. *Am J Obstet Gynecol* 1993;169: 120–121.

101 Miller DA, Mullin P, Hou D, et al. Vaginal birth after cesarean section in twin gestation. *Am J Obstet Gynecol* 1996;175: 194–198.

102 Suonio S, Huttunen M. Puerperal endometritis after abdominal twin delivery. *Acta Obstet Gynecol Scand* 1994;7:26–27.

103 Cahill A, Stamilio D, Pare E, et al. Vaginal birth after cesarean (VBAC) in twin gestation pregnancies: is it safe? *Am J Obstet Gynecol* 2005;184:97.

104 Weissman A, Achiron R, Lipitz S, et al. The first trimester growth-discordant twin: an ominous prenatal finding. *Obstet Gynecol* 1994;84:110–114.

105 Pandya PP, Hilbert F, Snijders RJM, et al. Nuchal translucency thickness and crown–rump length in twin pregnancies with chromosomally abnormal fetuses. *J Ultrasound Med* 1995;14: 565–568.

106 Johnson JM, Harman CR, Evans JA, et al. Maternal serum α-fetoprotein in twin pregnancy. *Am J Obstet Gynecol* 1990; 162:1020–1025.

107 Ghidini A, Lynch L, Hicks C, et al. The risk of second-trimester amniocentesis in twin gestations: a case–control study. *Am J Obstet Gynecol* 1993;169:1013–1016.

108 Pruggmayer MR, Jahoda MG, Van der Pol JG, et al. Genetic amniocentesis in twin pregnancy: results of a multicenter study of 529 cases. *Ultrasound Obstet Gynecol* 1992;2:6–10.

109 Evans MI, Goldberg JD, Horenstein J, et al. Selective termination for structural, chromosomal, and mendelian abnormalities: international experience. *Am J Obstet Gynecol* 1999;181: 893–897.

110 Eddleman K, Stone J, Lynch L, et al. Selective termination of anomalous fetuses in multiple pregnancies: 200 cases at a single center. *Am J Obstet Gynecol* 2001;185:S79.

111 Quintero RA, Goncalves L, Johnson MP, et al. Percutaneous umbilical-cord ligation in complicated monochorionic multiple gestations. *Am J Obstet Gynecol* 1996;174:326.

112 Taylor MJO, Shalev E, Tanawattanacharoen S, et al. Ultrasound-guided umbilical cord occlusion using bipolar diathermy for stage III/IV twin–twin transfusion syndrome. *Prenat Diagn* 2002;22:70–76.

113 Nicolini U, Poblete A, Boschetto C, et al. Complicated monochorionic twin pregnancies: experience with bipolar cord coagulation. *Am J Obstet Gynecol* 2001;185:703–707.

114 Deprest JA, Audibert F, Van Schoubroeck D, et al. Bipolar coagulation of the umbilical cord in complicated monochorionic twin pregnancy. *Am J Obstet Gynecol* 2000;182:340–345.

115 Meyer B, Elimian A, Royek A. Comparison of clinical and financial outcomes of triplet gestations managed by maternal-fetal medicine versus community physicians. *Am J Obstet Gynecol* 2001;185:S102.

116 Luke B, Mislunas R, Anderson E, et al. Specialized prenatal care and maternal and infant outcomes in twin pregnancy. *Am J Obstet Gynecol* 2003;189:934–938.

117 Sharma G, Ziubrank K. Nutritional adaptation. In: Blickstein I, Keith LG, eds. *Multiple pregnancy: epidemiology, gestation and perinatal outcome.* Abingdon: Taylor and Francis; 2005: 427–435.

118 Brown JE, Carlson M. Nutrition and multifetal pregnancy. *J Am Diet Assoc* 2000;100:343–348.

119 Luke B, Hediger ML, Nugent C, et al. Body mass index-specific weight gain associated with optimal weights in twin pregnancies. *J Reprod Med* 2003;48(4):217–224.

120 Goldenberg RL, Iams JD, Miodovnik M, et al. The preterm birth prediction study: risk factors in twin gestations. National Institute of Child Health and Human Development Maternal–Fetal Medicine Units Network. *Am J Obstet Gynecol* 1996;175: 1047–1053.

121 Newman RB, Krombach RS, Myers MC, et al. Effect of cerclage on obstetric outcome in twin gestations with a shortened cervical length. *Am J Obstet Gynecol* 2002;186:634–640.

122 Souka AP, Heath V, Flint S, et al. Cervical length at 23 weeks in twins in predicting spontaneous preterm delivery. *Obstet Gynecol* 1999;94:450–454.

123 McElrath T, Kaimal A, Benson C. Gestational age at delivery of pregnancies as a function of cervical length throughout gestation. *Am J Obstet Gynecol* 2001;185:S250.

124 Yang JH, Kuhlman K, Daly S, et al. Prediction of preterm birth by second trimester cervical sonography in twin gestations. *Ultrasound Obstet Gynecol* 2000;15:288–291.

125 Newman RB, Gill PJ, Campion S, et al. The influence of fetal number on antepartum uterine activity. *Obstet Gynecol* 1989;73:695–699.

126 Dyson DC, Danbe KH, Bamber JA, et al. Monitoring women at risk of preterm labor. *N Engl J Med* 1998;338:15–19.

127 Oliviera T, de Souza E, Mariani-Neto C, et al. Fetal fibronectin as a predictor of preterm delivery in twin gestations. *Int J Gynecol Obstet* 1998;62;135–139.

128 Dor J, Shalev J, Mashiach S, et al. Elective cervical suture of twin pregnancies diagnosed ultrasonically in the first trimester following induced ovulation. *Gynecol Obstet Invest* 1982;13: 55–60.

129 Goldman GA, Dicker D, Peleg A, et al. Is elective cerclage justified in the management of triplet and quadruplet pregnancy? *Aust NZ J Obstet Gynecol* 1989;29:9–12.

130 MacLennan AH, Green RC, O'Shea R. Routine hospital admission in twin pregnancy between 26 and 30 weeks gestation. *Lancet* 1990;335:267–269.

131 Crowther CA. Hospitalization and bedrest for multiple pregnancies (a Cochrane review). In: *The Cochrane Library*, Issue 4. Oxford: Update Software, 2003.

132 Ashworth MF, Spooner SF, Verkuyl DA, et al. Failure to prevent preterm labor and delivery in twin pregnancy using prophylactic oral salbutamol. *Br J Obstet Gynecol* 1990;97:878–882.

133 Rayburn W, Piehl E, Schork MA, et al. Intravenous ritodrine therapy: a comparison between twin and singleton gestations. *Obstet Gynecol* 1986;67:243–248.

134 National Institutes of Health Consensus Development Conference Statement. Effect of corticosteroids for fetal maturation on perinatal outcomes, February 28–March 2. 1994. *Am J Obstet Gynecol* 1995;173:246–252.

135 Ballabh P, Lo ES, Kumari J, et al. Pharmacokinetics of betamethasone in twins and singleton pregnancy. *Clin Pharmacol Ther* 2002;71:39–45.

136 Devoe LD, Ware DJ. Antenatal assessment of twin gestation. *Semin Perinatol* 1995;19(5):413–423.

137 Sairam S, Costeloe K, Thilaganathan B. Prospective risk of stillbirth in multiple-gestation pregnancies: a population-based analysis. *Obstet Gynecol* 2002;100:638–641.

138 Kim ES, Croom CS, Devoe LD. Prognostic accuracy of fetal testing in twin pregnancies. *Am J Obstet Gynecol* 1994;170:320.

139 Elliott JP, Finberg JH. Biophysical profile testing as an indicator of fetal well-being in high-order multiple gestations. *Am J Obstet Gynecol* 1995;172:508–512.

140 Degani S, Gonen R, Shapiro I, et al. Doppler flow velocimetry waveforms in fetal surveillance of twins: a prospective longitudinal study. *J Ultrasound Med* 1992;11:537–541.

141 Gaziano EP, Knox E, Bebdel RP. Is pulsed Doppler velocimetry useful in the management of multiple gestation pregnancies? *Am J Obstet Gynecol* 1991;164:1426–1433.

142 Whitworth NS, Magann EF, Morrision JC. Evaluation of fetal lung maturity in diamniotic twins. *Am J Obstet Gynecol* 1999; 180:1438–1441.

143 Peek MJ, McCarthey A, Kyle P, et al. Medical amnioreduction with sulindac to reduce cord complications in monoamniotic twins. *Am J Obstet Gynecol* 1997;176:334–336.
144 Quintero RA, Morales WJ, Allen MH, et al. Staging of twin–twin transfusion syndrome. *J Perinatol* 1999;19:550–555.
145 Mari G, Roberts A, Detti L, et al. Perinatal morbidity and mortality rates in severe twin-twin transfusion syndrome: results of the international amnioreduction registry. *Am J Obstet Gynecol* 2001;185:708–715.
146 Johnson JR, Rosi KQ, O'Shaughnessy RW. Amnioreduction versus septostomy in twin–twin transfusion syndrome. *Am J Obstet Gynecol* 2001;185:1044–1047.
147 Ville Y, Hecher K, Gagnon A, et al. Endoscopic laser coagulation in the management of severe twin-to-twin transfusion syndrome. Br J *Obstet Gynecol* 1998;105:446–453.
148 Senat MV, Deprest J, Boulvain M, et al. Endoscopic laser surgery versus serial amnioreduction for severe twin-to-twin transfusion syndrome. *N Engl J Med* 2004;351:136–144.
149 Quintero RA, Bornick PW, Allen MH, et al. Selective laser photocoagulation of communicating vessels in severe twin-twin transfusion syndrome in women with an anterior placenta. *Obstet Gynecol* 2001;97:477–481.
150 Moise KJ Jr, Dorman KF, Lamvu G, et al. A randomized trial of septostomy versus amnioreduction in the treatment of twin–twin transfusion syndrome. *Am J Obstet Gynecol* 2005; 193:2183.
151 Blickstein I. The definition, diagnosis, and management of growth discordant twins: an international consensus survey. *Acta Genet Med Gemellol* 1991;40:345–351.
152 Gaucherand P, Rudigoz RC, Piacenza JM. Monofetal death in multiple pregnancies: risks for the co-twin, risk factors and obstetrical management. *Eur J Obstet Gynecol Reprod Biol* 1994;55:111–115.
153 Farkouh LJ, Sabin ED, Heybourne KD, et al. Delayed interval delivery: extended series from a single maternal–fetal medicine practice. *Am J Obstet Gynecol* 2000;183:1499.
154 Platt JS, Rosa C. Delayed interval delivery in multiple gestations. *Obstet Gynecol Surv* 1998;54:343–348.
155 Udom-Rice I, Skupski DW, Chervenak FA. Intrapartum management of multiple gestation. *Semin Perinatol* 1995;19(5): 424–434.
156 Chervenak FA, Johnson RE, Youcha S, et al. Intrapartum management of twin gestation. *Obstet Gynecol* 1985;65:119–124.
157 Prins RP. The second-born twin: can we improve outcomes? *Am J Obstet Gynecol* 1994;170:1649–1656.
158 Leung TY, Tam WH, Leung TN, et al. Effect of twin-to-twin delivery interval on umbilical cord blood gas in the second twins. *Br J Obstet Gynaecol* 2002;109:63–67.
159 Fishman A, Grubb DK, Kovacs BW. Vaginal delivery of nonvertex second twin. *Am J Obstet Gynecol* 1993;168:861–864.
160 Tchabo JG, Tomao T. Selected intrapartum external cephalic version of the second twin. *Obstet Gynecol* 1992;79:421–423.
161 Davidson L, Easterling T, Jackson JC, et al. Breech extraction of low-birthweight second twins: can cesarean section be justified: *Am J Obstet Gynecol* 1992;166:497–502.
162 Mauldin JG, Newman RB, Mauldin PD. Cost-effective delivery management of the vertex and nonvertex twin gestation. *Am J Obstet Gynecol* 1998;179(4):864–869.
163 Winn HN, Cimino J, Powers J, Intrapartum management of nonvertex second-born twins: A critical analysis. *Am J Obstet Gynecol* 2001;185:1204–1208.
164 Blickstein I, Goldman RD, Kupfermine M. Delivery of breech-first twins: a multicenter retrospective study. *Obstet Gynecol* 2000;95:37–42.
165 Dommerques M, Mahieu-Caputo D, Mandelbrot L, et al. Delivery of uncomplicated triplet pregnancies: is the vaginal route safer? *Am J Obstet Gynecol* 1995;172:513–517.
166 Alamia V, Royek AB, Jaekle RK, et al. Preliminary experience with a prospective protocol for planned vaginal delivery of triplet gestations. *Am J Obstet Gynecol* 1998;179:1133–1135.

14 Biology of normal and deviant fetal growth

Andrée Gruslin and the late Carl A. Nimrod

Fetal growth is the result of a complex interplay of various factors, which include genetic, environmental, maternal, nutritional, placental, and endocrine influences. Over 40 specific factors have been shown, through animal studies, epidemiological, and observational data, to influence fetal growth.[1] The importance of identifying the determinants of fetal growth is highlighted by the fact that fetal growth restriction remains the second leading cause of perinatal mortality, and is further enhanced by the association between low birthweight (LBW) and adult-onset diseases.[2] Epidemiologic studies have demonstrated that individuals born with a LBW have an increased risk of cardiovascular diseases and diabetes in adulthood. Conversely, there has also been a positive association reported between high birthweight and breast cancer risk as, for instance, women who weighed more than 4000 g at birth have been shown to have a risk of breast cancer 3.5 times higher than those who weighed less than 3000 g.[3–5] These associations between birthweight and adult-onset diseases support the hypothesis that *in utero* events may result in alterations in the programming of the fetus itself or of its metabolic milieu, thereby resulting in significant adult diseases. Increasing laboratory and epidemiologic evidence of the *in utero* origins of these diseases makes it necessary that we understand the factors involved in fetal growth regulation and examine how they may interact as they carry long-term consequences for future health. This chapter will focus on the current literature describing the influences of maternal, genetic, environmental, endocrine, and placental factors on fetal growth, and will examine how these factors are involved in aberrant growth patterns such as growth restriction and macrosomia.

Genetic influences

Elements from both the maternal and the paternal genome are required for normal fetal growth and development. Recent data have demonstrated that, for certain genes, only one allele is functional. This is referred to as genetic imprinting, an epigenetic mechanism by which one of the two alleles of a gene is expressed according to its parental origin. The allele that is silenced is called imprinted. In the murine model, over 60 imprinted genes have been identified, and the majority influence fetal growth directly. This has led to the suggestion that imprinting may also be an important regulatory factor in human fetal growth. In fact, recent human studies have demonstrated that most maternally imprinted genes act as growth suppressors (e.g., H19, p57), whereas paternal ones act as growth promoters (e.g., insulin-like growth factor 2, IGF-2).[6] It has been postulated that imprinting occurs because of conflicts between the maternal and paternal genome and nutrient transfer to the fetus from the mother. Thus, paternally expressed genes result in fetal growth promotion at the expense of the mother, whereas genes that are maternally expressed would have the opposite effect. The most striking evidence of the importance of this mechanism lies in the influence of IGF-2 imprinting and its disorder on human fetal growth (Table 14.1). It has been shown that biallelic expression of IGF-2 leads to overgrowth of the fetus, which is recognized clinically as Beckwith–Wiedemann syndrome (Fig. 14.1), characterized by large birthweight, organomegaly, macroglossia, and neonatal hypoglycemia.[7] Conversely, in the mouse, deletion of the paternal IGF-2 allele has been shown to cause fetal growth restriction.[8] The mechanisms by which imprinting is altered include chromosomal deletion/duplication, point mutations, and uniparental disomy (UPD). The last refers to a situation in which chromosome fragments originate from a single parent. Murine studies have shown that, for some specific fragments, abnormal fetal growth occurred, suggesting that this portion of the chromosome carried an imprinted gene.[6,9,10] There are several examples of human imprinted genes associated with UPD. In humans, UPD has been observed for most chromosomes, although only a few are associated with an abnormal phenotype (often growth restriction), again suggesting that these carry an imprinted gene.[7] Specific examples include Prader–Willi syndrome, Angelman syndrome, and Silver–Russell syndrome (see Table 14.2).

There is evidence from the literature of an influence of maternal genotype on fetal growth. These genetic influences

Table 14.1 Evidence of a role for the IGF system in human fetal growth.

Homozygous deletion of exons 4 and 5 in the IGF-1 gene results in severe intrauterine growth restriction (IUGR) and postnatal growth failure
Biallelic expression of the IGF-2 gene leads to Beckwith–Wiedemann syndrome
Both IGFs are present in the fetal circulation very early and expressed in the placenta
Positive correlation between cord serum IGF-1 concentration and fetal size
Birthweight positively correlated with IGFBP-3 and negatively with IGFBP-1
Human IUGR associated with increased IGFBP-1 and -2 and decreased IGFBP-3
↑ IGFBP-1 at decidual–placental interface in severe preeclampsia/IUGR
↑ Circulatory levels of IGFBP-1 up to six times in severe preeclampsia
↑ IGFBP-1 in IUGR at term and antenatally (cordocentesis)
↓ PAPP-A leads to ↓ birthweight (PAPP-A protease of IGFBPs)

Summary of various evidence from human studies supporting the role of the IGF system in the regulation of fetal growth. This includes the involvement of IGF-1 and -2 as well as their binding proteins and the proteases, which themselves modulate these binding proteins. IGFBP, insulin-like growth factor binding protein; PAPP-A, pregnancy associated plasma protein A.

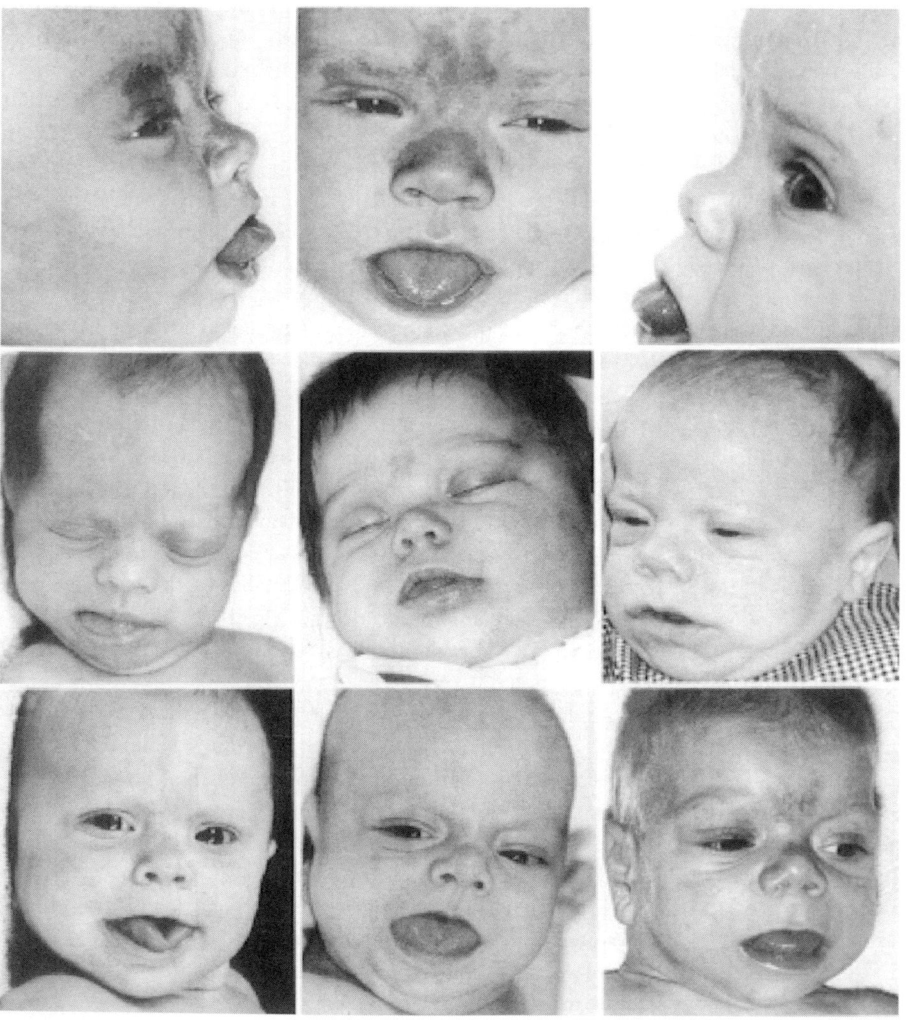

Figure 14.1 Infant with Beckwith–Wiedemann syndrome. Note the obvious macrosomia related to overexpression of IGF. From Wiedemann HR, Kunze J. *Clinical syndromes*, 3rd edn. Mosby-Wolfe Publishers; 1997:148–149.

are likely those involved in maternal size determination and metabolism, as evidenced by the fact that maternal height is correlated with birthweight and probably reflects its influence on uterine size and perhaps blood flow.[11] What is however becoming clear is that maternal phenotype, which results in physical constraints, probably plays an even more important role in fetal growth regulation.[12] This is evidenced by the cross-breeding studies between horses and ponies in which it was shown that, given the same fetal genotype, growth was greater when occurring in a large animal compared with a

Table 14.2 Clinically relevant outcomes of uniparental disomy in the human.

UPD	Outcome
Maternal UPD2	IUGR
Paternal UPD6q24	Diabetes (transient neonatal)
Maternal UPD7	Silver–Russell syndrome
Paternal UPD11p15	Beckwith–Wiedemann syndrome
Maternal UPD14	IUGR
Paternal UPD14	Short-limbed dwarfism
Maternal UPD15	Prader–Willi syndrome
Paternal UPD15	Angelman syndrome
Maternal UPD16	IUGR
Maternal UPD20	IUGR

Uniparental disomy represents one mechanism that can influence gene imprinting and therefore fetal growth.

small one.[13] Furthermore, studies of outcomes from assisted reproductive technologies using ova donation clearly demonstrated that birthweight correlated with the height and weight of the birth mother and not the donor.[14] From an evolutionary standpoint, this represents an adaptive mechanism preventing fetal overgrowth and the resulting maternal and fetal complications. This also suggests to the clinician that the interplay between maternal genotype and phenotype that influences birthweight must be recognized as a significant confounding variable in the interpretation of data from pregnancies that are the result of assisted reproductive technologies.

Conversely, paternal factors are thought to have very little influence over fetal growth. Human pedigree studies have demonstrated very little effect of paternal factors on birthweight. Studies of paternal height and weight have also concluded that only a very small effect on fetal weight was present. In a more recent report, paternal height was related to birthweight, with a small effect, an increase of 10 g/cm increase in paternal height, being apparent.[15] This therefore accounted for a very small amount of the variation in birthweight. As paternal weight and body mass index (BMI), which are acquired characteristics, did not influence birthweight, it was suggested that it was paternal genotype (a determinant of height) that played a small role in fetal growth. Again, the fact that this effect is small is highly desirable from an evolutionary standpoint as it prevents fetal overgrowth in mothers whose physical determinants would not allow it.

Fetal genotype, on the other hand, is an important regulator of growth. This is supported by the aberrant birthweight seen in chromosomally abnormal fetuses. Indeed, the average birthweight of fetuses with trisomy 13 is 2400 g; for those with trisomy 18, it is 2240 g and, finally, for trisomy 21, 2894 g.[16] This is believed to be mediated by a decrease in cellular proliferation leading to generalized hypoplasia. The cell cycle of trisomic fetuses has been shown to be slower, with a 50% reduction in the G2 phase and a generally decreased rate of DNA synthesis.[17] Other evidence of the importance of fetal genotype lies in the fact that fetal gender influences birthweight, as male fetuses are approximately 175 g heavier than females at term. Confined placental mosaicism (CPM) results from a chromosomal error located only in the placenta and has been shown to increase the risk of fetal growth restriction. It has been reported that up to 20% of cases of fetal growth restriction are associated with CPM, which can itself be associated with UPD.[14] Therefore, in cases of unexplained fetal growth restriction, a placental examination looking for CPM may provide useful information.

Maternal influences

Various maternal factors affect fetal growth. These include maternal anthropometry, overall health, nutritional status, and genotype as described above. Several studies have clearly demonstrated correlations between birthweight and maternal height, prepregnant weight, and weight gain during gestation.[11,18] However, the absence of a correlation between maternal weight gain and birthweight in very obese patients is noteworthy. This also applies to women with gestational diabetes possibly resulting from decreased maternal insulin sensitivity. In addition, birthweight has also been shown to increase with increasing parity, perhaps secondary to the cumulative effects of previous pregnancies on maternal metabolism.

Good maternal health is essential for proper placental implantation and normal fetal growth and development, as it allows the woman to respond and adapt appropriately to changes related to the establishment and maintenance of pregnancy.

In a recent review of the effect of exercise in pregnancy, Clapp[19] demonstrated that, in healthy, fit pregnant women, exercise (particularly regular, weightbearing, strenuous) was associated with improved maternal and fetal outcomes. It was proposed that regular physical activity improved placental growth as well as the normal physiologic changes of pregnancy. Furthermore, as exercise resulted in intermittent decreases in uterine blood flow along with a very small decrease in nutrient supply, those fetuses were leaner at birth but more tolerant of the physiologic stresses of pregnancy and labor.

Conversely, maternal health factors limiting oxygen and nutrient delivery to the fetus do have a significant negative impact on fetal growth. For instance, women with cyanotic heart disease, preeclampsia, or significant pulmonary diseases tend to have smaller infants as well as an increased risk of LBW infants. One of the most common maternal medical conditions worldwide that alters fetal growth is anemia.[20–22] In a recent study involving 629 women, 313 of whom were anemic, the risk of LBW and intrauterine growth restriction (IUGR) was increased by 2.2 times and 1.9 times respectively.[20] This is consistent with many other studies in which severe anemia was associated with a 200- to 400-g decrease in birthweight. Several mechanisms have been proposed to explain this association[23] including:

- Norepinephrine/cortisol: others have shown that iron deficiency anemia increases norepinephrine release, which can stimulate CRH and cortisol, known to have a negative effect on fetal growth. Furthermore, norepinephrine infusion in the sheep model results in a reduction in fetal protein synthesis and accretion.
- Chronic hypoxia: severe anemia may result in a reduction in oxygen transfer to the fetus, thereby impacting on fetal growth.
- Increased oxidative stress: through this mechanism, oxidative damage to erythrocytes could result as well as endothelial dysfunction, further impeding fetal growth.
- Increased infection; iron deficiency anemia has been shown to have a negative influence on B and T cells, neutrophils, and natural killer (NK) cells, thereby increasing susceptibility to infection. Maternal infection itself has been shown to activate the fetal hypothalamic–pituitary axis, as evidenced by increased cord blood concentrations of cortisol and dehydroepiandrostenedione sulfate, thereby again negatively affecting fetal growth.

Maternal nutrition is responsible for the availability of nutrients for the fetoplacental unit. Its importance is highlighted by the fact that fetal growth restriction is seen as a result of severe maternal undernutrition in many developing countries and that the incidence of LBW is higher in women with eating disorders.[1,24] Women exposed to the Dutch famine of 1944–1945 delivered LBW infants, but only if exposed in the third trimester of pregnancy. Placental growth was also reduced with the same exposure, but was increased in women exposed to the famine during their first trimester. This suggested that the influence of maternal nutrition on fetal growth depends upon the severity of the insult and its timing, as well as its influence on placental growth. Human and animal studies of maternal undernutrition have shown significant alterations in placental size and development, thereby affecting fetal growth directly. For instance, human maternal undernutrition has been associated with decreased placental volume, chorionic villous area, fetal capillary surface area, and volume density of trophoblasts.[25,26] These changes all correlated with LBW and thus represent a mechanism by which fetal growth is altered. Furthermore, in a recent study of maternal food restriction in the guinea pig model, a decrease in the total surface area of the placenta available for substrate exchange was demonstrated.[27] This correlated with fetal weight, suggesting that impaired placental transfer of nutrients to the fetus is involved in the process of growth restriction. In addition, the same study also reported an increase in the thickness of the placental barrier for diffusion, also contributing to altered growth through a decrease in substrate transfer to the fetus. It has been suggested that some of these changes may be mediated through alterations in growth factors such as IGF-2.[26,28]

At this time, it remains unclear whether nutritional deficiencies in specific dietary components have a greater impact on fetal growth compared with an overall deficiency. What is becoming more evident, however, is the importance of micronutrient intake on fetal growth and the role that nutrient–gene interactions may have in this process.[29] Some of the more important micronutrients studied to date include folate, zinc, iron, copper, as well as vitamins E and A. Of these, zinc has been shown to be critical for insulin packaging and secretion, and its deficiency has resulted in fetal growth restriction.[24,30] Both copper and iron can alter fetal development by the generation of free radicals, whereas their deficiency results in an accumulation of antioxidant enzymes. Vitamin E, an important regulator of insulin sensitivity, also contributes to fetal growth regulation, whereas vitamin A's role is through the stimulation of growth hormone postnatally and possibly of placental growth hormone prenatally.[29] Although this last mechanism is not entirely clear, the effects of vitamin A deficiency on prenatal growth are supported by its association with asymmetrical fetal organ growth as well as reductions in the relative masses of fetal lungs, heart, and liver in animal models.[29] The influence of micronutrients on human fetal growth has recently been investigated in a study of 797 pregnant women in rural India.[31] The authors showed that supplementation of their diet with micronutrient-rich foods such as green leafy vegetables, fruits, and milk was associated with improved birthweight. Interestingly, the intake of green leafy vegetables and fruits at 28 weeks correlated with birthweight, whereas a positive correlation with birthweight was shown for fat and milk intakes at 18 weeks. This suggests that there are likely different nutrient requirements for fetal growth at different stages of development, possibly owing to developmentally regulated tissue growth.

Interestingly, more evidence is accumulating suggesting an interaction between gene expression during fetal growth and nutrient availability.[1,32] For instance, folate deficiency leads to a decrease in remethylation of homocysteine to methionine. As *S*-adenosylmethionine is a methyl donor, its absence or decrease results in dysregulation of important developmental genes (imprinting defects) and defective DNA synthesis. This is further supported by animal studies including that by Gluckman and Pinal et al.[24] in which methyl-supplemented diets fed to pregnant mice altered the expression of an imprinted gene specific to the coat color of their offspring. As DNA methylation is important in the regulation of gene imprinting, it is likely that folic acid, through this process, is involved in fetal growth determination.

Several studies have also examined the influence of maternal fish and seafood consumption on fetal growth.[33–35] This potential association originated from the observation that birthweights tend to be higher in regions of the world such as the Faroe and Orkney Islands where there is a high maternal intake of marine foods. It has been proposed that the n-3 fatty acids from fish and seafood might enhance fetal growth by improving placental perfusion through an increase in the ratio of prostacyclins to thromboxanes, which itself reduces blood viscosity.[35] To date, two large epidemiological studies (Denmark and Faroe Islands) have shown a positive correlation between fish intake and birthweight.[36] In agreement with this, a more recent report from south-west England revealed a decrease in the incidence of fetal growth restriction with increasing fish consumption, but failed to show an association between birthweight and fish intake after adjusting for confounding variables.[35] Conversely, others have shown either no effect or even a reduction in birthweight associated with fish consumption.[33] These conflicting reports may be explained by the lack of adjustments for confounding variables, and may also result from the presence of pollutants in marine foods from certain regions. Indeed, fish is known to be a major source of polychlorinated biphenyls (PCBs), which have been shown to lead to fetal growth restriction in animal models.[33] Research in this area is therefore required and needs to take into account all the variables affecting fetal growth such as smoking, as well as evaluating the presence of pollutants in fish and seafood.

Finally, in the context of maternal influences on fetal growth, caffeine intake has also been examined with much discrepancy between studies.[37,36] This again often resulted from difficult and imprecise evaluation of maternal intake and failure to control for other important variables. The effect of caffeine on fetal growth is supported by the fact that it can cross the placental barrier and has a slow metabolism in pregnancy with a half-life of 10 hours at 17 weeks increasing to 18 hours in the third trimester. Finally, the fact that neither the placenta nor the fetus can metabolize caffeine further supports its negative influence on fetal growth. Although the exact mechanism by which this might occur has not been fully elucidated, it is likely that it involves a reduction in intervillous blood flow[37] and possibly an increase in oxygen consumption, as noted in preterm infants treated with caffeine for apnea.[36] Although, again, more information is needed on the impact of maternal caffeine intake, it appears so far that at least moderate consumption does not significantly decrease fetal growth, but that a negative impact could be seen with maternal consumption of over 600 mg daily.[37] The literature also suggests synergism between caffeine and cigarette smoke, as evidenced by a more significant influence of caffeine in women who smoke.[37]

Growth factors

IGF family

Adequate fetal growth is dependent upon a balanced interplay of positive and negative regulators originating from the fetal, placental, and maternal compartments. Of these, the IGF family plays an important role. The components of this family include IGF-1 and IGF-2, as well as two receptors (type 1 and 2) and six high-affinity binding proteins (IGFBP 1–6) and their proteases (e.g., PAPP-A), which ultimately regulate the bioavailability of these two growth factors. IGF-1 and -2 are peptides, produced mostly by the adult and fetal livers. They are both potent mitogens and important regulators of tissue growth and differentiation.[1,24] However, they are developmentally regulated in a different manner and have different actions. For instance, IGF-2 is an imprinted gene, expressed from the paternal allele, and is important for embryonic as well as placental growth and likely involved in cellular differentiation of specific organs such as the fetal pancreas. Biallelic expression of IGF-2 leads to overgrowth syndromes such as Beckwith–Wiedemann, whereas deletion of IGF-2 in the mouse is associated with decreased placental and fetal growth.[9] In the murine model again, Constancia et al.[8] have demonstrated that deletion of the placental transcript of IGF-2 resulted in decreased passive permeability of nutrients, leading to restricted placental and, subsequently, fetal growth. More recently, the same model was used to demonstrate that the placental IGF-2 gene is directly involved in the regulation of the diffusional characteristics of the placenta. The authors suggested that decreased IGF-2 expression might indeed be responsible for cases of idiopathic fetal growth restriction that are characterized by decreased placental diffusion capacity.[28]

Conversely, IGF-1 regulates fetal growth in the later part of pregnancy. It has been shown that IGF-1 promotes fetal substrate uptake, inhibits catabolism, and alters placental metabolism through an inhibition of lactate production, thereby improving placental transfer of nutrients.[24] The importance of IGF-1 in human fetal growth regulation is highlighted by a report of an infant born with homozygous deletions of exons 4 and 5 in this gene. This resulted in severe fetal growth restriction as well as postnatal growth failure.[38] In addition, deletion of IGF-1 in the mouse has also been shown to lead to fetal growth deficiency which persists postnatally, contrary to animals with IGF-2 deletions that are born at 60% of the size of wild-type controls but whose postnatal growth normalizes.[8] This suggests that IGF-2 is the dominant regulator during early intrauterine life, whereas IGF-1 influences the process later in gestation and postnatally.

Several factors influence IGF's actions, including their binding proteins and associated proteases, their receptor status, the presence of other hormones and, most importantly, maternal nutrition. Indeed, fetal IGF-1 is sensitive to fetal insulin levels, which are regulated by glucose concentrations (Figs 14.2 and 14.3). This is well illustrated by a series of sheep experiments in which maternal undernutrition was associated with a decrease in fetal IGF-1 and resulted in absent fetal growth. However, upon glucose or insulin infusion, fetal IGF-1 levels returned to normal.[24] In addition, it has been demonstrated in numerous studies that a positive correlation exists between cord blood IGF-1 levels and birthweight and

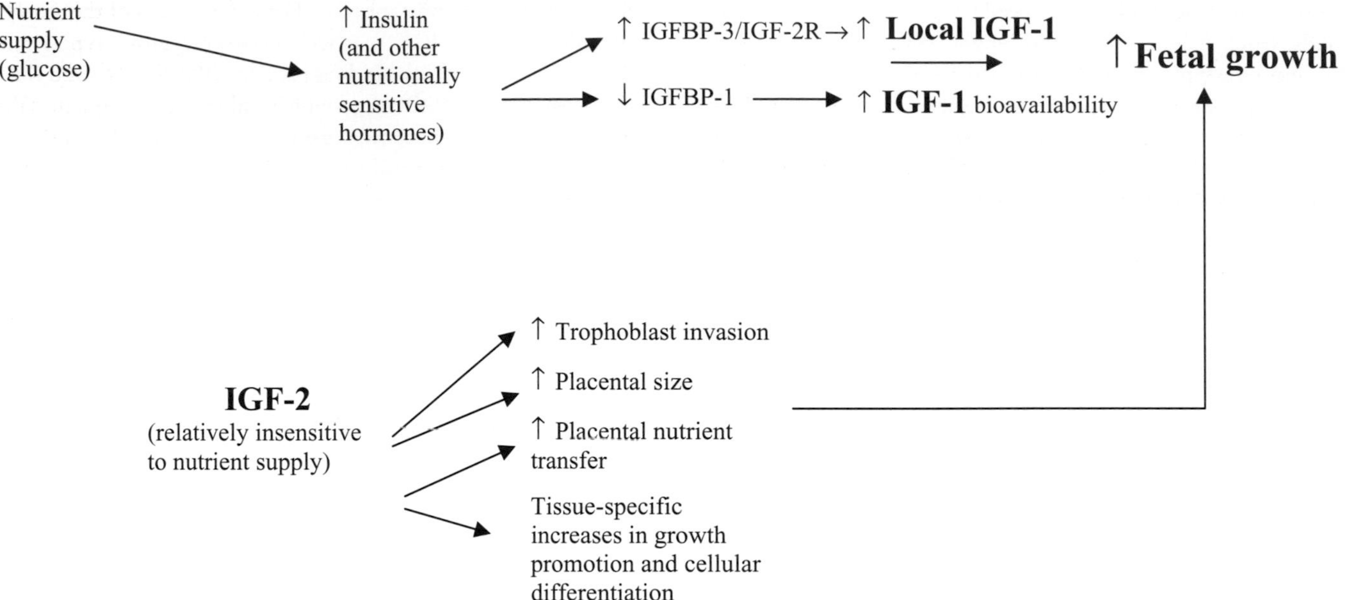

Figure 14.2 Simplification of the mechanism by which the IGF system regulates fetoplacental growth during development. As seen here, nutrient supply, although a direct influence on insulin (which itself regulates binding proteins and IGF-2 receptor), results in an increase in IGF-1, thereby promoting fetal growth. Conversely, IGF-2 is relatively insensitive to nutrient supply and plays a role in placental growth and development as well as promoting cellular differentiation in specific tissues.

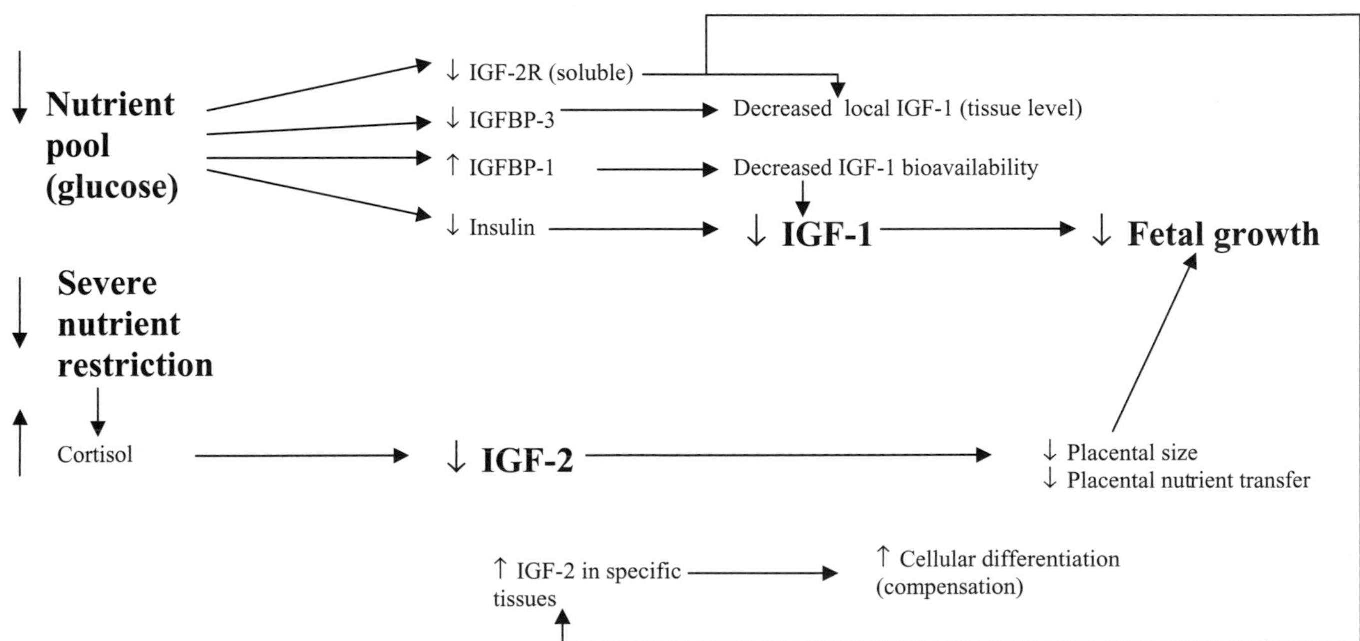

Figure 14.3 Simplified mechanism involving the IGF system in the induction of fetal growth restriction following decreased nutrient and oxygen supply. The lower glucose concentration results in several alterations including ↓ insulin with modulation in receptor concentration and binding proteins status, which all lead to decreased IGF-1 and therefore decreased fetal growth. With ongoing severe nutrient restriction and associated hypoxemia, cortisol concentration increases and IGF-2 decreases, which leads to a decrease in placental growth and function, further impeding fetal growth. Note that the decrease in IGF-2 receptor (IGF-2R; soluble form) results in a local increase in IGF-2 concentration in specific tissues. This is believed to promote cellular differentiation and provide some positive stimulus for fetal growth in order to attempt to compensate for the above changes.

that fetuses small for gestational age display lower IGF-1 concentrations.[39–42] This is consistent with an influence of insulin (as stimulated by glucose) over IGF-1 release in the fetus. As no correlation existed between maternal concentrations of IGF-1 and cord levels or birthweight, this suggested that IGF-1 in cord blood originated from the fetoplacental unit and that there was no placental transfer of maternal IGF-1 to the fetus. Conversely, IGF-2 expression is much less sensitive to nutrient supply. Indeed, it has been shown to be reduced only under circumstances of severe malnutrition. In the IUGR fetus, IGF-2 levels vary from organ to organ and have been noted to be elevated in brain and lungs, for example, likely in an effort to promote differentiation and maturation in the context of inadequate growth (see Figs 14.2 and 14.3).

Finally, placental production of IGF-1 should also be noted; although its exact role at this point has not been clearly elucidated, it is likely to be largely intraplacental as described in the above experiments in the murine model.

IGFBPs modulate the actions of IGFs by altering their half-life or simply through their transport to specific tissues. Of these proteins, IGFBP-1 has been shown to be negatively correlated with birthweight in humans.[40,43] There is increasing evidence to support an important role for IGFBP-1 in fetal growth.[44,45] For instance, it has been shown that trophoblast invasion, a step crucial to normal placentation and therefore fetal growth, is inhibited by IGFBP-1.[45] Furthermore, human fetuses that are growth restricted have been shown to display higher blood concentrations of IGFBP-1.[41] Interestingly, another study has demonstrated an inverse relationship between cord blood pO_2 and IGFBP-1. Taken together, these data suggest that hypoxia may stimulate fetal IGFBP-1 production, which decreases IGF-1 bioavailability, thereby minimizing fetal growth when supply is clearly limited.[46]

Compartmentalization of nutrients is essential to the maintenance of fetal growth. This process requires that fetal nutrient supply be maintained as a priority over maternal and even placental demands. Indeed, by secreting placental growth hormone (GH-v) and prolactin, a state of relative maternal insulin resistance is created in which glucose is preferentially transported across the placenta while maternal lipolysis is facilitated in order to respond to the demands of the mother.[24]

Leptin

Leptin is a product of the *ob/ob* gene located on chromosome 7. It is synthesized by adipocytes as well as placenta (trophoblast and amnion), stomach, bone cartilage, and teeth.[1] It is an important regulator of body weight, and its effect is mediated through a negative feedback mechanism between adipose tissues and specific satiety receptors located in the hypothalamus. Its production has been shown to be stimulated by various hormones including cortisol and insulin.[47] Under conditions of starvation, leptin levels decrease, which results in induction of food-seeking behavior as mediated by the hypothalamus. It is therefore not surprising that, in adults, leptin concentrations have been shown to be related to fat mass.

What is less clear is the role that this protein plays in fetal growth. Leptin is known to be produced by the maternal, fetal, and placental units, but whether or not it can cross the placenta has yet to be determined clearly.[1] Current studies have provided conflicting results when examining correlations between leptin concentrations and birthweight.[48,49] There is evidence for a positive correlation between cord blood leptin and birthweight in appropriately grown fetuses; however, this same relationship could not be consistently demonstrated in small for gestational age (SGA) fetuses and was also influenced by the presence or absence of maternal diabetes. Others have reported a significant decrease in fetal leptin levels in IUGR neonates, consistent with their marked reduction in fat tissue.[49] However, at this time, the exact mechanism by which fetal weight and fat mass are regulated and how leptin is involved in this process remains unclear.

Placental influences

The placenta influences fetal growth through its functional size, capacity to transport oxygen and nutrients, and its own metabolism. Placental growth is crucial to fetal growth. This is supported by the fact that, throughout gestation, placental growth closely parallels fetal growth. In addition, it has been demonstrated recently that placental volume measured at 14 weeks was directly related to fetal anthropometric measurements at 35 weeks.[11] Furthermore, placental villous area (the functional area) continues to increase throughout gestation along with vascularization of terminal villi and thinning of the syncytial layer, which optimizes exchange at the fetoplacental level.

Transport capacity

Fetal growth relies on glucose as a major fuel and, as there is no significant gluconeogenesis in the fetus, it must be obtained from maternal blood directly. Placental transfer of glucose depends on the total surface area of the syncytium available for exchange, the thickness of the placental barrier, the placenta's own metabolic needs, the concentration gradient of glucose between maternal and fetal blood, maternal blood supply and, finally, the presence of transporters.[50] Indeed, as the syncytial membrane is not very permeable to glucose, the placenta facilitates this process with the synthesis of specific transporters that are members of the GLUT gene family of facilitated diffusion transporters, which are located in the microvillous and basal membranes. Of these, GLUT3 is likely to be the major functional transporter in early pregnancy, whereas GLUT1 is more important near term.[50] The inverse relationship shown *in vitro* between extracellular glucose concentration and the presence and activity of GLUT1 suggests that glucose itself may be involved in the regulation of

GLUT1. However, it has been shown that, despite the consistent findings of low glucose in IUGR fetuses, their transporter density was not affected. How this applies to the human fetus remains to be elucidated as it is likely that glucose transfer *in vivo* is very complex and relies on various mechanisms.

The fetus also requires amino acids for protein synthesis, interconversion to other substrates, and oxidation. The transfer of amino acids is also a complex process and involves significant placental metabolism as the placenta can use, produce, and interconvert several amino acids.[51] However, in contrast to glucose, which is transferred across a gradient, amino acids are actively transported across the placenta, as supported by their higher concentrations in the fetus compared with the mother. This involves the presence of several transport systems that are all distinct from each other but exhibit some overlapping substrate specificity.[51,52] The importance of amino acid transport for fetal growth is highlighted by the observations made in IUGR. These fetuses display a decrease in amino acid concentration, an impairment of some transport systems, a decrease in surface area for exchange, decreased placental perfusion, and specific demonstrations of decreased transfer of taurine, phenylalanine, and leucine.[52]

Placental substrate delivery is also dependent on perfusion. As fetal nutrient demands increase throughout gestation, there is a 20-fold increase in maternal flow into the intervillous spaces. This process depends in part on adequate invasion of spiral arteries by trophoblasts, as supported by the marked reduction in transformed spiral arteries seen in IUGR,[1] which may result from impaired release of nitric oxide and carbon monoxide (two vasoactive substances) by trophoblasts.[1] Normal placental development also requires an early change from a relatively hypoxic to a relatively normoxic environment, resulting from spiral artery transformation and exposure of villi to maternal blood. Failure of this process leads to aberrant expression of several important growth factors involved in trophoblast migration, survival, and proliferation, function, and overall placental growth. Invasion may also be altered by external factors such as maternal smoking, which we have demonstrated to result in increased apoptotic cell death of first-trimester trophoblasts[53] and impairment of growth factor/cytokine-mediated trophoblast migration such as epidermal growth factor (EGF). It also requires adequate vascularization of villi, a complex mechanism that appears to be mediated partly by angiogenic factors that may include vascular endothelial growth factor (VEGF) and placental growth factor (PIGF).[54,55] IUGR fetuses have been shown to have decreased branching angiogenesis in villi, therefore supporting the importance of this process for fetal growth (Fig. 14.4). Finally, factors that alter maternal blood flow to the uteroplacental unit are also of significance in fetal growth. For instance, vessel obliterations have been demonstrated in placentas of mothers with antiphospholipid antibody syndrome, leading to restricted flow and potentially restricted fetal growth regulation. Similarly, women with significant cardiac or vascular disease also have altered uteroplacental blood flow as a result of decreased output or uterine and placental vascular lesions.

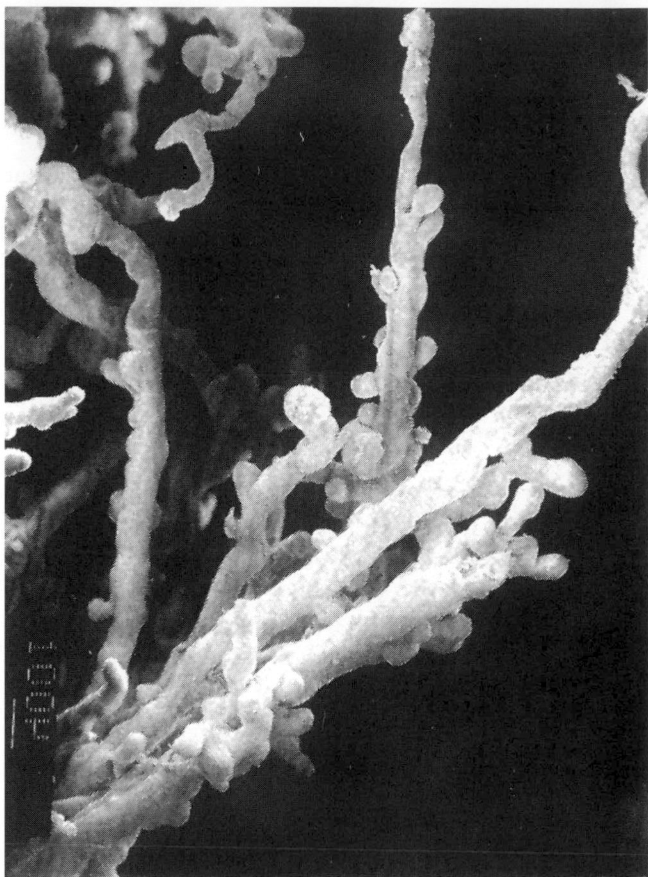

Figure 14.4 Placenta from a patient with fetal growth restriction and absent/reverse end-diastolic flow in the umbilical arteries. Note the unusually long, poorly branched terminal villi resulting from hypoxemia. From Bernishke, Kaufmann, eds. *Pathology of the human placenta*, 4th edn. Springer; 1999:457.

Placental growth hormones

The IGF family plays multiple roles in placental growth and development including an influence of IGF-2 in trophoblast invasion, a step crucial to adequate placentation and to the establishment of maternofetal exchange.[14] In addition, as discussed earlier, placental IGF-2 is involved in placental growth and transport.

GH-v gradually replaces maternal pituitary growth hormone throughout the first trimester. It exerts its biologic effects on the mother and placenta, as it is not detected in the fetus. It has high somatogenic and low lactogenic activities and has been shown to modulate maternal metabolism by stimulating gluconeogenesis, lipolysis, and anabolism.[56] The end result is to increase nutrient supply to the fetus and therefore indirectly influence fetal growth. It is responsive to changes in glucose concentration in the maternal circulation and is a key regulator of maternal IGF-1 as well as a mediator of insulin resistance in the mother, thereby having an important role in compartmentalization.

Conclusion

Fetal growth regulation is a complex process influenced by a multitude of factors, some of which have been explored here (Table 14.3). To date, we only have a limited knowledge of what these factors are and how they interact to influence growth *in utero*. Our incomplete understanding of this process in the human partly explains our current difficulties in identifying adequate therapeutic approaches for those fetuses that suffer from growth anomalies such as restriction and macrosomia. The adult consequences of these aberrant growth patterns *in utero* further highlight the importance of understanding the mechanisms behind fetal growth regulation.

Table 14.3 Determinants of fetal growth.

Maternal	Genotype (maternal height)	+++
	Physical constraints	+++++
Paternal	Genotype (paternal height)	+
	Paternal weight	No effect
Fetal	Genotype	+++
Placental	Size	++
	Transport capacity	++
	Metabolism	++

Key points

1 Abnormal fetal growth is associated with adult-onset diseases. Growth restriction increases the risk of cardiovascular diseases and diabetes, whereas fetal macrosomia appears to result in an increase in the incidence of certain types of cancer in the adult.

2 Genetic imprinting is a mechanism by which one of the two alleles of a gene is expressed according to its parental origin. Insulin-like growth factor (IGF)-2 is an example of an imprinted gene that plays an important role in fetal growth. Biallelic expression of IGF-2 results in fetal overgrowth (Beckwith–Wiedemann syndrome).

3 Uniparental disomy (UPD) is a situation in which chromosome fragments originate from a single parent. In the human fetus, UPD has been observed to be associated with aberrant growth (e.g., Prader–Willi syndrome).

4 Maternal phenotype is a very important determinant of fetal growth and, therefore, when evaluating this process, the interplay between maternal phenotype and genotype must be taken into consideration. There is a suggestion that paternal genotype plays a very small role in fetal growth.

5 Trisomic fetuses have a decrease in cellular proliferation leading to generalized hypoplasia.

6 Exercise in fit, pregnant individuals may improve placental growth. Fetuses tend to be leaner at birth but appear to be much more tolerant of the stresses of labor.

7 Maternal anemia is one of the most important medical conditions worldwide that is associated with fetal growth restriction. The mechanism involved may include increased catecholamines, hypoxia, increased oxidative stress and/or infections.

8 The influence of maternal undernutrition on fetoplacental growth depends on the severity and timing of the insult.

9 Micronutrients such as folate, zinc, iron, copper, and vitamins A and E play a role in the regulation of fetal growth.

10 It is controversial at the present time whether n-3 fatty acid consumption from marine foods promotes fetal growth.

11 Moderate consumption of caffeine does not significantly alter fetal growth. However, there appears to be synergism between caffeine intake and cigarette smoke resulting in inadequate fetal growth.

12 IGFs (IGF-1, -2) are important mitogens and play important roles in growth of the placenta and the fetus.

13 IGF-2 is important in embryonic growth and is involved in promoting cellular differentiation. Placental IGF-2 plays a role in the regulation of diffusion capacity and, therefore, in fetal growth.

14 IGF-1 regulates growth in the latter part of pregnancy and is partly regulated by insulin (as mediated by glucose). It is highly sensitive to nutrient supply.

15 Leptin is produced by the maternal, placental, and fetal units. Its cord concentrations are positively correlated with birthweight. However, the exact mechanism by which fetal fat mass may be regulated by leptin remains unknown.

16 The placenta influences fetal growth through its functional size, transport capacity, and metabolism.

17 Glucose is the major fuel for fetal growth. Specific transporters such as GLUT1 and 3 are expressed in the placenta and facilitate glucose transport to the fetus.

18 Amino acid transfer in the fetus relies on a variety of different placental transport systems. Growth-restricted fetuses have a decrease in amino acid concentration along with an impairment in some of these transport systems.

19 Normal fetal growth partly depends on placental growth, which itself initially requires adequate trophoblast invasion. Failure of this process may lead to abnormal expression of important growth factors, which may result in poor placental growth and function.

20 Placental growth hormone gradually replaces maternal pituitary growth hormone. It appears to be involved in the promotion of nutrient supply to the fetus through modulations in maternal metabolism.

References

1 Sacks D. Determinants of fetal growth. *Curr Diabetes Rep* 2004;4:281–287.

2 Barker DJP. In utero programming of chronic disease. *Clin Sci* 1998;95:115–128.

3 Ahlgren M, Sorensen T, Wohlfahrt J, et al. Birth weight and risk of breast cancer in a cohort of 106,504 women. *Int J Cancer* 2003 20;107:997–1000.

4 Vatten LJ, Nilsen TI, Tretli S, et al. Size at birth and risk of breast cancer: prospective population-based study. *Int J Cancer* 2005; 114:461–464.

5 Ahlgren M, Melbye M, Wohlfahrt J, Sorensen TI. Growth patterns and the risk of breast cancer in women. *N Engl J Med* 2004;351:1619–1626.

6 Wutz A, Theussl HC, Dausman J, et al. Non-imprinted Igf2r expression decreases growth and rescues the Tme mutation in mice. *Development* 2001;128:1881–1887.

7 Devriendt K. Genetic control of intra-uterine growth. *Eur J Obstet Gynecol Reprod Biol* 2000;92:29–34.

8 Constancia M, Hemberger M, Hughes J, et al. Placental-specific IGF-II is a major modulator of placental and fetal growth. *Nature* 2002;417:945–948.

9 Reik W, Constancia M, Dean W, et al. Igf2 imprinting in development and disease. *Int J Dev Biol* 2000;44:145–150.

10 Cetin I, Foidart JM, Miozzo M, et al. Fetal growth restriction: a workshop report. *Placenta* 2004;25:753–757.

11 Thame M, Osmound C, Bennett F, et al. Fetal growth is directly related to maternal anthropometry and placental volume. *Eur J Clin Nutr* 2004;58:894–900.

12 Price KC, Coe CL. Maternal constraint on fetal growth patterns in the rhesus monkey (*Macaca mulatta*): the intergenerational link between mothers and daughters. *Hum Reprod* 2000;15: 452–457.

13 Walton A, Hammond J. Maternal effects on growth and conformation in Shire horse–Shetland pony crosses. *Proc R Soc* 1938;125B:B11–B34.

14 Cetin I, Cozzi V, Antonazzo P. Fetal development after assisted reproduction – a review. *Placenta* 2003;24:S104–S113.

15 Nahum GG, Stanislaw H. Relationship of paternal factors to birth weight. *J Reprod Med* 2003;48:963–968.

16 Lin CC, Evans MI. *Intrauterine growth retardation*. New York: McGraw-Hill, 1984.

17 Kaback MM, Bernstein LH. Biologic studies of trisomic cells growing in vitro. *Ann NY Acad Sci* 1970;171:526–536.

18 Catalano PM, Kirwan JP. Maternal factors that determine neonatal size and body fat. *Curr Diabetes Rep* 2001;1:71–77.

19 Clapp JF, III. Exercise during pregnancy. *The Athletic Women* 2000;19:273–286.

20 Lone FW, Qureshi RN, Emanuel F. Maternal anaemia and its impact on perinatal outcome. *Trop Med Int Health* 2004;9: 486–490.

21 Hou J, Cliver SP, Tamura T, et al. Maternal serum ferritin and fetal growth. *Obstet Gynecol* 2000;95:447–452.

22 Michailidis GD, Morris RW, Mamopoulos A, et al. The influence of maternal hematocrit on placental development from the first to the second trimesters of pregnancy. *Ultrasound Obstet Gynecol* 2002;20:351–355.

23 Allen LH. Biological mechanisms that might underlie iron's effect on fetal growth and preterm birth. *J Nutr* 2001;131:581S–589S.

24 Gluckman PD, Pinal CS. Regulation of fetal growth by the somatotropic axis. *J Nutr* 2003;133:1741S–1746S.

25 Osgerby JC, Wathes DC, Howard D, Gadd TS. The effect of maternal undernutrition on the placental growth trajectory and the uterine insulin-like growth factor axis in the pregnant ewe. *J Endocrinol* 2004;182:89–103.

26 Roberts CT, Sohlstrom A, Kind KL, et al. Nutrition, genetics and placental development. Altered placental structure induced by maternal food restriction in guinea pigs: a role for circulating IGF-II and IGFBP-2 in the mother. *Placenta* 2001;22(Suppl. A): S77–S82.

27 Roberts CT, Sohlstrom A, Kind KL, et al. Maternal food restriction reduces the exchange surface area and increases the barrier thickness of the placenta in the guinea-pig. *Placenta* 2001;22: 177–185.

28 Sibley CP, Coan PM, Ferguson-Smith AC, et al. Placental-specific insulin-like growth factor 2 (Igf2) regulates the diffusional exchange characteristics of the mouse placenta. *Proc Natl Acad Sci USA* 2004;101:8204–8208.

29 Ashworth CJ, Antipatis C. Micronutrient programming of development throughout gestation. *Reproduction* 2001;122:527–535.

30 Yue-Xin Y, Xue-Cun C, Jian-Yu L, et al. Effect of zinc intake on fetal and infant growth among Chinese pregnant and lactating women. *Biomed Environ Sci* 2000;13:280–286.

31 Kinare AS, Natekar AS, Chinchwadkar MC, et al. Low midpregnancy placental volume in rural Indian women: a cause for low birth weight? *Am J Obstet Gynecol* 2000;182:443–448.

32 Steegers-Theunissen RPM, Steegers EAP. Nutrient–gene interactions in early pregnancy: a vascular hypothesis. *Eur J Obstet Gynecol Reprod Biol* 2003;106:115–117.

33 Buck GM, Tee GP, Fitzgerald EF, et al. Maternal fish consumption and infant birth size and gestation: New York state angler cohort study. *Environ Health* 2003;2:7.

34 Oken E, Kleinman KP, Olsen SF, et al. Associations of seafood and elongated n-3 fatty acid intake with fetal growth and length of

gestation: results from a US pregnancy cohort. *Am J Epidemiol* 2004;160:774–783.

35 Rogers I, Emmett P, Ness A, Golding J, ALSPAC study team. Maternal fish intake in late pregnancy and the frequency of low birth weight and intrauterine growth retardation in a cohort of British infants. *J Epidemiol Commun Health* 2004;58:486–492.

36 Vik T, Bakketeig LS, Trygg KU, et al. High caffeine consumption in the third trimester of pregnancy: gender-specific effects on fetal growth. *Paediatr Perinatal Epidemiol* 2003;17:324–331.

37 Bracken MB, Triche EW, Belanger K, et al. Association of maternal caffeine consumption with decrements in fetal growth. *Am J Epidemiol* 2003;157:456–466.

38 Woods KA, Camacho-Hubner C, Barter D, et al. Insulin-like growth factor I gene deletion causing intrauterine growth retardation and severe short stature. *Acta Paediatr Suppl* 1997;423: 39–45.

39 Vatten LJ, Nilsen ST, Odegard RA, et al. Insulin-like growth factor I and leptin in umbilical cord plasma and infant birth size at term. *Pediatrics* 2002;109:1131–1135.

40 Yang SW, Yu JS. Relationship of insulin-like growth factor-I, insulin-like growth factor binding protein-3, insulin, growth hormone in cord blood and maternal factors with birth height and birth weight. *Pediatr Int* 2000;42:31–36.

41 Ali O, Cohen P. Insulin-like growth factors and their binding proteins in children born small for gestational age: implication for growth hormone therapy. *Horm Res* 2003;60(Suppl. 3):115–123.

42 Orbak Z, Darcan S, Coker M, Goksen D. Maternal and fetal serum insulin-like growth factor-I (IGF-I), IGF binding protein-3 (IGFBP-3), leptin levels and early postnatal growth in infants born asymmetrically small for gestational age. *J Pediatr Endocrinol Metab* 2001;14:1119–1127.

43 Boyne MS, Thame M, Bennett FI, et al. The relationship among circulating insulin-like growth factor (IGF)-I, IFG-binding proteins-1 and -2 and birth anthropometry: a prospective study. *J Clin Endocrinol Metab* 2003;88:1687–1691.

44 Reece EA, Wiznitzer A, Le E, et al. The relation between human fetal growth and fetal blood levels of insulin-like growth factors I and II, their binding proteins, and receptors. *Obstet Gynecol* 1994;84:88–95.

45 Crossey PA, Pillai CC, Miell JP. Altered placental development and intrauterine growth restriction in IGF binding protein-1 transgenic mice. *J Clin Invest* 2002;110:411–418.

46 Nayak NR, Giudice LC. Current Topic. Comparative biology of the IGF system in endometrium, deciduas, and placenta, and clinical implications for fœtal growth and implantation disorders. *Placenta* 2003;24:281.

47 Kirel B, Tekin N, Tekin B, et al. Cord blood leptin levels: relationship to body weight, body mass index, sex and insulin and cortisol levels of maternal-newborn pairs at deliver. *J Pediatr Endocrinol Metab* 2000;13:71–77.

48 Oktem O, Dedeoglu N, Oymak Y, et al. Maternal serum, amniotic fluid and cord leptin levels at term: their correlations with fetal weight. *J Perinat Med* 2004;32:266–271.

49 Sooranna SR, Ward S, Bajoria R. Fetal leptin influences birth weight and twins in discordant growth. *Pediatr Res* 2001;49: 667–672.

50 Baumann MU, Deborde S, Illsley NP. Placental glucose transfer and fetal growth. *Endocrine* 2002;19:13–22.

51 Regnault TRH, de Vrijer B, Battaglia FC. Transport and metabolism of amino acids in placenta. *Endocrine* 2002;19:23–41.

52 Cetin I. Placental transport of amino acids in normal and growth-restricted pregnancies. *Eur J Obstet Gynecol Reprod Biol* 2003; 110:S50–S54.

53 Gruslin A, Qiu Q, Tsang BK. Influence of maternal smoking on trophoblast apoptosis throughout development: possible involvement of xiap regulation. *Biol Reprod* 2001;65:1164–1169.

54 Regnault TRH, de Vrijer B, Galan HL, et al. The relationship between transplacental O_2 diffusion and placental expression of PIGF, VEGF and their receptors in a placental insufficiency model of fetal growth restriction. *J Physiol* 2003;550:641–656.

55 Torry DS, Hinrichs M, Torry RJ. Determinants of placental vascularity. *Am J R I* 2004;51:257–268.

56 Chellakooty M, Skibsted L, Skouby SO, et al. Longitudinal study of serum placental GH in 455 normal pregnancies: correlation to gestational age, fetal gender, and weight. *J Clin Endocrinol Metab* 2002;87:2734–2739.

Part V

Fetal Infections and Teratogenesis

15 Developmental toxicology, drugs, and fetal teratogenesis

Robert L. Brent and Lynda B. Fawcett

Reproductive problems encompass a multiplicity of diseases including sterility, infertility, abortion (miscarriage), stillbirth, congenital malformations (resulting from environmental or hereditary etiologies), fetal growth retardation, and prematurity. These clinical problems occur commonly in the general population and, therefore, environmental causes are not always easy to corroborate (Table 15.1). Severe congenital malformations occur in 3% of births; according to the Center for Disease Control, they include those birth defects that cause death, hospitalization, and mental retardation, and those that necessitate significant or repeated surgical procedures, are disfiguring, or interfere with physical performance. This means that each year in the USA, 120 000 babies are born with severe birth defects. Genetic disease occurs in approximately 11% of births, and spontaneous mutations account for approximately 2–3% of genetic disease. This spontaneous mutation rate presents difficulties when determining the proportion of mutations that are induced from preconception exposure to environmental mutagens.

There have been dramatic advances in our understanding of the causes of human birth defects. In earlier times, superstition, ignorance, and prejudice played a major role in explaining why birth defects occurred. Reproductive problems have been viewed throughout history as diseases of affliction, along with cancer, psychiatric illness, and hereditary diseases. The stigma associated with birth defects has primitive beginnings and persists today; in the minds of many, even the most sophisticated, a birth defect is felt to be some form of punishment for previous misdeeds.[1–4] Ancient Babylonian writings recount tales of mothers being put to death because they delivered malformed infants. In the seventeenth century, one George Spencer was slain by the Puritans in New Haven having been convicted of fathering a cyclopean pig; the Puritans were unable to differentiate between George Spencer's cataract and the malformed pig's cloudy cornea.[1] More recently, the situation has been reversed and the responsibility for reproductive problems such as congenital malformations, infertility, abortions, and hereditary diseases is often blamed on others, for example, environmental agents dispensed by healthcare providers or utilized by employers.[1,2]

Reproductive problems alarm the public, the press, and scientists to a greater degree than many other diseases. Severely malformed children are disquieting to healthcare providers, especially if they are not experienced in dealing with such problems; no physician will be comfortable informing a family that their child was born without arms and legs. The objective evaluation of the environmental causes of reproductive diseases is clouded by the emotional climate that surrounds these diseases, resulting in the expression of partisan positions that either diminish or magnify the environmental risks. These nonobjective opinions can be expressed by scientists, the laity, or the press.[5,6] It is the responsibility of every physician to be aware of the emotionally charged situation when a family has a child with a birth defect; an inadvertent comment from medical staff attending delivery can have grave consequences for the physician and the family. Comments such as, "Oh, you had a radiograph during your pregnancy," or "You did not tell me that you were prescribed tetracycline while you were pregnant," can direct the patient's family to an attorney rather than to a teratology or genetic counselor.

At present, the etiology of congenital malformations can be divided into three categories: unknown, genetic, and environmental. Unfortunately, the largest group (65–75%) has an unknown etiology, whereas the most common known cause is genetic (15–25%).[7–9] Environmental factors account for 10% of congenital malformations. Over 50 teratogenic environmental drugs, chemicals, and physical agents have been described[9–12] by clinical dysmorphologists using modern epidemiological tools.[13–19] The basic science and clinical rules for evaluating teratogenic risks have been established.[20] The purpose of this chapter is to inform clinicians about environmental drugs, chemicals, and physical agents that have been documented to produce congenital malformations and reproductive effects, and to indicate that the multitude of teratogenic agents accounts for only a small proportion of malformations.

Table 15.1 Background reproductive risks in pregnancy.

Reproductive risk	Frequency
Immunologically and clinically diagnosed spontaneous abortions per million conceptions	350 000
Clinically recognized spontaneous abortions per million clinically recognized pregnancies	150 000
Genetic diseases per million births:	110 000
Multifactorial or polygenic genetic environmental interactions (i.e., neural tube defects, cleft lip, hypospadias, hyperlipidemia, diabetes)	90 000
Dominantly inherited disease (i.e., achondroplasia, Huntington's chorea, neurofibromatosis)	10 000
Autosomal and sex-linked genetic disease (i.e., cystic fibrosis, hemophilia, sickle-cell disease, thalassemia)	1 200
Cytogenetic (chromosomal abnormalities) (i.e., Down syndrome (trisomy 21), trisomies 13 and 18, Turner syndrome, 22q deletion, etc.)	5 000
New mutations*	3 000
Severe congenital malformations† per million births (resulting from all causes of birth defects: genetic, unknown, environmental)	30 000
Prematurity per million births	40 000
Fetal growth retardation per million births	30 000
Stillbirths (> 20 weeks) per million births	2000–20 900
Infertility	7% of couples

Modified from ref. 11.
*The mutation rate for many genetic diseases can be calculated; this can be readily performed with dominantly inherited diseases when offspring are born with a dominant genetic disease and neither parent has the disease.
†Congenital malformations have multiple etiologies including a significant proportion that are genetic.

Basic principles of teratology

To label an environmental agent as teratogenic it is necessary to characterize the dose, route of exposure, and stage of pregnancy when the exposure occurred. A 50-mg dose of thalidomide administered on the 26th day post conception has a significant risk of malforming the embryo. The same dose taken during the 10th week of gestation will not result in congenital malformations, and 1 mg of thalidomide taken at any time during pregnancy will have no effect on the developing embryo. X-ray irradiation can be teratogenic;[21–23] however, if the dose is too low or the X-ray does not directly expose the embryo, there is no increased risk of congenital malformations.[3] Therefore a list of teratogens indicates only teratogenic potential; evaluation of the dose and time of exposure may indicate that there is no teratogenic risk or that the risk is significant.

Physicians must be careful to carry out a thorough evaluation of the risks faced by a woman exposed to drugs and chemicals during pregnancy, and before alleging that a child's malformations result from exposure to an environmental agent. Clinical teratology and genetics is not emphasized in medical schools and residency education programs. However, clinicians have a multitude of educational aids to assist them in their evaluations; these include consultations with clinical teratologists and geneticists, the medical literature, and the Online Mendelian Inheritance of Man (OMIM) website.[24]

The analysis of human and animal studies on the reproductive effects of environmental agents should be guided by the basic principles of teratology and developmental biology;[3] these principles are outlined in Table 15.2.[25–32]

The etiology of congenital malformations

As mentioned earlier, the etiology of congenital malformations can be divided into three categories: unknown, genetic, and environmental (Table 15.3). A significant proportion of congenital malformations of unknown etiology are likely to have an important genetic component. Malformations with an increased recurrent risk such as cleft lip and palate, anencephaly, spina bifida, certain congenital heart diseases, pyloric stenosis, hypospadias, inguinal hernia, talipes equinovarus, and congenital dislocation of the hip fit into the category of multifactorial disease as well as that of polygenic inherited disease.[33,34] The multifactorial/threshold hypothesis postulates the modulation of a continuum of genetic characteristics by intrinsic and extrinsic (environmental) factors.

A significant percentage of spontaneous errors of development can occur without apparent abnormalities of the genome or environmental influences; these are due to the statistical probability of errors in the developmental process, similar to the concept of spontaneous mutation, and mean that we may never achieve our goal of eliminating birth defects. It is estimated that the majority of all miscarriages occur early in pregnancy, many within the first 3 weeks of development. The World Health Organization estimated that 15% of all clinically recognizable pregnancies end in spontaneous abortion,

Table 15.2 Basic scientific principles of teratology.

Principle	Description
Exposure to teratogens follows a toxicological dose–response curve	There is a threshold below which no teratogenic effect will be observed. As the dose of the teratogen is increased, both the severity and frequency of reproductive effects will increase (Fig. 15.1)
The embryonic stage at which exposure occurs will determine what effects, if any, a teratogen will have	Some teratogens have a broad period of embryonic sensitivity while others have a very narrow period of sensitivity
Most teratogens have a confined group of congenital malformations referred to as the syndrome of the agent's effects	Known teratogens may be presumptively implicated by the spectrum of malformations they produce. It is easier to exclude an agent as a cause of a birth defect than to definitively prove it was responsible because of the existence of genocopies of some teratogenic syndromes
No teratogen can produce every type of malformation	The presence of certain malformations can eliminate the possibility that a particular teratogenic agent was responsible because those malformations have not been demonstrated to be part of the syndrome caused by the teratogen, or because production of the malformation is not biologically plausible for that particular alleged teratogen

Based on concepts from ref. 20.

Table 15.3 Etiology of human congenital malformations observed during the first year of life.

Suspected cause	Percent of total
Unknown	65–75
Polygenic	
Multifactorial (gene–environment interactions)	
Spontaneous errors of development	
Synergistic interactions of teratogens	
Genetic	15 25
Autosomal and sex-linked inherited genetic disease	
Cytogenetic (chromosomal abnormalities)	
New mutations	
Environmental	10
Maternal conditions: alcoholism, diabetes, endocrinopathies, phenylketonuria, smoking and nicotine, starvation, nutritional deficits	4
Infectious agents: rubella, toxoplasmosis, syphilis, herpes simplex, cytomegalovirus, varicella zoster, Venezuelan equine encephalitis, parvovirus B19	3
Mechanical problems (deformations): amniotic band constrictions, umbilical cord constraint, disparity in uterine size and uterine contents	1–2
Chemicals, prescription drugs, high-dose ionizing radiation, hyperthermia	< 1

Modified from ref. 8.

many (50–60%) resulting from chromosomal abnormalities.[35–38] Finally, 3–6% of offspring are malformed, which represents the background risk for abnormal human development (Table 15.1).

Factors that affect susceptibility to developmental toxicants

A basic tenet of environmentally produced malformations is that teratogens or a teratogenic milieu have certain characteristics in common and follow certain basic principles. These principles determine the quantitative and qualitative aspects of environmentally produced malformations.

Embryonic stage

The risk of an exposure to a developmental toxicant resulting in morphological anomalies or intrauterine death depends on the dose and the embryonic or fetal stage at which exposure occurs. The period when an exposure occurs will determine which structures are most susceptible to the deleterious effects

Table 15.4 Developmental stage sensitivity to thalidomide-induced limb reduction defects in the human.

Days from conception for induction of defects	Limb reduction defects
21–26	Thumb aplasia
22–23	Microtia, deafness
23–34	Hip dislocation
24–29	Amelia, upper limbs
24–33	Phocomelia, upper limbs
25–31	Preaxial aplasia, upper limbs
27–31	Amelia, lower limbs
28–33	Preaxial aplasia, lower limbs; phocomelia, lower limbs; femoral hypoplasia; girdle hypoplasia
33–36	Triphalangeal thumb

Modified from ref. 4.

of the drug or chemical and to what extent the embryo can repair the damage. The period of sensitivity may be narrow or broad, depending on the environmental agent and the malformation in question. Limb defects produced by thalidomide have a very short period of susceptibility[4] (2 weeks; Table 15.4), whereas microcephaly, produced by radiation, has a long period of susceptibility (weeks 8–15 of pregnancy).[3]

The embryo is most sensitive to the lethal effects of drugs and chemicals during the period of embryonic development, from fertilization through the early postimplantation stage. Surviving embryos have malformation rates that are similar to those of control subjects because significant cell loss or chromosome abnormalities at these stages has a high likelihood of resulting in embryonic death, not because malformations cannot be produced at this stage. Because of the omnipotentiality of early embryonic cells, surviving embryos have a high probability of having malformation rates that are similar to embryos that have not been exposed.

The period of organogenesis (from day 18 through about day 40 post conception in the human) is the period of greatest sensitivity to teratogenic insults and when most gross anatomic malformations can be induced. Most environmentally produced major malformations occur before the 36th day post conception in the human. The exceptions are malformations of the genito-urinary system, the palate, and the brain, or deformations due to problems of constraint, disruption or destruction.

The fetal period is characterized by histogenesis involving cell growth, differentiation, and migration. Agents that result in cell depletion, vascular disruption, necrosis, specific tissue or organ pathology, physiological decompensation, or severe growth retardation have the potential to cause deleterious effects throughout gestation. The fetus is most sensitive to the induction of mental retardation and microcephaly at the end of the first and the beginning of the second trimester. Other permanent neurological effects can be induced in the second and third trimesters. Effects such as cell depletion or functional abnormalities, not readily apparent at birth, may give rise to changes in behavior or fertility which are only apparent later in life. The last gestational day on which certain malformations may be induced in the human is presented in Table 15.5.

Dose or magnitude of the exposure

The quantitative correlation between the magnitude of the embryopathic effects and the dose of a drug, chemical, or other agent is referred to as the dose–response relationship. This is extremely important when comparing effects among different species because the use of mg/kg doses are, at best, rough approximations. Dose equivalence for drugs and chemicals between humans and other species can be accomplished only by performing pharmacokinetic studies, metabolic studies, and dose–response investigations, whereas ionizing radiation exposures in rads or sieverts (Sv) are similar in most mammalian species.[3] The response should be interpreted carefully. For example, a substance given in large enough amounts to cause maternal toxicity is also likely to have deleterious effects on the embryo such as death, growth retardation, or retarded development. Also, it is unlikely that progesterone or its synthetic analogues are involved in congenital teratogenesis because the steroid receptors that are necessary for naturally occurring and synthetic progestin action are absent from nonreproductive tissues early in development.[7,39–41] Several considerations affect the interpretation of dose–response relationships and these are outlined in Table 15.6.

Threshold dose

The threshold dose is the dose below which the incidence of death, malformation, growth retardation, or functional deficit is not statistically greater than that of control subjects (Fig. 15.1). The threshold level of exposure usually varies between less than one and up to two orders of magnitude below the teratogenic or embryopathic dose for drugs and chemicals that kill or malform one-half of the embryos. An exogenous teratogenic agent, therefore, has a no-effect dose compared with mutagens or carcinogens, which have a stochastic dose–response curve (Table 15.7, Fig. 15.1). The incidence and severity of malformations produced by all exogenous teratogenic agents that have been appropriately studied have exhibited threshold phenomena during organogenesis.[7] The threshold concept stems from the principle that manifestations of developmental toxicity occur because the processes of repair and regeneration have been overwhelmed by a particular exposure to a developmental toxicant. It does not predicate that no effect occurs at lower exposures, just that there is no deleterious or irreversible effect.

Table 15.5 Estimated outcome of pregnancy vs. time from conception.

Time from conception	Percent survival to term*	Percent loss during interval*	Last time for induction of selected malformations†
Pre-implantation			–
0–6 days	25	54.55	–
Postimplantation			–
7–13 days	55	24.66	–
14–20 days	73	8.18	–
3–5 weeks	79.5	7.56	22–23 days: cyclopia, sirenomelia, microtia 26 days: anencephaly 28 days: meningomyelocele 34 days: transposition of great vessels
6–9 weeks	90	6.52	36 days: cleft lip 6 weeks: diaphragmatic hernia, rectal atresia, ventricular septal defect, syndactyly 9 weeks: cleft palate
10–13 weeks	92	4.42	10 weeks: omphalocele; 12 weeks: hypospadias
14–17 weeks	96.26	1.33	–
18–21 weeks	97.56	0.85	–
22–25 weeks	98.39	0.31	–
26–29 weeks	98.69	0.30	–
30–33 weeks	98.98	0.30	–
34–37 weeks	99.26	0.34	–
38+ weeks	99.32	0.68	38+ weeks: CNS cell depletion

*An estimated 50–70% of all human miscarriages occur in the first 3 weeks of gestation.[36,72]
†Modified from ref. 60.

Table 15.6 Considerations that affect the interpretation of dose–response relationships.

Concept	Description	Example
Active metabolites	Metabolites may be the proximate teratogen rather than the administered drug or chemical	The metabolite phosphoramide mustard and acrolein may produce abnormal development resulting from the metabolism of cyclophosphamide
Duration of exposure	A chronic exposure to a prescribed drug can contribute to an increased teratogenic risk	Anticonvulsant therapy; in contrast an acute exposure to the same drug may present little or no teratogenic risk
Fat solubility	Fat-soluble substances can produce fetal malformations for an extended period after the last ingestion or exposure because they have an unusually long half-life	Polychlorinated biphenyls (PCBs). Etretinate may present a similar risk but the data are not conclusive

Pharmacokinetics and metabolism of the drug or chemical

Physiological alterations during pregnancy as well as the bioconversion of compounds can significantly influence the teratogenic effects of drugs and chemicals by affecting absorption, body distribution, the active form(s), and excretion of the compound. Tables 15.8 and 15.9 outline the pregnancy-related physiological alterations in the mother and fetus, respectively, that affect the pharmacokinetics of drugs.[42–44]

Although other organs, including the placenta, can be involved in the metabolism of drugs or chemicals, the major site of bioconversion of chemicals *in vivo* is likely to be the maternal liver. Placental P450-dependent monooxygenation of xenobiotics will occur at low rates unless induced by compounds such as those found in tobacco smoke.[45] However, the rodent embryo and yolk sac have been shown to possess functional P450-oxidative isozymes capable of converting proteratogens to active metabolites during early organogenesis.[46] In addition, P450-independent bioactivation has been

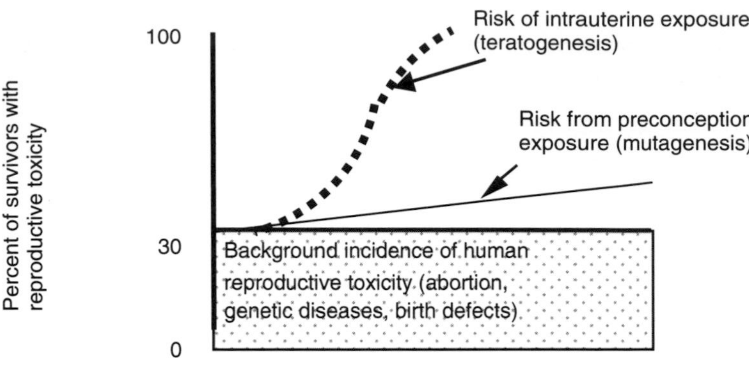

Figure 15.1 Dose–response relationship of reproductive toxins comparing preconception and postconception risks.

Table 15.7 Stochastic and threshold dose–response relationships of diseases produced by environmental agents.

Relationship	Pathology	Site	Diseases	Risk	Definition
Stochastic phenomena	Damage to a single cell may result in disease	DNA	Cancer, mutation	Some risk exists at all dosages; at low exposures the risk is below the spontaneous risk	The incidence of the disease increases with the dose but the severity and nature of the disease remain the same
Threshold phenomena	Multicellular injury	High variation in etiology, affecting many cell and organ processes	Malformation, growth retardation, death, chemical toxicity, etc.	No increased risk below the threshold dose	Both the severity and incidence of the disease increase with dose

Modified from ref. 73.

Table 15.8 Pregnancy-related physiological alterations in the mother that affect the pharmacokinetics of drugs.

Alteration	Effect on drug pharmacokinetics
Decreased gastrointestinal motility; increased intestinal transit time	Results in delayed absorption of drugs in the small intestine owing to increased stomach retention and enhanced absorption of slowly absorbed drugs
Decreased plasma albumin	Alters the kinetics of compounds normally bound to albumin
Renal elimination	Generally increased but is influenced by body position later in pregnancy
Increased plasma and extracellular fluid volumes	Affects concentration-dependent transfer of compounds
Inhibition of metabolic inactivation in the maternal liver	Increases half-life of drug in plasma
Variation in uterine blood flow	May afect transfer across the placenta (although little is known concerning this)

Based on concepts from refs 42–44.

Table 15.9 Pregnancy-related physiological alterations in the fetus that may affect the pharmacokinetics of drugs.

Alteration	Effect on drug pharmacokinetics
Amount and distribution of fat	Affects distribution of lipid-soluble drugs and chemicals
Lower plasma protein concentrations	Results in a higher concentration of unbound drug in the fetal circulation
Functional development of pharmacological receptors	Likely to proceed at different rates in the various tissues of the developing fetus
Extent of amniotic fluid swallowing	Drugs that are excreted by the fetal kidneys may be recycled through the fetus via swallowing of amniotic fluid

Based on concepts from refs 42–44.

suggested; for example, there is strong evidence that the rat embryo can reductively convert niridazole to an embryotoxic metabolite.[47]

Bioconversion of xenobiotics has been shown to be important in their teratogenic activity. There is strong evidence that the reactive metabolites of cyclophosphamide, 2-acetylaminofluorene, and nitroheterocycles (niridazole) are the proximate teratogens.[48] There is also experimental evidence suggesting that other chemicals undergo conversion to intermediates that have deleterious effects on embryonic development, for example, phenytoin, procarbazine, rifampicin, diethylstilbestrol, some benzhydrylpiperazine antihistamines, adriamycin, testosterone, benzo(a)pyrene, methoxyethanol, caffeine, and paraquat.[45,48]

Juchau[48] has defined several experimental criteria to suggest that a suspected metabolite is responsible for the *in vivo* teratogenic effects of a chemical or drug (Table 15.10). These criteria may explain why there are marked qualitative and quantitative differences in the species response to a teratogenic agent.

Table 15.10 Criteria to suggest that a suspected metabolite is responsible for the *in vivo* teratogenic effects of a drug or chemical.

The chemical must be convertible to the intermediate
The intermediate must be found in, or have access to, the tissue(s) affected
The embryotoxic effect should increase with the concentration of the metabolite
Inhibiting the conversion should reduce the embryotoxic effect of the agent
Promoting the conversion should increase the embryotoxicity of the agent
Inhibiting or promoting conversion should not alter the target tissues
Inhibiting the conversion should increase the embryotoxicity of the agent

Based on concepts from ref. 48.

Placental transport

It has been suggested that the placental barrier is protective and that harmful substances do not reach the embryo; however, it is now clear that there is no "placental barrier" *per se*. The package inserts on many drugs state that "this drug crosses the placental barrier"[6] and the uninitiated may infer from this statement that this characteristic of a drug is both unusual and hazardous. However, most drugs and chemicals cross the placenta, and only selected proteins, whose actions are species specific, will cross the placental barrier in one species but not another.

The role that the placenta plays in drug pharmacokinetics has been reviewed by Juchau and Rettie[45] and involves: (1) transport; (2) the presence of receptor sites for a number of endogenous and xenobiotic compounds (β-adrenergic agents, glucocorticoids, epidermal growth factor, IgG-Fc, insulin, low-density lipoproteins, opiates, somatomedin, testosterone, transcobalamin II, transferrin, folate, retinoid);[49] and (3) the bioconversion of xenobiotics.

The factors which determine the ability of a drug or chemical to cross the placenta and reach the embryo include molecular weight, lipid affinity or solubility, polarity or degree of ionization, protein binding, and receptor mediation. Compounds with a low molecular weight and lipid affinity, nonpolarity, and without protein-binding properties will cross the placenta rapidly and with ease. For example, ethyl alcohol reaches the embryo rapidly and in concentrations equal to or greater than the level in the mother. High-molecular-weight compounds like heparin (20 000 daltons) do not cross the placenta readily and, therefore, during pregnancy, heparin is used instead of warfarin-like compounds for the treatment of hypercoagulation conditions. Rose Bengal does not cross the placenta at all. In general, compounds with molecular weights of 1000 daltons or more do not readily cross the placenta, whereas those less than 600 daltons usually do; most drugs are 250–400 daltons and do cross the placenta.[50]

Genetic differences

The genetic constitution of an organism is an important factor in the susceptibility of a species to a drug or chemical. More than 30 disorders of increased sensitivity to drug toxicity or effects in the human result from an inherited trait.[51] Maternal and fetal genotypes determine the types of bioconversion route, the rate at which bioconversions take place, and the extent to which a compound is metabolized.

Environmental agents resulting in reproductive toxicity following exposure during pregnancy

Table 15.11 lists environmental agents that have resulted in reproductive toxicity and/or congenital malformations in humans. The list should not be used in isolation because many other parameters must be considered when analyzing reproductive risks in individual patients. Many of these agents represent a very small risk while others may represent substantial risks; the risks will vary with the magnitude, timing, and length of exposure. Further information can be obtained from more extensive reviews or summary articles. Table 15.12 lists agents that have had concerns raised about their reproductive effects but which, after a careful and complete evaluation, have not been found to represent an increased reproductive risk.[41,52–55] References for the environmental agents can be found in review articles and texts on teratogenesis.[13,18,24,38,51,56–61]

Interpretation of animal study data for assessment of reproductive risks in humans

As human studies are expensive and take years to complete, scientists have investigated the issue of whether appropriate animal models can be used to evaluate the reproductive and toxicological risks of environmental agents in humans (teratogenesis, growth retardation, pregnancy loss, stillbirth, and infertility).

Whole animal teratology studies are helpful in raising concerns about the reproductive effects of drugs and chemicals; however, negative animal studies do not guarantee that these agents are free from reproductive effects in humans. There are examples in which drug testing was negative in animals (rat and mouse), but was teratogenic in the human (thalidomide).[27] Similarly, there are examples in which a drug was teratogenic in an animal model but not in humans (diflunisal). Therefore, while chemicals and drugs can be evaluated for their toxic potential by utilizing *in vivo* animal studies and *in vitro* systems, it should be recognized that these testing procedures are only one component in the process of evaluating the potential toxic risk of drugs and chemicals. Well-performed epidemiology studies still represent the best methodology for determining the risks and effects of environmental toxicants on humans. Indeed, most human teratogens have been discovered by alert physicians or during epidemiology studies, not animal studies.[62] *In vitro* studies play an even less important role, although they are helpful in describing the cellular or tissue-specific effects of drugs and chemicals.

One useful aspect of animal studies is in corroborating findings reported in epidemiological studies. Attempts at risk assessment can be made by utilizing toxicokinetic data that have been obtained in an animal model, and exposure levels of the alleged toxicant and its metabolites that have been determined in humans. Studies to elucidate whether the mechanism of action of a drug or chemical in the animal model is the same as that in humans would further add to the toxicologist's ability to estimate human risks. This is not a simple process and explains why good-quality epidemiological studies are so valuable in determining human risks and toxicity.

Clinicians are given little training in medical school and during residency training on how to interpret animal toxicology studies. This is probably more true of reproductive

Table 15.11 Proven human teratogens or embryotoxins: drugs, chemicals, milieu, and physical agents that have resulted in human congenital malformations.

Reproductive toxin	Alleged effects
Aminopterin, methotrexate	Growth retardation, microcephaly, meningomyelocele mental retardation, hydrocephalus, and cleft palate
Androgens	Along with high doses of some male-derived progestins, can cause masculinization of the developing fetus
Angiotensin-converting enzyme (ACE) inhibitors	Fetal hypotension syndrome in second and third trimester resulting in fetal kidney hypoperfusion and anuria, oligohydramnios, pulmonary hypoplasia, and cranial bone hypoplasia. No effect in the first trimester
Antituberculous therapy	The drugs isoniazid (INH) and paraaminosalicylic acid (PAS) have an increased risk for some CNS abnormalities
Caffeine	Moderate exposure not associated with birth defects; high exposures associated with an increased risk of abortion but data are inconsistent
Chorionic villus sampling (CVS)	Vascular disruptive malformations, i.e., limb reduction defects
Cobalt in hematemic multivitamins	Fetal goiter
Cocaine	Very low incidence of vascular disruptive malformations, pregnancy loss
Corticosteroids	High exposures administered systemically have a low risk for cleft palate in some epidemiological studies; however, this is not a consistent finding
Coumarin derivative	Exposure during early pregnancy can result in nasal hypoplasia, stippling of secondary epiphysis, and intrauterine growth retardation. Exposure in late pregnancy can result in CNS malformations as a result of bleeding

Table 15.11 *Continued.*

Cyclophosphamide and other chemotherapeutic and immunosuppressive agents, e.g., cyclosporine, leflunomide	Many chemotherapeutic agents used to treat cancer have a theoretical risk of producing fetal malformations, as most of these drugs are teratogenic in animals; however, the clinical data are not consistent. Many have not been shown to be teratogenic but the numbers of cases in the studies are small; caution is the byword
Diethylstilbestrol	Genital abnormalities, adenosis, and clear cell adenocarcinoma of the vagina in adolescents. The risk of adenosis can be quite high; the risk of adenocarcinoma is 1:1000 to 1:10 000
Ethyl alcohol	Fetal alcohol syndrome (microcephaly, mental retardation, growth retardation, typical facial dysmorphogenesis, abnormal ears, and small palpebral fissures)
Ionizing radiation	A threshold greater than 20 rad (0.2 Gy) can increase the risk of some fetal effects such as micocephaly or growth retardation. The threshold for mental retardation is higher
Insulin shock therapy	Microcephaly and mental retardation
Lithium therapy	Chronic use for the treatment of manic depressive illness has an increased risk for Ebstein's anomaly and other malformations, but the risk appears to be very low
Minoxidil	Hirsutism in newborns (led to the discovery of the hair growth-promoting properties of minoxidil)
Methimazole	Aplasia cutis has been reported*
Methylene blue intraamniotic instillation	Fetal intestinal atresia, hemolytic anemia, and jaundice in the neonatal period. This procedure is no longer utilized to identify one twin
Misoprostol	Low incidence of vascular disruptive phenomenon, such as limb reduction defects and Mobius syndrome, has been reported in pregnancies in which this drug was used to induce an abortion
Penicillamine (D-penicillamine)	This drug results in the physical effects referred to as lathyrism, the results of poisoning by the seeds of the genus *Lathyrus*. It causes collagen disruption, cutis laxa, and hyperflexibility of joints. The condition appears to be reversible and the risk is low
Progestin therapy	Very high doses of androgen hormone-derived progestins can produce masculinization. Many drugs with progestational activity do not have masculinizing potential. None of these drugs has the potential for producing congenital malformations
Propylthiouracil	Along with other antithyroid medications can result in an infant born with a goiter
Radioactive isotopes	Tissue- and organ-specific damage is dependent on the radioisotope element and distribution, i.e., high doses of ^{131}I administered to a pregnant woman can cause fetal thyroid hypoplasia after the 8th week of development
Retinoids, systemic	Systemic retinoic acid, isotretinoin, and etretinate can result in an increased risk of CNS, cardio-aortic, ear, and clefting defects, microtia, anotia, thymic aplasia and other branchial arch and aortic arch abnormalities, and certain congenital heart malformations
Retinoids, topical	This is very unlikely to have teratogenic potential because teratogenic serum levels are not achieved from topical exposure
Streptomycin	Streptomycin and a group of ototoxic drugs can affect the eighth nerve and interfere with hearing; it is a relatively low-risk phenomenon. Children are even less sensitive to the ototoxic effects of these drugs than adults
Sulfa drug and vitamin K	Hemolysis in some subpopulations of fetuses
Tetracycline	Bone and teeth staining
Thalidomide	Increased incidence of deafness, anotia, preaxial limb reduction defects, phocomelia, ventricular septal defects, and GI atresias during susceptible period from the 22nd to the 36th day post conception
Trimethoprim	This drug was frequently used to treat urinary tract infections and has been linked to an increased incidence of neural tube defects. The risk is not high, but it is biologically plausible because of the drug's lowering effect on folic acid levels. This has also resulted in neurological symptoms in adults taking this drug
Vitamin A (retinol)	Very high doses of vitamin A have been reported to produce the same malformations as those reported for the retinoids. Dosages sufficient to produce birth defects would have to be in excess of 25 000 to 50 000 units per day
Vitamin D*	Large doses given in vitamin D prophylaxis are possibly involved in the etiology of supravalvular aortic stenosis, elfin facies, and mental retardation
Warfarin (coumarin)	Exposure during early pregnancy can result in nasal hypoplasia, stippling of secondary epiphysis, and intrauterine growth retardation. Exposure in late pregnancy can result in CNS malformations as a result of bleeding
Anticonvulsants	
Carbamazepine	Used in the reatment of convulsive disorders; increases the risk of facial dysmorphology

(Continued)

Table 15.11 *Continued.*

Diphenylhydantoin	Used in the treatment of convulsive disorders; increases the risk of fetal hydantoin syndrome, consisting of facial dysmorphology, cleft palate, ventricular septal defect (VSD), and growth and mental retardation
Trimethadione and paramethadione	Used in the treatment of convulsive disorders; increases the risk of characteristic facial dysmorphology, mental retardation, V-shaped eyebrows, low-set ears with anteriorly folded helix, high-arched palate, irregular teeth, CNS anomalies, and severe developmental delay
Valproic acid	Used in the treatment of convulsive disorders; increases the risk of spina bifida, facial dysmorphology, and autism
Chemicals	
Carbon monoxide poisoning*	CNS damage has been reported with very high exposures, but the risk appears to be low
Gasoline addiction embryopathy	Facial dysmorphology, mental retardation
Lead	Very high exposures can cause pregnancy loss; intrauterine teratogenesis is not established
Methyl mercury	Causes Minamata disease consisting of cerebral palsy, microcephaly, mental retardation, blindness, and cerebellum hypoplasia. Endemics have occurred from adulteration of wheat with mercury-containing chemicals that are used to prevent grain spoilage. Present environmental levels of mercury are unlikely to represent a teratogenic risk, but reducing or limiting the consumption of carnivorous fish has been suggested in order not to exceed the Environmental Protection Agency's (EPA's) maximum permissible exposure (MPE), which is far below the toxic effects of mercury
Polychlorinated biphenyls	Poisoning has occurred from adulteration of food products (cola-colored babies, CNS effects, pigmentation of gums, nails, teeth and groin, hypoplastic deformed nails, intrauterine growth retardation, abnormal skull calcification). The threshold exposure has not been determined, but it is unlikely to be teratogenic at the present environmental exposures
Toluene addiction embryopathy	Facial dysmorphology, mental retardation
Embryonic and fetal infections	
Cytomegalovirus	Retinopathy, CNS calcification, microcephaly, mental retardation
Herpes simplex virus	Fetal infection, liver disease, death
Human immunodeficiency virus (HIV)	Perinatal HIV infection
Parvovirus B19 infection	Stillbirth, hydrops
Rubella virus	Deafness, congenital heart disease, microcephaly, cataracts, mental retardation
Syphilis	Maculopapular rash, hepatosplenomegaly, deformed nails, osteochondritis at joints of extremities, congenital neurosyphilis, abnormal epiphyses, chorioretinitis
Toxoplasmosis	Hydrocephaly, microphthalmia, chorioretinitis, mental retardation
Varicella zoster virus	Skin and muscle defects, intrauterine growth retardation, limb reduction defects, CNS damage (very low increased risk)
Venezuelan equine encephalitis	Hydranencephaly, microphthalmia, CNS destructive lesions, luxation of hip
Maternal disease states	
Corticosteroid-secreting endocrinopathy	Mothers with Cushing's disease can have infants with hyperadrenocortism, but anatomical malformations do not appear to be increased
Iodine deficiency	Iodine deficiency can result in embryonic goiter and mental retardation
Intrauterine problems of constraint and vascular disruption	Defects such as club feet, limb reduction, aplasia cutis, cranial asymmetry, external ear malformations, midline closure defects, cleft palate and muscle aplasia, cleft lip, omphalocele, and encephalocele. More common in multiple-birth pregnancies, pregnancies with anatomical defects of the uterus, placental emboli, and amniotic bands
Maternal androgen endocrinopathy (adrenal tumors)	Masculinization
Maternal diabetes	Caudal and femoral hypoplasia, transposition of great vessels
Folic acid insufficiency in the mother	Increased incidence of neural tube defects (NTDs)
Maternal phenylketonuria	Abortion, microcephaly, and mental retardation. Very high risk in untreated patients
Maternal starvation	Intrauterine growth retardation, abortion, NTDs
Tobacco smoking	Abortion, intrauterine growth retardation, and stillbirth
Zinc deficiency*	NTDs

*Controversial.

Table 15.12 Agents erroneously alleged to have caused human malformations.

Agent	Alleged effect
Doxylamine succinate (Bendectin)	Alleged to cause numerous types of birth defects including limb reduction defects and heart malformations
Diagnostic ultrasonography	No significant hyperthermia, therefore no reproductive effects
Electromagnetic fields (EMF)	Alleged to cause abortion, cancer, and birth defects
Progestational drugs	Alleged to cause numerous types of congenital birth defects, including limb reduction defects and heart malformations
Trichloroethylene (TCE)	Alleged to cause cardiac defects

toxicology studies than of any other area of animal testing. For physicians the best source of information concerning animal testing comes from the drug package insert or the Physicians' Desk Reference (PDR).[63] The PDR utilizes the Food and Drug Administration's (FDA's) classification of reproductive risks (categories A, B, C, D, and X), which is partly based on animal testing. Category A includes drugs that present no risk of reproductive effects. Category B, C and D drugs show increasing risks and category X includes drugs such as methotrexate, isotretinoin (Acutane), or thalidomide that should not be used in pregnant women or women of reproductive age who are not taking contraceptives. However, these categories are often more misleading than helpful. Teratologists, obstetricians, and other clinicians who counsel pregnant women have been very critical of the FDA's classification[6] because it ignores the basic principles of teratology[3] and the importance of modern pharmacokinetics in evaluating animal studies.[29] In 1990, an article was published which indicated that of the 200 most frequently prescribed drugs, none represented a significant teratogenic risk.[64] However, only a small proportion of these drugs was placed in category A by the FDA, the most important reason being the misapplication of animal testing results. When a new drug is marketed or a new environmental toxicant is discovered, however, often the only information that is available are the animal data.

Evaluating animal studies to determine the potential risk in humans

When utilizing animal data to assess the potential risk of a drug or chemical exposure in humans, it is important to critically evaluate the studies using the basic principles of teratology guidelines (Table 15.2). As discussed previously, one of the most critical factors for consideration is the dose or magnitude of the exposure, and the concept of the threshold-dose effect for reproductive toxicants. A major shortcoming in many studies is the use of weight (mg/kg) as a measure of dose, as dose comparisons based on mg/kg doses are, at best, rough approximations. Instead, testing in animals could be improved if drugs and chemicals were administered to achieve pharmacokinetically equivalent serum levels in the animal and human. Dose equivalence between species can be accomplished only by performing pharmacokinetic studies, metabolic studies, and dose–response investigations in the human and the species being studied. Dose equivalence must also be determined for the drug-specific effects at the cellular level, to account for species differences in the molecular targets of chemicals or drugs. An excellent example of the importance of the use of pharmacological, rather than weight-based, dose equivalence in interpreting animal study data is illustrated by animal and epidemiological studies performed on leflunomide.[32]

Leflunomide is a relatively new drug (1998) which is used to treat rheumatoid arthritis. It contains a warning for reproductive effects (teratogenesis) and has been placed in category X. This classification was based on animal studies as there were no human data available at the time of marketing.

Leflunomide is a novel isoxazole immunomodulatory agent that has antiproliferative activity. It inhibits mitogen-stimulated proliferation of human peripheral blood mononuclear cells (PBMCs) in a dose-dependent fashion. It has been demonstrated that the active metabolite binds to, and is a potent inhibitor of, dihydroorotate dehydrogenase (DHODH), an enzyme important for DNA synthesis in the *de novo* pyrimidine synthesis pathway. Together, these data suggest that at serum concentrations achievable in patients, leflunomide inhibits *de novo* pyrimidine synthesis in activated lymphocytes and other rapidly dividing cell populations, resulting in reversible cell cycle arrest.

In oral embryotoxicity and teratogenicity studies in rats and rabbits, leflunomide was embryotoxic (growth retarding, embryolethal, and teratogenic). The no-effect level for embryotoxicity and teratogenicity in rats and rabbits was 1 mg/kg body weight, which resulted in serum levels of 3.7 and 4.1 μg/mL respectively. In patients being treated with leflunomide, the active metabolite (the pyrimidine antagonist), is maintained at a blood level of 40 μg/mL. The decision to label leflunomide as having a teratogenic risk was based on the fact that the human serum level was in the range of the teratogenic blood level in the animal models, and, therefore, the initial labeling was an appropriate precaution to prevent birth defects.

After 4 years of treating rheumatoid arthritic patients with leflunomide there was no indication of an increase in teratogenesis in a very small group of pregnant patients who continued their pregnancy to term. The animal data were, therefore, reanalyzed as follows (referred to as the method of action (MOA) approach). The most likely mechanism of leflunomide teratogenicity is the suppression of DNA synthesis and cell proliferation by the inhibition of pyrimidine synthesis. This is based on the assumption that, at the same serum levels of the active metabolite of leflunomide, suppression of DNA synthesis, pyrimidine synthesis, and cell proliferation is equal in the rat, rabbit, and human. There would then be concurrence and the risks would be determined to be identical in all three species; this was the basis of the X-category labeling. However, *in vitro* studies on the active metabolite of leflunomide revealed that the rat was 40 and 328 times more sensitive to the suppression of DHODH and cell proliferation, respectively, than the human.[32] This means that if enzyme suppression or antiproliferative activity is the mechanism (MOA) of teratogenicity in the rat, then the clinical use of leflunomide in pregnant women would probably not be teratogenic. It is important that this drug is subjected to ongoing epidemiological surveillance to confirm these findings. This is an example of how modern pharmacokinetic studies can improve risk assessment, making it easier to understand the epidemiological studies.

Examples of *in vivo* animal studies

In the past 2 years, many excellent *in vivo* animal studies have been carried out. Two particular studies demonstrate the importance, differences, and the usefulness of animal studies as well as the difficulties inherent in drawing inferences from animal studies to describe human risk. Dam and coauthors[65] used an *in vivo* animal model to study the effect of chlorpyrifos (CPF), an organophosphate insecticide whose domestic use has been curtailed in the USA because of concerns about its neurotoxicity, on gene expression. Newborn animals were injected subcutaneously with one of two different doses of CPF on postnatal days 1–4 or 11–14. Studies of the forebrain using molecular biological techniques revealed a significant elevation in one protein that persisted for 5 days after cessation of the exposure regimen. This is an interesting study; however, the results are of little use in determining the human risks of CPF for the following reasons:

1 CPF exposure in humans does not occur via subcutaneous injection but by ingestion or skin absorption of contaminated food or water.
2 The serum concentration of CPF was not determined for the two different exposures used.
3 There was no discussion of the range of levels of CPF that have occurred in human populations.
4 The threshold dose and the no-observed adverse effect level (NOAEL) were not determined.
5 The authors performed toxicogenomics without toxicokinetics.

In contrast, the *in vivo* study by Tyl and coauthors[66] on the reproductive toxicity of dietary bisphenol in rats is considered to be a modern, animal toxicology study for the following reasons:

1 The bisphenol was placed in the diet *ad libitum.*
2 There were seven exposure groups.
3 The exposures were listed in ppm and mg/kg.
4 The range of exposures used was very large: 0.001–500 mg/kg or a 500 000-fold range.
5 The following were not affected at any of the lower exposures although some effects were observed in the 500 mg/kg group: mating, fertility, gestational indices, ovarian primordial follicle counts, estrous cyclicity, precoital interval, gestational length, offspring sex ratios, postnatal survival, nipple/areolae retention in pre-weanling males, epididymal sperm number, motility, and morphology, daily sperm production, and efficiency of production
6 The adult NOAEL was 5 mg/kg/day and the reproductive NOAEL was 50 mg/kg/day. There was a reduction in total body weight and some reduction in organ weight at the higher exposures.

To perform a risk analysis for bisphenol in the human population, some additional information is required that was not reported in this study but which is available in other studies. Yamada and coauthors[67] obtained bisphenol exposure data in humans from the mother and amniotic fluid. The average concentration of bisphenol was 0.32 ng/mL of serum, with a range of 0.0–1.6 ng/mL, levels which appear to be far below the threshold exposure determined by Tyl and coauthors. However, Tyl and coauthors did not obtain the same pharmacokinetic data in the rat that Yamada and coauthors reported in the human, and therefore the serum concentration of bisphenol in the rat at the threshold exposure is not known. Furthermore, it is not known whether the metabolism and effects of bisphenol are similar in the human and the rat.

These studies[66,67] on the risk analysis for bisphenol in the human population indicate the difficulties that can be faced in achieving an accurate and complete interpretation of the data. Combining such studies may appear to be a rare occurrence in the field of risk analysis; fortunately, however, it is occurring more often.[68]

In vitro testing

In vitro tests can be utilized for preliminary screening procedures, and to study the mechanisms of teratogenesis and embryogenesis. However, *in vitro* studies will never be able to predict human teratogenic risks at particular exposures without additional data obtained from whole animal and epidemiological studies.[25,29,31,60] In spite of the advances in *in vitro* and *in vivo* testing for teratogenicity, human epidemiological surveillance by various methodologies is, and will continue to be, our most powerful tool for discovering human reproductive toxins and teratogens. It may be difficult for experimental teratologists to accept the fact that alert physicians and scientists have been the most prominent contributors to the discovery of the environmental causes of birth defects.[26]

The role of the physician in counseling families regarding the etiology of a child's congenital malformation

The clinician must be cognizant of the fact that many patients believe that most congenital malformations are caused by a drug or medication taken during pregnancy. Counseling patients about reproductive risks requires a significant degree of knowledge and skill. Physicians must also realize that erroneous counseling by inexperienced health professionals may result in nonmeritorious litigation.[2]

Unfortunately, it has sometimes been assumed that if a drug or chemical causes birth defects in an animal model or *in vitro* system at a high dose, then it has the potential for producing birth defects at any dose.[27,29] This may be reinforced by the fact that many teratology studies reported in the literature investigate the effects of several doses but do not determine the no-effect dose.

Ignoring the basic tenets of teratology appears to occur most commonly in the evaluation of environmental toxic exposures when the exposure is very low or unknown, and the agent has been reported to be teratogenic at a very high dose or a maternally toxic dose. In most instances, the actual population exposure is orders of magnitude below the threshold dose, the doses that were used in animal studies, or those received during toxic exposures in the population. This has been the case with 2,4,5-trichlorophenoxyacetic acid (2,4,5-T), polychlorinated biphenyls (PCBs), lead, cadmium, arsenic, pesticides, herbicides, veterinary hormones, and industrial exposures.

Unfortunately, there are examples where environmental disasters have been responsible for birth defects or pregnancy loss in exposed populations (methyl mercury in Japan, PCBs in the Far East, organic mercury in the Middle East, and lead poisoning in the nineteenth and early twentieth centuries) and examples where teratogenic drugs have been inadvertently introduced (Table 15.11). Therefore, it is not possible to determine whether a chemical or drug is safe or hazardous unless the magnitude of the exposure is known.

Scholarly evaluation

The physician should respond to a parent's query into the cause of a child's birth defect using the same professional and methodical approach that would be used in a differential diagnosis for any clinical problem. Physicians have a protocol for evaluating complex clinical problems, for example, "fever of unknown origin," "failure to thrive," "congestive heart failure," or "respiratory distress." If a mother of a malformed infant had some type of exposure during pregnancy, for example, medication or a diagnostic radiological examination, the consulting physician should not support or suggest the possibility of a causal relationship before performing a complete evaluation. This is also true if a pregnant woman is exposed to a drug, chemical, or physical agent. As mentioned previously, only a small percentage of birth defects result from exposure to prescribed drugs, chemicals, and physical agents[12,64] (Table 15.3). Even when the drug is listed as a teratogen, to exert a teratogenic effect it has to be administered during the sensitive period of development for that drug, and above the threshold dose. Furthermore, the malformations in a child should be the same as the malformations in the teratogenic syndrome produced by that particular drug. It should be emphasized that in a recent analysis of the 200 most prescribed drugs in the USA, none were found to have measurable teratogenic potential.[64]

After a complete examination of the child and a review of the genetic and teratology medical literature, the clinician must decide whether the child's malformations are genetic or result from exposure to an environmental toxin or agent. It may not be possible to definitively or presumptively conclude the etiology of the child's birth defects. This information must then be conveyed to the patient in an objective and compassionate manner. A similar situation exists if a pregnant woman has been exposed to a drug, chemical, or physical agent, as the mother will want to know the risk of the exposure to her unborn child. A formal approach is recommended to determine whether a particular environmental drug, chemical or physical agent is a reproductive toxicant; this should include, where possible, data obtained from a number of investigative approaches (Table 15.13[20]) including: (1) epidemiological studies,[25,26] (2) secular trend or ecological trend analysis, (3) animal reproductive studies,[27–31] (4) dose response relationships and pharmacokinetic, toxicokinetic, pharmacodynamic, and toxicodynamic studies comparing human and animal metabolism, (5) MOA studies that pertain specifically to the agent and include receptor affinity, cytotoxicity, genotoxicity, organ toxicity, neurotoxicity, etc.,[25,28,30,32] (6) biological plausibility.

Some typical analyses of the reproductive risks of doxylamine succinate (Bendectin), sex steroids, diagnostic ultrasound, and electromagnetic fields demonstrate the usefulness of an organized approach to determine whether an environmental agent has been demonstrated to be a reproductive toxin.[41,52–55,69]

Clinical evaluation

There are many articles and books that can assist the physician with the evaluation of the medical literature and the clinical evaluation of the patient,[13,18,24,38,51,56–61] although training programs do not usually prepare generalists to perform sophisticated genetic or teratology counseling. In addition to the usual history and physical evaluation, the physician has to obtain information about the nature, magnitude, and timing of the exposure. The physical examination should include descriptive and quantitative information about the physical

Table 15.13 Proof of developmental toxicity in humans.

Epidemiological studies

Controlled epidemiological studies consistently demonstrate an increased incidence of a particular spectrum of embryonic and/or fetal effects in exposed human populations

Secular trend data

Secular trends demonstrate a positive relationship between the changing exposures to a common environmental agent in human populations and the incidence of a particular embryonic and/or fetal effect

Animal developmental toxicity studies

An animal model that mimics the human developmental effect at clinically comparable exposures can be developed. Because mimicry may not occur in all animal species, animal models are more likely to be developed once there is good evidence for the embryotoxic effects reported in the human. Developmental toxicity studies in animals are indicative of a potential hazard in general rather than the potential for a specific adverse effect on the fetus when there are no human data on which to base the animal experiments

Dose–response relationship (pharmacokinetics and toxicokinetics)

Developmental toxicity in the human increases with dose (exposure), and the developmental toxicity in animals occurs at a dose that is pharmacokinetically (quantitatively) equivalent to the human exposure

Biological plausibility

The mechanisms of developmental toxicity are understood, and the effects are biologically plausible

Modified from refs 20 and 74.

characteristics of the child. While some growth measurements are routine, many measurements taken by specialized counselors are not part of the usual physical examination, e.g., palpebral fissure size, ear length, intercanthal distances, and total height-to-trunk ratio. Important physical variations in facial, hand, and foot structure as well as other anatomical structures may be suggestive of known syndromes, either teratological or genetic.

Evaluation of the reproductive risk or cause of a child's malformation after an environmental exposure during pregnancy

The vast majority of consultations involving pregnancy exposures conclude that the exposure does not change the reproductive risks for that pregnancy. In many instances, the information that is available is so vague that the counselor cannot reach a definitive conclusion about the magnitude of the risk. The following information is necessary to evaluate any risk:

1 What was the nature of the exposure?

2 Is the exposure agent identifiable? If so, has it been definitively identified as a reproductive toxin with a recognized range of malformations or other reproductive effects?

3 At what stage during embryonic and fetal development did the exposure occur?

4 If the agent is known to produce reproductive toxic effects, was the exposure above or below the threshold for these effects?

5 Were there other significant environmental exposures or medical problems during the pregnancy?

6 Is this a wanted pregnancy or is the family ambivalent about carrying this baby to term?

7 What is the medical and reproductive history of the mother with regard to prior pregnancies and the reproductive history of the family lineage?

After obtaining this information, the counselor is able to provide the family with an estimate of the reproductive risks of the exposure. Some examples of consultations that have been referred to our clinical teratology service are listed below.

Patient 1

A 34-year-old pregnant laboratory worker dropped and broke a reaction vessel containing a mixture of chemical reagents. She proceeded to clean the floor with paper towels and later became concerned about the potential harmful effects of the exposure. This was a planned, wanted pregnancy; she was in the sixth week of pregnancy and, therefore, the embryo was in the period of early organogenesis. The chemicals in the spill were tetrahydrofuran (70%), pyridine (20%), and iodine (1%). It was not possible to quantitatively estimate the exposure to these agents, but the laboratory worker experienced no symptoms from the exposure. There have been no epidemiological studies of tetrahydrofuran and pyridine in pregnant women but iodine has been shown to interfere with fetal thyroid development; in this situation, however, the exposure would have been inconsequential because, at this stage of pregnancy, the thyroid is not yet present. No other exposure to reproductive toxins occurred in this pregnancy and the family history for congenital malformations was negative. The woman was advised that it would be very unlikely that her teratogenic risk would be increased because the exposures to the embryo would be extremely low. She was told that she still faced the background risks for birth defects and miscarriage and, therefore, her reproductive risks would be the same as that of the general population (Table 15.1).

Patient 2

A 26-year-old pregnant woman was in an automobile accident in the 10th week of her pregnancy and sustained a severe concussion. Although she did not convulse post injury, the treating neurosurgeon prescribed 300 mg of diphenylhydantoin during her first 24 h in hospital. Fortunately, she recovered from the injury without any sequelae but her primary physician was concerned that she had received an anticonvulsant associated with a teratogenic syndrome. No other exposure to reproductive toxins occurred in this pregnancy and the family history for congenital malformations was negative, except for an uncle with neurofibromatosis. The primary physician requested a consultation with regard to the teratogenic risk. While diphenylhydantoin administered chronically throughout pregnancy has been associated with a low incidence of characteristic facial dysmorphogenesis, reduced mentation, cleft palate, and digital hypoplasia, there are no data to indicate that 24 h of therapy would cause any of these features. In addition, the development of the lip and palate are complete by the 10th week of pregnancy. This was a wanted pregnancy and the mother chose to continue her pregnancy; she delivered a normal 3370-g boy at term.

Patient 3

A 25-year-old woman was seen in the emergency service of her local hospital with nausea, vomiting, and diarrhea, on return from a cruise on which a number of the passengers became ill with similar symptoms. The emergency-ward physician ordered a pregnancy test followed by a flat-plate radiograph of the abdomen as there was evidence of peritoneal irritation; however, both of these tests were negative. One week later she missed her menstrual period and a subsequent pregnancy test was positive. Her obstetrician was concerned because she had been exposed to a radiological examination at a time when she was pregnant; he referred the patient for counseling after obtaining an ultrasound that indicated that the embryo was approximately 7 days post conception at the time of the examination. The patient advised the counselor that she was ambivalent about the pregnancy because of the "dangers" of the X-rays to her embryo. The estimated exposure to the embryo was less than 500 mrad (0.005 Sv), an exposure that is far below that known to affect the developing embryo. Also, the embryo was exposed during the first 2 weeks post conception, a time that is less likely to increase the risk of teratogenesis, even at much higher exposures.[3,70] After an evaluation of the family history and after receiving counseling about the risks of the radiological examination, the woman decided to continue the pregnancy; she delivered a normal 3150-g baby.

Evaluation of the cause of a child's congenital malformations: unknown, genetic, or environmental

Patient 4

The mother of a 30-year-old man born in the Azores in 1960 with a congenital absence of the right leg below the knee had pursued compensation for her son because she was certain that she must have received thalidomide during her pregnancy.[4] The German manufacturer of thalidomide refused compensation, claiming that thalidomide had never been distributed in the Azores. The mother fervently believed that thalidomide was responsible for her son's malformations and asked for my opinion; she sent me the radiograph studies of his hips and legs and his complete evaluation performed at the local hospital in the Azores. He had none of the other stigmata of thalidomide embryopathy (preaxial limb defects, phocomelia, facial hemangioma, ear malformations, deafness, crocodile tears, ventricular septal defect, intestinal or gallbladder atresia, and kidney malformations) and, most importantly, his limb malformations were not of the thalidomide type; he had a unilateral congenital amputation with no digital remnants at the end of the limb, his pelvic girdle was completely normal, and his limb defect involved only one leg with the other leg being normal. In this particular case, the man had a congenital amputation probably resulting from vascular disruption of an unknown etiology (known causes of vascular disruptive malformations are cocaine, misoprostol and chorionic villous sampling). It is difficult to determine whether any amount of appropriate counseling will give closure to this mother.

Patient 5

The family of a malformed boy claimed that the antinausea medication doxylamine succinate (Bendectin),[52,53,71] taken by the mother during pregnancy, was responsible for the child's congenital limb reduction defects. Bendectin was taken after the period of limb organogenesis; however, some limb malformations can be produced by teratogens after this time. The boy's malformation was the classical split-hand, split-foot syndrome, which is dominantly inherited; it was unaccompanied by any other dysmorphogenetic effects. Although significant number of cases of this syndrome result from a new mutation, neither parent manifested the malformation and this suggested that a new mutation had occurred in the sex cells of one of the parents. Therefore, the risk of this malformation occurring in the offspring of this boy would be 50%. It was concluded that Bendectin was not responsible for this child's malformation; however, in spite of the obvious genetic etiology of the birth defect, a legal suit was filed. A jury decided for the defendant, namely, that Bendectin was not responsible for the child's malformation.

Patient 6

A woman visited a hospital emergency ward with severe lower abdominal pain; as she had had a previous ectopic pregnancy that necessitated the removal of her ovary and fallopian tube, she was seen by an obstetrical resident. A pregnancy test was positive and she returned to the obstetrical clinic a week later when her chorionic gonadotropin level was retested. It had not changed from its previous level and, without performing an ultrasound, a diagnosis of ectopic pregnancy was made; in order to preserve the patient's reproductive potential, it was decided to treat the ectopic pregnancy with methotrexate rather than remove the remaining fallopian tube and ovary. However, following the administration of methotrexate, a laboratory report was received which indicated that the gonadotropin level had increased fivefold, and a subsequent ultrasound revealed a normally implanted embryo; the laboratory report received earlier in the day was found to be a copy of the original report performed a week earlier. The mother was counseled that the baby was at an increased risk of having congenital malformations because of the exposure to methotrexate; however, she refused to abort the pregnancy. The obstetrical department therefore offered to provide care for the pregnancy and delivery that included a number of ultrasound examinations. At 28 weeks, the patient went into labor and delivered a premature liveborn infant, and during infancy, the child was diagnosed with hydrocephalus, developmental delay, and spastic cerebral symptomatology. The family filed a lawsuit against the doctors and hospital and I was asked to evaluate the allegation that the abnormalities in the child were due to the administration of methotrexate. Methotrexate has been reported to cause growth retardation, microcephaly, developmental delay, and hydrocephalus, but not prematurity. The clinical care provided by the resident doctor was unfortunate; however, the provision of care by the obstetrical department turned out to be fortunate for the defendants in this case. A review of the records revealed two important findings: first, an ultrasound examination taken a week before the premature delivery revealed that there was no evidence of hydrocephalus and, second, the birthweight was appropriate for the gestational stage. Therefore, the exposure to methotrexate was not responsible for the serious problems in this infant; the hydrocephalus and neurological symptoms resulted from a central nervous system (CNS) bleed in the postnatal period as a complication of the prematurity.

These examples show that it is not a simple process to determine the reproductive risks of an exposure during pregnancy or to determine the etiology of a child's congenital malformations. It requires careful analysis of the medical and scientific literature on the reproductive toxic effects of exogenous agents in humans and animals, as well as an evaluation of the exposure and biological plausibility of an increased risk or a causal connection between the exposure and a child's congenital malformation. It also involves a careful physical examination, and a review of the scientific literature regarding the genetic and environmental causes of the malformations in question. Abridged counseling, based on superficial and incomplete analyses, is a disservice to the families involved.

Conclusion

Approximately 10% of human malformations are due to environmental causes and fewer than 1% are related to prescription drug exposure, chemicals, or radiation. However, malformations caused by drugs and other therapeutic agents are important because these exposures may be preventable. Advances in animal research and epidemiology have enabled scientists to gain a better understanding of the mechanisms of teratogenesis.

Concerns about environmental chemicals and physical agents are clearly justified because, in most cases, not enough information is available on the potentially differential effects on the fetus and child. Such information, for example, the population exposure and the NOAEL, can only be obtained from high-quality human and animal toxicology and epidemiological studies which include toxicokinetic and toxicodynamic data and, therefore, it is essential that we expand our research programs in these areas. Ecological studies that do not measure exposures in the human population are more confusing than helpful in determining human risks, and studying exposures to groups of agents, e.g., solvents and pesticides, does not allow a risk assessment for individual toxicants.

All chemicals and drugs have the potential for developmental toxicity if the exposure is high enough; it would therefore be beneficial if humans were not exposed to chemicals in the workplace or home, or if chemicals were not dispersed into the environment. To address this problem now, and in the future, an extensive program of monitoring, reducing, and eliminating the delivery of chemicals to the environment and the exposure of populations to chemicals is needed. Introducing or banning chemicals that expose the human population is an extremely difficult task that needs to be carefully planned on the basis of risks and benefits.

Key points

1. Severe congenital malformations (including those birth defects that cause death, hospitalization, and mental retardation, and those that necessitate significant or repeated surgical procedures, are disfiguring, or interfere with physical performance) occur in 3% of all births.
2. Only a small percentage of birth defects are due to prescribed drugs, chemicals, and physical agents. Even when a drug is listed as a teratogen, it has to be administered during the sensitive period of development for that drug, and above the threshold dose for producing teratogenesis. Environmental causes account for approximately 10% of human birth malformations, and fewer than 1% of all human malformations are related to prescription drug exposure, chemicals, or radiation.
3. The etiology of congenital malformations can be divided into three categories: unknown (65–75%), genetic (15–25%), and environmental (10%).
4. Reproductive problems alarm the public, press, and some scientists, to a greater degree than most other diseases.
5. Physicians must recognize the consequences of providing erroneous reproductive risks to pregnant women exposed to drugs and chemicals during pregnancy, or of alleging that a child's malformations are caused by an environmental agent without performing a complete and scholarly evaluation.
6. Labeling an environmental exposure as teratogenic is inappropriate unless one characterizes the exposure with regard to the dose, route of exposure, and stage of pregnancy when the exposure occurred.
7. The application of the basic scientific principles of teratology is extremely important in evaluating studies on the reproductive effects of an environmental agent. These principles include the following criteria: exposure to teratogens follows a toxicological dose–response curve; the embryonic stage at which exposure occurs determines what effects (if any) a teratogen has; most teratogens have a confined group of congenital malformations (syndrome of agent's effects) and; no teratogen can produce every type of malformation.
8. The risk of morphological anomalies or intrauterine death resulting from exposure to a developmental toxicant varies depending on the dose and the embryonic or fetal stage at which exposure occurs.
9. The threshold dose for an environmental toxicant is the dose below which the incidence of death, malformation, growth retardation, or functional deficit is not greater than that of control subjects. The severity and incidence of malformations produced by every exogenous agent that has been appropriately studied have exhibited threshold phenomena during organogenesis.
10. Teratogens follow a threshold dose–response curve, whereas mutagens and carcinogens tend to follow a stochastic dose–response curve.
11. Physiological alterations in pregnancy and the bioconversion of compounds can significantly influence the teratogenic effects of drugs and chemicals by affecting absorption, body distribution, active form(s), and excretion of the compound.
12. Interpretation of dose–response relationships for teratogens must take into account the active metabolites, when metabolites might be the proximate teratogen rather than the administered drug or chemical, the duration of the exposure (chronic versus acute), and the fat solubility of the agent.
13. The role that the placenta plays in drug pharmacokinetics involves transport, the presence of receptors for a number of endogenous and xenobiotic compounds, and the bioconversion of xenobiotics.
14. The genetic constitution of an individual is an important factor that affects the susceptibility of a species to a drug or chemical.
15. Animal teratology studies are helpful in raising concerns about the reproductive effects of drugs and chemicals, but negative animal studies do not guarantee that these agents are free from reproductive effects.
16. Well-performed epidemiology studies represent the best methodology for determining the human risk and the effects of environmental toxicants.
17. *In vitro* tests can be used to study the mechanisms of teratogenesis and embryogenesis, and for preliminary screening procedures. However, *in vitro* studies cannot predict human teratogenic risks at particular exposures without the benefit of data obtained from whole animal studies and epidemiological studies.
18. The clinician must be cognizant of the fact that many patients believe that most congenital malformations are caused by a drug or medication taken during pregnancy.
19. Ignoring the basic tenets of teratology appears to occur most commonly in the evaluation of environmental exposures when the exposure was very low or unknown and the agent has been reported to be teratogenic at a very high dose or maternally toxic dose.
20. The evaluation of the toxicity of drugs and chemicals should (when possible) use data obtained from investigative approaches including: (1) epidemiological studies, (2) secular trend analysis, (3) animal reproductive studies, (4) dose–response relationships, (5) mechanisms of action (MOA) studies that pertain specifically to the agent and include receptor affinity, cytotoxicity, genotoxicity, organ toxicity, and neurotoxicity, and (6) biological plausibility.

References

1 Brent RL. Medicolegal aspects of teratology. *J Pediatr* 1967;71: 288–298.

2 Brent RL. Litigation-produced pain, disease and suffering: an experience with congenital malformation lawsuits. *Teratology* 1977; 16:1–14.

3 Brent RL. Utilization of developmental basic science principles in the evaluation of reproductive risks from pre- and postconception environmental radiation exposures. *Teratology* 1999;59:182–204.

4 Brent RL, Holmes L. Clinical and basic science lessons from the thalidomide tragedy: what have we learned about the causes of limb defects? *Teratology* 1988;38:241–251.

5 Brent RL. The irresponsible expert witness: a failure of biomedical graduate education and professional accountability. *Pediatrics* 1982;70:754–762.

6 Brent RL. Drugs and pregnancy: are the insert warnings too dire? *Contemp Ob-Gyn* 1982;20:42–49.

7 Wilson J. *Environment and birth defects*. New York: Academic Press, 1973.

8 Brent RL. Environmental factors: miscellaneous. In: Brent RL, Harris M, eds. *Prevention of embryonic, fetal and perinatal disease*. Bethesda, MD: John E. Fogarty International Center for Aduanced Study in the Health Sciences, NIH; 1976:211.

9 Heinonen O, Slone D, Shapiro S. *Birth defects and drugs in pregnancy*. Littleton, MA: Publishing Sciences Group, 1977.

10 Brent RL, Beckman D. *Environmental teratogens*. New York: New York Academy of Medicine, 1990.

11 Beckman D, Fawcett L, Brent RL. Developmental toxicity. In: Massaro E, ed. *Handbook of human toxicology*. New York: CRC Press; 1997:1007–1084.

12 Brent RL, Beckman D. Prescribed drugs, therapeutic agents, and fetal teratogenesis. In: Reece E, Hobbins J, eds. *Medicine of the fetus and mother*, 2nd edn. Philadelphia, PA: Lippincott-Raven Publishers; 1999:289–313.

13 Aase J. *Diagnostic dysmorphology*. New York: Plenum Medical Book Co., 1990.

14 Beckman D, Brent RL. Fetal effects of prescribed and self-administered drugs during the second and third trimester. In: Avery G, Fletcher M, MacDonald M, eds. *Neonatology: pathophysiology and treatment*, 4th edn. Philadelphia, PA: JB Lippincott Co.; 1994:197–206.

15 Brent RL. What is the relationship between birth defects and pregnancy bleeding? New perspectives provided by the NICHD workshop dealing with the association of chorionic villous sampling and the occurrence of limb reduction defects. *Teratology* 1993;48: 93–95.

16 Brent RL, Beckman D. Teratogens: an overview. In: Knobil E, Neill J, eds. *Encyclopedia of reproduction*. New York: Academic Press; 1999:735–750.

17 Graham JJ, Jones K, Brent RL. Contribution of clinical teratologists and geneticists to the evaluation of the etiology of congenital malformations alleged to be caused by environmental agents, ionizing radiation, electromagnetic fields, microwaves, radionuclides, and ultrasound. *Teratology* 1999;59:307–313.

18 Jones K. *Smith's recognizable pattern of human malformations*, 5th edn. Philadelphia, PA: WB Saunders Co., 1994.

19 Brent RL, Beckman D. Angiotensin-converting enzyme inhibitors, an embryopathic class of drugs with unique properties: information for clinical teratology councilors. *Teratology* 1991;43:543–545.

20 Brent RL. Methods of evaluating the alleged teratogenicity of environmental agents. In: Sever J, Brent RL, eds. *Teratogen update: environmentally induced birth defect risks*. New York: Alan R Liss; 1986:199–201.

21 Brent RL. Effects and risks of medically administered isotopes to the developing embryo. In: Fabro S, Scialli A, eds. *Drug and chemical action in pregnancy*. New York: Marcel Dekker; 1986:427–439.

22 Brent RL. Radiation teratogenesis. *Teratology* 1980;21:281–298.

23 Brent RL, Beckman D. Developmental effects following radiation of embryonic and fetal exposure to x-ray and isotopes: counseling the pregnant and nonpregnant patient about these risks. In: Hendee W, Edwards F, eds. *Health effects of low levels exposure to ionizing radiation*. Bristol & Philadelphia: Institute of Physics Publishing; 1996:169–213.

24 Online Mendelian Inheritance in Man, OMIM™. McKusick-Nathans Institute for Genetic Medicine, Johns Hopkins University (Baltimore, MD) and National Center for Biotechnology Information, National Library of Medicine (Bethesda, MD), 2000. World Wide Web URL: http://www.ncbi.nlm.nih.gov/omim/

25 Brent RL. Evaluating the alleged teratogenicity of environmental agents. In: Brent RL, Beckman D, eds. *Clinics in perinatology*. Philadelphia, PA: WB Saunders; 1986:609–613.

26 Brent RL. Protecting the public from teratogenic and mutagenic hazards. *J Clin Pharmacol* 1972;12:61–70.

27 Brent RL. Drug testing in animals for teratogenic effects: thalidomide in the pregnant rat. *J Pediatr* 1964;64:762–770.

28 Brent RL. The prediction of human diseases from laboratory and animal tests for teratogenicity, carcinogenicity, and mutagenicity. In: Lasagna L, ed. *Controversies in therapeutics*. Philadelphia, PA: WB Saunders; 1980:134–150.

29 Brent RL. Predicting teratogenic and reproductive risks in humans from exposure to various environmental agents using *in vitro* techniques and *in vivo* animal studies. *Cong Anomalies* 1988; 28(Suppl.):41-55.

30 Christian M, Brent RL. Teratogen update: evaluation of the reproductive and developmental risks of caffeine. *Teratology* 2001;64: 51–78.

31 Brent RL. Scientific frontiers in developmental toxicology and risk assessment (Review). *Teratology* 2002;65:88–96.

32 Brent RL. Teratogen update: reproductive risks of leflunomide (Avara). A parimidine synthesis inhibitor: counseling women lacking leflunomide before or during pregnancy and men taking leflunomide who are contemplating fathering a child. *Teratology* 2001;63:106–112.

33 Carter C. Genetics of common single malformations. *Br Med Bull* 1976;32:21–26.

34 Fraser F. The multifactorial/threshold concept: uses and misuses. *Teratology* 1976;14:267–280.

35 Boue J, Boue A, Lazar P. Retrospective and prospective epidemiological studies of 1500 karyotyped spontaneous abortions. *Teratology* 1975;12:11–26.

36 Hertig A. The overall problem in man. In: Benirschke K, ed. *Comparative aspects of reproductive failure*. Berlin: Springer-Verlag; 1967:11.

37 Simpson J. Genes, chromosomes and reproductive failure. *Fertil Steril* 1980;33:107–116.

38 Sever J. Infections in pregnancy: highlights from the collective perinatal project. *Teratology* 1982;25:227–237.

39 Briggs M, Briggs M. Sex hormone exposure during pregnancy and malformations. *Adv Steroid Biochem Pharmacol* 1979;7:51–89.

40 Hochner-Celnikier D, Marandici A, Iohan F, Monder C. Estrogen and progesterone receptors in the organs of prenatal Cynomolgus monkey and laboratory mouse. *Biol Reprod* 1986;35:633–640.
41 Wilson J, Brent RL. Are female sex hormones teratogenic? *Am J Obstet Gynecol* 1981;141:567–580.
42 Jackson M. Drug absorption. In: Fabro S, Scialli A, eds. *Drug and chemical action in pregnancy: pharmacologic and toxicologic principles.* New York: Marcel Dekker; 1986:15.
43 Mattison D. Physiologic variations in pharmacokinetics during pregnancy. In: Fabro S, Scialli A, eds. *Drug and chemical action during pregnancy: pharmacologic and toxicologic principles.* New York: Marcel Dekker; 1986:37–102.
44 Sonawane B, Yaffe S. Physiologic disposition of drugs in the fetus and newborn. In: Fabro S, Scialli A, eds. *Drug and chemical action in pregnancy: pharmacologic and toxicologic principles.* New York: Marcel Dekker; 1986:103.
45 Juchau M, Rettie A. The metabolic role of the placenta. In: Fabro S, Scialli A, eds. *Drug and chemical action in pregnancy: pharmacologic and toxicologic principles.* New York: Marcel Dekker; 1986:153–169.
46 Yang H, Namkung M, Juchau M. Cytochrome P450-dependent biotransformation of a series of phenoxazone ethers in the rat conceptus during early organogenesis: evidence for multiple P450 isozymes. *Mol Pharmacol* 1988;34:67–73.
47 Fantel A, Person R, Juchau M. Niridazole metabolism by rat embryos in vitro. *Teratology* 1988;37:213–221.
48 Juchau M. Bioactivation in chemical teratogenesis. *Annu Rev Pharmacol Toxicol* 1989;29:165–187.
49 Miller R. Placental transfer and function: the interface for drugs and chemicals in the conceptus. In: Fabro S, Scialli A, eds. *Drug and chemical action in pregnancy: pharmacologic and toxicologic principles.* New York: Marcel Dekker; 1986:123.
50 Mirkin B. Maternal and fetal distribution of drugs in pregnancy. *Clin Pharmacol Ther* 1973;14:643–647.
51 McKusic V. Medelian inheritance in man: catalogs of autosomal dominant, autosomal recessive, and x-linked phenotypes, 8th edn. Baltimore, MD: Johns Hopkins University Press, 1988.
52 Brent RL. Bendectin: review of the medical literature of a comprehensively studied human non-teratogen and the most prevalent tortigen-litigen. *Reprod Toxicol* 1995;9:337–349.
53 Brent RL. Review of the scientific literature pertaining to the reproductive toxicity of bendectin. In: Faigman D, Kaye D, Saks M, et al., eds. *Modern scientific evidence: the law and science of expert testimony.* St. Paul, MN: West Publishing Group; 1997: 373–393.
54 Brent RL. Microwaves and ultrasound. In: Queenan J, Hobbins J, eds. *Protocols for high risk pregnancies*, 3rd edn. Cambridge: Blackwell Scientific; 1995:37–43.
55 Brent RL, Gordon W, Bennett W, Beckman D. Reproductive and teratogenic effects of electromagnetic fields. *Reprod Toxicol* 1993;7:535–580.
56 Friedman J, Polifka J. TERIS. The teratogen information system. Seattle, WA: University of Washington, 1999.
57 Scialli A, Lione A, Padget GKB. Reproductive effects of chemical, physical and biologic agents. Baltimore, MD: Johns Hopkins University Press, 1995.
58 Sever J, Brent RL. Teratogen update: environmentally induced birth defect risks. New York: Alan R Liss, 1986.
59 Sheperd T. *Catalogue of teratogenic agents*, 8th edn. Baltimore, MD: Johns Hopkins University Press, 1995.
60 Schardein J. *Chemically induced birth defects.* New York: Marcel Dekker, 1993.
61 Briggs G, Freeman R, Yaffe S. *Drugs in pregnancy and lactation*, 3rd edn. Baltimore, MD: Williams and Wilkins, 1990.
62 Miller R. How environmental hazards have been discovered: carcinogens, teratogens, neurotoxins, and others. *Pediatrics* 2004; 113:945–951.
63 *Physicians Desk Reference*, 57th edn: Medical Economics Co. Montvale, NJ: Thomson Healthcare; 2003.
64 Friedman J, Little B, Brent RL, et al. Potential human teratogenicity of frequently prescribed drugs. *Obstet Gynecol* 1990;75: 594–599.
65 Dam K, Seidler F, Slotkin T. Transcriptional biomarkers distinguish between vulnerable periods for developmental neurotoxicity of chlorpyrifos: implications for toxicogenomics. *Brain Res Bull* 2003;59:261–265.
66 Tyl R, Myers C, Thomas B, et al. Three-generation reproductive toxicity study of dietary bisphenol A in CD Sprague-Dawley rats. *Toxicol Sci* 2002;68:121–146.
67 Yamada H, Furuta I, Kato E, et al. Maternal serum and amniotic fluid bisphenol A concentrations in the early second trimester. *Reprod Toxicol* 2002;16:735–739.
68 Holson J, DeSesso J, Jacobson C, Farr C. Appropriate use of animal models in the assessment of risk during prenatal development: an illustration using inorganic arsenic. *Teratology* 2000;62:51–71.
69 Brent RL, Jensh R, Beckman D. Medical sonography: reproductive effects and risks. *Teratology* 1991;44:123–146.
70 Wilson J, Brent RL, Jordan H. Differentiation as a determinant of the reaction of rat embryos to x-irradiation. *Proc Soc Exp Biol Med* 1953;82:67–70.
71 Brent RL. Commentary on bendectin and birth defects: hopefully the final chapter. *Birth Defects Res* 2003;67:79–87.
72 Roberts C, Lowe C. Where have all the conceptions gone? *Lancet* 1975;1:498–499.
73 Brent RL. Editorial: definition of a teratogen and the relationship of teratogenicity to carcinogenicity. *Teratology* 1986;34:359–360.
74 Brent RL. Method of evaluating alleged human teratogens. *Teratology* 1978;17:83.

16 Drugs, alcohol abuse, and effects in pregnancy

Stephen R. Carr and Donald R. Coustan

Determining the developmental toxicity of a drug or chemical requires an understanding of the mechanism of action and pharmacology of the substance as well as an understanding of embryology. Drugs, both legal and illicit, exert fetal developmental effects that are dependent on the dose, route of administration, physiologic handling by both the pregnant woman and the fetus, genetic predisposition, and the timing of the exposure in the pregnancy. The type of abnormality seen following drug exposure during pregnancy may give valuable clues about when in the pregnancy that drug had its effect. Thalidomide is perhaps the best known example of a substance with a very narrow window of toxic effect in developing humans.[1] Exposure of human fetuses to thalidomide between days 22 and 36 after conception is associated with characteristic limb reduction defects, as well as other structural anomalies. Complete understanding of the above-named factors may not in many cases be possible, so providers who care for pregnant women must rely on published experience of the agent in question. In the course of a busy practice, exhaustive research is neither practical nor possible but, fortunately, there are convenient alternatives including the Physician's Desk Reference (PDR), online resources such as Reprotox, traditional texts, and those for portable use on a personal digital assistant (PDA). When agents are new to the pharmacopeia, caution is necessary. Data in animal models may not present the full spectrum of toxicity in human pregnancy. Responsible pharmaceutical companies sponsor registries to more rapidly amass clinically significant data concerning the fetal impact of drug exposure during pregnancy. Even given that, frequently it is many years after the introduction of an agent before any degree of certainty about the appropriateness of an agent for use in pregnancy can be established. These registries benefit from being part of an organized effort to present comprehensive information concerning legal medications. Such organized registries are rare for illicit drug use and, as a result, practitioners rely on animal models and analyses of case series.

In spite of well-intentioned efforts at education, prevention, and intervention, the use and abuse of drugs, both legal and illi-cit, continue to cause maternal and fetal problems during pregnancy.

Alcohol

Ethanol is a social drug that offers no apparent benefit to the pregnant woman or her fetus. In spite of this, more than 500 000 fetuses per year in the US are exposed to ethanol *in utero*.[2] In total, infants born with fetal alcohol syndrome (FAS) cost approximately US$40 billion yearly (in 1998 dollars), or approximately US$2 million as a lifetime cost per individual.[3] The term FAS was coined to describe 11 children of alcoholic mothers with characteristic features (Table 16.1).[4,5] In 1980, specific criteria for FAS were proposed by the Fetal Alcohol Study Group of the Research Society on Alcoholism, requiring that at least one feature from each of the three categories be present for the diagnosis to be made.[6] More recently, the Institute of Medicine defined five categories of alcohol-related birth effects[7] (Table 16.2). The average IQ of children with FAS is 70.[8] The original FAS children were followed for 10 years, and their growth deficiency and mental handicaps persisted.

It is difficult to estimate the prevalence of FAS or construct a dose–response curve for levels of alcohol exposure necessary to produce this problem, because it is difficult to accurately quantify alcohol intake; the amount of alcohol used is invariably underestimated. In addition, specific features of FAS may be caused by exposure to alcohol at different times in gestation. Craniofacial anomalies may occur during embryogenesis, disorders of central nervous system function may be brought about later in gestation, and growth disturbances may reflect alcohol exposure over a broad range of gestational ages.

The prevalence of FAS among offspring of heavy drinkers ranges from 2.5% to 10% in prospective studies.[9] Recent work estimates FAS prevalence in the US at 0.3–0.4 per 1000 live births.[10] Although it is difficult to obtain more specific data, it is clear that all cases of full-blown FAS occurred in chronic alcoholic mothers who drank heavily throughout pregnancy. It is also clear that binge drinking increases the risks of affected children having IQs in the mentally retarded range.[11] Studies have attempted to identify a threshold level of maternal ethanol ingestion above which effects are seen, and below which effects are not seen, without notable success. One analysis of the Spanish Collaborative Study of Congenital

Table 16.1 Alcohol and the fetus.

Fetal alcohol syndrome – at least one from each of the following categories:
Growth restriction, either prenatal or postnatal in onset
SGA/IUGR
Failure to thrive/short stature
Craniofacial abnormalities
Small eyes
Epicanthal folds
Long philtrum
Midface hypoplasia
Central nervous system abnormalities
Microcephaly
Developmental delay
Mental retardation
Learning disabilities
Alcohol-related birth defects – any of the preceding problems in the offspring of an alcoholic individual

SGA, small for gestational age; IUGR, intrauterine growth restriction.

Table 16.2 Categories of alcohol-related birth defects.

FAS: with confirmed maternal alcohol use and a characteristic pattern of malformations
FAS: without confirmed maternal alcohol use, but with the characteristic pattern of malformations
Partial FAS: with confirmed maternal alcohol use and some components of the characteristic malformations
Alcohol-related birth defects: the presence of congenital anomalies resulting from prenatal alcohol exposure
Alcohol-related neurodevelopmental disorder (ARND): central nervous system neurodevelopmental abnormalities, neurological hard or soft signs, or behavioral/cognitive abnormalities not consistent with background or environment

Malformations determined that even low and sporadic alcohol ingestion during pregnancy increased the risk of congenital anomalies.[12] Recent work has demonstrated increased neurodegeneration via apoptosis during synaptogenesis,[13] defects in neuronal migration and decreased numbers of neurons in the mature cortex,[14] and effects on myelination leading to decreases in white matter volume.[15]

The pathophysiologic mechanism for the adverse effects of alcohol on the developing fetus is poorly understood. Ethanol levels in maternal and fetal blood are identical in sheep, and studies in sheep demonstrate a time lag before ethanol's appearance in amniotic fluid.[16] A similar time lag has been found in the appearance of ethanol in human amniotic fluid.[17] There are increased c-myc protein levels and decreased growth-associated protein 43 levels after exposure of neural cell lines to ethanol.[18,19] Normal cellular morphologic differentiation requires decreases in c-myc and increases in growth-associated protein 43. Ethanol effects the production of these differentiation modulators and inhibits normal neuronal growth and differentiation. These studies describe changes in neuronal development/migration, apoptosis, and myelinization that are likely to be at the root of the neurobehavioral changes seen in children exposed to ethanol *in utero*. Acetaldehyde, a toxic metabolic product of ethanol, behaves similarly with respect to the amniotic fluid. Alcohol is metabolized via a number of different systems, including alcohol dehydrogenase in the cytosol fraction of the liver, the hepatic microsomal ethanol-oxidizing system, and the peroxisomal catalase system. There are genetic differences in some of these enzymes, and different individuals may induce them at different rates when exposed to the same concentrations of ethanol. Differential enzyme induction may lead to differential susceptibility to cell injury or disruption by other agents.[20] Alternatively, ethanol or acetaldehyde may interfere with placental transport of vital nutrients such as amino acids, leading to fetal malnutrition.[21] Either interference with normal cellular development or fetal malnutrition may result in the 150-g lower birthweight of babies exposed to one to three drinks per day seen in a study of 10 539 women.[22]

Alcohol ingestion by the gravida decreases fetal breathing movements but not gross body movements or fetal heart rate.[23] Alcohol withdrawal effects have been described, even in infants without the stigmata of FAS.[24] The fetal effects of alcohol appear to be multifactorial.

There is no treatment or cure for FAS or alcohol-related birth effects. One study suggested a protective effect of antioxidants (alpha-tocopherol and N-acetylcysteine) in the rat model, but this has not been confirmed in humans.[25] The best strategy is prevention, and the first component of prevention is education, so that women of childbearing age are aware of the risks of drinking during pregnancy. Educational campaigns have been carried out in the US at all levels. An epidemiologic study in Seattle reported that any alcohol use in early pregnancy fell from 81% in 1974–75 to 42% in 1980–81, and this was attributed to educational programs.[26] Although the prevalence of heavy drinking (defined in this study as 30 mL or more of absolute alcohol per day) before the discovery of pregnancy was unchanged at 6–7% during each time period, such use after pregnancy was discovered fell from 2.3% to 0.8%. In a population-based study in Finland from 1983 to 1985, 55% of women drank at least 2 oz of absolute alcohol during the week in which conception occurred, and only 16% were totally abstinent during the first trimester.[27] By 32 weeks, 50% were totally abstinent and, by term, 80% took no alcohol at all.

To prevent FAS, it is first necessary to identify mothers at risk. The CAGE[28] (Table 16.3), T-ACE[29] (Table 16.4), and TWEAK[30] (Table 16.5) questionnaires are all brief and effective. Several basic questions are asked in each of these questionnaires. Two or more positive answers on the CAGE questionnaire indicate a high probability of being a risk drinker. In the T-ACE questionnaires, the ability to hold a

Table 16.3 CAGE.

1. Have you ever felt the need to Cut down drinking?
2. Have you ever felt Annoyed by criticism of your drinking?
3. Have you ever had Guilty feelings about drinking?
4. Have you ever taken a morning "Eye-opener"?

Table 16.4 T-ACE.

1. How many drinks can you hold? (Tolerance)
2. Have you ever felt Annoyed by criticism of your drinking?
3. Have you ever felt the need to Cut down drinking?
4. Have you ever taken a morning "Eye-opener"?

Table 16.5 TWEAK.

Tolerance: how many drinks does it take before you feel the effects of alcohol? (2 points for ≥ 3 drinks)
Worry: have close friends or family worried or complained about your drinking in the past year? (2 points for yes)
Eye-opener: do you sometimes take a drink in the morning when you wake up? (1 point for yes)
Amnesia: are there times when you drink and afterwards can't remember what you said or did? (1 point for yes)
Cut down: do you sometimes feel the need to cut down on your drinking? (1 point for yes)

six-pack of beer or a bottle of wine scores two points on the tolerance question; affirmative answers on the others each score one point. A cumulative score of more than 2 indicates a high probability of being a risk drinker. A total of ≥ 2 points on the TWEAK questionnaire also indicates a high probability of problem drinking. One of these questionnaires should be administered to every patient when obtaining a history.

Recent research suggests that meconium fatty acid ethyl esters are a sensitive and specific marker for suspected but unreported maternal alcohol abuse in pregnancy.[31] This remains to be confirmed in clinical practice.

Once the individual at increased risk for having a child with alcohol-related birth defects is identified, attention should be turned to intervention. Rosett and co-workers[32] found that 67% of 49 pregnant problem drinkers reduced their alcohol intake when enrolled in a counseling program. Work in both the US and Finland found that cessation of heavy alcohol intake before the third trimester benefits the fetus.[33,34] A randomized trial, although not specific to pregnancy, demonstrated that two brief (10–15 min each using scripted advice and educational information) interventions decreased both chronic and binge drinking.[35]

Disulfiram use to increase the motivation of alcoholics to avoid consumption of alcohol is generally contraindicated in pregnancy.[36] Not a proven teratogen, disulfiram, when taken in combination with alcohol, leads to very high circulating acetaldehyde concentrations.

Table 16.6 Reported effects of cocaine on the fetus and pregnancy.

Placental abruption
Intrauterine growth restriction
Preterm labor
Premature rupture of the membranes with meconium
Spontaneous abortion
Intrauterine cerebral infarctions
Genitourinary tract anomalies
Neurobehavioral disorders

Pregnant women should be advised to avoid alcohol, but this advice should not be construed as suggesting interruption of pregnancy when a history of alcohol consumption has been elicited; the risks of low-level alcohol consumption, or even occasional binges of marked consumption, have not been clearly quantified to date.

Cocaine

Pharmacology

Cocaine is an alkaloid[37] and can be administered intranasally, orally, vaginally, sublingually, rectally, and by intravenous, subcutaneous, or intramuscular injection.

At one time, the most popular form of administration was the intranasal route. Use of "crack" cocaine, an inexpensive, pure, and portable form of cocaine that gives an immediate effect, has superseded snorting. Cocaine is detoxified by cholinesterases, and cocaine and its metabolites are excreted in the urine, where they may be present for up to 3 days. Cocaine blocks the presynaptic reuptake of norepinephrine and dopamine, with accumulation of these neurotransmitters at postsynaptic receptor sites. Vasoconstriction, hypertension, myocardial irritability, and seizures may result. Euphoria results from the accumulation of dopamine, a mechanism that may also be responsible for addiction. In the pregnant ewe, cocaine induces vasoconstriction, decreased uterine blood flow, maternal and fetal hypertension, and fetal hypoxemia due to impaired oxygen transfer.[38,39]

Adverse effects on the mother

Medical complications reported with cocaine include acute myocardial infarction, cardiac arrhythmias, aortic rupture, subarachnoid hemorrhage, strokes, ischemic bowel damage, and various other problems.[37] These same complications occur in pregnant women, and a report of intracerebral hemorrhage during the postpartum period confirms that expectation[40] (Table 16.6). The altered hormonal milieu of pregnancy may provide a setting in which the cardiovascular effects of cocaine are exaggerated.[41]

Adverse effects on pregnancy

Acker and associates[42] in 1983 reported two cases of abruptio placentae occurring 30 min to a few hours after intravenous or intranasal administration of cocaine. Although it is likely that the acute vasoconstrictive effects of cocaine are responsible for causing abruptions, a chronic effect also exists. Chasnoff et al.[43] found that women who used cocaine only in the first trimester demonstrated a high rate of abruption (9%), as did women who used the drug throughout gestation (15%). They suggested that cocaine alters the placental or uterine vasculature early in pregnancy, with adverse effects showing up near term. Other reports of perinatal morbidity in cocaine users have appeared. Morbidities include IUGR, preterm labor and delivery, premature rupture of membranes, and spontaneous abortion.[44–48] Cerebral infarcts occurring *in utero* have been reported in the offspring of cocaine users.[49] The major methodologic problem of these studies has been the issue of polydrug abuse. The majority of substance-abusing individuals abuse multiple substances, any one of which can adversely affect fetal growth and development. As a result, it is difficult to know whether a given effect is the result of abuse of a given substance or the abuse of a combination of substances. The teratogenic effects of cocaine have, as a result, proved difficult to evaluate, and patterns of cocaine use during the time of organogenesis are difficult to document. One study found major malformations (mostly cardiac anomalies) in five offspring of 50 cocaine users, compared with seven of 340 drug-free pregnancies ($P < 0.01$).[50] Chavez et al.[51] and Ferris et al.[52] found increased odds ratios for urogenital malformations among cocaine-abusing gravidae compared with noncocaine-abusing gravidae. A meta-analysis of 45 investigations into cocaine's teratogenic effects found a nonsignificant trend toward an increase in all malformations [odds ratio (OR) 4.08; 95% confidence interval (CI), 0.70–23.6] and cardiovascular malformations (OR 2.36; 95% CI, 0.83–6.74), but a significant increase in genitourinary malformations (OR 4.97; 95% CI, 1.05–23.6).[53] The proposed mechanisms by which cocaine exerts its teratogenic effects include vasoconstriction and reperfusion directly[39] and the generation of oxygen free radicals during the reperfusion that follows vasoconstriction.[54]

Adverse effects on the neonate

Withdrawal has been reported in neonates exposed to cocaine,[43,55,56] as well as electroencephalogram (EEG) abnormalities and abnormal visual evoked potentials.[56,57] The confounding effects of polysubstance abuse make it difficult to determine whether it is the unique effects of cocaine or the effects of cocaine acting in concert with other drugs that generate the effects seen. Overall, however, studies have not generally found that cocaine adversely affects mental and motor outcomes.[58,59] Recent work suggests that, while fetal cocaine exposure is associated with abnormalities in arousal, attention, and neurologic and neurophysiologic function, the effects appear to be short-lived phenomena seen in infancy and early childhood, and are correlated with other factors, including prenatal exposure to alcohol, tobacco, and marijuana.[60,61]

Cocaine use among pregnant women varies widely depending on the study. Two reports found that cocaine use was seen in 8–24% of pregnant women.[62,63] Better birth outcomes for cocaine-abusing gravidae can be achieved by a combination of specialized prenatal care and drug treatment.[64] Prenatal care by itself is associated with a marked decrease in the rate of low birthweight (less than 2500 g; 34.3% versus 52.3%, $P < 0.05$) and very low birthweight (less than 1500 g; 5.2% versus 18.2%, $P = 0.01$). Stopping cocaine after the first trimester appears to decrease some (low birthweight, preterm delivery) but not all of the risk.[43] The challenge remaining is to insure that these women continue to have access to care.

Heroin

Pharmacology

Heroin's effects are similar to those of morphine, except that it appears to cross the blood–brain barrier more quickly. This is an effect of the greater lipid solubility of heroin. Heroin is hydrolyzed to monoacetylmorphine and morphine, and is excreted in the urine. Its effects are similar to those of other opioids, and physical dependence leading to abstinence-related withdrawal symptoms is induced with chronic use. Gynecologic problems such as galactorrhea–amenorrhea have been reported in female heroin addicts.[65] Although cocaine use has shifted attention away from perinatal heroin addiction, this problem remains a challenge for obstetricians and other caregivers (Table 16.7).

Fetal effects

Heroin crosses the placenta, and addiction is common among fetuses of heroin-addicted mothers. Fetal withdrawal with intrauterine convulsions has been postulated.[66,67] The issue of low birthweight is confounded by elements of maternal lifestyle also known to affect fetal growth. Heroin-addicted mothers are more likely to deliver infants of low birthweight.[68] The relative risk of delivering low birthweight babies in heroin users is 4.61 (95% CI, 2.78–7.65) in pregnant heroin users, 1.36 (95% CI, 0.83–2.22) in methadone users, and 3.28 (95% CI, 2.47–4.39) in women who used both. Respiratory

Table 16.7 Reported effects of heroin on pregnancy.

Fetal addiction
Intrauterine withdrawal/neonatal abstinence syndrome
Low birthweight
Behavioral teratogenesis
Sudden infant death syndrome

distress syndrome may actually occur with less frequency in such children.[69] It is uncertain whether the 28% prematurity rate associated with heroin use seen in some studies is due to the drug use itself or to the influence of other factors. There are few convincing data to indicate an increased incidence of preterm delivery among pregnant heroin users. Teratogenicity has not been conclusively demonstrated, but behavioral teratogenicity is likely, with neonates of heroin addicts demonstrating impaired interactive abilities and motor changes.[70] Sudden infant death syndrome (SIDS) occurs with greater frequency among offspring of heroin-addicted mothers, but the mechanism is unclear.[71,72] Chasnoff[70] suggested that this high rate of SIDS may be associated with sleep apnea and has used theophylline treatment to prevent it.

Neonatal abstinence syndrome

The most striking finding with perinatal heroin addiction is neonatal withdrawal. It occurs in 50–80% of infants born to mothers addicted to heroin or treated with methadone.[60] This syndrome includes tremors, restlessness, hyperreflexia, high-pitched cry, sneezing, sleeplessness, tachypnea, yawning, sweating, fever, and, in severe cases, seizures.[73] The onset of symptoms occurs anywhere from birth to as long as 2 weeks of age and may persist for up to 4–6 months.[74] Treatment has ranged from supportive measures to the use of medications such as diazepam, barbiturates, and opioids such as paregoric and methadone.[69] There is some evidence that withdrawal is less severe in infants whose mothers' methadone dose was down to 20 mg/day or less before delivery.[75]

Treatment in pregnancy

Heroin-addicted mothers are usually treated with methadone maintenance. Specific programs for management of drug dependency during pregnancy have met with success in lowering the various morbidities encountered in such extremely high-risk pregnancies. Well-designed studies have demonstrated a threefold decrease in heroin use as well as a threefold increase in maintenance of treatment among women treated with methadone or buprenorphine when compared with women not so treated.[76] In addition, enrollment in a methadone maintenance program with adequate prenatal care results in an incidence of low birthweight infants similar to that of nondrug-using women with good prenatal care.[77] Heroin withdrawal during pregnancy has been associated with stillbirth in humans.[78] As a result, detoxification should be attempted only in a highly motivated patient.

Infection

The comorbidities of heroin use are similar whether or not the woman is pregnant. The most significant of these are infectious. Twelve percent of heroin addicts tested positive for hepatitis B surface antigen in one study,[79] and another study reported a 43.5% infection rate of infants within 6 months of delivery when born to asymptomatic carrier mothers.[80] When acute infection occurred in the first trimester, 76% of infants were infected.[81] The most significant problem facing intravenous drug users and their offspring now is the danger of acquired immunodeficiency syndrome (AIDS). Intravenous drug use accounts for the majority of human immunodeficiency virus (HIV) positivity among women, with some areas at one time reporting a 50% seropositivity rate among intravenous drug users.[82] Significantly increased rates of infection with syphilis are also present in heroin users.

Hallucinogens

Hallucinogenic drugs such as LSD were commonly taken recreationally in the 1960s and 1970s, but few credible studies were performed regarding the effects of such chemicals on pregnant women and their fetuses. Even retrospective studies were confounded by polydrug use, lifestyle differences, and reporting bias. Chromosome damage from *in vitro* exposure of leukocytes to LSD, increased prevalence of chromosome breaks *in vivo*, and a malformation rate of 10% have been reported in fetuses exposed to this agent,[83] but teratogenicity for LSD has not been confirmed. Little recent data are available because LSD use has declined in recent years.

Phencyclidine (PCP) use has continued to a greater extent than LSD. In a prospective epidemiologic study of 2327 pregnant women, women were assessed by questionnaire and urinary assays. Twelve (0.5%) admitted PCP use during the index pregnancy, and an additional seven (0.3%) tested positive for this drug in their urine.[84] Mouse studies demonstrated that PCP crosses the placenta and appears in breast milk in concentrations 10 times those in maternal plasma.[85] PCP appears in umbilical cord plasma and amniotic fluid from human pregnancies, and the human placenta is an active site for conversion of PCP to its metabolic products *in vitro*.[86,87] One case measured both maternal and umbilical cord levels and found the concentration of PCP in the fetus was double that in the mother.[88] Case reports describe abnormal neonatal behavior, abnormal brain wave patterns, depressed interactive behaviors, and diminished organizational responses to stimuli in infants exposed to PCP *in utero*, but no epidemiologic studies have quantified the risk.[89–92] Finally, one study demonstrated an increased rate of preterm delivery and meconium-stained amniotic fluid in children exposed to PCP *in utero*.[93]

Tobacco

Maternal smoking is associated with a wide variety of increased obstetric morbidities (Table 16.8). The major effects of tobacco present in the first trimester of pregnancy as decreased fecundity and increased spontaneous pregnancy loss, and in the second and third trimester as increased growth

Table 16.8 Obstetric morbidities among pregnant smokers.

Spontaneous abortion
Ectopic pregnancy
Preterm delivery
Placenta previa
IUGR/low birthweight
Placental abruption
PPROM
Sudden infant death syndrome

IUGR, intrauterine growth restriction; PPROM, preterm premature rupture of membranes.

restriction and preterm labor and delivery.[94,95] Maternal smoking during pregnancy decreases birthweight by 10–15 g per cigarette smoked daily. This may be due to direct effects of smoking on fetal growth, to decreased maternal caloric intake seen in pregnant smokers, or to the decreased intervillous volume and decreased number and surface area of fetal capillaries seen in the placentas of pregnant smokers.[96–98] The increased incidence of low birthweight and premature delivery associated with maternal smoking results in a 33% increase in overall perinatal and neonatal mortality.[99] Overall, perinatal mortality for infants of nonsmokers was 23.3 per 1000 births in the Ontario Perinatal Mortality Study.[100] Among smokers of more than one pack per day, that figure increased to 33.4 per 1000 births, and half of that increase was due to smoking-related increases in placental abruption and placenta previa. There are conflicting data on the effects of maternal smoking on human uterine and umbilical blood flow. Morrow et al.[101] found that smoking increased maternal heart rate and blood pressure and fetal heart rate without any changes in uterine artery systolic-to-diastolic ratios. They did note, however, smoking-dependent changes in the umbilical artery systolic-to-diastolic ratio. It remains unclear whether the effects seen were the result of the nicotine in the smoke or the carbon monoxide. Some animal literature suggests that maternal nicotine exposure is associated with decreased uterine blood flow,[102] but the evidence for a similar effect in primates and humans is less compelling. Nicotine administered to the mother has been associated with decreased uterine blood flow in rhesus monkeys but, in the human fetus, it has been associated with increased umbilical blood flow.[103,104] Both standard cigarette smoke and smoke from nicotine-free cigarettes were associated with decreased fetal Po_2 when inhaled by pregnant rhesus monkeys.[105] This effect may be attributed to carbon monoxide, because carboxyhemoglobin is preferentially trapped on the fetal side of the placenta. The relative hypoxia induced by increased carboxyhemoglobin levels in the fetus could induce a wide variety of adverse effects. Clinical studies have demonstrated variable effects on fetal breathing[106] and increased fetal heart rate with decreased beat-to-beat variability[107] during acute maternal exposure to cigarette smoke, but no effect was seen on nonstress test reactivity.[108] Chronic cigarette exposure was associated with lower Apgar scores in some but not all studies.[109,110] Intimal injury of the umbilical arteries of newborns from smoking mothers has been demonstrated, as have placental changes.[111–113] Maternal smoking has also been associated with a failure in expansion of total body water and mean plasma volume during pregnancy.[114] Maternal smoking has been associated with changes in hemostatic and platelet function,[115,116] but it is difficult to determine whether these changes are due to the effects of nicotine, carbon monoxide, or some other substance(s). Studies in rats have demonstrated damage to the fetal brainstem[117] and both a decrease in the number of neonatal type I pneumocytes and an increase in the number of type II pneumocytes in rats.[118] The type II pneumocytes were morphologically abnormal, with no microvilli on their alveolar surface.

The teratogenic potential of maternal cigarette smoking is becoming manifest. One study found increased mutations in the gene for hypoxanthine–guanine phosphoribosyltransferase in the cord blood T-cell lymphocytes of neonates exposed to maternal smoking as fetuses.[119] One epidemiologic study suggested that isolated oral clefts are increased in the offspring of cigarette smokers,[120] but an analysis of the Swedish Medical Birth Registry found that the association between smoking and facial clefts depended on the type of analysis done: an association between cleft palate and smoking was seen in all case designs, but the association between cleft lip with or without cleft palate and smoking was seen only in case–control analyses.[121] Lammer et al.[122] found that orofacial clefts are increased among smokers whose fetuses have polymorphic variants of NAT1, an enzyme involved in detoxification of smoke components, possibly explaining the discrepancy in study findings. Maternal smoking during pregnancy has been associated with a decreased risk of respiratory distress syndrome in the prematurely delivered offspring, an effect that has generally been attributed to enhanced pulmonic maturation secondary to intrauterine hypoxic stress.[123] Children exposed *in utero* to smoking consistently score lower on scores of expressive language and conceptual understanding and have a greater incidence of behavioral difficulties.[99,124,125]

Although it is possible to detect the effects of household smoking exposure on infants, one study was unable to demonstrate maternal–fetal transmission of thiocyanate acquired passively by the mother exposed to a smoking environment, but not herself a smoker.[126] Another study was able to show such an effect,[127] and one report demonstrated a significant reduction in birthweight among the offspring of mothers exposed passively to cigarette smoke, as evidenced by increased maternal cotinine levels during the second trimester.[128] A case-controlled study of 91 children found a dose-dependent relationship between maternal exposure to second-hand smoke and risk of childhood brain tumors,[129] and an adverse effect on language skills, visual, and spatial abilities was seen in children exposed prenatally to second-hand smoke when compared with children not exposed.[130]

Table 16.9 Fetal tobacco syndrome.

1. A mother who smoked five or more cigarettes a day throughout the pregnancy
2. No evidence of hypertension during the pregnancy
3. Symmetric growth retardation at term
4. No other obvious cause of growth retardation

Table 16.10 Intervention to promote smoking cessation during pregnancy.

Ask: ask the patient to choose a statement that best describes her smoking status:
- I've smoked < 100 cigarettes in my lifetime
- I quit smoking before I found out I was pregnant
- I quit smoking after I found out I was pregnant
- I still smoke, but I've cut down
- I still smoke and I haven't cut down

Advise: give clear, firm advice to quit smoking. Stress the benefits to her and the fetus.

Assess: investigate her willingness to quit.

Assist: offer and encourage coping mechanisms for quitting smoking (identify trigger situations):
- Provide support as part of the treatment
- Arrange for social support; involve family and friends
- Pregnancy-specific smoking cessation programs

Arrange: follow-up is essential. Reassess and re-encourage.

Attempts to modify smoking behavior during pregnancy have met with mixed success. Nieburg and colleagues[131] suggested the term fetal tobacco syndrome to describe infants meeting four conditions (Table 16.9). In 2000, the American College of Obstetricians and Gynecologists published a Technical Bulletin recommending that pregnant women be encouraged to stop smoking.[132] Identification of the smoker at the first prenatal visit should be coupled with intensive education about the risks of smoking during pregnancy. A brief 5- to 15-min intervention will increase smoking cessation by 30–70% in smoking gravidae. It is most effective in women who smoke < 20 cigarettes per day[133] and consists of Ask, Advise, Assess, Assist, and Arrange[134] (Table 16.10).

Although there have been great strides in American society in prohibiting smoking in public areas and in decreasing the number of cigarette-smoking citizens, smoking during pregnancy continues to be a problem. Statistics suggest that 15–29% of women continue to smoke during pregnancy.[135] Pregnant smoking women treated with a cessation program demonstrated a significant increase in birthweight and length of their offspring when compared with untreated smoking control subjects,[136] and quitting at any point in pregnancy is helpful.[134] We must find out if our patients are smoking, educate them about the risks, and refer them to smoking cessation programs in our communities. Behavioral therapies are the first line of intervention. If these therapies fail, then pharmacological treatment with either bupropion or nicotine replacement treatments (NRTs) can be considered. Buproprion is Food and Drug Administration (FDA) class B, and all the NRTs are FDA class C. A careful assessment of risks and benefits is necessary before starting these therapies.

Caffeine

Caffeine is a xanthine. The xanthines exert their systemic effects by increasing intracellular cyclic adenosine monophosphate, altering ionized calcium levels, and potentiating the action of catecholamines. These systemic effects include central nervous system excitation, smooth muscle relaxation, increased heart rate, increased cardiac output, an increase in gastric acid secretion, and increased diuresis. Caffeine is contained in coffee and tea (100–150 mg per average cup), cola drinks (35–55 mg per 12-oz serving), and cocoa (200 mg of theobromine per average cup). Pregnant women near term eliminate caffeine considerably more slowly than nonpregnant control subjects, and ingestion of two cups of coffee by these women was associated with a small but significant decrease in intervillous blood flow.[137,138] Caffeine is fat soluble and crosses the placenta in sheep and humans. Chronic coffee drinkers have increased fetal breathing activity, but acute ingestion of 200 mg of caffeine had no significant effect on fetal breathing.[139]

Caffeine is teratogenic in rodents. Doses of 50–75 mg/kg in mice, and greater than 80 mg/kg in rats induce malformations of limbs and digits.[140] These are levels higher than those likely to be achieved in human pregnancies. Additionally, if caffeine doses are given in split doses instead of in bolus fashion, 330 mg/kg/day is required to cause teratogenicity in rats. A report of three human pregnancies in which high maternal caffeine intake was associated with ectrodactyly in the offspring created a great deal of interest in the possibility of teratogenicity, but each mother had consumed between 1100 and 1777 mg of caffeine on an average day during her pregnancy.[141] Three large epidemiologic studies in humans detected no increase in congenital anomalies related to caffeine intake among pregnant women.[142–144] A recent review of the effect of caffeine on spontaneous abortion concluded that, while many epidemiologic studies have observed a positive association between caffeine intake and spontaneous pregnancy loss rates, the evidence should be considered equivocal because of the many methodologic flaws.[145] The data on the effect of caffeine on birthweight are similarly conflicting. Fortier et al.[146] found a dose-dependent effect of increasing caffeine consumption on decreasing birthweight in a population-based study of over 7000 women, but Mills et al.,[147] in their study on moderate caffeine intake, were unable to confirm this finding.

There is no convincing evidence supporting a teratogenic or other adverse role of caffeine in pregnancy when taken in amounts equivalent to less than 10 cups of coffee per day. Pregnant women should be advised to use moderation in their caffeine intake, but it need not be avoided altogether.

Key points

1 Drug effects on fetal development depend on the dose, the route of administration, physiologic handling of the drug by both the pregnant woman and the fetus, genetic predisposition, and timing of the exposure in the pregnancy.

2 Fetal alcohol syndrome (FAS) occurs in 2.5–10% of offspring of heavy drinkers, and includes growth restriction (either prenatal or postnatal in onset), craniofacial anomalies (small eyes, epicanthal folds, long philtrum, or midface hypoplasia), and central nervous system abnormalities (microcephaly, developmental delay, mental retardation, learning disabilities).

3 The categories of alcohol-related birth defects include: (1) FAS with confirmed maternal alcohol use; (2) FAS without confirmed maternal alcohol use but with characteristic malformations; (3) partial FAS with confirmed maternal alcohol use and some components of FAS; (4) alcohol-related birth defects with the presence of congenital anomalies resulting from prenatal alcohol exposure; and (5) alcohol-related neurodevelopmental abnormalities.

4 Women at risk for problem drinking during pregnancy can be identified using the "CAGE", "T-ACE," or "TWEAK" questionnaires. Interventions in women so identified can decrease problem drinking by more than 50%.

5 Drinking cessation before the third trimester of pregnancy will benefit the fetus, so it is never "too late."

6 All studies of the impact and effects of a particular illicit drug on developing fetuses are complicated by problems in accurately quantifying the exposure, and the fact that polysubstance abuse is the rule and not the exception.

7 Cocaine blocks presynaptic reuptake of norepinephrine and dopamine, resulting in vasoconstriction, hypertension, myocardial irritability, and euphoria.

8 Cocaine use during pregnancy is associated with an increased incidence of placental abruption (a side-effect of vasoconstriction and hypertension), and this effect persists even if the pregnant cocaine user stops using in the first trimester.

9 Maternal medical effects of cocaine use include acute myocardial infarction, cardiac arrhythmias, hypertension, aortic rupture, subarachnoid hemorrhage, and ischemic bowel damage.

10 Fetal/neonatal effects of cocaine use in pregnancy include placental abruption, intrauterine growth restriction, preterm labor and delivery, increased incidence of genitourinary birth defects, and withdrawal.

11 The features previously ascribed to the so-called "crack baby syndrome" (abnormalities in arousal, attention, and neurologic and neuropsychologic function) are short-lived and correlate with other factors including exposure to alcohol, tobacco, and marijuana.

12 Convincing a woman to use methadone instead of heroin decreases the relative risk of delivering a low birthweight baby from 4.61 to 1.36.

13 Structural teratogenicity has not been associated with heroin use during pregnancy, but behavioral teratogenicity is likely.

14 Neonatal abstinence occurs in 50–80% of infants born to mothers using heroin or methadone, and includes tremors, restlessness, hyperreflexia, high-pitched cry, sneezing, sleeplessness, tachypnea, yawning, sweating, fever, and sometimes seizures.

15 Neonatal abstinence and withdrawal is less severe if the maternal methadone dose is < 20 mg/day at delivery.

16 The major effects of tobacco present in the first trimester as decreased fecundity and increased pregnancy loss, and in the second and third trimester as increased growth restriction and preterm labor and delivery.

17 The increased incidence of low birthweight and preterm labor and delivery explains the 33% increase in overall perinatal and neonatal morbidity seen in pregnant smokers.

18 Cigarette smoking during pregnancy is associated with an increased incidence of orofacial clefts.

19 Smoking cessation interventions during pregnancy will increase smoking cessation by 30–70% in smoking gravidae.

20 Caffeine is teratogenic in rodents, but probably only in doses that are exceedingly difficult to achieve in humans (i.e., > 10 cups of coffee per day).

References

1 Koren G, Pastuszak A, Ito S. Drugs in pregnancy. *N Engl J Med* 1998;338:1128.
2 Centers for Disease Control. Alcohol use among women of child-bearing age – United States, 1991–1999. *Morbidity Mortality Weekly Rep* 2002;51:273.
3 Lupton C, Burd L, Harwood R. Cost of fetal alcohol spectrum disorders. *Am J Med Gen (Part C)* 2004;127C:42.
4 Jones KL, Smith DW. Recognition of the fetal alcohol syndrome in early infancy. *Lancet* 1973;1:999.
5 Jones KL, Smith DW, Uelland CN, et al. Pattern of malformation in offspring of chronic alcoholic mothers. *Lancet* 1973;1: 1267.
6 Rosett HL. Editorial: a clinical perspective on the fetal alcohol syndrome. *Alcohol Clin Exp Res* 1980;2:119.
7 Stratton K, Howe C, Bataglia F, eds. *Fetal alcohol syndrome: diagnosis, epidemiology, prevention and treatment*. Washington, DC: Institute of Medicine National Academy Press; 1996:4.
8 Hankin JR, Sokol RJ. Identification and care of problems associated with alcohol ingestion in pregnancy. *Semin Perinatol* 1995;19:286.
9 Rosett HL, Weiner L. Fetal alcohol syndrome. In: Rosett HL, Weiner L, eds. *Alcohol and the fetus: a clinical perspective*. New York: Oxford University Press; 1984:3.
10 Centers for Disease Control and Prevention. Fetal Alcohol Syndrome – Alaska, Arizona, Colorado and New York. *Morbidity Mortality Weekly Rep* 2002;51:433.
11 Bailey BN, Delaney-Black V, Covington CY, et al. Prenatal exposure to binge drinking and cognitive and behavioral outcomes at age 7 years. *Am J Obstet Gynecol* 2004;193:1037.
12 Martinez-Frias ML, Bermejo E, Rodriguez-Pinilla E, et al. Risk for congenital anomalies associated with different sporadic and daily doses of alcohol consumption: a case–control study. *Birth Defects Res (Part A)* 2004;70:194.
13 Ikonomidou C, Bittigau P, Ishimaru J, et al. Ethanol-induced apoptotic neurodegeneration and fetal alcohol syndrome. *Science* 2000;287:1056.
14 Miller MW. Effects of alcohol on the generation and migration of cerebral cortical neurons. *Science* 1986;233:1308.
15 Archibald SL, Gamst A, Riley EP, et al. Brain dysmorphology in individuals with severe prenatal alcohol exposure. *Dev Med Child Neurol* 2001;43:148.
16 Brien JF, Clarke DW, Richardson B, et al. Disposition of ethanol in maternal blood, fetal blood, and amniotic fluid in third-trimester pregnant ewes. *Am J Obstet Gynecol* 1985;152: 583.
17 Brien JF, Loomis CW, Tranmer J, et al. Disposition of ethanol in human maternal venous blood and amniotic fluid. *Am J Obstet Gynecol* 1983;146:181.
18 Penn U, Laufer EM, Land H. C-myc: evidence for multiple regulatory functions. *Semin Cancer Biol* 1990;1:69.
19 Saunders DE, Hannigan H, Zajac CS, et al. Reversal of alcohol's effects on neurite extension and on neuronal GAP43/B50, N-myc, and c-myc protein levels by retinoic acid. *Brain Res Dev Brain Res* 1995;86:16.
20 Lieber C. Biochemical and molecular basis of alcohol-induced injury to liver and other tissues. *N Engl J Med* 1988;319: 1639.
21 Fisher SE. Selective fetal malnutrition: the fetal alcohol syndrome. *Am Coll Nutr* 1988;7:101.
22 Passaro KT, Little RE, Savitz DA, et al. The effect of maternal drinking before conception and in early pregnancy on infant birth weight. The ALSPAC study team, Avon Longitudinal Study of Pregnancy and Childhood. *Epidemiology* 1996;7:377.
23 McLeod W, Brien J, Loomis C, et al. Effect of maternal ethanol ingestion on fetal breathing movements, gross body movements, and heart rate at 37 to 40 weeks' gestational age. *Am J Obstet Gynecol* 1983;145:251.
24 Coles CD, Smith IE, Fernhoff PM, et al. Neonatal ethanol withdrawal: characteristics in clinically normal, nondysmorphic neonates. *J Pediatr* 1984;105:445.
25 Guerri C, Pascual M, Garcia-Minguillan MC. Antioxidants prevent ethanol-induced cell death in developing brain and in cultured neural cells. *Alcohol Clin Exp Res* 2004;28(Suppl.):61A.
26 Streissguth AP, Darby BL, Barr HM, et al. Comparison of drinking and smoking patterns during pregnancy over a six year period. *Am J Obstet Gynecol* 1983;145:716.
27 Halmesmaki E, Raivio KO, Ylikorkala O. Patterns of alcohol consumption during pregnancy. *Obstet Gynecol* 1987;69:594.
28 Ewing JA. Detecting alcoholism: the CAGE questionnaire. *JAMA* 1984;252:1905.
29 Sokol RJ, Martier SS, Ager JW. The T-ACE questions: practical prenatal detection of risk drinking. *Am J Obstet Gynecol* 1989;160:863.
30 Russell M, Martier SS, Sokol R, et al. Screening for pregnancy risk-drinking. *Alcohol Clin Exp Res* 1994;18:1156.
31 Chan D, Klein J, Karaskov T, et al. Fetal exposure to alcohol as evidenced by fatty acid ethyl esters in meconium in the absence of maternal drinking history in pregnancy. *Ther Drug Monit* 2004;26:474.
32 Rosett HL, Weiner L, Edeline KC. Treatment experience with pregnant problem drinkers. *JAMA* 1983;249:2029.
33 Sisenwein FE, Tejani NA, Boxer HS, et al. Effects of maternal ethanol infusion during pregnancy on the growth and development of children at four to seven years of age. *Am J Obstet Gynecol* 1983;147:52.
34 Halmesmaki E. Alcohol counselling of 85 pregnant problem drinkers: effect on drinking and fetal outcome. *Br J Obstet Gynaecol* 1988;95:243.
35 Fleming MF, Barry KL, Manwell LB, et al. Brief physician advice for problem alcohol drinkers. *JAMA* 1997;277:1039.
36 Coustan DR, Mochizuki TK. *Handbook for prescribing medications during pregnancy*, 3rd edn. Boston, MA: Little, Brown; 1998:157.
37 Creigler LL, Mark H. Special report: medical complications of cocaine abuse. *N Engl J Med* 1986;315:1495.
38 Moore TR, Sorg J, Miller L, et al. Hemodynamic effects of intravenous cocaine on the pregnant ewe and fetus. *Am J Obstet Gynecol* 1986;155:883.
39 Woods JR, Jr, Plessinger MA, Clark KE. Effect of cocaine on uterine blood flow and fetal oxygenation. *JAMA* 1987;157:957.
40 Mercado A, Johnson G, Jr, Calver D, et al. Cocaine, pregnancy, and postpartum intracerebral hemorrhage. *Obstet Gynecol* 1989;73:467.
41 Chao C. Cardiovascular effects of cocaine during pregnancy. *Semin Perinatol* 1996;20:107.
42 Acker D, Sachs BP, Tracey KJ, et al. Abruptio placentae associated with cocaine use. *Am J Obstet Gynecol* 1983;146: 220.
43 Chasnoff D, Griffith DR, MacGregor S, et al. Temporal patterns of cocaine use in pregnancy: perinatal outcome. *JAMA* 1989;261:1741.

44 Bada HS, Das A, Bauer CR, et al. Low birth weight and preterm births: etiologic fraction attributable to prenatal drug exposure. *J Perinatol* 2005;25:631.

45 Chouteau M, Namerow PB, Leppert P. The effect of cocaine abuse on birth weight and gestational age. *Obstet Gynecol* 1988; 72:351.

46 Little BB, Snell LM, Klein VR, et al. Cocaine abuse during pregnancy: maternal and fetal implications. *Obstet Gynecol* 1989;73: 157.

47 Chasnoff D, Burns KA, Burns WJ. Cocaine use in pregnancy: perinatal morbidity and mortality. *Neurotoxicol Teratol* 1987; 9:291.

48 Bandstra ES, Morrow CE, Anthony JC, et al. Intrauterine growth of full-term infants: impact of prenatal cocaine exposure. *Pediatrics* 2001;108:1309.

49 Chasnoff D, Bussey ME, Savich R, et al. Perinatal cerebral infarction and maternal cocaine use. *J Pediatr* 1986;108:456.

50 Bingol N, Fuchs M, Diaz V, et al. Teratogenicity of cocaine in humans. *J Pediatr* 1987;110:93.

51 Chavez GC, Mulinare J, Cordero JF. Maternal cocaine use during early pregnancy as a risk factor for congenital urogenital anomalies. *JAMA* 1989;262:795.

52 Ferris EF, Mendoza SA, Griswold WR, et al. Prenatal risk factors for urinary tract anomalies. *Pediatr Res* 1992;31:92A.

53 Lutiger B, Graham K, Einarson TR, et al. Relationship between gestational cocaine use and pregnancy outcome: a meta-analysis. *Teratology* 1991;44:405.

54 Fantel AG, Barber CV, Mackkler B. Ischemial reperfusion: a new hypothesis for the developmental toxicity of cocaine. *Teratology* 1992;46:285.

55 Cherukuri R, Minkoff H, Feldman J, et al. A cohort study of alkaloidal cocaine ("crack") in pregnancy. *Obstet Gynecol* 1988; 72:147.

56 Doberczak TM, Shanzer S, Senie RT, et al. Neonatal neurologic and electroencephalographic effects of intrauterine cocaine exposure. *J Pediatr* 1988;113:354

57 Dixon SD, Coen R, Crutchfield S. Visual dysfunction in cocaine exposed infants. *Pediatr Res* 1987;21:359.

58 Coles C, Platzman K, Smith L. Effects of cocaine and alcohol use in pregnancy on neonatal growth and neurobehavioral status. *Neurotoxicol Teratol* 1992;14:23.

59 Griffith D, Freier C. Methodological issues in the assessment of the mother-child interactions of substance-abusing women and their children. *NIDA Res Monogr* 1992;117:228.

60 Chiriboga CA. Fetal alcohol and drug effects. *Neurologist* 2003;9:267.

61 Frank DA, Augustyn M, Knight WG, et al. Growth, development and behavior in early childhood following prenatal cocaine exposure: a systematic review. *JAMA* 2001;285: 1613.

62 Neerhof MG, MacGregor SN, Retzky SS, et al. Cocaine abuse during pregnancy: peripartum prevalence and perinatal outcome. *Am J Obstet Gynecol* 1989;161:633.

63 Matera C, Warren WB, Moomjy M, et al. Prevalence of use of cocaine and other substances in an obstetric population. *Am J Obstet Gynecol* 1990;163:797.

64 Chazotte C, Youchah J, Freda MC. Cocaine use in pregnancy and low birth weight: the impact of prenatal care and drug treatment. *Semin Perinatol* 1995;19:293.

65 Pelosi MA, Sama JC, Caterini H, et al. Galactorrhea–amenorrhea syndrome associated with heroin addiction. *Am J Obstet Gynecol* 1974;118:966.

66 Rementeria JL, Nunag NN. Narcotic withdrawal in pregnancy: stillbirth incidence with a case report. *Am J Obstet Gynecol* 1973;116:1152.

67 Zuspan FP, Gumpel JA, Mejia-Zelaya A, et al. Fetal stress from methadone withdrawal. *Am J Obstet Gynecol* 1975;122: 43.

68 Hulse GK, Milne E, English DR et al. The relationship between maternal use of heroin and methadone and infant birth weight. *Addiction* 1997;92:1571.

69 Glass L, Rajegowda BK, Evarls HE. Absence of respiratory distress syndrome in premature infants of heroin-addicted mothers. *Lancet* 1971;2:685.

70 Chasnoff U. Perinatal addiction: consequences of intrauterine exposure to opiate and nonopiate drugs. In: Chasnoff U, ed. *Drug use in pregnancy: mother and child.* Boston, MA: MTP Press; 1986:52.

71 Pierson PS, Howard P, Klaber HD. Sudden deaths in infants born to methadone-maintained addicts. *JAMA* 1972;220:1733.

72 Chavez CJ, Ostrea EM, Jr, Stryker JC, et al. Sudden infant death syndrome among infants of drug-dependent mothers. *J Pediatr* 1979;95:407.

73 Finnegan LP, Connoughton IF, Kron RE, et al. Neonatal abstinence syndrome: assessment and management. In: Harbison RD, ed. *Perinatal addiction.* New York: Spectrum; 1975:141.

74 Chasnoff U, Hatcher R, Burns WJ. Early growth patterns of methadone-addicted infants. *Am J Dis Child* 1980;134:1049.

75 Madden JD, Chappel IN, Zuspan F, et al. Observation and treatment of neonatal narcotic withdrawal. *Am J Obstet Gynecol* 1977;127:199.

76 Mattick RP, Breen C, Kimber J, et al. Buprenorphine maintenance versus placebo or methadone maintenance for opioid dependence. *Cochrane Database Syst Rev* 2002;2: CD002207.

77 Connaughton IF, Reeser D, Schut J, et al. Perinatal addiction: outcome and management. *Am J Obstet Gynecol* 1977;129:679.

78 Rementeria JL, Nunag NN. Narcotic withdrawal in pregnancy: stillbirth incidence with a case report. *Am J Obstet Gynecol* 1973;116:1152.

79 Kreek MJ, Doqcs L, Kane S, et al. Long-term methadone maintenance therapy: effects on liver function. *Ann Intern Med* 1972;222:811.

80 Shiraki K, Yoshihara N, Kawana T, et al. Hepatitis B surface antigen and chronic hepatitis in infants born to asymptomatic carrier mothers. *Am J Dis Child* 1977;131:644.

81 Schweitzer IL, Dunn AE, Peters RL, et al. Viral hepatitis B in neonates and infants. *Am J Med* 1973;55:762.

82 Weinberg DS, Murray HW. Coping with AIDS: the special problems of New York City. *N Engl J Med* 1987;317:1469.

83 Jacobson CB, Berlin CM. Possible reproductive detriment in LSD users. *JAMA* 1972;222:1367.

84 Golden NL, Kuhnert BR, Sokol RI, et al. Phencyclidine use during pregnancy. *Am J Obstet Gynecol* 1984;148:254.

85 Nicholas IM, Lipshitz J, Schreiber EC. Phencyclidine: its transfer across the placenta as well as into breast milk. *Am J Obstet Gynecol* 1982;143:143.

86 Kaufman KR, Petrucha RA, Pitts FN, Jr, et al. Phencyclidine in umbilical cord blood: preliminary data. *Am J Psychol* 1983;140: 450.

87 Rayburn WF, Holsztynska EF, Domino EF. Phencyclidine: biotransformation by the human placenta. *Am J Obstet Gynecol* 1984;148:111.

88 Petrucha RA, Kaufman KR, Pitts FN. Phencyclidine in pregnancy: a case report. *J Reprod Med* 1982;27:301.

89 Chasnoff D, Burns KA, Burns WJ, et al. Prenatal drug exposure: effects on neonatal and infant growth and development. *Neurotoxicol Teratol* 1986;8:357.
90 Golden NL, Sokol RI, Rubin IL. Angel dust: possible effects on the fetus. *Pediatrics* 1980;65:18.
91 Van Dyke DC, Fox AA. Fetal drug exposure and its possible implications for learning in the preschool and school aged population. *J Learn Disabil* 1990;23:160.
92 Strauss AA, Modanlou HD, Bosu SK. Neonatal manifestations of maternal phencyclidine (PCP) abuse. *Pediatrics* 1981;68:550.
93 Tabor BL, Smith-Wallace T, Yonekura ML. Perinatal outcome associated with PCP versus cocaine use. *Am J Drug Alcohol Abuse* 1990;16:337.
94 Shiverick KT, Salafia C. Cigarette smoking and pregnancy. I: ovarian, uterine and placental effects. *Placenta* 1999;20:265.
95 Wisborg K, Henriksen TB, Hedegaard M, et al. Smoking during pregnancy and preterm birth. *Br J Obstet Gynaecol* 1996;103:800.
96 Davies DP, Gray OP, Ellwood PC, et al. Cigarette smoking in pregnancy: associations with maternal weight gain and fetal growth. *Lancet* 1976;1:385.
97 Papoz L, Eschwege E, Pequignot G, et al. Maternal smoking and birth weight in relation to dietary habits. *Am J Obstet Gynecol* 1982;142:870.
98 Bush PG, Mayhew TM, Abramovich DR, et al. A quantitative study on the effects of maternal smoking on placental morphology and cadmium concentration. *Placenta* 2000;21:247.
99 Walsh RA. Effects of maternal smoking on adverse pregnancy outcomes: examination of the criteria of causation. *Hum Biol* 1994;66:1059.
100 Meyer MB, Tonascia JB. Perinatal events associated with maternal smoking during pregnancy. *Am J Epidemiol* 1976;1103:464.
101 Morrow RI, Ritchie JW, Bull SB. Maternal cigarette smoking: the effects on umbilical and uterine blood flow velocity. *Am J Obstet Gynecol* 1988;159:1069.
102 Resnik R, Brinnk GW, Wilkes M. Catecholamine mediated reduction in uterine blood flow after nicotine infusion in the pregnant ewe. *J Clin Invest* 1979;63:1133.
103 Suzuki K, Minei U, Johnson EE. Effect of nicotine upon uterine blood flow in the pregnant rhesus monkey. *Am J Obstet Gynecol* 1980;136:1009.
104 Lindblad A, Marsal K, Anderson KE. Effect of nicotine on human fetal blood flow. *Obstet Gynecol* 1988;72:371.
105 Socol ML, Manning FA, Murata Y, et al. Maternal smoking causes fetal hypoxia: experimental evidence. *Am J Obstet Gynecol* 1982;142:214.
106 Thaler I, Goodman IDS, Dawes GS. Effects of maternal cigarette smoking on fetal breathing and fetal movements. *Am J Obstet Gynecol* 1980;138:282.
107 Kariniemi V, Lehtovirta P, Rauramo I, et al. Effects of smoking on fetal heart rate variability during gestational weeks 27 to 32. *Am J Obstet Gynecol* 1984;149:575.
108 Barrett JM, Vanhooydonk JE, Boehm FH. Acute effect of cigarette smoking on the fetal heart rate nonstress test. *Obstet Gynecol* 1981;57:422.
109 Gam SM, Johnston M, Ridella SA, et al. Effect of maternal cigarette smoking on Apgar scores. *Am J Dis Child* 1981;135:503.
110 Hingson R, Gould M, Morelock S, et al. Maternal cigarette smoking, psychoactive substance use, and infant Apgar scores. *Am J Obstet Gynecol* 1982;144:959.
111 Asmussen I, Kjeldsen K. Intimal ultrastructure of human umbilical arteries: observations on arteries from newborn children of smoking and nonsmoking mothers. *Clin Res* 1975;36:579.
112 Rush D, Kristal A, Blanc W, et al. The effects of maternal cigarette smoking on placental morphology, histomorphometry, and biochemistry. *Am J Perinatol* 1986;3:263.
113 Brown HL, Miller LM, Jr, Khawli O, et al. Premature placental calcification in maternal cigarette smokers. *Obstet Gynecol* 1988;71:914.
114 Pirani BBK, MacGillivray I. Smoking during pregnancy: its effect on maternal metabolism and fetoplacental function. *Obstet Gynecol* 1978;52:257.
115 Condie RG, Pirani BBK. The influence of smoking on the haemostatic mechanism in pregnancy. *Acta Obstet Gynecol Scand* 1977;56:5118.
116 Leuschen MP, Davis RB, Boyd D, et al. Comparative evaluation of antepartum and postpartum platelet function in smokers and nonsmokers. *Am J Obstet Gynecol* 1986;155:1276.
117 Krous HF, Campbell GA, Fowler MW, et al. Maternal nicotine administration and fetal brain stem damage: a rat model with implications for sudden infant death syndrome. *Am J Obstet Gynecol* 1981;140:743.
118 Maritz GS, Thomas RA. Maternal nicotine exposure: response of type II pneumocytes of neonatal rat pups. *Cell Biol Int* 1995;19:323.
119 Finette BA, O'Neil JP, Vacek PM, et al. Gene mutations with characteristic deletions in cord blood T lymphocytes associated with passive maternal exposure to tobacco smoke. *Nature Med* 1998;4:1144.
120 Khoury MI, Gomez-Farias M, Mulinare J. Does maternal cigarette smoking during pregnancy cause cleft lip and palate in offspring? *Am J Dis Child* 1989;143:333.
121 Meyer KA, Williams P, Hernandez-Diaz S, et al. Smoking and oral clefts: exploring the impact of study designs. *Epidemiology* 2004;15:671.
122 Lammer EJ, Shaw GM, Iovannisci DM, et al. Maternal smoking and the risk of orofacial clefts: susceptibility with NAT1 and NAT2 polymorphisms. *Epidemiology* 2004;15:150.
123 White E, Shy KK, Dating JR, et al. Maternal smoking and infant respiratory distress syndrome. *Obstet Gynecol* 1986;67:365.
124 Naeye RL, Peters EC. Mental development of children whose mothers smoked during pregnancy. *Obstet Gynecol* 1984;64:601.
125 Fried PA, Watkinson B, Dillon RF. Neonatal neurological status in a low-risk population after prenatal exposure to cigarettes, marijuana, and alcohol. *Dev Behav Pediatr* 1987;8:318.
126 Hauth JC, Hauth J, Brawbaugh RB, et al. Passive smoking and thiocyanate concentrations in pregnant women and newborns. *Obstet Gynecol* 1984;63:519.
127 Bottoms SF, Kuhnert BR, Kuhnert PM, et al. Maternal passive smoking and fetal serum thiocyanate levels. *Am J Obstet Gynecol* 1982;144:787.
128 Haddow JE, Knight GJ, Palomaki GE, et al. Second trimester serum cotinine levels in nonsmokers in relation to birth weight *Am J Obstet Gynecol* 1988;159:481.
129 Filippini G, Farinotti M, Lovicu G, et al. Mothers active and passive smoking during pregnancy and risk of brain tumors in children. *Int J Cancer* 1994;15:769.
130 Makin J, Fried PA, Watkinson B. A comparison of active and passive smoking during pregnancy: long term effects. *Neurotoxicol Teratol* 1991;13:5.

131 Nieburg P, Marks JS, McLaren NM, et al. The fetal tobacco syndrome. *JAMA* 1985;253:2998.
132 American College of Obstetricians and Gynecologists. *Smoking cessation during pregnancy*. ACOG Educational Bulletin No. 260; 2000.
133 Melvin C, Dolan Mullen P, Windsor RA, et al. Recommended cessation counseling for pregnant women who smoke: a review of the evidence. *Tobacco Control* 2000;9:1.
134 Fiore MC, Bailey WC, Cohen SJ et al. *Treating tobacco use and dependence*. Clinical Practice Guideline. Rockville, MD: US Department of Health and Human Service, June 2000.
135 Andres RL, Day MC. Perinatal complications associated with maternal tobacco use. *Semin Neonatol* 2000;5:231.
136 Li CQ, Windsor RA, Perkins L, et al. The impact on infant birth weight and gestational age of cotinine-validated smoking reduction during pregnancy. *JAMA* 1993;269:1519.
137 Parsons WD, Pelletier JG. Delayed elimination of caffeine by women in the last 2 weeks of pregnancy. *Can Med Assoc J* 1982;127:377.
138 Kirkinen P, Jouppila P, Koivula A, et al. The effect of caffeine on placental and fetal blood flow in human pregnancy. *Am J Obstet Gynecol* 1983;147:939.
139 McGowan J, Devoe LD, Searle N, et al. The effects of long- and short-term maternal caffeine ingestion on human fetal breathing and body movements in term gestations. *Am J Obstet Gynecol* 1987;157:726.
140 Nehlig A, Debry G. Potential teratogenic and neurodevelopmental consequences of coffee and caffeine exposure: a review on human and animal data. *Neurotoxicol Teratol* 1994;16:531.
141 Jacobson MF, Goldman AS, Syme RH. Coffee and birth defects. *Lancet* 1981;1:1415.
142 Linn S, Schoenbaum SC, Monson RR, et al. No association between coffee consumption and adverse outcomes of pregnancy. *N Engl J Med* 1982;306:141.
143 Rosenberg L, Mitchell AA, Shapiro S, et al. Selected birth defects in relation to caffeine-containing beverages. *JAMA* 1982;247:1429.
144 Furuhashi N, Sato S, Suzuki M, et al. Effects of caffeine ingestion during pregnancy. *Gynecol Obstet Invest* 1985;19:187.
145 Signorello LB, McLaughlin JK. Maternal caffeine consumption and spontaneous abortion: a review of the epidemiologic evidence. *Epidemiology* 2004;15:229.
146 Fortier I, Marcoux S, Beaulac-Baillargeon L. Relation of caffeine intake during pregnancy to intrauterine growth retardation and preterm birth. *Am J Epidemiol* 1993;137:931.
147 Mills JL, Holmes LB, Aarons JR, et al. Moderate caffeine use and the risk of spontaneous abortion and intrauterine growth retardation. *JAMA* 1993;269:593.

17 Teratogenic viruses

Antonio V. Sison

A teratogen is an agent that induces malformations in humans, from the Greek word "teras" meaning monster. Teratogenic viruses include the following: cytomegalovirus (CMV), herpes simplex virus (HSV), varicella zoster virus (VZV), rubella virus, and Venezuelan equine encephalitis (VEE) virus. The role of parvovirus B19 in congenital malformations has been questioned but is briefly included in this chapter. The chapter reviews each individual virus's epidemiology, biology, pathogenesis, diagnosis and management in pregnancy, effects on the fetus and infant, and prevention of spread. Other viruses have been shown to cause fetal damage but are not considered to be teratogenic; these viruses and their specific fetal effects are summarized in Table 17.1. Epidemiological studies using clinical data, virus isolation techniques, and serology have provided estimates of the frequency of teratogenic viral infections in pregnant women and their children (Table 17.2). Factors that influence these data include the population sampled, the occurrence of epidemics, the methods of diagnoses used, the use of vaccines for rubella and varicella, delivery by Cesarean section when maternal herpes infection is present, and changing social behaviors.

The first major development in the control of viral infections was the introduction of the rubella virus vaccine in 1969. Over the following 25 years, other significant developments in the management and treatment of perinatal viral infections have included: (1) the introduction of vaccines against the hepatitis B virus and VZV; (2) the universal administration of hepatitis B vaccine to all newborns; (3) the dramatic reduction of perinatally acquired infection with human immunodeficiency virus (HIV) by administration of antiretroviral medication at the time of delivery; and (4) the application of modern molecular biological techniques, such as *in situ* hybridization and the polymerase chain reaction (PCR), in the prenatal diagnosis of viral infection. A vaccine against hepatitis B virus first became commercially available in 1981, whereas the VZV vaccine became available in Europe in 1984 and in the USA in 1995. Use of the rubella vaccine resulted in a 99% reduction in the incidence of congenital rubella syndrome (CRS) in the USA.[1] The vaccination of children with the VZV vaccine resulted in a 93% reduction in the expected number of cases compared with a historical attack rate of 87% in a cohort of unvaccinated children. Investigational vaccines against CMV, HSV, VEE, and HIV have been used in humans, although results of their efficacy are discouraging at present.

Cytomegalovirus

Biology

CMV is a DNA virus belonging to the Herpesviridae family. It is the most common congenitally acquired infection (Table 17.2). The name of the virus is derived from the characteristic "owl's eye" appearance of cells seen in histological sections of tissues which have been infected by the virus; this appearance is due to massive viral cytoplasmic replications, creating the distinct viral or cytomegalic inclusions. In 1956, Rowe and coauthors[2] were the first to successfully isolate the virus in tissue culture and describe its cytopathic effects. The following year, Weller and coauthors[3] independently reported the isolation of the same agent from infected infants.

Epidemiology

Seroprevalence studies of pregnant and nonpregnant women worldwide have consistently shown wide variations in seropositivity to CMV antibodies. These rates range from 40% to 80%, with higher rates related to lower socioeconomic status and an increase in patient age, gravidity, parity, and number of sexual partners. In general, the seroprevalence rate in the USA is approximately 60%. Studies using PCR have shown a cervical excretion rate of CMV of 13–40% and a urinary excretion rate of 1–13% throughout pregnancy.[4] Using nested PCR techniques, viral nucleic acid has been detected in other fluids such as nasopharyngeal secretions, urine, breast milk, and amniotic fluid.[5]

Congenital infection with CMV occurs at a frequency of approximately 0.5–2.5% of all newborns. In the USA,

Table 17.1 Viruses which are perinatally acquired and which can cause fetal/neonatal damage.

Virus	Perinatal/neonatal effects
Known teratogenic viruses	See text for perinatal effects
Cytomegalovirus	
Rubella virus	
Varicella zoster virus	
Herpes simplex virus (HSV1, HSV2)	
Parvovirus B19	
Venezuelan equine encephalitis virus	
Viruses that have been shown to cause fetal damage after transmission	
Coxsackieviruses (group B)	Myocarditis, meningoencephalitis, pleurodynia
Dengue virus	Fever, leucopenia, thrombocytopenia
Echovirus (14 and 19)	Apneic spells, hepatitis, thrombocytopenia
Hepatitis B virus	Hepatitis
Hepatitis C virus	Hepatitis
Human immunodeficiency virus	Growth restriction, leukopenia, failure to thrive, hypogammaglobulinemia, AIDS-related infections
Human papillomavirus	Laryngeal papilloma
Influenza virus	Endocardial fibroelastosis (?)
Mumps virus	Pneumonitis, endocardial fibroelastosis (?)
Parvovirus B19	Nonimmune fetal hydrops, anemia
Poliovirus	Paralysis
Rubeola (measles) virus	Premature delivery, measles, otitis media
Vaccinia virus	Spontaneous miscarriage, fetal death
Variola virus	Spontaneous miscarriage, fetal death
Western equine encephalitis virus	Meningitis
Viruses that have not been shown to cause fetal damage after transmission or when data on fetal transmission are inconclusive	
Coxsackieviruses (group A)	
Epstein–Barr virus	
Hepatitis A virus	
Non-A, non-B, non-C hepatitis viruses	
Rabies virus	
Smallpox virus	

Table 17.2 Frequency of teratogenic viral infections in pregnant women and their children.

Virus	Mother (per 10 000)	Child (per 10 000)
Cytomegalovirus	300–500	50–150
Rubella virus		
Epidemic	200–400	20–40
Nonepidemic	10–20	1–2
Currently in the USA	< 1	< 0.1
Herpes simplex virus	50–150	0.5–5.0
Parvovirus B19	25	5–10
Varicella zoster virus	1–2	< 0.01–1.0
Venezuelan equine encephalitis	With epidemics	With epidemics

approximately 40 000 infants are born annually with either clinical or laboratory evidence of CMV infection. Worldwide, it is estimated that 1% of all newborns are infected with CMV. Severe damage from congenital infection, such as the classic cytomegalic inclusion disease (CID), occurs at a rate of approximately 1 in 5000 to 1 in 20 000 births.

Perinatal transmission of CMV has been demonstrated in cases where the pregnant woman develops either a primary or recurrent CMV infection. Transmission rates of CMV after primary infection range from 15% to 50%,[6] whereas neonatal infection occurs in approximately 0.5–1.0% of cases where there is a recurrent infection in the mother. In general, the following principles apply to fetal infection with CMV: (1) severe damage, such as that seen in fully developed CID, results almost exclusively from primary maternal infection, and (2) clinically evident manifestations in the newborn are more common following primary infection in the mother.

Clinical manifestations

In general, maternal infection with CMV is asymptomatic. Symptomatic patients develop fever, pharyngitis, lymphadenopathy, and other generalized symptoms of viral illness. Primary CMV infection has been described as a

Table 17.3 Clinical manifestations of CMV in newborns and adults.

Birth defects
Cytomegalic inclusion disease (CID), which includes any of the following findings:
Early: petechiae, hepatosplenomegaly, jaundice, microcephaly, hemolytic anemia, cerebral calcifications, seizures, cerebellar or cortical atrophy, microphthalmia, intrauterine growth retardation, interstitial pneumonia, pneumonitis, mononucleosis-like illness, cardiovascular disease (e.g., ventriculomegaly, cardiomegaly), gastrointestinal defects, thrombocytopenia, ascites
Late: mental retardation, sensorineural hearing loss, learning disability, neuromuscular defects, psychomotor retardation
Early or late: chorioretinitis, optic atrophy, dental defects, spasticity

Clinical findings
Mother: mostly asymptomatic; when symptoms are present, heterophile-negative mononucleosis-like syndrome; laboratory diagnoses include CMV-specific IgG and IgM, viral culture
Infant: mostly asymptomatic; when symptoms are present, see above; laboratory diagnoses include CMV-specific IgM, viral culture, viral antigen, detection of viral DNA using *in situ* hybridization or PCR

heterophile-negative, mononucleosis-like syndrome. Following initial primary infection, CMV becomes latent; reactivation of latent infection is often asymptomatic and the factors that control reactivation are poorly understood at present. Fetal and neonatal infections can be acquired from mothers with either primary or recurrent infection; in general, the risk of fetal transmission and severity of the infection from reactivated disease in the mother is lower than with primary maternal infection.[7]

The clinical and laboratory manifestations of congenital CMV infection, summarized in Table 17.3, are divided into early and late findings. Most infected neonates are asymptomatic at birth, although 10% of these infants present with clinical manifestations later in life. In the USA, fully developed CID occurs at a rate of 1 case per 10 000 births; it involves multiorgan damage and is almost always a result of primary infection in the mother. The most common findings in CID include petechial rash (79%), hepatosplenomegaly (74%), jaundice (63%), and microcephaly (50%).[8]

Diagnosis

CMV infections usually go unrecognized unless symptoms develop. The presence of CMV-specific IgG antibodies in the mother confirms a recent or past infection; however, because CMV becomes latent in the mother, previous infection in the mother does not confer immunity against infection in the infant. CMV-specific IgM is detectable in both maternal and neonatal primary infections in 80% of cases.

Viral culture is the most accurate method of diagnosing CMV infection, although culture positivity cannot distinguish between primary and recurrent infection. Culture sites in the mother include the nasopharynx, cervix, vagina, and urine; in the infant, they include the nasopharynx, conjunctiva, and urine. Modern techniques, such as detection of viral DNA using PCR or *in situ* hybridization, have also been used in the prenatal diagnosis of CMV. Table 17.4 summarizes methods for the prenatal diagnosis of *in utero* infection with CMV.

Table 17.4 Prenatal methods of CMV detection.

Site/compartment	Method of detection
Amniotic fluid	CMV-specific IgM Viral culture Nucleic acid using PCR
Chorionic villus	Nucleic acid using PCR Nucleic acid using *in situ* hybridization
Fetal blood (from percutaneous umbilical blood sample)	CMV-specific IgM Viral culture Nucleic acid using PCR Viral antigen

Treatment and prevention

The treatment of CMV infection in the mother and infant is directed toward the symptoms, when they are present. Agents that have been used in the treatment of CMV include adenosine arabinoside, cytosine arabinoside, acyclovir, ganciclovir, and foscarnet (phosphonoformic acid). Unfortunately, they have had limited success; the first two agents are very toxic and the remainder have only been used in a very small number of studies. For example, ganciclovir has been used in the treatment of chorioretinitis and been shown to reduce viral shedding among infected infants; however, the reduction is only present for the duration of the treatment. Immunoprophylaxis with a live attenuated CMV vaccine has been used in seronegative kidney transplant recipients with some success.[9] Vaccine recipients were significantly less susceptible to acquiring primary CMV infection than those who received a placebo.

To date, the most effective method of reducing primary CMV infection in all pregnant women who are at high risk is to observe: (1) proper handwashing techniques, particularly when handling infants and young children, who are frequently infected and shed virus for extended periods of time, and (2) proper handling of infected body fluids and secretions in high-risk areas.

Rubella virus

In 1941, the Australian ophthalmologist, Gregg,[10] was the first physician to report congenital defects in children whose mothers had suffered an acute rubella (German measles) infection while pregnant. In total, 68 of the 78 infants who were studied developed cataracts and many also had congenital heart defects. Out of all the known teratogenic viruses, infection with rubella results in the most severe malformations.

Epidemiology

The most recent rubella pandemic was from 1962 to 1964, when 12.5 million cases of rubella and 20 000 cases of CRS were reported worldwide. In 1969, the introduction of the rubella vaccine in the USA reduced the annual incidence of rubella by 99% and, over the next two decades, the annual incidence of rubella decreased to 0.05 cases per 100 000 live births.

In the USA, up to 10% of women are susceptible to acute rubella infection in pregnancy despite routine and mandatory vaccination programs in children. At present, the single most important source of serosusceptible individuals in the USA are foreign-born immigrants who have not been vaccinated in their countries of origin, primarily Mexico and Central America.[11] Less than 5% of countries worldwide offer routine vaccination against rubella. In addition, specific groups in the USA, such as the Amish communities in Pennsylvania, do not commonly accept the vaccine and have a high serosusceptibility to rubella.

Biology and pathogenesis

Rubella is a member of the Togaviridae family, genus *Rubivirus*. The clinical manifestations of rubella infection in humans were first described in the mid-eighteenth century but the virus was only successfully isolated in tissue culture in 1962.[12] Humans acquire rubella infection primarily through infected respiratory droplets that are inoculated through the nasopharynx of the host. Infection is followed by the rapid spread of virus to regional lymph nodes and the bloodstream. Patients are viremic within 7 days of inoculation, although incubation periods are typically from 14 to 21 days, and viremia ceases 1–2 days before the onset of the rash. Viral shedding from the nasopharynx of infected individuals begins 7 days before, and up to 5 days after, onset of the rash.

When pregnant women develop acute rubella, congenital infection occurs through the transplacental route. Evidence of perinatal transmission through the birth canal has not been substantiated even though virus has been recovered from cervical secretions. Most fetal damage occurs in the first trimester and, in general, the earlier in gestation that the infection occurs, the more severe the fetal damage and malformation.

Clinical manifestations

Children and adults with primary rubella infection present with malaise, fever, lassitude, and headaches. A fine, macular, "rubelliform" rash develops within 1–5 days after these initial symptoms. The rash generally starts on the face and neck, extending to the trunk and extremities. Lymph node enlargement in the posterior auricular and suboccipital regions is common. Less common symptoms include arthralgias, tenosynovitis, myalgia, and peripheral neuritis.

Congenital manifestations of rubella are summarized in Table 17.5, with hearing loss the most common clinical finding in newborns. Late-onset clinical findings commonly present as endocrinological abnormalities, such as diabetes mellitus and thyroid disorders.

Table 17.5 Clinical manifestations of rubella infection in newborns and adults.

Birth defects
Congenital rubella syndrome (CRS), which includes any of the following findings:
Neurological: meningoencephalitis, microcephaly, intracranial calcifications, psychomotor retardation, behavioral disorders, autism, chronic progressive panencephalitis, hypotonia, speech defects
Otic: hearing loss
Ophthalmological: cataracts, retinopathy, glaucoma, cloudy cornea, microphthalmia, subretinal neovascularization
Cardiac: patent ductus arteriosus, pulmonary artery stenosis, pulmonary artery hyperplasia, coarctation of the aorta, ventricular septal defect, atrial septal defect, myocarditis, myocardial necrosis
Miscellaneous: thrombocytopenia purpura, chronic rubelliform rash, dermatoglyphic abnormalities, jaundice, hepatosplenomegaly, hepatitis, hemolytic anemia, interstitial pneumonia, bone defects, genitourinary abnormalities (cryptorchidism, polycystic kidneys)

Clinical findings
Mother: macular rubelliform rash, lymphadenopathy (posterior auricular, suboccipital), prodromal symptoms (malaise, fever, headaches), arthralgias, peripheral neuritis; laboratory diagnoses include rubella-specific IgG and IgM, virus isolation from nasopharynx, viral antigen
Infant: CRS (as above); laboratory diagnoses include rubella-specific IgG and IgM, virus isolation from nasopharynx

Diagnosis

The rubelliform rash on the face accompanied by posterior auricular lymphadenopathy and viral illness is virtually diagnostic of acute rubella infection in adults and children. Rubella-specific IgM can be detected a week after the onset of the rash, and typically persists for up to 2 months; it is detectable by culture of nasopharyngeal swabs, urine, blood, amniotic fluid, placenta, and synovial fluid.[13] Diagnosis of acute rubella infection is also made by the observation of a rise in acute and convalescent titers of rubella-specific IgG over a period of 3–4 weeks.

Congenital infection is diagnosed by the range of symptoms noted in Table 17.5. The Centers for Disease Control recently published a classification of CRS based on both clinical and laboratory findings.[11] Rubella-specific IgM is detectable for up to 6 months in infected newborns, and rubella IgG may remain elevated beyond this 6-month period. As in the mother, rubella is detectable by culture of infant blood, stools, cerebrospinal fluid, and urine. Daffos and coauthors[14] used cordocentesis to test fetal blood from pregnancies complicated by acute rubella in the first 20 weeks; the study demonstrated rubella-specific IgM in virtually all of the infants who were later shown to be infected at birth. Rubella viral RNA has also been detected using nested PCR techniques in chorionic villus samples, amniotic fluid, and fetal blood obtained by cordocentesis.[15]

Treatment and prevention

The treatment of acute rubella in adults and children is based on the symptoms. Most adults have complete recovery from the rash and lymphadenopathy within a week, although one-third may develop late-onset arthralgias. At present, there is no standard method of treating acute congenital rubella infections with antiviral therapy.

Since it was first introduced in the USA in 1969, the use of the rubella vaccine has been the most important factor in the worldwide management of rubella. The current strain of the live attenuated vaccine is still the original Wistar RA27/3 strain grown in human diploid fibroblasts; immunization with this vaccine induces rubella hemagglutination-inhibiting antibodies in approximately 97% of susceptible individuals. Two other live rubella vaccine strains were licensed in 1969, the Cendehill and HPV77 (DE-5 and DK-12) strains; however, the RA27/3 strain elicits a broader antibody response after vaccination.

Immunity against rubella is considered to be lifelong and enzyme-linked immunosorbent assay (ELISA) antibody levels persist for at least 10 years after vaccination. The American College of Obstetricians and Gynecologists (ACOG) currently recommends the following vaccination schedules: (1) all children from 12 to 15 months of age or older should be vaccinated against rubella and their mothers given a record of the vaccination; (2) all adults should be vaccinated, especially women who are known to be susceptible to rubella or who have a negative history of being immunized against rubella but whose serology status is unknown; however, pregnant women should not be vaccinated; (3) all prenatal patients should be tested for rubella IgG; and (4) all pregnant women identified as being susceptible to rubella should be advised about the potential risk of congenital rubella infection and be vaccinated after delivery.[16] In 2001, the interval between the administration of rubella vaccine and attempting pregnancy was reduced from 3 months to 1 month.[17] These guidelines also recommend that breastfeeding is not a contraindication to vaccine administration.

Varicella zoster virus

Congenital varicella syndrome is a collection of fetal abnormalities, primarily of the skin, eyes, and limbs, which were first described by Laforet and Lynch[18] in an infant born to a mother who contracted chickenpox at 8 weeks' gestation. VZV infection in adults and children presents as two different clinical conditions: as a primary infection (chickenpox), or as herpes zoster (shingles) resulting from reactivation of a latent infection.

Epidemiology

Chickenpox is one of the most contagious and, therefore, common infectious diseases of childhood. From 1980 through 1994, approximately 3.5 million cases of chickenpox were reported in the USA every year.[19] Chickenpox has an annual incidence of approximately 1500 cases per 100 000 of the population and around 85% of adults show serological evidence of immunity to chickenpox. However, despite the high number of serosusceptible individuals (15%), the incidence of primary VZV during pregnancy is only 0.013–0.07%.[20] In around 10–20% of adults, VZV infection may present later in life as shingles by reactivation of a latent viral infection; this is more frequent in older individuals.

In one study, the risk of fully developed congenital varicella syndrome following acute VZV infection in the first 20 weeks of pregnancy was shown to be approximately 2–5%.[21] However, more recently, a study of 347 pregnant women with acute VZV infection showed the frequency of congenital varicella syndrome to be only 0.4%.[22]

Biology

VZV is a member of the Herpesviridae family; its genetic structure is therefore similar to that of other herpesviruses. Horizontal transmission of VZV occurs via passage of infectious respiratory droplets from the nasopharynx of an infected host or from vesicular fluid expressed from the characteristic skin lesions. Following inoculation, the incubation period for VZV is approximately 1–3 weeks. The virus replicates at the site of entry, usually the nasopharynx; hence, patients are commonly viremic 1 week before, and up to 2 days after, the onset of clinical symptoms. This period of viremia is accompanied by prodromal symptoms.

Clinical manifestations

Most infections with VZV are symptomatic; acute VZV infections commonly present with painless, multiple, vesicular lesions starting on the head and face, then extending to the truck and extremities. The vesicles, ranging from 250 to 500 lesions during the acute stage, eventually rupture and develop a scab within several days. New vesicles may form as others heal, therefore the acute phase may involve lesions in different stages of development. The virus is detectable from skin lesions until the scab forms. The attack rates in susceptible individuals after exposure is approximately 90%.

After the primary infection, VZV remains latent in dorsal root ganglia and may present later in life as reactivated disease in the form of shingles. In both adults and children, shingles

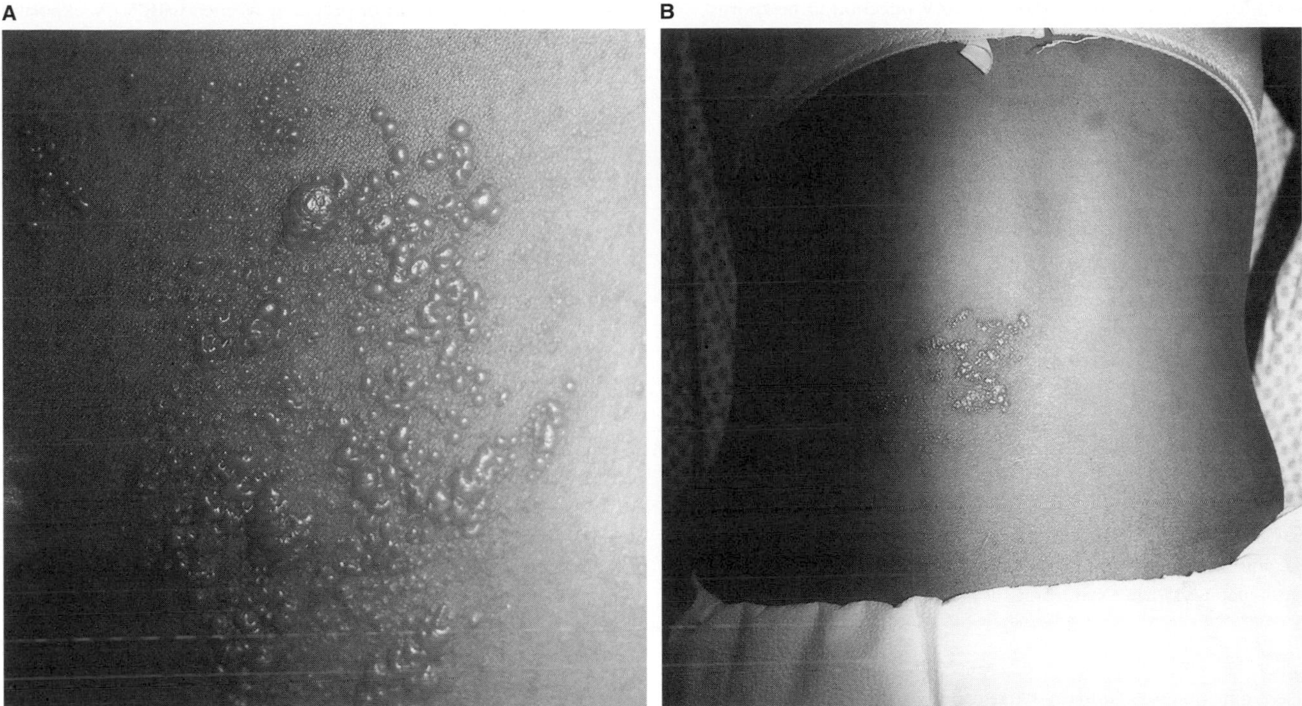

Figure 17.1 Vesiculopapular rash (A) and unilateral rash (B) of shingles (herpes zoster).

presents as very painful, vesicular lesions that typically follow the dermatomal pattern of the involved dorsal root ganglia (Fig. 17.1). The lesions are almost always unilateral. Peripheral neuralgia, which presents as hypesthesia on the skin around the lesions, precedes the lesions by several days. Virus is also recoverable from the lesions of shingles, although the viral load in the vesicular fluid is significantly lower than with primary infection. Shingles is a sequela in around 10% of acute VZV infections; this rate is higher among immunocompromised patients such as those with Hodgkin's disease or HIV infection.[23]

Vertical transmission of VZV has been well documented. *In utero* infection is the predominant method of transmission; the presence of virus in cervicovaginal secretions and the ability to transmit the virus through the birth canal have not been described. Congenital infection with VZV presents as one of four distinct clinical conditions: (1) fully developed congenital varicella syndrome; (2) disseminated varicella; (3) neonatal varicella; and (4) neonatal zoster (Table 17.6). The timing of maternal infection determines which clinical syndrome the newborn develops. Congenital varicella syndrome occurs following perinatal infection in the first 20 weeks of gestation. Infants born to women who develop clinical infection between 20 and 5 days before delivery are at risk of developing neonatal varicella. In contrast, those born to women who develop clinical infection from 5 days before and up to 2 days after delivery are at a 30% risk of developing disseminated varicella.

The most common findings in congenital varicella syndrome include skin, eye, and limb malformations, such as cicatricial scarring, chorioretinitis, anisocoria, cortical atrophy, limb paresis, and limb hypoplasia ipsilateral to the scarred limb. Intracranial calcifications have also been demonstrated in congenital VZV infections. Disseminated varicella presents with generalized vesicular skin lesions, pneumonia, and hepatitis; one-third of these infants die from this severe infection. Neonatal varicella is generally a mild course of chickenpox. Finally, Paryani and Arvin have reported a case of neonatal zoster in a 7-month-old infant without a prior history of chickenpox whose mother developed an acute infection while pregnant.[24]

Diagnosis

In adults and children, the characteristic rash (lesion) of VZV, which presents in multiple stages, is virtually diagnostic of primary infection. Virus is recoverable by culture of, and antigen detection in, scrapings of skin lesions. VZV-specific IgM becomes positive within several days of the onset of the rash. VZV-specific IgG confirms previous immunity to VZV and is present in 85–95% of adults. Approximately 70–90% of patients whose serology status to VZV is uncertain, or whose history of chickenpox in childhood is unknown, demonstrate previous seroimmunity.[25]

Congenital infections present with clinical findings as shown in Table 17.6. VZV-specific IgM in cord blood or infant blood confirms the diagnosis of fetal infection. Virus can also be isolated by culture of lesion scrapings from newborns. PCR has been used to detect viral DNA in the amniotic fluid from pregnancies complicated by VZV infection. Interestingly, infected newborns, even when asymptomatic, show evidence of

Table 17.6 Clinical manifestations of VZV infection in newborns and adults.

Birth defects
General: spontaneous abortion, fetal demise, premature delivery, low birthweight
Congenital varicella syndrome, which includes any of the following findings:
Neurological: cerebral cortical atrophy, microcephaly, encephalitis, seizures, mental retardation, intracranial calcifications, bulbar palsy, cerebellar hypoplasia, ventriculomegaly, neurodevelopmental delay, nystagmus
Ophthalmological: microphthalmia, optic atrophy, cataracts, chorioretinitis, anisocoria, corneal opacification, hydrocephalus, meningocele
Dermatological: cicatricial scarring of limb, vesicular lesions over dermatomal pattern
Limb disorder: limb hypoplasia ipsilateral to skin scarring, limb paresis, hypotonia, areflexia, flexion contracture deformities
Gastrointestinal: duodenal stenosis, colon atresia
Miscellaneous: Horner syndrome, hydroureter

Clinical findings
Mother: chickenpox, pneumonia, encephalitis, Reye syndrome, aseptic meningitis, Guillain–Barré syndrome, ophthalmological complications (conjunctivitis, uveitis), hepatitis, shingles (zoster), pneumonitis, esophagitis, myocarditis, herpes gangrenosum; laboratory diagnoses include VZV-specific IgG and IgM, virus culture, viral antigen, detection of viral DNA using PCR
Infant: four distinct clinical presentations:
(1) Congenital varicella syndrome
(2) Disseminated varicella; generalized lesions, pneumonia, hepatitis, viremia
(3) Neonatal varicella
(4) Neonatal zoster (shingles)
Laboratory diagnoses include VZV-specific IgG and IgM, virus culture, detection of viral DNA using PCR

Table 17.7 Management of pregnant women with VZV exposure and infection.

Pregnant women with VZV exposure, within 96 h of exposure
Test for VZV IgG
If IgG positive, confirms previous immunity, discontinue evaluation
If IgG negative, administer VZIG, 0.125 mg/kg i.m.
Observe for symptoms of chickenpox

Pregnant women with VZV exposure, more than 96 h after exposure
Test for VZV IgG
If IgG negative, efficacy of VZIG questionable, weigh risks and benefits of vaccine administration
Observe for symptoms of chickenpox

Pregnant women with primary chickenpox
Isolate from susceptible persons
Test for VZV IgG
Treat symptoms
Infection within the first 20 weeks of gestation:
  Counsel approximately 2–5% risk of congenital varicella syndrome, miscarriage, prematurity, low birthweight
  Observe for complications (e.g., varicella pneumonia)
  Consider acyclovir for pneumonia
  VZIG not necessary
Infection from 20 to 5 days before delivery:
  Counsel about risk for neonatal chickenpox
  Observe infant for chickenpox
  VZIG not necessary
Infection from 5 days before and up to 2 days after delivery
  Counsel approximately 30% risk of disseminated varicella
  Observe infant for disseminated varicella
  Administer VZIG to infant at birth, 1.25–2 mL i.m.
  Consider acyclovir for symptomatic infant
  Consider delaying birth until mother recovers from acute infection

Pregnant women with herpes zoster (shingles)
Counsel theoretical risk of neonatal infection
Isolate from susceptible persons (vesicular fluid is infectious)
Treat symptoms
Administer famciclovir for postherpetic neuralgia

lymphocyte transformation after stimulation with different VZV antigens.[24]

Treatment and prevention

In adults and children, acute infection with VZV is self-limited and treatment is generally directed at the symptoms. Table 17.7 summarizes the management of pregnant women who have been exposed to, or who develop, acute chickenpox. Pregnant women exposed to chickenpox should have their immune status identified; within 96 h of exposure, those found to be susceptible should receive varicella zoster immunoglobulin (VZIG) at a dose of 0.125 mg/kg of body weight. Of pregnant women exposed to VZV who were administered VZIG, only 20% developed primary varicella compared with 89% of patients who did not receive VZIG.[18] When administered more than 96 h after exposure, the efficacy of VZIG is questionable. Infants born to women who develop chickenpox from 5 days before and up to 2 days after delivery should be given VZIG.

Both pregnant and nonpregnant patients with herpes zoster benefit from a short course of antiviral therapy to shorten the duration of postherpetic neuralgia. These antiviral agents include acyclovir, valaciclovir, and famciclovir.

The VZV vaccine is the Oka strain of a live attenuated virus obtained from a child in Japan with a natural chickenpox infection, which was introduced into human embryonic lung cell cultures, and propagated in human diploid cell cultures. The vaccine was first introduced to high-risk children in Europe in 1984, in Japan in 1986, and in Korea in 1988; it was subsequently licensed in the USA in 1995. Seroimmunity is conferred 4–6 weeks after vaccination in 97% of susceptible children. The reported annual attack rate of chickenpox among vaccinated children is 0.2–1.0%, compared with 8–9%

in unvaccinated children. This represents a 93% reduction in acute VZV cases.

The Centers for Disease Control has the following recommendations regarding the VZV vaccine: (1) all children from 12 to 18 months of age should be routinely vaccinated regardless of VZV infection; (2) VZV vaccine is recommended for all susceptible children by 13 years of age; and (3) susceptible persons older than 13 years of age who are at high risk of acquiring VZV should receive the vaccine. The vaccine is contraindicated in pregnancy as it is a live virus; the teratogenic potential of the vaccine given inadvertently to pregnant women is not known. Women who receive the vaccine should be advised not to become pregnant for 1 month after administration. Early studies show no evidence of active VZV in breast milk in postpartum mothers who received the vaccine,[26] therefore there is no clear evidence that breastfeeding should be discontinued after administration of the vaccine.

Herpes simplex virus

Epidemiology

The first neonatal cases of HSV infection were reported independently by Batignani in 1934[27] and Hass in 1935.[28] In adults, HSV is one of the most widely disseminated and prevalent infections worldwide. In the USA, an estimated 45 million adults and adolescents are infected with HSV,[29] and approximately one in four women of reproductive age has antibodies to HSV2.[30] Large-scale epidemiological studies have consistently shown that an increased incidence of HSV infection correlates with increased sexual activity, early age of first sexual contact, and increased number of sexual contacts. Asymptomatic shedding of virus in cervicovaginal secretions occurs at a rate of 0.02–4% in nonpregnant women.

In the USA, the incidence of neonatal HSV infection is approximately 1 case per 7500 live births. Congenital infections with HSV have increased in the last three decades; the annual incidence of neonatal HSV increased from 2.6 per 100 000 live births in 1966 to 11.9 per 100 000 live births in 1981.[31]

Biology

Herpes simplex is a member of the Herpesviridae family of viruses. There are two subtypes of herpes simplex, HSV1 and HSV2. These subtypes are difficult to distinguish serologically as they share very close genomic homology and produce similar glycoproteins. At present, detection methods for HSV are based on the antibody response to glycoprotein G-2 for HSV2 and glycoprotein G-1 for HSV1; most other immune responses are similar for both HSV subtypes.[30]

Like other herpesviruses, HSV is neurotropic; after primary infection, HSV becomes latent in the infected host and virus is stored in the dorsal root ganglia. HSV is reactivated later in life and presents with recurrent episodes. Both HSV subtypes present with clinical symptoms in the genitals although most genital infections are due to HSV2. Infections with HSV2 are also associated with higher recurrence rates than infections with HSV1, in both the first and subsequent years following primary infection.

Clinical manifestations

Adults and children with HSV2 infection present with three distinct clinical syndromes: (1) first-episode primary infection; (2) first-episode nonprimary infection; and (3) recurrent infection. Following transmission from an actively shedding individual to a susceptible host, first-episode primary infections occur after an incubation of 3–7 days. These infections classically present with multiple, exquisitely painful, vesicular lesions at the site of inoculation. The vesicles rupture within 48–72 h, become ulcerated, indurated, and then resolve completely within 3–4 weeks. Virus is easily recoverable from the primary lesions. Viral shedding from both male and female asymptomatic patients has been well documented.[32] Lesions may be accompanied by fever, inguinal lymphadenopathy, malaise, and neuralgia. The majority of patients who show serological evidence of previous infection to HSV2 are asymptomatic, and up to 75% of patients with primary infection go unrecognized. Atypical clinical manifestations of genital HSV infection include genital fissures, furuncles and excoriations in the genitalia, aseptic meningitis, sacral autonomic nervous system dysfunction, and extragenital lesions. In rare instances, primary infection may progress into a more fulminant course, characterized by fever, anicteric hepatitis, and ulcerative pharyngitis.

After primary infection, HSV becomes latent. Reactivation of virus presents clinically as a first-episode, nonprimary infection or as a recurrent infection after a primary symptomatic outbreak. These reactivations are characterized by multiple, vesicular lesions of the genitals that are less painful, often without accompanying lymphadenopathy and generalized symptoms. Patients with first-episode, nonprimary infections and those with reactivation produce HSV2-specific IgG antibodies. Immunocompromised patients (e.g., those with HIV infection) may experience a more severe or protracted course of recurrent disease.

Nearly all HSV infection of neonates and infants occurs at delivery, through exposure to virus present in the birth canal. *In utero* transmission through transplacental passage of virus accounts for approximately 5% or less of all cases of congenital HSV.[33] For infants, the risks of acquiring HSV from the mother are summarized in Table 17.8.

Congenital infection with HSV manifests as one of three distinct clinical syndromes: (1) infection involving the skin, eyes, and mouth (SEM disease); (2) infection of the central nervous system (CNS), with or without SEM findings; and (3) disseminated HSV, when multiple organ damage is involved (Tables 17.9 and 17.10). Clinical disease is further classified as either early or late, depending on the timing of infection and onset of clinical manifestations. Infants infected transplacentally present with symptoms within the first 24–48 h of life. In contrast, infants who acquire HSV at the time of birth become clinically symptomatic within 1–2 weeks. One-half of the infants with CNS manifestations will also have SEM characteristics. CNS complications in infants, such as herpes encephalitis, can be life-threatening and carry a mortality rate of approximately 50%. Disseminated HSV with encephalitis carries the worst prognosis for infants, with a mortality rate of approximately 80%.

Table 17.8 Risk factors for transmission of HSV from mother to infant.

Incidence of neonatal HSV	1/3000–1/20 000 live births
Primary methods of infection	
Transplacental (*in utero*)	5%
Intrapartum	85%
Postpartum	10%
Risk of perinatal transmission	
Primary infection	30–50%
Nonprimary first episode	33%
Recurrent	< 5%
Percentage of infants with clinical syndrome at birth	
SEM disease	30%
CNS disease only	30%
Disseminated HSV	30%

SEM, neonatal herpes involving skin, eyes, and mouth.

Diagnosis

In adults and adolescents, genital infections with HSV are usually diagnosed clinically. Up to one-fourth of patients who present with a first-episode infection show serological evidence of a previous infection; these patients are, in fact, experiencing a recurrent infection. Commercial assays for HSV2-specific antibodies are useful in confirming a previous infection; however, cross-reactivity with HSV1 antibodies is possible. HSV2-specific IgG is detectable 2–12 weeks after exposure, with a mean seroconversion time of 22 days.[29] Therefore, many patients with primary infections do not demonstrate serological evidence of infection at the time of symptomatic clinical presentation. Virus isolation from vesicle fluid obtained from fresh lesions or from the cervix is the most specific laboratory method for detection of HSV.

Diagnosis of neonatal herpes includes a maternal history of HSV infection (primary or recurrent), clinical symptoms in the

Table 17.9 Clinical manifestations HSV infection in infants.

Site	Early symptoms	Late symptoms
Skin	Vesicles Exanthem Skin scarring	Recurrent cutaneous lesions
Eye	Chorioretinitis Keratoconjunctivitis Microphthalmia Cataracts	Chorioretinitis Blindness Cataracts Retinal dysplasia
Mouth	Oral ulcerations	
CNS	Microcephaly Cerebral atrophy Hydrancephaly Intracranial calcifications Encephalitis (bulging fontanelles, pyramidal tract signs, poor feeding, temperature instability)	Microcephaly Psychomotor retardation Learning disability Spasticity Seizures Porencephalic cysts Hydrancephaly
Disseminated HSV	Shock Disseminated intravascular coagulopathy Jaundice Respiratory distress Seizures Irritability Thrombocytopenia	
Miscellaneous	Hepatosplenomegaly Pneumonitis Purpura/petechiae	Hearing loss Dental anomalies Pneumonitis

infant (Table 17.9), and laboratory evidence of infection in both mother and infant. Because viral shedding may be asymptomatic in the cervix of pregnant women, symptomatic disease in the mother is not a requisite for the diagnosis of infection in the newborn. Detection of HSV1- and HSV2-specific IgM in the newborn may be helpful in the diagnosis of congenital infection. As in adults, virus isolation from skin vesicles, conjunctiva, nasopharynx, and cerebrospinal fluid remains the gold standard in the diagnosis of HSV in infants. Unfortunately, however, virus isolation carries a false-negative rate as high as 20% in primary infection and even higher in recurrent disease. Recent data on the detection of viral DNA using PCR show that this technique has greater specificity and sensitivity than classical virus isolation techniques.[34]

Table 17.10 Clinical manifestations of HSV infection in mothers and infants.

Birth defects
General: miscarriage, preterm delivery
Early and late symptoms: see Table 17.9
Clinical findings
Mother: mostly asymptomatic; when symptoms are present, genital and extragenital lesions (painful, vesicular to ulcerative lesions), gingivostomatitis, pharyngitis, herpetic whitlow, keratitis, penumonitis, hepatitis; disseminated HSV; laboratory diagnoses include HSV1- and HSV2-specific IgG and IgM, viral antigen, virus isolation, detection of viral DNA using PCR
Infant: see Table 17.9; laboratory diagnoses include HSV1- and HSV2-specific IgG and IgM, virus isolation, detection of viral DNA using PCR

Treatment

HSV infections in adults and adolescents are treated symptomatically. Antiviral therapy with aciclovir has been shown to be effective in: (1) reducing both the severity and duration of symptoms in primary infection; (2) preventing the occurrence and reducing the frequency of recurrent outbreaks; and (3) treating fulminant, disseminated HSV in adults and infants.

Aciclovir is a synthetic thymidine analog that acts as a competitive inhibitor of HSV1 and HSV2 DNA polymerase. The drug has also been shown to have *in vitro* and *in vivo* antiviral activity against CMV, VZV, and Epstein–Barr virus. HSV thymidine kinase phosphorylates aciclovir and the resulting triphosphate derivative terminates the elongating chain, thus inhibiting further viral replication. Second-generation thymidine analogs (famciclovir and valaciclovir) are also approved treatments for HSV; *in vivo*, valaciclovir is converted to aciclovir, while the active antiviral agent in famciclovir is penciclovir. Table 17.11 summarizes treatment options using these three antiviral drugs. Topical treatments for both genital and oral lesions have not been shown to be effective.

Acyclovir has been shown to be effective in the treatment of neonatal HSV infections. Vidarabine, another nucleoside

Table 17.11 Antiviral treatment options for HSV infection in adults.[29]

Type of infection	Drug	Dosage	Pregnancy category
First episode (primary or nonprimary)			
Treat for 7–10 days	Acyclovir	400 mg p.o. t.i.d.	B
	Acyclovir	200 mg p.o. 5 × /day	
	Valaciclovir	1 g p.o. b.i.d.	B
	Famciclovir	250 mg p.o. t.i.d.	B
Recurrent disease			
Treat for 5 days	Acyclovir	400 mg p.o. t.i.d.	
	Acyclovir	200 mg p.o. 5 × /day	
	Valaciclovir	500 mg p.o. b.i.d.	
	Valaciclovir	1 g po q.d.	
	Famciclovir	125 mg p.o. b.i.d.	
Suppressive therapy			
May be given for several years	Acyclovir	400 mg p.o. b.i.d.	
	Valaciclovir	0.5–1 g p.o. b.i.d.	
	Famciclovir	250 mg p.o. b.i.d.	
Herpes zoster (recurrent VZV)			
Treat for 7–10 days	Acyclovir	800 mg p.o. 5 × /day	
	Valaciclovir	1 g p.o. t.i.d.	
	Famciclovir	500 mg p.o. t.i.d.	

analog, has also been used successfully to reduce mortality in neonates with HSV encephalitis and disseminated HSV. A prospective, randomized trial comparing the efficacy of aciclovir and vidarabine in neonatal HSV showed no significant differences between the two treatments with regard to reduction of mortality and adverse sequelae.[35]

Prevention

In 1999, ACOG established guidelines for the management of HSV infection in pregnancy to help prevent perinatal transmission.[36] Previous management protocols, which advocated weekly testing of the cervix for HSV using culture methods, are now obsolete; recent data have demonstrated a poor correlation between antepartum shedding of HSV and shedding at the time of delivery and, therefore, perinatal transmission. Approximately 1.4% of neonatal infection occurs in pregnancies where antepartum cultures were negative. The current ACOG guidelines for management of HSV in pregnant women in labor are summarized in Table 17.12. Cesarean delivery is recommended for patients in labor with active genital lesions resulting from HSV infection (primary or recurrent). Patients with lesions that may be due to HSV infection or those with prodromal symptoms (e.g., tingling in the vulva) are also recommended to undergo a Cesarean delivery. Asymptomatic patients and those with HSV lesions that are remote from the vagina (e.g., thigh or buttock) should be allowed to deliver vaginally.[36] Also, a Cesarean delivery would be considered beneficial for patients at term who have active lesions and whose membranes have ruptured for longer than 4 h.

There are no conclusive data on the management of patients with active lesions who experience preterm premature rupture of membranes. The current recommendation for these patients is to weigh up the benefits of delivery in order to prevent the perinatal transmission of HSV against the risks of delivering a premature infant. There are no contraindications to the use of antenatal corticosteroid therapy in this setting.

Table 17.12 Guidelines for the management of HSV infection in pregnancy.

Pregnant women with a previous known history of HSV infection
Recommend prophylaxis against asymptomatic cervical shedding with antiviral therapy at 35 weeks
Allow vaginal delivery if asymptomatic in labor
Cesarean delivery for obstetric indications only
Weekly cervical cultures for HSV are not indicated
Perform culture in labor if symptomatic
Observe infant for HSV
Pregnant women with herpetic genital lesions, clinically suspicious for HSV
Culture lesions to confirm diagnosis
Recommend Cesarean delivery
Observe infant for HSV

A meta-analysis by Sheffield and coauthors,[37] using large multicenter studies, demonstrated that prophylaxis of asymptomatic pregnant women at term, who have a history of HSV and antiviral therapy, significantly reduced the incidence of HSV viral shedding at delivery. The use of acyclovir prophylaxis, starting at 36 weeks, effectively reduced the clinical recurrence and asymptomatic shedding of HSV at the time of delivery, and the need for Cesarean delivery for recurrent disease.

Parvovirus B19 infections

Erythema infectiosum, or fifth disease, is the major clinical presentation of parvovirus B19 infection in children and was first described in 1983.[38] The disease was named fifth disease as it is the fifth most common exanthema of childhood. The classic "slapped cheek" appearance of fifth disease typically presents in children; adults present with a generalized macular rash, anemia, and arthralgias. The teratogenic effects of parvovirus B19 infection have not been clearly defined although there have been several reports which identify parvovirus B19 as a teratogen.

The rash of erythema infectiosum is macular and reticulate; it typically starts on the face and extends to the trunk and extremities. Constitutional symptoms include fever, coryza, pharyngitis, and malaise; viremia occurs up to a week before the onset of the rash. Adult infections may be accompanied by a transient anemia; patients with hemoglobinopathies may precipitate a transient aplastic crisis. Fetal infection can lead to fetal death, miscarriage, and nonimmune hydrops fetalis; few reports have demonstrated fetal malformations following congenital infections, such as microphthalmia, bilateral cleft lip and palate, micrognathia, and hydrocephalus. The fetal hydrops is thought to result from the transient fetal anemia caused by the infection. A recent report by Enders and coauthors[39] has shown that the rate of development of fetal hydrops following acute infection in pregnancy is 3.9%. This study also revealed a high fetal death rate (6.3%), with the highest rates observed when hydrops developed before 20 weeks' gestation.

Acute infections with parvovirus B19 are diagnosed by the clinical presentation (e.g., macular facial rash, arthralgias, anemia). Diagnosis is confirmed by the presence of parvovirus-specific IgM, which is detectable 7–10 days after the onset of constitutional symptoms. Parvovirus-specific IgG is produced shortly afterwards and persists for years; immunity to parvovirus is permanent. Because IgM does not cross the placenta, parvovirus IgM in cordocentesis samples, cord blood, or neonatal blood, should indicate congenital infection.

Parvovirus infections in children and adults are self-limited and treatment is therefore symptomatic. Following diagnosis of acute parvovirus in pregnancy, weekly ultrasonography to detect fetal hydrops should be performed for 15 weeks. Because fetal anemia is the physiological cause of the hydrops, *in utero* transfusion has been shown to significantly improve fetal morbidity and mortality in severe cases. A study by Rodis and coauthors[40] of 5349 cases of fetal hydrops, secondary to acute parvovirus infection in the mother, showed a survival rate of 83%. Most cases of fetal hydrops revert back to normal within 4 weeks. There is clearly no risk of hydrops in mothers who have previous immunity to parvovirus B19. Following intrauterine fetal transfusion, Enders and coauthors[39] reported a survival rate of approximately 85% of hydrops cases.

Venezuelan equine encephalitis (VEE)

VEE is a member of the larger group *Alphavirus encephalitides*, which includes Western equine encephalitis, Eastern equine encephalitis, and chikungunya virus. VEE infections occur mostly in the Caribbean, southern USA, and South and Central America. Although VEE can result in an epidemic in horses, it usually causes only mild infections in humans. However, in October 1995, during a 6-week epidemic/epizootic in the Guajira state of Colombia, a total of 12403 patient visits for VEE were reported.[41] The mosquito of the genus *Culex* is the most common vector, while humans and other wild mammals (monkeys, rats, opossums, and jackrabbits) are common hosts.

After an incubation period of 2–5 days, adults with VEE infection present with fever, headaches, malaise, and myalgia. Severe complications include seizures, mental confusion, coma, and tremors. Symptoms last for 3–8 days and virus is recoverable from the serum of symptomatic individuals by culture. VEE-specific antibody can be used to confirm previous infection. Congenital infection has been associated with pregnancy loss and fetal malformations including microphthalmia, absent cerebellum, and other CNS damage. Inoculation of pregnant rhesus monkeys with VEE has been shown to result in congenital microcephaly, hydrocephalus, cataracts, and porencephalic cysts.[42]

VEE can be controlled by proper immunization and quarantine of animals, as well as by reducing the spread of mosquitoes in endemic areas. There is presently no effective vaccine against VEE in humans.

Key points

1. Cytomegalovirus (CMV) is currently the most common congenitally acquired infection in humans. In the USA, approximately 40000 infants are born annually with evidence of perinatally acquired CMV infection.
2. Most infections with CMV in adults and newborns are asymptomatic; classic cytomegalovirus inclusion disease (CID) occurs in approximately 1 in 50000 births.
3. Unlike other infections, congenital CMV can be acquired from mothers who develop either primary or recurrent infection; however, severe damage in the infant occurs principally from mothers who have primary infection.
4. Appropriate hand washing techniques are still the most effective method of preventing acute primary CMV infection among serosusceptible individuals, especially those who work in very high-risk areas.
5. The introduction of the rubella vaccine in the USA in 1969 has been the single most important factor in reducing the incidence of rubella infection in adults and children, and congenital rubella syndrome (CRS) in neonates. In 1999, the incidence of rubella was 0.1 case per 100000 individuals.
6. The single most common source of individuals serosusceptible to rubella is foreign-born immigrants who have not been vaccinated in their country of origin.
7. Rubella is most commonly transmitted transplacentally; there is no definitive evidence that rubella is acquired perinatally through the birth canal.
8. Acute rubella most commonly presents in adults and children with a triad of symptoms: macular, rubelliform rash, lymphadenopathy of the head and neck, and generalized flu-like illness.
9. Characteristic congenital infections with varicella zoster virus (VZV) include malformations of the skin (cicatricial formation), eye (chorioretinitis, microphthalmia), and limb (limb hypoplasia and deformities).
10. Approximately 10–20% of individuals who acquire chickenpox will develop shingles (zoster) later on in life.
11. Clinical manifestations of congenitally acquired VZV infection correlate with the timing of infection in pregnancy. Infections in the first trimester result in birth defects while those in the third trimester result in chickenpox or disseminated varicella in the newborn.
12. There is no evidence that VZV infection is acquired perinatally through the birth canal. Horizontal transmission occurs through transfer of infectious respiratory droplets or from infectious fluid expressed from the skin lesions of chickenpox.
13. Varicella zoster immunoglobulin (VZIG) is indicated for serosusceptible pregnant women within 96h of exposure to chickenpox. VZIG is also indicated for newborns whose mothers develop acute chickenpox from 5 days before and up to 2 days after delivery.
14. The highest risk of fetal infection with VZV occurs when the mother develops acute chickenpox from 5

days before and up to 2 days after delivery. In this case, the risk of neonatal disseminated varicella is approximately 30%.

15 The incidence of herpes simplex virus (HSV) infection correlates directly with increased sexual activity, early age of first sexual contact, and increased number of sexual contacts. Approximately one out of four women of reproductive age has serological evidence of HSV2 infection.

16 Transmission of HSV occurs primarily through exposure of the infant to the virus in the birth canal; *in utero* or transplacental infection rarely occurs.

17 The management of pregnant women with HSV includes the following: (1) Cesarean delivery for women with active *or* suspicious lesions; (2) in pregnant women with a history of HSV, consider aciclovir prophylaxis at term, to reduce recurrent infections; and (3) antiviral therapy for patients with primary HSV.

18 Acyclovir is a synthetic thymidine analogue that competes with thymidine for binding sites in HSV DNA polymerase. Other agents which are active against HSV include famciclovir and penciclovir; penciclovir is metabolized to aciclovir *in vivo*.

19 Patients with suspicious lesions or prodromal symptoms at the time of delivery are also recommended to undergo a Cesarean delivery to prevent neonatal transmission of HSV.

20 Vaccines have dramatically reduced the incidence of perinatal infection with rubella and VZV. Although being developed, there are currently no effective vaccines available for CMV, HSV, and parvovirus B19.

Further reading (key points)

Adler SP, Finney JW, Manganello AM, et al. Prevention of child-to-mother transmission of cytomegalovirus among pregnant women. *J Pediatr* 2004;145:485.

Brown ZA, Benedetti J, Ashley R, et al. Neonatal herpes simplex virus infection in relation to asymptomatic maternal infection at the time of labor. *N Engl J Med* 1991;324:1247.

Brown ZA, Selke S, Zeh J, et al. The acquisition of herpes simplex virus during pregnancy. *N Engl J Med* 1997;337:509.

Centers for Disease Control and Prevention. 2002 guidelines for treatment of sexually transmitted diseases. *Morb Mort Wkly Rep* 2002;51(RR-6):1.

Jim WT, Shu CH, Chiu NC, et al. Transmission of cytomegalovirus from mothers to preterm infants by breast milk. *Pediatr Infect Dis J* 2004;23:848.

Karakoc GB, Altintas DU, Kiline B, et al. Seroprevalence of rubella in school girls and pregnant women. *Eur J Epidemiol* 2003;18:81.

Revello MG, Gerna G. Pathogenesis and prenatal diagnosis of human cytomegalovirus infection. *J Clin Virol* 2004;29:71.

Schrag SJ, Arnold KE, Mohle-Boetani JC, et al. Prenatal screening for infectious diseases and opportunities for prevention. *Obstet Gynecol* 2003;102:753.

References

1 Centers for Disease Control and Prevention. Rubella and congenital rubella: United States, 1984–1986. *Morb Mort Wkly Rep* 1987;36:664.

2 Rowe WP, Hartlet JW, Waterman S, et al. Cytopathogenic agents resembling human salivary gland virus recovered from tissue culture of human adenoids. *Proc Soc Exp Biol Med* 1956;92:418.

3 Weller TH, Macauley JC, Craig JM et al. Isolation of intranuclear inclusion producing agents from infants with illnesses resembling Cytomegalic inclusion disease. *Proc Soc Exp Biol Med* 1957;94:4.

4 Shen CY, Chang SF, Yen MS, et al. Cytomegalovirus excretion in pregnant and nonpregnant women. *J Clin Microbiol* 1993;31:1635.

5 Borg KL, Nordbo SA, Winge P, Dalen A. Detection of cytomegalovirus using "boosted" nested PCR. *Mol Cell Probes* 1995;9:251.

6 Morris DJ, Sims D, Chiswick M, et al. Symptomatic congenital cytomegalovirus infection after maternal recurrent infection. *Pediatr Infect Dis J* 1994;12:61.

7 Fowler KB, Stagno S, Pass RF, et al. The outcome of congenital cytomegalovirus infection in relation to maternal antibody status. *N Engl J Med* 1992;326:663.

8 Stano S, Pass RF, Dworsky ME, Alford CA. Congenital and perinatal cytomegalovirus infection. *Semin Perinatol* 1983;7:30.

9 Plotkin SA, Friedman HM, Fleisher GR. Towne-vaccine induced prevention of cytomegalovirus disease after renal transplants. *Lancet* 1984;1:528.

10 Gregg NM. Congenital cataract following German measles in the mother. *Trans Ophthalmol Soc Aust* 1941;3:35.

11 Centers for Disease Control and Prevention. Control and prevention of rubella: evaluation and management of suspected outbreaks, rubella in pregnant women, and surveillance for congenital rubella syndrome. *Morb Mort Wkly Rep* 2001;50 (RR-12):1.

12 Parkman PD, Buescher EL, Artenstein MA. Recovery of rubella virus from army recruits. *Proc Soc Exp Biol Med* 1962;111:225.

13 Cradock-Watson JE, Miller E, Ridehalgh MK, et al. Detection of rubella virus in fetal and placental tissue and in the throats of neonates after serologically confirmed rubella in pregnancy. *Prenat Diagn* 1989;9:91.

14 Daffos F, Forestier F, Grangeot-Keros L, et al. Prenatal diagnosis of congenital rubella. *Lancet* 1984;2:1.

15 Tanemura M, Suzumori K, Yagami Y, Kartow S. Diagnosis of fetal rubella infection with reverse transcription and nested polymerase chain reaction: a study of 34 cases diagnosed in fetuses. *Am J Obstet Gynecol* 1996;174:578.

16 American College of Obstetricians and Gynecologists. Rubella and pregnancy. *Technical Bulletin* 1992;171.

17 American College of Obstetricians and Gynecologists. Rubella vaccination. *Committee Opinion* 2002;281.

18 Laforet EG, Lynch C. Multiple congenital defects following maternal varicella. *N Engl J Med* 1947;236:534.

19 Enders G. Varicella zoster virus in pregnancy. *Prog Med Virol* 1984;29:166.

20 Jones KL, Johnson KA, Chambers CD. Offspring of women infected with varicella during pregnancy: a prospective study. *Teratology* 1994;49:29.

21 Pastuszak AL, Levy M, Schick B, et al. Outcome after maternal varicella infection in the first 20 weeks of pregnancy. *N Engl J Med* 1994;330:901.

22 Harger JH, Ernest JM, Thurnau GR, et al. Frequency of congenital varicella syndrome in a prospective cohort of 347 pregnant women. *Obstet Gynecol* 2002;100:260.

23 Friedman-Kien AE, LaFleur FL, Gendler E, et al. Herpes zoster: a possible early clinical sing for development of acquired immunodeficiency syndrome in high-risk individuals. *J Am Acad Dermatol* 1986;14:1023.

24 Paryani SG, Arvin AM. Intrauterine infection with varicella-zoster virus after maternal varicella. *N Engl J Med* 1986;314:1452.

25 Streuwing JP, Hyams KC, Tueller JE, Gray GC. The risk of measles, mumps, and varicella among young adults: a serosurvey of US Navy and Marine Corps recruits. *Am J Pub Health* 1993;83:1717.

26 Bohlke K, Galil K, Jackson LA, et al. Postpartum varicella vaccination: is the vaccine virus excreted in breast milk? *Obstet Gynecol* 2003;102:970.

27 Batignani A. Conjunctivite de virus erpetico in neonato. *Bull Ocul* 1934;13:1217.

28 Hass M. Hepatoadrenal necrosis with intranuclear inclusion bodies: report of a case. *Am J Pathol* 1935;11:127.

29 Fleming DT, McQuillan GM, Johnson RE, et al. Herpes simplex virus type 2 in the United States, 1976–1994. *N Engl J Med* 1997;337:1105.

30 American College of Obstetricians and Gynecologists Practice Bulletin. Clinical management guidelines for obstetrician-gynecologists, No. 57, 2004. Gynecologic herpes simplex virus infections. *Obstet Gynecol* 2004;104:1111.

31 Sullivan-Bolyai J, Hull HF, Wilson C, Corey L. Neonatal herpes simplex infection in King County, Washington. Increasing incidence and epidemiological correlates. *JAMA* 1983;250:3059.

32 Rooney JF, Felser JM, Ostrove JM et al. Medical intelligence: acquisition of genital herpes from an asymptomatic sexual partner. *N Engl J Med* 1986;314:1561.

33 Whitley RJ. Neonatal herpes simplex virus infections: is there a role for immunoglobulin in disease prevention and therapy? *Pediatr Infect Dis J* 1994;13:432.

34 Jerome KR, Huang ML, Wald A, et al. Quantitative stability of DNA after extended storage of clinical specimens as determined by real-time PCR. *J Clin Microbiol* 2002;40:2609.

35 Whitley RJ, Arvin A, Prober C et al. A controlled trial comparing vidarabine with aciclovir in neonatal herpes simplex virus infection. *N Engl J Med* 1991;324:444.

36 American College of Obstetricians and Gynecologists Practice Bulletin. Clinical management guidelines for obstetrician-gynecologists, No. 8, 1999. Management of herpes in pregnancy. *Int J Gynecol Obstet* 2000;68:165.

37 Sheffield JS, Hollier LM, Hill JB, et al. Aciclovir prophylaxis to prevent herpes simplex virus recurrence at delivery: a systematic review. *Obstet Gynecol* 2004;102:1396.

38 Anderson MJ, Jones SE, Fisher-Hoch SP, et al. Human parvovirus, the cause of erythema infectiosum (fifth disease)? *Lancet* 1983;1: 1378.

39 Enders M, Weidner A, Zoellner I, et al. Fetal morbidity and mortality after human parvovirus B19 infection in pregnancy: prospective evaluation of 1018 cases. *Prenat Diagn* 2004;24: 513.

40 Rodis JF, Borgida AF, Wilson M et al. Management of parvovirus infection in pregnancy and outcomes of hydrops: a survey of members of the Society of Perinatal Obstetricians. *Am J Obstet Gynecol* 1998;179:985.

41 Centers for Disease Control and Prevention. Venezuelan equine encephalitis: Colombia, 1995. *Morb Mort Wkly Rep* 1995;44: 775.

42 London WT, Levitt NH, Kent SG, et al. Congenital cerebral and ocular malformations induced in rhesus monkeys by Venezuelan equine encephalitis virus. *Teratology* 1977;16:285.

18 Transplacentally acquired microbial infections in the fetus

Santosh Pandipati and Ronald S. Gibbs

Group B streptococcal infection

Group B streptococcus (GBS) is a bacterial member of a group of β-hemolytic streptococci that includes group A (*Streptococcus pyogenes*) and group D, which includes enterococci. Group B streptococci are facultative, Gram-positive diplococci with the vast majority causing complete (β) hemolysis on blood agar plates. Group B streptococci can be found as a colonizing organism in the gastrointestinal and genital tracts of humans. It can cause stillbirth, preterm labor, and chorioamnionitis. In the mother, GBS can cause urinary tract infection, endometritis, and septicemia; in the neonate, it is responsible for early- and late-onset sepsis, pneumonia, meningitis and, less frequently, osteomyelitis, septic arthritis, and cellulitis. There are several serotypes of GBS that cause human disease, and they can all be found in genital isolates; serotype III is the predominant cause of late-onset neonatal sepsis.

Epidemiology

Group B streptococci were first recognized as causing perinatal disease in the 1960s and, by the 1970s, they were recognized as a leading cause of neonatal and maternal infection. Neonatal fatality ranged from 20% to a staggering 50%. There were approximately 6100 early-onset and 1400 late-onset cases of neonatal disease in the pre-prevention era, with an incidence of early-onset disease in the 1980s and early 1990s of 1.5–2 cases per 1000 live births. Subsequent to the implementation of national prevention strategies in the mid-1990s, neonatal GBS disease incidence has declined to 0.4–0.5 cases per 1000 live births.

While it is possible that GBS colonizes all women at some point in their lifetimes, when cultured on their vaginas, rectums, or both, 20–30% of pregnant mothers are found to be rectovaginal GBS carriers. African–American women have higher colonization rates than Caucasians or Asians.[1] Colonization can be transient or intermittent, resulting in potentially different culture statuses between pregnancies.

Neonatal disease

Early-onset disease occurs within 1 week of life (with most cases being identified within 72 h of birth), while late-onset disease occurs after the first week of life. Owing to the dramatic decline in early-onset disease in the 1990s, early- and late-onset disease now have similar occurrence rates, with case fatality rates of 4.7% for the former and 2.8% for the latter.[2] Survival is largely dependent upon gestational age at birth, with 98% survival for greater than 37 weeks' gestation, 90% for 34–36 weeks, and 70% for infants less than 33 weeks old.[2]

Risk factors for early-onset disease include maternal GBS colonization, prolonged rupture of membranes, preterm delivery, GBS bacteriuria during pregnancy, birth of a previous infant with invasive GBS disease, maternal clinical chorioamnionitis, young maternal age, African–American race, Hispanic ethnicity, and low levels of antibody to type-specific, capsular polysaccharide antigens. Colonization with GBS, preterm delivery, maternal race, and young maternal age are also independent risk factors for late-onset disease. There is an increased risk of long-term neurologic sequelae in late-onset neonatal disease as up to one-third of these cases include neonatal meningitis.

Apart from neonatal disease, 9–15% of stillbirths have been attributed to infection, with GBS isolated in a large number of these cases. This is especially true of early stillbirths, i.e., those that occur at less than 28 weeks' gestation, as opposed to term stillbirths.

Maternal disease

In maternal infection, GBS is often found to be one of multiple miscreant organisms. In chorioamnionitis, group B streptococcal isolates can be found in as many as 15% of cases, often along with other organisms.[3] Endometritis is similarly a polymicrobial infection, with similar culture rates to GBS.[4] Group B streptococci can also be found in 2–15% of infected postCesarean section incisions. After *Escherichia coli*, GBS is the second most common bacteria found in maternal bacteremia, including cases of pyelonephritis. Clinical presentation of GBS infection can include a maternal fever and elevated white blood cell count.

GBS has rarely been shown to cause fatal infections, necrotizing fasciitis, and maternal meningitis.[5,6]

Diagnosis

The optimal culture site for lower genital tract colonization has been rectovaginal. Recently, GBS has been isolated from vaginoperianal, anorectal, and perianal specimens with equal rates of positivity. To optimize yield, swabs from the rectogenital tract should be inoculated in selective growth media (commercially available) to suppress competing bacteria. However, blood agar is adequate for GBS recovery from endometrial, amniotic fluid, urine, and blood specimens.

Rapid identification tests, including Gram stain, immunofluorescent antibody, colorimetric assay using starch serum media, and antigen detection (e.g., coagglutination, latex agglutination, enzyme immunoassay) all lack sufficient sensitivity or positive predictive value (PPV). Polymerase chain reaction (PCR) is a new technology that has not yet been widely implemented for rapid detection, but has been shown to be 97% sensitive and 100% specific, with a PPV of 100% and a negative predictive value (NPV) of 98.8%.[7] Under ideal conditions, test results have been available in 40–100 min. There are several limitations of PCR technology, including the inability to test for GBS sensitivity to various antibiotics, which is something that would be necessary in patients who have a history of anaphylaxis to penicillin. It is also unclear whether such rapid turnaround is adequate for routine use intrapartum, and whether all hospital laboratories can provide rapid results at night or at weekends. For now, screening should continue to rely upon genitorectal cultures as delineated in the 2002 Centers for Disease Control (CDC) guidelines (explained below).

Treatment

Fortunately, GBS continues to be susceptible to penicillin and ampicillin. However, as of 2003, 37% of invasive GBS isolates were noted to be resistant to erythromycin and 17% to clindamycin (Active Bacterial Core Surveillance/Emerging Infections Program Network, unpublished data). Resistance to cefoxitin, a second-generation cephalosporin, has also been detected.[8]

In 2002, the CDC, the American Academy of Pediatrics, and the American College of Obstetricians and Gynecologists produced new GBS chemoprophylaxis guidelines. These guidelines are predicated upon the GBS carrier status in the pregnant mother, which should have been obtained via a rectovaginal swab at approximately 36 weeks' gestation or within 5 weeks of delivery (see Fig. 18.1). In a circumstance in which one is testing a patient who has a history of penicillin allergy, especially anaphylaxis, upon obtaining a screening specimen, it is necessary to notify the laboratory to test for sensitivity to erythromycin and clindamycin if GBS is detected.[9] Multistate data from 2003 showed a 34%

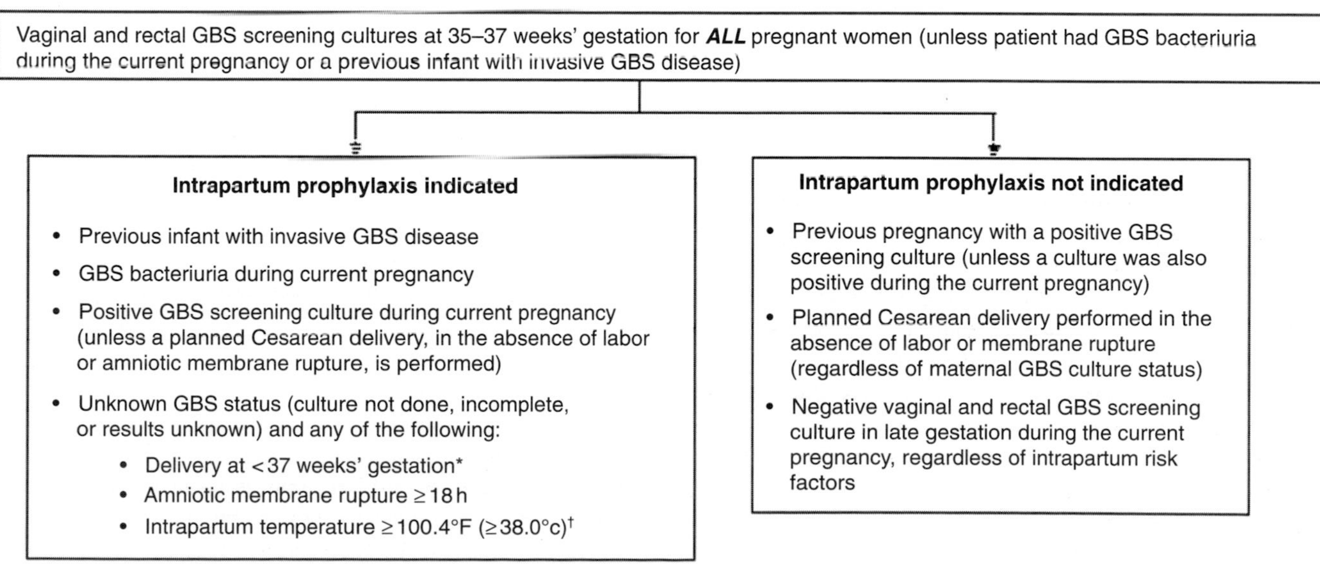

* If onset of labor or rupture of amniotic membranes occurs at < 37 weeks' gestation and there is a significant risk for preterm delivery (as assessed by the clinician), a suggested algorithm for GBS prophylaxis management is provided.
† If amnionitis is suspected, broad-spectrum antibiotic therapy that includes an agent known to be active against GBS should replace GBS prophylaxis.

Figure 18.1 Guidelines for prophylaxis and treatment regimens (from ref. 9).

reduction in early-onset neonatal GBS disease incidence in the year following the issuing of these new guidelines.[10]

For maternal infection, penicillin G is the drug of choice; this is usually administered at 5 million units intravenously initially, followed by 2.5 million units intravenously every 4–6h (see Fig. 18.2). For GBS prophylaxis intrapartum, the dosing interval should be 4h. In cases of shortage, as has been seen recently in the United States, ampicillin is a suitable alternative at 2g intravenously initially followed by 1g intravenously every 4–6h; again, note that intrapartum GBS prophylaxis necessitates dosing every 4h until delivery.

In the case of chorioamnionitis, a polymicrobial condition, it is prudent to use broad-spectrum coverage that includes treatment for GBS and common Gram-negative organisms such as *E. coli*. Such an intrapartum regimen might be ampicillin (2g i.v. every 6h) along with gentamicin (1.5mg/kg i.v. every 8h). Treatment should be initiated as soon as the diagnosis is made, as intrapartum therapy will treat the fetus and reduce neonatal sepsis.[11]

Postpartum endometritis is similarly a polymicrobial infection and deserves broad-spectrum treatment, preferably with i.v. antibiotics. Coverage should include anaerobic organisms and, hence, a triple antibiotic regimen of ampicillin, clindamycin, and gentamicin is commonly used.

For neonates suspected of having GBS sepsis, empiric treatment is initiated with i.v. ampicillin and i.v. aminoglycoside to provide coverage similar to that offered in the treatment of chorioamnionitis. If there is bacteremia without meningitis, the treatment is extended to 48–72h. In the case of GBS as the sole isolate, then i.v. penicillin G is administered to complete a 10-day course of antibiotics. In the case of meningitis, i.v. ampicillin and gentamicin are administered until cerebrospinal fluid is sterile; i.v. penicillin G is continued to complete a 14-day course of antibiotic treatment.

Recommended	Penicillin G, 5 million units i.v. initial dose, then 2.5 million units i.v. every 4h until delivery
Alternative	Ampicillin, 2g i.v. initial dose, then 1g i.v. every 4h until delivery
If penicillin allergic†	
Parients not at high risk for anaphylaxis	Cefazolin, 2g i.v. initial dose, then 1g i.v. every 8h until delivery
Patients at high risk for anaphylaxis§	
GBS susceptible to clindamycin and erythromycin ¶	Clindamycin, 900mg i.v. every 8h until delivery
	OR
	Erythromycin, 500mg i.v. every 6h until delivery
GBS resistant to clindamycin or erythromycin or susceptibility unknown	Vancomycin.** 1g i.v. every 12h until delivery

† History of penicillin allergy should be assessed to determine whether a high risk for anaphylaxis is present. Penicillin-allergic patients at high risk for anaphylaxis are those who have experienced immediate hypersensitivity to penicillin including a history of penicillin-related anaphylaxis; other high-risk patients are those with asthma or other diseases that would make anaphylaxis more dangerous or difficult to treat, such as persons being treated with beta-adrenergic-blocking agents.

§ If laboratory facilities are adequate, clindamycin and erythromycin susceptibility testing should be performed on prenatal GBS isolates from penicillin-allergic women at high risk for anaphylaxis.

¶ Resistance to erythromycin is often but not always associated with clindamycin resistance. If a strain is resistant to erythromycin but appears susceptible to clindamycin, it may still have inducible resistance to clindamycin.

** Cefazolin is preferred over vancomycin for women with a history of penicillin allergy other than immediate bypersensitivity reactions, and pharmacologic data suggest it achieves effective intra-amniotic concentrations. Vancomycin should be reserved for penicillin-allergic women at high risk for anaphylaxis.

Figure 18.2 Recommended regimens for intrapartum antimicrobial prophylaxis for perinatal group B streptococci disease prevention (from ref. 9). Broader-spectrum agents, including an agent active against GBS, may be necessary for treatment of chorioamnionitis.

Toxoplasmosis

The organism responsible for toxoplasmosis is *Toxoplasma gondii*, an obligate intracellular protozoan parasite that exhibits a complex life cycle. It exists in three forms: trophozoite (or tachyzoite), cyst, and oocyst. Trophozoites are the proliferative and invasive forms, whereas cysts are the latent forms, persisting in tissue for the lifetime of the host. Oocysts are found in cats that have ingested rodents infected with cysts. Humans become infected if they eat uncooked or undercooked fresh (never frozen) meat from infected animals. Human infection may also occur with hand-to-mouth contact with oocysts excreted in cat feces, most commonly due to poor handling of cat litter. Inhalation of aerosolized oocysts is another possible mechanism for infection. Parasitemia in a pregnant woman with acute toxoplasmosis may result in transplacental migration of the parasites, with subsequent fetal infection.

Epidemiology

The prevalence of toxoplasmosis varies throughout the world, and is dependent upon the geographic location and age of the population under consideration. Hot, arid climates are associated with low prevalence; in the United States and Europe, the prevalence, based on serologic status, increases with age and exposure. Infection during pregnancy also varies by geography; acute antenatal infection occurs in 10 in 1000 pregnancies in France,[12] whereas it occurs in only 1.1 in 1000 pregnancies in the United States.[13] The incidence of congenital infection is between 1 in 10 000 to 10 in 10 000 live births in the United States, or approximately 400–4000 births per year.[14] It is believed that half of these congenital infections are due to the consumption of contaminated meat.[14]

Fetal infection only occurs with acute maternal toxoplasmosis. The likelihood of transmission and the severity of risk to the fetus vary with gestational age. Congenital toxoplasmosis is more frequent, but usually less apparent, when maternal infection occurs in later gestations. In France, Desmonts and Couvreur[15] found that 17% of first-trimester pregnancies with acute maternal toxoplasmosis, 24% of the second-trimester pregnancies, and 62% of the third-trimester pregnancies resulted in infected infants at a time before treatment was available. However, severe infections or stillbirths occurred in 75% of the cases in the first trimester, 20% in the second trimester, and 0% in the third trimester.

Clinical manifestations

Maternal

An immunocompetent adult with acute toxoplasmosis is often only minimally symptomatic or completely asymptomatic. When the disease is clinically apparent, symptoms similar to infectious mononucleosis, including malaise, myalgias, sore throat, and fever, may be present. Painful, but nonsuppurative, lymph node enlargement, most commonly involving the posterior cervical lymph nodes, is a frequent finding in acute toxoplasmosis. Other associated findings include maculopapular rash, hepatosplenomegaly, and lymphocytosis. Ocular symptoms such as blurred vision, photophobia, and eye pain may be present with chronic disease. In the immunocompromised patient, severe disease with pulmonary and central nervous system involvement can be seen.

Fetal

Some investigators have reported an increased incidence of spontaneous abortion and preterm delivery in acute primary toxoplasmosis.[16,17] Clinical manifestations that may prompt suspicion of infection include intrauterine growth restriction, nonimmune hydrops, hydrocephaly, microcephaly, anencephaly, and hydrancephaly.[18,19] Ultrasound often fails to identify fetuses affected *in utero*. If ultrasonographic findings are present, they may include intracranial calcifications, ventricular dilation, hepatic enlargement, ascites, and increased placental thickness.[20]

Neonatal

The most common finding is a normal infant. In fact, more than half of infants with congenital toxoplasmosis have no signs or symptoms in the newborn period. Chorioretinitis is the most common abnormal finding. The classic triad of periventricular calcifications, chorioretinitis, and hydrocephaly is actually uncommon. Other findings can include growth restriction, low birthweight, hydrocephalus, microcephaly, intracranial calcifications, jaundice, hepatosplenomegaly, cataracts, microphthalmia, strabismus, blindness, epilepsy, psychomotor or mental retardation, petechia secondary to thrombocytopenia, anemia, maculopapular rash, pneumonia, vomiting, and diarrhea.[20] Serious long-term complications include mental retardation, severe visual deficits, and seizures. Adverse sequelae have been detected in long-term follow-up of infants with subclinical infection at birth.[19]

Diagnosis

Detection can be achieved via direct and indirect methods. Indirect techniques should be used in immunocompetent patients, as these methods rely upon serologic analysis, specifically the detection of organism-specific IgG and IgM antibodies. Direct detection is with PCR, hybridization, isolation, and histology, and is largely reserved for diagnosis in immunocompromised individuals.

Detection of IgG and IgM antibodies should be performed in pregnant women who are suspected of having had toxoplasmosis exposure. IgM can appear as early as 1 week after an acute infection, increases rapidly, and then wanes, persisting for several weeks to months; in rare circumstances, IgM may even persist for years. IgG does not appear until several weeks after the IgM increase, but low titers usually persist for years. Traditionally, the Sabin–Feldman dye test, indirect fluorescent assays, indirect hemagglutination assays, and complement fixation tests have been used. More recently, enzyme-linked immunosorbent assay (ELISA), IgG avidity test, and agglutination and differential agglutination tests have been used for the detection of IgG antibodies.[20] Most laboratories no longer use the Sabin–Feldman dye test. Avidity, i.e., functional affinity, testing of IgG antibodies is now routinely performed to help to distinguish acute from chronic infection. High-avidity antibodies are not seen in cases of infections acquired in the most recent 3–4 months. The differential agglutination (AC/HS) test is useful in distinguishing between a probable acute or chronic infection in pregnant women.

The presence of *Toxoplasma*-specific IgG would indicate protection from further infection. The presence of a high *Toxoplasma* IgG titer with the presence of IgM is suggestive of a recent infection, especially if the IgM titer is high, but it must be remembered that IgM may persist for months or even years in some instances following acute infection. A negative IgM test, if found within the first 24 weeks of gestation, especially if associated with low titers of IgG, essentially rules out an acute infection during gestation and points to a chronic infection antedating conception. However, a negative IgM titer in the third trimester does not negate the possibility of an acute infection in the first trimester with a subsequent decline. In this circumstance, additional testing, such as IgG avidity testing as explained above, can be helpful. Finally, women who test positive for IgM antibody in a nonreference laboratory should always undergo confirmatory testing in a reference laboratory, as 60% of these women are actually found to be chronically infected.[21]

Prenatal diagnosis of congenital toxoplasmosis is possible. Initially, ultrasound, cordocentesis, and amniocentesis were recommended. Serologic tests for specific IgM and IgG were performed on fetal blood, as were nonspecific tests, including white blood cell count and hepatic enzymes. Also, there was isolation of the organism by inoculation into mice.[22] However, IgM-specific antibodies may not be detected even in culture-proven cases because antibody synthesis may be delayed in the fetus and neonate. Isolation of parasites may also be unsuccessful because parasitemia may be intermittent, and the samples of fetal blood or amniotic fluid may be limited in quantity.[23] More recently, prenatal diagnosis using PCR technology on amniotic fluid obtained by amniocentesis has essentially eliminated the need for periumbilical fetal blood sampling or serologic testing of amniotic or fetal specimens as this approach has greater sensitivity and is simpler. Sensitivity for PCR analysis of amniotic fluid depends on gestational age, but overall has a rate of 64% (and in some studies has been noted to be as high as 98.8%), with a specificity of 100%, a PPV of 100%, and a NPV of 87.8%.[20, 21]

Treatment and prevention

In some European countries, large-scale seroscreening and specific therapy are used to prevent congenital toxoplasmosis. The efficacy of medication is approximately 50% in reducing congenital infection. If acute maternal toxoplasmosis is contracted between 2 and 10 weeks' gestation or if there are major lesions documented by ultrasound, the option of termination should be discussed. The combination of pyrimethamine (a folic acid antagonist) and sulfa drugs (sulfadiazine or triple sulfonamides) is the only effective medication generally available in the United States. Folinic acid should be used with pyrimethamine to minimize its potential side-effects of bone marrow suppression and pancytopenia. Spiramycin, a macrolide antibiotic, is used extensively in Europe, but is available for use in the United States only through the CDC. Spiramycin reduces the rate of fetal infection, but not the severity of infection. In Western Europe, spiramycin is used from diagnosis to delivery, and pyrimethamine plus sulfadiazine are used to protect against progressive fetopathy.

The primary method of prevention of congenital toxoplasmosis is the application of certain hygienic measures.[24] The pregnant woman should be advised to wash her hands thoroughly after contact with raw meat, cats, and materials potentially contaminated by cat feces. She should also eat meat only when it has been cooked to more than 66°C (about 151°F). The brown color of well-done meat is due to myoglobin turning to metmyoglobin at this temperature, which is also the temperature at which the cysts are rendered noninfectious. It is too early to tell whether a primary prevention program will significantly reduce the incidence of acquired toxoplasmosis. A prospectively evaluated prevention program reduced the rate of seroconversion by 34%, but this was not statistically significant.[25]

Mandatory serologic screening for toxoplasmosis during pregnancy is required by law in France and Austria, and has been advocated as a means of improving treatment and prenatal diagnosis in the United States.[26] Because of the low prevalence of disease in the United States, the high cost of a systematic screening program, and concern about the reliability of serologic testing, routine toxoplasmosis testing is still not widely recommended in the US.

Another approach is simply to screen infants and treat them when there is serologic infection. In New England, this approach identified 52 infected infants among approximately 600 000 newborns. After 1 year of treatment, only one child in 46 had a neurologic deficit, and 4 of 39 had eye lesions. Thus, neonatal screening and early treatment may reduce serious infections.[27]

Rubella

Rubella, or German measles, is caused by a single-stranded RNA virus that is a member of the togaviridae. There are two major genotypes, with European, North American, and Japanese isolates differing from some found in India and China. Given the stability of the viral genome, and the protective effect of IgG antibody, the humoral-mediated response confers immunity against future reinfection. The success of vaccination against rubella, and the subsequent decline of congenital rubella infection (CRI), stands as one of the major achievements of twentieth-century perinatal and neonatal medicine.

Epidemiology

The epidemiology of rubella infection was altered by the introduction of the vaccine in 1969. Before this, immunity to rubella through primary infection was acquired by 85% of the population by adolescence. The highest incidence was in the group aged 5–9 years, accounting for 38.5% of cases from 1966 to 1968. The incidence of rubella has declined by 99% from 57 686 cases in 1969 to 271 cases in 1999 (CDC, unpublished data, 2000, available at www.CDC.gov). The age distribution of rubella infection changed during the mid-1990s, with those aged 15 years or older now accounting for the majority of cases, whereas this was the opposite in the early 1990s. By 1999, 86% of cases occurred in adults and, since 1992, outbreaks have occurred among young adults from specific groups such as Hispanics and Asians and Pacific Islanders as well as individuals who have immigrated from countries such as Mexico. Seventy-three percent of rubella cases in 1999 occurred in Hispanics, with the majority of patients having been foreign born.[28] Despite widespread immunization programs, 10–20% of the United States population is susceptible to rubella.[29] After the initial decrease in the incidence of congenital rubella syndrome (CRS), the incidence has plateaued at approximately 0.05 cases per 100 000 live births for the past 10 years because of continued rubella infection in women of childbearing age. Similar to the distribution of rubella infection in adults, during 1997–1999 in the United States, 81% of infants reported to have CRI were Hispanic, with 92% of their mothers having been foreign born (CDC, unpublished data, 2000).

Before the implementation of large-scale vaccination policies in the United States, epidemics of rubella occurred every 6–9 years. The last epidemic before the introduction of the vaccine was in 1964. It is estimated that more than 20 000 cases of CRS and 11 000 pregnancy losses occurred as a result of this epidemic. The vaccine was originally targeted at young children, but this had little effect on attack rates in the group aged over 15 years. Now efforts are also made to vaccinate susceptible adults,[29] but opportunities to do so are missed, including in the postpartum period. According to data from CRS surveillance, almost half of mothers of CRS infants have had a previous live birth. All these cases of CRS could presumably have been prevented by postpartum vaccination after the birth of the first child.[29]

Transmission

Rubella virus is spread by respiratory droplets. This requires prolonged, close exposure. The virus is present in the nasopharynx and spreads via the lymphatics and then blood. It is less communicable than varicella, with an 80% attack rate. Fetal infection requires maternal viremia and placental transmission. Viremia has been thought to occur only with primary infection. Rare cases of reinfection leading to CRS have been reported.[30] Serologic evidence of fetal exposure to rubella has been documented after inadvertent vaccination in pregnancy. To date, no cases of congenital defects secondary to CRS have been reported due to vaccine.[31,32] Nevertheless, vaccine administration is contraindicated in pregnancy because the theoretical risk of CRS after vaccination, although low, may not be zero.[33] Virus is shed in breast milk as well. Neonatal exposure to rubella during breastfeeding has not been associated with morbidity.[34] Prolonged viral shedding from the CRS infant may be a source of infection. Virus has been isolated in the urine, cerebrospinal fluid, and even the lens of CRS patients.

The variable risk of CRS at different gestational ages has long been recognized. Rubella infection before implantation has been implicated in spontaneous abortion, stillbirth, neonatal death, and CRS. Enders and co-workers[35] reported that rubella occurring from 12 days to 12 weeks after the last menstrual period (LMP) resulted in an 81–90% fetal infection rate. No infection was noted if the rash appeared before the LMP or up to 11 days after the LMP. Cradock-Watson and Ridehalgh[36] reviewed rates of rubella infection after the first trimester. The overall rate of CRI (seropositivity, with or without clinical disease) was 29% based on rubella-specific IgM and 49% based on persistence of rubella-specific IgG after 8 months of age. Gestational age-specific rates of CRI ranged from 12% when infection occurred at 24–28 weeks to 58% at 36–40 weeks.

Clinical manifestations

Maternal

Postnatally acquired rubella is a mild or asymptomatic infection. The incubation period is 14–21 days, with viral shedding beginning 1 week before the onset of rash. The rash is macular and lasts 3 days, hence the name 3-day measles. Malaise, fever, and postauricular and suboccipital adenopathy are also common. Arthralgias are common in adult women; arthritis, neuritis, encephalitis, and thrombocytopenia are rare in postnatal infection. Because these symptoms are nonspecific, diagnosis should be made on serologic rather than clinical grounds.[37]

Fetal and neonatal

The pathogenesis of congenital defects includes impairment in organogenesis due to decreased mitosis and damage secondary to scarring and persistent infection.[38] Abnormalities resulting from impaired organogenesis occur with maternal infection in the first trimester. Other abnormalities, such as progressive hearing loss and pulmonic or aortic stenosis, are due to ongoing damage caused by persistent infection and immune response. In addition, first-trimester rubella infection is believed to cause abortion. This was difficult to confirm during the 1964 epidemic because of the small numbers of women who were both exposed in the first trimester and registered early in pregnancy. Current surveillance practices do not provide information on the incidence of pregnancy loss.[29]

Congenital infection may be divided into three categories based on its manifestations: CRS, extended CRS, and delayed CRS. Newborn rubella, or CRS, and extended CRS are apparent at birth. Delayed manifestations of congenital infection may not be apparent for years or decades.

Four major defects in CRS, in order of decreasing frequency, are deafness, mental retardation, heart lesions, and ophthalmologic abnormalities. Types of malformation are gestational-age specific. Cataracts and cardiac lesions are present when infection occurs before 8 weeks. Deafness occurs with infection before 16 weeks, and retinopathy with infection before

130 days. Timing of fetal exposure is at best estimated because of difficulties in dating gestational age and lack of information regarding the incubation period of fetal rubella infection. Sever and associates,[38] in the Collaborative Perinatal Research Study (CPRS) of 1964, reported that deafness was the most common single defect and was present in 100% of infants with multiple defects resulting from first-trimester infection. Conversely, eye defects, with cataracts and glaucoma being most frequent, were present only with other abnormalities. Cardiac lesions include ventricular septal defect, patent ductus arteriosus, and peripheral pulmonic stenosis. Thrombocytopenic purpura (blueberry muffin rash), hepatosplenomegaly, osseous lesions, meningoencephalitis, and rubelliform rash may also be present in CRS. Contrary to the previously held perception that second- and third-trimester rubella infections are without clinical consequence in the fetus, abnormalities (including developmental delay, hearing loss, growth retardation, pulmonic stenosis, and thrombocytopenia) have been found in 15 out of 24 infants exposed to rubella at between 14 and 31 weeks' gestation.[39]

The spectrum of extended CRS includes cerebral palsy, mental retardation, developmental and language delay, seizures, cirrhosis, growth retardation, and immunologic disorders (e.g., hypogammaglobulinemia). Delayed manifestations of CRI include endocrinopathies, late-onset deafness and ocular damage, renovascular hypertension, and encephalitis. Long-term follow-up of CRS patients revealed a 20% incidence of diabetes mellitus by the age of 35 years.[38] Other endocrinopathies include thyroid dysfunction and growth hormone deficiency. Deafness and ocular and vascular damage may be due to ongoing infection with scarring and inflammation.

Delayed manifestations of CRS are thought to be due to circulating immune complexes.[40,41] Delayed manifestations occur in more than 20% of those with initially symptomatic CRS.[38] The incidence of delayed defects in those with asymptomatic CRI and their gestational age-related risk are not clear. Data from the CPRS showed delayed effects in almost two-thirds of those infected in the third trimester.[42] Although major malformations due to infection in the first trimester may be devastating, the adverse effects from later infection are clearly not minor.

Progressive panencephalitis has been likened to subacute sclerosing panencephalitis due to rubeola infection and is a different entity from the encephalitis present at birth. Hypogammaglobulinemia may be a delayed result of CRI; altered cell-mediated immunity is necessary for continued latent viral infection. Because of altered cell-mediated immunity, the rubella virus persists in the congenitally infected person for up to a year, and perhaps longer.[37]

Diagnosis

Clinical diagnosis of postnatal infection is unreliable and must be confirmed by serology. Before the availability of serologic tests of rubella infection and immunity, virus isolation was attempted. The rubella virus is difficult to isolate. Serologic evidence of maternal primary infection includes the presence of rubella-specific IgM, which can persist for 8–12 weeks following acute infection. In the past, the presence of a fourfold increase in hemagglutination inhibition titer on acute and convalescent sera also provided evidence of a primary infection; commercially available enzyme immunoassays for rubella IgM and IgG are now routinely performed by most laboratories.[43] Indirect antibody assays are more prone to false-positive IgM results, due in part to crossreactivity with other IgM antibodies or with rheumatoid factor; hence, a second confirmatory test for rubella IgM by a different modality should be performed, especially before 20 weeks' gestation.

Prenatal diagnosis of CRI is possible. The presence of rubella-specific IgM in fetal blood confirms infection. Fetal immunocompetence is attained in the mid-second trimester; therefore, to avoid a false-negative result, fetal blood sampling to detect IgM must be delayed until 20–22 weeks' gestation.[42,44,45] First-trimester confirmation of fetal infection was described by Terry and colleagues[46] by detecting virus-specific antigen and RNA in a chorionic villus sample. This method is superior to virus isolation in the products of conception.[47] Nevertheless, the presence of rubella virus in the placenta may not correlate with fetal infection. More recently, the development of PCR technology has the potential of rendering fetal blood sampling virtually unnecessary. With reverse transcriptase PCR (RT PCR), amniotic fluid obtained via amniocentesis (when performed at least 8 weeks after acute maternal infection or at 15 weeks of gestation) can be evaluated for virus-specific RNA; this has a sensitivity of 87–100%.[43] However, cases have been reported of finding rubella RNA and IgM in fetal blood following negative PCR analysis of amniotic fluid at 19 and 23 weeks.

Prevention and treatment

Prevention of *in utero* rubella infection requires the acquisition of immunity by all persons before the childbearing years. Programs to ensure vaccination of all schoolchildren, susceptible college students, and military personnel help, but do not eradicate CRI. Missed opportunities for vaccination of adults still occur and contribute to the continued existence of CRS.[48] Congenitally infected neonates are also a source of virus. The rubella vaccine is a live-attenuated virus that yields immune responses similar to native infection; the rate of seroconversion is as high as 95% in individuals older than 11 months of age.[43] Long-term efficacy exceeds 90%, but antibody titers can decline over time. As mentioned previously, administration of the vaccine is contraindicated in pregnancy as there is a theoretical risk of acquiring CRS, although there have never been such cases documented worldwide.

There is no specific antiviral therapy for rubella infection. If *in utero* exposure to rubella virus is documented, the woman should be counseled as to the risks and consequences of CRI.

Prenatal diagnosis, even in the first trimester, is possible. With the potentially devastating effects of first-trimester infection, a patient may choose to terminate the affected pregnancy if the diagnosis is made in a timely manner.

Herpes simplex virus

Herpes simplex virus (HSV) is a double-stranded DNA virus, primarily of two subtypes (1 and 2), that is responsible for a variety of infections involving mucocutaneous surfaces, the central nervous system (CNS), and visceral organs. Taking up residence in sensory neuronal ganglia, genital HSV infection is a recurrent, lifelong infection.

Systemic symptoms are more common in primary occurrences, and can include fever, malaise, myalgia, and headache. Local symptoms include pain, discharge, adenopathy, dysuria, and urinary retention secondary to pain or local nerve involvement. Painful vesicles, which may emerge 2–10 days following primary exposure, ulcerate and heal without scarring. Viral shedding persists until the lesions heal. Cervical shedding is present with primary infection in more than 80% of patients and in up to 30% of recurrences. Asymptomatic shedding occurs in 0.35–1.4% of pregnancies.[49]

Genital HSV infection can lead to a number of complications that can profoundly affect the developing fetus and/or the neonate. Perinatal transmission has been linked with spontaneous abortion, preterm labor, and congenital malformations.[50] Anomalies linked to HSV are similar to those seen with congenital cytomegalovirus (CMV) infection: microcephaly, periventricular calcifications, chorioretinitis, intrauterine growth restriction, and vesicular eruptions.[51] While evidence for the teratogenic potential of HSV is circumstantial, neonatal disease can be devastating. This can range from infection of the skin, eyes and mouth, which, though rarely fatal, can lead to neurologic impairment in 30% of affected children, to CNS infection (symptoms include seizures, poor feeding, and irritability; mortality is more than 50% if untreated), and disseminated infection, which is often complicated by encephalitis and can be fatal in over 80% of cases if left untreated, with neurologic impairment in nearly all survivors.[49]

Epidemiology

HSV infection is ubiquitous. Among HSV infections, genital herpes is widely prevalent, affecting at least 50 million Americans. Seropositivity to type 1 HSV (HSV-1) is acquired by a majority of people by the age of 7 years. The incidence of seropositivity to HSV-2 varies with age, sexual habits, and economic status.[52] HSV-1 is the serotype most often found in oral lesions, while HSV-2 causes most lesions below the waist. Eighty-five percent of adult genital HSV is due to HSV-2. From 1988 to 1994, overall adult prevalence of HSV-2 infection was 21.9%, and it was slightly higher at 25.6% among females.[53] The prevalence of HSV-2 infections in the US is rising, with approximately 1.6 million new infections acquired annually.[54] Among adults, 5–10% have a history of symptomatic genital HSV-2 infection. However, another 20–30% who have never had symptomatic genital infection demonstrate type-specific antibodies against glycoprotein G (gG) of the HSV-2 virion. Thus, because HSV-2 infections rarely cause ulcerative lesions, most HSV-2-seropositive individuals are unaware of their exposure. Clearly then, much must be done toward prevention.

There are three primary types of genital herpes syndromes. Primary infection occurs with initial infection with either HSV-1 or -2 and without prior exposure to either. Recurrent infection is due to reactivation of latent virus, and is therefore not a reinfection. Finally, nonprimary first-episode genital herpes occurs when a patient has had a prior exposure to the other viral serotype.

Transmission

Transmission of genital HSV requires intimate contact of infectious secretions with susceptible mucous membranes or skin. Mechanical friction provides for more efficient transfer.[55] Unfortunately, clinical history does not provide reliable information regarding the likelihood of sexual transmission.[56] Although analysis of the survival characteristics of the herpes simplex virion in water and on plastic surfaces supports the possibility of fomite transfer, there are no documented cases of such transmission.[55] Essentially all cases of genital herpes are spread via sexual contact; genital HSV-1 is usually due to oral–genital contact.[57]

Transmission to the fetus or neonate can occur antenatally, intrapartum, or postnatally. In the US, neonatal transmission occurs in 1 in 3200 to 1 in 15000 live births. The highest risk is at the time of delivery, responsible for 85% of all neonatal herpes cases.[49] Intrauterine infection, resulting mainly from transplacental passage or ascension via the cervix, accounts for 5–8% of cases. Intrapartum transmission is not necessarily dependent upon maternal symptoms, but rather upon maternal viral shedding, especially when that shedding occurs in the context of first-episode genital herpes as opposed to reactivation disease. The risk of intrapartum transmission with a vaginal delivery in HSV-2-seropositive, asymptomatic women is 0.02%, with symptomatic recurrence it is 1–3%, and with asymptomatic seroconversion, i.e., with primary infection, or with nonprimary first episode near the time of delivery it is 40%.

Diagnosis

Diagnosis can be made by viral culture, Pap smear, monoclonal antibody testing, ELISA, or PCR. Cultures are widely used in persons with ulcers, but sensitivity declines within a few days of ulcer occurrence. PCR testing is highly sensitive. Pap smear findings indicating disease are usually incidental, and should not serve as a primary diagnostic modality.

Monoclonal antibody and ELISA testing have limited sensitivity in the absence of lesions and do not allow for the distinguishing of HSV type. Serologic diagnosis with Western blotting of gG can identify types 1 and 2. Food and Drug Administration (FDA)-approved commercially available gG-based type-specific assays for HSV have sensitivities ranging from 80% to 98%, with specificity ≥ 96%.

Prevention

While adult genital HSV is problematic, transmission to the fetus or neonate can be far more tragic. Prevention of transmission to the fetus, and especially the neonate, is an important goal. Efforts toward this goal include recognition of lesions, elective Cesarean delivery, suppression of viral shedding during the peripartum period, and maintenance of neonatal skin integrity.

In the largest prospective study of its kind, Brown et al.[58] looked at over 58 000 women in the state of Washington who underwent collection of genital secretions for HSV culture at the time of their presentation in labor. None of these women received or were receiving suppressive viral therapy. Of these women, 202 had HSV-positive cultures. Fifty-eight percent of these women were delivered vaginally, and 42% were delivered via Cesarean section, with 71% of the latter having recognized genital lesions as the indication for surgical delivery. Although not quite reaching statistical significance, the odds ratio (OR) for neonatal HSV infection was 0.14 (95% CI, 0.02–1.08), tending towards favoring Cesarean delivery. Based on previous studies, and the lack of a randomized, prospective, controlled trial to evaluate Cesarean delivery versus vaginal delivery even in the case of active genital lesions, the American College of Obstetricians and Gynecologists, in a 1999 Practice Bulletin, recommended Cesarean delivery in women "with active genital lesions or symptoms of vulvar pain or burning, which may indicate an impending outbreak," but did not recommend such a delivery modality in cases of recurrent disease with lesions distant from the perineum (such as the buttocks or the thigh).

Brown et al.[58] also found a statistically significant increase of nearly sevenfold for the development of neonatal HSV with the use of invasive fetal monitoring intrapartum. It is recommended that these monitors be avoided if possible, as should rupture of the membranes more than 4–6 h prior to delivery. Based on this finding, forceps and vacuum-assisted delivery should also be minimized. All these recommendations should of course be mitigated by concerns for fetal safety, and thus decisions should be made that are appropriate for the clinical situation at hand.

Oral suppressive therapy with the antiviral agent acyclovir in primary infection has been shown to decrease duration of shedding, pain, new lesion formation, and time to complete healing.[59] Duration of shedding may be decreased by 80%. Oral acyclovir is also effective in suppressing recurrences with long-term use.[60] Furthermore, among 601 acyclovir-exposed pregnancies (425 in the first trimester), there was no notable increase in the rate of birth defects compared with background, and there was no notable pattern of anomalies.[61] In a systematic review of acyclovir prophylaxis administered in five different trials that included women with first-episode disease, recurrent disease, and all HSV disease, Sheffield et al.[62] were able to demonstrate that prophylactic use of acyclovir starting at 36 weeks' gestation reduced the rate of clinical recurrence at delivery (OR 0.25; 95% CI 0.15–0.40), the rate of Cesarean delivery for HSV (OR 0.3; 95% CI 0.13–0.67), the overall Cesarean delivery rate (OR 0.61; 95% CI 0.43–0.86), and the rate of asymptomatic HSV shedding (OR 0.09; 95% CI 0.02–0.39). Thus, acyclovir (or, alternatively, famcyclovir or valacyclovir) suppressive therapy starting at 36 weeks' gestation should be considered in genital HSV patients, especially those with first-episode disease occurring during pregnancy, as there may not be adequate time for the generation of homologous maternal IgG antibodies that seem to protect the neonate from congenital acquisition of disease.

Cytomegalovirus

Human cytomegalovirus (CMV), otherwise known as human herpes virus 5 (HHV-5), is an enveloped double-stranded DNA virus and a member of the Herpesviridae family. CMV-specific IgG and IgM antibodies may be detectable several weeks after infection. Many different strains of CMV have been identified by restriction endonuclease analysis. Owing to its ubiquity, CMV is the most common viral cause of intrauterine and congenital infection as well as of sensorineural deafness.[45] Unfortunately, CMV can be spread to the fetus with either primary infection or reactivation disease and, in most instances, with the mother remaining asymptomatic.

Epidemiology

An estimated 0.2–2.2% of all neonates are infected *in utero*, with only 5–10% of these infants symptomatic at birth.[63] Affecting approximately 1 in 40 000 liveborn infants in the United States annually, CMV causes 30 000–40 000 cases of congenital infection every year.[64,65] Primary CMV infection occurs in 1–2% of pregnant women;[66] it is estimated that about 50% of reproductive-age women are susceptible to CMV infection. The rate of seropositivity, the risk of congenital infection, and the incidence of recurrent infection are greater in women of lower socioeconomic status. CMV infection is spread through infected secretions or body fluids such as endocervical mucus, semen, blood, urine, saliva, breast milk, and tears. High-risk environments for exposure to CMV include childcare centers, newborn nurseries, renal dialysis units, and areas of hospitals providing care for immunocompromised individuals.

Transmission

Fetal infection can occur with both primary and recurrent maternal infection; however, the likelihood and severity of congenital disease is greater with a primary infection.[67,68] Transmission to the fetus occurs in approximately 20–50% of pregnancies with primary maternal CMV infection.[65,69] Congenital infection can occur as a result of recurrent maternal infection, but the risk is less (approximately 1% detected in the newborn period and up to 8% if followed for 5 years) and the manifestations milder (mainly hearing loss). Transmission can occur at any time during pregnancy, with the lowest risk of transmission associated with primary CMV acquired periconceptionally, and an equal risk of transmission in the first and second trimesters; the third trimester poses the greatest risk of vertical transmission. However, there is evidence to indicate that fetuses that acquire infection earlier in gestation are at higher risk for worse outcomes compared with infection acquired later in gestation.[68] Studies indicate that recurrent infections and transmission to the fetus in immune women are more frequently due to reactivation than to reinfection.[70]

Clinical manifestations

Maternal

CMV infection in the immunocompetent mother is usually asymptomatic. In some patients, a heterophile-negative mononucleosis-like syndrome may be present. Fever, malaise, myalgias, mild pharyngitis, minimal lymphadenopathy, lymphocytosis, and abnormal liver function test results may be present in such cases.

Fetal

Major target organ systems include the hematopoietic and central nervous systems and general development. Characteristics of fetal infection that may aid in prenatal diagnosis include intrauterine growth retardation, cerebral ventriculomegaly, ascites, microcephaly, hydrocephaly, periventricular calcifications, hepatosplenomegaly, cardiomegaly, hyperechogenic bowel, and oligo- or polyhydramnios. CMV may cause nonimmune hydrops. CMV has also been implicated in myocarditis; there have been reports of fetal heart block and of fetal supraventricular tachycardia.[71–73] Ultrasound visualization of periventricular calcifications due to CMV has been reported, even in the second trimester.[74]

Neonatal

Approximately 10% of infants with congenital infection are symptomatic at birth. From the CDC registry, the most common clinical findings of congenital infection are hematologic (petechiae/purpura, 54%; hepatosplenomegaly, 40%; jaundice, 38%; hemolytic anemia, 11%), neurologic (intracranial calcifications, 37%; microcephaly, 36%; hearing impairment, 25%; chorioretinitis, 11%; seizures, 11%; one or more neurologic findings, 68%), small for gestational age (47%), pneumonia (8%), and death (9%).[75] Approximately 5–15% of the initially asymptomatic infants develop evidence of disease by 2 years of age, with sensorineural hearing deficits (5–10% of cases) and subsequent learning disabilities being the most important long-term sequelae.[64]

Diagnosis

The most definitive method of diagnosis of CMV infection is by isolation of the virus from the blood, urine, or cervix. Several years ago, virus was often not detectable in culture for 2–6 weeks, but with newer techniques the virus is now detectable usually within days. A number of serologic studies are available for the detection of antibody to CMV, including indirect hemagglutination assay, ELISA, immunofluorescent assay, neutralization tests, and complement fixation (CF). CF assays are often inaccurate because of a high false-positive rate due to crossreactivity with other herpesviruses. CMV-specific IgM antibody tests are helpful but of limited value because 30% of women with primary infections are initially seronegative, and the test result is positive in 10% of women with recurrent infections.[66] Acute and convalescent paired specimens demonstrating a significant increase in titer are suggestive of a primary infection.

When maternal primary infection is suspected, or there are findings on ultrasonography that are suspicious of congenital CMV infection, prenatal diagnosis can be carried out by amniocentesis or fetal blood sampling. Ideally, prenatal diagnosis should occur beyond 21 weeks' gestation, as this optimizes the sensitivity of diagnostic tests. PCR and/or viral culture of amniotic fluid can be performed to detect CMV. PCR, including nested PCR, has been shown to have a sensitivity of 77–100%, specificity of 67–99%, PPV of 100% and NPV of 93%.[76–78] Viral isolation has a sensitivity ranging from 50% to 72%, and a specificity of 97–100%.[79] PCR of amniotic fluid, when combined with viral isolation, has been shown to have a sensitivity of 84% and a specificity of 100%.[76]

Fetal blood can be tested for the presence of fetal IgM after 20 weeks' gestation, and has a sensitivity of 51–58% and a specificity of 100%.[77] The presence of cord blood CMV-specific IgM, which is detectable in 60% of infants with congenital infection, establishes the diagnosis.[67] It is possible to obtain false-negative IgM titers when cordocentesis is performed early in the course of fetal infection; IgM levels correlate positively with abnormal fetal ultrasound findings and hematologic test results. PCR analysis of fetal blood for the presence of CMV DNA has a sensitivity of 41%, whereas viral culture is only 7% sensitive. Additional tests include searching for the presence of viremia (i.e., infectious CMV in leukocytes; sensitivity of 0–55%), antigenemia (i.e., pp65-positive leukocytes; sensitivity 16–64%), and messenger RNA (sensitivity 82%).[68] On the whole, fetal blood sampling and amniotic fluid analysis has sensitivity, specificity, PPV and NPV of

80%, 99%, 98%, and 93% respectively.[78] As fetal blood sampling adds little additional value to amniotic fluid sampling, it should now be considered only for possible confirmatory testing of the fetus.

Treatment and prevention

No treatment other than symptomatic therapy is necessary for the immunocompetent adult with CMV infection. A variety of therapeutic agents – ganciclovir, adenosine arabinoside, acyclovir, idoxuridine, cytosine arabinoside, 5-fluoro-2′-deoxyuridine, leukocyte interferon, and transfer factor – have been administered for the treatment of congenital CMV infection, but none has been found to be satisfactory because of toxicity or recurrence of infection after drug administration is terminated. Currently, there is no role for antenatal treatment of fetal CMV infection.[77]

Vaccines have been investigated.[80] As the vast majority of congenital CMV infections occur in instances of maternal primary infection, a reasonable strategy is to vaccinate seronegative women prior to conception. Vaccine development has included investigations into live-attenuated vaccines, recombinant virus vaccines, subunit vaccines, DNA vaccines, and peptide vaccines.[77] None has been established as a superior method, and none has been adopted for routine use in humans.

Routine antepartum serologic screening for CMV is not recommended at this time. The detection of maternal CMV antibody before conception indicates prior infection, but the degree of protection that this immunity provides against congenital infection in subsequent pregnancies is unclear. The implications of a single antibody titer obtained during pregnancy are difficult to interpret. Even in a high-risk environment, the extent of risk for a seronegative pregnant woman by exposure is uncertain. One effective prevention strategy is the use of good handwashing, especially in high-risk settings such as daycare facilities or neonatal intensive care units.[81]

Parvovirus

Parvovirus B19, discovered in 1974, is the only member of the virus family Parvoviridae known to cause human pathology. B19, a ubiquitous single-stranded DNA virus with a predilection to infect erythroid precursor cells, causes variable disease dependent upon the immunologic and hematologic status of its host. In immunocompetent children, it is known to cause erythema infectiosum (Fifth disease or "slapped cheek syndrome"); in some individuals, especially adults, an acute symmetric polyarthropathy may develop.[82,83] Underlying hemolytic disorders predispose to the development of a transient aplastic crisis. Red cell aplasia and chronic anemia can result from persistent infection in the immunocompromised host. In the fetus, B19 infection can result in *in utero* demise, hydrops fetalis, and congenital anemia.

Clinical features

Erythema infectiosum is characterized by a facial rash commonly referred to as "slapped cheek" in appearance.[82] There is also a lace-like rash on the trunk and extremities. The rash may also reappear several weeks later, after exposure to temperature, sunlight, or emotional stress. Otherwise, the patient is well at the onset of the rash, but may have a history of mild systemic symptoms a few days before the rash's onset. Pruritus may be a common feature in some outbreaks. Erythema infectiosum is more common in the winter and spring and usually lasts approximately 5–9 days in children. Headache, fever, anorexia, sore throat, and gastrointestinal symptoms occur in a minority of children. Complications such as lymphadenopathy, arthralgia, or arthropathy rarely occur in children. As with other viral infections (such as rubella), erythema infectiosum tends to be more severe in adults. In adults, fatigue, fever, adenopathy, and arthritis are common. There have also been reports of more serious complications, such as encephalitis, pneumonia, and hemolytic anemia.

In investigations of outbreaks, asymptomatic infection has been reported in up to 20% of adults and children. B19 infection is also associated with a condition known as transient aplastic crisis with asymmetrical peripheral polyarthroplasty and with severe chronic anemia in patients who are immunodeficient.

Epidemiology

The major concern for the obstetrician is infection with B19 in pregnant women.[84–94] The incidence of primary B19 infection during pregnancy is approximately 1–5%, with transmission to the fetus occurring in 24–33% of cases. Thus, in most of the reported B19 infections during pregnancy, there has been no adverse outcome. The risk of developing hydrops fetalis in the case of congenital infection is approximately 1–1.6%, and B19 is estimated to cause 15–20% of all non-immune hydrops fetalis cases. The hepatic period of fetal hematopoeisis, 11–23 weeks of gestation, seems to be the most critical period of gestation that is prone to adverse fetal outcome; the fetus appears to be especially vulnerable to B19 infection because fetuses have a short blood cell survival time and the fetal red cell volume expands rapidly.[83]

Studies in both the United States and the United Kingdom have suggested that the risk of fetal death in a pregnant woman with documented B19 infection and an infected fetus is less than 10%.[95] The CDC estimates that the risk of fetal death after exposure of a pregnant woman to a household member with a documented infection is less than 2.5%, while the upper limit of the risk of fetal death would be less than 1.5% in a pregnant woman who has prolonged exposure to B19 infection in the workplace. Further, it is estimated that the upper limit of risk of fetal death occurring in pregnant women with other types of exposure (e.g., limited exposure to students with erythema infectiosum) would be substantially less. The mechanism of fetal death is undetermined, but it is likely that either severe anemia or direct myocarditis may precipitate congestive heart failure and hydrops. Once hydrops sets in, case fatality rates may be as high as 50% if untreated, but can improve to as low as 18% with fetal transfusions via cordocentesis.[83]

Transmission

DNA specific for B19 has been identified in the respiratory secretions of viremic patients, suggesting this as a major mode of spread. At the time that erythema infectiosum develops, however, patients are probably past the point of greatest infectiousness. After close contact exposure, the virus appears to be transmitted effectively; during school outbreaks, 10–60% of students develop erythema infectiosum. In the setting of outbreaks, it is not clear whether the major mode of transmission involves direct contact, person-to-person contact, or large particle droplets, small particle droplets, or fomites. It is also known that the virus can be transmitted parenterally through transfusion and vertically from mother to fetus.

Diagnosis

Diagnostic testing is available through commercial and reference laboratories such as the CDC.[85] B19 antibody assays are available, with the most sensitive test to detect recent infection being the IgM antibody assay. This can be performed by a captured antibody radioimmunoassay or by enzyme immunoassay. There is also an IgG B19 antibody assay that is usually positive by the seventh day of illness. IgG persists for years. The IgM antibody, on the other hand, begins to decline after 30–60 days. Prior to the advent of PCR technology, the most sensitive test for detecting the virus was B19 DNA nucleic acid hybridization.[83] Because DNA can persist for some time in serum, synovial membranes, and basement membranes, detection of low levels of B19 DNA is not sufficient to make the diagnosis of acute infection.

Treatment and prevention

Currently, no specific treatment is available to individuals with presumed B19 infection. They are treated with supportive measures. In otherwise healthy individuals, B19 infection usually produces a mild self-limited infection. Further, there is no vaccine to prevent B19 infection, and no studies have been conducted to assess the value of commercially available immunoglobulin. At this point, the CDC does not recommend routine prophylaxis with immunoglobulin. In healthcare settings where exposures to B19 may be possible through contact with patients with B19 infection (such as transient aplastic crisis), the CDC has recommended infection control measures such as admission to private rooms of patients with transient aplastic crisis due to chronic B19 infection. It is noteworthy that most patients with erythema infectiosum are past the period of infectiousness by the time that clinical symptoms develop, and these individuals do not present a risk for further transmission. Thus, isolation precautions are not necessary.[82]

Hospital personnel who may be pregnant should know about the potential risks to their fetus from exposure to B19 infection. In homes, school, and the workplace, the greatest risk of transmitting B19 occurs before the symptoms of erythema infectiosum develop. Therefore, transmission cannot truly be prevented by excluding contact with persons who have erythema infectiosum. The only measure that is currently recommended is handwashing.

In the past several years, the advancement of Doppler ultrasound technology has led to the development of monitoring of fetal middle cerebral artery peak systolic velocities (MCA PSV). Presumably, in the setting of fetal infection and subsequent anemia, the reduced blood viscosity leads to a greater cardiac output, and hence increased MCA PSV values. In a recent multicenter, prospective study evaluating weekly MCA PSV for the prediction of anemia in patients referred for acute maternal B19 infection based upon the presence of IgM antibody, sensitivity, specificity, PPV, and NPV, utilizing a cutoff of greater than 1.50 multiples of the median (MoM), were 94.1%, 93.3%, 94.1%, and 93.3% respectively.[95] In this study, no fetuses that had MCA PSV values less than 1.50 MoM had anemia at the time of birth, and none of these fetuses died; all cases of moderate to severe anemia were detected by the 1.50 MoM cutoff. The two fetal deaths were in the setting of hydrops.

This method of detecting clinically significant anemia has led to a drastic reduction in the number of diagnostic cordocenteses and is rapidly becoming the standard of care. Weekly ultrasound evaluation for up to 12 weeks following exposure is necessary to insure that the potentially affected fetus does not develop hydrops or elevated MCA PSV values that would indicate moderate to severe anemia. Surveillance frequency should be increased for MCA PSV > 1.50 MoM or for hydrops fetalis. Once there is clinically significant anemia, or overt fetal hydrops, intrauterine blood transfusions, sometimes weekly, are necessary for improving the chances of fetal survival. It has been estimated that, in the setting of hydrops, fetal transfusions increase survival rates from 15% to 30% when no intervention is attempted to 60–80%.

Varicella

Varicella zoster virus (VZV) is a member of the human herpesvirus group. VZV is a DNA virus that exhibits viral latency. Primary infection usually occurs in childhood, presenting clinically as chickenpox. As a highly contagious disorder, VZV infection is acquired by most children in the United States before reproductive age and is generally a self-limited disease characterized by typical skin lesions.[96] It is recognized that, when adults contract the disease, both constitutional and pulmonary symptoms may be severe. Reactivation of latent zoster infection presents clinically as shingles, generally occurring in the older population or in immunocompromised individuals. Zoster presents as painful crops of vesicular lesions occurring along the distribution of a segmental dermatome.

The remainder of this discussion is limited to the effects of VZV infection in pregnancy. There are two major concerns for the perinatologist. The first is the risk that the infection imposes upon the mother; the second is the risk of either teratogenesis in or perinatal acquisition by the fetus or neonate.

Epidemiology

More than 50 000 cases of chickenpox occur annually in the United States.[97] Yet, because of widespread under-reporting, it is estimated that the actual number of cases is 2–3 million.[98,99] More than 90% of the population has been infected during childhood. The incidence of VZV infection in pregnancy is estimated at approximately 5 in 10 000 pregnancies.

Diagnosis

Because the clinical presentation is usually characteristic, serology is not usually indicated to confirm the clinical diagnosis. In adults with a positive history of varicella, 97–99% are seropositive.[100] However, 71–93% of adults with negative or uncertain histories are also seropositive. Serologic testing is indicated in a pregnant woman with exposure but with a negative or uncertain history of varicella. Many methods are used including CF, indirect fluorescent antibody, fluorescent antibody to membrane antigen, radioimmunoassay, latex agglutination, and ELISA. These tests vary in sensitivity. CF is widely used, but is the least sensitive. Fluorescent antibody to membrane antigen is sensitive, but cumbersome. Commercial ELISA tests range in sensitivity from 86% to 97%.[100]

Clinical presentation

After an incubation period from 10 to 20 days (usually 13–17 days), fever and rash commonly occur simultaneously in children. In adults, fever and generalized malaise usually precede the rash by several days. The rash usually begins on the face and scalp and then spreads to the trunk. There is usually minimal involvement of the extremities. The skin lesions begin as macules and proceed to a vesicular and then a pustular stage. Healing is heralded by the presentation of crusts and scabs. The prominent feature of the disease is itching. Over a period of 2–5 days, new crops of lesions occur, and lesions in various stages of progression are usually present at the same time.

Bacterial infection of the skin is the common secondary complication of chickenpox.[96] Encephalitis, meningitis, myocarditis, glomerulonephritis, and arthritis are all rare complications in childhood. The most serious complication of varicella infection is pneumonia. It occurs more commonly in adults, but pneumonia does not appear to have an increased prevalence in pregnant women as opposed to other adults.[98,99,101] Currently, it is estimated that approximately 5–10% of adults with chickenpox develop pneumonia. In a review of the literature on varicella pneumonia in pregnancy, Young and Gershon[96] noted that, of 77 cases of chickenpox in pregnancy, 29% developed pneumonia. Because of selectivity, we estimate that this incidence of varicella pneumonia in pregnancy is high. Ten deaths occurred, all in women who had pneumonia. The mortality of varicella pneumonia in this series was 45%. There were no severe complications in women who did not develop pneumonia.[96]

For the clinician, the main objective is to maintain a high index of suspicion for pneumonia in women who have varicella infection in pregnancy. Pulmonary symptoms usually begin on the second to sixth day after the appearance of the rash, and usually present with mild nonproductive cough. If the disease is more severe, there may be additional symptoms, including hemoptysis, dyspnea, pleuritic chest pain, or progression to frank cyanosis. Physical examination in women who develop pneumonia would include looking for signs of fever, rales, and wheezes. Chest radiography characteristically shows a miliary pattern or a diffuse nodular pattern. On chest radiography, the perihilar regions are more likely to be involved. Women who have varicella infection without complications in pregnancy do not need to be hospitalized. However, women with this infection must be warned to contact their physician immediately in the event of any pulmonary symptoms, including a mild cough. At this point, hospitalization with full respiratory support, if necessary, should be indicated.

In a series of 43 pregnancies complicated by maternal varicella, Paryani and Arvin[102] noted that nine women had developed associated morbidity. Varicella pneumonia developed in four of these women (9%), one of whom died. Premature labor developed in 4 out of 42 (10%), with premature delivery occurring in two (5%). Another woman developed herpes zoster infection.

If a pregnant woman is exposed to varicella, it is likely that she is immune but, if she is not immune, it is most probable that she will be infected. McGregor and colleagues[103] pointed out that most pregnant women have detectable antibodies even if they have a negative history of chickenpox. In their series, 12 out of 17 (71%) such women were already antibody positive. Of those women with indeterminate histories, approximately 90% were immune. On the basis of these data, it appears appropriate and cost-effective to test for maternal antibody by any of the following tests: fluorescent antibody to membrane antigen, ELISA, enhanced neutralization test, and immune adherence hemagglutination. A reliable history of varicella is a valid measure of immunity, according to the CDC.[100]

If it is found that a woman has been exposed and is susceptible, varicella zoster immune globulin (VZIG) should be strongly considered. When administered intramuscularly within 96 h of exposure, it is likely that VZIG ameliorates the course of the maternal disease as it does in children.[104] However, it is not at all certain that passive immunity with

VZIG prevents fetal infection. Currently, there is no reason to believe that VZIG in pregnancy is harmful. Thus, the only disadvantage of providing VZIG to nonimmune pregnant women with exposure to varicella is the cost, currently US$400 for the adult dose.[100]

Acyclovir is a synthetic nucleoside analog that was introduced into clinical practice in the early 1980s. Its activity against VZV is considerably less than its activity against HSV. The safety of acyclovir therapy in pregnancy has not been established, but considerable experience to date (mainly in women with genital herpes infection) has been reassuring. Accordingly, in instances of serious complications of varicella infection such as pneumonia, use of intravenous acyclovir should be strongly considered. Use of acyclovir orally for the treatment of milder manifestations of varicella infection is controversial. Clinical trials among adolescents and adults have shown that acyclovir is effective in reducing the duration of severity of illness if the drug is initiated within 24 h of the onset of the varicella rash. Although the CDC does not recommend oral acyclovir for pregnant women, consideration should be given to its use early in the course of infection, provided the limited benefits and hypothetical risks are considered.[100]

In 1995, a live-attenuated varicella vaccine virus (Varivax) was introduced by Merck and Company. It is recommended that vaccination should be considered for susceptible women of childbearing age who are not pregnant. Varicella immunity may be ascertained at any routine healthcare visit, and women should be asked if they are pregnant and advised to avoid pregnancy for 1 month after each dose of the vaccine. The effects of the varicella vaccine on the fetus are unknown. It is recommended that pregnant women should not be vaccinated. Wild-type varicella poses only a small risk to the fetus and, because the virulence of the attenuated virus is less than that of the wild-type virus, the risk to the fetus, if any, is estimated to be even lower. In most circumstances, the decision to terminate a pregnancy should not simply be based on vaccine administration during pregnancy.[100]

Varicella in the newborn

Acquisition by the fetus of maternal antibody is usually protective. However, an infant born after maternal viremia, but before maternal development of antibodies, is at high risk of potentially life-threatening neonatal varicella infection. Infants at risk are those whose mothers develop clinical varicella within 5 days prior to birth or within the first 5 days after delivery. Congenital varicella infection has been reported in approximately 20% of term infants born to mothers with varicella within this time-frame, and the case fatality has been reported at approximately 30%. Infants born five or more days after maternal development of clinical illness develop either a mild varicella infection or none whatsoever. Both zoster immunoglobulin and VZIG have been shown to modify or prevent varicella infection in children, leading Brunell[104] to recommend their use in preventing severe neonatal infections.

Accordingly, infants at risk, as outlined earlier, should receive VZIG as passive immunization at a dose of 125 units. Weibel and colleagues[105] have reported excellent results using a live-attenuated varicella vaccine. The seroconversion rate was 94%, and the vaccine was 100% effective in preventing varicella. In a placebo-controlled group, approximately 10% of children developed varicella.

Effect of varicella zoster infection in early pregnancy

Congenital birth defects due to varicella in early pregnancy were not recognized until 1947.[106] The syndrome of congenital varicella infection consists of limb hypoplasia, cicatricial skin lesions, atrophic digits, psychomotor retardation, and even bilateral cortical atrophy.[106] Ultrasound findings can include dermatomal skin scarring, limb hypoplasia, ventriculomegaly, microcephaly, gastrointestinal and genitourinary abnormalities, and cortical atrophy.[45] We now recognize that maternal varicella infection in the first trimester of pregnancy may be responsible for such a syndrome, but the risk of the fetus developing these anomalies with first-trimester chickenpox has only recently been recognized. The highest risk of transmission is between 13 and 20 weeks' gestation and occurs through viremic seeding of the placenta and subsequent fetal infection.[107] Of 11 infants of women with first-trimester varicella, one (9%) developed findings consistent with congenital varicella syndrome.[102] More recent estimates have downgraded the risk to anywhere from 0.4% to approximately 1–2%.[45,108,109] Fetal infection can be determined by either culture of or PCR detection in amniotic fluid, with PCR being the more sensitive method.[45]

Effect of zoster in pregnancy

Herpes zoster infection, as noted, is caused by the same virus that causes clinical chickenpox. Zoster occurs rarely in pregnancy and, because it is a reactivation, maternal antibodies are already present. In healthy women, zoster poses no special threat to the fetus or newborn.

Influenza

Influenza viruses belong to the myxovirus group and cause the clinical entity of influenza that occurs in epidemics. Type A influenza is responsible for most epidemics and is associated with more severe disease, whereas types B and C occur less frequently.[110]

Epidemiology

The frequency and severity of influenza outbreaks have been related to changes in the viral antigens.[110] The major antigenic changes occur at 10- to 30-year intervals and are associated with severe infection because of the absence of protective antibodies. Two major pandemics occurred in 1918 and in 1957–1958. More than 20 million deaths occurred worldwide during the pandemic of 1918.[111]

Clinical presentation

With a short incubation period of 1–4 days, influenza presents with abrupt onset of an upper respiratory infection, fever, malaise, myalgia, and headache. With wide clinical variability, the major portion of the disease lasts approximately 3 days in most cases.

Definitive diagnosis can be made by isolation of the virus from throat washings during acute illness or by serologic confirmation of a fourfold rise in antibody. Although these antibodies are of the CF or hemagglutination inhibition types, they are rarely indicated clinically.

Effects on the mother

For the obstetrician, the major concern of influenza infection in pregnancy is the increased likelihood of potentially life-threatening pneumonia. From reports from the epidemics of 1918 and 1957, it appears that pregnant women were disproportionately represented in individuals dying of influenza. In addition, reported estimates of overall maternal mortality were approximately 27%, with a mortality of up to 61% in cases complicated by pneumonia prior to the era of treatment.[112] It is not certain, however, whether pregnant women are more likely to develop influenza or whether they are more likely to develop influenza pneumonia. Yet, if influenza pneumonia develops in pregnancy, it is more severe. Deaths among pregnant women with influenza may result from secondary bacterial infection and from primary influenza pneumonia without secondary superinfection.

Effects on the fetus

Contradictory data exist on the effects of influenza on abortion, prematurity, and congenital anomalies.[113] These studies may be summarized as noting that the vast majority of women who have influenza in pregnancy have normal outcomes and that there seems to be little influence on congenital abnormalities, intrauterine growth, prematurity, or stillbirth.

Hepatitis

Viral hepatitis is a common infection that predominantly affects the liver. Of all cases of hepatitis in pregnancy, approximately 50% are caused by hepatitis B. Hepatitis A is responsible for approximately 25% of cases, and hepatitis C (most of which was formerly nonA, nonB hepatitis) is responsible for most of the remainder. Laboratory diagnosis can now confirm the presence of hepatitis A, B, or C infection. Hepatitis A is also referred to as infectious hepatitis or short-incubation hepatitis, and hepatitis B has been referred to as serum hepatitis, long-incubation hepatitis, and hepatitis B surface antigen-positive hepatitis. Other infections that may cause a secondary hepatitis include Epstein–Barr virus (EBV) infection, coxsackie B infection, CMV infection, and others. In this chapter, the main emphasis is on the consequences of hepatitis B infection in pregnancy.

Epidemiology

Hepatitis B is a worldwide problem with an estimated 5% prevalence. Thus, it is estimated that there are more than 200 million carriers throughout the world. In the United States, which is a low-prevalence area, it is estimated that the prevalence is from 0.01% to 0.5% of the population [an estimated 1 million hepatitis B virus (HBV) carriers].[110] Women in the United States most at risk for hepatitis B surface antigenemia (HBsAg) are characterized as follows:

- Asian Pacific Basin or Native Alaskan women, whether immigrants or born in the United States, 15%;
- Haitian, subSaharan African, Eastern European, Middle Eastern, Caribbean, Central or South American women, 15%;
- Women with occupational exposure (e.g., medical or dental), 0.5–1.0%;
- Women working or residing in custodial institutions, 3%;
- Women with acute or chronic liver disease, illicit drug users, or women with multiple blood transfusions, 7–10%;
- Women living in a household with an HBV-infected person, 6–13%.

The impact of HBV infection is immense. Its consequences include chronic hepatitis, cirrhosis, and primary hepatocellular carcinoma. Of an estimated 300 000 new cases yearly in the United States, 75 000 of these patients become clinically ill, including 15 000 requiring hospitalization. A small number, estimated at 375, die of fulminant disease. Some 6–10% become chronic carriers, and as many as 25% of these HBV carriers eventually die of cirrhosis or hepatocellular carcinoma. Despite the availability of an effective vaccine, the incidence of HBV reported to the CDC has remained high. The incidence of hepatitis B infection in pregnant women is the same as that in the general population, and the course of the disease in pregnancy is probably not altered.

HBV infection is spread by sexual transmission, blood transfusion, intravenous drug abuse, and intrauterine or perinatal transmission from the mother to the fetus or newborn. The major concern in pregnancy is transmission to the infant. In the Far East, approximately 40% of HBV cases in mothers result in vertical transmission to the fetus or newborn.[114] In the United States, the reported overall risk of perinatal HBV transmission from HBV surface antigen-positive mothers ranges from 20% to 50%, with the rate of transmission depending on population characteristics. These influencing characteristics include ethnic background, lifestyle, and persistence of the HBe antigen (HBeAg). Nonfulminant hepatitis probably does not increase fetal wastage, but may be associated with an increased risk of prematurity. Finally, there is no apparent increase in congenital anomalies associated with maternal hepatitis B infection in pregnancy.

For hepatitis C, the principal risk factors include intravenous drug use and multiple blood transfusions. Approximately 90% of cases of post-transfusion hepatitis now result from hepatitis C infection. Other risk factors include heterosexual contact, organ donation, needlestick injury, and vertical transmission from mother to fetus. The overall prevalence of hepatitis C infection has been reported to be approximately 2–7%, but these are data from at-risk populations, including those from sexually transmitted disease clinics and intravenous drug users.

Determining the rate of perinatal transmission of hepatitis C virus (HCV) has been problematic, as initial reports were highly variable. Two groups appear to be at high risk for perinatal transmission: women who are coinfected with human immunodeficiency virus (HIV)[115] and women who have a large viral inoculum.[116] When the viral inoculum is low and when the mother is not coinfected with HIV, the likelihood of perinatal transmission is approximately 4.5%, whereas it is about 18% in the presence of HIV co-infection. In mothers with circulating levels of HCV RNA of 10 million copies or greater, the risk of perinatal transmission seems to be as high as 36%, but perinatal transmission virtually does not occur when levels are below this viral load.[117]

Virology and serology

HBV is a DNA virus that is 42 nm in diameter. The outer protein coat is the so-called surface, the HBsAg. This antigen is produced in excess by the virus and appears in the serum of individuals with active infection. The central core contains DNA, a DNA polymerase, and the core antigen, HBcAg. The core antigen is found only in infected liver cells, not in the serum. The third antigen, HBeAg, is found in the serum and is a marker of high rates of perinatal transmission.

Each of these three antigens has a corresponding antibody: anti-HBs, anti-HBc, and anti-HBe. The serologic pattern that is followed in 90% of cases of HBV infection is that, within 6 months of infection, all antigens are cleared from the serum. This individual becomes noninfectious. The antibodies to HBs and to HBc are lifelong markers of prior infection. [For further details, see the two figures in the hepatitis B section (diagnosis) in the following viral hepatitis website: http://web.uct.ac.za/depts/mmi/jmoodie/dihep.html.]

In the remaining 10% of individuals with HBV infection, there is persistence of HBsAg beyond 6 months. Approximately 60% of these women with persistence of infection develop chronic persistent hepatitis. Approximately 10% have asymptomatic HBsAg antigenemia, and approximately 30% have chronic active hepatitis. All these groups are potentially infective to others including, in pregnant women, transmission to the offspring. This is a group that is the target for prenatal screening. Transmission rates from mother to fetus or neonate are as follows:[118,119]

- Acute HBV in third trimester or within 1 month of delivery: 80–90% infection rate in infant;
- Asymptomatic, HBeAg positive: 90% infection rate in infant;
- Asymptomatic, HBeAg negative: 10–30% infection rate in infant;
- Asymptomatic, HBsAg positive: 0–10% infection rate in infant.

HCV is a single-stranded RNA virus that is 30–38 nm in diameter. The antigen is the hepatitis C antigen (HCAg), and the antibody is the anti-hepatitis C antibody (anti-HC). Anti-HC antibody is identified by third-generation tests, including the enzyme immunoassay for screening and the recombinant immunoblot assay as the confirmatory test. The antibody may not be present until 6–16 weeks after the onset of clinical illness. PCR methodology is now used to detect hepatitis C RNA, with high levels denoting a high likelihood of infectivity.

Clinical manifestations

After an incubation period of 45–160 days, hepatitis B may become clinically evident. Initial symptoms often include fever, headache, and abdominal pain, followed in several days by spontaneous resolution. At this point, the urine may become dark, and jaundice may be evident. The liver is usually somewhat enlarged and tender. As the jaundice resolves, the patient spontaneously feels better and usually recovers rapidly. As noted, in approximately 10% of patients with hepatitis B, a form of chronic disease continues. Hepatitis B may present as an acute fulminated form that may become fatal, although this is quite rare in well-nourished Western populations. Fulminant hepatitis is heralded by a rapidly shrinking liver, rapidly rising bilirubin level, and abnormalities in prothrombin time, with development of encephalopathy and ascites. The mortality rate in such cases of fulminant hepatitis is greater than 80%.

In neonates, the most frequent presentation of hepatitis infection is an asymptomatic child with chronic infection. Clinical illness is relatively infrequent with congenital hepatitis, but approximately 10% of neonates with asymptomatic disease become jaundiced within the first 3–4 months of life.

Treatment

Most women with hepatitis B infection during pregnancy can be managed on an outpatient basis. There is no specific treatment, but supportive measures include increased bedrest and a high-protein, low-fat diet. Specific indications for hospitalization of women with viral hepatitis include severe anemia, diabetes, protracted nausea and vomiting, abnormalities in prothrombin time, a rapidly falling or low serum albumin level, and a high serum bilirubin greater than approximately 15 mg/dL.

Table 18.1 Other microbial infections.

Organism	Congenital infection?	Maternal effects	Fetal and neonatal effects	Diagnosis	Treatment
Epstein–Barr virus (EBV)[107,127–132]	Rare to have primary infection in pregnancy, even among serosusceptible women; no reported cases of antenatal diagnosis of EBV congenital infection and only rare case reports of possible association with fetal anomalies	Asymptomatic (>50% of patients) to sore throat, fever, malaise, lymphadenopathy (rare: splenic rupture, meningitis, Guillain–Barré syndrome, death)	Possible association with cardiovascular defects and cataracts, as well as thrombocytopenia, hepatosplenomegaly, seizures, microcephaly, cerebral calcifications in rare case reports only	Maternal: in symptomatic patient detection of heterophil antibodies or EBV-specific serology Fetal: identification of umbilical cord blood lymphocyte transformation or EBV detection in oropharyngeal secretions	Supportive care in symptomatic patients; in cases with severe complications, corticosteroids and acyclovir have been used
Measles[110,133]	Rarely causes congenital measles (disease becomes clinically apparent within 10 days of neonatal life)	Fever, cough, coryza, conjunctivitis, maculopapular rash, malaise, Koplik's spots (complications: bacterial pneumonia, otitis media, encephalitis; rare: thrombocytopenic purpura, myocarditis, subacute sclerosing panencephalitis)	Increased risk of prematurity, especially with third-trimester disease; no constellation of anomalies	Based on clinical history and clinical presentation	Uncomplicated measles is treated symptomatically; antibiotics for secondary otitis media or pneumonia; susceptible exposed pregnant women, neonates (including those born to women who have measles in the last week of pregnancy), and contacts should receive passive immunization with immune serum globulin
Mumps[134–137]	No	Prodrome of fever, malaise, myalgia, anorexia, (bilateral) parotitis (rare: oophoritis, aseptic meningitis, pancreatitis, mastitis, thyroiditis, myocarditis, arthritis, nephritis)	Twofold increase in spontaneous abortion when occurring in the first trimester; possible association with congenital endocardial fibroelastosis	Based on clinical presentation	Symptomatic, supportive treatment; avoid vaccination with MMR vaccine during pregnancy
Listeriosis[138–142]	Yes	Illness usually in third trimester. May be asymptomatic. Fever, flu-like syndrome, abdominal/back pain, vomiting, diarrhea, headache, myalgia, sore throat. Preterm labor	Fetal and neonatal infection as evidenced by electronic fetal monitoring abnormalities (tachycardia, decreased variability, absence of accelerations), stillbirth; in neonates: respiratory distress, fever, meningismus, seizures, rash, jaundice	Culture and Gram stain of maternal blood, vagina, amniotic fluid (with finding of brown-stained fluid), and neonatal throat, skin, conjunctiva, cerebrospinal fluid	Intravenous antibiotics, usually ampicillin plus/minus gentamicin
Tuberculosis[143–148]	Yes, most commonly following maternal miliary disease; maternal active pulmonary disease is more likely to lead to postnatal infection	May be asymptomatic. Cough, weight loss, fever, malaise, fatigue, hemoptysis. Increased rate of preeclampsia, placental abruption/vaginal bleeding	Spontaneous abortion, stillbirth; no increase in anomalies. In neonate: low birthweight, hepatosplenomegaly, respiratory distress, fever, lymphadenopathy	Mother and neonate: purified protein derivative (PPD) testing, chest X-ray, possible lumbar puncture, and culture of appropriate sites. Placental examination and culture including acid-fast staining	In pregnant mother: antibiotic therapy for 9 months with rifampin, isoniazid, ethambutol, pyridoxine; pyrazinamide controversial

Prevention

Women with a definite exposure to HBV should be given hepatitis B immune globulin (HBIG) as soon as possible within a 7-day period of exposure, with a second dose 30 days after the first. Such passive immunization would be indicated for hospital exposures and inoculation with contaminated needles. Until June 1988, the CDC had recommended screening of pregnant women for asymptomatic hepatitis B infection on a selective basis. However, in mid-1988, the CDC[120] overhauled these recommendations based on several studies demonstrating that selective screening only identified 50% of women who were HBsAg positive.[120–123] The study populations were medically indigent women in Cleveland, New Orleans, and Miami, for example. In middle-class populations, the sensitivity of selective screening has not been well studied. Yet, a cost-analysis study carried out at the CDC concluded that, even in extremely low-prevalence populations (with a prevalence of less than 0.1%), the universal screening program would be cost-effective.[124]

The purpose of universal screening is to allow treatment of newborns of HBsAg-positive women with HBIG and hepatitis B vaccine, a regimen that is 90% effective in preventing the development of an HBV chronic carrier state in the newborn. The specifics of the recommendation are that women should be tested for HBsAg during an early prenatal visit. Testing for additional markers is considered unnecessary. Even though women who have HBeAg are at a much higher risk of perinatal transmission, there is still a risk of about 10–15% of perinatal transmission in women who do not have HBeAg but who have HBsAg. If a woman is identified as being HBsAg positive, she should be evaluated for active liver disease. Infants born to HBsAg-positive women should receive HBIG (0.5 mL intramuscularly) once they are stable, preferably within 12 h of birth. In addition, these infants should receive the recombinant HBV (Recombivax HB) vaccine (5 μg per dose), or they may receive the plasma-derived (Engerix-B) vaccine (10 μg per dose).[125] Either of these vaccines should be given intramuscularly in the following sequence of three doses: the first at birth and the second and third at 1 and 6 months of age respectively. It is estimated that the direct cost to prevent one newborn from becoming a chronic HBV carrier would be approximately US$12 700 if the prevalence of HBsAg in a given population is approximately 5 in 1000.[12] In infants born to seronegative mothers, HBIG is not indicated, but active vaccination is now recommended for all neonates.

Household members and sexual partners of women identified as being HBsAg positive should be tested to determine susceptibility to HBV infection. Susceptible individuals should receive the HBV vaccine.[126]

Women who deliver without prenatal care should be tested as early as possible on delivery admission so that infants at risk can begin to receive their prophylaxis within 48 h after birth. It is further recommended that hospitals that cannot rapidly test for HBsAg either develop this capability or offer testing to another laboratory.[126]

As a further preventive measure, it is recommended that universal precautions be applied, including the use of gloves, masks, and glasses or goggles by delivery room personnel to keep infectious fluids away from the mouth, nose, eyes, and breaks in the skin. These precautions are equally important in guarding against HBV infection and in preventing the transmission of HIV. Thus, to prevent both these serious infections, as well as hepatitis C infection, universal blood and body fluid precautions are the best measures for preventing nosocomial transmission.[126] Finally, all healthcare personnel are required to undergo hepatitis B vaccination in most healthcare facilities.

With hepatitis C, there does not appear to be any prophylaxis against perinatal transmission, and there does not appear to be a protective benefit from Cesarean delivery over vaginal delivery. As a result, even routine screening of otherwise asymptomatic pregnant women for hepatitis C is not recommended.[117]

Other microbial infections

Details of these can be found in Table 18.1.

Key points

1 Group B streptococcus (GBS) is a significant contributor to neonatal morbidity and mortality. GBS prophylaxis is highly effective in reducing perinatal infection and is the standard of care in women known to be GBS carriers or who are considered to be high risk.

2 GBS prophylaxis should be with penicillin. In penicillin-allergic patients without anaphylaxis, intravenous cephazolin is the preferred treatment. In patients who have a history of anaphylaxis with penicillin exposure, sensitivities should be obtained for the GBS isolate with regard to erythromycin and clindamycin. If the isolate is resistant to either antibiotic or both, then intravenous vancomycin is the preferred antibiotic for prophylaxis.

3 Diagnosis of intrauterine (fetal) toxoplasmosis is clinically available in the form of PCR analysis of amniotic fluid obtained via amniocentesis.

4 Many maternal "*Toxoplasma*-specific" IgM antibodies reported from commercial laboratories are false-positives.

5 Congenital rubella infection is possible in women who are not appropriately vaccinated against the virus, and fetal diagnosis can be performed by the detection of rubella-specific IgM in fetal blood beyond 20–22 weeks' gestation, or by PCR analysis of amniotic fluid.

6 In patients with a history of genital HSV infection, prophylactic oral acyclovir administration beginning at 36 weeks' gestation reduces the rates of clinical recurrence at delivery as well as the rates of Cesarean delivery.

7 The correct classification of the type of HSV infection (primary, nonprimary, recurrence) cannot be made clinically, but requires type-specific antibodies and HSV viral type.

8 For the prevention of perinatal transmission of HSV, Cesarean delivery is still indicated in women who present with signs and symptoms of a genital outbreak of HSV.

9 Congenital CMV infection can occur with primary and recurrent maternal infection with attributable fetal effects including growth retardation, cerebral ventriculomegaly, microcephaly, hepatosplenomegaly, and periventricular calcifications.

10 Primary CMV infection occurs in 1–2% of all pregnant women. Diagnosis can be made by PCR or viral culture of amniotic fluid.

11 Parvovirus can cause a fetal hemolytic anemia and nonimmune hydrops fetalis. Treatment in such circumstances depends upon intrauterine blood transfusions.

12 Congenital varicella infection can lead to fetal limb hypoplasia, psychomotor retardation, cerebral ventriculomegaly, and microcephaly, as well as quite severe maternal disease including pneumonia.

13 Acute varicella exposure or infection in pregnancy can be treated with VZIG and/or acyclovir.

14 Influenza is not known to cause congenital infection.

15 Hepatitis B and C can be transmitted perinatally. Hepatitis B vaccination outside of pregnancy is the mainstay of prevention.

16 In neonates born to mothers who are HBsAg positive and are known to have chronic disease, treatment with HBIG and hepatitis B vaccination is the standard for prevention of neonatal transmission.

17 There are only rare case reports of congenital EBV infection.

18 Measles rarely causes congenital disease, which is apparent within 10 days of neonatal life and is associated with an increased risk of prematurity.

19 Listeriosis can cause congenital infection and can lead to preterm labor and stillbirth. Intravenous ampicillin with or without gentamicin is the treatment of choice.

20 Tuberculosis can be a cause of congenital infection, most commonly following maternal miliary disease, and can lead to preeclampsia, placental abruption, spontaneous abortion, and stillbirth.

References

1 Regan JA, Klebanoff MA, Nugent RP. The epidemiology of group B streptococcal colonization in pregnancy. Vaginal infections and Prematurity Study Group. *Obstet Gynecol* 1991; 77(4):604.

2 Schrag SJ, Zywicki S, Farley MM, et al. Group B streptococcal disease in the era of intrapartum antibiotic prophylaxis. *N Engl J Med* 2000;342(1):15.

3 Sweet RL, Gibbs RS. Intraamniotic infection. In: Sweet RL, Gibbs RS, eds. *Infectious diseases of the female genital tract*, 4th edn. Philadelphia, PA: Lippincott Williams & Wilkins; 2002: 516.

4 Sperling RS, Newton E, Gibbs RS. Intra-amniotic infection in low birth-weight infants. *J Infect Dis* 1988;157(1):113.

5 Edwards MS, Baker CJ. Group B streptococcal infections. In: Remington JS, Klein JO, eds. *Infectious diseases of the fetus and newborn infant*, 3rd edn. Philadelphia: W.B. Saunders Company; 2001:1091.

6 Blanco JD, Gibbs RS. Infections following classical cesarean section. *Obstet Gynecol* 1980;55(2):167.

7 Yancey MK, Armer T, Clark P, et al. Assessment of rapid identification tests for genital carriage of group B streptococci. *Obstet Gynecol* 1992;80:1038.

8 Bland HL, Vermillion ST, Soper DE, et al. Antibiotic resistance patterns of group B streptococci in pregnant women. *J Clin Microbiol* 1990;28(1):5.

9 Centers for Disease Control and Prevention. Prevention of perinatal group B streptococcal disease. *MMWR Morbid Mortal Wkly Rep* 2002:51:1.

10 Schrag SJ, Arnold KE, Mohle-Boetani JC, et al. Diminishing racial disparities in early-onset neonatal group B streptococcal disease – United States 2000–2003. *MMWR Morbid Mortal Wkly Rep* 2004;53:502.

11 Pearlman M. Prevention of early-onset group B streptococcal disease in newborns (letter). *Obstet Gynecol* 2003;102:414.

12 Hohlfeld P, Daffos F, Costa JM, et al., Prenatal diagnosis of congenital toxoplasmosis with a polymerase-chain-reaction test on amniotic fluid. *N Engl J Med* 1994;331:695.

13 Sever JL, Elienberg JH, Ley AC, et al. Toxoplasmosis: maternal and pediatric findings in 23,000 pregnancies. *Pediatrics* 1988;82:181.

14 The Centers for Disease Control. Preventing congenital toxoplasmosis. *MMWR Morbid Mortal Wkly Rep* 2000; 49:57–75.

15 Desmonts G, Couvreur J. Congenital toxoplasmosis. A prospective study of 378 pregnancies. *N Engl J Med* 1974;290:1110.

16 Alford CA, Stagno S, Reynolds DW. Congenital toxoplasmosis: clinical, laboratory, and therapeutic considerations, with special

reference to subclinical disease. *Bull NY Acad Med* 1974;50: 160.

17 Stray-Pederson B, Lorentzen-Styr AM. Uterine *Toxoplasma* infections and repeated abortions. *Am J Obstet Gynecol* 1977;128:716.

18 Stagno S, Reynolds D, Amos C. Auditory and visual defects resulting from symptomatic and subclinical congenital cytomegalovirus and *Toxoplasma* infections. *Pediatrics* 1977; 59:699.

19 Wilson CB, Remington JS, Stagno S, Reynolds DW. Development of adverse sequelae in children born with subclinical congenital *Toxoplasma* infection. *Pediatrics* 1980;66:767.

20 Montoya JG, Liesenfeld O. Toxoplasmosis. *Lancet* 2004;363: 1965.

21 Montoya. Laboratory diagnosis of *Toxoplasma gondii* infection and toxoplasmosis. *J Infect Dis* 2002;185:S73.

22 Daffos F, Forestier F, Capella-Pavlovsky M, et al. Prenatal management of 746 pregnancies at risk for congenital toxoplasmosis. *N Engl J Med* 1988;318:271.

23 Desmonts G, Forestier F, Thulliez P, et al. Prenatal diagnosis of congenital toxoplasmosis. *Lancet* 1985;1:500.

24 Wong SY, Remington JS. Toxoplasmosis in pregnancy. *Clin Infect Dis* 1994;18:853.

25 Foulon W, Naessens A, Lauwers S, et al. Impact of primary prevention on the incidence of toxoplasmosis during pregnancy. *Obstet Gynecol* 1988;72:363.

26 McCabe R, Remington JS. Toxoplasmosis: the time has come. *N Engl J Med* 1988;318:313.

27 Guerina NG, Hsu HW, Meissner HC, et al. Neonatal serologic screening and early treatment for congenital *Toxoplasma gondii* infection. *N Engl J Med* 1994;330:1858.

28 Centers for Disease Control. Control and prevention of rubella: evaluation and management of suspected outbreaks, rubella in pregnant women, and surveillance for congenital rubella syndrome. *MMWR Morbid Mortal Wkly Rep* 2001;50:1.

29 Centers for Disease Control. Rubella and congenital rubella – United States, 1984 to 1986. *MMWR Morbid Mortal Wkly Rep* 1987;36:664.

30 Saule H, Enders G, Bemsau U. Congenital rubella infection after previous immunity of the mother. *Eur J Pediatr* 1988; 147:195.

31 Levine IB, Berkowitz CD, St Geme JW. Rubella virus reinfection during pregnancy leading to late-onset congenital rubella syndrome. *J Pediatr* 1982;100:589.

32 Preblud SR, Williams NM. Fetal risk associated with rubella vaccine: implications for vaccination of susceptible women. *Obstet Gynecol* 1985;66:121.

33 Bart SW, Stetier HC, Preblud SR, et al. Fetal risk associated with rubella vaccine: an update. *Rev Infect Dis* 1985;7:S95.

34 Losonsky GA, Fishaut JM, Strussenberg J, Ogra PL. Effect of immunization against rubella on lactation products. II. Maternal–neonatal interactions. *J Infect Dis* 1982;145: 661.

35 Enders G, Nickeri-Pacher U, Miller E, Cradock-Watson JE. Outcome of confirmed periconceptional maternal rubella. *Lancet* 1988;1:1445.

36 Cradock-Watson JE, Ridehalgh MKS. Fetal infection resulting from maternal rubella after the first trimester of pregnancy. *J Hyg (Camb)* 1980;85:381.

37 Freij BJ, South MA, Sever JL. Maternal rubella and the congenital rubella syndrome. *Clin Perinatol* 1988;15:247.

38 Sever JL, South MA, Shaver KA. Delayed manifestations of congenital rubella. *Rev Infect Dis* 1985;7:S164.

39 Hardy JB, McCracken GH Jr, Gilkeson MR, Sever JL. Adverse fetal outcome following maternal rubella after the first trimester of pregnancy. *JAMA* 1969;207:2414.

40 Verder H, Dickmeiss E, Haahr S, et al. Late-onset rubella syndrome: coexistence of immune complex disease and defective cytotoxic effector cell function. *Clin Exp Immunol* 1986;63: 367.

41 Tardieu M, Grospierre B, Durandy A, Griscelli C. Circulating immune complexes containing rubella antigens in late-onset rubella syndrome. *J Pediatr* 1980;97:370.

42 Daffos F, Forestier F, Grangeot-Keros, et al. Prenatal diagnosis of congenital rubella. *Lancet* 1984;2:1.

43 Banatvala JE, Brown DWG. Rubella. *Lancet* 2004;363: 1127.

44 Enders G, Jonathan W. Prenatal diagnosis of intrauterine rubella. *Infection* 1987;15:12.

45 Andrews JI. Diagnosis of fetal infections. *Curr Opin Obstet Gynecol* 2004;16:163.

46 Terry GM, Ho-Terry L, Warren RC, et al. First trimester prenatal diagnosis of congenital rubella: a laboratory investigation. *Br Med J* 1986;292:930.

47 Cradock-Watson JE, Miller E, Ridehalgh MKS, et al. Detection of rubella in fetal and placental tissues and in the throats of neonates after serologically confirmed rubella in pregnancy. *Prenatal Diag* 1989;9:91.

48 Centers for Disease Control. Rubella and congenital rubella syndrome – United States, 1985 to 1988. *MMWR Morbid Mortal Wkly Rep* 1989;38:173.

49 Brown Z. Preventing herpes simplex virus transmission to the neonate. *Herpes* 2004;11(Suppl.):175A.

50 Nahmias AJ, Josey WE, Naib ZM, et al. Perinatal risk associated with maternal genital herpes simplex virus infection. *Am J Obstet Gynecol* 1971;110:825.

51 Honig PJ, Holzwanger J, Leyden JJ. Congenital herpes simplex virus infections. Report of three cases and review of the literature. *Arch Dermatol* 1979;115:1329.

52 Nahmias AJ, Josey WE, Naib ZM, et al. Antibodies to Herpesvirus hominis types 1 and 2 in humans. I. Patients with genital herpetic infections. *Am J Epidemiol* 1970;91:539.

53 Fleming DT, McQuillan GM, Johnson RE, et al. Herpes simplex virus type 2 in the United States, 1976 to 1994. *N Engl J Med* 1997;337(16):1105.

54 Brown ZA, Wald A, Morrow RA, et al. Effect of serologic status and cesarean delivery on transmission rates of herpes simplex virus from infant to mother. *JAMA* 2003;289:203.

55 Nerurkar LS, West F, May M, et al. Survival of herpes simplex virus in water specimens collected from hot tubs in spa facilities and on hot plastic surfaces. *JAMA* 1983;250:3081.

56 Becker TM, Stone KM, Cates W, Jr. Epidemiology of genital herpes in the Unites States. The current situation. *J Reprod Med* 1986;31:359.

57 Harger JH, Pazin GJ, Breinig MC. Current understanding of the natural history of genital herpes simplex infections. *J Reprod Med* 1986;31:365.

58 Brown ZA, Wald A, Morrow RA, et al. Effect of serological status and cesarean delivery on transmission rates of herpes simplex virus from mother to infant. *JAMA* 2003;289:203.

59 Comy L, Adams HG, Brown ZA, et al. Genital herpes simplex virus infections: clinical manifestations, course, and complications. *Ann Intern Med* 1983;98:958.

60 Baker DA, Blythe JG, Kaufman R, et al. One-year suppression of frequent recurrences of genital herpes with oral acyclovir. *Obstet Gynecol* 1989;73:84.

61 Eldridge R, Andrews E, Tilson H, et al. Pregnancy outcomes following systemic prenatal acyclovir. *MMWR Morbid Mortal Wkly Rep* 1993;42:806.
62 Sheffield JS, Hollier LM, Hill JB, et al. Acyclovir prophylaxis to prevent herpes simplex virus recurrence at delivery: a systematic review. *Obstet Gynecol* 2003;102:1396.
63 Stagno S, Pass RF, Dworsky ME, Alford CA. Maternal cytomegalovirus infection and perinatal transmission. *Clin Obstet Gynecol* 1982;25:563.
64 Stagno S, Whitney RJ. Herpesvirus infections of pregnancy. Part 1: cytomegalovirus and Epstein–Barr virus infections. *N Engl J Med* 1985;313:1270.
65 Reddy U, Fry A, Pass R, Ghidini A. Infectious diseases and perinatal outcomes. *Emerg Infect Dis* [serial on the Internet], 2004 Nov 23. Available from http://www.cdc.gov/ncidod/EID/vol10no11/04-0623_10.
66 Sever JL, Larsen JW, Grossman JH. *Handbook of perinatal infections*, 2nd edn. Boston, MA: Little, Brown; 1989:38.
67 Stagno S, Pass RF, Dworsky ME, et al. Congenital cytomegalovirus infection: the relative importance of primary and recurrent maternal infection. *N Engl J Med* 1982;306:945.
68 Revello MG, Gerna G. Pathogenesis and prenatal diagnosis of human cytomegalovirus infection. *J Clin Virol* 2004;29:71.
69 Stagno S, Pass RF, Cloud G, et al. Primary cytomegalovirus infection in pregnancy. *JAMA* 1986;256:1904.
70 Huang E, Alford CA, Reynolds DW, et al. Molecular epidemiology of cytomegalovirus infections in women and their infants. *N Engl J Med* 1980;303:958.
71 Lewis PE, Cefalo RC, Zaritsky AL. Fetal heart block caused by cytomegalovirus. *Am J Obstet Gynecol* 1980;136:967.
72 Karn K, Julian TM, Ogbum PL. Fetal heart block associated with congenital cytomegalovirus infection. *J Reprod Med* 1984;29: 278.
73 Filloux F, Kelsey DK, Bose CL, et al. Hydrops fetalis with supraventricular tachycardia and cytomegalovirus infection. *Clin Pediatr* 1985;24:534.
74 Ghidini A, Sirtori M, Vergani P, et al. Fetal intracranial calcifications. *Am J Obstet Gynecol* 1989;160:86.
75 Istas AS, Demmler GJ, Dobbins JG. Surveillance for congenital cytomegalovirus disease: a report from the National Cytomegalovirus Disease Registry. *Clin Infect Dis* 1995;20: 665.
76 Gaytant MA, Steegers EA, Semmekrot BA, et al. Congenital cytomegalovirus infection: review of the epidemiology and outcome. *Obstet Gynecol Surv* 2002;57(4):245.
77 Revello MG, Gerna G. Diagnosis and management of human cytomegalovirus infection in the mother, fetus, and newborn infant. *Clin Microbiol Rev* 2002;15(4):680.
78 Liesnard C, Donner C, Brancart F, et al. Prenatal diagnosis of congenital cytomegalovirus infection: prospective study of 237 pregnancies at risk. *Obstet Gynecol* 2000;95(6 Pt 1):881.
79 Grangeot-Keros L, Cointe D. Diagnosis and prognosis of HCMV infection. *J Clin Virol* 2001;21:213.
80 Osbum JE. Cytomegalovirus: pathogenicity, immunology, and vaccine initiatives. *J Infect Dis* 1981;143:618.
81 Balfour CL, Balfour HH. Cytomegalovirus is not an occupational risk for nurses in renal transplant and neonatal units. *JAMA* 1986;256:1909.
82 Centers for Disease Control. Risks associated with human parvovirus B19 infection. *MMWR Morbid Mortal Wkly Rep* 1989;38:81.
83 Heegaard ED, Brown KE. Human parvovirus B19. *Clin Microbiol Rev* 2002;15(3):485.
84 Kinney JS, Anderson U, Farrar J, et al. Risk of adverse outcomes of pregnancy and human parvovirus B19 infection. *J Infect Dis* 1968;157:663.
85 Anand A, Gray ES, Brown T, et al. Human parvovirus infection in pregnancy and hydrops fetalis. *N Engl J Med* 1987;316: 183.
86 Woernle CH, Anderson LJ, Tatersall P. Human parvovirus B19 infection during pregnancy. *J Infect Dis* 1987;156:17.
87 Anderson U, Hurwitz ES. Human parvovirus B19 and pregnancy. *Clin Perinatol* 1989;15:273.
88 Poner HJ, Khong TY, Evans MF, et al. Parvovirus as a cause of hydrops fetalis: detection by in situ DNA hybridization. *J Clin Pathol* 1988;41:381.
89 Anderson MJ, Khousam MN, Maxwell DJ, et al. Human parvovirus B19 and hydrops fetalis (letter). *Lancet* 1988;1:535.
90 Weiland HT, Vermey-Keers C, Salimans MM, et al. Parvovirus B19 associated with fetal abnormality (letter). *Lancet* 1987;1: 682.
91 Carrington D, Gilmore DH, Whittle MJ, et al. Maternal serum α-fetoprotein – a marker of fetal aplastic crisis during intrauterine human parvovirus infection. *Lancet* 1987;1:433.
92 Brond PR, Caul EO, Usher J, et al. Intrauterine infection with human parvovirus (letter). *Lancet* 1986;1:448.
93 Maeda H, Shimokawa H, Satoh S, et al. Nonimmunologic hydrops fetalis resulting from intrauterine human parvovirus B-19 infection: report of two cases. *Obstet Gynecol* 1988;72: 482.
94 Schwarz TF, Roggendorf M, Hottentrager B, et al. Human parvovirus B19 infection in pregnancy (letter). *Lancet* 1988;2: 566.
95 Cosmi E, Mari G, Delle Chiaie L, et al. Noninvasive diagnosis by Doppler ultrasonography of fetal anemia resulting from parvovirus infection. *Am J Obstet Gynecol.* 2002;187(5): 1290.
96 Young NA, Gershon AA. Chicken pox, measles, and mumps. In: Remington JS, Klein JO, eds. *Infectious diseases of the fetus and newborn.* Philadelphia: W.B. Saunders; 1983:375.
97 Centers for Disease Control. Annual summary 1982. Reported morbidity and mortality in the United States. *MMWR Morbid Mortal Wkly Rep* 1983;31:21.
98 Hemann KL. Congenital and perinatal varicella. *Clin Obstet Gynecol* 1982;25:605.
99 Preblud SR, D'Angelo U. Chickenpox in the United States 1972 to 1977. *J Infect Dis* 1979;140:257.
100 Centers for Disease Control. Prevention of varicella. *MMWR Morbid Mortal Wkly Rep* 1996;45:1.
101 Brunell PA. Varicella zoster infections in pregnancy. *JAMA* 1967; 199:315.
102 Paryani SG, Arvin AM. Intrauterine infection with varicella zoster virus after maternal varicella. *N Engl J Med* 1986;314: 1542.
103 McGregor JA, Mark S, Crawford GP, et al. Varicella zoster antibody testing in the care of pregnant women exposed to varicella. *Am J Obstet Gynecol* 1987;157:281.
104 Brunell PA. Fetal and neonatal varicella-zoster infections. *Semin Perinatol* 1983;7:47.
105 Weibel RE, Neff BJ, Kuter BJ, et al. Live attenuated varicella virus vaccine. Efficacy trial in healthy children. *N Engl J Med* 1994;310:1409.
106 LaForet E, Lynch CL. Multiple congenital defects following maternal varicella. *N Engl J Med* 1947;236:534.
107 Schleiss MR. Vertically transmitted herpesvirus infections. *Herpes* 2003;10(1):4.

108 Pastuszak AL, Levy M, Schick B, et al. Outcome after maternal varicella infection in the first 20 weeks of pregnancy. *N Engl J Med* 1994;330:901.

109 Enders G, Miller E, Cradock-Watson J, et al. Consequences of varicella and herpes zoster in pregnancy: prospective study of 1739 cases. *Lancet* 1994;343:1547.

110 Sever JL, Larsen JW, Jr, Grossman JH, III. *Handbook of perinatal infections*. Boston, MA: Little, Brown; 1979:37.

111 Finland M. Influenza complicating pregnancy. In: Charles D, Finland M, eds. *Obstetrics and perinatal infections*. Philadelphia, PA: Lea & Febiger; 1973:355.

112 Ie S, Rubio ER, Alper B, Szerlip HM. Respiratory complications of pregnancy. *Obstet Gynecol Surv* 2002;57(1):39.

113 Griffiths PD, Ronalds CJ, Heath RB. A prospective study of influenza infections during pregnancy. *J Epidemiol Commun Health* 1980;34:1224.

114 Derso A, Boxafl EH, Tarlow MJ, Fiewett TH. Transmission of HBsAg from mother to infant in four ethnic groups. *Br Med J* 1978;1:949.

115 Novati R, Thiers V, Monforte AD, et al. Mother-to-child transmission of hepatitis C virus detected by nested polymerase chain reaction. *J Infect Dis* 1992;165:720.

116 Ohto H, Terazawa S, Sasaki N, et al. Transmission of hepatitis C virus from mothers to infants. The Vertical Transmission of Hepatitis C Virus Collaborative Study Group. *N Engl J Med* 1994;330:744.

117 Dienstag JL. Sexual and perinatal transmission of hepatitis C. *Hepatology* 1997;26(3 Suppl. 1):66S.

118 Stevens CE, Neurath RA, Beasley RP, Szmuness W. HBeAg and anti-HBe detection by radioimmunoassay: correlation with vertical transmission of hepatitis B virus in Taiwan. *J Med Virol* 1979;3:237.

119 Lee AKY, Ip HMH, Wong VCW. Mechanisms of maternal-fetal transmission of hepatitis B virus. *J Infect Dis* 1978;138:668.

120 Jonas MM, Schiff ER, O'Sullivan MJ, et al. Failure of Centers for Disease Control to identify hepatitis B infection in large municipal obstetrical populations. *Ann Intern Med* 1987;107:335.

121 Summers PR, Biswas MK, Pastorek JG, et al. The pregnant hepatitis B carrier: evidence favoring comprehensive antepartum screening. *Obstet Gynecol* 1987;69:701.

122 Kumar ML, Dawson NV, McCullough AJ, et al. Should all pregnant women be screened for hepatitis B? *Ann Intern Med* 1987;107:273.

123 Wetzel AM, Kirz DS. Routine hepatitis screening in adolescent pregnancies: is it cost effective? *Am J Obstet Gynecol* 1987;156:166.

124 Arevalo JA, Washington AE. Cost-effectiveness of prenatal screening and immunization for hepatitis B virus. *JAMA* 1998;259:365.

125 Poland GA, Jacobson RM. Clinical practice: prevention of hepatitis B with the hepatitis B vaccine. *N Engl J Med.* 2004;351(27):2832.

126 Prevention of perinatal transmission of hepatitis B virus: prenatal screening of all pregnant women for hepatitis B surface antigen. *MMWR Morbid Mortal Wkly Rep* 1988;37:341.

127 Miller HC, Clifford SH, Smith CA, et al. Study of the relation of congenital malformation to maternal rubella and other infections: preliminary report. *Pediatrics* 1949;3:259.

128 Radetsky M. A diagnostic approach to Epstein–Barr virus infections. *Pediatr Infect Dis* 1982;1:425.

129 Andiman WA. The Epstein–Barr virus and EB virus infections in childhood. *J Pediatr* 1979;95:171.

130 Freij BJ, Sever JL. Herpesvirus infections in pregnancy: risks to embryo, fetus, and neonate. *Clin Perinatol* 1988;15:203.

131 Sumaya CV. Epstein–Barr virus serologic testing: diagnostic indications and interpretations. *Pediatr Infect Dis* 1986;5:337.

132 Chang RS, Le CT. Failure to acquire Epstein–Barr virus infection after intimate exposure to the virus. *Am J Epidemiol* 1984;119:392.

133 Siegal M. Congenital malformations following chicken pox, measles, mumps, and hepatitis. Results of a cohort study. *JAMA* 1973;226:1521.

134 Siegal M, Fuerst HT, Peress NS. Comparative fetal mortality in maternal virus disease. A prospective study on rubella, measles, mumps, chicken pox, and hepatitis. *N Engl J Med* 1966;274:768.

135 St Geme JW, Jr, Peralta H, Farias E, et al. Experimental gestational mumps virus infection and anocardial fibroelastosis. *Pediatrics* 1971;48:82.

136 St Geme JW, Jr, Noren GR, Adams P. Proposed embryopathic relation between mumps virus and primary endocardial fibroelastosis. *N Engl J Med* 1966;275:339.

137 Bowers D. Mumps during pregnancy. *West J Surg Obstet Gynecol* 1953;61:72.

138 Mylonakis E, Paliou M, Hohmann EL, et al. Listeriosis during pregnancy: a case series and review of 222 cases. *Medicine (Baltimore)* 2002;81(4):260.

139 Weinberg ED. Pregnancy-associated depression of cell-mediated immunity. *Rev Infect Dis* 1984;6:814.

140 Linnan MJ, Mascola L, Lou XD, et al. Epidemic listeriosis associated with Mexican-style cheese. *N Engl J Med* 1988;319:823.

141 Teberg AJ, Yonekura ML, Salminen C, Pavlova Z. Clinical manifestations of epidemic neonatal listeriosis. *Pediatr Infect Dis J* 1987;6:817.

142 Cruikshank DP, Warenski JC. First-trimester maternal *Listeria monocytogenes* sepsis and chorioamnionitis with normal neonatal outcome. *Obstet Gynecol* 1989;73:469.

143 Frieden TR, Sterling TR, Munsiff SS, et al. Tuberculosis. *Lancet.* 2003;362(9387):887.

144 Ormerod P. Tuberculosis in pregnancy and the puerperium. *Thorax* 2001;56(6):494.

145 Bothamley G. Drug treatment for tuberculosis during pregnancy: safety considerations. *Drug Safety* 2001;24(7):553.

146 Monif GRG. *Infectious diseases in obstetrics and gynecology*, 2nd edn. Philadelphia, PA: Harper & Row; 1982:310.

147 Peter G, Hall CB, Halsey NA, et al. *Report of the committee on infectious diseases*, 24th edn. Elk Grove Village, IL: American Academy of Pediatrics; 1997:557.

148 Huber GL. Tuberculosis. In: Remington JS, Klein JO, eds. *Infectious diseases of the fetus and newborn infant*, 2nd edn. Philadelphia, PA: W.B. Saunders; 1983:577.

19 Antibiotics and other antimicrobial agents in pregnancy and during lactation

Janet I. Andrews and Jennifer R. Niebyl

Antibiotics are widely used during pregnancy. Because of the potential for maternal and fetal side-effects, they should be used only when the indication is clear and the risk–benefit ratio justifies their use. Pregnant patients should be warned that they are particularly susceptible to yeast infections and may need therapy later with antifungal agents. Free samples of the newest drugs should not be given to women who might become pregnant, as there is often no human pregnancy information on recently marketed drugs.

Penicillins

The penicillins have a wide margin of safety and lack toxicity in both the pregnant woman and the fetus.[1] There is no evidence that penicillin or its derivatives are teratogenic. In the Collaborative Perinatal Project, 3546 mothers took penicillin derivatives during the first trimester of pregnancy, with no increased risk of anomalies.[1] In a separate study, there was no increase in birth defects in 86 women exposed to dicloxacillin during the first trimester.[2]

Several studies have revealed that, in patients receiving equivalent dosages, the serum level of penicillins is lower and renal clearance higher throughout pregnancy than in the nonpregnant state.[3] Because of an increase in both renal blood flow and glomerular filtration rate, the increase in maternal renal function results in a higher renal excretion of drugs. The expansion of the maternal intravascular volume during the late stages of pregnancy is another factor that affects antibiotic blood levels.

The transplacental passage of penicillin occurs by simple diffusion. Maternal administration of penicillins with a high protein-binding capacity (e.g., oxacillin, cloxacillin, dicloxacillin, and nafcillin) results in lower fetal tissue and amniotic fluid levels than the administration of penicillins with a low protein-binding capacity (e.g., penicillin G, ampicillin, and methicillin).[4] The antibiotic is ultimately excreted in the fetal urine and thus into the amniotic fluid. At term, maternal serum and amniotic fluid concentrations of penicillin G, ampicillin, and methicillin are equal at 60 min after intravenous administration, representing rapid passage into the fetal circulation and amniotic fluid.

Most penicillins are primarily excreted in the urine unchanged, with only small amounts being inactivated in the liver. This requires a reduction in dosage in patients with impaired renal function, and an increase in dosage during pregnancy.

Clavulanate is added to penicillin derivatives to broaden their antibacterial spectrum. In a study of 556 infants exposed to clavulanate during the first trimester, no increased risk of birth defects was observed.[5] Amoxicillin/clavulanate was studied in randomized controlled trials as potential therapy for chorioamnionitis in women with preterm premature rupture of membranes.[6] During this trial, amoxicillin/clavulanate was compared with both placebo and erythromycin. An increased incidence of necrotizing enterocolitis was found in the amoxicillin/clavulanate group compared with both the placebo and erythromycin groups.[6] It has been suggested that amoxicillin/clavulanate selects for specific pathogens, which leads to abnormal microbial colonization of the gastrointestinal tract and ultimately initiation of necrotizing enterocolitis. Therefore, amoxicillin/clavulanate should be avoided in women at risk of preterm delivery.[7]

Penicillin G, ampicillin, and amoxicillin are excreted into breast milk in low concentrations.[4,8] Oxacillin and dicloxacillin[9] are highly protein bound and are excreted into breast milk in particularly small amounts. Although no adverse effects are attributable to penicillin in breast milk, three theoretical problems might be seen in the nursing infant: modification of bowel flora (possible diarrhea, candidiasis), allergic response, or interference with the interpretation of culture results. The benefits of continued breastfeeding usually outweigh these potential risks; when these drugs are used to treat mastitis or other infections in breastfeeding mothers, continued nursing is recommended.

Cephalosporins

In a study of 5000 Michigan Medicaid recipients, it was suggested that there was a teratogenic risk (25% increase in birth defects) following exposure to cefaclor, cephalexin, and cephradine but not other cephalosporins.[10] A separate study of 308 pregnant women exposed to cephalosporins during the first trimester showed no increased risk of malformations.[11] However, because other antibiotics (e.g., penicillin, ampicillin, amoxicillin, erythromycin) that have been used extensively have not been associated with an increased risk of congenital defects, they should be first-line therapy when antibiotic treatment is required during the first trimester.

Maternal serum levels of cephalosporins during pregnancy are lower than those in nonpregnant patients receiving equivalent dosages owing to a shorter half-life in pregnancy and an increased volume of distribution. Renal elimination is also increased in pregnancy.[12] These drugs readily cross the placenta into the fetal bloodstream and, ultimately, the amniotic fluid.

The cephalosporins are excreted into breast milk in sufficiently low concentrations that the infant receives an insignificant dose. Although the same theoretical concerns exist as with penicillins, the advantages of continued breastfeeding during treatment usually outweigh any potential risks.

Sulfonamides

Studies of several thousand human infants to investigate the potential risk of exposure to sulfonamides during the first trimester of pregnancy have found no evidence of teratogenic effects.[1,13]

Sulfonamides cause no known damage to the fetus *in utero* because the fetus can clear free bilirubin through the placenta. However, these drugs might theoretically have deleterious effects if present in the blood of the neonate after birth. The sulfonamides compete with bilirubin for binding sites on albumin, thus raising the levels of free bilirubin in the serum and increasing the risk of hyperbilirubinemia or kernicterus in the neonate.[14] For that reason, it is recommended that an alternative antibiotic is used during the third trimester if possible. However, kernicterus in the neonate has been reported only with neonatal administration, not following *in utero* exposure.

The sulfonamides are easily absorbed orally and readily cross the placenta, achieving fetal plasma levels that are 50–90% of those attained in the maternal plasma. The maternal serum levels of the drug are similar to those in nonpregnant individuals.[15]

Trimethoprim, a folate antagonist in bacterial systems, is often given with a sulfa drug for the treatment of urinary tract infections. Two small trials including 131 women failed to show any increased risk of birth defects after first-trimester exposure.[16,17] However, in 2296 Michigan Medicaid recipients, first-trimester trimethoprim exposure was associated with an increased risk of birth defects, particularly cardiovascular,[18] and in retrospective studies the risk of cardiovascular defects and oral clefts was increased two- to threefold.[19,20]

Sulfonamides are excreted into breast milk in low concentrations.[13] The amount of sulfonamide ingested by an infant is sufficiently low not to have any toxicity (less than 2% of the maternal dose) and so breastfeeding is usually continued during administration of these drugs. However, the administration of sulfa drugs to infants who are ill, stressed, or jaundiced, or who have glucose-6-phosphate dehydrogenase (G6PD) deficiency, is best avoided.[13] With these precautions, the American Academy of Pediatrics considers sulfonamides compatible with breastfeeding.[21] Trimethoprim is also excreted in breast milk in small amounts, and is compatible with breast feeding.

Nitrofurantoin

A link between the use of nitrofurantoin and congenital defects has not been reported. In the Collaborative Perinatal Project,[1] no significantly increased risk of anomalies or other adverse effects were seen in 590 infants exposed to nitrofurantoin during pregnancy (83 during the first trimester). In the Michigan Medicaid data,[22] 1292 infants were exposed during the first trimester with no increased risk of birth defects.

Nitrofurantoin absorption from the gastrointestinal tract varies depending on the form of drug administered. The macrocrystalline form is absorbed more slowly than the crystalline form and is associated with less gastrointestinal intolerance. Therapeutic serum levels are not achieved; therefore, this drug is not indicated when there is a possibility of bacteremia, such as with pyelonephritis.

Nitrofurantoin is excreted into breast milk in very low concentrations; the drug could not be detected in 20 samples taken from mothers receiving a dose of 100 mg, four times a day.[23,24]

Tetracyclines

The tetracyclines readily cross the placenta and are firmly bound by chelating to calcium in developing bone and tooth structures.[25] This causes brown discoloration of the teeth, hypoplasia of the enamel, inhibition of bone growth,[26] and other skeletal abnormalities. The yellowish-brown staining of the teeth usually occurs after 24 weeks' gestation, during the second or third trimester, whereas bone incorporation can occur earlier. Depression of skeletal growth is particularly common among premature infants treated with tetracycline. At present, alternative antibiotics are recommended during pregnancy.

Hepatotoxicity has been reported in pregnant women treated with large doses (2.4–4 g daily) of intravenous tetracyclines. This is dose related and has not been reported with brief courses of therapy.

First-trimester exposure to tetracycline was not found to have any teratogenic risk in 341 pregnant women in the Collaborative Perinatal Project,[1] or in 174 women in a second study.[2] A third study looking at the effect of exposure to doxycycline in 63 women also found no teratogenic risk.[27]

Tetracycline is excreted into breast milk in low concentrations. It is not detectable in the serum of breastfeeding infants, and delayed bone growth from tetracycline has not been reported in breastfed infants. This may be the result of the high binding capacity of the drug for calcium and protein, limiting absorption from the milk. The American Academy of Pediatrics considers tetracycline to be compatible with breastfeeding.[21]

Aminoglycosides

Gentamicin is preferred to tobramycin and amikacin, as it has been more extensively studied in pregnancy. Streptomycin and kanamycin have been associated with congenital deafness in the offspring of mothers who took these drugs during pregnancy. In one study,[28] the administration of 1 g of streptomycin twice weekly for 8 weeks during the first trimester resulted in ototoxicity. A second study[29] found that, out of the children born to 391 mothers who had received 50 mg/kg of kanamycin for prolonged periods during pregnancy, nine had hearing loss (2.3%).

Nephrotoxicity may be increased when aminoglycosides are given in combination with cephalosporins, and this should be avoided. Neuromuscular blockade may be potentiated by the combined use of these drugs and curariform drugs; therefore, the dosages should be reduced appropriately. Potentiation of magnesium sulfate-induced neuromuscular weakness has been reported in a neonate exposed to magnesium sulfate and gentamicin.[30]

Ototoxicity is the only known teratogenic effect associated with the use of these drugs during the first trimester of pregnancy.[31] No teratogenic effects were observed in 135 infants exposed to streptomycin in the Collaborative Perinatal Project.[1] In addition, in a group of 1619 newborns whose mothers were treated with multiple drugs, including streptomycin, for tuberculosis during pregnancy, the incidence of congenital defects was the same as that of the healthy control group.[32]

The aminoglycosides are poorly absorbed after oral administration and are rapidly excreted by the normal kidney. Because the rate of clearance is related to the glomerular filtration rate, dosage must be reduced in cases of abnormal renal function and increased during pregnancy.

The serum aminoglycoside levels are usually lower in pregnant than in nonpregnant patients receiving equivalent doses because of more rapid elimination. Thus, it is important to monitor levels to prevent subtherapeutic dosing,[33,34] as wide interpatient variation in gentamicin levels has been observed in obstetric patients. At full term, the concentrations of gentamicin in fetal blood are lower than those in maternal blood.[35]

Once-a-day dosing (7 mg/kg ideal body weight every 24 h) is recommended for gentamicin because this increases efficacy[36] while decreasing toxicity and cost.[37] This dosing schedule has been studied in patients with chorioamnionitis and endometritis and has been shown to be safe and effective.[38]

Small amounts of gentamicin are excreted into breast milk;[39] because oral absorption of these drugs by the infant is poor, side-effects are not expected.

Macrolides

There have been no reports of a link between the use of erythromycin and teratogenicity. Furthermore, there was no increased risk of birth defects noted in 79 patients in the Collaborative Perinatal Project[1] nor in 6972 patients in the Michigan Medicaid data.[40,41] There was no increased risk of birth defects in a study of 122 infants exposed during the first trimester to clarithromycin.[42]

Erythromycin and its salts are not consistently absorbed from the gastrointestinal tract of pregnant women, and transplacental passage is unpredictable. Both maternal and fetal serum levels achieved after the administration of the drug in pregnancy vary considerably and may be low.[43] For the treatment of syphilis in pregnancy, desensitization and administration of penicillin is still the method of choice because erythromycin therapy often fails.[44] Fetal plasma concentrations are 5–20% of those in maternal plasma. The usual oral dose is 250–500 mg every 6 h, although the higher dose may not be tolerated well in pregnant women, who are susceptible to nausea and gastrointestinal symptoms.

Erythromycin is excreted into breast milk in small amounts; however, no reports of adverse effects have been noted in infants exposed to erythromycin in breast milk.[40]

Lincosamides

Of 647 infants exposed to clindamycin during the first trimester, no increased risk of birth defects was noted.[45] Clindamycin crosses the placenta, achieving maximum cord serum levels of approximately 50% of the maternal serum.[43] When assessed at various stages of pregnancy, maternal serum levels after dosing were found to be similar to those of nonpregnant patients.[33]

Clindamycin is excreted into breast milk in low levels, and nursing is usually continued during administration of this drug.[45] The American Academy of Pediatrics considers the use of clindamycin to be compatible with breastfeeding.[21]

Fluoroquinolones

The fluoroquinolones (e.g., ciprofloxacin, levofloxacin, norfloxacin) have a high affinity for bone tissue and cartilage and may cause arthropathies in children. However, no malformations or musculoskeletal problems were noted in 38 infants exposed *in utero* during the first trimester in one study,[46] or in 134 cases in a second study.[47] An international multicenter study[48] prospectively followed 200 pregnant women exposed to quinolones and compared them with a control group of pregnant women exposed to nonteratogenic antimicrobials. The rates of teratogenicity and achievement of developmental milestones were reported. There were no differences in the major malformations or musculoskeletal dysfunctions between the two groups; however, the manufacturer recommends that fluoroquinolones are not used during pregnancy or in children. Gatifloxacin and moxifloxacin have not been studied in pregnant women.

Ciprofloxacin is excreted in breast milk in small amounts, and the use of quinolones during breastfeeding has not been recommended because of the theoretical potential for arthropathy in the infant. The manufacturer recommends that, before breastfeeding is resumed, 48 h elapse after administration of the last dose;[49] however, the American Academy of Pediatrics considers the use of ciprofloxacin to be compatible with breastfeeding.[21]

Metronidazole

Controversy regarding the use of metronidazole during pregnancy began when the drug was shown to be positive in the Ames test, which correlates with carcinogenicity in animals. However, the doses used were much higher than the doses used clinically, and carcinogenicity in humans has not been confirmed.[50]

Studies have failed to show any increase in the incidence of congenital defects among the newborns of mothers treated with metronidazole during early or late gestation. In a study of 1387 prescriptions filled, the risk of birth defects could not be determined;[51] a subsequent meta-analysis confirmed no teratogenic risk.[52]

Metronidazole is excreted into breast milk in small amounts. The American Academy of Pediatrics recommends interrupting breastfeeding for 12–24 h after a single oral dose of 2 g to allow clearance of the drug.[21]

Acyclovir and valaciclovir

The Acyclovir in Pregnancy Registry recorded 1695 exposures during pregnancy from 1984 to 1998 (including 756 during the first trimester), with no increased risk of abnormalities in the infants.[53] In addition, maternal systemic acyclovir treatment has been used near term to prevent recurrent genital herpes, with no adverse effects on the infants.[54,55] The Centers for Disease Control and Prevention (CDC) recommends that pregnant women with disseminated infection, e.g., herpetic encephalitis or hepatitis or varicella pneumonia, be treated with acyclovir.[56]

Valaciclovir is rapidly converted to acyclovir, and the level in breast milk is 2% of that of the maternal serum level, which is far less than the therapeutic dose for neonates.[57]

Antiretrovirals

In general, pregnancy should not preclude using the optimal regimen of antiviral therapy. Combination antiretroviral therapy, usually consisting of two nucleoside analog reverse transcriptase inhibitors and a protease inhibitor, is the recommended therapy for HIV-infected nonpregnant adults. However, it is important to take account of the circumstances before selecting the appropriate antiretroviral regimen during pregnancy.

Zidovudine (ZDV) should be included in the regimen whenever possible because of its excellent safety record and efficacy. In a prospective cohort study,[58] children exposed to ZDV during the perinatal period as a result of the Pediatric AIDS Clinical Trials Group Protocol 076 were studied up to a median age of 4.2 years, with no adverse effects observed in these children. The International Antiretroviral Registry was established in 1989 to detect any major teratogenic effects of antiretroviral drugs. Up to January 2004, over 1000 pregnancies had first-trimester exposures to ZDV and lamivudine with no reported increase in teratogenicity.[59]

Concerns have been raised regarding the use of some antiretroviral therapies in pregnancy. Efavirenz is not recommended during pregnancy because of reports of significant fetal malformations in monkeys who received efavirenz during the first trimester of pregnancy, and also three case reports of fetal neural tube defects in women who received the drug.[60] In 2001, Bristol–Myers Squibb issued a warning advising against the use of didanosine and stavudine in pregnant women because of case reports of lactic acidosis, including fatalities.[61] These two drugs should be used only if no alternatives are available.

Breastfeeding is not recommended in women with HIV infection, as the virus is transmitted in milk. However, one study has shown that women who received ZDV during pregnancy, labor, and for a week postpartum had a 38% reduction in the vertical transmission of HIV, despite breastfeeding, compared with control subjects.[62]

Anti-influenza drugs

Four drugs are currently recommended for the prevention or treatment of influenza in the USA: amantadine, rimantadine,

Table 19.1 Teratogenic effects of antibiotics and anti-infective agents.

Drug	First-trimester teratogen	Perinatal effects	Compatible with lactation
Penicillins	No	No	Yes
Amoxicillin/clavulanate	No	Necrotizing enterocolitis in premature infants	Yes
Cephalosporins	Unclear: may be specific to cephalosporin	No	Yes
Sulfamethoxazole	No	Competes with bilirubin for albumin binding sites; increased risk of jaundice	Yes, except in ill or premature infants
Trimethoprim	Possible	No	Yes
Nitrofurantoin	No	No	Yes
Tetracyclines	No	Tooth discoloration, decreased bone growth	Yes
Aminoglycosides	No	Ototoxicity (deafness)	Yes
Erythromycin	No	No	Yes
Clindamycin	No	No	Yes
Fluoroquinolones	No	Arthropathies in exposed children?	Yes
Metronidazole	No	No	Unknown
Acyclovir	No	No	Yes
Zidovudine	No	No	Yes
Amantidine	Possible	Unknown	Unknown
Isoniazid	No	Maternal hepatitis	Yes

zanamivir, and oseltamivir. In a surveillance study of Medicaid recipients, 64 pregnant women were exposed to amantadine during the first trimester.[63] Five of their infants were diagnosed with congenital anomalies, which was higher than the expected number of three. The CDC states that, because of the unknown effects of influenza antiviral drugs on pregnant women and their fetuses, they should be used during pregnancy only if the potential benefit justifies the potential risk to the embryo or fetus.[64]

Amantadine is excreted into breast milk in low concentrations. The manufacturer recommends that it is not used in nursing mothers; it has not been evaluated by the American Academy of Pediatrics.[65]

Isoniazid

There is no evidence of any teratogenic effect of isoniazid (INH).[66] The American Thoracic Society and the American College of Obstetricians and Gynecologists state that treatment with INH for patients with a positive purified protein derivative (PPD) test with a negative chest radiograph should be delayed until after delivery because of a small risk of maternal liver toxicity.[67] A recent decision analysis recommends starting treatment at 20 weeks antepartum.[68] However, if the probability of active tuberculosis is moderate to high, the American Thoracic Society and CDC recommend initiating therapy with INH, rifampin, and ethambutol during pregnancy.[69]

Isoniazid is concentrated in breast milk; however, the American Academy of Pediatrics considers it to be compatible with breastfeeding.[21] The infant should be periodically examined for signs of peripheral neuritis or hepatitis.[70]

Conclusions

Most antibiotics are safe to use during pregnancy but, as there is the potential for fetal effects that are still unrecognized, they should be used only when clearly indicated. A summary of drug effects in pregnancy and lactation is presented in Table 19.1.

Key points

1 Penicillin and its derivatives are safe for use in pregnancy.
2 Amoxicillin/clavulanic acid should be avoided in women at risk for preterm delivery as it increases the risk of necrotizing enterocolitis in the premature infant.
3 Sulfonamides cause no harm to the fetus *in utero* as the fetus can clear free bilirubin through the placenta. In the neonate, they increase the risk of hyperbilirubinemia.
4 Trimethoprim should not be given during the first trimester of pregnancy as it is a weak folic acid antagonist and has been associated with a threefold increased risk of cardiovascular defects and oral clefts.
5 Nitrofurantoin does not achieve therapeutic serum levels and is inadequate therapy for pyelonephritis.
6 The tetracyclines bind to and inhibit developing bones and teeth during the second and third trimesters of pregnancy and are contraindicated at that time.
7 Once-a-day dosing is recommended for gentamicin as it increases efficacy and decreases toxicity and cost.
8 Erythromycin is inadequate therapy for syphilis. For penicillin-allergic patients, desensitization and treatment with penicillin is recommended.
9 Fluoroquinolones have a high affinity for bone and cartilage and the manufacturer recommends against their use in pregnancy.
10 Studies have failed to show any risks of metronidazole in pregnancy.
11 In patients with recurrent herpetic infections of the vulva, prophylactic acyclovir in the last month of pregnancy can prevent recurrences and the need for Cesarean sections.
12 Pregnant women with varicella pneumonia should receive acyclovir.
13 Pregnant women with HIV should receive combination antiretroviral therapy that includes zidovudine (ZDV).
14 Breastfeeding is not recommended in women with HIV as the virus is transmitted through breast milk.
15 A combination antiretroviral regimen that includes both didanosine and stavudine should be avoided because of the risks of lactic acidosis.
16 Pregnant women with a positive purified protein derivative (PPD) and a negative chest radiograph should have therapy with isoniazid (INH) postponed until after delivery because of a small risk of maternal liver toxicity.
17 Treatment of active tuberculosis during pregnancy should be initiated with INH, rifampin and ethambutol.
18 Efavirenz is not recommended during pregnancy because of reports of malformations in monkeys and fetal neural tube defects in women who received the drug.
19 All antibiotics are compatible with breastfeeding except for sulfonamides when the infant is ill or premature, and possibly metronidazole and amantadine, whose effects are unknown.
20 Gentamicin is poorly absorbed orally by the infant and is safe during lactation.

References

1 Heinonen PO, Slone D, Shapiro S. *Birth defects and drugs in pregnancy*. Littleton, MA: Publishing Sciences Group, 1977.
2 Aselton P, Jick H, Milunsky A, et al. First-trimester drug use and congenital disorders. *Obstet Gynecol* 1985;65:451.
3 Heikkila AM, Erkkola RU. The need for adjustment of dosage regimen of penicillin V during pregnancy. *Obstet Gynecol* 1993; 81:919.
4 Briggs GG, Freeman RK, Yaffe SJ. *Drugs in pregnancy and lactation*, 6th edn. Baltimore, MD: Williams and Wilkins; 2002:1078.
5 Briggs GG, Freeman RK, Yaffe SJ. *Drugs in pregnancy and lactation*, 6th edn. Baltimore, MD: Williams and Wilkins; 2002:284.
6 Kenyon S, Boulvain M, Neilson J. Antibiotics for preterm rupture of the membranes: a systematic review. *Obstet Gynecol* 2004;104:1051.
7 Kenyon SL, Taylor DJ, Tarnow-Mordi W. Broad-spectrum antibiotics for preterm, prelabour rupture of fetal membranes: the ORACLE I randomised trial. ORACLE Collaborative Group. *Lancet* 2001;357:979.
8 Kafetzis D, Siafas C, Georgakopoulos P, Papadatos C. Passage of cephalosporins and amoxicillin into the breast milk. *Acta Paediatr Scand* 1981;70:285.
9 Depp R, Kind A, Kirby W, Johnson W. Transplacental passage of methicillin and dicloxacillin into the fetus and amniotic fluid. *Am J Obstet Gynecol* 1970;107:1054.
10 Briggs GG, Freeman RK, Yaffe SJ. *Drugs in pregnancy and lactation*, 6th edn. Baltimore, MD: Williams and Wilkins; 2002:222.
11 Czeizel AE, Rockenbauer M, Sorensen HT, et al. Use of cephalosporins during pregnancy and in the presence of congenital abnormalities: a population-based, case–control study. *Am J Obstet Gynecol* 2001;184:1289.
12 Nathorst-Boos J, Philipson A, Hedman A, et al. Renal elimination of ceftazidime during pregnancy. *Am J Obstet Gynecol* 1995;172:163.
13 Briggs GG, Freeman RK, Yaffe SJ. *Drugs in pregnancy and lactation*, 6th edn. Baltimore, MD: Williams and Wilkins; 2002:1293.
14 Harris RC, Lucey JF, MacLean JR. Kernicterus in premature infants associated with low concentration of bilirubin in the plasma. *Pediatrics* 1950;23:878.
15 Ylikorkala O, Sjostedt E, Jarvinen PA, et al. Trimethoprim-sulfonamide combination administered orally and intravaginally

in the first trimester of pregnancy: its absorption into serum and transfer to amniotic fluid. *Acta Obstet Gynecol Scand* 1973; 52:229.
16 Colley DP, Kay J, Gibson GT. A study of the use in pregnancy of co-trimoxazole and sulfamethizole. *Aust J Pharm* 1982;63:570.
17 Bailey RR. Single-dose antibacterial treatment for bacteriuria in pregnancy. *Drugs* 1984;27:183.
18 Briggs GG, Freeman RK, Yaffe SJ. *Drugs in pregnancy and lactation*, 6th edn. Baltimore, MD: Williams and Wilkins; 2002:1393.
19 Czeizel A. A case–control analysis of the teratogenic effects of co-trimoxazole. *Reprod Toxicol* 1990;4:305.
20 Hernandez-Diaz S, Werler MM, Walker AM, et al. Folic acid antagonists during pregnancy and the risk of birth defects. *N Engl J Med* 2000;343:1608.
21 Committee on Drugs. American Academy of Pediatrics. The transfer of drugs and other chemicals into human milk. *Pediatrics* 2001;108:776.
22 Briggs GG, Freeman RK, Yaffe SJ. *Drugs in pregnancy and lactation*, 6th edn. Baltimore, MD: Williams and Wilkins; 2002:1000.
23 Hosbach RE, Foster RB. Absence of nitrofurantoin from human milk. *JAMA* 1967;202:1057.
24 Varsano I, Fischl J, Shochet SB. The excretion of orally ingested nitrofurantoin in human milk. *J Pediatr* 1973;82:886.
25 Kline AH, Blattner RJ, Lunin M. Transplacental effects of tetracycline on teeth. *JAMA* 1964;118:178.
26 Cohlan SQ, Bevelander G, Tiamsic T. Growth inhibition of prematures receiving tetracycline. *Am J Dis Child* 1963;105:453.
27 Czeizel AE, Rockenbauer M. Teratogenic study of doxycycline. *Obstet Gynecol* 1997;89:524.
28 Robinson GC, Cambon KG. Hearing loss in infants of tuberculous mothers treated with streptomycin during pregnancy. *N Engl J Med* 1964;271:949.
29 Nishimura H, Tanimura T. *Clinical aspects of the teratogenicity of drugs*. Amsterdam: Excerpta Medica; 1976:131.
30 L'Hommedieu CS, Nicholas D, Armes DA, et al. Potentiation of magnesium sulfate-induced neuromuscular weakness by gentamicin, tobramycin, and amikacin. *J Pediatr* 1983;102:629.
31 Czeizel AE, Rockenbauer M, Olsen J, et al. A teratological study of aminoglycoside antibiotic treatment during pregnancy. *Scand J Infect Dis* 2000;32:309.
32 Marynowski A, Sianozecka E. Comparison of the incidence of congenital malformations in neonates from healthy mothers and from patients treated because of tuberculosis. *Ginekol Pol* 1972; 43:713.
33 Weinstein AJ, Gibbs RS, Gallagher M. Placental transfer of clindamycin and gentamicin in term pregnancy. *Am J Obstet Gynecol* 1976;124:688.
34 Zaske DE, Cipolle RJ, Strate RG, et al. Rapid gentamicin elimination in obstetric patients. *Obstet Gynecol* 1980;56:559.
35 Yoshioka H, Monma T, Matsuda S. Placental transfer of gentamicin. *J Pediatr* 1972;80:121.
36 Nicolau DP, Freeman CD, Belliveau PP, et al. Experience with a once-daily aminoglycoside program administered to 2,184 adult patients. *Antimicrob Agents Chemother* 1995;39:650.
37 Munckhof WJ, Grayson ML, Turnidge JD. A meta-analysis of studies on the safety and efficacy of aminoglycosides given either once daily or as divided doses. *J Antimicrob Chemother* 1996; 37:645.
38 Mitra AG, Whitten K, Laurent SL, et al. A randomized, prospective study comparing once-daily gentamicin versus thrice-daily gentamicin in the treatment of puerperal infection. *Am J Obstet Gynecol* 1997;177:786.
39 Celiloglu M, Celiker S, Guven H, et al. Gentamicin excretion and uptake from breast milk by nursing infants. *Obstet Gynecol* 1994;84:263.
40 Briggs GG, Freeman RK, Yaffe SJ. *Drugs in pregnancy and lactation*, 6th edn. Baltimore, MD; Williams and Wilkins; 2002:502.
41 Louik C, Werler MM, Mitchell AA. Erythromycin use during pregnancy in relation to pyloric stenosis. *Am J Obstet Gynecol* 2002;186:288.
42 Einarson A, Phillips E, Mawji F, et al. A prospective controlled multicentre study of clarithromycin in pregnancy. *Am J Perinatol* 1998;15:523.
43 Philipson A, Sabath LD, Charles D. Transplacental passage of erythromycin and clindamycin. *N Engl J Med* 1973;288:1219.
44 South MA, Short DH, Knox JM. Failure of erythromycin estolate therapy in *in utero* syphilis. *JAMA* 1964;190:70.
45 Briggs GG, Freeman RK, Yaffe SJ. *Drugs in pregnancy and lactation*, 6th edn. Baltimore, MD; Williams and Wilkins; 2002:286.
46 Berkovitch M, Pastuszak A, Gazarian M, et al. Safety of the new quinolones in pregnancy. *Obstet Gynecol* 1994;84:535.
47 Pastuszak A, Andreou R, Schick B, et al. New postmarketing surveillance data supports a lack of association between quinolone use in pregnancy and fetal and neonatal complications. *Reprod Toxicol* 1995;9:584.
48 Loebstein R, Addis A, Ho E, et al. Pregnancy outcome following gestational exposure to fluoroquinolones: a multicenter prospective controlled study. *Antimicrob Agents Chemother* 1998;42: 1336.
49 Briggs GG, Freeman RK, Yaffe SJ. *Drugs in pregnancy and lactation*, 6th edn. Baltimore, MD; Williams and Wilkins; 2002:271.
50 Beard CM, Noller KL, O'Fallon WM, et al. Lack of evidence for cancer due to use of metronidazole. *N Engl J Med* 1979;301:519.
51 Piper JM, Mitchel EF, Ray WA. Prenatal use of metronidazole and birth defects: no association. *Obstet Gynecol* 1993;82:348.
52 Burtin P, Taddio A, Ariburnu O, et al. Safety of metronidazole in pregnancy: A meta-analysis. *Am J Obstet Gynecol* 1995;172:525.
53 Stone KM, Reiff-Eldridge R, White AD, et al. Pregnancy outcomes following systemic prenatal acyclovir exposure: conclusions from the international acyclovir pregnancy registry, 1984–1999. *Birth Defects Res Part A Clin Mol Teratol* 2004;70:201.
54 Scott LL, Sanchez PJ, Jackson GL, et al. Acyclovir suppression to prevent cesarean delivery after first-episode genital herpes. *Obstet Gynecol* 1996:87:69.
55 Watts HD, Brown ZA, Money D, et al. A double-blind, randomized, placebo-controlled trial of acyclovir in late pregnancy for the reduction of herpes simplex virus shedding and cesarean delivery. *Am J Obstet Gynecol* 2003;188:836.
56 Andrews EB, Yankaskas BC, Cordero JF, et al. Acyclovir in pregnancy registry: six years' experience. *Obstet Gynecol* 1992;79:7.
57 Sheffield JS, Fish DN, Hollier LM. Acyclovir concentrations in human breast milk after valaciclovir administration. *Am J Obstet Gynecol* 2002;186:100.
58 Culnane M, Fowler MG, Lee SS, et al. Lack of long-term effects of *in utero* exposure to zidovudine among uninfected children born to HIV-infected women. *JAMA* 1999;281:151.
59 Antiretroviral Pregnancy Registry Steering Committee. Antiretroviral Pregnancy Registry International Interim Report for 1 January 1989 through 31 January 2004. Wilmington, NC: Registry Coordinating Center; 2004. World Wide Web URL: www.apregristry.com.
60 Perinatal HIV Guidelines Working Group. Public Health Service Task Force. Recommendations for use of antiretroviral drugs in pregnant HIV-1-infected women for maternal health and interventions to reduce perinatal HIV-1 transmission in the United

States. June 23, 2004. World Wide Web URL: http://AIDSinfo.nih.gov.

61 Bristol-Myers Squibb. Important drug warning. World Wide Web URL: http://www.fda.gov/medwatch/safety/2001/zerit&videx letter.htm.

62 Dabis F, Msellati P, Meda N, et al. 6-month efficacy, tolerance, and acceptability of a short regimen of oral zidovudine to reduce vertical transmission of HIV in breastfed children in Côte d'lvoire and Burkina Faso: a double-blind placebo-controlled multicentre trial. DITRAME Study Group. *Lancet* 1999;353:786.

63 Rosa F. Amantadine pregnancy experience. *Reprod Toxicol* 1994;8:531.

64 Centers for Disease Control and Prevention. Prevention and control of influenza. Recommendations of the advisory committee on immunization practices. *Morb Mort Wkly Rep* 2000; 49(RR-03):1.

65 Briggs GG, Freeman RK, Yaffe SJ. *Drugs in pregnancy and lactation*, 6th edn. Baltimore, MD; Williams and Wilkins; 2002:45.

66 Briggs GG, Freeman RK, Yaffe SJ. *Drugs in pregnancy and lactation*. 6th edn. Baltimore, MD; Williams and Wilkins; 2002:731.

67 American Thoracic Society. Treatment of tuberculosis and tuberculosis infection in adults and children. *Am J Respir Crit Care Med* 1994;149:1359.

68 Boggess KA, Myers ER, Hamilton CD. Antepartum or postpartum isoniazid treatment of latent tuberculosis infection. *Obstet Gynecol* 2000;96:757.

69 Blumberg HM, Burman WJ, Chaisson RE, et al. American Thoracic Society/Centers for Disease Control and Prevention/Infectious Diseases Society of America: treatment of tuberculosis. *Am J Respir Crit Care Med* 2003;167:603.

70 Briggs GG, Freeman RK, Yaffe SJ. *Drugs in pregnancy and lactation*, 6th edn. Baltimore, MD; Williams and Wilkins; 2002:732.

Part VI

Fetal Diseases

20 Principles of human genetics: chromosomal and single-gene disorders

Joe Leigh Simpson and Maurice J. Mahoney

Genetic disorders can result from any one of several mechanisms: numerical or structural alterations in chromosomal constitution, mutation involving a single genetic locus (mendelian), or the cumulative effect of several genes (polygenic), possibly interacting with environmental factors (multifactoral). In this chapter, the major principles underlying these genetic mechanisms are reviewed. Perturbations of these mechanisms are responsible for most of the disorders whose diagnosis is considered elsewhere in Part VI.

Chromosomal analysis

Chromosomal analyses are usually performed on peripheral blood (lymphocytes) or fibroblasts cultured from skin, gonads, chorionic villi (mesenchyme), or amniotic fluid cells. Very rapidly dividing cells (e.g., bone marrow, chorionic villus trophoblasts, fetal cord blood, newborn cord blood, or cancer cells) may sometimes be analyzed without culturing. Rapid techniques have been developed for the analysis of cord blood or percutaneous umbilical cord blood. Fluorescence *in situ* hybridization (FISH) analysis using chromosome-specific probes can produce results within hours (see below), but it provides information only on the chromosomes or chromosome regions tested. This may suffice if a specific disorder (e.g., trisomy 21 or 18) must be excluded; however, the information obtained is obviously more limited than that resulting from a complete chromosomal analysis.

If cultures are necessary, cells are grown in nutrient media to which various growth factors are usually added. A specified period of growth is typical for a given tissue: overnight for bone marrow, cord blood, and chorionic villus trophoblasts; 48–72 h for peripheral blood; and 7–14 days for chorionic villus mesenchyme or amniotic fluid cells. The preparation of cells for chromosomal analysis usually requires the sequential addition of: (1) colchicine or desoxymethylcolchicine to accumulate metaphases; (2) a hypotonic solution that causes cells to swell; (3) an acetic acid–methanol solution to fix cells permanently; and (4) a dye to enhance chromosome visibility. Traditionally, metaphases were photographed, prints developed, and individual chromosomes aligned (Fig. 20.1) Automated systems can now produce karyotypes directly from metaphases. Published karyotypes usually portray realigned chromosomes rather than the original metaphase. Analysis generally requires counting 15–20 cells and karyotyping 2–5 of them. Not all cells are intact; some will have been damaged ("broken") in preparation and have hypodiploid counts. This technical point is clinically relevant because approximately 2% of chorionic villi or amniotic fluid specimens contain one or more spurious cells. A single hypodiploid cell is unlikely to have clinical significance.

Sometimes, two or more cell lines exist in a single individual, a phenomenon called *mosaicism*. Because mosaicism arises during embryogenesis, not all tissues show the same complements. Of additional relevance to the obstetrician is that the complements in chorionic villus trophoblasts may differ not only from the complements of cultured chorionic villus mesenchyme but also from those of the embryo.[1]

Routine cytogenetic analysis usually reveals approximately 450–500 bands per haploid set of chromosomes. Using high-resolution chromosomal analysis, it is often possible to obtain a resolution of about 1000 bands. At this level, each band consists of approximately 3000–4000 kilobases (kb) of DNA, which are capable of translating about 30–40 genes. Therefore, deletions, duplications, and rearrangements involving considerable stretches of DNA can pass undetected, even with high-resolution chromosomal analysis.

Molecular cytogenetic analysis and fluorescence *in situ* hybridization

Exciting and useful advances have resulted from merging molecular techniques with traditional cytogenetics. The basic principle involves identifying a DNA sequence specific for a given chromosome and then making the sequence fluorescent for the purpose of cytological identification. In FISH analysis, a single-stranded DNA probe hybridizes to its complementary

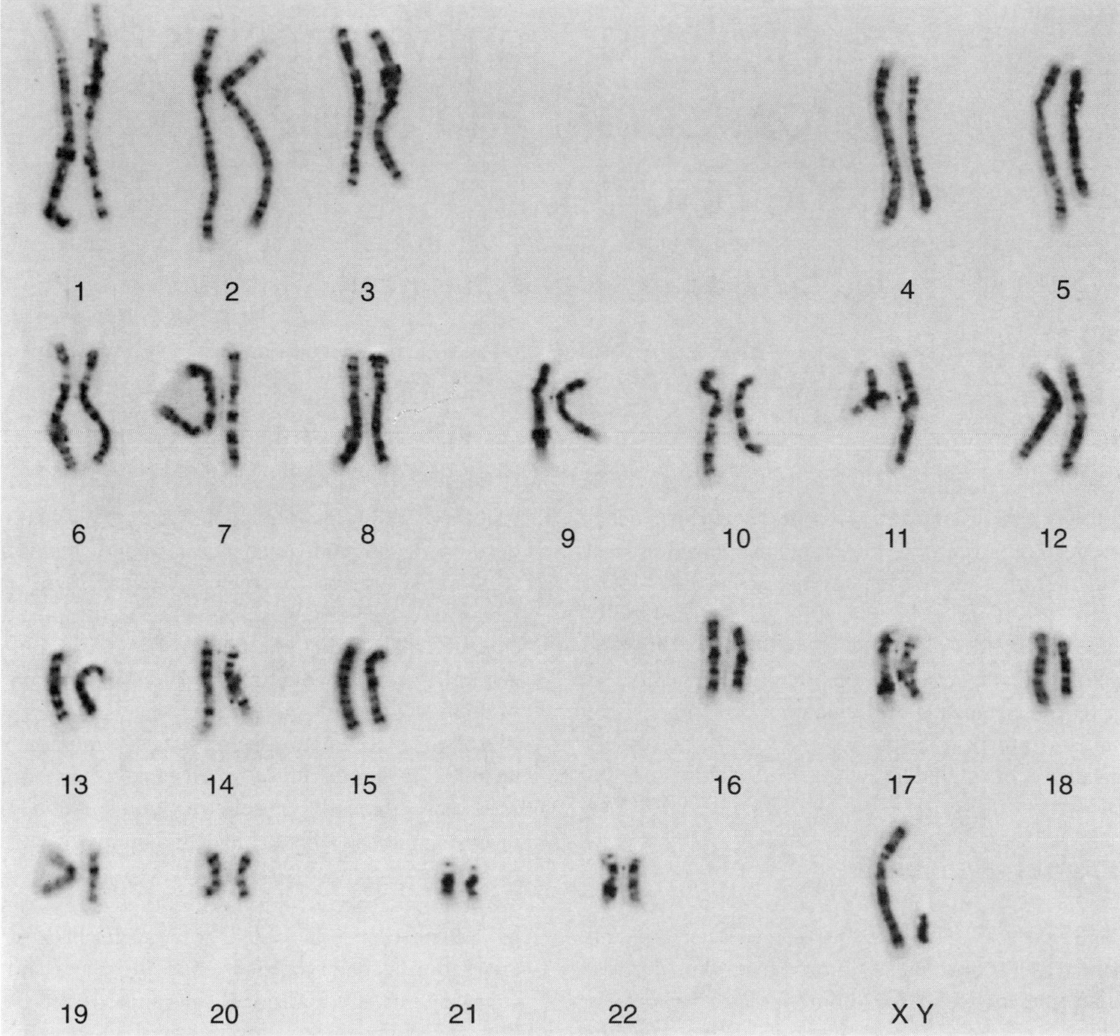

Figure 20.1 Karyotype of normal male (46,XY) G bands. (From ref. 26, with permission.)

DNA sequence when that specific sequence is present (Fig. 20.2). The DNA probe may be labeled directly with a fluorochrome or indirectly by adding another compund (e.g., biotin) that is then conjugated secondarily with a fluorochrome. If the probe is labeled directly, the fluor intercalates into the host (unknown) DNA. FISH can be used to derive information from interphase cells (e.g., uncultured amniotic fluid cells).

Using composite probes coupled with suppressive hybridization, whole chromosomes or chromosome segments can be "painted" and uniquely visualized.

Definitions and cytological origin of numerical chromosomal abnormalities

Aneuploidy is the lack of expected number of chromosomes (n or $2n$) in a haploid gamete or diploid cell. If an additional chromosome is present ($2n + 1$), *trisomy* exists. The term *polysomy* is sometimes applied if the additional chromosome is a sex chromosome (e.g., 47,XXY).

There are several cytological mechanisms that can result in trisomy, but in humans it usually arises *de novo* after meiotic or mitotic nondisjunction. Nondisjunction may originate after the failure of homologous chromosomes to disjoin in meiosis I or the failure of sister chromatids to disjoin in either meiosis II or mitosis. In humans, maternal meiosis I is by far the most common cytological origin of autosomal trisomy.[2] Nondisjunction in maternal meiosis I is usually associated with a maternal age effect (Table 20.1), whereas paternal nondisjunction is minimally associated with paternal age.

Irrespective of cytological origin, nondisjunction during meiosis produces aneuploid gametes and the resulting zygote has the identical chromosomal constitution in all cells. By contrast, nondisjunction during mitosis produces two or more cell lines (mosaicism).

Monosomy ($2n - 1$) arises by mechanisms that are similar to those which result in trisomy. Indeed, meiotic nondisjunc-

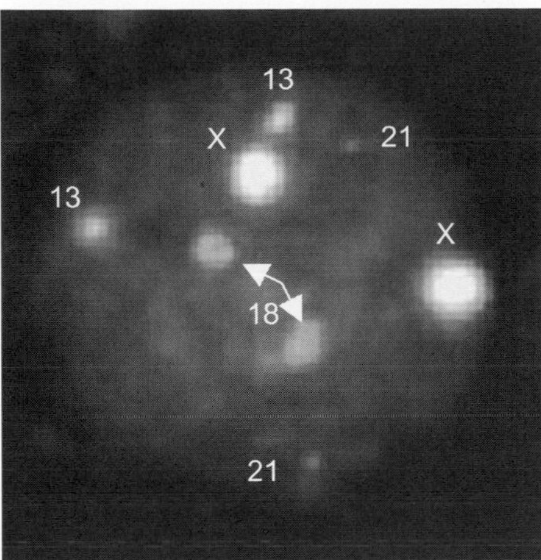

Figure 20.2 Fluorescence *in situ* hybridization (FISH) on a human blastomere biopsied from an eight-cell stage embryo. Fluorescent signals corresponding to specific chromosomes 13, 18, 21, and X are shown, demonstrating detection of a normal female (XX) embryo. Courtesy of Farideh Z. Bischoff, Department of Obstetrics and Gynecology, Baylor College of Medicine, Houston, TX, USA.

tion leading to a disomic gamete also produces a complementary gamete lacking that chromosome. In addition, monosomy may result from a chromosome merely lagging behind and failing to pass to daughter cells *(anaphase lag)*.

In *polyploidy*, more than two haploid sets of chromosomes exist. The most common form of polyploidy is triploidy ($3n = 69$), which may be characterized by either two maternal or two paternal haploid complements. In humans, dispermy is the most common mechanism resulting in polyploidy. Polyploidy is frequently detected among human abortuses but rarely among neonates. Triploidy accounts for 25% of chromosomally abnormal abortuses, or around 10–15% of all first-trimester abortuses.

Table 20.1 Chromosomal abnormalities in liveborns.

Maternal age	Risk of Down syndrome	Total risk of chromosomal abnormalities
20	1/1667	1/526*
21	1/1667	1/526*
22	1/1429	1/500*
23	1/1429	1/500*
24	1/1250	1/476*
25	1/1250	1/476*
26	1/1176	1/476*
27	1/1111	1/455*
28	1/1053	1/435*
29	1/1000	1/417*
30	1/952	1/384*
31	1/909	1/385*
32	1/769	1/322*
33	1/625	1/317
34	1/500	1/260
35	1/385	1/204
36	1/294	1/164
37	1/227	1/130
38	1/175	1/103
39	1/137	1/82
40	1/106	1/65
41	1/82	1/51
42	1/64	1/40
43	1/50	1/32
44	1/38	1/25
45	1/30	1/20
46	1/23	1/15
47	1/18	1/12
48	1/14	1/10
49	1/11	1/7

From ref. 25. Because sample size for some intervals is relatively small, confidence limits are sometimes relatively large. Nonetheless, these figures are suitable for genetic counseling.

*47,XXX excluded for ages 20–32 (data not available).

Definitions and cytological origin of structural chromosomal abnormalities

Minor structural variation (polymorphism) exists among human chromosomes without any apparent phenotypic consequences. Examples include prominent satellites on acrocentric chromosomes (nos. 13, 14, 15, 21, and 22) and variation in the length of the Y long arm. Such "variants" are transmitted in a dominant fashion.

On the other hand, major structural alterations clearly cause phenotypic abnormalities. It can be assumed that many genes are duplicated or deficient; phenotypic abnormalities might also result if the position of a gene is altered with respect to its neighbors *(position effect)*. Several types of chromosomal abnormalities are of clinical relevance.

Chromosomal deletion involves the loss of a portion of a chromosome, either terminal or interstitial. Deficiencies usually result from breakage and loss of an acentric fragment, but may also arise after crossing over within a pericentric inversion loop (see below). Autosomal deficiency usually leads to embryonic death or malformation, but deficiency in a sex chromosome is not necessarily as damaging.

A *translocation* occurs when, after chromosome breakage, material is exchanged between two or more chromosomes (Fig. 20.3). Rearrangement of genes need not necessarily be deleterious, provided that genes are neither lost nor gained. If the individual is phenotypically normal, it is assumed that no genetic material is lost; such a translocation is said to be balanced. If a translocation has led to a deficiency or excess of genetic material, the rearrangement is said to be unbalanced. Even if it is not evident on a karyotype, an unbalanced rearrangement can be assumed if the individual is phenotypically abnormal. If a fetus or offspring shows the same

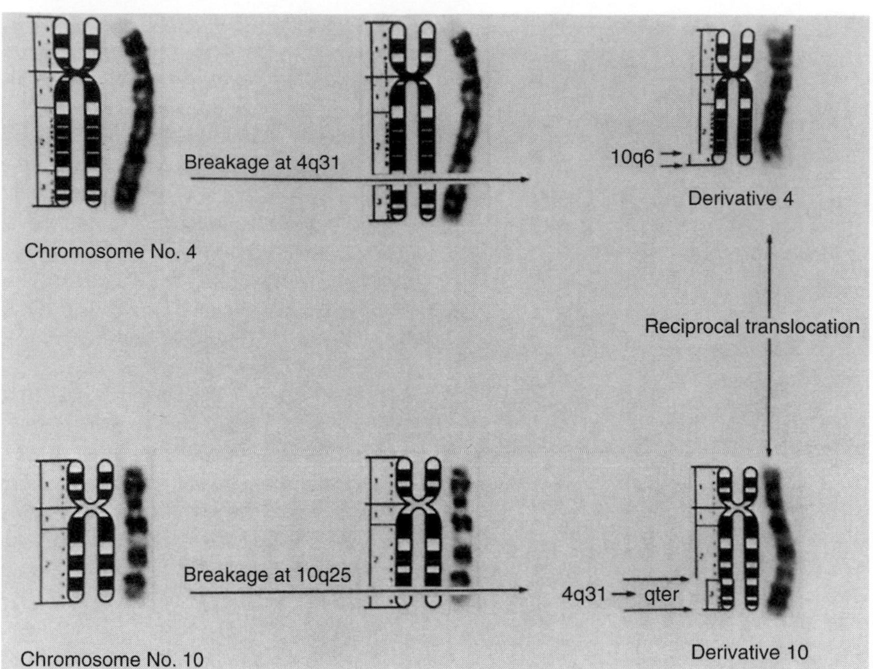

Figure 20.3 A reciprocal translocation between chromosomes 4 and 10. Origin of derivative chromosomes is shown. (From ref. 26, with permission.)

translocation as a normal parent, it can be assumed that the translocation is balanced and the fetus is normal. When a *de novo* translocation is detected in villi or amniotic fluid cells, it is hazardous to assume normalcy even if the translocation seems balanced. A subtle rearrangement may not be recognized, and this accounts for the 10–15% risk of phenotypic abnormality.

Translocations may be either reciprocal or robertsonian. In *reciprocal* translocations, breaks and rearrangements occur in two or more chromosomes but do not involve centromeres (see Fig. 20.3). Thus, translocation heterozygotes still have 46 chromosomes, although two pairs of homologous chromosomes differ in morphology and composition. In *robertsonian* translocations, two of the acrocentric chromosomes (nos. 13, 14, 15, 21, and 22) fuse at their centromere. Because no single acrocentric short arm is essential, heterozygotes are phenotypically normal. These individuals have only 45 chromosomes (centromeres) as a result of the fusion.

Robertsonian translocations

Robertsonian translocations involve the acrocentric chromosomes 13, 14, 15, 21, and 22. The most common single translocation involves chromosomes 14 and 21 (Fig. 20.4); 2–3% of Down syndrome cases result from this translocation. Theoretically, one-third of the viable offspring of translocation heterozygotes should have Down syndrome; however, of the viable offspring of female and male heterozygotes, empirical data reveal that only 10–15% and 2–4%, respectively, have Down syndrome.[3,4] Liveborn normal offspring have an equal likelihood of showing either translocation heterozygosity ($2n = 45$) like their parents or normal chromosomal complements ($2n = 46$).

In translocations involving chromosomes 21 and 22 [t(21;22)], female and male heterozygotes appear to be at a relatively high risk for Down syndrome offspring (10–15%).[3,4] Abnormal liveborn infants are uncommon in most other robertsonian translocations involving two different chromosomes, e.g., in t(13;14) less than 1% of offspring have trisomy 13. These findings are not surprising, given that trisomies 13 and 14 are lethal and rarely result in liveborns. Nonetheless, individuals with any robertsonian translocation should be counseled about antenatal chromosomal studies.

Robertsonian translocations involving homologous chromosomes have a bleak prognosis. Translocations involving chromosome 13 [t(13;13)] or chromosome 21 [t(21;21)] yield only abnormal liveborns or abortions (trisomy 13 or trisomy 21). Homologous translocations involving chromosomes 14, 15, and 22 almost always result in abortions; liveborns with these trisomies have been reported but are very rare. Thus, females with homologous translocations should be counseled about sterilization or donor oocytes, whereas donor sperm can be offered for male heterozygotes.

Reciprocal translocations

Many different reciprocal translocations exist, involving every chromosome, including the acrocentrics. Ideally, empirical data should be available for each translocation; however, at present, only data for general categories exist. Counseling requires attention to the mode of ascertainment.

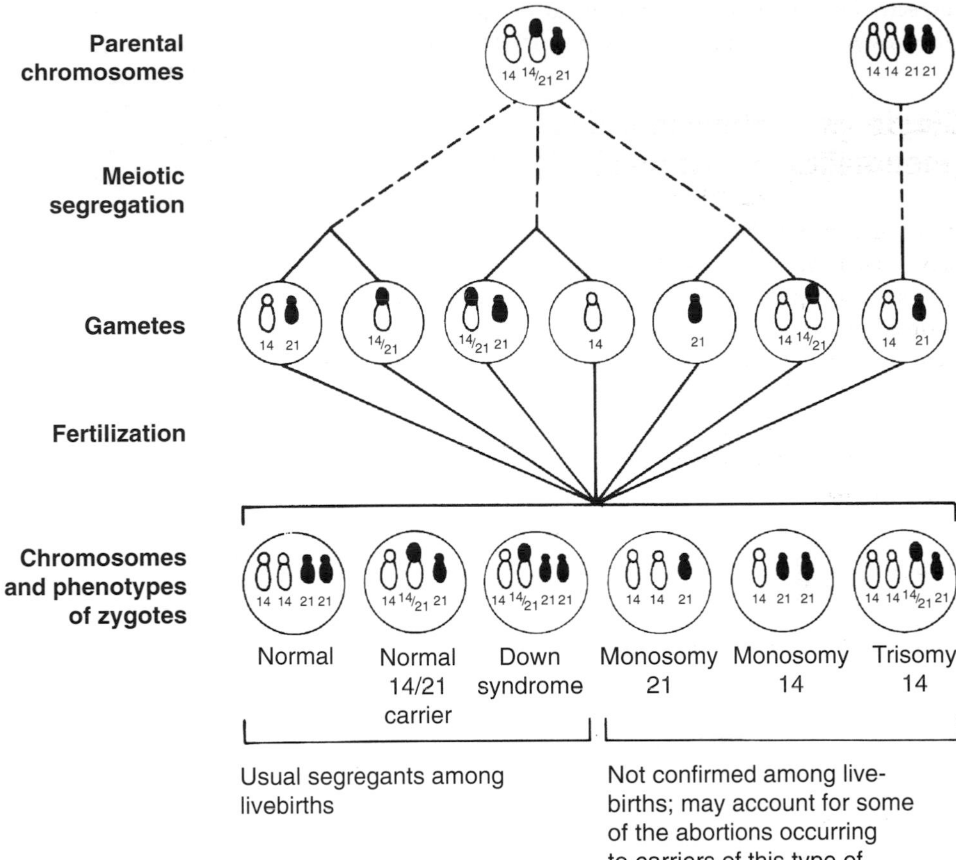

Figure 20.4 Diagram of possible gametes and progeny of a phenotypically normal individual heterozygous for a translocation between chromosomes 14 and 21. Three of the six possible gametes are incompatible with life. The likelihood that an individual with such a translocation would have a child with Down syndrome is thus 33%. However, the empirical risk is considerably less. (From ref. 27.)

A reciprocal translocation may be ascertained in one of several ways: through a balanced (clinically normal) proband that is coincidentally detected (e.g., in a survey), through phenotypically normal couples having repeated abortions, or through an abnormal fetus or infant having an unbalanced karyotype. The risk of a parent having a liveborn child with a chromosomal duplication or deficiency is higher in the last situation than in the first two.[4,5] The lower risk in the first situation presumably reflects selection against unbalanced segregants at the level of the gametes or, more likely, of the embryo. Overall, prenatal diagnosis and surveillance of couples where either the male or female shows a reciprocal translocation indicates that the risk of an unbalanced fetus is approximately 10%.[3,4] Although substantial, these risks are still less than the theoretical risks, which are as high as 50–60% (proportion of unbalanced gametes), assuming random segregation and no crossing over. Daniel and coauthors[6] found that, if ascertained through a full-term unbalanced neonate, the risks in unbalanced amniotic fluid specimens are 19% and 24% for female and male carriers respectively. If ascertained through a couple with repeated abortions, the risks are 3.5% and 1.5%. If ascertained coincidentally, the risks are 5% and 4%. Liveborn offspring who are phenotypically normal are equally likely to have either normal chromosomes (46,XY or 46,XX) or the same two balanced translocation chromosomes that are present in the carrier parent. Although most reciprocal translocations carry an empirical risk of only approximately 10%, the risk is higher for complex rearrangements involving more than two chromosomes[6] and for situations in which 3:1 segregation occurs.

An unresolved question is whether a translocation ascertained through repeated abortions carries a risk for abnormal liveborns that is as high as the risk ascertained through an abnormal liveborn. In the study by Daniel and coauthors,[6] the risks appear to be lower. The question frequently arises because approximately 2–3% of couples who experience repeated abortions show a translocation.[7] The clinician should assume that the risks are similar, irrespective of ascertainment, although this is probably conservative advice.

Sometimes it is not clear whether a *de novo* translocation is balanced or not. An infant with an abnormal phenotype is assumed to have an unbalanced rearrangement. With a normal phenotype, the converse can be assumed. However, such reasoning is hazardous if a *de novo* translocation (or supernumerary marker chromosome) is detected at prenatal diagnosis, even with a normal ultrasound. Warburton[8,9] has provided empirical data showing that the risks for *de novo* reciprocal or robertsonian translocations are 6.7% and 3.7%

respectively. For *de novo* nonsatellited or satellited marker chromosomes, the risks are 14.7% and 10.9% respectively.

Single gene abnormalities (mendelian inheritance)

In mendelian inheritance, a gene mutation usually involves only a single genetic locus. A chromosome carrying a single mutant gene with no other abnormality appears structurally normal because the change involves only a minute deletion or a change in a single nucleotide sequence. Analysis of a mutant gene is therefore not ordinarily facilitated by cytogenetic studies. Instead, the geneticist studies pedigrees, measures a gene product or its metabolite, or examines the DNA coding for the gene.

Definitions

Chromosomes exist in pairs, with one maternally derived and one paternally derived. Chromosomes contain genes; thus, genes, or more properly alleles (different states of a single gene), exist in pairs. Alleles occupy identical places on homologous chromosomes and can become interchanged during meiotic recombination.

The state of possessing a pair of identical alleles at a given position is termed *homozygosity*; if alleles are dissimilar, *heterozygosity* exists. An allele capable of expression in its heterozygous state is dominant, whereas an allele capable of expression only in homozygous form is recessive. These definitions apply only to autosomal loci; different circumstances exist for X-linked loci. A recessive trait whose allele is located on the X chromosome is expressed by all males (46,XY) carrying the recessive allele. Affected males are said to be *hemizygous*.

An important concept of particular relevance to autosomal recessive inheritance is *compound heterozygosity*, in which the two alleles are dissimilar but both abnormal (dysfunctional). Compound heterozygosity is often clinically indistinguishable from homozygosity for a single mutant allele. In autosomal recessive disorders, analysis using molecular techniques has shown that compound heterozygosity is the rule rather than the exception (the exception arises in consanguineous matings). In cystic fibrosis, some affected individuals are homozygous for deletion of three nucleotides at position 508 (ΔF508), but others have one such mutant allele and one other dysfunctional allele at the same locus (e.g., the missense mutation producing the premature stop (X) codon W1282X).

Transmission of mutant genes in families

The familial patterns followed by mendelian traits depend not only on whether the mutant gene is dominant or recessive but also on whether the gene is located on an autosome or a sex chromosome. There are five potential patterns of transmission: autosomal dominant, autosomal recessive, X-linked dominant, X-linked recessive, and Y-linked. The concept of mitochondrial inheritance, which for some genes yields maternal transmission exclusively, is not discussed here. Y-linked inheritance is of relevance here with respect to transmission of male gender and transmission of certain genes necessary for spermatogenesis.

Autosomal dominant inheritance

An autosomal dominant allele is recognized by its ability to be expressed in more than one generation (Fig. 20.5). In autosomal dominant traits, equal numbers of males and females are usually affected; the likelihood is 50% that an individual

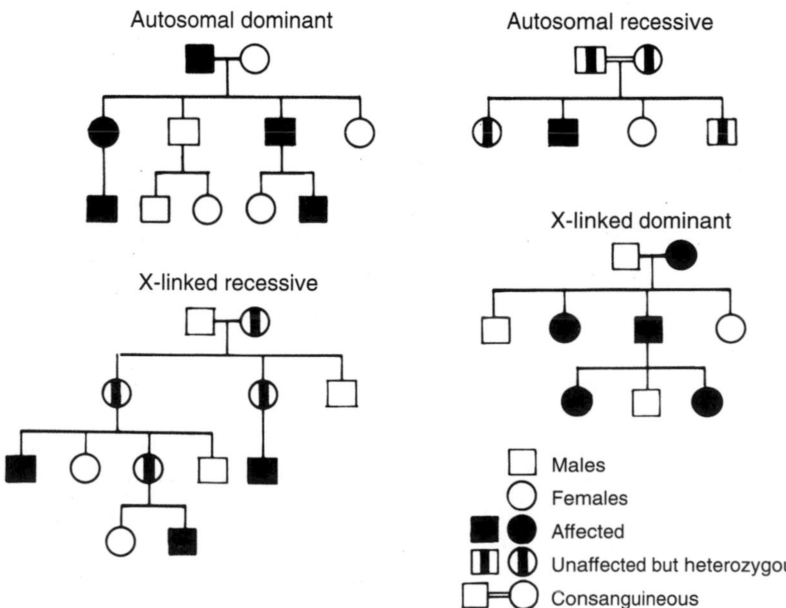

Figure 20.5 Idealized pedigree of common modes of mendelian inheritance. From ref. 28.

carrying a mutant autosomal dominant gene (allele) will transmit that allele to any given offspring, male or female. If penetrance (see below for definition) is complete, an unaffected individual will not have an affected offspring.

However, autosomal dominant patterns are not always associated with these idealized characteristics. Some individuals may be more severely affected than others, a phenomenon known as *variable expression.* This characteristic has been known clinically for decades, but the molecular basis has only recently been elucidated. In a given gene, the exact mutation may vary, e.g., a deletion or single-nucleotide substitution; this is called *molecular heterogeneity*. Some molecular changes are more deleterious than others; a mutation resulting in loss of a gene product (protein) is likely to be more serious than a mutation in which a single amino acid substitution has occurred. Variable expression occurs not only between families but also among affected members of a single family (intrafamilial *variability).* A single mutant gene may also be responsible for several ostensibly distinct phenotypic effects *(pleiotropy).* Occasionally, an autosomal dominant allele may exert its effect only on individuals of one sex *(sex limitation).* Another characteristic of autosomal dominant inheritance is that some individuals may be phenotypically normal yet carry a mutant autosomal dominant allele. Such a mutant allele is said to show *lack of penetrance* in the phenotypically normal individual. Lack of penetrance probably reflects our inability to study gene products or DNA directly; if molecular analysis was possible in all disorders, "nonpenetrant" individuals would probably show an abnormality in their DNA.

In the absence of an ability to measure DNA or its gene products, an autosomal dominant allele in humans must be recognized clinically. Usually, one of the following clinical characteristics must exist for dominant inheritance to be recognized:

1 a lack of interference with reproductive ability (e.g., polydactyly);

2 manifestation only after reproduction is completed (e.g., Huntington's disease);

3 a lack of penetrance or variable expressivity (i.e., a minimally affected parent might have severely affected progeny).

Dominant disorders need not always have been transmitted from an affected parent. The disorder may have arisen *de novo,* as result of a new mutation in a sperm or oocyte. The more severe the trait, the more likely it is that an affected individual has a new mutation. Approximately 90% of achondroplasia cases occur as a result of new mutations, whereas this occurs in relatively few cases of polydactyly. All individuals with a dominant trait conferring sterility must represent a new mutation.

Autosomal recessive inheritance

An autosomal recessive trait is expressed when an individual is homozygous for the mutant allele, i.e., at a given genetic locus both alleles show an identical mutation. As noted above, different but equally dysfunctional alleles can also exist (compound heterozygosity) and, for most disorders, this is usually the case. An individual with a recessive trait is usually the product of parents who are both heterozygous (carriers) for a mutation at the same locus. If two heterozygotes mate, the likelihood is 25% that a given offspring will be affected (see Fig. 20.5). If multiple siblings of both sexes are affected, autosomal recessive inheritance should definitely be considered. Consanguineous parents are more likely to carry an identical allele (mutant or normal) than nonconsanguineous parents. Thus, an individual with a recessive trait is relatively more likely to arise from a consanguineous than from a nonconsanguineous union. The rarer a trait, the higher the proportion of affected individuals who arise from consanguineous unions. For common traits (e.g., cystic fibrosis, sickle cell anemia), parents of affected offspring are usually not consanguineous.

Autosomal recessive inheritance can also occur if a homozygous individual mates with a heterozygous individual, in which case 50% of the offspring will be affected (pseudo-autosomal dominant inheritance). This phenomenon is becoming more frequent as survival to reproduction becomes less unusual for serious autosomal recessive traits (e.g., cystic fibrosis, sickle cell anemia).

The mathematical relationship between the frequencies of homozygotes and heterozygotes is clinically important and is expressed by the Hardy–Weinberg equilibrium. To illustrate, suppose that the normal allele is A and the mutant allele is a; A is said to have the frequency p, and a has the frequency q. Because the frequencies of alleles at a given locus add up to 1, $p + q = 1$. Squaring both sides of the equation gives $p^2 + 2pq + q^2 = 1$. In this binomial expansion, p^2 becomes the frequency of individuals homozygous for allele A (AA); q^2 is the frequency of individuals homozygous for allele a (aa); and $2pq$ is the frequency of the heterozygote (Aa). The frequency of a mutant allele (q) is usually much less than the frequency of a normal allele (p). If q is much less than 0.5, q^2 will be much less than $2pq$ because p will be nearly equal to 1.

The relative magnitudes of $2pq$ and q^2 make it clear that the "load" for deleterious recessive traits is carried mostly by heterozygotes; relatively few homozygotes exist. To illustrate, suppose the incidence of a trait (q^2) is 1 in 10 000. Thus, $q = 1$ in 100; $p = 99$ out of 100, or almost 1; and $2pq = 2 \times 1 \times 1$ in $100 = 1$ in 50, which is much more frequent than 1 in 10 000 (q^2). This mathematical exercise becomes clinically relevant when addressing proposals for eliminating mutant alleles from the population by selecting against homozygous fetuses. Theoretically, eliminating heterozygous individuals might also be unwise because they may possess an advantage over those normal homozygous individuals who may have been responsible for maintaining the mutant allele in the population. In fact, "normal" individuals may be heterozygous for at least five or six deleterious recessive genes.

Clinically unaffected individuals who have a sibling with an autosomal recessive disorder often inquire about the risk that their own offspring will have the disorder. Assuming that they and their mate are not related, the risk of having affected offspring can usually be shown to be low. If heterozygote detection tests are not available (less often the case, fortunately, with the use of molecular techniques), the a priori likelihood that the unaffected individual is a heterozygote can be calculated if the incidence of the trait is known. The unaffected sibling will have one of three equally likely genotypes: two will be heterozygous and one homozygous for the normal allele; the fourth genotype (homozygous mutant) is excluded on clinical grounds. Thus, the likelihood of the sibling being heterozygous is two in three. The likelihood of the sibling's mate being heterozygous for the same mutant gene reflects gene frequency in the general population, as determined by the Hardy–Weinberg equilibrium. If the trait were to have an incidence of 1 in 8100 births, the heterozygote frequency is 1 in 45 ($q^2 = 1/8100$; $q = 1/90$; $2pq = 1/45$). Thus, the likelihood that any given offspring will be affected is $2/3 \times 1/45 \times 1/4 = 2/540 = 1/270$. Rarer traits naturally confer a correspondingly lower likelihood. Most patients are surprised to find the risks so low. Risks for other family members can be calculated, assuming that a heterozygous individual has an equal likelihood of either transmitting or not transmitting a mutant gene. Thus, for example, a normal individual whose uncle is affected will have only a 1 in 3 chance of being heterozygous (i.e., $2/3 \times 1/2 = 2/6 = 1/3$).

X-linked recessive inheritance

A mutant recessive gene located on the X chromosome is expressed by all males (46,XY) who carry it. Such individuals are said to be hemizygous. X-linked recessive alleles are usually transmitted through phenotypically normal females who are heterozygous (see Fig. 20.5). In a family in which an X-linked recessive mutant allele is segregating, affected individuals might include male siblings, maternal uncles, nephews, male first cousins, and certain other maternal male relatives.

For a heterozygous female to transmit an X-linked recessive allele to any given offspring, the probability is 0.5. Males inheriting the allele will be affected, whereas females inheriting the allele will be heterozygous, like their mothers. An affected man will transmit the allele to all of his daughters but none of his sons; male-to-male transmission thus excludes X-linked inheritance. All offspring of an affected man will be phenotypically normal, unless the mother is heterozygous for the same mutant gene. In such a case, four genotypes are possible and females may be affected. This is unlikely for severe traits (e.g., Duchenne muscular dystrophy) but quite possible for mild traits (e.g., color blindness) or successfully treatable traits (e.g., hemophilia).

Women may occasionally manifest X-linked recessive traits: 46,XX individuals can be affected if they are homozygous, a circumstance that could result if their mother were heterozygous and their father hemizygous. Vicissitudes of X inactivation (preferential inactivation of normal X) can be so extreme that phenotypic effects exist which approximate those present in hemizygous men. Mutant genes also exist that skew X-inactivation away from randomization between the maternal X and paternal X in a given cell. Finally, women with only one X chromosome (45,X) may be affected if the X chromosome has a mutant allele.

The possibility of new mutations must be considered. It should not be assumed that the mother of a child with an X-linked recessive mutation is heterozygous because the child may represent a new mutation arising in the ovum. If the trait is lethal with respect to fertility, and if no other relatives are affected, the likelihood that a mutation is new can be shown to be one in three.

In counseling individuals at risk for X-linked recessive traits, it is frequently helpful to utilize Bayesian calculations. Conceptually simple, but sometimes complex in application, Bayesian calculations take into account all available data, not just a priori calculations. For example, common sense dictates that a woman at theoretical risk of having offspring with an X-linked recessive trait is actually less likely to be heterozygous if four consecutive sons prove unaffected. The following example illustrates this point. A prospective mother (proband) has two brothers who have an X-linked disorder for which neither metabolic nor DNA analysis is possible. It can be deduced that her own mother is an obligate heterozygote; thus, the likelihood of the prospective mother being heterozygous is 50%. This is known as the proband's a priori risk or prior probability. Suppose that the woman has three unaffected sons: if she is heterozygous, the probability of her having three consecutive unaffected sons is one in eight. However, it is more likely that she is, in fact, not heterozygous. Table 20.2 illustrates how to account for the three unaffected sons. The newly calculated likelihood of the woman being heterozygous is only one in nine, considerably lower than the likelihood calculated from a priori expectations alone.

X-linked dominant inheritance

In X-linked dominant traits, women are twice as likely to be affected as men; however, women are usually less severely affected and, in fact, some X-linked dominant traits are lethal in men. A man carrying an X-linked dominant allele transmits the mutant to all of his daughters but none of his sons (Table 20.3). There is a probability of 0.5 that a woman with an X-linked dominant allele will pass that allele to any offspring, male or female. Relatively few X-linked dominant traits are known.

Causes of gene mutation

Although specific gene mutations are rare, at least 1% of all infants have a disorder resulting from a single mutant gene. Some affected individuals inherit a mutant gene, whereas

Table 20.2 Bayesian analysis.

	Proband heterozygous	Proband not heterozygous
Prior probability	$\frac{1}{2}$	$\frac{1}{2}$
Conditional probability	$\left(\frac{1}{2}\right)^3 = \frac{1}{8}$	1
Joint probability (prior and conditional)	$\frac{1}{16}$	$\frac{1}{2}$
Posterior probability (joint and prior)	$\dfrac{\frac{1}{16}}{\frac{1}{16}+\frac{1}{2}\left(\text{or } \frac{9}{16}\right)}$	$\dfrac{\frac{1}{2} \text{ or } \frac{8}{16}}{\frac{1}{16}+\frac{1}{2}\left(\text{or } \frac{9}{16}\right)}$
	$= \dfrac{\frac{1}{16}}{\frac{9}{16}}$	$= \dfrac{\frac{8}{16}}{\frac{9}{16}}$
	$= \frac{1}{9}$	$= \frac{8}{9}$

This analysis calculates the likelihood of heterozygosity for a woman whose two brothers have an X-linked recessive disorder. The a priori risk (prior probability) of heterozygosity is 1/2, in as much as the woman's mother is an obligate heterozygote. Supposing the woman has three unaffected sons, what is the likelihood that she is nevertheless heterozygous? Multiplying prior by conditional probability yields joint probability. The posterior probability (1/9) is the newly derived heterozygosity risk, taking into account the three unaffected sons. (From ref. 30.)

Table 20.3 X-linked dominant inheritance.

Parents	Offspring
Affected male (Xy) and normal female (xx)	Xx, Xx, xy, xy
Normal male (xy) and affected female (Xx)	Xx, xx, Xy, xy

X carries an X-linked dominant allele; x does not carry the allele. For offspring of affected males, all females are affected, but no males. For offspring of affected females, 50% of females and 50% of males are affected. (From ref. 30.)

others are the first in their family to have the disorder. Spontaneous mutation rates average from 10^{-5} to 10^{-6} per locus per gamete per generation. Overall, each gamete is estimated to contain 20–30 mutations. Most mutations are neutral or lethal; otherwise, many more than 2–3% of liveborns would be abnormal.

Mutation rates increase with increasing paternal age, with fathers in their fifth or sixth decade having an increased likelihood of certain gene mutations arising in their germ cells. This applies to some but not all X-linked recessive and autosomal dominant disorders. This increase is believed to reflect the continuous germ cell replication (spermatogenesis) that occurs throughout a man's fertile lifetime, although the exact manner by which repeated replication leads to mutation remains obscure. Unlike the situation for chromosomal abnormalities, advanced maternal age is not associated with an increase in gene mutations.

Ionizing irradiation is a well-established mutagen. X-rays are the major source of ionizing irradiation, although ultraviolet light also causes mutations. An X-ray exposure of 50–100 rads (50–100 cGg) only doubles the mutation rate; therefore, the absolute risk is relatively low unless an individual is subjected to a massive exposure. Ultrasound and microwaves are not ionizing and probably not mutagenic.

Numerous chemicals cause mutations in animals and in *in vitro* testing systems, and many of these can be mutagenic in humans. Well-known examples include alkylating agents, DNA base analogs (e.g., 5-bromouracil), antimetabolites, nitrous acid, and acridine dyes. Inorganic salts, caffeine, nitrites, and other ubiquitous agents are also mutagenic under certain circumstances. It is difficult to determine the likelihood of particular compounds being mutagenic in humans in a given circumstance; retrospective clinical data cannot provide satisfactory information. However, even substantive exposure to alkylating agents or antimetabolites leads to little if any increase in abnormal liveborns. Individuals treated with chemotherapeutic agents before pregnancy show no increased abnormalities in subsequent progeny. This suggests that most induced mutations are lethal.

Linkage

Genes are located on chromosomes at given locations and in a definite linear relationship to one another. Genes on the same chromosome are said to be linked or to exhibit linkage. Specifically, genes show linkage if during meiosis, with its opportunity for recombination, they are more likely to remain on the same chromosome in parental combination than to behave as if they were on different chromosomes.

If the frequency of recombination between two linked genes is 1%, those genes are defined to be one map unit or one centimorgan apart (percentage recombination = centimorgans). Genes that are 50 centimorgans apart on the same chromosome fail, by definition, to show linkage because such genes segregate indistinguishably from genes on nonhomologous chromosomes. Linkage analysis is increasingly useful in antenatal diagnosis as a more complete map of the human genome becomes available. Linkage analysis in prenatal diagnosis usually relies on a polymorphic locus. Polymorphism exists when two or more alleles are present at a given locus, such that the less frequent allele is still present in 1% of the population. The polymorphism may be some aspect of a gene product, such as electrophoretic mobility. However, the type of polymorphism increasingly used diagnostically is that of DNA variants.

Nonmendelian inheritance: imprinting and uniparental disomy

Autosomal loci usually display biallelic gene expression, with both alleles of a pair (one paternally and one maternally derived) being active. Sometimes, however, only one of a pair of alleles is active (monoallelic expression), and the active allele must be derived from a particular parent (mother or father). An abnormal phenotype develops if the allele is not inherited from the appropriate parent, even if the other parent transmits a gene with a typically normal allele. In monoallelic expression, the allele not required must be inactivated; this process is well known in the case of inactivation of X chromosomes in excess of one, and is called imprinting. An imprinted gene is not expressed as a result of hypermethylation.

The prototypic disorders that led to the elucidation of autosomal imprinting in humans were Prader–Willi syndrome (PWS) and Angelman syndrome (AS). These two recognizable malformation syndromes are controlled by contiguous regions on the long arm of chromosome 15. A paternally derived critical region prevents the expression of PWS; a maternally derived region does not suffice because it is inactive. Conversely, in AS, a maternally derived critical region must be expressed because the paternal region is inactive. PWS and AS may manifest themselves under a variety of circumstances. In PWS, the paternally derived critical region may be deleted or two copies of the maternal region (both inactive) may be present, as a result of both copies of chromosome 15 being maternal in origin. The latter circumstance can result if a paternal chromosome 15 is expelled from a trisomic zygote consisting of two maternal and one paternal chromosome 15. Uniparental disomy (UPD) is then said to exist. If, in contrast, one of the two maternal chromosomes is expelled, a normal situation arises (zygotic correction).

UPD is a clinically relevant phenomenon. In total, 1–2% of chorionic villi contain trisomic cells, usually as a very low percentage. If the zygote had been trisomic and correction occurred by expulsion of one of the three chromosomes present in triplicate, the likelihood of UPD occurring is one in three. Whether UPD exerts a phenotypic effect depends on whether a given chromosome displays monoallelic expression for any of its genes. A special concern in prenatal diagnosis is that UPD can follow asymmetric segregation in a parent having a balanced robertsonian translocation.[10] Both maternal and paternal UPD exists for chromosome 14;[10] however, UPD does not seem to have a deleterious effect for all chromosomes, including chromosomes 13, 21, and 22.[11–14]

Imprinting is also relevant to entire haploid sets of chromosomes. If both haploid sets in a diploid zygote are maternal in origin, an ovarian teratoma (dermoid) results, whereas if both haploid sets are paternal a hydatidiform mole results. The general principle is that paternal chromosomes govern placental growth, whereas maternal chromosomes control embryonic growth. In triploidy, if two of the three haploid sets of chromosomes are paternal, a hydatidiform mole results; if two of the three sets are maternal, the placenta is small.

The relevance of imprinting to human pathology is only now being unraveled. The extent of its importance could be enormous not only for pregnancy loss and malformations, but also for somatic processes such as cancer.

Molecular basis of the gene

DNA exists in the form of a double helix, which may be envisioned as a twisted ladder. Each vertical column consists of alternating phosphate and deoxyribose carbohydrate residues. The carbohydrate and phosphate residues on opposite sides are connected by nitrogenous bases called nucleotides. The DNA nucleotides consist of the purines, adenine (A) and guanine (G), and the pyrimidines, thymine (T) and cytosine (C). Adenine is always connected to thymine by forming two hydrogen bonds (base pairing). Similarly, guanine is always connected to cytosine by three hydrogen bonds. As a result, the two DNA strands are complementary. If the sequence of bases on one strand is ATTGC (adenine–thymine–thymine–guanine–cytosine), the sequence on the opposite strand must be TAACG. The ratio of adenine to thymine is always 1:1, as is the ratio of guanine to cytosine. However, the ratio of adenine–thymine (AT) pairs to guanine–cytosine (GC) pairs varies not only in different parts of a single chromosome but also between different chromosomes. This variation is one basis for chromosomal banding.

Genetic information, specifically the amino acid sequence, is determined by the sequence of nucleotides on one of the two DNA strands. A sequence of three adjacent bases forms a codon; most codons specifically code for one of the 20 amino acids but a few code for a stop signal (i.e., cessation of transcription). Specifically, the message is said to be read from the *sense* strand of DNA, with the *antisense* strand being the complementary strand. The complementary strand corresponds to the messenger RNA (mRNA) sequence, although uracil is incorporated in mRNA rather than thymine.

Structural organization of the gene

Along the chromosome, genes are made up of *unique* sequences of DNA, which are able to code for protein, interspersed with *repetitive* or noncoding sequences. Other sequences are also present which are essential for DNA transcription and RNA translation, or which code for only part of a protein (e.g., *pseudogenes*); these types of DNA are less immediately relevant to this discussion.

Fig. 20.6 shows the sequence of events in which DNA is first transcribed into mRNA and then translated into protein. Upstream from the nucleotide sequence which codes for amino acids are sequences assumed to be involved in transcription regulation. Knowledge about gene regulation in humans is incomplete, but some intriguing observations have been made. The

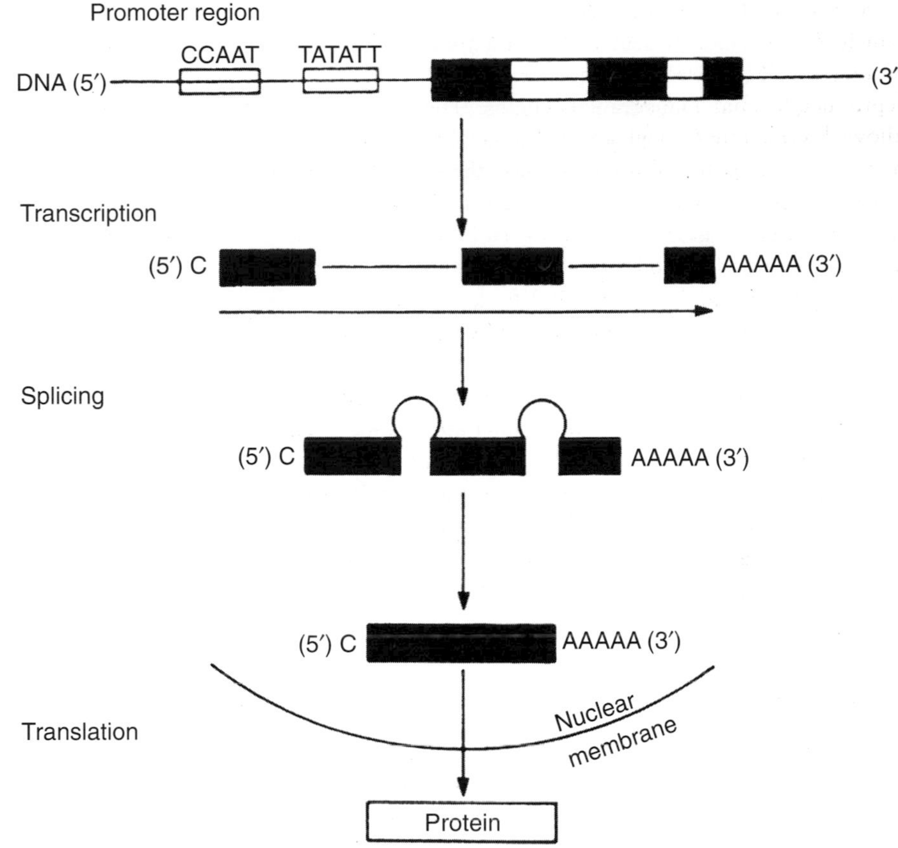

Figure 20.6 Transcription and translation. Intervening sequences (introns) must be excised, leaving exons to be translated to proteins. (From ref. 30.)

nucleotide sequence TATA ("TATA box") is consistently found 30 base pairs (bp) before (5′ to) the site at which transcription begins. The TATA box may be involved in positioning RNA polymerase II, the enzyme essential for transcribing mRNA from DNA. Another pivotal sequence is CAAT, located 50–75 bp upstream from the transcription site. The CAAT box may be the site at which RNA polymerase II actually binds. Transcription proceeds in the 5′ to 3′ direction, extending beyond the region of unique-sequence DNA. The signal terminating transcription is unknown, but the sequence AATAAA is consistently observed 15–30 bases 5′ to the site at which the polyadenylated [poly(A)] tail will be added.

Post-transcriptional events

The entire sequence (5′ region, unique-sequence region with its intervening repetitive sequences, 3′ region) is transcribed into mRNA in a 5′ to 3′ direction. Several post-transcriptional processes are necessary before the protein can be translated because the nucleotide sequence is discontinuous with respect to sequences coding for amino acids. A precise splicing mechanism exists to excise the noncoding intervening sequences (introns); the nucleotides GT on the 5′ side of the intervening sequence are removed (intron) along with nucleotides AG on the 3′ side (see Fig. 20.6). The remaining sequences are thus the coding sequences (exons).

Translation

Once the introns are excised, the transcribed mRNA can direct polypeptide synthesis (translation). The first step in translation is that mRNA moves into the cytoplasm to associate with ribosomes, which are structures consisting of both protein and a special high-molecular-weight RNA (ribosomal RNA, or rRNA). Adenosine triphosphate next reacts with the carboxyl end of specific amino acids to form an amino acid-specific transfer RNA that lines up on the ribosome complex at the point signified by its appropriate codon. The amnio acids that make up the polypeptide chain are thus brought into correct sequence.

Molecular analysis of the gene and its clinical applicability

Analytical techniques

Understanding how molecular genetics can be used for prenatal diagnosis requires a knowledge of analytical techniques. Here, several pivotal techniques are briefly described.

Southern blotting

DNA fragments of differing size can be distinguished using a technique called *Southern blotting*. DNA is digested by restriction endonucleases (see Restriction endonucleases), which are enzymes present in bacteria that are capable of cutting specific nucleotide sequences to yield fragments of reproducible (and manageable) lengths. The fragments are allowed to migrate through an agarose gel; heavier DNA fragments are less mobile and remain near the origin of the gel, whereas lighter fragments migrate faster and thus are further from the origin (Fig. 20.7). The gel is laid on a piece of nitrocellulose filter paper, and buffer is allowed to flow through the gel into the nitrocellulose filter. DNA fragments concomitantly migrate out of the gel and bind to the filter, creating a replica of the DNA fragment pattern. The nitrocellulose replicate is exposed to a specific gene probe (see Gene probes), which hybridizes only to the portion of the filter containing its complementary DNA. To identify the bound fragment and its length, the probe is made radioactive or, more commonly, is biotinylated. Thus, a gene (or, more specifically, a DNA sequence that is part of a gene) can be identified among thousands of fragments that have been categorized according to length.

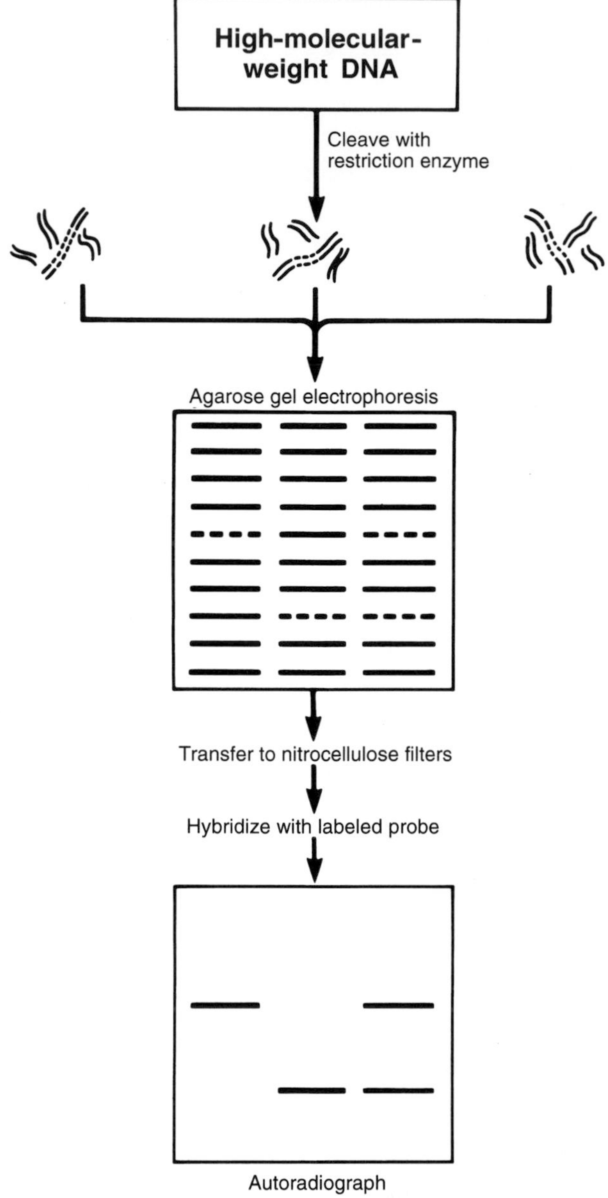

Figure 20.7 Southern blotting. DNA is cleaved with restriction enzymes, and the DNA fragments are separated by size, using agarose gel electrophoresis. The gel is then laid on a piece of nitrocellulose, and buffer allowed to flow through the gel onto the nitrocellulose. DNA fragments migrate out of the gel and bind to the filter. A replica of the DNA fragment pattern of the gel is thus created on the filter. The filter can then be hybridized to a suitably labeled probe, with DNA fragments that hybridize to the probe signaled by autoradiography or other techniques. (From ref. 29.)

Gene probes

For a specific gene (or, more precisely, a specific DNA sequence) to be located among thousands of DNA fragments, DNA probes are created from cloned DNA. Probes of unknown sequence (anonymous) can be generated, but, in the present context, we are concerned with diagnostically useful probes. If purified mRNA is available, single-stranded DNA probes can be generated using an enzyme called *reverse transcriptase*. This enzyme, present in viruses whose hereditary information is RNA not DNA, directs the synthesis of DNA from RNA (the reverse of the situation in humans). Exposing human mRNA to viral reverse transcriptase produces *complementary* single-stranded human DNA called *cDNA*. This cDNA is injected into a vector that is able to replicate the foreign DNA as well as its own. Bacteriophages, various synthetic systems (plasmids and cosmids), and yeast artificial chromosomes can all be used as vectors. The presence of a disorder that is characterized by the absence of DNA can be detected by determining whether or not a DNA probe for the normal gene hybridizes to an individual's DNA. If it does not, the DNA sequence must be missing (gene deletion) and the individual must be affected. It is also possible to construct short oligonucleotide- or allele-specific DNA probes of usually 15–20 nucleotides in length. These sensitive probes hybridize only to sequences that are complementary for every single nucleotide. If only a single nucleotide is absent (or altered), the oligonucleotide probe will fail to hybridize.

Polymerase chain reaction

The polymerase chain reaction (PCR) has revolutionized molecular biology. In PCR, a target sequence of up to 1 kb can be quickly amplified by 10^5 to 10^6 times. The prerequisite for this amplification is the identification of unique DNA primers that flank and are specific for the DNA region to be amplified. This region may consist of a part of a gene (e.g., that containing a mutation), a polymorphic DNA sequence closely linked to a given locus, or a repetitive DNA sequence characteristic of a chromosomal region (e.g., the Y long arm).

A heat-stable DNA polymerase extracted from *Thermus aquaticus* is traditionally used in PCR (thus, the term *Taq* polymerase), but other enzymes can also be used. The target DNA, unique primers, and *Taq* polymerase are added together. When the temperature is raised, denaturation into single-stranded DNA occurs. On cooling, amplification occurs. Repetition of this cycle results in the DNA between primers increasing in logarithmic fashion. Other sequences are amplified but only increase linearly; thus, they are soon inundated by the exponential increase in the sequence flanked by the primers.

Restriction endonucleases and restriction fragment length polymorphisms

Restriction endonucleases are bacterial enzymes that recognize and cut specific nucleotide sequences in double-stranded DNA molecules. The sites at which DNA is cut are called *restriction sites*. Over 200 restriction enzymes have been identified, each recognizing a unique sequence of bases. DNA fragments resulting from digestion with restriction enzymes differ in length according to the distance between recognition sites; the greater the distance between sites, the longer the length of intervening DNA. *Restriction fragments* are specified according to the numbers of bases (e.g., 8000 bases or 8 kb). Usually, there is more than one restriction site per gene, but occasionally the sites are situated in such a way that an entire gene lies between two sites. If a gene contains more than one restriction site, its DNA will be digested into fragments of different lengths.

DNA from ostensibly normal individuals does not always show the same spectrum of DNA fragments after exposure to a particular restriction enzyme. Among individuals in the general population, differences in DNA sequence exist which confer no advantage or disadvantage. Thus, polymorphism exists with respect to the presence or absence of restriction sites (these polymorphisms contrast with differences in DNA sequence that cause disorders such as sickle cell anemia). This phenomenon is termed *restriction fragment length polymorphism* (RFLP). RFLPs provide markers for linkage analysis. If a given RFLP is closely linked to a locus that confers a disease, linkage analysis to detect the presence or absence of a disorder may be possible. Because RFLPs exist every few centimorgans, linkage analysis allows prenatal diagnosis for all loci in which the family is informative and the gene has been localized. RFLP linkage analysis forms the basis for prenatal diagnosis for many disorders in which the molecular basis is either not known or cannot practically be sought.

The types of DNA polymorphism now most commonly used for linkage analysis are dinucleotide repeats. For example, does a given locus on a particular chromosome have 5, 7, 10, 12, or more repeat sequences of cytosine–adenine (CA)? The number of repeats is inherited in a mendelian fashion.

RFLPs can be used in prenatal diagnosis to detect mutations if a mutation alters a specific restriction enzyme site, or results in a new site. For example, in sickle cell anemia, codon 6 (the triplet signifying the sixth amino acid) has undergone a mutation from adenine to thymine. The restriction enzyme *Mst*II recognizes the normal nucleotide sequence but not the mutant sequence. After digestion with *Mst*II, hybridization of the digested DNA to a β-globin DNA probe can differentiate DNA containing the mutant gene from DNA containing the normal gene. The probe highlights a longer fragment in the mutant DNA as a result of the missing restriction site.

If the nucleotide sequence responsible for a given disorder is not known, a combination of linkage analysis and molecular techniques is used. If the mutant gene has been localized to a chromosome but not isolated, a nearby RFLP can serve as a marker. It is also possible to use polymorphic markers, such as the number of tandem repeats of nucleotides. To apply linkage analysis, one must determine whether an informative situation exists in the family. Figure 20.8 illustrates the approach used when an informative RFLP polymorphism does exist. The normal allele is signified by the presence of a 5700-bp fragment, whereas the mutant is signified by the presence of 3300- and 2400-bp fragments. Recall that the RFLP pattern that connotes an affected fetus in this family may show just the opposite in another family. The RFLP merely serves as a marker; its presence or absence is functionally independent from the disease. The same principles would apply if the polymorphic locus being used for linkage were a varying number of tandem repeats.

Polygenic–multifactorial inheritance

Genetic tendencies, rather than shared environmental factors, are very often responsible for physiological and anatomical variation, as well as for common anomalies affecting a single organ system (e.g., cleft palate); most of the latter show recurrence risks of 1–5% for first-degree relatives (siblings, offspring, parents). This can also be deduced from twin studies; monozygotic twins are much more likely to be concordant for any given anomaly than dizygotic twins. Both monozygotic and dizygotic twins are exposed to the same intrauterine environment; thus, genetic factors must be invoked to explain the differences.

Basis of polygenic inheritance

The logical explanation for either anatomical or physiological variation in a trait whose recurrence risk is 1–5% is the involvement of several genes. To illustrate, let us consider how the number of genotypic classes changes as the number of genes influencing a single characteristic increases. Suppose that only one gene controls a trait and that this gene has only two alleles, A and a. In the simplest case, the frequency of allele A equals the frequency of allele a. Thus, 25% of the population is AA ($p = q = 0.5$; $p^2 = q^2 = 0.25$), 25% is aa, and 50% is Aa ($2pq = 0.5$). If two genes influence the trait, alleles B and b

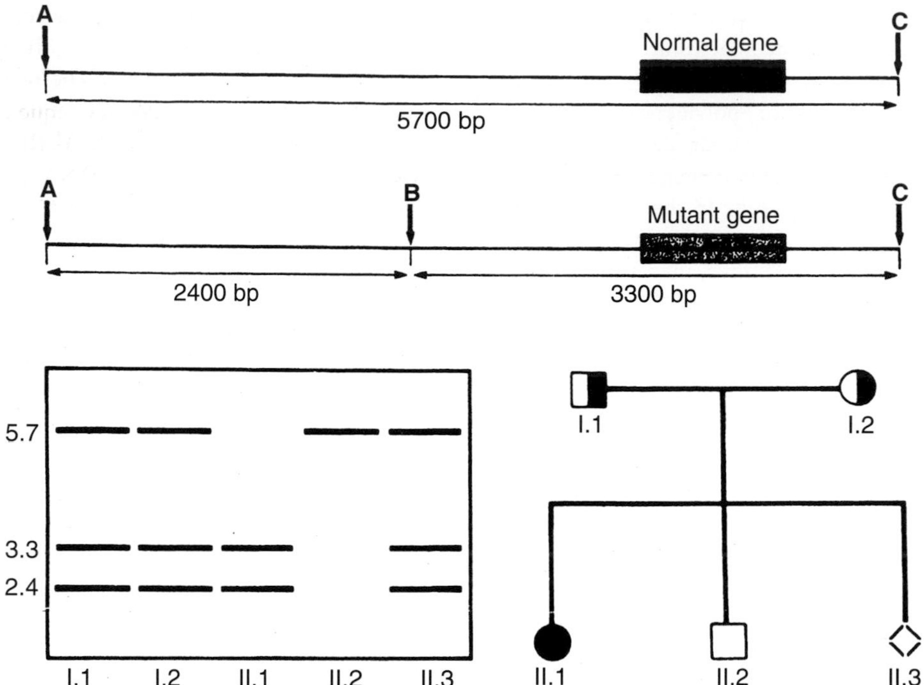

Figure 20.8 Prenatal diagnosis is achieved by use of a restriction fragment length polymorphism linked to the locus causing a disease. Suppose a restriction site (B) is closely linked to a gene. This restriction site is present in some individuals but not in others (polymorphism). A probe that hybridizes to DNA containing the polymorphic site identifies 2400-bp and 3300-bp fragments in individuals with the restriction site but identifies only a single 5700-bp fragment in those without the restriction site. On agarose gel electrophoresis, individuals homozygous for the restriction site display two bands (II.1). Homozygous individuals lacking the restriction site display only one band (II.2). In this family, parents (I.1, I.2) are doubly heterozygous. They are each heterozygous both for the restriction site and for an autosomal recessive mutant (pedigrees). DNA analysis of the affected child (II.1) shows only two bands (3300 and 2400 kb). We can conclude that, in both parents, the mutant gene is located on the chromosome characterized by the presence of restriction site B. DNA analysis reveals that their unaffected son (II.2) is not heterozygous but homozygous normal. DNA analysis from amniotic fluid cells or chorionic villi reveals that the fetus (II.3) is normal but heterozygous. (From ref. 29.)

will be present at the second locus. Nine genotypes are now possible: AABB, AABb, AAbb, AaBB, AaBb, Aabb, aaBB, aaBb, and aabb. The population will contain nine distinct classes of individuals if A, B, a, and b all exert dissimilar influences (Table 20.4). Therefore, as the number of genes controlling a trait increases, the number of genotypic classes increases rapidly. If one gene has two alleles, there are three classes. If two genes exist, each with two alleles, there will be nine classes and thus nine histographic bars. If one continues to represent histographically the proportion of individuals in each genotypic class, normal distribution will be approximated as more and more genotypes become possible (Fig. 20.9). Thus, continuous variation is approximated in the population. A trait controlled by more than one gene is said to be inherited in polygenic fashion (Table 20.5). With the availability of molecular techniques, the scientific validity of these assumptions has been substantiated. Infrequently, one gene exists which has a major effect, with several other genes having lesser effects.

Although the term *polygenic inheritance* is often used synonymously with continuous variation, the latter may also result from other mechanisms, namely a single multiple-allele locus influenced by environmental factors. If environmental as well as genetic factors influence a trait, the term *multifactorial* is more appropriate. Polygenic and multifactorial inheritance cannot usually be distinguished in humans, although comparisons between monozygotic and dizygotic twins theoretically permits such a distinction.

Table 20.4 Relationship between the number of genes controlling a trait and the number of classes of individuals in a population.

Number of genes	Classes of individuals	Number of classes
1 (A, a)	AA, Aa, aa	3
2 (A, a; B, b)	AABB, AABb, AAbb, AaBB, AaBb, Aabb, aaBB, aaBb, aabb	9
n		3^n

From ref. 28.

Polygenic–multifactorial inheritance is invoked to explain the inheritance of normal anatomical and physiological variables that display *continuous variation*, such as height, skin color, hair color, blood pressure, age at menarche, and ability

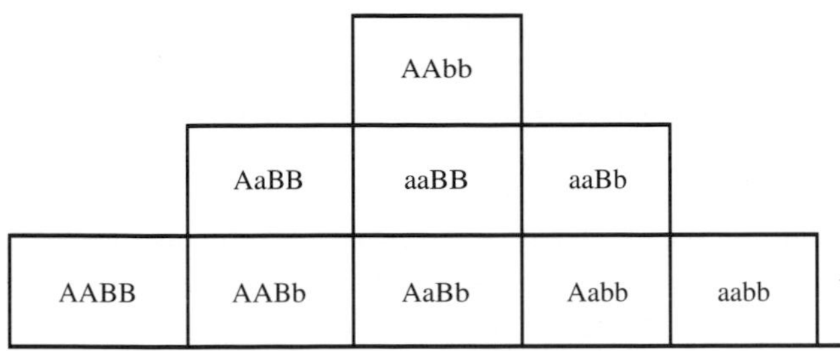

Figure 20.9 Histographs showing relative proportions in the population of individuals having the different genotypes that would be produced if two genes influence a trait and if each gene has two alleles. Further, each gene is comparable in effect, that is, A = B and a = b. However, A and B exert a different effect than a and b. The graph approximates normal distribution. (From ref. 28.)

Table 20.5 Common polygenic–multifactorial traits.

Neural tube defects (most cases)
Hydrocephaly (most cases)
Cleft lip, with or without cleft palate
Cleft lip (alone)
Cardiac defects (most types)
Diaphragmatic hernia
Omphalocele and gastroschisis
Renal agenesis
Ureteral anomalies
Hypospadias
Posterior urethral valves
Uterine (müllerian fusion) defects (probably)
Hip dislocation
Limb reduction defects
Talipes equinovarus (clubfoot)

to metabolize a given drug or toxin. However, polygenic inheritance alone does not explain discontinuous variation in which the population consists of two discrete groups, one affected (e.g., cleft palate) and one unaffected. There exists no continuum in the population for such traits. To explain such dichotomy (discontinuity), one must postulate a threshold beyond which the accrued genetic liability for developing a specific trait becomes so great that a malformation is manifested (Fig. 20.10). Phenotypically normal parents delivered of a child with a polygenic–multifactorial trait (anomaly) are assumed to have genetic liabilities nearer the threshold than most other individuals in the general population. This model is biologically reasonable if "liability" reflects the rate of embryonic growth. A slow rate of growth may preclude a key embryonic step from occurring by a crucial time, thus leading to anomalous development.

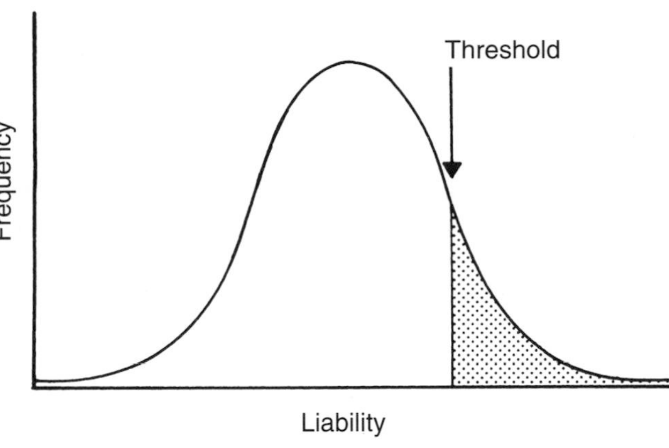

Figure 20.10 Schematic presentation of one model for polygenic or multifactorial inheritance, assuming a threshold beyond which liability is so great that an abnormality is manifested. Parents of affected individuals presumably have a greater liability (i.e., are closer to the threshold) than most other individuals in the population.[28]

Diagnosis of single-gene disorders

The previous sections of this chapter have reviewed the major mechanisms that result in genetic disorders and general approaches to their diagnosis. The following sections will examine specific approaches to the diagnosis of single-gene or mendelian disorders.

Single-gene disorders represent a large group of conditions that number in the hundreds and that are individually infrequent and often rare. Diagnosis depends mostly on gene analysis (i.e., DNA analysis) or analysis of a gene product, and occasionally on effects secondary to deficient gene function.

Multifactorial or polygenic disorders have complex etiologies, often depicted as combining small effects of several hypothetical factors. Neural tube defects, facial clefts, and dysplastic kidneys are examples of disorders in this category. At present, successful prenatal diagnosis of a multifactorial disorder is usually accomplished by sonographic imaging of altered anatomy. It may be that, eventually, a small number of genetic or nongenetic factors, perhaps as few as one or two, may be recognized as having the major causative role in generating an anomaly; that factor or factors could then become the target for diagnostic efforts. Prenatal diagnosis of multifactorial disorders may come to resemble the laboratory-based diagnosis of chromosomal and single-gene disorders if progress is made in this direction.

The continuing and rapid progress in molecular and biochemical genetics means that it is futile to make any attempt to compile a complete list of either possible diagnoses or the appropriate methodology to make a specific diagnosis. The list changes continually, especially as new genes are discovered. When an obstetrician or genetic counselor is faced with questions in this area, it is necessary to consult with specialists or refer to a prenatal diagnosis center.

Screening for recessive disorders

Most recessive disorders are rare, especially those associated with severe morbidities. Except in inbred communities, they often appear in a family as a first occurrence without other members being affected. When they recur, they do so in siblings. For several disorders, screening programs have been developed for potential parents; this will allow them to be prewarned about first occurrences and enable decisions to be made about prenatal diagnosis. Different paradigms have evolved for these programs in different locales. Some programs address both members of a couple simultaneously; other programs address one member initially, and the second only when the first person is shown to be a carrier. Although carrier screening and the counseling that must accompany it are ideally accomplished before conception, very often they occur in the early months of an ongoing pregnancy.

The frequency of recessive mutations among population groups depends on the disorder. These differences may result in targeting certain population groups that have a high carrier frequency for an autosomal recessive disease. The first carrier screening programs addressed Tay–Sachs disease in people of Ashkenazi Jewish heritage, and hemoglobinopathies (sickle cell disorders and thalassemias) in people of African, Mediterranean, and South Asian heritages. In the case of X-linked disorders, a screening program would test only women because hemizygous men would show obvious morbidities.

Methods of diagnosis

This section will describe the major methods used in diagnosis and the groups of disorders that are diagnosable today, with specific examples from each. For further details, the reader is referred to textbooks on prenatal diagnosis,[15,16] online resources for single-gene disorders,[17,18] and a catalog that lists prenatally diagnosed conditions.[19]

The primary abnormality in a single-gene disorder lies in the structure of the gene or, less often, in a controlling element of that gene. The simplest method of diagnosis is usually analysis of the gene, and this has become possible for over 200 genes. For many disorders, however, the gene is either not known or has not yet been isolated and studied, so other diagnostic strategies are necessary. These parallel the methods of postnatal genetic diagnosis that have been established for many decades. Even when a gene has been isolated and studied, at times a more efficient diagnosis of a disease state will be made by analysis of the gene product or some other effect secondary to the primary gene defect. This is the case, for example, when a disease state arises from a large number of different mutations in a specific gene (allelic variation or allelic heterogeneity) or when the disease state arises from mutations in more than one gene, each affecting a final common pathway that leads to disease expression (genetic heterogeneity). Thus, a number of strategies that are one or more steps away from the primary gene defect have been used.

At present, most prenatal diagnoses of single-gene disorders require tissue or cells that contain the fetal genome and fetal gene products, usually cells external to the fetus itself but within the womb. These are recovered by amniocentesis or chorionic villus sampling. Occasionally, cells obtained directly from the fetus via fetal blood sampling (cordocentesis) or fetal organ biopsy (from skin, liver, or muscle) are required. Use of the least dangerous approach that will achieve accurate information is axiomatic to the discipline of prenatal diagnosis. Thus, fetal organ biopsy is rarely used, being reserved for situations in which a disease is expressed in that organ but not in amniotic fluid cells or chorionic villi. Diagnostic techniques that avoid entry into the uterus altogether are preferable. This has become possible with progress in the isolation of fetal cells and fetal nucleic acids (DNAs and RNAs), which cross into the maternal circulation and can be recovered from a small sample of the pregnant woman's blood.[20,21]

The field of pre-implantation diagnosis, in conjunction with *in vitro* fertilization, is also being developed. In this technique, the diagnosis of a single-gene disorder is based on DNA analysis of either polar bodies or a single cell aspirated from an embryo before that embryo is transferred into the womb. Many aspects remain under active investigation, including the diagnostic accuracy, success of the methods, and safety of the procedures. A few errors have occurred, but over 1500 babies have now been born with correct pre-implantation diagnoses. Of mendelian disorders, cystic fibrosis has been the most frequently addressed.

In addition to the analysis of genes and gene products, several other approaches are used that depend on expression of the disease phenotype. Sometimes, they are not applicable at the early stages of pregnancy but must await expression of the disease as the fetus develops. These approaches include sonographic imaging and magnetic resonance imaging (MRI), embryo fetoscopic imaging, measurement of metabolite concentrations, histology of biopsies, and chromosomal analysis.

Sonographic imaging

Pedigree analysis has established single-gene mutations as the presumed or probable etiology of a large number of malformations and birth defect syndromes.[22] Pathogenetic events take place during embryogenesis, leaving malformations as evidence of an earlier cell malfunction. Visualization of altered anatomy by sonographic imaging or MRI can be used to reach a diagnosis.

Certain genetic malformation syndromes will always manifest an anatomical abnormality. For example, type II osteogenesis imperfecta, which is most often a dominant disorder resulting from mutations in type I collagen genes, results in compacted, deformed limb bones by the second trimester. In other syndromes, one particular manifestation is much less constant than another. A cardinal feature of the recessive disorder chondroectodermal dysplasia (Ellis–van Creveld syndrome) is the presence of six fingers, whereas heart defects occur in only approximately one-half of cases. The recessive disorder Meckel–Gruber syndrome usually shows the triad of encephalocele, polydactyly, and cystic kidneys, but any one of the three may be absent or rudimentary in a specific case. The variability in disease expression, and the time during gestation at which altered anatomy occurs and can be visualized, become crucial factors in diagnosis by ultrasound or MRI. Thorough knowledge of the disease and its expression are important. In many circumstances, positive findings can be accepted as establishing a diagnosis but negative findings will not exclude a diagnosis. When family history shows a high risk for an inherited malformation syndrome, that specific diagnosis can be inferred from an abnormal finding. Without the family history, the same finding can result in several considerations in a differential diagnosis.

Embryo fetoscopic imaging

Direct optical visualization of the fetus in the second trimester by fetoscopy was introduced in the 1970s. It had the capacity to visualize the surface of the fetus and allow diagnoses based on anatomical findings. The advantage of fetoscopy over sonographic imaging was in viewing small areas of anatomy such as the tips of the digits, details of the genitalia, or features of facial anatomy. Syndactyly, hypospadias, or preauricular sinuses could be visualized, enabling the diagnosis of a malformation syndrome that was beyond the capability of ultrasound. The embryo can now be visualized with an embryoscope during the first trimester.[23] Today, these techniques are rarely used for prenatal diagnosis because of the risks associated with them and the increasing sophistication of sonographic imaging and MRI.

Metabolite analysis

Inborn errors of metabolism, in which there is typically a block in a metabolic pathway, can usually be characterized by an accumulation or deficiency of one or more metabolites. Measurements of metabolites in the blood or urine of the pregnant woman have not been useful, but analysis of fluids or tissues from the fetal compartment offer a much better opportunity for diagnosis. Here, metabolites can be obtained before they are acted on by maternal dilution or metabolism. Several disorders, including methylmalonic acidemias and propionic acidemia, have been accurately diagnosed solely through measurements of metabolites in amniotic fluid. Canavan disease, galactosemia, and adrenogenital syndrome resulting from 21-hydroxylase deficiency are also diagnosable in this way. However, extensive efforts are required to establish these diagnostic methods. The range of concentrations of metabolites from normal fetuses and fetuses with disease must be established although the number of pregnancies at risk for most inborn errors of metabolism is very small.

Histological examination

Tissue biopsies have played a limited role in prenatal diagnosis. The two tissues that are usually available with low risk to the fetus are cells from the amniotic fluid and chorionic villi (placenta), neither of which is part of the fetus *per se*. Unfortunately, uncultured amniotic fluid cells are a variable mixture of many cell types which, in the second trimester, are dominated by desquamated epithelial cells in varying stages of disintegration. Fetal blood sampling and skin, liver, and muscle biopsy increase the risks of miscarriage and fetal demise. Diagnoses based on histology have come from skin biopsies that can be used to assess the presence of inherited skin diseases, including ichthyoses, epidermolysis bullosa syndromes, and ectodermal dysplasias. Because these and other diseases with distinctive histopathology are often defined by abnormal genes, DNA tests are supplanting biopsies for many diagnoses.

Chromosomal analysis

A few single-gene disorders show chromosomal abnormalities when cells are examined by cytogenetic techniques, e.g., chromosome breakage syndromes, Fanconi pancytopenia syndrome, and Roberts–SC phocomelia syndrome, which is characterized by the premature separation of dividing chromosomes at centromeres.

Small chromosomal deletions have been described that are associated with defined clinical syndromes. The underlying defect is the absence of several contiguous genes. One of the absent genes may be largely responsible for the phenotype, or the disease expression may reflect the absence of two or more genes. Examples of contiguous gene deletion syndromes are Miller–Dieker syndrome, with a microdeletion on chromosome 17p, and DiGeorge velocardiofacial syndrome, with a microdeletion on chromosome 22q. If the disorder does not preclude reproduction, dominant transmission can be seen in a family. Increasingly, diagnosis utilizes DNA probes and hybridization with single probes or microarrays.

Another situation involving an unusual status of chromosomes is that of uniparental disomy (UPD), in which both members of a chromosome pair have originated from a single parent. Prader–Willi syndrome can be caused either by a microdeletion on the paternally inherited chromosome 15q when there is biparental disomy for chromosome 15 or by maternal uniparental disomy. In either case, the result is the absence of paternal genes in the Prader–Willi region of chromosome 15; these genes are imprinted and the absence of paternal copies leads to the syndrome. Diagnosis of UPD requires DNA analysis that compares the DNA of each parent with that of the fetus.

Gene products

Single-gene disorders are most often defined by a deficiency, alteration, or excess of a gene product. The analysis of gene products continues to be important in both postnatal and prenatal diagnosis, even in this age of gene analysis and description of specific gene mutations. Gene product analysis has a major advantage when a disease shows important allelic or genetic heterogeneity.

Today, most gene products that are associated with a disease process are proteins or peptides. Abnormal RNAs as gene products have not yet become important in genetic diagnosis. In single-gene disorders, protein analysis usually involves the measurement of enzyme activity; occasionally, physical attributes of the protein, such as electrophoretic mobility or recognition of the protein by antibodies, are analysed. The large majority of prenatal diagnoses based on protein gene products use amniotic fluid cells and chorionic villi. Occasionally, another specialized tissue, such as liver or blood cells, is required because of limited expression of the gene, e.g., globins are expressed only in red blood cells.

Healthy, living tissue is usually necessary for accurate protein analysis. Amniotic fluid cells, obtained by amniocentesis, are almost always cultured to provide this healthy tissue. Biopsies of chorionic villi or blood cell aspirates, on the other hand, consist almost entirely of healthy cells and thus can be used without being cultured as well as being used as a source of cultured cells. Because the culture process takes many days, analyses on uncultured biopsies have the advantage of providing a more rapid diagnosis.

Gene analysis

To understand a genetic disease at the molecular level, the gene responsible for the disease must be isolated and molecular abnormalities demonstrated in that gene. This has been successful for many single-gene disorders; thus, DNA analysis has become the dominant method for prenatal diagnosis of these conditions. Examples of common disorders include cystic fibrosis, fragile X syndrome, Duchenne–Becker muscular dystrophy, and most hemoglobinopathies.

Gene analysis usually begins with an initial phase of gene mapping, in which the gene's approximate location on a chromosome or its relation to neighboring genetic material is determined, followed by the eventual isolation of the gene and documentation of its mutations. During the first phase, DNA analysis depends on linkage relationships to neighboring markers that can be followed from the parents to the fetus. These markers are known as RFLPs or tandem repeat polymorphisms. Because linked markers rather than the disease gene itself are being followed, the relationship of these markers to the mutant and normal alleles of the disease gene must be established individually for each family that requests prenatal diagnosis. Major limitations include the possibility that RFLPs may be unavailable in a given family to distinguish mutant and normal alleles (e.g., if all family members have the same polymorphic allele, the polymorphism is not informative in that family), a family member who is crucial to establishing linkage relationships is not available, and meiotic crossover events occur between the linked marker and the gene of interest. The last limitation becomes minimized if informative markers are sought on both sides, thus flanking the gene of interest.

When the gene and its structure are known and mutations have been discovered, there is a possibility of direct DNA diagnosis based on the mutations present in the family. Family studies should be initiated well before prenatal diagnosis is necessary, although direct gene analysis can sometimes be accomplished during pregnancy for disorders in which there has been intensive study of the gene and its mutations. In most circumstances, fetal DNA is obtained from chorionic villi or amniotic fluid cells. Sometimes, uncultured amniotic fluid cells will not provide sufficient DNA of requisite quality, and diagnosis must await a period of cell culture. This delay is usually not necessary when chorionic villi are used. The polymerase chain reaction provides a method of amplifying tiny amounts of DNA and can help to minimize the time to diagnosis. In the future, fetal cells or fetal nucleic acids (DNA or RNA) recovered from the maternal circulation will probably become an alternative to chorionic villi and amniotic fluid cells.

Prenatal diagnosis of specific disorders

The following sections list specific disorders that can be diagnosed prenatally. The lists are not complete, and new information is constantly appearing. It is especially important to consult with specialists in prenatal diagnosis when dealing with single-gene disorders, because there are hundreds of disorders and sometimes several possible methods by which a diagnosis may be made. Texts relating to this specialty and on-line sources are also available.[15–19] As more and more genes are isolated and previously unknown gene products discovered, it is becoming possible to diagnose disorders for the first time. In addition, different and improved methods may become available to improve the accuracy, safety, or timing of a diagnosis.

Another caveat for the diagnosis of single-gene disorders is the absolute requirement for an accurate diagnosis in a proband or gene carrier in the family, in order to apply many of the diagnostic tests. For example, if an enzyme assay or a mutation analysis is to be used, it must already be known from prior studies in the family that the proposed test is the appropriate one. Correct information about paternity is also required, sometimes for several matings in the family, if a DNA linkage method is being used.

Malformation syndromes

Sonographic imaging and MRI can detect malformations of many organ systems. When a specific diagnosis is being sought because of a previously affected child, a specific demonstrable malformation can be essentially diagnostic. The absence of a demonstrable malformation is often much less reassuring about the absence of the disorder. Examples of malformation syndromes are presented in Table 20.6.

Table 20.6 Malformation syndrome.

Syndrome	Inheritance pattern*
Aqueductal stenosis	XL (and others)
Walker–Warburg syndrome	AR
Craniofacial dysostosis and craniosynostosis syndrome	AD
Holoprosencephaly	AR (and others)
Achondrogenesis	AD, AR?
Ellis–van Creveld syndrome	AR
Asphyxiating thoracic dystrophy	AR
Thanatophoric dysplasia	AD
Short-rib polydactyly syndromes	AR
Thrombocytopenia–absent radius syndrome	AR
Adult polycystic kidney disease	AD
Arthrogryposis	AR, AD
Multiple pterygium syndrome	AR, XL
Meckel–Gruber syndrome	AR
Noonan syndrome	AD
Roberts syndrome	AR

AD, autosomal dominant; AR, autosomal recessive; XL, X-linked.

*Some malformation syndromes occur sufficiently often in families to warrant designation of an inheritance pattern; they may occur sporadically as well, raising possibilities of AD inheritance if reproduction is sharply limited, or have multifactorial etiologies.

Table 20.7 Skin disorders.

Disorders	Inheritance pattern
Epidemolysis bullosa syndrome	AR, AD
Ichthyosis syndromes	AR
Anhidrotic ectodermal dysplasia	XL, AR
Sjögern–Larsson syndrome	AR
Oculocutaneous albinism	AR

AD, autosomal dominant; AR, autosomal recessive; XL, X-linked.

Skin disorders

Severe skin disorders have previously been diagnosed using skin biopsies (Table 20.7). Specific proteins and the genes associated with these diseases are being discovered so that DNA or other biochemical assays now replace histological examination of biopsies in most circumstances.

Chromosome breakage syndromes and DNA repair defects

Fanconi pancytopenia syndrome has been successfully diagnosed many times; however, the diagnosis of Bloom syndrome and ataxia-telangiectasia, which also show increased chromosome breakage, has been limited. Xeroderma pigmentosum syndromes show faulty repair of induced DNA damage; prenatal diagnosis based on this phenomenon has had some success. For all of these conditions, it is likely that a gene-based diagnosis will be available in the near future.

Table 20.8 Hematological disorders.

Disorder	Inheritance pattern
β-thalassemias	AR
α-thalassemias	AR
Sickle cell disorders	AR
Hemophilia A	XL
Hemophilia	XL
von Willebrand's disease	AD
Wiskott–Aldrich syndrome	XL
Chronic granulomatous disease	XL, AR
Severe combined immunodeficiency diseases	AR, XL
Hereditary elliptocytosis	AR

AD, autosomal dominant; AR, autosomal recessive; XL, X-linked.

Hematological disorders

Several different types of hematological disorder have been diagnosed prenatally (Table 20.8). These include globin abnormalities (especially the thalassemias and sickle cell disorders), hemophilias, and immune deficiency syndromes. Increasingly, DNA analysis has become available for this group of disorders. Before this, fetal blood, obtained by cordocentesis, was necessary for diagnosis and this is still used occasionally, e.g., to analyze a gene product or enumerate a class of cells. Some gene products, for example the globins, are present only in red blood cells. Because fetal red blood cells are significantly larger than maternal red blood cells, an automated cell size analyzer, such as the Coulter counter and Channelyser, is used to distinguish fetal and maternal blood cells in the aspirates obtained during fetal blood sampling (Fig. 20.11).

Fragile X syndrome

After Down syndrome, fragile X syndrome is the second most frequent genetic cause of significant mental retardation in most populations. The underlying gene defect is almost always an expansion of the number of trinucleotide repeats (strings of CGGs) in the *FMR-1* gene. Normal genes have fewer than 40–55 repeats, depending upon the authority. Men and boys with more than 200 repeats (defined as a full mutation) usually show moderate to severe retardation. One-half of women and girls with full mutations show few, if any, symptoms, whereas the other one-half have severe learning disabilities or mild retardation. Some asymptomatic women and men have a fragile X allele with an intermediate number of repeats, i.e., between 55 and 200. Such premutation alleles are unstable on transmission from mother to offspring; they have a tendency

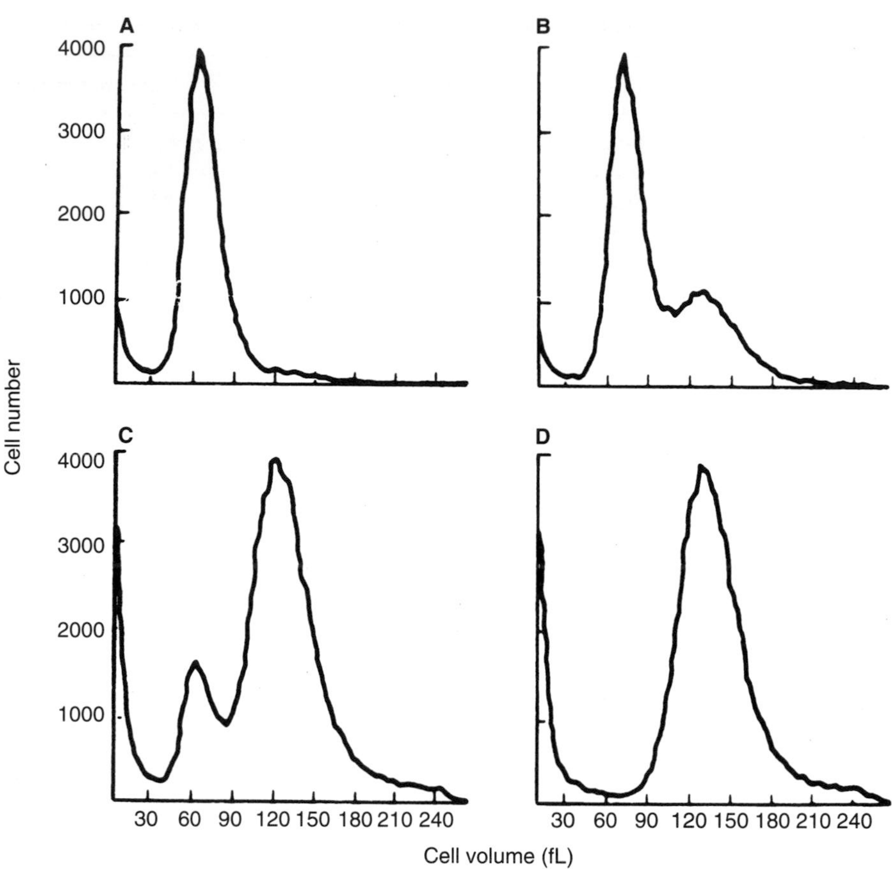

Figure 20.11 Coulter Channelyser analysis of fetal and maternal red blood cells. (A) 100% maternal; (B) 30% fetal, 70% maternal; (C) 80% fetal, 20% maternal; and (D) 100% fetal. (From ref. 30.)

to enlarge, sometimes into the full mutation with associated symptoms. This tendency to expand is not observed when a premutation allele is transmitted by a man.

Limited population screening has begun to try and identify women who carry premutation or full mutation alleles and enable them the opportunity to undergo prenatal diagnosis. Diagnosis is accomplished using DNA from chorionic villi or amniotic fluid cells. Counseling is complex given the spectrum of disease expression and a varying probability of expansion, which is dependent on the size of the mother's allele; the larger the allele, the more likely it is to expand. A further complication has been the recognition that carriers of permutation alleles may face symptoms in adulthood. Approximately 20% of women show premature ovarian failure, and older men may develop a syndrome of tremor, ataxia, and possible dementia.

Cystic fibrosis

The gene and gene product for cystic fibrosis were discovered simultaneously. There is a common mutation in the cystic fibrosis gene that is present in 30–70% of people from different ethnic populations who carry cystic fibrosis mutations. The most common mutation in non-Ashkenazi Jewish Caucasians is a deletion of the three nucleotides coding for a phenylalanine (F) at position 508 of the cystic fibrosis protein (ΔF508). In Ashkenazi Jews, the most common mutation is W1282X, the X connoting a stop codon that produces a truncated protein. Today, over 1000 disease-causing mutations in the cystic fibrosis gene are known. For a person carrying two mutant alleles, disease is usually expressed as a severe lung, or lung and pancreatic malfunction. For some people, however, disease is expressed as a mild lung disorder or, sometimes, solely as atresia of the vas deferens. Population screening for carriers has begun in some countries. Most protocols test for a limited number of mutations although sequencing of the entire gene is becoming increasingly available. In the USA, it is recommended to test for a panel of 23 mutations; this panel identifies 94.04% of cystic fibrosis carriers in Ashkenazi Jews. 82.29% in other non-Hispanic Caucasians, 71.72% in Hispanic Americans, 64.46% in African Americans, and 48.93% in Asian Americans.[24] The absence of complete carrier detection and the recognition of a much wider spectrum of disease expression than previously realized has complicated prenatal diagnosis and counseling for cystic fibrosis.

Inborn errors of metabolism

Most inborn errors of metabolism that are diagnosable prenatally are detected by measuring enzyme activities. A few disorders are diagnosed by other types of protein analysis or by the measurement of secondary effects of the metabolic block. DNA analysis is beginning to play an important role as well. Tables 20.9–20.12 list many of the inborn errors that have been diagnosed.

Table 20.9 Inborn errors of lipid metabolism.

Disorder	Inheritance pattern
Fabry's disease	XL
Gaucher's disease	AR
Tay–Sachs disease	AR
Sandhoff's disease	AR
Metachromatic leukodystrophy	AR
Adrenoleukodystrophy	XL, AR
Zellweger syndrome	AR
Krabbe's disease	AR
Mucolipidoses	AR

AR, autosomal recessive; XL, X-linked. (From ref. 31.)

Table 20.10 Inborn errors of amnio acid and fatty acid metabolism.

Disorder	Inheritance pattern
Ornithine transcarbamylase deficiency	XL
Citrullinemia	AR
Argininosuccinic acidemia	AR
Propionic acidemias	AR
Methylmalonic acidemias	AR
Isovaleric acidemia	AR
Glutaric acidurias	AR
Phenylketonuria	AR
Maple syrup urine disease	AR
Biotinidase deficiency	AR
Tyrosinemia	AR
Nonketotic hyperglycinemia	AR
Cystinosis	AR
Homocystinuria	AR
Medium-chain acyl-CoA dehydrogenase deficiency and other fatty acid oxidation disorders	AR
Canavan disease	AR

AR, autosomal recessive; XL, X-linked. (From ref. 31.)

Muscle and nerve disorders

Mapping and cloning of genes have made possible the prenatal diagnosis of several muscle and nerve disorders for which little basic information had previously been known (Table 20.13). Most of the diagnostic activity has involved Duchenne–Becker muscular dystrophy, and its gene product (dystrophin) has proved useful in clarifying the presence or absence of disease in muscle obtained by biopsy or autopsy. Spinal muscular atrophy is usually caused by mutations in the survival motor neuron (*SMN*) gene. This is true for the severe infantile presentation (Werdnig–Hoffmann disease) as well as for the juvenile- and adult-onset forms. Several adult- (or juvenile-) onset neurological disorders, including myotonic dystrophy and Huntington's disease, result from the expansion of trinucleotide repeats, as occurs in the fragile X syndrome.

Table 20.11 Inborn errors of carbohydrate metabolism and related disorders.

Disorder	Inheritance pattern
Galactosemia	AR
Glycogen storage diseases	AR
Sialidoses	AR
Mucopolysaccharidoses	AR, XL
Pyruvate carboxylase deficiency	AR
Mannosidosis	AR
Fucosidosis	AR

AR, autosomal recessive; XL, X-linked. (From ref. 31.)

Table 20.12 Miscellaneous inborn errors of metabolism.

Disorder	Inheritance pattern
Lesch–Nyhan disease	XL
Smith–Lemli–Opitz syndrome	AR
Menkes' disease	XL
Osteogenesis imperfecta	AD, AR
Porphyrias	AD, AR
Adrenogenital syndrome due to 21-hydroxylase deficiency	AR
Hypophosphatasia	AR

AD, autosomal dominant; AR, autosomal recessive; XL, X-linked. (From ref. 31.)

Table 20.13 Muscle and nerve disorders.

Disorder	Inheritance pattern
Duchenne-Becker muscular dystrophy	XL
Spinal muscular atrophy	AR
Myotonic dystrophy	AD
Spinocerebellar ataxia	AD
Friedreich's ataxia	AR
Huntington's disease	AD
Neurofibromatosis type 1	AD

AD, autosomal dominant; AR, autosomal recessive; XL, X-linked. (From ref. 31.)

Mitochondrial genes

In mitochondrial disorders, one or more of the functions of mitochondria are seriously impaired as a result of either abnormal nuclear genes inherited in the usual mendelian manner, or abnormal mitochondrial genes. Mitochondrial genes, which reside within the mitochondrion, are inherited solely from the mother via the cytoplasm of the oocyte.

Common mutations of these genes include point mutations, and small and large deletions. A pattern of maternal transmission of disease may be evident in a family pedigree. Satisfactory methods for the prenatal diagnosis of diseases caused by mutant mitochondrial genes are still being developed. The situation is complicated by the fact that cells contain many mitochondria and, hence, many copies of mitochondrial genes, and by the fact that there is a mixture of inherited mutant mitochondrial genes and normal mitochondrial genes. The distribution of mutant and normal genes in various tissues and organs gives rise to a wide range of symptoms, age of onset of disease, and organs primarily affected. This complexity presents a major challenge for prenatal diagnosis.

Conclusion

Single-gene disorders represent an extremely heterogeneous category of inherited problems. Many of the features that define a disorder in postnatal life can be sought in prenatal diagnosis, but extreme care must be taken to examine the variability of expression and onset of the disorder, possible genetic heterogeneity underlying the phenotype, and accuracy of diagnosis for the family that is requesting a prenatal diagnosis. Increasingly, these disorders are being defined by genes and their mutations, and prenatal diagnosis is relying on analysis of those genes.

Key points

1 Genetic disorders can result from any one of several mechanisms: numerical or structural alterations in chromosomal constitution, a mutation involving a single genetic locus (mendelian), or the cumulative effect of several genes (polygenic–multifactoral).

2 Routine cytogenetic analysis usually reveals 450–500 bands per haploid set of chromosomes. At this level, each band consists of approximately 1500–2000 kilobases (kb) of DNA (1 500 000–2 000 000 bases).

3 Trisomy may arise by several cytological mechanisms, but in humans it usually arises *de novo* after maternal meiotic nondisjunction.

4 In a couple in which one parent has a balanced robertsonian translocation involving chromosomes 14 and 21, Down syndrome will arise in 10–15% of viable offspring of female heterozygotes and 2–4% of viable offspring of male heterozygotes.

5 In a couple in which one parent has an unbalanced translocation, the risk is 10–15% for offspring of either female or male carrier.

6 When a nonfamilial (*de novo*) translocation that is apparently balanced is detected in amniotic fluid or chorionic villi, the risk of the fetus being abnormal is still increased over background: 7% for reciprocal translocations and less for robertsonian translocations.

7 In autosomal dominant traits, equal numbers of males and females are usually affected. The likelihood that an individual carrying a mutant autosomal dominant gene (allele) will transmit that allele to any given offspring, male or female, is 50%.

8 An individual with an autosomal recessive trait is usually the product of parents who are both heterozygous (carriers) for mutation at the same locus. The likelihood that a given offspring will be affected is 25%.

9 In a family in which an X-linked recessive mutant allele is segregating, individuals at risk include male siblings, maternal uncles, maternal nephews, maternal male first cousins, and certain other maternal male relatives.

10 Anomalies affecting a single organ system (e.g., cleft palate) show recurrence risks of 1–5% for first-degree relatives (siblings, offspring, parents).

11 The multiple contributing causes of presumed multifactorial disorders are poorly understood. Prenatal diagnosis depends largely on some phenotypic feature, usually altered sonographic anatomy, and not on gene analysis.

12 Screening potential parents to identify carriers of serious recessive disorders has evolved because most of these disorders are infrequent and the disease has yet to appear in the family.

13 By 2006, recessive gene screening programs were commonly available for cystic fibrosis, hemoglobinopathies, and Tay–Sachs disease. Several other disorders characterized by an increased frequency in the Ashkenazi Jewish population along with a limited number of common mutations also had screening available.

14 Fetal diagnosis using gene analysis (DNA analysis) can be carried out using cells from chorionic villi (placenta) or amniotic fluid. In the future, it may be possible to separate fetal DNA or RNA from maternal blood for fetal diagnosis.

15 Many gene products (proteins) are present in chorionic villi or amniotic fluid cells and, therefore, fetal diagnosis can use these tissues for assays of enzyme activities and other protein characteristics.

16 Most single-gene disorders that are expressed as anatomical abnormalities cause abnormalities that are also seen as isolated birth defects which are not part of a genetic syndrome (e.g., cleft lip, omphalocele, heart defect). If the a priori risk for a genetic syndrome is high based on family history, the diagnosis of a syndrome from the anatomical finding is very likely;

if the a priori risk is low, diagnosis is much less likely.

17 For mendelian disorders that are expressed by abnormal anatomy, there is usually considerable variability in the abnormalities in both structure and time of appearance during development; there is even variability in whether a given abnormality will be present or not.

18 Microdeletions or microduplications of small chromosomal segments that cause contiguous gene syndromes are diagnosable using DNA hybridization, often with microarray technology.

19 Uniparental disomy (UPD), when both members of a chromosome pair come from one parent (e.g., in Prader–Willi or Angelman syndromes), requires comparison of fetal DNA with parental DNA.

20 When gene mutations cannot be determined in a family at risk for a single-gene disorder, yet mapping of the causative gene has been accomplished, linkage analysis using restriction fragment length polymorphisms (RFLPs) or single nucleotide polymorphisms (SNPs) can often provide a very accurate diagnosis. A careful study of the family, often involving several members, is an absolute requirement in these circumstances.

References

1 Ledbetter DH, Martin AO, Verlinsky Y, et al. Cytogenetic results of chorionic villus sampling: high success rate and diagnostic accuracy in the United States Collaborative Study. *Am J Obstet Gynecol* 1990;162:495.

2 Hassold TJ, Jacobs PA. Trisomy in man. *Annu Rev Genet* 1984;18:69.

3 Boué A, Gallano P. A collaborative study of the segregation of inherited chromosome structural rearrangements in 1356 prenatal diagnoses. *Prenat Diagn* 1984;4:45.

4 Daniel A, Hook EB, Wulf G. *Am J Hum Genet* 1988;43: 918,A230.

5 Jacobs PA, Frackiewicz A, Law P, et al. The effect of structural aberrations of the chromosomes on reproductive fitness in man. Ii. Results. *Clin Genet* 1975;8:169.

6 Daniel A, Hook EB, Wulf G. Risks of unbalanced progeny at amniocentesis to carriers of chromosome rearrangements: data from United States and Canadian laboratories. *Am J Med Genet* 1989;33:14.

7 Simpson JL, Meyers CM, Martin AO, et al. Translocations are infrequent among couples having repeated spontaneous abortions but no other abnormal pregnancies. *Fertil Steril* 1989;51:811.

8 Warburton D. De novo structural rearrangements diagnosed at amniocentesis. *Prenat Diagn* 1984;4:69.

9 Warburton D. De novo balanced chromosome rearrangements and extra marker chromosomes identified at prenatal diagnosis: clinical significance and distribution of breakpoints. *Am J Hum Genet* 1991;49:995.

10 Antonarakis SE, Blouin JL, Maher J, et al. Maternal uniparental disomy for human chromosome 14, due to loss of a chromosome 14 from somatic cells with T(13;14) Trisomy 14. *Am J Hum Genet* 1993;52:1145.

11 Schinzel AA, Basaran S, Bernasconi F, et al. Maternal uniparental disomy 22 has no impact on the phenotype. *Am J Hum Genet* 1994;54:21.

12 Slater H, Shaw JH, Bankier A, et al. Upd 13: no indication of maternal or paternal imprinting of genes on chromosome 13. *J Med Genet* 1995;32:493.

13 Stallard R, Krueger S, James RS, et al. Uniparental isodisomy 13 in a normal female due to transmission of a maternal T(13q13q). *Am J Med Genet* 1995;57:14.

14 Blouin JL, Avramopoulos D, Pangalos C, et al. Normal phenotype with paternal uniparental isodisomy for chromosome 21. *Am J Hum Genet* 1993;53:1074.

15 Milunsky A. *Genetic disorders and the fetus: diagnosis, prevention, and treatment.* Baltimore, MD: John Hopkins University Press, 2004.

16 Rodeck C, Whittle MJ. *Fetal medicine: basic science and clinical practice.* London: Churchill Livingstone, 1999.

17 Online Mendelian Inheritance in Man, OMIM. McKusick-Nathans Institute for Genetic Medicine, Johns Hopkins University (Baltimore, MD) and National Center for Biotechnology Information, National Library of Medicine (Bethesda, MD), 1998. World Wide Web URL: http://www.ncbi.nlm.nih.gov/omim/.

18 Gene Tests. University of Washington (Seattle, WA), 2005. World Wide Web URL: http://www.genetests.org/.

19 Weaver DD. *Catalog of prenatally diagnosed conditions.* Baltimore, MD: Johns Hopkins University Press, 1998.

20 Lo YM, Tein MS, Lau TK. Quantitative analysis of fetal DNA in maternal plasma and serum: implications for noninvasive prenatal diagnosis. *Am J Hum Genet* 1998;62:768.

21 Poon LL, Leung TN, Lau TK, et al. Presence of fetal RNA in maternal plasma. *Clin Chem* 2000;46:1832.

22 Jones KL. *Smith's recognizable patterns of human malformation*, 6th edn. New York, W. B. Saunders Co. 2005.

23 Quintero RA, Puder KS, Cotton DB. Embryoscopy and fetoscopy. *Obstet Gynecol Clin North Am* 1993;20:563.

24 Watson MS, Cutting GR, Desnick RJ, et al. Cystic fibrosis population carrier screening: 2004 revision of American College of Medical Genetics Mutation Panel. *Genet Med* 2004;6: 387.

25 Hook EB. Rates of chromosome abnormalities at different maternal ages. *Obstet Gynecol* 1981;58:282.

26 Simpson JL, Tharapel AT. Principles of cytogenetics. In: Phillip E, Barnes J, eds. *Scientific foundations of obstetrics and gynecology*, 4th edn. London: Butterworth-Heinemann; 1991:4; 49.

27 Gerbie AB, Simpson JL. Antenatal detection of genetic disorders. *Postgrad Med* 1976;59:129.

28 Simpson JL. *Disorders of sexual differentiation: etiology and clinical delineation.* New York: Academic Press; 1976:1.

29 Gabbe SG, Niebyl JR, Simpson JL. *Obstetrics: normal and problem pregnancies*, 4th edn. New York: Churchill Livingstone; 2002.

30 Simpson JL. Principles of human genetics. In: Reece EA, Hobbins JC, eds. *Medicine of the fetus and mother.* Philadelphia, PA: Lippincott, 1999.

31 Mahoney MJ. Single gene disorders. In: Reece EA, Hobbins JC, eds. *Medicine of the fetus and mother.* Philadelphia, PA: Lippincott, 1999.

21

Genetic counseling in prenatal and perinatal medicine

Jeff Milunsky and Aubrey Milunsky

There is no family, and hence no pregnancy, in which genetic factors can be ignored. Normal body structure and function are direct consequences of multiple gene action that is frequently conditioned by environmental interaction. Indeed the maternal milieu of the fetus is now increasingly recognized as not only influencing growth and development but also in some way seeding the origins of disease in adulthood.[1] Hypertension, type 2 diabetes, obesity, breast and prostate cancer, and coronary artery disease are but a few examples of disorders causally connected to fetal influences. Not unexpectedly, genetics has a role in virtually every illness: in causation, predisposition and susceptibility, immune response, modulation, or reaction to medical treatment. Determination of genetic susceptibilities reflects the widening scope of molecular diagnostics, which, in turn, has increased opportunities for predictive, preconception, preimplantation, and prenatal diagnosis. These advances are important as each of us carries some disadvantageous (and advantageous) genes. About one in 13 conceptions results in a conceptus with a chromosome abnormality and about 50% of first-trimester spontaneous abortions are associated with chromosome anomalies.[2] Liveborn infants have a 0.4% rate of clinically significant chromosome defects and an additional 0.2% rate of balanced chromosomal rearrangements.[3,4] Some 3–4% of all births are associated with a major congenital malformation, mental retardation, or genetic disorder, a rate that doubles by 7–8 years of age, given late-appearing and/or late-diagnosed genetic disorders.[5] The burden of genetic disease is sufficiently significant in childhood to account for 71% of hospital admissions in a major North American Children's Hospital.[6] Cataloged single-gene traits or disorders now approximate 10 000.[7] The extent and importance of the role of genetics in disease causation becomes apparent immediately when one includes later-onset disease, such as heart disease, hypertension, diabetes, and the polygenic disorders in general. If chromosomal, monogenic, and polygenic disorders are combined, about 60% of all sick individuals have genetically influenced diseases.[8] It is appropriate and important that parents are fully informed of the risks they normally undertake in having a child[9] and about any significant additional risks of 0.5–1.0% or more.

Preconception care and counseling

Major and continuing efforts must be made to educate the public at large about the importance of pregnancy planning and, in particular, of preconception care and counseling.[9] Our knowledge of embryonic and fetal development and the sophisticated developments of the "new genetics" make the matter more compelling than ever. Physicians need to inculcate the wisdom not only of planning pregnancy, but also of initiating care in the preconception period. Many issues that influence fetal development and maternal welfare need to be addressed at the preconception visit.

Careful attention is necessary in eliciting the *medical history and examination*. Medical disorders may be detected that have a bearing on pregnancy, fetal development, delivery, and the newborn. For example, the significance of excessive joint laxity may be recognized for the first time at the preconception visit and point to diagnoses such as the Ehlers–Danlos syndrome, with its associated complications of premature delivery and tissue fragility.[10] Excess bruisability may reflect a disorder of coagulation and a history of recurrent fetal loss may signal the presence of a factor V Leiden gene mutation.[11] A history of unexplained syncope or a family history of sudden death should alert the physician to the possibility of the long QT syndrome.[12] In these few examples, early detection affords the opportunity to avoid potential later complications and facilitates anticipatory obstetric and perinatal management.

The preconception visit is also the time to secure *control and treatment of specific disorders* that may affect an otherwise successful pregnancy. Prospective mothers with type 1 and type 2 diabetes need help and advice to achieve tight control of their hyperglycemia. They need to understand that the poorer the control of their diabetes, the higher the frequency of congenital malformations and the more severe they may be.[13] Women with epilepsy, in particular, require review by their own neurologists concerning anticonvulsant medication. When appropriate, anticonvulsants could be changed to those that might pose lesser risks of fetal anomalies without risking maternal health. Women with sickle cell disease[14] or cystic fibrosis,[15,16] who face serious personal and fetal risks, need special attention and treatment to secure the best chance for successful pregnancy and survival. Recognition of systemic lupus erythematosus allows appropriate careful medical surveillance and later monitoring of the fetal and neonatal heart for early detection and treatment of congenital heart block, which occurs much more frequently in this condition.[17]

The *obstetric and gynecologic* history, taken at the preconception visit, provides important opportunities again for intervention. Patients with prolonged infertility of unknown cause or recurrent spontaneous abortion, who may face a 3–8% risk of a parental chromosome abnormality,[18,19] require chromosome analysis, as do their spouses. Failure to detect a parental chromosome translocation or other rearrangement may later be followed by the conception and birth of a child with an unbalanced karyotype.

History of a previous stillbirth should raise questions about the need for parental chromosome analysis. Between 6% and 11% of stillbirths have a chromosome abnormality,[20] and a small portion of such cases indeed may have a transmitting parent with a chromosome rearrangement or disorder. The preconception visit, in addition, facilitates determination of whether the prospective mother is susceptible to rubella, cytomegalovirus, or toxoplasmosis, or has herpes or AIDS. Timely vaccination for rubella, where indicated, should be provided well before conception.

Nutritional considerations that bear on fetal development have become more important. Our original data indicated that multivitamins containing folic acid taken during the preconception period and continuing at least through the first 6 weeks of pregnancy reduce the frequency of neural tube defects by 70%,[21] a conclusion confirmed by definitive double-blind randomized control studies.[22,23] Notwithstanding uncertainty about the precise mechanism by which folic acid exerts its protective effects, there are now clear indications that 0.4 mg daily provides the necessary supplementation dose. In pregnancies that follow the conception of offspring with a neural tube defect, a dose of *4 mg* daily is recommended, taken while planning pregnancy and at least through the first 6 weeks post conception.[22,24] For the 30% of cases of spina bifida that are resistant to folic acid supplementation, additional supplementation with the B-complex vitamin inositol may eventually be shown to add protective effects.[25]

The *clinical genetic history* focuses first on analysis of the family pedigree. An obvious pattern of inheritance may emerge without a known named disorder. For example, a *maternal* history of nephews, brothers, or uncles with unexplained mental retardation may point to sex-linked mental retardation including the fragile X syndrome. A previous living child with a specified genetic defect might require additional diagnostic studies, parental examination, or other appropriate investigations. Carrier detection tests using DNA analysis for conditions such as Duchenne or Becker muscular dystrophy, spinal muscular atrophy, chronic granulomatous disease, and ornithine transcarbamylase deficiency are among the many disorders now approachable through molecular analysis.[4]

Attention to the patient's *ethnicity* may be the only warning to the obstetrician of potential genetic risks. Virtually all ethnic groups carry some "genetic burden."[9] For example, Caucasians have a risk of about 1 in 25 of carrying a cystic fibrosis gene mutation. Over 1300 cystic fibrosis mutations[26] have been reported and screening panels for the most common mutations detect between 85% and 90% of Caucasian carriers. Physicians are now expected to offer cystic fibrosis DNA carrier tests to all couples in their reproductive years.[27] Laboratory standards and guidelines now exist for population-based cystic fibrosis carrier screening.[28] The cystic fibrosis carrier screening panel has recently been revised to reflect more current data and exclude a polymorphism that was previously thought to be a mutation.[29] Prenatal diagnosis can be offered only if the parental mutations are known or if the pregnancy is suspected to be at risk for cystic fibrosis (i.e., presence of echogenic fetal bowel). About 1 in 12 individuals of Mediterranean extraction carry a gene mutation for β-thalassemia. Once again, a simple blood examination for mean corpuscular volume and for hemoglobins A_2 and F will assist in carrier detection. About 1 in 30 Ashkenazi Jews carry the gene for Tay–Sachs disease, and should be routinely offered the necessary carrier detection test for this lethal degenerative neurological disorder. DNA analysis for the three most common Tay–Sachs disease mutations in this ethnic group yields a detection rate of over 98%, without the problem of false-negatives or -positives and repeat sampling that hampers the hexosaminadase assay.[30] About 1 in 40 Ashkenazi Jews carries a gene mutation for Canavan disease and similarly should be routinely offered the necessary DNA carrier detection tests for this severe neurodegenerative condition.[31] For all the autosomal recessive disorders just mentioned, only if both parents are carriers would there be a 25% risk of bearing an affected child. In all these instances, prenatal diagnosis would be available.[4] This information becomes important for individuals who might select prenatal or preimplantation diagnosis as an option or for couples who could select other reproductive choices, such as artificial insemination or ovum donation, from donors who test negative for *detectable* gene mutations.

Dramatic and continuing advances in molecular genetics increasingly enable *predictive tests* for disorders not previously detectable by any method. Hence, even asymptomatic individuals may be able to determine whether they have a particular dominant gene for which there is a risk of 50% for transmission in each pregnancy, or whether they carry autosomal or X-linked genes, with their associated risks. Selected examples of such disorders for which presymptomatic and

Table 21.1 Examples of monogenic disorders for which DNA diagnostic tests facilitate presymptomatic and prenatal diagnosis as well as carrier detection.

Autosomal dominant disorders	
Adult polycystic kidney disease	Multiple endocrine neoplasia
Charcot–Marie–Tooth disease type 1A	Myotonic muscular dystrophy
Familial adenomatous polyposis	Spinocerebellar ataxia type 1
Huntington's disease	Tuberous sclerosis
Long QT syndrome	Von Hippel–Lindau disease
Machado–Joseph disease (SCA III)	
Autosomal recessive disorders	
α-Thalassemia	Phenylketonuria
β-Thalassemia	Sickle cell anemia
Cystic fibrosis	Spinal muscular atrophy
Canavan disease	Tay–Sachs disease
Familial dysautonomia	Wilson's disease
Friedreich's ataxia	
Sex-linked disorders	
Adrenoleukodystrophy	
Charcot–Marie–Tooth disease	
Chronic granulomatous disease	
Duchenne/Becker muscular dystrophy	
Hemophilia A	
Lesch–Nyhan syndrome	
X-linked lymphoproliferative disease	
Menkes' disease	
Myotubular myopathy	
Ornithine transcarbamylase deficiency	
Spinal and bulbar muscular atrophy	

prenatal diagnosis and carrier detection are feasible are listed in Table 21.1. Hence, for example, once a parent is shown to carry the dynamic gene mutation for myotonic muscular dystrophy, accurate prenatal diagnosis by direct DNA analysis can be accomplished. These tests allow detection of maternal myotonic dystrophy, facilitating prenatal diagnosis, anticipation,[32] optimal surveillance, and possible early intervention or prevention of the frequently serious intrapregnancy, labor, delivery, and postpartum and neonatal complications (Table 21.2).

Discovery of disorders with mutations resulting from the unstable expansion of trinucleotide repeats has rapidly escalated. The first such reports in 1991 described unstable CGG triplet repeats in males with the fragile X syndrome.[36] Thus far, 17 such disorders with dynamic mutations have been described and are outlined in Table 21.3. Friedreich's ataxia is the first autosomal recessive disorder that has been described with a triplet repeat expansion in about 96% of cases.[37] The remaining cases are due to other mutations within the gene. It is noteworthy that the typical carrier will have one normal allele and a second expanded allele.

The genetic mechanism of anticipation refers to progressively earlier manifestation and/or more severe expression of

Table 21.2 Myotonic muscular dystrophy: potential pregnancy, neonatal, and other complications.

Potential abortion
Fetal death
Polyhydramnios
Prolonged labor
Fetal distress
Uterine atony
Postpartum hemorrhage
Cardiac arrhythmias
Increased sensitivity to anesthetic and relaxant agents
Postoperative respiratory depression
Neonatal death
Arthrogryposis
Mental retardation

Data from refs 32–34.

a disorder with succeeding generations. Anticipation is seen in several of these disorders, and can be explained by the further expansion of the specific triplet repeat. In addition to expansions, triplet repeat reversions (decrease in number of repeats) have been documented in a small percentage of cases.[38] When interpreting test results, the number of such repeats may be used in genetic counseling to estimate the risk of recurrence and disease severity.

Advances in human genetics continue to escalate rapidly following the completion of the Human Genome Project. Obstetricians and all physicians who care for patients in their childbearing years should remain alert to these advances. In a growing number of centers, preimplantation diagnosis may require discussion during the preconception visit. Worldwide, over 5000 cases have been accomplished, and for some individuals this is an expensive, but possible, option.[39,40] Finally, among the more important aspects of the preconception visit is the provision of *genetic counseling,* the details of which now follow.

Genetic counseling

Genetic counseling is a communication process concerning the occurrence and the risks of recurrence of genetic disorders within a family. The aim of such counseling is to provide the patient with a clear and comprehensive understanding of all the important implications of the disorder in question, as well as the possible options. The purpose is also to help families through their problems, necessary decision making, and emotional adjustments and adaptations, where indicated. Although the physician may wish to prevent or minimize the suffering of both patient and family and to decrease the incidence of serious genetic disease, the primary strategy must be to achieve clear understanding by prospective parents, facilitating rational decision making.[8,9,41] All prospective parents

Table 21.3 Dynamic mutations with triplet repeat expansions.

Disease	Chromosome	Repeat sequence	Size in normal*	Size in carrier*	Size in affected*
Dentatorubral pallidoluysian atrophy	12p12–13	CAG	7–34	–	49–75
Fragile X syndrome†	Xq27.3	CGG	5–54	50–200	200 to 2000
Fragile XE	Xq27.3	GGC	6–25	116–133	200 to > 850
Friedreich's ataxia†	9q13	GAA	7–40	50–200	200 to > 1200
Huntington's disease	4p16.3	CAG	6–36	–	35–121
Kennedy's disease (spinal bulbar muscular atrophy)	Xq11–12	CAG	12–34	–	40–62
Machado–Joseph disease	14q32.1	CAG	13–36	–	68–79
Myotonic dystrophy type 1	19q13.3	CTG	5–37	–	50 to > 2000
Myotonic dystrophy type 2‡	3q21.3	CCTG	< 44	–	75–11 000
Spinocerebellar ataxia type I	6p22–23	CAG	6–39	–	41–81
Spinocerebellar ataxia type II	12q24.1	CAG	15–29	–	35–59
Spinocerebellar ataxia type VI	19p13	CAG	4–16	–	21–27
Spinocerebellar ataxia type VII	3p21.1	CAG	4–18	–	37–130
Spinocerebellar ataxia type VIII	13q21	CTG	16–37	–	> 90
Spinocerebellar ataxia type X§	22q13–qter	ATTCT	10–22	–	> 19 000
Spinocerebellar ataxia type XII	5q31–33	CAG	7–28	–	66–78
Spinocerebellar ataxia type XVII	6q27	CAG	27–44	–	> 45

*Variable ranges reported and overlapping sizes may occur.
†Mutation may not involve an expansion.
‡Expansion involves four nucleotides.
§Expansion involves five nucleotides.

have a right to know if they have an increased risk of having children with a genetic disorder, or other defect, and what their options are. The physician's duty is to communicate this information clearly and in simple language (with a translator if required), to offer specific tests (serially, if necessary), or to refer couples for second expert opinion and to document the consultation and recommendations.

The primary reasons couples seek genetic counseling in the context of risks and prenatal diagnosis are circumscribed:

1 Advanced maternal age. An arbitrary age of 35 years has long functioned as the standard of expected care, at which maternal age-related risks of chromosome defects should be discussed and prenatal genetic studies recommended.[4] Increasingly, geneticists consider it appropriate to inform parents of their risks that the fetus has a chromosome disorder based on first- and second-trimester maternal serum multiple analyte screening. Indeed, the decision about amniocentesis reflects the balance of risks between fetal loss and fetal defects. Although decisions made for or against such studies should be primarily parental, based on appropriate consultation with their physician, third-party payers continue to influence many of these decisions through cost considerations.

2 Maternal serum screening using four analytes. These assays yield increased odds for Down syndrome, trisomy 18, and other chromosome defects[42–45] or indicate increased risks for neural tube defects[46] necessitating ultrasound studies that may be followed by amniocentesis.

3 A previous fetus or child with a chromosomal, monogenic, or polygenic disorder.

4 A family history of a specific familial disorder.

5 One prospective parent with a suspected or known chromosomal, monogenic, or polygenic disorder.

6 A maternal disorder with or without specific drug treatment, associated with an increased risk of congenital defects.

7 A known or suspected carrier state for a certain genetic disorder on the basis of previous or required tests or ethnicity.

8 Exposure during, or prior to, pregnancy, to potentially hazardous medications, infectious organisms, X-rays, toxins, or occupational hazards.

9 Known or suspected consanguinity.

10 The background risk of congenital defects and genetic disorders.

In general, genetic counseling is best provided by a clinical geneticist or certified genetic counselor under supervision of a clinical geneticist. In both the USA and Canada, board-certified specialists in clinical genetics and medical genetics are available for referral. If an obstetrician is well informed, he or she should be able to provide the necessary counseling for advanced maternal age and, increasingly, for abnormal maternal serum screening results. Caution should guide the physician in avoiding areas outside expected expertise. Quotation of risk figures through intuitive judgments is strictly contraindicated. Clinical geneticists who provide counseling are expected to provide a letter to the referring physician, with a copy to the patient (or two separate letters, if preferred). Either way, documentation of the key elements transmitted during counseling would be regarded as mandatory, regardless of who provides such services.

The genetic basis for counseling

Genetic disorders that affect fetal development may be chromosomal, monogenic, or multifactorial in origin. Acquired disorders that complicate fetal development (e.g., infectious diseases, medications, toxins) will not be discussed here, even although their actions may be mediated through individual genetic susceptibility. Chromosomal disorders arise as a consequence of abnormal chromosome number or from structural rearrangements of one or more chromosomes. Single-gene disorders may be inherited or arise *de novo* as a consequence of mutation. The modes of inheritance for single-gene disorders are classified as autosomal dominant, autosomal recessive, X-linked, or mitochondrial. Multifactorial disorders result from an interaction between multiple genes and one or more environmental factors. The arbitrary distinction between chromosomal and single-gene inheritance should be understood, as many examples exist in which structural alteration of a chromosome results in deletion or interruption of one or more genes. Notwithstanding such arbitrary classifications, it is simpler, when trying to determine the origin of a specific phenotype, to think in terms of the preceding categorical classification.

Chromosomal disorders

Each of our somatic cells contains 46 chromosomes, with 23 derived from each parent. There are 44 nonsex chromosomes (called autosomes) and two sex chromosomes. Females have two X chromosomes (XX) and males have one X chromosome and one Y chromosome (XY). The chromosomes can be distinguished from each other on the basis of size, location of the centromere (which divides a chromosome into long and short arms), and the unique banding pattern. Not only can subtle details of chromosome structure now be delineated (e.g., deletions), but also the origin of an extra or abnormal chromosome can be determined frequently and precisely. For example, the extra chromosome 18 in trisomy 18 derives from a maternal source in 95% of cases, whereas the structurally abnormal chromosome (with a deletion) in Prader–Willi syndrome appears to be uniformly of paternal origin. High-resolution chromosome analysis of prophase chromosomes, rather than metaphase, allows easier recognition of structural defects.

It is now recognized that individuals can inherit two copies of part or all of a chromosome from one parent and no copy from the other parent. This process, called uniparental disomy (UPD), is uncommon, but contributes to the occurrence of some well-known clinical disorders. Uniparental heterodisomy refers to the inheritance of two homologous chromosomes that originate from one parent. Uniparental isodisomy indicates that the two chromosomes inherited from one parent are identical.[47] This derivation of a pair of homologs from one parent cannot be detected cytogenetically. Molecular cytogenetic techniques using fluorescence *in situ* hybridization (FISH), painting probes, and DNA markers facilitate detection. UPD has been described most commonly in the Prader–Willi[48] and Angelman syndromes,[49] and in addition has been reported in cystic fibrosis,[50] spinal muscular atrophy,[51] mosaic trisomy 15,[52] and robertsonian translocations.[53] About two-thirds of Prader–Willi syndrome patients have a recognizable cytogenetic deletion in one chromosome 15q11–q13 region. Another approximately 30% of cases are due to maternal UPD.[48] A newly recognized concern is the increased likelihood of inheriting a severe or lethal form of recessive disease in cases of uniparental isodisomy. UPD has been identified for 12 autosomes (e.g., chromosome 7 and cystic fibrosis) and the X chromosome. The indication for UPD study in most instances has been either a genetic disorder such as Prader–Willi syndrome or Angelman syndrome or an abnormality found on prenatal diagnosis, especially involving chromosomes 11, 14, and 15.[54,55] UPD is caused primarily by meiotic nondisjunction events, followed by trisomy or monosomy "rescue."[56]

Chromosomal disorders are classified as either numerical or due to structural rearrangements. Numerical disorders are characterized by extra or absent chromosomes. For example, the most common numerical chromosome disorder in newborns is characterized by an entire extra chromosome 21, resulting in trisomy 21 (Down syndrome). Among first-trimester abortuses, an absent sex chromosome, resulting in a 45,X fetus, is the most common numerical chromosome disorder. A single cell division, soon after fertilization, may go awry, resulting in a numerical chromosome abnormality in the daughter cells of that division and, consequently, in chromosomally abnormal cells from that original stem cell. These abnormal cells continue to divide and multiply alongside the subjacent chromosomally normal cells and eventually result in an individual who has two or more different cell lines – a chromosomal mosaic. Chromosomal mosaicism is found most frequently among the sex chromosome disorders.

Sex chromosome aneuploidy is the most common chromosome abnormality present at birth, with an overall incidence of 1 in 400.[57] Its incidence at amniocentesis is even greater and is estimated to be 1 in 250 in women over 35 years of age.[58] Genetic counseling after the prenatal diagnosis of sex chromosome aneuploidy often presents a challenge even for the experienced genetics professional. Knowledge of the phenotypic variability and the range of associated developmental and behavioral problems is essential to provide the most complete counseling. Linden et al.[59] reviewed the literature and summarized current knowledge on the intrauterine diagnosis of sex chromosome aneuploidy based on seven prospective studies. Sex chromosome mosaic karyotypes are most often 45,X/46,XX, 46,XX/47,XXX, or 46,XY/47,XXY, but many other combinations are possible. The presence of a normal 46,XX or 46,XY cell line tends to modify the effects of the aneuploid cells. On evaluations of intelligence, educational intervention, motor skills, and behavioral problems, those with mosaicism scored similarly to control subjects, and no significant differences were determined.[60,61] Fertility may vary, depending on the chromosomal constitution. Although 46,XX/47,XXX women usually are fertile, the prognosis for 45,X/46,XX and 46,XY/47,XXY mosaics is less definite.[59] When a prenatal diagnosis of sex chromosome mosaicism is made, a thorough discussion of the expected phenotype, developmental issues and probable learning disabilities should be tempered with the statement that a specific prognosis based on karyotype for any affected child is not possible. It should be explained that mental retardation is not typically associated with sex chromosome aneuploidy, but that the affected individual's IQ is often 10–15 points less than that of siblings. Owing to the information gleaned from these important prospective studies, genetic counselors can now better assist obstetricians in providing accurate and comprehensive information to parents of affected fetuses, thereby facilitating informed decision making about pregnancy management.

Chromosome mosaicism detected prenatally may also reflect confined placental mosaicism (CPM). CPM refers to the discrepancy between the chromosomal complement of the fetus and its placenta, due to postzygotic mitotic errors during embryonic development. CPM can be detected prenatally in about 2% of viable human pregnancies at 10–12 weeks of gestation.[62] CPM may be caused by the trisomic zygote rescue, which may then result in either a liveborn trisomic fetus or a diploid fetus. A diploid cell line, the product of the random loss of a trisomic chromosome, is expected to have UPD for the chromosome pair involved in the original trisomy in one-third of these cases.[63,64] The most common placental–fetal dichotomy involves placental trisomy for chromosome 16.[65] In pregnancies with CPM, a general effect of trisomy in the placenta may result in some degree of placental insufficiency, which may lead to intrauterine growth restriction, pregnancy associated hypertension, or intrauterine fetal death.[66] Ultrasound monitoring of fetal growth in such cases would be appropriate.

Structural chromosome defects may result from the breakage and loss of a variable-sized piece of a long or short arm (deletion) or the breakage of two chromosomes and transfer with fusion of parts of the broken fragments onto the residual chromosomes (translocation). About 1 in 500 liveborns has a balanced chromosomal translocation, whereas an unbalanced translocation occurs in about 1 in 1675 liveborn infants.

Translocations involving the acrocentric chromosomes in one parent are associated with risks of an unbalanced translocation, ranging mostly from 4% to 20%, with higher risks for maternal carriers (Table 21.4). Reciprocal translocations between autosomes are associated, almost invariably, with much lower risks for unbalanced karyotypes, mostly below 3% and frequently around 1%. An isochromosome is formed by abnormal splitting of a centromere during meiosis. This occurs infrequently but may cause the loss of an entire chromosome arm and duplication of the remaining arm, resulting in a single symmetric chromosome with two genetically identical arms. Duplications of either an entire region (resulting in partial trisomy of the long or short arm of a specific chromosome) or a tiny segment of a chromosome arm may result in congenital malformations, with or without mental retardation.

Chromosome inversions, which occur following breakage at two sites along a chromosome length, followed by inversion and reattachment, are not uncommon. Such inversions, which involve the centromere (called pericentric inversions)[66] or do not involve the centromere (called paracentric inversions),[67] are generally thought to be associated with a risk of 5% for congenital defects, with or without mental retardation, when they occur *de novo* (see Table 21.4). The exception is the pericentric inversion involving the long arm of chromosome 9, which appears to have no clinical significance. This "normal" chromosomal variation is present in about 1% of individuals.[72]

Subtle chromosome deletions pose serious diagnostic difficulties when they occur *de novo*.

High-resolution chromosome analysis (prometaphase chromosomes) and FISH have increased the recognition of these microdeletion syndromes. Virtually all microdeletion syndromes are associated with serious or fatal genetic disease (Table 21.5). The finding of a microdeletion in an infant should lead automatically to chromosome analysis of both parents seeking a translocation or other chromosomal rearrangement. Individuals with mental retardation of unknown etiology need to be assessed by a geneticist, who may test for one of these microdeletion syndromes. The most common microdeletion involving chromosome 22q11.2 has been associated with several distinct genetic disorders that are known to have overlapping clinical features. These disorders include DiGeorge syndrome, velocardiofacial syndrome, isolated conotruncal cardiac defects, Cayler syndrome, and Opitz syndrome. The expanding, variable phenotype of individuals with 22q11 deletions is now recognized. These advances pose additional diagnostic and counseling challenges.

Indications for chromosome analysis

1 For *both* prospective parents with infertility or three or more spontaneous abortions, or two or more stillbirths.

2 When one parent has a chromosome abnormality[66] (most commonly a sex chromosome defect) or is a known carrier of a chromosomal translocation or other structural rearrangement.

3 For all of the offspring of one parent who carries a structural chromosome rearrangement.

4 For the prospective parent who has genital malformations or abnormalities of sexual development.

5 On all stillborns (with or without dysmorphic features or malformations) or babies following neonatal death without a specific diagnosis.

6 In newborns with dysmorphic features, or those who exhibit serious growth restriction, with or without a single major congenital malformation.

Table 21.4 Recurrence risks for the more common chromosome disorders.

Chromosome disorders	Risk of recurrence (%)	Notes
Numerical abnormalities		
A previous child born with trisomy 21	1–1.5	Includes risks for all aneuploidy and applies to all women < 30 years. Those > 30 have maternal age-associated risks of aneuploidy
A previous child born with trisomy 18	< 1	
A previous child born with trisomy 13	< 1	
A previous child with Turner syndrome (45X)	Population risk	As long as mother is not a Turner syndrome mosaic, risks of recurrence will approximate population risk (1 in 2500 females)
A previous child with XXX syndrome	Population risk	As long as neither parent has sex chromosome mosaicism and mother is < 35 years, risks of recurrence will approximate population risk (1 in 1000 females)
A previous child with Klinefelter syndrome (47,XXY)	Population risk	As long as neither parent has sex chromosome mosaicism and mother is < 35 years, risk of recurrence will approximate population risk (1 in 1000 males)
A previous child with 47,XYY	Population risk	Population risk approximates 1 in 1000 males
Structural rearrangements		
Robertsonian translocations		
t(13;14) (14;21) maternal		
t(14;21) paternal	Rare	
t(13;21) maternal	11–15	
t(13;21)	1–2	
t(15;21) maternal	11–15	
t(15;21) paternal	1–2	
Reciprocal translocation in general maternal	5–20	Risks depend on how original case was ascertained – if through recurrent miscarriage lower figure applies
In general paternal	3–30	Risks depend on how original case was ascertained – if through recurrent miscarriage lower figure applies
t(11;22) maternal	6	
t(11;22) paternal	5	
Inversions (autosomal)		
Pericentric	5–10	If original case ascertained through a previous child with a structural rearrangement
Pericentric	1–3	If original case ascertained fortuitously and without phenotypic abnormality
Paracentric	< 1	

Data from refs 66–70.

7 In infants or children with developmental delay, with or without dysmorphic features or associated malformations.

FISH allows for the microscopic visualization of specific regions of the genome in metaphase chromosomes and interphase nuclei.[73] Examples of the many clinical applications of FISH are illustrated in Table 21.6. Diagnostic limitations exist when an additional molecular mechanism is responsible for the disorder (see details on uniparental disomy and Prader–Willi, above). FISH has been applied to neonatal and prenatal detection of aneuploidy and structural aberrations in chorionic villus cells and amniocytes. The use of multicolor FISH has enabled the identification of cryptic translocations previously not elucidated by routine cytogenetic analysis. These translocations may be the etiology of multiple miscarriages, stillbirths, or prolonged infertility. Using this technology, the identification of microdeletions/duplications and marker chromosomes has become routine. Additional cryptic chromosome rearrangements either at the subtelomeric ends of chromosomes or along the length of the chromosome have now been identified in patients with mental retardation with or without additional congenital abnormalities. Subtelomeric FISH and comparative genomic hybridization have identified the etiology of previously idiopathic mental retardation in up to 10% of cases.[74–76] Once a specific abnormality has been

Table 21.5. Examples of chromosome microdeletion syndromes.

Disorder	Clinical features	Deletion site
Angelman	Severe mental retardation, ataxia, jerky movements, inappropriate laughter, absent speech	15q11–q13
Langer–Giedion	Variable mental retardation, dysmorphic facies, multiple exostoses, sparse scalp hair, cone-shaped epiphyses	8q24.1
Miller–Dieker	Severe mental retardation, lissencephaly, dysmorphic facies, vertical furrowing in forehead when crying	17p13.3
Prader–Willi	Mild mental retardation, infantile hypotonia, obesity, hypopigmentation, hypogonadism	15q11–q13
Retinoblastoma	Retinal malignancy, typical facies, possible mental retardation	13q14
Rubinstein–Taybi	Variable mental retardation, dysmorphic facies, broad thumbs/toes	16p13.3
Smith–Magenis	Mental retardation, dysmorphic facies, self-destructive behavior, microcornea, renal abnormalities, hearing impairment	17p11.2
Steroid sulfatase deficiency	Frequent stillbirths, ichthyosis, low maternal estriol in urine and plasma	Xp22
Velocardiofacial/DiGeorge	Overlapping clinical features: mental retardation, cleft palate, cardiac defects, learning disabilities, hypocalcemia, hypoplastic lymphoid tissue, T-cell deficiency, dysmorphic facies	22q11.2
WAGR	Wilms tumor, aniridia, genitourinary abnormalities, mental retardation	11p13
Williams	Mental retardation, dysmorphic "elfin" facies, cardiac defect, renal anomalies, infantile hypercalcemia	7q11.23

Table 21.6 Examples of clinical application of FISH.

Identification of microdeletion syndromes
Prader–Willi
Angelman
Velocardiofacial/DiGeorge
Miller–Dieker
Williams
Steroid sulfatase deficiency
Smith-Magenis

Identification of duplications
Charcot–Marie–Tooth type 1a
Beckwith–Wiedemann

Identification of subtelometric rearrangements

Identification of cryptic translocations

Identification of marker chromosomes

Prenatal and postnatal identification of chromosome aneuploidy

Cancer cytogenetics

determined, further testing of family members including parents may yield specific recurrence risks and prenatal diagnosis opportunities.

The frequency of chromosomal anomalies in liveborn infants is illustrated in Table 21.7. Careful consideration should be given to such anomalies in all cases of aberrant fetal development, including those detected in the third trimester (i.e., intrauterine growth restriction, IUGR). Advancing maternal age is associated with an increasing frequency of numerical chromosome disorders resulting from nondisjunction and includes not only trisomy 21, but also trisomies 13 and 18, triple-X, and the 47,XXY male (Klinefelter syndrome). The

Table 21.7 Frequency of chromosome abnormalities in liveborn infants.

Chromosome abnormality	Approximate frequency
Numerical disorders	
Autosomal trisomies	
47,+21 (Down syndrome)	1:800
47,+18 (Edward syndrome)	1:7500
47,+13 (Patau syndrome)	1:22 700
Other	1:34 000
Sex chromosome abnormalities	
47,XYY	1:1000 males
47,XXY	1:1000 males
Other (males)	1:1300 males
45,X	1:2500 females
47,XXX	1:1000 females
Other (females)	1:2700 females
Structural rearrangements	
Structural balanced	All 1:500
Robertsonian translocation	
Reciprocal and insertional translocation	
Inversion	
Structural unbalanced	All 1:1600
Robertsonian	
Reciprocal and insertional	
Inversion	
Deletion	
Supernumerary	
Other	

Data from refs 3 and 30.

risks of recurrence, following the birth of babies with different trisomies, are shown in Table 21.4. Certainly, one numerical chromosome abnormality, caused by nondisjunction, may be followed by a different one caused by the same basic mechanism. Hence, following conception of an offspring with trisomy 21, recurrence of a numerical abnormality has been different in some 50% of subsequent chromosomally abnormal offspring.[4] Available data suggest no increased risk of chromosome abnormality in future pregnancies after spontaneous abortions of lethal trisomies or recurrent abortion with normal parental karyotypes.[77]

Monogenic disorders

Single-gene disorders occur in approximately 10 per 1000 live births, with about 7 in 1000 being due to autosomal dominant genes, about 2.5 in 1000 being due to recessive genes, and 0.4 per 1000 being due to X-linked genes. Thus far, hundreds of genetic disorders with biochemical defects have been recognized.[78] Their single mutant genes have involved mainly abnormalities in enzymes and, increasingly, specific proteins. A reduced lifespan is associated with over half of all monogenic disorders, whereas reproductive capacity is reduced in about 69% of such disorders.[78]

Clinically, dominant disorders are viewed as those in which symptomatic individuals are heterozygotes, whereas those with autosomal recessive disorders are symptomatic and are considered homozygotes. The distinction between dominant and recessive disorders is largely arbitrary, but useful clinically. It is known, for example, that for the autosomal recessive sickle cell disease, heterozygotes have subtle physiologic abnormalities, affecting renal concentrating ability as well as demonstrating a selective advantage for resistance to malaria. Heterozygotes for ataxia telangiectasia are known to be at an increased risk for developing malignancy. Hence, carriers of recessive genes may manifest disorders, just as do those individuals with dominant genes. Concerning the concept of dominant and recessive genes, other subtleties are recognized. For example, in retinoblastoma (typically transmitted as an autosomal dominant disorder with virtually full penetrance) the deletion, or point mutation, on one chromosome 13 has to be associated with another mutation in the homologous allele on the other chromosome 13 for retinoblastoma to develop. In other words, "two hits" are necessary, although for this classical, dominant disorder, a recessive gene mechanism is effective. Notwithstanding continued progress in understanding complex mechanisms resulting in genetic disorders due to dominant or recessive genes, it still remains useful to consider them clinically in their well-established categories.

Autosomal dominant disorders

As the genes for autosomal dominant disorders exist on one of the 22 autosomes, both males and females may be affected. An individual who is affected has a 50% risk of transmitting the gene to each of his or her offspring. The phenomenon of pleiotropy is especially important in this category of disorders. A single gene that has several different effects is regarded as pleiotropic (e.g., either of the genes causing tuberous sclerosis may result in retardation, achromic spots, and subungual fibromas). In contrast, genetic heterogeneity means that several genes have the same effect. A good example is deafness, which can result from many different single-gene disorders. New mutations commonly cause autosomal dominant disorders. For example, about seven out of eight individuals with achondroplasia are due to a dominant *de novo* gene mutation. Moreover, the frequency of such mutations rises with advancing paternal age. Variability in clinical expression (called expressivity) is also especially important in dominantly inherited disorders. One excellent example is the multiple endocrine neoplasia syndrome, in which individual affected family members may have either hyperplasia or malignancy or both, in various endocrine organs. Also typical of autosomal dominant disorders is the variation seen in the age of onset, even for the same condition. Hence, Huntington's disease may manifest in childhood or not until old age, even although the mutant gene has been present from the time of conception. Molecular analysis allows determination of the presence of the mutant gene, but does not usually provide any ability to predict onset time (except for several triplet repeat disorders). Some guidance on this point is likely to emerge from a study of disease onset ages within specific families. Predictive prenatal diagnostic testing for presymptomatic adult-onset disorders poses significant challenges. Disorders such as Huntington's disease, familial breast/ovarian cancer syndromes, long QT syndrome, familial adenomatous polyposis, multiple endocrine neoplasia and Von Hippel–Lindau syndrome all are amenable to presymptomatic and prenatal diagnosis. Prenatal testing for these serious disorders that may only manifest years to decades after birth, may also reveal the presymptomatic affected status of an at-risk parent. Preconception/prenatal genetic counseling is critically important in such cases to consider the complex issues of diagnosis, penetrance, expressivity, anticipation, heterogeneity, risks, as well as available and future treatment.

Autosomal recessive disorders

The mutant genes that cause this group of disorders are located on one of the 22 autosomes, and therefore both males and females may be affected. Clinically obvious autosomal recessive disorders exist only in the homozygous state (each parent contributing one of the mutant genes). Hence, when both parents are carriers, they have a 25% risk of having affected offspring in each pregnancy. An autosomal recessive disorder can result in an offspring inheriting the same harmful gene from each parent, even although the site of the mutation within the gene may be different. These so-called compound heterozygotes still develop the disease, but the nature of its clinical manifestations and time of onset may be altered.

Important examples include cystic fibrosis, Tay–Sachs disease, and metachromatic leukodystrophy.

Typically, the rarer the mutant recessive gene, the greater the likelihood that those affected will result from consanguineous unions, or those where the couple has ethnicity in common. Although new mutations that result in recessive disorders may occur, they have not been easy to distinguish clinically. With increasing use of DNA analysis, the frequency and nature of recessive mutations are likely to be better understood. Meanwhile, for the more common autosomal recessive disorders, the physician needs to recognize the patient's ethnicity and provide the straightforward carrier detection tests for that specific group. Hence, couples who share Mediterranean, Ashkenazi Jewish, Black, or Asian extraction should be routinely offered indicated preconception carrier detection tests for at least β-thalassemia, Tay–Sachs and Canavan disease, sickle cell disease, and α-thalassemia, respectively.

X-linked disorders

The mutant genes that result in X-linked disorders are located on the X chromosome. Given that the male has only one X chromosome and the female has two, both the risk and severity of X-linked disease will vary between the sexes. Males will usually manifest the fullest expression of the disorder, whereas random X inactivation will largely influence expression in females. In contrast to females who carry autosomal recessive genes, those heterozygous for X-linked genes frequently manifest some sign(s) of the disease in question (Table 21.8). An important example is female carriers of Duchenne muscular dystrophy (DMD), who are at significant risk for developing either cardiomyopathy or cardiac conduction defects.[79] A careful surveillance protocol for these life-threatening conditions is warranted.

Male-to-male transmission does not occur in X-linked disease. This is because a male never contributes his X chromosome to a son. An affected male, by contributing his only X chromosome to all his daughters, will render them all carriers of the trait in question. In examining the pedigree of a family with possible X-linked disease, attention is usually given to whether the disease has occurred in maternal nephews, uncles, or first cousins and through the female line. Female heterozygotes have a 50% risk of having affected male offspring.

X-linked dominant traits are characterized by an affected male transmitting the condition to all his daughters and none of his sons, and by an affected female, with a 50% likelihood of transmitting the disorder to her sons *or* daughters. X-linked dominant disorders occur about twice as often in females as in males and may be less severe in affected females. Rarely, an X-linked dominant trait may be lethal in affected males, resulting in a disorder that appears to occur, clinically, only in females and in which an affected female has a 50% likelihood of transmitting the trait to her daughters. These affected women have an increased frequency of miscarriage, representing affected male fetuses (e.g., incontinentia pigmenti). Mutations of X-linked genes are not uncommon and are most often associated with the occurrence of a sporadic affected male within a family. Because of advances in molecular genetics, we now know that even in some of these families, despite the presence of a normal gene in the mother of such an affected male, germline mosaicism may account for recurrence in a future pregnancy. The birth of a male with DMD, no family history, and no detectable mutation by DNA analysis of maternal peripheral leukocytes might lead to counseling based on spontaneous mutation rates. Once again, germline mosaicism is now well recognized in mothers of apparently sporadic DMD sons, and the risk of recurrence in such cases approximates 7–14% if the at-risk X-haplotype is determined.[80] Hence, genetic counseling following sporadic occurrence of a male with X-linked DMD should include the recommendation of prenatal genetic studies in all subsequent pregnancies notwithstanding negative DNA carrier testing of the mother.

Table 21.8 Signs in females who are X-linked recessive disease carriers.

Achromatopsia	Decreased visual acuity and myopia
Adrenoleukodystophy	Neurological and adrenal dysfunction
Alport syndrome	Hematuria and hearing impairment
Choroideremia	Chorioretinal dystrophy
Chronic granulomatous disease	Cutaneous and mucocutaneous lesions
Duchenne muscular dystrophy	Pseudohypertrophy, weakness, cardiomyopathy/conduction defects
Dyskeratosis congenita	Retinal pigmentation
Fabry's disease	Angiokeratomas, corneal dystrophy, "burning hands and feet"
Fragile X syndrome	Mild-moderate mental retardation; behavioral aberrations; schizoaffective disorders; premature ovarian failure, fragile X tremor ataxia syndrome
G6PD deficiency	Hemolytic crises, neonatal hyperbilirubinemia
Hypohidrotic ectodermal dysplasia	Sparse hair, decreased sweating
Omithine transcarbamylase deficiency	Hyperammonemia, psychiatric/neurological manifestations
Spondyloepiphyseal dysplasia, late onset	Arthritis

Modified from ref. 30.

Fragile X syndrome

Special attention must be given to the X-linked disorder known as fragile X syndrome, which represents the most common single cause of inherited mental retardation in males. Typical features include mental retardation of varying severity, macroorchidism, typical facial features (including a large head, prominent ears, forehead, and jaw), signs suggestive of a connective tissue disorder (including hyperextensibility, pectus excavatum, flat feet, possible mitral valve prolapse, and dilation of the aortic root) and behavioral disorders, seizures, stereotypies, speech disorders, autistic signs, and other neurological features. The fragile X syndrome occurs in 1 out of every 4500 males, and about 1 in 250 females carry the gene. About one-third of female heterozygotes may be variably mentally retarded. This disorder is named for the appearance of the chromosomal fragile site, located on the distal long arm of the X chromosome and demonstrated by using folic acid-depleted culture medium for blood chromosome study. Detection of the unstable CGG triplet repeat with concurrent ascertainment of the methylation status is the standard diagnostic test for fragile X syndrome. Where before two-thirds of fragile X carrier females were not detected cytogenetically, DNA analysis of triplet repeats will facilitate detection of 96% of carriers. In addition, females with the dynamic fragile X premutation may also develop premature ovarian failure.[81] Normal transmitting males are those who carry a premutation, do not have fragile X syndrome, and transmit this premutation to their daughters. Although thought to be phenotypically normal, studies have now shown that a subgroup of older men with the fragile X premutation develop a progressive neurodegenerative syndrome that includes intention tremor, parkinsonism, ataxia, cognitive decline, and generalized brain atrophy.[82] This disorder has been named the fragile X tremor ataxia syndrome and has also been shown to manifest in a subgroup of elderly women with the fragile X premutation.[83,84]

A careful family history and pedigree analysis is important when considering testing for fragile X. Special awareness is needed for the manifesting carrier female, a family history of mental retardation or learning disabilities on the maternal side, and of the "unaffected" transmitting male. Prenatal diagnosis can now identify not only the affected male, but also the female with this X-linked disorder. Carrier females can mostly be distinguished from clinically manifesting females by the number of triplet repeats and the degree of methylation.

Interpretation of the methylation assay can be complicated, especially when chorionic villus samples are assayed.[85] Methylation is not well correlated with fragile X gene expression based on assays of chorionic villi.

Mitochondrial disorders

Mitochondrial disorders have protean manifestations, which include neurologic, multisystem, and tissue-specific conditions that are primarily maternally inherited. One specific characteristic of mitochondrial disorders is called *heteroplasmy*, which is the coexistence of normal and mutant mitochondrial DNA molecules within each cell. Although possible, prenatal diagnosis for specific mitochondrial point mutations may be affected by heteroplasmy, resulting in many uncertainties including severity, type, and age of onset of symptoms, thus complicating prenatal counseling.

Multifactorial genetic disorders

Many disorders result from the interaction of multiple genes with one or more environmental factors. Typical birth defects in this category include cleft lip and palate, congenital heart disease, and neural tube defects. Generally, risks of recurrence tend mostly to range between 3% and 5%; important exceptions (such as pyloric stenosis) are well known. For example, if the mother had pyloric stenosis, the risk is 16–20% for having an affected son and 7% for having an affected daughter. If the father had pyloric stenosis, the risk is about 5% for having an affected son and about 2.5% for having an affected daughter.[86] Recurrence risks typically vary from family to family and are particularly influenced by the number of affected family members and the severity of the condition in the index case. In general, if there are more affected relatives with more severe disease, the risk to their other relatives will be higher.

Consideration of phenocopies is particularly important in determining the etiology of what might be considered a multifactorial disorder. For example, cleft lip and palate may also occur as a consequence of a monogenic disorder, a chromosome abnormality, or a specific teratogenic medication.

Evaluating the cause of stillbirth or perinatal death

The full spectrum of grief can be expected to attend all stillbirths and perinatal deaths. Therefore, the physician can, and should, anticipate feelings of denial, expressions of guilt, experience of depression, and expressed or contained anger from the parents. Although the intensity and duration of such *normal* responses by parents may vary, active steps to evaluate the cause(s) of their loss serves to assist in turning anguish into action and to possibly providing important information that would help alleviate the grieving process. A summary protocol for such evaluation is suggested in Table 21.9.

Genetic etiologies of stillbirth need to be considered as they may lead to increased risks for miscarriage, stillbirth, or abnormality in future offspring. Genetic causes include thrombophilias, chromosome abnormalities, or single-gene disorders, including X-linked dominant, lethal autosomal recessive, and lethal *de novo* autosomal dominant conditions. Following stillbirth or perinatal death, careful review of the family (genetic) history and of the medical and obstetric history is

Table 21.9 Protocol for evaluating the cause of stillbirth or perinatal death.

Review genetic, medical, and obstetric history
Determine possible consanguinity
Gently and persistently recommend that parents permit a complete autopsy
Obtain photographs, including full face and profile, whole body, and, where applicable, detailed pictures of any specific abnormality (e.g., of digits)
Obtain full-body skeletal radiographs
Consider full-body magnetic resonance imaging,[87] if autopsy not permitted
Carefully document any dysmorphic features
Obtain heparinized cord or fetal blood sample for chromosomal or DNA analysis
Obtain fetal serum for infectious disease studies (e.g., parvovirus, cytomegalovirus, toxoplasmosis)
Obtain fetal tissue sample (sterile fascia best) for cell culture aimed at chromosome analysis, biochemical, or DNA studies
Obtain parental bloods for chromosome analysis, where indicated
Communicate final autopsy results and conclusions of special analyses
Provide follow-up counseling, including a summary letter

recommended. Assessment of consanguinity should include determination of possible common ancestral origins of the parents, as well as consideration of last names of grandparents or great-grandparents. Autopsy should automatically be recommended in all such cases, unless an absolute and definitive diagnosis is already known. During the overwhelming grief at such times, one or both parents frequently are not inclined to allow an autopsy. Experience has taught that many such parents later regret having lost the opportunity to determine specific answers to very definite questions. If the ward, medical, and nursing staffs have been unable to obtain permission for autopsy, judicious action would include requesting the senior attending physician to meet with the parents immediately, lending experience and authority to the recommendation, urging that information gained at autopsy may benefit their other or future children. Keeping the deceased child on the ward for a few hours pending this decision will sometimes prove helpful. Photographs of the face, including profile views, and whole-body pictures, including detailed photographs of any specific abnormality (e.g., of digits) would be helpful to a dysmorphologist later. Full-body skeletal X-rays may prove similarly important later. Any dysmorphic features should be carefully documented. Heparinized cord or fetal blood samples should be obtained for chromosome analysis in all cases. Between 6% and 11% of all such offspring will have a chromosome abnormality, whether or not an abnormal physical phenotype is present.[19] A fetal serum sample should also be obtained for infectious disease studies, which might include, for example, parvovirus, cytomegalovirus, and toxoplasmosis.

Fetal tissue samples should be obtained for cell culture (internal fascia of the thigh) to determine the chromosome complement, to determine the biochemical phenotype, where applicable, or to analyze DNA (liver tissue frozen without preservative), where indicated. The obstetrician is expected to ensure that sterile culture medium is kept available for these often-unexpected circumstances, thereby avoiding submission to the laboratory of pieces of fetal tissue in dry gauze or in a container, without any culture medium whatsoever. Parental blood samples for chromosome analysis may be useful if fetal karyotyping fails or if a specific chromosomal anomaly is detected (e.g., translocation). Results of the autopsy, as well as those of any special tests performed, should be communicated directly to the parents. Many weeks may elapse before such communication can occur. Nevertheless, face-to-face consultation with *both* parents is recommended to reiterate any previous counseling, especially as anxiety block to the reception of information may have lessened somewhat by that time. This communication and counseling should be followed by a summary letter explaining their future risks and options and emphasizing any necessary recommendations.

Guidelines to genetic counseling

The principles guiding the delivery of genetic counseling have been discussed extensively elsewhere.[4,41,88] The quintessential points will be summarized briefly here.

Accurate diagnosis

Current expectations demand that a careful and sharp focus be kept on fetal development throughout pregnancy. Discrepancy between gestational age and fetal growth, disparity in specific measurements (e.g., femur length, size of lateral ventricles), or questions of organ presence or normality (e.g., large or absent kidneys) will alert the perinatologist to the need for further study, including serial examinations, in order to seek accurate diagnosis. Reliable genetic counseling cannot begin if an accurate diagnosis has not been established. This same exhortation applies to the history obtained at the first obstetric visit (ideally the preconception visit), when pregnancy planning has been initiated. At this visit, expectations include careful review of the family pedigree and formal confirmation of specific congenital defects or genetic disorders that bear on the risk of the proband in the current or future pregnancies. Examination of previous autopsy reports, X-rays, and photographs – including those of previous stillborns – is often necessary for confirmation or for help in establishing a diagnosis not made earlier. Now more than ever, the advent of molecular genetic diagnosis makes it incumbent on the physician to determine precisely whether a history of "muscular dystrophy" was, in fact, Duchenne, myotonic, or some other type. Failure to check a history of "encephalocele" in a previous deceased newborn could result in counseling with an approximate 3% risk estimate. The autopsy record, however, may have revealed polydactyly and polycystic kidneys, which, in combination with the encephalocele, constitute Meckel syndrome, an autosomal recessive disorder with a 25% risk of recurrence.

Nondirective counseling

Most therapeutic medicine involves paternalistic management, with directions to the patient to take a specific medication that will restore him or her to good health. The consensus among medical geneticists in the Western world is to provide nondirective genetic counseling, where the physician is expected to dispense the most complete information available while remaining impartial and objective. In contrast, a directive approach invites, consciously or subconsciously, the opportunity for the physician to insinuate his or her own religious, racial, eugenic, or other beliefs or dictates of conscience into the counseling process. Hence, whether they have antiabortion views or personal judgments of the estimated burden of a specific disease on a family, physicians are strongly encouraged to avoid directing patients' decisions. Efficacy in genetic counseling means helping the clients to rational decision making, which may not necessarily result in a reduction in the frequency of a genetic disease.

Concern for the individual

A physician's paramount concern is for the individual patient. The physician is *not* an advocate for society when in the midst of patient care and counseling. Hence, if a patient does not wish to terminate a pregnancy in the face of a serious fetal genetic disease, it is inappropriate for the physician to try to influence that decision, either on behalf of other family members or because of the "cost to society." This principle does not, however, preclude the requirement to inform the patient fully about all aspects, both advantageous and disadvantageous, of the decision he or she is making. An informative discussion, therefore, should range over issues that the patient may not be cognizant of to include future interrelationships of the couple, the effect on their other children, the suffering of the affected child, anticipated reactions by relatives and the public at large, and the many economic and other societal implications.

Truth in counseling

There are relatively few instances in genetic counseling when the abiding principle of telling the truth is threatened. Detection of unexpected nonpaternity perhaps ranks first in frequency and is likely to retain its favored status with increasing use of DNA diagnostic studies. Detection of nonpaternity during routine prenatal chromosome studies is not at all uncommon. Such discoveries are usually predicated on recognition or suspicion of a potential fetal chromosome abnormality, necessitating blood samples from both "parents." Determination of what might appear to be a *de novo* translocation, rather than an inherited one, brings the issue into sharp relief. Because risk counseling for fetal normality will be decidedly different for the *de novo* versus inherited translocation and because the other male is invariably unaware of his possible translocation, every effort needs to be made to arrange a face-to-face consultation with the pregnant patient herself. These not-infrequent encounters raise tricky ethical and legal questions and require considerable finesse in management.

Discovery of nonpaternity during DNA diagnostic studies in members of the family distant to the proband (her own father, an uncle, a first cousin) represents the same thematic challenge. Once again, considerable judgment and insight is required by the physician in determining whether to transmit such information; ethical and legal issues exist and cannot be ignored. Nevertheless, where sufficient information (e.g., to set "phase" for genotype evaluation through DNA studies) is available, communication concerning nonpaternity might best be avoided. Only in situations in which life-threatening circumstances are clear is there an absolute need for communication and disclosure. Even then great sensitivity and finesse are required.

Confidentiality and trust

The traditional and expected confidentiality and trust relationship between physician and patient is no different in the genetics arena. This principle may be challenged, for example, when the need arises to inform the sisters of a proven X-linked disease carrier about their own risks and need for testing. Difficulty arises if the patient insists on not communicating with her family and specifically instructs the physician also to desist. Although statutes of conditional immunity cover physicians communicating private information concerning highly infectious diseases (e.g., meningococcemia), such immunity may not safeguard the physician transmitting genetic risk information. Notwithstanding this difference in informing about germs and genes, the advent of AIDS and the associated privacy issues further add to the dilemma in managing these kinds of genetic cases.

Information transmitted to the physician's or institution's employees about patients' serious genetic neurological genetic disorders (e.g., Huntington's disease) add a further dimension in which confidentiality and trust may be questioned. The physician's first and clearest duty is to the patient, and great caution must be exercised to safeguard this critical relationship and to secure all the elements of absolute privacy.

Timing of genetic counseling

The need for preconception counseling has been emphasized. Notwithstanding this frequently repeated recommendation, huge numbers of couples emerge for genetic counseling *during* pregnancy. Professional and public education is needed to reverse this practice if couples are to benefit from available options (not to have children, adoption, *in vitro* fertilization, artificial insemination by donor, ovum donation, embryo transfer, surrogacy, vasectomy, tubal ligation, carrier detection tests, preimplantation diagnosis, prenatal diagnosis, treatment, and selection or avoidance of abortion).

The timing of genetic counseling following the birth of a child with a serious congenital defect is also important. Although communication and support are critical during these first unhappy days, formal genetic counseling should not be attempted. Anxiety block effectively prevents anguished parents from assimilating or comprehending the important information being communicated. Essential diagnostic information must be communicated, but not in a corridor, not to the patient alone without her partner, and not to the patient who is still under the effects of anesthesia. Sadly, examples of all of these practices are well known. Although a formal appointment should be scheduled with such a couple within 6 weeks of the birth, access by telephone should also be made available for response to urgent questions and concerns.

Parental counseling

Contribution of one-half of the genome by the father is not the only reason the physician should insist on the father accompanying his mate for genetic counseling. Not only may outright diagnostic information be obtained from such a face-to-face visit, but also a more reliable paternal family history may be obtainable. Moreover, issues to be discussed are frequently complex and invariably involve questions of guilt, family prejudices, religious obstacles, fear, and serious differences of opinion between mates. Physicians should systematically insist, at the time appointments are made, that a couple attend together for counseling. Even although a letter summarizing the essential points made during counseling should be routinely sent to the referring doctor and the parents being counseled, the male partner must be urged to attend.

Knowledge, jargon, and empathy

Enormous advances in human genetics over the past three decades have led to a huge and exponentially increasing body of specialized knowledge. As a consequence of these developments, a board-certified specialty in medical genetics was initiated in 1982 in the USA and, shortly thereafter, in Canada. Physicians who are not medical geneticists need to be especially careful about venturing into areas in which they lack expertise. Communication concerning risks, based on DNA studies for a rapidly increasing number of prenatally detectable disorders, serves as one example for which caution and referral would be appropriate. Understanding the full expression of a disease not only in the fetus or newborn, but also in the child and adult, and its wider consequences for the family, requires special knowledge and experience.

Communications concerning genetic disorders are frequently based on complex information. An important principle is to avoid technical jargon in communication and to make no assumptions about a patient's basic knowledge or understanding. Some patients, especially professionals, are embarrassed to reveal their ignorance or lack of understanding even after an explanation has been provided. Great sensitivity is always necessary, and sufficient insight in these circumstances may encourage repetition of the communication then and there, or at a subsequent planned appointment.

The birth of a child with a fatal or serious genetic defect is invariably associated with complex responses and reactions from both parents. After the anticipated shock, self-incrimination or guilt, anger, and (one hopes) final adaptation will come the associated dashed expectations and dreams, fear of recurrence, anxiety about disability and/or death, economic woes, concern about social stigmatization, and stress between partners (often for not planning). The physician should be able to dispense empathy and sensitivity, not be judgmental, and to project warmth, understanding, and support. Together with knowledge, these prerequisites take time – the final ingredient for effective counseling. Genetic counseling cannot be brief and hurried.

Do no harm

The classical exhortation *primum non nocere* ("do no harm") is no less pertinent to clinical genetics than to medicine generally. In this context, perinatologists may offer predictive diagnosis from chorion villi or amniotic fluid cells for disorders that will manifest decades after birth. Prime examples include Huntington's disease,[89] myotonic muscular dystrophy,[32] and Friedreich's ataxia.[90] Recommendations and guidelines concerning predictive testing for the presymptomatic detection of Huntington's disease have been published by the International Huntington Association and the World Federation of Neurology Research Group on Huntington's disease.[91,92] These recommendations propose rigorous pre- and post-test counseling and state that the test should not be available to individuals under the age of 18 years. The inherent danger in such presymptomatic testing (as opposed to prenatal predictive testing) is the potential depression and possible demoralization that a patient might experience. For a disorder without curative, let alone meaningful palliative, treatment the wisdom of providing presymptomatic diagnoses must be seriously considered. Although 50% of individuals at risk will receive good news, relieving them of anxiety, the other 50% face an effective death sentence. Given the high suicide rate in individuals at risk for Huntington's disease, it may reasonably be questioned whether one does more harm than good by providing this 50% with a death sentence years before manifestations appear.[93] Given the pace of advances in human genetics, it might well be possible in the foreseeable future to develop a therapy that enhances the mechanism already in place and to delay the manifestations of Huntington's disease for decades after birth. It would be sad to find a life ruined by severe depression or suicide, only to be followed shortly thereafter by discoveries that delay the manifestations of Huntington's disease by decades or permanently. Difficult as these decisions may be for individual patients at risk, such undertakings can only be regarded as acceptable if performed with extreme care, concern, and professionalism. Although patients retain the right to make the choice for presymptomatic testing, there is reason to remain concerned about the wisdom of such choices for those who find themselves affected. On the other hand, an increasing number of examples already exist in which presymptomatic testing is possible and important to either the patient or the future offspring, or both. Use of DNA linkage analysis and mutation analysis[94] for autosomal dominant polycystic kidney disease may lead to unsuspected diagnosis of an associated intracranial aneurysm and pre-emptive surgery with avoidance of a life-threatening sudden cerebral hemorrhage. In a study of 141 affected individuals, 11% decided against bearing children on the basis of risk.[95] These authors noted that only 4% of at-risk individuals between 18 and 40 years of age would seek elective abortion for an affected fetus. The importance of accurate presymptomatic tests for potential at-risk donors has been emphasized.[96]

Duty

The physician has a duty to inform the patient, impartially, fully, and in a nondirective way, providing a clear delineation of available risks and options. Where facts are uncertain or new advances possible, there is a clear duty for the physician to refer the patient to or consult with a medical geneticist. All communications with the patient must be documented and, preferably, summarized in a letter to the patient. Physicians have a duty to support patients and to remain nonjudgmental about their decisions. An additional duty is to remain aware of new advances and progress in human genetics so that patients may benefit from them in a timely manner. In 1991, Pelias[97] discussed the geneticist's duty to recontact patients when new relevant information concerning their diagnosis, or possible treatment, becomes available. This daunting task to recontact patients, perhaps years after their initial visit to the genetics clinic, can be tempered by initially informing the client of the expanding nature of genetic knowledge and the need to remain in at least annual contact with the clinical geneticist. This theme should be recorded in clinic notes and reiterated in follow-up letters to the patient and to referring and consulting physicians. Given the many millions who move each year and change their physicians, it would be judicious to vest the responsibility with both the primary care doctor and the patient to remain in contact with a clinical geneticist.

Key points

1 The preconception period is important for control and treatment of specific disorders that may affect an otherwise successful pregnancy.

2 Infertility may have a genetic basis for which genetic testing and counseling are indicated.

3 Stillbirths and/or multiple miscarriage may have a genetic etiology for which genetic counseling and testing are indicated.

4 Family history of a specific disorder may enable carrier testing and prenatal diagnosis and is an indication for genetic counseling.

5 Carrier testing for specific genetic disorders based on ethnicity is a recognized standard of care.

6 Identification of maternal myotonic muscular dystrophy will enable prenatal diagnosis, optimal surveillance, and possible early intervention or prevention of the frequently serious intrapregnancy, labor, delivery, postpartum, and neonatal complications.

7 Genetic counseling is a communication process concerning the occurrence and the risks of recurrence of genetic disorders within a family.

8 The physician should be aware of the multiple indications for a genetic counseling referral in the context of risks and prenatal diagnosis.

9 Uniparental disomy molecular testing may be indicated in the prenatal diagnosis of robertsonian translocations.

10 Sex chromosome aneuploidy is a frequent finding in prenatal diagnosis and may present genetic counseling challenges due to the phenotypic and developmental variability within each karyotype group.

11 The use of FISH has increased the identification of the etiology of previously idiopathic mental retardation allowing more accurate recurrence risk counseling and prenatal diagnosis opportunities.

12 Autosomal dominant disorders are characterized by pleiotropy, variable expressivity, variable age of onset, and often new mutations and heterogeneity.

13 Consanguinity increases the risk of autosomal recessive disorders.

14 Female carriers of X-linked genes often manifest sign(s) of the disorder due to random X inactivation.

15 Germline mosaicism complicates recurrence risk counseling in apparently sporadic cases of an increasing number of disorders.

16 Fragile X female carriers are at risk of developing premature ovarian failure, whereas both male and

female premutation carriers are at risk to develop the fragile-X tremor ataxia syndrome.

17 Heteroplasmy complicates the prenatal diagnostic interpretation of some mitochondrial disorders.

18 Reviewing the genetic, medical, and obstetric history as well as a complete autopsy are critical in evaluating the cause of stillbirth and may be invaluable in future genetic counseling.

19 Reliable genetic counseling cannot occur if an accurate diagnosis has not been established.

20 Genetic counseling is best provided by a clinical geneticist or certified genetic counselor under supervision of a clinical geneticist.

References

1 Barker DJP: *Mothers, babies, and disease in later life*. London: BMJ Publishing Group, 1994.

2 Boue J, Boue A, Lazar P. Retrospective and prospective epidemiological studies of 1500 karyotyped spontaneous human abortions. *Teratology* 1975;12:11.

3 Hook EB, Hamerton JL. The frequency of chromosome abnormalities detected in consecutive newborn studies – differences between studies – results by sex and by severity of phenotypic involvement. In: Hook FB, Porter IH, eds. *Population cytogenetics: studies in humans*. New York: Academic Press, 1977.

4 Milunsky A, ed. *Genetic disorders and the fetus: diagnosis, prevention and treatment*. Baltimore, MD: Johns Hopkins University Press, 2004.

5 Myrianthopoulos NC. *Malformations in children from one to seven years*. New York: Alan R Liss, 1985.

6 McCandless SE, Brunger JW, Cassidy SB. The burden of genetic disease on inpatient care in a children's hospital. *Am J Hum Genet* 2004;74:788.

7 Online Mendelian Inheritance in Man, OMIM™. McKusick-Nathans Institute for Genetic Medicine, Johns Hopkins University (Baltimore, MD) and National Center for Biotechnology Information, National Library of Medicine (Bethesda, MD), 2000. World Wide Web URL: http://www.ncbi.nlm.nih.gov/omim/

8 Baird PA, Anderson TW, Newcombe HB, et al. Genetic disorders in children and young adults: a population study. *Am J Hum Genet* 1988;42:677.

9 Milunsky A. *Your genetic destiny: know your genes, secure your health, save your life*. Cambridge, MA: Perseus Publishing, 2001.

10 Lind J, Wallenburg HC. Pregnancy and the Ehlers–Danlos syndrome: a retrospective study. *Acta Obstet Gynecol Scand* 2002; 81:293–300.

11 Dudding TE, Attia J. The association between adverse pregnancy outcomes and maternal factor V Leiden genotype: a meta-analysis. *Thromb Haemost* 2004 ;91:700–711.

12 Towbin JA. Molecular genetic basis of sudden cardiac death. *Pediatr Clin North Am* 2004 ;51:1229–1255.

13 Penney GC, Mair G, Pearson DW, et al. Outcomes of pregnancies in women with type 1 diabetes in Scotland: a national population-based study. *Br J Obstet Gynaecol* 2003;110:315.

14 Rappaport VJ, Velazquez M, Williams K. Hemoglobinopathies in pregnancy. *Obstet Gynecol Clin North Am* 2004;31:287–317, vi.

15 Goss CH, Rubenfeld GD, Otto K, Aitken ML. The effect of pregnancy on survival in women with cystic fibrosis. *Chest* 2003; 124:1460–1468.

16 Gillet D, de Braekeleer M, Bellis G, et al. Cystic fibrosis and pregnancy. Report from French data (1980–1999). *Br J Obstet Gynaecol* 2002;109:912–918.

17 Chameides L, Truex RC, Vetter V, et al. Association of maternal systemic lupus erythematosus with congenital complete heart block. *N Engl J Med* 1977;297:1204.

18 Tharapel AT, Tharapel SA, Bannerman RM. Recurrent pregnancy losses and parental chromosomeabnormalities: a review. *Br J Obstet Gynaecol* 1985;92:899.

19 Sachs ES, Jahoda MG, Van Hemel JD, et al. Chromosome studies of 500 couples with two or more abortions. *Obstet Gynecol* 1985;65:375.

20 Alberman ED, Creasy MR. Frequency of chromosomal abnormalities in miscarriages and perinataldeaths. *J Med Genet* 1977;14:313.

21 Milunsky A, Jick H, Jick SS, et al. Multivitamin/folic acid supplementation in early pregnancy reduces the prevalence of neural tube defects. *JAMA* 1989;262:2847.

22 MRC Vitamin Study Research Group. Prevention of neural tube defects: results of the MRC Vitamin Study. *Lancet* 1991;338: 132–137.

23 Creizel AE, Dudas I. Prevention of the first occurrence of neural tube defects by periconceptional vitamin supplementation. *N Engl J Med* 1992;327:1832–1835.

24 Centers for Disease Control. *Recommendations for the use of folic acid to reduce the number of cases of spina bifida and other neural tube defects*. September 11, 1992. Vol. 41/no. RR–14.

25 Cogram P, Tesh S, Tesh J, et al. D-Chiro-inositol is more effective than myo-inositol in preventing folate-resistant mouse neural tube defects. *Hum Reprod* 2002;17:2451–2458.

26 CF Mutation Database, 2004. World Wide Web URL: http://genet.sickkids.on.ca/cgi-bin/WebObjects/MUTATION.woa

27 American College of Obstetricians and Gynecologists and American College of Medical Genetics. *Preconception and prenatal carrier screening for cystic fibrosis: clinical and laboratory guidelines*. Washington DC; American College of Obstetricians and Gynecologists, 2001.

28 Grody WW, Cutting GR, Klinger KW, et al. Laboratory standards and guidelines for population-based cystic fibrosis carrier screening. *Genet Med* 2001;3:149–154.

29 Watson MS, Cutting GR, Desnick RJ, et al. Cystic fibrosis population carrier screening: 2004revision of American College of Medical Genetics mutation panel. *Genet Med* 2004;6:387–391.

30 Triggs-Raine BL, Feigenbaum ASJ, Natowicz M, et al. Screening for carriers of Tay–Sachs disease among Ashkenazi Jews. *N Engl J Med* 1990;323:6–12.

31 ACOG committee on genetics. ACOG committee opinion. Number 298, August 2004. Prenatal and preconceptional carrier screening for genetic diseases in individuals of Eastern European Jewish descent. *Obstet Gynecol* 2004;104:425–428.

32 Milunsky JM, Skare JS, Milunsky A. Presymptomatic and prenatal diagnosis of myotonic musculardystrophy with linked DNA probes. *Am J Med Sci* 1991;301:231.

33 Milunsky A, Skare JC, Milunsky JM, et al. Diagnosis of myotonic muscular dystrophy with linked deoxyribonucleic acid probes. *Am J Obstet Gynecol* 1991;164:751.
34 Sarnat HB, O'Connor T, Byrne PA. Clinical effects of myotonic dystrophy on pregnancy and the neonate. *Arch Neurol* 1976; 33:459.
35 Webb D, Muir I, Faulkner J, Johnson G. Myotonia dystrophica: obstetric complications. *Am J Obstet Gynecol* 1978;132:265.
36 Verkerk AJHM, Pieretti M, Sutcliffe JS, et al. Identification of a gene (FMR1) containing a CGG repeat coincident with a breakpoint cluster region exhibiting length variation in fragile X syndrome. *Cell* 1991;65:905–914.
37 Campuzano V, Montermini L, Molot MD, et al. Friedreich's Ataxia: autosomal recessive disease caused by an intronic gaa triplet repeat expansion. *Science* 1996;271:1423–1427.
38 O'Hoy KL, Tsilfidis C, Mahadevan MS, et al. Reduction in size of the myotonic dystrophytrinucleotide repeat mutation during transmission. *Science* 1993;259:809–812.
39 Verlinsky Y, Kuliev A. Preimplantation diagnosis for aneuploidies in assisted reproduction. *Minerva Ginecol* 2004;56:197–203.
40 Sampson JE, Ouhibi N, Lawce H, et al. The role for preimplantation genetic diagnosis in balanced translocation carriers. *Am J Obstet Gynecol* 2004;190:1707–1711.
41 Milunsky A, ed. *The prevention of genetic disease and mental retardation*. Philadelphia, PA: WB Saunders, 1975.
42 Wald NJ, Cuckle HS, Densem JW, et al. Maternal serum screening for Down's syndrome in early pregnancy. *BMJ* 1988b;297:883–888.
43 Palomaki GE, Haddow JE, Knight GJ, et al. Risk-based prenatal screening for trisomy 18 using alpha-fetoprotein, unconjugated oestriol and human chorionic gonadotrophin. *Prenat Diagn* 1995;15:713–723.
44 Milunsky A, Nebiolo L. Maternal serum triple analyte screening and adverse pregnancy outcome. *Fetal Diag Ther* 1996;11: 249–253.
45 Cuckle HS, Holding S, Jones R, et al. Combining inhibin A with existing second-trimester markers in maternal serum screening for Down's syndrome. *Prenat Diagn* 1996;16:1095–1100.
46 Candenas M, Villa R, Fernandez Collar R, et al. Maternal serum alpha-fetoprotein screening for neural tube defects. Report of a program with more than 30000 screened pregnancies. *Acta Obstet Gynecol Scand* 1995;74:266–269.
47 Engel E. A new genetic concept: uniparental disomy and its potential effect, isodisomy. *Am J Med Genet* 1980;6:137.
48 Nicholls RD, Knoll JHM, Butler MG, et al. Genetic imprinting suggested by maternal uniparental heterodisomy in nondeletion Prader–Willi syndrome. *Nature* 1989;342:281–285.
49 Malcolm S, Clayton-Smith J, Nichols M, et al. Uniparental paternal disomy in Angelman's syndrome. *Lancet* 1991;337:694.
50 Spence JE, Perciaccante, RG, Greig GM, et al. Uniparental disomy as a mechanism for human genetic disease. *Am J Hum Genet* 1988;42:217–226.
51 Brzustowicz LM, Alitto BA, Matseoane D, et al. Paternal isodisomy for chromosome 5 in a child with spinal muscular atrophy. *Am J Hum Genet* 1994;54:482–488.
52 Milunsky JM, Wyandt HE, Huang X-L, et al. Trisomy 15 mosaicism and uniparental disomy (UPD) in a liveborn infant. *Am J Med Genet* 1996;61:269–273.
53 Stevenson DA, Brothman AR, Chen Z, et al. Paternal uniparental disomy of chromosome 14: confirmation of a clinically-recognizable phenotype. *Am J Med Genet* 2004;130A(1):88–91.
54 Kalousek DK, Barrett I. Genomic Imprinting Related to Prenatal Diagnosis. *Prenatal Diag* 1994;14:1191–1201.
55 Sensi A, Cavani S, Villa N, et al. Nonhomologous Robertsonian translocations (NHRTs) and uniparental disomy (UPD) risk: an Italian multicentric prenatal survey. *Prenat Diagn* 2004;24: 647–652.
56 Ledbetter DH, Engel E. Uniparental disomy in humans: development of an imprinting map and its implications for prenatal diagnosis. *Hum Mol Genet* 1995;4:1757–1764 (Review).
57 Milunsky JM. Prenatal diagnosis of sex chromosome abnormalities. In: Milunsky A, ed. *Genetic disorders and the fetus*, 5th edn. Baltimore, MD: Johns Hopkins University Press, 2004;297.
58 Benn PA, Hsu LYF. Prenatal diagnosis of chromosomal abnormalities through amniocentesis. In: Milunsky A, ed. *Genetic disorders and the fetus*, 5th edn. Baltimore, MD: Johns Hopkins University Press; 2004:214–296.
59 Linden MG, Bender BG, Robinson A. Intrauterine diagnosis of sex chromosome aneuploidy. *Obstet Gynecol* 1996;87:468–475.
60 Evans JA, Hamerton JL, Robinson A, eds. Children and young adults with sex chromosome aneuploidy: Follow-up, clinical, and molecular studies. *March of Dimes, Birth Defects: Original Article Series*. New York: Wiley-Liss, 1990.
61 Ratcliffe SG, Paul NP, eds. Prospective studies on children with sex chromosome aneuploidy. *March of Dimes, Birth Defects: Original Article Series*. New York: Alan R. Liss, 1986.
62 Ledbetter DH, Zachery DH, Simpson JM, et al. Cytogenetic results from the U.S. collaborative study on CVS. *Prenat Diagn* 1992;12:317–354.
63 Engel and Delozier-Blanchet. Uniparental disomy, isodisomy, and imprinting: probable effects in man and strategies for their detection. *Am J Med Genet* 1991;40:437–439.
64 Hall JG. Genomic imprinting: Review and relevance to human diseases. *Am J Hum Genet* 1990;46:857–873.
65 Simoni G, Brambati B, Maggi F, et al. Trisomy 16 confined to chorionic villi and unfavourable outcome of pregnancy. *Ann Genet* 1992;35:110–112.
66 Kalousek DK. Confined Placental Mosaicism and Uniparental Disomy. *Func Dev Morph* 1994;4:93–98.
67 Groupe de cytogénéticiens français. Pericentric inversions in man. A French collaborative study. *Ann Genet* 1986;29:129.
68 Groupe de cytogénéticiens français. Paracentric inversions in man. A French collaborative study. *Ann Genet* 1986;29:169.
69 Daniel A, ed. *The cytogenetics of mammalian autosomal rearrangements*. New York: Alan R Liss, 1988.
70 Gardner RJM, Sutherland GR. *Chromosome abnormalities and genetic counseling*. New York: Oxford University Press, 2004.
71 Sybert VP, McCauley E. Turner's syndrome. *N Engl J Med* 2004;351:1227–1238.
72 de la Chapella A, Schroder J. Stenstrand K, et al. Pericentric inversions of human chromosomes 9 and 11. *Am J Hum Genet* 1974; 26:746–766.
73 Gray JW, Kallioniemi A, Kallioniemi O, et al. Molecular cytogenetics: diagnosis and prognostic assessment. *Curr Opin Biotechnol* 1992;3:623–631.
74 Kirchhoff M, Pedersen S, Kjeldsen E, et al. Prospective study comparing HR-CGH and subtelomeric FISH for investigation of individuals with mental retardation and dysmorphic features and an update of a study using only HR-CGH. *Am J Med Genet* 2004;127A:111–117.
75 Anderlid BM, Schoumans J, Anneren G, et al. Subtelomeric rearrangements detected in patients with idiopathic mental retardation. *Am J Med Genet* 2002;107:275–284.
76 Oostlander A, Meijer G, Ylstra B. Microarray-based comparative genomic hybridization and its applications in human genetics. *Clin Genet* 2004; :488–495.

77 Warburton D, Kline J, Stein Z, et al. Does the karyotype of a spontaneous abortion predict the karyotype of a subsequent abortion? Evidence from 273 women with two karyotyped spontaneous abortions. *Am J Hum Genet* 1987;41:465.

78 Scriver CR, Beaudet AL, Sly WS, Valle D, eds. *The metabolic basis of inherited disease*, 8th edn. New York: McGraw-Hill, 2001.

79 Politano L, Nigro V, Giovannani N, et al. Development of cardiomyopathy in female carriers of duchenne and becker muscular dystrophies. *JAMA* 1996;275:1335–1338.

80 Bakker E, Veenama H, Den Dunnen JT, et al. Germinal mosaicism increases the recurrence risk for "new" Duchenne muscular dystrophy mutations. *J Med Genet* 1989;26:553.

81 Letters to the Editor. Dizygous twinning and premature menopause in fragile X syndrome. *Lancet* 1994;344:1500.

82 Hagerman PJ, Hagerman RJ. Fragile X-associated tremor/ataxia syndrome (FXTAS). *Ment Retard Dev Disabil Res Rev* 2004; 10(1):25–30.

83 Jacquemont S, Hagerman RJ, Leehy MA, et al. Penetrance of the fragile X–associated tremor/ataxiasyndrome in a premuation carrier population. *JAMA* 2004;291:460–469.

84 Hagerman RJ, Leavitt BR, Farzin F, et al. Fragile-X-associated tremor/ataxia syndrome (FXTAS) in females with the FMR1 premutation. *Am J Hum Genet* 2004;74:1051–1056.

85 Scriver CR, Beaudet AL, Sly WS, Valle D. *The metabolic and molecular basis of inherited disease*, vol. 1, 8th edn. New York: McGraw-Hill; 2001:1275.

86 Milunsky A. *Know your genes*. Boston, MA: Houghton-Mifflin; 1977.

87 Brookes JAS, Hall-Craggs MA, Sams VR, Lees WR. Non-invasive perinatal necropsy by magnetic resonance imaging. *Lancet* 1996; 348:1139–1141.

88 sia YE, Hirschhorn K, Silverberg RL, Godmilow L, eds. *Counseling in genetics*. New York: Alan R Liss, 1979.

89 Brandt J, Quaid KA, Folstein SE, et al. Presymptomatic diagnosis of delayed-onset disease with linked DNA markers: the experience in Huntington's disease. *JAMA* 1989;261:3108.

90 Wallis J, Shaw J, Wilkes D, et al. Prenatal diagnosis of Friedrich ataxia. *Am J Med Genet* 1989;34:458.

91 International Huntington Association and World Federation of Neurology: Ethical issues, policy statement on Huntington disease molecular genetics, and predictive tests. *J Med Gen* 1990;27: 34–38.

92 International Huntington Association and World Federation of Neurology: Guidelines for the molecular genetics predictive test in Huntingtons disease. *Neurology* 1994;44:1533–1536.

93 Decruyenaere M, Evers-Kiebooms G, Cloostermans T, et al. Psychological distress in the 5-year period after predictive testing for Huntington's disease. *Eur J Hum Genet* 2003;11:30.

94 Harris PC, Ward CJ, Peral B, et al. Autosomal dominant polycystic kidney disease: molecular analysis (Review). *Hum Mol Gen* 1995;4:1745–1749.

95 Sujansky E, Kreutzer SB, Johnson AM, et al. Attitudes of at-risk and affected individuals regarding presymptomatic testing for autosomal dominant polycystic kidney disease. *Am J Med Genet* 1990;35:510.

96 Hannig VL, Hopkins JR, Johnson HK, et al. Presymptomatic testing adult onset polycystic kidney disease in at-risk kidney transplant donors. *Am J Med Genet* 1991;40:425.

97 Pelias MZ. Duty to disclose in medical genetics: a legal perspective. *Am J Med Genet* 1991;39:347–354.

22 Basic principles of ultrasound

Mladen Predanic, Frank A. Chervenak, and E. Albert Reece

Introduction

Ultrasound has had a profound influence on the practice of medicine, especially in obstetrics. Since its first introduction into medicine, almost half a century ago, ultrasound studies have shown a potential to provide information about the fetus in a noninvasive manner. Most importantly, it does not appear to be associated with any known adverse fetal bioeffects. Thus, diagnostic ultrasound gained wide clinical acceptance and become of considerable diagnostic value. The new powerful ultrasound machines, with superb resolution, three-dimensional capabilities, and various Doppler modalities, are convenient to use, comfortable for the patient, and not very expensive. It is an unquestionable fact that prenatal ultrasound provides information that allows diagnosis and treatment of fetal malformations that otherwise could be diagnosed only postnatally and often in an untimely fashion. However, a major question still remains unequivocally unanswered: Is prenatal diagnostic ultrasound safe? Although no known human epidemiologic data or unquestionable evidence exist to demonstrate any deleterious effect of diagnostic ultrasound in neonates over the last 40–50 years of clinical use, there are some tissue biological effects generated by ultrasound. Even more, the acoustic output of modern equipment constantly changes with the advancement of the technology, whereas investigations into the possibility of subtle or transient fetal adverse ultrasound bioeffects are still at an early stage. Therefore, diagnostic prenatal ultrasound should only be considered safe if used prudently.

Basic physics

Sound consists of waves and is described by frequency, wavelength, amplitude, intensity, and the propagation of speed. An *ultrasound* is a sound with a frequency higher than the human ear can detect. The frequency of ultrasound used in medicine for fetal imaging is in the range of 3–7.5 million cycles per second (megahertz, MHz). Such high-frequency ultrasound is generated by high mechanical deformation of certain materials (e.g., crystals or ceramics), caused by electrical stimulation, which produces a generation of waves at ultrasound frequencies. This is described as the *piezoelectric* phenomenon, and it also works in reverse.[1] An ultrasound "receptor" will resonate at certain frequencies, creating electrical impulses when stimulated by reflected ultrasonic waves (echoes).

Materials amenable to the piezoelectric phenomenon make up the core of the ultrasound transducer. These "crystals" are arrayed at the tip of the ultrasound probe. An ultrasound wave is generated by the electric pulse, transmitted through the tissue, and at some tissue depth is reflected and returned to the transducer. Returned "echoes" are detected and converted by the same transducer into electric impulses of equivalent amplitude that corresponds to the depth of the returned ultrasonic wave. The array of the electric impulses is analyzed by the computer software and converted into the image. Depending on the mode of data analysis, we are able to demonstrate tissue structures by B-mode two-dimensional real-time sonography; M-mode (e.g., used for assessment of heart motion); a pulsed Doppler modality that pictures blood flow in the form of waveforms that correspond to the systolic and diastolic components of the cardiac cycle; color and power Doppler modes (superimposed blood flow in the form of colored dots/areas over the B-mode picture); and, more recently, three-dimensional sonography that renders analyzed structures in a static three-dimensional image, or four-dimensional ultrasound, which demonstrates a three-dimensional image in real time (Table 22.1). All of these advances were possible because of the tremendous advancements in computer technology and software systems that enable quick and accurate analysis of the received ultrasound data.[1]

Ultrasound image and resolution

It is imperative to understand that ultrasound images are generated from an ultrasound beam that is three-dimensional in

Table 22.1 Basic ultrasound modes and images.

Ultrasound mode	Ultrasound image	Brief description	Comment
A-mode (one-dimensional)	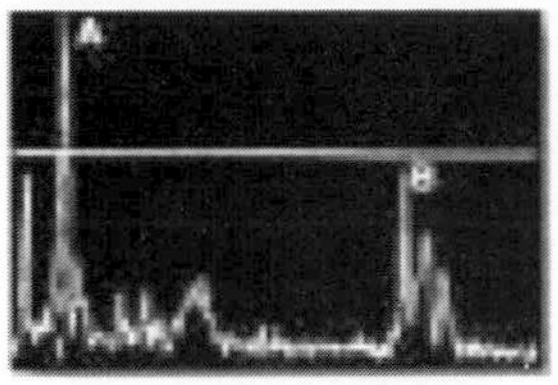	Wave spikes occur when a *single* beam passes through objects of different consistency and hardness	Of historical value, now obsolete in medical imaging
B-mode (one-dimensional, 1-D)	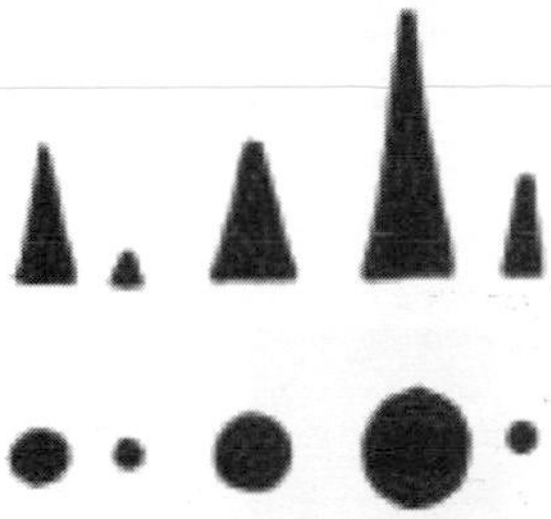	Same as A-mode, but wave spikes (upper row) are replaced with *dots* (lower row) where "brightness" corresponds to amplitude of reflected sound	Of historical value, now obsolete in medical imaging
B-mode (two-dimensional) (in real time)	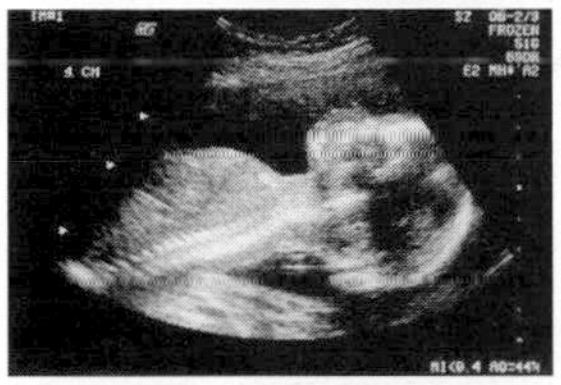	B-mode generated from multiple crystals (array) in real time (up to 100 images per second)	Today's standard of ultrasound imaging, utilized by almost any ultrasound machine
M-mode	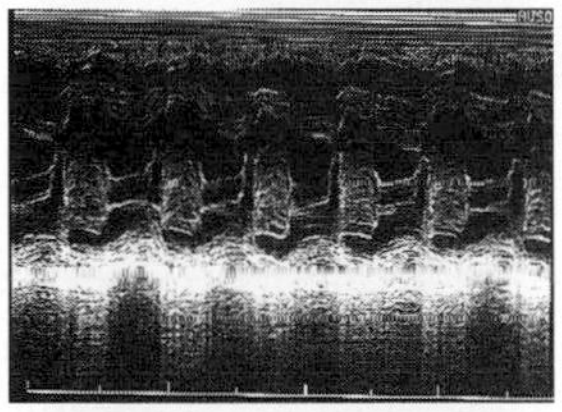	Combination of B-mode one-dimensional (vertical axis) and time (horizontal axis)	Fetal cardiac imaging
Pulsed Doppler	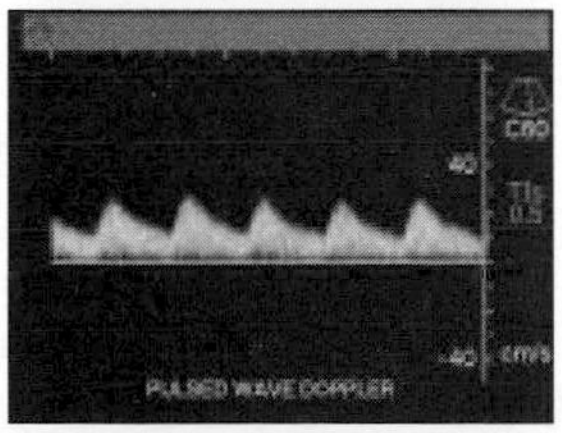	Based on Doppler principle* demonstrates blood flow in real time (wave spikes are systolic component of the blood flow)	Used to analyze blood flow characteristics (e.g., velocities and resistance to blood flow)
Color Doppler	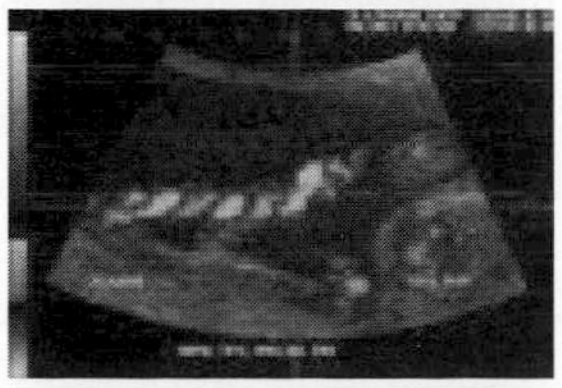	Codes blood flow (or any motion) by Doppler principle, into two colored dots according to the direction and blood flow velocities; it is superimposed over B-mode image	Used to map blood flow spots within the investigated tissue or organ
Power (color) Doppler	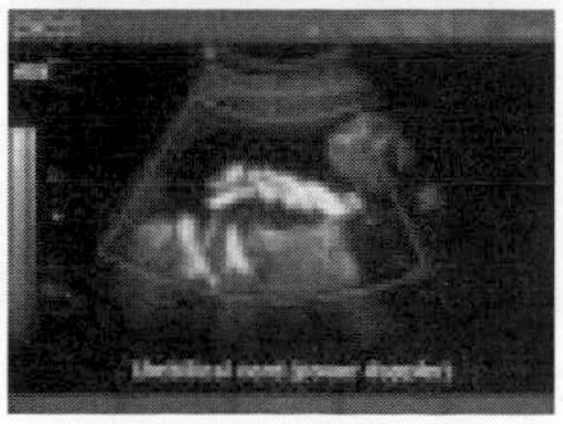	Similar to color Doppler, but codes all blood flow into one color (no directional information) – more sensitive to slow blood flow than color Doppler	Used to enhance blood flow mapping in tissue with slow blood flow states

Table 22.1 *Continued.*

Ultrasound mode	Ultrasound image	Brief description	Comment
Three- and four-dimensional (four-dimensional is three-dimensional ultrasound in real time)		Two-dimensional B-mode with third dimension (depth) analyzed by powerful computer software to render three-dimensional image; three-dimensional image is static, whereas four-dimensional image is the three-dimensional image in real time	Diagnostic value of three- over two-dimensional B-mode real-time ultrasound is controversial, although may significantly reduce scanning time

*Doppler principle. Source moving toward the receiver has higher frequency than source moving away from receiver, which has lower frequency.

A

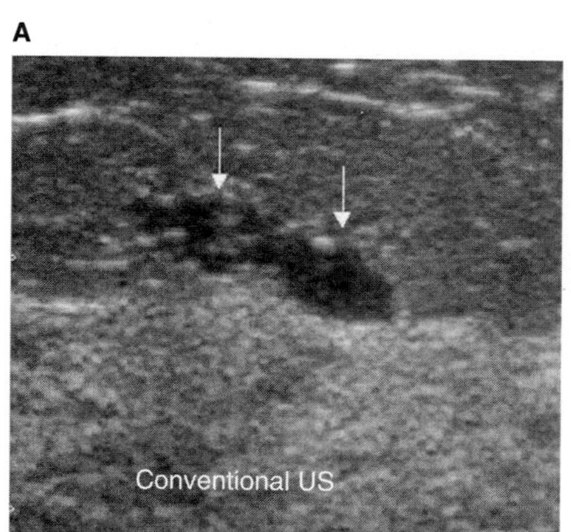

B

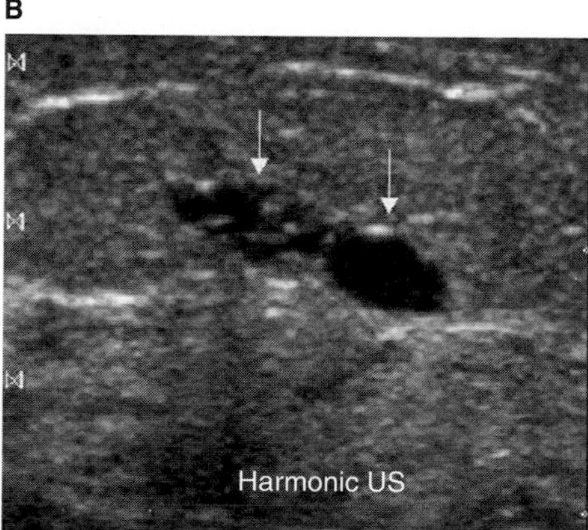

Figure 22.1 Comparison between conventional (A) and harmonic ultrasound imaging (B).

form. The three dimensions are thickness (*azimuthal* resolution), width, and depth (*lateral* and *axial* resolution). Any transducer that generates an ultrasound beam is capable of focusing that beam at certain depths via an "electromagnetic lens." Generated ultrasound beams are unevenly thick, with the narrowest part at the level of their focus. If the beam is thick, the reflected echoes from the same plane at a certain depth will be unified in one two-dimensional image that may appear blurry. It is especially true for the images that are closest and farthest away from the probe where the ultrasound beam is the thickest. At the same time, the image is most clear at the focus level where the beam is narrowest. *Axial* resolution, or parallel to the direction of the sound waves leaving the transducer, is related to the length of the ultrasound pulse. Shorter ultrasound wavelengths or higher frequencies will produce better axial resolution. In contrast, *lateral* resolution is equal to the beam diameter in millimeters, is perpendicular to the axial, and inevitably poorer that axial resolution. Because it is related to the beam diameter, it is significantly affected in curved transducers where the beam diameter increases with depth and becomes equivalent in thickness to the azimuthal resolution. Thus, the image that is away from the probe appears not only blurry, but also distorted sometimes as well.

Although the image quality directly depends on the frequency of the ultrasound probe, resolution has been significantly improved by an increase in the number of transducer crystals (or channels); improvements in transducer crystal technology (creating broadband and high-dynamic-range images); increased array aperture (more crystals firing in a single time-frame); faster computational capabilities (faster computer chipsets); improved technical algorithms for focusing on received ultrasound beam (increasing the number of focal zones along the beam); incorporating automatic time-gain controls, and progressively replacing analog portions of the signal path to digital. The signal path of the beam former (transducer), in the older analog processing data chain ultrasound machines, was analyzed based on the axial resolution formed by the use of the one or multifocuses. With the employment of more powerful computers, the whole process became digitized. Super-fast digital beam formers allowed significantly increased numbers of focal points (microfine focuses) along the beam to the size of a screen pixel. This technology reduced signal–noise ratio in data processing by several hundred-fold and created a significantly clearer picture. The most recent advent in use is the so-called *harmonic* imaging (Fig. 22.1). Tissue harmonic imaging utilizes lower frequency echoes for the ultrasound penetration that receives and processes only the higher frequency echoes generated by the body's inherent characteristics. The final product is dramatically cleaner contrast between adjacent tissue structures that is particularly useful in obese patients.

Ultrasound safety

The diagnostic ultrasound has widespread acceptance due to its clinical utility, convenience, and noninvasiveness. In the USA, approximately 65% of pregnant women have at least one ultrasound examination.[2] We usually reassure any prospective mother that ultrasound is safe and does not have any harmful effects on the baby; therefore, it is of paramount importance to be familiar with ultrasound safety.[3] Some evidence exists that high-energy ultrasound may produce biological effects in exposed tissues. The most studied effects are the local increase in temperature (thermal changes), and oscillatory and potentially catastrophic motions of bubbles, if present, in the tissues (microcavitation).[4]

The nature of ultrasound is such that, during its propagation through the tissue, portions of its energy are absorbed and converted into heat. Although the heat is dissipated by the adjacent tissues and blood flow through the insonated area, tissue temperature may rise a fraction of a degree Celsius.[5] Such temperature aberrations normally occur during the human diurnal cycle, and temperature may increase by 3–4°C in febrile states. Hyperthermia is a proven teratogenic agent in various animals (mouse, rat, hamster, monkey, sheep, and others) and is considered so in humans. In addition, certain stages of embryonic and fetal development may be more susceptible to thermal effects.[6] Effects appear to be a threshold phenomenon when temperature increases of 1.5°C or higher are considered necessary for damage to occur. However, the energy output of the diagnostic ultrasound is of such low intensity that it is unlikely to induce temperature changes of such a degree to produce adverse pregnancy effects.[7] In addition, no recently published study has demonstrated unequivocal adverse effects of diagnostic ultrasound. However, it is a theoretical possibility and should not be completely ignored.

The interaction of sound with microscopic gas bubbles that pre-exist in tissues may cause a bioeffect termed *microcavitation* or acoustic cavitation.[4] Because of the succession of positive and negative pressures that can cause oscillatory motions of bubbles, several outcomes may result: (1) stable cavitation or (2) implosion of the bubbles described as transient cavitation. These can result in cell membrane disruption and even the release of free radicals that are cell toxic. Another potential effect is radiation stress, caused by acoustic streaming in liquid media secondary to the pressure gradient generated by the moving sound wave. These biological effects have been produced in plants, insects, and some mammalian tissues. Although there is no direct evidence to suggest that in humans, under clinical conditions, ultrasound-induced microcavitation produces biological effects, the Food and Drug Administration (FDA), together with the American Institute of Ultrasound in Medicine (AIUM), the American College of Obstetrics and Gynecologists (ACOG), and the National Electrical Manufacturers Association, introduced a method of displaying ultrasonic output that would control and minimize possible bioeffects in insonated fetal tissues.[5,7–10] If an ultrasound machine exceeds predetermined limits for output, either a thermal index or mechanical index must be displayed on the screen. If the thermal index, which is appropriate for Doppler applications, exceeds 1.0, there is a potential for the tissue temperature to rise. If the mechanical index, which is appropriate for scale imaging, exceeds 1.0, there is a potential for cavitational effects.[5,8] It is important to note that although the more recent epidemiologic studies were published in 1998 through 2002, ultrasound examinations consisted exclusively of B-mode, and all machines used predated 1992, i.e., the "new" FDA regulations, allowing output to rise to more than 94 mW/cm^2, the then-accepted upper limit for fetal application. Those acoustic outputs can be considered "low" by today's standards. Still, available published evidence showed no difference in the prevalence of delayed speech or motor development, impaired neurological development, growth, vision, or hearing, low birthweight, dyslexia, or childhood cancer among children exposed to ultrasound *in utero*.[11–13] The only well-designed study showing some effect was a recent article that presented a small increase in the frequency of non-right-handedness (ambiguity) in male infants of mothers exposed to diagnostic ultrasound.[14] Nevertheless, in general, it is safe to say that when sonography is performed for a valid medical indication by a well-trained individual who respects the basic rules of time and exposure, the information that can be obtained is of such great value that it clearly overshadows the remote risks that may exist.[15–19] In contrast with medical indications, performing ultrasound for "keepsake" records of the fetus, especially in the first trimester of the pregnancy, should be discouraged. Embryonic tissue may not have the tensile strength of fetal or adult tissue secondary to underdevelopment of the intercellular matrix to withhold cellular damage due to biological effects caused by ultrasound, especially if the energy output is above recommendations, or if it is used for prolonged periods of time. The risk of thermal bioeffects is increased when imaging is advanced from simple grayscale B-mode (in which the risk may be nonexistent) to pulsed Doppler. Doppler examinations present the highest risk of thermal *bioeffects* owing to their high pulse repetition frequency and longer pulses.[17,18] It also appears that the risks of appreciable harmful *bioeffects* may increase with increasing scanning time, ultrasound frequency (increases thermal risks but decreases cavitation risks), and output power (increasing the gain on the "output" knob, an "energy" trackball, or a "power" cursor) (Table 22.2). However, we believe that newer technologies, such as harmonic imaging and three-dimensional sonography, may be safer. Both modalities are based on data post processing; therefore, one might speculate that time used for ultrasound scanning may be significantly reduced and thereby decrease the potential for adverse ultrasound biological effects.

In conclusion, the duration of exposure and output levels should be kept at a minimum, which is the basis of the ALARA (*a*s *l*ow *a*s *r*easonably *a*chievable) principle, endorsed, among

Table 22.2 A summary of the recommendations published by several national and international organizations, including the American Institute of Ultrasound in Medicine (AIUM), International Society for Ultrasound in Obstetrics and Gynecology, Australasian Society for Ultrasound in Medicine, British Society for Medical Ultrasound, and World Federation for Ultrasound in Medicine and Biology.

Ultrasound induces biological effects (bioeffects) in the tissues but is generally considered safe if properly used – no epidemiologic studies have shown, so far, harmful effects in humans
A clear medical indication should be present for performance of diagnostic sonography; when a clear medical indication exists, the benefits outweigh the risks potentially caused by performing sonography
Ultrasound services should be provided by people with adequate training, including knowledge of safety and bioeffects issues
An elevation of fetal body temperature above 41°C for 5 min or more is considered hazardous
Nonthermal bioeffects (microcavitation) may result in capillary bleeding, particularly in the lungs and bowels when gas bubbles are present; fetal lungs and bowels do not contain gas, therefore a mechanical risk is probably nonexistent
B- and M-mode sonography appears entirely safe in pregnancy
Pulsed Doppler and color Doppler sonography with a small region of interest have the greatest potential for bioeffects; these should be carried out with particular care in the first trimester
New technologies, such as harmonic imaging and three-dimensional sonography, do not present more risk than native B-mode imaging
Sonographic examination, particularly spectral Doppler sonography, in a pregnant patient with an elevated temperature might pose additional risks to the fetus
The duration of exposure and output energy levels should be kept at a minimum – ALARA (*as low as reasonably achievable*) principle
Continuous research and education in ultrasound safety and biological effects are strongly encouraged

Modified from Abramowicz JS. Ultrasound in obstetrics and gynecology: is this hot technology too hot? *J Ultrasound Med* 2002;21:1327–1333.

Table 22.3 Indications for ultrasonography during pregnancy.

Estimation of gestational age
Evaluation of fetal growth
Vaginal bleeding
Abdominal and pelvic pain
Incompetent cervix
Determination of fetal presentation
Suspected multiple gestation
Adjunct to amniocentesis
Significant uterine size and clinical dates discrepancy
Pelvic mass
Suspected hydatidiform mole
Adjunct to cervical cerclage placement
Suspected ectopic pregnancy
Suspected fetal death
Suspected uterine abnormality
Evaluation for fetal well-being
Suspected amniotic fluid abnormalities
Suspected placental abruption
Adjunct to external cephalic version
Premature rupture of membranes and/or premature labor
Abnormal biochemical markers
Follow-up evaluation of a fetal anomaly
Follow-up evaluation of placental location for suspected placenta previa
History of previous congenital anomaly
Evaluation of fetal condition in late registrants for prenatal care

Modified from American Institute of Ultrasound in Medicine (AIUM). Practice guideline for the performance of an antepartum obstetric ultrasound examination. *J Ultrasound Med* 2003;22: 1116–1125.

others, by the American Institute of Ultrasound in Medicine, the National Electrical Manufacturers Association, and the FDA.[5] Nevertheless, continuous research and education on ultrasound safety are strongly encouraged.

Ultrasound examination

The current standpoint of ACOG is that ultrasound in pregnancy should be performed only when there is a valid medial indication (Table 22.3).[20] Therefore, physicians are not obligated to perform ultrasonography in patients who are at low risk and have no indications. However, if a patient requests ultrasonography, it is reasonable to honor the request – the final decision to have an ultrasound scan rests with the physician and patient jointly.[15,20]

It is our belief that the benefits of routine ultrasound in pregnancy outweigh the risks associated with potential adverse ultrasound effects. The early recognition of fetal anomalies may introduce *in utero* treatment, or at least prepare parents for the emotional ordeal that follows delivery of the fetus with a major malformation. Although 90% of infants with congenital anomalies are born to women with no risk factors, a controversy about routine ultrasound use exists.[21] A minimal and inconsistent impact on perinatal morbidity or mortality was observed with the use of routine ultrasound screening in the second trimester of pregnancy.[22–24] However, there are data that support its cost-effectiveness when performed in tertiary centers.[25]

The ACOG, in its most recent clinical management guidelines for obstetricians and gynecologists, has defined three types of ultrasound examinations performed during the second or third trimester of pregnancy.[20] The *standard* examination includes an evaluation of fetal presentation, amniotic fluid volume, cardiac activity, and placental position, fetal biometry, and an anatomic survey. Fetal anatomy may be assessed adequately at 16–20 weeks of gestation (Table 22.4).

Table 22.4 Essential elements of the fetal anatomic ultrasound survey.

Head and neck
Cerebellum
Choroid plexus
Cisterna magna
Lateral cerebral ventricles
Midline falx
Cavum septi pellucidi

Chest
The basic cardiac examination includes a four-chamber view of the fetal heart. If technically feasible, an extended basic cardiac examination can also be attempted to evaluate both outflow tracts

Abdomen
Stomach (presence, size, and situs)
Kidneys
Bladder
Umbilical cord insertion site into the fetal abdomen
Umbilical cord vessel number

Spine
Cervical, thoracic, lumbar, and sacral spine

Extremities
Legs and arms (presence or absence)

Gender
Medically indicated in low-risk pregnancies only for evaluation of multifetal gestations

Modified from American Institute of Ultrasound in Medicine (AIUM). Practice guidelines for the performance of an antepartum obstetric ultrasound examination. *J Ultrasound Med* 2003;22: 1116–1125.

If technically feasible, the uterus and adnexae should also be examined. A *limited* examination is performed when a specific question requires investigation. For example, it may be employed to verify fetal presentation in a laboring patient, or to confirm heart activity in a patient with absent fetal movements. A *specialized* examination is a detailed or targeted anatomic examination that is performed when an anomaly is suspected on the basis of patient history, biochemical abnormalities, or clinical evaluation. Other specialized examinations include fetal Doppler studies, biophysical profile, fetal echocardiography, or additional biometric studies.

In addition to indications in the second and third trimester of pregnancy, Table 22.5 demonstrates indications for the use of ultrasound in the first trimester of pregnancy. The first trimester is a time of rapid embryonic–fetal development. Highly accurate first-trimester dating can be obtained by measuring the crown–rump length (CRL) of the fetus (Fig. 22.2). A number of studies have demonstrated that fetal CRL is the most accurate measurement for the sonographic dating of pregnancy. It has a high reproducibility and can be used reliably until approximately 12 weeks' gestation. Beyond this period, a variety of sonographic parameters, such as biparietal diameter (BPD), abdominal circumference, and femoral diaphysis length can be used to estimate gestational age. However, the variability of gestational age estimations increases with advancing pregnancy. As early as the late first trimester, separate fetal body structures can be examined.

Table 22.5 Indications for ultrasound in the first trimester of pregnancy.

To confirm the presence of an intrauterine pregnancy
To evaluate a suspected ectopic pregnancy
To define the cause of vaginal bleeding
To evaluate pelvic pain
To estimate gestational age
To diagnose or evaluate multiple gestations
To confirm cardiac activity
As an adjunct to chorionic villus sampling, embryo transfer, or localization and removal of an intrauterine device
To evaluate maternal pelvic masses or uterine abnormalities
To evaluate suspected hydatidiform mole

Modified from American Institute of Ultrasound in Medicine (AIUM). Practice guideline for the performance of an antepartum obstetric ultrasound examination. *J Ultrasound Med* 2003;22:1116–1125.

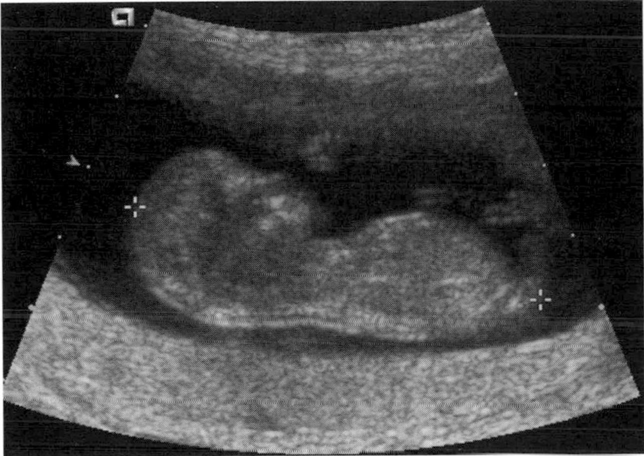

Figure 22.2 Transverse image of the embryo at 12 weeks and 1 day of gestational age depicting the crown–rump length measurement of 5.43 mm.

Head

The oval outline of the fetal head should be sought in all examinations. The intracranial anatomy should be examined to ascertain that major midline structures are present, such as thalami, intrahemispheric fissure, and cavum septi pellucidi (Fig. 22.3). Advanced head evaluation includes other head measurements, such as the extra- and intraorbital distances, ventricular diameters, as well as the occipital frontal

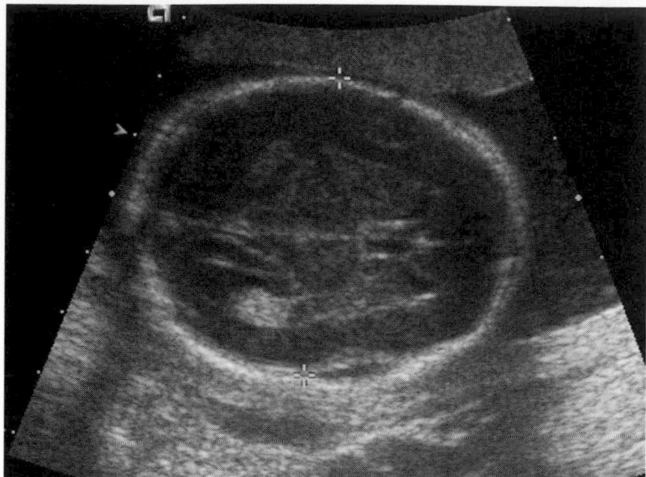

Figure 22.3 Transverse ultrasound image at the level of the biparietal diameter, demonstrating thalami (T) and septum cavum pellucidum (SCP).

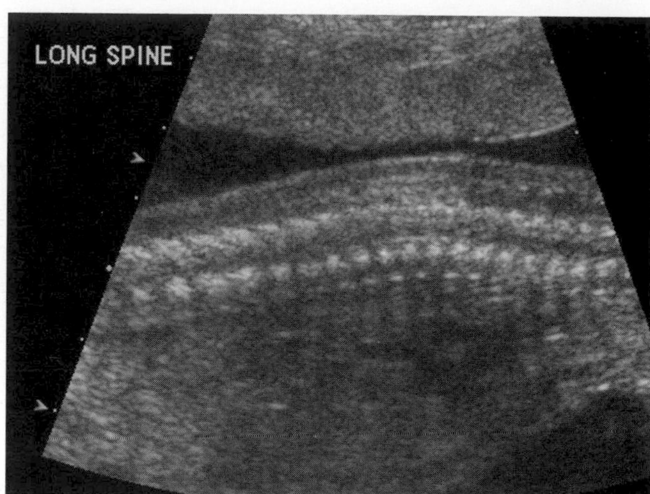

Figure 22.5 Longitudinal image of the fetal spine.

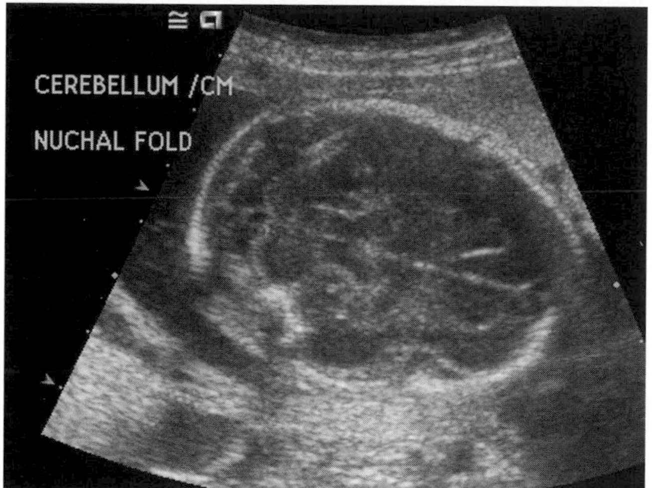

Figure 22.4 Posterior fossa with cerebellar diameter, fourth ventricle, and cisterna magna.

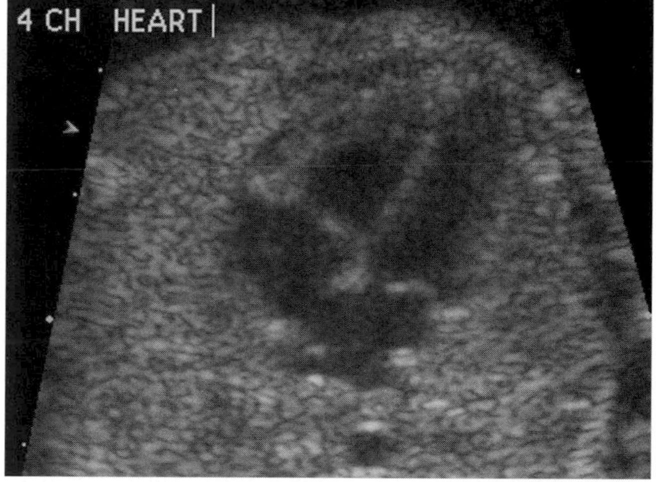

Figure 22.6 Four-chamber view of the fetal heart.

distance and the cephalic index. The cephalic index is the ratio of BPD to occipital front distance, which is normally in the range of 0.75–0.85. The posterior fossa reveals information about the cerebellar diameter, which correlates with gestational age, presence of the cerebellar vermis, and the size of the cisterna magna (Fig. 22.4).

Fetal spine

The fetal spine ossifies as early as 10 weeks and is seen as parallel sets of echoes representing the articulating vertebral facets. It is usually examined in the longitudinal (coronal) plane, although in a targeted examination for neural tube defects, the transverse view of the total spine should be demonstrated (Fig. 22.5).

Fetal heart

A four-chamber heart view (Fig. 22.6) is a basic part of all examinations after 18 to 20 week's gestation. It is fast and easy to perform a screening test for congenital heart disease because the majority of heart structural anomalies may be detected using this single view. However, outflow tract anomalies (e.g. transposition of the great vessels) can be easily missed if "long" and "short" axis heart views are not performed (Fig. 22.7).

Abdomen

The fetal abdomen and stomach, as a single cystic area, can be visualized as early as 14 weeks' gestation. Ventral wall

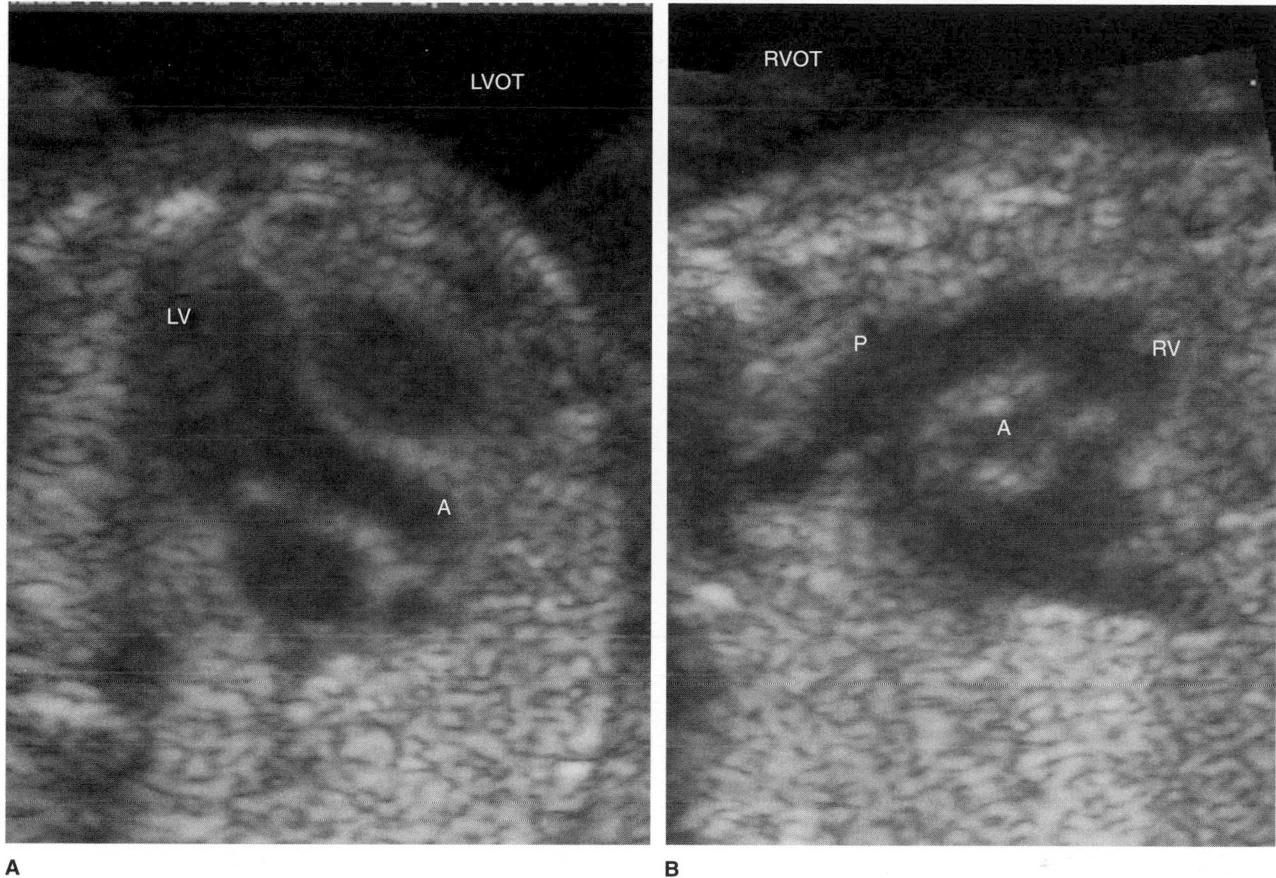

Figure 22.7 Left and right ventricle outflow tracts of the fetal heart: (A) LVOT, left ventricle and aorta; (B) RVOT, right ventricle and pulmonary artery.

defects can be excluded by the demonstration of an intact abdominal umbilical cord insertion (Fig. 22.8). Fetal kidneys (Fig. 22.9) and other upper abdomen organs can be easily demonstrated, such as gallbladder and liver. Fetal bladder is usually visible as a fluid-filled structure in the midline of the pelvis.

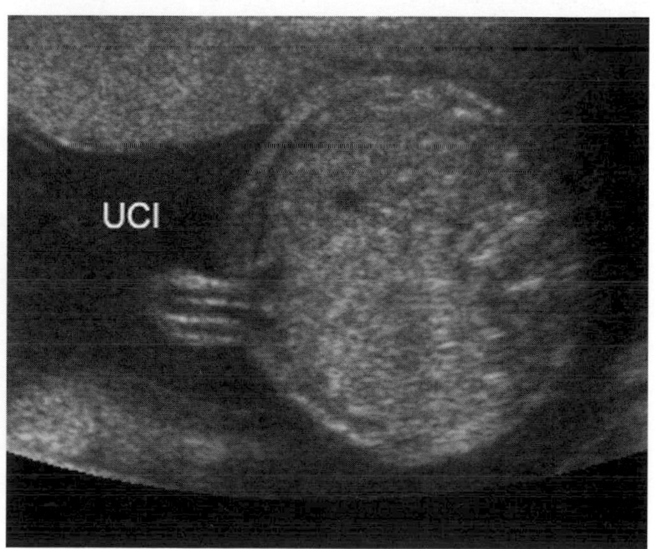

Figure 22.8 Fetal abdominal umbilical cord insertion.

Extremities

The four fetal limbs are identified routinely during ultrasound examination. Although it is not necessary to measure all six tubular bones in every fetus, measurements of at least one or two segments (femur and humerus) are performed. Both bones of the normal distal segments should be present. An image of the fetal hands and feet are also highly desirable, but are not required for a basic ultrasound examination (Fig. 22.10).

Fetal biometry

Fetal biometry is used to assess the size or estimated fetal weight that is usually plotted against a growth curve (generated from the large portion of general fetal population) to evaluate fetal growth characteristics. The estimated fetal weight is derived from various combinations of fetal measurements at certain gestational age, and mainly includes BPD, head circumference, abdominal circumference, and femoral diaphysis length, described elsewhere in this text. However, it is important to ascertain caution with the results of the fetal biometry, because there is large inter- and intraobserver variation in measurements at extremes of the fetal age (e.g., less than 24 or beyond 36 weeks' gestation).

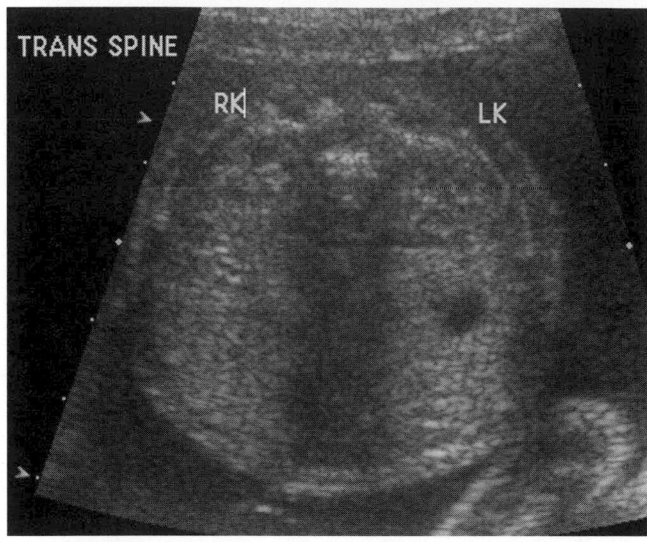

Figure 22.9 Transverse image through the fetal kidneys.

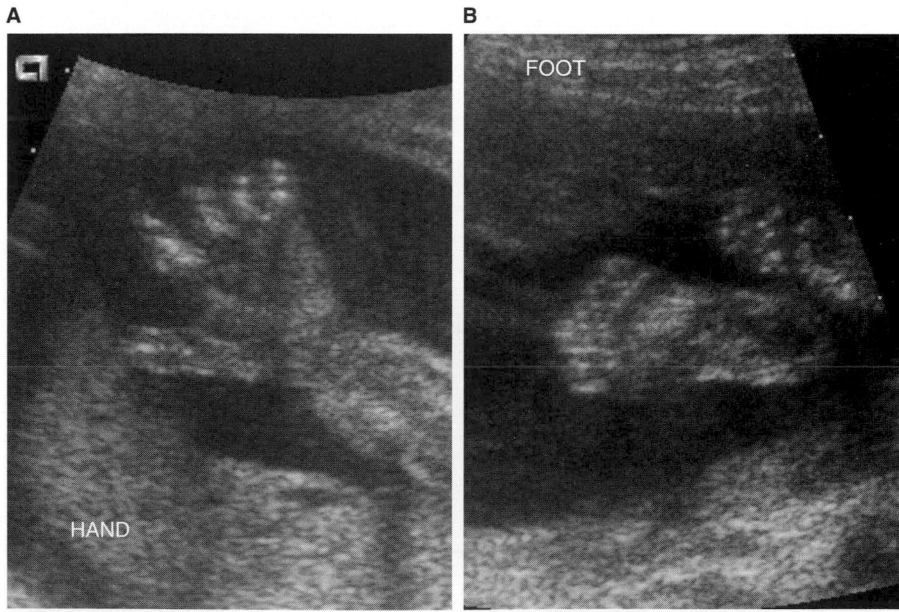

Figure 22.10 Fetal open hand (A) and a foot (B).

Key points

1 Sonography principles are based on the *piezoelectric phenomenon* and generated ultrasound waves. These ultrasound waves are reflected from tissue boundaries of different density, and processed by powerful computer software to generate real-time two- or three-dimensional images.

2 Recent advances in ultrasound data processing, such as "harmonic" imaging and super-fast digital beamers, permit significantly improved ultrasound resolution.

3 Although three- and four-dimensional (real-time three-dimensional) ultrasound produce excellent fetal images, their clinical superiority over conventional real-time two-dimensional ultrasound is controversial.

4 Ultrasound waves may produce certain biological tissue effects, e.g., thermal changes and mechanical effects (microcavitation), if used for prolonged periods of time with extremely high-energy outputs. However, these ultrasound energy output levels are *not* used with diagnostic ultrasound at present time.

5 To ensure ultrasound safety, it is the general consensus that the thermal and mechanical indexes are displayed on the screen if the ultrasound machine exceeds predetermined limits for energy output.

6 At the present time, diagnostic ultrasound is considered safe for the fetus when used appropriately and prudently. However, casual use of ultrasound, especially during the first trimester of pregnancy, should be avoided, especially implementation of pulsed Doppler ultrasound, which, theoretically, may produce a high thermal index.

7 Ultrasound examination in pregnancy is an accurate method of evaluating viability of the pregnancy, fetal number, and placental location, as well as gestational dating, which is most accurately determined in the first trimester of pregnancy.

8 Ultrasound is also able to accurately diagnose major fetal anomalies; however, the diagnosis of fetal growth abnormalities is less precise.

9 The optimal timing for a single ultrasound examination (if performed in the absence of specific indications) is at 18–20 weeks of gestation.

10 Appropriate patient counseling before the ultrasound examination regarding its limitations for diagnosis is of paramount importance and should be exercised routinely.

References

1 Kremkau FW. *Diagnostic ultrasound: principles and instruments*, 6th edn. Philadelphia, PA: WB Saunders, 2002.

2 Martin JA, Hamilton BE, Sutton PD, et al. Births: final data for 2002. *Natl Vital Stat Rep* 2003;52:1–113.

3 Reece EA, Assimakopoulos E, Zhen X, Hobbins JC. The safety of obstetrical ultrasound: Concerns for the fetus. *Obstet Gynecol* 1990;76: 139–146.

4 Dalecki D. Mechanical bioeffects of ultrasound. *Ann Rev Biomed Eng* 2004;6:229–248.

5 American Institute of Ultrasound in Medicine. Mechanical bioeffects from diagnostic ultrasound: AIUM consensus statements. *J Ultrasound Med* 2000;19:69–168.

6 Duck FA. Is it safe to use diagnostic ultrasound during the first trimester? (Editorial). *Ultrasound Obstet Gynecol* 1999;13: 385–388.

7 Abramowicz JS, Kossoff G, Marsal K, ter Haar G. International Society of Ultrasound in Obstetrics and Gynecology (ISUOG) Safety and Bioeffects Committee: safety statement. *Ultrasound Obstet Gynecol* 2000;16:594–596.

8 American Institute of Ultrasound in Medicine. *Official statement: clinical safety*. Laurel, MD: AIUM, 1997.

9 British Medical Ultrasound Society. Guidelines for the safe use of diagnostic ultrasound equipment. *BMUS Bulletin*, August, 2000.

10 Seeds JW. The routine or screening obstetrical ultrasound examination. *Clin Obstet Gynecol* 1996;39:814–830.

11 Kieler H, Ahlsten G, Haglund B, et al. Routine ultrasound screening in pregnancy and the children's subsequent neurologic development. *Obstet Gynecol* 1998;91:750–756.

12 Kieler H, Haglund B, Waldenstrom U, Axelsson O. Routine ultrasound screening in pregnancy and the children's subsequent growth, vision and hearing. *Br J Obstet Gynaecol* 1997;104: 1267–1272.

13 Kieler H, Cnattingius S, Haglund B, et al. Sinistrality, a side-effect of prenatal sonography: a comparative study of young men. *Epidemiology* 2001; 12:618–623.

14 Kieler H, Axelsson O, Haglund B, et al. Routine ultrasound screening in pregnancy and the children's subsequent handedness. *Early Hum Dev* 1998;50:233–245.

15 American Institute of Ultrasound in Medicine. AIUM Practice Guideline for the Performance of an Antepartum Obstetric Ultrasound Examination. *J Ultrasound Med* 2003;22:1116–1125.

16 Barnett SB, Kossoff G, Edwards MJ. Is diagnostic ultrasound safe? Current international consensus on the thermal mechanism. *Med J Aust* 1994;160:33–37.

17 Barnett SB, Maulik D, International Perinatal Doppler Society. Guidelines and recommendations for safe use of Doppler ultrasound in perinatal applications. *J Maternal Fetal Med* 2001;10: 75–84.

18 Kurjak A. Are color and pulsed Doppler sonography safe in early pregnancy? *J Perinat Med* 1999;27:423–430.

19 Ter Haar G, Duck F (eds). *The safe use of ultrasound in medical diagnosis*. London: British Medical Ultrasound Society/British Institute of Radiology, 2000.

20 American College of Obstetricians and Gynecologists. *Clinical management guidelines for obstetrician–gynecologists*, no. 58, December 2004.

21 Saari-Kemppainen A, Karjalainen O, Ylostalo P, Heinonen OP. Fetal anomalies in a controlled one-stage ultrasound screening

trial. A report from the Helsinki Ultrasound Trial. *J Perinatal Med* 1994;22:279–289.

22 Long G, Sprigg A. A comparative study of routine versus selective fetal anomaly ultrasound scanning. *J Med Screen* 1998;5:6–10.

23 Bucher H, Schmidt JG. Does routine ultrasound scanning improve outcome of pregnancy? Meta-analysis of various outcome measures. *Br Med J* 1993; 307:13–17.

24 Vintzileos AM, Ananth CV, Smulian JC, et al. Routine second-trimester ultrasonography in the United States: a cost-benefit analysis. *Am J Obstet Gynecol* 2000; 182:655–660.

25 Leivo T, Tuominen R, Saari-Kemppainen A, et al. Cost-effectiveness of one-stage ultrasound screening in pregnancy: a report from the Helsinki ultrasound trial. *Ultrasound Obstet Gynecol* 1996;7:309–314.

23 Prenatal diagnosis of central nervous system malformations

Gianluigi Pilu and Sandro Gabrielli

Only a small proportion of congenital anomalies of the central nervous system (CNS) are clinically recognizable and are therefore identified at birth. Long-term follow-up studies suggest that the prevalence of these conditions is much greater than expected for epidemiologic survey of neonates and is about 1 in 100 births.[1] Modern high-resolution ultrasound equipment has a unique potential for evaluating normal and abnormal anatomy of the fetal neural axis from the very early stages of development. Yet, identification of selected anomalies, such as ventriculomegaly and spina bifida, remains a challenge in many cases. In this chapter, the sonographic investigation of the fetal brain and the identification of CNS anomalies will be reviewed.

Normal sonographic anatomy of the fetal central nervous system

The fetal cerebrum undergoes major developmental changes throughout gestation. Fetal neurosonography demands a thorough knowledge of the ontogenesis of the brain. The interested reader is referred to specific publications on this subject.[2,3] Starting from 7 weeks' gestation, the primary cerebral vesicles can be identified with transvaginal sonography as fluid-filled areas. From 11 weeks' gestation, the brightly echogenic choroid plexuses filling the large lateral ventricles are the most prominent intracranial structures. In the second trimester, a detailed sonographic examination of the already well-developed cerebral structures allowing the detection of most anomalies is feasible. However, the results of an obstetric sonogram depend greatly upon the level of expertise of the sonographer and the time dedicated to the scan. In evaluating the fetal brain, a distinction must be made between a standard scan (frequently referred to as a level 1 scan) and an expert (or level 2) scan. The standard scan is fundamentally a screening examination for low-risk patients, and there is a general consensus that it is conveniently carried out with two axial views of the head, demonstrating the lateral ventricles, basal ganglia, and posterior fossa.[4] Measurement of the biparietal diameter, head circumference, internal diameter of the atrium and cisterna magna depth, and choroid plexuses is recommended.

A level 2 scan is a diagnostic examination, usually performed in a patient at increased risk of fetal anomalies, and may include coronal and sagittal views of the head that are more difficult to obtain, but have the advantage of delineating more clearly subtle details of intracranial anatomy, particularly by using a vaginal probe in vertex fetuses.[5] Three-dimensional ultrasound (Fig. 23.1) is a useful adjunct to the bidimensional examination in that it allows visualization of scanning planes that are difficult or impossible to obtain directly.[6]

Magnetic resonance of the fetal brain

Magnetic resonance imaging (MRI) has been used in obstetric patients for the diagnosis of fetal cerebral anomalies. The MRI procedure is not believed to be hazardous to the fetus, and the new equipment allows fast scanning at a reasonable level of resolution. In general, the anatomy is well depicted in fetuses older than 20 weeks' gestation. Compared with ultrasound, MRI allows a better discrimination between the cortex and the liquid spaces, and is particularly valuable in the assessment of migrational disorders, intracranial hemorrhage, and complex cerebral anomalies (Fig. 23.2). Furthermore, it is not influenced by fetal position, skull calcification, and oligohydramnios. There is a controversy in the current literature as to whether or not MRI provides valuable information to the sonographic examination when it is performed by an expert.[7–9] Nevertheless, the use of MRI in obstetric patients is becoming widespread. It should be stressed that, with current technology, this technique gives the best results only after fetal viability, when in most countries termination of pregnancy is no longer possible.

Ventriculomegaly

Enlargement of the lateral cerebral ventricles can be regarded as a specific marker of abnormal brain development, and is

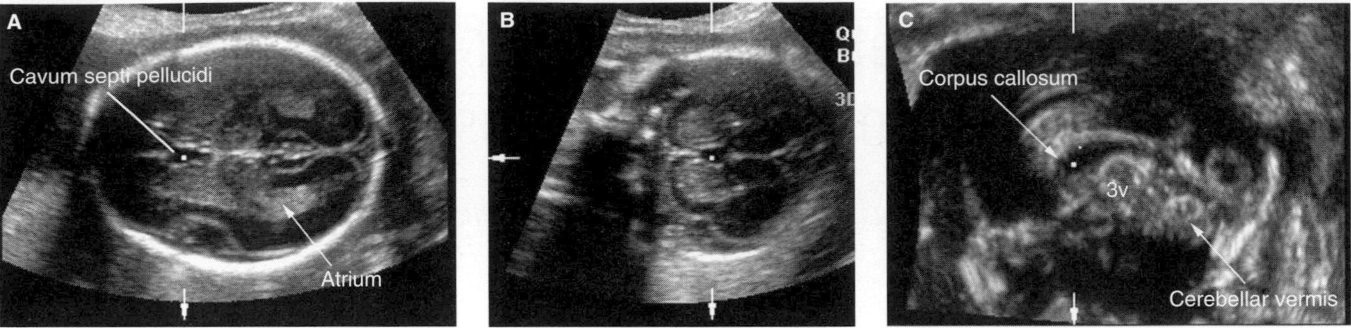

Figure 23.1 Multiplanar imaging of the fetal brain using three-dimensional sonography. The data volume has been obtained with the probe aligned along the axial plane (A). Two orthogonal sections have been reconstructed, simultaneously demonstrating the coronal (B) and midsagittal plane (C). The corpus callosum and cerebellar vermis are easily recognized. 3v, third ventricle.

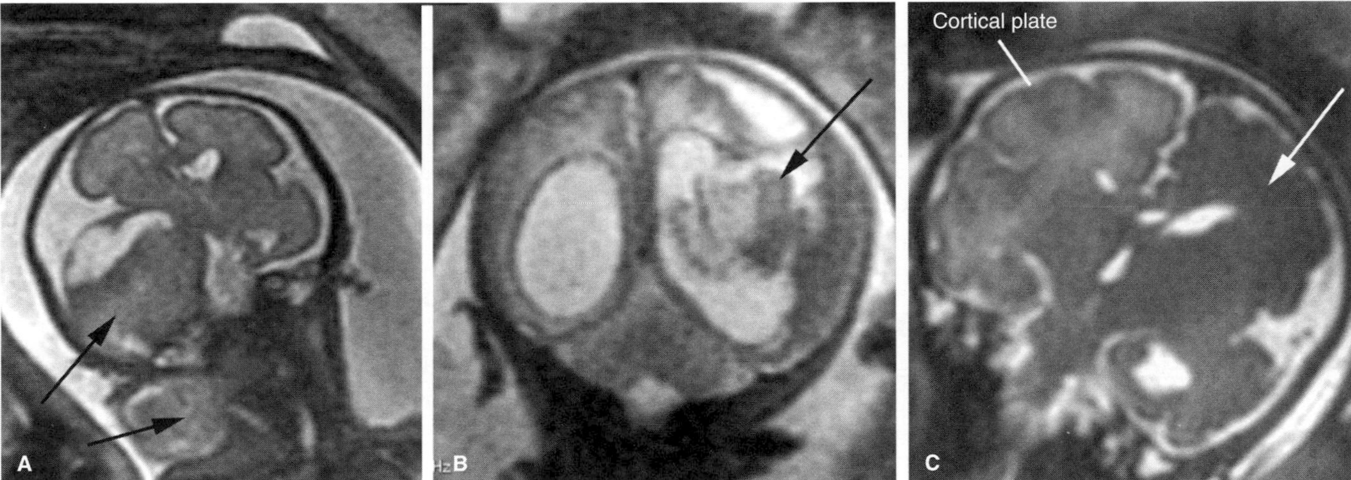

Figure 23.2 Magnetic resonance imaging of fetal cerebral anomalies. (A) Large teratoma with an intracranial and an extracranial component (arrows); (B) grade 4 intraventricular hemorrhage with destruction of the surrounding cortex (arrow); (C) unilateral megalencephaly: this anomaly is the consequence of a migrational abnormality affecting one hemisphere (arrow) that is overgrown, has abnormal convolutions, and lacks a well-developed cortical plate. Note the normally developed cortical plate in the ipsilateral hemisphere.

encountered with many different cerebral anomalies. Evaluation of the integrity of the cerebral lateral ventricles is therefore of particular importance while screening for fetal cerebral anomalies. Although many different approaches to the evaluation of the integrity of lateral ventricles have been proposed, measurement of the internal width of the atrium of the lateral ventricle at the level of the glomus of the choroid plexus is currently favored (Fig. 23.3). Under normal conditions, the measurement is less than 10mm, while a value of more than 15mm indicates severe ventriculomegaly, almost always associated with an intracranial malformation.[4,10,11] The outcome of these fetuses is variable and depends largely upon the underlying etiology of the ventricular dilatation. The available studies suggest that fetuses with isolated severe ventriculomegaly have an increased risk of perinatal death and a probability of severe neurologic sequelae in the range of 50% of

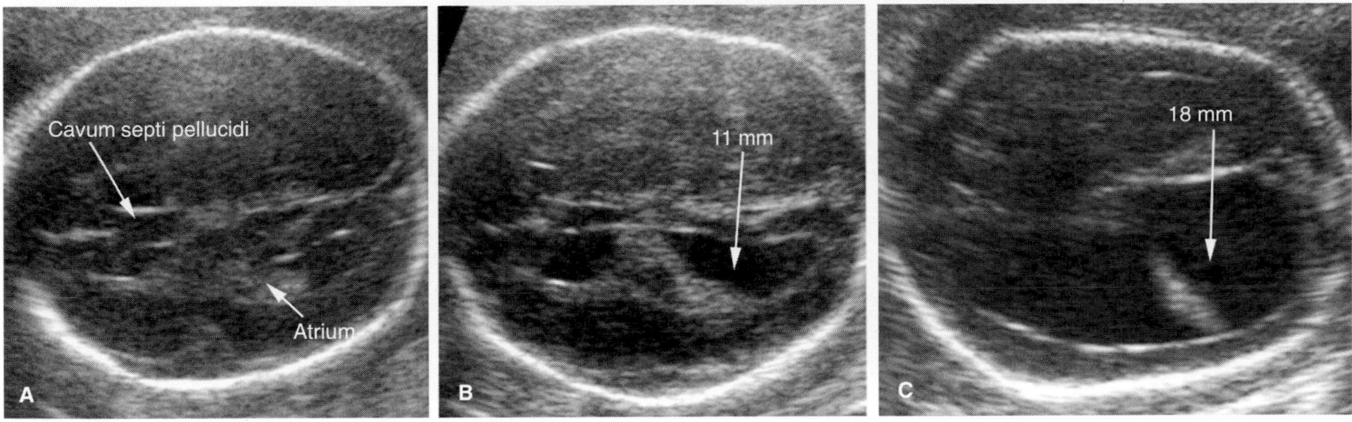

Figure 23.3 (A) Normal transventricular scan demonstrating an atrium of lateral ventricle of normal size; (B) mild ventriculomegaly; (C) severe ventriculomegaly.

survivors.[10] An intermediate value of the atrial width, 10–15 mm, is commonly referred to as mild ventriculomegaly and is associated with a much increased probability of cerebral and extracerebral malformations, aneuploidies, and infections, and therefore should be carefully evaluated in an expert center. Fetuses with isolated mild ventriculomegaly usually have a good outcome and, in most instances, the ventricles return to normal size during gestation. However, these infants run an increased risk of neurologic compromise and, in some cases, develop severe cerebral anomalies in the last part of gestation or after birth, including hydrocephalus, white matter injury, and cortical plate abnormalities. The risk is particularly increased when the atrial width is greater than 12 mm, when the dilation affects both lateral ventricles, and in females.[11]

Congenital hydrocephalus has genetic implications. It should be stressed that the experience thus far indicates that antenatal ultrasound is unreliable for predicting the recurrence of isolated ventriculomegaly, particularly of the X-linked variety, because in many cases enlargement of the lateral ventricles only develops late in gestation or after birth.[12] DNA analysis for the X-linked variety is now available and should be considered, although the exact sensitivity remains uncertain.[12–14]

When the diagnosis of severe ventriculomegaly is made prior to viability, many parents would probably request termination of pregnancy. In continuing pregnancies, no modifications of standard obstetric management are required. A Cesarean section is recommended only in those cases with associated macrocrania. Cephalocentesis to reduce cranial size is associated with significant morbidity, and is indicated only in cases with a presumption of a severe prognosis.

Neural tube defects

The average incidence of neural tube defects is 1–2 in 1000 births, with a peak of 7 in 1000 in South Wales. The multifactorial etiology of this anomaly is well established.

Anencephaly is characterized by the absence of the cranial vault and telencephalon. Necrotic remnants of the brain stem and rhomboencephalic structures are covered by a vascular membrane. Associated malformations are common and include spina bifida, cleft lip palate, clubfoot, and omphalocele. Polyhydramnios is frequently found. The diagnosis is easy in the midtrimester, and relies upon the demonstration of the absence of the cranial vault. Although the fetal head can be positively identified by vaginal sonography as early as the 7th week of gestation, the diagnosis may be difficult in the first trimester.[15] Anencephaly is considered to be the final stage of acrania, as a consequence of disruption of abnormal brain tissue unprotected by the calvarium.[16,17] A cephalic pole, albeit overtly abnormal, is therefore usually present in early gestation, and may be difficult to identify prior to 11 weeks' gestation (Fig. 23.4).

Spina bifida is commonly subdivided into open and closed forms.[18] Open spina bifida is predominant at birth and is a full-thickness defect of the skin, underlying soft tissues, and vertebral arches exposing the neural canal. The defect may be covered by a thin meningeal membrane (meningocele). In the presence of neural tissue inside the sac, the lesion is defined as a myelomeningocele, a term often used to indicate all cases of spina bifida aperta. The defect may vary considerably in size. The lumbar, thoracolumbar, or sacrolumbar areas are most frequently affected. Leakage of cerebrospinal fluid through the defect causes an increased concentration of alpha-fetoprotein (AFP) in the amniotic fluid and maternal serum.[19] Closed spina bifida is characterized by a vertebral schisis covered by skin. The skin is usually pigmented, dimpled, or presents areas of hypertrichosis. A subcutaneous mass, a meningocele, or lipoma may be present. Maternal serum and amniotic fluid AFP are usually within normal limits.

The diagnosis of open spina bifida is possible from midgestation, but it is often difficult and requires meticulous scanning (Fig. 23.5). The accuracy depends heavily on the experience of the operator, the quality of the equipment, and the amount

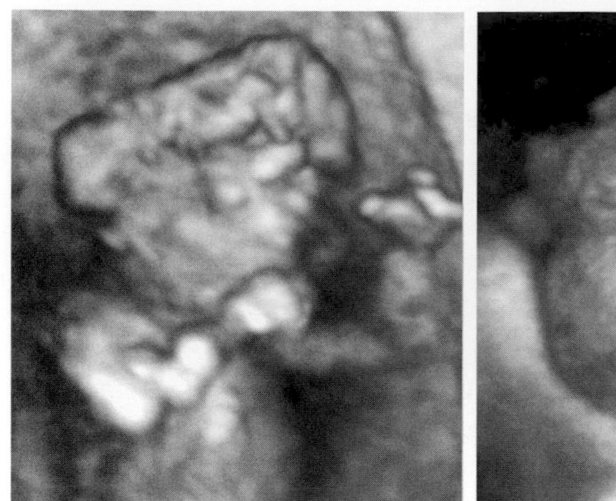
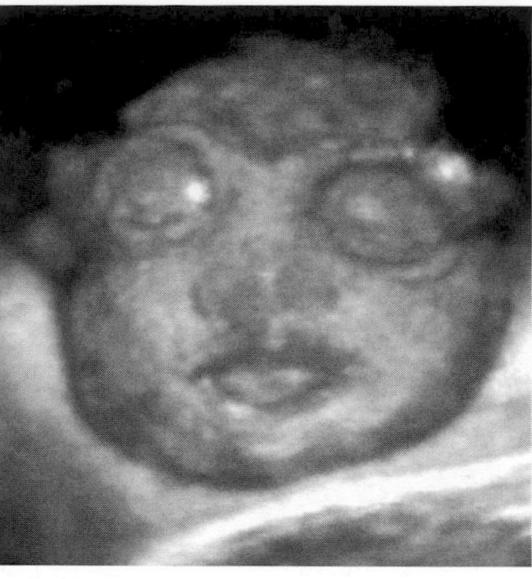

Figure 23.4 Three-dimensional ultrasound of anencephaly at different gestational ages: on the left, a 12-week-old fetus with an abnormal cephalic pole; on the right, absence of the cephalic pole in the third trimester (courtesy of Dr R. Ximenez, Sao Paulo, Brazil).

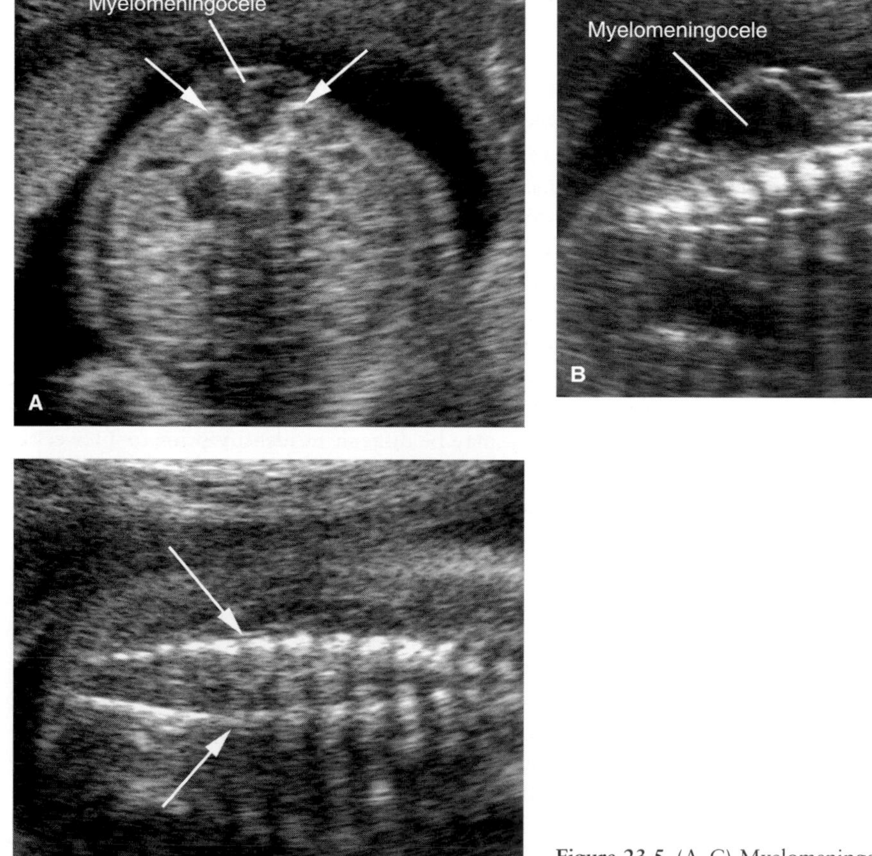

Figure 23.5 (A–C) Myelomeningocele in a midtrimester fetus.

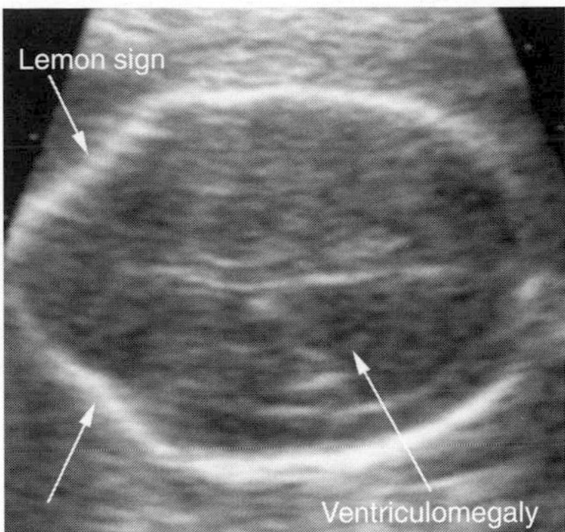

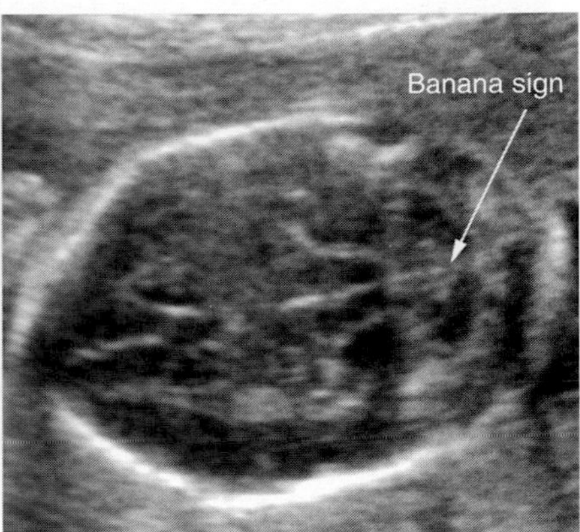

Figure 23.6 The cranial signs associated with open spina bifida.

of time dedicated to the scan. The accuracy of referral centers is close to 100%.[19–21] The accuracy of routine nontargeted examinations is uncertain. Examination of the fetal head can assist the sonologist, as open spina bifida is consistently associated with easily recognizable cranial lesions (Fig. 23.6). Leakage of cerebrospinal fluid leads to displacement of the cerebellar vermis, fourth ventricle, and medulla oblongata through the foramen magnum inside the upper cervical canal (Chiari type II or Arnold–Chiari malformation). Sonographically, this results in a small head measurement at midgestation, obliteration of the cisterna magna, small size and abnormal shape of the cerebellum that is impacted deep into the posterior fossa (banana sign), and frontal bossing (lemon sign).[22] Hydrocephalus of variable degrees is present in virtually all cases of spina bifida aperta at birth, but in less than 70% of cases in the midtrimester.

Closed spina bifida is associated with normal intracranial anatomy and normal AFP levels and is therefore usually unpredictable, with the possible exception of cases associated with large subcutaneous lesions.

Anencephaly is invariably fatal. The outcome for infants with open spina bifida is dictated by the site and extension of the lesion.[23] The mortality rate is high, the 7-year survival rate being only 40% despite early treatment. Many of the survivors will suffer from significant disabilities such as lower limb paralysis or dysfunction and incontinence. The association of spina bifida and severe hydrocephalus was traditionally considered a poor prognostic factor for intellectual development. More recent studies indicate that, in many cases, control of intracranial hypertension by shunting results in normal intelligence.

Recently, attempts have been made at intrauterine repair of spina bifida, and it has been suggested that these operations may reduce the morbidity of the affected infants.[24]

The outcome of closed spina bifida is difficult to predict *in utero*. These infants usually do not develop Arnold–Chiari malformation and hydrocephalus. However, particularly those with subcutaneous masses may suffer from neurologic sequelae of variable degrees.[18]

The term cephalocele indicates a protrusion of intracranial contents through a bony defect of the skull. In most cases, the lesion arises from the midline, in the occipital area, and less frequently from the parietal or frontal bones. Encephaloceles are characterized by the presence of brain tissue inside the lesion. When only meninges protrude, the term cranial meningocele should be used. Cephaloceles often cause impaired cerebrospinal fluid circulation and hydrocephalus. Massive encephaloceles may be associated with microcephaly.

Fetal cephaloceles should be suspected when a paracranial mass is seen on sonography. The diagnosis of encephaloceles is easy, as the presence of brain tissue inside the sac is striking on ultrasound. Differentiation of a cranial meningocele from soft tissue edema or a cystic hygroma of the neck may be difficult. Demonstration of the bony defect in the skull would allow a proper diagnosis, but cranial meningoceles are often associated with extremely small (a few millimeters) defects that are not amenable to antenatal sonographic recognition. Indirect clues can assist the diagnosis. Cranial cephaloceles are very often associated with ventriculomegaly. Cystic hygromas arise from the region of the neck, have multiple internal septations and a thick wall, and are often associated with generalized soft tissue edema and hydrops.

The pediatric literature suggests that the outcome of cephaloceles is mainly related to the presence or absence of brain tissue inside the lesion. However, the largest available antenatal series reports a dismal prognosis for both varieties.[25,26]

Midline anomalies

Midline cerebral anomalies include a group of brain defects that encompass a wide spectrum of severity and are typically associated with craniofacial malformations (Fig. 23.7).

The holoprosencephalies are complex abnormalities of the forebrain that share in common an incomplete separation of the cerebral hemispheres and formation of diencephalic structures.[27] The most widely accepted classification of these

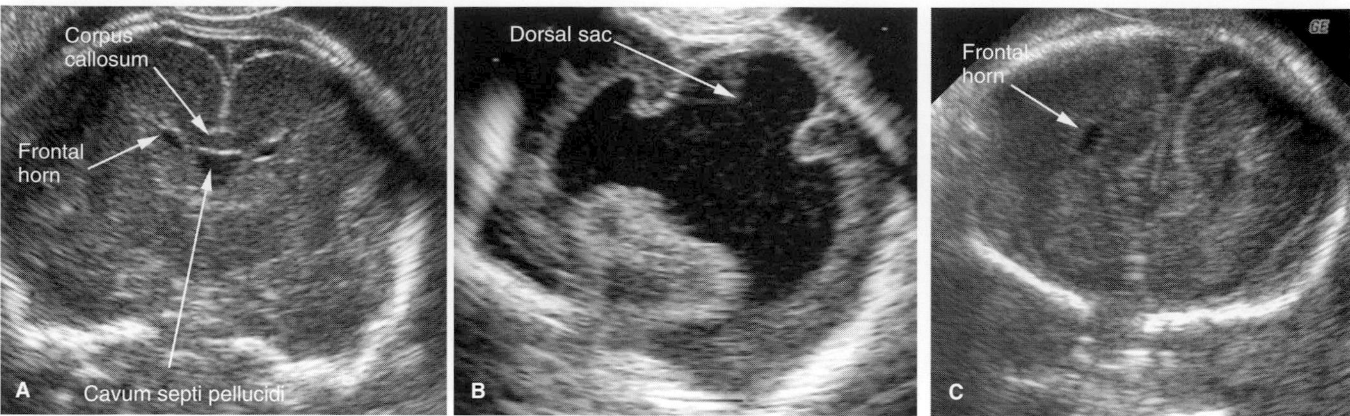

Figure 23.7 (A) Normal coronal scan at mid-gestation; (B) alobar holoprosencephaly; (C) complete agenesis of corpus callosum.

disorders recognizes three major varieties: the alobar, semilobar, and lobar types. In the alobar variety, the most pronounced one, the interhemispheric fissure and the falx cerebrii are totally absent, there is a single primitive ventricle (holoventricle), the thalami are fused on the midline, and there is absence of the third ventricle, neurohypophysis, olfactory bulbs and tracts. In semilobar holoprosencephaly, the two cerebral hemispheres are partially separated posteriorly, but there is still a single ventricular cavity. In both alobar and semilobar forms, the roof of the ventricular cavity, the thela choroidea, normally enfolded within the brain, may balloon out between the cerebral convexity and the skull to form a cyst of variable size – the dorsal sac. Alobar and semilobar holoprosencephaly are often associated with microcephaly, and less frequently with macrocephaly, which is invariably due to internal obstructive hydrocephalus. In the lobar variety, the interhemispheric fissure is well developed posteriorly and anteriorly, but there is still a variable degree of fusion of the cyngulate gyrus and of the lateral ventricles, and absence of the septum pellucidum. The facial anomalies are pleomorphic, but can be regarded as the consequence of hypoplasia of the midfacial structures. They span between cyclopia and severe hypotelorism with median cleft lip–palate. The nose can be absent, replaced by a proboscis or extremely flattened.

The incidence of holoprosencephaly at birth is uncertain. This anomaly was, however, found in 1 of 250 voluntary terminations of pregnancy.[28] This observation suggests a high intrauterine fatality rate. The etiology is heterogeneous. In most cases, the anomaly is isolated and sporadic. In other cases, chromosomal abnormalities (trisomy 13 and polyploidy), and/or anatomic abnormalities are found.

Prenatal diagnosis of alobar holoprosencephaly depends upon the demonstration of a single rudimentary cerebral ventricle.[27] Additional findings include the presence of typical facial anomalies.[29,30] Similar findings are expected with the semilobar type. Recognition of the lobar variety has also been reported. Diagnosis requires a midcoronal scan, demonstrating absence of the cavum septum pellucidum and central fusion of the frontal horns, which have a flat squared roof and communicate amply with the inferior third ventricle.[27,31] The presence of the fused fornices, which appear as a linear structure running within the third ventricle from the anterior to the posterior commissure, is a frequent and very specific finding with this condition.[32] As in lobar holoprosencephaly, the interhemispheric fissure is shallow anteriorly as a result of the fusion of the frontal lobes; the branches of the anterior cerebral artery run along the surface of the brain giving rise on color Doppler to a typical sign that has been referred to as the serpent crawling under the skull.[33]

The invariably poor prognosis for infants affected by alobar and semilobar holoprosencephaly is well established. Thus far, cases diagnosed *in utero* have had extremely poor neurologic development.[31]

Agenesis of the corpus callosum (ACC) is an anomaly of uncertain prevalence and clinical significance. Estimates of 0.3–0.7% in the general population and 2–3% in the developmentally disabled are usually quoted.[34] The etiology is heterogeneous. Genetic factors are probably predominant. The high frequency of associated malformations and chromosomal aberrations suggest that ACC is often part of a widespread developmental disturbance.

ACC may be either complete or partial. In the latter case, also referred to as dysgenesis of the corpus callosum, the caudad portion (splenium and body) is missing to varying degrees.

The diagnosis of ACC is possible from mid-gestation, but is a challenge even for expert sonologists.[34] In routine examinations, an increased atrial width with a "tear-drop configuration" of the lateral ventricles and/or failure to visualize the cavum septum pellucidum (which is always absent with complete ACC) should alert to the possibility of fetal ACC.

Once a suspicion has been formulated, a direct diagnosis is possible by demonstrating the absence of the corpus callosum by coronal and sagittal scans. These views are at times difficult to obtain, in particular in vertex fetuses. However, vaginal sonography is of great advantage in such cases. Abnormal branching of the anterior cerebral artery can also be demonstrated with the use of color Doppler ultrasound.[34]

Diagnosis of partial ACC has also been reported, but the sonographic findings are even more elusive than with the complete form.[34]

The outcome of ACC is mainly dictated by the associated anomalies. Isolated ACC is associated with a normal to borderline intellectual development in most cases.[35] However, long-term studies indicate a progressive decrease in intellectual capacity over time, and most infants tend to have significant difficulties at school.[36] ACC has also been linked to psychosis.[37]

The term Dandy–Walker syndrome was originally introduced to indicate the association of: (1) ventriculomegaly of variable degree; (2) a large cisterna magna; and (3) a defect in the cerebellar vermis through which the cyst communicates with the fourth ventricle. At present, the term Dandy–Walker complex (or continuum) is used to indicate a spectrum of anomalies of the posterior fossa that share in common a cystic posterior fossa and/or hypoplasia of the cerebellar vermis.[38]

The classic type of Dandy–Walker malformation has an estimated incidence of about 1:30 000 births, and is found in 4–12% of all cases of infantile hydrocephalus. The frequency of minor variants of this condition is unknown.

Dandy–Walker malformation is frequently associated with other neural defects, mostly with other midline anomalies, such as ACC and holoprosencephaly. Other deformities include encephaloceles, polycystic kidneys, cardiovascular defects, and facial clefting. Postnatal studies indicate a frequency of associated malformations ranging between 50% and 70%.[38,39]

The sonographic landmark of the Dandy–Walker complex is an enlarged cisterna magna (by common definition, a depth greater than 10 mm),[40,41] usually associated with a midline cleft of the vermis (Fig. 23.8). The classic type of Dandy–Walker malformation is associated with a large cisterna magna and severe ventriculomegaly, and tends to have a poor prognosis. However, minor variations are encountered more frequently.[38,42,43] The clinical significance of these findings is uncertain, and no clear-cut prognostic data exist. Recent neuropediatric series suggest an association between the size of the cerebellar vermis and intellectual development.[39] Under normal conditions, it is usually possible with either sonography or MRI to obtain a midsagittal view of the fetal cerebellar vermis demonstrating the fastigium of the fourth ventricle and the two main fissures from about mid-gestation.[39] With hypoplasia of the vermis, these landmarks cannot be identified. Nomograms of the normal size of the vermis throughout gestation are also available[44] (Fig. 23.9).

Caution is warranted while making the diagnosis of a minor variety of the Dandy–Walker continuum. Development of the cerebellar vermis is incomplete prior to 20 weeks' gestation, and this frequently creates an artifact mimicking a vermian defect.[45]

When the classic form of Dandy–Walker malformation is found prior to viability, pregnancy termination can be offered to the parents. In continuing pregnancies, no modification of standard obstetric management exists. Cesarean delivery is indicated only if macrocrania is present. A careful search for associated malformations is indicated when the cisterna magna is greater than 10 mm or there is the impression of a vermian defect after 20 weeks.[40,43]

As the diagnosis of midline anomalies depends mostly upon scans of sagittal and coronal planes of the fetal head that are sometimes difficult to obtain, we have found that three-dimensional ultrasound is frequently of considerable help. Multiplanar slicing of a volume obtained from axial scans usually provides images of diagnostic quality (Fig. 23.10).

Destructive cerebral lesions

Many congenital anomalies of the brain are not the consequence of an embryogenetic malformative process, but are due to a destructive process. The pathophysiology is frequently

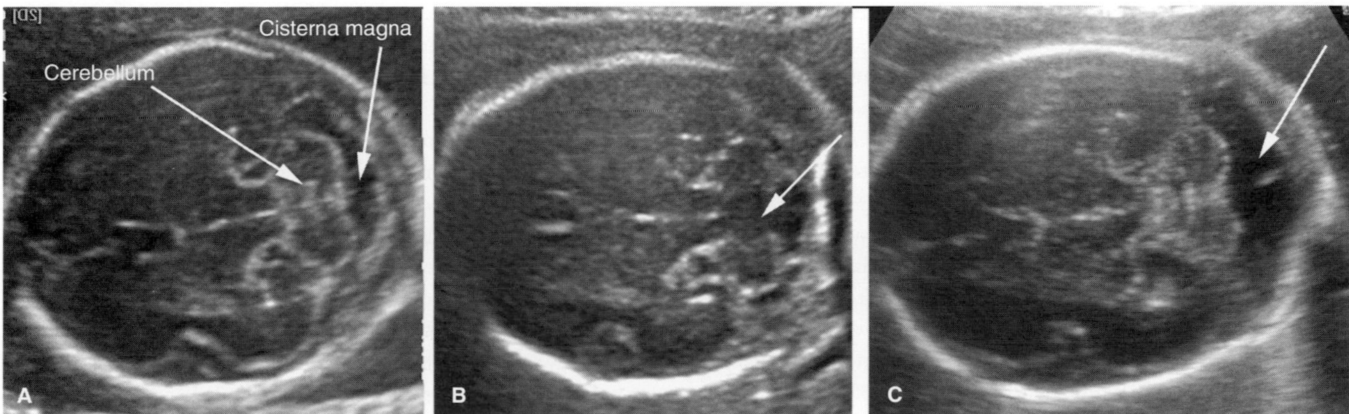

Figure 23.8 The normal transcerebellar scan (A) compared with variations of the Dandy–Walker continuum; (B) a cerebellar "cleft" (arrow) suggesting a vermian defect; (C) an enlarged cisterna magna (arrow) with a seemingly normal vermis.

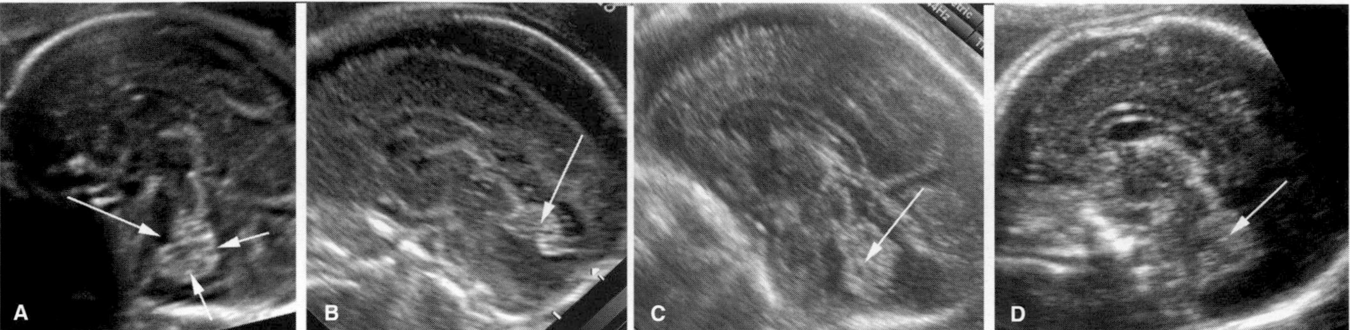

Figure 23.9 The normal midsagittal view (A) demonstrating the main landmarks of the cerebellar vermis (fastigium of fourth ventricle and the two main scissures) (arrows) is compared with variations of the Dandy–Walker continuum: (B) upward rotation of a hypoplastic vermis; (C) upward rotation of a seemingly intact vermis; (D) enlargement of the cisterna magna with an intact vermis (megacisterna magna). Although the outcome cannot be clearly predicted, a hypoplastic vermis (B) is a poor prognostic factor, while the upward rotation of a seemingly intact vermis and a megacisterna magna (C and D), when isolated, may be asymptomatic.

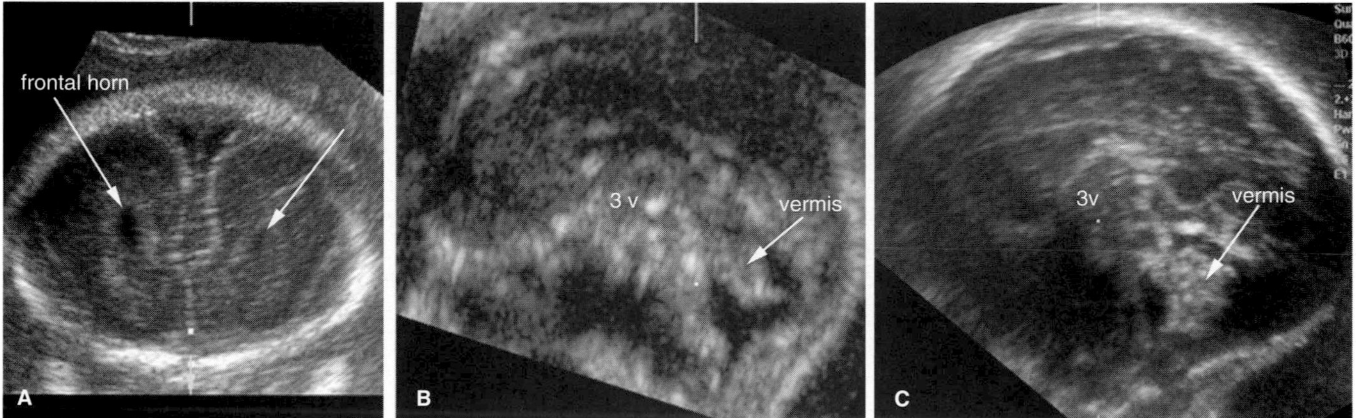

Figure 23.10 Multiplanar imaging of the fetal brain using three-dimensional ultrasound. (A) Complete agenesis of the corpus callosum; (B) upward rotation of a hypoplastic cerebellar vermis; (C) upward rotation of an intact vermis. The images are of comparable quality to those obtained with direct bidimensional scanning (compare with Figs 23.7C, 23.9B, and 23.9D respectively). 3v, third ventricle.

unclear, and the conditions remain idiopathic. A link with obstetric complications of a different nature is however frequently found.[46–48]

Intracranial hemorrhage (ICH) is usually found at the level of the lateral ventricles, although it can occur in other anatomical locations. It is a frequent complication in premature infants. Although rarely, it may occur antenatally, as a consequence of coagulopathy or trauma, or other as yet unexplained factors.[46] The sonographic appearance of an ICH is extremely variable depending upon the severity and the time since it occurred (Fig. 23.11). Blood accumulated into the ventricles appears as an echogenic collection. With time, the blood clot retracts, demonstrates an anechoic core, and is frequently associated with ventricular dilation (grade 3 hemorrhage). Large hemorrhagic collections may be complicated by infarct and destruction of the surrounding white matter (grade 4 hemorrhage).

The prognosis is severe. In a review of the literature,[46] perinatal death occurred in about 50% of cases, and 50% of survivors had neurologic compromise at long-term follow-up. There was a correlation between the outcome and the grade of the hemorrhage. The prognosis was more favorable with grade 1 and 2 hemorrhages (hemorrhage limited to the germinal matrix or lateral ventricles without ventriculomegaly), which at times may even resolve *in utero*, and was usually severe with grade 3 and 4 lesions (intraventricular hemorrhage associated with severe ventriculomegaly and white matter destruction respectively).

Congenital porencephaly is defined as the presence of cystic cavities within the brain matter (Fig. 23.12). The cavities usually communicate with the ventricular system, the subarachnoid space, or both. Loss of cerebral tissue may derive from a morphogenetic disorder (true porencephaly or schizencephaly). More frequently, it is the consequence of an

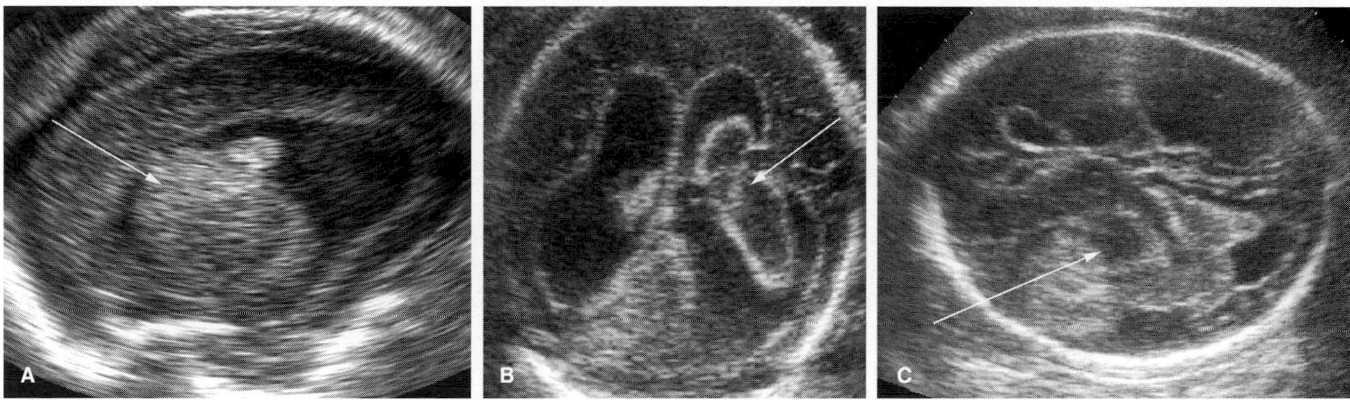

Figure 23.11 Types of intracranial hemorrhage. (A) Soon after the hemorrhage, the blood is intensely echogenic (arrow); this is a grade 2 hemorrhage. (B) An old hemorrhage (arrow); the coronal scan demonstrates a typical blood clot and ventricular enlargement (grade 3 hemorrhage). (C) Hemorrhage (arrow) associated with destruction of the cortex (grade 4 hemorrhage).

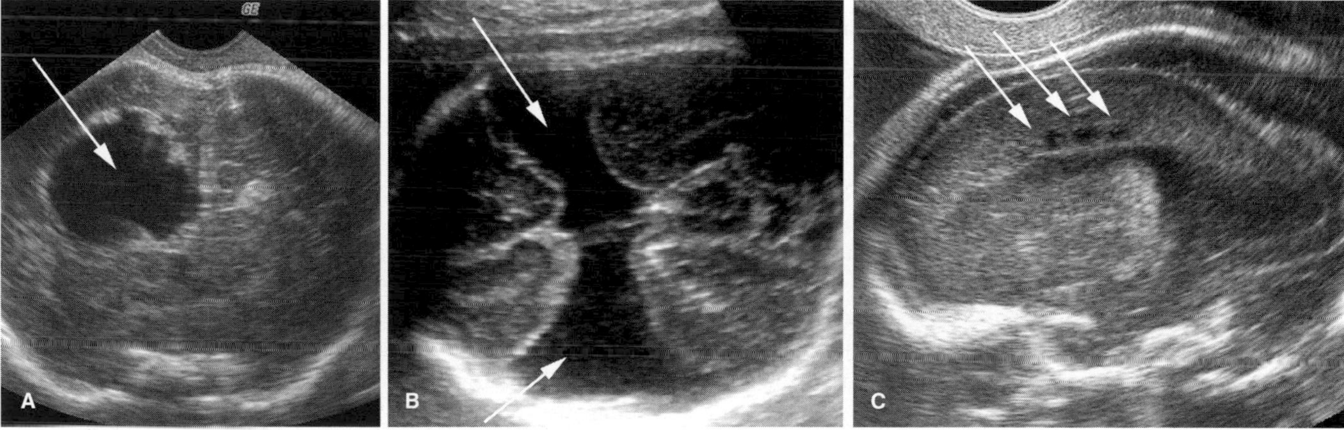

Figure 23.12 Destructive lesions of the fetal brain: (A) porencephalic cyst (arrow); (B) schizencephaly (arrows); (C) periventricular leukomalacia (arrows).

intrauterine disruption (pseudoporencephaly or encephaloclastic porencephaly). The developmental form is typically bilateral and symmetrical, and is frequently associated with microcephaly. In pseudoporencephaly, a unilateral lesion is usually found. In both cases, there is wide variability in the size of the lesion. Cerebrospinal fluid turnover is often impaired, and hydrocephalus is present. Hydranencephaly can be regarded as an extreme form of pseudoporencephaly. Most of the cerebral hemispheres are replaced by fluid. The brain stem and rhomboencephalic structures are usually spared. The head may be small, of normal size, or extremely enlarged. The etiology is heterogeneous. Congenital infections, including toxoplasmosis and cytomegalovirus, and intrauterine strangulation or occlusion of the internal carotid arteries have been reported. Accurate antenatal diagnosis of both schizencephaly and porencephaly has been reported.[49] It should be stressed, however, that porencephaly is a disruption that usually occurs only in the third trimester.

The outcome of infants with congenital destructive process of the brain is dictated by the size and location of the lesion. Extensive porencephaly, particularly if associated with hydrocephalus or microcephaly, and hydranencephaly have a uniformly poor outcome.

Periventricular leukomalacia is a degenerative disorder of the white matter that is most frequently encountered in premature infants and is frequently associated with a severe prognosis. The cystic variety of this condition has been described recently in the fetus.[48] The diagnosis is made by demonstrating multiple small cysts close to the upper corner of the lateral ventricles (Fig. 23.12).

Disorders of nerve cell proliferation

The association between decreased head size and reduction in both brain mass and total cell number in microcephalic infants is well established. However, the threshold of abnormality is uncertain. Some authors suggest employing a head circumference below –2 standard deviations from the mean as the diagnostic criterion. Others prefer to consider head circumference below –3 standard deviations as abnormal. The incidence of microcephaly obviously varies in different surveys, depending upon the definition used to identify the lesion.

Microcephaly should not be considered as a single clinical entity, but rather as a symptom of many etiologic disturbances, including both environmental and genetic factors. Microcephaly features a typical disproportion in size between the skull and the face. The forehead is sloping. The brain is small, with the cerebral hemispheres affected to a greater extent than the diencephalic and rhomboencephalic structures. Abnormal convolutional patterns, including macrogyria, microgyria, and agyria, are frequently found. The ventricles may be enlarged. Microcephaly is frequently found in cases of porencephaly, lissencephaly, and holoprosencephaly.

Many difficulties arise in attempting to identify fetal microcephaly.[50] The utility of head measurements alone may be hampered by incorrect dating or intrauterine growth retardation. Furthermore, the natural history of fetal microcephaly is largely unknown. A progressive development of the lesion interfering with early recognition has been described. A comparison of biometric parameters such as the head circumference:abdominal circumference ratio and the femur length:biparietal diameter ratio has been suggested. Nevertheless, both false-positive and false-negative diagnoses occur frequently. It is clear that the predictive value of ultrasound biometry has significant limitations. A qualitative evaluation of the intracranial structures is a very useful adjunct to biometry because many cases of microcephaly are associated with morphologic derangement, particularly with ventriculomegaly, schizencephaly, and disorders of ventral induction. Demonstration of a sloping forehead also increases the index of suspicion.[51]

The final outcome of microcephaly is uncertain. Infants with small heads have a much increased risk of neurologic compromise, and this correlates with head size. When the head circumference is extremely small, 4 standard deviations or more below the mean, and/or there are associated abnormalities, the prognosis tends to be severe.

Megalencephaly, that is, an abnormally large brain, is usually found in individuals of normal and even superior intelligence, but it may be associated with mental retardation and neurologic impairment.[52] Megalencephaly is also part of congenital anomalies and syndromes such as Beckwith–Wiedemann syndrome, achondroplasia, neurofibromatosis, and tuberous sclerosis. Obstetric and pediatric sonographers are frequently challenged by the problem of megalencephaly, a condition that should be suspected in the presence of abnormally large head measurements without evidence of hydrocephalus or intracranial masses. In such cases, examination of the parents may be of help, as asymptomatic megalencephaly is frequently familial.

Anomalies of neuronal migration

The neuronal cells that form the gray matter originate internally to the brain, on the surface of the lateral ventricles, and only later migrate along radially aligned glial cells to the surface of the brain. The migration occurs in different waves that last for several weeks. Most of the process takes place between 8 weeks' and 16 weeks' gestation, but continues up to 25 weeks. Once the neuronal cells have reached their destination on the surface of the brain, they undergo a process of maturation and differentiation, grow axons and dendrites, and develop synapses with other neurons, giving rise to a well-ordered, six-layer cortex. Migrational abnormalities are characterized by the incomplete formation of the cortical layers, with abnormal locations of neurons that have failed to reach their final destination. In general, the cortex is thickened by a large, disorganized layer of neurons. Conversely, the white matter underneath the cortex is thinned by failure in production of axons by the disorganized neuronal cells. Macroscopically, the main finding is an alteration in the convolutional pattern of the brain, which may be associated with modifications in brain mass and the size of the ventricles.

Failure of neuronal migration includes a broad spectrum of anomalies: absence to severe reduction of convolutions (lissencephaly), increased number of small convolutions (polymicrogyria), unilateral megalencephaly, schizencephaly, and gray matter heterotopias. The migrational process may be arrested by environmental factors (ischemia, teratogens), but a genetic predisposition is clearly present at least for some anomalies.

Postnatally, the technique of choice for the diagnosis of this condition is MRI, which allows a clear discrimination between white and gray matter. Sonographic detection of typical macroscopic abnormalities of brain anatomy (clefts in the cortex, gyral anomalies, etc.) has led to the diagnosis of these conditions antenatally, although usually only in late gestation[8,53,54] (Fig. 23.2).

Choroid plexus cysts

Choroid plexus cysts are sonolucent spaces within the choroid plexus, with well-defined walls. The cysts may be unilateral or bilateral and are occasionally multiple. They are typically found at the level of the atrium of lateral ventricles, and less frequently within the bodies. When examined with high-resolution ultrasound equipment, the choroid plexus of the lateral ventricle often appears slightly dishomogeneous. A choroid plexus cyst should measure at least 2 mm in diameter. Large cysts up to 14 mm may be seen, and usually contain internal sediments.

Fetal choroid plexus cysts are benign findings that are however associated with an increased likelihood of trisomy

18.[55,56] The available data do not indicate an association with other chromosomal aberrations, including trisomy 21.[57,58] In 80–90% of fetuses with trisomy 18, anatomic deformities will be detected by ultrasound.[59] On the basis of these data, a prudent approach is to perform a thorough sonographic examination of the fetus when a choroid plexus cyst is identified. This examination should include evaluation of the hands, feet, and heart. If an additional ultrasound abnormality is identified, chromosomal analysis should be offered to the patient. Otherwise, the patient may be counseled with the figures suggested by Snijders and co-workers,[58] that is, that the risk of trisomy 18 is increased 1.5 times over the baseline.

Isolated choroid plexus cysts do not modify standard obstetrical management. As no deleterious effect on the fetus has been reported with this finding thus far, there is no need in our opinion for follow-up scans. A handful of very large cysts of the choroid plexuses causing intracranial hypertension has been described in the neurosurgical literature, but these probably represent a separate clinical entity.[60]

Conclusions

Modern ultrasound equipment yields a unique potential for the evaluation of the normal and abnormal fetal CNS. A large number of congenital anomalies can be consistently recognized. Transvaginal sonography is extending antenatal diagnosis to very early gestation.[61–63] MRI can be used to improve the accuracy of the diagnosis in selected cases.

Nevertheless, it is important to stress that development of the brain continues throughout gestation and that a significant number of anomalies cannot be predicted even by an expert examiner at mid-gestation. In a recent study, 17% of fetal cerebral abnormalities could not be diagnosed prior to viability.[64] Furthermore, when an anomaly is identified, counseling the parents and deciding on a sensible obstetric management is frequently difficult. Some cerebral anomalies have outcomes that can be predicted with reasonable precision. This is certainly the case with catastrophic lesions such as anencephaly and severe holoprosencephaly, as well as with anomalies that are invariably detected at birth, such as spina bifida. There are, however, a large number of conditions that can be accurately identified *in utero* and yet have an unclear natural history. ACC, mild ventriculomegaly, and minor variations of the Dandy–Walker continuum are remarkable examples in this regard. It has to be appreciated that, at present, there is quite a dramatic discrepancy between the diagnostic capability of antenatal ultrasound (which is potentially very high) and our understanding of the prognostic implications of anatomic alterations (which is limited by many points of view).

Eventually, the diagnosis of acquired brain lesions owing to hemorrhagic or ischemic causes will be possible, and it is likely to become part of the management of selected high-risk pregnancies.[46–48]

Key points

1 The incidence of central nervous system malformations is in the range of 1:100 births.

2 Ultrasound allows the diagnosis of many malformations from mid-gestation; the results of the examination depend partly upon the expertise of the sonologist and the time dedicated to the examination; a standard sonogram is performed in low-risk patients by the use of two scanning planes demonstrating the lateral ventricles and posterior fossa; an expert sonogram is performed by using other scanning planes oriented along the sutures and fontanelles of the fetal head that allow the identification of other details; the use of three-dimensional ultrasound facilitates the examination.

3 Some cerebral malformations may not be detected antenatally by ultrasound, particularly in early gestation.

4 Magnetic resonance is frequently used in fetuses at high risk of cerebral malformations, particularly to assess hemorrhage, abnormalities of cortical development, and complex cerebral anomalies.

5 Under normal conditions, the internal diameter of the atrium of the lateral ventricles is less than 10 mm; a value of 10 mm greatly increases the likelihood of a cerebral anomaly.

6 An atrial diameter of more than 15 mm is usually associated with an intracranial malformation.

7 An atrial diameter of 10–15 mm, a condition usually referred to as mild ventriculomegaly, may represent a normal variant, but greatly increases the likelihood of cerebral anomalies and extracerebral anomalies, chromosomal aberrations, and abnormal neurodevelopment.

8 Anencephaly is easily diagnosed sonographically at mid-gestation and may be identified as early as 12 weeks' gestation.

9 Spina bifida is one of the most frequent anomalies of the central nervous system; the most severe type, the open variety, can be identified sonographically by mid-gestation, although the diagnosis is at times difficult; obstetric patients usually undergo screening by assay of maternal serum alpha-fetoprotein; the

sonographic diagnosis is assisted by the demonstration of typical cranial alterations, the lemon and banana signs, that are usually easier to identify than the spinal defect.

10 Closed spina bifida is usually unpredictable sonographically.

11 The most severe varieties of holoprosencephaly, the alobar and semilobar forms, are usually recognized by mid-gestation by the demonstration of the absence of the midline echo and the presence of a single rudimentary ventricular cavity.

12 The less severe variety of holoprosencephaly is more difficult to identify and diagnose; the main clue is the absence of the cavum septi pellucidi and the central fusion of the frontal horns.

13 Agenesis of the corpus callosum may be one of the most frequent congenital anomalies; in a standard examination, it may be suspected by indirect findings, such as mild ventriculomegaly and/or the absence of the cavum septi pellucidi; a specific sonographic diagnosis is possible but requires an expert examination; agenesis of the corpus callosum is an important risk factor for mental retardation; infants with isolated agenesis of the corpus callosum may have a normal, albeit frequently low, intellect.

14 The term Dandy–Walker complex is used to define cases in which the cisterna magna is large (more than 10 mm) and/or there is hypoplasia of the cerebellar vermis; many variations exist, and the prognosis is difficult to predict.

15 Many congenital anomalies of the cerebrum are not the consequence of an embryogenetic malformative process but are due to a destructive antenatal event, usually hemorrhagic or ischemic; fetal intracranial hemorrhage may be recognized by sonography, but the findings vary depending upon the time the lesion has occurred and the severity of the hemorrhage; most intracranial bleeding occurs at the level of the ventricles; a recent hemorrhage appears as an echogenic collection that may be associated with ventricular enlargement; in the weeks following the hemorrhage, the blood clot retracts and develops a sonolucent core; severe forms of intraventricular hemorrhage (those associated with either hydrocephalus and/or destruction of the nearby cortex) are associated with an excess of perinatal deaths and neurologic compromise.

16 Destructive insults of the brain result in cystic cavities (porencephaly) of the cortex; cystic degeneration of the white matter (periventricular leukomalacia) has also been described in the fetus; in some cases, these lesions are the consequence of obstetric complications such as intrauterine hypoxia/ischemia, infections, or congenital coagulopathy.

17 Microcephaly is associated with an increased risk of neurologic compromise; the fetal head can be effectively measured with sonography, but the diagnosis of microcephaly is hampered by an overlap with normal variations (there is no clear quantitative threshold) and particularly by intrauterine progressive development, which occurs in many cases; when the head is small, a specific antenatal diagnosis may be difficult; as microcephaly is associated with intracranial abnormalities in many cases, a careful inspection of cerebral anatomy may be helpful.

18 Disorders of neuronal migration include a wide spectrum of disorders characterized by abnormal sulcation of the brain; they may be diagnosed sonographically and/or with magnetic resonance, but usually only in late gestation.

19 Choroid plexus cysts are small fluid collections within the choroid plexus of lateral ventricles; they are identified in 1% or more of fetuses at mid-gestation, and are transient and benign findings that however increase the risk of trisomy 18; as most cases of trisomy 18 are associated with anomalies that are readily identified with sonography, there is a general consensus that a careful inspection of fetal anatomy is indicated; amniocentesis may not be necessary.

20 Any time that a sonographic examination is performed in the second or third trimester, a survey of intracranial anatomy should be performed; the sensitivity of antenatal sonography remains uncertain; certainly, many even severe anomalies are associated with subtle antenatal findings or become manifest only in late gestation and therefore escape antenatal detection.

References

1 Myrianthopoulos NC. Epidemiology of central nervous system malformations. In: Vinken PJ, Bruyn GW, eds. *Handbook of clinical neurology*. Amsterdam: Elsevier; 1977:139–171.

2 Blaas HG, Eik-Nes SH, Kiserud T, Hellevik LR. Early development of the hindbrain: a longitudinal ultrasound study from 7 to 12 weeks of gestation. *Ultrasound Obstet Gynecol* 1995;5(3):151–160.

3 Blaas HG, Eik-Nes SH, Kiserud T, et al. Three-dimensional imaging of the brain cavities in human embryos. *Ultrasound Obstet Gynecol* 1995;5(4):228–232.

4 Filly RA, Cardoza JD, Goldstein RB, Barkovich AJ. Detection of fetal central nervous system anomalies: a practical level of effort for a routine sonogram. *Radiology* 1989;172(2):403–408.

5 Timor-Tritsch IE, Monteagudo A. Transvaginal fetal neurosonography: standardization of the planes and sections by anatomic landmarks. *Ultrasound Obstet Gynecol* 1996;8(1):42–47.

6 Timor-Tritsch IE, Monteagudo A, Mayberry P. Three-dimensional ultrasound evaluation of the fetal brain: the three horn view. *Ultrasound Obstet Gynecol* 2000;16(4):302–306.

7 Malinger G, Lev D, Lerman-Sagie T. Is fetal magnetic resonance imaging superior to neurosonography for detection of brain anomalies? *Ultrasound Obstet Gynecol* 2002;20(4):317–321.

8 Malinger G, Ben-Sira L, Lev D, et al. Fetal brain imaging: a comparison between magnetic resonance imaging and dedicated neurosonography. *Ultrasound Obstet Gynecol* 2004;23(4):333–340.

9 Timor-Tritsch IE, Monteagudo A. Magnetic resonance imaging versus ultrasound for fetal central nervous system abnormalities. *Am J Obstet Gynecol* 2003;189(4):1210–1211; author reply 1211–122.

10 Gupta JK, Bryce FC, Lilford RJ. Management of apparently isolated fetal ventriculomegaly. *Obstet Gynecol Surv* 1994;49(10): 716–721.

11 Pilu G, Falco P, Gabrielli S, et al. The clinical significance of fetal isolated cerebral borderline ventriculomegaly: report of 31 cases and review of the literature. *Ultrasound Obstet Gynecol* 1999; 14(5):320–326.

12 Serville F, Benit P, Saugier P, et al. Prenatal exclusion of X-linked hydrocephalus-stenosis of the aqueduct of Sylvius sequence using closely linked DNA markers. *Prenat Diagn* 1993;13(6):435–439.

13 Rogers JG, Danks DM. Prenatal diagnosis of sex-linked hydrocephalus. *Prenat Diagn* 1983;3(3):269.

14 Lyonnet S, Pelet A, Royer G, et al. The gene for X-linked hydrocephalus maps to Xq28, distal to DXS52. *Genomics* 1992;14(2): 508–510.

15 Johnson SP, Sebire NJ, Snijders RJ, et al. Ultrasound screening for anencephaly at 10–14 weeks of gestation. *Ultrasound Obstet Gynecol* 1997;9(1):14–16.

16 Bronshtein M, Ornoy A. Acrania: anencephaly resulting from secondary degeneration of a closed neural tube: two cases in the same family. *J Clin Ultrasound* 1991;19(4):230–234.

17 Timor-Tritsch IE, Greenebaum E, Monteagudo A, Baxi L. Exencephaly–anencephaly sequence: proof by ultrasound imaging and amniotic fluid cytology. *J Matern Fetal Med* 1996;5(4):182–185.

18 Tortori-Donati P, Rossi A, Cama A. Spinal dysraphism: a review of neuroradiological features with embryological correlations and proposal for a new classification. *Neuroradiology* 2000;42(7): 471–491.

19 Filly RA, Callen PW, Goldstein RB. Alpha-fetoprotein screening programs: what every obstetric sonologist should know. *Radiology* 1993;188(1):1–9.

20 Platt LD, Feuchtbaum L, Filly R, et al. The California Maternal Serum alpha-Fetoprotein Screening Program: the role of ultrasonography in the detection of spina bifida. *Am J Obstet Gynecol* 1992;166(5):1328–1329.

21 Watson WJ, Chescheir NC, Katz VL, Seeds JW. The role of ultrasound in evaluation of patients with elevated maternal serum alpha-fetoprotein: a review. *Obstet Gynecol* 1991;78(1):123–128.

22 Nicolaides KH, Campbell S, Gabbe SG, Guidetti R. Ultrasound screening for spina bifida: cranial and cerebellar signs. *Lancet* 1986;2(8498):72–74.

23 Bruner JP, Tulipan N. Tell the truth about spina bifida. *Ultrasound Obstet Gynecol* 2004;24(6):595–596.

24 Bruner JP, Tulipan N, Reed G, et al. Intrauterine repair of spina bifida: preoperative predictors of shunt-dependent hydrocephalus. *Am J Obstet Gynecol* 2004;190(5):1305–1312.

25 Budorick NE, Pretorius DH, McGahan JP, et al. Cephalocele detection in utero: sonographic and clinical features. *Ultrasound Obstet Gynecol* 1995;5(2):77–85.

26 Goldstein RB, LaPidus AS, Filly RA. Fetal cephaloceles: diagnosis with US. *Radiology* 1991;180(3):803–808.

27 Blaas HG, Eriksson AG, Salvesen KA, et al. Brains and faces in holoprosencephaly: pre- and postnatal description of 30 cases. *Ultrasound Obstet Gynecol* 2002;19(1):24–38.

28 Matsunaga E, Shiota K. Holoprosencephaly in human embryos: epidemiologic studies of 150 cases. *Teratology* 1977;16(3): 261–272.

29 Pilu G, Reece EA, Romero R, et al. Prenatal diagnosis of craniofacial malformations with ultrasonography. *Am J Obstet Gynecol* 1986;155(1):45–50.

30 Pilu G, Romero R, Rizzo N, et al. Criteria for the prenatal diagnosis of holoprosencephaly. *Am J Perinatol* 1987;4(1):41–49.

31 Pilu G, Sandri F, Perolo A, et al. Prenatal diagnosis of lobar holoprosencephaly. *Ultrasound Obstet Gynecol* 1992;2(2):88–94.

32 Pilu G, Ambrosetto P, Sandri F, et al. Intraventricular fused fornices: a specific sign of fetal lobar holoprosencephaly. *Ultrasound Obstet Gynecol* 1994;4(1):65–67.

33 Bernard JP, Drummond CL, Zaarour P, et al. A new clue to the prenatal diagnosis of lobar holoprosencephaly: the abnormal pathway of the anterior cerebral artery crawling under the skull. *Ultrasound Obstet Gynecol* 2002;19(6):605–607.

34 Pilu G, Sandri F, Perolo A, et al. Sonography of fetal agenesis of the corpus callosum: a survey of 35 cases. *Ultrasound Obstet Gynecol* 1993;3(5):318–329.

35 Gupta JK, Lilford RJ. Assessment and management of fetal agenesis of the corpus callosum. *Prenat Diagn* 1995;15(4):301–312.

36 Moutard ML, Kieffer V, Feingold J, et al. Agenesis of corpus callosum: prenatal diagnosis and prognosis. *Childs Nerv Syst* 2003;19(7–8):471–476.

37 Lewis SW, Reveley MA, David AS, Ron MA. Agenesis of the corpus callosum and schizophrenia: a case report. *Psychol Med* 1988;18(2):341–347.

38 Adamsbaum C, Moutard ML, Andre C, et al. MRI of the fetal posterior fossa. *Pediatr Radiol* 2005;35(2):124–140.

39 Boddaert N, Klein O, Ferguson N, et al. Intellectual prognosis of the Dandy–Walker malformation in children: the importance of vermian lobulation. *Neuroradiology* 2003;45(5):320–324.

40 Nyberg DA, Mahony BS, Hegge FN, et al. Enlarged cisterna magna and the Dandy–Walker malformation: factors associated with chromosome abnormalities. *Obstet Gynecol* 1991;77(3): 436–442.

41 Mahony BS, Callen PW, Filly RA, Hoddick WK. The fetal cisterna magna. *Radiology* 1984;153(3):773–776.

42 Pilu G, Visentin A, Valeri B. The Dandy–Walker complex and fetal sonography. *Ultrasound Obstet Gynecol* 2000;16(2):115–117.

43 Ecker JL, Shipp TD, Bromley B, Benacerraf B. The sonographic diagnosis of Dandy–Walker and Dandy–Walker variant: associated findings and outcomes. *Prenat Diagn* 2000;20(4):328–332.

44 Malinger G, Ginath S, Lerman-Sagie T, et al. The fetal cerebellar vermis: normal development as shown by transvaginal ultrasound. *Prenat Diagn* 2001;21(8):687–692.

45 Bromley B, Nadel AS, Pauker S, et al. Closure of the cerebellar vermis: evaluation with second trimester US. *Radiology* 1994;193(3):761–763.

46 Ghi T, Simonazzi G, Perolo A, et al. Outcome of antenatally diagnosed intracranial hemorrhage: case series and review of the literature. *Ultrasound Obstet Gynecol* 2003;22(2):121–130.

47 Malinger G, Lev D, Zahalka N, et al. Fetal cytomegalovirus infection of the brain: the spectrum of sonographic findings. *Am J Neuroradiol* 2003;24(1):28–32.

48 Ghi T, Brondelli L, Simonazzi G, et al. Sonographic demonstration of brain injury in fetuses with severe red blood cell alloimmunization undergoing intrauterine transfusions. *Ultrasound Obstet Gynecol* 2004;23(5):428–431.

49 Pilu G, Falco P, Perolo A, et al. Differential diagnosis and outcome of fetal intracranial hypoechoic lesions: report of 21 cases. *Ultrasound Obstet Gynecol* 1997;9(4):229–236.

50 Bromley B, Benacerraf BR. Difficulties in the prenatal diagnosis of microcephaly. *J Ultrasound Med* 1995;14(4):303–306.
51 Pilu G, Falco P, Milano V, et al. Prenatal diagnosis of microcephaly assisted by vaginal sonography and power Doppler. *Ultrasound Obstet Gynecol* 1998;11(5):357–360.
52 DeMyer W. Megalencephaly: types, clinical syndromes, and management. *Pediatr Neurol* 1986;2(6):321–328.
53 Malinger G, Lev D, Lerman-Sagie T. Abnormal sulcation as an early sign for migration disorders. *Ultrasound Obstet Gynecol* 2004;24(7):704–705.
54 Fong KW, Ghai S, Toi A, et al. Prenatal ultrasound findings of lissencephaly associated with Miller–Dieker syndrome and comparison with pre- and postnatal magnetic resonance imaging. *Ultrasound Obstet Gynecol* 2004;24(7):716–723.
55 Gupta JK, Khan KS, Thornton JG, Lilford RJ. Management of fetal choroid plexus cysts. *Br J Obstet Gynaecol* 1997;104(8): 881–886.
56 Gupta JK, Cave M, Lilford RJ, et al. Clinical significance of fetal choroid plexus cysts. *Lancet* 1995;346(8977):724–729.
57 Bromley B, Lieberman R, Benacerraf BR. Choroid plexus cysts: not associated with Down syndrome. *Ultrasound Obstet Gynecol* 1996;8(4):232–235.
58 Snijders RJ, Shawa L, Nicolaides KH. Fetal choroid plexus cysts and trisomy 18: assessment of risk based on ultrasound findings and maternal age. *Prenat Diagn* 1994;14(12):1119–1127.
59 Nyberg DA, Kramer D, Resta RG, et al. Prenatal sonographic findings of trisomy 18: review of 47 cases. *J Ultrasound Med* 1993;12(2):103–113.
60 Neblett CR, Robertson JW. Symptomatic cysts of the telencephalic choroid plexus. *J Neurol Neurosurg Psychiatr* 1971;34:324–331.
61 Blaas HG, Eik-Nes SH, Vainio T, Isaksen CV. Alobar holoprosencephaly at 9 weeks gestational age visualized by two- and three-dimensional ultrasound. *Ultrasound Obstet Gynecol* 2000;15(1): 62–65.
62 Blaas HG. Holoprosencephaly at 10 weeks 2 days (CRL 33 mm). *Ultrasound Obstet Gynecol* 2000;15(1):86–87.
63 Blaas HG, Eik-Nes SH, Isaksen CV. The detection of spina bifida before 10 gestational weeks using two- and three-dimensional ultrasound. *Ultrasound Obstet Gynecol* 2000;16(1):25–29.
64 Malinger G, Lerman-Sagie T, Watemberg N, et al. A normal second-trimester ultrasound does not exclude intracranial structural pathology. *Ultrasound Obstet Gynecol* 2002;20(1): 51–56.

24 Prenatal diagnosis of thoracic and cardiac abnormalities

Gianluigi Pilu, Philippe Jeanty, and Juliana M.B. Leite

Cardiac anomalies

Abnormalities of the heart and great arteries are among the most common congenital abnormalities, with an estimated incidence of 5 per 1000 births and about 30 per 1000 stillbirths. In general, about one-half are either severe or require surgery early in life and are generally referred to as major cardiac abnormalities.

Fetal echocardiography is the primary diagnostic tool used to assess fetal cardiac structure and function.[1,2] This is a specialized sonogram that is certainly indicated when there is an increased risk of fetal cardiac abnormalities, and is usually performed at 18–22 weeks' gestation. When the risk of a fetal cardiac anomaly is particularly high, an earlier evaluation, at around 13–15 weeks, by either transabdominal or vaginal sonography, may be considered, as many cardiac anomalies are already demonstrable at this stage. This early examination should, however, be corroborated by a repeat evaluation around mid-gestation.

A complete fetal echocardiographic examination should incorporate the following standard views: a demonstration of the visceral and cardiac situs, a four-chamber view, ventriculo-arterial connections, and course of the great arteries (Fig. 24.1). Real-time examination of cardiac structures is enhanced by the use of color Doppler. Different approaches are possible to visualize these anatomical details, and the interested reader is referred to specific works on this subject.[3,4]

Fetal echocardiography allows the detection of many cardiac malformations, but the precise accuracy is difficult to establish. Antenatal studies have a tendency to detect the more severe anomalies and miss the more benign lesions.[2] Defects that have commonly been missed include ventricular septal defects, atrial septal defects, semilunar valve stenosis, and tetralogy of Fallot, among others. Lesions that affect the four-chamber view are more commonly detected than conotruncal lesions. Finally, the natural evolution of some anomalies may be such that they only appear in the third trimester. Examples of this include premature occlusion of the foramen ovale, aortic and pulmonary stenosis with intact ventricular septum, and cardiac tumors, among others. Most studies in which a detailed fetal echocardiogram was performed report sensitivities in the range of 70–85%.[5]

The sensitivity of the four-chamber view, which should always be included in any standard sonographic examination performed from mid-gestation on, is controversial. Albeit in some studies it has been found to be as high as 80%, others have reported disappointing results, with sensitivities of 5–15%[6,7] – most likely the experience of the sonologist performing the examination is critical from this point of view.

A new technique for the sonographic evaluation of the fetal heart, based upon the use of three-dimensional ultrasound, has been recently introduced, commonly referred to as STIC (*spa*tio*te*mporal *i*mage *c*orrelation technology (Fig. 24.2). The use of this technology has provided many potential advantages, both for diagnostic use (e.g., to reconstruct scanning planes that cannot be directly obtained)[8–11] and for screening and teleconsultation,[12,13] which have been only partially investigated thus far.

Septal defects

Defects of the atrial and ventricular septum represent about 10% and 30%, respectively, of all cardiac defects. Prenatal diagnosis is based upon demonstration of a gap of the septa (Fig. 24.3). In general, identification is difficult and is impossible in most cases. Most atrial defects involve the *septum secundum*, which is difficult to analyze owing to the physiologic presence of the foramen ovale. Most ventricular septal defects are small and equally difficult to demonstrate antenatally. As they are usually associated with blood shunting across the septum, color Doppler may aid in the diagnosis, which remains nevertheless difficult, and is very rarely made.[14] When a ventricular septal defect is identified, STIC technology has been suggested to be useful in that it allows visualization of the septal gap in three orthogonal planes, allowing demonstration of both dimensions and position[8,15] (see Fig. 24.2).

Atrial and ventricular septal defects are not a cause of

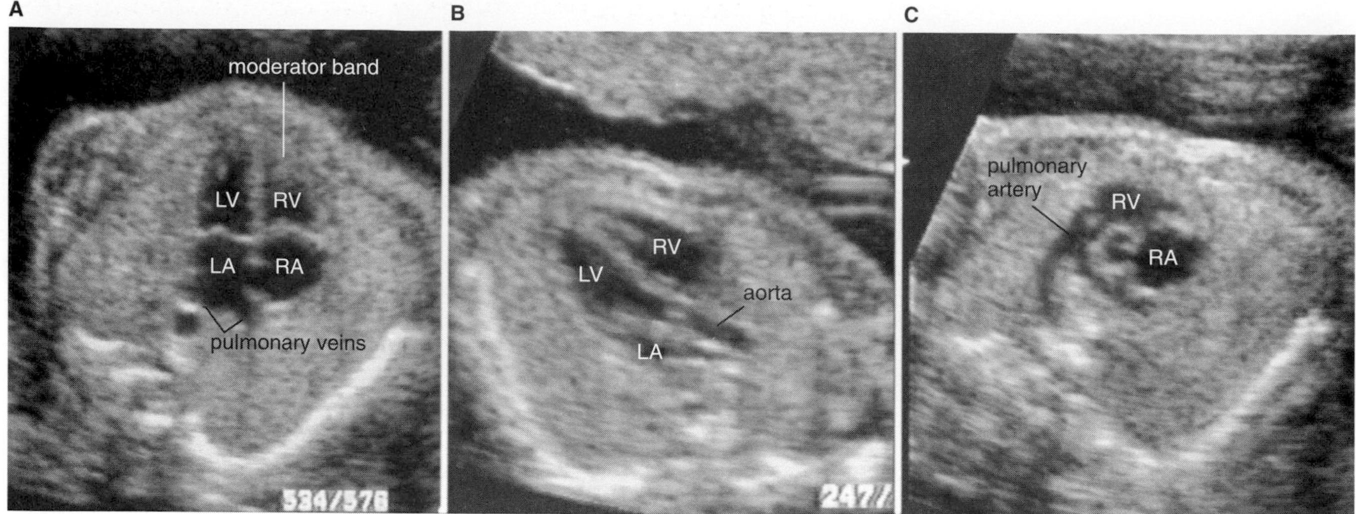

Figure 24.1 The essential views used for an echocardiographic examination in a normal fetus at 22 weeks' gestation. (A) Four-chamber view. (B) View of the left ventricle demonstrating the left ventriculoarterial connection. (C) Transverse section of great vessels demonstrating the right ventriculoarterial connection and the crossing of great arteries. (RA/LA, right/left atrium; RV/LV, right/left ventricle.)

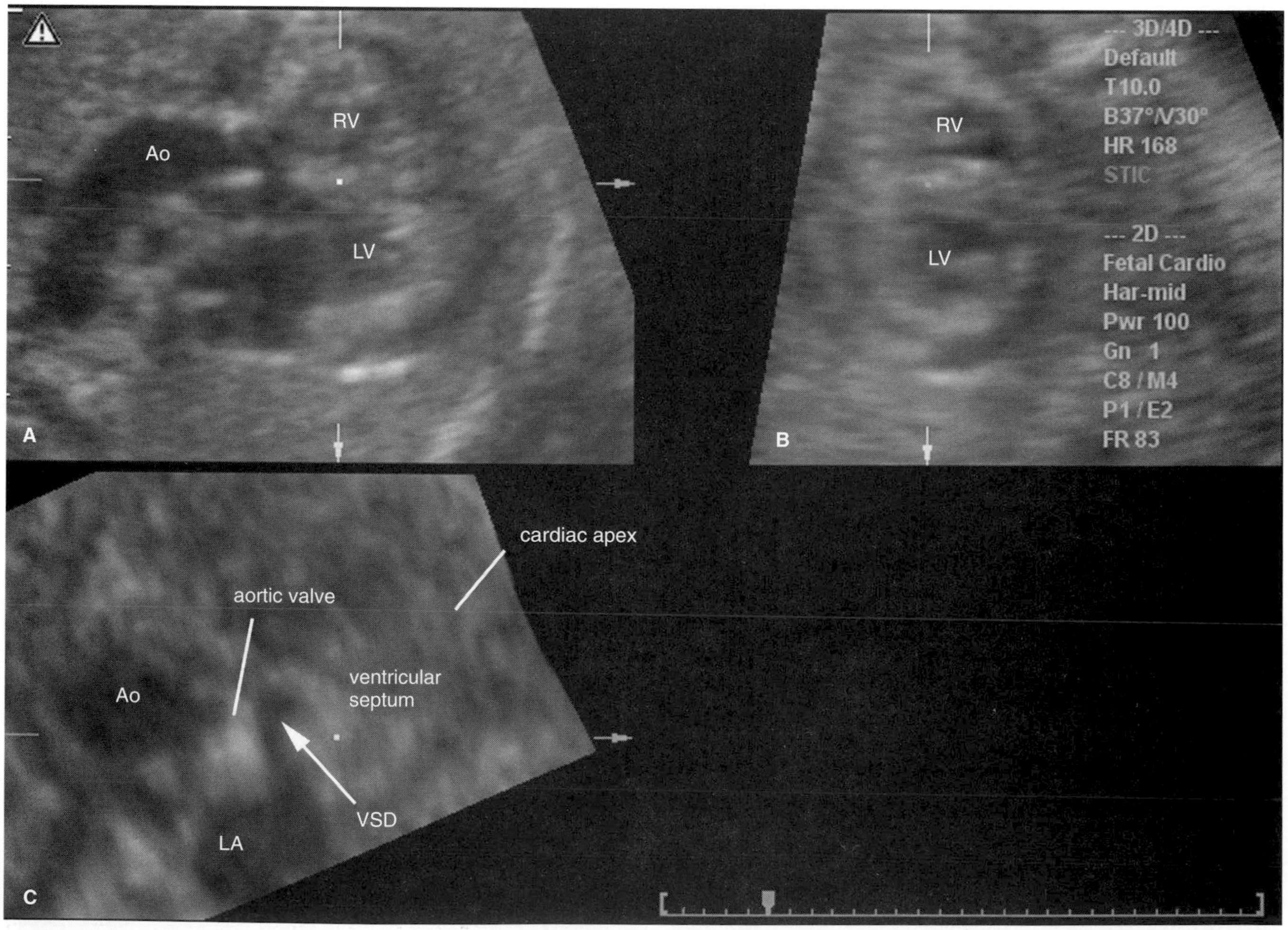

Figure 24.2 Sonogram of fetal tetralogy of Fallot obtained with three-dimensional technology and STIC technology. Three orthogonal planes are simultaneously visualized and can be observed in motion during one reconstructed cardiac cycle. (A) Axial view of the chest demonstrating the aorta (Ao) overriding by about 50% the ventricular septum. (B) Coronal view demonstrating a short axis of both ventricle.
(C) Reconstructed sagittal view of the chest demonstrating a lateral view of the entire ventricular septum and ascending aorta; this view demonstrates the subaortic location and extent of the ventricular septal defect.

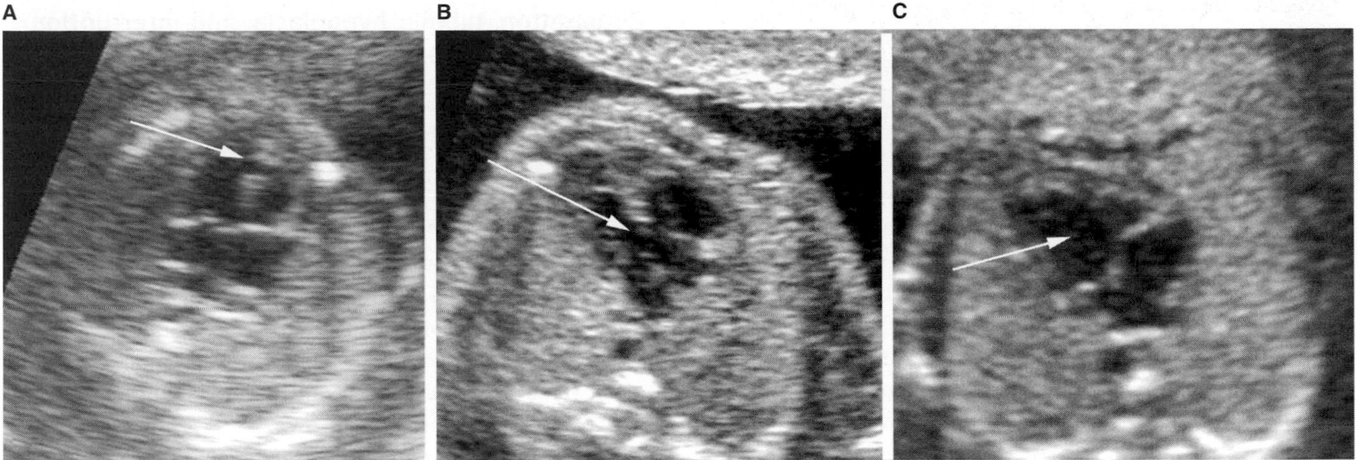

Figure 24.3 Four-chamber views demonstrating abnormalities of cardiac septa: (A) muscular ventricular septal defect; (B) complete atrioventricular septal defect; (C) double-inlet single ventricle.

impaired cardiac function *in utero*, as a large intracardiac right-to-left shunt is a physiologic condition in the fetus. Most affected infants are asymptomatic even in the neonatal period. When they are not associated with other cardiac anomalies, the prognosis is excellent. Spontaneous closure is frequent. *Primum* atrial septal defect is the simplest of the atrioventricular septal defects and will be considered below.

The core of the heart, being the apical portion of the atrial septum, the basal portion of the interventricular septum and the medial portion of atrioventricular valves, develops from the mesenchymal masses, or endocardial cushions. Abnormal development of these structures, commonly referred to as endocardial cushion defects, atrioventricular canal, or atrioventricular septal defects, represents about 7% of all cardiac anomalies. In the complete form, *persistent common atrioventricular canal*, the tricuspid and mitral valve are fused in a large single atrioventricular valve that opens above and bridges the two ventricles (see Fig. 24.3). In the complete form of atrioventricular canal, the common atrioventricular valve may be incompetent and systolic blood regurgitation from the ventricles to the atria may give rise to congestive heart failure. In the partial form, there is a defect in the apical portion of the atrial septum (septum primum defect). There are two separate atrioventricular valves, but they are inserted at the same level on the ventricular septum.

Antenatal diagnosis of complete atrioventricular septal defects is not always easy. When the atrial and septal defects are large, the four-chamber view reveals an obvious deficiency of the central core structures of the heart.[16] Color Doppler ultrasound can be useful in that it facilitates the visualization of the central opening of the single atrioventricular valve. The atria may be dilated as a consequence of atrioventricular insufficiency. In such cases, color and pulsed Doppler ultrasound allow the identification of the regurgitant jet. However, we have seen cases in which the defects of the septa were so small that they presented a real diagnostic challenge. False-negatives have also been reported.[17] The incomplete forms are even more difficult to recognize. A useful hint is the demonstration that the tricuspid and mitral valves attach at the same level at the crest of the septum. The low detection rate of fetal atrioventricular septal defects is attested by several large studies of low-risk patients.[7,18] To improve the sensitivity of ultrasound, the ratio of the atria to the ventricular portion of the heart has been recently suggested.[19]

Atrioventricular septal defects do not impair the fetal circulation *per se*. However, the presence of atrioventricular valve insufficiency may lead to intrauterine heart failure. The prognosis of atrioventricular septal defects is poor when detected *in utero*, probably because of the high frequency of associated anomalies in antenatal series.[16,20] Atrioventricular septal defects will usually be encountered either in fetuses with chromosomal aberrations (50% of cases are associated with aneuploidy, 60% being trisomy 21, 25% trisomy 18) or in fetuses with cardiosplenic syndromes. In the former cases, an atrioventricular septal defect is frequently found in association with extracardiac anomalies. In the latter cases, complex cardiac anomalies and abnormal disposition of the abdominal organs are almost the rule. Survival after surgical closure is more than 90%, but in about 10% of patients a second operation for atrioventricular valve repair or replacement is necessary. Long-term prognosis is good.[16,20]

Univentricular heart

This term defines a group of anomalies characterized by the presence of an atrioventricular junction that is entirely connected to only one chamber in the ventricular mass. Therefore, univentricular heart includes both those cases in which two atrial chambers are connected, by either two distinct atrioventricular valves or a common one to a main ventricular chamber (*double-inlet single ventricle*) (see Fig. 24.3), and those in which, because of the absence of one atrioventricular connection (tricuspid or mitral atresia), one of the ventricular chambers is either rudimentary or absent. Univentricular heart is rare; it represents about 1.5% of all congenital cardiac defects. Tricuspid atresia is by far the most frequent variety.

In double-outlet single ventricle, two separate atrioventricular valves are seen opening into a single ventricular cavity without evidence of the interventricular septum. In tricuspid atresia, there is only one atrioventricular valve connected to a main ventricular chamber. A small rudimentary ventricular chamber lacking an atrioventricular connection is a frequent but not constant finding.

Surgical treatment (the Fontan procedure) involves separation of the systemic circulations by anastomosing the superior and inferior vena cava directly to the pulmonary artery. The survivors from this procedure may develop several complications including arrhythmias, thrombus formation, and protein-losing enteropathy. The 5-year survival is about 70% and the long-term outcome is uncertain.[21]

Aortic stenosis

Aortic stenosis represents about 3% of all cardiac defects and is commonly divided into supravalvar, valvar, and subaortic forms. Supravalvar and subaortic are rare and usually cannot be detected antenatally. The valvar form of aortic stenosis can be due to dysplastic, thickened aortic cusps or fusion of the commissure between the cusps. With severe valvar aortic stenosis, the left ventricle may be either hypertrophic or dilated and hypocontractile. The ascending aorta is frequently enlarged. Hyperechogenicity of the aortic valve and pulsed Doppler demonstration of increased peak velocity (usually in excess of 1 m/s) support the diagnosis. At the color Doppler examination, high velocity and turbulence usually results in aliasing, with a mosaic of colors within the ascending aorta. Severe aortic stenosis may result in atrioventricular valve insufficiency and intrauterine heart failure. Most cases of mild to moderate aortic stenosis are probably not amenable to early prenatal diagnosis. Asymmetric septal hypertrophy and hypertrophic cardiomyopathy of fetuses of diabetic mothers resulting in subaortic stenosis has been diagnosed occasionally by demonstrating an unusual thickness of the ventricular septum.

Depending upon the severity of the aortic stenosis, the association of left ventricular pressure overload and subendocardial ischemia, due to decrease in coronary perfusion, may lead to intrauterine impairment of cardiac function. Subvalvar and subaortic forms are not generally manifested in the neonatal period. Conversely, the valvar type can be a cause of congestive heart failure in the newborn and fetus as well. The neonatal outcome depends on the severity of the obstruction. If the left ventricular function is adequate, balloon valvoplasty is carried out in the neonatal period, and in about 50% of cases surgery is necessary within the first 10 years of life because of aortic insufficiency or residual stenosis. If left ventricular function is inadequate, a Norwood type of repair is necessary (see Hypoplastic left heart syndrome, below).

Coarctation, tubular hypoplasia, and interruption of the aortic arch

Coarctation is a localized narrowing of the juxtaductal arch, most commonly between the left subclavian artery and the ductus. Cardiac anomalies are frequently present and include aortic stenosis and insufficiency, ventricular septal defect, atrial septal defect, transposition of the great arteries, and truncus and double-outlet right ventricle. Noncardiac anomalies include diaphragmatic hernia and Turner syndrome but not Noonan syndrome. Interrupted aortic arch is typically associated with chromosome 22 microdeletion.[22]

Coarctation or interruption of the aortic arch should be suspected when the right ventricle is enlarged (right ventricle–left ventricle ratio of more than 1:3 (Fig. 24.4). Narrowing of the isthmus, or the presence of a shelf, is often difficult to demonstrate because in the fetus the aortic arch and ductal arch are close and are difficult to distinguish. In most cases, coarctation can only be suspected *in utero* and a definite diagnosis must be delayed until after birth.[21] The characteristic finding of an ascending aorta that is more vertical than usual and the impossibility of demonstrating a connection with the descending aorta suggests the diagnosis of interrupted aortic arch. Coarctation/interrupted aortic arch should always be considered when intracardiac lesions diverting blood flow from the left to the right heart are encountered (aortic stenosis and atresia in particular).

Critical coarctation and interruption are fatal in the neonatal period after closure of the ductus and therefore prostaglandin therapy is necessary to maintain a patent ductus. Surgery (which involves excision of the coarcted segment and end-to-end anastomosis) is associated with a mortality of about 10% and the incidence of restenosis in survivors (requiring further surgical repair) is about 15%.

Interrupted aortic arch should always be considered when intracardiac lesions diverting blood flow from the left to the right heart are encountered (aortic stenosis and atresia in particular). Isolated interruption of the aortic arch is often encountered with enlargement of the right ventricle (right ventricle–left ventricle ratio of more than 1:3).

Interrupted aortic arch is one of the lesions most frequently associated with a microdeletion of chromosome 22, and represents an indication for prenatal diagnosis of this condition. In the most typical case, there is aortic arch interruption and a small or absent thymus.[22] Recent reports suggest an overall late survival of more than 70% after surgery.

Hypoplastic left heart syndrome

Hypoplastic left heart syndrome accounts for 4% of all cardiac anomalies at birth, but it is one of the most frequent cardiac malformations diagnosed antenatally. It is a spectrum of anomalies characterized by a very small left ventricle with mitral and/or aortic atresia or hypoplasia. Blood flow to the

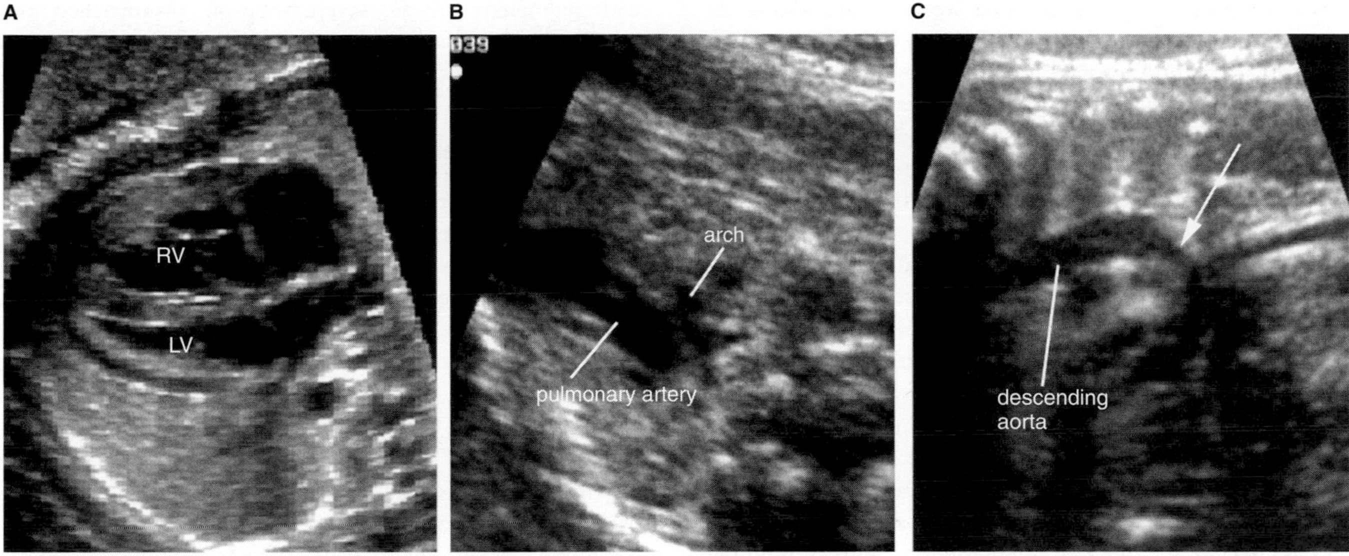

Figure 24.4 Aortic coarctation in a third-trimester fetus. (A) Four-chamber view demonstrating a disproportion in the size of the ventricles with predominance of the right cavities. (B) Transverse section of the upper thorax demonstrating a discrepancy in the size of the great vessels with a narrow transverse aortic arch. (C) Sagittal view of the chest demonstrating narrowing of the aortic arch.

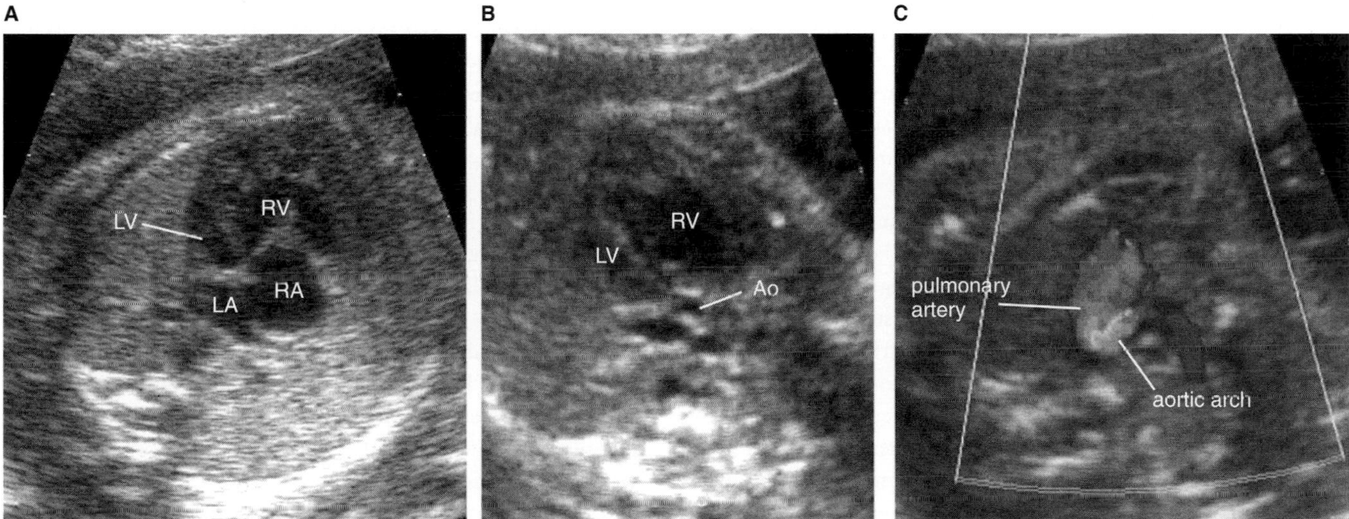

Figure 24.5 Hypoplastic left heart syndrome at mid-gestation. (A) Four-chamber view demonstrating a small left ventricle that does not reach the apex of the heart. (B) View of the left ventricle demonstrating a very small ascending aorta. (C) Color Doppler demonstrates reverse blood flow into the small aortic arch.

head and neck vessels and coronary artery is supplied in a retrograde manner via the ductus arteriosus.

Prenatal echocardiographic diagnosis of the syndrome depends on the demonstration of a diminutive left ventricle and ascending aorta (Fig. 24.5). In most cases, the ultrasound appearance is self-explanatory, and the diagnosis an easy one. There is, however, a broad spectrum of hypoplasia of the left ventricle and in some cases the ventricular cavity is almost normal in size. We anticipate that these cases will certainly be missed in most routine surveys of fetal anatomy. At closer scrutiny, however, the movement of the mitral valve appears severely impaired to nonexistent, ventricular contractility is decreased, and the ventricle often displays an internal echogenic lining owing to endocardial fibroelastosis. The definitive diagnosis depends on the demonstration of hypoplasia of the ascending aorta and atresia of the aortic valve. Color flow mapping is an extremely useful adjunct to the real-time examination, in that it allows the demonstration of retrograde blood flow within the ascending aorta and aortic arch (see Fig. 24.5).

Hypoplastic left heart is well tolerated *in utero*. The patency of the ductus arteriosus allows adequate perfusion of the head and neck vessels. Intrauterine growth may be normal, and the onset of symptoms most frequently occurs after birth. The prognosis for infants with hypoplastic left heart syndrome, however, is extremely poor and this lesion is responsible for

25% of cardiac deaths in the first week of life. Almost all affected infants die within 6 weeks if they are not treated. In the neonatal period, prostaglandin therapy is given to maintain ductal patency but still congestive heart failure develops within 24 h of life. Options for surgery include cardiac transplantation in the neonatal period and the two-staged Norwood repair. *Stage 1* involves anastomosis of the pulmonary artery to the aortic arch for systemic outflow, placement of systemic–pulmonary arterial shunt to provide pulmonary blood flow, and arterial septectomy to ensure unobstructed pulmonary venous return; the survival rate of fetuses diagnosed *in utero* is in the range of 40%. *Stage 2* (usually carried out in the sixth month of life) involves anastomosis of the superior vena cava to the pulmonary arteries. Neurodevelopmental abnormalities have been reported in survivors of the Norwood operation. The survival rate for hypoplastic left heart diagnosed *in utero* at 3 years of life is in the range of 30%.[21,23] Although there is controversy in the literature, some reports indicate that prenatal diagnosis increases the likelihood of survival, presumably by optimizing perinatal treatment.[24,25]

Pulmonary stenosis and pulmonary atresia

Pulmonary stenosis and pulmonary atresia with intact ventricular septum (also known as *hypoplastic right ventricle*) represent 9% and about 2% of all cardiac anomalies, respectively.

The most common form of pulmonary stenosis is the valvar type, due to the fusion of the pulmonary leaflets. Hemodynamics are altered proportionally to the degree of the stenosis. The work of the right ventricle is increased, as well as the pressure, leading to hypertrophy of the ventricular walls. The same considerations formulated for the prenatal diagnosis of aortic stenosis are valid for pulmonary stenosis as well. A handful of cases recognized *in utero* have been reported in the literature thus far, mostly severe types with enlargement of the right ventricle and/or poststenotic enlargement or hypoplasia of the pulmonary artery.

Pulmonary atresia with intact ventricular septum in infants is usually associated with a hypoplastic right ventricle. However, cases with enlarged right ventricle and atrium have been described with unusual frequency in prenatal series.[26] Enlargement of the ventricle and atrium is probably the consequence of tricuspid insufficiency. Prenatal diagnosis of pulmonary atresia with intact ventricular septum relies on the demonstration of a small pulmonary artery with an atretic pulmonary valve. The considerations previously formulated for the diagnosis of hypoplastic left heart syndrome apply to this condition as well.

Patients with mild stenosis are asymptomatic and there is no need for intervention. Patients with severe stenosis and right ventricular overload may develop congestive heart failure and require balloon valvoplasty in the neonatal period with excellent survival and normal long-term prognosis. Fetuses with pulmonary atresia, severe tricuspid insufficiency, and an enlarged right heart have a very high degree of perinatal mortality.

Ebstein's anomaly and tricuspid valve dysplasia

Ebstein's anomaly results from the faulty implantation of the tricuspid valve. The posterior and septal leaflets are elongated and tethered below their normal level of attachment on the annulus or displaced apically, away from the annulus, down to the junction between the inlet and trabecular portion of the right ventricle. The anterior leaflet is normally inserted but deformed. The resulting configuration is that of a considerably enlarged right atrium at the expense of the right ventricle. The portion of the right ventricle that is protruding into the right atrium is called the *atrialized* inlet of the right ventricle. It has a thin wall that may even be membranous and is commonly dilated. The tricuspid valve is usually both incompetent and stenotic. Associated anomalies include atrial septal defect, pulmonary atresia, ventricular septal defect, and supraventricular tachycardia. Ebstein's anomaly may be associated with trisomies 13 and 21, and Turner, Cornelia de Lange and Marfan syndromes. Maternal ingestion of lithium has also been incriminated as a causal factor.

The characteristic echocardiographic finding is that of a massively enlarged right atrium, a small right ventricle, and a small pulmonary artery. Doppler can be used to demonstrate regurgitation in the right atrium.[27] About 25% of the cases have supraventricular tachycardia (from re-entrant impulse), atrial fibrillation, or atrial flutter. Similar findings are encountered with dysplasia of a normally implanted tricuspid valve (Fig. 24.6).

Although the disease has a variable severity, with some cases discovered only late in life, Ebstein's anomalies and tricuspid dysplasia detected prenatally have a dismal prognosis, with a very high perinatal mortality rate.[27] This probably reflects that the prenatal variety is more severe than the forms detected in children or adults.

Conotruncal malformations

Conotruncal malformations are a heterogeneous group of defects that involve two different segments of the heart: the conotruncus and the ventricles. Conotruncal anomalies are relatively frequent. They account for 20–30% of all cardiac anomalies and are the leading cause of symptomatic cyanotic heart disease in the first year of life. Prenatal diagnosis is of interest for several reasons.[28] Given the parallel model of fetal circulation, conotruncal anomalies are well tolerated *in utero*. The clinical presentation occurs usually hours to days after delivery, and is often severe, representing a true emergency and leading to considerable morbidity and mortality. Yet, these malformations have a good prognosis when promptly treated. Two ventricles of adequate size and two great vessels are commonly present, giving the premise for biventricular surgical

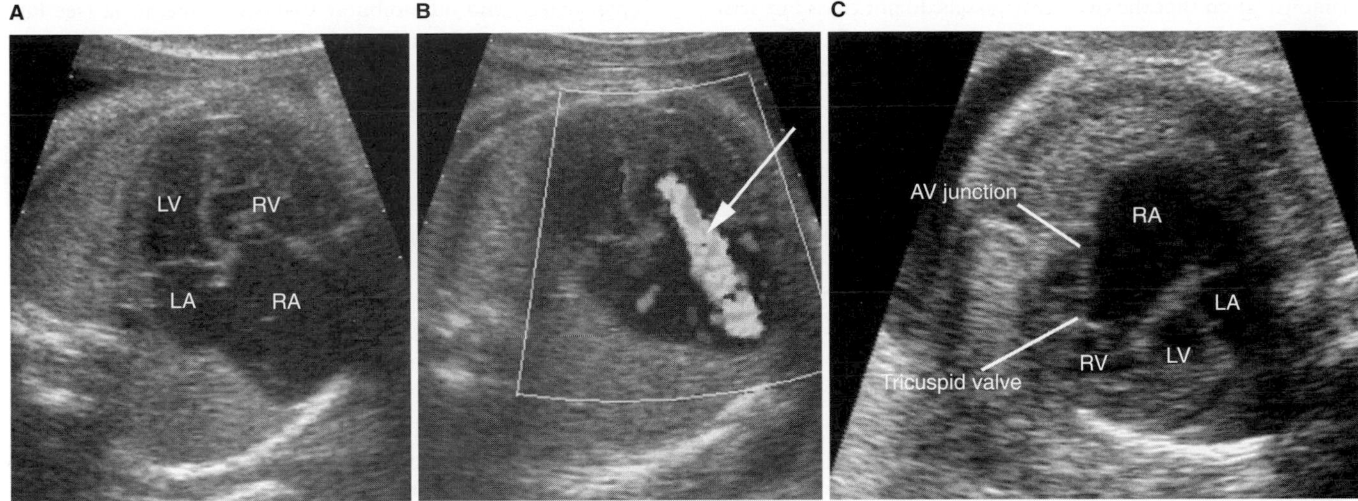

Figure 24.6 Tricuspid abnormalities associated with severe insufficiency and cardiomegaly: (A and B) tricuspid dysplasia with a very large right atrium and severe insufficiency at the color Doppler examination; (C) Ebstein's anomaly of the tricuspid valve: note that the tricuspid valve inserts at a much lower level than the AV junction.

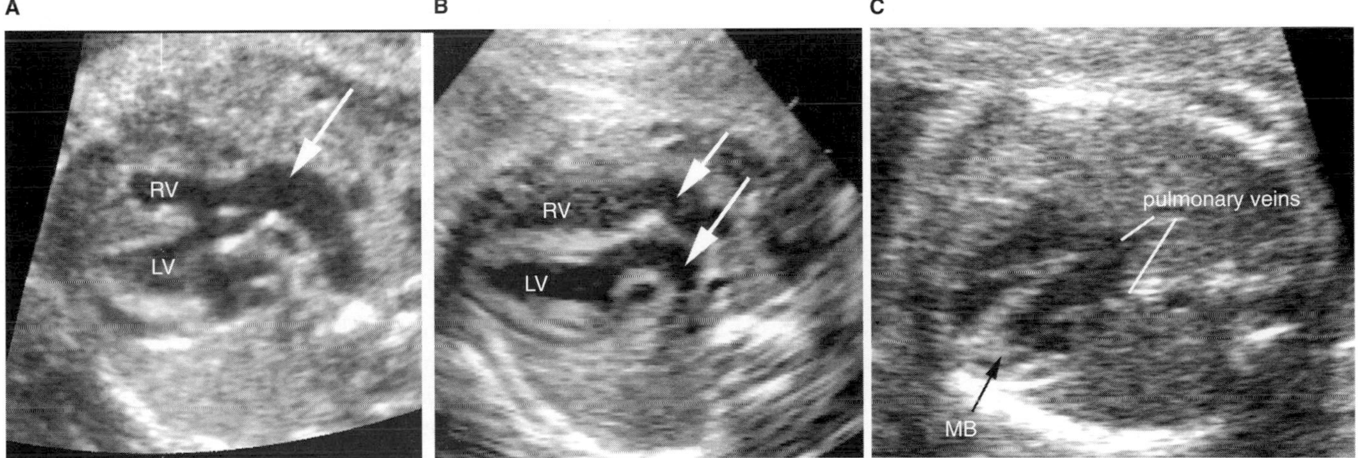

Figure 24.7 Conotruncal anomalies. (A) Tetralogy of Fallot: a large vessel (arrow) overrides the ventricular septum by about 50% and forms the aortic arch; similar findings are expected with truncus arteriosus and some types of double outlet right ventricle, and meticulous scanning is required for a differential diagnosis. (B) Complete transposition of the great vessels; the great arteries (arrows) arise from the base of the heart in parallel fashion without crossing. (C) Corrected transposition: the four-chamber view demonstrates that the posterior ventricle, which is connected to an atrial chamber, which, in turn, is connected to the pulmonary veins, has a moderator band (MB) that is a characteristic feature of the morphologic right ventricle; an increased deviation of the cardiac axis is also noted; compare this image with the normal four-chamber view demonstrated in Fig. 24.1.

correction. The outcome is indeed much more favorable than with most of the other cardiac defects that are detected antenatally.[21] Unfortunately, the recognition of these anomalies remains difficult. The four-chamber view is frequently unremarkable in these cases. A specific diagnosis requires meticulous scanning and at times may represent a challenge even for experienced sonologists (Fig. 24.7). Recently, an association has been demonstrated between conotruncal anomalies and microdeletion of chromosome 22. This association is particularly frequent with truncus arteriosus and tetralogy of Fallot, and, in particular, in those cases with absence of the pulmonary valve. A small or absent thymus in these cases greatly increases the likelihood of the association.[22]

Transposition of the great arteries (TGA) is an abnormality in which the aorta arises entirely or in large part from the right ventricle and the pulmonary artery arises from the left ventricle. Associated cardiac lesions are present in about 50% of cases, including ventricular septal defects (which can occur anywhere in the ventricular septum), pulmonary stenosis, unbalanced ventricular size ("complex transpositions"), and anomalies of the mitral valve, which can be straddling or overriding.

Complete transposition is probably one of the most difficult cardiac lesions to recognize *in utero*. In most cases the four-chamber view is normal, and the cardiac cavities and the vessels have normal dimensions. A clue to the diagnosis is the demonstration that the two great vessels do not cross but arise parallel from the base of the heart (see Fig. 24.7). The most useful echocardiographic view, however, is the left-heart view, demonstrating that the vessel connected to the left ventricle has a posterior course and bifurcates into the two pulmonary arteries. Conversely, the vessel connected to the right ventricle has a long upward course and gives rise to the brachiocephalic vessels. *Corrected transposition* is characterized by a double discordance, at the atrioventricular and ventriculo-arterial level. The left atrium is connected to the right ventricle, which is in turn connected to the ascending aorta. Conversely, the right atrium is connected with the right ventricle, which, in turn, is connected to the ascending aorta. The derangement of the conduction tissue secondary to malalignment of the atrial and ventricular septa may result in dysrhythmias, namely complete atrioventricular block. For diagnostic purposes, the identification of the peculiar difference of ventricular morphology (moderator band, papillary muscles, insertion of the atrioventricular valves) has a prominent role (see Fig. 24.7). Demonstration that the pulmonary veins are connected to an atrium, which, in turn, is connected with a ventricle that has the moderator band at the apex, is an important clue, which is furthermore potentially identifiable even in a simple four-chamber view. Diagnosis requires meticulous scanning to carefully assess all cardiac connections, using the same views described for the complete form. The presence of atrioventricular block increases the index of suspicion.

As anticipated from the parallel model of fetal circulation, complete transposition is uneventful *in utero*. After birth, survival depends on the amount and size of the mixing of the two otherwise independent circulations. Patients with transposition and an intact ventricular septum present shortly after birth with cyanosis and deteriorate rapidly. When a large ventricular septal defect is present, cyanosis can be mild. Clinical presentation may be delayed for 2–4 weeks, and usually occurs with signs of congestive heart failure. When severe stenosis of the pulmonary artery is associated with a ventricular septal defect, symptoms are similar to patients with tetralogy of Fallot. The time and mode of clinical presentation with corrected transposition depend upon the concomitant cardiac defects.

Surgery (which involves arterial switch to establish anatomic and physiologic correction) is usually carried out within the first 2 weeks of life. Operative mortality is about 10% and 10-year follow-up studies report normal function in the vast majority of cases. It has been suggested recently that prenatal diagnosis reduces perinatal mortality presumably by allowing early treatment avoiding heart failure and hypoxemia.[29] The outcome of corrected transposition depends largely upon the associated cardiac defects that are variable. As the systemic ventricle is the right ventricle, there is a high chance of cardiac failure in adulthood.

The essential features of *tetralogy of Fallot* are a subaortic ventricular septal defect, aorta overriding the ventricular septal defect, and infundibular stenosis of the aorta (see Fig. 24.5). In about 20% of cases there is atresia of the pulmonary valve, a condition that is commonly referred to as *pulmonary atresia with ventricular septal defect*. Tetralogy of Fallot can be associated with other specific cardiac malformations, defining peculiar entities. These include atrioventricular septal defects (found in 4% of cases) and absence of the pulmonary valve (found in less than 2% of cases). Hypertrophy of the right ventricle, one of the classic elements of the tetrad, is always absent in the fetus and only develops after birth.

Echocardiographic diagnosis of tetralogy of Fallot relies on the demonstration of a ventricular septal defect in the outlet portion of the septum and an overriding aorta (see Figs 24.2 and 24.7). Color and pulsed Doppler can be used to identify the patency of the pulmonary valve and exclude pulmonary atresia. Diagnostic problems arise at the extremes of the spectrum of tetralogy of Fallot. In cases with minor forms of right outflow obstruction and aortic overriding differentiation from a simple ventricular septal defect can be difficult. In those cases in which the pulmonary artery is not imaged, a differential diagnosis between pulmonary atresia with ventricular septal defect and truncus arteriosus communis is similarly difficult. Abnormal enlargement of the right ventricle and main pulmonary trunk and artery suggests absence of pulmonary valve.

Tetralogy of Fallot does not result in cardiac failure in fetuses. Even in cases of tight pulmonary stenosis or atresia, the wide ventricular septal defect provides adequate combined ventricular output, while the pulmonary vascular bed is supplied in a retrograde manner by the ductus. The only exception to this rule is represented by cases with an absent pulmonary valve, which may result in massive regurgitation to the right ventricle and atrium. When severe pulmonic stenosis is present, cyanosis tends to develop immediately after birth. With lesser degrees of obstruction to pulmonary blood flow, the onset of cyanosis may not appear until later in the first year of life. When there is pulmonary atresia, rapid and severe deterioration follows ductal constriction. Survival after complete surgical repair (which is usually carried out in the third month of life) is more than 90%, and about 80% of survivors have normal exercise tolerance.

In *double outlet right ventricle* (DORV), most of the aorta and pulmonary valve arise completely, or almost completely, from the right ventricle. The relation between the two vessels may vary, ranging from a Fallot-like to a TGA-like situation (the Taussig–Bing anomaly). DORV is not a single malformation from a pathophysiologic point of view. The term refers only to the position of the great vessels that is found in association with ventricular septal defects, tetralogy of Fallot, transposition, and univentricular hearts. Pulmonary stenosis is very common in all types of DORV, but left-outflow obstructions, from subaortic stenosis to coarctation and interruption of the aortic arch, can also be seen.

Prenatal diagnosis of DORV can be reliably made in the fetus but differentiation from other conotruncal anomalies can be very difficult, especially with tetralogy of Fallot and transposition of the great arteries with ventricular septal defect. The main echocardiographic features include (1) alignment of the two vessels totally or predominantly from the right ventricle and (2) presence in most cases of bilateral coni (subaortic and subpulmonary). The hemodynamics are dependent upon the anatomic type of DORV and the associated anomalies. As the fetal heart works as a common chamber where the blood is mixed and pumped, DORV is not associated with intrauterine heart failure. However, DORV, in contrast with other conotruncal malformations, is commonly associated with extracardiac anomalies and/or chromosomal defects. Usually, DORV does not interfere with hemodynamics in fetal life. The early operative mortality is about 10%.

A single arterial vessel that originates from the heart overrides the ventricular septum and supplies the systemic, pulmonary, and coronary circulations, characterizing truncus arteriosus. The single arterial trunk is larger than the normal aortic root and is predominantly connected with the right ventricle in about 40% of cases, with the left ventricle in 20%, and is equally shared in 40%. The truncal valve may have one, two, or three cusps and is rarely normal. It can be stenotic or, more frequently, insufficient. A misaligned ventricular septal defect, usually wide, is an essential part of the malformation. There are three types based on the morphology of the pulmonary artery. In *type 1*, the pulmonary arteries arise from the truncus within a short distance from the valve, as a main pulmonary trunk, which then bifurcates. In *type 2*, there is no main pulmonary trunk. In *type 3*, only one pulmonary artery (usually the right) originates from the truncus, whereas a systemic collateral vessel from the descending aorta supplies the other. Similar to tetralogy of Fallot, and unlike the other conotruncal malformations, truncus is frequently (about 30%) associated with extracardiac malformations.

Truncus arteriosus can be reliably detected with fetal echocardiography. The main diagnostic criteria are: (1) a single semilunar valve overrides the ventricular septal defect and (2) there is direct continuity between one or two pulmonary arteries and the single arterial trunk. The semilunar valve is often thickened and moves abnormally. Doppler ultrasound is of value to assess incompetence of the truncal valve. A peculiar problem found in prenatal echocardiography is the demonstration of the absence of pulmonary outflow tract and the concomitant failure to image the pulmonary arteries. In these situations a differentiation between truncus and pulmonary atresia with ventricular septal defect may be impossible.

Similar to the other conotruncal anomalies truncus arteriosus is not associated with alteration of fetal hemodynamics. Truncus arteriosus is frequently a neonatal emergency. These patients usually have unobstructed pulmonary blood flow and show signs of progressive congestive heart failure with the postnatal fall in pulmonary resistance. Many patients will present with cardiac failure in the first 1 or 2 weeks of life. Surgical repair (usually before the sixth month of life) involves closure of the ventricular septal defect and creation of a conduit connection between the right ventricle and the pulmonary arteries. Survival after surgery is about 90%, but the patients require repeated surgery for replacement of the conduit.

Heterotaxy

In heterotaxy, also referred to as cardiosplenic syndromes, the fetus is made of either two left or two right sides. Other terms commonly used include left or right isomerism, asplenia, and polysplenia. Unpaired organs (liver, stomach, and spleen) may be absent, midline, or duplicated. Because of left atrial isomerism (thus absence of the right atrium, which is the normal location for the pacemaker) and abnormal atrioventricular junctions, atrioventricular blocks are very common. Heterotaxy represents about 2% of all congenital heart defects.

In polysplenia, the fetus has two left sides (one in the normal position and the other as a mirror image); this is called left isomerism. Multiple small spleens (usually too small to be detected by antenatal ultrasound) are found posterior to the stomach. The liver is midline and symmetric but the stomach and aorta can be on opposite sides. In asplenia, the fetus has two right sides (right isomerism). The liver is generally midline and the stomach right- or left-sided. The aorta and cava are on the same side (either left or right) of the spine.

Cardiac malformations are almost invariably present and are usually severe, with a tendency towards a single structure replacing normal paired structures: single atrium, single atrioventricular valve, single ventricle, and single great vessel.

The main clue for the diagnosis of fetal heterotaxy is the demonstration of complex cardiac anomalies associated with abnormal disposition of the thoracic and/or abdominal organs.[30,31] In polysplenia, a typical finding is interruption of the inferior vena cava with azygous continuation (there is failure to visualize the inferior vena cava and a large venous vessel, the azygos vein, runs to the left and close to the spine and ascends into the upper thorax). Symmetry of the liver can be sonographically recognized *in utero* by the abnormal course of the portal circulation, which does not display a clearly defined portal sinus bending to the right.

The heterogeneous cardiac anomalies found in association with heterotaxy are usually easily seen, but a detailed diagnosis often poses a challenge; in particular, assessment of connection between the pulmonary veins and the atrium (an element that has a major prognostic influence) can be extremely difficult. Associated anomalies include absence of the gallbladder, malrotation of the guts, duodenal atresia, and hydrops.

The outcome depends on the number of cardiac anomalies, but it tends to be poor. Atrioventricular insufficiency and severe fetal bradycardia due to atrioventricular block may lead to intrauterine heart failure.[30,31]

Fetal dysrhythmias

Irregular patterns of fetal heart rhythms are a frequent finding. Short periods of tachycardia, bradycardia, and ectopic beats as well are very commonly seen, and in the vast majority of cases have no clinical significance. A sustained bradycardia of less than 100 beats per minute (bpm), a sustained tachycardia of more than 200 bpm and irregular beats occurring more than one in 10 should be considered abnormal and require further investigation.[32] The fetal electrocardiogram is of little value in the prenatal diagnosis of dysrhythmias, as a satisfactory transabdominal recording can be obtained in a minority of cases. At present, M-mode and pulsed Doppler ultrasound are the best available techniques for the assessment of irregular fetal heart rhythm.[32,33] The study of the mechanical events of the sequence of contraction may be accomplished in different ways. Simultaneous visualization of atrioventricular valves and ventricular wall motion, aortic valve opening and atrial wall movement with M-mode, and sampling of the ventricular inlet or inferior vena cava with M-mode can be used from time to time. The sequence of excitation can be reasonably inferred by the sequence of contraction (Fig. 24.8).

Premature atrial and ventricular contractions are the most frequent fetal dysrhythmias. Repeated premature contractions can give rise to complex rhythm patterns. Premature atrial contractions may be either conducted to the ventricles or blocked, depending upon the time of the cardiac cycle in which they occur, thus resulting in either an increased or a decreased ventricular rate. Blocked premature atrial contractions should be differentiated from atrioventricular block. Premature atrial and ventricular contractions are considered a benign condition. They probably do not induce any hemodynamic perturbance, do not appear to be associated with an increased risk of structural abnormalities, and usually disappear *in utero* or soon after birth. However, as there is at least a theoretical possibility that in a few cases an ectopic beat triggers a re-entrant tachyarrhythmia, serial monitoring of the fetal heart during pregnancy is suggested.[33]

Supraventricular tachyarrhythmias include supraventricular paroxysmal tachycardia (SVT), atrial flutter, and atrial fibrillation. SVT is characterized by an atrial frequency between 200 and 300 bpm and a 1:1 atrioventricular conduction rate. It can occur by one of two mechanisms: automaticity and re-entry. In the former case, an irritable ectopic focus discharges at high frequency. In the latter case, an electrical impulse re-enters the atria giving rise to repeated electrical activity. Re-entry may occur at the level of the sinoatrial node, inside the atrium, the atrioventricular node and the His–Purkinje system. Re-entry may also occur along an anomalous atrioventricular connection such as the Kent bundle in the Wolff–Parkinson–White (WPW) syndrome. In atrial flutter, the atrial rate ranges from 300 to 400 bpm. Owing to variable degrees of atrioventricular block, the ventricular rate ranges between 60 and 200 bpm. In atrial fibrillation, the atrial rate is more than 400 bpm and the ventricular rate ranges between 120 and 200 bpm. Atrial flutter and fibrillation often alternate, and are thought to arise from similar mechanisms, which include circus movement of the electrical impulse, ectopic formation, multiple re-entry, and multifocal

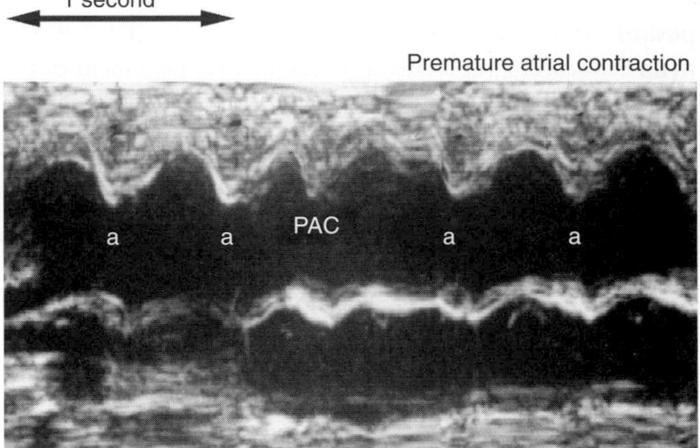

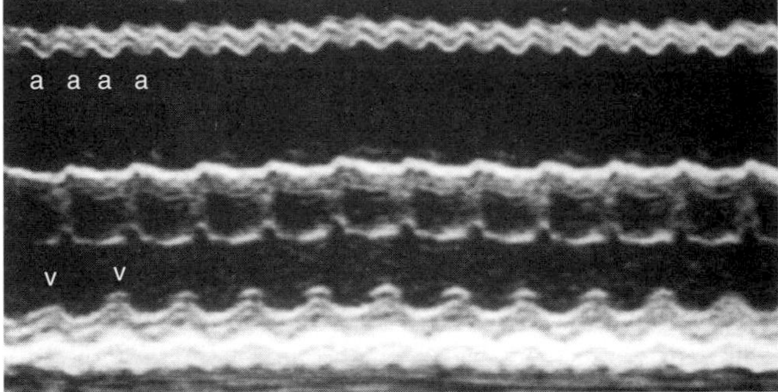

Complete AV block

a a a a a a

v v

Figure 24.8 Diagnosis with M-mode of fetal dysrhythmias: *a* indicates atrial contractions, *v* ventricular contractions. In the upper panel, a premature atrial contraction (PAC) is seen. In the middle panel, the atria contract rapidly with a frequency of about 440/s and the ventricle respond with a frequency of 220/s. This is atrial flutter with 2:1 atrioventricular block. In the lower panel, the atria contract regularly with a frequency of about 120/s. The ventricle contract with a frequency of about 50/s, independently from atrial contractions. This is complete atrioventricular block.

impulse formation. SVT is by far the most common tachyarrhythmia in children. The most frequent form is the one caused by atrioventricular nodal re-entry.

The association between fetal tachyarrhythmia and nonimmune hydrops is well established. It has been postulated that a fast ventricular rate results in suboptimal filling of the ventricles. This would lead to decreased cardiac output, right atrial overload, and congestive heart failure. The frequency of nonimmune hydrops is variable. We have seen fetuses with SVT that did well *in utero* and were successfully treated after birth. It can be postulated that in those cases in which a re-entry mechanism is involved, the fetus alternates phases of tachycardia and phases of normal rhythm. Intrauterine pharmacologic cardioversion of fetal tachyarrhythmia by maternal administration of drugs has been attempted with success in many cases. Transplacental passage of antiarrhythmic drugs is limited when fetal hydrops is present, and under these conditions a direct administration by ultrasound-guided funipuncture has been proposed. The optimal approach to the treatment of this condition is still uncertain. Digoxin, verapamil, propranolol, quinidine, procainamide, flecainide, and amiodarone have all been used from time to time. The interested reader is referred to specific works in this subject. Independent of the therapeutic regimen employed, the largest available series suggests a survival rate in the range of 90%.[33–36]

Atrioventricular (AV) block can result from immaturity of the conduction system, absence of connection to the AV node or abnormal anatomic position of the AV node. AV block is commonly classified into three types. First-degree AV block corresponds to a simple conduction delay, which is associated with prolongation of the PR interval on the ECG. Second-degree AV block is subdivided into Mobitz types 1 and 2. Mobitz type 1 consists of a progressive prolongation of the PR interval that finally leads to the blocking of one atrial impulse (Luciani–Wenckebach phenomenon). In Mobitz type 2 the ventricular rate is a submultiple of the atrial rate (e.g., 2:1, 3:1). In third-degree or complete AV block, there is a complete dissociation of the atria and ventricles, usually with independent and slow activation of the ventricles. Third-degree AV block is associated in over one-half of the cases with cardiac structural anomalies, mostly atrioventricular discordance. In cases without structural cardiac disease, the etiology of AV block mostly depends upon the presence of maternal antibodies against SSA and SSB antigens (anti-Ro and anti-La). Transplacental passage of these antibodies would lead to inflammation of and damage to the conduction system. Anti-SSA antibodies have been reported in over 80% of mothers who delivered infants with AV block, although only 30% had clinical evidence of connective tissue disease, mostly lupus erythematosus.

First- and second-degree AV block are not usually associated with any significant hemodynamic perturbation. Third-degree AV block may lead to important bradycardia, determining a decreased cardiac output and congestive heart failure *in utero*. Outcome is poor when there are associated cardiac anomalies and/or hydrops. Conversely most fetuses with isolated block will survive.[37–39]

The use of maternal steroids to limit the inflammatory response in the fetal cardiac conducting system has been postulated to carry an advantage. The use of immunosuppressive agents has also been advocated.[37]

Thoracic anomalies

Hyperechogenic and cystic lungs

The typical finding is that of enlarged brightly echogenic lungs displacing the mediastinum and causing an inversion of the diaphragm (Fig. 24.9).[40,41] Most frequently, part of one lung, or one entire lung, is affected, causing lateral displacement of the heart and mediastinum. Rarely, both lungs are affected,

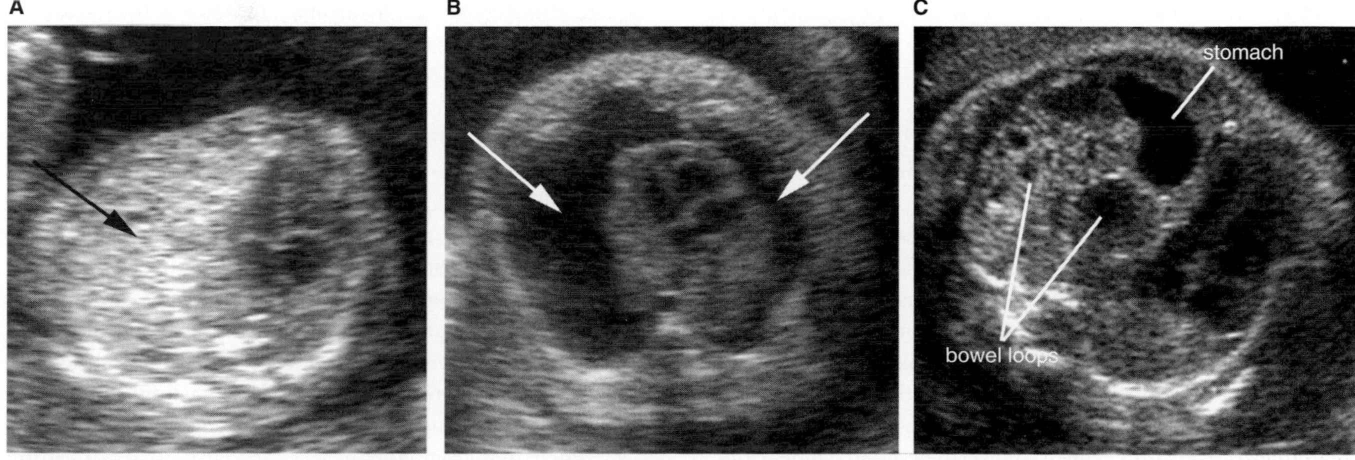

Figure 24.9 Thoracic anomalies. (A) Echogenic lung (arrow). (B) Bilateral pleural effusions (arrows) associated with hydrops and polyhydramnios. (C) Left diaphragmatic hernia: the heart is shifted to the right side of the chest and the left hemithorax is occupied by a complex area in which stomach and bowel loops can be recognized.

compressing both sides of the mediastinum. The pathophysiology is related to obstruction of the respiratory tree, which causes accumulation of fluid and secretions in the lungs. The effects of respiratory obstruction on the lungs are variable. Accumulation of fluid may lead to lung hyperplasia. Early and longstanding obstruction is probably responsible for the histological alterations that are commonly referred to as *cystic adenomatoid malformation* of the lungs. The etiology is variable. Obstruction may result from primary atresia or be the consequence of a mucus plug. A further possibility is pulmonary sequestration. With this condition, part of the lung develops separately from the bronchi and the pulmonary circulation, and is supplied through arteries that arise from the descending aorta. A differential diagnosis between these three conditions is often difficult. With lung sequestration, a specific diagnosis is possible by demonstrating the abnormal vessels connecting the aorta to the abnormal lung using color Doppler. Spontaneous regression or resolution of the increased echogenicity indicates that a mucus plug is the most likely hypothesis. When both lungs are affected, the most likely diagnosis is an obstruction of the upper airways, usually atresia of the trachea. Polyhydramnios and fetal hydrops may occur, particularly with bilateral echogenic lungs and large sequestration. Lung sequestration may also be associated with cardiac and diaphragmatic defects.

In some cases, macroscopic cysts may be associated with increased echogenicity. Occasionally, large and multiple cysts are the dominant finding. Cystic adenomatoid malformation is usually found at birth in these cases (macrocystic variety) and the pathophysiology probably overlaps that of echogenic lungs.

Unilateral echogenic and/or cystic lungs, without other anomalies or hydrops, have a very good outcome. The lesions usually decrease in size with gestation, and the infants are asymptomatic at birth. However, dysplastic lung tissue, is usually present and must be surgically removed.[42,43] Conversely, bilateral lesions or those associated with hydrops usually have a poor outcome. In these cases, drainage, or shunting of the cysts may be attempted.

Pleural effusions

Fetal pleural effusions may be an isolated finding or they may occur in association with generalized edema and ascites (Fig. 24.9).[44] Irrespective of the underlying cause, infants affected by pleural effusions usually present in the neonatal period with severe, and often fatal, respiratory insufficiency. This is either a direct result of pulmonary compression caused by the effusions or due to pulmonary hypoplasia secondary to chronic intrathoracic compression. Isolated pleural effusions in the fetus may either resolve spontaneously or they can be treated effectively after birth. Nevertheless, in some cases severe and chronic compression of the fetal lungs can result in pulmonary hypoplasia and neonatal death. In others, mediastinal compression leads to the development of hydrops and polyhydramnios, which are associated with a high risk of premature delivery and perinatal death. Attempts at prenatal therapy by repeated thoracocenteses for drainage of pleural effusions have been generally unsuccessful in reversing the hydropic state, because the fluid reaccumulates within 24–48 h of drainage. A better approach is chronic drainage by the insertion of thoracoamniotic shunts. This is useful both for diagnosis and treatment. First, the diagnosis of an underlying cardiac abnormality or other intrathoracic lesion may become apparent only after effective decompression and return of the mediastinum to its normal position. Second, it can reverse fetal hydrops, resolve polyhydramnios and thereby reduce the risk of preterm delivery, and may prevent pulmonary hypoplasia. Third, it may be useful in the prenatal diagnosis of pulmonary hypoplasia because in such cases the lungs often fail to expand after shunting. Furthermore, it may help distinguish between hydrops due to primary accumulation of pleural effusions, in which case the ascites and skin edema may resolve after shunting, and other causes of hydrops such as infection, in which drainage of the effusions does not prevent worsening of the hydrops. Survival after thoracoamniotic shunting is in the range of 50% and is more likely with isolated pleural effusions than with generalized hydrops.[45]

Diaphragmatic hernia

Diaphragmatic hernia is found in about 1 in 4000 births. Development of the diaphragm is usually completed by the ninth week of gestation. In the presence of a defective diaphragm there is herniation of the abdominal viscera into the thorax at about 10–12 weeks, when the intestines return to the abdominal cavity from the umbilical cord. However, at least in some cases intrathoracic herniation of viscera may be delayed until the second or third trimesters of pregnancy. Diaphragmatic hernia is usually a sporadic abnormality. However, in about 50% of affected fetuses there are associated chromosomal abnormalities (mainly trisomy 18, trisomy 13, and Pallister–Killian syndrome – mosaicism for tetrasomy 12p), other defects (mainly craniospinal defects, including spina bifida, hydrocephaly, and the otherwise rare iniencephaly, and cardiac abnormalities) and genetic syndromes (such as Fryns syndrome, de Lange syndrome, and Marfan syndrome).

Prenatally, the diaphragm is imaged by ultrasonography as an echo-free space between the thorax and abdomen. However, the integrity of the diaphragm is usually inferred from the normal disposition of the thoracic and abdominal organs. Diaphragmatic hernia is usually diagnosed by the ultrasonographic demonstration of stomach, intestines, or liver in the thorax and the associated mediastinal shift to the opposite side. Herniated abdominal contents, associated with a left-sided diaphragmatic hernia, are easy to demonstrate because the echo-free fluid-filled stomach and small bowel contrast dramatically with the more echogenic fetal lung (see Fig. 24.9). In contrast, a right-sided hernia is more difficult to identify because the echogenicity of the fetal liver is similar to that of the lung.

Antenatal prediction of pulmonary hypoplasia remains one of the challenges of prenatal diagnosis because this would be vital both in counseling parents and also in selecting those cases that may benefit from prenatal surgery. Poor prognostic signs include herniation of the liver into the fetal chest and a lung–head ratio (area of the demonstrable lung divided by head circumference) < 1.00.[46]

In the human, the bronchial tree is fully developed by the 16th week of gestation, at which time the full adult number of airways is established. In diaphragmatic hernia the reduced thoracic space available to the developing lung leads to reduction in airways, alveoli, and arteries. Thus, although isolated diaphragmatic hernia is an anatomically simple defect that is easily correctable, the mortality rate is high in cases with severe hernia.

In a few cases of diaphragmatic hernia, hysterotomy and fetal surgery were carried out but these interventions have now been abandoned. Endoscopic occlusion of the fetal trachea has also been carried out in human fetuses with diaphragmatic hernia but the preliminary experience thus far has not been encouraging.[47]

Conclusions

Sonography allows the detection of many congenital anomalies of the heart and thorax. Congenital heart defects are among the most common malformations and a major cause of perinatal death. Evaluation of the fetal heart allows a precise diagnosis of most major cardiac anomalies beginning early in gestation. However, a specific expertise is required. The outcome of some severe cardiac abnormalities may be ameliorated by prenatal diagnosis. Thoracic anomalies are rare. Echogenic lungs and diaphragmatic hernia are the most frequent entities. The former are usually benign, and although they may have a dramatic sonographic presentation, in general, they have a good prognosis. Diaphragmatic hernia continues to be associated with significant mortality and long-term morbidity. Despite many attempts, the value of antenatal treatment remains highly uncertain.

Acknowledgment

This chapter first appeared in thefetus.net and has been reproduced here with permission.

Key points

1 Congenital heart disease occurs in approximately 0.5% of births. In general, about one-half are either severe or require surgery early in life and are generally referred to as major cardiac abnormalities. Despite advances in pediatric cardiology and cardiac surgery heart defects remain a major cause of perinatal and infantile death.

2 Diagnosis of cardiac defects is possible; however, a specific examination is required (fetal echocardiogram) and this is usually performed in pregnancies with an increased risk. The sensitivity is in the range of 80%. Most of the severe cardiac anomalies can be recognized by at least mid-gestation.

3 While performing a standard sonogram from mid-gestation on, it is recommended to obtain a four-chamber view of the heart; the sensitivity of this approach varies in different studies, but the general consensus is that it is an acceptable approach.

4 Septal defects are the most common form of congenital heart disease. In most cases the lesions are small and prenatal diagnosis is not possible; these anomalies may have little clinical significance but at times require surgical correction.

5 Atrioventricular septal defects (or atrioventricular canal) are a more relevant entity mostly because of the very frequent association with other anomalies such as trisomy 21; diagnosis of this defect is simpler although false-negatives may occur.

6 The term univentricular heart applies to anomalies in which the atria are connected with one single ventricular chamber. These anomalies constitute the lion's share of the cardiac malformations diagnosed *in utero*. These conditions can be treated after birth with a likelihood of survival at 3 years in the range of 60%; only complex palliative procedures are possible, however, and the long-term outcome remains difficult to predict.

7 Hypoplastic left heart syndrome includes a continuum of malformations that share in common atresia or extreme hypoplasia of the aorta; it is one of the major causes of perinatal and infant death. The most important clue to the diagnosis is the presence of a very small left ventricle and ascending aorta, typically with inversion of blood flow into the aortic arch. Survival may be increased by prenatal diagnosis. Only 30% of infants diagnosed *in utero* are alive, however, at follow-up in 3 years.

8 A disproportion in the size of the ventricles with a predominance of the right side is very frequently a presenting sign of fetal coarctation or interrupted aortic arch; a definitive diagnosis may be difficult *in utero* and at times can only be made after birth.

9 Aortic and pulmonary stenosis are among the most frequent cardiac anomalies; however, mild and moderate cases go usually undetected *in utero*. Prenatal diagnosis is limited to the severe varieties that may

progress *in utero* toward hypoplastic left heart or pulmonary atresia with intact septum.

10 Tricuspid dysplasia and Ebstein's malformation of the tricuspid valve may be complicated by severe tricuspid insufficiency, cardiomegaly, and hydrops; such combination is most frequently lethal, with very few infants surviving.

11 Conotruncal anomalies include transposition of the great arteries, tetralogy of Fallot, double outlet right ventricle, and truncus arteriosus communis. They represent about 30% of congenital heart defects and usually have a good outcome if adequately treated after birth in that usually biventricular repair is possible. Diagnosis is difficult because assessing the connections between ventricles and great arteries requires meticulous scanning; however, prenatal diagnosis would be important because at times these conditions (complete transposition in particular) represent neonatal emergencies.

12 Heterotaxy, or cardiosplenic syndromes, includes a group of anomalies characterized by the association between cardiac defects and anomalous disposition of abdominal organs; cardiovascular malformations are frequently complex and the prognosis tends to be poor.

13 Irregular patterns of fetal heart rhythms are frequent. Short periods of tachycardia, bradycardia, and ectopic beats as well are very commonly seen, and in the vast majority of cases have no clinical significance. A sustained bradycardia of less than 100 bpm, a sustained tachycardia of more than 200 bpm and irregular beats occurring more than 1 in 10 should be considered abnormal and require further investigation. The techniques of choice for the diagnosis of fetal dysrhythmias are M-mode and/or spectral Doppler ultrasound.

14 Premature atrial or ventricular beats are by far the most frequent fetal arrhythmias. They are benign, are not associated with an increased risk of cardiac malformations, and tend to disappear throughout gestation. Serial monitoring has been recommended because, although rare, they sometimes can evolve toward fetal tachycardia.

15 Fetal tachycardias (frequency greater than 200 bpm) are potentially serious dysrhythmias that may cause fetal hydrops and perinatal death. Treatment is possible, however, usually by maternal administration of antiarrhythmic agents, and the survival rate exceeds 90%.

16 Congenital complete heart block may occur either as a consequence of a cardiac malformation (heterotaxy or corrected transposition) or because of transplacental passage of maternal autoimmune (anti-Ro and anti-La) antibodies. In the former case, prognosis is poor; in the latter, most infants survive. Maternal administration of steroids has been proposed for the treatment of immune heart block.

17 Echogenic lungs arise as a consequence of cystic adenomatoid malformation of the lungs, airway obstruction, or lung sequestration. There is clinical as well as pathophysiological overlapping among these entities, however, when they are not complicated by hydrops they have a good outcome generally.

18 Pleural effusion may be isolated or a part of fetal hydrops. Primitive pleural effusions may evolve toward hydrops, probably because they compress the mediastinum and obstruct venous return to the heart; prenatal treatment is possible by implantation of a thoracoamniotic shunt; survival rate is in the range of 50%.

19 Diaphragmatic hernia is a severe fetal anomaly that can be treated after birth but continues to be associated with significant mortality and morbidity as a consequence of lung hypoplasia. Diagnosis is possible and is based upon demonstration of abdominal organs into the fetal chest. The identification of cases with only bowel loops herniated in the second trimester and of the right diaphragmatic hernias remains difficult; some sonographic findings including the herniation of the liver into the chest and the ratio of the demonstrable lung to the head have prognostic implications.

20 Prenatal treatment of diaphragmatic hernia has been attempted using different strategies. Open fetal surgery had been abandoned. More recently attempts have been made by tracheal occlusion using endoscopic techniques but the first series has not been encouraging.

References

1 Allan L. Antenatal diagnosis of heart disease. *Heart* 2000; 83(3):367.

2 Allan L, Benacerraf B, Copel JA, et al. Isolated major congenital heart disease. *Ultrasound Obstet Gynecol* 2001;17:370–379.

3 Chaoui R, McEwing R. Three cross-sectional planes for fetal color Doppler echocardiography. *Ultrasound Obstet Gynecol* 2003; 21(1):81–93.

4 Yagel S, Cohen SM, Achiron R. Examination of the fetal heart by five short-axis views: a proposed screening method for comprehensive cardiac evaluation. *Ultrasound Obstet Gynecol* 2001;17: 367–9.

5 Randall P, Brealey S, Hahn S, et al. Accuracy of fetal echocardiography in the routine detection of congenital heart disease among unselected and low risk populations: a systematic review. *Br J Gynaecol* 2005;112(1):24–30.

6 Copel JA, Pilu G, Green J, et al. Fetal echocardiographic screening for congenital heart disease: the importance of the four-chamber view. *Am J Obstet Gynecol* 1987;157: 648–655.

7 Tegnander E, Eik-Nes SH, Johansen OJ, Linker DT. Prenatal detection of heart defects at the routine fetal examination at 18

weeks in a non-selected population. *Ultrasound Obstet Gynecol* 1995;5:372–380.

8 Goncalves LF, Espinoza J, Lee W, et al. A new approach to fetal echocardiography: digital casts of the fetal cardiac chambers and great vessels for detection of congenital heart disease. *J Ultrasound Med* 2005;24(4):415–424.

9 Espinoza J, Goncalves LF, Lee W, et al. A novel method to improve prenatal diagnosis of abnormal systemic venous connections using three- and four-dimensional ultrasonography and 'inversion mode'. *Ultrasound Obstet Gynecol* 2005;25(5):428–434.

10 Chaoui R, Hoffmann J, Heling KS. Three-dimensional (3D) and 4D color Doppler fetal echocardiography using spatio-temporal image correlation (STIC). *Ultrasound Obstet Gynecol* 2004;23: 535–545.

11 DeVore GR, Falkensammer P, Sklansky MS, Platt LD. Spatio-temporal image correlation (STIC): new technology for evaluation of the fetal heart. *Ultrasound Obstet Gynecol* 2003;22: 380–387.

12 Vinals F, Mandujano L, Vargas G, Giuliano A. Prenatal diagnosis of congenital heart disease using four-dimensional spatio-temporal image correlation (STIC) telemedicine via an Internet link: a pilot study. *Ultrasound Obstet Gynecol* 2005;25(1): 25–31.

13 Vinals F, Poblete P, Giuliano A. Spatio-temporal image correlation (STIC): a new tool for the prenatal screening of congenital heart defects. *Ultrasound Obstet Gynecol* 2003;22:388–394.

14 Paladini D, Palmieri S, Lamberti A, et al. Characterization and natural history of ventricular septal defects in the fetus. *Ultrasound Obstet Gynecol* 2000;16:118–122.

15 Yagel S, Valsky DV, Messing B. Detailed assessment of fetal ventricular septal defect with 4D color Doppler ultrasound using spatio-temporal image correlation technology. *Ultrasound Obstet Gynecol* 2005;25(1):97–98.

16 Allan LD. Atrioventricular septal defect in the fetus. *Am J Obstet Gynecol* 1999;181:1250–1253.

17 Bronshtein M, Egenburg S, Auslander R, Zimmer EZ. Atrioventricular septal defect in a fetus: a false negative diagnosis in early pregnancy. *Ultrasound Obstet Gynecol* 2000;16(1):98–99.

18 Grandjean H, Larroque D, Levi S. The performance of routine ultrasonographic screening of pregnancies in the Eurofetus Study. *Am J Obstet Gynecol* 1999;181(2):446–454.

19 Machlitt A, Heling KS, Chaoui R. Increased cardiac atrial-to-ventricular length ratio in the fetal four-chamber view: a new marker for atrioventricular septal defects. *Ultrasound Obstet Gynecol* 2004;24(6):618–622.

20 Machado MV, Crawford DC, Anderson RH, Allan LD. Atrioventricular septal defect in prenatal life. *Br Heart J* 1988;59: 352–355.

21 Perolo A, Prandstraller D, Ghi T, et al. Diagnosis and management of fetal cardiac anomalies: 10 years of experience at a single institution. *Ultrasound Obstet Gynecol* 2001;18:615–618.

22 Chaoui R, Kalache KD, Heling KS, et al. Absent or hypoplastic thymus on ultrasound: a marker for deletion 22q11.2 in fetal cardiac defects. *Ultrasound Obstet Gynecol* 2002;20:546–552.

23 Allan LD, Sharland G, Tynan MJ. The natural history of the hypoplastic left heart syndrome. *Int J Cardiol* 1989;25:341–343.

24 Tworetzky W, McElhinney DB, Reddy VM, et al. Improved surgical outcome after fetal diagnosis of hypoplastic left heart syndrome. *Circulation* 2001;103:1269–1273.

25 Copel JA, Tan AS, Kleinman CS. Does a prenatal diagnosis of congenital heart disease alter short-term outcome? *Ultrasound Obstet Gynecol* 1997;10:237–241.

26 Allan LD, Crawford DC, Tynan MJ. Pulmonary atresia in prenatal life. *J Am Coll Cardiol* 1986;8:1131–1136.

27 Hornberger LK, Sahn DJ, Kleinman CS, et al. Tricuspid valve disease with significant tricuspid insufficiency in the fetus: diagnosis and outcome. *J Am Coll Cardiol* 1991;17(1):167–173.

28 Paladini D, Rustico M, Todros T, et al. Conotruncal anomalies in prenatal life. *Ultrasound Obstet Gynecol* 1996;8:241–246.

29 Bonnet D, Coltri A, Butera G, et al. Detection of transposition of the great arteries in fetuses reduces neonatal morbidity and mortality. *Circulation* 1999;99:916–918.

30 Phoon CK, Villegas MD, Ursell PC, Silverman NH. Left atrial isomerism detected in fetal life. *Am J Cardiol* 1996;77:1083–1088.

31 Atkinson DE, Drant S. Diagnosis of heterotaxy syndrome by fetal echocardiography. *Am J Cardiol* 1998;82:1147–1149, A10.

32 Allan LD, Anderson RH, Sullivan ID, et al. Evaluation of fetal arrhythmias by echocardiography. *Br Heart J* 1983;50:240–245.

33 Kleinman CS, Copel JA, Weinstein EM, et al. In utero diagnosis and treatment of fetal supraventricular tachycardia. *Semin Perinatol* 1985;9:113–129.

34 Hansmann M, Gembruch U, Bald R, et al. Fetal tachyarrhythmias: transplacental and direct treatment of the fetus: a report of 60 cases. *Ultrasound Obstet Gynecol* 1991;1:162–168.

35 Maxwell DJ, Crawford DC, Curry PV, Tynan MJ, Allan LD. Obstetric importance, diagnosis, and management of fetal tachycardias. *Br Med J* 1988;297:107–110.

36 van Engelen AD, Weijtens O, Brenner JI, et al. Management outcome and follow-up of fetal tachycardia. *J Am Coll Cardiol* 1994;24:1371–1375.

37 Friedman DM, Buyon JP. Complete atrioventricular block diagnosed prenatally: anything new on the block? *Ultrasound Obstet Gynecol* 2005;26(1):2–3.

38 Jaeggi ET, Hornberger LK, Smallhorn JF, Fouron JC. Prenatal diagnosis of complete atrioventricular block associated with structural heart disease: combined experience of two tertiary care centers and review of the literature. *Ultrasound Obstet Gynecol* 2005;26(1):16–21.

39 Berg C, Geipel A, Kohl T, Breuer J, Germer U, Krapp M, et al. Atrioventricular block detected in fetal life: associated anomalies and potential prognostic markers. *Ultrasound Obstet Gynecol* 2005;26(1):4–15.

40 Achiron R, Strauss S, Seidman DS, Lipitz S, Mashiach S, Goldman B. Fetal lung hyperechogenicity: prenatal ultrasonographic diagnosis, natural history and neonatal outcome. *Ultrasound Obstet Gynecol* 1995;6(1):40–2.

41 Achiron R, Zalel Y, Lipitz S, Hegesh J, Mazkereth R, Kuint J, et al. Fetal lung dysplasia: clinical outcome based on a new classification system. *Ultrasound Obstet Gynecol* 2004;24(2): 127–33.

42 Cacciari A, Ceccarelli PL, Pilu GL, Bianchini MA, Mordenti M, Gabrielli S, et al. A series of 17 cases of congenital cystic adenomatoid malformation of the lung: management and outcome. *Eur J Pediatr Surg* 1997;7(2):84–9.

43 Davenport M, Warne SA, Cacciaguerra S, Patel S, Greenough A, Nicolaides K. Current outcome of antenally diagnosed cystic lung disease. *J Pediatr Surg* 2004;39(4):549–56.

44 Estoff JA, Parad RB, Frigoletto FDJ, Benacerraf B. The natural history of isolated fetal hydrothorax. *Ultrasound Obstet Gynecol* 1992;2(3):162–5.

45 Smith RP, Illanes S, Denbow ML, Soothill PW. Outcome of fetal pleural effusions treated by thoracoamniotic shunting. *Ultrasound Obstet Gynecol* 2005;26(1):63–66.

46 Lipshutz GS, Albanese CT, Feldstein VA, et al. Prospective analysis of lung-to-head ratio predicts survival for patients with prenatally diagnosed congenital diaphragmatic hernia. *J Pediatr Surg* 1997;32:1634–1636.

47 Cortes RA, Keller RL, Townsend T, et al. Survival of severe congenital diaphragmatic hernia has morbid consequences. *J Pediatr Surg* 2005;40(1):36–45; discussion 45–6.

25 Gastrointestinal and genitourinary anomalies

Sandro Gabrielli, Nicola Rizzo, and E. Albert Reece

Gastrointestinal anomalies

Structural anomalies of the gastrointestinal (GI) tract are relatively common. Fetuses with GI anomalies, which often allow a good quality of life after postnatal surgical correction, largely benefit from prenatal diagnosis.[1] Anomalies can be subdivided into two groups: intestinal obstructions and ventral wall defects.

Normal ultrasound anatomy of gastrointestinal and urinary tract

The liver occupies most of the upper abdomen, showing a homogeneous, echogenic ultrasound pattern. The portal circulation, the hepatic veins, the hepatic arteries, and the biliary ducts represent the ductal system crossing into the liver. The gallbladder is often distended *in utero*, appearing as a pear-shaped, fluid-filled structure arising from the hilum, and angles from the anteroposterior axis of the abdomen at 45°. The intra-abdominal umbilical vein can be confused with the gallbladder. The left umbilical vein (the right umbilical vein is reabsorbed before 6–7 weeks' gestation) penetrates into the abdomen through the umbilical ring; it runs centrally and cranially, entering the liver and receiving the venae advehentes, and then anastomoses with the left portal vein. From the junction with the left portal vein, the oxygenated blood may reach the heart through the ductus venosus or the hepatic veins. The stomach is almost constantly distended and, in a transverse scan, appears as a semilunar, fluid-filled, and neatly outlined area. Stomach dimensions can vary significantly at each gestational age, due to the filling and emptying state. An axial section, in which the intrahepatic umbilical vein, the stomach, and the liver are simultaneously visualized, is used to measure the abdominal circumference (Fig. 25.1).[2] The spleen appears as a triangular area posterior to the stomach, with a similar structure to the liver. The study of the visceral situs is of great importance as structural cardiac defects are frequently associated with abnormal location of abdominal viscera (polysplenic and asplenic syndromes). Normally, the stomach and spleen are located on the left side, while the portal sinus, which corresponds to the hepatic hilum, is on the right side; the descending aorta can be visualized close to the vertebrae and slightly on the left, the inferior vena cava more anteriorly and on the right. The fetal bowel is usually uniformly echogenic, and it may be difficult to distinguish bowel from liver, particularly in the second and early third trimester. Late in pregnancy, loops distended by the accumulating meconium are easily visualized. In the second trimester, a diffuse hyperechogenicity is quite often seen in the lower abdomen (Fig. 25.2). This finding is of no clinical significance when isolated. It has been reported, however, in association with trisomy 21, cystic fibrosis, and intrauterine growth retardation (IUGR).[3] Hyperechogenicity seems to be a consequence of intra-amniotic bleeding.[4] During the third trimester, as meconium accumulates in the lumen of the bowel, a suspicion of pathological obstructive dilation is sometimes raised. Loops of small and large bowel measuring less than 7 and 20 mm, respectively, seem to be perfectly normal. Therefore, ultrasound diagnosis of bowel obstruction is rather difficult. An increased fluid content in the lumen of the bowel, giving a clearly anechoic picture, is another useful criterion for diagnosis.

All components of the urinary system, except ureters, can be visualized *in utero* from the beginning of the early second trimester. Viewing a cross-section of the abdomen, as early as 14 weeks' and up to 20 weeks' gestation, the kidneys appear circular and slightly hypoechoic, compared with the liver and bowel loops, at both sides of the vertebral bodies.[5]

At 20 weeks, the kidneys show a hyperechoic capsule, the parenchyma is less hyperechoic, and calices sometimes surround a minimally physiologically dilated pelvis. This dilated pelvis has nothing to do with hydronephrosis, and is probably due to a more efficient diuresis than in later gestation. At this gestational age, the cortical area is slightly more echogenic than the medulla.[6]

With progressing gestation, fat tissue accumulates around the kidneys, enhancing the borders of the kidneys in contrast

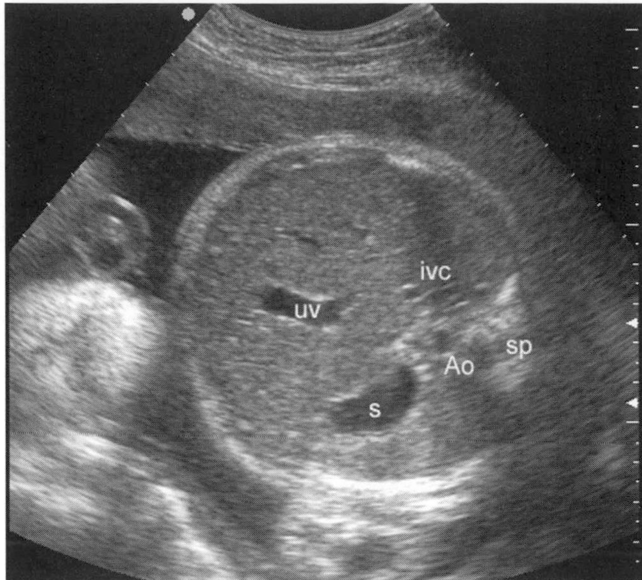

Figure 25.1 Cross-section of the fetal trunk during the second trimester of pregnancy, showing the intrahepatic umbilical vein (uv). Ao, aorta; ivc, inferior vena cava; s,stomach; sp, spine.

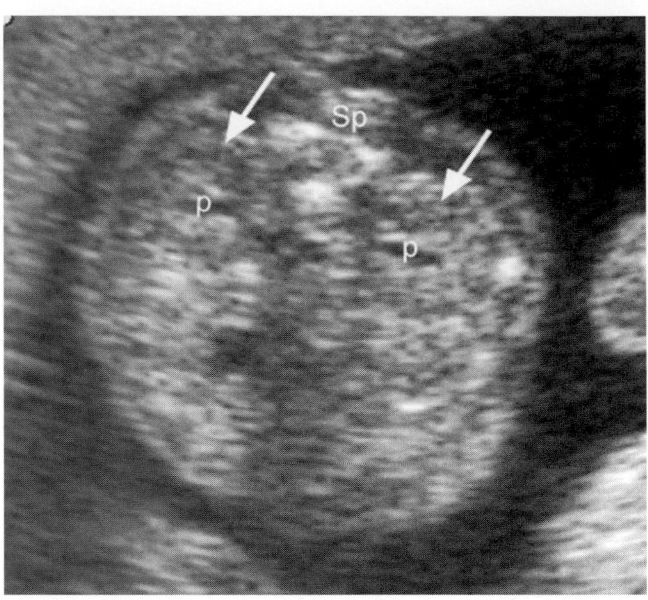

Figure 25.3 Cross-section of the abdomen of a fetus during the second trimester, demonstrating normal kidneys (k) at both sides of the spine (Sp); p, pelvis.

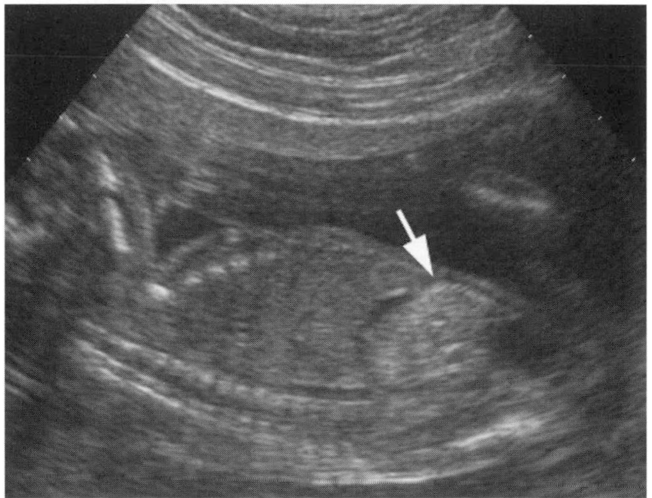

Figure 25.2 Longitudinal scan of the fetal trunk at 22 weeks' gestation showing diffuse hyperechogenicity of the lower abdomen (arrow).

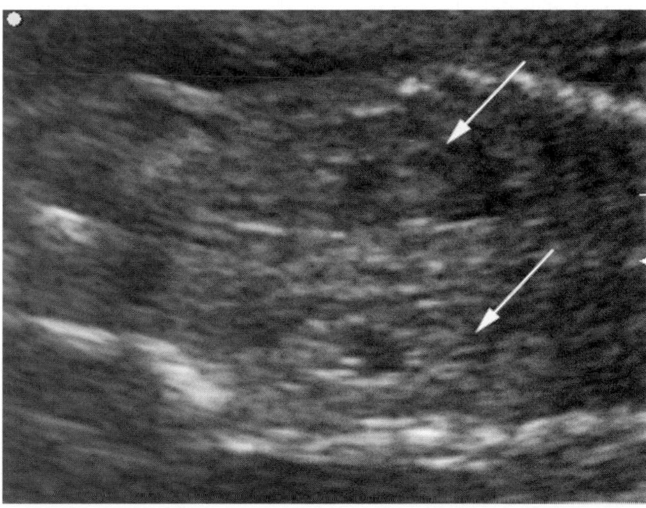

Figure 25.4 Coronal scan of the fetal trunk at 21 weeks' gestation, demonstrating the kidneys (k) as elliptical masses.

with the other splanchnic organs. Around 26–27 weeks' gestation, renal pyramids can be detected, and the arcuate arteries can be seen pulsating in their proximity in real-time ultrasonography.

During the midtrimester, kidneys should be differentiated from adrenals by looking for the renal pelvis.

Transverse and coronal sections of the abdomen can be used to study the kidneys. In a transverse scan, kidneys appear as roundish structures at both sides of the spine, while on coronal scans, they appear as elliptical areas (Figs 25.3 and 25.4). On a cross-section of the abdomen, kidneys cover less than one-third of the surface of the entire abdomen. Biometry of the kidneys has been suggested by various authors to diagnose congenital anomalies.[7] Moreover, on coronal scans, renal arteries are clearly seen with color power Doppler (Fig. 25.5).

The fetal bladder can be detected as a fluid-filled area in the anterior lower abdomen from early midtrimester, when urine formation begins. At both sides of the bladder, branches of the umbilical artery are visualized with color power Doppler

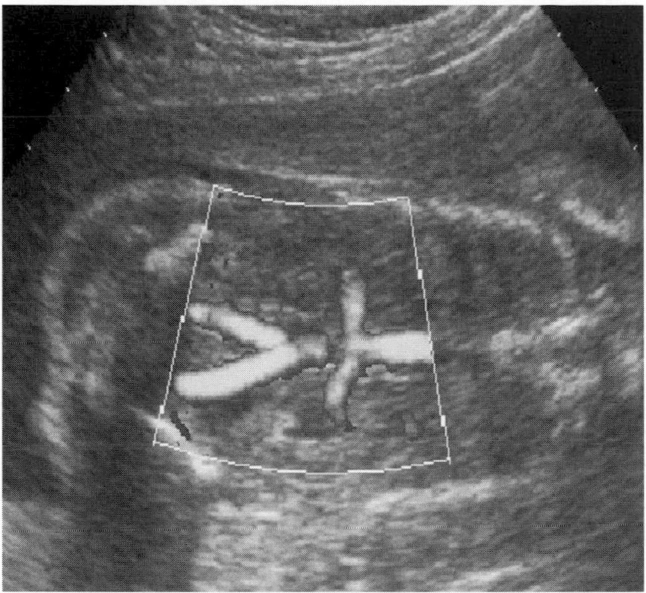

Figure 25.5 Renal arteries are visualized on coronal scans with color power Doppler.

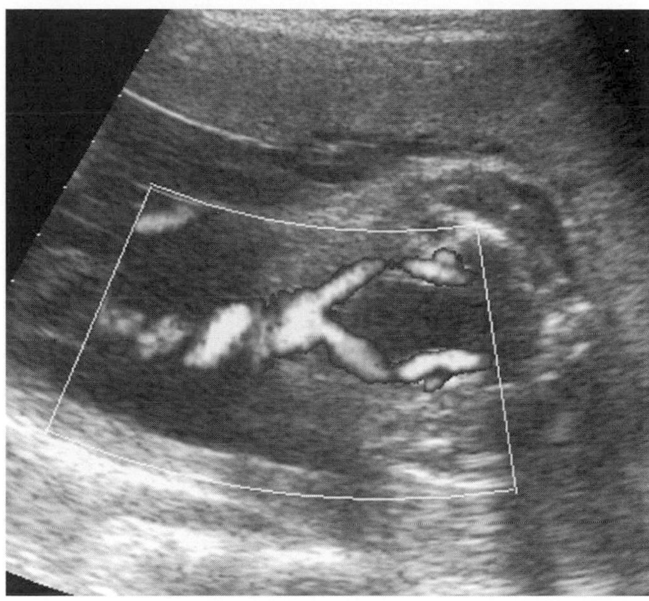

Figure 25.6 Branches of the umbilical artery are clearly seen at both sides of the urinary bladder.

(Fig. 25.6). The contribution of the kidneys to the amniotic fluid dynamics is little before 16 weeks, but it increases steadily throughout gestation so that, in the second half of gestation, amniotic fluid is formed mostly by urine.[8] Change in shape and volume depends on alternate emptying and filling. It has been demonstrated that micturition occurs approximately every 110 min.[9] The fetal bladder, however, should always be visualized, because of incomplete emptying.

Obstructions

The echo-free areas resulting from fluid collection and progressive dilation of the bowel cephalad to the obstruction site are easily detected by ultrasound.[10] Furthermore, a GI obstruction is often associated with hydramnios, allowing a better visualization. A proximal obstruction can be expected in approximately 1 in 15 pregnancies with polyhydramnios.[11] GI obstructions can involve the esophagus, duodenum, and small bowel; they can be intrinsic or extrinsic (e.g., intrathoracic cyst or annular pancreas). Conversely, distal obstructions are not usually associated with hydramnios, and their detection is rather more difficult.

Esophageal atresia

Esophageal atresia is a relatively frequent anomaly, occurring in 1 in 3000–3500 live births. It is caused by an impairment in the process of recanalization of the primitive esophagus. An abnormal connection between trachea and esophagus is usually derived from an imperfect development of the respiratory diverticulum. In the most common type of fistula (90–95%), the upper portion of the esophagus ends blindly (esophageal atresia), and the lower portion develops from the trachea near the bifurcation. The two portions of the esophagus may be connected by a solid cord. Less common are: (1) the upper portion ending in the trachea, the lower portion being of variable length; (2) double fistula, in which upper and lower portions end in the trachea; (3) tracheo-esophageal fistula without esophageal atresia; (4) esophageal atresia without tracheo-esophageal fistula; and (5) tracheal aplasia (lethal).

Severe structural anomalies are associated in nearly 50% of cases, including heart, GI, and genitourinary (GU) tract anomalies, skeletal deformities, cleft defects of the face, and central nervous system (CNS) lesions such as meningoceles or hydrocephalus. Chromosomal anomalies, particularly trisomy 21,[12] are also commonly present. The VACTERL syndrome refers to a condition where vertebral, anorectal, and cardiac anomalies, tracheo-esophageal fistula, esophageal atresia, renal anomalies, and limb anomalies are associated.[13]

Prenatal diagnosis is suspected when, in the presence of polyhydramnios (usually after 25 weeks), serial ultrasound examinations fail to demonstrate the fetal stomach, or the stomach appears permanently small (< 15% of the abdominal circumference) (Fig. 25.7);[14] gastric secretions, however, may be sufficient to distend the stomach and make it visible. Also, in the case of an associated fistula, the stomach may look normal. Occasionally, after 25 weeks, the dilated proximal esophageal pouch can be seen as an elongated upper mediastinal and retrocardiac anechoic structure (Fig. 25.8). The

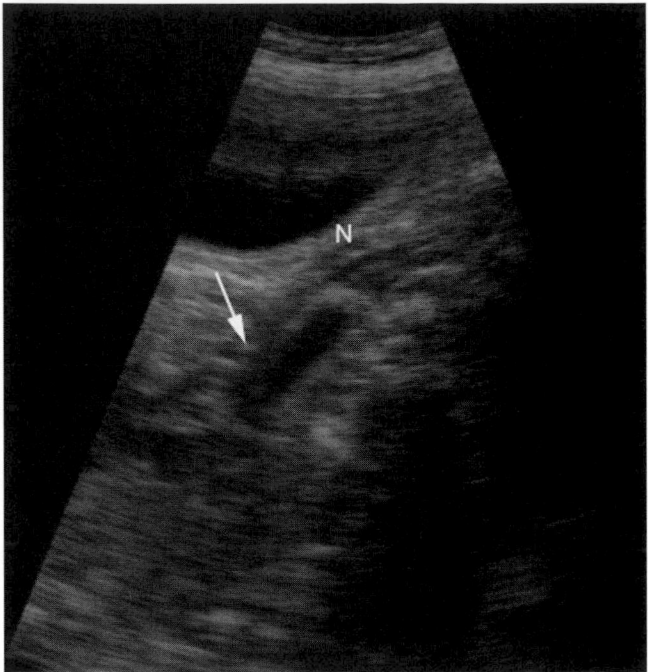

Figure 25.7 Coronal section of the neck in a fetus with esophageal atresia, showing the blind end of the esophagus (arrow). N, neck.

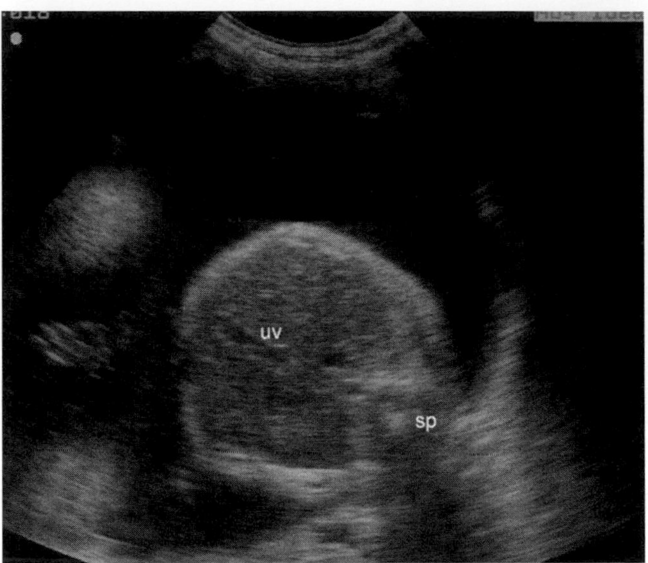

Figure 25.8 Cross-section of the fetal abdomen in a fetus with esophageal atresia. Stomach is not visualized. sp, spine; uv, umbilical vein.

differential diagnosis for the combination of absent stomach and polyhydramnios includes intrathoracic compression, from conditions such as diaphragmatic hernia, and musculoskeletal anomalies, causing inability of the fetus to swallow.

Factors such as associated anomalies, respiratory complications at birth, gestational age at delivery, and neonatal weight play the most important prognostic role. Thus, for babies with an isolated tracheo-esophageal fistula, born after 32 weeks, when an early diagnosis is made, avoiding reflux and aspiration pneumonitis, the postoperative survival rate is more than 95%. In the case of fetal weight < 2.5 kg and in the presence of respiratory complications or other anomalies, the survival rate decreases to 6%.[15] Drainage of fluid can be performed in cases of severe polyhydramnios. Time and mode of delivery are not influenced by prenatal diagnosis. Delay in postnatal recognition, however, results in increased neonatal morbidity and mortality.[16] Prenatal diagnosis alerts the pediatrician, facilitates prompt neonatal diagnostic confirmation, and enables the prevention of potentially severe complications, such as aspiration pneumonia.

Duodenal obstruction

Duodenal obstruction occurs in approximately 1 in 7500–10 000 live births. It is a sporadic abnormality, although in some cases there is an autosomal-recessive pattern of inheritance. The anomaly can be either extrinsic or intrinsic. Extrinsic lesions are mainly the consequence of a compression of the duodenum by the surrounding annular pancreas or by peritoneal fibrous bands. Duodenal atresia or stenosis (intrinsic lesions) derives from an incomplete developmental process during the second and third month of fetal life.[17] As the intestine turns from a solid structure into an empty tubular one, the persistence of one or more septa, resulting in a diaphragm, is defined as stenosis. Complete atresia develops from the separation of solid intestine into two or more blind portions, which can be either totally isolated from each other or connected by fibrous bands.

Approximately half of the fetuses with duodenal atresia have associated abnormalities, including trisomy 21 in about 40% of the cases and skeletal defects (vertebral and rib anomalies, sacral agenesis, radial abnormalities, and talipes), gastrointestinal abnormalities (esophageal atresia/tracheo-esophageal fistula, intestinal malrotation, Meckel diverticulum, and anorectal atresia), and cardiac and renal defects.

Detection of two echo-free areas inside the abdomen ("double-bubble" sign), representing the dilated stomach and the first portion of the duodenum, is crucial for prenatal diagnosis[18] (Fig. 25.9). Polyhydramnios is invariably associated. However, obstruction due to a central web may result in only a "single bubble," representing the fluid-filled stomach. Sonographic demonstration of continuity of the duodenum with the stomach enables differentiation of a distended duodenum from other cystic masses, including choledocal or hepatic cysts (Fig. 25.10).[19] Potential pitfalls derive from visualization of a double bubble on a longitudinal scan of the fetal trunk in cases of intense peristaltic activity. By performing axial scans of the trunk, one should avoid a misdiagnosis. Prenatal diagnosis is not usually made until after

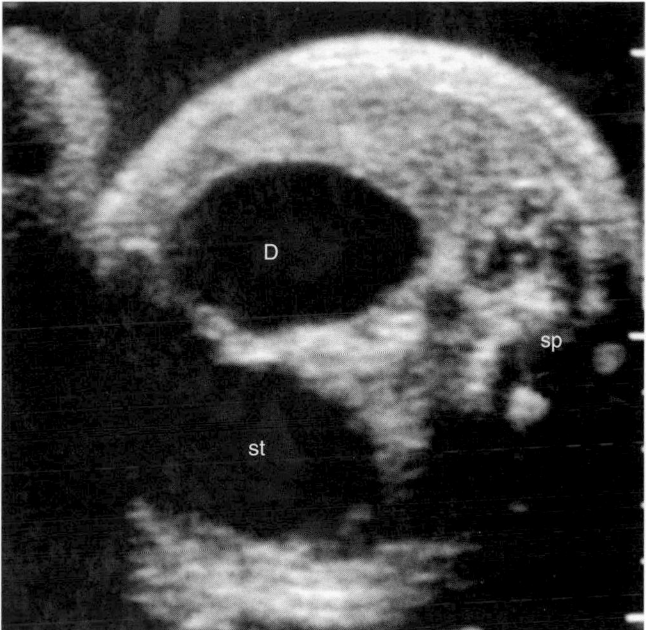

Figure 25.9 Cross-section of the upper fetal abdomen in a case of duodenal atresia, showing the pathognomonic "double-bubble" sign. D, dilated duodenal bulb; sp, spine; st, stomach.

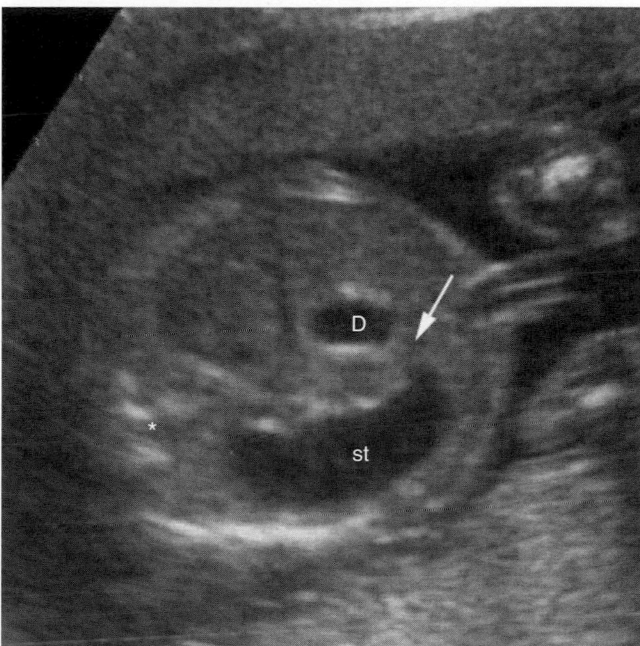

Figure 25.10 Oblique scan of the abdomen in a fetus with duodenal atresia. Notice the thin connection between stomach and duodenum (arrow). D, duodenum; st, stomach.

25 weeks, suggesting that the fetus is unable to swallow a sufficient volume of amniotic fluid for bowel dilation to occur before midtrimester. Diagnosis has occasionally been reported in the second trimester. Recently, a case of duodenal atresia has been recognized in the first trimester.[20]

Postnatal prognosis of duodenal atresia depends mainly on the following: associated anomalies, birthweight, and prompt confirmation of prenatal diagnosis.

Survival after surgery in patients with an isolated anomaly is more than 95%. Obstetric management is not influenced by prenatal diagnosis; however, spontaneous premature labor is frequent due to polyhydramnios. Prenatal diagnosis allows prevention of neonatal vomiting or aspiration pneumonia through early aspiration of gastric contents.

Intestinal obstructions (below the level of the duodenum)

Intestinal obstructions occur in about 1 in 2000 births. In about half of the cases, there is small bowel obstruction and, in the other half, anorectal atresia. Small bowel obstruction may derive from primary atresia or stenosis of the bowel, meconium ileus, and extrinsic constriction from adhesions. The most frequent site of small bowel obstruction is the distal ileus, followed by the proximal jejunum. In about 5% of cases, obstructions occur in multiple sites. Although the condition is usually sporadic, in multiple intestinal atresias, familial cases have been described.

Associated abnormalities and chromosomal defects are rare. However, in the case of anorectal atresia, associated defects such as genitourinary, vertebral, cardiovascular, and gastrointestinal anomalies are found in about 80% of cases. Meconium ileus may be associated with cystic fibrosis.

The lumen of the small bowel and colon does not normally exceed 7 mm and 20 mm respectively. Diagnosis of obstruction is usually made late in pregnancy, after 25 weeks, because dilation of the intestinal lumen is slow and progressive. Jejunal and ileal obstructions are imaged as multiple fluid-filled loops of bowel in the abdomen (Fig. 25.11).[21] The more distal the site of the obstruction, the greater the number of anechoic structures (Fig. 25.12). The abdomen is usually distended, and active peristalsis may be observed. If bowel perforation occurs, transient ascites, meconium peritonitis, and meconium pseudocysts may ensue. Polyhydramnios, usually after 25 weeks, is common, especially with proximal obstructions.[22] Similar bowel appearances and polyhydramnios may be found in fetuses with Hirschprung disease, the megacystis–microcolon–intestinal hypoperistalsis syndrome, and chloride diarrhea. The differential diagnosis of small bowel obstruction includes renal tract abnormalities and other intra-abdominal cysts such as mesenteric, ovarian, or duplication cysts. A specific clue for bowel obstruction is the presence of peristalsis. Prenatal diagnosis of anorectal atresia is rather difficult, because the proximal bowel may not demonstrate significant dilation, and the amniotic fluid volume is usually normal; occasionally, calcified intraluminal meconium may be seen in the fetal pelvis.

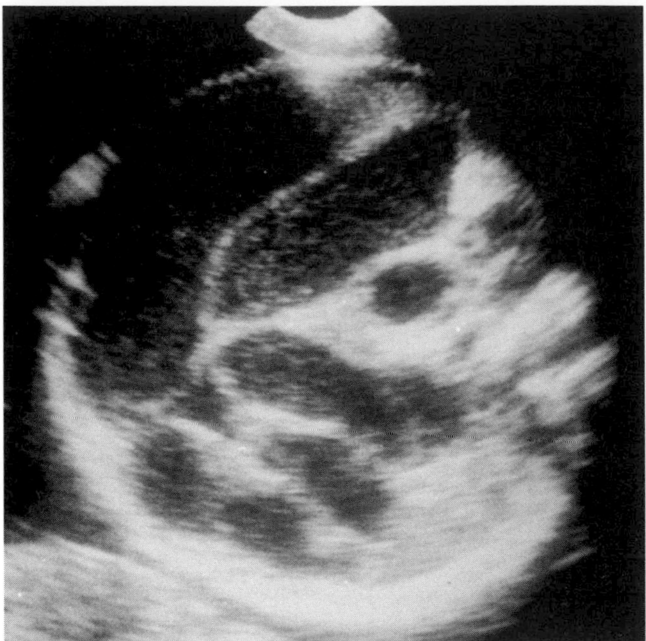

Figure 25.11 Cross-section of the abdomen in a fetus with small bowel atresia. Dilated bowel is visible.

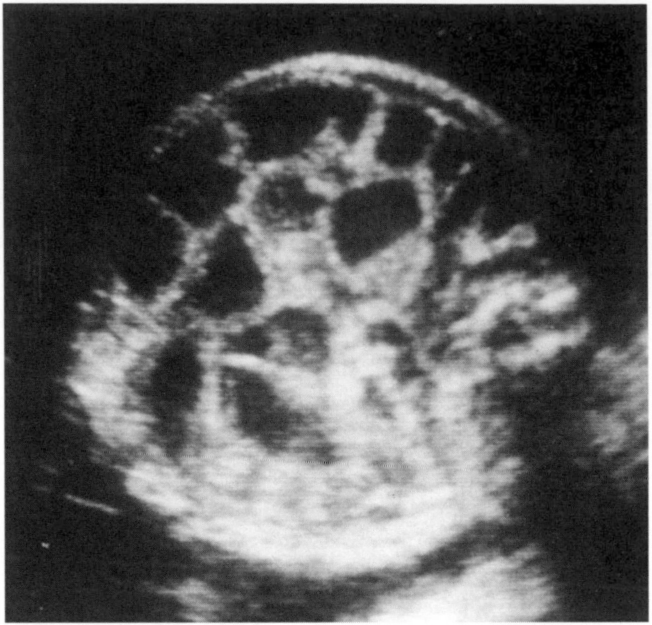

Figure 25.12 Cross-section of the abdomen in a fetus with small bowel atresia. Multiple distended loops of bowel are visible.

The prognosis is related to gestational age at delivery, associated abnormalities, and the site of obstruction.[23] In those born after 32 weeks with isolated obstruction requiring resection of only short segments of bowel, the survival rate is more than 95%. Loss of large segments of bowel can lead to short gut syndrome, which is a lethal condition.

Fetuses with uncomplicated intestinal obstruction can be delivered vaginally at term. Induction should be considered when perforation with ascites occurs. In these cases, fetal paracentesis to decrease abdominal pressure on the diaphragm, thus allowing expansion of the lungs, may be indicated.[24] If perforation and bleeding into the abdominal cavity occur, delay in delivery may cause hydrops fetalis, owing to severe anemia, decreased oncotic pressure, and loss of plasma volume.[25]

Meconium peritonitis

Meconium peritonitis is a chemically sterile peritonitis consequent to intestinal perforation *in utero*. Various conditions may be the cause: intestinal atresia, vulvulus, meconium ileus, etc. In 25–40% of cases, it is secondary to perforation of a meconium ileus such as in the case of cystic fibrosis. In a minority of cases, the cause remains unknown.

As meconium begins to accumulate in fetal bowel at 4 months, any perforation occurring after that time could bring the outflow of meconium into the peritoneal cavity. As a result, an intense reaction occurs, leading to extensive adhesions. If it is localized at the site of perforation, a calcified mass develops (fibroadhesive type). In other cases (cystic type), the continuous outflow of intestinal content into a cavity (pseudocyst) determines the formation of a highly echogenic mass at the site of the perforation (Fig. 25.13). Polyhydramnios is a frequent finding; ascites may also be present.[26]

A peritonitis can be suspected when a fetus affected by intestinal obstruction suddenly shows the presence of ascites or generalized hydrops. Differential diagnosis should be made with other abdominal masses, in particular with abdominal teratomas and gallbladder calcifications. However, teratomas are complex masses, and gallbladder calcifications are strictly connected with the gallbladder.

Prognosis is generally severe. Only a few cases have been described in the literature; therefore, the most suitable management of pregnancy is still questioned. Serial ultrasound examinations are indicated. In stable conditions, without ascites, obstetric management should not change. In case of a deteriorating condition, with developing ascites, preterm delivery could be considered to avoid damage to the bowel. Pregnancies that continue until term should be monitored intensively to assess fetal well-being. Cesarean section does not seem to ameliorate the prognosis; the risk of abdominal dystocia, however, should always be considered. Delivery in a tertiary-care facility allows immediate postnatal surgical intervention.[27]

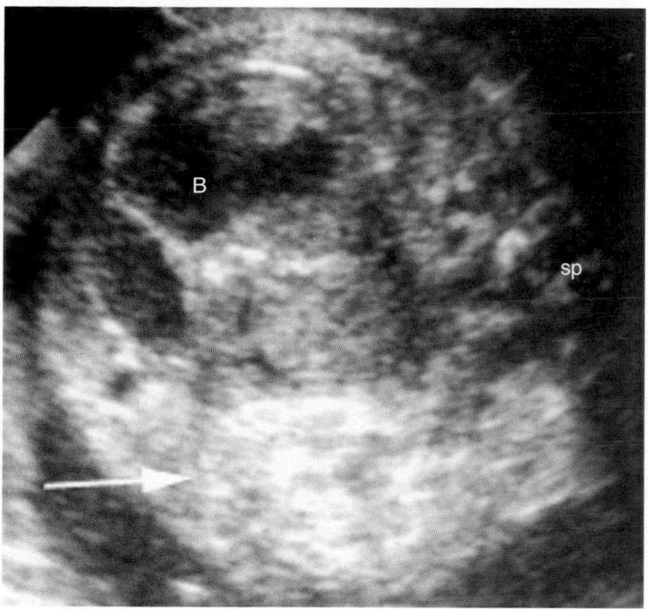

Figure 25.13 Cross-section of the fetal abdomen showing a highly hyperechogenic mass (arrow) of meconium peritonitis (cystic type). B, distended loops of bowel; sp, spine.

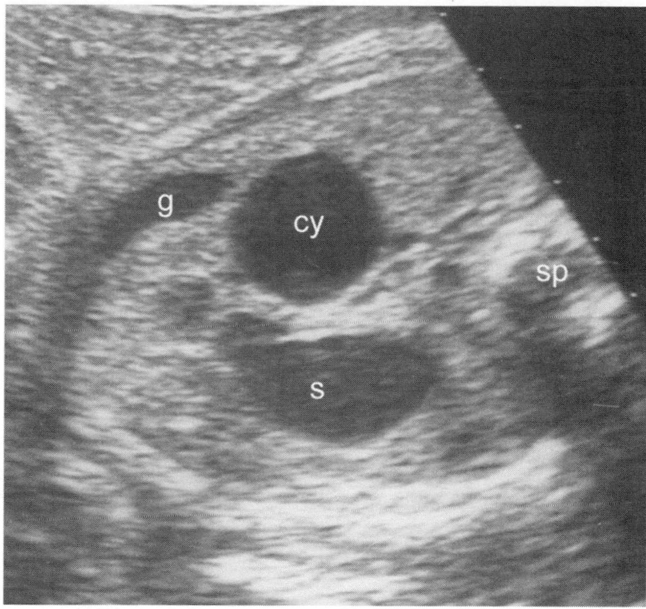

Figure 25.14 Oblique scan at the level of the right upper abdomen in a fetus with choledocal cyst (cy) close to the gallbladder (g). sp, spine; s, stomach.

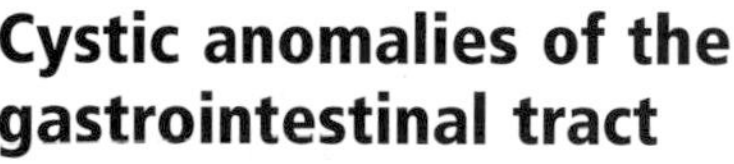

Cystic anomalies of the gastrointestinal tract

Choledochal cysts

The etiology is unknown. The presence of a cyst in the upper side of the fetal abdomen suggests the diagnosis of choledochal cyst. They represent cystic dilation of the common biliary duct. Differential diagnosis includes intestinal duplication cysts, hepatic cysts, situs inversus, and duodenal atresia. The absence of the connection with the stomach, which does not appear dilated, enables the exclusion of duodenal atresia (Fig. 25.14). The absence of polyhydramnios or peristalsis suggests a nonintestinal disorder. A prompt diagnosis and surgical postnatal removal (although, carrying a 10% mortality rate) could avoid complications such as biliary cirrhosis, portal hypertension, calculus formation, and adenocarcinoma.

Mesenteric, omental, and retroperitoneal cysts

Cystic structures located in the small or large bowel mesentery, the omentum, or the retroperitoneal space are caused by obstruction of the lymphatic drainage system or may represent lymphatic hamartomas. Quite rare, these cystic lesions are usually anechoic, multi- or unilocular, median, and of variable size. The fluid contents may be serous, chylous, or hemorrhagic. Obstetric management is unchanged; surgical removal is required in the case of bowel obstruction or acute abdominal pain following torsion or hemorrhage into a cyst.

Hepatic cysts

Hepatic cysts are typically located in the right lobe of the liver. They are quite rare and result from obstruction of the hepatic biliary system. They appear as unilocular, intrahepatic cysts, and they are usually asymptomatic, although they may rarely show complications such as infections or hemorrhages. In 30% of the cases of polycystic kidneys (adult type), asymptomatic hepatic cysts may be associated.[28]

Intestinal duplication cysts

These are quite rare, and may be located along the entire GI tract. They appear sonographically as tubular or cystic structures of variable size. They may be isolated or associated with other GI malformations.[29] Thickness of the muscular wall of the cysts and the presence of peristalsis may facilitate the diagnosis. Complications in the first months of postnatal life are represented by bowel obstruction and respiratory complications.

Anomalies of the umbilical vein

These are very rare anomalies. They can be divided into three groups: persistence of the right umbilical vein with ductus venosus and presence or absence of left umbilical vein; absent ductus venosus with extrahepatic insertion of umbilical vein; dilated umbilical vein with normal insertion and decurrence.[30] Normally, the umbilical vein enters the abdomen almost centrally at the level of the liver and courses on the left of the gallbladder. Persistence of the right umbilical vein is demonstrated by the fact that it is localized on the right of the gallbladder, bending toward the stomach.[31] Color Doppler may help to diagnose these anomalies and may allow the differential diagnosis with other cystic abdominal lesions. Associated anomalies are frequent in the first two groups, and this influences the prognosis. These anomalies include cardiac, skeletal, GI, and urinary anomalies. IUGR is also present, together with single umbilical artery. The anomalies of the third group are rarely associated with other defects, and prognosis depends upon the time of diagnosis and dimension of the varicosity.

Gallbladder anomalies

Agenesis of the gallbladder is associated with biliary atresia in 20% of cases. Prenatal diagnosis has not yet been described. Gallstones may be visualized as minute hyperechogenic intraluminal structures. Conservative management is indicated, as they may disappear postnatally.

Hepatosplenomegaly

Isolated hepatomegaly or splenomegaly is rare. Causes of hepatosplenomegaly are immune and nonimmune hydrops, hemolytic anemia, congenital infection, metabolic disorders, and hepatic tumors. Hepatic hemangioma, despite its benign nature, is associated with a high mortality rate (81%) secondary to congestive heart failure due to arterial–venous shunting. The sonographic finding is usually a hypoechogenic intrahepatic structure. The tumor may be pulsating and recognizable with Doppler ultrasound. The presence of hepatic calcifications and a hyperechogenic solid mass may suggest a diagnosis of hepatoblastoma, which represents the most frequent malignant tumor during fetal life. Hamartomas usually present as a multilocular cystic mass. Hepatic hyperechogenicity, unrelated to infections or tumors, seems to carry a favorable prognosis when other anomalies are absent and the karyotype is normal.[32]

Abdominal wall defects

Defects of the abdominal wall including omphalocele and gastroschisis (defect of the upper abdominal wall) and bladder and cloacal exstrophy (defect of the lower abdominal wall) are recognizable owing to the protrusion of abdominal contents into the amniotic fluid cavity. Prognosis largely depends on associated anomalies and complications such as fetal growth restriction.

Omphalocele

Omphalocele, or exomphalos, occurs in about 1 in 4000 births, and results from failure of normal embryonic regression of the midgut from the umbilical stalk into the abdominal coeloma. The abdominal contents, including intestines and liver or spleen covered by a sac of parietal peritoneum and amnion, are herniated into the base of the umbilical cord.[33] When omphalocele is small, the umbilical cord is inserted into its apex; in cases of large defects, the cord is attached inferiorly, and the umbilical vein and arteries are splayed out in the wall of the sac. If the sac ruptures *in utero*, its remnants, with the umbilical vessels, are still visible on the border of the lesion. The defect varies greatly in size, from a small opening through which only one or two loops of the small intestine or a Meckel's diverticulum protrude to an enormous defect containing most of the abdominal contents.

The majority of cases of omphalocele are sporadic, and the recurrence risk is usually less than 1%. However, in some cases, there may be an associated genetic syndrome.

Omphalocele is often associated with other abnormalities, as a result of general interference with embryonic development during early gestation.[34] Malrotation of the gut and duodenal obstruction are frequent. GU anomalies, including exstrophy of the bladder, penile anomalies, and undescended testes, are also very common. Congenital heart diseases are frequent and represent the most important cause of death for the affected child. Craniofacial anomalies are quite rare. Chromosomal abnormalities (mainly trisomy 18 or 13) are found in about 30% of cases at mid-gestation and in 15% of neonates.[35] If macrosomia is present, one should suspect Beckwith–Wiedemann syndrome (EMG syndrome), which includes multiple abnormalities such as omphalocele, macroglossia, occasionally requiring partial glossectomy to prevent mandibular prognathism, and macrosomia with hyperplastic fetal visceromegaly; a severe resistant neonatal hypoglycemia may be expected in 50% of cases. In some cases, Beckwith–Wiedemann syndrome is associated with mental handicap, which is thought to be secondary to inadequately treated hypoglycemia. About 5% of affected individuals develop tumors during childhood, most commonly nephroblastoma and hepatoblastoma. In Beckwith–Wiedemann syndrome, most cases are sporadic, although autosomal-dominant, recessive, X-linked, and polygenic patterns of inheritance have been described. Omphalocele is also present in pentalogy of Cantrell, which includes a large upper abdominal omphalocele, an anterior diaphragmatic hernia, a sternal cleft, ectopia cordis, and various cardiac anomalies such as ventricular septal defect or tetralogy of Fallot. A low omphalocele is frequently associated with bladder or cloacal exstrophy and other anomalies, including anal atresia or myelomeningocele, and lower limb anomalies.[36]

Prenatal diagnosis of omphalocele is based on the demonstration of the midline anterior abdominal wall defect, the herniated sac with its visceral contents, and the umbilical cord insertion at the apex of the sac (Figs 25.15 and 25.16).[37,38] As normal migration of the midgut back into the abdomen occurs between the 9th and the 12th gestational weeks, the diagnosis of ventral wall defects should not be made before 14 weeks.[39] Exceptionally, heart and bladder are contained in the herniated sac.[40] In small defects, umbilical cord insertion is on top of the mass, whereas in large lesions, the cord is attached to its lower border. A cystic structure associated with the umbilical cord, representing an allantoic cyst often associated with omphalocele, can be interpreted as protrusion of abdominal contents through a defect in the abdominal wall.[41] Polyhydramnios is often present. The differential diagnosis includes mainly gastroschisis, in which the only herniated abdominal contents are bowel loops, not contained by an amnioperitoneal membrane.

Isolated lesions have a good prognosis with a survival rate after surgery of higher than 90%.[42,43] The volume of the protruded viscera is crucial for determining fetal prognosis: giant defects associated with liver evisceration and ectopia cordis may have a much worse prognosis than small defects, in which only bowel loops are extruded.[44,45] In cases of small defects or an isolated anomaly, if omphalocele is intact, there is no need to anticipate delivery.[46] When omphalocele has gone into a rupture, a preterm Cesarean section has been suggested to avoid the exposure of the bowel to the amniotic fluid, which may compromise the outcome of postnatal surgical correction.[47] However, risks of prematurity should be taken into account. Large or ruptured omphalocele should probably be delivered by Cesarean section, in strictly sterile conditions, to avoid trauma and infection of the herniated viscera and to decrease the risk of dystocia. However, it has yet to be demonstrated whether this management improves fetal outcome. In 1983, in a large retrospective study of 112 cases of abdominal wall defects, Kirk and Wah[48] found no adverse effects related to vaginal delivery or to the success of surgical postnatal correction. However, because the mortality rate of newborns affected by abdominal wall defects largely depends on the clinical condition of the malformed baby on admission,[49] maternal transport to a tertiary center and an accurately planned Cesarean delivery would probably avoid the risks of a sudden, unexpected delivery leading to a delay in surgical care.

Gastroschisis

Gastroschisis is found in about 1 in 4000 births. In gastroschisis, the primary body folds and the umbilical ring develop normally, and evisceration of the intestine occurs through a small abdominal wall defect located just lateral and usually to the right of an intact umbilical cord.[50] Other pathogenetic theories suggest that gastroschisis results from an intrauterine rupture of an incarcerated hernia into the cord,[51] or from a vascular accident involving the omphalomesenteric artery, leading to disruption of the umbilical ring and herniation of abdominal contents.[52] The loops of intestine lie uncovered in the amniotic fluid. Occasionally, only a short tract of the intestine is herniated; in most cases, however, all the small and large intestines protrude. Stomach, gallbladder, urinary bladder, testes or uterus, and adnexae are also prolapsed. Chemical peritonitis is an ominous complication due to

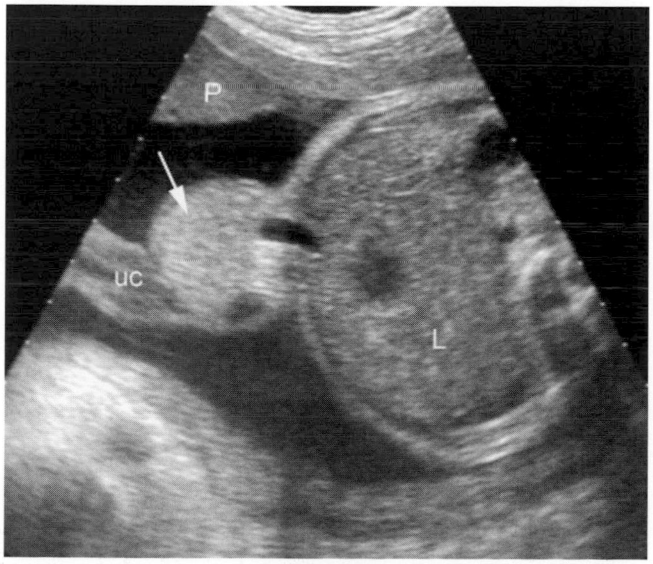

Figure 25.15 Cross-section of a fetus with omphalocele. Note the herniated hyperechogenic mass (arrow) at the level of cord insertion. L, liver; P, placenta; uc, umbilical cord on top of the defect.

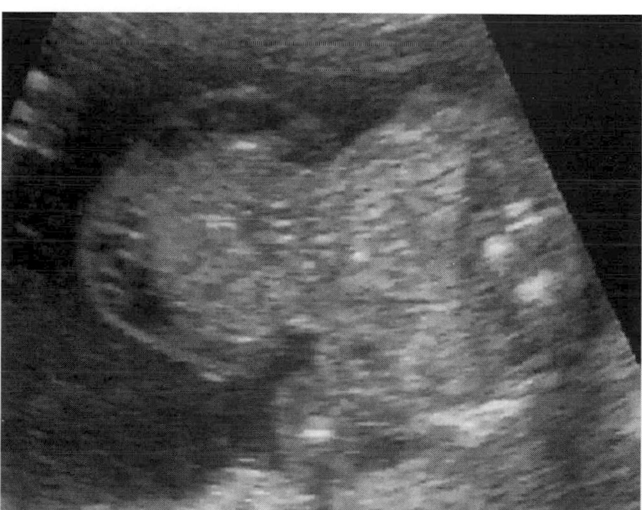

Figure 25.16 Cross-section of a 20-week fetus with a large omphalocele. The liver protrudes from the abdominal wall defect covered by an amnioperitoneal membrane.

amniotic fluid exposure of eviscerated abdominal contents. In such cases, the intestine shows marked dilation of the lumen and increased thickness of the walls, which appear edematous, of leathery consistency, and matted together and encased in a net of fibrinous material. In many cases, the intestine reveals an abnormal shortening. Single or multiple atretic sites of the protruded gut can be detected. Gastroschisis is a sporadic abnormality.

Associated anomalies are uncommon compared with omphalocele, and usually involve the intestinal tract (malrotation). Occasionally, intestinal obstruction due to angulation of gut, adhesions, or atresia secondary to vascular impairment of the wall can be seen as ancillary complications.

Prenatal diagnosis is based on the demonstration of the normally situated umbilicus and the herniated loops of intestine, which are free-floating and widely separated (Fig. 25.17).[53]

Hypoechogenic areas can sometimes be identified within the bubble-like structures, suggesting the presence of meconium. The extruded structures are not covered by amnioperitoneal membrane, and normal umbilical cord insertion is present (Fig. 25.18). Polyhydramnios is common, as well as increased amniotic fluid alpha-fetoprotein (AFP) levels. About 30% of fetuses are growth restricted, but the diagnosis can be difficult because gastroschisis as such is associated with a small abdominal circumference.[54] In these cases, the volume of amniotic fluid is often reduced and visualization suboptimal.

Prognosis has improved dramatically during the last three decades.[55] Decreased perinatal mortality from 82% in 1960 to less than 10% in 1984 is likely to be attributable to improved surgical technique and the use of parenteral nutrition. Mortality is usually the consequence of short gut syndrome. It is still debated whether sonographic findings such as dilation and thickening of the bowel wall can predict infant outcome.[56–58] Dilation of the stomach seems to be associated with increased perinatal morbidity and mortality.[59]

Gastroschisis is less frequently associated with other congenital anomalies than omphalocele. As with omphalocele, it can be part of amniotic band syndrome. Unlike omphalocele, gastroschisis is often associated with IUGR[60] and oligohydramnios; in these cases, risks related to prematurity should be balanced against benefits of the shortened exposure time to the action of amniotic fluid.

In cases with associated growth restriction, strict surveillance of fetal well-being is recommended between 34 and 36 weeks.[61]

As with omphalocele, the impact of route of delivery on outcome is still debated. Some authors show that babies born from elective Cesarean section had less sepsis and less short-term morbidity,[62] while other groups do not demonstrate the benefit of Cesarean section versus vaginal delivery.[63,64]

It seems crucial, however, that delivery takes place in tertiary-care centers where the neonate can receive intensive care and where neonatal surgical correction is promptly available. Delay in pediatric care, in fact, increases the risk of sepsis and may be the cause of severe dehydration and rapid heat loss, which may compromise the outcome of surgical correction. Long-term follow-up of survivors is excellent: children show normal growth and development in follow-up to 5 years of age.[65]

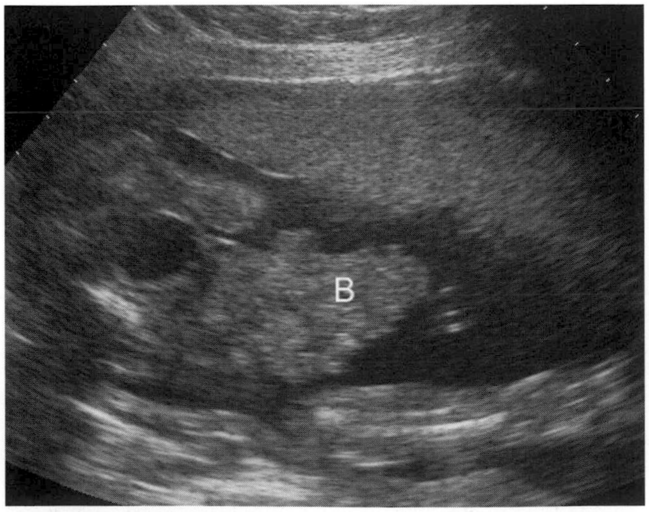

Figure 25.17 A case of gastroschisis diagnosed at 22 weeks' gestation: free-floating loops of bowel (B) herniated through a lateral abdominal wall defect.

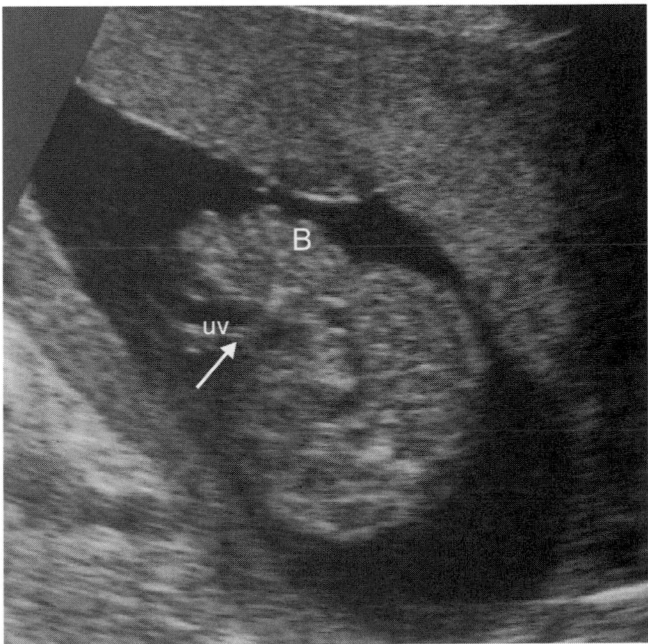

Figure 25.18 Loops of bowel protruding through a lateral defect of the abdominal wall. See the intact insertion of the cord (arrow). B, bowel; uv, umbilical vein.

Body stalk anomaly

Body stalk anomaly is a rare fatal disease with a birth incidence of 1 in 14 000.[66] It is characterized by a defect of the anterior abdominal wall with absence of the umbilicus and umbilical cord. The placenta appears to be fused with the herniated viscera, and consequent skeletal kyphosis is a common feature. This anomaly derives from failure of the cephalic, caudal, and lateral body folds to develop, together with the abnormal persistence of the coelomatic cavity, which usually obliterates by the fourth week of embryonic life. Prenatal diagnosis is based upon demonstration of a vast defect in the anterior abdominal wall, through which herniated viscera protrude and fuse with the placenta.[67] Major anomalies of any apparatus may be associated.

Bladder exstrophy and cloacal exstrophy

Bladder and cloacal exstrophy are rare sporadic anomalies, even if familial cases have been described. Incidence of bladder exstrophy is 1 in 30 000 live births, while incidence of cloacal exstrophy is 1 in 200 000 live births. Bladder exstrophy is a consequence of impaired development of the caudal fold of the anterior abdominal wall. The anterior wall is absent, and exposure of the posterior bladder wall is common. Omphalocele is frequently associated, as well as epispadias, incomplete descent of the testicles, and imperforate anus. In cloacal exstrophy, both GI and GU tracts are involved. Cloacal exstrophy (also referred to as OEIS complex) is the association of an omphalocele, exstrophy of the bladder, imperforated anus, and spinal defects such as meningomyelocele. The hemibladders are on either side of the intestines.

Bladder exstrophy should be suspected when the fetal bladder is not visualized in the presence of normal amniotic fluid (the filling cycle of the bladder is normally about 15 min) or when an echogenic mass is seen protruding from the lower abdominal wall in close association with umbilical arteries.[68] In cloacal exstrophy, the findings are similar to bladder exstrophy (large infraumbilical defect that extends to the pelvis), but a posterior anomalous component is present.[69] Other findings include single umbilical artery, ascites, vertebral anomalies, clubfoot, and ambiguous genitalia. In boys, the penis is divided and duplicated. With aggressive reconstructive bladder, bowel, and genital surgery, the survival rate is more than 80%.[70] Bladder exstrophy is compatible with complete repair, although permanent urinary tract diversion becomes necessary in some cases. Cloacal exstrophy is a much more severe disease involving the lower abdominal tract as well, and is associated with significant sequelae.

Genitourinary tract anomalies

Congenital malformations of the GU tract are relatively frequent, probably due to the complexity of embryologic development, representing the major cause of neonatal abdominal masses. Prenatal diagnosis is crucial to choose the most appropriate prenatal and postnatal management, and has greatly improved the prognosis of affected children.[71] The volume of amniotic fluid should be carefully evaluated. A significant decrease in amniotic fluid volume heralds the presence of many GU anomalies and, when detected after the second trimester, is an ominous prognostic factor because of the association with pulmonary hypoplasia.[72] Owing to the paucity of amniotic fluid, the diagnosis of GU tract anomalies is sometimes a difficult task; recently, magnetic resonance imaging (MRI) has been proposed as a useful tool to provide adequate visualization of renal and bladder regions, despite a reduced volume of amniotic fluid.[73]

Bilateral renal agenesis

Bilateral renal agenesis is found in 1 in 5000 births, while unilateral disease is found in 1 in 2000 births. Renal agenesis derives from failure of development of the ureteric bud or nephrogenic blastema, because both components occur at the formation of normal kidneys.

This abnormality is usually isolated and sporadic, although it may rarely be secondary to a chromosomal abnormality or part of a genetic syndrome such as Fraser syndrome, or a developmental defect such as VACTERL association. In nonsyndromic cases, the risk of recurrence is approximately 3%. However, in about 15% of cases, one of the parents has unilateral renal agenesis and, in these families, the risk of recurrence is increased.[74]

Renal agenesis can be part of Potter's syndrome, which includes pulmonary hypoplasia, skeletal deformities, and typical facies, characterized by low-set ears. Oligohydramnios is considered to be responsible for pulmonary hypoplasia and skeletal deformities, which are also present in some cases of prolonged rupture of membranes or IUGR.[75] Conversely, when oligohydramnios is not severe, the characteristic features of Potter's syndrome are uncommon.[76] Other structural anomalies, such as cardiac and GI tract anomalies, are associated with variable incidence.

Failed visualization of kidneys and bladder, associated with oligohydramnios, prompts the diagnosis of bilateral renal agenesis. Additionally, adrenals are usually hypertrophic and can be confused with normal kidneys (Fig. 25.19). Prenatal diagnosis can be rather difficult owing to the lack of amniotic fluid and the "crumpled" position adopted by these fetuses. Identification of the renal capsule and renal pelvis enables the two structures to be distinguished.[77]

The differential diagnosis includes premature rupture of the membranes, severe uteroplacental insufficiency, and obstructive uropathy or bilateral multicystic or polycystic kidneys. Vaginal sonography with a high-resolution probe is useful in these cases. Failure to visualize the renal arteries with color Doppler is sometimes crucial to the diagnosis (Fig. 25.20A and B). Prenatal diagnosis of unilateral renal agenesis is difficult as there are no major features, such as anhydramnios and empty bladder, to alert the sonographer.

Bilateral renal agenesis is a lethal condition. Amniotic fluid enables normal development of the lungs up to 22–24 weeks. Early severe oligohydramnios invariably leads to pulmonary hypoplasia, and infants die in the neonatal period owing to respiratory insufficiency. Unilateral agenesis has a favourable prognosis.

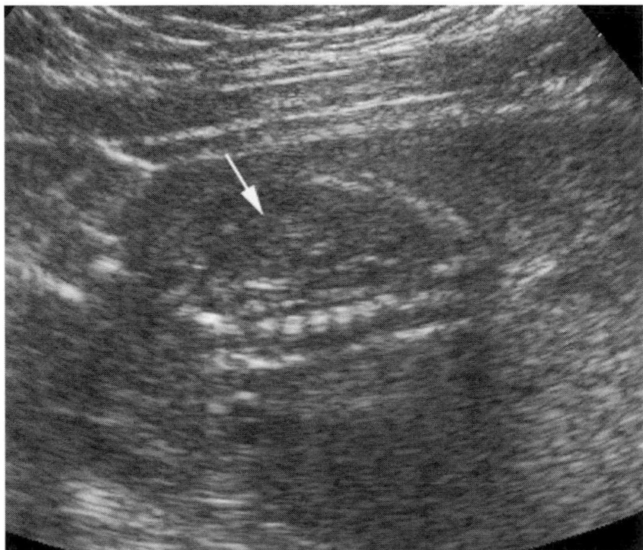

Figure 25.19 No demonstrable kidneys and flattened adrenal gland in a 20-week fetus with bilateral renal agenesis.

Cystic kidneys

Four main categories of cystic dysplastic kidneys are recognized. Two different entities can be identified with certainty via antenatal ultrasonography: multicystic kidney and cystic dypslasia occurring as a consequence of early and longstanding obstructive uropathy.

Multicystic kidneys

Multicystic kidneys are usually unilateral, although bilateral renal involvement has been reported.[78] The dysplastic process is usually limited to the medulla, but can involve the cortex as well. The prevalence of the unilateral type is unknown; bilateral involvement is estimated to occur in 1 in 1000 live births.[79]

In the majority of cases, this is a sporadic abnormality, but a few examples of familial cases have been described.[79] Pathogenesis of the anomaly is controversial; it is most likely secondary to atresia of the ureter, the pelvis, or both during the metanephric stage of development.[81]

Multicystic kidney is often associated with other congenital anomalies, including mainly congenital heart diseases and chromosomal aberrations (mainly trisomy 18), and it is often part of genetic syndromes. It may frequently be associated with contralateral renal agenesis and hydronephrosis.[82] Misdiagnosis can occur when the contralateral kidney is ectopic.

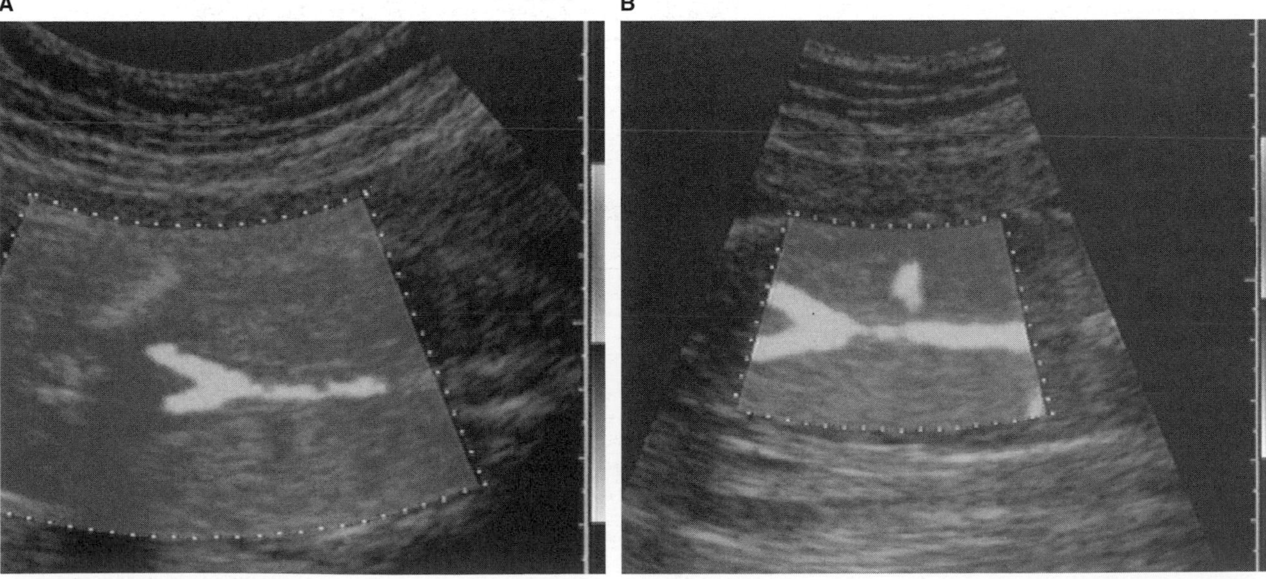

Figure 25.20 Color Doppler failed to demonstrate the renal arteries in the case of bilateral (A) and unilateral (B) renal agenesis.

In 10% of cases, the anomaly is associated with contralateral hydronephrosis, usually from obstruction at the ureteropelvic junction (UPJ). Because the obstructed kidney is the only functioning one, serial examination should be planned to monitor dilation of the pelvis and the amount of amniotic fluid.

Multicystic kidneys are usually unilateral and appear as a cluster of multiple irregular cysts of variable size with little intervening hyperechogenic stroma (Fig. 25.21).[83,84] Affected kidneys are usually extremely enlarged. The hypoplastic or atretic collecting system is undetectable by ultrasound. In the unilateral variant, contralateral kidney and bladder are normal, as is the amount of amniotic fluid. Occasionally, the contralateral renal pelvis appears slightly enlarged owing to compensatory urine flow. Distinction between multicystic kidneys and obstructions at the UPJ in prenatal sonograms can be extremely difficult.[85] Coronal scans seem to be the most specific because, in UPJ obstructions, they clearly demonstrate the connection between the renal pelvis and the dilated caliceal system. Conversely, in cystic lesions, the cysts are separated. Such a distinction is much easier when ultrasound examination is performed in early pregnancy. Isolated unilateral multicystic kidneys have a good prognosis. The need for postnatal nephrectomy is currently under discussion: it is required when the size of the kidney is inconvenient to the patient, but it should be considered in all cases, because complications, including GI infections, hypertension, and malignant mixed tumors, may originate from a retained affected kidney.[86,87] Bilateral multicystic dysplastic kidney disease (MDKD) invariably has a poor prognosis.

Cystic dysplasia

Early and persistent obstruction of the lower GU tract is associated with secondary cystic dysplasia of the kidneys, which appear hyperechogenic, increased in size, and present small cysts that spread through the parenchyma. In these cases, the diagnosis is made by the simultaneous demonstration of obstructive uropathy (distended bladder, convoluted ureters, pyelectasia, oligohydramnios), and these findings can be part of genetic renal disorders.[88]

Autosomal-recessive cystic kidney

Autosomal-recessive cystic kidney (also referred to as infantile polycystic kidney) invariably involves both kidneys, and occursin 1 in 20 000 live births. A defect in the collecting system seems to be responsible for the anomaly. Kidneys are symmetrically enlarged, and the parenchyma is totally occupied by numerous cysts of minute dimensions. At section, the cysts present a cubic epithelium.

Sonographically, both kidneys usually appear extremely enlarged and hyperechogenic (Fig. 25.22).[89] In severe cases, the bladder is absent and oligohydramnios is extreme. However, these sonographic appearances may be manifest only in late gestation.[90] Molecular genetics helps in the diagnosis only when the index case has been clearly identified, and only if DNA from the case is available and can be screened in order to identify the familial mutations.

The prognosis is variable. Cases appearing early in

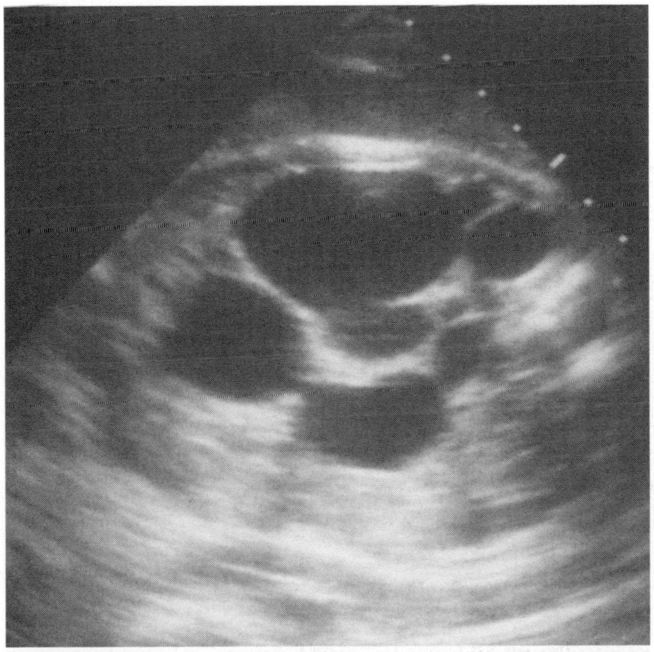

Figure 25.21 Coronal scan of the trunk of a 33-week fetus with unilateral multicystic dysplastic kidney disease. The cysts are clearly separated by echoic tissue.

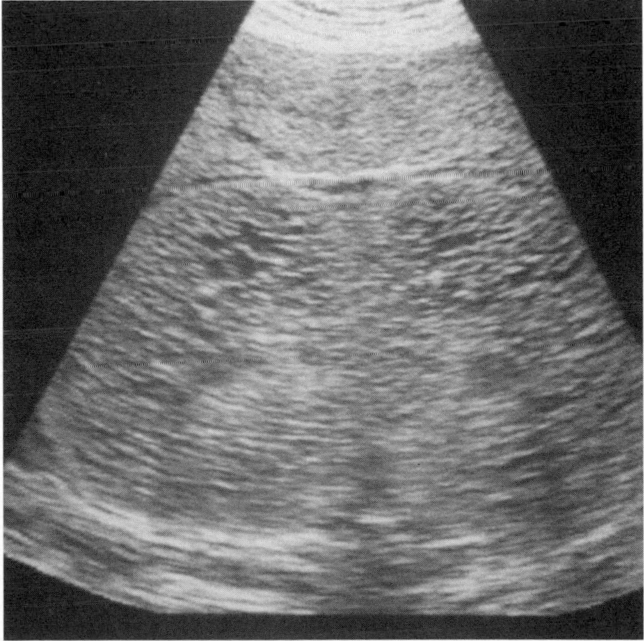

Figure 25.22 Coronal section of a fetus with recessive-type polycystic kidneys. Kidneys appear extremely enlarged and hyperechogenic.

gestation are associated with oligohydramnios in the second trimester and are usually lethal owing to a combination of renal failure and pulmonary hypoplasia.[91,92] In other cases, the onset of the disease occurs later in gestation or after birth, and there is variable progression toward renal failure. The infantile and juvenile types result in chronic renal failure, hepatic fibrosis, and portal hypertension; many survive into their teens but require renal transplantation.

Autosomal-dominant cystic kidney

Autosomal-dominant cystic kidney (also referred to as adult polycystic kidney) almost invariably affects both kidneys, although often asymmetrically.[93,94] It is usually asymptomatic until the third or fourth decade of life.

Autosomal-dominant cystic kidney is a common inherited nephropathy affecting more than 1 in 1000 live births. It may be inherited as an autosomal-dominant trait, or it may be a feature of genetic and nongenetic syndromes. Sporadic diseases have also been reported in the literature.[95]

Using a highly polymorphic DNA probe genetically linked to the mutant gene, prenatal diagnosis is possible.[96]

Sonography does not usually demonstrate abnormalities prior to the second or third decade of life. In a handful of cases, however, affected fetuses have demonstrated findings similar to the autosomal-recessive variety, including enlarged and echogenic kidneys.[93,95] Kidneys appear grossly enlarged with multiple cysts of variable size intermixed with well-represented, hyperechogenic solid tissue (Fig. 25.23). Dissection shows multiple cysts of variable size filled with fluid within both the medulla and the cortex. Histology demonstrates the presence of normal renal parenchyma. Nephrons and collecting tubules are poorly defined, as are papillae and calices. The cysts are lined by cuboidal cells.

It is clear that this disease covers a wide spectrum. The experience with prenatal diagnosis is limited. It would not seem that intrauterine presentation is necessarily associated with a poor prognosis.

Cystic kidneys are also found with many mendelian disorders, such as tuberous sclerosis, Jeune syndrome, Sturge–Weber syndrome, Zellweger syndrome, Laurence–Moon–Biedl syndrome, and Meckel–Gruber syndrome.

Obstructive uropathies

Enlargement of the GU tract usually occurs, albeit not exclusively, as a consequence of obstruction. When the obstruction is complete and occurs early in fetal life, cystic renal dysplasia ensues. On the other hand, where intermittent obstruction allows for normal renal development, or when obstruction occurs in the second half of pregnancy, hydronephrosis will result, and the severity of renal damage will depend on the degree and duration of the obstruction. Different entities with variable findings and clinical implications exist depending on the location and severity of the dilatation.[97]

Hydronephrosis refers to dilation of the renal pelvis (Fig. 25.24 and 25.25). Mild hydronephrosis, or pyelectasia, is defined by the presence of an anteroposterior diameter of the pelvis of more than 4 mm at mid-gestation and more than 7 mm in the third trimester. Transient hydronephrosis may be

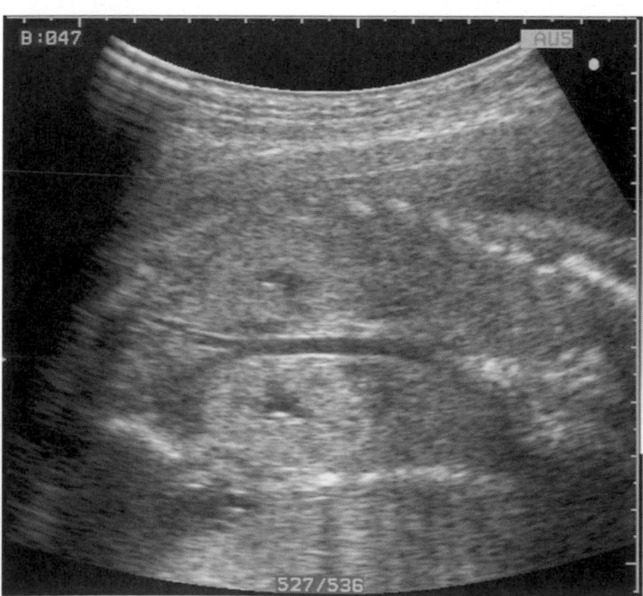

Figure 25.23 Coronal scan of the fetal trunk demonstrating the polycystic kidneys (PK).

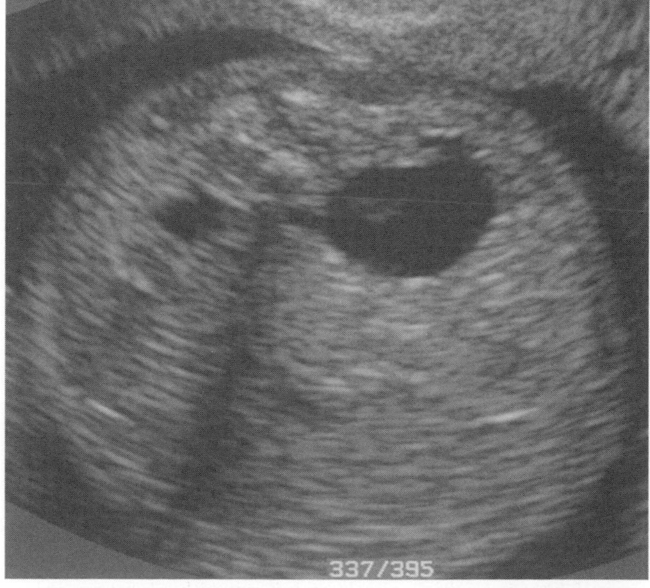

Figure 25.24 Cross-section of the fetal abdomen showing a mildly enlarged renal pelvis and a contralateral normal pelvis.

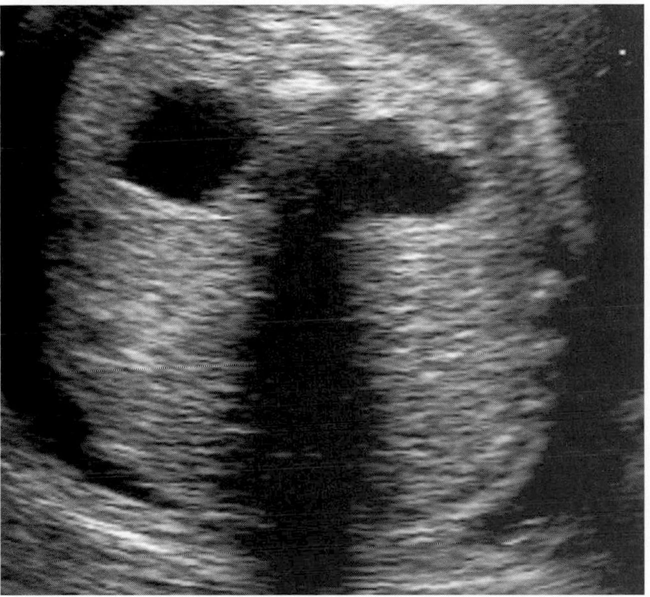

Figure 25.25 Cross-section of the fetal abdomen showing mild dilation of both pelves.

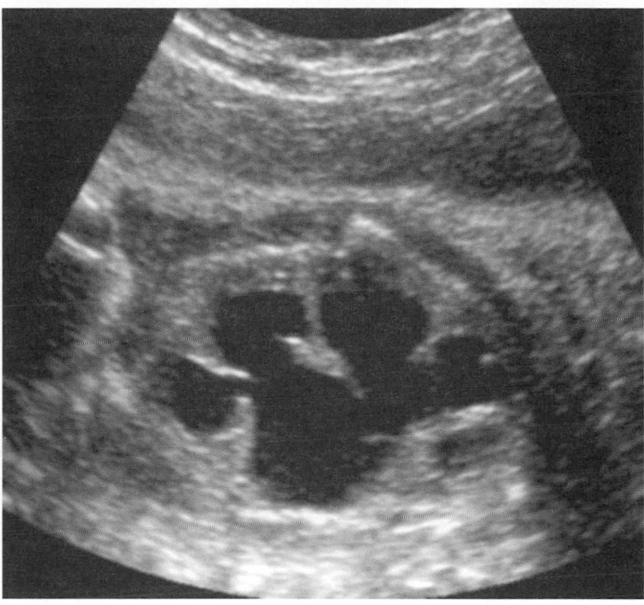

Figure 25.26 Coronal view of the kidney in a case of ureteropelvic junction obstruction. Pelves and calices appear fairly dilated.

due to relaxation of smooth muscle of the GU tract by high levels of progesterone or maternal–fetal overhydration. In the majority of cases, the condition remains stable or resolves in the neonatal period. In about 20% of cases, there may be an underlying pathology that requires postnatal follow-up and possible surgery. The incidence of surgery with a renal pelvis of 5–10 mm is in the range of 3–4%. Moderate hydronephrosis, characterized by an anteroposterior pelvic diameter of more than 10 mm, is almost invariably associated with caliceal dilation, is usually progressive and, in more than 50% of cases, requires surgery during the first 2 years of life. Sonographically, it may be be difficult at times to distinguish severe hydronephrosis with significant caliceal enlargement from a multicystic kidney. A scan oriented along the coronal plane of the kidney is required to demonstrate the radial projection of the calices around the enlarged pelvis (Fig. 25.26). Sections oriented in different planes may create the false impression of multiple cysts separated by parenchymal tissue that is typical of multicystic kidney.

Mild pyelectasia (anteroposterior diameter between 4 and 10 mm) has recently been suggested as a sonographic marker for chromosomal abnormalities[98] and, in some cases, may reveal vesicoureteric reflux at birth.[99]

Hydroureteronephrosis is the combination of hydronephrosis and an enlarged ureter (Fig. 25.27). Of course, these findings are generally present with megacystis. However, the following discussion refers to hydroureteronephrosis with a normal bladder, which may result from either ureterovesical reflux or ureterovesical junction obstruction. Under normal conditions, the small ureter cannot be visualized with antenatal ultrasonography. The dilated ureter appears as a tortuous fluid-filled tubular structure interposed between the renal pelvis, which is variably dilated, and the bladder.[100,101] Sometimes, it is clearly visible as a ureterocele, which is represented by a thin-walled and fluid-filled small circular area inside the bladder (Fig. 25.28). Amniotic fluid is present in normal amounts. Rarely, a primary megaureter will be present, with a normal renal pelvis. The outcome and management principles are similar to those outlined for hydronephrosis.

Ureteral duplication can be associated with hydronephrosis and megaureter. A specific diagnosis is possible when two distinct renal pelves can be seen within one kidney (Fig. 25.29). Typically, there is some degree of dilation of the upper renal pole.[102,103]

Megacystis

Megacystis is defined as an abnormal enlargement of the urinary bladder, and is most frequently the consequence of urethral obstruction. Typically, it is seen in the early midtrimester and has been visualized as early as 11 weeks' gestation.[104] The bladder is usually greatly enlarged, occupying most of the abdomen and distending it. Urethral obstruction can be caused by urethral agenesis, persistence of the cloaca, urethral stricture, or posterior urethral valves. Posterior urethral valves occur only in males and are the most common cause of bladder outlet obstruction. The condition is generally sporadic and is found in about 1 in 3000 male fetuses; however, in some cases, it has a genetic basis.[105] In the

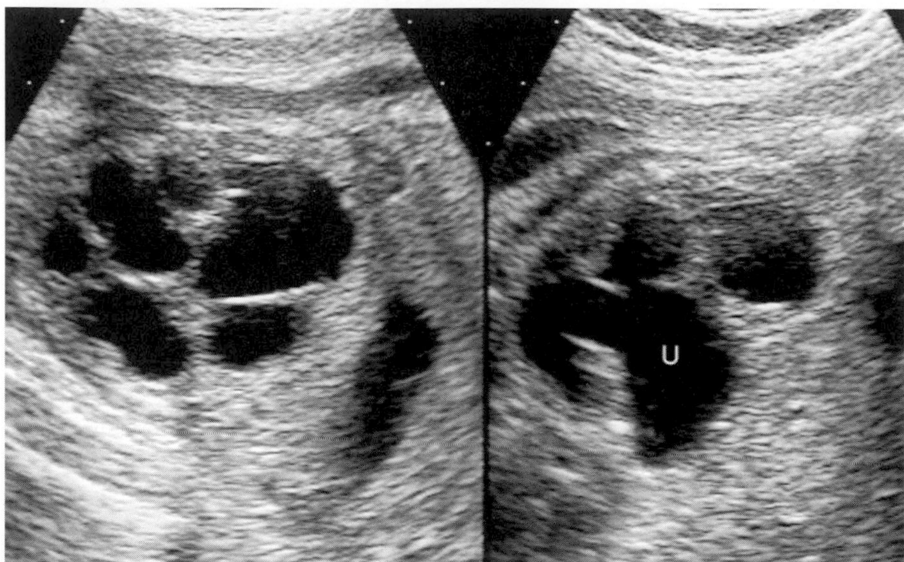

Figure 25.27 Coronal scan of the lower abdomen in a fetus with unilateral ureterovesical junction obstruction. Calices and pelvis are dilated, as well as the proximal portion of the ureter (U).

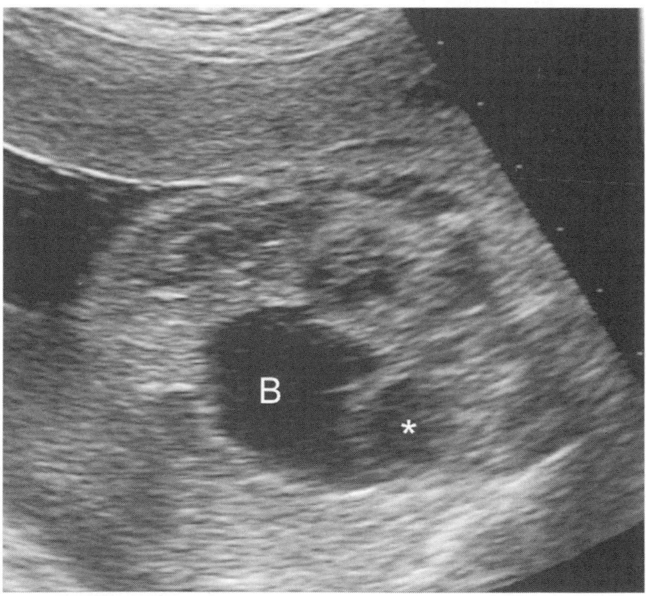

Figure 25.28 Thin-walled, fluid-filled, small, circular area (*) inside the bladder (B), representing a ureterocele in a fetus with ureterovesical junction obstruction.

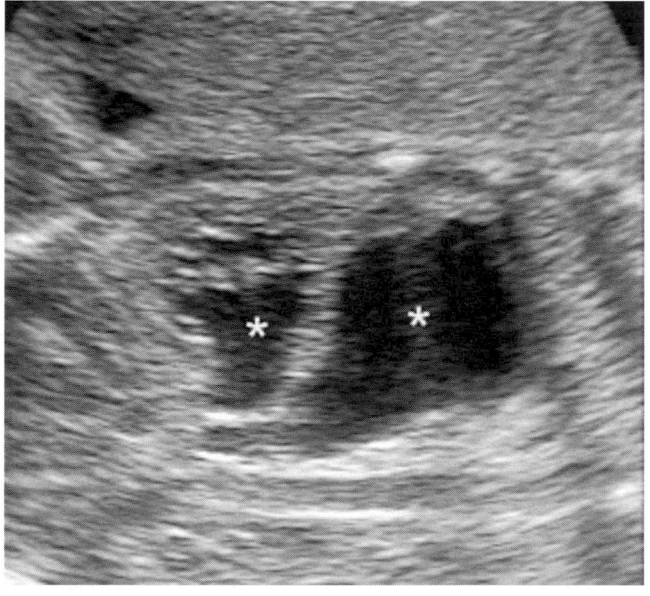

Figure 25.29 Coronal scan of the abdomen of a fetus with duplication of the kidneys. The two renal pelves (*) appear moderately dilated.

majority of cases, obstruction is caused by two semicircular membranous plicae at the level of the verumontanum.[74] As urine flows from the bladder, these plicae adhere and close the upper portion of the urethra.

With posterior urethral valves, there is usually incomplete or intermittent obstruction of the urethra, resulting in an enlarged and hypertrophied bladder with varying degrees of hydroureters, hydronephrosis, a spectrum of renal hypoplasia and dysplasia, oligohydramnios, and pulmonary hypoplasia[106,107] (Figs 25.30–25.33). Diagnosis has been made from as early as 12 weeks' gestation (Fig. 25.34).

In some cases, urinary ascites is associated with rupture of the bladder or transudation of urine into the peritoneal cavity.

When megacystis is found in association with an increased amount of amniotic fluid, the possibility of a megacystis–microcolon–intestinal hypoperistalsis syndrome should be considered. This is a sporadic abnormality characterized by a massively dilated bladder and hydronephrosis in the presence

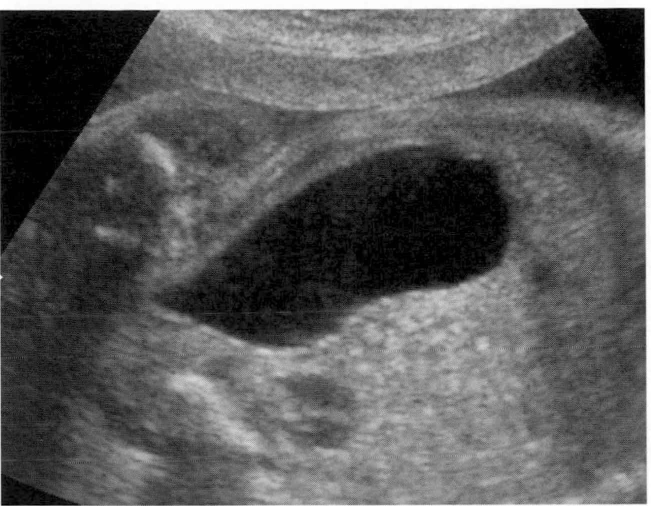

Figure 25.30 Longitudinal scan of the lower abdomen in a fetus with megacystis. The proximal tract of the ureter is dilated.

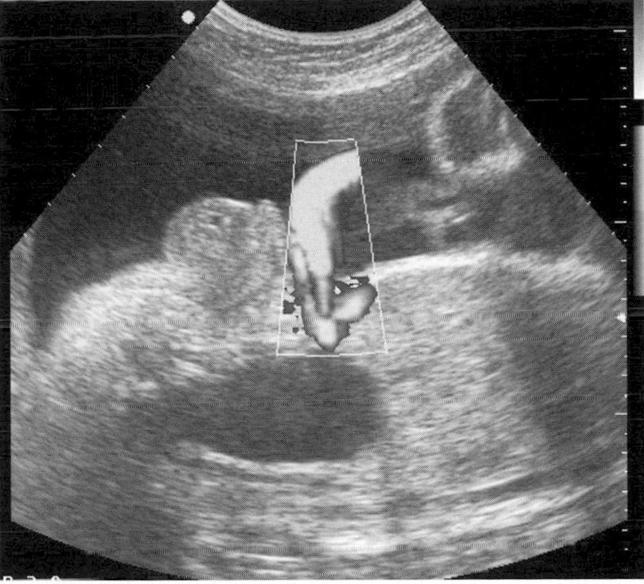

Figure 25.31 Longitudinal scan of the trunk of a male fetus affected by megacystis. The insertion of the umbilical vessels on the anterior abdominal wall is demonstrated with color Doppler.

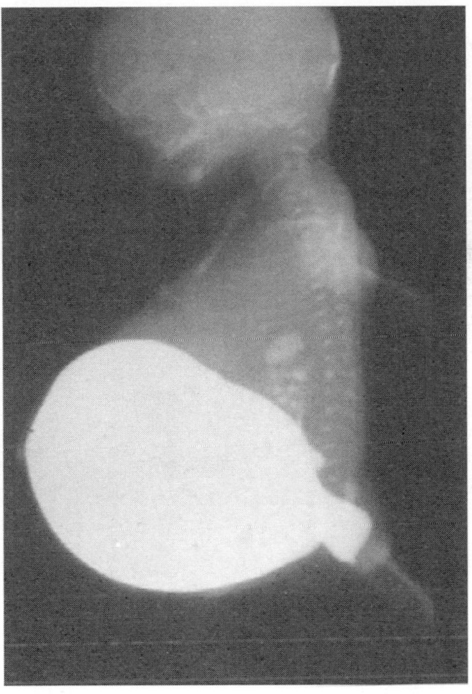

Figure 25.32 Severe megacystis. Radiograph of neonate with severe dilation of the urinary bladder.

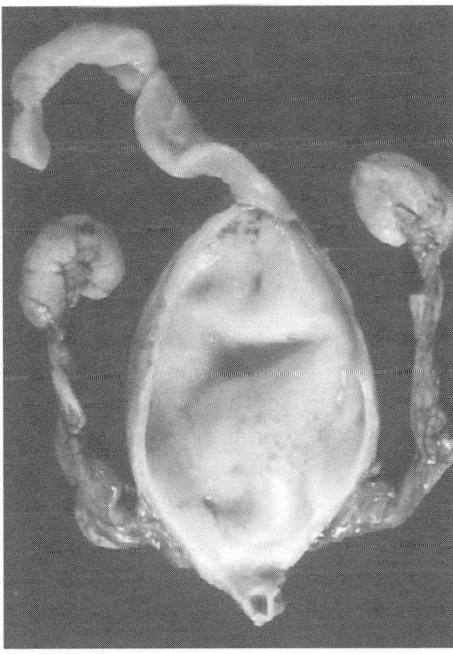

Figure 25.33 Megacystis: pathological specimen of the urinary bladder which appeared enlarged with thickened walls.

of normal or increased amniotic fluid; the fetuses are usually female. There is associated shortening and dilation of the proximal small bowel, and microcolon with absent or ineffective peristalsis. The condition is usually lethal owing to bowel and renal dysfunction.

The outcome of urethral obstruction depends on how severe it is and how early it occurs. Complete persistent obstruction occurring in the early midtrimester (e.g., urethral atresia, early posterior urethral valves) results in massive distention of the bladder and abdominal wall (prune-belly abdomen), severe oligohydramnios, dysplastic kidneys, and pulmonary hypoplasia.[108] Obstruction occurring in late gestation may be associated with oligohydramnios and hydronephrosis, but does not result in pulmonary hypoplasia and dysplastic kidneys. The management of early-appearing megacystis has been debated.[109–112] Shunting of the fetal bladder is feasible, although there is no

A

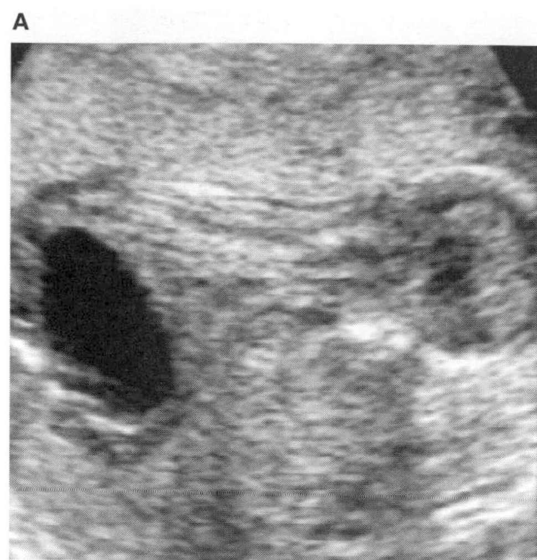

B

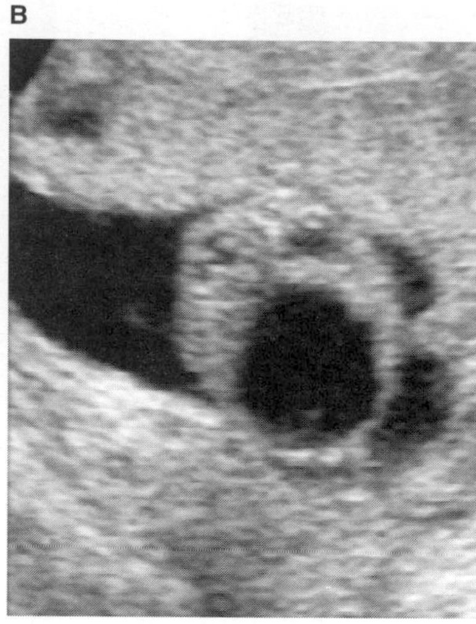

Figure 25.34 Longitudinal scan of a 12-week fetus with megacystis, obtained using a 6.5-MHz transvaginal probe.

conclusive evidence that such intervention improves renal or pulmonary function beyond what can be achieved by postnatal surgery. Antenatal evaluation of renal function relies on a combination of ultrasonographic findings and analysis of fetal urine obtained by puncture of the bladder or renal pelvis. An attempt to assess the severity of renal compromise should be made before embarking on fetal therapy. Poor prognostic signs are: (1) the presence of bilateral multicystic or severely hydronephrotic kidneys with increased parenchymal echogenicity, suggestive of renal dysplasia; (2) anhydramnios, implying complete urethral obstruction; and (3) decreased output (< 2 mL/h) of isotonic urine (osmolarity > 210 mOsm; sodium > 100 mEq/mL; chloride > 90 mEq/mL, and high levels of beta-2 microglobulin). In these cases, there is little chance of the infant surviving. Conversely, potential candidates for intrauterine surgery are fetuses with: (1) bilateral moderately severe pelvicaliceal dilation and normal cortical echogenicity; and (2) normal levels of urinary sodium, calcium and beta-2 microglobulin. One must remember, however, that normal values cannot exclude renal failure in childhood.[113]

Fetal ovarian cysts

Ovarian cysts are one of the most common causes of abdominal masses in the female neonate.[114,115] They are the most significant genital anomaly presenting in the prenatal period.

Although classically related to hormonal stimulation, the cause of the anomaly is still uncertain. Interestingly, congenital ovarian cysts occur in association with hypothyroidism.[116]

Prenatal ultrasound diagnosis is possible from the second trimester of pregnancy.[117–119] Cystic mass in the fetal lower abdomen, integrity of GI and GU tracts, and female sex are the main ultrasound criteria for diagnosis of fetal ovarian cyst. The cyst may be completely fluid or septated,[120] and sometimes presents with a fluid-solid level (Fig. 25.35). Diagnosis, however, is always presumptive, as mesenteric and urachal cysts, enteric duplication anomalies, cystic teratoma, and low intestinal obstructions cannot be ruled out with certainty *in utero*. Serial examinations of the anomaly allow the detection of structural changes in the cyst, which prompt the diagnosis of a complication of the cyst.[121]

Associated anomalies are uncommon, although increased amniotic fluid is often present, probably secondary to partial GI obstruction.[122]

Prognosis and management of fetal ovarian cysts depend largely on the natural history of the mass.[123] The cyst may increase in size, decrease, or even disappear, or lead to complications such as torsion, infarction, and rupture. In this light, once prenatal ultrasound diagnosis has been made, serial examinations should be performed throughout gestation to detect any structural changes in the mass. Enlargement of the mass, causing distention of the fetal abdomen, is an indication for Cesarean section to avoid the risk of soft tissue dystocia. Ultrasound-guided fine-needle aspiration of large fetal ovarian cysts may eliminate the need for a Cesarean section, theoretically reducing the risk of intrauterine torsion. However, the benefit of such an invasive procedure is unclear, possibly being a cause of intraperitoneal bleeding. Sudden development of intense hyperechogenicity within the mass, followed by a complex, heterogeneous appearance, should be considered to result from an intrauterine torsion of the cyst with infarction. When this occurs, immediate delivery is recommended. Conversely, small cysts detected *in utero* can subsequently disappear and may not be present on a postnatal ultrasound evaluation.

In summary, prenatal diagnosis of fetal ovarian cysts *per se* does not modify standard obstetric management, whereas complications occurring during gestation, such as torsion and rupture, may require active obstetric intervention. Neonates with confirmed diagnosis often require postnatal ovariectomy soon after birth.

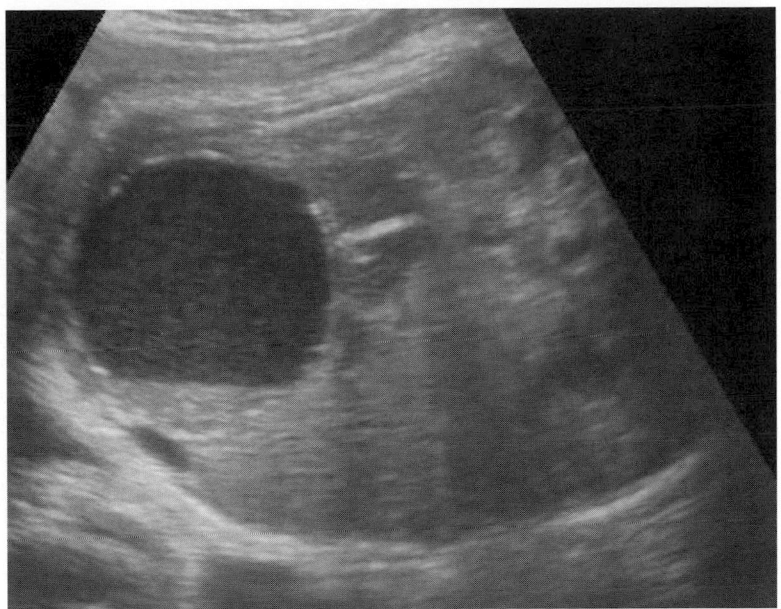

Figure 25.35 Cross-section of the abdomen of a 28-week fetus showing a cystic mass. A diagnosis of ovarian cyst was made.

Key points

1 Esophageal atresia is suspected when polyhydramnios is present and serial ultrasound examinations fail to demonstrate the fetal stomach, or the stomach appears permanently small (< 15% of the abdominal circumference). Prenatal diagnosis cannot be made at times, as gastric secretions may be enough to distend the stomach and make it visible. Moreover, in cases of associated tracheal fistula, the stomach may look normal.

2 Approximately half of fetuses with duodenal atresia have associated abnormalities, including trisomy 21 in about 40% of cases, skeletal defects (vertebral and rib anomalies, sacral agenesis, radial abnormalities, and talipes), gastrointestinal abnormalities (esophageal atresia/tracheo-esophageal fistula, intestinal malrotation, Meckel diverticulum, and anorectal atresia), and cardiac and renal defects.

3 Jejunal and ileal obstructions are imaged as multiple fluid-filled loops of bowel in the abdomen. The more distal the site of the obstruction, the greater the number of anechoic structures. The abdomen is usually distended, and active peristalsis may be observed. In cases of bowel perforation, transient ascites, meconium peritonitis, and meconium pseudocysts can be seen. After 25 weeks, polyhydramnios is rather common, particularly in proximal obstructions.

4 As meconium begins to accumulate in fetal bowel at 4 months, any perforation occurring after that time could bring the outflow of meconium into the peritoneal cavity. As a result, an intense reaction occurs, leading to extensive adhesions. If it is localized at the site of perforation, a calcified mass develops (fibroadhesive type). In other cases (cystic type), the continuous outflow of intestinal content into a cavity (pseudocyst) determines the formation of a highly echogenic mass at the site of the perforation. A peritonitis can be suspected when a fetus with intestinal obstruction suddenly shows the presence of ascites or generalized hydrops. Prognosis is generally severe. In stable conditions, without ascites, obstetric management should not change. In case of a deteriorating condition, with developing ascites, preterm delivery should be considered to avoid damage to the bowel.

5 Omphalocele is often associated with other abnormalities, such as gut and duodenal obstructions, exstrophy of the bladder, penile anomalies, and undescended testes, and particularly congenital heart diseases, which represent the most important cause of death for the affected child. Chromosomal abnormalities (mainly trisomy 18 or 13) are found in about 30% of cases at midgestation and in 15% of neonates. Beckwith–Wiedemann syndrome (EMG syndrome) is a mostly sporadic genetic syndrome, which includes omphalocele, macroglossia, and macrosomia with hyperplastic fetal visceromegaly; a severe resistant neonatal hypoglycemia and mental handicap are sometimes present. Pentalogy of Cantrell includes a large upper abdominal omphalocele, an anterior diaphragmatic hernia, a sternal cleft, an ectopia cordis, and cardiac anomalies such as ventricular septal defect or tetralogy of Fallot.

6 Prenatal diagnosis of omphalocele is based on the demonstration of the midline anterior abdominal wall

defect, the herniated sac with its visceral contents, and the umbilical cord insertion at the apex of the sac. As normal migration of the midgut back into the abdomen occurs between the 9th and the 12th gestational weeks, the diagnosis of ventral wall defects should not be made before 14 weeks. Exceptionally, heart and bladder are contained in the herniated sac. In small defects, umbilical cord insertion is on top of the mass, whereas in large lesions, the cord is attached to its lower border.

7 In gastroschisis, the loops of intestine lie uncovered in the amniotic fluid. Occasionally, only a short tract of the intestine is herniated; in most cases, however, all the small and large intestines protrude. Stomach, gallbladder, urinary bladder, testes or uterus, and adnexae are also prolapsed. Chemical peritonitis is an ominous complication due to amniotic fluid exposure of eviscerated abdominal contents. In such cases, the intestine shows marked dilation of the lumen and increased thickness of the walls.

8 The impact of the route of delivery on outcome is still debated in the case of gastroschisis and omphalocele. As babies born from elective Cesarean section seem to have a lower risk of sepsis and short-term morbidity, the benefit of Cesarean section versus vaginal delivery is not yet clearly demonstrated. It seems crucial, however, that delivery takes place in tertiary care centers where the neonate can receive intensive care and prompt surgical correction. Long-term follow-up of survivors is excellent.

9 Bladder exstrophy is a consequence of impaired development of the caudal fold of the anterior abdominal wall. The anterior wall is absent, and exposure of the posterior bladder wall is common. Omphalocele, as well as epispadias, is frequently associated with incomplete descent of the testicles and imperforate anus. Cloacal exstrophy is associated with omphalocele, exstrophy of the bladder, imperforated anus, and spinal defects such as meningomyelocele.

10 Failed visualization of kidneys and bladder, associated with oligohydramnios, prompts the diagnosis of bilateral renal agenesis. Prenatal diagnosis can be rather difficult due to the lack of amniotic fluid and the "crumpled" position adopted by these fetuses. Additionally, adrenals are usually hypertrophic and can be confused with normal kidneys. Identification of the renal capsule and renal pelvis enables the two structures to be distinguished. Failure to visualize the renal arteries with color Doppler is another important clue to the diagnosis. The differential diagnosis includes premature rupture of the membranes, severe uteroplacental insufficiency, and obstructive uropathy or bilateral multicystic or polycystic kidneys. Vaginal sonography with a high-resolution probe may be useful in these cases.

11 Multicystic kidneys are usually unilateral and appear as a cluster of multiple irregular cysts of variable size with little intervening hyperechogenic stroma. Affected kidneys are usually extremely enlarged. Distinction between MDKD and obstructions at the UPJ in prenatal sonograms can be extremely difficult. Coronal scans may demonstrate the connection between the renal pelvis and the dilated caliceal system in UPJ, and separation of the cysts in MDKD. Such a distinction is much easier when ultrasound examination is performed in early pregnancy, as the progression of obstructive uropathy results in a sonographic appearance similar to that of MDKD.

12 Early and persistent obstruction of the lower urinary tract is associated with secondary cystic dysplasia of the kidneys that appear enlarged, hyperechogenic, and present small cysts that spread through the parenchyma. In these cases, the diagnosis is made by the simultaneous demonstration of obstructive uropathy (distended bladder, convoluted ureters, pyelectasia, oligohydramnios), and the prognosis is poor.

13 Autosomal-recessive cystic kidneys (also referred to as infantile polycystic kidney) invariably involves both kidneys, with a recurrence risk of 1 in 20 000 live births. A defect in the collecting system seems to be responsible for the anomaly. Kidneys are symmetrically enlarged, and the parenchyma is totally occupied by numerous cysts of minute dimensions. Sonographically, both kidneys usually appear extremely enlarged and hyperechogenic. The hyperechogenicity seems to be due to multiple minute cysts, which fall below the resolution power of the ultrasound equipment, thus increasing the acoustic transmission. In severe cases, the bladder is absent and oligohydramnios is extreme.

14 Autosomal-dominant cystic kidneys is a common inherited nephropathy affecting more than 1 in 1000 live births. It may be inherited as an autosomal-dominant trait, and it may be a feature of genetic and nongenetic syndromes. Sporadic cases have also been reported in the literature.

15 Hydronephrosis refers to dilatation of the renal pelvis. Mild hydronephrosis, or pyelectasia, is defined by the presence of an anteroposterior diameter of the pelvis of more than 4 mm at mid-gestation and more than 7 mm in the third trimester. Transient hydronephrosis may be due to relaxation of smooth muscle of the urinary tract by high levels of progesterone or maternal–fetal overhydration. In the majority of cases, the condition remains stable or resolves in the neonatal period. In about 20% of cases, there may be an underlying pathology that requires postnatal follow-up and possible surgery.

16 Sonographically, it may be be difficult to distinguish severe hydronephrosis with significant caliceal enlargement from a multicystic kidney. Coronal scans demonstrate the radial projection of the calices around the enlarged pelvis enabling the diagnosis. Duplication

of the kidney is commonly associated with dilation of one or both renal pelves.

17 Megacystis is defined as an abnormal enlargement of the urinary bladder, and is most frequently the consequence of urethral obstruction. It is usually seen in the early midtrimester and has been visualized as early as 11 weeks' gestation. A more or less severe oligohydramnios is present.

18 Megacystis associated with an increased amount of amniotic fluid raises the suspicion of a megacystis–microcolon–intestinal hypoperistalsis syndrome. This is a sporadic abnormality characterized by a massively dilated bladder and hydronephrosis in the presence of normal or increased amniotic fluid; the fetuses are usually female. There is associated shortening and dilation of the proximal small bowel and microcolon with absent or ineffective peristalsis. The condition is usually lethal owing to bowel and renal dysfunction.

19 Prenatal surgical treatment of bilateral urinary obstructive uropathies relies on antenatal evaluation of renal function. Potential candidates for intrauterine surgery are fetuses with: (1) bilateral moderately severe pelvicaliceal dilation and normal cortical echogenicity; (2) normal levels of urinary sodium, calcium, and beta-2 microglobulin. One must remember, however, that normal values cannot exclude renal failure in childhood.

20 Prenatal diagnosis of fetal ovarian cyst is based on the ultrasound finding of a cystic mass in the fetal lower abdomen, integrity of GI and GU tracts, and female sex. In the majority of cases, the cyst is completely fluid; sometimes it is septated. Polyhydramnios is often present. Differential diagnosis should be made with other abdominal cystic lesions such as mesenteric and urachal cysts, enteric duplication anomalies, cystic teratoma, and low intestinal obstructions. Serial examinations of the anomaly allow the detection of structural changes in the cyst, which prompt the diagnosis of a complication of the cyst.

References

1 Touloukian RJ, Hobbins JC. Maternal ultrasonography on the antenatal diagnosis of surgically correctable fetal abnormalities. *J Pediatr Surg* 1980;15:373.

2 Campbell S, Wilkin D. Ultrasonic measurement of fetal abdominal circumference in estimation of fetal weight. *Br J Obstet Gynaecol* 1975;82:689.

3 Sepulveda W, Nicolaidis P, Mai AM, et al. Is isolated second-trimester hyperechogenic bowel a predictor of suboptimal fetal growth? *Ultrasound Obstet Gynecol* 1996;7:104.

4 Sepulveda W, Hollingsworth J, Bower S. Fetal hyperechogenic bowel following intramniotic bleeding. *Obstet Gynecol* 1994;83:947.

5 Lawson TL, Foley WD, Berland LL, et al. Ultrasonic evaluation of fetal kidneys: analysis of normal size and frequency of visualization as related to stage of pregnancy. *Radiology* 1981;138: 153.

6 Bowie JD, Rosemberg ER, Andreotti MD, et al. The changing sonographic appearance of fetal kidneys during pregnancy. *J Ultrasound Med* 1983;2:505.

7 Jeanty P, Dramaix-Wilmet M, Elkhazen N. Measurement of fetal kidney growth on ultrasound. *Radiology* 1982;144: 159.

8 Abramovich DR. The volume of amniotic fluid and its regulating factors. In: Fairweather DVI, Eskes TKA, eds. *Amniotic fluid research and clinical application*, 2nd edn. Amsterdam: Excerpta Medica; 1978:31.

9 Campbell S, Wladimiroff JW, Dewhurst CJ. The antenatal measurement of fetal urine production. *J Obstet Gynaecol Br Commonw* 1973;80:680.

10 Haeusler MC, Berghold A, Stoll C, et al. Prenatal ultrasonographic detection of gastrointestinal obstruction: results from 18 European congenital anomaly registries. *Prenat Diagn* 2002;22: 616.

11 Duenholter JH, Santos-Ramos R, Rosenfeld CR, et al. Prenatal diagnosis of gastrointestinal tract obstruction. *Obstet Gynecol* 1976;47:976.

12 Chittmittrapap S, Spitz L, Kiely EM, et al. Oesophageal atresia and associated anomalies. *Arch Dis Child* 1989;64:364.

13 Smith DW. *Recognizable patterns of human malformation*, 4th edn. Philadelphia, PA: W.B. Saunders; 1989:602–603.

14 Eyheremendy E, Pfister M. Antenatal real-time diagnosis of esophageal atresia. *J Clin Ultrasound* 1983;11:395.

15 Grybowski J, Walker WA. *Gastrointestinal problems in the infant*, 2nd edn. Philadelphia, PA: W.B. Saunders; 1983:877–895.

16 Andrassy RJ, Mahour GH. Gastrointestinal anomalies associated with oesophageal atresia or tracheoesophageal fistula. *Arch Surg* 1979;114:1125.

17 Gross RE. *The surgery of infancy and childhood*. Philadelphia: W.B. Saunders, 1953.

18 Loveday BJ, Barr JA, Aitken J. The intrauterine demonstration of duodenal atresia by ultrasound. *Br J Radiol* 1975;48:1031.

19 Romero R, Ghidini A, Gabrielli S, et al. Gastrointestinal tract and abdominal wall defects. In: Brock DJH, Rodeck CH, Ferguson-Smith MA, eds. *Prenatal diagnosis and screening*. Edinburgh: Churchill Livingstone; 1992:227.

20 Petrikowski BM. First trimester diagnosis of duodenal atresia. *Am J Obstet Gynecol* 1994;171:569.

21 Wrobleski D, Wesselhoef C. Ultrasonic diagnosis of prenatal intestinal obstruction. *J Pediatr Surg* 1979;14:598.

22 Nikapota VLB, Loman C. Gray-scale sonographic demonstration of fetal small bowel atresia. *J Clin Ultrasound* 1979;7:307.

23 Basu R, Burge DM. The effect of antenatal diagnosis on the management of small bowel atresia. *Pediatr Surg Int* 2004;20: 177.

24 Baxi LV, Yeh MN, Blanc WA, et al. Antepartum diagnosis and management of in utero intestinal volvulus with perforation. *N Engl J Med* 1983;308:1519.

25 Seward JF, Zusman J. Hydrops fetalis associated with small bowel volvulus. *Lancet* 1978;i52.

26 Blumenthal DH, Rushovich AM, Williams RK, et al. Prenatal sonographic findings of meconium peritonitis with pathological correlations. *J Clin Ultrasound* 1982;10:350.
27 Konye JC, de Chazal R, MacFayden U, et al. Antenatal diagnosis and management of meconium peritonitis: a case report and review of the literature. *Ultrasound Obstet Gynecol* 1995;6:66.
28 Avni EF, Rypens F, Donner C, et al. Hepatic cysts and hyperechogenicities: perinatal assessment and unifying theory on their origin. *Pediatr Radiol* 1994;24:569.
29 Richards DS, Langham MR, Anderson CD. The prenatal sonographic appearance of enteric duplication cysts. *Ultrasound Obstet Gynecol* 1996;7:17.
30 Moore L, Toi A, Chitayat D. Abnormalities of the intra-abdominal fetal umbilical vein: report of four cases and a review of the literature. *Ultrasound Obstet Gynecol* 1996;7:21.
31 Shen O, Tadmor OP, Yagel S. Prenatal diagnosis of persistent right umbilical vein. *Ultrasound Obstet Gynecol* 1996;8:31.
32 Achiron R, Seidman DS, Afek A, et al. Prenatal ultrasonographic diagnosis of fetal hepatic hyperechogenicities: clinical significance and implications for management. *Ultrasound Obstet Gynecol* 1996;7:251.
33 Morison JE. *Fetal and neonatal pathology*, 2nd edn. London: Butterworths, 1963.
34 Mayer T, Black R, Matlak M, et al. Gastroschisis and omphalocele. An eight year review. *Ann Surg* 1980;192:783.
35 Snijders RJM, Sebire NJ, Souka A, et al. Fetal exomphalos and chromosomal defects: relationship to maternal age and gestation. *Ultrasound Obstet Gynecol* 1995;6:250.
36 Meizner I, Bar-Ziv J. In utero prenatal ultrasound diagnosis of a rare case of cloacal exstrophy. *J Clin Ultrasound* 1985;13:500.
37 Paidas MJ, Crombleholme TM, Robertson FM. Prenatal diagnosis and management of fetus with an abdominal wall defect. *Semin Perinatol* 1994;18:196.
38 Achiron R, Soriano D, Lipitz S, et al. Fetal midgut herniation into the umbilical cord: improved definition of ventral abdominal anomaly with the use of transvaginal sonography. *Ultrasound Obstet Gynecol* 1995;6:256.
39 Schmidt W, Jarkoni S, Crelin ES, et al. Sonographic visualization of physiologic anterior abdominal wall hernia in the first trimester. *Obstet Gynecol* 1987;69:911.
40 Harrison MR, Filly RA, Stauger P, et al. Prenatal diagnosis and management of omphalocele and ectopia cordis. *J Pediatr Surg* 1982;17:64.
41 Fink IJ, Filly RA. Omphalocele associated with umbilical cord allantoic cyst: sonographic evaluation in utero. *Obstet Gynecol* 1983;149:473.
42 Heider AL, Strauss RA, Kuller JA. Omphalocele: clinical outcomes in cases with normal karyotypes. *Am J Obstet Gynecol* 2004;190:135.
43 Blazer S, Zimmer EZ, Gover A, et al. Fetal omphalocele detected early in pregnancy: associated anomalies and outcomes. *Radiology* 2004;232:191.
44 Tsakayannis DE, Zurakowski D, Lillehei CW. Respiratory insufficiency at birth: a predictor of mortality for infants with omphalocele. *J Pediatr Surg* 1996;31:1088.
45 Biard JM, Wilson RD, Johnson MP, et al. Prenatally diagnosed giant omphaloceles: short- and long term outcomes. *Prenat Diagn* 2004;24:434.
46 Nakajama DK. Management of the fetus with an abdominal wall defect. In: Harrison MR, Golbus MS, Filly RA, eds. *The unborn patient: prenatal diagnosis and treatment*. Orlando, FL: Grune & Stratton; 1984:217.
47 Harrison MR, Golbus MS, Filly RA. The management of the fetus with a correctable congenital defect. *JAMA* 1981;246:744.
48 Kirk EP, Wah RM. Obstetrics management of a fetus with omphalocele or gastroschisis. *Am J Obstet Gynecol* 1983;146:512.
49 Klein MD, Kosloske AM, Hertzier JH. Congenital defects of abdominal wall. A review of the experience in New Mexico. *JAMA* 1981;245:1643.
50 Shaw A. The myth of gastroschisis. *J Pediatr Surg* 1975;10:235.
51 Thomas DFM, Atwell JD. The embryology and surgical management of gastroschisis. *Br J Surg* 1976;63:893.
52 Hoyme EH, Higginbotton CM, Jones LK. The vascular pathogenesis of gastroschisis: intrauterine interruption of the omphalomesenteric artery. *J Pediatr* 1981:98:228.
53 Giulian BB, Alvear DT. Prenatal ultrasonographic diagnosis of fetal gastroschisis. *Radiology* 1978;129:473.
54 Colombani PM, Cunningham MD. Perinatal aspects of omphalocele and gastroschisis. *Am J Dis Child* 1977;131:1386.
55 Mabogunje OOA, Mahour GH. Omphalocele and gastroschisis: trends in survival across two decades. *Am J Surg* 1984;148:679.
56 Langer JC, Khanna J, Caco C, et al. Prenatal diagnosis of gastroschisis: development of objective sonographic criteria for predicting outcome. *Obstet Gynecol* 1993;81:53.
57 Pryde PG, Bardicef M, Treadwell MC, et al. Gastroschisis: can antenatal ultrasound predict infant outcomes? *Obstet Gynecol* 1994;84:505.
58 Baerg J, Kaban G, Tonita J, et al. Gastroschisis: a sixteen-year review. *J Pediatr Surg* 2003;38:771.
59 Aina-Mumuney AJ, Fischer AC, Blakemore KJ, et al. A dilated fetal stomach predicts a complicated postnatal course in cases of prenatally diagnosed gastroschisis. *Am J Obstet Gynecol* 2004;190:1326.
60 Fries MH, Filly RA, Callen PW, et al. Growth retardation in prenatally diagnosed cases of gastroschisis. *J Ultrasound Med* 1993;12:583.
61 Brantberg A, Blaas HG, Salvesen KA, et al. Surveillance and outcome of fetuses with gastroschisis. *Ultrasound Obstet Gynecol* 2004;23:4.
62 Sakala EP, Erhard LN, White JJ. Elective cesarean section improves outcomes of neonates with gastroschisis. *Am J Obstet Gynecol* 1993;169:1050.
63 Adra AM, Landy HJ, Nahmias J, Gomez-Marin O. The fetus with gastroschisis: impact of route of delivery and prenatal ultrasonography. *Am J Obstet Gynecol* 1996;174:540.
64 Quirk JG, Fortney J, Collins HB, et al. Outcomes of newborns with gastroschisis: the effects of mode of delivery, site of delivery, and interval from birth to surgery. *Am J Obstet Gynecol* 1996;174:1134.
65 Swartz KR, Harrison MW, Campbell JR, Campbell TJ. Long-term follow-up of patients with gastroschisis. *Am J Surg* 1986;151:546.
66 Mann L, Ferguson-Smith MA. Prenatal assessment of anterior abdominal wall defects and their prognosis. *Prenat Diagn* 1984;4:427.
67 Grybowski J, Walker WA. *Gastrointestinal problems in the infant*. Philadelphia, PA: W.B. Saunders; 1983:284–287.
68 Meizner I, Levy A, Barnhard Y. Cloacal exstrophy sequence: an exceptional ultrasound diagnosis. *Obstet Gynecol* 1995;86:446.
69 Warne S, Chitty LS, Wilcox DT. Prenatal diagnosis of cloacal anomalies. *Br J Urol Int* 2002;89:78.
70 Lund DP, Hendren WH. Cloacal exstrophy: experience with 20 cases. *J Pediatr Surg* 1993;28:1360.

71 Schwoebel MG, Sacher P, Bucher HU, et al. Prenatal diagnosis improves the prognosis in children with obstructive uropathy. *J Pediatr Surg* 1984;19:187.

72 Barss VA, Benacerraf BR, Frigoletto FD. Second trimester oligohydramnios, a predictor of poor fetal outcome. *Obstet Gynecol* 1984;64:608.

73 Caire JT, Ramus RM, Magee K, et al. MRI of fetal genitourinary anomalies. *Am J Roentgenol* 2003;181:1381.

74 Osathanondh V, Potter EL. Pathogenesis of polycystic kidneys. *Arch Pathol* 1964;77:459.

75 Pashayan H, Dowd T, Nigro AV. Bilateral absence of the kidneys and ureters. Three cases reported in one family. *J Med Genet* 1977;14:205.

76 Perlman M, Levin M. Fetal pulmonary hypoplasia, anuria and oligohydramnios: clinico-pathologic observations and review of the literature. *Am J Obstet Gynecol* 1974;118:1119.

77 Dubbins PA, Kurtz AB, Wapner RJ, et al. Renal agenesis: spectrum of in utero findings. *J Clin Ultrasound* 1981;9:189.

78 Johannessen JV, Haneberg B, Moe PJ. Bilateral multicystic dysplasia of the kidneys. *Beitr Pathol Bd* 1973;148:290.

79 Sanders RC, Hartman DS. The sonographic distinction between neonatal multicystic kidney and hydronephrosis. *Radiology* 1984;151:621.

80 Bernstein J, Kissane JM. Hereditary disorders of the kidney. *Perspect Pediatr Pathol* 1973;1:117.

81 Potter EL, Craig JM. *The pathology of the fetus and infant*, 3rd edn. Chicago: Yearbook Medical Publishers, 1975.

82 Aubertin G, Cripps S, Coleman G, et al. Prenatal diagnosis of apparently isolated unilateral multicystic kidney: implications for counseling and management. *Prenat Diagn* 2002;22: 388.

83 Friedberg JE, Mitnick JS, David DA. Antepartum ultrasonic detection of multicystic kidney. *Radiology* 1979;131:198.

84 Rizzo N, Gabrielli S, Pilu G, et al. Prenatal diagnosis and obstetrical management of multicystic dysplastic kidney disease. *Prenat Diagn* 1987;7:109.

85 Beretsky I, Laukin DH, Rusoff JH, Phelan L. Sonographic differentiation between the multicystic dysplastic kidney and the uretero-pelvic junction obstruction in utero using high-resolution real-time scanners employing digital detection. *J Clin Ultrasound* 1984;12:429.

86 Kelalis PP, King LR. *Clinical pediatric urology*. Philadelphia: W.B. Saunders, 1976.

87 King LR. Editorial comment. In: *Yearbook of urology*. Chicago: Yearbook Medical Publishers; 1974:61.

88 Roume J, Ville Y. Prenatal diagnosis of genetic renal diseases: breaking the code. *Ultrasound Obstet Gynecol* 2004;24:10.

89 Romero R, Cullen M, Jeanty P, et al. The diagnosis of congenital renal anomalies with ultrasound. II: infantile polycystic renal disease. *Am J Obstet Gynecol* 1984;150:259.

90 Simpson JL, Sabbagha RE, Elias S, et al. Failure to detect polycystic kidneys in utero by second trimester ultrasonography. *Hum Genet* 1982;60:295.

91 Madewell JE, Hartman DS, Lichtenstein JE. Radiologic–pathologic correlations in cystic disease of the kidney. *Radiol Clin North Am* 1979;133:580.

92 Spence HM, Singleton R. Cysts and cystic disorders of the kidneys: types, diagnosis and treatment. *Urol Surv* 1972;22: 131.

93 Zerres K, Weiss H, Bulla M. Prenatal diagnosis of an early manifestation of autosomal dominant adult-type polycystic kidney disease. *Lancet* 1982;2:988.

94 Zerres K, Volpel MC, Weiss H. Cystic kidneys. Genetics, pathologic anatomy, clinical picture, and prenatal diagnosis. *Hum Genet* 1984;68:104.

95 Main D, Mennuti MT, Cornfeld D, et al. Prenatal diagnosis of adult polycystic kidney disease. *Lancet* 1983;2:337.

96 Reeders ST, Zerres K, Ga IA, et al. Prenatal diagnosis of autosomal dominant polycystic kidney disease with a DNA probe. *Lancet* 1986;2:6.

97 Sairam S, Al-Habib A, Sasson S, Thilaganathan B. Natural history of fetal hydronephrosis diagnosed on mid-trimester ultrasound. *Ultrasound Obstet Gynecol.* 2001;17:191.

98 Wickstrom E, Maizels M, Sabbagha RE, et al. Isolated fetal pyelectasis: assessment of risk for postnatal uropathy and Down syndrome. *Ultrasound Obstet Gynecol* 1996;8:236.

99 Persutte WH, Koyle M, Lenke RR, et al. Mild pyelectasis ascertained with prenatal ultrasonography is pediatrically significant. *Ultrasound Obstet Gynecol* 1997;10:12.

100 Jeffrey RB, Laing FC, Wing VW, et al. Sonography of the fetal duplex kidney. *Radiology* 1984;153:123.

101 Montana MA, Cyr DR, Lenke RR, et al. Sonographic detection of fetal ureteral obstruction. *Am J Roentgenol* 1985;145: 595.

102 Whitten SM, McHoney M, Wilcox DT, et al. Accuracy of antenatal fetal ultrasound in the diagnosis of duplex kidneys. *Ultrasound Obstet Gynecol* 2003;21:342.

103 Abuhamad AZ, Horton CEJ, Horton SH, et al. Renal duplication anomalies in the fetus: clues for prenatal diagnosis. *Ultrasound Obstet Gynecol* 1996;7:174.

104 Liao AW, Sebire NJ, Geerts L, et al. Megacystis at 10–14 weeks of gestation: chromosomal defects and outcome according to bladder length. *Ultrasound Obstet Gynecol* 2003;21:338.

105 Levine PM, Delaune J, Gonzales ET, Jr. Genetic etiology of posterior urethral valves. *J Urol* 1983;130:781.

106 Beck AD. The effect of intrauterine urinary obstruction upon the development of fetal kidney. *J Urol* 1971;105:784.

107 Mahony BS, Callen PW, Filly RA. Fetal urethral obstruction: US evaluation. *Radiology* 1985;157:221.

108 Jouannic J, Hyett Jon A, Pandya PP, et al. Perinatal outcome in fetuses with megacystis in the first half of pregnancy. *Prenat Diagn* 2003;23:340.

109 Harrison MR, Golbus MS, Filly RA. Congenital hydronephrosis. In: Harrison MR, Golbus MS, Filly RA, eds. *The unborn patient*. Orlando, FL: Grune & Stratton; 1984:277.

110 Krueger RP, Hardy BE, Churchill BM. Growth in boys with posterior urethral valves. Primary valve resection vs. upper tract diversion. *Urol Clin North Am* 1980;7:265.

111 Evans M. Newsletter, International Fetal Medicine and Surgery Society, 1989.

112 Crombleholme TM, Harrison MR, Langer JC, et al. Early experience with open fetal surgery for congenital hydronephrosis. *J Pediatr Surg* 1988;23:1114.

113 Muller S, Dreux S, Audibert F, et al. Fetal serum β2-microglobulin and cystatin C in the prediction of post-natal renal function in bilateral hypoplasia and hyperechogenic enlarged kidneys. *Prenat Diagn* 2004;24:327.

114 Ahmed S. Neonatal and childhood ovarian cyst. *J Pediatr Surg* 1971;6:702.

115 Carlson DH, Griscom NT. Ovarian cysts in the newborn. *J Roentgenol Radium Ther Nucl Med* 1972;116:664.

116 Jafri SZ, Bree RL, Silver TM, et al. Fetal ovarian cysts: sonographic detection and association with hypothyroidism. *Radiology* 1984;150:809.

117 Valenti C, Kassner EG, Yermankov V, et al. Antenatal diagnosis of a fetal ovarian cyst. *Am J Obstet Gynecol* 1975;123:216.
118 Lee TG, Blake S. Prenatal fetal abdominal ultrasonography and diagnosis. *Radiology* 1977;124:475.
119 Kirkinen PJP, Tuononen S. Ultrasonic detection of bilateral ovarian cyst in the fetus. *Eur J Obstet Gynecol Reprod Biol* 1982;131:87.
120 Sandler MA, Smith SJ, Pope SG, et al. Prenatal diagnosis of septated ovarian cysts. *J Clin Ultrasound* 1985;13:55.
121 Rizzo N, Gabrielli S, Perolo A, et al. Prenatal diagnosis and management of fetal ovarian cysts. *Prenat Diagn* 1989;9:97.
122 Tabsh KMA. Antenatal sonographic appearance of a fetal ovarian cyst. *J Clin Ultrasound* 1982;1:329.
123 Preziosi P, Pariello G, Maiorana A, et al. Antenatal sonographic diagnosis of complicated ovarian cysts. *J Clin Ultrasound* 1986;14:196.

26

Fetal skeletal anomalies

Luís F. Gonçalves, Patricia L. Devers, Jimmy Espinoza, and Roberto Romero

Skeletal dysplasias are a heterogeneous group of disorders that affect the development of chondro-osseous tissues, resulting in abnormalities in the size and shape of various segments of the skeleton. Despite recent advances in imaging modalities and molecular genetics,[1–3] accurate prenatal diagnosis of skeletal dysplasias remains a clinical challenge.[4] Although 253 osteochondrodysplasias and 45 genetically determined dysostoses have been included in the most recent revision of the International Nosology and Classification of Constitutional Disorders of Bone,[5] the number that can be recognized with the use of sonography in the antepartum period is considerably smaller. This chapter reviews the birth prevalence, classification, and molecular genetics, and provides an approach to prenatal diagnosis of skeletal dysplasias identifiable at birth.

Birth prevalence and contribution to perinatal mortality

Table 26.1 presents a summary of the published prevalence of skeletal dysplasias abstracted from 12 studies.[6–17] Estimated prevalences ranged from 1.1 to 9.5 per 10 000 births, with the highest prevalence reported from a greatly inbred population.[17]

In a large multicentric Italian study, the birth prevalence of skeletal dysplasias recognizable in the neonatal period, excluding limb amputations, was estimated as 2.4 per 10 000 births.[7] In this large series, 23% of affected infants were stillborn and 32% died during the first week of life. The overall frequency of skeletal dysplasias among perinatal deaths was 9.1 per 1000. This study also reported the birth prevalence of the different skeletal dysplasias and their relative frequency among perinatal deaths (Table 26.2). The four most common skeletal dysplasias were thanatophoric dysplasia, achondroplasia, osteogenesis imperfecta, and achondrogenesis. Thanatophoric dysplasia and achondrogenesis accounted for 62% of all lethal skeletal dysplasias, whereas the most common nonlethal skeletal dysplasia was achondroplasia.[7]

In another larger series reporting the prevalence and classification of lethal neonatal skeletal dysplasias in the west of Scotland, the prevalence was 1.1 per 10 000 births, and the most frequently diagnosed conditions were thanatophoric dysplasia (1 per 42 000), osteogenesis imperfecta (1 per 56 000), chondrodysplasia puntacta (1 per 84 000), campomelic syndrome (1 per 112 000), and achondrogenesis (1 per 112 000).[8] Rasmussen and colleagues[15] reported a prevalence of 2.14 cases per 10 000 deliveries in a longitudinal study that included elective pregnancy termination, stillborn infants at more than 20 weeks of gestation, and liveborn infants diagnosed by the fifth day of life. The rate of lethal cases was 0.95 per 10 000 deliveries.[15]

Classification of skeletal dysplasias

Nosology

Over the past 30 years, the classification of skeletal dysplasias has evolved from one based upon clinical/radiological/pathological descriptions to one that also includes the underlying molecular abnormality for conditions in which the defect is known.[18] In an attempt to develop a uniform terminology, a group of experts met in Paris in 1977 and proposed an International Nomenclature for Skeletal Dysplasias based purely on descriptive findings of either a clinical or radiologic nature.[19] This nomenclature was revised in 1992,[20–22] when it was reoriented on radiodiagnostic and morphologic criteria, grouping morphologically similar disorders into families of disorders based on presumed pathogenetic similarities. The International Working Group on Constitutional Diseases of Bone met in Los Angeles, California, in 1997, to perform the third revision of the Paris Nomenclature of Constitutional Disorders of Bone.[23,24] Families of disorders were rearranged based on etiopathogenetic information concerning the gene and/or protein defect. Disorders in which the defect was well docu-

Table 26.1 Birth prevalence of osteochondrodysplasias: summary of 12 studies.

Reference	Rate per 10 000	Comment
Gustavson and Jorulf[6]	4.7	In newborns
Camera and Mastroiacovo[7]	2.4	In neonates
Connor and colleagues[8]	1.1	Lethal skeletal dysplasias in neonates
Weldner and colleagues[9]	7.5	–
Orioli and colleagues[10]	2.3	First 3 days of life
Stoll and colleagues[11]	3.2	First 8 days of life
Andersen and Hauge[12]	7.6	Diagnosed in all ages
Andersen[13]	1.5	Lethal chondrodysplasias only
Kallen and colleagues[14]	1.6	No details about age
Rasmussen and colleagues[15]	–	–
All cases	2.1	In first 5 days of life
Lethal chondrodysplasias	0.95	–
Gordienko and colleagues[16]	3.1	–
Al Gazali and colleagues[17]	9.5	Newborns and stillbirths > 500 g; prevalence of consanguinity 72%

Table 26.2 Birth prevalence (per 10 000 total births) of skeletal dysplasias.

Skeletal dysplasias	Birth prevalence (per 10 000)	Frequency among perinatal deaths
Thanatophoric dysplasia	0.69	1:246
Achondroplasia	0.37	–
Achondrogenesis	0.23	1:639
Osteogenesis imperfecta type II	0.18	1:799
Osteogenesis imperfecta (other types)	0.18	–
Asphyxiating thoracic dysplasia	0.14	1:3196
Chondrodysplasia puntacta	0.09	–
Campomelic dysplasia	0.05	1:3196
Chondroectodermal dysplasia	0.05	1:3196
Larsen syndrome	0.05	–
Mesomelic dysplasia (Langer's type)	0.05	–
Others	0.46	1:800

Reproduced with permission from ref. 7.

mented were regrouped into distinct families based on the mutations. These include the "achondroplasia group" of disorders with mutations in the fibroblast growth factor receptor 3 (*FGFR3*) gene, the "diastrophic dysplasia group" of disorders with mutations in diastrophic dysplasia sulfate transporter gene, the "type II collagenopathies" with mutations in the type II collagen gene, and the "type XI collagenopathies" with mutations in the cartilage oligomeric protein (*COMP*) gene. Several new groups were added, including the "lethal skeletal dysplasias," the group with fragmented bones, and the "miscellaneous neonatal severe dysplasia" group. Other groups were renamed. The classification was revised in 2001 and is now called the International Nosology and Classification of Constitutional Disorders of Bones (2001).[5] Although the classification remains a combination of morphological and molecular groupings of disorders, genetically determined dysostoses were added to the skeletal dysplasias, as in clinical practice these two groups overlap. Genetically determined dysostoses have been divided into three groups: those with predominant cranial and facial involvement (e.g., Crouzon syndrome), those with predominant axial involvement (e.g., spondylocostal dysplasia), and those with predominant involvement of the extremities (e.g., Fanconi syndromes). The full version of the 2001 classification[5] can be downloaded from the website of the International Skeletal Dysplasia Society (http://www.isds.ch/ISDSframes.html, last accessed on 06/11/2006).

Nosology of lethal skeletal dysplasias

Of special interest to perinatologists are the lethal osteochondrodysplasias, which were classified by Spranger and Maroteaux[25] into 11 groups based on the radioanatomical manifestations (Table 26.3). The purpose of this classification is to facilitate differential diagnosis, and the groups do not necessarily constitute pathogenetic "families."

Table 26.3 Nosology of lethal osteochondrodysplasias.

Hypophosphatasia and morphologically similar disorders	Short rib–polydactyly syndrome, type IV (Yang)
Hypophosphatasia	Short rib–polydactyly syndromes
Probable hypophosphatasia	Short rib–polydactyly syndrome, type VI (Majewski)
Lethal metaphyseal dysplasia	Short rib–polydactyly syndrome, type VII (Beemer)
Chondrodysplasia punctata and similar disorders	*Lethal metatropic dysplasia and similar disorders*
Rhizomelic chondrodysplasia punctata	Lethal metatropic dysplasia (hyperchondrogenesis)
Lethal chondrodysplasia punctata, X-linked dominant	Fibrochondrogenesis
Greenberg dysplasia	Schneckenbecken dysplasia
Dappled diaphysis dysplasia	*Kniest-like disorders*
Achondrogenesis and similar disorders	Dyssegmental dysplasia, Silverman type
Achondrogenesis IA (Houston–Harris)	Dyssegmental dysplasia, Rolland–Desbuquois
Achondrogenesis IB (Fraccaro)	Lethal Kniest disease
New lethal osteochondrodysplasia	Chondrodysplasia resembling Kniest dysplasia
Achondrogenesis II (Langer–Saldino)	Blomstrand chondrodysplasia
Hypochondrogenesis	*Lethal osteochondrodysplasias with pronounced diaphyseal abnormalities*
Thanatophoric dysplasia and similar disorders	Campomelic syndrome
Thanatophoric dysplasia, type I	Stuve–Wiedemann syndrome
Thanatophoric dysplasia, type II	Boomerang dysplasia
Homozygous achondroplasia	Atelosteogenesis
Lethal achondrodysplasia	Disorder resembling atelosteogenesis
Glasgow variant	de la Chappelle dysplasia
Platyspondylic lethal chondrodysplasias	McAlister dysplasia
Platyspondylic chondrodysplasia, Torrance type	Pseudodystrophic dysplasia
Platyspondylic chondrodysplasia, San Diego type	*Osteogenesis imperfecta and similar disorders*
Platyspondylic chondrodysplasia, Luton type	Osteogenesis imperfecta type IIA
Platyspondylic chondrodysplasia, Shiraz type	Osteogenesis imperfecta type IIB
Opsismodysplasia	Osteogenesis imperfecta type IIC
Sixth form of platyspondylic chondrodysplasia	Astley–Kendall dysplasia
Seventh form of platyspondylic chondrodysplasia	*Lethal disorders with gracile bones*
Short rib–polydactyly syndromes	Fetal hypokinesia phenotype
Short rib–polydactyly syndrome, type I (Saldino–Noonan)	Lethal osteochondrodysplasia with gracile bones
Short rib–polydactyly syndrome, type II (Verma–Naumoff)	Lethal osteochondrodysplasia with intrauterine overtubulation
Short rib–polydactyly syndrome, type III (Le Marec)	

Reproduced with permission from ref. 25.

Molecular–pathogenetic classification of skeletal dysplasias

The process of skeletal formation and growth includes differentiation of mesenchymal cells to form cartilage for future bone endochondral ossification. Long bone growth occurs through differentiation of chondrocytes in the growth plates, whereas the craniofacial skeleton and clavicles develop by intramembranous ossification.[26,27] Disruption in any of these processes results in skeletal abnormalities.[28] A wide range of phenotypes has been described in osteochondrodysplasias. However, recent advances in the understanding of the molecular basis of skeletal dysplasias indicate that a spectrum of phenotypes share a similar genetic basis.[29,30] Although the familial tendency of chondrodysplasias has been known for many years, the molecular basis for a number of conditions has only recently been clarified.[2,3,31,31,32]

Therefore, it is anticipated that two parallel but interacting classifications will evolve, one clinical, and the other molecular, to help further understand the pathogenesis of individual disorders. Indeed, a classification of genetic disorders of the skeleton based on the structure and function of implicated genes and proteins has recently been proposed (Molecular–Pathogenetic Classification of Genetic Disorders of the Skeleton – Table 26.4)[2] to complement the existing International Nosology and Classification of Constitutional Disorders of Bone[5]. In this classification skeletal disorders with a well-documented genetic and biochemical basis were assigned to one of seven groups: (1) defects in extracellular structural

Table 26.4 Molecular–pathogenetic classification of genetic disorders of the skeleton.

Gene or protein	Inheritance	Clinical phenotype	References
Group 1: Defects in extracellular structural proteins			
COL1A1, COL1A2 (collagen 1 α1, α2 chains)	AD	*Family:* Osteogenesis imperfecta	Byers 1990;[834] Prockop and colleagues, 1994[835]
COL2A1 (collagen 2 α1 chain)	AD	*Family:* achondrogenesis 2, hypochondrogenesis, congenital spondyloepiphyseal dysplasia (SEDC), Kniest dysplasia, Stickler artho-ophthalmopathy, familial osteoarthritis, other variants	Spranger and colleagues, 1994[836]
COL9A1, COL9A2, COL9A3 (collagen 9 α1, α2, α3 chains)	AD	Multiple epiphyseal dysplasia (MED, two or more variants)	Lohiniva and colleagues, 2000;[837] Spayde and colleagues, 2000[838]
COL10A1 (collagen 10 α chain)	AD	Metaphyseal dysplasia Schmid	Wallis and colleagues, 1996[839]
Col11A1, Col11A2 (collagen 11 α1, α2 chains)	AR, AD	Otospondylomegaepiphyseal dysplasia (OSMED), Stickler (variant), Marshall syndrome	Melkoniemi and colleagues, 2000;[840] Spranger, 1998[841]
COMP (cartilage oligomeric matrix protein)	AD	Pseudoachondroplasia, multiple epiphyseal dysplasia (MED, one form)	Briggs and colleagues, 1998[842]
MATN3 (matrilin-3)	AD	Multiple epiphyseal dysplasia (MED, one variant)	Chapman and colleagues, 2001[843]
Perlecan	AR	Schwartz–Jampel type 1, dyssegmental dysplasia	Arikawa-Hirasawa and colleagues, 2001[441]
Group 2: Defects in metabolic pathways (including enzymes, ion channels, and transporters)			
TNSALP (tissue nonspecific alkaline phosphatase)	AR, AD	Hypophosphatasia (several forms)	Mornet and colleagues, 1998[407]
ANKH (pyrophosphate transporter)	AD	Craniometaphyseal dysplasia	Nurnberg and colleagues, 2001;[844] Reichenberger and colleagues, 2001[845]
DTDST/SLC26A2 (diastrophic dysplasia sulfate transporter)	AR	*Family:* achondrogenesis 1B, atelosteogenesis 2, diastrophic dysplasia, recessive multiple epiphyseal dysplasia (rMED)	Rossi and Superti-Furga, 2001;[414] Superti-Furga and colleagues, 1996a, b[846,847]
PAPSS2, phosphoadenosine-phosphosulfate-synthase 2	AR	Spondyloepimetaphyseal dysplasia Pakistani type	ul Haque and colleagues, 1998[848]
TCIRGI, osteoblast proton pump subunit	AR	Severe infantile osteopetrosis	Frattini and colleagues, 2000[849]
CIC-7 (chloride channel 7)	AR	Severe osteopetrosis	Kornak and colleagues, 2001[850]
Carboanhydrase II	AR	Osteopetrosis with intracranial calcifications and renal tubular acidosis	Venta and colleagues, 1991[851]
Vitamin K–epoxide reductase complex	AR	Chondrodysplasia punctata with vitamin K-dependent coagulation defects	Oldenburg and colleagues, 2000;[852] Pauli, 1988;[853] Pauli and colleagues, 1987[854]
MGP (matrix Gla protein)	AR	Keutel syndrome (pulmonary stenosis, brachytelephalangism, cartilage calcifications and short stature)	Munroe and colleagues, 1999[855]
ARSE (arylsulfatase E)	XLR	X-linked chondrodysplasia punctata (CDPX1)	Franco and colleagues, 1995[856]
3-β-hydroxysteroid-dehydrogenase	XLD	CHILD syndrome	Konig and colleagues, 2000[583]
3-β-hydroxysteroid Δ(8)Δ(7) isomerase	XLD	X-linked chondrodysplasia punctata, Conradi–Hünermann type (CDPX2), CHILD syndrome	Braverman and colleagues, 1999;[857] Grange and colleagues, 2000[858]

Table 26.4 *Continued*

Gene or protein	Inheritance	Clinical phenotype	References
PEX7 (peroxisomal receptor/ importer)	AR	Rhizomelic chondrodysplasia punctata 1	Motley and colleagues, 1997[859]
DHAPAT (dihydroxyacetonphosphate-acyltransferase, peroxisomal enzyme)	AR	Rhizomelic chondrodysplasia punctata 2	Ofman and colleagues, 1998[860]
Alkyldihydroxydiacetonphosphate synthase (AGPS; peroxisomal enzyme)	AR	Rhizomelic chondrodysplasia punctata 3	de Vet and colleagues, 1998[861]
Group 3: Defects in folding and degradation of macromolecules			
Sedlin (endoplasmic reticulum protein with unknown function)	XR	X-linked spondyloepiphyseal dysplasia (SED-XL)	Gedeon and colleagues, 1999[862]
Cathepsin K (lysosomal proteinase)	AR	Pycnodysostosis	Hou and colleagues, 1999[863]
Lysosomal acid hydrolases and transporters (sulfatase, glycosidase, translocase, etc.)	AR, XLR	Lysosomal storage diseases: mucopolysaccharidoses, oligosaccharidoses, glycoproteinoses (several forms)	Leroy and Wiesmann, 1993[864]
Targeting system of lysosomal enzymes (GlcNAc-1-phosphotransferase)	AR	Mucolipidosis II (I cell disease), mucolipidosis III	Leroy and Wiesmann, 1993[864]
MMP2 (matrix metalloproteinase 2)	AR	Torg-type osteolysis (nodulosis arthropathy and osteolysis syndrome)	Martignetti and colleagues, 2001[865]
Group 4: Defects in hormones and signal transduction mechanisms			
25-α-Hydroxycholecalciferol-1-hydroxylase	AR	Vitamin D-dependent rickets type 1 (VDDR1)	Kitanaka and colleagues, 1998[866]
1,25-α-Dihydroxy-vitamin D_3 receptor	AR	Vitamin D-resistant rickets with end organ unresponsiveness to vitamin D_3 (VDDR2)	Hughes and colleagues, 1988[867]
CASR (calcium "sensor"/receptor)	AD	Neonatal severe hyperparathyroidism with bone disease (if affected fetus in unaffected mother); familial hypocalciuric hypercalcemia	Bai and colleagues, 1997[868]
PTH/PTHrP receptor	AD (activating mutations), AR (inactivating mutation)	Metaphyseal dysplasia Jansen, lethal dysplasia Blomstrand	Schipani and colleagues, 1996;[869] Zhang and colleagues, 1998[870]
GNAS1 (stimulatory Gs alpha protein of adenylate cyclase)	AD	Pseudohypoparathyroidism (Albright hereditary osteodystrophy and several variants) with constitutional haploinsufficiency mutations, McCune–Albright syndrome with somatic mosaicism for activating mutations	Patten and colleagues, 1990[871]
PEX proteinase	XL	Hypophosphatemic rickets, X-linked semidominant type (impaired cleavage of FGF23)	The HYP Consortium, 1995;[872] Sabbagh and colleagues, 2000[873]
FGF23, fibroblasts growth factor 23	AD	Hypophosphatemic rickets, autosomal dominant type (resistance to PEX cleavage)	The ADHR Consortium, 2000[874]

Table 26.4 *Continued*

Gene or protein	Inheritance	Clinical phenotype	References
FGFR1 (fibroblast growth factor receptor 1)	AD	Craniosynostosis syndromes (Pfeiffer, other variants)	Wilkie, 1997[875]
FGFR2	AD	Craniosynostosis syndromes (Apert, Crouzon, Pfeiffer, several variants)	Wilkie, 1997[875]
FGFR3	AD	Thanatophoric dysplasia, achondroplasia, hypochondroplasia, SADDAN; craniosynostosis syndromes (Crouzon with acanthosis nigricans, Muenke nonsyndromic craniosynostosis)	Passos–Bueno and colleagues, 1999;[228] Wilkie, 1997[875]
ROR-2 ("orphan receptor tyrosine kinase")	AR	Robinow syndrome	Afzal and colleagues, 2000;[876] Van Bokhoven and colleagues, 2000[877]
	AD	Brachydactyly type B	Oldridge and colleagues, 2000[878]
TNFRSF11A (receptor activator of nuclear factor κB; RANK)	AD	Familial expansile osteolysis	Hughes and colleagues, 2000[879]
TGFβ1	AD	Diaphyseal dysplasia (Camurati–Engelmann)	Janssens and colleagues, 2000[880]
CDMP1 (cartilage-derived morphogenetic protein 1)	AR	Acromesomelic dysplasia Grebe/ Hunter–Thompson	Thomas and colleagues, 1997;[630] Thomas and colleagues, 1996[881]
	AD	Brachydactyly type C	Polinkovsky and colleagues, 1997[882]
Noggin ("growth factor," TGF antagonist)	AD	Multiple synostosis syndrome, synphalangism and hypoacusis syndrome	Gong and colleagues, 1999[883]
DLL3 (*delta-like 3*, intercellular signaling)	AR	Spondylocostal dysostosis (one form)	Bulman and colleagues, 2000[884]
IHH (Indian hedgehog signal molecule)	AD	Brachydactyly A1	Gao and colleagues, 2001[885]
C7orf2 (orphan receptor)	AR	Acheiropodia	Ianakiev and colleagues, 2001[886]
SOST (sclerostin; cystine knot secreted protein)	AR	Sclerosteosis, van Buchem disease	Balemans and colleagues, 2001[887]
LRP5 (LDL receptor- related protein 5)	AR	Osteoporosis–pseudoglioma syndrome	Gong and colleagues, 2001[888]
WISP3 (growth regulator/growth factor)	AR	Progressive pseudorheumatoid dysplasia	Hurvitz and colleagues, 1999[889]
Group 5: Defects in nuclear proteins and transcription factors			
SOX9 (HMG-type DNA binding protein/ transcription factor)	AD	Campomelic dysplasia	Wagner and colleagues, 1994[890]
GlI3 (zinc finger gene)	AD	Greig cephalopolysyndactyly, polydactyly type A and others, Pallister–Hall syndrome	Kalff–Suske and colleagues, 1999;[891] Radhakrishna and colleagues, 1999[892]
TRPS1 (zinc finger gene)	AD	Trichorhinophalangeal syndrome (types 1–3)	Momeni and colleagues, 2000[893]
EVC (leucine zipper gene)	AR	Chondroectodermal dysplasia (Ellis–van Creveld)	Ruiz-Perez and colleagues, 2000[548]
TWIST (helix–loop–helix transcription factor)	AD	Craniosynostosis Saethre–Chotzen	el Ghouzzi and colleagues, 1997[894]
P63 (p53-related transcription factor)	AD	EEC syndrome, Hay–Wells syndrome, limb–mammary syndrome, split hand–split foot malformation (some forms)	Celli and colleagues, 1999;[895] McGrath and colleagues, 2001;[896] Van Bokhoven and colleagues, 2001[897]
CBFA-1 (core binding factor A-1; runt-type transcription factor)	AD	Cleidocranial dysplasia	Mundlos and colleagues, 1997[898]
LXM1B (LIM homeodomain protein)	AD	Nail–patella syndrome	Dreyer and colleagues, 1998[899]

Table 26.4 *Continued*

Gene or protein	Inheritance	Clinical phenotype	References
DLX3 (distal-less 3 homeobox gene)	AD	Trichodento-osseous syndrome	Price and colleagues, 1998[900]
HOXD13 (homeobox gene)	AD	Synpolydactyly	Akarsu and colleagues, 1996[901]
MSX2 (homeobox gene)	AD (gain of function) AD (loss of function)	Craniosynostosis, Boston-type parietal foramina	Jabs and colleagues, 1993;[902] Wilkie and colleagues, 2001[903]
ALX4 (homeobox gene)	AD	Parietal foramina (cranium bifidum)	Mavrogiannis and colleagues, 2001[904]
SHOX (short stature-homeobox)	Pseudoautosomal	Léri–Weill dyschondrosteosis, idiopathic short stature?	Shears and colleagues, 1998[905]
TBX3 (T-box 3, transcription factor)	AD	Ulnar–mammary syndrome	Bamshad and colleagues, 1997[906]
TBX5 (T-box 5, transcription factor)	AD	Holt–Oram syndrome	Li and colleagues, 1997[733]
EIF2AK3 (transcription initiation factor kinase)	AR	Wolcott–Rallison syndrome (neonatal diabetes mellitus and spondyloepiphyseal dysplasia)	Delepine and colleagues, 2000[907]
NEMO (NFκB essential modulator; kinase activity)	XL	Osteopetrosis, lymphedema, ectodermal dysplasia and immunodeficiency (OLEDAID)	Doffinger and colleagues, 2001;[908] Smahi and colleagues, 2000[909]
Group 6: Defects in oncogenes and tumor suppressor genes			
EXT1, EXT2 (exostosin-1, exostosin-2; heparan sulfate polymerases)	AD	Multiple exostoses syndrome types 1 and 2	Cheung and colleagues, 2001;[910] Duncan and colleagues, 2001;[911] Lind and colleagues, 1998[912]
SH3BP2 (c-Abl-binding protein)	AD	Cherubism	Ueki and colleagues, 2001[913]
Group 7: Defects in RNA and DNA processing and metabolism			
RNAse MRP–RNA component	AR	Cartilage–hair–hypoplasia	Ridanpaa and colleagues, 2001;[914] Bonafé and colleagues, 2002[915]
ADA (adenosine deaminase)	AR	Severe combined immunodeficiency (SCID) with (facultative) metaphyseal changes	Hirschhorn, 1995[916]

Reproduced with permission from ref. 2.

proteins, (2) defects in metabolic pathways (including enzymes, ion channels, and transporters), (3) defects in folding and degradation of macromolecules, (4) defects in hormones and signal transduction mechanisms, (5) defects in nuclear proteins and transcription factors, (6) defects in oncogenes and tumor-suppressor genes, and (7) defects in RNA and DNA processing and metabolism.

Table 26.4 presents a comprehensive list of mutations associated with skeletal dysplasias and the clinical phenotypes associated with them.[2] The reader is reminded that approximately only one-third of bone dysplasias have had their molecular basis elucidated, and that new genes involved in skeletal dysplasias are continually being discovered.[3] We will review the significant mutations associated with each phenotype in subsequent sections of this chapter.

Terminology frequently used in the description of bone dysplasias

Shortening of the extremities can involve the entire limb (micromelia), the proximal segment (rhizomelia), the intermediate segment (mesomelia), or the distal segment (acromelia). The diagnosis of rhizomelia or mesomelia requires the comparison of the dimensions of the bones of the legs and forearm with those of the thigh and arm. Figures 26.1 and 26.2 display the relationship between the humerus and ulna, and the femur and tibia, and can be used in the assessment of rhizomelia and mesomelia. Table 26.5 presents the skeletal dysplasias characterized by rhizomelia, mesomelia, and micromelia.

Several skeletal dysplasias feature alterations of the hands

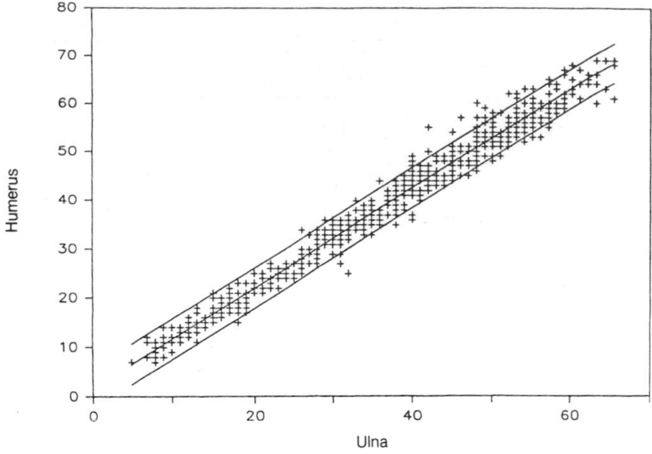

Figure 26.1 Relationship between the lengths of the ulna and the humerus.

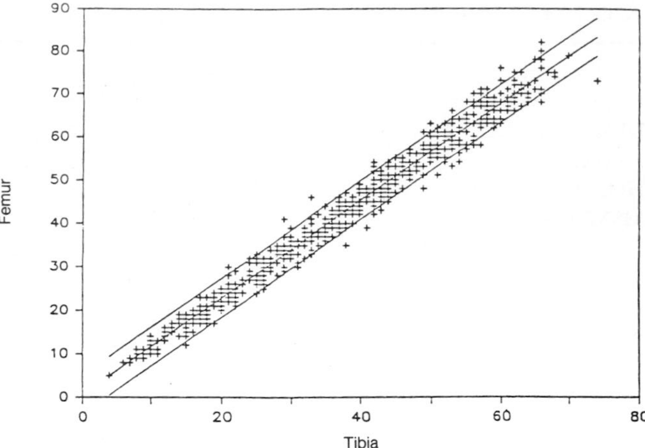

Figure 26.2 Relationship between the lengths of the tibia and femur.

Table 26.5 Skeletal dysplasias characterized by rhizomelia, mesomelia, and micromelia.

Rhizomelia
Thanatophoric dysplasia
Atelosteogenesis
Chondrodysplasia puntacta (rhizomelic type)
Congenital short femur
Achondroplasia
Mesomelia
Mesomelic dysplasia (Langer, Reinhardt, and Robinow types)
Acromelia
Ellis–van Creveld syndrome (chondroectodermal dysplasia)
Micromelia
Achondrogenesis
Atelosteogenesis
Short rib–polydactyly syndrome
Diastrophic dysplasia
Fibrochondrogenesis
Osteogenesis imperfecta (type II)
Kniest dysplasia
Dyssegmental dysplasia
Roberts syndrome

and feet. The term "polydactyly" refers to the presence of more than five digits. It is classified as *postaxial* if the extra digits are on the ulnar or fibular side, and *preaxial* if they are located on the radial or tibial side. Syndactyly refers to soft-tissue or bony fusion of adjacent digits. Clinodactyly consists of deviation of a finger (or fingers).

The most common spinal abnormality seen in skeletal dysplasias is platyspondyly, which consists of flattening of the vertebrae (Fig. 26.3).[33–39] Kyphosis and scoliosis can also be identified *in utero* (Fig. 26.4).[40–44] Prenatal diagnosis of hemivertebra (Fig. 26.5)[40,45,46] and coronal clefting of vertebral bodies has been made.[43,47]

Biometry of the fetal skeleton in the diagnosis of bone dysplasias

Long-bone biometry has been used extensively for the prediction of gestational age. Nomograms for this purpose use the long bone as the independent variable and the estimated fetal age as the dependent variable. However, the type of nomogram required to assess the normality of bone dimensions uses gestational age as the independent variable and the long bone as the dependent variable. For the proper use of these nomograms, the clinician must accurately know the gestational age of the fetus. Therefore, patients at risk for skeletal dysplasias should be advised to seek prenatal care at an early gestational age to assess all clinical estimators of gestational age. Tables 26.6 and 26.7 present nomograms for the assessment of limb biometry for the upper and lower extremities, respectively. Comparisons between limb dimensions and the head perimeter can be used for patients presenting with uncertain gestational age (Figs 26.6 and 26.7). Although some investigators have employed the biparietal diameter for this purpose, the head perimeter has the advantage of being shape independent. A limitation of this approach is that it assumes that the cranium is not involved in the dysplastic process, and this may not be the case in some skeletal dysplasias.

The nomograms and figures in this chapter provide the mean and the 5th and the 95th percentiles of limb biometric parameters. The reader should be aware that 5% of the general population would fall outside these boundaries. Ideally, a more stringent criterion, such as the 1st percentile of limb growth for gestational age, should be used for diagnosis. Unfortunately, none of the currently available nomograms has been based on enough patients to provide an

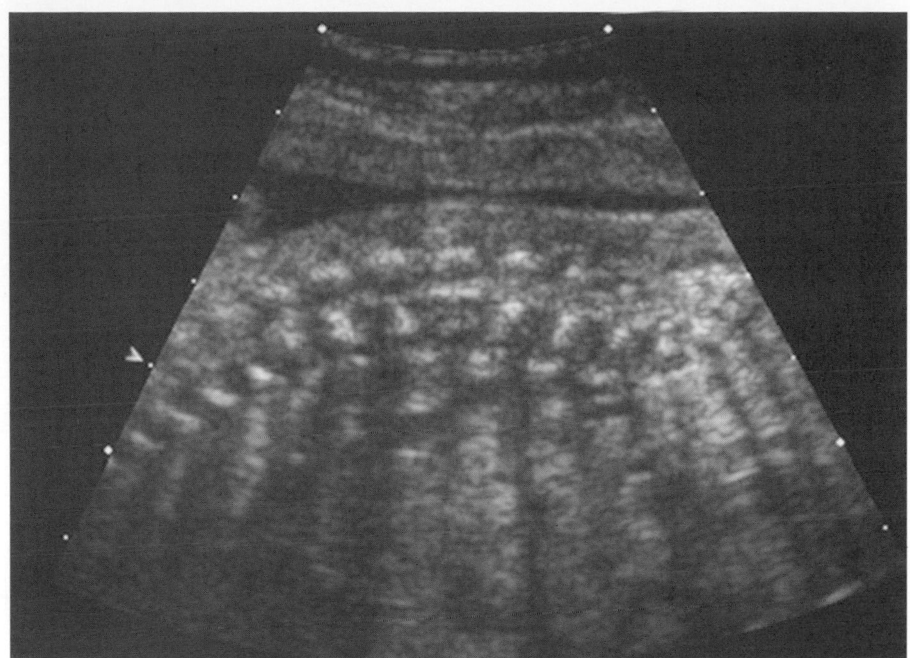

Figure 26.3 Sagittal scan of the lumbar spine in a fetus with platyspondyly.

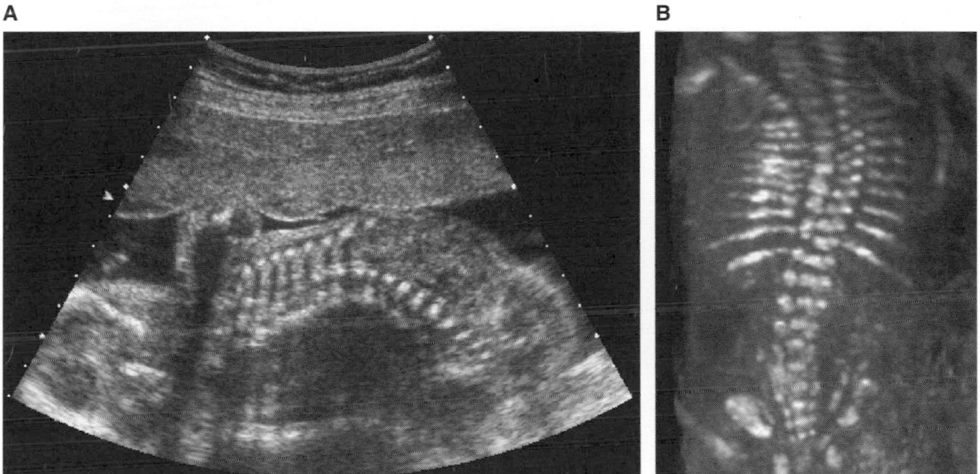

Figure 26.4 (A) Coronal scan of the fetal spine by two-dimensional ultrasound, showing scoliosis. (B) Three-dimensional rendered images of the fetal spine, showing scoliosis.

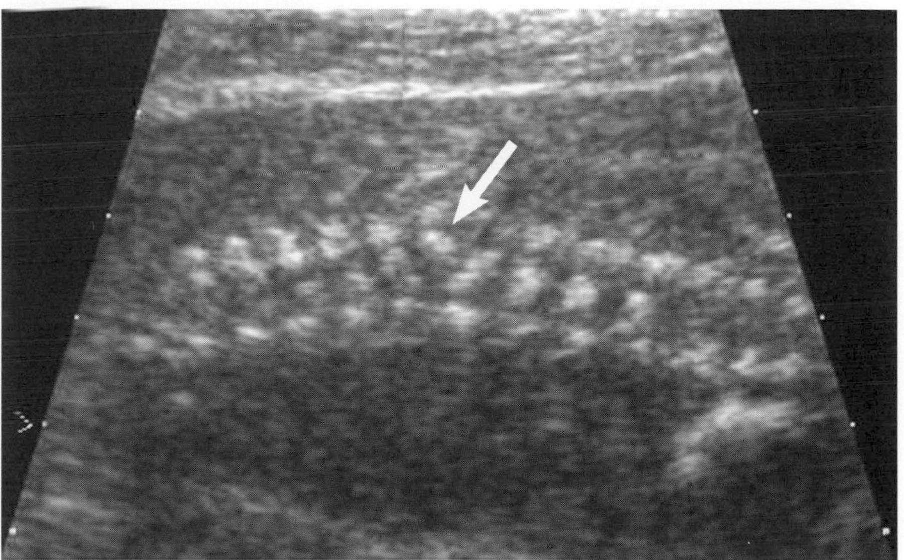

Figure 26.5 Coronal scan of the fetal spine showing lateral hemivertebra in the thoracic segment.

Table 26.6 Normal values for the leg (mm).

Week	Tibia			Fibula			Femur		
	5th percentile	50th percentile	95th percentile	5th percentile	50th percentile	95th percentile	5th percentile	50 percentile	95th percentile
12	–	7	–	–	6	–	4	8	13
13	–	10	–	–	9	–	6	11	16
14	7	12	17	6	12	19	9	14	18
15	9	15	20	9	15	21	12	17	21
16	12	17	22	13	18	23	15	20	24
17	15	20	25	13	21	28	18	23	27
18	17	22	27	15	23	31	21	25	30
19	20	25	30	19	26	33	24	28	33
20	22	27	33	21	28	36	26	31	36
21	25	30	35	24	31	37	29	34	38
22	27	32	38	27	33	39	32	36	41
23	30	35	40	28	35	42	35	39	44
24	32	37	42	29	37	45	37	42	46
25	34	40	45	34	40	45	40	44	49
26	37	42	47	36	42	47	42	47	51
27	39	44	49	37	44	50	45	49	54
28	41	46	51	38	45	53	47	52	56
29	43	48	53	41	47	54	50	54	59
30	45	50	55	43	49	56	52	56	61
31	47	52	57	42	51	59	54	59	63
32	48	54	59	42	52	63	56	61	65
33	50	55	60	46	54	62	58	63	67
34	52	57	62	46	55	65	60	65	69
35	53	58	64	51	57	62	62	67	71
36	55	60	65	54	58	63	64	68	73
37	56	61	67	54	59	65	65	70	74
38	58	63	68	56	61	65	67	71	76
39	59	64	69	56	62	67	68	73	77
40	61	66	71	59	63	67	70	74	79

Table 26.7 Normal values for the arm (mm).

Week	Humerus			Ulna			Radius		
	5th percentile	50th percentile	95th percentile	5th percentile	50th percentile	95th percentile	5th percentile	50th percentile	95th percentile
12	–	9	–	–	7	–	–	7	–
13	6	11	16	5	10	15	6	10	14
14	9	14	19	8	13	18	8	13	17
15	12	17	22	11	16	21	11	15	20
16	15	20	25	13	18	23	13	18	22
17	18	22	27	16	21	26	14	20	26
18	20	25	30	19	24	29	15	22	29
19	23	28	33	21	26	31	20	24	29
20	25	30	35	24	29	34	22	27	32
21	28	33	38	26	31	36	24	29	33
22	30	35	40	28	33	38	27	31	34
23	33	38	42	31	36	41	26	32	39
24	35	40	45	33	38	43	26	34	42
25	37	42	47	35	40	45	31	36	41
26	39	44	49	37	42	47	32	37	43
27	41	46	51	39	44	49	33	39	45
28	43	48	53	41	46	51	33	40	48
29	45	50	55	43	48	53	36	42	47
30	47	51	56	44	49	54	36	43	49
31	48	53	58	46	51	56	38	44	50
32	50	55	60	48	53	58	37	45	53
33	51	56	61	49	54	59	41	46	51
34	53	58	63	51	56	61	40	47	53
35	54	59	64	52	57	62	41	48	54
36	56	61	65	53	58	63	39	48	57
37	57	62	67	55	60	65	45	49	53
38	59	63	68	56	61	66	45	49	54
39	60	65	70	57	62	67	45	50	54
40	61	66	71	58	63	68	46	50	55

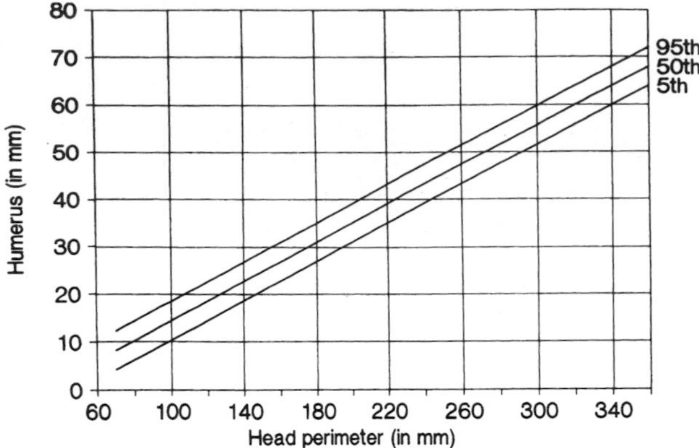

Figure 26.6 Relationship between the head perimeter and the length of the humerus.

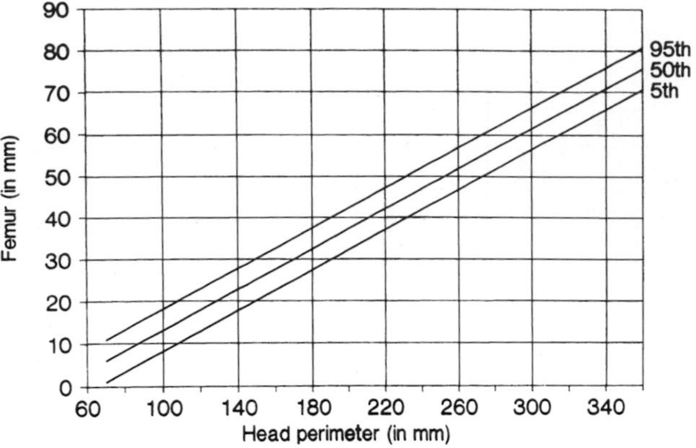

Figure 26.7 Relationship between the head perimeter and the length of the femur.

accurate discrimination between the 5th and the 1st percentiles. However, most skeletal dysplasias diagnosed *in utero* or at birth are associated with dramatic long bone shortening, and, under these circumstances, the precise boundary used (1st or 5th percentile) is not critical. An exception to this is achondroplasia, in which limb biometry is mildly affected until the third trimester, when abnormal growth can be detected by examining the slope of growth of femur length.[48] In a study including 127 cases of 17 skeletal dysplasias, Gonçalves and Jeanty[49] conducted discriminant analysis and showed that the femur length is the best biometric parameter to distinguish among the five most common disorders: thanatophoric dysplasia, osteogenesis imperfecta type II, achondrogenesis, achondroplasia, and hypochondroplasia. Gabrielli and colleagues[50] evaluated the possibility of an early diagnosis of skeletal dysplasias in high-risk patients. A total of 149 consecutive, uncomplicated singleton pregnancies at 9–13 weeks after amenorrhea were included in the study. Transvaginal ultrasound was used to establish the relationship between biparietal diameter and crown–rump length using polynomial regression. Eight patients with previous skeletal dysplasias were evaluated with serial examinations every 2 weeks between 10 and 11 weeks, and femur length correlated significantly with both biparietal diameter and crown–rump length. Of the five cases with skeletal dysplasias, only two (one with recurrent osteogenesis imperfecta and one with recurrent achondrogenesis) were diagnosed in the first trimester. This study suggests that an early evaluation of the fetus and the correlation of femur length with crown–rump length and of femur length with biparietal diameter may be useful for early diagnosis of severe skeletal dysplasias. In less severe cases, biometric evaluation appears to be of limited value. Nomograms have recently been published for long bone measurements according to crown–rump length in a large population of normal fetuses that were examined between 11 and 14 weeks of gestation, and they may help in the early assessment of pregnancies at risk for skeletal dysplasias.[51]

Clinical presentation

The challenge of antenatal diagnosis of skeletal dysplasias generally presents itself in one of two ways: (1) a patient who has delivered an infant with a skeletal dysplasia and desires antenatal assessment of a subsequent pregnancy or (2) the incidental finding of a shortened, bowed, or anomalous extremity during a routine sonographic examination. In patients at risk, the examination is easier when the particular phenotype is known. The inability to obtain reliable information about skeletal mineralization and the involvement of other systems (e.g., skin) using sonography is a limiting factor in the establishment of an accurate diagnosis after the identification of an incidental finding. Another limitation is the paucity of information about the *in utero* natural history of these disorders.

Despite these difficulties and limitations, there are good medical reasons for attempting an accurate prenatal diagnosis of skeletal dysplasias. A number of these disorders are uniformly lethal (Table 26.3), whereas others are associated with mental retardation.[52] In addition, there is a group of disorders associated with thrombocytopenia in which vaginal delivery may expose these infants to the risk of intracranial hemorrhage. Therefore, accurate diagnosis of skeletal dysplasias is important for prenatal counseling.

Diagnostic imaging and the prenatal diagnosis of skeletal dysplasias

Despite the increasing availability of molecular testing, a comprehensive molecular diagnostic search for all skeletal dysplasias is not possible at this time. Indeed, only about one-third of skeletal dysplasias have had their molecular basis defined.[3] Therefore, the roles of diagnostic imaging in the prenatal investigation of skeletal dysplasias are: (1) to narrow the differential diagnosis of skeletal dysplasias so that appropriate confirmatory molecular tests can be selected; (2) to predict lethality; and (3) to identify the fetus with a skeletal dysplasia early enough in pregnancy so that the diagnostic workup can be completed before the limit of fetal viability.[53–57]

Ultrasound is the primary imaging modality used for the initial diagnostic evaluation of an affected fetus, and several studies have explored the role of ultrasound in the detection of skeletal dysplasias.[33,48,58–68] A prospective analysis of a high-risk population (15 women, 16 cases) carrying a genetic risk for skeletal dysplasias was conducted by Kurtz and Wapner.[48] Based on ultrasonographic findings in the second trimester, they were able to diagnose five abnormal fetuses among the 16 fetuses at risk. Weldner et al.[9] screened 12453 patients in the second and third trimesters and estimated the prevalence of skeletal dysplasias as 7.5 per 10000. Sharony and colleagues[64] studied fetuses and stillbirths referred from other centers for suspected skeletal dysplasia. Most of the cases were sporadic, and the most common final diagnoses were osteogenesis imperfecta (16%) and thanatophoric dysplasia (14%). Table 26.8 summarizes the diagnostic accuracy of two-dimensional ultrasound for prenatal diagnosis of skeletal dysplasias.[4,16,68–71] An accurate diagnosis was made in 31–73% of cases.

The introduction of three-dimensional ultrasound and rendering algorithms to reconstruct the fetal skeleton may improve diagnostic accuracy as additional phenotypic features not detectable by two-dimensional ultrasound may be identified.[72–84] For example, Garjian and colleagues[75] and Krakow and colleagues[82] reported the diagnosis of additional facial[75,82] and scapular anomalies,[75] as well as abnormal calcification patterns[82] in fetuses with skeletal dysplasias, whereas Moeglin and Benoit[78] used the multiplanar visualization method to demonstrate the "pointed appearance" of the upper femoral diaphysis in a case of achondroplasia. Three-dimensional reconstruction of the fetal bones is best performed using the "maximum intensity projection" mode, a rendering algorithm that prioritizes the display of voxels with the highest gray levels contained within a region of interest selected by the user.[75,78] If the fetus is examined early enough during pregnancy, the entire skeleton can be included within the region of interest of the three-dimensional volume dataset and, therefore, panoramic visualization can be achieved.[75] However, the diagnosis may be missed as the phenotypic characteristics of some skeletal dysplasias do not manifest until later in pregnancy. Case reports and small series of several skeletal dysplasias have been published describing phenotypic characteristics or skeletal features (Table 26.9).[73,75–78,80–83,85]

Three-dimensional helical computed tomography (3DHCT) has recently been proposed as an adjunctive imaging

Table 26.8 Accuracy of prenatal ultrasound for diagnosis of skeletal dysplasias.

Author	Year	No. of cases	Correct diagnosis*
Gordienko and colleagues[16]	1996	26	73% (9)
Gaffney and colleagues[68]	1998	35	31% (11)
Tretter and colleagues[70]	1998	27	48% (13)
Hersh and colleagues[71]	1998	23	48% (11)
Doray and colleagues[69]	2000	47	60% (28)
Parilla and colleagues[4]	2003	31	65% (20)

*Numbers in parentheses indicate the number of fetuses with the correct diagnosis.

Table 26.9 Additional phenotypic findings and improved visualization in cases of skeletal dysplasias by prenatal three-dimensional ultrasound compared with two-dimensional ultrasound in published reports.

Skeletal dysplasia	Phenotypic characteristics identified better by three- rather than two-dimensional ultrasound
Platylospondylic lethal chondrodysplasia[73]	Enhanced visualization of femoral and tibial bowing, better characterization of the facial soft tissues with surface rendering
Campomelic dysplasia[75,83]	Micrognathia, flat face, hypoplastic scapulae, bifid foot
Thanatophoric dysplasia[75–77,82]	Improved characterization of frontal bossing and depressed nasal bridge, demonstration of redundant skinfolds, low-set dysmorphic ears
Achondroplasia[78,82]	Improved characterization of frontal bossing and depressed nasal bridge; superior evaluation of the epiphyses and metaphyses of the long bones, with demonstration of a vertical metaphyseal slope; caudal narrowing of the interpedicular distance; clear visualization of trident hand; better visualization of disproportion between limb segments
Chondrodysplasia puntacta, rhizomelic form[82]	Improved characterization of the Binder facies (depressed nasal bridge, midface hypoplasia, small nose with upturned alae); identification of laryngeal stippling
Achondrogenesis[82]	Panoramic demonstration of short neck and severe shortening of all segments of the limbs
Jarcho–Levin syndrome[81]	Vertebral defects with absence of ribs and transverse process
Larsen syndrome[85]	Genu recurvatum, midface hypoplasia, low-set ears

Phenotypic characteristics of osteogenesis imperfecta,[75] short rib–polydactyly syndrome,[80] and Apert syndrome[82] have also been described using three-dimensional ultrasound, although no additional findings with two-dimensional ultrasound were observed.

modality for the prenatal diagnosis of skeletal dysplasias (Fig. 26.8).[86] Similar to three-dimensional ultrasound, postprocessing techniques such as "maximum intensity projection," "surface rendering," and "volume rendering" can be used for three-dimensional reconstruction.[87–89] Long bone measurements obtained by postmortem helical computed tomography studies have been compared with those obtained within 24 h of delivery by ultrasound, and a significant correlation between the two methods was observed.[90] Excellent panoramic images of the fetal skeleton can be obtained by 3DHCT without superimposition of the maternal skeleton (which occurs with radiography). Ruano and colleagues[86] compared the phenotypic characteristics of three skeletal dysplasias [achondroplasia (n = 3), osteogenesis imperfecta (n = 2), and chondrodysplasia puntacta (n = 1)] visualized by prenatal 3DHCT, and three-/two-dimensional ultrasound. Deformation of the fetal pelvis and an increase in the intervertebral space of the lumbar vertebrae were diagnosed more often using 3DHCT than two-and three-dimensional ultrasound. In contrast, some phenotypic characteristics of fetuses with skeletal dysplasias were demonstrated only by ultrasound: phalangeal hypoplasia (by both two- and three-dimensional ultrasound), facial dysmorphism (by three-dimensional ultrasound only), and point-calcified epiphysis (by both two- and three-dimensional ultrasound). Although the overall count of correct phenotypic characteristics detected prenatally favored 3DHCT over three-dimensional ultrasound [94.3% (33 out of 35) vs. 77.1% (27 out of 35), P = 0.03, McNemar's test for correlated samples], the diagnostic performance of 3DHCT was not superior to that of three-dimensional ultrasound, as the correct prenatal diagnosis was established by both modalities in all cases. Provided that the two diagnostic methods have similar diagnostic accuracy, three-dimensional ultrasound has two important advantages over 3DHCT, namely lack of radiation exposure and wider availability in the clinical setting. It is also noteworthy that the overall experience with three-dimensional ultrasound for the diagnosis of skeletal dysplasias is still limited.[72–85] Nevertheless, even in this study, three-dimensional ultrasound performed better than two-dimensional ultrasound, both in the identification of phenotypic characteristics [77.1% (27 out of 35) vs. 51.4% (18 out of 35), P = 0.004, McNemar's test] as well as in establishing an accurate diagnosis.

Approach to the diagnosis of skeletal dysplasias

Our proposed systematic approach to the prenatal diagnosis of skeletal dysplasias is summarized in Table 26.10.

Evaluation of long bones

Measurements

All long bones should be measured in all extremities. Comparisons with other segments should be performed to establish whether the limb shortening is predominantly rhizomelic, mesomelic, or acromelic, or whether it involves all segments (Fig. 26.9). A detailed examination of each bone is necessary to exclude the absence or hypoplasia of individual bones (fibula, tibia, scapula, radius).[65,91–94]

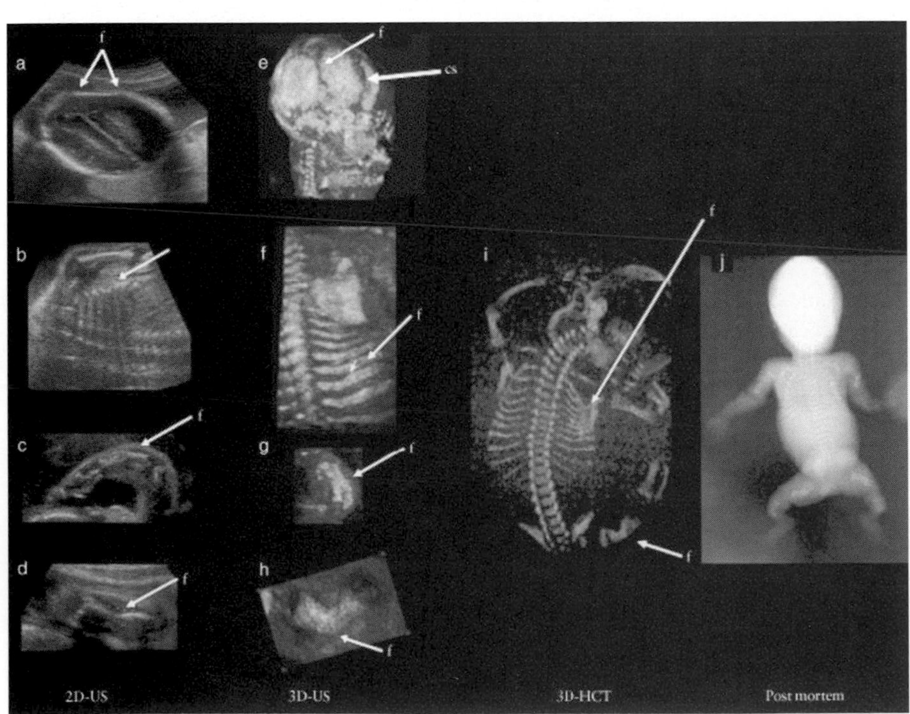

Figure 26.8 Comparison of phenotypic features of osteogenesis imperfecta by 3DHCT, three- and two-dimensional ultrasound, and postmortem radiographs.

Table 26.10 Steps for examination of the fetus with a suspected skeletal dysplasia by two- and three-dimensional ultrasound.

1. Measure all long bones
2. Compare with other segments and classify the limb shortening as:
   Rhizomelia
   Mesomelia
   Acromelia
   Severe micromelia
3. Qualitative assessment of long bones:
   Demineralization
   Fractures
   Bowing
   Metaphyseal flaring
   Absence of bones
4. Measure chest dimensions to determine risk of pulmonary hypoplasia
5. Evaluate hands and feet:
   Digits (polydactyly/syndactyly)
   Positional deformities
6. Evaluate the cranium:
   Macrocrania
   Frontal bossing
   Cloverleaf skull
   Hypertelorism/hypotelorism
7. Evaluate for facial clefts
8. Examine the spine:
   Platyspondyly
   Demineralization
   Hemivertebrae
   Coronal clefts
   Vertebral disorganization
9. Evaluate internal organs, including echocardiography
10. Evaluate fetal motion
11. Evaluate amniotic fluid volume

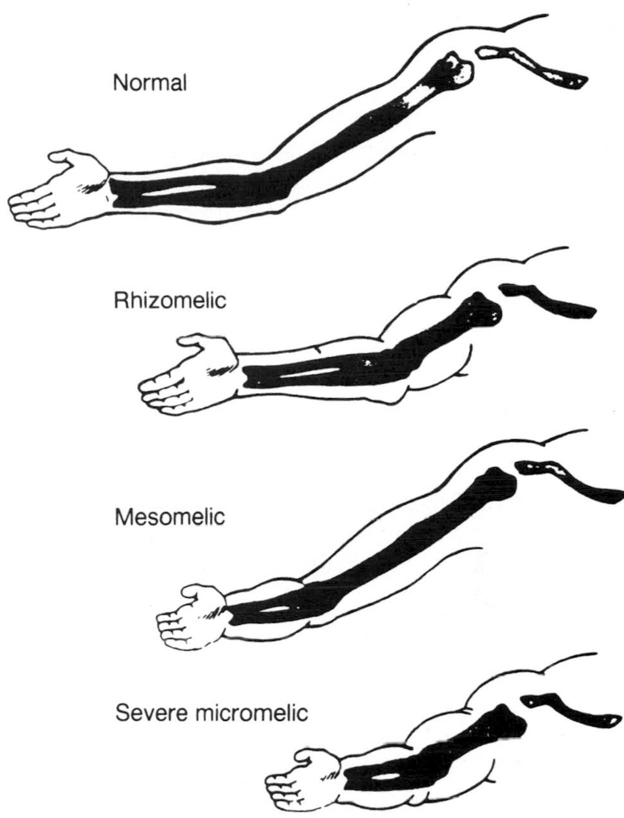

Figure 26.9 Varieties of short limb dysplasia according to the segment involved.

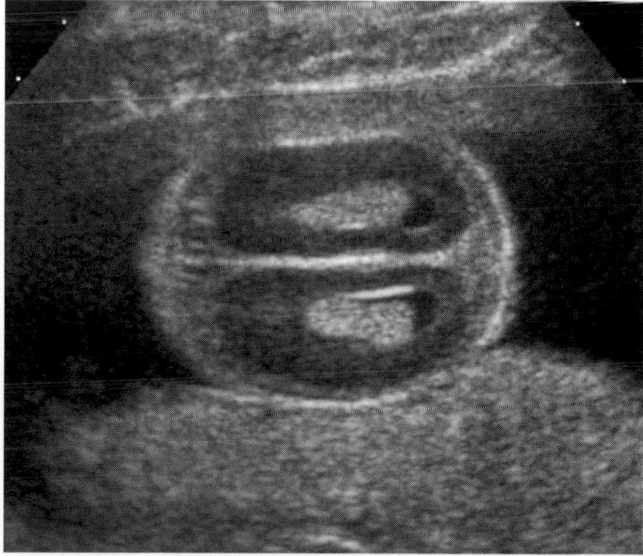

Figure 26.10 Demineralization of the skull in a case of osteogenesis imperfecta.

Degree of mineralization

An attempt should be made to characterize the degree of mineralization. This can be assessed by examining the acoustic shadow behind the bone and the echogenicity of the bone itself. Signs of demineralization include the visualization of an unusually prominent falx and the absence of or decreased echogenicity of the spine. It should be stressed that there are limitations in the sonographic evaluation of mineralization of long bones and that other structures, such as the skull, may be better suited for this assessment (Fig. 26.10).

Degree of long bone curvature

At present, there is no objective means of assessing long bone curvature, and experience is the only tool to assist the operator to discern the boundary between normality and abnormality. Campomelia (excessive bowing) (Fig. 26.11) is a characteristic of certain disorders (e.g., campomelic dysplasia).

Metaphyseal flaring

Metaphyseal flaring denotes widening at the level of the metaphyseal growth plate. It can be observed in many conditions, including achondroplasia, hypochondroplasia, hypochondrogenesis, asphyxiating thoracic dysplasia, chondrodysplasia puntacta, diastrophic dysplasia, hypophosphatasia, Kniest dysplasia, kyphomelic dysplasia, metatropic dysplasia, and osteogenesis imperfecta.[95]

Fractures

The possibility of fractures should be considered, as they can be present in some conditions (e.g., osteogenesis imperfecta) (Fig. 26.12). The fractures may be extremely subtle or may lead to angulation and separation of the segments of the affected bone (Fig. 26.13).

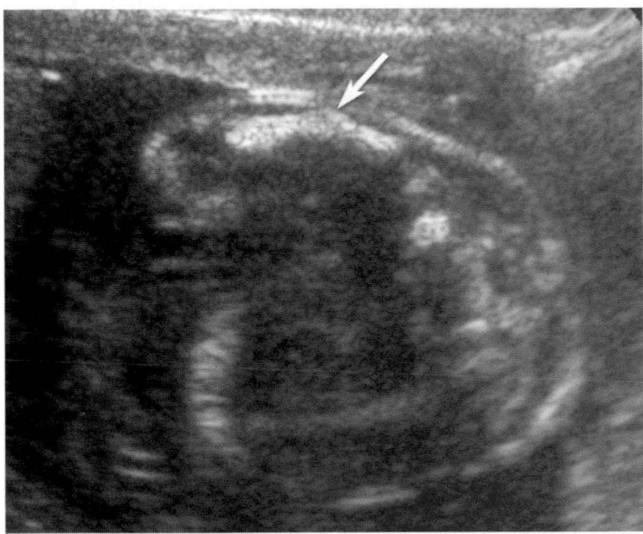

Figure 26.11 Femur bowing (arrow) in a case of proximal focal femoral deficiency syndrome.

Prediction of pulmonary hypoplasia

Several skeletal dysplasias are associated with a hypoplastic thorax. This finding is extremely important because chest

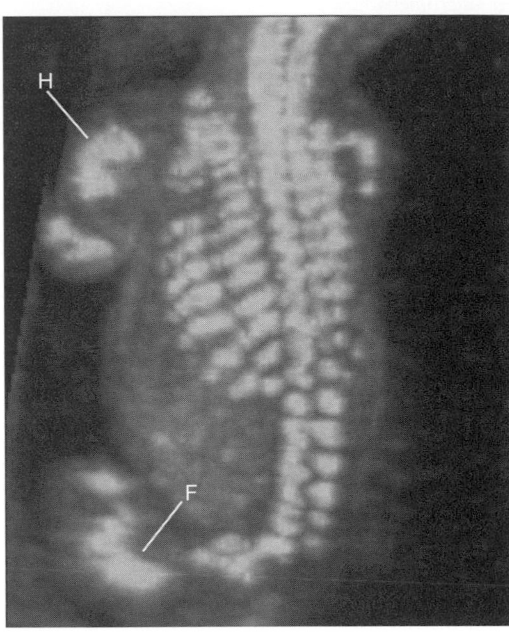

Figure 26.12 Three-dimensional ultrasonography in a case of osteogenesis imperfecta type II. The volume dataset was rendered using the maximum intensity (skeletal) mode. Multiple fractures in the ribs are present. Note the severe bowing and shortening of the left femur (F) and humerus (H).

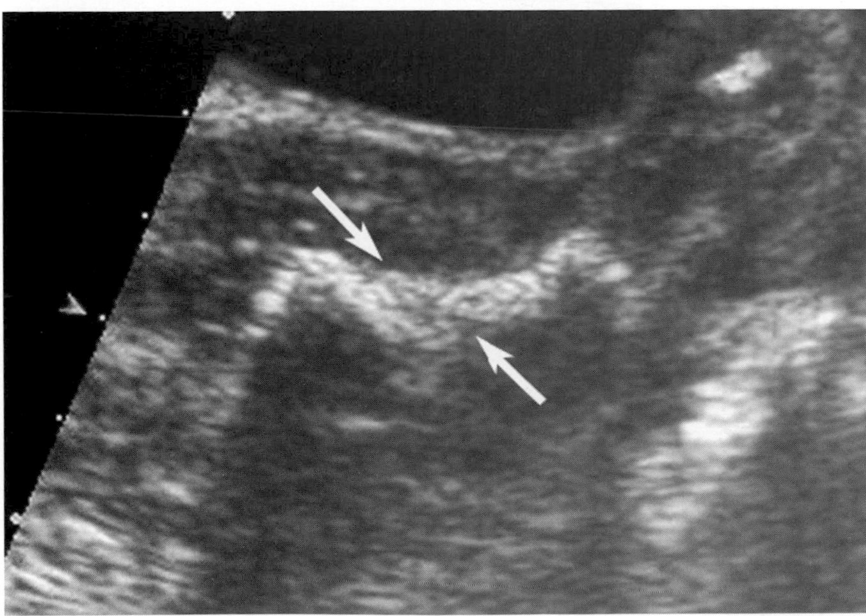

Figure 26.13 *In utero* fracture in a case of osteogenesis imperfecta. The arrows indicate the hypoechogenic fracture line.

restriction leads to pulmonary hypoplasia, a frequent cause of death in these conditions (Table 26.3). A number of ultrasonographic parameters have been investigated for the prediction of pulmonary hypoplasia. These include measurements of the thorax and lungs, a series of ratios between thoracic measurements and other biometric parameters, Doppler velocimetry of the pulmonary arteries, Doppler evaluation of tracheal fluid flow, and, more recently, three-dimensional volumetric measurements of the fetal lungs by either ultrasound or MRI. Below we briefly review studies that have attempted to use ultrasonographic or MRI parameters for prenatal prediction of lung hypoplasia.

Evaluation of thoracic and lung dimensions by two-dimensional ultrasound

Thoracic and lung biometry have been extensively studied to identify fetuses at high risk for pulmonary hypoplasia.[96–107] Table 26.11 lists skeletal dysplasias associated with altered thoracic dimensions, and Figs 26.14 and 26.15 illustrate features associated with a hypoplastic thorax.

The methods used to measure the bony thorax, chest, lungs, and heart by two-dimensional ultrasound are illustrated in Fig. 26.16. Thoracic dimensions in fetuses with known gestational age can be evaluated by the nomograms in Tables 26.12 and 26.13. When gestational age is uncertain, age-independent ratios, such as the thoracic–abdominal circumference ratio (normal value 0.77:1.01) and the thoracic–head circumference ratio (normal value 0.56:1.04), can be used.[97]

Table 26.11 Skeletal dysplasias associated with altered thoracic dimensions.

Long, narrow thorax
Asphyxiating thoracic dysplasia (Jeune)
Chondroectodermal dysplasia (Ellis–van Creveld)
Metatropic dysplasia
Fibrochondrogenesis
Atelosteogenesis
Campomelic dysplasia
Jarcho–Levin syndrome
Achondrogenesis
Osteogenesis imperfecta congenita
Hypophosphatasia
Dyssegmental dysplasia
Cleidocranial dysplasia
Short thorax
Osteogenesis imperfecta (type II)
Kniest dysplasia (metatropic dysplasia type II)
Pena–Shokeir syndrome
Hypoplastic thorax
Short rib–polydactyly syndrome (type I and type II)
Thanatophoric dysplasia
Cerebrocostomandibular syndrome
Cleidocranial dysostosis syndrome
Homozygous achondroplasia
Melnick–Needles syndrome (osteodysplasty)
Fibrochondrogenesis
Otopalatodigital syndrome type II

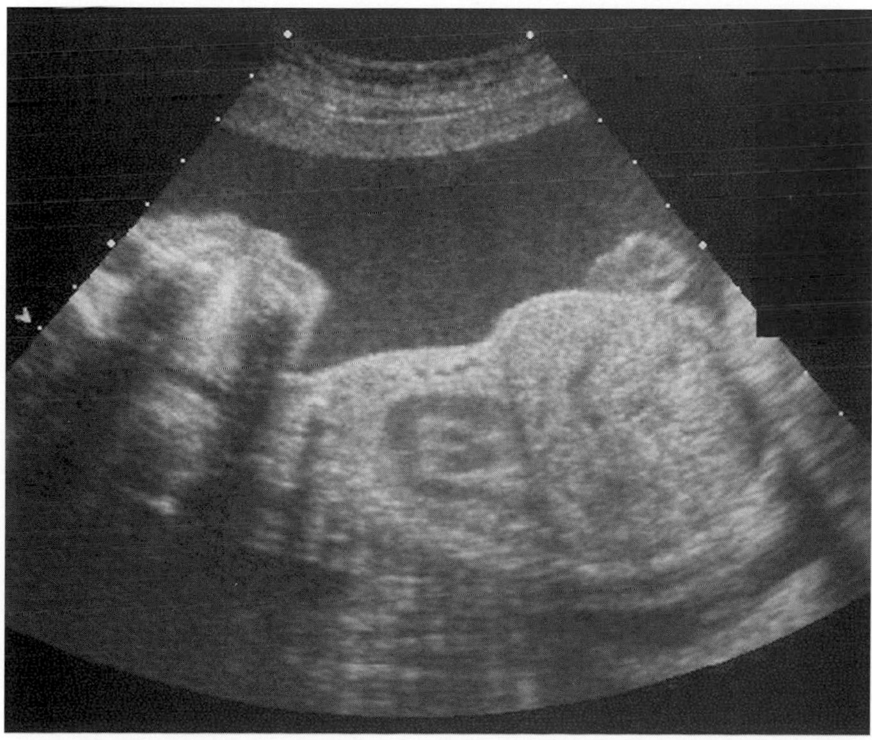

Figure 26.14 Longitudinal section of a fetus with thanatophoric dysplasia. Note the significant disproportion between the chest and abdomen.

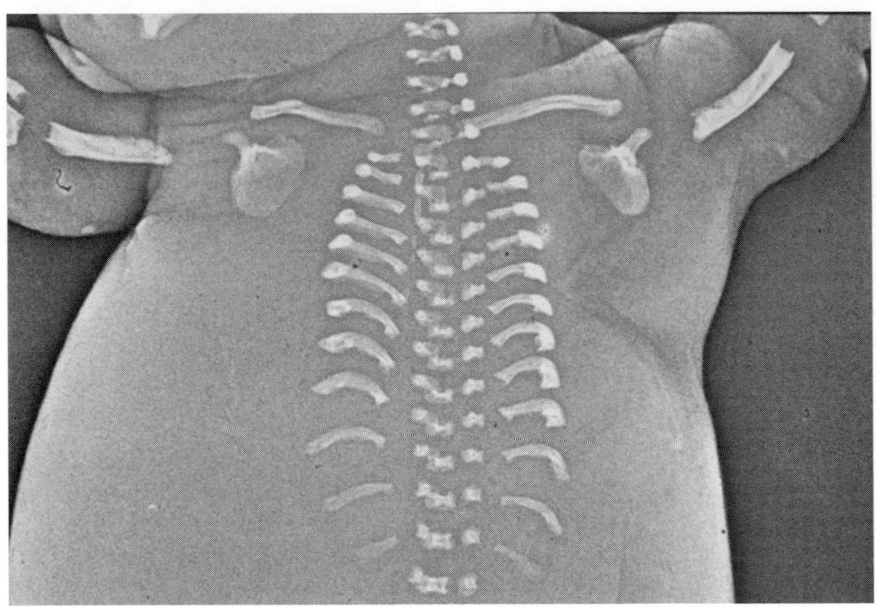

Figure 26.15 Extremely short ribs in a fetus with short rib–polydactyly syndrome.

Table 26.12 Fetal thoracic circumference measurements (cm).

Gestational age (weeks)	No.	Predictive percentiles								
		2.5	5	10	25	50	75	90	95	97.5
16	6	5.9	6.4	7.0	8.0	9.1	10.3	11.3	11.9	12.4
17	22	6.8	7.3	7.9	8.9	10.0	11.2	12.2	12.8	13.3
18	31	7.7	8.2	8.8	9.8	11.0	12.1	13.1	13.7	14.2
19	21	8.6	9.1	9.7	10.7	11.9	13.0	14.0	14.6	15.1
20	20	9.5	10.0	10.6	11.7	12.8	13.9	15.0	15.5	16.0
21	30	10.4	11.0	11.6	12.6	13.7	14.8	15.8	16.4	16.9
22	18	11.3	11.9	12.5	13.5	14.6	15.7	16.7	17.3	17.8
23	21	12.2	12.8	13.4	14.4	15.5	16.6	17.6	18.2	18.8
24	27	13.2	13.7	14.3	15.3	16.4	17.5	18.5	19.1	19.7
25	20	14.1	14.6	15.2	16.2	17.3	18.4	19.4	20.0	20.6
26	25	15.0	15.5	16.1	17.1	18.2	19.3	20.3	21.0	21.5
27	24	15.9	16.4	17.0	18.0	19.1	20.2	21.3	21.9	22.4
28	24	16.8	17.3	17.9	18.9	20.0	21.2	22.2	22.8	23.3
29	24	17.7	18.2	18.8	19.8	21.0	22.1	23.1	23.7	24.2
30	27	18.6	19.1	19.7	20.7	21.9	23.0	24.0	24.6	25.1
31	24	19.5	20.0	20.6	21.6	22.8	23.9	24.9	25.5	26.0
32	28	20.4	20.9	21.5	22.6	23.7	24.8	25.8	26.4	26.9
33	27	21.3	21.8	22.5	23.5	24.6	25.7	26.7	27.3	27.8
34	25	22.2	22.8	23.4	24.4	25.5	26.6	27.6	28.2	28.7
35	20	23.1	23.7	24.3	25.3	26.4	27.5	28.5	29.1	29.6
36	23	24.0	24.6	25.2	26.2	27.3	28.4	29.4	30.0	30.6
37	22	24.9	25.5	26.1	27.1	28.2	29.3	30.3	30.9	31.5
38	21	25.9	26.4	27.0	28.0	29.1	30.2	31.2	31.9	32.4
39	7	26.8	27.3	27.9	28.9	30.0	31.1	32.2	32.8	33.3
40	6	27.7	28.2	28.8	29.8	20.9	32.1	33.1	33.7	34.2

Reproduced with permission from ref. 97.

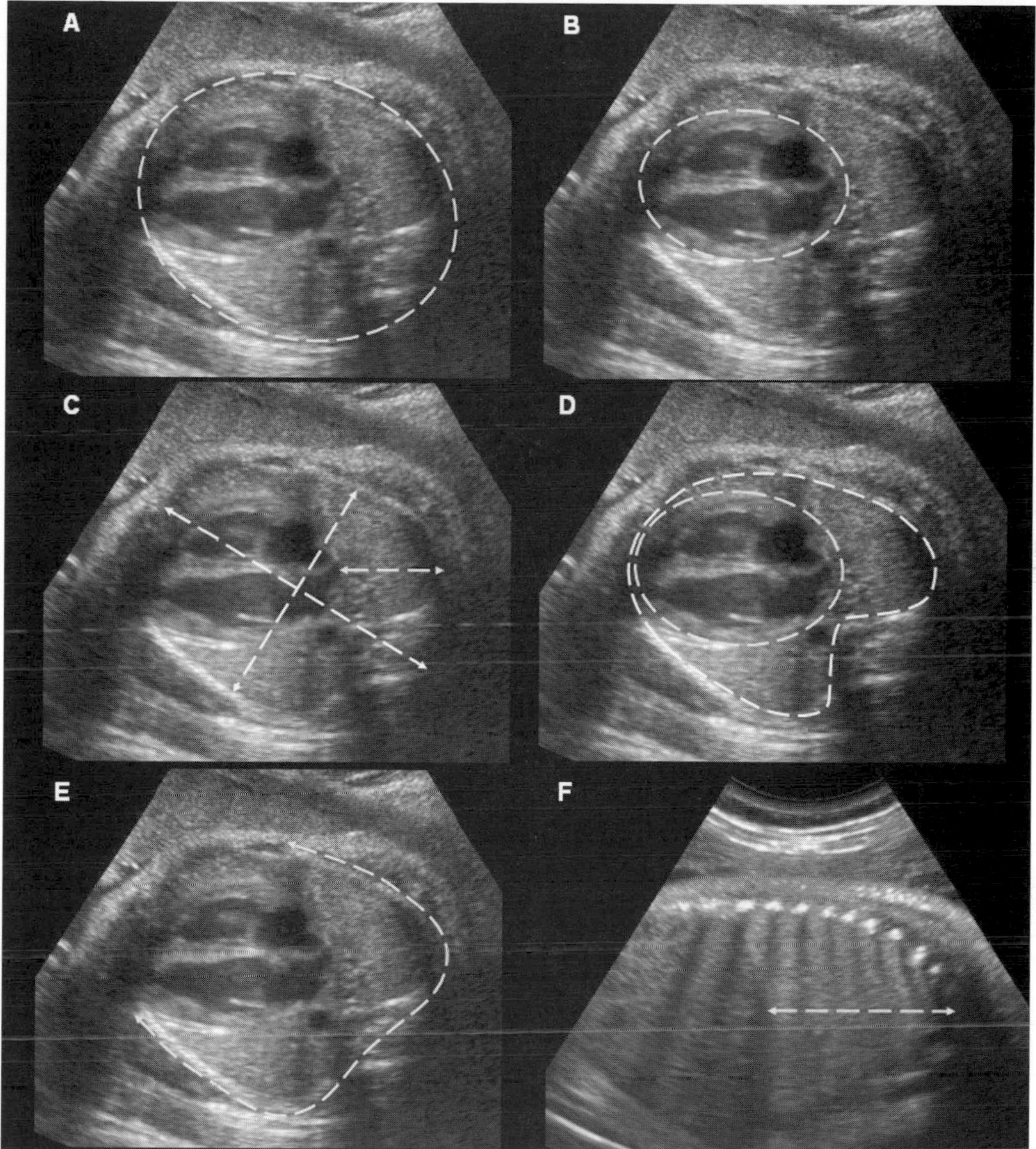

Figure 26.16 The various methods to measure thoracic, lung, and heart dimensions.

A summary of the diagnostic accuracy of biometric parameters for the diagnosis of pulmonary hypoplasia is presented in Table 26.14.[98–104,107–113] Of particular interest are the measurements of the right lung diameter or the ratio between right lung diameter and bony thoracic circumference proposed by Merz and colleagues.[105] In a study of 32 fetuses with a postnatal diagnosis of pulmonary hypoplasia (skeletal dysplasias, $n = 7$; renal agenesis, $n = 11$; diaphragmatic hernia, $n = 7$; and hydrothorax, $n = 2$), all had a right lung diameter below the 5th percentile for age, regardless of the primary disorder.[110] In a subsequent study of 19 fetuses with congenital diaphragmatic hernia, Bahlmann and colleagues[111] demonstrated that the right lung diameter–bony thoracic circumference ratio detected all fetuses with pulmonary hypoplasia with 100% sensitivity and 100% specificity. Whether the same degree of accuracy for this test can be replicated in a uniform population of fetuses with osteochondrodysplasias remains to be determined.

Short femur length and the prediction of lethality in skeletal dysplasias

Rahemtullah and colleagues[114] studied 18 cases of skeletal dysplasias and all lethal cases were associated with a femur length–abdominal circumference ratio ≤ 0.16. Although the test detected lethal cases with 100% sensitivity, two cases of achondroplasia were erroneously identified as lethal with this method. A less pragmatic approach has been proposed by Hersh and colleagues,[71] who correctly predicted lethality in 23

Table 26.13 Fetal thoracic length measurements (cm).

Gestational age (weeks)	No.	Predictive percentiles								
		2.5	5	10	25	50	75	90	95	97.5
16	6	0.9	1.1	1.3	1.6	2.0	2.4	2.8	3.1	3.2
17	22	1.1	1.3	1.5	1.8	2.2	2.6	3.0	3.2	3.4
18	31	1.3	1.4	1.7	2.0	2.4	2.8	3.2	3.4	3.6
19	21	1.4	1.6	1.8	2.2	2.7	3.0	3.4	3.6	3.8
20	20	1.6	1.8	2.0	2.4	2.8	3.2	3.6	3.8	4.0
21	30	1.8	2.0	2.2	2.6	3.0	3.4	3.7	4.0	4.1
22	18	2.0	2.2	2.4	2.8	3.2	3.6	3.9	4.1	4.3
23	21	2.2	2.4	2.6	3.0	3.4	3.8	4.1	4.3	4.5
24	27	2.4	2.6	2.8	3.1	3.5	3.9	4.3	4.5	4.7
25	20	2.6	2.8	3.0	3.3	3.7	4.1	4.5	4.7	4.9
26	25	2.8	2.9	3.2	3.5	3.9	4.3	4.7	4.9	5.1
27	24	2.9	3.1	3.3	3.7	4.1	4.5	4.9	5.1	5.3
28	24	3.1	3.3	3.5	3.9	4.3	4.7	5.0	5.4	5.4
29	24	3.3	3.5	3.7	4.1	4.5	4.9	5.2	5.5	5.6
30	27	3.5	3.7	3.9	4.3	4.7	5.1	5.4	5.6	5.8
31	24	3.7	3.9	4.1	4.5	4.9	5.3	5.6	5.8	6.0
32	28	3.9	4.1	4.3	4.6	5.0	5.4	5.8	6.0	6.2
33	27	4.1	4.3	4.5	4.8	5.2	5.6	6.0	6.2	6.4
34	25	4.2	4.4	4.7	5.0	5.4	5.8	6.2	6.4	6.6
35	20	4.4	4.6	4.8	5.2	5.6	6.0	6.4	6.6	6.8
36	23	4.6	4.8	5.0	5.4	5.8	6.2	6.5	6.8	7.0
37	22	4.8	5.0	5.2	5.6	6.0	6.4	6.7	7.0	7.1
38	21	5.0	5.2	5.4	5.8	6.2	6.5	6.9	7.1	7.3
39	7	5.2	5.4	5.6	6.0	6.4	6.7	7.1	7.3	7.5
40	6	5.4	5.6	5.8	6.1	6.5	6.9	7.3	7.5	7.7

Reproduced with permission from ref. 97.

out of 25 cases of skeletal dysplasias with a femur length below the 1st percentile for age by combining this information with other sonographic findings (i.e., bell-shaped thorax, decreased bone echogenicity, or both).

Doppler velocimetry of the pulmonary arteries for the prediction of pulmonary hypoplasia

Underdevelopment and structural changes of the pulmonary vascular bed in cases of pulmonary hypoplasia may result in increased pulmonary vascular resistance and reduced pulmonary arterial compliance.[115] Therefore, several investigators have attempted to use Doppler measurements of the pulmonary arteries and/or its branches as a test to identify fetuses at risk for pulmonary hypoplasia.[113,116–120] Mitchell and colleagues[116] evaluated the resistance index of the peripheral pulmonary arteries for the prediction of pulmonary hypoplasia in 10 fetuses with bilateral multicystic dysplastic kidneys. The resistance index of the peripheral pulmonary arteries was above the 95th percentile for gestational age in 80% of the cases with pulmonary hypoplasia.

Subsequent studies have yielded contradictory results. For example, Achiron and colleagues[117] found that the pulsatility index of the peripheral pulmonary arteries was within normal limits in four fetuses with proven pulmonary hypoplasia, suggesting that the pulsatility index of the lung circulation is a poor test to predict lung hypoplasia. Chaoui and colleagues[118] reported that only six out of nine fetuses with lung hypoplasia had an elevated pulsatility index in the main branches of the left and right pulmonary arteries. Similarly, Laudy and colleagues[113] studied 40 fetuses at risk for pulmonary hypoplasia and found that Doppler velocimetry indices of the proximal and middle pulmonary branches were not better than chest biometry to predict pulmonary hypoplasia.

In contrast, Yoshimura and colleagues[119] reported low peak systolic velocities in four out of five fetuses and an increased pulsatility index in five out of five fetuses with confirmed pulmonary hypoplasia (thanatophoric dysplasia, $n = 2$; nonimmune hydrops, $n = 2$; and bilateral renal agenesis, $n = 1$). Rizzo and colleagues,[120] in a population of 20 fetuses with prolonged preterm premature rupture of the membranes, found that an elevated pulsatility index in a peripheral pulmonary artery observed 2 weeks after membrane rupture detected the subsequent development of pulmonary hypoplasia with a sensitivity of 62.5%, a specificity of 94.6%, a

Table 26.14 Biometric parameters proposed by different authors for the evaluation of lung hypoplasia.

Author, year	Parameter	Fetuses at risk	Prevalence	Sensitivity (%)	Specificity (%)	Accuracy (%)	Population
Nimrod and colleagues, 1986[98]	TC	45	38	88	96	93	PROM, oligohydramnios, pleural effusion, other conditions affecting lung growth
Fong and colleagues 1988[100]	TC	18	50	60	88	72	Prolonged PROM, oligohydramnios, fetal malformations associated with lung hypoplasia
Songster and colleagues, 1989[101]	FL/TC	26	42	80	92	88	PROM, urinary tract anomalies, fetal skeletal dysplasias, intrauterine growth restriction, twin–twin transfusion syndrome
Vintzileos and colleagues, 1989[102]	TC	13	69	33	57	46	Severe oligohydramnios > 5 weeks' duration
	TA			33	71	54	
	TA-HA			50	71	62	
	(TC × 100)/AC			33	86	62	
	CA/HA			67	86	77	
	(TA-HA) × 100/CA			83	86	85	
Roberts and Mitchell, 1990[108]	LL	20	60	92	100	95	PROM < 25 weeks of gestation and > 7 days' duration
	TC			67	100	80	
D'Alton and colleagues, 1992[103]	TC/AC	16	44	75	100	88	PROM < 26 weeks of gestation
Ohlsson and colleagues, 1992[109]	TC	58	28	80	90	87	PROM < 30 weeks and 19 cases of congenital anomalies
	TC/CA			80	97	91	
	TC/FL			55	97	90	
Maeda and colleagues, 1993[104]	LA	19	79	100	75	95	Non-immune hydrops, polycystic kidneys, PROM, diaphragmatic hernia, immune hydrops, trisomy 18
Yoshimura and colleagues, 1996[107]	TC	21*	*	100	83	90	Case–control study: 21 patients at risk for pulmonary hypoplasia (renal anomalies associated with pulmonary hypoplasia; thanatophoric
	TA			100	87	92	

Table 26.14 *Continued*

Author, year	Parameter	Fetuses at risk	Prevalence	Sensitivity (%)	Specificity (%)	Accuracy (%)	Population
	TC/AC			90	90	90	dysplasia; prolonged PROM < 26 weeks' gestation), 30 PROM patients with normal lung function
	LA	16*		81	100	93	
	TA-HA			100	87	91	
	TA/HA			69	100	89	
	TA-HA/TA			69	97	87	
	LA/TA			31	100	76	
Merz and colleagues, 1999[110]	LD	32	†	100	†	†	Skeletal dysplasias (n = 7), renal agenesis (n = 11), diaphragmatic hernia (n = 7), hydrothorax (n = 2)
	TTD			53			
	TSD			47			
	TC			47			
Bahlmann and colleagues, 1999[111]	TC	17	82	14	100	29	Diaphragmatic hernia
	LD			100	100	100	
	LD/TC			100	100	100	
Heling and colleagues, 2001[112]	TTD	29	55	44	50	46	Bilateral renal agenesis, bilateral multicystic kidneys, chronic PROM < 25 weeks of gestation, hydrothorax
	APTD			57	42	52	
	LL			29	66	42	
Laudy and colleagues, 2002[113]	TC	40	43	94	38	61	Prolonged oligohydramnios due to PROM or congenital renal disease
	CC/TC			76	50	61	
	TC/AC			69	71	70	

AC, abdominal circumference; APTD, anteroposterior thoracic diameter; CC, cardiac circumference; FL, femur length; HA, heart area; LA, lung area; LL, lung length; TA, thoracic area; TLD, lung diameter; TSD, thoracic sagittal diameter; TTD, transverse thoracic diameter; TC, thoracic circumference; PROM, premature rupture of membranes.

Only the papers for which data to calculate at least the sensitivity were included.

*Case–control study: all fetuses in the column "Fetuses at risk" had pulmonary hypoplasia; 30 gestational age-matched control fetuses were studied.

†All fetuses had pulmonary hypoplasia.

positive predictive value of 83.3%, and a negative predictive value of 78.5%. Finally, Fuke and colleagues[121] proposed the use of acceleration time/ejection time at the main branches of the pulmonary arteries to identify fetuses at risk for pulmonary hypoplasia. The normal ratio is 0.17 ± 0.04 for the right and 0.15 ± 0.04 for the left pulmonary arteries, and this ratio did not change with gestational age. Five out of six fetuses with pulmonary hypoplasia among 17 fetuses at risk were correctly identified by the test. All 11 normal fetuses had a normal acceleration time/ejection time of the pulmonary arteries.

Evaluation of lung volume by three-dimensional ultrasound

Fetal lung volumetry by three-dimensional ultrasonography has been performed using two techniques: multiplanar[122–126] (Fig. 26.17) and VOCAL (Virtual Organ Computer-aided AnaLysis, General Electric Medical Systems, Kretztechnik, Zipf, Austria) techniques (Fig. 26.18).[127–132]

Kalache and colleagues[127] demonstrated that both the three-dimensional multiplanar and three-dimensional VOCAL modes can be used to measure pulmonary volumes in fetuses, an observation that has been subsequently confirmed by Moeglin and colleagues[132] A potential advantage of the VOCAL technique is the possibility of obtaining fine contours of the lungs, which may be particularly valuable when the outline of the lung is irregular, such as in cases of congenital diaphragmatic hernia. In contrast, lung volume measurements obtained by the three-dimensional multiplanar technique are faster, usually taking less than 5 min to perform.[132] Volumes are best estimated when datasets are acquired using a transverse view of the fetal thorax.[124]

Nomograms for lung volume by three-dimensional ultrasound have been proposed by several investigators.[122–124,129,132–134] A brief description of the studies with the largest number of cases is described herein. Ruano and colleagues[129] determined nomograms for lung volume calculated using the VOCAL technique in 109 normal fetuses. The observed/expected fetal lung volume ratio was significantly lower in fetuses with congenital diaphragmatic hernia than in control subjects (median 0.34, range 0.15–0.66, vs. median 1.02, range 0.62–1.97, $P < 0.001$). Moeglin and colleagues[132] proposed an alternative approach to calculate lung volumes using two-dimensional ultrasound. The method uses the assumption that the lung is a geometrical

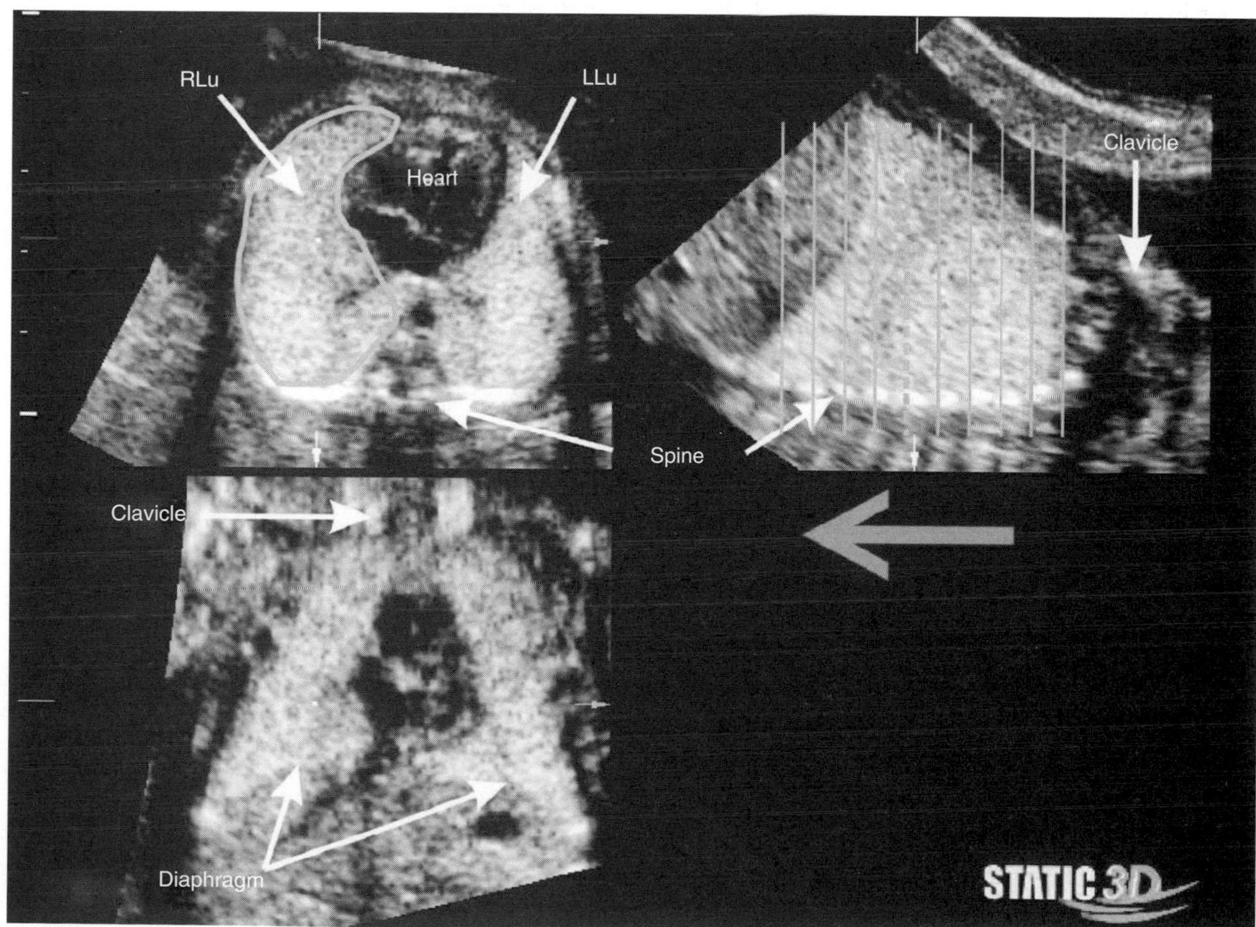

Figure 26.17 Measurement of fetal lung volume using three-dimensional multiplanar ultrasonography.

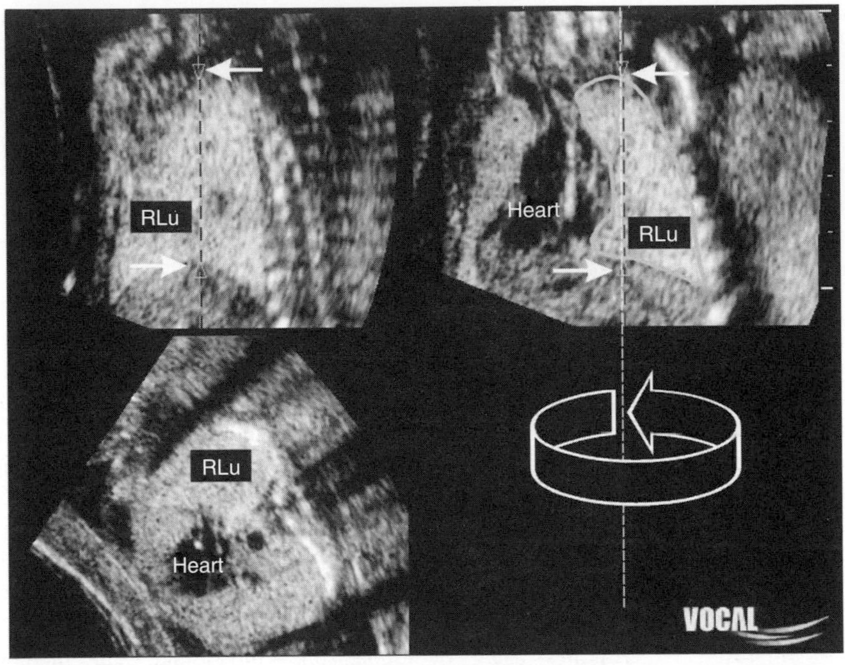

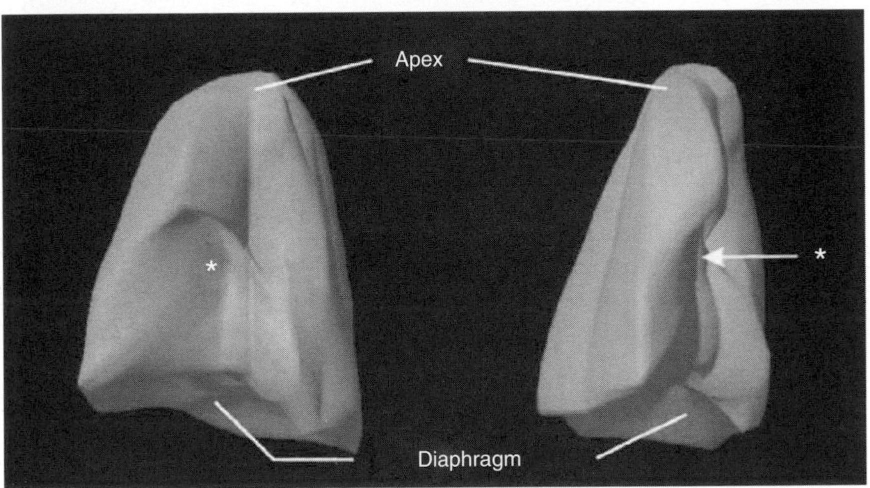

Figure 26.18 Fetal lung volume measurement using the VOCAL technique.

pyramid and the total pulmonary volume is calculated as: [surface area of right lung base (cm^2) + surface area of left lung base (cm^2)] × (height of right lung/3) (cm). Surface area of lung bases is measured on the transverse thoracic view containing the four chambers of the heart, and the height of the right lung is measured on a right sagittal paramedical view. Although lung volumes calculated by this method are significantly smaller than volumes calculated using the VOCAL technique, Moeglin and colleagues[132] have proposed an equation to extrapolate three-dimensional volumes from two-dimensional measurements using the formula RPVE (mL) = 4.24 + (1.53 × 2DGPV), where RPVE is the re-evaluated pulmonary volume equation. Preliminary results in nine fetuses with pulmonary hypoplasia are encouraging, with all of them having lung volume estimates below the 1st percentile for gestational age.[132]

Evaluation of lung volume or signal intensity by MRI

Parameters proposed to evaluate lung volume by MRI include the relative lung volume (observed lung volume–expected lung volume ratio), lung volume–estimated fetal weight ratio (LV/EFW), and the lung–spinal fluid signal intensity ratio (L/SF).[135–142]

Rypens and colleagues[135] determined normal lung volume biometry across gestational age in 336 fetuses with normal lungs. Normal fetal lung volume increased with gestational age. However, there was a constant ratio between the volume of the left and right volumes, with right lung volume accounting for 56% of the total fetal lung volume. MRI volumes corresponded to 90% of the volumes measured by pathologic examination.

Williams and colleagues[138] calculated relative lung volume in a group of 91 fetuses with sonographically normal lungs and compared the measurements with 28 fetuses at risk for pulmonary hypoplasia. The mean relative lung volume was significantly smaller in the group of fetuses at risk for pulmonary hypoplasia (34% ± 15% vs. 102% ± 17%, $P < 0.0.01$). Tanigaki and colleagues[139] compared the diagnostic performance of LV/EFW determined by MRI with three ultrasonographic parameters commonly used to assess the risk of pulmonary hypoplasia at birth. In a population of 17 fetuses at risk for pulmonary hypoplasia, a fetal LV/EFW below the 5th percentile for age was the most accurate diagnostic parameter.

Signal intensity ratios to predict lung hypoplasia have also been evaluated.[140–142] Kuwashima and colleagues[140] proposed that the lungs of fetuses with pulmonary hypoplasia would have low-intensity signals compared with fetuses with normal lung development. Osada and colleagues[141] compared LV/EFW between 58 normal fetuses and 29 fetuses at risk for pulmonary hypoplasia. In addition to LV/EFW, the authors also evaluated lung signal intensities expressed as a proportion of the spinal fluid signal intensity (L/SF). Although diagnostic indices were not reported in this study, receiver–operator characteristic (ROC) curve analysis showed that simultaneous measurement of fetal lung volume and signal intensity by MRI had an area under the curve of 0.990 to predict lung hypoplasia, compared with 0.930 and 0.955 for lung volume or L/SF ratio alone. Keller and colleagues[142] evaluated signal intensities of lung/liver, lung/amniotic fluid, lung/muscle, liver/fluid, and liver/muscle for the prediction of lung hypoplasia. In contrast with the study of Osada and colleagues,[141] these signal intensity ratios did not differ significantly from those in the normal population.

Doppler assessment of tracheal fluid flow

Kalache and colleagues[143] have proposed that the volume of lung fluid displaced in the trachea could be useful for the analysis of fetal lung function. The investigators tested this hypothesis in a case–control study that included six cases of congenital diaphragmatic hernia diagnosed prenatally and a control group of five healthy fetuses matched for gestational age to each case. Parameters analyzed included: (1) the length of the inspiratory phase, (2) the length of the expiratory phase, (3) the peak velocities during inspiration and expiration, and (4) the volume estimation of the displaced fluid in the trachea during breathing [calculated as volume = velocity time integral (VTI) $\times \pi \times (d \times 0.5)^2$]. The estimated breathing-related tracheal volume flow in uncomplicated pregnancies increased with gestational age (from 0.21 ± 0.10 mL/breath at 26 weeks to 1.37 ± 0.48 mL/breath at 36 weeks of gestation), and was significantly lower in fetuses with diaphragmatic hernia who died of pulmonary hypoplasia. Tracheal volume flow in survivors was similar to that in control subjects.

Evaluation of hands and feet

Hands and feet should be examined to exclude polydactyly (Fig. 26.19), brachydactyly, and extreme postural deformities such as those seen in diastrophic dysplasia. Table 26.15 shows a nomogram of the fetal foot size throughout gestation. Table 26.16 displays disorders associated with hand and foot deformities. Disproportion between hands and feet and the other parts of the extremity may also be a sign of a skeletal dysplasia. Figure 26.20 illustrates the relationship between femur

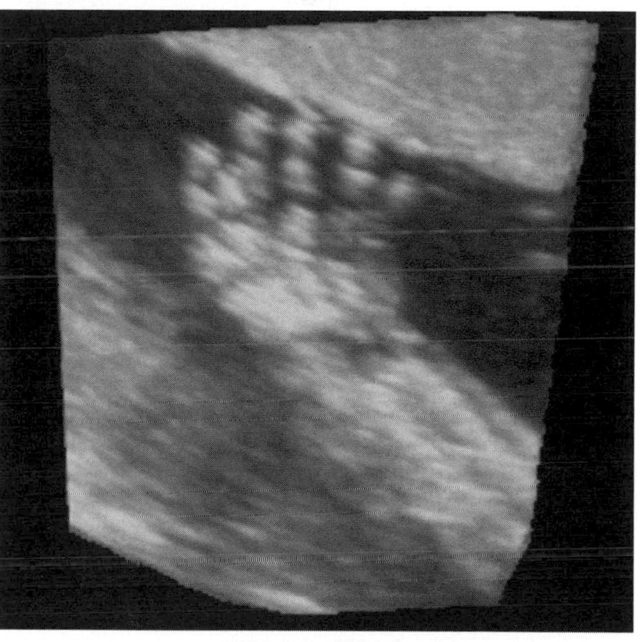

Figure 26.19 Three-dimensional rendered volume using the maximum intensity (skeletal) mode showing postaxial polydactyly.

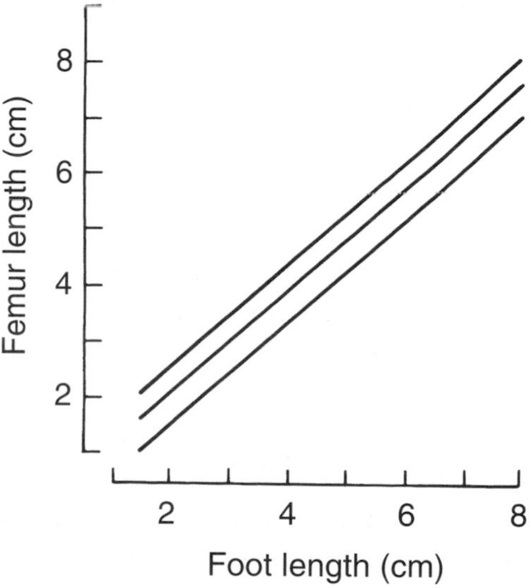

Figure 26.20 Relationship between femur and foot length.

Table 26.15 Nomogram of fetal foot size throughout gestation (cm).

Gestational age (weeks)	No.	5th percentile	10th percentile	50th percentile	90th percentile	95th percentile
15	18	1.4	1.5	1.8	2.2	2.3
16	146	1.6	1.7	2.1	2.5	2.6
17	375	1.9	2.0	2.4	2.8	2.9
18	613	2.2	2.3	2.7	3.1	3.2
19	1160	2.5	2.6	3.0	3.3	3.4
20	929	2.8	2.9	3.2	3.6	3.7
21	552	3.1	3.2	3.5	3.9	4.0
22	360	3.4	3.5	3.9	4.2	4.3
23	222	3.7	3.8	4.2	4.6	4.7
24	177	4.0	4.1	4.5	4.9	5.0
25	125	4.3	4.4	4.8	5.1	5.2
26	123	4.6	4.7	5.1	5.4	5.5
27	108	4.8	4.9	5.3	5.7	5.8
28	74	5.1	5.2	5.6	5.9	6.0
29	66	5.3	5.4	5.8	6.2	6.3
30	65	5.6	5.7	6.1	6.4	6.5
31	62	5.8	5.9	6.3	6.7	6.8
32	65	6.0	6.1	6.5	6.9	7.0
33	39	6.3	6.4	6.8	7.1	7.2
34	37	6.5	6.6	7.0	7.4	7.5
35	24	6.8	6.9	7.3	7.6	7.7
36	15	7.0	7.1	7.5	7.9	8.0
37	17	7.3	7.4	7.7	8.1	8.2

Reproduced with permission from ref. 917.

length and foot length. The femur–foot length ratio is nearly constant from 14 to 40 weeks of gestation, with a mean value of 0.99 ± 0.06 (SD). A ratio below 0.87 is considered abnormal.[144] Although fetuses with skeletal dysplasias have been reported to have abnormally low ratios, more experience is required to test the diagnostic value of this method.[145] It is expected that a small proportion of normal fetuses may have an abnormal ratio. As in the case of other limb biometric parameters, large deviations from the lower limit of normal are likely to be significant.

Evaluation of the fetal cranium

Several skeletal dysplasias are associated with defects of membranous ossification and, therefore, affect skull bones. Examination of the skull bones may reveal poor ossification (see Fig. 26.10), frontal bossing (Fig. 26.21), or cloverleaf deformity (Fig. 26.22). Table 26.17 presents abnormalities of the skull and face in the different skeletal dysplasias.

Evaluation of the fetal face

Sonographic examination of fetal facial features is of major importance in the assessment and diagnosis of fetuses with skeletal dysplasias as many of these disorders are associated with typical facial abnormalities.[146] Sonographic evaluation of the fetal face is easily performed in a high percentage of patients from 16 to 20 weeks of gestation onward. The single most reliable view in detecting facial abnormalities is the sagittal view. This view permits determination of midface hypoplasia, which occurs in several skeletal dysplasias, such as thanatophoric dysplasia, achondroplasia, campomelic dysplasia, osteogenesis imperfecta type I, and spondyloepiphyseal dysplasia congenita.[61,147]

In median clefting, the central portion of the upper lip is absent, and on the midline sagittal view no upper lip will be demonstrated. In bilateral cleft lip, the midline view will show a variable appearance, depending on the amount of residual premaxillary tissue present in the midline. In unilateral cleft lip, the midline sagittal scan may be relatively normal; the parasagittal view will reveal the cleft. This should subsequently be confirmed by scanning the coronal plane.

Cleft palate occurs in 66% of patients with cleft lip. Isolated cleft palate is more difficult to diagnose with ultrasound because of shadowing of facial bones. Three-dimensional ultrasonography has been shown to be superior to two-dimensional ultrasonography for the prenatal diagnosis of cleft lip and palate.[148–150] Potential advantages of three- over two-dimensional ultrasound include: (1) a true coronal view of the lips can be displayed, even when the original scanning plane was obtained from a different orientation; (2) three-

Table 26.16 Skeletal dysplasias associated with polydactyly and syndactyly.

Postaxial polydacytly
Chondroectodermal dysplasia
Short rib–polydactyly syndrome (type I, type II)
Asphyxiating thoracic dysplasia
Otopalatodigital syndrome
Mesomelic dysplasia, Werner type (associated with absence of thumbs)
Preaxial polydactyly
Chondroectodermal dysplasia
Short rib–polydactyly syndrome type II
Carpenter syndrome
Syndactyly
Poland syndrome
Acrocephalosyndactylies (Carpenter syndrome, Apert syndrome)
Otopalatodigital syndrome type II
Mesomelic dysplasia, Werner type
TAR syndrome
Jarcho–Levin syndrome
Brachydactyly
Mesomelic dysplasia, Robinow type
Otopalatodigital syndrome
Hitchhiker thumb
Diastrophic dysplasia
Clubfoot deformity
Diastrophic dysplasia
Osteogenesis imperfecta
Kniest dysplasia
Spondyloepiphyseal dysplasia

dimensional standardized multiplanar imaging makes it easier to successfully demonstrate the maxillary tooth-bearing alveolar ridge in suspected cases; and (3) the maxillary tooth-bearing alveolar ridge can be more accurately localized by the multiplanar technique because this region can be easily mistaken for the mandibular ridge.[151,152] Rendered views of the cleft lip/palate have been described as being particularly useful for patient counseling.[151,153,154] A novel technique for visualization of the fetal palate, the "three-dimensional reverse face view," has been proposed recently for the antenatal characterization of facial clefting, in particular for clefting of the hard palate.[155] This technique entails rotating the volume dataset 180° around the vertical axis in order to examine the secondary palate. Campbell and colleagues[156] reported preliminary results of this technique in eight cases of suspected orofacial clefting. A cleft in the soft palate was missed in only one case.

Micrognathia is also frequent in cases of skeletal dysplasia (Table 26.18).[157–159] The jaw index [(anteroposterior mandibular diameter/BPD) × 100] has been proposed as an objective and accurate parameter to diagnose micrognathia *in utero*. In a population of 198 malformed fetuses, 11 of which had micrognathia at necropsy or birth, a jaw index below 23 detected 100% of the cases with micrognathia with 98.1% specificity. In comparison, only 72.7% of the cases were detected by subjective evaluation of the fetal profile.

Intraorbital and interorbital diameters should be measured as hypertelorism may occur in cases of skeletal dysplasia (Table 26.19).

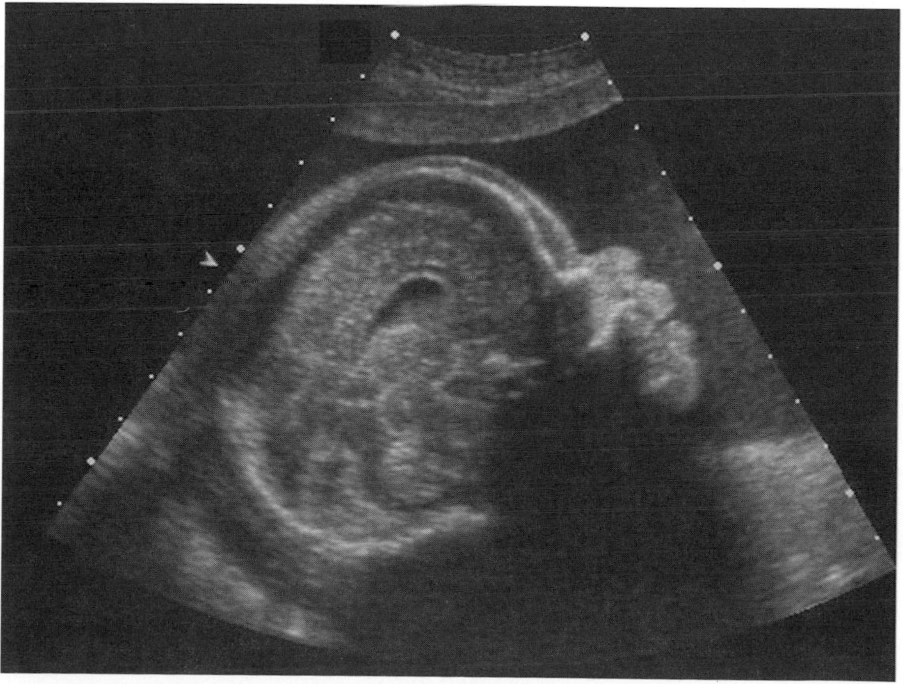

Figure 26.21 Frontal bossing in a sagittal scan in a fetus with achondroplasia.

Table 26.17 Skeletal dysplasias associated with skull and face deformities.

Large head
Achondroplasia
Achondrogenesis
Thanatophoric dysplasia
Osteogenesis imperfecta
Cleidocranial dysplasia
Hypophosphatasia
Campomelic dysplasia
Short rib–polydactyly syndrome, type III
Robinow mesomelic dysplasia
Otopalatodigital syndrome
Cloverleaf skull
Thanatophoric dysplasia
Campomelic dysplasia
Other craniostenosis
Apert syndrome
Carpenter syndrome
Congenital cataracts
Chondrodysplasia punctata
Cleft palate
Asphyxiating thoracic dysplasia
Kniest dysplasia
Dystrophic dysplasia
Spondyloepiphyseal dysplasia
Campomelic dysplasia
Jarcho–Levin syndrome
Ellis–van Creveld syndrome
Short rib–polydactyly syndrome, type II
Metatropic dysplasia
Otopalatodigital syndrome, type II
Dyssegmental dysplasia
Roberts syndrome
Short upper lip
Chondroectodermal dysplasia
Micrognathia
Campomelic dysplasia
Distrophic dysplasia
Weissenbacher–Zweymuller syndrome
Otopalatodigital syndrome
Pena–Shokeir syndrome
Thrombocytopenia with absent radii (TAR) syndrome
Langer syndrome

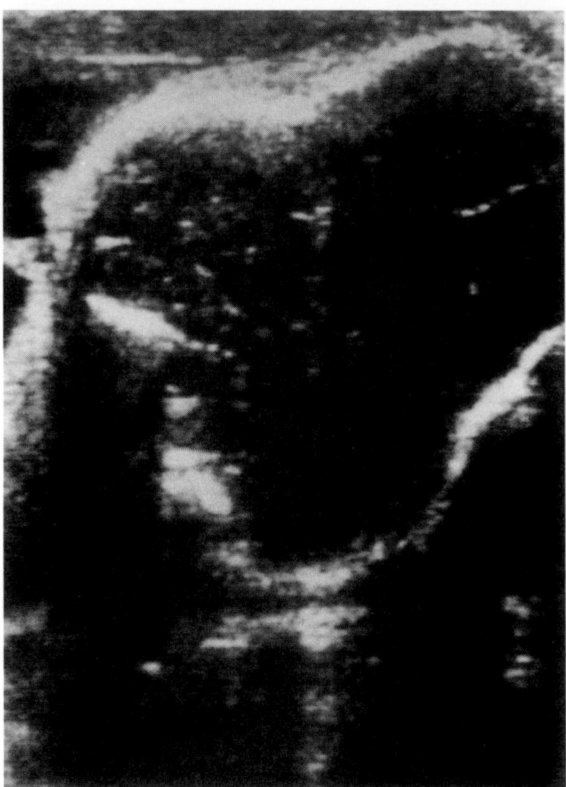

Figure 26.22 Coronal scan of the head of a fetus with thanatophoric dysplasia with a cloverleaf skull.

Table 26.18 Skeletal dysplasias associated with micrognathia.

Campomelic dysplasia
Diastrophic dysplasia
Otopalatodigital syndrome
Achondrogenesis
Mesomelic dysplasia
Pena–Shokeir syndrome
Treacher–Collins syndrome
Nager acrofacial dysostosis
Oromandibular limb hypogenesis
Goldenhar syndrome
Atelosteogenesis
Hydrolethalus syndrome

Evaluation of the fetal spine

Sonographic assessment of the fetal spine is a component in the examination of a fetus with suspected skeletal dysplasia. The following parameters should be assessed.

Vertebral bodies

Fetal vertebral bodies are composed of three ossification centers representing the vertebral body and two laminae.[160–163] Abnormalities of the ossification center of the fetal vertebral body may result in bony defects, such as hemivertebrae (see Fig. 26.5), butterfly vertebrae, or block vertebrae causing congenital scoliosis (see Fig. 26.4). A study of the associated anomalies of 27 cases in which prenatal ultrasound detected hemivertebrae noted that, although 11 fetuses had no other abnormal findings, 16 fetuses had associated anomalies.[160] These anomalies included cardiac, gastrointestinal, renal, facial, extremity, and cranial malformations. Seven fetuses had bilateral renal agenesis (Potter sequence). Only five of the fetuses with additional anomalies survived. Usually these anomalies are not a risk factor for aneuploidy.

Table 26.19 Skeletal dysplasias associated with hypertelorism.

Otopalatodigital syndrome
Arthrogryposis multiplex congenital
Larsen syndrome
Roberts syndrome
Cleidocranial dysostosis
Achondroplasia
Campomelic dysplasia
Coffin syndrome
Klippel–Feil syndrome
Apert syndrome
Sprengel's deformity
Mesomelic dysplasia
Holt–Oram syndrome

Platyspondyly may be diagnosed with current high-resolution sonography (Fig. 26.3).[164] Objective evaluation may be performed by computing a ratio between measurements of the vertebral interspace to vertebral body height.[33] Rib defects are often associated with thoracic vertebral body anomalies.

Clefting of the vertebrae may be complete or incomplete, coronal, or sagittal.[43] Coronal vertebral clefts are a result of missed fusion between the anterior and posterior primary ossification centers beyond 16 weeks of gestation. It can be observed by sonography *in utero*.[165,166] Sagittal clefts in the vertebral bodies are believed to represent a localized splitting of the notochord due to adhesions between the ectoderm and endoderm during the embryonic period. These clefts range from a single cleft to multiple clefts as part of a malformation syndrome. The role of vertebral clefting in the diagnosis of skeletal dysplasias was assessed by searching the database at the International Skeletal Dysplasia Registry in a study conducted by Westvik and Lachman.[166] Coronal and sagittal clefts were present in 40 different conditions. Coronal clefts were more common than sagittal clefts and were mainly located in the thoracolumbar region. Clefts were most frequently observed in atelosteogenesis (88%), followed by chondrodysplasia punctata (79%), dyssegmental dysplasia (73%), Kniest dysplasia (63%), and short rib–polydactyly syndrome (53%).[166] The authors concluded that vertebral clefts are of major diagnostic value in these groups of skeletal dysplasia.

Spinal curvature

The most common osseous anomaly causing scoliosis is unilateral unsegmented bar with contralateral hemivertebrae.[160,167–170] Spinal dysraphism may occur with congenital scoliosis and this possibility should be examined carefully. An apparent etiologic relationship exists between neural tube defects and other vertebral anomalies. Siblings of infants with congenital scoliosis have a 4% risk of neural tube defects.[171] This increased risk is present in siblings of children with a single hemivertebra as well as multiple vertebral anomalies (with or without neural arch defects). The differential diagnosis of fetal scoliosis includes neural tube defects, large abdominal wall defects, amniotic band syndrome, caudal regression, and hemivertebrae. Nonossification of the lumbar vertebral bodies has been detected in achondrogenesis and other diseases.[172–174]

Evaluation of the internal organs

A detailed examination of the cardiovascular, genitourinary, gastrointestinal, and central nervous system organs should be performed in all fetuses with skeletal anomalies. Some syndromes present with specific abnormalities of the internal organs, thus helping in the differential diagnoses of these entities. For example, congenital heart disease is a prominent feature of Ellis–van Creveld and Holt–Oram syndromes.

Newborn evaluation

Despite all efforts to establish an accurate prenatal diagnosis, a careful study of the newborn is always required.[67] The evaluation should include a detailed physical examination performed by a geneticist or an individual with experience in the field of skeletal dysplasias and radiographs of the skeleton. The latter should include anterior, posterior, lateral, and Towne views of the skull and anteroposterior views of the spine, extremities, and scapula,[175] with separate films of the hands and feet. Examination of the skeletal radiographs will permit precise diagnoses in a large proportion of cases, since the classification of skeletal dysplasias is largely based on radiographic findings. In lethal skeletal dysplasias, histologic examination of the chondro-osseous tissue should be performed, as this information may help reach a specific diagnosis. Chromosomal studies should be included, as there is a specific group of constitutional bone disorders associated with cytogenetic abnormalities. Biochemical studies are helpful in rare instances (e.g., hypophosphatasia). DNA restriction and enzymatic activity assays should be considered in cases in which the phenotype suggests a metabolic disorder, such as a mucopolysaccharidosis. The recent significant advance in identifying several mutations responsible for dysplasias is useful for prenatal diagnosis by amniocentesis or chorionic villus sampling (CVS) in patients at risk.[2,3,176] DNA should be saved in all cases.

Increased nuchal translucency and skeletal dysplasia

In chromosomally normal pregnancies, increased nuchal translucency thickness is associated with increased risk of major anomalies.[177–180] Skeletal dysplasias have been associated with increased nuchal translucency thickness in fetuses with a normal karyotype.[180–184] In the multicenter screening project for trisomy 21 using the combination of maternal age and nuchal translucency, 100 000 pregnancies were included.[177] An association between nuchal translucency and a wide range of skeletal dysplasias was found among these patients. Several case reports and small series have also suggested that in chromosomally normal fetuses there may be an association between increased nuchal translucency thickness and skeletal anomalies. Table 26.20 summarizes these data.

Osteochondrodysplasias

A growing number of skeletal dysplasias have been recognized *in utero*. A complete account of each disorder is beyond the scope of this chapter. The following discussion presents only a few of the most common disorders relevant to prenatal diagnosis.

Achondroplasia, thanatophoric dysplasia, and hypochondroplasia

These three chondrodysplasias are discussed in the same section since they are caused by different mutations in the *FGFR3* gene.[185–192] Mutations in *FGFR3* are gain-of-function mutations that produce a constitutively active protein capable of initiating intracellular signal pathways in the absence of ligand binding.[193,194] This activation leads to premature maturation of the bone.[194]

Achondroplasia

The most common nonlethal skeletal dysplasia is achondroplasia, an autosomal dominant condition with a prevalence of 1 per 66 000. It is characterized by rhizomelic shortening, limb bowing, lordotic spine, and enlarged head.[195] This disease is the result of anomalous growth of cartilage, followed by abnormal endochondral ossification, which is responsible for the shortness of long bones. The bones of the hands and feet are short (brachydactyly). The head is large; a flattened nasal bridge, frontal bossing, and broad mandible are frequent features. The problems in the prenatal diagnosis of this condition have been discussed in detail by Kurtz and colleagues.[196] Moreover, Modaff and colleagues[197] provided data about the frequency of prenatal misdiagnosis of achondroplasia and illustrated the difficulty of making this specific prenatal diagnosis. They collected data retrospectively from 37 consecutive referrals of infants with achondroplasia in whom ultrasound was performed prenatally: 9 out of 37 (24%) had a positive family history of achondroplasia; all nine were correctly diagnosed prenatally. Out of the 28 with no family history of achondroplasia, 16 (57%) were recognized to have abnormalities on ultrasound but none was diagnosed with certainty. Five received an appropriate diagnosis of "most likely" achondroplasia and four others were given a nonspecific (but appropriate) diagnosis of some skeletal dysplasia, not otherwise specified. In seven instances (25%), an incorrect diagnosis of a lethal or very severe disorder was assigned.

Table 26.20 Skeletal dysplasias associated with increased thickness of nuchal translucency.

Skeletal dysplasia	Author (year)
Achondrogenesis	Hewitt, 1993;[918] Soothill and Kyle, 1997;[919] Fisk and colleagues, 1991[327]
Achondroplasia	Fukada and colleagues, 1997;[920] Hernadi and Torocsik, 1997[921]
Asphyxiating thoracic dysplasia	Ben Ami and colleagues, 1997;[486] Hsieh and colleagues, 1999[477]
Blomstrand osteochondrodysplasia	den Hollander and colleagues, 1997[922]
Campomelic acamptomelic dysplasia	Michel-Calemard and colleagues, 2004[184]
Campomelic dysplasia	Hafner and colleagues, 1998[923]
Cleidocranial dysplasia	Hiippala and colleagues, 2001[924]
Chondroectodermal dysplasia (Ellis–van Creveld)	Venkat-Raman and colleagues, 2005[925]
Ectrodactyly ectodermal dysplasia	Leung and colleagues, 1995[926]
Fanconi anemia	Tercanli and colleagues, 2001[688]
Fetal akinesia deformation sequence	Souka and colleagues, 1998;[180] Hyett and colleagues, 1997;[927] Madazli and colleagues, 2002;[829] Makrydimas and colleagues, 2004[831]
Hypophosphatasia	Souka and colleagues, 2002[182]
Jarcho–Levin syndrome	Eliyahu, 1997;[928] Souka, 1998[180]
Osteogenesis imperfecta II	Makridymas and colleagues, 2001[181]
Short rib–polydactyly syndrome	Hill and Leary, 1998[512]
Sirenomelia	Hewitt, 1993[918]
Smith–Lemli–Opitz syndrome	Souka, 1998;[180] Hyett and colleagues, 1995;[929] Maymon and colleagues, 1999;[930] Sharp and colleagues, 1997;[931] Hobbins and colleagues, 1994[932]
Thanatophoric dysplasia	Souka, 1998;[180] Ferreira and colleagues, 2004[933]
VACTREL association	Souka, 1998[180]

The major difficulty in the antenatal diagnosis is that the long bone growth in this disease is not recognized in most cases until the third trimester of pregnancy.[49,198] Therefore, it is usually not possible to detect this disorder in time to allow for pregnancy termination.[199] However, prenatal diagnosis of achondroplasia is possible and has been reported.[200–202] The trident hand is a specific finding for achondroplasia.[203,204] A distinct difference in the femoral length growth curves of homozygous, heterozygous, and unaffected children of achondroplastic parents has been described by Patel and Filly.[205]

More than 99% of individuals with achondroplasia have one of two mutations in the *FGFR3* gene. The more common mutation, found in approximately 98% of patients, is a G → A point mutation at nucleotide 1138. About 1% of affected individuals have a G → C point mutation at the same nucleotide. The G380R mutation has been shown to result in constitutive activation of the fibroblast growth factor receptor. Prenatal diagnosis in pregnancies in which one or both parents has achondroplasia is possible by molecular diagnosis, using CVS or amniocentesis.[206–208] Molecular analysis can also be used to identify mutations in fetuses suspected to have achondroplasia based on ultrasound findings. As discussed, achondroplasia would typically present in the late second or third trimester of pregnancy, limiting available methods of prenatal diagnosis to amniocentesis.

Heterozygous achondroplasia is compatible with a normal life and intellectual development. However, cervicomedullary junction abnormalities, which may lead to compression, put the infant with achondroplasia at risk for lethal sequelae.[209] Although the disease is lethal in the homozygous state, a case of a 37-month survivor has been reported.[210] The radiologic characteristics of homozygous achondroplasia lie between those of thanatophoric dysplasia and heterozygous achondroplasia. Administration of growth hormone has been proposed for the treatment of achondroplasia.[211]

SADDAN (severe achondroplasia with developmental delay and acanthosis nigricans)

Tavormina and colleagues[212] identified a *FGFR3* missense mutation in four unrelated individuals with skeletal dysplasias, which approaches the severity observed in thanatophoric dysplasia type I. Three out of the four individuals developed extensive areas of acanthosis nigricans (beginning in early childhood), suffered from severe neurological impairments, and have survived past infancy without prolonged life-support measures. The *FGFR3* mutation (A1949T:Lys650Met) occurs at the nucleotide adjacent to the thanatophoric dysplasia type II mutation (A1948G:Lys650Glu) and results in a different amino acid substitution. They referred to the phenotype caused by the Lys650Met mutation as "severe achondroplasia with developmental delay and acanthosis nigricans" (SADDAN) because it differs significantly from the phenotypes of other known *FGFR3* mutations. It is also associated with unusual bone deformities, such as femoral bowing with reverse (i.e., posterior apex), tibial and fibular bowing, and "ram's horn" bowing of the clavicle. This condition has not been associated with cloverleaf skull or craniosynostosis.[213]

Thanatophoric dysplasia

Thanatophoric dysplasia is the most common lethal skeletal dysplasia in fetuses and neonates.[7] It is characterized by extreme rhizomelia, a normal trunk length with a narrow thorax, and a large head featuring a prominent forehead. It occurs in 0.24–0.69 of 10 000 births.[8,15,187,214] Two subtypes have been identified: type I, with typical bowed "telephone receiver" femurs[215] (Fig. 26.23) and without cloverleaf skull; and type II, with severe cloverleaf skull (Fig. 26.22) and short, straight long bones.[21,216] However, mild cloverleaf skull has been described in type I.[217–219] Cloverleaf skull may result from premature closure of the coronal and lambdoid sutures, defective development of the cranial base with secondary synostosis, or a primary developmental disorder of the brain with secondary deformation of the skull. The differential diagnosis between the two types depends on the radiographic findings and histology. Both types of thanatophoric dysplasia are inherited in an autosomal dominant manner.[220] The majority of cases of thanatophoric dysplasia (all type I and most cases of type II) are sporadic. Some familial cases of type II have been reported.[220–225]

Distinct mutations in *FGFR3* cause each one of the two types of thanatophoric dysplasia.[221,222,226,227] Three common mutations (R248C, Y373C, and S249C) are found in approximately 90% of the patients with thanatophoric dysplasia type I.[193,228] One mutation, K650E, is found in almost all cases of thanatophoric dysplasia type II.[229–231] Camera and col-

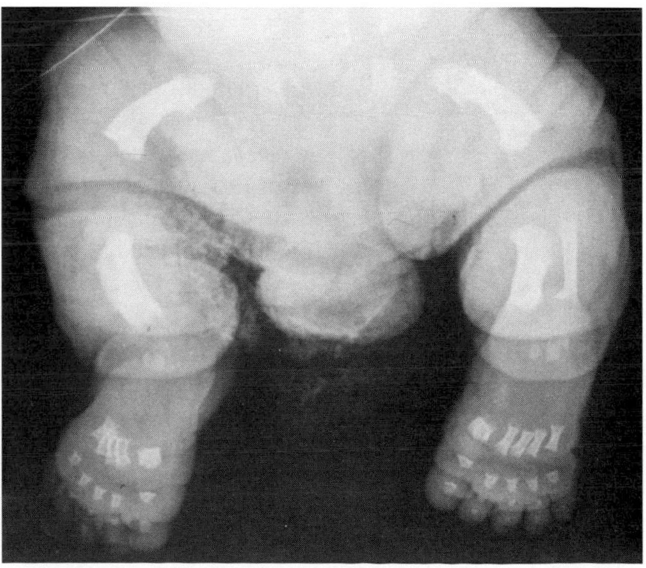

Figure 26.23 Bowed and short femurs in thanatophoric dysplasia.

leagues[232] reported an individual with the common thanatophoric dysplasia type I mutation and the clinical phenotype of achondroplasia. Mosaicism was thought to be a possible explanation for the milder phenotype. However, mosaicism was not found in buccal mucosal cells or blood.

The prenatal sonographic findings depend on the specific type of thanatophoric dysplasia.[165] The association of cloverleaf skull and micromelia is specific for thanatophoric dysplasia. Campomelic syndrome is also associated with cloverleaf skull. Micromelia, however, is not a feature of that condition. Ventriculomegaly, macrocranium, and polyhydramnios are frequently seen. There is a relatively large calvarium with a prominent forehead (Fig. 26.21), a saddle nose, and hypertelorism. Additional findings are short ribs, platyspondyly (see Fig. 26.3), and short and broad tubular bones in the hands and feet. The differential diagnoses include short rib–polydactyly syndrome, homozygous achondroplasia (in which both parents are typically affected), and asphyxiating thoracic dysplasia (differentiated by slight shortening of long bones and normal vertebrae). On review of the radiologic findings of several cases of thanatophoric dysplasia, Horton and colleagues[233] were able to discern a group of distinct entities characterized by severe platyspondyly. These disorders include the Torrance, San Diego, Lutton, and Shiraz types of platyspondylic lethal osteochondrodysplasias. Differential diagnosis among these entities is based on histologic and radiologic characteristics. Individuals with platyspondylic lethal skeletal dysplasia – San Diego type – have been reported to have *FGFR3* mutations that were previously reported in association with thanatophoric dysplasia type I.[234]

Thanatophoric dysplasia is a uniformly lethal disorder, although survival of several months has been reported in some isolated cases.[225,233,235–238] Prenatal sonographic diagnosis has been documented on several occasions,[77,173,239–256] and in one case of a triplet pregnancy.[192] Prenatal diagnosis by CVS or amniocentesis is available.[76,257–259]

Hypochondroplasia

Hypochondroplasia is an autosomal dominant disorder that resembles achondroplasia.[260] It can result from a mutation in the *FGFR3* gene,[261,262] although genetic heterogeneity is suspected.[263] The incidence and prevalence have not been determined, at least in part because of lack of agreement on a definitive set of diagnostic criteria, which makes it difficult to review data from many studies reported in the literature. Most cases occur sporadically as a result of a new mutation.[264]

Two *FGFR3* mutations (C1620A and C1620G) result in a lysine for asparagine substitution at codon 540 (N5400K0) and have been shown to cause hypochondroplasia.[186,265] Several other *FGFR3* mutations have been proposed to cause a small number of cases of hypochondroplasia. In addition, the insulin-like growth factor-1 (IGF-1) gene has been proposed to be linked to hypochondroplasia in a subset of cases, although no pathogenetic mutations have been reported.[263]

The differential diagnosis between this condition and achondroplasia is based on the sparing of the head and the lack of tibial bowing in hypochondroplasia.[260,266–270] Although this condition is generally first detected during childhood, prenatal diagnosis has been reported in fetuses at risk for the condition.[267,271] DNA-based diagnosis via CVS or amniocentesis may be possible.

Fibrochondrogenesis and atelosteogenesis

Fibrochondrogenesis and atelosteogenesis have a clinical presentation similar to that of thanatophoric dysplasia. The differential diagnosis between these disorders *in utero* is extremely difficult. Fibrochondrogenesis and atelosteogenesis are extremely rare, and only a few cases of each have been reported.

Fibrochondrogenesis

Fibrochondrogenesis is a very rare lethal chondrodysplasia inherited with an autosomal recessive pattern and characterized by micromelia with significant metaphyseal flaring, normal head size, undermineralized skull, platyspondyly, clefting of the vertebral bodies, and narrow, bell-shaped thorax.[272,273] Metaphyseal flaring is not a feature of thanatophoric dysplasia.[274–277] This condition has been described in a consanguineous family.[278] Other conditions to be considered in the differential diagnosis include metatropic dysplasia and Kniest dysplasia. Prenatal diagnosis of fibrochondrogenesis by ultrasound has been reported as early as 17 weeks of gestation.[279–281] The molecular defect involved in fibrochondrogenesis is not known.[282]

Atelosteogenesis

Atelosteogenesis is also a lethal chondrodysplasia characterized by severe micromelia (with hypoplasia of the distal segments of the humerus and femur), bowing of long bones, narrow chest with short ribs, coronal and sagittal vertebral clefts,[43] and dislocations at the level of the elbow and knee. Clubfoot deformities may also be present.[283] Three subtypes of atelosteogenesis have been described based on radiologic and pathologic findings.[284–287] Atelosteogenesis types I and III are sporadic and caused by mutations in the gene encoding filamin B.[288] Atelosteogenesis type II is inherited with an autosomal recessive pattern and is caused by mutation in DTDST.[289–292] It overlaps phenotypically and genetically with diastrophic dysplasia and achondrogenesis type IB.[287,293,294]

Differential diagnosis includes diastrophic dysplasia and de la Chapelle dysplasia.[295,296] Three cases of a lethal dysplasia termed *boomerang syndrome* ("boomerang-like tibia") may actually represent the same disorder as atelosteogenesis type I.[297] There are now more than three reported cases.[43,298–302]

Achondrogenesis

Achondrogenesis, or anosteogenesis, is a lethal chondrodystrophy that is characterized by extreme micromelia, short trunk, and macrocrania. The birth prevalence is 0.09–0.23 in 10 000 births.[8,15,64,68,70] Traditionally, this disorder has been classified into two types: the more severe form, which is type I achondrogenesis (Parenti–Fraccaro), and type II achondrogenesis (Langer–Saldino). In 1998, type I was subdivided into two subtypes: type IA (Houston–Harris) and type IB (Fraccaro).[303,304] Hypochondrogenesis had been considered a separate disorder from achondrogenesis. However, evidence now suggests that hypochondrogenesis and achondrogenesis type II are phenotypic variants of the same disorder.[305–307] Indeed, clinically and radiologically, achondrogenesis type II, hypochondrogenesis, and neonatal spondyloepiphyseal dysplasia congenita form a continuous spectrum of disease.[308] The fundamental biochemical disorder seems to be allelic mutations of the gene coding for type II procollagen.[309] A different classification dividing achondrogenesis into four types has been proposed by Whitley and Gorlin,[309] but this proposal has not gained wide acceptance.

Type IA achondrogenesis (Houston–Harris) is characterized by micromelia, lack of ossification of vertebral bodies but ossification of the pedicles in the cervical and upper thoracic region, and short ribs with multiple fractures. The calvarium is demineralized. Type IB (Fraccaro), which is a recessively inherited chondrodysplasia, is caused by mutation in the *DTDS* gene[310–312] and is similar to type IA, but the calvarium is ossified, and fractured ribs are not seen. Although the vertebral bodies are minimally or not at all ossified, the pedicles show some ossification. Type II achondrogenesis is characterized by micromelia, lack of mineralization of all or many of the vertebral bodies, sacrum, and ischium, enlarged calvarium with normal ossification, variable shortening of the ribs, and absence of fractures (Fig. 26.24).[313] Table 26.21 illustrates the characteristics of the different types of achondrogenesis.[305,314,315]

Prenatal diagnosis should be suspected on the basis of micromelia, lack of vertebral ossification, and a large head with various degrees of ossification of calvarium.[172,313–326] Polyhydramnios and hydrops have been associated with achondrogenesis. However, sonographic examinations of affected fetuses do not demonstrate fluid accumulation in body cavities. The hydropic appearance of these fetuses and neonates is probably attributable to redundancy of soft-tissue mass over a limited skeletal frame. An association between cystic hygromas and achondrogenesis has been reported in a fetus with normal chromosomal constitution.[313,314,327]

Achondrogenesis type IA and IB are inherited in an autosomal recessive pattern, whereas most cases of achondrogenesis type II and hypochondrogenesis have been sporadic (new autosomal dominant mutations). Some severe cases of type II achondrogenesis follow an autosomal recessive pattern.[328]

The primary defect in achondrogenesis type IA has not been identified. The only gene known to be associated with achondrogenesis type IB is *SLC26A2* (*DTDST*), which encodes a sulfate transporter protein.[329] As the basic defect in achondrogenesis type IB is known, molecular diagnosis is possible. The distinction between achondrogenesis type IB (which has a risk of 25% for recurrence) and the more frequent

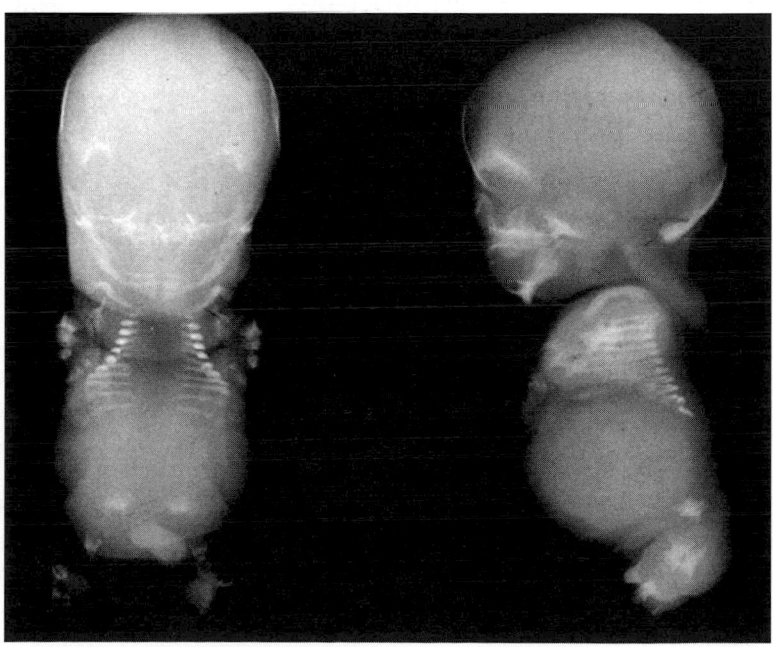

Figure 26.24 Frontal and lateral views in a case of achondrogenesis type II. There is no mineralization of the spine and ischial bones. The thorax is bell shaped, with short and straight ribs and no fractures. Long bones are short, with metaphyseal flaring and cupping.

Table 26.21 Radiologic differences of achondrogenesis types IA/IB, type II, and hypochondrogenesis.

Site	Type IA (Houston–Harris)	Type IB (Fraccaro)	Type II (Langer–Saldino)	Hypochondrogenesis
Skull	Membranous calvarium	All parts of ossified skull well seen	Normal ossification	Normal ossification
Long bones	Extremely shortened with metaphyseal cupping and spurs, "rectangular bones"	Arms and legs shorter than with type IA with minimal ossification; abundant metaphyseal spiking or spurring in lower leg bones, "square or stellate bones"	Short and bowed with metaphyseal flaring and cupping, "mushroom stem bones"	Less bowed and shortened with irregular or smooth metaphyses
Spine	Vertebral bodies unossified, with partly ossified pedicles	Vertebral bodies minimally or not ossified, pedicles ossified	Variable pattern of ossified or unossified vertebral bodies and pedicles	Thoracic and upper lumbar vertebral bodies ossified but still platyspondylic Cervical and lower lumbar bodies unossified
Pelvis	Poorly formed and ossified, with crenated iliac bones, ischial bones poorly ossified, pubic bones unossified	Iliac bones same aspect as in type IA, ischial and pubic bones unossified	Halberd-like iliac bones with unossified ischial and pubic bones	Near normally developed iliac bones with partial ossification of ischial bones and unossified pubic bones
Thorax	Short and barrel shaped, short ribs with cupped metaphyses and multiple fractures	Same as in type IA with unfractured ribs	Short and barrel/bell shaped with short unfractured ribs	Near normal but shallow cage with short unfractured ribs

autosomal dominant achondrogenesis type II, which has a lower recurrence risk, is important for genetic counseling. A couple at risk of having a child with achondrogenesis type IB may take the advantage of molecular prenatal diagnosis by CVS or amniocentesis.[289,293,310] Achondrogenesis type II and hypochondrogenesis result from mutations in the *COL2A1* gene.[330] Prenatal diagnosis by molecular analysis of the *COL2A1* gene is available.

Osteogenesis imperfecta and hypophosphatasia

Osteogenesis imperfecta and hypophosphatasia are discussed together because they are characterized by skeletal demineralization.

Osteogenesis imperfecta

The term "osteogenesis imperfecta" was introduced over a century ago to describe a newborn with extremely brittle bones (see Figs 26.12 and 26.13). At present, the term refers to a heterogeneous group of disorders caused in most cases by mutations in one or two structural genes for type I procollagen.[331–337] Extraskeletal malformations are variably associated with the disorder and include blue sclera, dentinogenesis imperfecta, hyperlaxity of ligaments and skin, hearing impairment, and presence of wormian bones on skull radiographs.[337] Advanced paternal age is a risk factor for osteogenesis imperfecta,[338] and its prevalence is 0.18 per 10 000 births.[8,15]

The most popular classification is that proposed by Sillence and colleagues.[339] A modification of this classification has been recently reported by Rauch and Glorieux[337] and includes three additional types (V, VI, and VII; Table 26.22). Clinically, the most relevant characteristic of osteogenesis imperfecta is bone fragility, with severity increasing in the following order: (1) type I; (2) types IV, V, VI, and VII; (3) type III; and (4) type II.[337]

In type I (autosomal dominant), patients have bone fragility, blue sclerae (all ages), and hearing loss. There is osteoporosis, a normal calvarium, and no dentinogenesis imperfecta; fractures range from none to multiple. Mutations that cause type I osteogenesis imperfecta result in premature termination codons that lead to decreased production of type I procollagen.[333]

Type II is an autosomal dominant condition.[340] It is also known as the perinatal variety and is uniformly lethal. There is almost no ossification of the skull, beaded ribs, shortened, crumpled long bones, and multiple fractures *in utero* (see Figs 26.12 and 26.13). The thorax is short but not narrow. Type

Table 26.22 Expanded Sillence classification of osteogenesis imperfecta.

Type	Clinical severity	Typical features	Typically associated mutations
I	Mild non-deforming osteogenesis imperfecta	Normal height or mild short stature, blue sclerae, no dentinogenesis imperfecta	Premature stop codon in *COLIAI*
II	Perinatal lethal	Multiple rib and long bone fractures at birth, pronounced deformities, broad long bones, low density of skull bones on radiographs, dark sclerae	Glycine substitutions in *COLIAI* or *COLIA2*
III	Severely deforming	Very short, triangular face, severe scoliosis, grayish sclerae, dentinogenesis imperfecta	Glycine substitutions in *COLIAI* or *COLIA2*
IV	Moderately deforming	Moderately short, mild to moderate scoliosis, grayish or white sclerae, dentinogenesis imperfecta	Glycine substitutions in *COLIAI* or *COLIA2*
V	Moderately deforming	Mild to moderate short stature, dislocation of radial head, mineralized interosseous membrane, hyperplastic callus, white sclerae, no dentinogenesis imperfecta	Unknown
VI	Moderately to severely deforming	Moderately short, scoliosis, accumulation of osteoid in bone tissue, fish-scale pattern of bone lamellation, white sclerae, no dentinogenesis imperfecta	Unknown
VII	Moderately deforming	Mild short stature, short humeri and femora, coxa vara, white sclerae, no dentinogenesis imperfecta	Unknown

Reproduced with permission from ref. 337.

II is subclassified into three subtypes (IIA, IIB, and IIC) according to radiologic criteria: group A – short, broad, 'crumpled' long bones, angulation of tibias, and continuously beaded ribs; group B – short, broad, crumpled femurs, angulation of tibias but normal ribs or ribs with incomplete beading; and group C – long, thin, inadequately modeled long bones with multiple fractures and thin beaded ribs.[341]

Type III (autosomal recessive, rare) is a nonlethal variety characterized by blue sclerae and multiple fractures present at birth. The sclerae become white with time. The membranous skull is severely deossified and the long bones are mildly shortened but with marked angulations. Type IIB and type III osteogenesis imperfecta are difficult to distinguish and may represent different degrees of severity of the same disorder.[342]

In type IV (autosomal dominant) the long bones and sclerae are normal. There is mild to moderate osseous fragility, and 25% of the newborns have fractures. There is significant heterogeneity in the expression of the disease even within the same family.[343] From this heterogeneous group, Rauch and Glorieux and colleagues[337,344–346] have recently identified three separate clinical entities based on distinct clinical and bone histological features. These disorders have been classified as osteogenesis imperfecta types V, VI, and VII (Table 26.22).

Osteogenesis imperfecta type I is caused by a premature stop codon in *COL1A1*.[332] Types II, III, and IV typically result from mutations that lead to substitutions for glycine within the triple-helical domain of the pro-alpha chain, disrupting the normal folding of the molecule and leading to the production of abnormal collagen.[347,348] Approximately 90% of patients with a clinical diagnosis of osteogenesis imperfecta have a mutation in either the *COL1A1* or *COL1A2* gene, resulting in abnormal molecular constitution of procollagen type I.[337,349–351] Gene mutations associated with types V, VI, and VII have not been identified.[337]

Collagen biosynthesis in cell culture from chorionic villi has been demonstrated and may serve as a way for prenatal diagnosis.[352] In a large study, Pepin and colleagues[353] completed prenatal diagnosis of collagen synthesized by cells cultured from CVS in 107 cases, and in 22 cases they used direct mutation identification or analysis of polymorphic restriction sites in the *COL1A1* gene of type 1 collagen. There were neither false-negative nor false-positive results. The time needed for diagnosis was 20–30 days when the biopsy was taken using biochemical techniques and 10–14 days when molecular strategies were used.

The natural history of osteogenesis imperfecta *in utero* is quite variable. Prenatal diagnosis of type II osteogenesis imperfecta has been reported several times,[75,354–375] even as early as 12 weeks of gestation by either two- or three-dimensional ultrasonography.[376–379] It is important, however, to note that in some cases fractures and limb shortening may not be observed until the second or even the third trimester.[380–382] Prenatal diagnosis of osteogenesis imperfecta types I, III, and IV has also been reported using either ultrasound, biochemistry, or molecular techniques.[353,383–386]

Hypophosphatasia

Hypophosphatasia is a rare autosomal recessive inherited disorder characterized by demineralization of bones and low alkaline phosphatase in serum and other tissues.[387] Alkaline phosphatase acts on pyrophosphate and other phosphate esters, leading to the accumulation of inorganic phosphates that are critical for the formation of bone crystals. Bone fragility is thought to be the result of deficient generation of bone crystals.[388]

Hypophosphatasia is a condition that has been subdivided into three clinical types according to the age of onset: congenital/infantile, childhood, and adult.[389,390] The congenital/infantile and childhood varieties have an autosomal recessive pattern of inheritance, whereas the adult form can be transmitted as either an autosomal dominant or autosomal recessive trait.[387] The congenital (neonatal) form is associated with early neonatal death or stillbirth.[391]

Fetuses with congenital hypophosphatasia have generalized demineralization of the skeleton, with shortening and bowing of tubular bones. Multiple fractures are present. The marked demineralization of the cranial vault results in deformation of the skull after external compression. This sonographic sign is also present in some cases of type II osteogenesis imperfecta and type IA achondrogenesis. Prenatal diagnosis of this condition has been reported with ultrasound[390,392–401] and by assaying alkaline phosphatase in tissue obtained by CVS[402] or amniotic fluid culture. Alkaline phosphatase measurement in amniotic fluid is not a reliable means of making a diagnosis of hypophosphatasia because most of the alkaline phosphatase in amniotic fluid is of intestinal origin.[403,404] The involved enzymes in hypophosphatasia are bone and liver alkaline phosphatases. These isoenzymes contribute only 16% of the total amniotic fluid enzymatic activity.[405]

Hypophosphatasia has been shown to be caused by mutations in the alkaline phosphatase liver gene [*ALPL*, also called the tissue non-specific alkaline phosphatase (*TNSALP*) gene] on chromosome 1.[406] There is a large spectrum of mutations in the Caucasion population.[407,408] Therefore, although prenatal diagnosis by DNA analysis is possible,[409] this requires sequencing the entire gene, which increases the complexity of the process. Missense mutations in the gene lead to variable residual enzymatic activity and the extremely high phenotypic heterogeneity observed in hypophosphatasia.[188,410]

Diastrophic dysplasia

Diastrophic dysplasia is characterized by micromelia, clubfoot, hand deformities, multiple joint flexion contractures, and scoliosis.[411] Because of phenotypic variability, the diagnosis may be difficult at birth, and milder cases are diagnosed later.[412] The clinical features include rhizomelic-type micromelia, contractures, hand deformities with abducted position of the thumbs ("hitchhiker thumb": Figs 26.25 and 26.26), and severe talipes equinovarus. The shape of the head is normal, but micrognathia and cleft palate may be present. This dysplasia is a generalized disorder of cartilage, involving destruction of the cartilage matrix with formation of fibrous scar tissue and subsequent ossification. The ossification is responsible for the contractures. Mutation in the diastrophic dysplasia sulfate transporter gene (*SLC26A2/DTDST*) is associated with impaired sulfation of proteoglycan and causes this disorder.[413–416] Five common *SLC26A2* mutations (*R279W*, *IVS1+2T→C*, *DELV340*, *R178X*, and *C653S*) account for approximately 65% of disease alleles.[414] Sequence analysis of the coding region can detect mutations in greater than 90% of alleles in individuals with typical clinical, radiologic, and histologic features.[414]

The prenatal diagnosis of diastrophic dysplasia has been made in patients at risk,[42,44,412,417–420] based on severe shortening and bowing of all long bones. Sepulveda and colleagues[421] reported clearer visualization of the limbs and face deformities using three-dimensional ultrasound. Prenatal diagnosis in at-risk pregnancies in which the familial mutations have been identified can be accomplished by DNA analysis of fetal cells obtained by CVS or amniocentesis.[422] Biochemical studies of fibroblasts and/or chondrocytes are available and may be useful for cases in which molecular genetic tests fail to identify *SLC26A2* mutations.[423] This disorder has a wide spectrum, and some cases may not be diagnosable *in utero*.

Diastrophic dysplasia is not universally lethal. Intelligence and sexual development are unaffected. However, death in the neonatal period due to respiratory/spinal abnormalities and mental retardation has been reported in some patients.

Differential diagnoses include arthrogryposis multiplex congenita, type II atelosteogenesis, and pseudodiastrophic dysplasia. Pseudodiastrophic dysplasia has a similar presentation as diastrophic dysplasia[424] and is inherited in an autosomal recessive pattern.[15] Histologic examination is required for a differential diagnosis. The distinctive morphologic abnormalities of the growth plate noted in diastrophic dysplasia have not been observed in pseudodiastrophic dysplasia. Cetta and colleagues[425] demonstrated that a patient with pseudodiastrophic dysplasia had no defect in the *DTDST* gene. Sulfate uptake by skin fibroblasts was normal, indicating normal sulfate transport. Sulfation of proteoglycans was also normal.

Kniest-like disorders

The term "Kniest-like disorders" is used to refer to a group of conditions that share histologic and radiologic characteristics with Kniest syndrome but differ in terms of clinical presentation and inheritance.[426]

Kniest syndrome

In 1952, Dr. Wilhelm Kniest[427] published a case of a 3.5-year-old girl with "skeletal changes showing a certain relationship

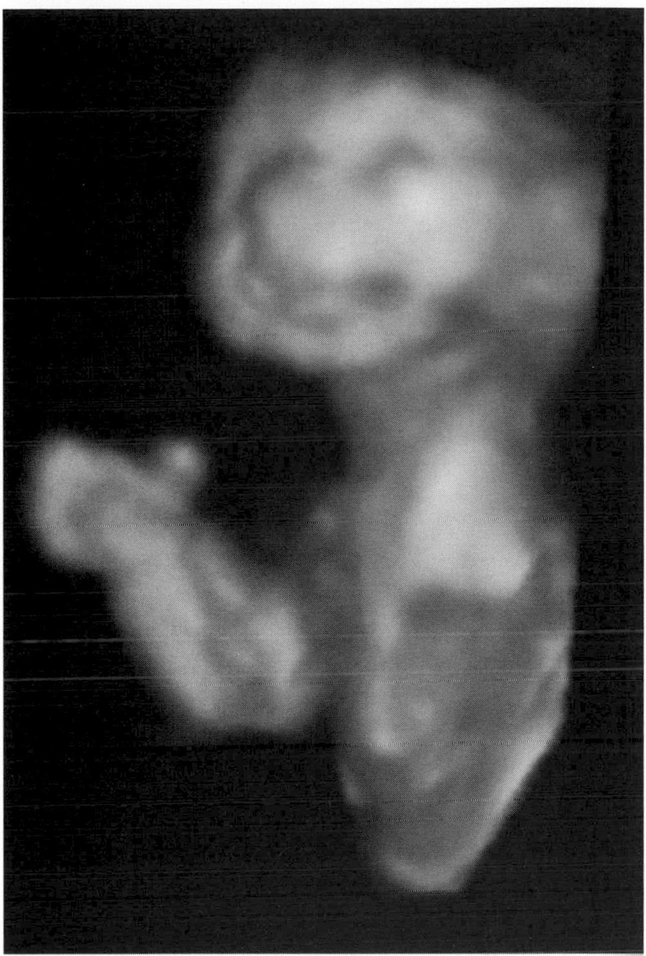

Figure 26.25 Three-dimensional rendered volume of a fetus with diastrophic dysplasia showing a hitchhiker thumb.

to classical chondrodystrophy but differing in many of its manifestations." His publication clarified the confusion of this disorder with other chondrodystrophies and it is known today as one of the type II collagenopathies.[428–431] Kniest dysplasia is characterized by involvement of the spine (platyspondyly and coronal clefts) and the tubular bones (shortened and metaphyseal flaring), with a broad and short thorax. There is a wide spectrum of disease.[432] The patient described by Dr. Kniest is still alive, although severely handicapped with short stature and blindness.[432] Molecular analysis of the patient's DNA showed a single base (G) deletion of the *COL2A1* gene. Most commonly, the disorder is compatible with life. However, lethality in the neonatal period has been reported.[433]

Abnormalities of type II collagen are involved in the pathogenesis of the disease.[434] The disorder is inherited in an autosomal dominant pattern.[220]

Dyssegmental dysplasia

Dyssegmental dysplasia is another entity related to Kniest dysplasia. Two distinct types of dyssegmental dysplasia have been recognized: the mild, Rolland–Desbuquois form and the lethal Silverman Handmaker.[435–438] The latter is characterized by anarchic ossification of the vertebral bodies, metaphyseal flaring, and severe bowing of the long bones. The Rolland–Desbuquois type has essentially the same features, but the defects are much milder. Prenatal identification has been made in patients at risk.[439,440] Other conditions associated with vertebral disorganization are Jarcho–Levin syndrome and mesomelic dysplasia. A cephalocele is present in 50% of cases of Silverman–Handmaker type and has been attributed to defective segmentation at the level of the occiput. The disease is autosomal recessive.[220] The Silverman–Handmaker type of dyssegmental dysplasia is caused by a functional null mutation in the gene encoding perlecan (*HSPG2*).[441]

Campomelic dysplasia

Campomelic dysplasia is a rare lethal disorder first described by Maroteaux in 1971.[442] The prevalence varies between 0.05 and 1.6 per 10 000.[443,444] A unique aspect of campomelic dysplasia is that 75% of affected infants with a male karyotype present sex reversal syndrome and have female or ambiguous genitalia.[445,446] The histology of the gonads

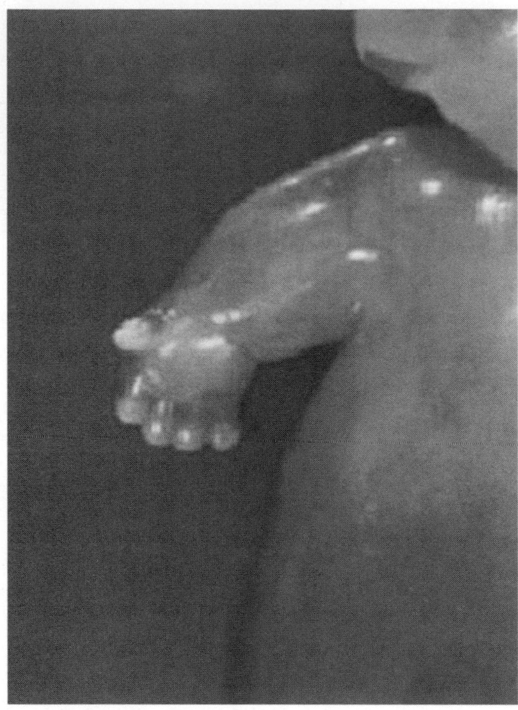

Figure 26.26 Hitchhiker thumb in diastrophic dysplasia.

varies from gonads with testicular differentiation to dysgenetic gonads with primary follicles. Mutations in the *SOX9* gene have been reported in several patients with this disorder.[445–449] Campomelic dysplasia arises by mutations that interfere with DNA binding by *SOX9* or truncate the C-terminal transactivation domain, and thereby impede the ability of *SOX9* to activate target genes during organ development.[449]

Campomelic syndrome is characterized by a bowing of the long bones of the lower extremities, an enlarged and elongated skull with a peculiar small facies, hypoplastic scapulae, and several associated anomalies such as micrognathia, cleft palate, talipes equinovarus, congenital dislocation of the hip, macrocephaly, hydrocephalus, hydronephrosis, and congenital heart defects.[340] The most significant features are bowing of the femur and tibia; other tubular bones are normal in length. The thorax is narrow and can be "bell shaped." Cervical vertebrae are hypoplastic and poorly ossified.[450] In the largest clinical and genetic study, which included 36 patients with this disorder, Mansour and colleagues[443] concluded that campomelic dysplasia is an autosomal condition, as females and males are both affected, and their data suggested a sporadic autosomal dominant mode of heritance.

There are two "short-bone varieties" of campomelic dysplasia, representing distinct syndromes: the normocephalic form is known as *kyphomelic dysplasia*, and the craniostenotic type appears to be identical to the Antley–Bixler syndrome. Differential diagnoses include osteogenesis imperfecta, thanatophoric dysplasia, and hypophosphatasia. Antenatal diagnosis of campomelic dysplasia has been reported many times in the literature, mainly in patients at risk.[70,451–459] At the time of this writing, only one laboratory offers prenatal molecular diagnosis for campomelic dysplasia.[460] The test is available for families in which a mutation has previously been identified. The difficulties in the diagnosis are discussed by Norgard[461] and by Sanders and colleagues.[458] The condition is frequently lethal in infancy, but some survivors have been reported.[451,462–466] The cause of death is respiratory distress due to tracheomalacia. However, cleft palate, micrognathia, hypotonia, and small chest are also associated with this condition.[451]

Skeletal dysplasias characterized by a hypoplastic thorax

The dysplastic process involves the ribs and other bones of the rib cages in many skeletal dysplasias. A reduction in thoracic dimensions leads to restriction of lung growth and, consequently, pulmonary hypoplasia. Lung hypoplasia is the main cause of death in lethal skeletal dysplasias. There are specific groups of dysplasias in which thoracic hypoplasia is a cardinal feature. These include asphyxiating thoracic dysplasia, Ellis–van Creveld syndrome, short rib–polydactyly syndrome, and campomelic syndrome. Table 26.23 illustrates the criteria for the differential diagnoses of the first three of these conditions. Other disorders presenting with altered thoracic dimensions are thanatophoric dysplasia, atelosteogenesis, fibrochondrogenesis, achondrogenesis, and Jarcho–Levin syndrome (Fig. 26.27).[467]

Asphyxiating thoracic dysplasia

Asphyxiating thoracic dysplasia, originally described by Jeune and Carron[468] and known as Jeune syndrome, is a rare autosomal recessive skeletal disorder. Its prevalence is 0.14 in 10 000 births.[469–471] It is characterized by a narrow and "bell-shaped" thorax, with short, horizontal ribs. Long bones are normal or mildly shortened. Polydactyly and cleft lip and/or palate can occur in association and the presence of a proximal femoral ossification center at birth is a characteristic finding.[472] Asphyxiating thoracic dysplasia has a wide spectrum of clinical manifestations, varying from lethal to mild forms; long-term survivors have been reported.[470,473,474] The clinical course of individuals surviving the neonatal period is complicated by respiratory distress of varying severity, nephropathy, and hepatic and pancreatic problems.[475–477] Prenatal diagnosis has been reported.[478–490] A locus for asphyxiating thoracic dystrophy maps to chromosome 15q13. However, mutation analysis of two candidate genes (*GREMLIN* and *FORMIN*) did not reveal pathogenic mutations.[491] Molecular diagnosis for this condition was not available clinically at the time of this writing.[460]

Table 26.23 Disorders with thoracic dysplasia and polydactyly.

	Asphyxiating thoracic dysplasia (Jeune)	Chondroectodermal dysplasia (Ellis–van Creveld)	Short rib–polydactyly syndrome type I (Saldino–Noonan)	Short rib–polydactyly syndrome type II (Majewski)	Short rib syndrome type III (Naumoff)	Short rib syndrome type IV (Beemer–Langer)
Relative prevalence	Common	Uncommon	Common	Extremely rare	Rare	Rare
Clinical features						
Thoracic constriction	+ +	+	+ + +	+ + +	+ + +	+ + +
Polydactyly	+	+ +	+ +	+ +	+ +	+ +
Limb shortening	+	+	+ + +	+	+ +	+ +
Congenital heart disease	–	+ +	+ +	+ +	–	–
Other abnormalities	Renal disease	Ectodermal dysplasia	Genitourinary and gastrointestinal anomalies	Cleft lip and palate	Renal abnormality	Cleft lip and palate and genitourinary and gastrointestinal anomalies
Radiographic features						
Tubular bone shortening	+	+	+ + +	+ +	+ + +	+ +
Distinctive features in femora	–	–	Pointed ends	–	Marginal spurs	
Short, horizontal ribs	+ +	+ +	+ + +	+ + +	+ + +	+ + +
Vertical shortening of ilia and flat acetabula	+ +	+ +	+ +	–	+ +	
Defective ossification of vertebral bodies	–	–	+ +	–	+	+ +
Shortening of skull base	–	–	–	–	+	–

+, Not common; + +, common; + + +, most common; –, absent.

Reproduced with permission from Cremim BJ. *Bone dysplasias of infancy. A radiological atlas*. Berlin: Springer–Verlag; 1978.

Short rib–polydactyly syndromes

Short rib–polydactyly syndromes are a group of disorders characterized by micromelia, constricted thorax, and post-axial polydactyly (Fig. 26.28).[492–495] Traditionally, three different types have been recognized (Saldino–Noonan, Majewski, and Naumoff). These conditions have been identified prenatally by two-[496–517] and three-dimensional[80] ultrasonography, as well as by fetoscopy.[518] Table 26.23 illustrates the differential diagnosis and features of these conditions. Recently, some authorities have expanded the definition of short rib–polydactyly syndrome to encompass at least seven disorders, including the three previously mentioned entities along with the Yang, Le Marec, and Beemer varieties, as well as asphyxiating thoracic dysplasia.[519–522] Spranger and Maroteaux[25] and colleagues[507,510,523] have indicated that the absence of polydactyly does not exclude the diagnosis of this entity.

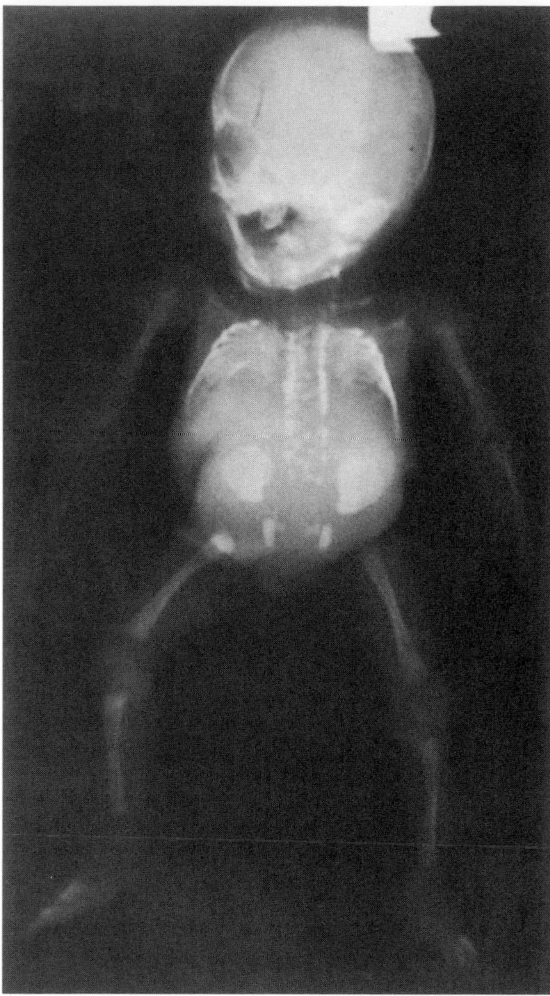

Figure 26.27 Jarcho–Levin syndrome. There is dramatic spinal shortening with disorganization of the vertebral bodies, a characteristic chest deformity ("crab-like appearance", with posterior fusion and anterior flaring of the ribs), and unaffected long bones.

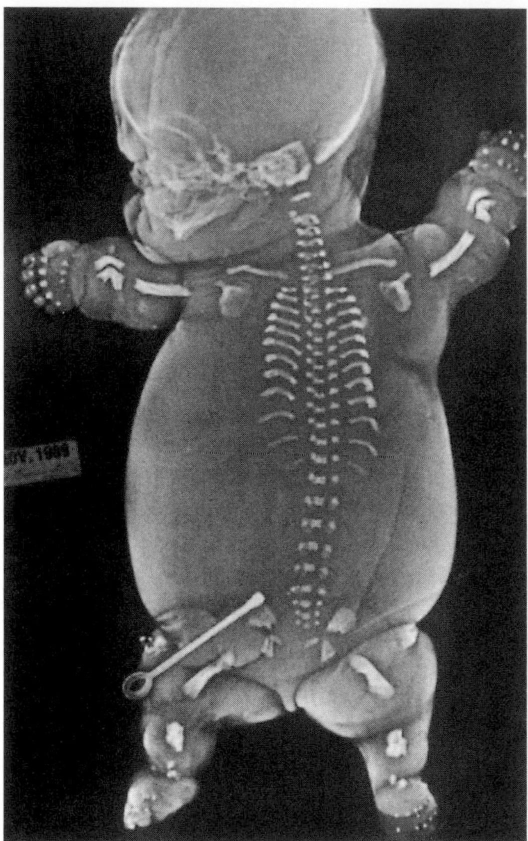

Figure 26.28 Short rib–polydactyly syndrome. There is severe shortening of all long bones, very short and horizontal ribs, and postaxial polydactyly in all four extremities. Note the angulation of the bones in the forearm.

Chondroectodermal dysplasia

Chondroectodermal dysplasia, also known as Ellis–van Creveld syndrome, is inherited with an autosomal recessive pattern.[524–529] It is characterized by acromesomelia, with normal spine and skull, postaxial polydactyly (Fig. 26.29), long and narrow thorax with short ribs, and congenital heart disease (60% of cases).[530–536] Polydactyly is a consistent finding. The supernumerary digit usually has well-formed metacarpal and phalangeal bones. Survivors who reach adulthood present with short stature but normal intelligence. Prenatal diagnosis has been reported.[535,537–547] One-third of affected individuals die in the postnatal period as a result of cardiopulmonary disease.[531–536,539–541,544–546]

Ellis–van Creveld syndrome is caused by mutations in the Ellis–van Creveld syndrome gene (*EVC* gene), which maps to the short arm of chromosome 4 in humans (4p16).[527,548] Ellis–van Creveld syndrome can also be caused by mutation in a nonhomologous gene, *EVC2*, located close to the *EVC* gene in a head-to-head configuration.[549,550]

Limb deficiency or congenital amputations

On occasion, the only identifiable anomaly is the absence of an extremity (limb deficiency) or a segment of an extremity (congenital amputation) (Table 26.24).[551] These constitute a group of disorders different from osteochondrodysplasias. The overall incidence of congenital limb reduction deformities is approximately 0.49 in 10 000 births (Table 26.25).[552] It has been estimated that 51% of these limb reduction defects are simple transverse reduction deficiencies of one forearm or hand without associated anomalies. The remainder consists of multiple reduction deficiencies, with an approximate 23%

Table 26.24 Congenital amputations.

Absent limbs only
Single absent limb
Multiple absent limbs
Absent limbs with rings
Congenital ring constriction syndrome
Absent limbs and face anomaly
Aglossia–adactylia syndromes
Möbius syndrome
Absent limbs with other anomalies
Ichthyosiform skin (CHILD syndrome)
Fibula agenesis complex brachydactyly (Du Pan syndrome)
Splenogonadal fusion
Skull and scalp defects (Adams–Oliver syndrome)
Phocomelia
Thalidomide syndrome
Thrombocytopenia with absent radii syndrome
Roberts pseudothalidomide-SC syndrome
Grebe syndrome
Proximal femoral focal deficiency
Femoral hypoplasia–unusual facies syndrome
Femur–fibula–ulna complex
Femur–tibia–radius complex
Split hand–split foot (SH/SF) syndromes
Only SH/SF
SH/SF and absent long bones
Ectrodactyly, ectodermal dysplasia, cleft lip and palate syndrome
Others
Split foot and triphalangeal thumb, autosomal dominant
Split foot, or split hand and central polydactyly (see central polydactyly)
SH/SF and congenital nystagmus (Karsch–Neugebauer syndrome)
SH/SF and renal malformations (acrorenal syndrome)
Split foot and mandibulofacial dysostosis (Fontaine syndrome), autosomal dominant

Reproduced with permission from ref. 551.

Table 26.25 Prevalence of different types of limb reduction malformations in Hungary, 1975–1977.

Type	Total	Population prevalence (per 1000 births)
Terminal transverse	79	0.14
Radial	13	0.09
Ulnar	41	0.11
Split hand and/or foot	20	0.04
Ring constriction	62	0.49
Total	274	0.49

Adapted from ref. 552.

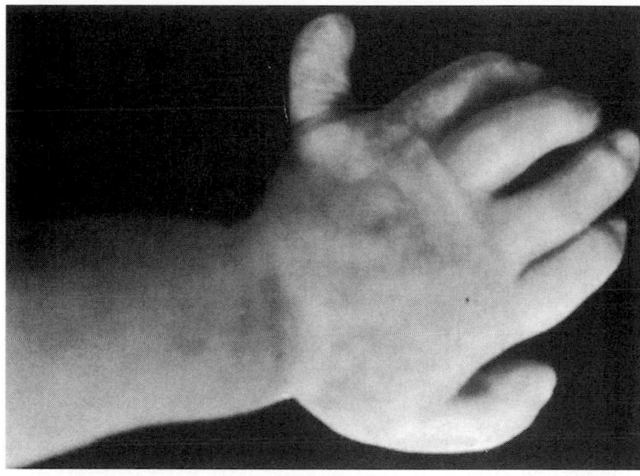

Figure 26.29 Postaxial polydactyly in a fetus with Ellis–van Creveld syndrome.

incidence of additional anomalies of the internal organs or craniofacial structures.[551]

Limb deficiencies can present alone or as part of a specific syndrome. An isolated limb deficiency of the upper extremity (e.g., distal segment of an arm) is generally an isolated anomaly. In contrast, congenital amputation of the leg generally occurs within the context of a syndrome, as do bilateral amputations or reduction of all limbs.[553]

Isolated amputation of an extremity can be due to amniotic band syndrome, exposure to a teratogen, or a vascular accident. In most cases, the anomaly is sporadic, and the risk of recurrence is negligible. The sonographic findings were reviewed recently.[554]

The following section reviews syndromes in which a limb amputation or deficiency is associated with other anomalies. We will follow the classification proposed by Goldberg.[551]

Syndromes with absent limbs and facial anomalies

The aglossia–adactylia syndrome consists of transverse amputations of the limbs and malformations of the mouth, including micrognathia, vestigial tongue (hypoglossia), dental abnormalities, as well as ankylosis of the tongue to the hard palate, the floor of the mouth, or the lips (glossopalatine ankylosis). The spectrum of anomalies of the extremities is variable, ranging from absent digits to severe deficiencies of all four extremities. Intelligence is generally normal. The condition is sporadic and has been attributed to a vascular accident.[555,556] It includes the Möbius sequence, Hanhart syndrome, glossopalatine ankylosis syndrome, limb deficiency–splenogonadal fusion syndrome, and Charlie M syndrome.[557–562] There is confusion in the classification of these patients because of the associated anomalies and the frequency of overlapping features. Although some authors have considered Hanhart syndrome and glossopalatine ankylosis syndrome as distinct entities, differential diagnosis is extremely difficult.[563]

The Möbius sequence consists of a number of facial anomalies attributed to paralysis of the sixth and seventh cranial nerves.[564] Limited jaw mobility and micrognathia are present.[565,566] Ptosis is also a common feature. The Möbius sequence is generally sporadic, but autosomal dominant, autosomal recessive, and X-linked recessive forms have been described.[567–569] The associated limb reduction anomalies (25% of cases) are generally present in the upper extremities and range from transverse deficiencies to absent digits. Mental retardation occurs in 10% of the cases.[567] The Möbius, Poland, and Klippel–Feil syndromes have been considered to occur as a result of subclavian artery supply disruption, based on the hypothesis that interruption of the early embryonic blood supply to the subclavian artery, vertebral artery, and/or their branches may lead to these conditions.[568,570–575]

Limb reduction defects associated with other anomalies

Congenital hemidysplasia with ichthyosiform erythroderma and limb defects (CHILD syndrome) is a defect characterized by strict demarcation of the skin lesions to one side of the midline.[576–578] The presence of unilateral defects of long bones is an important feature of the syndrome.[579] Limb deficiencies may vary from hypoplasia of phalanges or metacarpals to complete absence of an extremity. The calvarium, scapulae, or ribs may also be involved. Zellweger syndrome, chondrodysplasia punctata, and warfarin embryopathy may present with similar findings. Visceral anomalies include congenital heart disease,[579,580] unilateral hydronephrosis, hydroureter, and unilateral absence of the kidney, fallopian tube, ovaries, adrenal gland, and thyroid. CHILD syndrome predominantly affects females (by a ratio of 19:1)[581,582] and is caused by mutations in the gene *NSDHL* (NAD[P]H steroid dehydrogenase-like protein), located at Xq28 and encoding a β-hydroxysteroid dehydrogenase that is involved in the cholesterol biosynthetic pathway.[583–585]

Fibula aplasia complex brachydactyly (Du Pan syndrome) is an extremely rare condition characterized by bilateral agenesis of the fibula with abnormalities of the metacarpals and proximal phalanges. Limb reduction defects can involve the lower extremities.[586] An autosomal recessive pattern of inheritance has been suggested.[587] Faiyaz-Ul-Haque and colleagues[588] have recently examined genomic DNA from a family with Du Pan syndrome for mutations in the *CDMP1* gene. Affected individuals were homozygous for a missense mutation, T1322C, in the coding region of the *CDMP1* gene.

The splenogonadal fusion syndrome is characterized by limb reduction defects and splenogonadal fusion.[589,590] Most reported cases have occurred in males.[591] Typically, a mass is detectable in the scrotum, and an ectopic spleen is identified during surgery.[592] There is a continuous type in which the normally located spleen is connected to the gonad by bands or cords of splenic tissue.[593] A review of 14 reported cases indicates some overlap between this syndrome and the aglossia–adactylia syndrome or Hanhart syndrome.[594]

The Adams–Oliver syndrome is a group of disorders characterized by the association of limb reduction defects and scalp anomalies (aplasia cutis and deficiency of bony calvarium).[595] Sporadic and familial cases have been reported.[596] Other organ systems may be involved and there are reports of associated cardiovascular, brain, pulmonary, and renal anomalies.[597–603] Becker and colleagues[604] reported prenatal diagnosis, using ultrasound, of two cases of Adams–Oliver syndrome in the same family, the first at 13 weeks and the second at 23 weeks of gestation. Both cases showed limb reduction defects and, in the second case, the scalp defect was diagnosed as an echo-free space between the scalp and bone.

Phocomelia

In phocomelia the extremities resemble those of a seal. Typically, although the hands and feet are present, the intervening arms and legs are absent. Hands and feet may be normal or abnormal. Three syndromes must be considered in the differential diagnosis of phocomelia: Roberts syndrome, some varieties of the thrombocytopenia with absent radius (TAR) syndrome, and Grebe syndrome. Phocomelia also can be caused by exposure to thalidomide, but this is only of historical interest.[605] Prenatal diagnosis of phocomelia has been reported by three-dimensional ultrasound.[606]

Roberts syndrome

Roberts syndrome is an autosomal recessive disorder characterized by the association of tetraphocomelia and facial dysmorphisms (hypertelorism, facial clefting defects, hypoplastic nasal alae).[607–609] The upper extremities are generally more severely affected than the lower extremities. The spine is not involved. Polyhydramnios has been noted, and other anomalies associated with the syndrome include horseshoe kidney, hydrocephaly, cephalocele, and spina bifida.[610] Prenatal diagnosis has been reported.[4,610–619]

Grebe syndrome

Grebe syndrome (Grebe–Quelce-Salgado chondrodystrophy) is an autosomal recessive nonlethal disorder of limb development. It was first described in two girls by Grebe,[620] and in 47 Brazilian individuals by Quelce-Salgado.[621] The prevalence at birth has been estimated as 5 in 1 000 000.[622] Affected individuals have normal head, neck, and trunk skeleton, relatively normal humeri and femora, short and deformed radii, ulnae, tibiae, and fibulae, and severe abnormalities of hands and feet.

Polydactyly is frequent. Digits are very small and have been variously described as "bulbous,"[623] "bud-like,"[624] "mere knobs,"[625] "globular appendages,"[626] or "stubby toe-like fingers."[627] The proximal and middle phalanges of the fingers and toes are invariably absent, whereas the distal phalanges are present.[626] Radiographic documentation has provided information on subtle clinical characteristics for obligate heterozygotes: polydactyly, brachydactyly, hallux valgus, and metatarsus adductus.[626,628,629] The disease is caused by a missense mutation in the gene encoding cartilage-derived morphogenetic protein-1 (CDMP-1).[630] Most patients reported to date are from Brazil. Survivors have normal intelligence and develop normal secondary sexual characteristics. Prenatal diagnosis of Grebe syndrome by ultrasound has been reported.[623,631]

TAR syndrome is discussed in detail in the section on radial clubhand deformities.

Congenital short femur

Proximal femoral focal deficiency, or congenital short femur, refers to a group of disorders encompassing a wide range of congenital developmental anomalies of the femur. The disorder has been classified into five groups: type I, simple hypoplasia of the femur; type II, short femur with angulated shaft; type III, short femur with coxa vara (the most common); type IV, absent or defective proximal femur; and type V, absent or rudimentary femur.[632,633] One or both femurs may be affected. The right femur is more frequently involved. Anomalies of the upper limbs can also be present and do not exclude the diagnosis.[8] The proximal femoral focal deficiency syndrome may be associated with umbilical or inguinal hernias. If both femurs are affected, it is important to examine the face carefully, as the disorder may be bilateral femoral hypoplasia and unusual face syndrome,[634,635] which consists of bilateral femoral hypoplasia and facial defects, including short nose with broad tip, long philtrum, micrognathia, and cleft palate. Long bone abnormalities can extend to other segments of the lower extremities (absent fibula) and to the upper extremities. The syndrome is sporadic and has been associated with maternal diabetes mellitus. A familial form has been described. The diagnosis has been made *in utero*.[635–639]

If the defect is unilateral, it may correspond to the femur–fibula–ulna or femur–tibia–radius complex. These two syndromes have different implications for genetic counseling: the former is nonfamilial, whereas the latter has a strong genetic component.[640]

Split hand and foot deformities

The term "split hand and foot syndrome" is used to refer to a group of disorders characterized by splitting of the hand and foot into two parts. Other terms include "lobster claw deformity," "ectrodactyly," and "aborted fingers."[582,641] The conditions are classified into typical and atypical varieties.[642] The typical form consists of absence of both the finger and metacarpal bone, resulting in a deep, V-shaped central defect that clearly divides the hand into ulnar and radial parts. It occurs in 1 per 90 000 live births and has a familial tendency (usually inherited with an autosomal dominant pattern).[643] The atypical variety is characterized by a much wider cleft formed by a defect of the metacarpals and the middle fingers. As a consequence, the cleft is U-shaped and wide, with only thumb and small finger remaining. This occurs in 1 per 150 000 live births.[644]

A complex system for the classification of these disorders, based on the distribution of remaining fingers, has been proposed.[645] However, this system is not helpful in differential diagnosis and syndrome classification. Split hand and foot deformities can occur as isolated anomalies or as part of a more complex syndrome. The syndromic types are more frequently encountered.

The split hand and foot and absent long bones syndromes include two conditions in which there is split hand and aplasia of the tibia or split foot with aplasia of the ulna. However, skeletal anomalies are not limited to these bones; the clavicle, femur, and fibula can also be affected. The pattern of inheritance of these disorders has not been clearly determined. Autosomal dominant, recessive, and X-linked recessive patterns have been proposed.[646]

The ectrodactyly–ectodermal dysplasia–cleft lip/palate syndrome is an autosomal dominant condition which generally involves the four extremities, with more severe deformities of the hands.[647,648] The spectrum of ectodermal defects is wide, and includes hypopigmentation, dry skin, sparse hair, and dental defects.[649–652] Tear duct anomalies and decreased lacrimal secretions lead to chronic keratoconjunctivitis and severe loss of visual acuity.[653,654] The cleft lip is generally bilateral. Obstructive uropathy often occurs in this condition.[655] Intelligence is generally normal.[656]

A different group of syndromes involves associations of the split hand and foot deformity with other anomalies. These entities include split foot and triphalangeal thumb, split foot and hand and central polydactyly, Karsch–Neugebauer syndrome (split hand and foot with congenital nystagmus), acrorenal syndrome, and mandibulofacial dysostosis (Fontaine syndrome).[657]

Clubhands

Clubhand deformities are classified into two main categories: radial and ulnar. Radial clubhand includes a wide spectrum of disorders that encompass absent thumb, thumb hypoplasia, thin first metacarpal, and absent radius (Table 26.26). Ulnar clubhand is much less frequent than radial clubhand and ranges from mild deviations of the hand on the ulnar side of

Table 26.26 Radial ray defects: a differential diagnosis of congenital deficiency of the radius and radial ray.

Isolated: nonsydromatic

Syndromes with blood dyscrasias
Fanconi's anemia

Thrombocytopenia with absent radii syndrome

Aase syndrome: congenital anemia, nonopposable triphalangeal thumb, scaphoid and distal radius hypoplasia, radioulnar synostosis, short stature with narrow shoulders, autosomal recessive (see Diamond–Blackfan syndrome for a similar, perhaps identical, syndrome)

Syndromes with congenital heart disease
Holt–Oram syndrome

Lewis upper limb–cardiovascular syndrome: more extensive arm malformations and more complex heart anomalies than with Holt–Oram, but probably not a separate syndrome, autosomal dominant

Syndromes with craniofacial abnormalities
Nager acrofacial dysostosis

Radial clubhand and cleft lip and/or cleft palate: sporadic

Juberg–Hayward syndrome: cleft lip and palate, hypoplastic thumbs, short radius, radial head subluxation, autosomal recessive

Baller–Gerold syndrome: craniosynostosis, bilateral radial clubhand, absent/hypoplastic thumb, autosomal recessive

Rothmund–Thomson syndrome: prematurely aged skin changes, juvenile cataract, sparse gray hair, absent thumbs, radial clubhands, occasional knee dysplasia (see progeria syndromes)

Duane radial dysplasia syndrome: abnormal ocular movements, inability to abduct and eyeball retraction with adduction, radius and radial ray hypoplasia, vertebral anomalies, renal malformation, autosomal dominant (see Klippel–Feil variants)

IVIC syndrome (Instituto Venezolano de Investigaciones Cientificas): radial ray deficiency, hypoplastic or absent thumbs and radial clubhands, impaired hearing, abnormal movements of extraocular muscles with strabismus, autosomal dominant

LARD syndrome (lacrimo-auriculo-radial-dental; Levy–Hollister): absent lacrimal structures, protuberant ears, thumb and radial ray hypoplasia, abnormal teeth, autosomal dominant

Radial defects with ear anomalies and cranial nerve VII dysfunction

Radial hypoplasia, triphalangeal thumb, hypospadias, diastema of maxillary central incisors, autosomal dominant

Syndromes with congenital scoliosis
The VATER association
Goldenhar syndrome (oculoauriculovertebral dysplasia)
Kippel–Feil syndrome

Radial aplasia and chromosome aberrations

Syndromes with mental retardation
Seckel syndrome (bird-headed dwarfism): microcephaly, beak-like protrusion of nose, mental retardation, absent/hypoplastic thumbs, bilateral dislocated hips

Thalidomide embryopathy (of historical interest, but some 60% had radial clubhand)

Reproduced with permission from ref. 551.

the forearm to complete absence of the ulna. Although radial clubhand is frequently syndromic, ulnar clubhand is usually an isolated anomaly. Table 26.27 shows conditions that present with ulnar ray defects.

Whenever a clubhand is identified, it is important to conduct a thorough examination of the fetus and newborn to delineate associated anomalies that may suggest a syndrome. Fetal blood sampling procedures and fetal echocardiography are recommended. A complete blood cell count, including platelets, is important to establish the diagnoses of Fanconi's pancytopenia, TAR syndrome, and Aase syndrome. A fetal karyotype is indicated because several chromosomal abnormalities (e.g., trisomy 18, trisomy 21, and other structural aberrations) have been reported in association with clubhand deformities. Congenital heart disease is an important feature of the Holt–Oram syndrome, of the Lewis upper limb–cardiovascular syndrome, and of some cases of TAR syndrome.

Radial clubhand

The term "isolated radial clubhand" indicates that the clubhand is not part of a recognized syndrome.[658,659] However, this does not exclude the possibility that other anomalies may be

Table 26.27 Ulnar ray defects: a differential diagnosis of congenital deficiency of the ulna and ulnar ray.

Isolated: nonsyndromatic absent ulna

Ulna hypoplasia and skeletal deficiency elsewhere

Ulna aplasia with lobster claw deformity of hand and/or foot, autosomal dominant

Femur–fibula–ulna complex

Syndromes with ulna deficiency

Cornelia de Lange syndrome

Miller syndrome (postaxial acrofacial dysostosis): absent ulna and ulnar rays and absent fourth and fifth toes; Treacher–Collins mandibulofacial hypoplasia, autosomal recessive, distinguish from Nagar preaxial acrofacial dysostosis

Pallister ulnar–mammary syndrome: hypoplasia of ulna and ulnar rays, hypoplasia of the breast and absence of apocrine sweat glands, autosomal dominant

Pillay syndrome (ophthalmomandibulomelic dysplasia): absent distal third of ulna, absent olecranon, hypoplastic trochlea and proximal radius, fusion of interphalangeal joints in ulnar fingers, knee dysplasia, corneal opacities, fusion of temporomandibular joint, autosomal dominant

Weyers' oligodactyly syndrome: deficiency of ulna and ulnar rays, antecubital webbing, short sternum, malformed kidney and spleen, cleft lip and palate, sporadic

Schnizel syndrome: absent/hypoplastic fourth, fifth metacarpals and phalanges, hypogenitalism, anal atresia, autosomal dominant

Mesometic dwarfism, Reinhardt–Pfeiffer type (ulno-fibula dysplasia): a generalized bone dysplasia but with a disproportionate hypoplasia of the ulna and fibula, autosomal dominant

Mesomelic dwarfism, Langer's type: a generalized bone dysplasia, but with aplasia of the distal ulna and proximal fibula and hypoplasia of the mandible

Reproduced with permission from ref. 551.

present (e.g., scoliosis, congenital heart disease). Isolated nonsyndromic radial clubhand is generally a sporadic disorder.[659–662]

Radial clubhand may be part of the three syndromes characterized by hematologic abnormalities: Fanconi's pancytopenia, TAR syndrome, and Aase syndrome.

Fanconi's anemia

Fanconi's anemia (pancytopenia) is an autosomal recessive disease characterized by the association of bone marrow failure (anemia, leukopenia, and thrombocytopenia)[663] and skeletal anomalies, including a radial clubhand with absent thumbs, radial hypoplasia, and a high frequency of chromosomal instability (demonstrated in amniotic fluid cells or fetal lymphocytes as a high frequency of chromosomal breakage after incubation with diepoxybutane).[664–667] Approximately 25% of affected individuals do not have limb reduction anomalies. Associated findings include microcephaly, congenital dislocation of the hip, scoliosis, and cardiac/pulmonary/gastrointestinal anomalies.[668–670] Intrauterine growth restriction is common. Up to 25% of patients with this condition will show some degree of mental deficiency. It is assumed that the basic defect is related to the ability to repair DNA damage, in particular that of so-called DNA crosslinks. At present, at least 11 complementation groups have been defined in Fanconi's anemia (A, B, C, D1/BRCA2, D2, E, F, G, I, J, and L)[671] and eight associated genes have been identified: *FANCA*, *FANCC*, *FANCD2*, *FANCE*, *FANCF*, *FANCG/XRCC9*, *FANCL*, and *FANCD1* (*BRCA2*).[672–679] About 200 mutations have been described and, among these, mutations in the gene for complementation group FA-A (FANCA) account for approximately 65% of the cases.[671] Prenatal diagnosis has been reported many times.[639,680–688] Molecular genetic testing is currently available for mutation analysis of the common Ashkenazi Jewish *FANCC* mutation and sequence analysis for *FANCA*, *FANCC*, *FANCF*, and *FANCG*.[689]

Thrombocytopenia with absent radius (TAR syndrome)

TAR syndrome is an autosomal recessive disorder characterized by thrombocytopenia (platelet count of less than 100 000/mm^3) and bilateral absence of the radius.[690–694] The thumb and metacarpals are always present. The ulna and humerus may be absent, and clubfoot deformities may be present. Congenital heart disease is present in 33% of the cases (e.g., tetralogy of Fallot and septal defects). Delivery by Cesarean section is recommended, as these fetuses are at risk for intracranial hemorrhage.[695,696] TAR has been successfully diagnosed *in utero* many times.[695–708]

Aase syndrome

Aase syndrome is an autosomal recessive condition characterized by congenital hypoplastic anemia and a radial clubhand with bilateral triphalangeal thumb and a hypoplastic distal radius.[709–712] Cardiac defects (ventricular septal defects, coarctation of the aorta) may be present.[713] Triphalangeal thumbs are a feature of several bone dysostoses and malformation syndromes. They may also occur in random association with other defects, and as isolated, often familial, anomalies.[714] The differential diagnoses of this condition include Holt–Oram syndrome, Diamond–Blackfan syndrome,[715,716] chromosomal abnormalities, and the fetal hydantoin syndrome.

Holt–Oram syndrome

Holt–Oram syndrome is an autosomal dominant disorder characterized by congenital heart disease (mainly atrial septal defects, secundum type, and ventricular septal defects),[715,717–720] aplasia or hypoplasia of the radius, and triphalangeal or absent thumbs.[721,722] Limb defects are often asymmetric, with the left side being more affected than the right side. There is no correlation between the severity of the limb defects and the cardiac anomaly.[723,724] Indeed, some individuals only have a skeletal anomaly.[724] Other findings include hypertelorism, chest wall, and vertebral anomalies.[725–728] This condition has been diagnosed prenatally by two- and three-dimensional ultrasonography.[725,729–732] Holt–Oram syndrome is caused by mutations in the *TBX5* gene,[733,734] and pre-implantation diagnosis of this condition has been reported recently.[735] The upper limb–cardiovascular syndrome described by Lewis and colleagues[736] is probably not a separate entity from the Holt–Oram syndrome.

Radial clubhand and scoliosis

Radial clubhand is also associated with congenital scoliosis. The three syndromes that should be considered part of the differential diagnosis include VATER association, some cases of Goldenhar syndrome, and Klippel–Feil syndrome.[737]

VATER association

The VATER association is the result of defective mesodermal development during embryogenesis before the 35th day of gestation.[738–741] The typical findings are vertebral segmentation defects (70%), anal atresia (80%), tracheoesophageal fistula (70%), esophageal atresia, and radial and renal defects (65% and 53% respectively).[742,743] Other anomalies include a single umbilical artery (35%) and congenital heart disease, occurring in nearly 50% of the patients.[744–749] The VATER association occurs sporadically, although recurrence within a sibship has been reported.[747] Prenatal diagnosis using sonography has been reported.[46,749–759]

Goldenhar syndrome

Goldenhar syndrome is characterized by hemifacial microsomia, vertebral anomalies, and radial defects.[760–764] Alterations in the morphogenesis of the first and second brachial arches result in hypoplasia of the malar/maxillary/mandibular regions, microtia, and ocular/oropharyngeal anomalies.[764–769] Prenatal diagnosis has been reported.[765,770–773]

Klippel–Feil syndrome

The Klippel–Feil syndrome is characterized by fusion of any two of the cervical vertebrae, resulting in a short neck, a low posterior hairline, and restricted mobility of the upper spine. Several associated anomalies may be present, including spina bifida, cleft palate, rib abnormalities, lung disorders, congenital heart disease, and limb anomalies.[774] Prenatal diagnosis of this condition has not been reported.

Other conditions associated with radial clubhand

Radial clubhand has been reported in association with several chromosomal anomalies, including trisomies 18 and 21, deletion of the long arm of 13, and ring formation of chromosome 4.[667,775,776]

Some disorders present with craniofacial abnormalities and radial clubhand deformities. These conditions are sporadic and have common features that make a prenatal differential diagnosis difficult. The most common craniofacial anomaly is cleft lip and palate. Uuspaa's study[777] of 3225 cases with orofacial cleft showed a 2.8% association with upper extremity deformities.

Ulnar clubhand occurs as an isolated, nonsyndromic anomaly in most cases. It can also be associated with a variety of syndromes (e.g., Poland complex) (Table 26.27).[778]

Polydactyly

Polydactyly is the presence of an additional digit (Fig. 26.19).[779,780] The extra digit may range from a fleshy nubbin to a complete digit with controlled flexion and extension (Figs 26.29 and 26.30). Polydactyly can be classified as postaxial (the most common form), preaxial, or central (Table 26.16). Postaxial polydactyly occurs on the ulnar side of the hand and fibular side of the foot.[781–783] Preaxial polydactyly is present on the radial side of the hand and the tibial side of the foot (Fig. 26.31).[784] Central polydactyly consists of an extra digit that is usually hidden between the long and the ring finger.[785–787]

The majority of cases of polydactyly are isolated and inherited as an autosomal dominant trait. The preaxial type, especially a triphalangeal thumb, is most likely to be part of a syndrome. Central polydactyly is often bilateral and may be associated with other hand and foot malformations.[785–787]

Arthrogryposis

The term "arthrogryposis multiplex congenita" (AMC) refers to multiple joint contractures present at birth in an intact skeleton.[788–790] Normal fetal movement between 7 and 8 weeks of gestation onward is important for the development of the joints; limitation of the fetal joint motion leads to the development of contractures and AMC.[791,792] This has been confirmed in animal models,[793] for example chick and rat

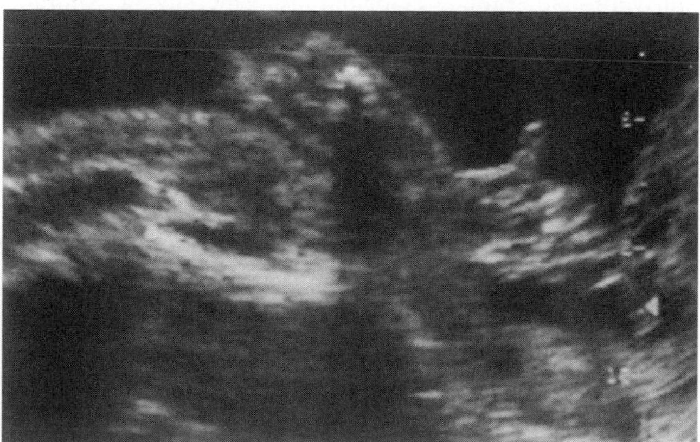

Figure 26.30 Sonographic image of the hand shown in Fig. 26.29. Note the abnormal angulation of the extra digit on the ulnar side of the forearm.

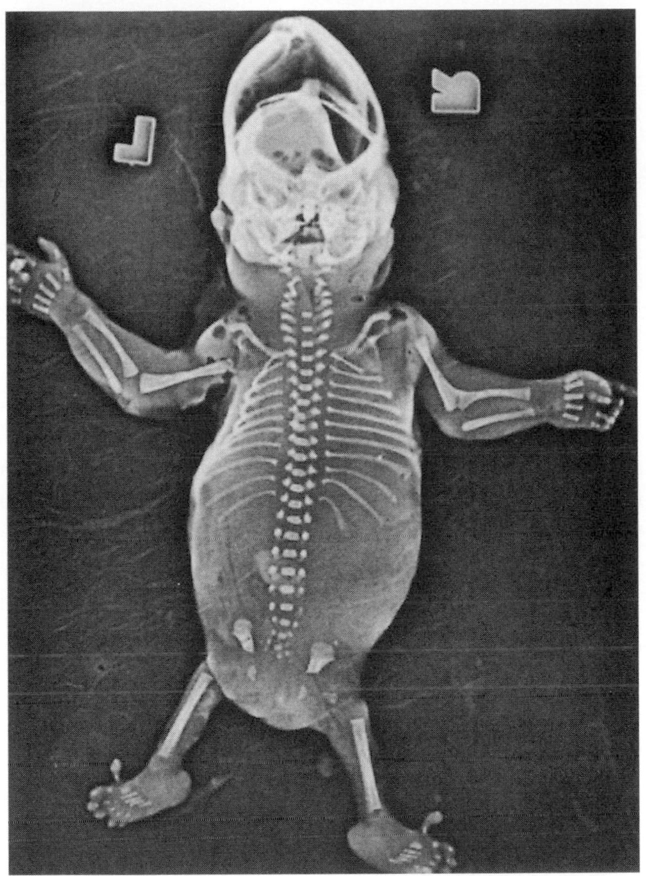

Figure 26.31 Unusual facies–femoral hypoplasia syndrome. Note the absence of the left femur and only a tiny portion of ossified bone on the right side. There is partial fusion of the tibia and fibula. Of interest is the presence of preaxial polydactyly in both feet.

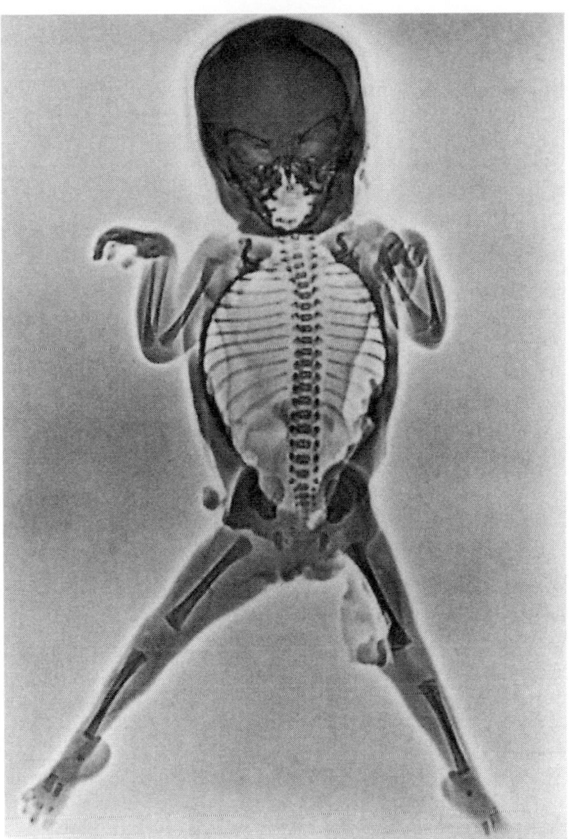

Figure 26.32 Arthrogryposis multiplex congenita. There is flexion of the upper limbs with hyperextension of the lower limbs.

embryos, using tubocurarine and botulism toxins,[794,795] inducing viral myopathy by coxsackie A viruses[796] and cross-section of the spinal cord.[797] Therefore, AMC is a syndrome, not a specific disorder. The incidences of the different underlying causes of AMC are variable in the literature. Neurological, muscular, connective tissue, or skeletal abnormalities or intrauterine crowding can lead to impaired fetal motion and AMC.[791,792] Table 26.28 shows motor systems that can lead to AMC. In a series of 74 children, Banker[798] found that the most common cause of AMC was a neurogenic disorder, followed by myopathic disorders. Swinyard and Bleck[799] reported CNS disorders as a cause in 75% and muscle disorders in 10–15%, based on autopsies of 75 cases of fetuses and newborns. Quinn and colleagues[800] reported that only 5 out of 21 cases of lethal AMC were of neurogenic cause, 11 were myogenic, and five were of uncertain pathology. The condition is present in 0.03% of live births.[801,802] The etiology of AMC may derive from hereditary conditions,[803–810] infectious agents, drugs, toxins, and fetal alcohol syndrome.[791,792,811] Maternal hyperthermia has also been associated with AMC.[812] Maternal antibodies specific for a fetal acetylcholine receptor have been reported to cause fetal AMC without evidence of maternal myasthenia gravis.[813,814] In addition, plasma from human mothers of fetuses with AMC, when injected into pregnant mice, causes deformities in the offspring.[815] The pattern of inheritance depends on the specific cause of AMC.[816] In a series of 350 cases, Hall[817] found that 46% of cases corresponded to a syndrome with no recurrence risk, 23% corresponded to disorders inherited with a mendelian pattern (autosomal dominant, recessive, or X linked), 20% were unknown conditions, 6% were associated with environmental disorders, 3% were chromosomal, and 2% were multifactorial in origin.

The recurrence risk varies depending on the underlying cause. Hall and Reed[811] found that in 20% of 350 patients no diagnosis was made. They concluded that, in this situation, the risk for recurrence is 4.7% if the limbs only were affected, 7% if the CNS was involved, and 1.4% if the limbs and another area were involved.

The deformities are usually symmetric. In most cases of AMC, all four limbs are involved (Fig. 26.32), followed by deformities of the lower extremities only, or bimelic involvement. The severity of the deformities increases distally in the

Table 26.28 Disorders of the developing motor system on all levels, leading to immobilization.

Disorders of the developing neuromuscular system
Loss of anterior horn cells
Radicular disease with collagen proliferation
Peripheral neuropathy with neurofibromatosis
Congenital myasthenia
Neonatal myasthenia (maternal myasthenia gravis)
Amyoplasia congenita
Congenital muscular dystrophy
Central core disease
Congenital myotonic dystrophy
Glycogen accumulation myopathy
Disorders of developing connective tissue or connective tissue disease
Muscular and articular connective tissue dystrophy
Articular defects by mesenchymal dysplasia
Increased collagen synthesis
Disorders of developing medulla or medullary disease
Congenital spinal epidural hemorrhage
Congenital duplication of the spinal canal
Disorders of brain development (e.g., porencephaly or brain disease)
Congenital encephalopathy

involved limb, with the hands and feet typically being the most deformed.

Many congenital anomalies are associated with AMC. The most frequent are cleft palate, Klippel–Feil syndrome, meningomyelocele, and congenital heart disease. In total, 10% of patients with AMC have associated anomalies of the central nervous system.[789]

The prenatal diagnosis of AMC with ultrasound has been reported.[818–831] The cardinal findings are absent fetal movement on real-time examination and severe flexion deformities.[821] Four-dimensional ultrasonography may help in better characterization of the phenotype prenatally.[832]

The prognosis of AMC depends on the specific cause. Although some cases are uniformly lethal, others are associated with mild to moderate handicap. Fahy and Hall,[833] in a retrospective study, included 828 cases of AMC and found that polyhydramnios is a poor prognostic sign.

Key points

1 Skeletal dysplasias are a heterogeneous group of disorders with an estimated prevalence of 1.1 to 9.5 per 10 000 births; the highest prevalence was reported in a greatly inbred population.

2 The most common skeletal dysplasias are achondroplasia, thanatophoric dysplasia, osteogenesis imperfecta type II, and achondrogenesis.

3 Despite the tremendous advances in the understanding of genetic causes and molecular mechanisms involved in skeletal dysplasias, approximately only one-third have had the molecular basis elucidated.

4 The role of diagnostic imaging in the prenatal investigation of skeletal dysplasias is (1) to narrow the differential diagnosis so that appropriate confirmatory molecular tests can be offered, (2) to predict lethality, and (3) to identify the fetus with a skeletal dysplasia early enough in pregnancy so that the diagnostic workup can be completed before the limit of fetal viability.

5 Three-dimensional reconstruction of the fetal bones is best performed using the maximum intensity mode (skeletal mode).

6 Panoramic images of the fetal skeleton without superimposition of maternal structures can be obtained by three-dimensional helical computed tomography.

7 No parameter has yet been identified to detect pulmonary hypoplasia with 100% sensitivity and specificity. Measurements of the right lung diameter and the ratio between the right lung diameter and the circumference of the bony thorax are easy to perform and have demonstrated good accuracy in the detection of pulmonary hypoplasia in preliminary studies. The role of three-dimensional ultrasound and MRI for the prediction of pulmonary hypoplasia remains to be determined.

8 Achondroplasia may not be diagnosed until the third trimester, as long bone shortening may not manifest until later in pregnancy.

9 Achondroplasia, hypochondroplasia, and thanatophoric dysplasia are caused by mutations in the *FGFR3* gene. Molecular diagnosis is possible.

10 The main differential findings between thanatophoric dysplasia types I and II are as follows: type I has typical bowed "telephone receiver" femur and no cloverleaf skull, whereas in type II cloverleaf skull is present and the long bones are straight.

11 The three most common mutations in the *FGFR3* gene in thanatophoric dysplasia type I are R248C, Y373C, and S249C.

12 The most common mutation in the *FGFR3* gene in thanatophoric dysplasia type II is K650E.

13 A peer-reviewed source with continuously updated information regarding availability of molecular diagnosis for skeletal dysplasias and contact

information for laboratories offering testing is available at the website of GeneTests (http://www.genetests.org).

14 The main differential diagnoses for thanatophoric dysplasia are fibrochondrogenesis and atelosteogenesis. Metaphyseal flaring is a feature of fibrochondrogenesis but not of thanatophoric dysplasia, and the molecular basis of fibrochondrogenesis is unknown. Coronal and sagittal vertebral clefts are a feature of atelosteogenesis.

15 In achondrogenesis, the spine is usually unossified or poorly ossified. Long bones are extremely short and the head is relatively large.

16 A hallmark of diastrophic dysplasia is the "hitchhiker thumb."

17 Anarchic ossification of the spine is observed in dyssegmental dysplasia.

18 Bowing of the long bones and hypoplastic scapulae are features of campomelic dysplasia. In this disorder, 75% of the affected infants with a male karyotype have female or ambiguous genitalia.

19 Short rib–polydactyly syndromes are characterized by micromelia, constricted thorax, and polydactyly.

20 In cases of congenital amputation, limb deficiencies of the upper extremity are generally isolated, whereas limb deficiencies involving the lower extremity, bilateral amputations, or reduction of all limbs generally occur in the context of a syndrome.

21 In unilateral femoral hypoplasia, consider the diagnosis of proximal femoral focal deficiency syndrome. In bilateral femoral hypoplasia, examine the face carefully and consider the possibility of femoral hypoplasia with unusual facies syndrome.

22 The differential diagnosis of radial clubhands includes Fanconi's anemia, thrombocytopenia with absent radius syndrome, Aase syndrome, and Holt–Oram syndrome.

23 In cases of radial clubhands associated with scoliosis, consider VATER association, Goldenhar syndrome and Klippel–Feil syndrome as differential diagnoses.

References

1 Maymon E, Romero R, Ghezzi F, et al.. Fetal skeletal anomalies. In: Fleischer A, Manning F, Jeanty P, Romero R, eds. *Sonography in obstetrics and gynecology: principles and practice*. New York: McGraw-Hill; 2001:445–506.

2 Superti-Furga A, Bonafe L, Rimoin DL. Molecular-pathogenetic classification of genetic disorders of the skeleton. *Am J Med Genet* 2001;106:282–293.

3 Superti-Furga A. Growing bone knowledge. *Clin Genet* 2004;66:399–401.

4 Parilla BV, Leeth EA, Kambich MP, et al. Antenatal detection of skeletal dysplasias. *J Ultrasound Med* 2003;22:255–258.

5 Hall CM. International nosology and classification of constitutional disorders of bone (2001). *Am J Med Genet* 2002;113: 65–77.

6 Gustavson KH, Jorulf H. Different types of osteochondrodysplasia in a consecutive series of newborns. *Helv Paediatr Acta* 1975;30:307–314.

7 Camera G, Mastroiacovo P. Birth prevalence of skeletal dysplasias in the Italian multicentric monitoring system for birth defects. In: Papadatos CJ, Bartsocas CS, eds. *Skeletal dysplasias*. New York: Alan R. Liss; 1982:441.

8 Connor JM, Connor RA, Sweet EM, et al. Lethal neonatal chondrodysplasias in the West of Scotland 1970–1983 with a description of a thanatophoric, dysplasialike, autosomal recessive disorder, Glasgow variant. *Am J Med Genet* 1985;22:243–253.

9 Weldner BM, Persson PH, Ivarsson SA. Prenatal diagnosis of dwarfism by ultrasound screening. *Arch Dis Child* 1985;60: 1070–1072.

10 Orioli IM, Castilla EE, Barbosa-Neto JG. The birth prevalence rates for the skeletal dysplasias. *J Med Genet* 1986;23:328–232.

11 Stoll C, Dott B, Roth MP, Alembik Y. Birth prevalence rates of skeletal dysplasias. *Clin Genet* 1989;35:88–92.

12 Andersen PE, Jr., Hauge M. Congenital generalised bone dysplasias: a clinical, radiological, and epidemiological survey. *J Med Genet* 1989;26:37–44.

13 Andersen PE, Jr. Prevalence of lethal osteochondrodysplasias in Denmark. *Am J Med Genet*1989;32:484–89.

14 Kallen B, Knudsen LB, Mutchinick O, et al. Monitoring dominant germ cell mutations using skeletal dysplasias registered in malformation registries: an international feasibility study. *Int J Epidemiol* 1993;22:107–115.

15 Rasmussen SA, Bieber FR, Benacerraf BR, et al. Epidemiology of osteochondrodysplasias: changing trends due to advances in prenatal diagnosis. *Am J Med Genet* 1996;61:49–58.

16 Gordienko IY, Grechanina EY, Sopko NI, et al. Prenatal diagnosis of osteochondrodysplasias in high risk pregnancy. *Am J Med Genet* 1996;63:90–97.

17 Al Gazali LI, Bakir M, Hamid Z, Varady E, et al. Birth prevalence and pattern of osteochondrodysplasias in an inbred high risk population. *Birth Defects Res* (Part A *Clin Mol Teratol*) 2003;67:125–132.

18 Savarirayan R, Rimoin DL. The skeletal dysplasias. *Best Pract Res Clin Endocrinol Metab* 2002;16:547–560.

19 International Nomenclature of Constitutional Diseases of Bone: revision, May 1977. *J Pediatr* 1978;93:614–616.

20 International Nomenclature of Constitutional Diseases of Bone: revision, May 1983. *Australas Radiol* 1986;30:163–167.

21 Spranger J. International classification of osteochondrodysplasias. The International Working Group on Constitutional Diseases of Bone. *Eur J Pediatr* 1992;151:407–415.

22 Lachman RS, Tiller GE, Graham JM, Jr., Rimoin DL. Collagen, genes and the skeletal dysplasias on the edge of a new era: a review and update. *Eur J Radiol* 1992;14:1–10.

23 Lachman RS. International nomenclature and classification of the osteochondrodysplasias (1997). *Pediatr Radiol* 1998;28: 737–744.

24 Lachman RS. Introduction and overview. *Pediatr Radiol* 1998;28:735–736.

25 Spranger J, Maroteaux P. The lethal osteochondrodysplasias. *Adv Hum Genet* 1990;19:1–2.
26 Mundlos S, Olsen BR. Heritable diseases of the skeleton. Part I: Molecular insights into skeletal development-transcription factors and signaling pathways. *FASEB J* 1997;11:125–132.
27 Mundlos S, Olsen BR. Heritable diseases of the skeleton. Part II: Molecular insights into skeletal development-matrix components and their homeostasis. *FASEB J* 1997;11:227–233.
28 Frassica FJ, Inoue N, Virolainen P, Chao EY. Skeletal system: biomechanical concepts and relationships to normal and abnormal conditions. *Semin Nucl Med* 1997;27:321–327.
29 Erlebacher A, Filvaroff EH, Gitelman SE, Derynck R. Toward a molecular understanding of skeletal development. *Cell* 1995;80:371–378.
30 Gilbert-Barness E, Opitz JM. Abnormal bone development: histopathology of skeletal dysplasias. *Birth Defects Orig Artic Ser* 1996;30:103–156.
31 Horton WA. Progress in human chondrodysplasias: molecular genetics. *Ann NY Acad Sci* 1996;785:150–159.
32 Reardon W. Skeletal dysplasias detectable by DNA analysis. *Prenat Diagn* 1996;16:1221–1236.
33 Rouse GA, Filly RA, Toomey F, Grube GL. Short-limb skeletal dysplasias: evaluation of the fetal spine with sonography and radiography. *Radiology* 1990;174:177–180.
34 Brodie SG, Lachman RS, Jewell AF, et al. Lethal osteosclerotic osteochondrodysplasia with platyspondyly, metaphyseal widening, and intracellular inclusions in sibs. *Am J Med Genet* 1998;80:423–428.
35 Chen CP, Chern SR, Shih SL, et al. Kyphomelic dysplasia in two sib fetuses. *J Med Genet* 1998;35:65–69.
36 Chitayat D, Gruber H, Mullen BJ, et al. Hydrops-ectopic calcification-moth-eaten skeletal dysplasia (Greenberg dysplasia): prenatal diagnosis and further delineation of a rare genetic disorder. *Am J Med Genet* 1993;47:272–277.
37 Seller MJ, Berry AC, Maxwell D, et al. A new lethal chondrodysplasia with platyspondyly, long bone angulation and mixed bone density. *Clin Dysmorphol* 1996;5:213–215.
38 Trajkovski Z, Vrcakovski M, Saveski J, Gucev ZS. Greenberg dysplasia (hydrops-ectopic calcification-moth-eaten skeletal dysplasia): prenatal ultrasound diagnosis and review of literature. *Am J Med Genet* 2002;111:415–419.
39 Wilcox WR, Lucas BC, Loebel B, et al. Pacman dysplasia: report of two affected sibs. *Am J Med Genet* 1998;77:272–276.
40 Benacerraf BR, Greene MF, Barss VA. Prenatal sonographic diagnosis of congenital hemivertebra. *J Ultrasound Med* 1986;5:257–259.
41 Song TB, Kim YH, Oh ST, et al. Prenatal ultrasonographic diagnosis of congenital kyphosis due to anterior segmentation failure. *Asia Oceania J Obstet Gynaecol* 1994;20:31–33.
42 Gembruch U, Niesen M, Kehrberg H, Hansmann M. Diastrophic dysplasia: a specific prenatal diagnosis by ultrasound. *Prenat Diagn* 1988;8:539–545.
43 Nores JA, Rotmensch S, Romero R, et al. Atelosteogenesis type II: sonographic and radiological correlation. *Prenat Diagn* 1992;12:741–753.
44 Tongsong T, Wanapirak C, Sirichotiyakul S, Chanprapaph P. Prenatal sonographic diagnosis of diastrophic dwarfism. *J Clin Ultrasound* 2002;30:103–105.
45 Ryu JK, Cho JY, Choi JS. Prenatal sonographic diagnosis of focal musculoskeletal anomalies. *Korean J Radiol* 2003;4:243–251.
46 Weisz B, Achiron R, Schindler A, et al. Prenatal sonographic diagnosis of hemivertebra. *J Ultrasound Med* 2004;23:853–57.
47 Herzberg AJ, Effmann EL, Bradford WD. Variant of atelosteogenesis? Report of a 20-week fetus. *Am J Med Genet* 1988;29:883–890.
48 Kurtz AB, Wapner RJ. Ultrasonographic diagnosis of second-trimester skeletal dysplasias: a prospective analysis in a high-risk population. *J Ultrasound Med* 1983;2:99–106.
49 Goncalves L, Jeanty P. Fetal biometry of skeletal dysplasias: a multicentric study. *J Ultrasound Med* 1994;13:977–985.
50 Gabrielli S, Falco P, Pilu G, et al. Can transvaginal fetal biometry be considered a useful tool for early detection of skeletal dysplasias in high-risk patients? *Ultrasound Obstet Gynecol* 1999;13:107–111.
51 De Biasio P, Prefumo F, Lantieri PB, Venturini PL. Reference values for fetal limb biometry at 10–14 weeks of gestation. *Ultrasound Obstet Gynecol* 2002;19:588–591.
52 Coffin GS, Siris E, Wegienka LC. Mental retardation with osteocartilaginous anomalies. *Am J Dis Child* 1966;112:205.
53 Baker ER, Goldberg MJ. Diagnosis and management of skeletal dysplasias. *Semin Perinatol* 1994;18:283–291.
54 Azouz EM, Teebi AS, Eydoux P, et al. Bone dysplasias: an introduction. *Can Assoc Radiol J* 1998;49:105–109.
55 Vanhoenacker FM, Van Hul W, Gielen J, De Schepper AM. Congenital skeletal abnormalities: an introduction to the radiological semiology. *Eur J Radiol* 2001;40:168–183.
56 Unger S. A genetic approach to the diagnosis of skeletal dysplasia. *Clin Orthop* 2002;401:32–38.
57 Goncalves LF, Espinoza J, Mazor M, Romero R. Newer imaging modalities in the prenatal diagnosis of skeletal dysplasias. *Ultrasound Obstet Gynecol* 2004;24:115–120.
58 Pretorius DH, Rumack CM, Manco-Johnson ML, Manchester D, Meier P, Bramble J et al. Specific skeletal dysplasias in utero: sonographic diagnosis. *Radiology* 1986;159:237–242.
59 Donnenfeld AE, Mennuti MT. Second trimester diagnosis of fetal skeletal dysplasias. *Obstet Gynecol Surv* 1987;42:199–217.
60 McGuire J, Manning F, Lange I, et al. Antenatal diagnosis of skeletal dysplasia using ultrasound. *Birth Defects Orig Artic Ser* 1987;23:367–384.
61 Escobar LF, Bixler D, Weaver DD, et al. Bone dysplasias: the prenatal diagnostic challenge. *Am J Med Genet* 1990;36:488–494.
62 Kurtz AB, Needleman L, Wapner RJ, et al. Usefulness of a short femur in the in utero detection of skeletal dysplasias. *Radiology* 1990;177:197–200.
63 Spirt BA, Oliphant M, Gottlieb RH, Gordon LP. Prenatal sonographic evaluation of short-limbed dwarfism: an algorithmic approach. *Radiographics* 1990;10:217–236.
64 Sharony R, Browne C, Lachman RS, Rimoin DL. Prenatal diagnosis of the skeletal dysplasias. *Am J Obstet Gynecol* 1993;169:668–675.
65 Bowerman RA. Anomalies of the fetal skeleton: sonographic findings. *Am J Roentgenol* 1995;164:973–979.
66 MacDonald MR, Welsh MP. Perinatal approach to skeletal dysplasia. *Nebr Med J* 1995;80:334–335.
67 Carvalho L, Soares M, Feijoo MJ, et al. A collaborative approach to the diagnosis of a lethal short limb skeletal dysplasia. *Genet Couns* 1997;8:139–143.
68 Gaffney G, Manning N, Boyd PA, et al. Prenatal sonographic diagnosis of skeletal dysplasias—a report of the diagnostic and prognostic accuracy in 35 cases. *Prenat Diagn* 1998;18:357–362.
69 Doray B, Favre R, Viville B, Langer B, Dreyfus M, Stoll C. Prenatal sonographic diagnosis of skeletal dysplasias. A report of 47 cases. *Ann Genet* 2000;43:163–169.

70 Tretter AE, Saunders RC, Meyers CM, et al. Antenatal diagnosis of lethal skeletal dysplasias. *Am J Med Genet* 1998;75: 518–522.

71 Hersh JH, Angle B, Pietrantoni M, Cook VD, et al. Predictive value of fetal ultrasonography in the diagnosis of a lethal skeletal dysplasia. *South Med J* 1998;91:1137–1142.

72 Merz E, Bahlmann F, Weber G, Macchiella D. Three-dimensional ultrasonography in prenatal diagnosis. *J Perinat Med* 1995; 23:213–222.

73 Steiner H, Spitzer D, Weiss-Wichert PH, Graf AH, Staudach A. Three-dimensional ultrasound in prenatal diagnosis of skeletal dysplasia. *Prenat Diagn* 1995;15:373–377.

74 Ploeckinger-Ulm B, Ulm MR, Lee A, Kratochwil A, Bernaschek G. Antenatal depiction of fetal digits with three-dimensional ultrasonography. *Am J Obstet Gynecol* 1996;175:571–574.

75 Garjian KV, Pretorius DH, Budorick NE, et al. Fetal skeletal dysplasia: three-dimensional US: initial experience. *Radiology* 2000;214:717–723.

76 Chen CP, Chern SR, Shih JC, et al. Prenatal diagnosis and genetic analysis of type I and type II thanatophoric dysplasia. *Prenat Diagn* 2001;21:89–95.

77 Machado LE, Bonilla-Musoles F, Raga F, et al. Thanatophoric dysplasia: ultrasound diagnosis. *Ultrasound Q* 2001;17:235–243.

78 Moeglin D, Benoit B. Three-dimensional sonographic aspects in the antenatal diagnosis of achondroplasia. *Ultrasound Obstet Gynecol* 2001;18:81–83.

79 Kos M, Hafner T, Funduk-Kurjak B, Bozek T, Kurjak A. Limb deformities and three-dimensional ultrasound. *J Perinat Med* 2002;30:40–47.

80 Viora E, Sciarrone A, Bastonero S, Errante G, Botta G, Campogrande M. Three-dimensional ultrasound evaluation of short-rib polydactyly syndrome type II in the second trimester: a case report. *Ultrasound Obstet Gynecol* 2002;19:88–91.

81 Clementschitsch G, Hasenohrl G, Steiner H, Staudach A. [Early diagnosis of a fetal skeletal dysplasia associated with increased nuchal translucency with 2D and 3D ultrasound]. *Ultraschall Med* 2003;24:349–352.

82 Krakow D, Williams J, III, Poehl M, et al. Use of three-dimensional ultrasound imaging in the diagnosis of prenatal-onset skeletal dysplasias. *Ultrasound Obstet Gynecol* 2003;21:467–472.

83 Seow KM, Huang LW, Lin YH, Pan HS, Tsai YL, Hwang JL. Prenatal three-dimensional ultrasound diagnosis of a camptomelic dysplasia. *Arch Gynecol Obstet* 2004;269:142–144.

84 Benoit B. The value of three-dimensional ultrasonography in the screening of the fetal skeleton. *Childs Nerv Syst* 2003;19: 403–409.

85 Shih JC, Peng SS, Hsiao SM, et al. Three-dimensional ultrasound diagnosis of Larsen syndrome with further characterization of neurological sequelae. *Ultrasound Obstet Gynecol* 2004;24:89–93.

86 Ruano R, Molho M, Roume J, Ville Y. Prenatal diagnosis of fetal skeletal dysplasias by combining two-dimensional and three-dimensional ultrasound and intrauterine three-dimensional helical computer tomography. *Ultrasound Obstet Gynecol* 2004;2004.

87 Wilting JE. Technical aspects of spiral-CT. *Medica Mundi* 1989;43:34–43.

88 Brink JA. Technical aspects of helical (spiral) CT. *Radiol Clin North Am* 1995;33:825–841.

89 Heiken JP, Brink JA, Vannier MW. Spiral (helical) CT. *Radiology* 1993;189:647–656.

90 Braillon PM, Buenerd A, Lapillonne A, Bouvier R. Skeletal and total body volumes of human fetuses: assessment of reference data by spiral CT. *Pediatr Radiol* 2002;32:354–359.

91 Pashayan H, Fraser FC, McIntyre JM, Dunbar JS. Bilateral aplasia of the tibia, polydactyly and absent thumb in father and daughter. *J Bone Joint Surg Br* 1971;53:495–499.

92 Luthy DA, Hall JG, Graham CB. Prenatal diagnosis of thrombocytopenia with absent radii. *Clin Genet* 1979;15:495–499.

93 Filkins K, Russo J, Bilinki I, et al. Prenatal diagnosis of thrombocytopenia absent radius syndrome using ultrasound and fetoscopy. *Prenat Diagn* 1984;4:139–142.

94 Graham M. Congenital short femur: prenatal sonographic diagnosis. *J Ultrasound Med* 1985;4:361–363.

95 Hall, C. M. and Washbrook, J. *REAMS: Radiological electronic atlas of skeletal malformation syndromes*, vol. 1. London: Oxford Press Electronic Publishing; 2000.

96 DeVore GR, Horenstein J, Platt LD. Fetal echocardiography. VI. Assessment of cardiothoracic disproportion: a new technique for the diagnosis of thoracic hypoplasia. *Am J Obstet Gynecol* 1986;155:1066–1071.

97 Chitkara U, Rosenberg J, Chervenak FA, et al. Prenatal sonographic assessment of the fetal thorax: normal values. *Am J Obstet Gynecol* 1987;156:1069–1074.

98 Nimrod C, Davies D, Iwanicki S, et al. Ultrasound prediction of pulmonary hypoplasia. *Obstet Gynecol* 1986;68:495–498.

99 Johnson A, Callan NA, Bhutani VK, et al. Ultrasonic ratio of fetal thoracic to abdominal circumference: an association with fetal pulmonary hypoplasia. *Am J Obstet Gynecol* 1987;157: 764–769.

100 Fong K, Ohlsson A, Zalev A. Fetal thoracic circumference: a prospective cross-sectional study with real-time ultrasound. *Am J Obstet Gynecol* 1988;158:1154–1160.

101 Songster GS, Gray DL, Crane JP. Prenatal prediction of lethal pulmonary hypoplasia using ultrasonic fetal chest circumference. *Obstet Gynecol* 1989;73:261–266.

102 Vintzileos AM, Campbell WA, Rodis JF, et al. Comparison of six different ultrasonographic methods for predicting lethal fetal pulmonary hypoplasia. *Am J Obstet Gynecol* 1989;161:606–612.

103 D'Alton M, Mercer B, Riddick E, Dudley D. Serial thoracic versus abdominal circumference ratios for the prediction of pulmonary hypoplasia in premature rupture of the membranes remote from term. *Am J Obstet Gynecol* 1992;166:658–663.

104 Maeda H, Nagata H, Tsukimori K, et al. Prenatal evaluation and obstetrical management of fetuses at risk of developing lung hypoplasia. *J Perinat Med* 1993;21:355–361.

105 Merz E, Wellek S, Bahlmann F, Weber G. [Normal ultrasound curves of the fetal osseous thorax and fetal lung]. *Geburtshilfe Frauenheilkd* 1995;55:77–82.

106 Abuhamad AZ, Sedule-Murphy SJ, Kolm P, et al. Prenatal ultrasonographic fetal rib length measurement: correlation with gestational age. *Ultrasound Obstet Gynecol* 1996;7:193–196.

107 Yoshimura S, Masuzaki H, Gotoh H, et al. Ultrasonographic prediction of lethal pulmonary hypoplasia: comparison of eight different ultrasonographic parameters. *Am J Obstet Gynecol* 1996;175:477–483.

108 Roberts AB, Mitchell JM. Direct ultrasonographic measurement of fetal lung length in normal pregnancies and pregnancies complicated by prolonged rupture of membranes. *Am J Obstet Gynecol* 1990;163:1560–1566.

109 Ohlsson A, Fong K, Rose T, et al. Prenatal ultrasonic prediction of autopsy-proven pulmonary hypoplasia. *Am J Perinatol* 1992;9:334–337.

110 Merz E, Miric-Tesanic D, Bahlmann F, et al. Prenatal sonographic chest and lung measurements for predicting severe pulmonary hypoplasia. *Prenat Diagn* 1999;19:614–619.

111 Bahlmann F, Merz E, Hallermann C, et al. Congenital diaphragmatic hernia: ultrasonic measurement of fetal lungs to predict pulmonary hypoplasia. *Ultrasound Obstet Gynecol* 1999;14: 162–168.

112 Heling KS, Tennstedt C, Chaoui R, et al. Reliability of prenatal sonographic lung biometry in the diagnosis of pulmonary hypoplasia. *Prenat Diagn* 2001;21:649–657.

113 Laudy JA, Tibboel D, Robben SG, et al. Prenatal prediction of pulmonary hypoplasia: clinical, biometric, and Doppler velocity correlates. *Pediatrics* 2002;109:250–258.

114 Rahemtullah A, McGillivray B, Wilson RD. Suspected skeletal dysplasias: femur length to abdominal circumference ratio can be used in ultrasonographic prediction of fetal outcome. *Am J Obstet Gynecol* 1997;177:864–869.

115 Laudy JA, Wladimiroff JW. The fetal lung. 2: Pulmonary hypoplasia. *Ultrasound Obstet Gynecol* 2000;16: 482–494.

116 Mitchell JM, Roberts AB, Lee A. Doppler waveforms from the pulmonary arterial system in normal fetuses and those with pulmonary hypoplasia. *Ultrasound Obstet Gynecol* 1998;11:167–172.

117 Achiron R, Heggesh J, Mashiach S, et al. Peripheral right pulmonary artery blood flow velocimetry: Doppler sonographic study of normal and abnormal fetuses. *J Ultrasound Med* 1998;17:687–692.

118 Chaoui R, Kalache K, Tennstedt C, et al. Pulmonary arterial Doppler velocimetry in fetuses with lung hypoplasia. *Eur J Obstet Gynecol Reprod Biol* 1999;84:179–185.

119 Yoshimura S, Masuzaki H, Miura K, et al. Diagnosis of fetal pulmonary hypoplasia by measurement of blood flow velocity waveforms of pulmonary arteries with Doppler ultrasonography. *Am J Obstet Gynecol* 1999;180:441–446.

120 Rizzo G, Capponi A, Angelini E, et al. Blood flow velocity waveforms from fetal peripheral pulmonary arteries in pregnancies with preterm premature rupture of the membranes: relationship with pulmonary hypoplasia. *Ultrasound Obstet Gynecol* 2000;15:98–103.

121 Fuke S, Kanzaki T, Mu J, Wasada K, et al. Antenatal prediction of pulmonary hypoplasia by acceleration time/ejection time ratio of fetal pulmonary arteries by Doppler blood flow velocimetry. *Am J Obstet Gynecol* 2003;188:228–233.

122 Lee A, Kratochwil A, Stumpflen I, et al. Fetal lung volume determination by three-dimensional ultrasonography. *Am J Obstet Gynecol* 1996;175:588–592.

123 Laudy JA, Janssen MM, Struyk PC, et al. Three-dimensional ultrasonography of normal fetal lung volume: a preliminary study. *Ultrasound Obstet Gynecol* 1998;11:13–16.

124 Pohls UG, Rempen A. Fetal lung volumetry by three-dimensional ultrasound. *Ultrasound Obstet Gynecol* 1998;11:6–12.

125 Bahmaie A, Hughes SW, Clark T, et al. Serial fetal lung volume measurement using three-dimensional ultrasound. *Ultrasound Obstet Gynecol* 2000;16:154–158.

126 Osada H, Iitsuka Y, Masuda K, et al. Application of lung volume measurement by three-dimensional ultrasonography for clinical assessment of fetal lung development. *J Ultrasound Med* 2002;21:841–847.

127 Kalache KD, Espinoza J, Chaiworapongsa T, et al. Three-dimensional ultrasound fetal lung volume measurement: a systematic study comparing the multiplanar method with the rotational (VOCAL) technique. *Ultrasound Obstet Gynecol* 2003;21:111–118.

128 Kalache KD, Espinoza J, Chaiworapongsa T, et al. Three-dimensional reconstructed fetal lung using VOCAL. *Ultrasound Obstet Gynecol* 2003;21:205.

129 Ruano R, Benachi A, Joubin L, et al. Three-dimensional ultrasonographic assessment of fetal lung volume as prognostic factor in isolated congenital diaphragmatic hernia. *Br J Gynaecology* 2004;111:423–429.

130 Ruano R, Joubin L, Sonigo P, et al. Fetal lung volume estimated by 3-dimensional ultrasonography and magnetic resonance imaging in cases with isolated congenital diaphragmatic hernia. *J Ultrasound Med* 2004;23:353–358.

131 Ruano R, Benachi A, Martinovic J, et al. Can three-dimensional ultrasound be used for the assessment of the fetal lung volume in cases of congenital diaphragmatic hernia? *Fetal Diagn Ther* 2004;19:87–91.

132 Moeglin D, Talmant C, Duyme M, Lopez AC. Fetal lung volumetry using two- and three-dimensional ultrasound. *Ultrasound Obstet Gynecol* 2005;25:119–127.

133 Chang CH, Yu CH, Chang FM, et al. Volumetric assessment of normal fetal lungs using three-dimensional ultrasound. *Ultrasound Med Biol* 2003;29:935–942.

134 Sabogal JC, Becker E, Bega G, et al. Reproducibility of fetal lung volume measurements with 3-dimensional ultrasonography. *J Ultrasound Med* 2004;23:347–352.

135 Rypens F, Metens T, Rocourt N, et al. Fetal lung volume: estimation at MR imaging initial results. *Radiology* 2001;219: 236–241.

136 Coakley FV, Lopoo JB, Lu Y, et al. Normal and hypoplastic fetal lungs: volumetric assessment with prenatal single-shot rapid acquisition with relaxation enhancement MR imaging. *Radiology* 2000;216:107–111.

137 Paek BW, Coakley FV, Lu Y, et al. Congenital diaphragmatic hernia: prenatal evaluation with MR lung volumetry: preliminary experience. *Radiology* 2001;220:63–67.

138 Williams G, Coakley FV, Qayyum A, et al. Fetal relative lung volume: quantification by using prenatal MR imaging lung volumetry. *Radiology* 2004;233:457–462.

139 Tanigaki S, Miyakoshi K, Tanaka M, et al. Pulmonary hypoplasia: prediction with use of ratio of MR imaging-measured fetal lung volume to US-estimated fetal body weight. *Radiology* 2004;232:767–772.

140 Kuwashima S, Nishimura G, Iimura F, et al. Low-intensity fetal lungs on MRI may suggest the diagnosis of pulmonary hypoplasia. *Pediatr Radiol* 2001;31:669–672.

141 Osada H, Kaku K, Masuda K, et al. Quantitative and qualitative evaluations of fetal lung with MR imaging. *Radiology* 2004;231:887–892.

142 Keller TM, Rake A, Michel SC, et al. MR assessment of fetal lung development using lung volumes and signal intensities. *Eur Radiol* 2004;14:984–989.

143 Kalache KD, Chaoui R, Hartung J, et al. Doppler assessment of tracheal fluid flow during fetal breathing movements in cases of congenital diaphragmatic hernia. *Ultrasound Obstet Gynecol* 1998;12:27–32.

144 Campbell J, Henderson A, Campbell S. The fetal femur/foot length ratio: a new parameter to assess dysplastic limb reduction. *Obstet Gynecol* 1988;72:181–184.

145 Hershey DW. The fetal femur/foot length ratio: a new parameter to assess dysplastic limb reduction. *Obstet Gynecol* 1989;73:682.

146 Turner GM, Twining P. The facial profile in the diagnosis of fetal abnormalities. *Clin Radiol* 1993;47:389–395.

147 Escobar LF, Bixler D, Padilla LM, Weaver DD. Fetal craniofacial morphometrics: in utero evaluation at 16 weeks' gestation. *Obstet Gynecol* 1988;72:674–679.

148 Chen ML, Chang CH, Yu CH, et al. Prenatal diagnosis of cleft palate by three-dimensional ultrasound. *Ultrasound Med Biol* 2001;27:1017–1023.

149 Chmait R, Pretorius D, Jones M, et al. Prenatal evaluation of facial clefts with two-dimensional and adjunctive three-dimensional ultrasonography: a prospective trial. *Am J Obstet Gynecol* 2002;187:946–949.

150 Mittermayer C, Blaicher W, Brugger PC, et al. Foetal facial clefts: prenatal evaluation of lip and primary palate by 2D and 3D ultrasound. *Ultraschall Med* 2004;25:120–125.

151 Johnson DD, Pretorius DH, Budorick NE, et al. Fetal lip and primary palate: three-dimensional versus two-dimensional US. *Radiology* 2000;217:236–239.

152 Lee W, Kirk JS, Shaheen KW, et al. Fetal cleft lip and palate detection by three-dimensional ultrasonography. *Ultrasound Obstet Gynecol* 2000;16:314–320.

153 Pretorius DH, Nelson TR. Fetal face visualization using three-dimensional ultrasonography. *J Ultrasound Med* 1995;14:349–356.

154 Mittermayer C, Lee A. Three-dimensional ultrasonographic imaging of cleft lip: the winners are the parents. *Ultrasound Obstet Gynecol* 2003;21:628–629.

155 Campbell S, Lees CC. The three-dimensional reverse face (3D RF) view for the diagnosis of cleft palate. *Ultrasound Obstet Gynecol* 2003;22:552–554.

156 Campbell S, Lees C, Moscoso G, Hall P. Ultrasound antenatal diagnosis of cleft palate by a new technique: the 3D "reverse face" view. *Ultrasound Obstet Gynecol* 2005;25:12–18.

157 Prows CA, Bender PL. Beyond Pierre Robin sequence. *Neonatal Netw* 1999;18:13–19.

158 Pilu G, Reece EA, Romero R, et al. Prenatal diagnosis of craniofacial malformations with ultrasonography. *Am J Obstet Gynecol* 1986;155:45–50.

159 Bromley B, Benacerraf BR. Fetal micrognathia: associated anomalies and outcome. *J Ultrasound Med* 1994;13:529–533.

160 Abrams SL, Filly RA. Congenital vertebral malformations: prenatal diagnosis using ultrasonography. *Radiology* 1985;155:762.

161 Zelop CM, Pretorius DH, Benacerraf BR. Fetal hemivertebrae: associated anomalies, significance, and outcome. *Obstet Gynecol* 1993;81:412–416.

162 Achiron R, Lipitz S, Grisaru D, et al. Second-trimester ultrasonographic diagnosis of segmental vertebral abnormalities associated with neurological deficit: a possible new variant of occult spinal dysraphism. *Prenat Diagn* 1996;16:760–763.

163 Kozlowski K, Bieganski T, Gardner J, Beighton P. Osteochondrodystrophies with marked platyspondyly and distinctive peripheral anomalies. *Pediatr Radiol* 1999;29:1–5.

164 Wells TR, Landing BH, Bostwick FH. Studies of vertebral coronal cleft in rhizomelic chondrodysplasia punctata. *Pediatr Pathol* 1992;12:593–600.

165 Lachman RS. Fetal imaging in the skeletal dysplasias: overview and experience. *Pediatr Radiol* 1994;24:413–417.

166 Westvik J, Lachman RS. Coronal and sagittal clefts in skeletal dysplasias. *Pediatr Radiol* 1998;28:764–770.

167 McMaster MJ. Occult intraspinal anomalies and congenital scoliosis. *J Bone Joint Surg Am* 1984;66:588–601.

168 McMaster MJ, David CV. Hemivertebra as a cause of scoliosis. A study of 104 patients. *J Bone Joint Surg Br* 1986;68:588–595.

169 McMaster MJ. Congenital scoliosis caused by a unilateral failure of vertebral segmentation with contralateral hemivertebrae. *Spine* 1998;23:998–1005.

170 McMaster MJ, Singh H. Natural history of congenital kyphosis and kyphoscoliosis. A study of one hundred and twelve patients. *J Bone Joint Surg Am* 1999;81:1367–1383.

171 Connor JM, Conner AN, Connor RA, et al. Genetic aspects of early childhood scoliosis. *Am J Med Genet* 1987;27:419–424.

172 Johnson VP, Yiu-Chiu VS, Wierda DR, Holzwarth DR. Midtrimester prenatal diagnosis of achondrogenesis. *J Ultrasound Med* 1984;3:223–226.

173 Mahony BS, Filly RA, Callen PW, Golbus MS. Thanatophoric dwarfism with the cloverleaf skull: a specific antenatal sonographic diagnosis. *J Ultrasound Med* 1985;4:151–154.

174 Sorge G, Ruggieri M, Lachman RS. Spondyloperipheral dysplasia. *Am J Med Genet* 1995;59:139–142.

175 Mortier GR, Rimoin DL, Lachman RS. The scapula as a window to the diagnosis of skeletal dysplasias. *Pediatr Radiol* 1997;27:447–451.

176 Francomano CA. The genetic basis of dwarfism. *N Engl J Med* 1995;332:58–59.

177 Nicolaides KH, Azar G, Byrne D, et al. Fetal nuchal translucency: ultrasound screening for chromosomal defects in first trimester of pregnancy. *BMJ* 1992;304:867–69.

178 Pandya PP, Kondylios A, Hilbert L, Snijders RJ, Nicolaides KH. Chromosomal defects and outcome in 1015 fetuses with increased nuchal translucency. *Ultrasound Obstet Gynecol* 1995;5:15–19.

179 Brady AF, Pandya PP, Yuksel B, et al. Outcome of chromosomally normal livebirths with increased fetal nuchal translucency at 10–14 weeks' gestation. *J Med Genet* 1998;35:222–224.

180 Souka AP, Snijders RJ, Novakov A, et al. Defects and syndromes in chromosomally normal fetuses with increased nuchal translucency thickness at 10–14 weeks of gestation. *Ultrasound Obstet Gynecol* 1998;11:391–400.

181 Makrydimas G, Souka A, Skentou H, et al. Osteogenesis imperfecta and other skeletal dysplasias presenting with increased nuchal translucency in the first trimester. *Am J Med Genet* 2001;98:117–120.

182 Souka AP, Raymond FL, Mornet E, et al. Hypophosphatasia associated with increased nuchal translucency: a report of two affected pregnancies. *Ultrasound Obstet Gynecol* 2002;20:294–295.

183 Clementschitsch G, Hasenohrl G, Steiner H, Staudach A. [Early Diagnosis of a Fetal Skeletal Dysplasia Associated with Increased Nuchal Translucency with 2D and 3D Ultrasound]. *Ultraschall Med* 2003;24:349–352.

184 Michel-Calemard L, Lesca G, Morel Y, et al. Campomelic acampomelic dysplasia presenting with increased nuchal translucency in the first trimester. *Prenat Diagn* 2004;24:519–523.

185 Shiang R, Thompson LM, Zhu YZ, et al. Mutations in the transmembrane domain of FGFR3 cause the most common genetic form of dwarfism, achondroplasia. *Cell* 1994;78:335–342.

186 Bellus GA, McIntosh I, Smith EA, et al. A recurrent mutation in the tyrosine kinase domain of fibroblast growth factor receptor 3 causes hypochondroplasia. *Nat Genet* 1995;10:357–359.

187 Wilcox WR, Tavormina PL, Krakow D, et al. Molecular, radiologic, and histopathologic correlations in thanatophoric dysplasia. *Am J Med Genet* 1998;78:274–281.
188 Ozono K. Recent advances in molecular analysis of skeletal dysplasia. *Acta Paediatr Jpn* 1997;39:491–498.
189 Climent C, Lorda-Sanchez I, Urioste M, et al. [Achondroplasia: molecular study of 28 patients]. *Med Clin (Barc.)* 1998;110: 492–494.
190 Cohen MM, Jr. Achondroplasia, hypochondroplasia and thanatophoric dysplasia: clinically related skeletal dysplasias that are also related at the molecular level. *Int J Oral Maxillofac Surg* 1998;27:451–455.
191 Wilkin DJ, Szabo JK, Cameron R, et al. Mutations in fibroblast growth-factor receptor 3 in sporadic cases of achondroplasia occur exclusively on the paternally derived chromosome. *Am J Hum Genet* 1998;63:711–716.
192 Lemyre E, Azouz EM, Teebi AS, et al. Bone dysplasia series. Achondroplasia, hypochondroplasia and thanatophoric dysplasia: review and update. *Can Assoc Radiol J* 1999;50:185–197.
193 Rousseau F, el Ghouzzi V, Delezoide AL, et al. Missense FGFR3 mutations create cysteine residues in thanatophoric dwarfism type I (TD1). *Hum Mol Genet* 1996;5:509–512.
194 Cohen MM, Jr. Some chondrodysplasias with short limbs: molecular perspectives. *Am J Med Genet* 2002;112:304–313.
195 Ramaswami U, Rumsby G, Hindmarsh PC, Brook CG. Genotype and phenotype in hypochondroplasia. *J Pediatr* 1998;133: 99–102.
196 Kurtz AB, Filly RA, Wapner RJ, et al. In utero analysis of heterozygous achondroplasia: variable time of onset as detected by femur length measurements. *J Ultrasound Med* 1986;5:137–140.
197 Modaff P, Horton VK, Pauli RM. Errors in the prenatal diagnosis of children with achondroplasia. *Prenat Diagn* 1996;16: 525–530.
198 Kurtz AB, Filly RA, Wapner RJ, et al. In utero analysis of heterozygous achondroplasia: variable time of onset as detected by femur length measurements. *J Ultrasound Med* 1986;5:137–140.
199 Elejalde BR, de Elejalde MM, Hamilton PR, Lombardi JM. Prenatal diagnosis in two pregnancies of an achondroplastic woman. *Am J Med Genet* 1983;15:437–439.
200 Huggins MJ, Mernagh JR, Steele L, et al. Prenatal sonographic diagnosis of hypochondroplasia in a high-risk fetus. *Am J Med Genet* 1999;87:226–229.
201 Chitayat D, Fernandez B, Gardner A, et al. Compound heterozygosity for the Achondroplasia-hypochondroplasia FGFR3 mutations: prenatal diagnosis and postnatal outcome. *Am J Med Genet* 1999;84:401–405.
202 Mesoraca A, Pilu G, Perolo A, et al. Ultrasound and molecular mid-trimester prenatal diagnosis of de novo achondroplasia. *Prenat Diagn* 1996;16:764–768.
203 Guzman ER, Day-Salvatore D, Westover T, et al. Prenatal ultrasonographic demonstration of the trident hand in heterozygous achondroplasia. *J Ultrasound Med* 1994;13:63–66.
204 Cordone M, Lituania M, Bocchino G, et al. Ultrasonographic features in a case of heterozygous achondroplasia at 25 weeks' gestation. *Prenat Diagn* 1993;13:395–401.
205 Patel MD, Filly RA. Homozygous achondroplasia: US distinction between homozygous, heterozygous, and unaffected fetuses in the second trimester. *Radiology* 1995;196:541–545.
206 Mesoraca A, Pilu G, Perolo A, et al. Ultrasound and molecular mid-trimester prenatal diagnosis of de novo achondroplasia. *Prenat Diagn* 1996;16:764–768.
207 James PA, Shaw J, du Sart D. Molecular diagnosis in a pregnancy at risk for both spondyloepiphyseal dysplasia congenita and achondroplasia. *Prenat Diagn* 2003;23:861–863.
208 Schrijver I, Lay MJ, Zehnder JL. Rapid combined genotyping assay for four achondroplasia and hypochondroplasia mutations by real-time PCR with multiple detection probes. *Genet Test* 2004;8:185–189.
209 Lachman RS. Neurologic abnormalities in the skeletal dysplasias: a clinical and radiological perspective. *Am J Med Genet* 1997;69:33–43.
210 Pauli RM, Conroy MM, Langer LO, Jr, et al. Homozygous achondroplasia with survival beyond infancy. *Am J Med Genet* 1983;16:459–473.
211 Seino Y, Moriwake T, Tanaka H, et al. Molecular defects in achondroplasia and the effects of growth hormone treatment. *Acta Paediatr* 1999;88(Suppl.):118–120.
212 Tavormina PL, Bellus GA, Webster MK, et al. A novel skeletal dysplasia with developmental delay and acanthosis nigricans is caused by a Lys650Met mutation in the fibroblast growth factor receptor 3 gene. *Am J Hum Genet* 1999;64:722–731.
213 Bellus GA, Bamshad MJ, Przylepa KA, et al. Severe achondroplasia with developmental delay and acanthosis nigricans (SADDAN): phenotypic analysis of a new skeletal dysplasia caused by a Lys650Met mutation in fibroblast growth factor receptor 3. *Am J Med Genet* 1999;85:53–65.
214 Spranger J. [International nomenclature of constitutional bone diseases (the Paris nomenclature)]. *Fortschr Geb Rontgenstr Nuklearmed* 1971;115:283–287.
215 Brodie SG, Kitoh H, Lipson M, et al. Thanatophoric dysplasia type I with syndactyly. *Am J Med Genet* 1998;80:260–262.
216 Weber M, Johannisson R, Carstens C, et al. Thanatophoric dysplasia type II: new entity? *J Pediatr Orthop B* 1998;7:10–22.
217 Brodie SG, Kitoh H, Lipson M, et al Thanatophoric dysplasia type I with syndactyly. *Am J Med Genet* 1998;80:260–262.
218 Iannaccone G, Gerlini G. The so-calle "cloverleaf skull syndrome": a report of three cases with a discussion of its relationships with thanatophoric dwarfism and the craniostenoses. *Pediatr Radiol* 1974;2:175–184.
219 Jasnosz KM, MacPherson TA. Perinatal pathology casebook. Thanatophoric dysplasia with cloverleaf skull. *J Perinatol* 1993;13:162–164.
220 Online Mendelian Inheritance in Man, OMIM (TM). McKusick-Nathans Institute for Genetic Medicine, Johns Hopkins University (Baltimore, MD) and National Center for Biotechnology Information, National Library of Medicine (Bethesda, MD), 2000.World Wide Web URL: http://www.ncbi.nlm.nih.gov/omim/; 2005.
221 Tavormina PL, Shiang R, Thompson LM, et al. Thanatophoric dysplasia (types I and II) caused by distinct mutations in fibroblast growth factor receptor 3. *Nat Genet* 1995;9:321–328.
222 Yang SS, Heidelberger KP, Brough AJ, et al. Lethal short-limbed chondrodysplasia in early infancy. In: Rosenberg HS, Bockland RP, eds. *Perspectives in pediatric pathology*. Chicago, IL: Year Book Medical Publishers; 1976. 1.
223 McKusick VA, Francomano CA, Antonarakis SE. *Mendelian inheritance in man: catalogs of autosomal dominant, autosomal recessive, and X-linked phenotypes*. Baltimore, MD: Johns Hopkins University Press, 1990.
224 Partington MW, Gonzales-Crussi F, Khakee SG, Wollin DG. Cloverleaf skull and thanatophoric dwarfism. Report of four cases, two in the same sibship. *Arch Dis Child* 1971;46:656–664.

225 Schild RL, Hunt GH, Moore J, Davies H, Horwell DH. Antenatal sonographic diagnosis of thanatophoric dysplasia: a report of three cases and a review of the literature with special emphasis on the differential diagnosis. *Ultrasound Obstet Gynecol* 1996;8:62–67.
226 Vajo Z, Francomano CA, Wilkin DJ. The molecular and genetic basis of fibroblast growth factor receptor 3 disorders: the achondroplasia family of skeletal dysplasias, Muenke craniosynostosis, and Crouzon syndrome with acanthosis nigricans. *Endocrinol Rev* 2000;21:23–39.
227 d'Avis PY, Robertson SC, Meyer AN, et al. Constitutive activation of fibroblast growth factor receptor 3 by mutations responsible for the lethal skeletal dysplasia thanatophoric dysplasia type I. *Cell Growth Differ* 1998;9:71–78.
228 Passos-Bueno MR, Wilcox WR, Jabs EW, et al. Clinical spectrum of fibroblast growth factor receptor mutations. *Hum Mutat* 1999;14:115–125.
229 Rousseau F, Saugier P, Le Merrer M, et al. Stop codon FGFR3 mutations in thanatophoric dwarfism type 1. *Nat Genet* 1995;10:11–12.
230 Gorlin RJ. Fibroblast growth factors, their receptors and receptor disorders. *J Craniomaxillofac Surg* 1997;25:69–79.
231 Bellus GA, Spector EB, Speiser PW, et al. Distinct missense mutations of the FGFR3 lys650 codon modulate receptor kinase activation and the severity of the skeletal dysplasia phenotype. *Am J Hum Genet* 2000;67:1411–1421.
232 Camera G, Baldi M, Strisciuglio G, et al. Occurrence of thanatophoric dysplasia type I (R248C) and hypochondroplasia (N540K) mutations in two patients with achondroplasia phenotype. *Am J Med Genet* 2001;104:277–281.
233 Horton WA, Rimoin DL, Hollister DW, Lachman RS. Further heterogeneity within lethal neonatal short-limbed dwarfism: the platyspondylic types. *J Pediatr* 1979;94:736–742.
234 Brodie SG, Kitoh H, Lachman RS, et al. Platyspondylic lethal skeletal dysplasia, San Diego type, is caused by FGFR3 mutations. *Am J Med Genet* 1999;84:476–480.
235 Moir DH, Kozlowski K. Long survival in thanatophoric dwarfism. *Pediatr Radiol* 1976;5:123–125.
236 Stensvold K, Ek J, Hovland AR. An infant with thanatophoric dwarfism surviving 169 days. *Clin Genet* 1986;29:157–159.
237 Baker KM, Olson DS, Harding CO, Pauli RM. Long-term survival in typical thanatophoric dysplasia type 1. *Am J Med Genet* 1997;70:427–436.
238 Dominguez R, Talmachoff P. Diagnostic imaging update in skeletal dysplasias. *Clin Imaging* 1993;17:222–234.
239 Fink IJ, Filly RA, Callen PW, Fiske CC. Sonographic diagnosis of thanatophoric dwarfism in utero. *J Ultrasound Med* 1982;1:337–339.
240 Chervenak FA, Blakemore KJ, Isaacson G, et al. Antenatal sonographic findings of thanatophoric dysplasia with cloverleaf skull. *Am J Obstet Gynecol* 1983;146:984–985.
241 Beetham FG, Reeves JS. Early ultrasound diagnosis of thanatophoric dwarfism. *J Clin Ultrasound* 1984;12:43–44.
242 Burrows PE, Stannard MW, Pearrow J, Sutterfield S, Baker ML. Early antenatal sonographic recognition of thanatophoric dysplasia with cloverleaf skull deformity. *Am J Roentgenol* 1984;143:841–843.
243 Elejalde BR, de Elejalde MM. Thanatophoric dysplasia: fetal manifestations and prenatal diagnosis. *Am J Med Genet* 1985;22:669–683.
244 Weiner CP, Williamson RA, Bonsib SM. Sonographic diagnosis of cloverleaf skull and thanatophoric dysplasia in the second trimester. *J Clin Ultrasound* 1986;14:463–465.
245 Meizner I, Levy A, Carmi R, Simhon T. Early prenatal ultrasonic diagnosis of thanatophoric dwarfism. *Isr J Med Sci* 1990;26: 287–289.
246 Kassanos D, Botsis D, Katassos Tet al. Prenatal sonographic diagnosis of thanatophoric dwarfism. *Int J Gynaecol Obstet* 1991;34:373–376.
247 Corsello G, Maresi E, Rossi C, et al. Thanatophoric dysplasia in monozygotic twins discordant for cloverleaf skull: prenatal diagnosis, clinical and pathological findings. *Am J Med Genet* 1992;42:122–126.
248 Gerihauser H, Schuster C, Immervoll H, Sochor G. [Prenatal diagnosis of thanatophoric dwarfism]. *Ultraschall Med* 1992; 13:41–45.
249 Camera G, Dodero D, Camandona F, Camera A. [Prenatal diagnosis of thanatophoric dysplasia at 21st week of pregnancy]. *Pathologica* 1993;85:215–219.
250 Marin-Ruiz R, Alarcon HC, Montiel RW, Gonzalez Moreno JM. [Thanatophoric dysplasia. Its prenatal ultrasonic diagnosis. A case report]. *Ginecol Obstet Mex* 1993;61:344–347.
251 van der Harten HJ, Brons JT, Dijkstra PF, et al. Some variants of lethal neonatal short-limbed platyspondylic dysplasia: a radiological ultrasonographic, neuropathological and histopathological study of 22 cases. *Clin Dysmorphol* 1993;2:1–19.
252 Szatmary FP, Szabo L, Toth T, Kristof A. [Prenatal diagnosis of thanatophoric dysplasia]. *Orv Hetil* 1995;136:75–78.
253 Todros T, Sciarrone A, Voglino G, et al. [Prenatal diagnosis of thanatophoric dysplasia at the 20th week of pregnancy using ultrasonography]. *Pathologica* 1995;87:723–725.
254 Yuce MA, Yardim T, Kurtul M, et al. Prenatal diagnosis of thanatophoric dwarfism in second trimester. A case report. *Clin Exp Obstet Gynecol* 1998;25:149–150.
255 Sun CC, Grumbach K, DeCosta DT, et al. Correlation of prenatal ultrasound diagnosis and pathologic findings in fetal anomalies. *Pediatr Dev Pathol* 1999;2:131–142.
256 Sahinoglu Z, Uludogan M, Gurbuz A, Karateke A. Prenatal diagnosis of thanatophoric dysplasia in the second trimester: ultrasonography and other diagnostic modalities. *Arch Gynecol Obstet* 2003;269:57–61.
257 Sawai H, Komori S, Ida A, et al. Prenatal diagnosis of thanatophoric dysplasia by mutational analysis of the fibroblast growth factor receptor 3 gene and a proposed correction of previously published PCR results. *Prenat Diagn* 1999;19:21–24.
258 De Biasio P, Prefumo F, Baffico M, et al. Sonographic and molecular diagnosis of thanatophoric dysplasia type I at 18 weeks of gestation. *Prenat Diagn* 2000;20:835–837.
259 Chen CP, Chern SR, Chang TY, et al. Second trimester molecular diagnosis of a stop codon FGFR3 mutation in a type I thanatophoric dysplasia fetus following abnormal ultrasound findings. *Prenat Diagn* 2002;22:736–737.
260 Hall BD, Spranger J. Hypochondroplasia: clinical and radiological aspects in 39 cases. *Radiology* 1979;133:95–100.
261 Cohn DH. Mutations affecting multiple functional domains of FGFR3 cause different skeletal dysplasias: a personal retrospective in honor of John Wasmuth. *Ann NY Acad Sci* 1996; 785:160–163.
262 Matsui Y, Yasui N, Kimura T, et al. Genotype phenotype correlation in achondroplasia and hypochondroplasia. *J Bone Joint Surg Br* 1998;80:1052–1056.

263 Mullis PE, Patel MS, Brickell PM, et al. Growth characteristics and response to growth hormone therapy in patients with hypochondroplasia: genetic linkage of the insulin-like growth factor I gene at chromosome 12q23 to the disease in a subgroup of these patients. *Clin Endocrinol (Oxf.)* 1991;34:265–274.
264 Bailey AJ, Sims TJ, Stanescu V, et al. Abnormal collagen cross-linking in the cartilage of a diastrophic dysplasia patient. *Br J Rheumatol* 1995;34:512–515.
265 Prinos P, Costa T, Sommer A, et al. A common FGFR3 gene mutation in hypochondroplasia. *Hum Mol Genet* 1995;4:2097–2101.
266 Scott CI, Jr. Achondroplastic and hypochondroplastic dwarfism. *Clin Orthop* 1976;18–30.
267 Stoll C, Manini P, Bloch J, Roth MP. Prenatal diagnosis of hypochondroplasia. *Prenat Diagn* 1985;5:423–426.
268 Stoilov I, Kilpatrick MW, Tsipouras P, Costa T. Possible genetic heterogeneity in hypochondroplasia. *J Med Genet* 1995;32: 492–493.
269 Angle B, Hersh JH, Christensen KM. Molecularly proven hypochondroplasia with cloverleaf skull deformity: a novel association. *Clin Genet* 1998;54:417–420.
270 Prinster C, Carrera P, Del Maschio M, et al. Comparison of clinical-radiological and molecular findings in hypochondroplasia. *Am J Med Genet* 1998;75:109–112.
271 Huggins MJ, Mernagh JR, Steele L, et al. Prenatal sonographic diagnosis of hypochondroplasia in a high-risk fetus. *Am J Med Genet* 1999;87:226–229.
272 Eteson DJ, Adomian GE, Ornoy A, et al. Fibrochondrogenesis: radiologic and histologic studies. *Am J Med Genet* 1984;19: 277–290.
273 Al Gazali LI, Bakalinova D, Bakir M, Dawodu A. Fibrochondrogenesis: clinical and radiological features. *Clin Dysmorphol* 1997;6:157–163.
274 Whitley CB, Langer LO, Jr, Ophoven J, et al. Fibrochondrogenesis: lethal, autosomal recessive chondrodysplasia with distinctive cartilage histopathology. *Am J Med Genet* 1984;19: 265–275.
275 Lazzaroni-Fossati F, Stanescu V, Stanescu R, et al. [Fibrochondrogenesis]. *Arch Fr Pediatr* 1978;35:1096–1104.
276 Hunt NC, Vujanic GM. Fibrochondrogenesis in a 17-week fetus: a case expanding the phenotype. *Am J Med Genet* 1998;75: 326–329.
277 Martinez-Frias ML, Garcia A, Cuevas J, et al. A new case of fibrochondrogenesis from Spain. *J Med Genet* 1996;33:429–431.
278 Al Gazali LI, Bakir M, Dawodu A, Haas D. Recurrence of fibrochondrogenesis in a consanguineous family. *Clin Dysmorphol* 1999;8:59–61.
279 Hunt NC, Vujanic GM. Fibrochondrogenesis in a 17-week fetus: a case expanding the phenotype. *Am J Med Genet* 1998;75: 326–329.
280 Megarbane A, Haddad S, Berjaoui L. Prenatal ultrasonography: clinical and radiological findings in a boy with fibrochondrogenesis. *Am J Perinatol* 1998;15:403–407.
281 Randrianaivo H, Haddad G, Roman H, et al. Fetal fibrochondrogenesis at 26 weeks' gestation. *Prenat Diagn* 2002;22:806–810.
282 Hall CM, Elcioglu NH. Metatropic dysplasia lethal variants. *Pediatr Radiol* 2004;34:66–74.
283 Maroteaux P, Spranger J, Stanescu V, et al. Atelosteogenesis. *Am J Med Genet* 1982;13:15–25.
284 Sillence DO, Lachman RS, Jenkins T, et al. Spondylohumerofemoral hypoplasia (giant cell chondrodysplasia): a neonatally lethal short-limbed skeletal displasia. *Am J Med Genet* 1982;13:7–14.
285 Yang SS, Roskamp J, Liu CT, et al. Two lethal chondrodysplasias with giant chondrocytes. *Am J Med Genet* 1983;15:615–625.
286 McAlister WH, Crane JP, Bucy RP, Craig RB. A new neonatal short limbed dwarfism. *Skeletal Radiol* 1985;13:271–275.
287 Sillence D, Worthington S, Dixon J, et al. Atelosteogenesis syndromes: a review, with comments on their pathogenesis. *Pediatr Radiol* 1997;27:388–396.
288 Krakow D, Robertson SP, King LM, et al. Mutations in the gene encoding filamin B disrupt vertebral segmentation, joint formation and skeletogenesis. *Nat Genet* 2004;36:405–410.
289 Hastbacka J, Superti-Furga A, Wilcox WR, et al. Atelosteogenesis type II is caused by mutations in the diastrophic dysplasia sulfate-transporter gene (DTDST): evidence for a phenotypic series involving three chondrodysplasias. *Am J Hum Genet* 1996;58:255–262.
290 Sillence DO, Kozlowski K, Rogers JG, et al. Atelosteogenesis: evidence for heterogeneity. *Pediatr Radiol* 1987;17:112–118.
291 Stern HJ, Graham JM, Jr, Lachman RS, et al. Atelosteogenesis type III: a distinct skeletal dysplasia with features overlapping atelosteogenesis and oto-palato-digital syndrome type II. *Am J Med Genet* 1990;36:183–195.
292 Superti-Furga A, Neumann L, Riebel T, et al. Recessively inherited multiple epiphyseal dysplasia with normal stature, club foot, and double layered patella caused by a DTDST mutation. *J Med Genet* 1999;36:621–624.
293 Rossi A, van der Harten HJ, Beemer FA, et al. Phenotypic and genotypic overlap between atelosteogenesis type 2 and diastrophic dysplasia. *Hum Genet* 1996;98:657–661.
294 Newbury-Ecob R. Atelosteogenesis type 2. *J Med Genet* 1998;35:49–53.
295 De la CA, Maroteaux P, Havu N, Granroth G. [A rare lethal bone dysplasia with recessive autosomic transmission]. *Arch Fr Pediatr* 1972;29:759–770.
296 Whitley CB, Burke BA, Granroth G, Gorlin RJ. de la Chapelle dysplasia. *Am J Med Genet* 1986;25:29–39.
297 Kozlowski K, Sillence D, Cortis-Jones R, Osborn R. Boomerang dysplasia. *Br J Radiol* 1985;58:369–371.
298 Chervenak FA, Isaacson G, Rosenberg JC, Kardon NB. Antenatal diagnosis of frontal cephalocele in a fetus with atelosteogenesis. *J Ultrasound Med* 1986;5:111–113.
299 Bejjani BA, Oberg KC, Wilkins I, et al. Prenatal ultrasonographic description and postnatal pathological findings in atelosteogenesis type 1. *Am J Med Genet* 1998;79:392–395.
300 Schultz C, Langer LO, Laxova R, Pauli RM. Atelosteogenesis type III: long term survival, prenatal diagnosis, and evidence for dominant transmission. *Am J Med Genet* 1999;83:28–42.
301 Ueno K, Tanaka M, Miyakoshi K, et al. Prenatal diagnosis of atelosteogenesis type I at 21 weeks' gestation. *Prenat Diagn* 2002;22:1071–1075.
302 Wessels MW, den Hollander NS, de Krijger RR, et al. Prenatal diagnosis of boomerang dysplasia. *Am J Med Genet* 2003;122:148–154.
303 Borochowitz Z, Ornoy A, Lachman R, Rimoin DL. Achondrogenesis II-hypochondrogenesis: variability versus heterogeneity. *Am J Med Genet* 1986;24:273–288.
304 Borochowitz Z, Lachman R, Adomian GE, et al. Achondrogenesis type I: delineation of further heterogeneity and identification of two distinct subgroups. *J Pediatr* 1988;112:23–31.

305 Spranger J. Pattern recognition in bone dysplasias. In: Papadatos CJ, Bartsocas CS, eds. *Endocrine genetics and genetics of growth*. New York: Alan R. Liss; 1985, 315.
306 Godfrey M, Keene DR, Blank E, et al. Type II achondrogenesis-hypochondrogenesis: morphologic and immunohistopathologic studies. *Am J Hum Genet* 1988;43:894–903.
307 van der Harten HJ, Brons JT, Dijkstra PF, et al. Achondrogenesis-hypochondrogenesis: the spectrum of chondrogenesis imperfecta. A radiological, ultrasonographic, and histopathologic study of 23 cases. *Pediatr Pathol* 1988;8:571–597.
308 Murray LW, Bautista J, James PL, Rimoin DL. Type II collagen defects in the chondrodysplasias. I. Spondyloepiphyseal dysplasias. *Am J Hum Genet* 1989;45:5–15.
309 Whitley CB, Gorlin RJ. Achondrogenesis: new nosology with evidence of genetic heterogeneity. *Radiology* 1983;148:693–698.
310 Superti-Furga A. Achondrogenesis type 1B. *J Med Genet* 1996;33:957–961.
311 Cai G, Nakayama M, Hiraki Y, Ozono K. Mutational analysis of the DTDST gene in a fetus with achondrogenesis type 1B. *Am J Med Genet* 1998;78:58–60.
312 Wenstrom KD, Williamson RA, Hoover WW, Grant SS. Achondrogenesis type II (Langer-Saldino) in association with jugular lymphatic obstruction sequence. *Prenat Diagn* 1989;9:527–532.
313 Won HS, Yoo HK, Lee PR, et al. A case of achondrogenesis type II associated with huge cystic hygroma: prenatal diagnosis by ultrasonography. *Ultrasound Obstet Gynecol* 1999;14:288–290.
314 Ozeren S, Yuksel A, Tukel T. Prenatal sonographic diagnosis of type I achondrogenesis with a large cystic hygroma. *Ultrasound Obstet Gynecol* 1999;13:75–76.
315 Golbus MS, Hall BD, Filly RA, Poskanzer LB. Prenatal diagnosis of achondrogenesis. *J Pediatr* 1977;91:464–466.
316 Anteby SO, Aviad I, Weinstein D. Prenatal diagnosis of achondrogenesis. *Radiol Clin (Basel)* 1977;46:109–114.
317 Smith WL, Breitweiser TD, Dinno N. In utero diagnosis of achondrogenesis, type I. *Clin Genet* 1981;19:51–54.
318 Mahony BS, Filly RA, Cooperberg PL. Antenatal sonographic diagnosis of achondrogenesis. *J Ultrasound Med* 1984;3:333–335.
319 Benacerraf B, Osathanondh R, Bieber FR. Achondrogenesis type I: ultrasound diagnosis in utero. *J Clin Ultrasound* 1984;12:357–359.
320 Glenn LW, Teng SS. In utero sonographic diagnosis of achondrogenesis. *J Clin Ultrasound* 1985;13:195–198.
321 Schramm T, Nerlich A. [Sonographic diagnosis of a case of type 1 achondrogenesis in the 2d trimester]. *Geburtshilfe Frauenheilkd* 1989;49:917–919.
322 Balakumar K. Antenatal diagnosis of Parenti-Fraccaro type achondrogenesis. *Indian Pediatr* 1990;27:496–499.
323 Jeeson UC, Prabhu S, Nambiar D. Prenatal diagnosis of achondrogenesis. *Indian Pediatr* 1990;27:190–193.
324 Mandjee D, Clement F, Belin M, et al. [Achondrogenesis. Ultrasonic diagnosis and clinical and anatomopathologic comparison]. *Rev Fr Gynecol Obstet* 1991;86:391–400.
325 Boudier E, Zurlinden B, Cour A, et al. [Antenatal diagnosis of achondrogenesis. Two successive cases in the same family]. *J Gynecol Obstet Biol Reprod (Paris)* 1991;20:623–626.
326 Tongsong T, Srisomboon J, Sudasna J. Prenatal diagnosis of Langer-Saldino achondrogenesis. *J Clin Ultrasound* 1995;23:56–58.
327 Fisk NM, Vaughan J, Smidt M, Wigglesworth J. Transvaginal ultrasound recognition of nuchal edema in the first-trimester diagnosis of achondrogenesis. *J Clin Ultrasound* 1991;19:586–590.
328 Chen H, Liu CT, Yang SS. Achondrogenesis: a review with special consideration of achondrogenesis type II (Langer-Saldino). *Am J Med Genet* 1981;10:379–394.
329 Superti-Furga A, Hastbacka J, Wilcox WR, et al. Achondrogenesis type IB is caused by mutations in the diastrophic dysplasia sulphate transporter gene. *Nat Genet* 1996;12:100–102.
330 Vissing H, D'Alessio M, Lee B, et al. Glycine to serine substitution in the triple helical domain of pro-alpha 1 (II) collagen results in a lethal perinatal form of short-limbed dwarfism. *J Biol Chem* 1989;264:18265–18267.
331 Kuivaniemi H, Tromp G, Prockop DJ. Mutations in collagen genes: causes of rare and some common diseases in humans. *FASEB J* 1991;5:2052–2060.
332 Willing MC, Pruchno CJ, Atkinson M, Byers PH. Osteogenesis imperfecta type I is commonly due to a COL1A1 null allele of type I collagen. *Am J Hum Genet* 1992;51:508–515.
333 Willing MC, Deschenes SP, Slayton RL, Roberts EJ. Premature chain termination is a unifying mechanism for COL1A1 null alleles in osteogenesis imperfecta type I cell strains. *Am J Hum Genet* 1996;59:799–809.
334 Wang Q, Orrison BM, Marini JC. Two additional cases of osteogenesis imperfecta with substitutions for glycine in the alpha 2(I) collagen chain. A regional model relating mutation location with phenotype. *J Biol Chem* 1993;268:25162–25167.
335 Dyne KM, Valli M, Forlino A, et al. Deficient expression of the small proteoglycan decorin in a case of severe/lethal osteogenesis imperfecta. *Am J Med Genet* 1996;63:161–166.
336 Byers PH, Steiner RD. Osteogenesis imperfecta. *Annu Rev Med* 1992;43:269–282.
337 Rauch F, Glorieux PF. Osteogenesis imperfecta. *Lancet* 2004;363:1377–1385.
338 Orioli IM, Castilla EE, Scarano G, Mastroiacovo P. Effect of paternal age in achondroplasia, thanatophoric dysplasia, and osteogenesis imperfecta. *Am J Med Genet* 1995;59:209–217.
339 Sillence DO, Senn A, Danks DM. Genetic heterogeneity in osteogenesis imperfecta. *J Med Genet* 1979;16:101–116.
340 Young ID, Thompson EM, Hall CM, Pembrey ME. Osteogenesis imperfecta type IIA: evidence for dominant inheritance. *J Med Genet* 1987;24:386–89.
341 Sillence DO, Barlow KK, Garber AP, Hall JG, Rimoin DL. Osteogenesis imperfecta type II delineation of the phenotype with reference to genetic heterogeneity. *Am J Med Genet* 1984;17:407–423.
342 Sillence DO, Barlow KK, Cole WG, et al. Osteogenesis imperfecta type III. Delineation of the phenotype with reference to genetic heterogeneity. *Am J Med Genet* 1986;23:821–832.
343 Andersen PE, Jr, Hauge M. Osteogenesis imperfecta: a genetic, radiological, and epidemiological study. *Clin Genet* 1989;36:250–255.
344 Glorieux FH, Rauch F, Plotkin H, et al. Type V osteogenesis imperfecta: A new form of brittle bone disease. *J Bone Miner Res* 2000;15:1650–1658.
345 Glorieux FH, Ward LM, Rauch F, et al. Osteogenesis imperfecta type VI: a form of brittle bone disease with a mineralization defect. *J Bone Miner Res* 2002;17:30–38.
346 Ward LM, Rauch F, Travers R, et al. Osteogenesis imperfecta type VII: an autosomal recessive form of brittle bone disease. *Bone* 2002;31:12–18.
347 Byers PH, Starman BJ, Cohn DH, Horwitz AL. A novel mutation causes a perinatal lethal form of osteogenesis imperfecta. An

insertion in one alpha 1(I) collagen allele (COL1A1). *J Biol Chem* 1988;263:7855–7861.
348 Wenstrup RJ, Cohn DH, Cohen T, Byers PH. Arginine for glycine substitution in the triple-helical domain of the products of one alpha 2(I) collagen allele (COL1A2) produces the osteogenesis imperfecta type IV phenotype. *J Biol Chem* 1988;263: 7734–7740.
349 Barsh GS, Byers PH. Reduced secretion of structurally abnormal type I procollagen in a form of osteogenesis imperfecta. *Proc Natl Acad Sci USA* 1981;78:5142–5146.
350 Barsh GS, Roush CL, Bonadio J, et al. Intron-mediated recombination may cause a deletion in an alpha 1 type I collagen chain in a lethal form of osteogenesis imperfecta. *Proc Natl Acad Sci USA* 1985;82:2870–2874.
351 Chu ML, Gargiulo V, Williams CJ, Ramirez F. Multiexon deletion in an osteogenesis imperfecta variant with increased type III collagen mRNA. *J Biol Chem* 1985;260:691–694.
352 Chamson A, Bertheas MF, Frey J. Collagen biosynthesis in cell culture from chorionic villi. *Prenat Diagn* 1995;15:165–170.
353 Pepin M, Atkinson M, Starman BJ, Byers PH. Strategies and outcomes of prenatal diagnosis for osteogenesis imperfecta: a review of biochemical and molecular studies completed in 129 pregnancies. *Prenat Diagn* 1997;17:559–570.
354 Chervenak FA, Romero R, Berkowitz RL, et al. Antenatal sonographic findings of osteogenesis imperfecta. *Am J Obstet Gynecol* 1982;143:228–230.
355 Milsom I, Mattsson LA, Dahlen-Nilsson I. Antenatal diagnosis of osteogenesis imperfecta by real time ultrasound: two case reports. *Br J Radiol* 1982;55:310–312.
356 Elejalde BR, de Elejalde MM. Prenatal diagnosis of perinatally lethal osteogenesis imperfecta. *Am J Med Genet* 1983;14: 353–359.
357 Griffin ER, III, Webster JC, Almario VP. Ultrasonic and radiological features of osteogenesis imperfecta congenita: case report. *Milit Med* 1983;148:157–158.
358 Patel ZM, Shah HL, Madon PF, Ambani LM. Prenatal diagnosis of lethal osteogenesis imperfecta (OI) by ultrasonography. *Prenat Diagn* 1983;3:261–263.
359 Stephens JD, Filly RA, Callen PW, Golbus MS. Prenatal diagnosis of osteogenesis imperfecta type II by real-time ultrasound. *Hum Genet* 1983;64:191–193.
360 Woo JS, Ghosh A, Liang ST, Wong VC. Ultrasonic evaluation of osteogenesis imperfecta congenita in utero. *J Clin Ultrasound* 1983;11:42–44.
361 Aylsworth AS, Seeds JW, Guilford WB, Burns CB, Washburn DB. Prenatal diagnosis of a severe deforming type of osteogenesis imperfecta. *Am J Med Genet* 1984;19:707–714.
362 Brown BS. The prenatal ultrasonographic diagnosis of osteogenesis imperfecta lethalis. *J Can Assoc Radiol* 1984;35:63–66.
363 Ghosh A, Woo JS, Wan CW, Wong VC. Simple ultrasonic diagnosis of osteogenesis imperfecta type II in early second trimester. *Prenat Diagn* 1984;4:235–20.
364 Bradley FJ, Essex T. Osteogenesis imperfecta: report of 2 cases. *J Am Osteopath Assoc* 1985;85:462–466.
365 Carpenter MW, Abuelo D, Neave C. Midtrimester diagnosis of severe deforming osteogenesis imperfecta with autosomal dominant inheritance. *Am J Perinatol* 1986;3:80–83.
366 Merz E, Goldhofer W. Sonographic diagnosis of lethal osteogenesis imperfecta in the second trimester: case report and review. *J Clin Ultrasound* 1986;14:380–383.
367 Brons JT, van der Harten HJ, Wladimiroff JW, et al. Prenatal ultrasonographic diagnosis of osteogenesis imperfecta. Am J *Obstet Gynecol* 1988;159:176–181.
368 Munoz C, Filly RA, Golbus MS. Osteogenesis imperfecta type II: prenatal sonographic diagnosis. *Radiology* 1990;174:181–185.
369 Pfutzenreuter N, Panzer F, Bastert G. Prenatal diagnosis of osteogenesis imperfecta congenita; a case report. *Eur J Obstet Gynecol Reprod Biol* 1990;34:189–194.
370 Constantine G, McCormack J, McHugo J, Fowlie A. Prenatal diagnosis of severe osteogenesis imperfecta. *Prenat Diagn* 1991;11:103–110.
371 Morin LR, Herlicoviez M, Loisel JC, et al. Prenatal diagnosis of lethal osteogenesis imperfecta in twin pregnancy. *Clin Genet* 1991;39:467–470.
372 D'Ottavio G, Tamaro LF, Mandruzzato G. Early prenatal ultrasonographic diagnosis of osteogenesis imperfecta: a case report. *Am J Obstet Gynecol* 1993;169:384–385.
373 Berge LN, Marton V, Tranebjaerg L, et al. Prenatal diagnosis of osteogenesis imperfecta. *Acta Obstet Gynecol Scand* 1995;74:321–323.
374 Chen FP, Chang LC. Prenatal diagnosis of osteogenesis imperfecta congenita by ultrasonography. *J Formos Med Assoc* 1996;95:386–389.
375 Tongsong T, Wanapirak C, Siriangkul S. Prenatal diagnosis of osteogenesis imperfecta type II. *Int J Gynaecol Obstet* 1998;61:33–38.
376 DiMaio MS, Barth R, Koprivnikar KE, et al. First-trimester prenatal diagnosis of osteogenesis imperfecta type II by DNA analysis and sonography. *Prenat Diagn* 1993;13:589–596.
377 Buisson O, Senat MV, Laurenceau N, Ville Y. [Update on prenatal diagnosis of osteogenesis imperfecta type II : an index case report diagnosed by ultrasonography in the first trimester]. *J Gynecol Obstet Biol Reprod (Paris)* 2002;31:672–676.
378 McEwing RL, Alton K, Johnson J, Scioscia AL, Pretorius DH. First-trimester diagnosis of osteogenesis imperfecta type II by three-dimensional sonography. *J Ultrasound Med* 2003;22: 311–314.
379 Ruano R, Picone O, Benachi A, et al. First-trimester diagnosis of osteogenesis imperfecta associated with encephalocele by conventional and three-dimensional ultrasound. *Prenat Diagn* 2003;23:539–542.
380 Bishop NJ. Osteogenesis imperfecta calls for caution. *Nat Med* 1999;5:466–467.
381 Bischoff H, Freitag P, Jundt G, et al. Type I osteogenesis imperfecta: diagnostic difficulties. *Clin Rheumatol* 1999;18:48–51.
382 Bulas DI, Stern HJ, Rosenbaum KN, et al. Variable prenatal appearance of osteogenesis imperfecta. *J Ultrasound Med* 1994;13:419–427.
383 Robinson LP, Worthen NJ, Lachman RS, et al. Prenatal diagnosis of osteogenesis imperfecta type III. *Prenat Diagn* 1987;7: 7–15.
384 Thompson EM. Non-invasive prenatal diagnosis of osteogenesis imperfecta. *Am J Med Genet* 1993;45:201–206.
385 Nuytinck L, Sayli BS, Karen W, De Paepe A. Prenatal diagnosis of osteogenesis imperfecta type I by COL1A1 null-allele testing. *Prenat Diagn* 1999;19:873–875.
386 Ries L, Frydman M, Barkai G, et al. Prenatal diagnosis of a novel COL1A1 mutation in osteogenesis imperfecta type I carried through full term pregnancy. *Prenat Diagn* 2000;20:876–880.
387 Mornet E, Muller F, Ngo S, et al. Correlation of alkaline phosphatase (ALP) determination and analysis of the tissue non-

specific ALP gene in prenatal diagnosis of severe hypophosphatasia. *Prenat Diagn* 1999;19:755–757.

388 Vandevijver N, Die-Smulders CE, Offermans JP, et al. Lethal hypophosphatasia, spur type: case report and fetopathological study. *Genet Couns* 1998;9:205–209.

389 Ramage IJ, Howatson AJ, Beattie TJ. Hypophosphatasia. *J Clin Pathol* 1996;49:682–684.

390 Pauli RM, Modaff P, Sipes SL, Whyte MP. Mild hypophosphatasia mimicking severe osteogenesis imperfecta in utero: bent but not broken. *Am J Med Genet* 1999;86:434–438.

391 Terada S, Suzuki N, Ueno H, et al. A congenital lethal form of hypophosphatasia: histologic and ultrastructural study. *Acta Obstet Gynecol Scand* 1996;75:502–505.

392 Wladimiroff JW, Niermeijer MF, van der Harten JJ, et al. Early prenatal diagnosis of congenital hypophosphatasia: case report. *Prenat Diagn* 1985;5:47–52.

393 Warren RC, McKenzie CF, Rodeck CH, Moscoso G, Brock DJ, Barron L. First trimester diagnosis of hypophosphatasia with a monoclonal antibody to the liver/bone/kidney isoenzyme of alkaline phosphatase. *Lancet* 1985;2:856–858.

394 Yagel S, Milwidsky A, Ornoy A, et al. Imaging case of the month. Hypophosphatasia. *Am J Perinatol* 1985;2:261–262.

395 DeLange M, Rouse GA. Prenatal diagnosis of hypophosphatasia. *J Ultrasound Med* 1990;9:115–117.

396 Hall C. Pre-natal diagnosis of lethal dwarfism using ultrasound. *Radiogr Today* 1991;57:22–23.

397 Kleinman G, Uri M, Hull S, Keene C. Perinatal ultrasound casebook. Antenatal findings in congenital hypophosphatasia. *J Perinatol* 1991;11:282–284.

398 Tongsong T, Sirichotiyakul S, Siriangkul S. Prenatal diagnosis of congenital hypophosphatasia. *J Clin Ultrasound* 1995;23: 52–55.

399 Moore CA, Curry CJ, Henthorn PS, et al. Mild autosomal dominant hypophosphatasia: in utero presentation in two families. *Am J Med Genet* 1999;86:410–415.

400 Gortzak-Uzan L, Sheiner E, Gohar J. Prenatal diagnosis of congenital hypophosphatasia in a consanguineous Bedouin couple. A case report. *J Reprod Med* 2000;45:588–590.

401 Tongsong T, Pongsatha S. Early prenatal sonographic diagnosis of congenital hypophosphatasia. *Ultrasound Obstet Gynecol* 2000;15:252–255.

402 Sato S, Matsuo N. Genetic analysis of hypophosphatasia. *Acta Paediatr Jpn* 1997;39:528–532.

403 Rudd NL, Miskin M, Hoar DI, et al. Prenatal diagnosis of hypophosphatasia. *N Engl J Med* 1976;295:146–148.

404 Rattenbury JM, Blau K, Sandler M, et al. Prenatal diagnosis of hypophosphatasia (Letter). *Lancet* 1976;1:306.

405 Orimo H, Nakajima E, Hayashi Z, et al. First-trimester prenatal molecular diagnosis of infantile hypophosphatasia in a Japanese family. *Prenat Diagn* 1996;16:559–563.

406 Weiss MJ, Cole DE, Ray K, et al. A missense mutation in the human liver/bone/kidney alkaline phosphatase gene causing a lethal form of hypophosphatasia. *Proc Natl Acad Sci USA* 1988;85:7666–7669.

407 Mornet E, Taillandier A, Peyramaure S, et al. Identification of fifteen novel mutations in the tissue-nonspecific alkaline phosphatase (TNSALP) gene in European patients with severe hypophosphatasia. *Eur J Hum Genet* 1998;6:308–314.

408 Spentchian M, Merrien Y, Herasse M, et al. Severe hypophosphatasia: characterization of fifteen novel mutations in the ALPL gene. *Hum Mutat* 2003;22:105–106.

409 Henthorn PS, Whyte MP. Infantile hypophosphatasia: successful prenatal assessment by testing for tissue-non-specific alkaline phosphatase isoenzyme gene mutations. *Prenat Diagn* 1995;15:1001–1006.

410 Zurutuza L, Muller F, Gibrat JF, et al. Correlations of genotype and phenotype in hypophosphatasia. *Hum Mol Genet* 1999;8:1039–1046.

411 Horton WA, Rimoin DL, Lachman RS, et al. The phenotypic variability of diastrophic dysplasia. *J Pediatr* 1978;93:609–613.

412 Kaitila I, Ammala P, Karjalainen O, et al. Early prenatal detection of diastrophic dysplasia. *Prenat Diagn* 1983;3:237–244.

413 Superti-Furga A, Hastbacka J, Rossi A, et al. A family of chondrodysplasias caused by mutations in the diastrophic dysplasia sulfate transporter gene and associated with impaired sulfation of proteoglycans. *Ann N Y Acad Sci* 1996;785:195–201.

414 Rossi A, Superti-Furga A. Mutations in the diastrophic dysplasia sulfate transporter (DTDST) gene (SLC26A2): 22 novel mutations, mutation review, associated skeletal phenotypes, and diagnostic relevance. *Hum Mutat* 2001;17:159–171.

415 Karniski LP. Mutations in the diastrophic dysplasia sulfate transporter (DTDST) gene: correlation between sulfate transport activity and chondrodysplasia phenotype. *Hum Mol Genet* 2001;10:1485–1490.

416 Megarbane A, Farkh I, Haddad-Zebauni S. How many phenotypes in the DTDST family chondrodysplasias? *Clin Genet* 2002;62:189–190.

417 Gollop TR, Eigier A. Prenatal ultrasound diagnosis of diastrophic dysplasia at 16 weeks. *Am J Med Genet* 1987;27: 321–324.

418 Jung C, Sohn C, Sergi C. Case report: prenatal diagnosis of diastrophic dysplasia by ultrasound at 21 weeks of gestation in a mother with massive obesity. *Prenat Diagn* 1998;18:378–383.

419 Wax JR, Carpenter M, Smith W, et al. Second-trimester sonographic diagnosis of diastrophic dysplasia: report of 2 index cases. *J Ultrasound Med* 2003;22:805–808.

420 Severi FM, Bocchi C, Sanseverino F, Petraglia F. Prenatal ultrasonographic diagnosis of diastrophic dysplasia at 13 weeks of gestation. *J Matern Fetal Neonatal Med* 2003;13:282–284.

421 Sepulveda W, Sepulveda-Swatson E, Sanchez J. Diastrophic dysplasia: prenatal three-dimensional ultrasound findings. *Ultrasound Obstet Gynecol* 2004;23:312–314.

422 Hastbacka J, Salonen R, Laurila P, et al. Prenatal diagnosis of diastrophic dysplasia with polymorphic DNA markers. *J Med Genet* 1993;30:265–268.

423 Bonafe L, Superti-Furga, A. Diastrophic dysplasia. GeneReviews at GeneTests: Medical Genetics Information Resource (database online), 2004. Copyright, University of Washington, Seattle, 1997–2005. Available at http://www.genetests.org. (18 February 2005).

424 Eteson DJ, Beluffi G, Burgio GR, et al. Pseudodiastrophic dysplasia: a distinct newborn skeletal dysplasia. *J Pediatr* 1986;109:635–641.

425 Cetta G, Rossi A, Burgio GR, Beluffi G. Diastrophic dysplasia sulfate transporter (DTDST) gene is not involved in pseudodiastrophic dysplasia. *Am J Med Genet* 1997;73:493–494.

426 Hooshang T, Ralph SL. *Radiology of syndromes, metabolic disorders, and skeletal dysplasias*. Chicago, IL: Year Book Medical Publishers, 1983.

427 Kniest W. Zur Abgrenzung der Dysostosis enchondralis von der Chondrodystrophie. *Z Kinderheilk* 1952;70:633–640.

428 Siggers CD, Rimoin DL, Dorst JP, et al. The Kniest syndrome. *Birth Defects Orig Artic Ser* 1974;10:193–208.

429 Winterpacht A, Hilbert M, Schwarze U, et al. Kniest and Stickler dysplasia phenotypes caused by collagen type II gene (COL2A1) defect. *Nat Genet* 1993;3:323–326.

430 Fernandes RJ, Wilkin DJ, Weis MA, et al. Incorporation of structurally defective type II collagen into cartilage matrix in kniest chondrodysplasia. *Arch Biochem Biophys* 1998;355:282–290.

431 Weis MA, Wilkin DJ, Kim HJ, et al. Structurally abnormal type II collagen in a severe form of Kniest dysplasia caused by an exon 24 skipping mutation. *J Biol Chem* 1998;273:4761–4768.

432 Spranger J, Winterpacht A, Zabel B. Kniest dysplasia: Dr. W. Kniest, his patient, the molecular defect. *Am J Med Genet* 1997;69:79–84.

433 Chen H, Yang SS, Gonzalez E. Kniest dysplasia: neonatal death with necropsy. *Am J Med Genet* 1980;6:171–178.

434 Poole AR, Rosenberg L, Murray L, Rimoin D. Kniest dysplasia: a probable type II collagen defect. *Pathol Immunopathol Res* 1988;7:95–98.

435 Handmaker SD, Campbell JA, Robinson LD, et al. Dyssegmental dwarfism: a new syndrome of lethal dwarfism. *Birth Defects Orig Artic Ser* 1977;13:79–90.

436 Andersen PE, Jr, Hauge M, Bang J. Dyssegmental dysplasia in siblings: prenatal ultrasonic diagnosis. *Skeletal Radiol* 1988;17:29–31.

437 Prabhu VG, Kozma C, Leftridge CA, Helmbrecht GD, France ML. Dyssegmental dysplasia Silverman-Handmaker type in a consanguineous Druze Lebanese family: long term survival and documentation of the natural history. *Am J Med Genet* 1998;75:164–170.

438 Stoll C, Langer B, Gasser B, Alembik Y. Sporadic case of dyssegmental dysplasia with antenatal presentation. *Genet Couns* 1998;9:125–130.

439 Kim HJ, Costales F, Bouzouki M, Wallach RC. Prenatal diagnosis of dyssegmental dwarfism. *Prenat Diagn* 1986;6:143–150.

440 Hsieh YY, Chang CC, Tsai HD, et al. Prenatal diagnosis of dyssegmental dysplasia. A case report. *J Reprod Med* 1999;44:303–305.

441 Arikawa-Hirasawa E, Wilcox WR, Le AH, et al. Dyssegmental dysplasia, Silverman-Handmaker type, is caused by functional null mutations of the perlecan gene. *Nat Genet* 2001;27:431–434.

442 Maroteaux P, Spranger J, Opitz JM, et al. [The campomelic syndrome]. *Presse Med* 1971;79:1157–1162.

443 Mansour S, Hall CM, Pembrey ME, Young ID. A clinical and genetic study of campomelic dysplasia. *J Med Genet* 1995;32:415–420.

444 Normann EK, Pedersen JC, Stiris G, van der Hagen CB. Campomelic dysplasia: an underdiagnosed condition? *Eur J Pediatr* 1993;152:331–333.

445 Foster JW, Dominguez-Steglich MA, Guioli S, et al. Campomelic dysplasia and autosomal sex reversal caused by mutations in an SRY-related gene. *Nature* 1994;372:525–530.

446 Wunderle VM, Critcher R, Hastie N, et al. Deletion of long-range regulatory elements upstream of SOX9 causes campomelic dysplasia. *Proc Natl Acad Sci USA* 1998;95:10649–10654.

447 Goji K, Nishijima E, Tsugawa C,et al. Novel missense mutation in the HMG box of SOX9 gene in a Japanese XY male resulted in campomelic dysplasia and severe defect in masculinization. *Hum Mutat* 1998; (Suppl. 1):114–116.

448 Hageman RM, Cameron FJ, Sinclair AH. Mutation analysis of the SOX9 gene in a patient with campomelic dysplasia. *Hum Mutat* 1998;(Suppl. 1):112–113.

449 McDowall S, Argentaro A, Ranganathan S, et al. Functional and structural studies of wild type SOX9 and mutations causing campomelic dysplasia. *J Biol Chem* 1999;274:24023–24030.

450 Houston CS, Opitz JM, Spranger JW, Macpherson RI, et al. The campomelic syndrome: review, report of 17 cases, and follow-up on the currently 17-year-old boy first reported by Maroteaux et al in 1971. *Am J Med Genet* 1983;15:3–28.

451 Fryns JP, van den Berghe K, van Assche A, van den Berghe H. Prenatal diagnosis of campomelic dwarfism. *Clin Genet* 1981;19:199–201.

452 Redon JY, Le Grevellec JY, Marie F,et al. [Prenatal diagnosis of camptomelic dysplasia]. *J Gynecol Obstet Biol Reprod (Paris)* 1984;13:437–441.

453 Slater CP, Ross J, Nelson MM, Coetzee EJ. The campomelic syndrome: prenatal ultrasound investigations. A case report. *S Afr Med J* 1985;67:863–866.

454 Winter R, Rosenkranz W, Hofmann H, et al. Prenatal diagnosis of campomelic dysplasia by ultrasonography. *Prenat Diagn* 1985;5:1–8.

455 Cordone M, Lituania M, Zampatti C, et al. In utero ultrasonographic features of campomelic dysplasia. *Prenat Diagn* 1989;9:745–750.

456 Tennstedt C, Bartho S, Bollmann R, et al. [Osteochondrodysplasias. Prenatal diagnosis and pathological-anatomic findings]. *Zentralbl Pathol* 1993;139:71–80.

457 Lachman RS. Fetal imaging in the skeletal dysplasias: overview and experience. *Pediatr Radiol* 1994;24:413–417.

458 Sanders RC, Greyson-Fleg RT, Hogge WA, et al. Osteogenesis imperfecta and campomelic dysplasia: difficulties in prenatal diagnosis. *J Ultrasound Med* 1994;13:691–700.

459 Tongsong T, Wanapirak C, Pongsatha S. Prenatal diagnosis of campomelic dysplasia. *Ultrasound Obstet Gynecol* 2000;15:428–430.

460 GeneTests: Medical Genetics Information Resource (database online). Copyright, University of Washington, Seattle, 1993–2005. Updated weekly. Available at http://www.genetests.org. (20 February 2005).

461 Norgard M, Yankowitz J, Rhead W, et al. Prenatal ultrasound findings in hydrolethalus: continuing difficulties in diagnosis. *Prenat Diagn* 1996;16:173–179.

462 Beluffi G, Fraccaro M. Genetical and clinical aspects of campomelic dysplasia. *Prog Clin Biol Res* 1982;104:53–68.

463 Ray S, Bowen JR. Orthopaedic problems associated with survival in campomelic dysplasia. *Clin Orthop* 1984;77–82.

464 Cooke CT, Mulcahy MT, Cullity GJ, et al. Campomelic dysplasia with sex reversal: morphological and cytogenetic studies of a case. *Pathology* 1985;17:526–529.

465 Offiah AC, Mansour S, McDowall S, et al. Surviving campomelic dysplasia has the radiological features of the previously reported ischio-pubic-patella syndrome. *J Med Genet* 2002;39:e50.

466 Mansour S, Offiah AC, McDowall S, et al. The phenotype of survivors of campomelic dysplasia. *J Med Genet* 2002;39:597–602.

467 Romero R, Ghidini A, Eswara MSet al. Prenatal findings in a case of spondylocostal dysplasia type I (Jarcho-Levin syndrome). *Obstet Gynecol* 1988;71:988–991.

468 Jeune M, Carron R. Dystrophic thoracique asphyxiante caractere familial. *Arch Fr Pediatr* 1955;12:276–279.

469 Maarup LP, Host A. [The Jeune syndrome, asphyxiating thoracic dysplasia. A review and description of 2 siblings.] *Ugeskr Laeger* 1985;147:1676–1678.

470 Capilupi B, Olappi G, Cornaglia AM, Novati GP. [Asphyxiating thoracic dysplasia or Jeune's syndrome. Description of 2 mild familial cases.] *Pediatr Med Chir* 1996;18:529–532.
471 Kozlowski K, Masel J. Asphyxiating thoracic dystrophy without respiratory disease: report of two cases of the latent form. *Pediatr Radiol* 1976;5:30–33.
472 Friedman JM, Kaplan HG, Hall JG. The Jeune syndrome (asphyxiating thoracic dystrophy) in an adult. *Am J Med* 1975;59:857–862.
473 Novakovic I, Kostic M, Popovic-Rolovic M, et al. [Jeune's syndrome (3 case reports)]. *Srp Arh Celok Lek* 1996;124(Suppl. 1):244–246.
474 Silengo M, Gianino P, Longo P, et al. Dandy–Walker complex in a child with Jeune's asphyxiating thoracic dystrophy. *Pediatr Radiol* 2000;30:430.
475 Katthofer B. [Asphyxiating thoracic dysplasia (Jeune-syndrome): a medical and nursing report]. *Kinderkrankenschwester* 1993;12:342–344.
476 Trabelsi M, Hammou-Jeddi A, Kammoun A, et al. [Asphyxiating thoracic dysplasia associated with hepatic ductal hypoplasia, agenesis of the corpus callosum and Dandy-Walker syndrome]. *Pediatrie* 1990;45:35–38.
477 Hsieh YY, Hsu TY, Lee CC, et al. Prenatal diagnosis of thoracopelvic dysplasia. A case report. *J Reprod Med* 1999;44: 737–740.
478 Lipson M, Waskey J, Rice J, et al. Prenatal diagnosis of asphyxiating thoracic dysplasia. *Am J Med Genet* 1984;18:273–277.
479 Elejalde BR, de Elejalde MM, Pansch D. Prenatal diagnosis of Jeune syndrome. *Am J Med Genet* 1985;21:433–438.
480 Schinzel A, Savoldelli G, Briner J, Schubiger G. Prenatal sonographic diagnosis of Jeune syndrome. *Radiology* 1985;154: 777–778.
481 Panero Lopez AL, Puyol Buil PJ, Belaustegui CA, Sotelo MT. [Asphyxiating thoracic dysplasia in 2 dizygotic twins]. *An Esp Pediatr* 1987;26:453–456.
482 Skiptunas SM, Weiner S. Early prenatal diagnosis of asphyxiating thoracic dysplasia (Jeune's syndrome). Value of fetal thoracic measurement. *J Ultrasound Med* 1987;6:41–43.
483 Kapoor R, Saha MM, Gupta NC. Antenatal diagnosis of asphyxiating thoracic dysplasia. *Indian Pediatr* 1989;26: 495–497.
484 Ardura FJ, Alvarez GC, Rodriguez FM, Andres dL. [Asphyxiating thoracic dysplasia associated with proximal myopathy and arachnoid cyst]. *An Esp Pediatr* 1990;33:592–596.
485 Chen CP, Lin SP, Liu FF, et al. Prenatal diagnosis of asphyxiating thoracic dysplasia (Jeune syndrome). *Am J Perinatol* 1996;13:495–498.
486 Ben Ami M, Perlitz Y, Haddad S, Matilsky M. Increased nuchal translucency is associated with asphyxiating thoracic dysplasia. *Ultrasound Obstet Gynecol* 1997;10:297–298.
487 Tongsong T, Chanprapaph P, Thongpadungroj T. Prenatal sonographic findings associated with asphyxiating thoracic dystrophy (Jeune syndrome). *J Ultrasound Med* 1999;18:573–576.
488 den Hollander NS, Robben SG, Hoogeboom AJ, et al. Early prenatal sonographic diagnosis and follow-up of Jeune syndrome. *Ultrasound Obstet Gynecol* 2001;18:378–383.
489 Das BB, Nagaraj A, Fayemi A, et al. Fetal thoracic measurements in prenatal diagnosis of Jeune syndrome. *Indian J Pediatr* 2002;69:101–103.
490 Chen SH, Chung MT, Chang FM. Early prenatal diagnosis of Jeune syndrome in a low-risk pregnancy. *Prenat Diagn* 2003;23:606–607.
491 Morgan NV, Bacchelli C, Gissen P, et al. A locus for asphyxiating thoracic dystrophy, ATD, maps to chromosome 15q13. *J Med Genet* 2003;40:431–435.
492 Wladimiroff JW, Niermeijer MF, Laar J, et al. Prenatal diagnosis of skeletal dysplasia by real-time ultrasound. *Obstet Gynecol* 1984;63:360–364.
493 Muller LM, Cremin BJ. Ultrasonic demonstration of fetal skeletal dysplasia. Case reports. *S Afr Med J* 1985;67:222–226.
494 Lavanya R, Pratap K. Short rib polydactyly syndrome: a rare skeletal dysplasia. *Int J Gynaecol Obstet* 1995;50:291–292.
495 Sarafoglou K, Funai EF, Fefferman N, et al. Short rib-polydactyly syndrome: more evidence of a continuous spectrum. *Clin Genet* 1999;56:145–148.
496 Thomson GS, Reynolds CP, Cruickshank J. Antenatal detection of recurrence of Majewski dwarf (short rib-polydactyly syndrome type II Majewski). *Clin Radiol* 1982;33:509–517.
497 Gembruch U, Hansmann M, Fodisch HJ. Early prenatal diagnosis of short rib-polydactyly (SRP) syndrome type I (Majewski) by ultrasound in a case at risk. *Prenat Diagn* 1985;5:357–362.
498 Meizner I, Bar-Ziv J. Prenatal ultrasonic diagnosis of short-rib polydactyly syndrome (SRPS) type III: a case report and a proposed approach to the diagnosis of SRPS and related conditions. *J Clin Ultrasound* 1985;13:284–287.
499 Steffelaar JW, Lankhorst PF, Reuss A, et al. [Prenatal diagnosis in a primigravida of the short rib-polydactyly syndrome using echography]. *Ned Tijdschr Geneeskd* 1988;132:405–407.
500 Meizner I, Bar-Ziv J. Prenatal ultrasonic diagnosis of short rib polydactyly syndrome, type I. A case report. *J Reprod Med* 1989;34:668–672.
501 de Sierra TM, Ashmead G, Bilenker R. Prenatal diagnosis of short rib (polydactyly) syndrome with situs inversus. *Am J Med Genet* 1992;44:555–557.
502 Benacerraf BR. Prenatal sonographic diagnosis of short rib-polydactyly syndrome type II, Majewski type. *J Ultrasound Med* 1993;12:552–555.
503 Cideciyan D, Rodriguez MM, Haun RL, et al. New findings in short rib syndrome. *Am J Med Genet* 1993;46:255–259.
504 Prudlo J, Stoltenburg-Didinger G, Jimenez E, et al. Central nervous system alterations in a case of short-rib polydactyly syndrome, Majewski type. *Dev Med Child Neurol* 1993;35: 158–162.
505 Meizner I, Barnhard Y. Short-rib polydactyly syndrome (SRPS) type III diagnosed during routine prenatal ultrasonographic screening. A case report. *Prenat Diagn* 1995;15:665–668.
506 Montemarano H, Bulas DI, Chandra R, Tifft C. Prenatal diagnosis of glomerulocystic kidney disease in short-rib polydactyly syndrome type II, Majewski type. *Pediatr Radiol* 1995;25:469–471.
507 Wu MH, Kuo PL, Lin SJ. Prenatal diagnosis of recurrence of short rib-polydactyly syndrome. *Am J Med Genet* 1995;55:279–284.
508 Fujisawa K. [Saldino-Noonan syndrome (short rib polydactyly syndrome type I)]. *Ryoikibetsu Shokogun Shirizu* 1996;297–299.
509 Majewski E, Ozturk B, Gillessen-Kaesbach G. Jeune syndrome with tongue lobulation and preaxial polydactyly, and Jeune syndrome with situs inversus and asplenia: compound heterozygosity Jeune-Mohr and Jeune-Ivemark? *Am J Med Genet* 1996;63:74–79.
510 Scarano G, Della MM, Capece G, et al. A case of short-rib syndrome without polydactyly in a stillborn: a new type? *Birth Defects Orig Artic Ser* 1996;30:95–101.

511 Dugoff L, Coffin CT, Hobbins JC. Sonographic measurement of the fetal rib cage perimeter to thoracic circumference ratio: application to prenatal diagnosis of skeletal dysplasias. *Ultrasound Obstet Gynecol* 1997;10:269–271.
512 Hill LM, Leary J. Transvaginal sonographic diagnosis of short-rib polydactyly dysplasia at 13 weeks' gestation. *Prenat Diagn* 1998;18:1198–1201.
513 den Hollander NS, van der Harten HJ, Laudy JA, et al. Early transvaginal ultrasonographic diagnosis of Beemer-Langer dysplasia: a report of two cases. *Ultrasound Obstet Gynecol* 1998;11:298–302.
514 Golombeck K, Jacobs VR, von Kaisenberg C, et al. Short rib-polydactyly syndrome type III: comparison of ultrasound, radiology, and pathology findings. *Fetal Diagn Ther* 2001; 16:133–38.
515 Sirichotiyakul S, Tongsong T, Wanapirak C, Chanprapaph P. Prenatal sonographic diagnosis of Majewski syndrome. *J Clin Ultrasound* 2002;30:303–307.
516 Naki MM, Gur D, Zemheri E, et al. Short rib-polydactyly syndrome. *Arch Gynecol Obstet* 2005;272:173–175.
517 Sridhar S, Kishore R, Thomas N, Jana AK. Short rib polydactyly syndrome-Type I. *Indian J Pediatr* 2004;71:359–361.
518 Toftager-Larsen K, Benzie RJ. Fetoscopy in prenatal diagnosis of the Majewski and the Saldino-Noonan types of the short rib-polydactyly syndromes. *Clin Genet* 1984;26:56–60.
519 Tsai FJ, Tsai CH, Wang TR. Beemer-Langer type short rib-polydactyly syndrome: report of two cases. *Zhonghua Min Guo Xiao Er Ke Yi Xue Hui Za Zhi* 1994;35:331–334.
520 Myong NH, Park JW, Chi JG. Short-rib polydactyly syndrome, Beemer-Langer type, with bilateral huge polycystic renal dysplasia: an autopsy case. *J Korean Med Sci* 1998;13:201–206.
521 Hentze S, Sergi C, Troeger J, et al. Short-rib-polydactyly syndrome type Verma-Naumoff-Le Marec in a fetus with histological hallmarks of type Saldino-Noonan but lacking internal organ abnormalities. *Am J Med Genet* 1998;80:281–285.
522 Elcioglu N, Karatekin G, Sezgin B, et al. Short rib-polydactyly syndrome in twins: Beemer-Langer type with polydactyly. *Clin Genet* 1996;50:159–163.
523 Shindel B, Wise S. Recurrent short rib-polydactyly syndrome with unusual associations. *J Clin Ultrasound* 1999;27:143–146.
524 McKusick VA, Egeland JA, Eldridge R, Krusen DE. Dwarfism in the Amish I. The Ellis-van Creveld syndrome. *Bull Johns Hopkins Hosp* 1964;115:306–336.
525 Ohdo S. [Ellis-van Creveld syndrome]. *Ryoikibetsu Shokogun Shirizu* 1996;261–263.
526 Wasant P, Waeteekul S, Rimoin DL, Lachman RS. Genetic skeletal dysplasia in Thailand: the Siriraj experience. *Southeast Asian J Trop Med Public Health* 1995;26(Suppl.)1:59–67.
527 Polymeropoulos MH, Ide SE, Wright M, et al. The gene for the Ellis-van Creveld syndrome is located on chromosome 4p16. Genomics 1996;35:1–5.
528 Alcalde MM, Castillo JA, Garcia UP, et al. [Ellis-van Creveld syndrome: an easy early diagnosis?]. *Rev Esp Cardiol* 1998;51: 407–409.
529 Ortega RJ, Ferrer FJ, Fernandez LA,et al. [The Ellis-van Creveld syndrome (chondroectodermal dysplasia). Apropos a clinical case]. *An Esp Pediatr* 1999;50:74–76.
530 Levin SE, Dansky R, Milner S, Benatar A, Govendrageloo K, du PJ. Atrioventricular septal defect and type A postaxial polydactyly without other major associated anomalies: a specific association. *Pediatr Cardiol* 1995;16:242–246.
531 Digilio MC, Marino B, Giannotti A, Dallapiccola B. Single atrium, atrioventricular canal/postaxial hexodactyly indicating Ellis-van Creveld syndrome. *Hum Genet* 1995;96:251–253.
532 Chang YC, Wu JM, Lin SJ, Wu MH. Common atrium with Ebstein's anomaly in a neonate with Ellis-van Creveld syndrome. *Zhonghua Min Guo Xiao Er Ke Yi Xue Hui Za Zhi* 1995;36:50–52.
533 Yapar EG, Ekici E, Aydogdu T, et al. Diagnostic problems in a case with mucometrocolpos, polydactyly, congenital heart disease, and skeletal dysplasia. *Am J Med Genet* 1996;66:343–346.
534 Digilio MC, Marino B, Giannotti A, Dallapiccola B. Atrioventricular canal defect and postaxial polydactyly indicating phenotypic overlap of Ellis-van Creveld and Kaufman-McKusick syndromes. *Pediatr Cardiol* 1997;18:74–75.
535 Horigome H, Hamada H, Sohda S, et al. Prenatal ultrasonic diagnosis of a case of Ellis-van Creveld syndrome with a single atrium. *Pediatr Radiol* 1997;27:942–944.
536 Gelb BD. Molecular genetics of congenital heart disease. *Curr Opin Cardiol* 1997;12:321–328.
537 Isajiw G. Prenatal diagnosis with fetoscopy. *N Engl J Med* 1977;297:949.
538 Hobbins JC, Mahoney MJ. Fetoscopy in continuing pregnancies. *Am J Obstet Gynecol* 1977;129:440–442.
539 Mahoney MJ, Hobbins JC. Prenatal diagnosis of chondroectodermal dysplasia (Ellis-van Creveld syndrome) with fetoscopy and ultrasound. *N Engl J Med* 1977;297:258–260.
540 Bui TH, Marsk L, Eklof O, Theorell K. Prenatal diagnosis of chondroectodermal dysplasia with fetoscopy. *Prenat Diagn* 1984;4:155–159.
541 Zimmer EZ, Weinraub Z, Raijman A, et al. Antenatal diagnosis of a fetus with an extremely narrow thorax and short limb dwarfism. *J Clin Ultrasound* 1984;12:112–114.
542 Berardi JC, Moulis M, Laloux V, et al. [Ellis-van Creveld syndrome. Contribution of echography to prenatal diagnosis. Apropos of a case]. *J Gynecol Obstet Biol Reprod (Paris)* 1985;14:43–47.
543 Frikiche A, Verloes A, Stassen M, et al. [Ellis-Van Creveld syndrome. Apropos of a case diagnosed in utero]. *Rev Med Liege* 1989;44:68–72.
544 Torrente I, Mangino M, De Luca A, et al. First-trimester prenatal diagnosis of Ellis-van Creveld syndrome using linked microsatellite markers. *Prenat Diagn* 1998;18:504–506.
545 Guschmann M, Horn D, Gasiorek-Wiens A, et al. Ellis-van Creveld syndrome: examination at 15 weeks' gestation. *Prenat Diagn* 1999;19:879–883.
546 Tongsong T, Chanprapaph P. Prenatal sonographic diagnosis of ellis-van creveld syndrome. *J Clin Ultrasound* 2000;28:38–41.
547 Dugoff L, Thieme G, Hobbins JC. First trimester prenatal diagnosis of chondroectodermal dysplasia (Ellis-van Creveld syndrome) with ultrasound. *Ultrasound Obstet Gynecol* 2001;17: 86–88.
548 Ruiz-Perez VL, Ide SE, Strom TM, et al. Mutations in a new gene in Ellis-van Creveld syndrome and Weyers acrodental dysostosis. *Nat Genet* 2000;24:283–286.
549 Galdzicka M, Patnala S, Hirshman MG, et al. A new gene, EVC2, is mutated in Ellis-van Creveld syndrome. *Mol Genet Metab* 2002;77:291–295.
550 Ruiz-Perez VL, Tompson SW, Blair HJ, et al. Mutations in two nonhomologous genes in a head-to-head configuration cause Ellis-van Creveld syndrome. *Am J Hum Genet* 2003;72:728–732.
551 Goldberg MJ. *The dysmorphic child: an orthopedic perspective.* New York: Raven Press, 1987.

552 Bod M, Czeizel A, Lenz W. Incidence at birth of different types of limb reduction abnormalities in Hungary 1975–1977. *Hum Genet* 1983;65:27–33.

553 Zhu J, Miao L, Xu C, Wang Y, Chen T. [Analysis of 822 infants with limb reduction defect in China]. *Hua Xi Yi Ke Da Xue Xue Bao* 1996;27:400–403.

554 Bromley B, Benacerraf B. Abnormalities of the hands and feet in the fetus: sonographic findings. *Am J Roentgenol* 1995;165: 1239–1243.

555 Lecannellier J, Vischer D. [The aglossia-adactylia syndrome]. *Helv Paediatr Acta* 1976;31:77–84.

556 Tuncbilek E, Yalcin C, Atasu M. Aglossia-adactylia syndrome (special emphasis on the inheritance pattern). *Clin Genet* 1977;11:421–423.

557 Marti-Herrero M, Cabrera-Lopez JC, Toledo L, et al. [Moebius syndrome. Three different forms of presentation]. *Rev Neurol* 1998;27:975–78.

558 Cuvelier B, Cousin J, Pauli A, et al [Aglossia-adactylia syndrome: two new cases (author's transl)]. *Ann Pediatr (Paris)* 1981;28: 433–435.

559 Canete ER, Gil RR, Alvarez MR, et al. [Hanhart syndrome (aglossia-adactylia syndrome). Report of 2 cases]. *An Esp Pediatr* 1990;33:465–468.

560 Deffez JP, Rostand B, Allain P, Brethaux J, Grimbert N, Van Cuc E. [An unusual aglossia-adactylia syndrome (author's transl)]. *Rev Stomatol Chir Maxillofac* 1981;82:241–246.

561 Grippaudo FR, Kennedy DC. Oromandibular-limb hypogenesis syndromes: a case of aglossia with an intraoral band. *Br J Plast Surg* 1998;51:480–483.

562 Robinow M, Marsh JL, Edgerton MT, et al. Discordance in monozygotic twins for aglossia-adactylia, and possible clues to the pathogenesis of the syndrome. *Birth Defects Orig Artic Ser* 1978;14:223–230.

563 Lammens M, Moerman P, Fryns JP, et al. Neuropathological findings in Moebius syndrome. *Clin Genet* 1998;54:136–141.

564 d'Orey C, Melo MJ, Costa A, et al. [Moebius syndrome in newborn infants]. *Arch Pediatr* 1997;4:897–898.

565 Baraitser M. Genetics of Mobius syndrome. *J Med Genet* 1977;14:415–417.

566 Bonanni P, Guerrini R. Segmental facial myoclonus in moebius syndrome. *Mov Disord* 1999;14:1021–1024.

567 Abramson DL, Cohen MM, Jr, Mulliken JB. Mobius syndrome: classification and grading system. *Plast Reconstr Surg* 1998;102:961–967.

568 Matsui A, Nakagawa M, Okuno M. Association of atrial septal defect with Poland-Moebius syndrome: vascular disruption can be a common etiologic factor. A case report. *Angiology* 1997;48:269–271.

569 Journel H, Roussey M, Le Marec B. MCA/MR syndrome with oligodactyly and Mobius anomaly in first cousins: new syndrome or familial facial-limb disruption sequence? *Am J Med Genet* 1989;34:506–510.

570 Bavinck JN, Weaver DD. Subclavian artery supply disruption sequence: hypothesis of a vascular etiology for Poland, Klippel-Feil, and Mobius anomalies. *Am J Med Genet* 1986;23:903–918.

571 Brill CB, Peyster RG, Keller MS, Galtman L. Isolation of the right subclavian artery with subclavian steal in a child with Klippel-Feil anomaly: an example of the subclavian artery supply disruption sequence. *Am J Med Genet* 1987;26:933–940.

572 Farina D, Gatto G, Leonessa L, et al. Poland syndrome: a case with a combination of syndromes. *Panminerva Med* 1999;41: 259–260.

573 Larrandaburu M, Schuler L, Ehlers JA, et al. The occurrence of Poland and Poland-Moebius syndromes in the same family: further evidence of their genetic component. *Clin Dysmorphol* 1999;8:93–99.

574 Lipson AH, Gillerot Y, Tannenberg AE, Giurgea S. Two cases of maternal antenatal splenic rupture and hypotension associated with Moebius syndrome and cerebral palsy in offspring. Further evidence for a utero placental vascular aetiology for the Moebius syndrome and some cases of cerebral palsy. *Eur J Pediatr* 1996;155:800–804.

575 St Charles S, DiMario FJ, Jr, Grunnet ML. Mobius sequence: further in vivo support for the subclavian artery supply disruption sequence. *Am J Med Genet* 1993;47:289–293.

576 Happle R, Koch H, Lenz W. The CHILD syndrome. Congenital hemidysplasia with ichthyosiform erythroderma and limb defects. *Eur J Pediatr* 1980;134:27–33.

577 Hebert AA, Esterly NB, Holbrook KA, Hall JC. The CHILD syndrome. Histologic and ultrastructural studies. *Arch Dermatol* 1987;123:503–509.

578 Hashimoto K, Topper S, Sharata H, Edwards M. CHILD syndrome: analysis of abnormal keratinization and ultrastructure. *Pediatr Dermatol* 1995;12:116–129.

579 Hoeger PH, Adwani SS, Whitehead BF, et al. Ichthyosiform erythroderma and cardiomyopathy: report of two cases and review of the literature. *Br J Dermatol* 1998;139:1055–1059.

580 Happle R, Effendy I, Megahed M, et al. CHILD syndrome in a boy. *Am J Med Genet* 1996;62:192–194.

581 Happle R, Mittag H, Kuster W. The CHILD nevus: a distinct skin disorder. *Dermatology* 1995;191:210–216.

582 Holmes LB, Redline RW, Brown DL, et al. Absence/hypoplasia of tibia, polydactyly, retrocerebellar arachnoid cyst, and other anomalies: an autosomal recessive disorder. *J Med Genet* 1995;32:896–900.

583 Konig A, Happle R, Bornholdt D, et al. Mutations in the NSDHL gene, encoding a 3beta-hydroxysteroid dehydrogenase, cause CHILD syndrome. *Am J Med Genet* 2000;90:339–346.

584 Bittar M, Happle R. CHILD syndrome avant la lettre. *J Am Acad Dermatol* 2004;50:S34–S37.

585 Hummel M, Cunningham D, Mullett CJ, et al. Left sided CHILD syndrome caused by a nonsense mutation in the NSDHL gene. *Am J Med Genet* 2003;122:246–251.

586 Lipson AH. Amelia of the arms and femur/fibula deficiency with splenogonadal fusion in a child born to a consanguineous couple. *Am J Med Genet* 1995;55:265–268.

587 Ahmad M, Abbas H, Wahab A, Haque S. Fibular hypoplasia and complex brachydactyly (Du Pan syndrome) in an inbred Pakistani kindred. *Am J Med Genet* 1990;36:292–296.

588 Faiyaz-Ul-Haque M, Ahmad W, Zaidi SH, et al. Mutation in the cartilage-derived morphogenetic protein-1 (CDMP1) gene in a kindred affected with fibular hypoplasia and complex brachydactyly (DuPan syndrome). *Clin Genet* 2002;61:454–458.

589 Vosshenrich R, Bartkowski R, Fischer U, Grone HJ. [Splenogonadal fusion]. *Rofo* 1991;155:191–193.

590 Bonneau D, Roume J, Gonzalez M, Toutain A, Carles D, Marechaud M et al. Splenogonadal fusion limb defect syndrome: report of five new cases and review. *Am J Med Genet* 1999;86:347–58.

591 Pauli RM, Greenlaw A. Limb deficiency and splenogonadal fusion. *Am J Med Genet* 1982;13:81–90.

592 Bearss RW. Splenic-gonadal fusion. *Urology* 1980;16:277–279.

593 Moore PJ, Hawkins EP, Galliani CA, Guerry-Force ML. Splenogonadal fusion with limb deficiency and micrognathia. *South Med J* 1997;90:1152–1155.
594 Bonafede RP, Beighton P. Autosomal dominant inheritance of scalp defects with ectrodactyly. *Am J Med Genet* 1979;3:35–41.
595 Fryns JP, Legius E, Demaerel P, van den BH. Congenital scalp defect, distal limb reduction anomalies, right spastic hemiplegia and hypoplasia of the left arteria cerebri media. Further evidence that interruption of early embryonic blood supply may result in Adams-Oliver (plus) syndrome. *Clin Genet* 1996;50:505–509.
596 Verdyck P, Holder-Espinasse M, Hul WV, Wuyts W. Clinical and molecular analysis of nine families with Adams-Oliver syndrome. *Eur J Hum Genet* 2003;11:457–463.
597 Ishikiriyama S, Kaou B, Udagawa A, Niwa K. Congenital heart defect in a Japanese girl with Adams-Oliver syndrome: one of the most important complications. *Am J Med Genet* 1992; 43:900–901.
598 Bamforth JS, Kaurah P, Byrne J, Ferreira P. Adams Oliver syndrome: a family with extreme variability in clinical expression. *Am J Med Genet* 1994;49:393–396.
599 Zapata HH, Sletten LJ, Pierpont ME. Congenital cardiac malformations in Adams-Oliver syndrome. *Clin Genet* 1995;47: 80–84.
600 Lin AE, Westgate MN, van der Velde ME, Lacro RV, Holmes LB. Adams-Oliver syndrome associated with cardiovascular malformations. *Clin Dysmorphol* 1998;7:235–241.
601 Savarirayan R, Thompson EM, Abbott KJ, Moore MH. Cerebral cortical dysplasia and digital constriction rings in Adams-Oliver syndrome. *Am J Med Genet* 1999;86:15–19.
602 Swartz EN, Sanatani S, Sandor GG, Schreiber RA. Vascular abnormalities in Adams-Oliver syndrome: cause or effect? *Am J Med Genet* 1999;82:49–52.
603 Amor DJ, Leventer RJ, Hayllar S, Bankier A. Polymicrogyria associated with scalp and limb defects: variant of Adams-Oliver syndrome. *Am J Med Genet* 2000;93:328–334.
604 Becker R, Kunze J, Horn D, Gasiorek-Wiens A, Entezami M, Rossi R et al. Autosomal recessive type of Adams-Oliver syndrome: prenatal diagnosis. *Ultrasound Obstet Gynecol* 2002;20:506–510.
605 Newman CG. The thalidomide syndrome: risks of exposure and spectrum of malformations. *Clin Perinatol* 1986;13:555–573.
606 Lee A, Kratochwil A, Deutinger J, Bernaschek G. Three-dimensional ultrasound in diagnosing phocomelia. *Ultrasound Obstet Gynecol* 1995;5:238–240.
607 Waldenmaier C, Aldenhoff P, Klemm T. The Roberts' syndrome. *Hum Genet* 1978;40:345–349.
608 Sinha AK, Verma RS, Mani VJ. Clinical heterogeneity of skeletal dysplasia in Roberts syndrome: a review. *Hum Hered* 1994;44:121–126.
609 de Ravel TJ, Seftel MD, Wright CA. Tetra-amelia and splenogonadal fusion in Roberts syndrome. *Am J Med Genet* 1997;68:185–189.
610 Benzacken B, Savary JB, Manouvrier S, et al. Prenatal diagnosis of Roberts syndrome: two new cases. *Prenat Diagn* 1996;16:125–130.
611 Grundy HO, Burlbaw J, Walton S, Dannar C. Roberts syndrome: antenatal ultrasound: a case report. *J Perinat Med* 1988;16: 71–75.
612 Robins DB, Ladda RL, Thieme GA, et al. Prenatal detection of Roberts-SC phocomelia syndrome: report of 2 sibs with characteristic manifestations. *Am J Med Genet* 1989;32:390–394.
613 Sherer DM, Shah YG, Klionsky N, Woods JR, Jr. Prenatal sonographic features and management of a fetus with Roberts-SC phocomelia syndrome (pseudothalidomide syndrome) and pulmonary hypoplasia. *Am J Perinatol*1991;8:259–262.
614 Hirschhorn K, Kaffe S. Prenatal diagnosis of Roberts syndrome. *Prenat Diagn* 1992;12:976.
615 Stioui S, Privitera O, Brambati B, et al. First-trimester prenatal diagnosis of Roberts syndrome. *Prenat Diagn* 1992;12:145–149.
616 Gruber A, Rabinerson D, Kaplan B, Ovadia Y. Prenatal diagnosis of Roberts syndrome. *Prenat Diagn* 1994;14:511–512.
617 Sharma AK, Jain A, Phadke SR, Srivastava S. Prenatal diagnosis of Roberts syndrome. *Indian Pediatr* 1994;31:1261–1264.
618 Otano L, Matayoshi T, Gadow EC. Roberts syndrome: first-trimester prenatal diagnosis. *Prenat Diagn* 1996;16:770–771.
619 Paladini D, Palmieri S, Lecora M, et al. Prenatal ultrasound diagnosis of Roberts syndrome in a family with negative history. *Ultrasound Obstet Gynecol* 1996;7:208–210.
620 Grebe H. Die Achondrogenesis: ein einfach rezessives. *Erbmerkmal Folia Hered Path* 1952;2:23–28.
621 Quelce-salGado A. A new type of dwarfism with various bone aplasias and hypoplasias of the extremities. *Acta Genet Stat Med* 1964;14:63–66.
622 Kumar D. Grebe syndrome. In: Buyse ML, edi. Birth defects encyclopedia. Cambridge: Blackwell Science; 1990: 813–814.
623 Kulkarni ML, Kulkarni BM, Nasser PU. Antenatal diagnosis of Grebe syndrome in a twin pregnancy by ultrasound. *Indian Pediatr* 1995;32:1007–1011.
624 Rittler M, Higa S. Grebe syndrome: a second case with extremely severe manifestations. *J Med Genet* 1997;34:1038.
625 Garcia-tcastro JM, Perez-Comas A. Nonlethal achondrogenesis (Grebe-Quelce-Salgado type) in two Puerto Rican sibships. *J Pediatr* 1975;87:948–952.
626 Costa T, Ramsby G, Cassia F, et al. Grebe syndrome: clinical and radiographic findings in affected individuals and heterozygous carriers. *Am J Med Genet* 1998;75:523–529.
627 Kumar D, Curtis D, Blank CE. Grebe chondrodysplasia and brachydactyly in a family. *Clin Genet* 1984;25:68–72.
628 Beighton P. Heterozygous manifestations in the heritable disorders of the skeleton. *Pediatr Radiol* 1997;27:397–401.
629 Curtis D. Heterozygote expression in Grebe chondrodysplasia. *Clin Genet* 1986;29:455–456.
630 Thomas JT, Kilpatrick MW, Lin K, et al. Disruption of human limb morphogenesis by a dominant negative mutation in CDMP1. *Nat Genet* 1997;17:58–64.
631 Munoz Rojas MV, Goncalves LF. Grebe-Quelce-Salgado chondrodystrophy: prenatal diagnosis of two new cases in unrelated families in Southern Brazil. *Am J Med Genet* 2002;113:193–199.
632 Hamanishi C. Congenital short femur. Clinical, genetic and epidemiological comparison of the naturally occurring condition with that caused by thalidomide. *J Bone Joint Surg Br* 1980; 62:307–320.
633 Daentl DL, Smith DW, Scott CI, Hall BD, Gooding CA. Femoral hypoplasia: unusual facies syndrome. *J Pediatr* 1975;86: 107–111.
634 Sanpera I, Jr, Fixsen JA, Sparks LT, Hill RA. Knee in congenital short femur. *J Pediatr Orthop B* 1995;4:159–163.
635 Makino Y, Inoue T, Shirota K, et al. A case of congenital familial short femur diagnosed prenatally. *Fetal Diagn Ther* 1998;13:206–208.
636 Hadi HA, Wade A. Prenatal diagnosis of unilateral proximal femoral focal deficiency in diabetic pregnancy: a case report. *Am J Perinatol* 1993;10:285–287.

637 Goncalves LF, De Luca GR, Vitorello DA, et al. Prenatal diagnosis of bilateral proximal femoral hypoplasia. *Ultrasound Obstet Gynecol* 1996;8:127–130.

638 Kalaycioglu A, Aynaci O. Proximal focal femoral deficiency, contralateral hip dysplasia in association with contralateral ulnar hypoplasia and clefthand: a case report and review of literatures of PFFD and/or FFU. *Okajimas Folia Anat Jpn* 2001;78:83–89.

639 Filly AL, Robnett-Filly B, Filly RA. Syndromes with focal femoral deficiency: strengths and weaknesses of prenatal sonography. *J Ultrasound Med* 2004;23:1511–1516.

640 Sen Gupta DK, Gupta SK. Familial bilateral proximal femoral focal deficiency. Report of a kindred. *J Bone Joint Surg (Am)* 1984;66:1470–1472.

641 Frey M, Williams J. What is your diagnosis? Radiographic diagnosis: ectrodactyly. *J Am Vet Med Assoc* 1995;206:619–620.

642 Miura T, Suzuki M. Clinical differences between typical and atypical cleft hand. *J Hand Surg (Br)* 1984;9:311–315.

643 Glicenstein J, Guero S, Haddad R. [Median clefts of the hand. Classification and therapeutic indications apropos of 29 cases]. *Ann Chir Main Memb Super* 1995;14:253.

644 Tada K, Yonenobu K, Swanson AB. Congenital central ray deficiency in the hand: a survey of 59 cases and subclassification. *J Hand Surg (Am)* 1981;6:434–441.

645 van den BH, Dequeker J, Fryns JP, David G. Familial occurrence of severe ulnar aplasia and lobster claw feet: a new syndrome. *Hum Genet* 1978;42:109–113.

646 Verma IC, Joseph R, Bhargava S, Mehta S. Split-hand and split-foot deformity inherited as an autosomal recessive trait. *Clin Genet* 1976;9:8–14.

647 Roelfsema NM, Cobben JM. The EEC syndrome: a literature study. *Clin Dysmorphol* 1996;5:115–127.

648 Rudiger RA, Haase W, Passarge E. Association of ectrodactyly, ectodermal dysplasia, and cleft lip-palate. *Am J Dis Child* 1970;120:160–163.

649 Miller CI, Hashimoto K, Shwayder T, et al. What syndrome is this? Ectrodactyly, ectodermal dysplasia, and cleft palate (EEC) syndrome. *Pediatr Dermatol* 1997;14:239–240.

650 Kasmann B, Ruprecht KW. Ocular manifestations in a father and son with EEC syndrome. *Graefes Arch Clin Exp Ophthalmol* 1997;235:512–516.

651 Buss PW, Hughes HE, Clarke A. Twenty-four cases of the EEC syndrome: clinical presentation and management. *J Med Genet* 1995;32:716–723.

652 Krunic AL, Vesic SA, Goldner B, et al. Ectrodactyly, soft-tissue syndactyly, and nodulocystic acne: coincidence or association? *Pediatr Dermatol* 1997;14:31–35.

653 Gershoni-Baruch R, Goldscher D, Hochberg Z. Ectrodactyly-ectodermal dysplasia-clefting syndrome and hypothalamo-pituitary insufficiency. *Am J Med Genet* 1997;68:168–172.

654 Maas SM, de Jong TP, Buss P, Hennekam RC. EEC syndrome and genitourinary anomalies: an update. *Am J Med Genet* 1996;63:472–478.

655 Leiter E, Lipson J. Genitourinary tract anomalies in lobster claw syndrome. *J Urol* 1976;115:339–341.

656 Penchaszadeh VB, de Negrotti TC. Ectrodactyly-ectodermal dysplasia-clefting (EEC) syndrome: dominant inheritance and variable expression. *J Med Genet* 1976;13:281–284.

657 Halal F, Homsy M, Perreault G. Acro-renal-ocular syndrome: autosomal dominant thumb hypoplasia, renal ectopia, and eye defect. *Am J Med Genet* 1984;17:753–762.

658 Chan KM, Lamb DW. Triphalangeal thumb and five-fingered hand. *Hand* 1983;15:329–334.

659 Wood VE. Congenital thumb deformities. *Clin Orthop* 1985;7–25.

660 Blauth W, Sonnichsen S. [Congenital clubhand]. *Orthopade* 1986;15:160–171.

661 Bujdoso G, Lenz W. Monodactylous splithand-splitfoot. A malformation occurring in three distinct genetic types. *Eur J Pediatr* 1980;133:207–215.

662 Goldberg MJ, Meyn M. The radial clubhand. *Orthop Clin North Am* 1976;7:341–359.

663 Carroll RE, Louis DS. Anomalies associated with radial dysplasia. *J Pediatr* 1974;84:409–411.

664 Alter BP. Bone marrow failure syndromes. *Clin Lab Med* 1999;19:113–133.

665 Glanz A, Fraser FC. Spectrum of anomalies in Fanconi anaemia. *J Med Genet* 1982;19:412–416.

666 Grill F, Freilinger W, Strobl W. [Treatment of a radial club hand]. *Z Orthop Ihre Grenzgeb* 1996;134:324–331.

667 Rotman MB, Manske PR. Radial clubhand and contralateral duplicated thumb. *J Hand Surg (Am)* 1994;19:361–363.

668 Bueno LO, Bueno M, I, Jimenez VA, et al. [A girl with pancytopenia, short stature and minor skeletal abnormalities]. *An Esp Pediatr* 1997;46:409–410.

669 Nilsson LR. Chronic pancytopenia with multiple congenital abnormalities (Fanconi's anaemia). *Acta Paediatr* 1960;49:518–529.

670 Prindull G, Stubbe P, Kratzer W. Fanconi's anemia. I. Case histories, clinical and laboratory findings in six affected siblings. *Z Kinderheilkd* 1975;120:37–49.

671 Levran O, Diotti R, Pujara K, et al. Spectrum of sequence variations in the FANCA gene: an International Fanconi Anemia Registry (IFAR) study. *Hum Mutat* 2005;25:142–149.

672 Lo TF, Jr., Rooimans MA, Bosnoyan-Collins L, et al. Expression cloning of a cDNA for the major Fanconi anaemia gene, FAA. *Nat Genet* 1996;14:320–323.

673 Digweed M. [Molecular basis of Fanconi's anemia]. *Klin Padiatr* 1999;211:192–197.

674 de Winter JP, Rooimans MA, van der WL, et al. The Fanconi anaemia gene FANCF encodes a novel protein with homology to ROM. *Nat Genet* 2000;24:15–16.

675 Howlett NG, Taniguchi T, Olson S, et al. Biallelic inactivation of BRCA2 in Fanconi anemia. *Science* 2002;297:606–609.

676 Meetei AR, de Winter JP, Medhurst AL, et al. A novel ubiquitin ligase is deficient in Fanconi anemia. *Nat Genet* 2003;35:165–170.

677 Timmers C, Taniguchi T, Hejna J, et al. Positional cloning of a novel Fanconi anemia gene, FANCD2. *Mol Cell* 2001;7:241–248.

678 Strathdee CA, Duncan AM, Buchwald M. Evidence for at least four Fanconi anaemia genes including FACC on chromosome 9. *Nat Genet* 1992;1:196–198.

679 Ianzano L, D'Apolito M, Centra M, et al. The genomic organization of the Fanconi anemia group A (FAA) gene. *Genomics* 1997;41:309–314.

680 Auerbach AD, Warburton D, Bloom AD, Chaganti RS. Preliminary communication: prenatal detection of the Fanconi Anemia gene by cytogenetic methods. *Am J Hum Genet* 1979;31:77–81.

681 Auerbach AD, Adler B, Chaganti RS. Prenatal and postnatal diagnosis and carrier detection of Fanconi anemia by a cytogenetic method. *Pediatrics* 1981;67:128–135.

682 Auerbach AD, Sagi M, Adler B. Fanconi anemia: prenatal diagnosis in 30 fetuses at risk. *Pediatrics* 1985;76:794–800.

683 Kwee ML, Lo TF, Jr, Arwert F, et al. Early prenatal diagnosis of Fanconi anaemia in a twin pregnancy, using DNA analysis. *Prenat Diagn* 1996;16:345–348.
684 Marx MP, Dawson B, Heyns AD. Prenatal diagnosis of Fanconi's anemia. *S Afr Med J* 1982;62:348.
685 Murer-Orlando M, Llerena JC, Jr, Birjandi F, et al. FACC gene mutations and early prenatal diagnosis of Fanconi's anaemia. *Lancet* 1993;342:686.
686 Voss R, Kohn G, Shaham M, et al. Prenatal diagnosis of Fanconi anemia. *Clin Genet* 1981;20:185–190.
687 Merrill A, Rosenblum-Vos L, Driscoll DA,et al. Prenatal diagnosis of Fanconi anemia (Group C) subsequent to abnormal sonographic findings. *Prenat Diagn* 2005;25:20–22.
688 Tercanli S, Miny P, Siebert MS, et al. Fanconi anemia associated with increased nuchal translucency detected by first-trimester ultrasound. *Ultrasound Obstet Gynecol* 2001;17:160–162.
689 Shimamura, A., Moreau, L., and D'Andrea, A. Fanconi anemia. Copyright, University of Washington, Seattle, 1993–2005. Updated weekly. GeneTests: Medical Genetics Information Resource (database online), 2004. 20 February 2005.
690 Hall JG, Levin J, Kuhn JP, et al. Thrombocytopenia with absent radius (TAR). *Medicine (Baltimore)* 1969;48:411–439.
691 de Alarcon PA, Graeve JA, Levine RF, et al. Thrombocytopenia and absent radii syndrome: defective megakaryocytopoiesis-thrombocytopoiesis. *Am J Pediatr Hematol Oncol* 1991;13: 77–83.
692 Ballmaier M, Schulze H, Strauss G, et al. Thrombopoietin in patients with congenital thrombocytopenia and absent radii: elevated serum levels, normal receptor expression, but defective reactivity to thrombopoietin. *Blood* 1997;90:612–619.
693 Sekine I, Hagiwara T, Miyazaki H, et al. Thrombocytopenia with absent radii syndrome: studies on serum thrombopoietin levels and megakaryopoiesis in vitro. *J Pediatr Hematol Oncol* 1998;20:74–78.
694 Miceli S, Jure MA, de Saab OA, et al. A clinical and bacteriological study of children suffering from haemolytic uraemic syndrome in Tucuman, Argentina. *Jpn J Infect Dis* 1999;52:33–37.
695 de Vries LS, Connell J, Bydder GM, et al. Recurrent intracranial haemorrhages in utero in an infant with alloimmune thrombocytopenia. Case report. *Br J Obstet Gynaecol* 1988;95:299–302.
696 Shelton SD, Paulyson K, Kay HH. Prenatal diagnosis of thrombocytopenia absent radius (TAR) syndrome and vaginal delivery. *Prenat Diagn* 1999;19:54–57.
697 Luthy DA, Mack L, Hirsch J, Cheng E. Prenatal ultrasound diagnosis of thrombocytopenia with absent radii. *Am J Obstet Gynecol* 1981;141:350–351.
698 Daffos F, Forestier F, Kaplan C, Cox W. Prenatal diagnosis and management of bleeding disorders with fetal blood sampling. *Am J Obstet Gynecol* 1988;158:939–946.
699 Hedberg VA, Lipton JM. Thrombocytopenia with absent radii. A review of 100 cases. *Am J Pediatr Hematol Oncol* 1988;10:51–64.
700 Donnenfeld AE, Wiseman B, Lavi E, Weiner S. Prenatal diagnosis of thrombocytopenia absent radius syndrome by ultrasound and cordocentesis. *Prenat Diagn* 1990;10:29–35.
701 Fromm B, Niethard FU, Marquardt E. Thrombocytopenia and absent radius (TAR) syndrome. *Int Orthop* 1991;15:95–99.
702 Delooz J, Moerman P, van den BK, Fryns JP. Tetraphocomelia and bilateral femorotibial synostosis. A severe variant of the thrombocytopenia-absent radii (TAR) syndrome? *Genet Couns* 1992;3:91–93.
703 Labrune P, Pons JC, Khalil M, et al. Antenatal thrombocytopenia in three patients with TAR (thrombocytopenia with absent radii) syndrome. *Prenat Diagn* 1993;13:463–466.
704 Donnenfeld AE. Prenatal diagnosis of thrombocytopenia in TAR syndrome. *Prenat Diagn* 1994;14:73–74.
705 Weinblatt M, Petrikovsky B, Bialer M, et al. Prenatal evaluation and in utero platelet transfusion for thrombocytopenia absent radii syndrome. *Prenat Diagn* 1994;14:892–896.
706 Boute O, Depret-Mosser S, Vinatier D, et al. Prenatal diagnosis of thrombocytopenia-absent radius syndrome. *Fetal Diagn Ther* 1996;11:224–230.
707 Ergur A, Yergok YZ, Ertekin A, et al. Prenatal diagnosis of an uncommon syndrome: thrombocytopenia absent radius (TAR). *Zentralbl Gynakol* 1998;120:75–78.
708 Urban M, Opitz C, Bommer C, et al. Bilaterally cleft lip, limb defects, and haematological manifestations: Roberts syndrome versus TAR syndrome. *Am J Med Genet* 1998;79:155–160.
709 Muis N, Beemer FA, van Dijken P, Klep-de Pater JM. The Aase syndrome. Case report and review of the literature. *Eur J Pediatr* 1986;145:153–157.
710 D'Avanzo M, Pistoia V, Tolone C, et al. Aase-Smith syndrome: report of a new case. *Br J Haematol* 1988;70:125–126.
711 Hing AV, Dowton SB. Aase syndrome: novel radiographic features. *Am J Med Genet* 1993;45:413–415.
712 Yetgin S, Balci S, Irken G, et al. Aase-Smith syndrome: report of a new case with unusual features. *Turk J Pediatr* 1994; 36:239–242.
713 Pfeiffer RA, Ambs E. [The Aase syndrome: hereditary autosomal recessive congenital erythropoiesis insufficiency and triphalangeal thumbs]. *Monatsschr Kinderheilkd* 1983;131:235–237.
714 Dror Y, Durie P, Marcon P, Freedman MH. Duplication of distal thumb phalanx in Shwachman-Diamond syndrome. *Am J Med Genet* 1998;78:67–69.
715 Schneider MD, Schwartz RJ. Heart or hand? Unmasking the basis for specific Holt-Oram phenotypes. *Proc Natl Acad Sci USA* 1999;96:2577–2578.
716 McLennan AC, Chitty LS, Rissik J, Maxwell DJ. Prenatal diagnosis of Blackfan-Diamond syndrome: case report and review of the literature. *Prenat Diagn* 1996;16:349–353.
717 Bennhagen RG, Menahem S. Holt-Oram syndrome and multiple ventricular septal defects: an association suggesting a possible genetic marker? *Cardiol Young* 1998;8:128–130.
718 Bohm M. Holt-Oram syndrome. Circulation 1998;98:2636–2637.
719 James MA, McCarroll HR, Jr, Manske PR. Characteristics of patients with hypoplastic thumbs. *J Hand Surg (Am)* 1996;21:104–113.
720 Wilson GN. Correlated heart/limb anomalies in Mendelian syndromes provide evidence for a cardiomelic developmental field. *Am J Med Genet* 1998;76:297–305.
721 Brockhoff CJ, Kober H, Tsilimingas N, et al. Holt-Oram syndrome. *Circulation* 1999;99:1395–1396.
722 Cachat F, Rapatsalahy A, Sekarski N, et al. [Three different types of atrial septal defects in the same family]. *Arch Mal Coeur Vaiss* 1999;92:667–669.
723 Elbaum R, Royer M, Godart S. Radial club hand and Holt-Oram syndrome. *Acta Chir Belg* 1995;95:229–236.
724 Sletten LJ, Pierpont ME. Variation in severity of cardiac disease in Holt-Oram syndrome. *Am J Med Genet* 1996;65:128–132.
725 Brons JT, van Geijn HP, Wladimiroff JW, et al. Prenatal ultrasound diagnosis of the Holt-Oram syndrome. *Prenat Diagn* 1988;8:175–181.

726 Matsuoka R. [Holt-Oram syndrome]. *Ryoikibetsu Shokogun Shirizu* 1996;267–270.
727 Newbury-Ecob RA, Leanage R, Raeburn JA, Young ID. Holt-Oram syndrome: a clinical genetic study. *J Med Genet* 1996;33:300–307.
728 Zhang KZ, Sun QB, Cheng TO. Holt-Oram syndrome in China: a collective review of 18 cases. *Am Heart J* 1986;111:572–577.
729 Muller LM, De Jong G, Van Heerden KM. The antenatal ultrasonographic detection of the Holt-Oram syndrome. *S Afr Med J* 1985;68:313–15.
730 Tongsong T, Chanprapaph P. Prenatal sonographic diagnosis of Holt-Oram syndrome. *J Clin Ultrasound* 2000;28:98–100.
731 Lehner R, Goharkhay N, Tringler B, et al. Pedigree analysis and descriptive investigation of three classic phenotypes associated with Holt-Oram syndrome. *J Reprod Med* 2003;48:153–159.
732 Sepulveda W, Enriquez G, Martinez JL, Mejia R. Holt-Oram syndrome: contribution of prenatal 3–dimensional sonography in an index case. *J Ultrasound Med* 2004;23:983–987.
733 Li QY, Newbury-Ecob RA, Terrett JA, et al. Holt-Oram syndrome is caused by mutations in TBX5, a member of the Brachyury (T) gene family. *Nat Genet* 1997;15:21–29.
734 Basson CT, Huang T, Lin RC, Bachinsky DR, et al. Different TBX5 interactions in heart and limb defined by Holt-Oram syndrome mutations. *Proc Natl Acad Sci USA* 1999;96:2919–2924.
735 He J, McDermott DA, Song Y, et al. Preimplantation genetic diagnosis of human congenital heart malformation and Holt-Oram syndrome. *Am J Med Genet* 2004;126:93–98.
736 Lewis KB, Bruce RA, Baum D, Motulsky AG. The upper limb-cardiovascular syndrome. An autosomal dominant genetic effect on embryogenesis. *JAMA* 1965;193:1080–1086.
737 Chemke J, Nisani R, Fischel RE. Absent ulna in the Klippel-Feil syndrome: an unusual associated malformation. *Clin Genet* 1980;17:167–170.
738 Masuno M. [VATER association (VACTERL association)]. *Ryoikibetsu Shokogun Shirizu* 1996;309–310.
739 Medina-Escobedo G, Ridaura-Sanz C. [The VATER association]. *Bol Med Hosp Infant Mex* 1992;49:231–240.
740 Temtamy SA, Miller JD. Extending the scope of the VATER association: definition of the VATER syndrome. *J Pediatr* 1974;85: 345–349.
741 Quillin SP, Gilula LA. Imaging rounds #111. VATER association. *Orthop Rev* 1992;21:85, 88–85, 89.
742 Corsello G, Maresi E, Corrao AM, et al. VATER/VACTERL association: clinical variability and expanding phenotype including laryngeal stenosis. *Am J Med Genet* 1992;44:813–815.
743 Quan L, Smith DW. The VATER association. Vertebral defects, Anal atresia, T-E fistula with esophageal atresia, Radial and Renal dysplasia: a spectrum of associated defects. *J Pediatr* 1973;82:104–107.
744 Botto LD, Khoury MJ, Mastroiacovo P, et al. The spectrum of congenital anomalies of the VATER association: an international study. *Am J Med Genet* 1997;71:8–15.
745 Unuvar E, Oguz F, Sahin K, et al. Coexistence of VATER association and recurrent urolithiasis: a case report. *Pediatr Nephrol* 1998;12:141–143.
746 Werner W, Beintker M, Schubert J, Kaiser WA. [The VATER syndrome from the urologic viewpoint]. *Urologe A* 1998;37: 203–205.
747 Auchterlonie IA, White MP. Recurrence of the VATER association within a sibship. *Clin Genet* 1982;21:122–124.
748 Ozbey H, Ozbey N. Association of ambiguous genitalia with VATER anomalies. *Pediatr Surg Int* 1997;12:230.
749 Tongsong T, Wanapirak C, Piyamongkol W, Sudasana J. Prenatal sonographic diagnosis of VATER association. *J Clin Ultrasound* 1999;27:378–384.
750 Claiborne AK, Blocker SH, Martin CM, McAlister WH. Prenatal and postnatal sonographic delineation of gastrointestinal abnormalities in a case of the VATER syndrome. *J Ultrasound Med* 1986;5:45–47.
751 Harris RD, Nyberg DA, Mack LA, Weinberger E. Anorectal atresia: prenatal sonographic diagnosis. *Am J Roentgenol* 1987; 149:395–400.
752 McGahan JP, Leeba JM, Lindfors KK. Prenatal sonographic diagnosis of VATER association. *J Clin Ultrasound* 1988;16: 588–591.
753 Froster UG, Wallner SJ, Reusche E, et al. VACTERL with hydrocephalus and branchial arch defects: prenatal, clinical, and autopsy findings in two brothers. *Am J Med Genet* 1996;62: 169–172.
754 Miller OF, Kolon TF. Prenatal diagnosis of VACTERL association. *J Urol* 2001;166:2389–2391.
755 Tercanli S, Troeger C, Fahnenstich H, et al. [Prenatal diagnosis and management in VACTERL association]. *Z Geburtshilfe Neonatol* 2001;205:65–70.
756 Tongsong T, Chanprapaph P, Khunamornpong S. Prenatal diagnosis of VACTERL association: a case report. *J Med Assoc Thai* 2001;84:143–148.
757 Krapp M, Geipel A, Germer U, et al. First-trimester sonographic diagnosis of distal urethral atresia with megalourethra in VACTERL association. *Prenat Diagn* 2002;22: 422–424.
758 Ardiet E, Houfflin-Debarge V, Besson R, et al. Prenatal diagnosis of congenital megalourethra associated with VACTERL sequence in twin pregnancy: favorable postnatal outcome. *Ultrasound Obstet Gynecol* 2003;21:619–620.
759 Chen CP, Shih JC, Chang JH, et al. Prenatal diagnosis of right pulmonary agenesis associated with VACTERL sequence. *Prenat Diagn* 2003;23:515–518.
760 Rollnick BR, Kaye CI, Nagatoshi K, et al. Oculoauriculovertebral dysplasia and variants: phenotypic characteristics of 294 patients. *Am J Med Genet* 1987;26:361–375.
761 Lal P, Agrawal P, Krishna A. Goldenhar syndrome. *Indian Pediatr* 1997;34:837–838.
762 Manfre L, Genuardi P, Tortorici M, Lagalla R. Absence of the common crus in Goldenhar syndrome. *Am J Neuroradiol* 1997;18:773–775.
763 Altamar-Rios J. [Goldenhar's syndrome: a case report]. *An Otorrinolaringol Ibero Am* 1998;25:491–497.
764 Ferraris S, Silengo M, Ponzone A, Perugini L. Goldenhar anomaly in one of triplets derived from in vitro fertilization. *Am J Med Genet* 1999;84:167–168.
765 Tamas DE, Mahony BS, Bowie JD, et al. Prenatal sonographic diagnosis of hemifacial microsomia (Goldenhar-Gorlin syndrome). *J Ultrasound Med* 1986;5:461–463.
766 Matsuo K. [Oculoauriculovertebral syndrome (Goldenhar syndrome)]. *Ryoikibetsu Shokogun Shirizu* 1996;287–288.
767 Tekkok IH. Syringomyelia as a complication of Goldenhar syndrome. *Childs Nerv Syst* 1996;12:291.
768 Araneta MR, Moore CA, Olney RS, et al. Goldenhar syndrome among infants born in military hospitals to Gulf War veterans. *Teratology* 1997;56:244–251.
769 Luchtenberg M, Blotiu A, Lindemann G, Emmerich KH. [Anomalies of the efferent lacrimal ducts in Goldenhar syndrome]. *Klin Monatsbl Augenheilkd* 1998;213:aA8–aA9.

770 Jeanty P, Zaleski W, Fleischer AC. Prenatal sonographic diagnosis of lipoma of the corpus callosum in a fetus with Goldenhar syndrome. *Am J Perinatol* 1991;8:89–90.
771 De Catte L, Laubach M, Legein J, Goossens A. Early prenatal diagnosis of oculoauriculovertebral dysplasia or the Goldenhar syndrome. *Ultrasound Obstet Gynecol* 1996;8:422–424.
772 Kita D, Munemoto S, Ueno Y, Fukuda A. Goldenhar's syndrome associated with occipital meningoencephalocele—case report. *Neurol Med Chir (Tokyo)* 2002;42:354–355.
773 Martinelli P, Maruotti GM, Agangi A, et al Prenatal diagnosis of hemifacial microsomia and ipsilateral cerebellar hypoplasia in a fetus with oculoauriculovertebral spectrum. *Ultrasound Obstet Gynecol* 2004;24:199–201.
774 Thompson GH. The neck. In: Behrman GH, Kliegman RM, Jenson HB, eds. *Behrman: Nelson textbook of pediatrics*. Philadelphia, PA: WB Saunders; 2004: 2288–2290.
775 Gausewitz SH, Meals RA, Setoguchi Y. Severe limb deficiency in Poland's syndrome. *Clin Orthop* 1984;9–13.
776 Swanson AB, Tada K, Yonenobu K. Ulnar ray deficiency: its various manifestations. *J Hand Surg (Am)* 1984;9:658–664.
777 Uuspaa V. Upper extremity deformities associated with the orofacial clefts. *Scand J Plast Reconstr Surg* 1978;12:157–162.
778 David TJ. Preaxial polydactyly and the Poland complex. *Am J Med Genet* 1982;13:333–334.
779 de la TJ, Simpson RL. Complete digital duplication: a case report and review of ulnar polydactyly. *Ann Plast Surg* 1998;40:76–79.
780 Graham TJ, Ress AM. Finger polydactyly. *Hand Clin* 1998; 14:49–64.
781 De Smet L. Ulnar dimelia. *Acta Orthop Belg* 1999;65:382–384.
782 Kaplan BS, Bellah RD. Postaxial polydactyly, ulnar ray dysgenesis, and renal cystic dysplasia in sibs. *Am J Med Genet* 1999;87:426–429.
783 Bader B, Grill F, Lamprecht E. [Polydactyly of the foot]. *Orthopade* 1999;28:125–132.
784 Kleanthous JK, Kleanthous EM, Hahn PJ, Jr. Polydactyly of the foot. Overview with case presentations. *J Am Podiatr Med Assoc* 1998;88:493–499.
785 Goodman RM, Sternberg M, Shem-Tov Y, Katznelson MB, et al. Acrocephalopolysyndactyly type IV: a new genetic syndrome in 3 sibs. *Clin Genet* 1979;15:209–214.
786 Lowry RB. Editorial comment: variability in the Smith-Lemli-Opitz syndrome: overlap with the Meckel syndrome. *Am J Med Genet* 1983;14:429–433.
787 Khaldi F, Bennaceur B, Hammou A, et al. An autosomal recessive disorder with retardation of growth, mental deficiency, ptosis, pectus excavatum and camptodactyly. *Pediatr Radiol* 1988;18:432–435.
788 Porter HJ. Lethal arthrogryposis multiplex congenital (fetal akinesia deformation sequence, FADS). *Pediatr Pathol Lab Med* 1995;15:617–637.
789 Gordon N. Arthrogryposis multiplex congenita. *Brain Dev* 1998;20:507–511.
790 Seringe R. [Congenital equinovarus clubfoot]. *Acta Orthop Belg* 1999;65:127–153.
791 Swinyard CA, Bleck EE. The etiology of arthrogryposis (multiple congenital contracture). *Clin Orthop* 1985;15–29.
792 Hall JG. Arthrogryposis multiplex congenita: etiology, genetics, classification, diagnostic approach, and general aspects. *J Pediatr Orthop B* 1997;6:159–166.
793 Jacobson L, Polizzi A, Vincent A. An animal model of maternal antibody-mediated arthrogryposis multiplex congenita (AMC). *Ann NY Acad Sci* 1998;841:565–567.
794 Drachman DB, Coulombre AJ. Experimental clubfoot and arthrogryposis multiplex congenita. *Lancet* 1962;2:523–526.
795 Moessinger AC. Fetal akinesia deformation sequence: an animal model. *Pediatrics* 1983;72:857–863.
796 Drachman DB, Weiner LP, Price DL, Chase J. Experimental arthrogryposis caused by viral myopathy. *Arch Neurol* 1976;33:362–367.
797 Drachman DA, Sokoloff L. The role of movement in embryonic joint development. *Development* 1966;14:401–420.
798 Banker BQ. Neuropathologic aspects of arthrogryposis multiplex congenita. *Clin Orthop* 1985;30–43.
799 Swinyard CA. Concepts of multiple congenital contractures (arthrogryposis) in man and animals. *Teratology* 1982;25: 247–258.
800 Quinn CM, Wigglesworth JS, Heckmatt J. Lethal arthrogryposis multiplex congenita: a pathological study of 21 cases. *Histopathology* 1991;19:155–162.
801 Thompson GH, Bilenker RM. Comprehensive management of arthrogryposis multiplex congenita. *Clin Orthop* 1985;6–14.
802 Burglen L, Amiel J, Viollet L, et al. Survival motor neuron gene deletion in the arthrogryposis multiplex congenita-spinal muscular atrophy association. *J Clin Invest* 1996;98:1130–1132.
803 Hall JG. Genetic aspects of arthrogryposis. *Clin Orthop* 1985;44–53.
804 Herva R, Leisti J, Kirkinen P, Seppanen U. A lethal autosomal recessive syndrome of multiple congenital contractures. *Am J Med Genet* 1985;20:431–439.
805 Lerman-Sagie T, Levi Y, Kidron D, et al. Syndrome of osteopetrosis and muscular degeneration associated with cerebro-oculo-facio-skeletal changes. *Am J Med Genet* 1987;28:137–412.
806 Illum N, Reske-Nielsen E, Skovby F, et al. Lethal autosomal recessive arthrogryposis multiplex congenita with whistling face and calcifications of the nervous system. *Neuropediatrics* 1988;19:186–192.
807 Hennekam RC, Barth PG, Van Lookeren CW, et al. A family with severe X-linked arthrogryposis. *Eur J Pediatr* 1991;150: 656–660.
808 Krakowiak PA, O'Quinn JR, Bohnsack JF, et al. A variant of Freeman-Sheldon syndrome maps to 11p15.5–pter. *Am J Hum Genet* 1997;60:426–432.
809 Shohat M, Lotan R, Magal N, et al. A gene for arthrogryposis multiplex congenita neuropathic type is linked to D5S394 on chromosome 5qter. *Am J Hum Genet* 1997;61:1139–1143.
810 Zori RT, Gardner JL, Zhang J, et al. Newly described form of X-linked arthrogryposis maps to the long arm of the human X chromosome. *Am J Med Genet* 1998;78:450–454.
811 Hall JG, Reed SD. Teratogens associated with congenital contractures in humans and in animals. *Teratology* 1982;25: 173–191.
812 Smith DW, Clarren SK, Harvey MA. Hyperthermia as a possible teratogenic agent. *J Pediatr* 1978;92:878–883.
813 Vincent A, Newland C, Brueton L, et al. Arthrogryposis multiplex congenita with maternal autoantibodies specific for a fetal antigen. *Lancet* 1995;346:24–25.
814 Riemersma S, Vincent A, Beeson D, et al. Association of arthrogryposis multiplex congenita with maternal antibodies inhibiting fetal acetylcholine receptor function. *J Clin Invest* 1996;98: 2358–2363.
815 Jacobson L, Polizzi A, Morriss-Kay G, Vincent A. Plasma from human mothers of fetuses with severe arthrogryposis multiplex congenita causes deformities in mice. *J Clin Invest* 1999;103: 1031–1038.

816 Rivera MR, Avila CA, Kofman-Alfaro S. Distal arthrogryposis type IIB: probable autosomal recessive inheritance. *Clin Genet* 1999;56:95–97.

817 Hall JG. An approach to research on congenital contractures. *Birth Defects Orig Artic Ser* 1984;20:8–30.

818 Dudkiewicz I, Achiron R, Ganel A. Prenatal diagnosis of distal arthrogryposis type 1. *Skeletal Radiol* 1999;28:233–235.

819 Goldberg JD, Chervenak FA, Lipman RA, Berkowitz RL. Antenatal sonographic diagnosis of arthrogryposis multiplex congenita. *Prenat Diagn* 1986;6:45–49.

820 Gorczyca DP, McGahan JP, Lindfors KK, et al. Arthrogryposis multiplex congenita: prenatal ultrasonographic diagnosis. *J Clin Ultrasound* 1989;17:40–44.

821 Kirkinen P, Herva R, Leisti J. Early prenatal diagnosis of a lethal syndrome of multiple congenital contractures. *Prenat Diagn* 1987;7:189–196.

822 Miskin M, Rothberg R, Rudd NL, et al. Arthrogryposis multiplex congenita—prenatal assessment with diagnostic ultrasound and fetoscopy. *J Pediatr* 1979;95:463–464.

823 Socol ML, Sabbagha RE, Elias S, et al. Prenatal diagnosis of congenital muscular dystrophy producing arthrogryposis. *N Engl J Med* 1985;313:1230.

824 Ajayi RA, Keen CE, Knott PD. Ultrasound diagnosis of the Pena Shokeir phenotype at 14 weeks of pregnancy. *Prenat Diagn* 1995;15:762–764.

825 Sepulveda W, Stagiannis KD, Cox PM, et al. Prenatal findings in generalized amyoplasia. *Prenat Diagn* 1995;15:660–664.

826 Scott H, Hunter A, Bedard B. Non-lethal arthrogryposis multiplex congenita presenting with cystic hygroma at 13 weeks gestational age. *Prenat Diagn* 1999;19:966–71.

827 Tongsong T, Chanprapaph P, Khunamornpong S. Prenatal ultrasound of regional akinesia with Pena-Shokeir phenotype. *Prenat Diagn* 2000;20:422–425.

828 Paladini D, Tartaglione A, Agangi A,et al. Pena-Shokeir phenotype with variable onset in three consecutive pregnancies. *Ultrasound Obstet Gynecol* 2001;17:163–165.

829 Madazli R, Tuysuz B, Aksoy F, et al. Prenatal diagnosis of arthrogryposis multiplex congenita with increased nuchal translucency but without any underlying fetal neurogenic or myogenic pathology. *Fetal Diagn Ther* 2002;17:29–33.

830 Witters I, Moerman P, Fryns JP. Fetal akinesia deformation sequence: a study of 30 consecutive in utero diagnoses. *Am J Med Genet* 2002;113:23–28.

831 Makrydimas G, Sotiriadis A, Papapanagiotou G, et al. Fetal akinesia deformation sequence presenting with increased nuchal translucency in the first trimester of pregnancy. *Fetal Diagn Ther* 2004;19:332–335.

832 Ruano R, Dumez Y, Dommergues M. Three-dimensional ultrasonographic appearance of the fetal akinesia deformation sequence. *J Ultrasound Med* 2003;22:593–599.

833 Fahy MJ, Hall JG. A retrospective study of pregnancy complications among 828 cases of arthrogryposis. *Genet Couns* 1990;1:3–11.

834 Byers PH. Brittle bones – fragile molecules: disorders of collagen gene structure and expression. *Trends Genet* 1990;6:293–300.

835 Prockop DJ, Kuivaniemi H, Tromp G. Molecular basis of osteogenesis imperfecta and related disorders of bone. *Clin Plast Surg* 1994;21:407–413.

836 Spranger J, Winterpacht A, Zabel B. The type II collagenopathies: a spectrum of *Eur* chondrodysplasias. *J Pediatr* 1994;153:56–65.

837 Lohiniva J, Paassilta P, Seppanen U, et al. Splicing mutations in the COL3 domain of collagen IX cause multiple epiphyseal dysplasia. *Am J Med Genet* 2000;90:216–222.

838 Spayde EC, Joshi AP, Wilcox WR, et al. Exon skipping mutation in the COL9A2 gene in a family with multiple epiphyseal dysplasia. *Matrix Biol* 2000;19:121–128.

839 Wallis GA, Rash B, Sykes B, et al. Mutations within the gene encoding the alpha 1 (X) chain of type X collagen (COL10A1) cause metaphyseal chondrodysplasia type Schmid but not several other forms of metaphyseal chondrodysplasia. *J Med Genet* 1996;33:450–457.

840 Melkoniemi M, Brunner HG, Manouvrier S, et al. Autosomal recessive disorder otospondylomegaepiphyseal dysplasia is associated with loss-of-function mutations in the COL11A2 gene. *Am J Hum Genet* 2000;66:368–377.

841 Spranger J. The type XI collagenopathies. *Pediatr Radiol* 1998;28:745–750.

842 Briggs MD, Mortier GR, Cole WG, et al. Diverse mutations in the gene for cartilage oligomeric matrix protein in the pseudoachondroplasia-multiple epiphyseal dysplasia disease spectrum. *Am J Hum Genet* 1998;62:311–319.

843 Chapman KL, Mortier GR, Chapman K, et al. Mutations in the region encoding the von Willebrand factor A domain of matrilin-3 are associated with multiple epiphyseal dysplasia. *Nat Genet* 2001;28:393–396.

844 Nurnberg P, Thiele H, Chandler D, et al. Heterozygous mutations in ANKH, the human ortholog of the mouse progressive ankylosis gene, result in craniometaphyseal dysplasia. *Nat Genet* 2001;28:37–41.

845 Reichenberger E, Tiziani V, Watanabe S, et al. Autosomal dominant craniometaphyseal dysplasia is caused by mutations in the transmembrane protein ANK. *Am J Hum Genet* 2001;68:1321–1326.

846 Superti-Furga A, Hastbacka J, Wilcox WR, et al. Achondrogenesis type IB is caused by mutations in the diastrophic dysplasia sulphate transporter gene. *Nat Genet* 1996;12:100–102.

847 Superti-Furga A, Rossi A, Steinmann B, Gitzelmann R. A chondrodysplasia family produced by mutations in the diastrophic dysplasia sulfate transporter gene: genotype/phenotype correlations. *Am J Med Genet* 1996;63:144–147.

848 ul Haque MF, King LM, Krakow D, et al. Mutations in orthologous genes in human spondyloepimetaphyseal dysplasia and the brachymorphic mouse. *Nat Genet* 1998;20:157–162.

849 Frattini A, Orchard PJ, Sobacchi C, et al. Defects in TCIRG1 subunit of the vacuolar proton pump are responsible for a subset of human autosomal recessive osteopetrosis. *Nat Genet* 2000;25:343–346.

850 Kornak U, Kasper D, Bosl MR, et al. Loss of the ClC-7 chloride channel leads to osteopetrosis in mice and man. *Cell* 2001;104:205–215.

851 Venta PJ, Welty RJ, Johnson TM, et al. Carbonic anhydrase II deficiency syndrome in a Belgian family is caused by a point mutation at an invariant histidine residue (107 His–Tyr): complete structure of the normal human CA II gene. *Am J Hum Genet* 1991;49:1082–1090.

852 Oldenburg J, von Brederlow B, Fregin A, et al. Congenital deficiency of vitamin K dependent coagulation factors in two families presents as a genetic defect of the vitamin K-epoxide-reductase-complex. *Thromb Haemost* 2000;84:937–941.

853 Pauli RM. Mechanism of bone and cartilage maldevelopment in the warfarin embryopathy. *Pathol Immunopathol Res* 1988;7:107–112.

854 Pauli RM, Lian JB, Mosher DF, Suttie JW. Association of congenital deficiency of multiple vitamin K-dependent coagulation factors and the phenotype of the warfarin embryopathy: clues to the mechanism of teratogenicity of coumarin derivatives. *Am J Hum Genet* 1987;41:566–583.
855 Munroe PB, Olgunturk RO, Fryns JP, Van Maldergem L, Ziereisen F, Yuksel B et al. Mutations in the gene encoding the human matrix Gla protein cause Keutel syndrome. *Nat Genet* 1999;21:142–44.
856 Franco B, Meroni G, Parenti G, et al. A cluster of sulfatase genes on Xp22.3: mutations in chondrodysplasia punctata (CDPX) and implications for warfarin embryopathy. *Cell* 1995;81:15–25.
857 Braverman N, Lin P, Moebius FF, et al. Mutations in the gene encoding 3 beta-hydroxysteroid-delta 8, delta 7-isomerase cause X-linked dominant Conradi-Hunermann syndrome. *Nat Genet* 1999;22:291–294.
858 Grange DK, Kratz LE, Braverman NE, Kelley RI. CHILD syndrome caused by deficiency of 3beta-hydroxysteroid-delta8, delta7-isomerase. *Am J Med Genet* 2000;90:328–335.
859 Motley AM, Hettema EH, Hogenhout EM, et al. Rhizomelic chondrodysplasia punctata is a peroxisomal protein targeting disease caused by a non-functional PTS2 receptor. *Nat Genet* 1997;15:377–380.
860 Ofman R, Hettema EH, Hogenhout EM, et al. Acyl-CoA:dihydroxyacetonephosphate acyltransferase: cloning of the human cDNA and resolution of the molecular basis in rhizomelic chondrodysplasia punctata type 2. *Hum Mol Genet* 1998;7:847–853.
861 de Vet EC, Ijlst L, Oostheim W, et al. Alkyl-dihydroxyacetonephosphate synthase. Fate in peroxisome biogenesis disorders and identification of the point mutation underlying a single enzyme deficiency. *J Biol Chem* 1998;273:10296–10301.
862 Gedeon AK, Colley A, Jamieson R, et al. Identification of the gene (SEDL) causing X-linked spondyloepiphyseal dysplasia tarda. *Nat Genet* 1999;22:400–404.
863 Hou WS, Bromme D, Zhao Y, et al. Characterization of novel cathepsin K mutations in the pro and mature polypeptide regions causing pycnodysostosis. *J Clin Invest* 1999;103:731–8.
864 Leroy JG, Wiesmann U. Disorders of lysosomal enzymes. In: Royce PM, Steinmann B, eds. *Connective tissue and its heritable disorders*. New York: Wiley-Liss; 1993: 613–640.
865 Martignetti JA, Aqeel AA, Sewairi WA, et al. Mutation of the matrix metalloproteinase 2 gene (MMP2) causes a multicentric osteolysis and arthritis syndrome. *Nat Genet* 2001;28:261–265.
866 Kitanaka S, Takeyama K, Murayama A, et al. Inactivating mutations in the 25-hydroxyvitamin D3 1alpha-hydroxylase gene in patients with pseudovitamin D-deficiency rickets. *N Engl J Med* 1998;338:653–661.
867 Hughes MR, Malloy PJ, Kieback DG, et al. Point mutations in the human vitamin D receptor gene associated with hypocalcemic rickets. *Science* 1988;242:1702–1705.
868 Bai M, Pearce SH, Kifor O, et al. In vivo and in vitro characterization of neonatal hyperparathyroidism resulting from a de novo, heterozygous mutation in the Ca^{2+}-sensing receptor gene: normal maternal calcium homeostasis as a cause of secondary hyperparathyroidism in familial benign hypocalciuric hypercalcemia. *J Clin Invest* 1997;99:88–96.
869 Schipani E, Langman CB, Parfitt AM, et al. Constitutively activated receptors for parathyroid hormone and parathyroid hormone-related peptide in Jansen's metaphyseal chondrodysplasia. *N Engl J Med* 1996;335:708–714.
870 Zhang P, Jobert AS, Couvineau A, Silve C. A homozygous inactivating mutation in the parathyroid hormone/parathyroid hormone-related peptide receptor causing Blomstrand chondrodysplasia. *J Clin Endocrinol Metab* 1998;83: 3365–368.
871 Patten JL, Johns DR, Valle D, et al. Mutation in the gene encoding the stimulatory G protein of adenylate cyclase in Albright's hereditary osteodystrophy. *N Engl J Med* 1990;322:1412–1419.
872 A gene (PEX) with homologies to endopeptidases is mutated in patients with X-linked hypophosphatemic rickets. The HYP Consortium. *Nat Genet* 1995;11:130–136.
873 Sabbagh Y, Jones AO, Tenenhouse HS. PHEXdb, a locus-specific database for mutations causing X-linked hypophosphatemia. *Hum Mutat* 2000;16:1–6.
874 Autosomal dominant hypophosphataemic rickets is associated with mutations in FGF23. *Nat Genet* 2000;26:345–348.
875 Wilkie AO. Craniosynostosis: genes and mechanisms. *Hum Mol Genet* 1997;6:1647–1656.
876 Afzal AR, Rajab A, Fenske CD, et al. Recessive Robinow syndrome, allelic to dominant brachydactyly type B, is caused by mutation of ROR2. *Nat Genet* 2000;25:419–422.
877 Van Bokhoven H, Celli J, Kayserili H, et al. Mutation of the gene encoding the ROR2 tyrosine kinase causes autosomal recessive Robinow syndrome. *Nat Genet* 2000;25:423–426.
878 Oldridge M, Fortuna AM, Maringa M, et al. Dominant mutations in ROR2, encoding an orphan receptor tyrosine kinase, cause brachydactyly type B. *Nat Genet* 2000;24:275–278.
879 Hughes AE, Ralston SH, Marken J, et al. Mutations in TNFRSF11A, affecting the signal peptide of RANK, cause familial expansile osteolysis. *Nat Genet* 2000;24:45–48.
880 Janssens K, Gershoni-Baruch R, Guanabens N, et al. Mutations in the gene encoding the latency-associated peptide of TGF-beta 1 cause Camurati-Engelmann disease. *Nat Genet* 2000;26: 273–275.
881 Thomas JT, Lin K, Nandedkar M, et al. A human chondrodysplasia due to a mutation in a TGF-beta superfamily member. *Nat Genet* 1996;12:315–17.
882 Polinkovsky A, Robin NH, Thomas JT, et al. Mutations in CDMP1 cause autosomal dominant brachydactyly type C. *Nat Genet* 1997;17:18–19.
883 Gong Y, Krakow D, Marcelino J, et al. Heterozygous mutations in the gene encoding noggin affect human joint morphogenesis. *Nat Genet* 1999;21:302–304.
884 Bulman MP, Kusumi K, Frayling TM, et al. Mutations in the human delta homologue, DLL3, cause axial skeletal defects in spondylocostal dysostosis. *Nat Genet* 2000;24:438–441.
885 Gao B, Guo J, She C, et al. Mutations in IHH, encoding Indian hedgehog, cause brachydactyly type A-1. *Nat Genet* 2001;28: 386–388.
886 Ianakiev P, van Baren MJ, Daly MJ, et al. Acheiropodia is caused by a genomic deletion in C7orf2, the human orthologue of the Lmbr1 gene. *Am J Hum Genet* 2001;68:38–45.
887 Balemans W, Ebeling M, Patel N, et al. Increased bone density in sclerosteosis is due to the deficiency of a novel secreted protein (SOST). *Hum Mol Genet* 2001;10:537–543.
888 Gong Y, Slee R. Group o-PC. Human bone mass accrual is affected by mutations in the low-density lipoprotein receptor-related protein 5 gene. *Am J Hum Genet* 2001;69(suppl.): S189.
889 Hurvitz JR, Suwairi WM, Van Hul W, et al. Mutations in the CCN gene family member WISP3 cause progressive pseudorheumatoid dysplasia. *Nat Genet* 1999;23:94–98.

890 Wagner T, Wirth J, Meyer J, et al. Autosomal sex reversal and campomelic dysplasia are caused by mutations in and around the SRY-related gene SOX9. *Cell* 1994;79:1111–1120.
891 Kalff-Suske M, Wild A, Topp J, et al. Point mutations throughout the GLI3 gene cause Greig cephalopolysyndactyly syndrome. *Hum Mol Genet* 1999;8:1769–1777.
892 Radhakrishna U, Bornholdt D, Scott HS, et al. The phenotypic spectrum of GLI3 morphopathies includes autosomal dominant preaxial polydactyly type-IV and postaxial polydactyly type-A/B; No phenotype prediction from the position of GLI3 mutations. *Am J Hum Genet* 1999;65:645–655.
893 Momeni P, Glockner G, Schmidt O, et al. Mutations in a new gene, encoding a zinc-finger protein, cause tricho-rhino-phalangeal syndrome type I. *Nat Genet* 2000;24:71–74.
894 el Ghouzzi, V, Le Merrer M, Perrin-Schmitt F, et al. Mutations of the TWIST gene in the Saethre-Chotzen syndrome. *Nat Genet* 1997;15:42–46.
895 Celli J, Duijf P, Hamel BC, et al. Heterozygous germline mutations in the p53 homolog p63 are the cause of EEC syndrome. *Cell* 1999;99:143–153.
896 McGrath JA, Duijf PH, Doetsch V, et al. Hay-Wells syndrome is caused by heterozygous missense mutations in the SAM domain of p63. *Hum Mol Genet* 2001;10:221–229.
897 Van Bokhoven H, Hamel BC, Bamshad M, et al. p63 Gene mutations in eec syndrome, limb-mammary syndrome, and isolated split hand-split foot malformation suggest a genotype-phenotype correlation. *Am J Hum Genet* 2001;69:481–492.
898 Mundlos S, Otto F, Mundlos C, et al. Mutations involving the transcription factor CBFA1 cause cleidocranial dysplasia. *Cell* 1997;89:773–779.
899 Dreyer SD, Zhou G, Baldini A, et al. Mutations in LMX1B cause abnormal skeletal patterning and renal dysplasia in nail patella syndrome. *Nat Genet* 1998;19:47–50.
900 Price JA, Bowden DW, Wright JT, et al. Identification of a mutation in DLX3 associated with tricho-dento-osseous (TDO) syndrome. *Hum Mol Genet* 1998;7:563–569.
901 Akarsu AN, Stoilov I, Yilmaz E, et al. Genomic structure of HOXD13 gene: a nine polyalanine duplication causes synpolydactyly in two unrelated families. *Hum Mol Genet* 1996;5:945–952.
902 Jabs EW, Muller U, Li X, et al. A mutation in the homeodomain of the human MSX2 gene in a family affected with autosomal dominant craniosynostosis. *Cell* 1993;75:443–450.
903 Wilkie AO, Tang Z, Elanko N, et al. Functional haploinsufficiency of the human homeobox gene MSX2 causes defects in skull ossification. *Nat Genet* 2001;24:387–390.
904 Mavrogiannis LA, Antonopoulou I, Baxova A, et al. Haploinsufficiency of the human homeobox gene ALX4 causes skull ossification defects. *Nat Genet* 2001;27:17–18.
905 Shears DJ, Vassal HJ, Goodman FR, et al. Mutation and deletion of the pseudoautosomal gene SHOX cause Leri-Weill dyschondrosteosis. *Nat Genet* 1998;19:70–73.
906 Bamshad M, Lin RC, Law DJ, et al. Mutations in human TBX3 alter limb, apocrine and genital development in ulnar-mammary syndrome. *Nat Genet* 1997;16:311–315.
907 Delepine M, Nicolino M, Barrett T, et al. EIF2AK3, encoding translation initiation factor 2–alpha kinase 3, is mutated in patients with Wolcott-Rallison syndrome. *Nat Genet* 2000;25:406–409.
908 Doffinger R, Smahi A, Bessia C, et al. X-linked anhidrotic ectodermal dysplasia with immunodeficiency is caused by impaired NF-kappaB signaling. *Nat Genet* 2001;27:277–285.
909 Smahi A, Courtois G, Vabres P, et al. Genomic rearrangement in NEMO impairs NF-kappaB activation and is a cause of incontinentia pigmenti. The International Incontinentia Pigmenti (IP) Consortium. *Nature* 2000;405:466–472.
910 Cheung PK, McCormick C, Crawford BE, et al. Etiological point mutations in the hereditary multiple exostoses gene EXT1: a functional analysis of heparan sulfate polymerase activity. *Am J Hum Genet* 2001;69:55–66.
911 Duncan G, McCormick C, Tufaro F. The link between heparan sulfate and hereditary bone disease: finding a function for the EXT family of putative tumor suppressor proteins. *J Clin Invest* 2001;108:511–516.
912 Lind T, Tufaro F, McCormick C, et al. The putative tumor suppressors EXT1 and EXT2 are glycosyltransferases required for the biosynthesis of heparan sulfate. *J Biol Chem* 1998;273: 26265–26268.
913 Ueki Y, Tiziani V, Santanna C et al. Mutations in the gene encoding c-Abl-binding protein SH3BP2 cause cherubism. *Nat Genet* 2001;28:125–126.
914 Ridanpaa M, van Eenennaam H, Pelin K, et al. Mutations in the RNA component of RNase MRP cause a pleiotropic human disease, cartilage-hair hypoplasia. *Cell* 2001;104:195–203.
915 Bonafé L, Schmitt K, Eich G, et al. RMRP gene sequence analysis confirms a cartilage hair hypoplasia variant with only skeletal manifestations and reveals a high density of single-nucleotide polymorphisms. *Clin Genet* 2002;61:146–151.
916 Hirschhorn R. Adenosine deaminase deficiency: molecular basis and recent developments. *Clin Immunol Immunopathol* 1995;76:S219–S227.
917 Meirowitz NB, Ananth CV, Smulian JC, et al. Foot length in fetuses with abnormal growth. *J Ultrasound Med* 2000;19: 201–205.
918 Hewitt B. Nuchal translucency in the first trimester. *Aust NZ J Obstet Gynaecol* 1993;33:389–391.
919 Soothill P, Kyle P. Fetal nuchal translucency test for Down's syndrome. *Lancet* 1997;350:1629–1622.
920 Fukada Y, Yasumizu T, Takizawa M, et al. The prognosis of fetuses with transient nuchal translucency in the first and early second trimester. *Acta Obstet Gynecol Scand* 1997;76:913–916.
921 Hernadi L, Torocsik M. Screening for fetal anomalies in the 12th week of pregnancy by transvaginal sonography in an unselected population. *Prenat Diagn* 1997;17:753–759.
922 den Hollander NS, van der Harten HJ, Vermeij-Keers C, et al. First-trimester diagnosis of Blomstrand lethal osteochondrodysplasia. *Am J Med Genet* 1997;73:345–350.
923 Hafner E, Schuchter K, Liebhart E, Philipp K. Results of routine fetal nuchal translucency measurement at weeks 10–13 in 4233 unselected pregnant women. *Prenat Diagn* 1998;18:29–34.
924 Hiippala A, Eronen M, Taipale P, et al. Fetal nuchal translucency and normal chromosomes: a long-term follow-up study. *Ultrasound Obstet Gynecol* 2001;18:18–22.
925 Venkat-Raman N, Sebire NJ, Murphy KW, et al. Increased first-trimester fetal nuchal translucency thickness in association with chondroectodermal dysplasia (Ellis-Van Creveld syndrome). *Ultrasound Obstet Gynecol* 2005;25:412–414.
926 Leung KY, MacLachlan NA, Sepulveda W. Prenatal diagnosis of ectrodactyly: the 'lobster claw' anomaly. *Ultrasound Obstet Gynecol* 1995;6:443–446.

927 Hyett J, Noble P, Sebire NJ, et al. Lethal congenital arthrogryposis presents with increased nuchal translucency at 10–14 weeks of gestation. *Ultrasound Obstet Gynecol* 1997;9:310–313.
928 Eliyahu S, Weiner E, Lahav D, Shalev E. Early sonographic diagnosis of Jarcho-Levin syndrome: a prospective screening program in one family. *Ultrasound Obstet Gynecol* 1997;9:314–318.
929 Hyett JA, Clayton PT, Moscoso G, Nicolaides KH. Increased first trimester nuchal translucency as a prenatal manifestation of Smith-Lemli-Opitz syndrome. *Am J Med Genet* 1995;58: 374–376.
930 Maymon R, Ogle RF, Chitty LS. Smith-Lemli-Opitz syndrome presenting with persisting nuchal oedema and non-immune hydrops. *Prenat Diagn* 1999;19:105–107.
931 Sharp P, Haan E, Fletcher JM, et al. First-trimester diagnosis of Smith-Lemli-Opitz syndrome. *Prenat Diagn* 1997;17: 355–361.
932 Hobbins JC, Jones OW, Gottesfeld S, Persutte W. Transvaginal ultrasonography and transabdominal embryoscopy in the first-trimester diagnosis of Smith-Lemli-Opitz syndrome, type II. *Am J Obstet Gynecol* 1994;171:546–549.
933 Ferreira A, Matias A, Brandao O, Montenegro N. Nuchal translucency and ductus venosus blood flow as early sonographic markers of thanatophoric dysplasia. A case report. *Fetal Diagn Ther* 2004;19:241–245.

27 First- and second-trimester prenatal diagnosis

John C. Hobbins

The recent emphasis on noninvasive prenatal diagnosis has evolved over a time when the average age of pregnant patients has crept upward. For example, in 1985, 5.6% of pregnant patients were 35 years of age or older in the United States.[1] This group of advanced maternal age (AMA) patients comprised 12.5% of the overall pregnant population in 2002 and, today, it is estimated that those aged 35 years or older comprise 20% of the pregnant population.

The older pregnant patient today is different from yesterday's AMA woman. She is often a nullipara with a career who, while postponing pregnancy well into her thirties, is inclined to want as much diagnostic information as possible before deciding upon whether or not to have an invasive procedure. In fact, at the University of Connecticut, the percentage of AMA patients having invasive testing decreased by 68% between 1991 and 2002. Interestingly, the number of invasive procedures per diagnosis of Down syndrome (DS; trisomy 21) dropped from 1:43 to 1:14 over a time when the number of detected cases of DS rose by 33%.[2]

With the trend toward fewer invasive procedures, Egan et al.[3] postulated that, if every patient over 34 years of age with a reassuring second-trimester biochemical screen were to forego amniocentesis, 1971 fetuses in the United States would be saved from procedure-related loss.

In this chapter, the rapidly changing panoply of noninvasive first- and second-trimester techniques will be summarized, along with a description of how these tests can be used in combination to provide a reasonably accurate adjusted risk of trisomy 18 and trisomy 21 for every patient. In addition, the latest information on invasive diagnostic procedures will be discussed.

Invasive procedures

Amniocentesis – second trimester

The labeling of a woman of 35 years of age as being AMA stemmed from the concept that her age-related risk for DS of 1:270 was about the same as the procedure-related risk of amniocentesis. It is interesting that this very arbitrary allocation has been so well ingrained that an individual of 34 years 11 months at the time of delivery would be considered "low risk" and a woman 2 months older would be designated as "high risk."

The risk of amniocentesis most often quoted is 1:200, and this seems to have come from a vintage National Institutes of Child Health and Human Development (NICHD) study[4] published in 1976, in which some of the amniocenteses were performed without ultrasound. Nevertheless, from the data presented below, this has become a very reasonable estimate of the procedure-related risk.

In order to arrive at a procedure-related risk, one has to determine what the chances are of a spontaneous fetal loss up until at least 24 weeks, when an ultrasound evaluation at the time of the amniocentesis shows a normal appearing fetus. In a study from Denmark,[5] 4066 women who were 34 years of age or younger were recruited. After an ultrasound examination suggested that their fetuses were normal, half were randomly allocated to have amniocenteses, and the other half were designated as control subjects. The patients were compulsively followed until 26 weeks. The loss rate in the control group was 7 per 1000 and in the amniocentesis group was 17 per 1000. The derived 1% procedure-related loss rate took some by surprise, but the study has stood up to heavy scrutiny because the numbers were reasonable, the operators were very experienced, and the procedures were all performed under ultrasound direction.

Several uncontrolled early studies (prior to 1992) have yielded loss rates after second-trimester amniocentesis that range from 1.9% to 4.9%. To evaluate the procedure-related loss rate from contemporary midtrimester amniocenteses, Seeds[6] analyzed data from 29 studies, each including more than 1000 patients having midtrimester amniocenteses. In this sampling, there were five controlled studies (two matched and three unmatched), totaling 8607 patients having amniocenteses and 6457 control patients. The difference in loss rate until 28 weeks between the amniocentesis group and the control group was 0.6%. In the entire sample of 33 795 patients having a second-trimester ultrasound-guided amniocentesis, the loss rate was 2.1% until 28 weeks, and the loss rate in the above 6457 control subjects was 1.4%, giving a procedure-related risk of 0.7%.

Given the lack of randomized data, it is difficult to precisely quote a risk for amniocentesis, but it is clear that:

- Experience plays a role in procedure-related losses.[7]
- With the exception of data from one large nonrandomized study[8] suggesting a lower amniocentesis risk, available published information points toward a procedure-related risk of about 1 in 200.
- There is a fixed spontaneous second-trimester loss rate of about 0.5%.

Early amniocentesis

When chorionic villus sampling (CVS) emerged as an option for early prenatal diagnosis, only a few operators were trained in this invasive technique. However, many were trained in amniocentesis. In order to comply with their patients' requests for earlier diagnostic information, some clinicians began offering amniocentesis between 11 and 14 weeks.

Many studies have shown that early amniocentesis is not a safe option. In a Canadian randomized trial, the Canadian Early and Mid-trimester Amniotic Fluid Trial (CEMAT),[9] the postprocedure loss rate for early amniocentesis was 2.9% versus 1.0% for the standard amniocentesis group. The most recent multicenter study, the Early Amniocentesis versus Transabdominal CVS (EATA) study,[10] showed a loss rate up to 20 weeks of 1.5% in the early amniocentesis group versus 0.8% after CVS. Also, Sundberg et al.[11] showed an unacceptable rate of clubfoot with early amniocentesis versus CVS (1.7% versus 0%), and the Canadian (CEMAT) study had a rate of clubbing of 1.3% compared with traditional second-trimester amniocentesis, which yielded a rate of 0.1%.

As the amnion and chorion are often not apposed between 12 and 14 weeks, the separated needle holes will allow fluid to track extramembranously to and through the cervix, as noted in 3.5% and 4% of cases in the Canadian and Sundberg studies respectively.

Because of a higher loss rate with early amniocentesis compared with standard amniocentesis or CVS, and as there is a higher rate of amniotic fluid leakage, respiratory distress syndrome (RDS), and clubbing of the extremities, this technique has been virtually abandoned.

Chorionic villus sampling (CVS)

Investigators in China and Russia first reported on the concept of sampling placental tissue in the first trimester for diagnostic purposes. Brambati et al.[12] were the first to exploit this idea by threading a catheter through the cervix and directing the tip under ultrasound guidance into the placenta. This extramembranous technique allowed small samples of chorionic villi to be obtained for karyotyping with seemingly modest risk.

The transabdominal method of CVS emerged to allow easier access to predominantly anterior placentas. Some investigators, however, have now chosen to use the transabdominal approach exclusively, while others select the approach that gains easiest access to the placenta.

Spontaneous loss rates in apparently normal pregnancies are about 15% at 5–6 menstrual weeks, about 2% at 11 weeks, and slightly less than 1% at 16 weeks. Raw loss rates after CVS have varied between 1.6% and 3.4% in five experienced centers in the United States (R. J. Wapner, personal communication) (Table 27.1).

There is no doubt that the more insertions, the greater the risk of the procedure, and the greater the experience of the operator, the less the need for multiple needle insertions. For example, Saura et al.[14] showed that the spontaneous loss rate was 6.6% in the first 200 cases carried out. This rate dropped to 3.4% in the next 300 cases and leveled off at 1.2% after 1000 cases.

CVS, which became a very popular option for AMA patients in the 1980s, was dealt a blow when a study[15] emerged citing an intolerably high rate of limb reduction defects with CVS (about 2%). When it was clear that this study had a heavy sampling of patients having very early CVS (≤ 9 weeks), an international registry of CVS (WHO CVS Registry)[16] involving 208 682 patients was accessed. This showed the rate of limb reduction defects to be 5.9 per 10 000, close to the incidence in the overall population of 6 per 10 000 (British Columbia birth statistics). Brambati et al.[12] reviewed their own data and found that, at 6–7 weeks, CVS was associated with a 1.6% incidence of limb reduction defects and, at 9–12 weeks, the incidence was 0.6%. From this, it is clear that CVS prior to 10 weeks should be avoided.

We have been quoting to our patients a procedure-related loss rate of CVS, performed at 10–13 weeks, of about 1%, and, realizing that the paucity of randomized data does not allow us to provide more precise information, we have indicated that this risk is slightly higher than that of amnio-

Table 27.1 Pregnancy loss rate in experienced US centers.

	Continued pregnancy	Spontaneous abortion	Spontaneous abortion (%)
Carolinas Medical Center	3545	117	2.4
Genetics and IVF	14 116	232	1.6
Illinois Masonic Medical Center	6580	195	3.0
Thomas Jefferson University	13 629	346	2.5
University of California, San Francisco	10 386	354	3.4
Wayne State University	6995	143	2.0
Total	55 251	1387	2.5

From ref. 13.

centesis, as concluded by the authors of a review of the Cochrane Database.[18]

Fetal blood sampling

Attempts to sample the fetal circulation emerged when it became clear that many fetal conditions could not be diagnosed by amniotic fluid analysis. The condition that catalyzed the first attempts at fetal blood sampling was beta-thalassemia, a devastating problem that could be identified by globin chain synthesis analysis.

In 1974, Hobbins et al.[19] reported their ability to obtain fetal blood endoscopically from the surface vessels coursing along the chorionic plate of the placenta. In 1979, Rodeck and Campbell[20] moved their endoscopic focus to the umbilical cord, which enabled them to sample blood directly from the umbilical vein.

The fetoscopic approach to blood sampling became instantly obsolete when, in 1983, Daffos et al.[21] demonstrated the capability to enter the umbilical vein percutaneously under ultrasound direction with less maternal and fetal morbidity.

However, through the 1990s, the need for blood sampling procedures diminished because more diagnoses could be made through new methods in the investigation of amniotic fluid, such as polymerase chain reaction (PCR) in cases of infection and fluorescent *in situ* hybridization (FISH) for rapid karyotyping, at less risk.

The risk of fetal blood sampling has varied widely between investigators. For example, in 1993, Ghidini et al.[22] pulled together data from the literature from various centers. The fetal loss rate was inversely proportional to the size of the series and was as high as 12% in studies with small numbers. With pooled data from centers with the greatest experience, the risk of fetal loss was 1.4% prior to 28 weeks and 1.4% after 28 weeks. This seemed like a very reasonable risk for some high-risk patients. However, one author who had an extremely low loss rate contributed almost half the cases. If these cases were removed, then data from the remaining centers indicated a 7.2% fetal loss rate for all patients and 3% for low-risk patients.[23]

Now, fetal blood sampling has been relegated to only a few indications, such as alloimmune thrombocytopenia (AIT) and fetal anemia. Even in rhesus (Rh) disease, fetal blood sampling has been largely supplanted by Doppler waveform analysis of the middle cerebral arteries, with cordocentesis being saved for those needing intrauterine transfusions.

Noninvasive prenatal diagnosis

AMA patients entering the first or second trimester come in three types:

1 Those who want to know with 100% accuracy whether their fetuses have a chromosomal abnormality or a major congenital anomaly.

2 Those who do not want invasive testing because termination of pregnancy would not be an option for them and the risk of the test would not be worth the reassurance it might provide.

3 Those who want the most accurate noninvasive information available regarding their risk of fetal aneuploidy, before deciding whether or not to undergo invasive testing.

As noted above, as more noninvasive diagnostic combinations have become available, the number of patients in the third category has increased substantially over the last 5 years, while the numbers of those in the first category have decreased.

This portion of the chapter will deal with noninvasive diagnostic options, most of which have only become available over the last few years, and basically involve two modalities: ultrasound and maternal serum biochemistry.

First trimester

In 1992, Nicolaides et al.[24] reported on the association between an enlarged nuchal translucency (NT) and fetal chromosome abnormalities. The measurement represented the distance between the inner portion of the nuchal membrane and the underlying tissue (Fig. 27.1). After compulsively organizing a multicenter screening program, which involved careful standardization of the methods and regimented operator training, the group reported their results in a prospective study involving 96 127 patients (Table 27.2).[25] The calculation of fetal DS risk was based on the patient's age, the fetal crown–rump length, and the NT measurement. At a false-positive rate of 5%, the detection rate for trisomy 21 was 77%, a sensitivity that exceeded that of the then widely used second-trimester triple screen.

Although the sensitivity figure was questioned initially because spontaneously aborting screen-negative trisomy 21 fetuses were not accounted for in the calculated results,[26] the detection rates from other centers, also involving large numbers of patients, have validated the results of Nicolaides and Snijders. The data from the First Trimester Maternal Serum Biochemistry and Fetal Nuchal Translucency Screening (BUN) study[27] involving 8514 patients and showing a 69% sensitivity at a 5% false-positive rate, and the results from the

Table 27.2 Down syndrome detection using nuchal translucency (NT) with age.

Year	Detection rate (%)	Screen-positive rate (%)
1996	84	6
1997	79	5
1998	77	5
1999	73	5
2002	79	5

Data from Fetal Medicine Foundation, London, UK.

First And Second Trimester Evaluation for Risk (FASTER) trial[28] involving 35 000 patients, bear out the concept that the screening test can be used in a US population.

It has been demonstrated that the accuracy of NT screening drops to nonefficacious levels when less experienced sonographers and sonologists are involved in the process. Therefore, properly trained individuals and carefully standardized protocols for performing the ultrasound examination are necessary for any NT screening program to be effective.

First-trimester biochemistry

As second-trimester biochemical combinations were the first to be used in screening for aneuploidy with obvious success, investigators began testing various analytes in the first trimester and, at the time of writing, the two that have seemed most effective are pregnancy-associated plasma protein A (PAPP-A), a product of the placenta that is a protease for insulin-like growth factor (IGF) binding protein, and the beta subunit of human chorionic gonadotropin (βhCG), another placental product.

In DS, the average PAPP-A is 0.39 multiples of the median (MoM) and βhCG is 1.83 MoM.[29] If these two analytes are used together, a risk for a given patient can be fashioned by adding the variables of the patient's age and the estimated gestational age. Based on this model, PAPP-A, by itself, has a sensitivity for trisomy 21 of 42% at a 5% screen-positive rate, and βhCG has a sensitivity of 24% at a screen-positive rate of 5%. However, together, they have a sensitivity of 62% at a 5% screen-positive rate.[27]

NT and biochemistry in combination

As adding a new testing variable to any of the screening protocols seems to enhance the testing sensitivity, it was a natural next step to combine NT with first-trimester biochemistry in a diagnostic algorithm ("combined test"). This combination has yielded sensitivities of between 62% and 90% with varying screen-positive rates. Malone and D'Alton[30] combined data from seven studies involving 85 482 patients in which the sensitivity of this combined approach was 82% at a screen-positive rate of 5% (Table 27.3).

Nasal bone

In 1866, Langdon Down noted that infants with a particular syndrome, ultimately named after him, had noses that were quite small. This stimulated Cicero et al.[31] to investigate the possibility that this observation could be used as an adjunctive diagnostic tool in the first trimester. The endpoint was quite simple – the presence or absence of a nasal bone. In their first publication,[31] they found that 73% of fetuses with DS had absent nasal bones, compared with only 0.5% of the normal fetal population. The updated experience of this group[32] was published in 2003 and involved 3788 patients. They found that:

1 They could adequately evaluate the nasal bones in 98.9% of cases.

2 Some 67% of DS fetuses had absent nasal bones.

3 There were ethnic variations in the results.

4 The nasal bone findings were independent of NT. In fact, the addition of nasal bone evaluation increased the sensitivity of the combined test from 89% to 97% with a screen-positive rate of 5%.

Recent data from Malone et al.[33] do not concur with the excellent results from Cicero and other authors,[34,35] although this could represent a difference in technique.

Second-trimester biochemistry

In 1984, Merkatz et al.[36] serendipitously noticed that pregnancies complicated with fetal DS were sometimes associated with low levels of maternal serum alpha-fetoprotein (MSAFP). Since then, it was found that adding total hCG, which tends to be elevated, and unconjugated estriol, which is generally

Table 27.3 First-trimester screening for trisomy 21 using nuchal translucency (NT), pregnancy-associated plasma protein A (PAPP-A), and free beta-human chorionic gonadotropin (βhCG) at 10–13 weeks' gestation.

	n	Trisomy 21					
		Prevalence per 1000	Sensitivity (*n*) (%)	FPR (%)	PPV (%)	LR (+)	LR (–)
1.	1467	8.9	11/13 (85)	3.3	18.6	26	0.2
2.	5809	5.7	30/33 (91)	5.0	9.4	18	0.1
3.	1602	3.1	4/5 (80)	8.3	2.9	10	0.2
4.	4939	2.8	12/14 (86)	5.0	4.7	17	0.2
5.	17299	2.6	28/45 (62)	5.0	3.1	12	0.4
6.	14383	5.7	75/82 (92)	7.1	6.8	13	0.1
7.	39983	2.1	68/85 (80)	3.4	4.8	24	0.2
Total	85482	3.1	228/277 (82.3)	4.7	5.4	17.5	0.18
(Pooled 95% CI)			(77, 87)	(4.6, 4.8)	(5.1, 5.7)	(16.6, 18.7)	(0.14, 0.24)

From ref. 30.
FPR, false-positive rate; PPV, positive predictive value; LR, likelihood ratio.

low, to MSAFP improved the screening sensitivity for DS from about 33% to 65%. Although many other analytes have been investigated, the additional analyte most commonly used to take the above "triple" screen to a "quad" screen is inhibin A, contributed by the placenta.

If one were to plot the individual analytes against gestational age and incorporate the patient's age into the calculation, the newest data from the BUN study[27] indicate a triple-screen sensitivity for DS of 67.2% at a screen-positive rate of 5%. This represents a substantial increase in diagnostic yield from using the patient's age and second-trimester MSAFP alone. In patients above 35 years of age, the triple-screen sensitivity can exceed 85% (but at a 14% screen-positive rate). Unpublished FASTER trial results show an even higher sensitivity with the quad screen than expected.

Prenatal diagnostic combination options

From the above-mentioned trials, sufficient data have emerged to fashion three different approaches to prenatal diagnosis using first-trimester ultrasound and first- and second-trimester biochemical information. As the titles for these programs below are descriptive and concepts are just now evolving, these names may well change.

Integrated (basic) screen

This represents the protocol pursued in the FASTER trial. It consists of a first-trimester NT and PAPP-A screen and a second-trimester quad screen. The controversial part of this scheme is that the patient is not informed of the first-trimester results until all the information is in; she gets one answer a few days after the second-trimester blood is drawn. Through analysis of existing data, this method gives a 96% sensitivity at a 5% screen-positive rate.

Independent sequential screen

This consists of a combined screen of NT, PAPP-A, and βhCG, which is performed in the first trimester with the patient being apprised of the results immediately. The result of second-trimester biochemistry is then given to the patient, which is independent of the first-trimester result and based on a pretest risk of age alone. The reported sensitivity of this technique in the BUN study[37] using a triple screen was 98% at an overall screen-positive rate of 17%. However, when using extrapolated data to give parallel results, this technique would have resulted in a sensitivity of 87% at a screen-positive rate of 5%. With a quad screen, the sensitivity figure would be higher.

Dependent sequential

In this case, risk is derived from the combined first-trimester test (NT and PAPP-A, with or without hCG), which is given to the patient. She then goes into her second-trimester quad screen with a new pretest risk that is not based on her age but on the result of the first-trimester test. The second result would then yield a lower false-positive rate than the independent screen described above. With modeling from FASTER data, this would yield a sensitivity of 95% at a total screen-positive rate of 5%.

A variation on the above dependent sequential theme is a "contingency" approach, in which a preset first-trimester numerical risk would be used as a threshold below which no further testing would be required.[38] This would make sense from a cost standpoint and could diminish patient angst.

Increased nuchal translucency in euploid fetuses

Fetuses with NT measurements that are above the 95th percentile need further diagnostic attention even if invasive procedures indicate a normal karyotype. A number of fetal abnormalities that are too long to list have been reported to be associated with an increased NT. Basic anomaly categories are noted in Table 27.4 along with the prevalence of each in the face of a normal fetal karyotype.[39]

The common denominator in many of these generally rare anomaly syndromes is a cardiac abnormality. One of the theories for increased NT is that nuchal fluid accumulates secondary to cardiac dysfunction, which is then accompanied by tricuspid regurgitation and an increase in ductus venosus backflow during atrial contraction, often noted in first-trimester fetuses with DS. In 1999, Hyett et al.[40] quantified the risk of a structural cardiac abnormality based on the size of the NT. The highest prevalence has been noted in abnormalities of the left heart, such as aortic stenosis, hypoplastic left heart syndrome, and coarctation of the aorta. Souka et al.[39] have put together data that will help in counseling patients whose euploid fetuses have increased NTs (Table 27.5).

The anomalies most commonly associated with this combination of NT and euploidy are diaphragmatic hernia, exomphalos, body stalk abnormality, skeletal dysplasia, and various syndromes such as fetal akinesia, Noonan syndrome, Smith–Lemli–Opitz syndrome, and spinal muscular atrophy. Those

Table 27.4 Increased nuchal translucency (NT) in euploid fetuses.

Abnormality	Prevalence
Fetal demise	1:19
Major cardiac defect	1:23
Limb: body wall	1:90
Omphalocele	1:120
Fetal akinesia	1:120
Skeletal dysplasia	1:190
Diaphragmatic hernia	1:220

From ref. 39.

Table 27.5 Relation between nuchal translucency thickness and prevalence of chromosomal defects, miscarriage, or fetal death and major fetal abnormalities.

Nuchal translucency	Chromosomal defects (%)	Fetal death (%)	Major fetal abnormalities (%)	Alive and well (%)
< 95th percentile	0.2	1.3	1.6	97
95th–99th percentile	3.7	1.3	2.5	93
3.5–4.4 mm	21.1	2.7	10.0	70
4.5–5.4 mm	33.3	3.4	18.5	50
5.5–6.4 mm	50.5	10.1	24.2	30
> 6.5 mm	64.5	19.0	46.2	15

From Souka AP, Von Kaisenberg CS, Hyett JA, et al. Increased nuchal translucency with normal karyotype. *Am J Obstet Gynecol* 2005;192:1005–1021.

not seemingly associated with increased NT and euploidy are neural tube defects, holoprosencephaly, gastroschisis, and renal anomalies.

Our approach to fetuses with large NTs and normal karyotypes is to do a very detailed ultrasound in the second trimester (after ruling out any obvious first-trimester structural abnormalities by transvaginal ultrasound) and to add a detailed fetal echocardiogram at about 20 weeks. If these examinations are negative, then the risk of fetal anomalies drops to almost baseline levels.

The genetic sonogram

In 1985, Benacerraf et al.[41] reported that about 40% of fetuses with DS had increased nuchal skinfold thickness (NSFT) in the second trimester and, around that time, she and others published an observed tendency toward shorter femurs in these fetuses when compared with the biparietal diameter[42] or the expected femur length.[43] This started a search for many other ultrasound-derived "soft" markers for DS that is still continuing. To date, at least 12 different soft markers have been investigated alone, in combination with other markers, or incorporated into a scoring system to adjust the risk of fetal DS for a given patient. Some markers are clearly superior performers, while others are not or are so new that their efficacy has not been adequately tested with large enough numbers. The most commonly used markers are summarized in Table 27.6.

Interestingly, the heart, which is a source of potent information about aneuploidy, has not been adequately investigated. For example, about 30% of DS infants have structural abnormalities at birth, but undoubtedly more have ventricular septal defects in the second trimester that close over later. Also, many more will have at least a transient functional right heart predominance that results in a larger right atrium with a deviated interatrial septum along with tricuspid regurgitation. By thoroughly scrutinizing the fetal heart, DeVore[44] has increased the sensitivity of the genetic sonogram to over 90%.

The concept with this noninvasive form of testing is to calculate a likelihood ratio based on an ultrasound examination that would allow a far more accurate adjusted risk for DS from an individual patient than with age alone. The idea is very workable but is dependent upon the predictive accuracy of the providers offering the genetic sonogram, which consists of: (1) ruling out major structural abnormalities by performing a standard fetal survey according to guidelines published by the American Institute of Ultrasound in Medicine and the American College of Radiology; (2) measuring femur and humerus length; and (3) looking for soft markers for DS. Although there are standards in place for the investigations of (1) and (2), there is no consensus regarding which soft markers to evaluate, with the exception of the NSFT, the best performer to date.

Table 27.6 Soft markers.

Nuchal skinfold thickness
Ear length
Frontal lobe length
Nasal bone length
Echogenic focus in the heart
Echogenic bowel
Iliac angle
Iliac bone length
"Sandal gap" feet
Absent or small middle phalanx of the fifth digit
Pyelectasis
Mild ventriculomegaly
Biometry: femur length (vs. biparietal diameter or against expected femur length for gestational age)

The most commonly investigated markers, in addition to the NSFT, are:

1 An echogenic intracardiac focus in the heart (EIF), which is noted in about 18% of fetuses with DS.[45]
2 An echogenic bowel, seen in about 13% of fetuses with DS.[46]
3 Modest pyelectasis, noted in about 20% of fetuses with DS.[47]

Other less commonly utilized markers are:

1 Fetal ear length[43] (sometimes small in DS).
2 Iliac angle[49] (often widened in DS).
3 Indirect measurements of the frontal lobe[50] (most often small in DS).

Table 27.7 The genetic sonogram experience.

Study	No. of patients	Sensitivity (%)	FPR (%)	LR (+)	LR (–)
Bromley	175	82	14.4	5.7	0.20
Vintzileos	34	82	9.0	9.1	0.20
Bromley	54	75	5.7	13.1	0.27
Benacerraf	45	73	4.4	16.5	0.28
Nyberg	142	74	14.7	5.0	0.30
Bahado-Singh	31	74	15.0	5.0	0.31
Nyberg	186	70	13.3	5.3	0.36
Sohl	55	67	19.4	3.5	0.41
Vergagni	22	59	5.3	11.1	0.43

4 The middle phalanx of the fifth digit[51] (sometimes absent or very small in DS).

The newest marker on the scene is fetal nasal bone length, which represents an extension of the observation noted in the first trimester mentioned above. Early investigation suggests that this marker may well be the best performer in the second trimester if measured compulsively and compared against a commonly used standard, the biparietal diameter. Bromley et al.[52] have demonstrated that, if using a nasal bone/biparietal cutoff of 10, 81% of fetuses with DS would be detected with a screen-positive rate of 11%. The addition of this marker to the genetic sonogram, although not yet tested prospectively, should enhance the sensitivity of the genetic sonogram well above the figures in the literature, which are summarized in Table 27.7.

The finding of a marker for DS can raise the risk, but much depends upon which marker is found and whether or not it is in isolation. For example, an enlarged NSFT increases the risk at least 11 times,[53] even in isolation, while minor markers, such as the fetal ear, middle bone of the fifth digit, and femur length, have a very modest effect on the adjustment of risk when isolated.

Choroid plexus cysts are clearly markers for trisomy 18, but it is unclear whether they are markers for DS. Bromley et al.[52] and unpublished FASTER data show no greater association with DS, whereas some smaller studies suggest a higher prevalence of this finding in DS than in the control populations studied.

At the time of writing, it seems reasonable not to change a pre-ultrasound risk for an isolated marker that most studies have shown to have likelihood ratios of ≤ 2.0, and to adjust the risk upward only when likelihood ratios are high, such as for NSFT, short humerus, and small nasal bone. However, once more than one marker is found, this catapults the risk upward. For example, Nyberg et al.[53] have shown that, with each additional "minor" marker found, the likelihood of DS goes up exponentially (Table 27.8).

Table 27.8 Comparison of the number of markers in fetuses with Down syndrome (DS) and control fetuses.

Markers (%)	DS (%) Nyberg $n = 186$	Normal (%) Nyberg $n = 8728$	LR Nyberg
0	31.2	86.7	0.36
1	22.6	11.3	2.0
2	15.1	1.6	9.7
3+	14.5	0.1	115.2
Majority	16.7	0.6	27.5

The beauty of the genetic sonogram is that, if the carefully performed examination fails to reveal any fetal anomalies, short limbs, or markers for DS, the risk can be adjusted downward. An eight-center study[54] pooling data from experienced diagnostic centers in the United States had an average sensitivity of 71.6% with a range of 63.6–80%. Also, this study, along with others,[55–57] showed that the genetic sonogram performed as well in those with an elevated biochemical risk for DS as in those of AMA, suggesting that the genetic sonogram and second-trimester biochemistry had independent diagnostic values.

At present, current results in the literature suggest that centers with large patient numbers and accurate outcome data can calculate their own likelihood ratios. Then, using Bayes' theorem, an adjusted risk can be estimated for a given patient after a negative genetic sonogram. For example, a 35-year-old woman with a pretest value of 1:280 having a reassuring sonogram in a center generating a likelihood ratio of 0.3 would be adjusted downward to a risk of 1:840 (0.3 × 280).

Programs yet to establish their own sensitivity and specificity values but following a carefully standardized protocol for a genetic sonogram could add a conservative "cushion" by simply adjusting the pretest risk downward by half after a negative genetic sonogram. The FASTER trial[58] has shown that the few trisomy 21 fetuses not screened in with the integrated test were picked up in over 8000 patients in the study having a genetic sonogram, giving a 100% sensitivity for DS when the ultrasound was added to the integrated testing scheme.

Trisomy 18

While the thrust of prenatal diagnosis has been directed toward DS because of its frequency, especially in AMA patients, progress in the noninvasive investigation of trisomy 18 has quietly moved forward to a point where the diagnosis can be made with ultrasound and biochemistry in the first and second trimesters in virtually every affected fetus. For example, the BUN study[27] showed a sensitivity for trisomy 18 of 91% at a 2% screen-positive rate using the "combined" first-trimester screen approach. One hundred percent of trisomy 18 fetuses were identified in those patients over 35 years old with a screen-positive rate of 2.6%.

With second-trimester biochemistry alone, the sensitivity quoted by most laboratories is around 65%. However, for some reason, this figure has been calculated for a screen-positive rate of 0.5%. If the screen-positive rate is raised to 5%, sensitivity would far exceed 90%.

As fetuses with trisomy 18, an ultimately lethal perinatal abnormality, are almost always phenotypically abnormal and usually have a cardiac defect (90%), very few fetuses with this condition will slip through a genetic sonogram unnoticed. Table 27.9 outlines the various markers known to be associated with trisomy 18.

Controversy still exists about whether or not to employ invasive sampling when common markers of trisomy 18, choroid plexus cysts, are found in isolation. First, it is important to be assured that the finding is truly in isolation by compulsively excluding every one of the markers in Table 27.9. If this is the case, and the biochemistry is reassuring, the chance of a fetus having trisomy 18 is close to zero and certainly far less than the risk of amniocentesis.

Table 27.9 Ultrasound signs for trisomy 18.

Symmetrical intrauterine growth retardation (IUGR)
Polyhydramnios
Cardiac anomaly (over 90%)
Other major anomalies
"Strawberry"-shaped calvarium
Small frontal lobe
Small and deformed ears
Small transcerebellar diameter
Large cisterna magna
Small mandible
Single umbilical artery
Overlapping fingers
"Rocker bottom" foot

Screening for fetal anomalies with ultrasound

About 28 per 1000 fetuses will have a major congenital anomaly, and many of these fetuses will have findings that can be identified with ultrasound. In the literature, there is a huge variation in the identification rates for fetal anomalies. As a standard (basic) fetal ultrasound survey is designed to screen for most anomalies, it is surprising how low the overall identification rate has generally been.

The RADIUS study,[59] published in 1994, was launched to assess the value of routine screening with ultrasound in the second and third trimesters. After excluding about half the patients who were enrolled in the study to concentrate on purely low-risk patients, 7685 patients were randomly assigned to have two ultrasound evaluations, and 7596 control subjects were designated not to have an ultrasound unless a clinical indication arose.

The study had virtually complete ascertainment; 6.5% of anomalies were diagnosed in the control group, and 15% were diagnosed in the ultrasound group before 24 weeks. Although it was heartening that three times more anomalies were identified when ultrasound was used routinely, the fact that 85% of major anomalies were missed was not. A similar randomized control trial (RCT) originating in Helsinki[60] showed an identification rate of 40%.

When simply evaluating the sensitivity of ultrasound in the identification of fetal anomalies, an RCT is not required. The largest of the observational studies is the multicenter Eurofetus study.[61] In pooled data from > 200 000 patients, the sensitivity for major anomalies was 73.7% and for minor anomalies was 45.7%. Prior to 24 weeks, the sensitivity was 55% for major anomalies, more than three times that of the RADIUS trial.

There are many variables that affect the efficacy of a fetal anatomic survey. For example, operator experience plays an important role. The RADIUS trial showed a sensitivity in identifying fetal anomalies at all gestational ages of 38% in tertiary centers, compared with 16% in the hands of local practitioners. The Helsinki study generated a sensitivity of 77% and 36% for the above categories respectively.

Results also vary according to the degree of risk assigned to patients being evaluated. If the risk is high, the practitioner might be more alert to subtle findings than when there is a lessened pre-examination chance of an anomaly.

Fetal cells in the maternal circulation

The placenta is an almost perfect gatekeeper with regard to restricting components of the fetal circulation from traversing into the maternal circulation. However, about one cell per 10 million maternal cells is fetal in origin but, in some patients, such as those destined to have preeclampsia, more fetal cells seem to get across the placenta. The concept of capturing these fetal cells is compelling as it would represent the ideal form of noninvasive diagnosis, requiring a simple blood draw. However, scientists have struggled for more than 10 years to isolate these cells of fetal origin.

In 1969, Walknowska et al.[62] first found lymphocytes carrying the Y chromosome in maternal blood. In 1990, Bianchi et al.[63] identified fetal nucleated red cells in the maternal circulation. Since then, many techniques have been employed for cell separation including magnetic-activated cell separation (MACS) and fluorescence-activated cell sorting (FACS). The chromosome analysis has been largely accomplished through FISH methodology.

Since 1990, such investigations have been in full swing but, to date, the largest study published is the NICHD Fetal Cell Isolation Study (NIFTY),[64] involving almost 3000 patients. In this study, the accuracy of predicting a male karyotype was 41% and, in the 60 samples from aneuploidy pregnancies, 79% were identified at a false-positive rate of 4.1%.

Until now, the process suffers from technical difficulties inherent in the job of finding the one cell per 10 million that contains the key to the fetal karyotype and from the cost of employing a very expensive, labor-intensive process with, thus far, disappointing results.

The investigation has turned up some ancillary, potentially useful information.

1 More fetal cells and fetal DNA are noted in the blood of mothers who later develop preeclampsia.
2 More fetal cells and DNA are found in patients with aneuploid fetuses.
3 Fetal free cell DNA has a short half-life compared with fetal cells that can remain in the maternal circulation into the next pregnancy (with obvious negative diagnostic implications).

At the time of writing, the ability to isolate free DNA from maternal serum has exciting potential. It can be found in the maternal plasma by 7 weeks of gestation, and levels increase as pregnancy progresses. It has a 16-min half-life.

In 1998, Lo et al.[65] published their ability to diagnose fetal RhD status by molecular analysis of maternal plasma and, in 2000, Lo et al.[66] and Zhang et al.[67] reported being able to determine fetal sex by DNA analysis using PCR. Then, these groups published their success in determining fetal Rh status with a sensitivity and specificity of 94% and 100%, respectively, in the first trimester, and 92% and 100%, respectively, in the second trimester.

At the moment, this approach to fetal diagnosis is passing through an embryonic stage in investigation. However, there is reason to believe that, with technical breakthroughs and expanded clinical investigation, coupled with strategies to cut costs, these methods could contribute hugely to large-scale screening for aneuploidy, X-linked conditions, and blood group disorders.

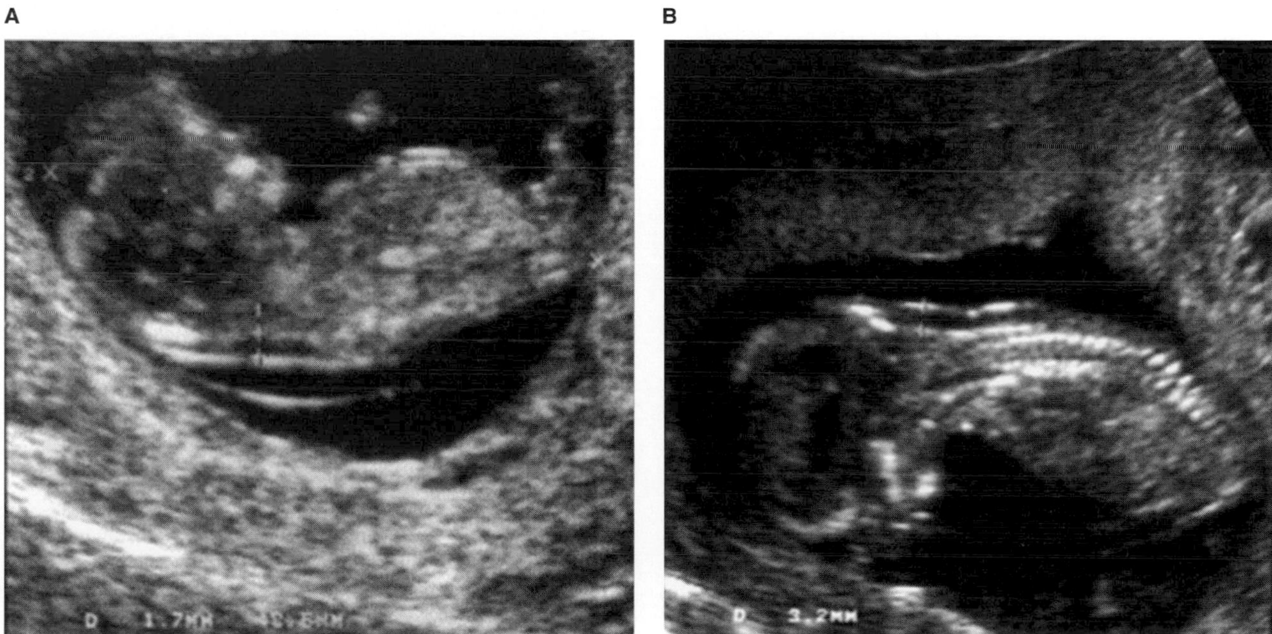

Figure 27.1 Nuchal translucency (NT) measurements. Notice separate amnion in (A).

Conclusions

Progress in prenatal diagnosis has been exponential over the last decade, and there is reason to believe that the "dots" of progress will continue to be connected along the same pathway in the next decade. Ultrasound technology is exploding, as evidenced by the recent advent of three- and four-dimensional methods, investigators are better trained, and "bench" science is becoming more automated. Soon, invasive techniques will be needed for patients who are only at the very highest risk for severe fetal abnormalities.

Acknowledgment

It is with deep appreciation that I acknowledge the substantial efforts contributed by Jane Berg in the preparation of this manuscript, as well as in many other endeavors over the past 7 years.

Key points

1 There is now a major emphasis on noninvasive prenatal diagnosis stimulated by patient desire for the best information with which to make decisions regarding invasive testing.

2 Standard second-trimester amniocentesis has a procedure-related risk that is difficult to pinpoint precisely but, according to the literature, is about 1 in 200.

3 The risk of CVS varies among investigators, but seems to be slightly higher than if a patient waits until the second trimester for an amniocentesis. However, with the emergence of first-trimester noninvasive testing, the need for CVS will increase in patients at high risk for fetal aneuploidy.

4 The risks of early amniocentesis (11–14 weeks) are generally not acceptable.

5 First-trimester nuchal translucency assessment, along with biochemistry, has a reasonable sensitivity in the adjustment of risk of trisomy 21 and trisomy 18.

6 The emergence of second-trimester biochemistry (triple screen and quad screen) has significant diagnostic benefit by itself but, when used adjunctively with first-trimester tests, has a very high predictive value.

7 Various combinations of first- and second-trimester ultrasound methods and biochemistry have sensitivities for Down syndrome that exceed 95% at a 5% screen-positive rate.

8 The genetic sonogram has an average sensitivity for trisomy 21 of about 75% in major centers and, when negative, can be used to adjust the risk of Down syndrome downward by at least 50%.

9 The accuracy of a second-trimester ultrasound examination for the identification of fetal anomalies had initially been a disappointment, but it now has the capability of diagnosing over 50% of major abnormalities.

10 During the last decade, little major progress has been made in the isolation of fetal cells in the maternal circulation. However, very recent inroads into the separation and analysis of fetal DNA in the maternal circulation have tremendous diagnostic potential in fetal aneuploidy, X-linked conditions, and blood group disorders.

11 The number of pregnant patients who are of advanced maternal age has soared steadily over the last decade to a point where it exceeds 20%.

12 Loss rates from second-trimester amniocentesis and CVS seem to be dependent upon the experience of the investigator.

13 Fetuses with increased nuchal translucency but with a normal karyotype have increased risks for various anomaly syndromes.

14 Once ultrasound rules out a major structural anomaly and a fetal echocardiogram has ruled out the presence of a major cardiac abnormality, fetuses with increased nuchal translucency and normal karyotypes do not have an increased risk for an adverse pregnancy outcome.

15 A genetic sonogram consists of a search for major anomalies and markers for DS in addition to assessing femur and humeral lengths.

16 With the exception of an increase in nuchal skinfold thickness, small nasal bone, or short humerus, it is unclear how to precisely adjust the risk for DS in a given patient who has other ultrasound markers in isolation.

17 Initial studies from the United States have shown a low sensitivity for ultrasound in the diagnosis of major congenital anomalies in the second trimester. However, European studies have shown a marked improvement in detection rates over the last 10 years.

18 The identification of anomalies is now dependent upon an enhanced ability to diagnose cardiac anomalies (perhaps through three- and four-dimensional technologies).

19 With more investigation in prenatal diagnosis techniques, patients will be able to make better informed decisions, which in turn should translate into fewer unnecessary invasive procedures.

References

1 National Center for Health Statistics. *Vital statistics of the United States, Natality, 1974–1993*. Hyattsville, MD: National Center for Health Statistics, 1977–1996.

2 Benn PA, Egan JFX, Fang M, et al. Changes in the utilization of prenatal diagnosis. *Obstet Gynecol* 2004;103:1255–1260.

3 Egan JFX, Benn P, Borgida AF, et al. Efficacy of screening for fetal Down syndrome in the United States from 1974 to 1997. *Obstet Gynecol* 2000;96:979–985.

4 National Institute of Child Health and Human Development National Institutes of Health, Bethesda, MD. Midtrimester amniocentesis for prenatal diagnosis. *JAMA* 1976;236:1471–1476.

5 Tabor A, Madesen M, Obel E, et al. Randomized controlled trial of genetic amniocentesis in 4606 low-risk women. *Lancet* 1986;1:1287–1293.

6 Seeds JW. Diagnostic mid-trimester amniocentesis: how safe? *Am J Obstet Gynecol* 2004;191:608–616.

7 Blessed WB, Lacoste H, Welch RA. Obstetrician–gynecologists performing genetic amniocentesis may be misleading themselves and their patients. *Am J Obstet Gynecol* 2001;184:1340–1344.

8 Eddleman K, Berkowitz R, Kharbutli Y, et al. for the First and Second Trimester Evaluation of Risk (FASTER) Study Group. Pregnancy loss rates after midtrimester amniocentesis: the FASTER trial. *Am J Obstet Gynecol* 2004;189:S111.

9 Anonymous. Randomised trial to assess safety and fetal outcome of early and midtrimester amniocentesis. The Canadian Early and Mid-trimester Amniocentesis Trial (CEMAT) Group. *Lancet* 1998;251:242–247.

10 Philip J, Silver RK, Wilson RD, et al. for the NICHD EATA Trial Group. Late first-trimester invasive prenatal diagnosis: results of an international randomized trial. *Obstet Gynecol* 2004;103: 1164–1173.

11 Sundberg K, Bang J, Smidt-Jensen S, et al. Randomised study of risk of fetal loss related to early amniocentesis versus chorionic villus sampling. *Lancet* 1997;350;697–703.

12 Brambati B, Simoni G, Travi M, et al. Genetic diagnosis by chorionic villus sampling before 8 gestational weeks: efficiency, reliability, and risks of 317 completed pregnancies. *Prenat Diagn* 1992;12:789–800.

13 Wapner R, Jackson L, Evans MI, et al. *Am J Obstet Gynecol* 1996; 174:310.

14 Saura R, Gauthier B, Taine L, et al. Operator experience and fetal loss rate in transabdominal CVS. *Prenat Diagn* 1994;14: 70–71.

15 Burton BK, Schultz CJ, Burd LI. Limb anomalies associated with chorionic villus sampling. *Obstet Gynecol* 1992;79:726–730.

16 Froster UG, Jackson L. Limb defects and chorionic villus sampling: results from an international registry, 1992–94. *Lancet* 1996;347:489–494.

17 Brambati B, Simoni G, Travi M, et al. Genetic diagnosis by chorionic villus sampling before 8 gestational weeks: efficiency, reliability, and risks of 317 completed pregnancies. *Prenat Diag* 1992;12:789–799.

18 Alfirevic Z, Sundberg K, Brigham S. Amniocentesis and chorionic villus sampling for prenatal diagnosis. *Cochrane Database Syst Rev* 2004;4.

19 Hobbins JC, Mahoney MJ, Goldstein LA. New method of intrauterine evaluation by the combined use of fetoscopy and ultrasound. *Am J Obstet Gynecol* 1974;118:1069–1072.

20 Rodeck CH, Campbell S. Umbilical-cord insertion as source of pure fetal blood for prenatal diagnosis. *Lancet* 1979;1:1244–1245.

21 Daffos F, Capella-Pavlovsky M, Forestier F. A new procedure for fetal blood sampling in utero: preliminary results of fifty-three cases. *Am J Obstet Gynecol* 1983;146:85–987.

22 Ghidini A, Sepulveda W, Lockwood CJ, et al. Complications of fetal blood sampling. *Am J Obstet Gynecol* 1993;168:1339–1344.

23 Yankowitz J, Weiner CP. Blood transfusion for haemolytic disease as a cause of leukocytosis in the fetus. *Prenat Diagn* 1996;16: 719–722.

24 Nicolaides KH, Azar G, Byme D, et al. Fetal nuchal translucency: ultrasound screening for chromosomal defects in first trimester of pregnancy. *Br Med J* 1992;304:867–869.

25 Snijders RJ, Nobel P, Sebire N, et al. UK multicentre project on assessment of risk of trisomy 21 by maternal age and fetal nuchal-translucency thickness at 10–14 weeks of gestation. Fetal Medicine Foundation First Trimester Screening Group. *Lancet* 1998;352:343–346.

26 Haddow JE, Palomaki GE, Knight GJ, et al. Screening of maternal serum for fetal Down's syndrome in the first trimester. *N Engl J Med* 1998;338:955–961.

27 Wapner R, Thom E, Simpson JL, et al. for the First Trimester Maternal Serum Biochemistry and Fetal Nuchal Translucency Screening (BUN) Study Group. First-trimester screening for trisomies 21 and 18. *N Engl J Med* 2003;349:1405–1413.

28 Malone FD, Wald NJ, Canick JA, et al. for the First- and Second-Trimester Evaluation of Risk (FASTER Trial. First- and Second-Trimester Evaluation of Risk (FASTER) trial: principal results of the NICHD multicenter Down syndrome screening study. *Am J Obstet Gynecol* 2003;189:S56.

29 Wald NJ, Hackshaw AK. Combining ultrasound and biochemistry in first-trimester screening for Down syndrome. *Prenat Diagn* 1997;17:821–829.

30 Malone FD, D'Alton ME. First-trimester sonographic screening for Down syndrome. *Obstet Gynecol* 2003;102:1066–1079.

31 Cicero S, Curcio P, Papageorghiou A, et al. Absence of nasal bone in fetuses with trisomy 21 at 11–14 weeks of gestation: an observational study. *Lancet* 2001;358:1665–1667.

32 Cicero S, Longo D, Rembouskos G, et al. Absent nasal bone at 11–14 weeks of gestation and chromosomal defects. *Ultrasound Obstet Gynecol* 2003;22:31–35.

33 Malone FD, Ball RH, Nyberg DA, et al. for the FASTER Study Consortium. First-trimester nasal bone evaluation for aneuploidy in an unselected general population: results from the FASTER Trial. *Am J Obstet Gynecol* 2003;189:S79.

34 Zoppi MA, Ibba RM, Axiana C, et al. Absence of fetal nasal bone and aneuploidies at first-trimester nuchal translucency screening in unselected pregnancies. *Prenat Diagn* 2003;23:496–500.

35 Orlandi F, Bilardo CM, Campogrande M, et al. Measurement of nasal bone length at 11–14 weeks of pregnancy and its potential role in Down syndrome risk assessment. *Ultrasound Obstet Gynecol* 2003;22:36–39.

36 Merkatz IR, Nitowsky HM, Macri JN, et al. An association between low maternal serum alpha-fetoprotein and fetal chromosomal abnormalities. *Am J Obstet Gynecol* 1984;148:886–894.

37 Platt LD, Greene N, Johnson A, et al. for the First Trimester Maternal Serum Biochemistry and Fetal Nuchal Translucency Screening (BUN) Study Group. Sequential pathways of testing after first-trimester screening for trisomy 21. *Obstet Gynecol* 2004;104:661–666.

38 Wright D, Bradbury I, Benn P, et al. Contingent screening for Down syndrome is an efficient alternative to non-disclosure sequential screening. *Prenat Diagn* 2004;24:762–766.

39 Souka AP, Krampl E, Bakalis S, et al. Outcome of pregnancy in chromosomally normal fetuses with increased nuchal translucency in the first trimester. *Ultrasound Obstet Gynecol* 2001;18:9–17.

40 Hyett J, Perdu M, Sharland G, et al. Using nuchal translucency to screen for major congenital cardiac defects at 10–14 weeks of gestation: population based cohort study. *Br Med J* 1999;318:81–85.

41 Benacerraf BR, Barss VA, Laboda LA. A sonographic sign for the detection in the second trimester of the fetus with Down's syndrome. *Am J Obstet Gynecol* 1985;151:1078–1079.

42 Persutte WH, Coury A, Hobbins JC. Correlation of fetal frontal lobe and transcervical diameter measurements: the utility of a new sonographic technique. *Ultrasound Obstet Gynecol* 1997;10:94–97.

43 Benacerraf BR, Cnann A, Gelman R, et al. Can sonographers reliably identify anatomic features associated with Down syndrome in fetuses? *Radiology* 1989;173:377–380.

44 DeVore GR. The role of fetal echocardiography in genetic sonography. *Semin Perinatol* 2003;27:160–172.

45 Bromley B, Lieberman E, Laboda L, et al. Echogenic intracardiac focus: a sonographic sign for fetal Down syndrome. *Obstet Gynecol* 1995;86:998–1001.

46 Egan JFX. The genetic sonogram in second trimester Down syndrome screening. *Clin Obstet Gynecol* 2003;46:897–908.

47 Benacerraf BR, Mandell J, Estroff JA, et al. Fetal pyelectasis: a possible association with Down syndrome. *Obstet Gynecol* 1990;76:58–60.

48 Chitkara U, Lee L, Oehlert JW, et al. Fetal ear length measurement: a useful predictor of aneuploidy? *Ultrasound Obstet Gynecol* 2002;19:131–135.

49 Shipp TD, Bromley B, Lieberman E, et al. The iliac angle as a sonographic marker for Down syndrome in second-trimester fetuses. *Obstet Gynecol* 1997;89:446–450.

50 Persutte WH, Coury A, Hobbins JC. Correlation of fetal frontal lobe and transcerebellar diameter measurements: the utility of a new prenatal sonographic technique. *Ultrasound Obstet Gynecol* 1997;10:94–97.

51 Benacerraf BR, Sathanondh R, Frigoletto FD. Sonographic demonstration of hypoplasia of the middle phalanx of the fifth digit: a finding associated with Down syndrome. *Am J Obstet Gynecol* 1988;159:181–183.

52 Bromley B, Lieberman E, Shipp TD, et al. Fetal nose bone length: a marker for Down syndrome in the second trimester. *J Ultrasound Med* 2002;21:1387–1394.

53 Nyberg DA, Souter VL, El-Bastawissi A, et al. Isolated sonographic markers for detection of fetal Down syndrome in the second trimester of pregnancy. *J Ultrasound Med* 2001;20:1053–1063.

54 Hobbins JC, Lezotte DC, Persutte WH, et al. An 8-center study to evaluate the utility of midterm genetic sonograms among high-risk pregnancies. *J Ultrasound Med* 2003;22:33–38.

55 Bahado-Singh RO, Rowther M, Bailey J, et al. Midtrimester nuchal thickness and the prediction of postnatal congenital heart defect. *Am J Obstet Gynecol* 2002;187:1250–1253.

56 Yeo L, Vintzileos AM. The use of genetic sonography to reduce the need for amniocentesis in women at high-risk for Down syndrome. *Semin Perinatol* 2003;27:152–159.

57 Benn PA, Kaminsky LM, Ying J, et al. Combined second-trimester biochemical and ultrasound screening for Down syndrome. *Obstet Gynecol* 2002;100:1168–1176.

58 Malone F, Nyberg DA, Vidaver J, et al. First and second trimester evaluation of risk (FASTER) trial: the role of second trimester genetic sonography. *Am J Obstet Gynecol* 2003;191:S3.

59 Crane JP, LeFevre ML, Winborn RC, et al. A randomized trial of prenatal ultrasonographic screening: impact on the detection, management, and outcome of anomalous fetuses. The RADIUS Study. *Am J Obstet Gynecol* 1994;171:392–399.

60 Saari-Kemppainen A, Karjalainen O, Ylostalo P, et al. Ultrasound screening and perinatal mortality: controlled trial of systematic one-stage screening in pregnancy. The Helsinki Ultrasound Trial. *Lancet* 1990;336:387–391.

61 Grandjean H, Larroque D, Levi S. The performance of routine ultrasonographic screening of pregnancies in the Eurofetus Study. *Am J Obstet Gynecol* 1999;181:445–454.

62 Walknowska J, Conte FA, Grumbach MM. Practical and theoretical implications of fetal–maternal lymphocyte transfer. *Lancet* 1969;1:1119–1122.

63 Bianchi DW, Flint AF, Pizzimenti MF, et al. Isolation of fetal DNA from nucleated erythrocytes in maternal blood. *Proc Natl Acad Sci USA* 1990;87:3279–3283.

64 NIFTY Study: Bianchi DW, Simpson JL, Jackson LG, et al. Fetal gender and aneuploidy detection using fetal cells in maternal blood: analysis of NIFTY I data. National Institute of Child Health and Development Fetal Cell Isolation Study. *Prenat Diagn* 2002;22:609–615.

65 Lo YM, Hjelm NM, Fidler C, et al. Prenatal diagnosis of fetal RhD status by molecular analysis of maternal plasma. *N Engl J Med* 1998;339:1734–1738.

66 Lo YM, Lau TK, Chan LY, et al. Quantitative analysis of the bidirectional fetomaternal transfer of nucleated cells and plasma DNA. *Clin Chem* 2000;46:1301–1309.

67 Zhang J, Fidler C, Murphy MF, et al. Determination of fetal RhD status by maternal plasma DNA analysis. *Ann NY Acad Sci* 2000;906:153–155.

28

First- and second-trimester screening for open neural tube defects and Down syndrome

James E. Haddow, Glenn E. Palomaki, and Ronald J. Wapner

Biochemical testing for fetal disorders dates from the discovery that amniotic fluid alpha-fetoprotein (AFP) levels are elevated in the presence of open neural tube defects (NTDs; open spina bifida and anencephaly) during the early second trimester.[1] This finding led to diagnostic testing for open NTDs in pregnant women with a previous affected pregnancy. An important limitation of the public health impact of such testing was that fewer than 5% of the annual births affected by open NTDs occurred among women known to be at high risk. Subsequently, maternal serum AFP (MSAFP) levels were also documented to be elevated in the presence of open NTDs, and such measurements were offered to all pregnant women for screening purposes. Women with elevated serum AFP levels were offered diagnostic amniotic fluid AFP (AFAFP) testing. Initially, the presence of open spina bifida could be confirmed only by ultrasound examination of the fetal spine; however, this was technically difficult. This has now been supplemented by more reliable and technically easier ultrasound observations of the fetal cranium and brain (the "lemon" and "banana" signs).[2,3]

Data accumulated during the early years of screening for open NTDs set the stage for the discovery that MSAFP levels were lower in the presence of Down syndrome. A combination of maternal age and AFP levels resulted in an improved prediction of Down syndrome risk, with amniotic fluid chromosome analysis offered to high-risk women. The subsequent discovery of other biochemical markers for Down syndrome greatly improved the efficiency of second-trimester screening. A further important breakthrough occurred with the identification of both biochemical [pregnancy-associated plasma protein A (PAPP-A); free beta subunit of human chorionic gonadotropin (βhCG)] and ultrasound (nuchal translucency, NT) markers for Down syndrome in the first trimester. When used together, these markers perform better than second-trimester screening and have the added advantage of early detection. At present, several strategies that combine first- and second-trimester biochemical measurements (with and without NT measurements) are being evaluated as a way of maximizing the rate of detection and minimizing the rate of false-positives.

Diagnostic testing for open NTDs in amniotic fluid

In 1956, Bergstrand and Czar[4] described a protein in fetal serum, located in the α1 region on electrophoresis [subsequently labeled α1-fetoprotein (AFP)], that was not present in adult serum. It is this unique fetal protein that serves as a marker for leakage of fetal serum into the amniotic fluid and which is therefore helpful in diagnosing open fetal lesions. The molecular weight and structure of AFP is similar to that of albumin (about 69 kDa),[5] but antibodies raised against AFP have virtually no cross-reactivity. This characteristic was critical in allowing the development of a variety of antibody-based assays for reliably measuring AFP in amniotic fluid and maternal serum. The bulk of amniotic fluid protein is now known to be maternally derived,[6,7] and AFP is the only marker that has been found to be helpful in identifying open NTDs.

Figure 28.1 illustrates the relationship between AFAFP values in unaffected pregnancies and AFAFP values in pregnancies affected with open spina bifida; there is a small degree of overlap. Most of that overlap, leading to false-positives in amniotic fluid, can be traced to procedure-related fetal blood contamination. Sometimes, before samples are sent for AFP analysis, they are centrifuged and the red cells are removed. In such cases, hemoglobin F can often be detected in the supernatant, leading to a heightened suspicion of a false-positive result. Once fetal blood contamination has been excluded, the likelihood of obtaining a false-positive result is considerably reduced.

Acetylcholinesterase (AChE) is a neuronally derived protein. Measurements of AChE in amniotic fluid[8] are also used to significantly improve the ability to distinguish between affected and unaffected pregnancies. This gel-electrophoretic approach has not only proved to be highly sensitive at detecting open NTDs (99% of anencephaly cases and 98% of open spina bifida cases with positive AFP results), but also yielded

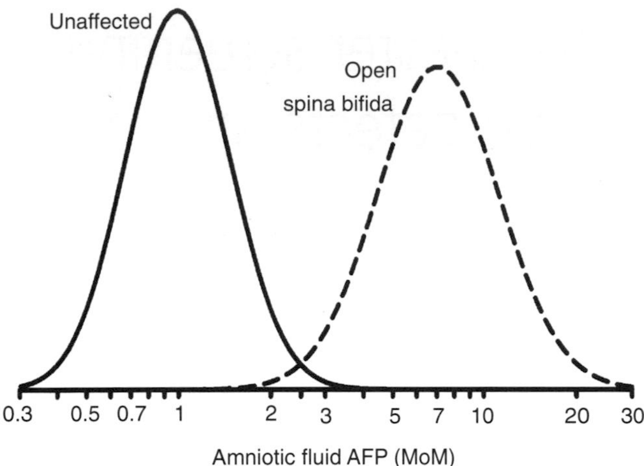

Figure 28.1 Amniotic fluid AFP distributions in singleton, unaffected pregnancies (solid line) and pregnancies affected by open spina bifida (dashed line) during the second trimester. AFP measurements are expressed as multiples of the unaffected population median (MoM) on a logarithmic scale. Distributions of AFP values are logarithmic Gaussian for both of the populations and a small degree of overlap is present. This forms the basis for defining detection and false-positive rates at various amniotic fluid AFP cut-off levels. The odds of being affected, given a positive AFP measurement, can also be estimated using these distributions and the population prevalence of open spina bifida.

negative results in 9 out of 10 cases when the AFAFP measurement was falsely elevated.[9]

Other fetal disorders are also associated with elevated AFAFP levels, including open ventral wall defects (omphalocele and gastroschisis), congenital nephrosis, and the presence of a severely distressed or recently dead fetus.[10] In the USA, open ventral wall defects are the second most common open fetal malformations identified by elevated AFAFP levels during the second trimester, occurring at a rate of three per 10 000 pregnancies.[11] These lesions may also be associated with the presence of AChE in amniotic fluid, probably secondary to leakage from intestinal nerve plexuses. Congenital nephrosis, an autosomal recessive disorder, is rare in most of the world but occurs frequently in Finland.[12]

Experienced laboratories can utilize the band densities of AChE to help distinguish between open ventral wall defects and open NTDs.[13] This distinction has previously been helpful in guiding follow-up sonographic studies in cases when a lesion is difficult to visualize. Presently, however, ultrasound imaging can almost always differentiate between these defects. Fetal death is frequently associated with both elevated AFP levels and the presence of AChE in amniotic fluid.[14] Gel electrophoresis of AChE in such cases often shows a characteristic smeared pattern. Small amounts of fetal calf serum, when accidentally introduced into an amniotic fluid sample prior to analysis, can produce a visible AChE band.[14] When this is suspected, testing for bovine serum albumin can identify the cause of the false-positive result.

Maternal serum screening for open NTDs in the second trimester

In 1974, it was discovered that, during the second trimester, AFP levels in maternal serum were, on average, higher when anencephaly or open spina bifida was present in the fetus.[15,16] A multicenter study in the UK[17] tested the feasibility of using MSAFP measurements for second-trimester screening purposes; pregnancies identified as high risk would then become candidates for diagnostic procedures, including amniocentesis and high-resolution ultrasound.

MSAFP concentrations rise by approximately 15% per week during the second trimester in unaffected singleton pregnancies, and it was therefore necessary to take this into account when establishing normative data. In addition, it was important to take into account any potential differences in assay standards among centers. For example, an MSAFP level measured as 40 ng/mL in one center might be measured as 75 ng/mL in a second center. Both of these measurements would be correct in relation to other measurements within the respective population, but it would be impossible to compare them without establishing a common currency. In analyzing data from the UK collaborative study, Wald and colleagues[17] began by converting data from each of the centers into multiples of the unaffected population's median. The median is the most stable and reliable measure of any given population's midpoint, and serves as the point of reference against which all other measurements can be expressed as multiples of the median (MoM). This conversion of the data allowed the different within-laboratory mass unit values for each gestational week to be taken into account, and made it possible to compare the median MSAFP values for pregnancies affected with open spina bifida (3.8 MoM) or anencephaly (7.7 MoM) with values from unaffected singleton pregnancies (1.0 MoM). Figure 28.2 demonstrates the distributions of MSAFP values in unaffected singleton pregnancies and in pregnancies affected by open spina bifida. Defining the distributions of MSAFP values in MoM also allowed the extent of overlap between unaffected and affected populations to be analyzed. With this information, both the individual and the collective odds that a pregnancy would be affected with a given fetal disorder could be estimated (Fig. 28.3).

The ability to estimate the individual and collective odds for open spina bifida provided a rational basis for deciding on a reasonable cut-off level for high-risk classification. For example, 3.4% of screened pregnancies from the general population and 75% of open spina bifida pregnancies were associated with MSAFP values of 2.5 MoM or above. At that time, the prevalence of open spina bifida in the UK was approximately two cases per 1000 births. Therefore, for every 10 000 pregnancies screened, 340 would initially be placed in the high-risk category and 17 of those (1 out of 20) would be affected with open spina bifida. In the USA, where the prevalence of open spina bifida was lower (one case per 1000

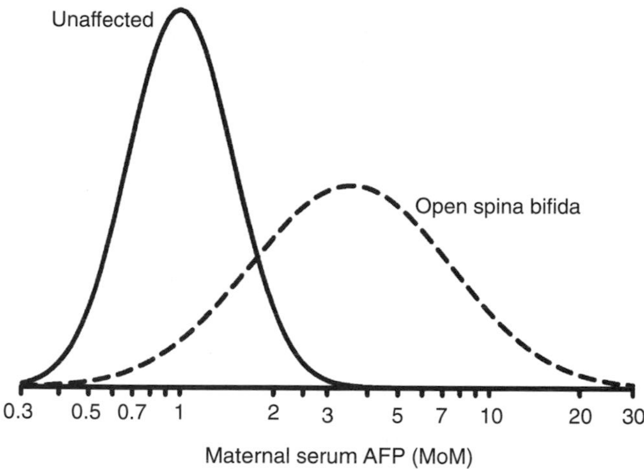

Figure 28.2 Maternal serum AFP distributions in singleton, unaffected pregnancies (solid line) and in pregnancies affected by open spina bifida (dashed line) during the second trimester. AFP measurements are expressed as multiples of the unaffected population median (MoM) on a logarithmic scale. Distributions of AFP values are logarithmic Gaussian for both of the populations and a moderate degree of overlap is present. These distributions form the basis for estimating both collective and individual odds for being affected with open spina bifida, once the maternal serum AFP value and the population prevalence are known.

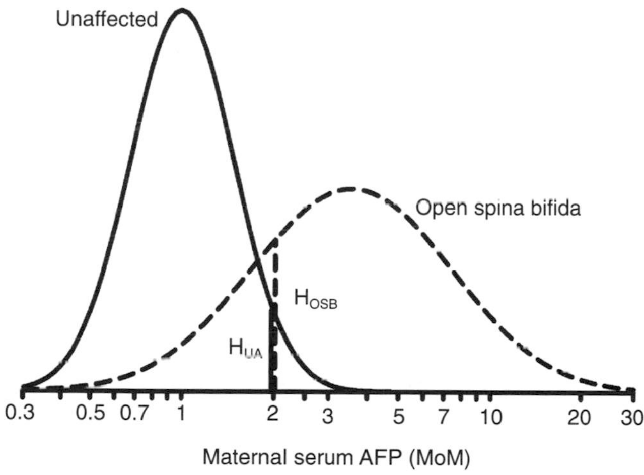

Figure 28.3 Estimation, during the second trimester, of a pregnant woman's individual odds of carrying a fetus affected by open spina bifida once her maternal serum AFP value has been determined. In this example, the woman's AFP level is 2.0 MoM, and the measurements from that point on the baseline to the intersection with the unaffected (H_{UA}) and affected (H_{OSB}) curves are approximately 4 units (solid vertical line) and 8 units (dashed vertical line) respectively, producing a likelihood ratio of 2. Based on her AFP level, the woman's individual odds of having a pregnancy affected by open spina bifida are now two times higher than those of the general population.

births), 1 out of 40 of the pregnancies in the high-risk category would be affected by open spina bifida. It also became possible to assign individual risk estimates for open spina bifida based on the initial MSAFP value. If pregnancies are dated by ultrasound measurement before screening, the overall screening performance is improved in that the rate of detection is increased and the false-positive rate is reduced. Improved MSAFP assay performance also influences the odds estimates. In contrast to the mid-1970s when coefficients of variation ranged from 8% to 25%, assays now have figures that are below 5%. This improvement substantially lowers the false-positive rate. Some believe that faulty assay performance is largely responsible for the less than complete detection of open lesions and that improvement in the assay will lead to better detection rates. This perception is incorrect as commercially available assays now perform very satisfactorily.[18] Detection is limited because the distribution of MSAFP levels in various open fetal lesions overlaps to varying degrees with that of the unaffected population. This characteristic needs to be understood by physicians, office personnel, and patients, so that expectations do not exceed the capacity of the screening test.

The original estimates for both detection rates and false-positive rates of MSAFP screening for open NTDs were based upon the date of the last menstrual period (LMP).[17] Even when LMP dates are carefully obtained, they are incorrect by more than 2 weeks in about 20% of cases.[19] Furthermore, there is a tendency to think that a pregnancy is further advanced than it really is, and this diminishes detection because normative data are based on a known rise in MSAFP measurements of about 15% per week during the second trimester. In 1980, the average biparietal diameter (BPD) of fetuses with spina bifida was found to be smaller than that of unaffected fetuses at any given gestational week in the second trimester.[20] Other ultrasound measurements did not differ. If BPD measurements were to be used routinely for dating in MSAFP screening, the MSAFP measurements would appear to be higher for pregnancies with open spina bifida, and sensitivity for detecting the lesion would be increased, possibly to above 90%. An abbreviated ultrasound study involving fetal biometry would correct the dates of pregnancies that are further advanced than predicted by LMP and would also identify twins, thereby reducing false-positive screening results. Cases of anencephaly would also be identified at this point. Systematically carrying out fetal biometry and dating pregnancies by BPD measurements would reduce screening program costs and increase screening performance, thereby avoiding unnecessary anxiety for many women.

As AFP screening became more widely used, factors were identified that influence the analyte level, the risks of open NTDs, or both. One of these factors is maternal weight. Heavier women tend to have lower concentrations of serum markers because of their increased blood volume. This factor has added significance in that very heavy women are reported to have a higher risk of having a fetus affected with open spina bifida.[21–28] Adjusting for a woman's weight has the overall effect of increasing detection while decreasing false-positives; the false-positive rate becomes similar for both lighter and heavier women. A second influencing factor is maternal race.[29] Among black women, MSAFP levels are about 10–15% higher than among white women.[30] If this is not taken into account, an inappropriately high proportion of black women will be identified as having positive screening results and will be sent for further diagnostic procedures. The inappropriateness of this action is compounded by the fact that black women have a lower risk (by about one-half) of open NTDs. A 16-center US collaborative study[31] confirmed the feasibility of adjusting the MSAFP values to reflect a more appropriate proportion of black women with positive screening results. A third influencing factor is maternal insulin-dependent diabetes, which is associated with a 20% lower MSAFP value than unaffected singleton pregnancies.[32,33] Women with insulin-dependent diabetes also have a higher risk of having a pregnancy affected by open NTDs. At present, a re-evaluation is in progress to determine whether the level of diabetic control, as measured by hemoglobin A_{1c}, influences the MSAFP concentration[34,35] but this issue is not yet completely resolved.

Use of ultrasound in the identification of open NTDs

Ultrasound is an invaluable complement to AFP measurements in the evaluation of NTDs. Advances in imaging now allow the diagnosis of all cases of anencephaly as early as 12 weeks' gestation, and the diagnosis of over 95% of fetuses with spina bifida in the second trimester. In addition, many other causes of elevated MSAFP levels are discernable by ultrasound. Accordingly, ultrasound can be used both in the definitive diagnosis of open NTDs in high-risk patients and as part of an AFP screening program.

Use of ultrasound as a component of open NTD screening

The efficacy of using MSAFP levels in screening for open NTDs is well documented[36,37] and has stood as a routine obstetrical test for almost 30 years. As physicians have become more skilled in the identification of fetal structural anomalies using ultrasound, and the resolution of the equipment has improved, experts have questioned whether AFP screening could be replaced by ultrasound. In expert centers this may be feasible. Wald and colleagues,[38,39] as well as others, have demonstrated that ultrasound evaluation of the fetal spine and head rivals MSAFP screening when performed in a high-risk population by experienced perinatal sonographers. However, there is little to suggest that ultrasound will perform as well in a general low-risk pregnant population, when the availability of sonographers with extensive experience of identifying open NTDs is limited. Detection rates in this population are approximately 60–80%. Therefore, MSAFP screening between 15 and 20 weeks' gestation (ideally between 16 and 18 weeks) remains the primary approach to open NTD screening.

Because only about 2% of women with an initially elevated MSAFP screen have a fetus with an open NTD, the initial step in the subsequent evaluation is the performance of a fetal ultrasound to rapidly identify other causes of the elevated screen. These include incorrect dating (see section on maternal serum screening for open NTDs in the second trimester, above), the presence of twins, oligohydramnios, fetal demise, and other more easily identifiable fetal anomalies such as omphalocele and gastroschisis. In up to 50% of cases, incorrect dating will be identified and subsequent adjustment of the MSAFP value will resolve the issue. If the cause of the elevation remains unknown after the initial scan, genetic counseling and additional testing by either ultrasound or amniocentesis will be required.

Until recently, the standard diagnostic test for high-risk patients (i.e., those with unexplained elevated MSAFP levels, those having a previously affected child, and those taking medications known to increase the risk of open NTDs) was amniocentesis with an evaluation of AFAFP and AChE levels. Measurement of this combination of amniotic fluid analytes has a greater than 99% detection rate for anencephaly and an approximately 95–99% detection rate for spina bifida with a 0.4% false-positive rate.[40–42] Recently, advances in high-resolution ultrasound have led to similar detection rates without the potential risk of an invasive procedure.[43,44] In the hands of the most experienced sonographers, targeted sonographic evaluation of high-risk cases has a sensitivity of 97–100% with 100% specificity.

Ultrasound detection of a meningomyelocele is frequently based on the finding of a small cystic mass protruding from the fetal lumbosacral or thoracic area. On other occasions, the findings may be more subtle and may only present as a widening of the posterior processes of the vertebral bodies. Although many open NTDs will be seen in the coronal or sagittal planes, others may not. The definitive views to identify or exclude spina bifida are transverse images of each individual vertebral body (Fig. 28.4).

The ultrasound diagnosis of open NTDs has been greatly enhanced by the recognition of associated anomalies of the fetal skull and brain,[2,45] which are present in over 95% of cases of spina bifida imaged in the second trimester. These findings include ventriculomegaly, microcephaly, frontal bone scalloping ("lemon" sign), and obliteration of the cisterna magna with either an absent or abnormal anterior curvature of the cerebellar hemisphere ("banana" sign). These last two findings are secondary to the presence of an Arnold–Chiari malformation and their appearance is related to gestational age. The lemon sign appears in approximately 90–98% of pregnancies with spina bifida imaged before 24 weeks' gestation but in significantly fewer of those imaged at a more advanced

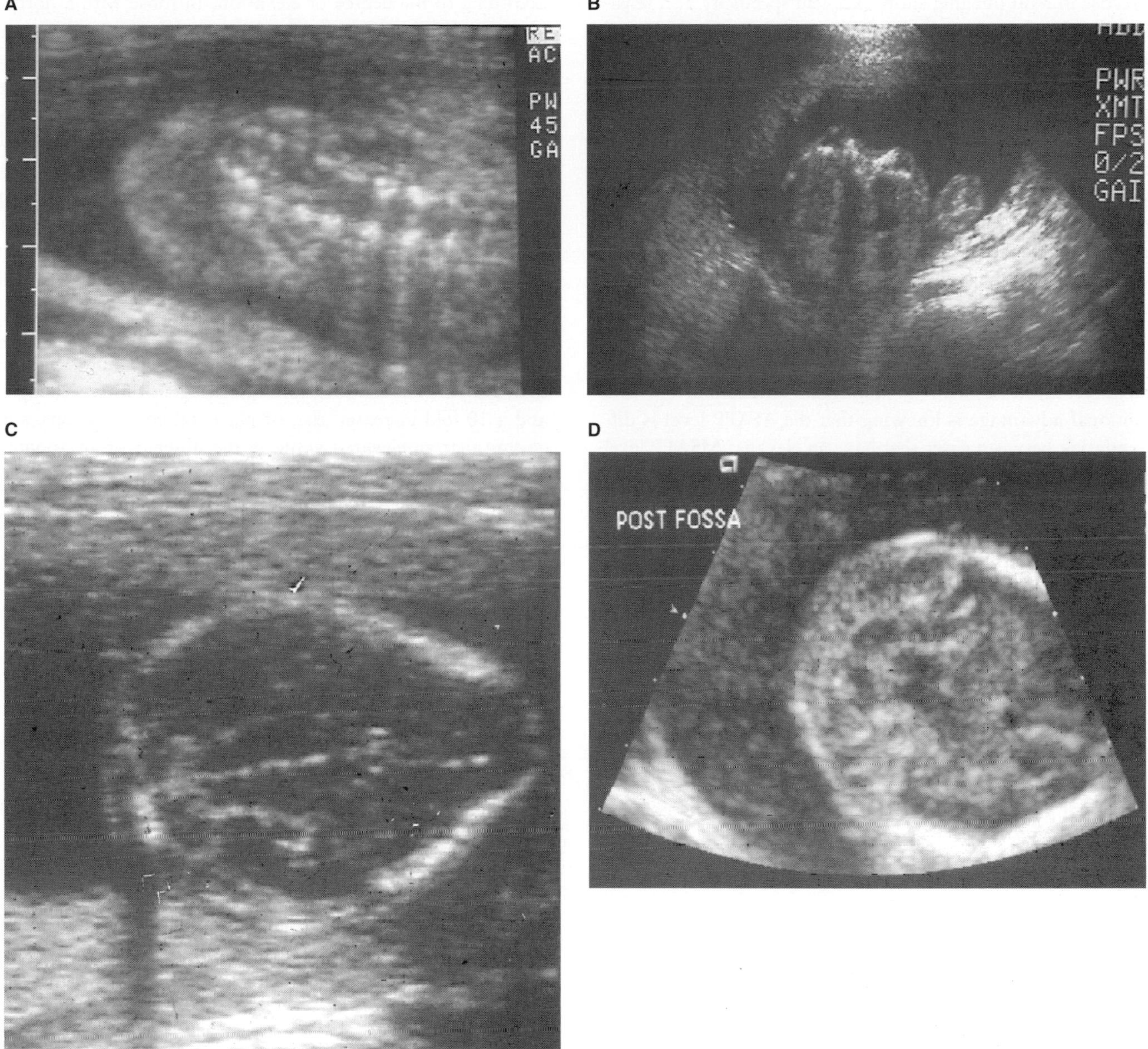

Figure 28.4 Ultrasound prenatal diagnosis of spina bifida. (A) Coronal view of lower lumbar spine demonstrating widening of the posterior processes and disruption of the vertebra; (B) a transverse view of a meningomyelocele (note that in this case the spinal defect is seen as an indentation with no sac); (C) head view of a fetus with spina bifida demonstrating the "lemon" sign secondary to frontal bone scalloping; and (D) typical "banana" sign, showing downward displacement of the cerebellum.

gestational age. Cerebellar abnormalities are present in 95% of fetuses irrespective of gestational age; however, they appear as the banana sign most frequently before 24 weeks and as cerebellar absence after 24 weeks.[3,45]

The cranial signs associated with spina bifida are frequently more easily attainable than the detailed transverse scans required to identify the specific spinal lesion. It is reassuring that the sacral lesions that are the most difficult to visualize appear to be the ones most frequently accompanied by cranial and cerebellar findings. In the series reported by Van den Hof[3] and Nyberg and colleagues,[45] all sacral lesions were accompanied by abnormalities of the head, whereas only lumbar lesions were associated with normally shaped heads.

Two schools of thought continue to exist as to whether ultrasound scanning alone is sufficient for high-risk patients or whether amniocentesis should continue to be the primary diagnostic procedure. Recent studies have confirmed that, with the addition of the cranial signs, centers with specialized expertise in fetal imaging show excellent specificity and sensitivity for the detection of open NTDs.[43,46] In less experienced hands, however, where both false-positive and false-negative results are obtained, ultrasound must still be considered a screening rather than a diagnostic procedure.[47–49]

Even in centers with expertise in sonography there may be additional value in performing an amniocentesis. In addition to the close to 100% detection rate reported with AFAFP and AChE measurements,[50] invasive testing has the additional advantage of enabling the fetal karyotype to be evaluated. Several studies suggest that elevated MSAFP levels independently increase the risk of fetal aneuploidy.[51] In pregnancies complicated by an elevated MSAFP, the incidence of fetal aneuploidy is 0.61% in fetuses with a normal ultrasound and 16% in those with an abnormal ultrasound.[52,53] One additional advantage is knowing that the AFAFP level is differentiating between cases that have an elevated MSAFP level secondary to placental leakage and those that also have an elevated AFAFP level. Those with only elevated maternal serum values have an increased risk of placental problems, including fetal growth retardation, stillbirth, and preeclampsia. Those with elevated amniotic fluid levels should be further evaluated for fetal anomalies. In the evaluation of a very high MSAFP level, amniocentesis may be of particular value because there is a direct relationship between the degree of MSAFP elevation and the occurrence of anomalies.[54,55] With an MSAFP of 2.5 MoM, there is a 3.4% risk of anomalies, whereas at 7 MoM, the risk increases to 40.3%.[55]

Although many of the congenital anomalies associated with elevated AFAFP levels are easily diagnosed with ultrasound (e.g., omphalocele, gastroschisis, bladder extrophy, and some cases of sacrococcygeal teratoma), other equally severe fetal problems may have no ultrasound findings. For example, fetal skin lesions such as epidermolysis bullosa may leak serum and be associated with elevated levels of both MSAFP and AFAFP. Very high levels of both MSAFP and AFAFP are also seen in congenital nephrosis,[56] frequently without any abnormalities identified on second-trimester ultrasound.

At present, the ideal management of an elevated MSAFP level should include both ultrasound and amniocentesis. If a high-quality ultrasound fails to identify a fetal defect, the risks and benefits of both amniocentesis and a specialized ultrasound examination should be discussed with the patient. The decision can then be based on the degree of AFP elevation, the patient's history, the quality and findings of the ultrasound examination, and the patient's age.

An elevated MSAFP level in which both the ultrasound scan and AFAFP and AChE levels are normal retains an increased risk of adverse pregnancy outcome; there is a 20–58% risk of poor pregnancy outcome with an unexplained raised MSAFP level.[57–59] Risks include low birthweight, growth restriction, placental abruption, fetal or neonatal death, and preeclampsia. Crandall and colleagues[60] studied 1002 women with MSAFP values greater than 2.5 MoM and stratified them according to the degree of elevation. In those with a normal ultrasound and amniocentesis, the risk of an adverse outcome was 27% overall but varied with the degree of elevation. An adverse outcome occurred in 16% of cases when the MSAFP was 2.5–2.9 MoM, 29% when the MSAFP was 3.0–5.0 MoM, and 70% when it was greater than 5.0 MoM. Wailer and co-workers[61] evaluated the predictive value of a high MSAFP level compared with a low level in 51 008 women screened for MSAFP. The risk of delivery before 28 weeks was 0.4% for those with low MSAFP values (< 0.81 MoM) and 3.2% for those with high values (> 2.5 MoM), an eightfold difference.[61–63] The rates of delivery before 37 weeks were 2.6% for the low MSAFP group and 24.3% for the high MSAFP group. Notably, women with MSAFP values greater than 2.5 MoM had a 10.5-fold increased risk of preeclampsia and a 10-fold increased risk of placental complications, suggesting that an elevated value in the absence of an anomaly may derive from a fetal–maternal hemorrhage of sufficient volume to have clinical significance. To date, no management protocol has been demonstrated to improve outcome in these cases. Despite this, such patients should be followed throughout the pregnancy, with serial testing of fetal growth and well-being.

Maternal serum screening for Down syndrome in the second trimester using AFP measurements

A new and unexpected association between low MSAFP levels and certain autosomal trisomies (Down syndrome, trisomy 18) was reported in 1984.[64] This discovery was rapidly confirmed and a method was proposed that would enable a patient-specific risk for Down syndrome to be obtained by combining a woman's age-related risk with the increase (or decrease) in risk as defined by her serum AFP level.[65] The additional information provided by MSAFP measurements had the potential to identify a subgroup of younger pregnant women whose individual risk of a Down syndrome-affected pregnancy was similar to that of women aged 35 and older.

An eight-center collaborative field trial was initiated in 1985 to determine the efficacy of applying MSAFP screening routinely to the pregnant population.[66] A total of 77 273 pregnancies were screened; 4.7% were initially classified as being at high risk for Down syndrome, and 2.7% remained at high risk after gestational dates had been confirmed. Of these high-risk women, 66% elected to have amniocentesis, and 18 fetuses with Down syndrome and four fetuses with trisomy 18 were identified. One case of Down syndrome was identified per 89 amniocenteses performed (among unscreened women aged 35 and older, the rate is approximately one case per 150 second-trimester pregnancies), and an additional three Down syndrome births were identified from among the women who refused amniocentesis. Thus, approximately 25% of the fetal Down syndrome cases were identified in pregnant women under 35, and the study concluded that this type of screening was feasible. A survey of screening centers carried out in 1988 in the USA reported that more than one million pregnancies were being screened for Down syndrome by MSAFP testing.[67]

Maternal serum screening for Down syndrome in the second trimester using multiple markers

In the late 1980s, the levels of hCG and unconjugated estriol (uE_3) in a pregnant woman's blood were found to be useful screening markers for Down syndrome during the second trimester.[68–71] Levels of uE_3 and AFP are lower in the presence of Down syndrome, whereas hCG levels are higher. These three markers in combination raised the detection rate for Down syndrome to approximately 60%, while keeping the false-positive rate at 5%. In the early 1990s, several successful trials were undertaken in Europe and the USA to determine the efficacy of multiple-marker screening under everyday conditions. The first trial, reported from the USA, was carried out by two centers in New England.[72] In this study, a risk cutoff of 1:190 was selected with the aim of initially identifying about 5% of the screened pregnancies as being at high risk for Down syndrome (i.e., a positive screening result was defined as being a risk of at least 1 in 190). Among the 25 207 women who were screened, 6.6% were initially classified as being at high risk. The revised positive rate was 3.8% after follow-up and reclassification of LMP dates by ultrasound. These women were offered amniocentesis and chromosome studies; 79% accepted. In this group of 720 women, 20 fetuses with Down syndrome (one per 38 amniocenteses) and seven fetuses with other chromosomal disorders were identified. It was determined from follow-up information that the Down syndrome detection rate was 58%, which was close to the expected rate.[71]

In the mid-1990s, dimeric inhibin-A (DIA) was discovered to be a useful second trimester marker for Down syndrome.[73] The median DIA level in maternal serum of affected pregnancies was twice that of unaffected pregnancies. A consensus estimate of performance data from eight case–control studies showed a univariate detection rate for Down syndrome of 41%, with a 5% false-positive rate.[73] An independent dataset that was reported in conjunction with this consensus analysis concluded that adding DIA to the three-marker screening panel would raise the detection rate for Down syndrome to 78% at a 5% false-positive rate (using ultrasound dating), a substantial improvement. This performance estimate has been confirmed in a recent multicenter study, which found an 81% detection rate with the same 5% false-positive rate.[74] DIA is now commonly included with AFP, uE_3, and hCG as part of routine second-trimester screening. Figure 28.5 provides overlapping distributions of these four second-trimester markers on a common scale to allow for direct comparisons.

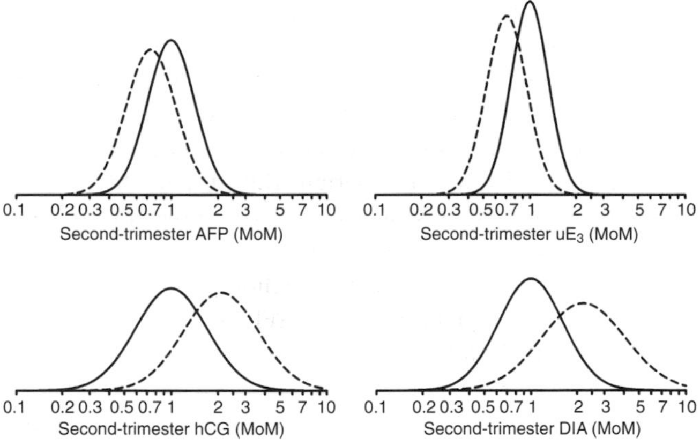

Figure 28.5 Overlapping distributions of second-trimester maternal serum AFP, uE_3, hCG, and DIA measurements in unaffected (solid line) and Down syndrome (dashed line) pregnancies. The four figures are drawn on the same scale. For AFP and uE_3 measurements, Down syndrome pregnancies have lower values, whereas hCG and DIA measurements are higher. These overlapping distributions show the relative frequencies, so those with less variability (i.e., smaller standard deviation) are higher. Overall, AFP is the least effective of the four screening markers for Down syndrome.

Adding trisomy 18 interpretations to second-trimester maternal serum screening

Trisomy 18 (Edwards syndrome) is a lethal chromosome disorder.[75] The birth prevalence of trisomy 18 increases with maternal age, similar to Down syndrome. In the general pregnant population, the second-trimester prevalence of trisomy 18 is approximately one out of 2400 pregnancies, whereas the birth prevalence is one out of 8000; this is because of a third-trimester spontaneous fetal loss rate of 70%.[76] More than one-half of the liveborn infants will die by the age of 10 days and over 90% by 100 days.[75] Prenatal detection can be medically and economically justified when performed in conjunction with Down syndrome screening if a high proportion of women offered amniocentesis have an affected fetus. Fetuses with trisomy 18 are growth retarded and this, along with a high rate of fetal loss in the third trimester, leads to a Cesarean section rate of 50% or higher when the condition is undiagnosed.[77] Approximately 25% of fetuses with trisomy 18 also have spina bifida or omphalocele.

Second-trimester maternal serum levels of AFP, uE_3, and hCG are all lower, on average, in the presence of trisomy 18. This pattern is not associated with incorrect gestational dating (unlike the pattern for Down syndrome) and, therefore, is rarely seen in unaffected pregnancies. Optimal screening performance requires a risk-based algorithm that treats the analyte measurements as continuous variables and includes maternal age, similar to the approach used for Down syndrome screening described earlier in this chapter. This algorithm was developed using data provided by nine prenatal screening centers in North America and Europe, which retrospectively provided maternal serum AFP, uE_3, and hCG measurements (expressed as MoM) and relevant pregnancy-related information on a total of 94 second-trimester trisomy 18 pregnancies.[78] In the 89 pregnancies without an accompanying open NTD, the median levels for AFP, uE_3, and hCG were 0.65, 0.43, and 0.36 MoM, respectively. Overall, 70% of uE_3 MoM values, 54% of hCG values, and 44% of AFP values from trisomy 18 pregnancies were equal to or less than those of the 5th percentile of unaffected pregnancies. At a risk cutoff level of 1:100, a combination of AFP, uE_3, and hCG measurements detected 60% of the trisomy 18 pregnancies with a false-positive rate of about 0.2%; one in every nine amniocenteses identified a fetus with trisomy 18. The risk-based screening protocol is now the preferred approach to screening for trisomy 18.

Abnormal analyte levels with normal karyotype

The association of elevated AFP levels with poor pregnancy outcome is discussed above. Similarly, there are clinical consequences of altered levels of the other analytes used in aneuploid screening.

Unexplained elevated hCG levels

The risk of an adverse pregnancy outcome with elevated hCG levels appears to be independent of the risks associated with elevated AFP levels. Studies have shown that an unexplained elevated hCG level is associated with an increased risk of preeclampsia, preterm birth, low birthweight, fetal demise, and possibly hypertension.[79] It appears that the higher the level of hCG, the greater the risk.

Elevated hCG and AFP levels

The combination of elevated MSAFP and hCG levels occurs rarely but may have an overall pregnancy complication rate exceeding 50%. A study of 66 singleton and 33 multiple pregnancies with an MSAFP of more than 2 MoM and an hCG of more than 3.0 MoM found that 60% of singletons and 81% of twins had at least one obstetric complication; these included preeclampsia, preterm birth, growth restriction, placental abnormalities, and fetal death.[80] Confined placental mosaicism for chromosome 16 has been reported to be associated with extremely high levels of both analytes and to have a very poor prognosis.[81,82]

Low second-trimester maternal serum uE_3 levels

Low maternal serum uE_3 levels have been linked to adverse pregnancy outcomes.[83,84] Very low or absent uE_3 levels of 0.0–0.15 MoM suggest biochemical abnormalities of the fetus or placenta, including placental steroid sulfatase deficiency, Smith–Lemli–Opitz syndrome, congenital adrenal hypoplasia, adrenocorticotropin deficiency, hypothalamic corticotropin deficiency, and anencephaly.

Smith–Lemli–Opitz syndrome is an autosomal recessive disorder secondary to a defect in 3-hydroxysteroid-7-reductase, which alters cholesterol synthesis and results in low cholesterol levels and the accumulation of the cholesterol precursor 7-dehydrocholesterol in blood and amniotic fluid. Because cholesterol is a precursor of E_3, the defect results in reduced or undetectable levels of E_3 in maternal serum and amniotic fluid. Smith–Lemli–Opitz syndrome is characterized by low birthweight, failure to thrive, and moderate to severe mental retardation. It is associated with multiple structural anomalies, including syndactyly of the second and third toes, microcephaly, ptosis, and typical-appearing facies.[85–87]

Bradley and colleagues[88] summarized findings in 33 women who delivered infants with Smith–Lemli–Opitz syndrome. Out of the 26 women whose second-trimester uE_3 values were determined, 24 had levels that were below the 5th percentile (< 0.5 MoM). The median level in this group was 0.23 MoM (below the 1st percentile). A risk assessment based on maternal serum uE_3 levels in combination with AFP and hCG has been suggested[89] and subsequently used prospectively in a cohort of 1 079 301 pregnancies.[90] Reliable and inexpensive prenatal diagnostic testing for Smith–Lemli–Opitz syndrome is available based on amniotic fluid cholesterol or 7-dehydrocholesterol levels.[91]

Placental steroid sulfatase deficiency is an X-linked recessive disorder resulting from deletion of Xp22.3. This enzyme deficiency prevents removal of the sulfate molecule from fetal estrogen precursors, preventing their conversion to E_3. The fetal phenotype depends on the extent of the deletion, with over 90% of cases presenting as X-linked ichthyosis that can be treated with topical keratolytic agents. However, in about 5% of cases, there can be a deletion of contiguous genes, causing mental retardation. The deletion can extend, on occasion, to cause Kallmann syndrome or chondrodysplasia punctata. The lack of estrogen biosynthesis may result in delayed onset of labor, prolonged labor, or stillbirth.

Prenatal diagnosis of the deletion that leads to placental sulfatase deficiency and congenital ichthyosis can be performed by karyotyping or fluorescence *in situ* hybridization.[92–94] Although very low uE_3 levels, usually below the level of detection, can detect males at risk for this disorder, testing in these cases is not routinely offered because the phenotype is usually mild. However, the rarer more serious cases of extensive deletions will be missed.[95]

Ultrasound in second-trimester aneuploid screening

Second-trimester ultrasound markers for Down syndrome

There are no single physical characteristics that are diagnostic for Down syndrome, rather the diagnosis is suspected when a combination of associated features (e.g., Simian crease, epicanthal folds, increased nuchal skinfold) are present. Similarly, the *in utero* probability of Down syndrome is increased when ultrasound imaging demonstrates anomalies or physical features that occur more frequently in Down syndrome fetuses than in the general population. Some of these are distinct congenital anomalies such as atrioventricular canal or duodenal atresia, which strongly suggest the possibility of Down syndrome and are independent indications to offer invasive testing. None of these occurs frequently enough, however, to be valuable in routine screening of a low-risk population. For example, although 40% of fetuses with duodenal atresia have Down syndrome, it is seen in only 8% of affected fetuses. More valuable for routine screening are the "soft markers," which are variations of normal that occur more commonly in fetuses with Down syndrome than in unaffected fetuses. By comparing the prevalence of these markers in Down syndrome fetuses with their prevalence in the unaffected population, a likelihood ratio can be calculated that can be used to modify the a priori age or serum-screen risk.

For a marker to be useful for screening, it should be present in a high proportion of Down syndrome pregnancies, infrequently seen in normal fetuses, easily imaged during routine sonographic examination, and present early enough in the second trimester that subsequent diagnostic testing by amniocentesis can be performed with results available when pregnancy termination remains an option. Markers commonly used to assess the risk of Down syndrome include the following:

- An *increased nuchal fold* is the most distinctive second-trimester marker. To obtain the correct image, the fetal head is scanned in a transverse plane similar to that used in measuring the BPD. The thalami and upper portion of the cerebellum should be in the plane of the image. The distance between the external surface of the occipital bone and the external surface of the skin is measured. About 35% of Down syndrome fetuses have a nuchal skinfold measurement that is greater than 6 mm compared with only 0.7% of unaffected fetuses. When fetuses with more than one marker are included, a measurement of greater than 6 mm yields a likelihood ratio for Down syndrome of 50. When an increased nuchal fold is an isolated finding, the likelihood ratio for Down syndrome is 20. Thus, the presence of an increased nuchal fold alone is an indication to offer invasive testing.[96–101]
- In the second trimester, Down syndrome fetuses may have *short proximal extremities*. An observed–expected ratio of less than 0.91 or a BPD–femur ratio of more than 1.5 has a reported likelihood ratio for Down syndrome of 1.5–2.7 when present as an isolated finding. A short humerus is more strongly related to Down syndrome than a short femur, with reported likelihood ratios ranging from 2.5 to 7.5.[102]
- *Echogenic intracardiac foci* are secondary to mineralization within the papillary muscle and occur in up to 5% of normal pregnancies and in approximately 13–18% of Down syndrome pregnancies.[103] When an echogenic focus is present as an isolated marker, the likelihood ratio for Down syndrome is approximately 2. The risk does not seem to vary if the focus is in the right or left ventricle or if it is unilateral or bilateral.
- *Increased echogenicity of the fetal bowel*, when brighter than the surrounding bone, has a likelihood ratio for Down syndrome of 5.5–6.7.[104–106] This finding can also be seen with fetal cystic fibrosis, congenital cytomegalovirus infection, swallowed bloody amniotic fluid, and severe intrauterine growth restriction. Therefore, if amniocentesis is performed for karyotype analysis in these cases, testing for other potential etiologies should be considered.
- Mild *fetal pyelectasis* (a renal anterior–posterior diameter of greater than 4 mm) has been suggested as a potential marker for Down syndrome. As an isolated marker, the likelihood ratio ranges from 1.5 to 1.9. More recently, Snijders and coworkers[107] did not find a significant increase in mild fetal pyelectasis in Down syndrome pregnancies compared with normal pregnancies, and its value in Down syndrome screening is questionable.
- Other markers that have been described include a hypoplastic fifth middle phalanx of the hand,[108] short ears, a sandal gap between the first and second toes,[109,110] an abnormal iliac wing angle,[111] an altered foot–femur ratio,[112] and a short or absent nasal bone.[113] These markers are inconsistently used because of the time and expertise required to obtain them.

Use of ultrasound to estimate the risk of Down syndrome

As with other screening modalities, second-trimester ultrasound can be used to alter the a priori risk in either direction. A benign second-trimester scan that finds none of the known markers and no anomalies has been suggested to have a likelihood ratio for Down syndrome of 0.4, assuming the image quality is satisfactory.[114] Nyberg and colleagues used this approach to calculate an age-adjusted ultrasound risk assessment for Down syndrome in 8914 pregnancies (186 fetuses with Down syndrome, 8728 control subjects). Some type of sonographic finding (major abnormality, minor marker, or both) was observed in 68.8% of fetuses with trisomy 21 compared with 13.6% of control fetuses ($P < 0.001$); about one-third of fetuses with Down syndrome have neither a marker nor an anomaly.

A positive finding on ultrasound can also be used to modify the risk of aneuploidy. The magnitude of the increase depends on the marker(s) or anomalies seen. Nyberg and colleagues[114,115] reviewed their own data and the data of others[116] to estimate a likelihood ratio for each marker when it is present as an isolated finding (see Table 28.1).

Combined ultrasound and multiple marker risk assessment in the second trimester

Ultrasound markers can be combined with serum markers, but a relatively small correlation between the two approaches needs to be taken into consideration if a quantitative approach is used.[117] Bahado-Singh and colleagues[118] combined ultrasound markers with maternal analytes, including urinary hyperglycosylated hCG and urinary β-core fragment of hCG. In a sample of 585 pregnancies, the sensitivity of this combined screening approach for trisomy 21 was 93.7%, with a false-positive rate of 5%.

Table 28.1 Likelihood ratios (LR) and 95% confidence intervals (CI) for isolated markers in three studies.

Sonographic marker	LR*	LR (95% CI)†	LR (95% CI)‡
Nuchal thickening	18.6	11 (5.2–22)	17 (8–38)
Hyperechoic bowel	5.5	6.7 (2.7–16.8)	6.1 (3–12.6)
Short humerus	2.5	5.1 (1.6–16.5)	7.5 (4.7–12)
Short femur	2.2	1.5 (0.8–2.8)	2.7 (1.2–6)
EIF	2	1.8 (1.0–3)	2.8 (1.5–5.5)
Pyelectasis	1.5	1.5 (0.6–3.6)	1.9 (0.7–5.1)

From ref. 115.

EIF, echogenic intracardiac focus.

*LR assumed by the original AAURA model, Nyberg et al.[114] (n = 1042).

†LR of analysis of Nyberg et al.[115] (n = 8830).

‡LR of meta-analysis by Smith-Bindman and colleagues[116] (n > 131 000).

Ultrasound screening for other chromosomal abnormalities

Fetal aneuploidy other than Down syndrome can be suspected based on the finding of specific ultrasound abnormalities. Table 28.2 demonstrates the association of specific ultrasound findings and chromosomal abnormalities.

Choroid plexus cysts deserve specific mention because they occur relatively frequently. They are seen in approximately 1% of fetuses between 16 and 24 weeks' gestation and have been associated with trisomy 18. About 30–35% of fetuses with trisomy 18 will have choroid plexus cysts. Alternatively, among fetuses with a choroid plexus cyst, about 3% will have trisomy 18, and most (65–90%) will also have other ultrasound findings. Early studies suggested that an isolated choroid plexus cyst might result in a probability of trisomy 18 of as high as 1 in 150. However, many of these series contained a high proportion of older women, resulting in the risk being overstated. Snijders and co-workers[119] more recently calculated that an isolated choroid plexus cyst has a likelihood ratio for trisomy 18 of 1.5. The size, location, or persistence of the cyst does not alter the risk.[120–124]

Maternal serum screening for Down syndrome in the first trimester

Within a few years of the 1984 report of the association between reduced AFP levels in the second trimester and Down syndrome,[64] researchers reported measurements of AFP and other second-trimester markers earlier in pregnancy.[125,126] The

Table 28.2 Association of ultrasound markers with aneuploidy.

US finding	Chromosomal abnormalities (%) when:		Trisomy 13	Trisomy 18	Trisomy 21	Other	45X
	Isolated	Multiple					
Holoprosencephaly (n = 132)	4	39	30	7	–	7	–
Choroid plexus cysts (n = 1806)	1	46	11	121	18	11	–
Facial cleft (n = 118)	0	51	25	16	–	6	–
Cystic hygroma (n = 276)	52	71	–	13	26	11	163
Nuchal skinfold	19	45	–	9	85	19	10
Diaphragmatic hernia (n = 173)	2	34	–	18	–	14	–
Ventriculomegaly (n = 690)	2	17	10	23	13	14	–
Posterior fossa cyst (n = 101)	0	52	10	22	–	8	–
Major heart defects (n = 829)	16	66	30	82	68	31	30
Duodenal atresia (n = 44)	38	64	–	–	21	2	–
Hyperechoic bowel (n = 196)	7	42	–	–	22	17	–
Omphalocele (n = 475)	13	46	28	108	–	31	–
Renal anomalies (n = 1825)*	3	24	40	52	48	62	–
Mild hydronephrosis (n = 631)	2	33	8	6	27	9	–
IUGR (early) (n = 621)	4	38	11	47	–	18	36 (triploidy)
Talipes (n = 127)	0	33	–	–	–	–	–

Adapted from Snijders and Nicolaides.

IUGR, intrauterine growth restriction; "isolated," isolated findings; "multiple," multiple findings.

*Renal anomalies defined as mild hydro, moderate hydro, severe hydro, multicystic kidney, obstruction, or renal agenesis

levels of AFP and uE_3 were found to differ only slightly between affected and unaffected pregnancies in the late first trimester.[71] Measurements of hCG and particularly its free β-subunit were found to have some utility; however, the serum marker PAPP-A was found to be the best single marker.[127–129] One factor leading to some early confusion in reported studies is that the strength of association of all of the known first-trimester markers changes week by week.[130] For example, PAPP-A measurements alone are a much better marker at 10 weeks' gestation (58% detection with a 5% false-positive rate) than at 13 weeks' gestation (27% detection with a 5% false-positive rate). This has required screening programs to have the ability to compute week-specific Down syndrome risks.[131] According to the SURUSS report,[131] the combination of maternal age, PAPP-A, and hCG (or the free β-subunit) at 12 weeks' gestation has a detection rate of about 63% with a 5% false-positive rate (less than the 81% found using quadruple markers in the second trimester). This led to a general agreement that stand-alone first-trimester biochemical screening should not be made available clinically. At present, few, if any, laboratories in the USA routinely provide Down syndrome risks based only on first-trimester biochemistry.

First-trimester ultrasound findings in Down syndrome pregnancies

In his initial description of the syndrome that bears his name, Langdon Down described skin which was so deficient in elasticity that it appeared to be too large for the body. This was particularly evident in the neck area of newborns. Since that time it has been clearly demonstrated that, as early as 10 weeks' gestation, the fetal neck area is expanded in Down syndrome. Although all fetuses demonstrate a small amount of fluid in the posterior nuchal area (called nuchal translucency, NT) at between 10 and 13 weeks' gestation (Fig. 28.6), fetuses with Down syndrome will, on average, have a larger amount. This difference allows measurement of NT to be converted to a likelihood ratio and used to modify the a priori maternal age risk of trisomy 21.

NT is defined as the maximum fluid-filled space between the skin of the posterior fetal neck area and the underlying structures. This area can be measured by transabdominal ultrasound in over 95% of cases and with transvaginal scanning in the remaining cases. Because the amount of fluid in euploid pregnancies increases with gestational age, no absolute "normal" value exists (Fig. 28.7); rather, the measurement is converted to either multiples of the gestational age median or the absolute deviation from the median (called delta NT) before conversion to a likelihood ratio. This manipulation is similar to that routinely used for gestational age standardization of biochemical analytes.

The performance of NT combined with maternal and gestational age in Down syndrome risk assessment has been well studied. In more than 100 000 pregnancies, NT measurements were greater than the 95th percentile in over 70% of fetuses

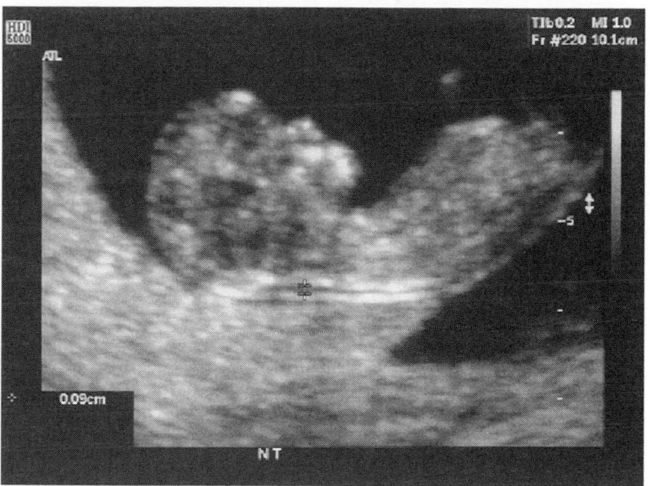

Figure 28.6 Correct measurement of NT in the first trimester.

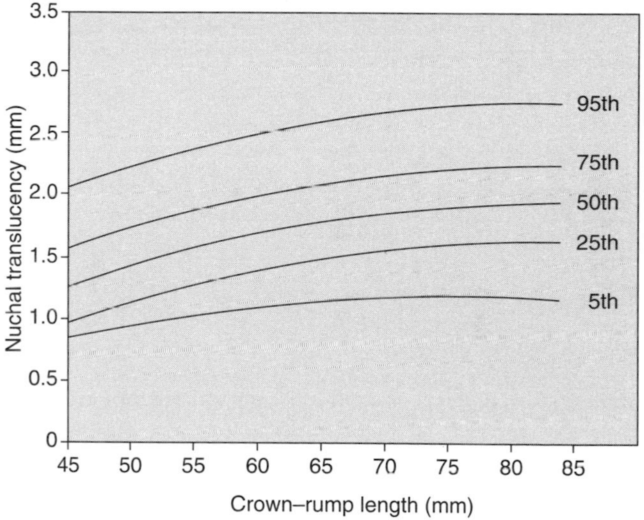

Figure 28.7 Median, 5th, and 95th percentile of NT by crown–rump length.

with trisomy 21.[132] Using a cutoff risk of 1:300, 82% of trisomy 21 pregnancies were screen positive with a total screen-positive rate of 8.3%. When a screen-positive rate of 5% was chosen, the sensitivity of screening was 77%. Subsequent studies have demonstrated similar rates of between 70% and 75%.[133,134]

Although NT appears to be a powerful first-trimester Down syndrome screening analyte, it will be efficacious only if all operators measure it in a standard fashion. To encourage this, the Fetal Medicine Foundation in London, UK, developed detailed guidelines for taking NT measurements, which include the following:

1 The crown–rump length should be between 45 mm and 84 mm.

2 Either transabdominal or transcervical scanning can be used. Transabdominal is successful in most cases and should

be the primary approach in order to minimize the time and expense.

3 A true sagittal scan of the fetus is required.

4 The image must be magnified so that the fetus occupies 75% of the image. This insures that each increment in the distance between calipers will be approximately 0.1 mm. It has been demonstrated that ultrasound measurements can be accurate to the nearest 0.1 or 0.2 mm.[135]

5 The fetal skin must be clearly separated from the amnion. When the fetus is lying directly on the amnion, separation can be accomplished either by waiting for fetal movement or by facilitating this (asking the mother to cough or tapping on her lower abdomen).

6 The maximum thickness of the subcutaneous translucency between the skin and the soft tissue overlying the cervical spine should be measured by placing the calipers as in Fig. 28.8. The measurement should be taken three times, and the maximum one used for the risk calculation

7 The NT should be measured with the fetal head in the neutral position. Hyperextension will increase the measurement by as much as 0.6 mm, and excessive flexion will decrease it by 0.4 mm.[136]

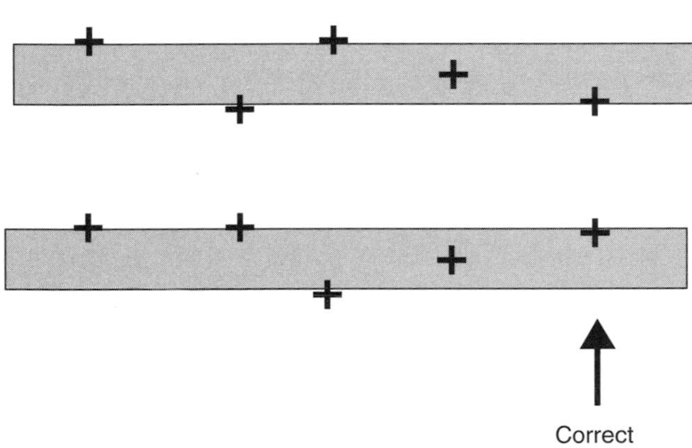

Figure 28.8 Appropriate placement of calipers for measuring NT. The arrow represents correct caliper location.

Although the above criteria assist in standardizing the technique used for measuring NT, consistently reliable results require sonographer training, image review, and ongoing quality management. In the USA, the Society of Maternal Fetal Medicine has developed a program of education and image review which leads to certification and indicates that individuals have mastered the technique (www.ntqr.org). Once sonographers and sonologists have completed this process, their clinical measurements are monitored and compared with expected standards. Centers or individuals demonstrating a deviation from the norm are alerted and remediation provided. This process is similar to those used by laboratories to ensure consistent values for biochemical analytes. A similar program is provided by the Fetal Medicine Foundation in London. Studies have demonstrated the efficacy of NT monitoring programs in assuring accurate results.[137]

Combining NT and biochemical markers to screen for Down syndrome in the first trimester

If first-trimester biochemical and NT measurements at 10–13 weeks' gestation are combined, the performance is at least as good as or better than the second-trimester quadruple test. Table 28.3 shows the expected Down syndrome detection rate at 11–13 weeks' gestation for a 'combined' first-trimester screening test (maternal age, ultrasound NT measurements, and maternal serum measurements of PAPP-A and the free β-

Table 28.3 Comparing the Down syndrome detection rate (DR) and false-positive rate (FPR) for first-trimester combined testing (by week of gestation) with second-trimester quadruple marker testing.

Performance	First-trimester combined test* at:			Second-trimester quadruple test†
	11 weeks	12 weeks	13 weeks	
DR of 80%‡				
FPR (%)	3.5	3.4	3.2	4.5
FPR of 5%‡				
DR (%)	83	83	84	81
Risk cutoff of 35-year-old woman§ (1:270)				
DR (%)	83	83	83	84‡
FPR (%)	4.7	4.6	4.6	5.7‡
OAPR¶ (1:n)	1:25	1:24	1:24	1:30‡

*Combined test: maternal age in combination with NT, PAPP-A, and free βhCG measurements (hCG can be substituted for free βhCG with little change in performance).

†Quadruple test: maternal age in combination with second-trimester measurements of AFP, uE_3, hCG, and DIA.

‡From SURUSS report.[131]

§Modeled for first trimester.

¶OAPR: the odds of being affected given a positive result.

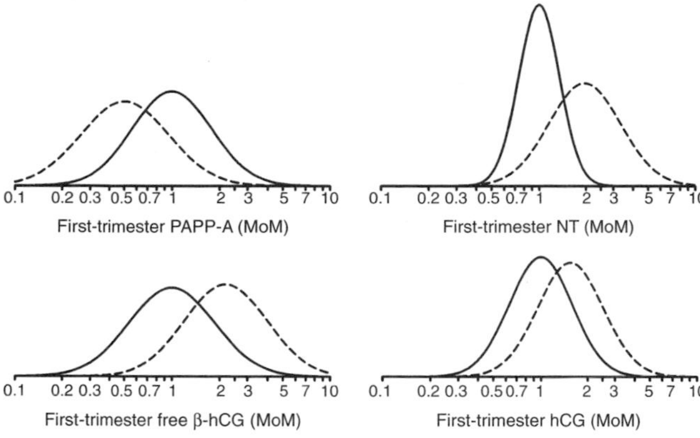

Figure 28.9 Overlapping distributions of first-trimester Down syndrome markers, including maternal serum PAPP-A, NT, free β-subunit of hCG, and hCG. These distributions vary by gestational week. The distributions correspond to the twelfth completed week, and the scales are the same as for Fig. 28.5 to allow for direct comparison. NT and PAPP-A measurements are more effective screening markers than hCG and free βhCG.

subunit of hCG). For comparison, the quadruple test performance is also provided. Either the free β-subunit of hCG or total hCG can be used as the fourth marker. Because PAPP-A and NT are the best discriminators, programs can choose, with minimal impact on performance, which form of hCG to use based on other factors, such as availability and cost of reagents.[138] Figure 28.9 provides overlapping distributions for NT measurements and for the three biochemical markers used for first-trimester screening.

Other first-trimester ultrasound markers

Individuals with Down syndrome are known to have midfacial flattening and hypoplasia of the nasal bridge, which most likely results from altered collagen formation. Pathologic studies of Down syndrome fetuses demonstrate this finding as early as the end of the first trimester.[139] Recently, Cicero and colleagues[113] reported that ultrasound can identify this abnormality in a high proportion of Down syndrome fetuses in the first trimester. This finding is present in approximately 65% of Down syndrome fetuses and only 2.5% of the unaffected population, which results in a Down syndrome likelihood ratio of approximately 30 when the nasal bone is absent and 0.3 when it is present.[140]

Although the initial reports on nasal bone imaging suggest that it may have an important role in Down syndrome risk assessment, many caveats remain before it can be recommended for routine use. It is difficult to routinely image, the frequency of absence varies depending on the patient's ethnic group (e.g., there is a much higher frequency in patients of African origin[141]), visualization is gestational-age dependent, and measurements of the nasal bone are not independent of the NT thickness. For these reasons, at the present time, the use of nasal bone imaging in a Down syndrome risk algorithm is not recommended as part of primary screening. Nicholaides and colleagues[142] have demonstrated its potential for secondary evaluation of patients initially identified as being at risk by more standard procedures. In his analysis, a first-trimester screening approach using NT, biochemical analytes, and nasal bone evaluation had a detection rate of 92% with a false-positive rate of 2.5%.[142]

Other first-trimester ultrasound findings have also been suggested to have a role in Down syndrome risk assessment. These include altered flow through the ductus venosus and the presence of tricuspid regurgitation.[143,144] At the present time, reports of these findings come from only a limited number of centers and their use for screening is still being investigated.

Integrating first- and second-trimester screening strategies for Down syndrome

Choosing an overall screening strategy for Down syndrome is complicated by the need to consider not only the performance of each strategy but also the ancillary issues of program implementation. This includes the timing and availability of diagnostic tests, adherence to risk cutoffs, concern about holding first-trimester test results until the second trimester, acceptability to women and healthcare providers, financial costs, medical costs, and second-trimester serum testing for open NTDs. Although there are clinical and programmatic advantages to screening in either the first or the second trimesters, the concept of combining markers from both trimesters into a single integrated interpretation provides the most accurate estimate of Down syndrome risk yet available.[145] Integrated screening calls for the holding of first-trimester information until the second-trimester results are also available. A single risk is then provided to the woman, and a single risk cutoff level is used to define screen-positive results (e.g., ≥ 1:200). Figure 28.10 demonstrates that integrated screening performs more effectively than any of the strategies applied in the first or second trimesters. However, it requires that information is withheld from patients until at least 16 weeks' gestation.

The potential advantages of a first-trimester diagnosis have led to the creation of screening strategies that combine the high performance of integrated screening with a high detection rate of Down syndrome pregnancies in the first trimester.[146] Two of these strategies, sequential screening and contingent screening, are reviewed below; both include NT measurements.

- Sequential screening[147] initially offers counseling and diagnostic testing to all women with a first-trimester risk at or above an initial risk cutoff level (e.g., ≥ 1:50); the remaining women are given a quadruple test (AFP, uE_3, hCG, and DIA) in the second trimester that is interpreted as an "integrated" test, using information from both trimesters. Those with a Down syndrome risk above a final second-trimester risk

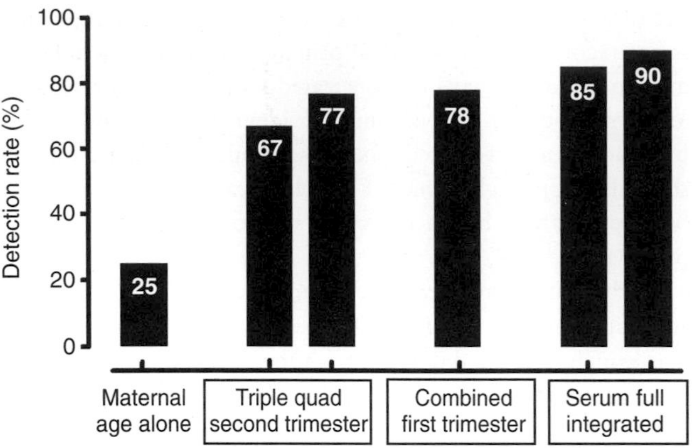

Figure 28.10 Comparative performance of several Down syndrome screening strategies. Numbers in the individual bar graphs indicate detection rates at a 5% false-positive rate. Maternal age alone results in a 25% detection rate, and each strategy after that is associated with successively higher detection rates. The highest detection rate is achieved with full integrated screening, followed by serum integrated screening.

cut-off level (e.g., ≥ 1:270) are also offered counseling and second-trimester diagnostic testing.

• Contingent screening[148,149] differs from sequential screening by having not only a high-risk cutoff level defined in the first trimester but also a low-risk cutoff level (e.g., ≥ 1:50 and < 1:1500). Women with Down syndrome risks below the low cutoff level are informed that they do not require further testing, as they are unlikely to become screen positive.

Given that integrated screening uses all of the informative markers before assigning a risk and determining who should be offered diagnostic testing, the other two strategies will, of necessity, be less efficient, as defined by detection and false-positive rates. This is because both sequential and contingent screening strategies assign an interim risk and make the offer of diagnostic testing in the first trimester based on only a subset of informative markers. Thus, the early detection of some affected pregnancies and the reduced need for second-trimester screening (contingent testing) must logically be "paid for" by having either a somewhat lower detection rate or more false-positives. Modeling these strategies shows that sequential and contingent screening performances can approach that of integrated screening if the proportion of women offered diagnostic testing in the first trimester is kept well below the proportion offered diagnostic testing in the second trimester. Both perform more effectively than either the first-trimester combined strategy or second-trimester stand-alone screening.[150]

Speculation

In the near future, Down syndrome screening programs will increasingly combine information from both trimesters as a way of reducing false-positives while simultaneously improving detection. Although NT measurements have been shown to be reliable in the research setting, it is not yet clear whether such testing can be reliably offered as a routine screening test.[134] Other improvements, such as repeated measures of biochemical markers,[149,151] are being investigated as ways of increasing performance even further, even when NT measurements are not available. Also, methods using multiple contingent policies are being promulgated.[152] Routinely available screening strategies, including those based on maternal serum alone, may soon be able to detect over 90% of Down syndrome pregnancies with only a 1–2% false-positive rate by combining information from first- and second-trimester screening tests. Research is also continuing in the area of collecting and testing individual fetal cells (or fetal DNA) in the maternal circulation as either a screening or a diagnostic test.[153]

Key points

1 In 1956, a fetal-specific protein (alpha-fetoprotein or AFP) was discovered in fetal serum.

2 Elevated AFP in second-trimester amniotic fluid is a strong indicator of the presence of a fetal open neural tube defect (NTD).

3 AFP levels in maternal serum can be used as a screening (but not diagnostic) test for open NTDs in the second trimester.

4 AFP measurements in both amniotic fluid and maternal serum vary with gestation. They are routinely expressed as a multiple of the median (MoM) AFP value found in unaffected pregnancies of the same gestational age.

5 In expert hands, ultrasound markers in the fetal brain at 18–21 weeks' gestation are diagnostic of open NTDs.

6 Beginning in the 1970s, a woman's age was used as a determinant in screening for Down syndrome, with those aged 35 and older being offered amniocentesis and karyotyping.

7 In 1984, reduced levels of maternal serum AFP in the second trimester were reported in Down syndrome pregnancies.

8 Combining maternal age and serum AFP measurements allowed diagnostic testing to be offered to younger women; this combination had a detection rate of 25%

(with a 5% false-positive rate) among women aged under 35 years.

9 Down syndrome risk, as defined by screening marker levels in combination with maternal age, is now used as the prime screening variable, and cutoff levels to determine detection and false-positive rates are based on risk.

10 Adding second-trimester serum markers (unconjugated estriol, uE_3; human chorionic gonadotropin, hCG; and dimeric inhibin-A, DIA) improved detection to 60–70% (with a 5% false-positive rate).

11 Second-trimester multiple marker screening is also able to identify 60% of trisomy 18 pregnancies (with a false-positive rate of less than 1%).

12 In the second trimester, significant ultrasound abnormalities can be seen in about three-fourths of all trisomy 18 pregnancies.

13 In the mid-1980s, pregnancy-associated plasma protein-A (PAPP-A) and free βhCG were found to be useful as Down syndrome markers in the late first trimester, but performance was not as good as second-trimester serum testing.

14 At about the same time, ultrasound measurements of nuchal translucency (NT) thickness (at between 11 and 13 completed gestational weeks) were found to be the best single marker for Down syndrome.

15 Combining NT measurements with biochemical markers (combined testing) in the first trimester yields equivalent performance to second-trimester quadruple marker testing.

16 Obtaining reliable NT measurements requires specific training, high-quality sonographic equipment, and participation in ongoing quality assurance.

17 In about 60% of Down syndrome fetuses and 1% of unaffected fetuses, it is not possible to visualize a nasal bone, but such measurements are difficult to achieve in routine screening.

18 Integrated testing fuses both first-trimester combined and second-trimester quadruple testing into a single second-trimester risk.

19 Integrated screening can have a detection rate of 90%, with a false-positive rate of less than 2%, depending on the gestational age at first-trimester sampling and the combination of markers used.

20 Sequential and contingent screening strategies are modifications of integrated screening that aim to preserve the high performance of integrated screening, and have the ability to diagnose a proportion of Down syndrome cases in the first trimester.

References

1 Brock DJ, Sutcliffe RG. Alpha-fetoprotein in the antenatal diagnosis of anencephaly and spina bifida. *Lancet* 1972;2:197.

2 Nicolaides KH, Campbell S, Gabbe SG, Guidetti R. Ultrasound screening for spina bifida: cranial and cerebellar signs. *Lancet* 1986;2:72.

3 Van den Hof MC, Nicolaides KH, Campbell J, Campbell S. Evaluation of the lemon and banana signs in one hundred thirty fetuses with open spina bifida. *Am J Obstet Gynecol* 1990;162:322.

4 Bergstrand CG, Czar B. Demonstration of a new protein fraction in serum from the human fetus. *Scand J Clin Lab Invest* 1956;8:174.

5 Ruoslahti E. Isolation and biochemical properties of alpha-fetoprotein. In: Crandall BR, Brazier MAB, eds. *Prevention of neural tube defects: the role of alpha-fetoprotein.* New York: Academic Press; 1978:9.

6 Haddow JE, Cowchock FS, Macri JN, et al. Second trimester amniotic fluid protein values from normal, neural tube defect, and fetal demise pregnancies after exclusion of material blood contaminated by testing for pregnancy-associated macroglobulin. *Pediatr Res* 1978;12:243.

7 Johnson AM, Umansky I, Alper CA, et al. Amniotic fluid proteins: maternal and fetal contributions. *J Pediatr* 1974;84:588.

8 Smith AD, Wald NJ, Cuckle HS, et al. Amniotic-fluid acetylcholinesterase as a possible diagnostic test for neural-tube defects in early pregnancy. *Lancet* 1979;1:685.

9 Collaborative Acetylcholinesterase Study. Amniotic fluid acetylcholinesterase electrophoresis as a secondary test in the diagnosis of anencephaly and open spina bifida in early pregnancy. *Lancet* 1981;2:321.

10 Wald N, Cuckle H. Open neural tube defects. In: Wald N, ed. *Antenatal and neonatal screening.* Oxford: Oxford University Press; 1984:53.

11 Goldfine C, Haddow JE, Knight GJ, Palomaki GE. Amniotic fluid alpha-fetoprotein and acetylcholinesterase measurements in pregnancies associated with gastroschisis. *Prenat Diagn* 1989;9:697.

12 Seppala M, Rapola J, Huttunen NP, et al. Congenital nephrotic syndrome: prenatal diagnosis and genetic counselling by estimation of amniotic-fluid and maternal serum alpha-fetoprotein. *Lancet* 1976;2:123.

13 Goldfine C, Miller WA, Haddow JE. Amniotic fluid gel cholinesterase density ratios in fetal open defects of the neural tube and ventral wall. *Br J Obstet Gynaecol* 1983;90:238.

14 Haddow JE, Goldfine C. The evolving role of amniotic fluid acetylcholinesterase analysis for identifying open fetal neural tube defects during the second trimester. In: Mizejewski GJ, Porter IH, eds. *Alpha-fetoprotein and congenital disorders.* San Diego, CA: Academic Press;1985:215.

15 Brock DJ, Bolton AE, Scrimgeour JB. Prenatal diagnosis of spina bifida and anencephaly through maternal plasma-alpha-fetoprotein measurement. *Lancet* 1974;1:767.

16 Wald NJ, Brock DJ, Bonnar J. Prenatal diagnosis of spina bifida and anencephaly by maternal serum-alpha-fetoprotein measurement. A controlled study. *Lancet* 1974;1:765.

17 Wald NJ, Cuckle H, Brock JH, et al. Maternal serum-alpha-fetoprotein measurement in antenatal screening for anencephaly and spina bifida in early pregnancy. Report of UK collaborative

study on alpha-fetoprotein in relation to neural-tube defects. *Lancet* 1977;1:1323.
18 Knight GJ, Palomaki GE, Haddow JE. Assessing the reliability of AFP test kits. *Contemp Obstet Gynecol* 1987;30:37.
19 Wald N, Cuckle H, Boreham J, Turnbull AC. Effect of estimating gestational age by ultrasound cephalometry on the specificity of alpha-fetoprotein screening for open neural-tube defects. *Br J Obstet Gynaecol* 1982;89:1050.
20 Wald N, Cuckle H, Boreham J, Stirrat G. Small biparietal diameter of fetuses with spina bifida: implications for antenatal screening. *Br J Obstet Gynaecol* 1980;87:219.
21 Haddow JE, Kloza EM, Knight GJ, Smith DE. Relation between maternal weight and serum alpha-fetoprotein concentration during the second trimester. *Clin Chem* 1981;27:133.
22 Haddow JE, Smith DE, Sever J. Effect of maternal weight on maternal serum alpha-fetoprotein. *Br J Obstet Gynaecol* 1982; 89:93.
23 Johnson AM, Palomaki GE, Haddow JE. The effect of adjusting maternal serum alpha-fetoprotein levels for maternal weight in pregnancies with fetal open spina bifida. A United States collaborative study. *Am J Obstet Gynecol* 1990;163:9.
24 Shaw GM, Velie EM, Schaffer D. Risk of neural tube defect-affected pregnancies among obese women. *JAMA* 1996;275: 1093.
25 Wald N, Cuckle H, Boreham J, et al. The effect of maternal weight on maternal serum alpha-fetoprotein levels. *Br J Obstet Gynaecol* 1981;88:1094.
26 Waller DK, Mills JL, Simpson JL, et al. Are obese women at higher risk for producing malformed offspring? *Am J Obstet Gynecol* 1994;170:541.
27 Watkins ML, Scanlon KS, Mulinare J, Khoury MJ. Is maternal obesity a risk factor for anencephaly and spina bifida? *Epidemiology* 1996;7:507.
28 Werler MM, Louik C, Shapiro S, Mitchell AA. Prepregnant weight in relation to risk of neural tube defects. *JAMA* 1996;275:1089.
29 Johnson AM. *Racial differences in maternal serum alpha-fetoprotein screening*. New York: Academic Press, 1985.
30 Baumgarten A. Racial difference and biological significance of maternal serum alpha-fetoprotein. *Lancet* 1986;2:573.
31 Johnson AM, Palomaki GE, Haddow JE. Maternal serum alpha-fetoprotein levels in pregnancies among black and white women with fetal open spina bifida: a United States collaborative study. *Am J Obstet Gynecol* 1990;162:328.
32 Milunsky A, Alpert E, Kitzmiller JL, et al. Prenatal diagnosis of neural tube defects. VIII. The importance of serum alpha-fetoprotein screening in diabetic pregnant women. *Am J Obstet Gynecol* 1982;142:1030.
33 Wald NJ, Cuckle H, Boreham J, et al. Maternal serum alpha-fetoprotein and diabetes mellitus. *Br J Obstet Gynaecol* 1979; 86:101.
34 Baumgarten A, Robinson J. Prospective study of an inverse relationship between maternal glycosylated hemoglobin and serum alpha-fetoprotein concentrations in pregnant women with diabetes. *Am J Obstet Gynecol* 1988;159:77.
35 Greene MF, Haddow JE, Palomaki GE, Knight GJ. Maternal serum alpha-fetoprotein levels in diabetic pregnancies. *Lancet* 1988;2:345.
36 Milunsky A, ed. *Genetic disorders and the fetus: diagnosis, prevention, and treatment*, 3rd edn. Baltimore, MD: John Hopkins University Press, 1998.
37 Cuckle HS, Wald NJ, Nanchahal K, et al. Repeat maternal serum alpha-fetoprotein testing in antenatal screening programmes for Down's syndrome. *Br J Obstet Gynaecol* 1989;96:52.
38 Wald N. Neural tube defects. In: Wald N, Leck I, eds. *Antenatal and neonatal screening*, 2nd edn. Oxford: Oxford University Press; 2000:61.
39 Wald N, Kennard A, Donnenfeld A, et al. Ultrasound scanning for congenital abnormalities. In: Wald N, Leck I, eds. *Antenatal and neonatal screening*, 2nd edn. Oxford: Oxford University Press; 2000:441.
40 Crandall BF, Matsumoto M. Routine amniotic fluid alphafetoprotein assay: experience with 40,000 pregnancies. *Am J Med Genet* 1986;24:143.
41 Ferguson-Smith MA, Yates JRW, Kelly D, et al. Hereditary persistence of alpha-fetoprotein: a new autosomal dominance trait identified in antenatal screening programme for spina bifida. *Cytogenet Cell Genet* 1985;40:628.
42 Wald N, Cucke H, Nanachahal K. Amniotic fluid acetylcholinesterase measurement in the prenatal diagnosis of open neural tube defects: second report of the Collaborative Acetylcholinesterase Study. *Prenat Diagn* 1989;9:813.
43 Lennon CA, Gray DL. Sensitivity and specificity of ultrasound for the detection of neural tube and ventral wall defects in a high-risk population. *Obstet Gynecol* 1999;94:562.
44 Boyd PA, Wellesley DG, De Walle HE, et al. Evaluation of the prenatal diagnosis of neural tube defects by fetal ultrasonographic examination in different centres across Europe. *J Med Screen* 2000;7:169.
45 Nyberg DA, Mack LA, Hirch J, et al. Abnormalities of fetal cranial contour in sonographic detection of spina bifida: evaluation of the lemon sign. *Radiology* 1988;167:387.
46 Nadel AS, Green JK, Holmes, LB, et al. Absence of need for amniocentesis in patients with elevated levels of maternal serum alpha-fetoprotein and normal ultrasonographic examinations. *N Engl J Med* 1990;323:557.
47 Schell DL, Drugan A, Brindley BA, et al. Combined ultrasonography and amniocentesis for pregnant women with elevated serum alpha-fetoprotein: revising the risk estimate. *J Reprod Med* 1990;35:543.
48 Lindfors KK, Gorczyca DP, Hanson FW, et al. The roles of ultrasonography and amniocentesis in evaluation of elevated maternal serum alpha-fetoprotein. *Am J Obstet Gynecol* 1991;164:1571.
49 Megerian G, Godmilow L, Donnenfeld AE. Ultrasound-adjusted risk and spectrum of fetal chromosomal abnormality in women with elevated maternal serum alpha-fetoprotein. *Obstet Gynecol* 1995;85:952.
50 Loft AG, Hogdall E, Larsen SO, Norgaard-Pedersen B. A comparison of amniotic fluid alpha-fetoprotein and acetylcholinesterase in the prenatal diagnosis of open neural tube defects and anterior abdominal wall defects. *Prenat Diagn* 1993;13:93.
51 James SJ, Pogribna M, Pogribny IP, et al. Abnormal folate metabolism and mutation in the methylenetetrahydrofolate reductase gene may be maternal risk factors for Down syndrome. *Am J Clin Nutr* 1999;70:495.
52 Watson WJ, Chescheir NC, Katz VL, Seeds JW. The role of ultrasound in evaluation of patients with elevated maternal serum alpha-fetoprotein: a review. *Obstet Gynecol* 1991;78:123.
53 Harmon JP, Hiett AK, Palmer CG, Golichowski AM. Prenatal ultrasound detection of isolated neural tube defects: is cytogenetic evaluation warranted? *Obstet Gynecol* 1995;86:595.
54 Crandall BF, Chua C. Risks for fetal abnormalities after very and moderately elevated AF-AFPs. *Prenat Diagn* 1997;17:837.
55 Reichler A, Hume RF, Jr, Drugan A, et al. Risk of anomalies as a function of level of elevated maternal serum alpha-fetoprotein. *Am J Obstet Gynecol* 1994;171:1052.

56 Seppala M, Ruoslahti E. Alpha fetoprotein in amniotic fluid: an index of gestational age. *Am J Obstet Gynecol* 1972;114;595.
57 Katz VL, Chescheir NC, Cefalo RC. Unexplained elevations of maternal serum alpha-fetoprotein. *Obstet Gynecol Surv* 1990;45:719.
58 Brazerol WF, Grover, S, Donnenfeld AE. Unexplained elevated maternal serum α-fetoprotein levels and perinatal outcome in an urban clinic population. *Am J Obstet Gynecol* 1994; 171.
59 Milunsky A, Jick SS, Bruell CL, et al. Predictive values, relative risks and overall benefits of high and low maternal serum alphafetoprotein screening in singleton pregnancies: new epidemiologic data. *Am J Obstet Gynecol* 1989;161:291.
60 Crandall BF, Robinson L, Grau P. Risks associated with an elevated maternal serum alpha-fetoprotein level. *Am J Obstet Gynecol* 1991;165:581.
61 Wailer DK, Lustig LS, Cunningham GC, et al. Second-trimester maternal serum alpha-fetoprotein levels and the risk of subsequent fetal death. *N Engl J Med* 1991;325:6.
62 Wailer DK, Lustig LS, Smith AH, et al. Alpha-fetoprotein: a biomarker for pregnancy outcome. *Epidemiology* 1993;4: 471.
63 Wailer DK, Lustig LS, Cunningham GC, et al. The association between maternal serum alpha-fetoprotein and preterm birth, small for gestational age infants, preeclampsia, and placental complications. *Obstet Gynecol* 1996;88:816.
64 Merkatz IR, Nitowsky HM, Macri JN, Johnson WE. An association between low maternal serum alpha-fetoprotein and fetal chromosomal abnormalities. *Am J Obstet Gynecol* 1984;148: 886.
65 Cuckle HS, Wald NJ, Lindenbaum RH. Maternal serum alpha-fetoprotein measurement: a screening test for Down syndrome. *Lancet* 1984;1:926.
66 New England Regional Genetics Group Prenatal Collaborative Study of Down Syndrome Screening. Combining maternal serum alpha-fetoprotein measurements and age to screen for Down syndrome in pregnant women under age 35. *Am J Obstet Gynecol* 1989;160:575.
67 Palomaki GE, Knight GJ, Holman MS, Haddow JE. Maternal serum alpha-fetoprotein screening for fetal Down syndrome in the United States: results of a survey. *Am J Obstet Gynecol* 1990; 162:317.
68 Bogart MH, Pandian MR, Jones OW. Abnormal maternal serum chorionic gonadotropin levels in pregnancies with fetal chromosome abnormalities. *Prenat Diagn* 1987;7:623.
69 Canick JA, Knight GJ, Palomaki GE, et al. Low second trimester maternal serum unconjugated oestriol in pregnancies with Down's syndrome. *Br J Obstet Gynaecol* 1988;95:330.
70 Wald NJ, Cuckle HS, Densem JW, et al. Maternal serum unconjugated oestriol as an antenatal screening test for Down's syndrome. *Br J Obstet Gynaecol* 1988;95:334.
71 Wald NJ, Cuckle HS, Densem JW, et al. Maternal serum screening for Down's syndrome in early pregnancy. *Br Med J* 1988;297:883.
72 Haddow JE, Palomaki GE, Knight GJ, et al. Prenatal screening for Down's syndrome with use of maternal serum markers. *N Engl J Med* 1992;327:588.
73 Haddow JE, Palomaki GE, Knight GJ, et al. Second trimester screening for Down's syndrome using maternal serum dimeric inhibin A. *J Med Screen* 1998;5:115.
74 Dugoff L, Hobbins JC, Malone FD, et al. Quad screen as a predictor of adverse pregnancy outcome. *Obstet Gynecol* 2005;106:260.
75 Carter PE, Pearn JH, Bell J, et al. Survival in trisomy 18. Life tables for use in genetic counselling and clinical paediatrics. *Clin Genet* 1985;27:59.
76 Hook EB, Cross PK, Schreinemachers DM. Chromosomal abnormality rates at amniocentesis and in live-born infants. *JAMA* 1983;249:2034.
77 Schneider AS, Mennuti MT, Zackai EH. High cesarean section rate in trisomy 18 births: a potential indication for late prenatal diagnosis. *Am J Obstet Gynecol* 1981;140:367.
78 Palomaki GE, Haddow JE, Knight GJ, et al. Risk-based prenatal screening for trisomy 18 using alpha-fetoprotein, unconjugated oestriol and human chorionic gonadotropin. *Prenat Diagn* 1995;15:713.
79 Yaron Y, Cherry M, Kramer RL, et al. Second-trimester maternal serum marker screening: maternal serum alpha-fetoprotein, beta-human chorionic gonadotropin, estriol, and their various combinations as predictors of pregnancy outcome. *Am J Obstet Gynecol* 1999;181:968.
80 Kuller JA, Sellati LE, Chescheir NC, et al. Outcome of pregnancies with elevation of both maternal serum alpha-fetoprotein and human chorionic gonadotropin. *Am J Perinatol* 1995;12:93.
81 Morssink LP, Kornman LH, Beekhuis JR, et al. Abnormal levels of maternal serum human chorionic gonadotropin and alpha-fetoprotein in the second trimester: relation to fetal weight and preterm delivery. *Prenat Diagn* 1995;15:1041.
82 Benn P. Trisomy 16 and trisomy 16 mosaicism: a review. *Am J Med Genet* 1998;79:121.
83 Santolaya-Forgas J, Jessup J, Burd LI, et al. Pregnancy outcome in women with low mid-trimester maternal serum unconjugated estriol. *J Reprod Med* 1996;41:87.
84 Kowalczyk TD, Cabaniss ML, Cusmano L. Association of low unconjugated estriol in the second trimester and adverse pregnancy outcome. *Obstet Gynecol* 1998;91:396.
85 Blitzer MG, Kelley RI, Schwartz MF. Abnormal maternal serum marker pattern associated with Smith–Lemli–Opitz (SLO) syndrome. *Am J Hum Genet* 1994;55:A277.
86 Canick JA, Abuelo DN, Bradley LA, et al. Maternal serum marker levels in two pregnancies affected with Smith–Lemli–Opitz syndrome. *Prenat Diagn* 1997;17:187.
87 Tint GS, Abuelo D, Till M, et al. Fetal Smith–Lemli–Opitz syndrome can be detected accurately and reliably by measuring amniotic fluid dehydrocholesterols. *Prenat Diagn* 1998;18: 651.
88 Bradley LA, Palomaki GE, Knight GJ, et al. Levels of unconjugated estriol and other maternal serum markers in pregnancies with Smith–Lemli–Opitz (RSH) syndrome fetuses. *Am J Med Genet* 1999;82:355.
89 Palomaki GE, Bradley LA, Knight GJ, et al. Assigning risk for Smith–Lemli–Opitz syndrome as part of 2nd trimester screening for Down's syndrome. *J Med Screen* 2002;9:43.
90 Craig WY, Haddow JE, Palomaki GE, et al. Identifying Smith–Lemli–Optiz syndrome in conjunction with prenatal screening for Down's syndrome. *Prenat Diagn* 2006;26:842.
91 Kratz LE, Kelley RI. Prenatal diagnosis of the RSH/Smith–Lemli–Opitz syndrome. *Am J Med Genet* 1999;82:376.
92 Zalel Y, Kedar I, Tepper R, et al. Differential diagnosis and management of very low second trimester maternal serum unconjugated estriol levels, with special emphasis on the diagnosis of X-linked ichthyosis. *Obstet Gynecol Surv* 1996;51:200.
93 Bradley LA, Canick JA, Palomaki GE, et al. Undetectable maternal serum unconjugated estriol levels in the second trimester: risk of perinatal complications associated with placental sulfatase deficiency. *Am J Obstet Gynecol* 1997;176:531.

94 Santolaya-Forgas J, Cohen L, Vengalil S, et al. Prenatal diagnosis of X-linked ichthyosis using molecular cryogenetics. *Fetal Diagn Ther* 1997;12:36.

95 Schleifer RA, Bradley LA, Richards DS, et al. Pregnancy outcome for women with very low levels of maternal serum unconjugated estriol on second-trimester screening. *Am J Obstet Gynecol* 1995;173:1152.

96 Benacerraf BR, Gelman R, Frigoletto FD, Jr. Sonographic identification of second-trimester fetuses with Down's syndrome. *N Engl J Med* 1987;317:1371.

97 Perella R, Duerinckx AJ, Grant EG, et al. Second-trimester sonographic diagnosis of Down syndrome: role of femur-length shortening and nuchal-fold thickening. *Am J Roentgenol* 1988;151:981.

98 Nyberg DA, Resta RG, Hickok DE, et al. Femur length shortening in the detection of Down syndrome: Is prenatal screening feasible? *Am J Obstet Gynecol* 1990;162:1247.

99 Crane JP, Gray DL. Sonographically measured nuchal skinfold thickness as a screening tool for Down syndrome: results of a prospective clinical trial. *Obstet Gynecol* 1991;77:533.

100 Donnenfeld AE. Sonographic screening for Down syndrome. *Genet Teratol* 1992;1:1.

101 Borrell A, Costa D, Martinez JM, et al. Early midtrimester fetal nuchal thickness: effectiveness as a marker of Down syndrome. *Am J Obstet Gynecol* 1996;175:45.

102 Bahado-Singh R, Deren O, Oz U, et al. An alternative for women initially declining genetic amniocentesis: individual Down syndrome odds on the basis of maternal age and multiple ultrasonographic markers. *Am J Obstet Gynecol* 1998;179:514.

103 Bromley B, Lieberman E, Shipp TD, et al. Significance of an echogenic intracardiac focus in fetuses at high and low risk for aneuploidy. *J Ultrasound Med* 1998;17:127.

104 Nyberg DA, Resta RG, Mahony BS, et al. Fetal hyperechogenic bowel and Down's syndrome. *Ultrasound Obstet Gynecol* 1993; 3:330.

105 MacGregor SN, Tamura R, Sabbagha R, et al. Isolated hyperechoic fetal bowel: significance and implications for management. *Am J Obstet Gynecol* 1995;173:1254.

106 Corteville JE, Gray DL, Langer JC. Bowel abnormalities in the fetus: correlation of prenatal ultrasonographic findings with outcome. *Am Obstet Gynecol* 1996;175:724.

107 Snijders RJ, Sebire NJ, Faria M, et al. Fetal mild hydronephrosis and chromosomal defects: relation to maternal age and gestation. *Fetal Diagn Ther* 1995;10:349.

108 Benacerraf BR, Osathanondh R, Frigoletto FD. Sonographic demonstration of hypoplasia of the middle phalanx of the fifth digit: a finding associated with Down syndrome. *Am J Obstet Gynecol* 1988;159:181.

109 Drugan A, Johnson MP, Evans MI. Ultrasound screening for fetal chromosome anomalies. *Am J Med Genet* 2000;90:98.

110 Shipp TD, Benacerraf BR. Second trimester ultrasound screening for chromosomal abnormalities. *Prenat Diagn* 2002; 22:296.

111 Paladini D, Tartaglione A, Agangi A, et al. The association between congenital heart disease and Down syndrome in prenatal life. *Ultrasound Obstet Gynecol* 2000;15:104.

112 Johnson MP, Barr M, Jr, Treadwell MC, et al. Fetal leg and femur/foot length ratio: a marker for trisomy 21. *Am J Obstet Gynecol* 1993;169:557.

113 Cicero S, Curcio P, Papageorghiou A, et al. Absence of nasal bone in fetuses with trisomy 21 at 11–14 weeks of gestation: an observational study. *Lancet* 2001;358:1665.

114 Nyberg DA, Luthy DA, Resta RG, et al. Age-adjusted ultrasound risk assessment for fetal Down's syndrome during the second trimester: description of the method and analysis of 142 cases. *Ultrasound Obstet Gynecol* 1998;12:8.

115 Nyberg DA, Sourer VL, El-Bastawissi A, et al. Isolated sonographic markers for detection of fetal Down syndrome in the second trimester of pregnancy. *Ultrasound Med* 2001;20: 1053.

116 Smith-Bindman R, Hosmer W, Feldstein VA, et al. Second-trimester ultrasound to detect fetuses with Down syndrome: a meta-analysis. *JAMA* 2001;285:1044.

117 Souter VL, Nyberg DA, El-Bastawissi A, et al. Correlation of ultrasound findings and biochemical markers in the second trimester of pregnancy in fetuses with trisomy 21. *Prenat Diagn* 2002;22:175.

118 Bahado-Singh R, Shahabi S, Karaca M, et al. The comprehensive midtrimester test: high-sensitivity Down syndrome test. *Am J Obstet Gynecol* 2002;186:803.

119 Snijders RJ, Shawa L, Nicolaides KH. Fetal choroid plexus cysts and trisomy 18: assessment of risk based on ultrasound findings and maternal age. *Prenat Diagn* 1994;14:1119.

120 Shunagshoti S, Netsky MG. Neuroepithelial (colloid) cysts of the nervous system. Further observation of pathogenesis, location, incidence and histochemistry. *Neurology* 1966;16:887.

121 Nadel AS, Bromley BS, Frigoletto FD, Jr, et al. Isolated choroid plexus cysts in the second-trimester fetus: is amniocentesis really indicated? *Radiology* 1992;185:545.

122 Riebel T, Nasir R, Weber K. Choroid plexus cysts: a normal finding on ultrasound. *Pediatr Radiol* 1992;22:410.

123 Porto M, Murata Y, Warneke LA, et al. Fetal choroid plexus cysts: an independent risk factor for chromosomal anomalies. *J Clin Ultrasound* 1993;21:103.

124 Nava S, Godmilow L, Reeser S, et al. Significance of sonographically detected second-trimester choroid plexus cysts: a series of 211 cases and a review of the literature. *Ultrasound Obstet Gynecol* 1994;4:448.

125 Brambati B, Simoni G, Bonacchi I, Piceni L. Fetal chromosomal aneuploidies and maternal serum alpha-fetoprotein levels in first trimester. *Lancet* 1986;2:165.

126 Ozturk M, Milunsky A, Brambati B, et al. Abnormal maternal serum levels of human chorionic gonadotropin free subunits in trisomy 18. *Am J Med Genet* 1990;36:480.

127 Wallace EM, Crossley JA, Ritoe SC, et al. Evolution of an inhibin A ELISA method: implications for Down's syndrome screening. *Ann Clin Biochem* 1998;35:656.

128 Knight GJ, Palomaki GE, Haddow JE, et al. Pregnancy associated plasma protein A as a marker for Down syndrome in the second trimester of pregnancy. *Prenat Diagn* 1993;13: 222.

129 Wald N, Stone R, Cuckle HS, et al. First trimester concentrations of pregnancy associated plasma protein A and placental protein 14 in Down's syndrome. *Br Med J* 1992:305:28.

130 Spencer K, Crossley JA, Aitken DA, et al. Temporal changes in maternal serum biochemical markers of trisomy 21 across the first and second trimester of pregnancy. *Ann Clin Biochem* 2002;39:567.

131 Wald NJ, Rodeck C, Hackshaw AK, et al. First and second trimester antenatal screening for Down's syndrome: the results of the Serum, Urine and Ultrasound Screening Study (SURUSS). *J Med Screen* 2003;10:56.

132 Snijders RJ, Noble P, Sebire N, et al. UK multicentre project on assessment of risk of trisomy 21 by maternal age and fetal

nuchal-translucency thickness at 10–14 weeks of gestation. Fetal Medicine Foundation First Trimester Screening Group. *Lancet* 1998;352:343.

133 Wapner R, Thom E, Simpson JL, et al. First-trimester screening for trisomies 21 and 18. First Trimester Maternal Serum Biochemistry and Fetal Nuchal Translucency Screening (BUN) Study Group. *N Engl J Med* 2003;349:1405.

134 Malone FD, Canick JA, Ball RH, et al. First-trimester or second-trimester screening, or both, for Down's syndrome. *N Engl J Med* 2005;353:2001.

135 Braithwaite JM, Morris RW, Economides DL. Nuchal translucency measurements: frequency distribution and changes with gestation in a general population. *Br J Obstet Gynaecol* 1996;103:1201.

136 Whitlow BJ, Chatzipapas IK, Economides DL. The effect of fetal neck position on nuchal translucency measurement. *Br J Obstet Gynaecol* 1998;105:872.

137 Snijders RJ, Thom EA, Zachary JM, et al. First-trimester trisomy screening: nuchal translucency measurement training and quality assurance to correct and unify technique. *Ultrasound Obstet Gynecol* 2002;19:353.

138 Reddy UM, Mennuti MT. Incorporating first-trimester Down syndrome studies into prenatal screening: executive summary of the National Institute of Child Health and Human Development workshop. *Obstet Gynecol* 2006;107:167.

139 Larose C, Massoc P, Hillon Y, et al. Comparison of fetal nasal bone assessment by ultrasound at 11–14 weeks and by postmortem X-ray in trisomy 21: a prospective observation study. *Ultrasound Obstet Gynecol* 2003;22:27.

140 Cicero S, Rembouskos G, Vandecruys H, et al. Likelihood ratio for trisomy 21 in fetuses with absent nasal bone at the 11–14 week scan. *Ultrasound Obstet Gynecol* 2004;23:218.

141 Cicero S, Bindra R, Rembouskos G, et al. Integrated ultrasound and biochemical screening for trisomy 21 using fetal nuchal translucency, absent fetal nasal bone, free beta-hCG and PAPP-A at 11 to 14 weeks. *Prenat Diagn* 2003;23:306.

142 Nicolaides KH, Spencer K, Avgidou K, et al. Multicenter study of first-trimester screening for trisomy 21 in 75 821 pregnancies: results and estimation of the potential impact of individual risk-orientated two-stage first-trimester screening. *Ultrasound Obstet Gynecol* 2005;25:221.

143 Huggon IC, DeFigueiredo DB, Allan LD. Tricuspid regurgitation in the diagnosis of chromosomal anomalies in the fetus at 11–14 weeks of gestation. *Heart* 2003;89:1071.

144 Faiola S, Tsoi E, Huggon IC, et al. Likelihood ratio for trisomy 21 in fetuses with tricuspid regurgitation at the 11 to 13 + 6-week scan. *Ultrasound Obstet Gynecol* 2005;26:22.

145 Wald NJ, Watt HC, Hackshaw AK. Integrated screening for Down's syndrome on the basis of tests performed during the first and second trimesters. *N Engl J Med* 1999;341:461.

146 Cuckle HS. Growing complexity in the choice of Down's syndrome screening policy. *Ultrasound Obstet Gynecol* 2002;19:323.

147 Wright D, Bradbury I, Benn P, et al. Contingent screening for Down syndrome is an efficient alternative to non-disclosure sequential screening. *Prenat Diagn* 2004;24:762.

148 Benn P, Wright D, Cuckle H. Practical strategies in contingent sequential screening for Down syndrome. *Prenat Diagn* 2005;25:645.

149 Wright DE, Bradbury I. Repeated measures screening for Down's syndrome. *Br J Obstet Gynaecol* 2005;112:80.

150 Palomaki GE, Steinort K, Knight GJ, Haddow JE. Comparing three screening strategies for combining first- and second-trimester Down syndrome markers. *Obstet Gynecol* 2006;107:367.

151 Palomaki GE, Wright DE, Summers AM, et al. Repeated measurement of pregnancy-associated plasma protein-A (PAPP-A) in Down syndrome screening: a validation study. *Prenat Diagn* 2006;26:730.

152 Wright D, Bradbury I, Cuckle H, et al. Three-stage contingent screening for Down syndrome. *Prenat Diagn* 2006;26:588.

153 Farina A, LeShane ES, Lambert-Messerlian GM, et al. Evaluation of cell-free fetal DNA as a second-trimester maternal serum marker of Down syndrome pregnancy. *Clin Chem* 2003;49:239.

Part VII

Methods of Evaluation of Fetal Development and Well-being

29 Prenatal diagnosis of deviant fetal growth

E. Albert Reece and Zion J. Hagay

Fetal growth is a fundamental characteristic of the continuity of life and fetal well-being. Cell divisions, cell hyperplasia, and cell hypertrophy are the cornerstones of fetal growth. Winick[1] has suggested that, early in pregnancy, growth of fetal organs takes place first by cell hyperplasia or cell division, then by hyperplasia and cell hypertrophy and, finally, by the cessation of hyperplasia, after which growth continues by cellular hypertrophy alone. Despite this apparent orderly sequence of events, fetuses grow at different rates, become different sizes, and have different shapes. It has been observed in sheep that, up until 130 days' gestation, growth seems to be very similar between fetuses but, after this point, varying patterns of growth may be recognized.

In this chapter, we discuss the two extreme types of deviant fetal growth – accelerated (macrosomia) and diminished [intrauterine growth restriction (IUGR)]. In addition, prenatal diagnosis of these conditions is discussed.

Intrauterine growth restriction

Etiology and definition

IUGR is an abnormality of fetal growth and development that affects 3–7% of all deliveries, depending on the diagnostic criteria used.[2–4] The growth-restricted fetus is at greater risk for mortality and morbidity. It is estimated that perinatal mortality is 5–10 times higher in the growth-restricted neonate than in the neonate who is sized appropriately for gestational age.[5] Several associated morbid conditions of serious concern occurring after different periods of growth failure *in utero* include birth asphyxia, neonatal hypoglycemia, hypocalcemia, polycythemia, meconium aspiration, and persistent fetal circulation. Investigators have reported poorer neurodevelopmental outcome in small-for-gestational-age (SGA) infants, particularly when there is also associated prematurity.[6–8] The incidence of major neurologic handicaps in preterm SGA infants may be 35%.[9]

There are several causes of IUGR. These may be conceptually divided into three main categories: maternal, fetal, and uteroplacental (Table 29.1). It should be stressed, however, that in almost half the cases of IUGR, the etiology is unknown. Furthermore, it has been found that the single most important maternal clinical risk factor is a previous history of IUGR.[10] Therefore, suspicion of IUGR should not be based only on the existence of clinical risk factors during the index pregnancy.

One point of confusion and disagreement is the criteria that are used to define IUGR. IUGR has been defined variously as an infant whose birthweight is below the 3rd,[11] 5th,[12] and 10th[13] percentiles for gestational age or whose birthweight is more than two standard deviations below the mean for gestational age.[14,15] The ponderal index is determined in the neonate by the following formula:

$$\text{Ponderal index} = [\text{birthweight (g)} \times 100]/[\text{crown–heel length (cm)}]^3$$

The ponderal index may identify a neonate who has a small amount of soft tissue clinically evident by loss of subcutaneous tissue and muscle mass, even though the birthweight is normal for gestational age. Neonates with a ponderal index below the 10th percentile for gestational age are probably suffering from malnutrition *in utero*. For example, a fetus of 2900 g born at 38 weeks' gestation would have been larger (e.g., 3500 g) under normal nutritional conditions. Such an infant may be identified as having IUGR only when using the ponderal index definition for this condition.

In an interesting study by Weiner and Robinson,[16] the results of sonographic diagnoses of IUGR were compared with the postnatal ponderal indices. The study showed that 40% of SGA infants identified by birthweight percentiles were not growth restricted according to their ponderal index. In contrast, 53% of the neonates diagnosed as IUGR by postnatal ponderal index were average for gestational age according to their birthweight percentile. Because the importance of antenatal diagnosis of IUGR is to identify those infants at high risk for intrapartum and neonatal complications, the ponderal index is more closely related to perinatal morbidity and mortality than the birthweight percentile.[17] Therefore, it would be useful to be able to employ the ponderal index in attempting

Table 29.1 Risk factors of intrauterine growth restriction.

Maternal risk factors
- Alcohol
- Smoking
- Drugs
  - Corticosteroids
  - Propranolol
  - Dilantin
  - Coumadin
  - Heroin
- Anemia
- Malnutrition
- Prepregnancy weight of < 50 kg
- Cyanotic heart disease
- Chronic hypertension
- Pregnancy-induced hypertension
- Diabetes mellitus (with vasculopathy)
- Connective tissue disease

Fetal risk factors
- Genetic disorders (e.g., dwarf syndromes)
- Chromosomal abnormalities (e.g., trisomies 13, 18, and 21)
- Congenital anomalies (e.g., gastroschisis)
- Fetal infection (e.g., viral, protozoan)

Uterine and placental risk factors
- Müllerian anomalies (e.g., septate uterus)
- Placental insufficiency due to
  - Infarctions
  - Infection
  - Chorioangioma
  - Multifetal pregnancy
  - Circumvallate placenta
  - Previa
  - Focal abruption
  - Marginal insertion of the cord

to diagnose IUGR *in utero*. Unfortunately, there is presently no practical method to evaluate ponderal index *in utero*. Hence, the most commonly used definition of IUGR is a fetal weight below the 10th percentile for gestational age.

Another index, the crown–heel length, has been used to evaluate neonatal size. Prediction from the femur length (FL) measurement, however, has been found to be too imprecise to be useful.[18]

One unresolved problem concerns which growth curve to use. Goldenberg and colleagues[19] have shown that the 10th percentile birthweights at each gestational age differ substantially among published charts, occasionally by more than 500 g. One of the most widely used birthweight curves is that of Battaglia and Lubchenco,[2] which was derived from 5635 liveborn white and Hispanic people living at approximately 8000 feet above sea level in Denver, CO, USA. Obviously, this growth curve cannot be applied to a different ethnic and geographic population.

It has been suggested that much of the confusion that presently surrounds IUGR would be eliminated, at least in the United States, if we used a clearly defined American population to derive the percentiles for defining IUGR.[19] In fact, discrepancies between different birthweight charts from different geographic areas underscore the need for generating birthweight curves from the population to which they will be applied.

Classification of intrauterine growth restriction

Clinically, three categories of IUGR may be recognized. Each reflects the time of onset of the pathologic process (Fig. 29.1).[20–23]

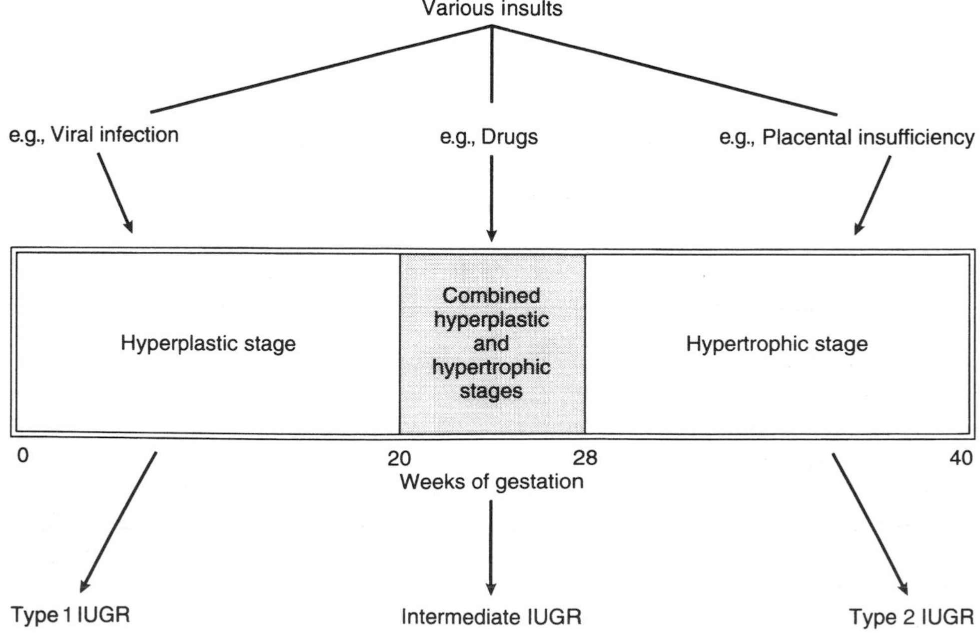

Figure 29.1 A schematic illustration of possible insults during the three stages of embryonic–fetal development and the corresponding intrauterine growth restriction (IUGR) that may develop.

Type 1, or symmetric, IUGR

Type 1 IUGR refers to the infant with decreased growth potential. This type of IUGR begins early in gestation, and the entire fetus is proportionally SGA.

Head and abdominal circumferences, length, and weight are all below the 10th percentile for gestational age. However, those infants have a normal ponderal index.

Type 1 IUGR is a result of growth inhibition early in gestation. This early stage of embryonic–fetal development is characterized by active mitosis from 4 to 20 weeks' gestation and is called the hyperplastic stage.[24–26] Any pathologic process during this stage may lead to a reduced number of cells in the fetus.

Symmetric IUGR accounts for 20–30% of growth-restricted fetuses.[22,27] This condition may result from the inhibition of mitosis, as is seen in intrauterine infection (e.g., herpes simplex, rubella, cytomegalovirus, toxoplasmosis), chromosomal disorders, and congenital malformations. It should be remembered, however, that symmetrically small fetuses may be constitutionally small and suffer from no abnormality at all.[20]

In general, type 1 IUGR is associated with a poor prognosis: this is in direct relation to the pathologic condition that causes it. Weiner and Williamson[28] showed that, in the absence of an identifiable maternal factor and sonographically detected abnormality, approximately 25% of fetuses evaluated for severe, early-onset growth restriction have aneuploidy. Therefore, the performance of percutaneous umbilical blood sampling is strongly recommended to search for karyotypic abnormality.

Type 2, or asymmetric, IUGR

Type 2, or asymmetric, IUGR refers to the neonate with restricted growth and is most frequently due to uteroplacental insufficiency.[21,29]

Type 2 IUGR is a result of a later growth insult than type 1 and usually occurs after 28 weeks' gestation. As has been shown by Vorherr,[26] in the late second trimester, normal fetal growth is characterized by a process of hypertrophy. In this hypertrophic stage, there is a rapid increase in cell size and the formation of fat, muscle, bone, and other tissues. In this phase, the process of hyperplasia is decreased (Fig. 29.2).

Symmetrically growth-restricted fetuses have a near normal total number of cells, but these cells are decreased in size. Asymmetric IUGR fetuses have low ponderal indices with below average infant weight but normal head circumference (HC) and fetal length. In these cases of asymmetric IUGR, fetal growth is normal until late in the second trimester or early in the third, when head growth remains normal, whereas abdominal growth slows ("brain-sparing effect"). This asymmetry is a result of a fetal compensatory mechanism that responds to a state of poor placental perfusion. Redistribution of fetal cardiac output occurs with increased flow to the brain, heart,

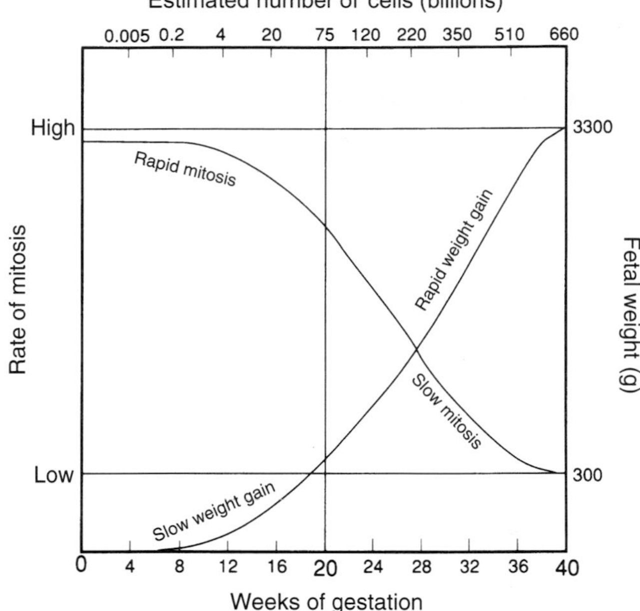

Figure 29.2 Cell number and rate of mitosis in relation to embryonic–fetal growth. Embryonic weight gain is slow (small initial cell number) even though the rate of mitosis is very high. At approximately weeks 16 to 20 of gestation, a substantial fetal cell mass is reached. Thereafter, however, mitosis is slowed (organ differentiation and function). Even though slowed, division of a large number of fetal cells produces a rapid fetal weight gain. (Redrawn from ref. 26.)

and adrenals and decreased glycogen storage and liver mass.[30] However, if placental insufficiency is aggravated during late pregnancy, the head growth may be flattened, and its size may drop below the normal growth curve.

It is estimated that 70–80% of growth-restricted fetuses are type 2 IUGR.[31] This form of IUGR is frequently associated with maternal diseases such as chronic hypertension, renal disease, diabetes mellitus with vasculopathy, and others (see Table 29.1).

Intermediate IUGR

Intermediate IUGR refers to growth restriction that is a combination of types 1 and 2 IUGR. The insult to fetal growth in intermediate IUGR most probably occurs during the middle phase of fetal growth – that of hyperplasia and hypertrophy (see Figs 29.1 and 29.2) – which corresponds to 20–28 weeks' gestation. At this stage, there is a decrease in mitotic rate and a progressive overall increase in cell size.

This form of IUGR is less common than types 1 and 2; it is estimated as being responsible for 5–10% of all growth-restricted fetuses. Chronic hypertension, lupus nephritis, or other maternal vascular diseases that are severe and begin early in the second trimester may result in an intermediate

IUGR with symmetric growth and no significant brain-sparing effect.

Ultrasonic measurements used in the diagnosis of IUGR

The intrauterine detection of restricted fetal growth by clinical means is possible in approximately 30% of affected pregnancies.[32] Ultrasonography offers an objective, reliable, and effective means of identifying restricted intrauterine fetal growth. However, to make a proper diagnosis and appropriately manage the growth-restricted fetus, it is crucial to determine the gestational age as accurately as possible.

Pregnancy dating has traditionally been based on historical and clinical clues. The certain date of a patient's last menstrual period had been regarded as the most reliable method of estimating a fetus' gestational age.[33] However, it has been reported that 20–40% of pregnant women fail to recall the exact date of their last menstrual period.[34]

Therefore, ultrasonography may be of help in dating a pregnancy. In the first trimester, crown–rump length measurement allows for an estimation of gestational age with a range of 4.7 days at the 95% confidence level. Between 12 and 24 weeks' gestation, the biparietal diameter (BPD) measurement provides reliable estimates comparable with that of the crown–rump measurement performed in the first trimester of pregnancy. Beyond 28–30 weeks' gestation, there is a progressive increase in BPD variations, and the establishment of accurate gestational age is less satisfactory.

The FL correlates with gestational age, particularly during 14–22 weeks' gestation, with a range of 6–7 days at the 95% confidence level.[35]

Accurate antenatal diagnosis of IUGR may prevent the high perinatal morbidity and mortality associated with this condition and permit appropriate management and obstetric intervention when fetal compromise is evident. Most authorities believe that, whenever IUGR is diagnosed after 37 weeks' gestation, delivery is indicated to decrease the risk of fetal death.[36]

Several sonographic parameters may be used in the diagnosis of IUGR. These parameters are critically reviewed in the following sections.

Biparietal diameter

Nomograms of BPD or HC are available to provide calculated estimates of weekly increments for the size of the fetal head (Tables 29.2–29.4).[37] Hence, when comparing the observed increase in BPD with the expected rate of growth, the physician should be able to identify growth-restricted fetuses when the head is affected in the growth curtailment. In fact, the BPD was the first ultrasonic parameter used for detection of IUGR.[23,38] The detection rates of IUGR with single and serial BPD measurements alone have been reported to be of poor value by most authors.[39,40–42] Reported accuracy rates have ranged from 43% to 82%.[40,43–47] Rosendahl and Kivinen[48] studied the efficiency of a single BPD measurement at 34 weeks' gestation to identify infants with birthweights below the 10th percentile. Single BPD measurements at 34 weeks' gestation detected only 26.9% of the SGA infants, with a positive predictive value of 30.9%, which means that 69% of the fetuses with restricted BPD actually proved to be normally grown. The study by Warsof and colleagues[49] indicates that a single BPD measurement in the third trimester is a poor predictor of IUGR.

Others studies used serial BPD determinations in the hope of improving accuracy; however, their results were equally disappointing. Kurjak and colleagues[43] have shown that only 48% of fetuses with a small BPD (below the 10th percentile) had birthweights below the 10th percentile and actually resulted in delivery of SGA infants.

From the previously mentioned data, it is clear that BPD alone cannot be used as a good predictor of IUGR. This is not surprising, because almost two-thirds of IUGR cases are of the asymmetric or late-flattening type, which have normal growth of the head until late in pregnancy as a consequence of the brain-sparing process. Therefore, BPD in asymmetric IUGR may be normal until late in gestation. Another reason for the low sensitivity of BPD measurements in detecting IUGR is the distortion of the fetal head shape that may occur, for example in dolichocephaly, or may be seen in cases of breech presentation when the BPD may be falsely small.

BPD determinations, when used singly, fail to identify approximately 20–50% of IUGR infants and, therefore, cannot be used as the only parameter in screening for IUGR.[39]

Transverse cerebellar diameter

The cerebellum can be easily visualized as early as the first trimester as a butterfly-shaped figure in the posterior fossa of the fetal head, behind the thalami and in front of the echolucent area (cisterna magna) (Fig. 29.3). The transverse cerebellar diameter (TCD) in millimeters has been shown to correlate with gestational age in weeks up to 24 weeks. After 24 weeks' gestation, the growth curves turn upward, and this uniform correlation no longer exists. Goldstein and colleagues[50] have constructed a nomogram of the TCD throughout pregnancy (Table 29.5).

Reece and colleagues[51] subsequently evaluated the TCD measurement in IUGR fetuses. They reported that the TCD measurement was not significantly affected by restricted fetal growth and, therefore, the TCD could be used as a reliable predictor of gestational age even in cases of IUGR. This parameter is particularly useful because it is a standard against which other parameters can be compared. Duchatel and colleagues[52] have corroborated these findings in their report of 12 cases of IUGR below the 3rd percentile in which the TCD remained unaltered. Other investigators have provided additional support for the usefulness of the TCD by constructing a nomogram of the ratio between TCD and abdominal circumference (AC).[53] In a small series, these investigators have

Table 29.2 Gestational age from the biparietal diameter.

BPD (mm)	5th percentile	50th percentile	95th percentile	BPD (mm)	5th percentile	50th percentile	95th percentile
10	7 + 0	10 + 1	13 + 1	39	14 + 0	17 + 1	20 + 1
11	7 + 2	10 + 2	13 + 3	40	14 + 2	17 + 3	20 + 3
12	7 + 3	10 + 4	13 + 4	41	14 + 4	17 + 5	20 + 5
13	7 + 5	10 + 5	13 + 5	42	14 + 6	18 + 0	21 + 0
14	7 + 6	10 + 6	14 + 0	43	15 + 1	18 + 2	21 + 2
15	8 + 1	11 + 1	14 + 1	44	15 + 3	18 + 4	21 + 4
16	8 + 2	11 + 2	14 + 3	45	15 + 6	18 + 6	21 + 6
17	8 + 4	11 + 4	14 + 4	46	16 + 1	19 + 1	22 + 1
18	8 + 5	11 + 5	14 + 6	47	16 + 3	19 + 3	22 + 4
19	9 + 0	12 + 0	15 + 0	48	16 + 5	19 + 5	22 + 6
20	9 + 1	12 + 2	15 + 2	49	17 + 0	20 + 1	23 + 1
21	9 + 3	12 + 3	15 + 3	50	17 + 3	20 + 3	23 + 3
22	9 + 4	12 + 5	15 + 5	51	17 + 5	20 + 5	23 + 6
23	9 + 6	12 + 6	16 + 0	52	18 + 0	21 + 0	24 + 1
24	10 + 1	13 + 1	16 + 1	53	18 + 2	21 + 3	24 + 3
25	10 + 2	13 + 3	16 + 3	54	18 + 5	21 + 5	24 + 5
26	10 + 4	13 + 4	16 + 5	55	19 + 0	22 + 0	25 + 1
27	10 + 6	13 + 6	17 + 0	56	19 + 2	22 + 3	25 + 3
28	11 + 0	14 + 1	17 + 1	57	19 + 5	22 + 5	25 + 6
29	11 + 2	14 + 3	17 + 3	58	20 + 0	23 + 1	26 + 1
30	11 + 4	14 + 4	17 + 5	59	20 + 3	23 + 3	26 + 3
31	11 + 6	14 + 6	18 + 0	60	20 + 5	23 + 6	26 + 6
32	12 + 1	15 + 1	18 + 1	61	21 + 1	24 + 1	27 + 1
33	12 + 3	15 + 3	18 + 3	62	21 + 3	24 + 4	27 + 4
34	12 + 4	15 + 5	18 + 5	63	21 + 6	24 + 6	27 + 6
35	12 + 6	16 + 0	19 + 0	64	22 + 1	25 + 2	28 + 2
36	13 + 1	16 + 2	19 + 2	65	22 + 4	25 + 4	28 + 5
37	13 + 3	16 + 4	19 + 4	66	22 + 6	26 + 0	29 + 0
38	13 + 5	16 + 6	19 + 6	67	23 + 2	26 + 2	29 + 3

Reprinted from Jeanty P, Remero R. *Obstetrical ultrasound*. New York: McGraw-Hill, 1984, with permission.

BPD, biparietal diameter.

Table 29.3 Estimated variability associated with determining menstrual age from biparietal diameter values.

Group (menstrual age)	Hadlock et al.*	Days	Kurtz et al.†	Days
1 (12–18 weeks)	± 0.85 weeks (r^2 = 90.4%)	5.9	± 0.80 weeks	5.6
2 (18–24 weeks)	± 1.29 weeks (r^2 = 87.6%)	9.03	± 1.70 weeks	11.9
3 (24–30 weeks)	± 1.40 weeks (r^2 = 89.1%)	9.8	± 1.34 weeks	9.38
4 (30–36 weeks)	± 1.96 weeks (r^2 = 76.5%)	13.7	± 1.42 weeks	9.94
5 (36–42 weeks)	± 2.06 weeks (r^2 = 25.6%)	14.42	± 1.23 weeks	8.61

Modified from Hadlock FP, Deter R, Harrist R, et al. Fetal biparietal diameter: a critical re-evaluation of the relation to menstrual age by means of real-time ultrasound. *J Ultrasound Med* 1982;1:91; and Kurtz AB, Wapher RJ, Kurtz RJ, et al. Analysis of biparietal diameter as an accurate indicator of gestational age. *J Clin Ultrasound* 1980;8:319.

* Ninety-five percent confidence interval.

† Ninety percent confidence interval (of mean values).

Table 29.4 Gestational age from the head circumference.

HC (mm)	5th percentile	50th percentile	95th percentile	HC (mm)	5th percentile	50th percentile	95th percentile
60	8 + 6	10 + 5	12 + 3	205	19 + 5	21 + 4	23 + 2
65	9 + 1	11 + 0	12 + 5	210	20 + 2	22 + 0	23 + 5
70	9 + 3	11 + 2	13 + 0	215	20 + 5	22 + 3	24 + 1
75	9 + 6	11 + 4	13 + 2	220	21 + 1	22 + 6	24 + 5
80	10 + 1	11 + 6	13 + 4	225	21 + 4	23 + 3	25 + 1
85	10 + 3	12 + 1	14 + 0	230	22 + 1	23 + 6	25 + 4
90	10 + 5	12 + 4	14 + 2	235	22 + 4	24 + 3	26 + 1
95	11 + 1	12 + 6	14 + 4	240	23 + 1	24 + 6	26 + 4
100	11 + 3	13 + 1	14 + 6	245	23 + 4	25 + 3	27 + 1
105	11 + 5	13 + 4	15 + 2	250	24 + 1	25 + 6	27 + 4
110	12 + 1	13 + 6	15 + 4	255	24 + 4	26 + 3	28 + 1
115	12 + 3	14 + 1	16 + 0	260	25 + 1	26 + 6	28 + 5
120	12 + 6	14 + 4	16 + 2	265	25 + 5	27 + 3	29 + 1
125	13 + 1	14 + 6	16 + 5	270	26 + 1	28 + 0	29 + 5
130	13 + 4	15 + 2	17 + 0	275	26 + 5	28 + 4	30 + 2
135	13 + 6	15 + 5	17 + 3	280	27 + 2	29 + 0	30 + 6
140	14 + 2	16 + 0	17 + 6	285	27 + 6	29 + 4	31 + 2
145	14 + 5	16 + 3	18 + 1	290	28 + 3	30 + 1	31 + 6
150	15 + 0	16 + 6	18 + 4	295	29 + 0	30 + 5	32 + 3
155	15 + 3	17 + 2	19 + 0	300	29 + 4	31 + 2	33 + 0
160	15 + 6	17 + 4	19 + 3	305	30 + 1	31 + 6	33 + 4
165	16 + 2	18 + 0	19 + 6	310	30 + 5	32 + 3	34 + 1
170	16 + 5	18 + 3	20 + 1	315	31 + 2	33 + 0	34 + 5
175	17 + 1	18 + 6	20 + 4	320	31 + 6	33 + 4	35 + 2
180	17 + 4	19 + 2	21 + 0	325	32 + 3	34 + 1	36 + 0
185	18 + 0	19 + 5	21 + 3	330	33 + 0	34 + 6	36 + 4
190	18 + 3	20 + 1	21 + 6	335	33 + 5	35 + 4	37 + 1
195	18 + 6	20 + 4	22 + 3	340	34 + 2	36 + 0	37 + 5
200	19 + 0	21 + 0	22 + 6				

Reprinted from Jeanty P, Remero R. *Obstetrical ultrasound*. New York: McGraw-Hill, 1984, with permission.

HC, head circumference.

shown that this ratio permits the identification of IUGR by demonstrating the fairly consistent growth of the TCD relative to the decrease in AC in cases of IUGR. In yet another study by Hill and colleagues,[54] the TCD was found to be within two standard deviations in only 40% of IUGR cases and, in 60% of cases, the TCD was more than two standard deviations below the mean. The results of this paper are at variance with the three reports discussed earlier. Nevertheless, the majority of data available would suggest that the use of the TCD when gestational age is unknown or IUGR is suspected is extremely valuable. The accuracy of the TCD can be enhanced by using biometric ratios, especially FL:AC, as well as amniotic fluid volume and the presence or absence of fetal ossification centers.

Abdominal circumference

The AC has been reported to be the best fetal biometric parameter that correlates with fetal weight and is the most sensitive parameter for detecting IUGR.[55] Warsof and colleagues[49] studied the effectiveness of three ultrasonic growth parameters – BPD, HC, and AC – in detecting IUGR in a large group of obstetric patients. They demonstrated that AC measurements are more predictive of IUGR than BPD or HC, singly or in combination. In this study, it was shown that screening at 34 weeks' gestation for IUGR results in a sensitivity of approximately 70% and a positive predictive value of 50%. However, the authors used the 25th rather than the 10th percentile measurement to determine a positive result to maximize sensitivity of the screening test.

It is noteworthy that the sensitivity and true positive rates are influenced by the incidence of IUGR in the population studied. This is demonstrated in the studies by Geirsson and colleagues,[56,57] who have shown that measuring the abdominal area at 36 weeks' gestation to detect fetuses below the 10th percentile for weight resulted in a sensitivity of 72% in a high-risk group, but only 56% when the entire obstetric population was screened. The positive predictive values were

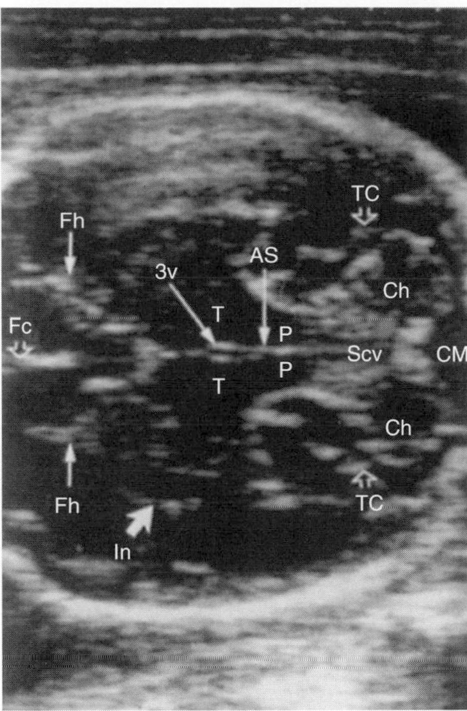

Figure 29.3 Intracranial anatomy of the fetal head. AS, aqueduct of Sylvius; Ch, cerebellar hemispheres; CM, cisterna magna; Fc, midline falx cerebri; Fh, frontal horn; In, insula; P, peduncle; 3v, third ventricle; Scv, superior cerebellar vermis; T, thalami; TC, cerebellar tonsils.

68% in the high-risk group and 50% in the unselected group.

Others have found results that further demonstrate that AC is the single best predictor of IUGR, with an accuracy that may reach 96% of cases.[43,58] In fact, in contrast to the BPD measurement, AC is smaller in both symmetric and asymmetric types of IUGR, and therefore its measurement has a higher sensitivity. Animal studies have shown that the liver is the most affected organ in IUGR. Because the liver is the largest intra-abdominal organ, assessment of the AC at the level of the liver is actually an indirect indication of the nutritional status of the fetus.

Unfortunately, AC has more intraobserver and interobserver variation than either BPD or FL.[36] Furthermore, AC variability may result from fetal breathing movements, compression, or position of the fetus. To obtain the proper AC, the section should be round and at the level of the fetal stomach and the portal umbilical vein (or the bifurcation of the main portal vein into the right and left branches). Normal values of AC are presented in Table 29.6.[59]

Long bones

The FL is another important parameter in evaluating fetal growth (Table 29.7). Long bones other than the femur can be equally useful in the assessment of gestational age (Tables 29.8 and 29.9). It has been demonstrated by several authors that there is a linear relationship between FL specifically and long bones in general and crown–heel length of a newborn.[18,60] These long bones are generally decreased in symmetrically growth-restricted fetuses, but may be of normal length in asymmetric IUGR. In fact, the fetal head and long-bone length in asymmetric IUGR tend to be affected late in gestation.[60] Because the measurement of most long bones is relatively simple, they become a useful means of estimating gestational age on a routine basis. Like most other biometric parameters, the standard deviation tends to expand with increasing gestational age. Hence, accuracy is greatest in early gestation.

Total intrauterine volume

The rationale for measuring total intrauterine volume derives from the fact that, in IUGR, intrauterine content is reduced (fetal, placental mass, and the amount of amniotic fluid). Gohari and colleagues[61] calculated total intrauterine volume using the formula of an ellipsoid volume. Although these results were encouraging because 75% of IUGR were correctly diagnosed, this method has been abandoned by most centers because of the widespread use of real-time ultrasonography and the fact that a static scanner is needed to measure total intrauterine volume.

Amniotic fluid volume assessment

In the growth-restricted fetus, decreased amounts of amniotic fluids may be observed. This is a direct result of decreased renal perfusion and reduced urine production. Manning and colleagues[62] have shown that oligohydramnios, determined by ultrasound as the absence of a pocket of amniotic fluid greater than 1 cm in its largest diameter, may predict with high accuracy that the fetus is growth restricted. Their study group included patients at high risk for IUGR. In this group, oligohydramnios was found to be highly sensitive (84% and 97%), with a predictive value approaching 90%. Unfortunately, progressive growth curtailment usually occurs without evidence of significant amniotic fluid reduction. Hence, this parameter is not very sensitive to evolving IUGR. As shown previously, its utility is greatest in diagnosing frank IUGR.

When amniotic fluid volume evaluation was tested as a screening method in the detection of IUGR in the general obstetric population, the results were quite disappointing. Philipson and colleagues[63] studied 2453 pregnant patients and found the oligohydramnios test to be poorly sensitive (16%); in other words, in 84% of IUGR infants, there was no evidence of oligohydramnios and therefore the problem would have been missed by this test. In summary, it seems that this ultrasonic method of detecting fetal growth restriction is unsatisfactory because of low accuracy.

Table 29.5 Nomogram of the transverse cerebellar diameter, biparietal diameter, and head circumference according to percentile distribution.

Gestational age (weeks)	Cerebellum (mm)					Biparietal diameter (mm)					Head circumference (mm)				
	10	25	50	75	90	10	25	50	75	90	10	25	50	75	90
15	10	12	14	15	16	30	31	33	34	35	12	12	126	128	128
16	14	16	16	16	17	34	34	35	36	38	123	125	130	136	141
17	16	17	17	18	18	36	37	38	40	43	134	136	138	149	160
18	17	18	18	19	19	38	40	42	43	44	142	147	154	158	160
19	18	18	19	19	22	42	43	45	46	48	147	154	159	170	178
20	18	19	20	20	22	45	46	47	48	53	146	164	173	190	190
21	19	20	22	23	24	48	49	50	52	57	185	185	191	208	211
22	21	23	23	24	24	50	51	53	54	55	193	193	193	200	203
23	22	23	24	25	26	53	54	56	58	60	203	203	206	222	222
24	22	24	25	27	28	56	59	60	61	64	219	220	224	228	230
25	23	21	28	28	29	61	61	63	66	68	219	224	234	248	251
26	25	28	29	30	32	63	64	65	66	67	235	237	241	246	246
27	26	28	30	31	32	64	67	68	69	70	237	237	243	246	246
28	27	30	31	32	34	68	69	70	71	72	246	247	253	261	264
29	29	32	34	36	38	71	72	74	76	79	254	264	274	288	301
30	31	32	35	37	40	72	74	75	75	79	253	261	277	288	298
31	32	35	38	39	43	75	78	76	81	84	274	277	291	301	303
32	33	36	38	40	42	75	78	80	81	83	275	280	298	307	308
33	32	36	40	43	44	80	80	81	82	87	292	292	297	316	322
34	33	38	40	41	44	81	82	84	86	91	326	326	326	327	327
35	31	37	40	43	47	78	83	87	89	93	300	300	301	303	303
36	36	29	43	52	55	84	85	88	89	91	309	309	313	318	318
37	37	37	45	52	55	87	87	89	92	92	303	303	313	324	324
38	40	40	48	52	55	87	87	90	93	94	–	–	–	–	–
39	52	52	52	55	55	92	92	92	92	92	–	–	–	–	–

Table 29.6 Normal values for the abdominal circumference.

Week number	Jeanty			Deter	Week number	Jeanty			Deter
	5th percentile	50th percentile	95th percentile	50th percentile		5th percentile	50th percentile	95th percentile	50th percentile
12	35	57	80	63	27	193	215	238	227
13	45	67	90	74	28	206	225	248	238
14	55	77	100	84	29	213	235	257	249
15	65	88	110	95	30	222	244	267	260
16	76	98	120	106	31	231	254	276	271
17	86	109	131	117	32	240	262	285	282
18	97	119	142	128	33	248	271	293	293
19	108	130	152	139	34	256	279	301	304
20	119	141	163	150	35	264	286	309	315
21	129	152	174	161	36	271	293	316	326
22	140	163	185	172	37	278	300	322	337
23	151	173	196	183	38	283	306	328	348
24	162	184	206	194	39	289	311	333	359
25	172	195	217	205	40	294	316	338	370
26	183	205	227	216					

Reprinted from ref. 56.

Table 29.7 Gestational age estimated from the femur length.

Femur length (mm)	5th percentile	50th percentile	95th length (mm)	Femur percentile	5th percentile	50th percentile	95th percentile
10	10 + 3	12 + 4	14 + 6	46	23 + 1	25 + 3	27 + 4
11	10 + 5	12 + 6	15 + 1	47	23 + 4	25 + 6	28 + 0
12	11 + 1	13 + 2	15 + 4	48	24 + 0	26 + 1	28 + 3
13	11 + 3	13 + 4	15 + 6	49	24 + 3	26 + 4	28 + 6
14	11 + 5	13 + 6	16 + 1	50	24 + 6	27 + 0	29 + 1
15	12 + 0	14 + 1	16 + 3	51	25 + 1	27 + 3	29 + 4
16	12 + 3	14 + 4	16 + 6	52	25 + 4	27 + 6	30 + 0
17	12 + 5	14 + 6	17 + 1	53	26 + 0	28 + 1	30 + 3
18	13 + 0	15 + 1	17 + 3	54	26 + 3	28 + 4	30 + 6
19	13 + 3	15 + 4	17 + 6	55	26 + 6	29 + 1	31 + 2
20	13 + 5	15 + 6	18 + 1	56	27 + 2	29 + 4	31 + 5
21	14 + 1	16 + 2	18 + 4	57	27 + 5	29 + 6	32 + 1
22	14 + 3	16 + 4	18 + 6	58	28 + 1	30 + 2	32 + 4
23	14 + 5	16 + 6	19 + 1	59	28 + 4	30 + 5	32 + 6
24	15 + 1	17 + 2	19 + 4	60	28 + 6	31 + 1	33 + 2
25	15 + 3	17 + 4	19 + 6	61	29 + 3	31 + 4	33 + 6
26	15 + 6	18 + 0	20 + 1	62	29 + 6	32 + 0	34 + 1
27	16 + 1	18 + 2	20 + 4	63	30 + 1	32 + 3	34 + 4
28	16 + 4	18 + 5	20 + 6	64	30 + 5	32 + 6	35 + 1
29	16 + 6	19 + 0	21 + 1	65	31 + 1	33 + 2	35 + 4
30	17 + 1	19 + 3	21 + 4	66	31 + 4	33 + 5	35 + 6
31	17 + 4	19 + 6	22 + 0	67	32 + 0	34 + 1	36 + 3
32	17 + 6	20 + 1	22 + 2	68	32 + 3	34 + 4	36 + 6
33	18 + 2	20 + 4	22 + 5	69	32 + 6	35 + 0	37 + 1
34	18 + 5	20 + 6	23 + 1	70	33 + 2	35 + 4	37 + 5
35	19 + 0	21 + 1	23 + 3	71	33 + 5	35 + 6	38 + 1
36	19 + 3	21 + 4	23 + 6	72	34 + 1	36 + 3	38 + 4
37	19 + 6	22 + 0	24 + 1	73	34 + 3	36 + 6	39 + 0
38	20 + 1	22 + 3	24 + 4	74	35 + 1	37 + 2	39 + 4
39	20 + 4	22 + 5	24 + 6	75	35 + 4	37 + 5	39 + 6
40	20 + 6	23 + 1	25 + 2	76	36 + 0	38 + 1	40 + 3
41	21 + 2	23 + 4	25 + 5	77	36 + 3	38 + 4	40 + 6
42	21 + 5	23 + 6	26 + 1	78	36 + 6	39 + 1	41 + 2
43	22 + 1	24 + 2	26 + 4	79	37 + 2	39 + 4	41 + 5
44	22 + 4	24 + 5	26 + 6	80	37 + 6	40 + 0	42 + 1
45	22 + 6	25 + 0	27 + 1	–	–	–	–

Reprinted from Jeanty P, Romero R. *Obstetrical ultrasound*. New York: McGraw-Hill, 1984, with permission.

Placental growth

Grannum and colleagues[64] were the first to present an ultrasonic classification of placental maturity. This classification grades placentas from 0 to 3 according to specific ultrasonic findings at the basal and chronic plates, as well as within substances of the organ itself (Table 29.10). It is noteworthy that placentas do not all necessarily go through the full maturation process during pregnancy. This is demonstrated by the fact that, in normal pregnancies at term, only 20% of placentas are classified as grade 3.[65] Furthermore, ultrasound examination of placental maturation, or examination after 42 weeks' gestation, shows that 45% of placentas are of grade 3 and all the others are grade 2.[66] Therefore, it has been assumed that the appearance of a grade 3 placenta before 35 weeks' gestation should alert the physician to the possibility of the presence or subsequent development of IUGR. However, there are still no substantial data to support this assumption. Kazzi and colleagues[67] studied the value of placental grading in the diagnosis of IUGR in a high-risk group of patients. They have shown that grade 3 placentas accurately diagnose IUGR in 62% of cases, with a positive predictive value of 59%. Therefore, the prenatal diagnosis of IUGR using placental grading is rather limited.

Table 29.8 Gestational age in weeks and days as obtained from the long bones.

Bone length (mm)	Humerus percentile			Ulna percentile			Tibia percentile		
	5th	50th	95th	5th	50th	95th	5th	50th	95th
10	9 + 6	12 + 4	15 + 2	10 + 1	13 + 1	16 + 1	10 + 4	13 + 3	16 + 2
11	10 + 1	12 + 6	15 + 4	10 + 4	13 + 4	16 + 4	10 + 6	13 + 5	16 + 4
12	10 + 3	13 + 1	15 + 6	10 + 6	13 + 6	16 + 6	11 + 1	14 + 1	17 + 0
13	10 + 6	13 + 4	16 + 1	11 + 1	14 + 1	17 + 2	11 + 4	14 + 3	17 + 2
14	11 + 1	13 + 6	16 + 4	11 + 4	14 + 4	17 + 5	11 + 6	14 + 6	17 + 5
15	11 + 3	14 + 1	16 + 6	11 + 6	15 + 0	18 + 0	12 + 1	15 + 1	18 + 0
16	11 + 6	14 + 4	17 + 2	12 + 2	15 + 3	18 + 3	12 + 4	15 + 4	18 + 3
17	12 + 1	14 + 6	17 + 4	12 + 5	15 + 5	18 + 6	13 + 0	15 + 6	18 + 6
18	12 + 4	15 + 1	18 + 0	13 + 1	16 + 1	19 + 1	13 + 2	16 + 1	19 + 1
19	12 + 6	15 + 4	18 + 2	13 + 4	16 + 4	19 + 4	13 + 5	16 + 4	19 + 4
20	13 + 1	15 + 6	18 + 5	13 + 6	16 + 6	20 + 0	14 + 1	17 + 0	19 + 6
21	13 + 4	16 + 2	19 + 1	14 + 2	17 + 2	20 + 3	14 + 4	17 + 3	20 + 2
22	13 + 6	16 + 5	19 + 3	14 + 5	17 + 5	20 + 6	14 + 6	17 + 6	20 + 5
23	14 + 2	17 + 1	19 + 6	15 + 1	18 + 1	21 + 1	15 + 1	18 + 1	21 + 1
24	14 + 5	17 + 3	20 + 1	15 + 4	18 + 4	21 + 4	15 + 4	18 + 4	21 + 3
25	15 + 1	17 + 6	20 + 4	16 + 0	19 + 0	22 + 1	16 + 0	18 + 6	21 + 6
26	15 + 4	18 + 1	21 + 0	16 + 3	19 + 3	22 + 4	16 + 3	19 + 2	22 + 1
27	15 + 6	18 + 4	21 + 3	16 + 6	19 + 6	22 + 6	16 + 6	19 + 5	22 + 4
28	16 + 2	19 + 0	21 + 6	17 + 2	20 + 2	23 + 3	17 + 1	20 + 1	23 + 0
29	16 + 5	19 + 3	22 + 1	17 + 5	20 + 6	23 + 6	17 + 4	20 + 4	23 + 4
30	17 + 1	19 + 6	22 + 4	18 + 1	21 + 1	24 + 2	18 + 1	21 + 0	23 + 6
31	17 + 4	20 + 2	23 + 0	18 + 4	21 + 5	24 + 6	18 + 4	21 + 3	24 + 2
32	18 + 0	20 + 5	23 + 4	19 + 1	22 + 1	25 + 1	18 + 6	21 + 6	24 + 5
33	18 + 3	21 + 1	23 + 6	19 + 4	22 + 5	25 + 5	19 + 2	22 + 1	25 + 1
34	18 + 6	21 + 4	24 + 2	20 + 1	23 + 1	26 + 1	19 + 5	22 + 4	25 + 4
35	19 + 2	22 + 0	24 + 6	20 + 4	24 + 4	26 + 5	20 + 1	23 + 1	26 + 0
36	19 + 5	22 + 4	25 + 1	21 + 1	24 + 1	27 + 1	20 + 4	23 + 4	26 + 3
37	20 + 1	22 + 6	25 + 5	21 + 4	24 + 4	27 + 5	21 + 0	23 + 6	26 + 6
38	20 + 4	23 + 3	26 + 1	22 + 1	25 + 1	28 + 1	21 + 4	24 + 3	27 + 2
39	21 + 1	23 + 6	26 + 4	22 + 4	25 + 4	28 + 5	21 + 6	24 + 6	27 + 5
40	21 + 4	24 + 2	27 + 1	23 + 1	26 + 1	29 + 1	22 + 3	25 + 2	28 + 1
41	22 + 0	24 + 6	27 + 4	23 + 4	26 + 5	29 + 5	22 + 6	25 + 5	28 + 4
42	22 + 4	25 + 2	28 + 0	24 + 1	27 + 1	30 + 2	23 + 2	26 + 1	29 + 1
43	23 + 0	25 + 5	28 + 4	24 + 5	27 + 5	30 + 6	23 + 5	26 + 4	29 + 4
44	23 + 4	26 + 1	29 + 0	25 + 1	28 + 2	31 + 2	24 + 1	27 + 1	30 + 0
45	24 + 0	26 + 5	29 + 4	25 + 6	28 + 6	31 + 6	24 + 4	27 + 4	30 + 4
46	24 + 4	27 + 1	30 + 0	26 + 2	29 + 3	32 + 3	25 + 1	28 + 0	30 + 6
47	25 + 0	27 + 5	30 + 4	26 + 9	29 + 6	33 + 0	25 + 4	28 + 4	31 + 3
48	25 + 4	28 + 1	31 + 0	27 + 3	30 + 4	33 + 4	26 + 1	29 + 0	31 + 6
49	26 + 0	28 + 6	31 + 4	28 + 0	31 + 1	34 + 1	26 + 4	29 + 3	32 + 2
50	26 + 4	29 + 2	32 + 0	28 + 4	31 + 4	34 + 5	27 + 0	29 + 6	32 + 6
51	27 + 1	29 + 6	32 + 4	29 + 1	32 + 1	35 + 2	27 + 4	30 + 3	33 + 2
52	27 + 4	30 + 2	33 + 1	29 + 5	32 + 6	35 + 6	28 + 0	30 + 6	33 + 6
53	28 + 1	30 + 6	33 + 4	30 + 2	33 + 3	36 + 3	28 + 4	31 + 3	34 + 2
54	28 + 5	31 + 3	34 + 1	30 + 6	34 + 0	37 + 0	29 + 0	31 + 6	34 + 6
55	29 + 1	32 + 0	34 + 5	31 + 4	34 + 4	37 + 5	29 + 4	32 + 3	35 + 2
56	29 + 6	32 + 4	35 + 2	32 + 1	35 + 1	38 + 2	30 + 0	32 + 6	35 + 6
57	30 + 2	33 + 1	35 + 6	32 + 6	35 + 6	38 + 6	30 + 4	33 + 3	36 + 2
58	30 + 6	33 + 4	36 + 3	33 + 3	36 + 3	39 + 4	31 + 0	33 + 6	36 + 6
59	31 + 1	34 + 1	36 + 6	34 + 0	37 + 1	40 + 1	31 + 4	34 + 3	37 + 2
60	32 + 0	34 + 6	37 + 4	34 + 4	37 + 5	40 + 6	32 + 0	34 + 6	37 + 6
61	32 + 4	35 + 2	38 + 1	35 + 2	38 + 2	41 + 3	32 + 4	35 + 4	38 + 2
62	33 + 1	35 + 6	38 + 5	35 + 6	39 + 0	42 + 0	33 + 0	35 + 6	38 + 6
63	33 + 6	36 + 4	39 + 2	36 + 4	39 + 4	42 + 5	33 + 4	36 + 4	39 + 3
64	34 + 3	37 + 1	39 + 6	37 + 1	40 + 2	43 + 2	34 + 1	37 + 0	39 + 6
65	35 + 0	37 + 5	40 + 4	–	–	–	34 + 4	37 + 4	40 + 3
66	35 + 4	38 + 2	41 + 1	–	–	–	35 + 1	38 + 0	41 + 0
67	36 + 1	38 + 6	41 + 5	–	–	–	35 + 5	38 + 4	41 + 4
68	36 + 6	39 + 4	42 + 4	–	–	–	36 + 1	39 + 1	42 + 0
69	37 + 3	40 + 1	42 + 6	–	–	–	36 + 6	39 + 5	42 + 4

Reprinted from Jeanty P, Rodesch F, Delbeke D, et al. Estimation of gestational age from measurements of fetal long bones. *J Ultrasound Med* 1984;3:75, with permission.

Table 29.9 Gestational age as obtained from clavicle length.

Clavicle length (mm)	Gestational age (weeks and days) percentile		
	5th	50th	95th
11	8 + 3	13 + 6	17 + 2
12	9 + 1	14 + 4	18 + 1
13	10 + 0	14 + 3	19 + 6
14	11 + 6	15 + 2	20 + 5
15	12 + 5	16 + 1	21 + 4
16	12 + 3	18 + 0	21 + 3
17	13 + 2	18 + 5	22 + 2
18	14 + 1	19 + 4	23 + 0
19	16 + 0	19 + 3	24 + 6
20	16 + 6	10 + 2	25 + 5
21	17 + 4	21 + 1	26 + 4
22	17 + 3	22 + 6	26 + 2
23	18 + 2	23 + 5	27 + 1
24	19 + 1	24 + 4	28 + 0
25	21 + 0	24 + 3	29 + 6
26	21 + 5	25 + 1	30 + 5
27	22 + 4	26 + 0	30 + 3
28	22 + 3	27 + 5	31 + 2
29	23 + 2	28 + 5	32 + 1
30	24 + 0	29 + 4	34 + 0
31	25 + 6	29 + 2	34 + 6
32	26 + 5	30 + 1	35 + 4
33	27 + 4	31 + 0	35 + 3
34	27 + 3	32 + 6	36 + 2
35	28 + 1	33 + 5	37 + 1
36	29 + 0	33 + 3	39 + 0
37	30 + 6	34 + 2	39 + 5
38	31 + 5	35 + 1	40 + 4
39	32 + 4	37 + 0	40 + 3
40	32 + 2	37 + 6	41 + 2
41	33 + 1	38 + 4	41 + 0
42	35 + 0	38 + 3	43 + 6
43	35 + 6	39 + 2	44 + 5
44	36 + 5	40 + 1	45 + 4
45	36 + 3	41 + 6	45 + 3

Reprinted from Yarkoni S, Schmidt W, Reece EA, et al. Clavicular measurement: a new biometric parameter for fetal evaluation. *J Ultrasound Med* 1985;4:467, with permission.

In fact, placental grading in general has been supplanted by more sensitive tests that are consequently used in clinical practice.

Body proportionality

Investigators examined the possibility that the use of fetal body proportionality might improve ultrasonic accuracy in the diagnosis of IUGR. Indices of body proportionality that have been studied and found clinically useful include the HC/AC ratio (Table 29.11) and the FL/AC ratio.

Head circumference (HC)–abdominal circumference (AC) ratio

The use of the ratio of HC to AC in determining IUGR was proposed by Campbell and Thoms in 1977.[37] The rationale for this was based on the observation that type 2 IUGR may have a disturbed HC/AC ratio as a result of the brain-sparing effect. Although this method has been shown to have a sensitivity of approximately 70% in detecting asymmetric IUGR, its use is limited by its high false-positive rate in screening a general population.[37,68]

Further limitations of this technique are its inability to detect asymmetric growth restriction and the need for accurate knowledge of gestational age to make the diagnosis of IUGR. It is therefore believed that the value of the HC/AC ratio lies in the assessment of proportionality, and thus it may assist the clinician in classifying IUGR as symmetric or asymmetric. Obviously, an elevated ratio suggests symmetric IUGR (see Table 29.11).

Femur length (FL)–abdominal circumference (AC) ratio

The ratio of FL to AC is the equivalent of the postnatal ponderal index and has been proposed as a useful method of detecting asymmetric IUGR.[69] This ratio has the advantage of being age independent and thus may help in the diagnosis of IUGR when gestational age is unknown. In fact, FL/AC ratios have a constant value of 22 ± 2% after 21 weeks' gestation. Hadlock and colleagues[69] evaluated this method in the diagnosis of IUGR and reported that 63% of growth-restricted fetuses were accurately diagnosed when a ratio of more than 23.5% was considered abnormal. However, these authors and others have indicated the poor predictive value of less than 25% of a positive test result.[70] In spite of this, the FL/AC ratio still has its merits, because it is the only ultrasonic technique that enables the physician to identify IUGR when gestational age is unknown.

Estimated fetal weight

Several formulas that use multiple ultrasonic parameters are used to estimate fetal weight.[71–73] The most widely used formula is that of Shepard and colleagues,[74] in which estimated fetal weight (EFW) is derived from the BPD and AC. This equation predicts fetal weight with an accuracy of 15–20%.[75] Hadlock and colleagues[76] and Warsof and colleagues[77] have also introduced equations to estimate fetal weight using combinations of BPD, AC, and FL.

Ott and Doyle[78] reported accurate predictions of IUGR in 90% of cases in a high-risk population when EFW was determined by BPD and AC. The use of this formula may introduce errors that are related to the variations in BPD that usually occur as a result of changes in head shape in the last weeks of pregnancy, in malpresentation, and in pregnancies complicated by spontaneous rupture of membranes.[79,80] BPD may be inaccurate if there is dolichocephaly or brachycephaly. We therefore strongly recommend that the physician calculates

Table 29.10 Summary of placental grading.

	Grade 0	Grade 1	Grade 2	Grade 3
Chorionic plate	Straight and well-defined	Subtle undulations	Indentations extending to, but not into, the basal layer	Indentations communicating with the basal layer
Placental substance	Homogeneous	Few scattered echogenic areas	Linear echogenic densities (comma-like densities)	Circular densities with echospared areas in center, large irregular densities that cast acoustic shadowing
Basal layer	No densities	No densities	Lineal arrangement of small echogenic areas (basal stippling)	Large and somewhat confluent basal echogenic areas can create acoustic shadows

Reprinted from ref. 66, with permission.

Table 29.11 Head circumference to abdominal circumference ratio compared with gestational age.

Gestational age (weeks)	Head circumference		
	−2 Standard deviations	Mean	+2 Standard deviations
14	1.085	1.230	1.375
15	1.080	1.225	1.365
16	1.075	1.215	1.350
17	1.070	1.205	1.340
18	1.065	1.195	1.330
19	1.060	1.185	1.320
20	1.055	1.178	1.305
21	1.050	1.177	1.295
22	1.045	1.165	1.285
23	1.040	1.155	1.275
24	1.030	1.145	1.265
25	1.025	1.135	1.255
26	1.050	1.125	1.245
27	1.010	1.120	1.235
28	1.000	1.110	1.225
29	0.999	1.095	1.215
30	0.975	1.085	1.200
31	0.965	1.075	1.190
32	0.945	1.060	1.175
33	0.935	1.045	1.163
34	0.925	1.030	1.150
35	0.915	1.020	1.135
36	0.910	1.005	1.120
37	0.905	0.995	1.100
38	0.900	0.980	1.085
39	0.896	0.970	1.065
40	0.895	0.965	1.046
41	0.894	0.960	1.025

Reprinted from Campbell S, Metreweli C, eds. *Practical abdominal ultrasound.* Chicago, IL: Year Book, 1978.

the cephalic index in each case. If the cephalic index is abnormal (< 75% or > 80%), one should not rely on estimated weight formulas that include the BPD.

Weiner and colleagues[81] have proposed the use of another formula for the prediction of fetal birthweight that incorporates HC and FL to avoid errors related to changes in head shape. The authors suggest that the prediction of IUGR fetuses may be more accurate using this formula.

In an effort to further increase the accuracy of ultrasonic estimation of fetal weight, Hadlock and colleagues[76] advocate the use of HC, AC, and FL measurements in combination. They have shown that the prediction of fetal weight has a standard deviation of ± 15% (two standard deviations). However, the accuracy in predicting fetal weight decreases in small fetuses (< 1500 g), and the error may approach ± 20%.

Various ultrasound methods are used to estimate fetal weight with essentially equal accuracy when low-risk obstetric populations are studied. It is thought that as many as 80% of IUGR fetuses can be detected; however, there is still a relatively low positive predictive value that approaches only 40%. Therefore, 60% of fetuses suspected of IUGR because of low EFW will actually be normally grown.

Doppler in IUGR

Maternal arterial uterine blood flow increases from 50 mL/min early in pregnancy to about 700 mL/min at term. The increase is secondary to a gradual decrease in vessel resistance to blood flow throughout the pregnancy. Doppler ultrasound gives us information on the vascular resistance and, indirectly, on the blood flow. Three indices are considered to be related to the vascular resistance: S/D ratio (systolic/diastolic ratio), resistance index (RI = systolic velocity–diastolic velocity/systolic velocity), and pulsatility index (systolic velocity–diastolic velocity/mean velocity). Doppler velocimetry uses ultrasound to measure peak-systolic and end-diastolic blood flow through the umbilical artery. As the pregnancy progresses, diastolic flow increases, and the systolic/diastolic ratio should gradually decrease. In a large number of IUGR pregnancies, an alteration in placental blood flow occurs. As a result, researchers have correlated an increased systolic/diastolic ratio with IUGR. The ratio is increased in about 80% of cases of IUGR diagnosed by ultrasound examination.[82] An average systolic/diastolic ratio of greater than three at 30 or more weeks of gestation has a sensitivity of 78% and a specificity of 85% in predicting IUGR.[83]

Doppler velocimetry, previously argued as a diagnostic technique for IUGR, has not found a place in routine antenatal surveillance. Nowadays, Doppler ultrasound has been shown to be useful in the assessment of growth-restricted fetuses.[84] It has helped physicians to understand the pathophysiology of IUGR with regard to diminished blood flow. The results of this procedure correlate with increased fetal morbidity and mortality: an absent or reversed end-diastolic umbilical flow is an ominous finding and may need intervention.[85–87] As a screening test, however, the procedure appears to be lacking in benefit; some studies[88] have shown that 40–60% of infants with IUGR had normal Doppler velocimetry results just before birth. However, normal umbilical flow is rarely associated with significant morbidity.[89]

Doppler velocimetry has been shown to reduce interventions and improve fetal outcome in pregnancies at risk for IUGR.[90] Randomized controlled trials have demonstrated that monitoring with Doppler velocimetry reduces the risk of perinatal morbidity.[90] Moreover, the IUGR fetuses seem to be at even greater risk of impending demise when Doppler abnormalities are observed in the venous circulation.[91]

Uterine circulation

The main uterine artery is the most commonly analyzed vessel. In normal pregnancy, the S/D ratio or RI values decrease significantly with advancing gestation until 24–26 weeks. In the absence of this physiologic decrease, a higher incidence of hypertensive diseases and/or IUGR has been widely documented. Chien and colleagues[92] published an overview of the efficacy of uterine artery Doppler as a predictor of preeclampsia, IUGR, and perinatal death. In low-risk women, an abnormal uterine artery Doppler result gave a likelihood ratio (LR) of developing IUGR of 3.6 (95% confidence interval (CI) 3.2–4.0), while a normal test reduced the risk to below background, with a LR of 0.8 (95% CI 0.08–0.09). For high-risk women, an abnormal test gave a LR of 2.7 (95% CI 2.1–3.4), while a normal result reduced the risk of LR to 0.7 (95% CI 0.6–0.9) (Fig. 29.4).

Umbilical artery

In the normal fetus, the pulsatility index decreases with advancing gestation. This reflects a decrease in the placental vascular resistance. In fetuses with IUGR, there is an increase in the pulsatility index secondary to the decrease, absence, or reversal of end-diastolic flow. The changes in these waveforms are thought to be indicative of increased placental resistance. The absent or reversed end-diastolic flows are strongly associated with an abnormal course of pregnancy and a higher incidence of perinatal complications, when compared with fetuses with IUGR but characterized by the presence of end-diastolic flow (Fig. 29.5).[93,94]

Fetal cerebral circulation

The middle cerebral artery is the vessel of choice to assess the fetal cerebral circulation because it is easy to identify, has a high reproducibility, and provides information on the brain-sparing effect. The circulation in the brain is normally high impedance. The middle cerebral artery (MCA) in the fetal brain carries more than 80% of cerebral flow.[95] When a fetus does not acquire enough oxygen, central redistribution of blood flow occurs, resulting in a preferentially increased blood flow to protect the brain, heart, and adrenals. This increase in blood flow can be evidenced by Doppler ultrasound of the MCA. This effect has been called the brain-sparing effect and is demonstrated by a lower value of the pulsatility index (Fig. 29.6).[95] In IUGR fetuses with a pulsatility index below the

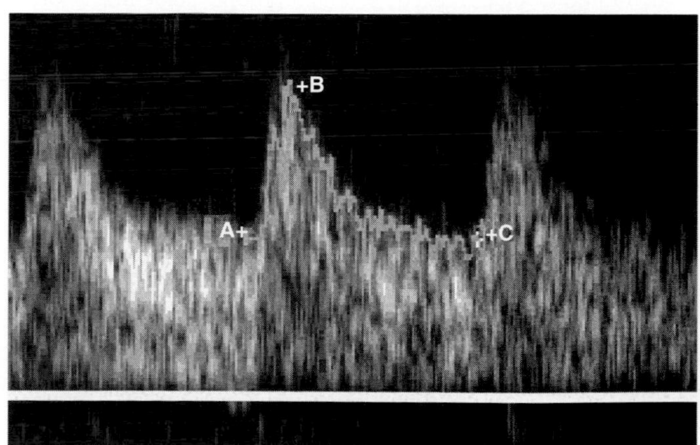

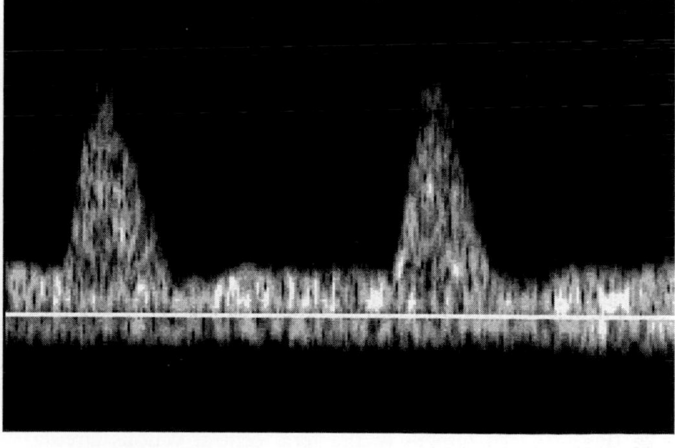

Figure 29.4 Uterine artery Doppler waveform showing normal (left) and abnormal (right) flow.

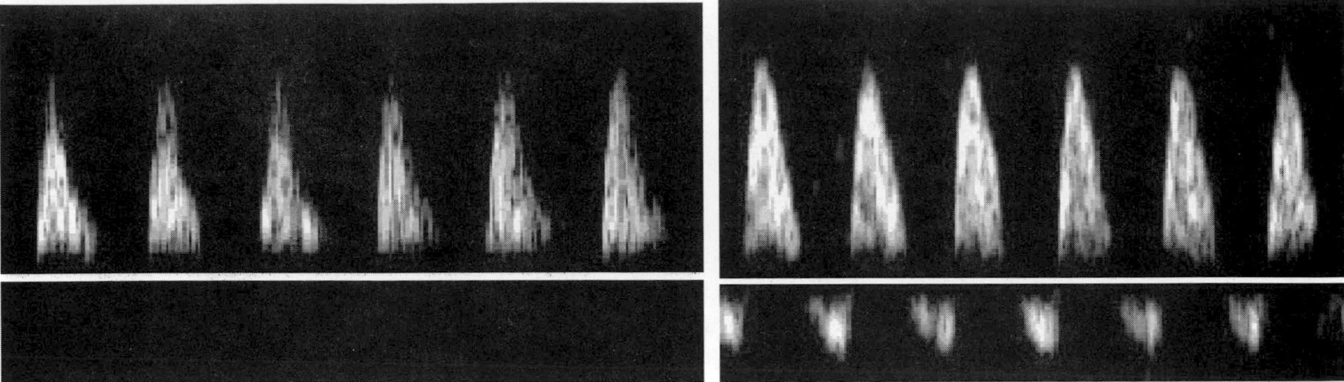

Figure 29.5 Abnormal umbilical artery Doppler waveform showing absent (left) and reversed (right) end-diastolic flow.

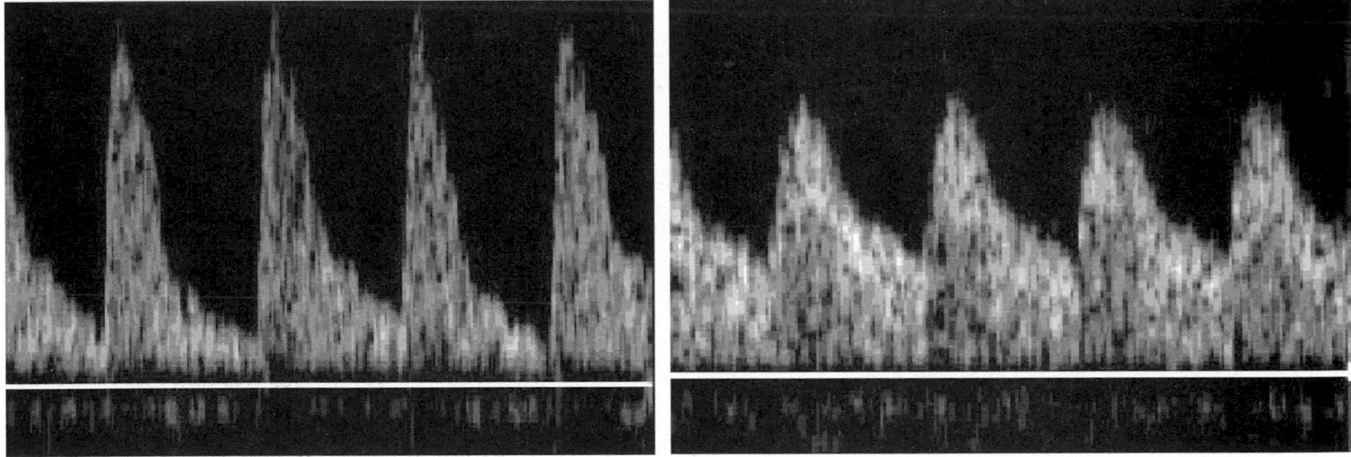

Figure 29.6 Doppler waveform of middle cerebral artery showing normal (left) and abnormal (right) flow.

normal range, there is a greater incidence of adverse perinatal outcome.[90] The brain-sparing effect may be transient, as reported during prolonged hypoxemia. The disappearance of the brain-sparing effect is a very critical event for the fetus, and appears to precede fetal death.[97,98]

Fetal venous Doppler

Doppler flow of the fetal inferior vena cava (IVC) and ductus venosus is practical and provides information about right ventrical preload, myocardial compliance, and right ventricular end-diastolic pressure.[99,100] Chronic fetal hypoxemia leads to decreased preload, decreased cardiac compliance, and elevated end-diastolic pressure in the right ventricle.[100] These changes raise central venous pressure in the chronically hypoxemic fetus, which shows up as an increased reverse flow in Doppler waveforms of the IVC and the ductus venosus during late diastole (Fig. 29.7). Changes in the fetal central venous circulation are associated with an advanced stage of fetal hypoxemia. At this late stage of fetal adaptation to hypoxemia, cardiac decompensation is often noted with myocardial dysfunction.[101] The presence of reversed flow in the ductus venosus is an ominous sign. Indeed, fetal metabolic acidemia is often present in association with Doppler waveform abnormalities of the IVC and ductus venosus.[102]

Macrosomia

The etiology of fetal macrosomia is believed to be multifactorial. Although this condition is often associated with diabetes mellitus in pregnancy, especially in women without vasculopathy, macrosomia may also occur in nondiabetics. Fetal macrosomia is defined as either an EFW of > 4000 g at term or an EFW of more than that of the 90th percentile for gestational age.

Macrosomic infants and their mothers are at increased risk for intrapartum injury, and perinatal mortality is more

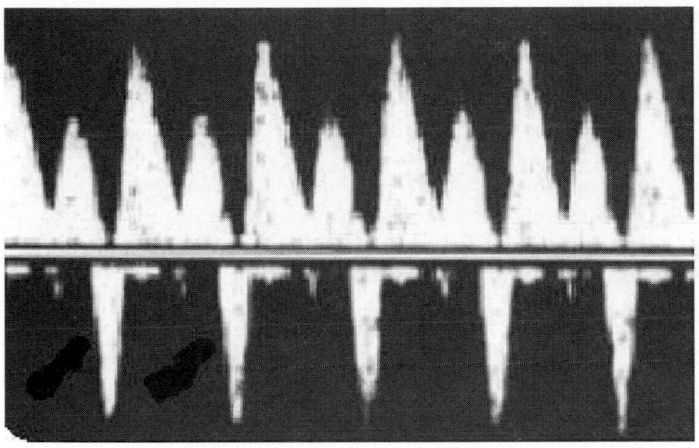

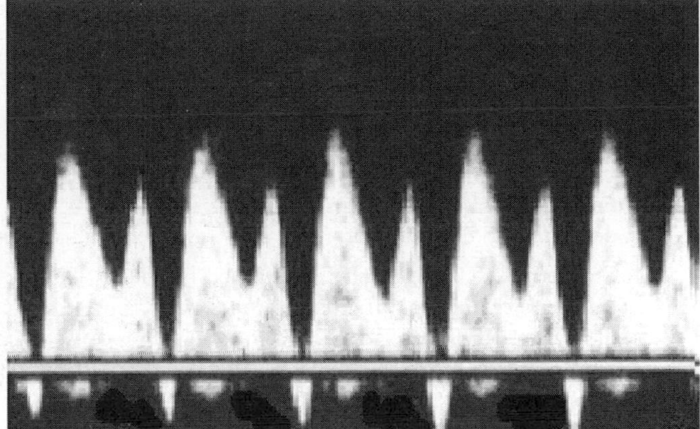

Figure 29.7 Adaptation for progressive fetal hypoxia.

common among these fetuses. The principal causes of injury include shoulder dystocia, fractures, and neurologic damage.[103–106]

Accurate prenatal diagnosis of fetal macrosomia would permit fetuses to be delivered by Cesarean section, thus obviating these complications. On the other hand, liberal Cesarean section may expose the mother to unnecessary operative risks.

Prenatal diagnosis of macrosomic fetuses is often difficult because less than 40% of such infants are born to mothers with identifiable risk factors for macrosomia.[107] A number of sonographic parameters have been used in an attempt to diagnose altered fetal growth, including the BPD, HC, HC/AC, or HC to thoracic circumference ratio, the macrosomic index, and the EFW. Miller and colleagues[108] conducted a study of 382 patients with singleton pregnancies whose infants were born outside 1 week of the ultrasound examination. Of the 382 pregnancies, 58 delivered macrosomic infants (> 4500 g). Ultrasonically determined BPD, FL, AC, and EFW were analyzed for their ability to predict the macrosomic newborn. EFW was found to be superior to BPD or FL in the prenatal diagnosis of fetal macrosomia. Elliott and colleagues[109] calculated a macrosomic index for 70 diabetic pregnancies by subtracting the BPD from the chest diameter. Thirty-three macrosomic infants (weighing more than 4500 g) were delivered. In this study, 20 of 23 (87%) infants weighing more than 4500 g had a chest BPD of more than 0.4 cm. The authors reported four cases of shoulder dystocia among 15 infants with macrosomic indices of more than 0.4 cm. They recommended Cesarean section for all fetuses with a chest BPD of more than 0.4 cm because this approach would decrease the incidence of traumatic morbidity from 27% to 9%.

In yet another study, Tamura and colleagues[110] showed that the EFW determined by Shepard and colleagues,[74] when greater than the 90th percentile, correctly predicted macrosomia at birth in 74% of cases. When both the AC and the EFW exceeded the 90th percentiles, macrosomia was correctly diagnosed in 88.8% of pregnant women with diabetes mellitus. The BPD and HC percentiles were significantly less predictive of macrosomia.

Summary

Although the etiology of IUGR is variable, prenatal diagnosis is possible using a variety of biometric parameters. When the gestational age is certain, IUGR is diagnosed if sonographic predictors of gestational age reflect an age significantly reduced from the expected, or an EFW less than the 10th percentile. Adjunctive indices that can enhance the prenatal diagnosis include reduced amniotic fluid volume, early third trimester grade 3 placenta, abnormal Doppler waveform analysis, and abnormal biometric ratios.

When the gestational age is unknown or uncertain, it is necessary to differentiate between the IUGR fetus and the normally grown fetus identified at an inaccurate gestational age. The TCD is a useful parameter for estimating gestational age even in IUGR fetuses and can be a parameter against which other biometric indices are compared. Biometric ratios, especially FL/AC, may also be useful adjuncts in the prenatal diagnosis of IUGR.

The prenatal diagnosis of macrosomia is best accomplished by the use of EFW. However, a certain amount of caution should be exercised in light of the fact that a margin of error exists with this method of weight estimation. EFW is reported to be accurate to within 10% of the actual birthweight 85% of the time. In the remaining 15% of cases, EFW is less accurate, and the error can range from 15% to 20% of the actual birthweight.

Key points

1 Definition: IUGR is defined as a fetus that weighs less than the 10th percentile for its gestational age.

2 Symmetric IUGR (intrinsic): normal head circumference/abdominal circumference ratio caused by genetic disease or fetal infection; poor prognosis.

3 Asymmetric IUGR (extrinsic): increased head circumference/abdominal circumference ratio caused by placental insufficiency; good prognosis with appropriate treatment.

4 Risk factors are multiple and include: chronic maternal disease including chronic maternal hypertension, pregnancy-induced hypertension, diabetes, cyanotic heart disease, collagen vascular disease, severe maternal anemia, renal disease, multifetal pregnancy, etc.; fetal genetic disorders or fetal malformations; intrauterine infections such as rubella, herpes, toxoplasmosis, syphilis, cytomegalovirus; previous history of small-for-gestational-age baby, smoking, drug, or alcohol abuse; and abnormalities of the placenta or placental blood flow.

5 Diagnosis: One should be suspicious when the fundal height does not exhibit the predicted 1 cm/week growth between 20 and 36 weeks of gestation. A lag in fundal height by 4 cm mandates ultrasonographic evaluation; otherwise, consider ultrasound on a clinical basis. Serial ultrasonic scanning may confirm the diagnosis.

6 Evaluation: Clinical indicators of IUGR are poor maternal weight gain (most sensitive indicator for IUGR) and fundal height less than expected for gestational age. Consider environmental and comorbid factors such as tobacco abuse (most significant individual risk), poor nutrition, illicit drug use, alcohol abuse, minimal to no prenatal care, traumatic stress.

7 Fetal assessment consists of following fetal movement counts, nonstress test, serial obstetric ultrasounds for growth, and biophysical profile.

8 Monitoring. Nonstress testing every week. Biophysical profile every week. This test uses ultrasound and a series of measurements to determine the health status of the developing fetus. Pregnancy ultrasound every 10–14 days.

9 Peripartum risks of IUGR include meconium aspiration, intrauterine asphyxia, polycythemia, hypoglycemia.

10 Long-term effects in the fetus before or during delivery include the following: premature delivery, poor tolerance of labor, increased rates of Cesarean section, increased risk of birth defects, asphyxia at birth, temperature instability, hypoglycemia, infections, death.

11 Management. The development of IUGR makes the pregnancy high risk. Stillbirth, oligohydramnios, and intrapartum fetal acidosis are common antepartum complications. Close antepartum surveillance is required, and the decision about when to deliver the infant is complex. Neonatal complications include persistent fetal circulation, meconium aspiration syndrome, hypoxic ischemic encephalopathy, hypoglycemia, hypocalcemia, hyperviscosity, and defective temperature regulation.

12 A perinatologist should manage these pregnancies.

13 Address risk factors: tobacco cessation, eliminate other negative habits, ensure adequate maternal weight gain, maximize prenatal care, reduce environmental stressors.

14 Perinatology consultation indications: poor nonstress test, decreasing biparietal diameter, oligohydramnios, abdominal circumference 4 weeks less than biparietal diameter.

15 Prognosis. Babies who suffer from IUGR are at an increased risk for death, hypoglycemia, hypothermia, and abnormal development of the nervous system. These risks increase with the severity of the growth restriction.

16 The growth that occurs after birth cannot be predicted with certainty based on the size of the baby when it is born. Infants with asymmetrical IUGR are more likely to catch up in growth after birth than infants who suffer from prolonged symmetrical IUGR.

References

1 Winick M. Fetal malnutrition. *Clin Obstet Gynaecol* 1970;13:3.

2 Battaglia FC, Lubchenco LO. A practical classification of newborn infants by weight and gestational age. *J Pediatr* 1967;71:159.

3 Berkowitz RL, Hobbins JC. Ultrasonography in the antepartum patient. In: Bolognese RJ, Schwartz R, eds. *Perinatal medicine: management of the high risk fetus and neonate*. Baltimore, MD: Williams & Wilkins; 1977:85.

4 Galbraith RS, Karchmar EJ, Pievey WN, et al. The clinical prediction of intrauterine growth retardation. *Am J Obstet Gynecol* 1979;133:281.

5 Ounsted M, Moar V, Scott WA. Perinatal morbidity and mortality in small-for-dates babies: the relative importance of some maternal factors. *Early Hum Dev* 1981;5:367.

6 Commey JOO, Fitzhardinge PM. Handicap in the preterm small-for-gestational age infants. *J Pediatr* 1979;94:779.

7 Pena IC, Teberg AJ, Finello K. Neurodevelopmental outcome of the small for gestational age preterm infant during the first year of life. *Pediatr Res* 1986;20:165 (abstract).

8 Pena IC, Teberg AJ, Finello K. Effect of intrauterine growth retardation on premature infants of similar gestational age. *Pediatr Res* 1987;21:183 (abstract).

9 Fitzhardinge PM, Kalman E, Ashby S, et al. Present status of the infant of very low birth weight treated in a referral neonatal intensive care unit in 1974. In: Elliott K, O'Connor M, eds. *Major mental handicap: methods and cost of prevention*. Ciba Foundation Symposium 59. Amsterdam: Elsevier; 1978:139.

10 Scott A, Moar V, Ounsted M. The relative contributions of different maternal factors in small-for-gestational age pregnancies. *Eur J Obstet Gynecol Reprod Biol* 1981;12:157.
11 Fitzhardinge PM, Steven EM. The small-for-date infant. II. Neurological and intellectual sequelae. *Pediatrics* 1972;50: 50.
12 Michaeleis R, Schulte F, Nolte R. Motor behavior of small for gestational age newborn infants. *J Pediatr* 1970;76:208.
13 Lubchenko LO, Hansman C, Dressler M, et al. Intrauterine growth as estimated from liveborn birth-weight data at 24 to 42 weeks of gestation. *Pediatrics* 1963;32:793.
14 Gruenwald P. Growth of the human fetus. *Am J Obstet Gynecol* 1966;94:1112.
15 Daikoku NH, Tyson JE, Graf C, et al. The relative significance of human placental lactogen in the diagnosis of retarded fetal growth. *Am J Obstet Gynecol* 1979;135:516.
16 Weiner CP, Robinson D. The sonographic diagnosis of intrauterine growth retardation using the postnatal ponderal index and the crown-heel length as standards of diagnosis. *Am J Perinatol* 1989;6:375.
17 Walther FJ, Ramaeker LHJ. The ponderal index as a measure of the nutritional status at birth and its relation to some aspects of neonatal morbidity. *J Perinat Med* 1982;10:42.
18 Hadlock FP, Deter RL, Roecker E, et al. Relation of fetal femur length to neonatal crown–heel length. *J Ultrasound Med* 1984;3:1.
19 Goldenberg RL, Gutter GR, Hoffman HJ, et al. Intrauterine growth retardation: standards of diagnosis. *Am J Obstet Gynecol* 1989;161:271.
20 Seeds JW. Impaired fetal growth: definition and clinical diagnosis. *Obstet Gynecol* 1984;64:303.
21 Johnson MP, Evans MI. Intrauterine fetal growth retardation pathophysiology and possibilities for intrauterine treatment. *Fetal Ther* 1987;2:109.
22 Mintz M, Landon M. Sonographic diagnosis of fetal growth disorders. *Clin Obstet Gynaecol* 1988;31:44.
23 Lockwood CJ, Weiner S. Assessment of fetal growth. *Clin Perinatol* 1986;13:3.
24 Enesca M, LeBlond CP. Increase in cell number as a factor in the growth of the organs and tissues of the young male rat. *J Embryol Exp Morphol* 1962;10:530.
25 Winick M, Noble A. Cellular response in rats during malnutrition at various ages. *J Nutr* 1966;89:300.
26 Vorherr H. Factors influencing fetal growth. *Am J Obstet Gynecol* 1982;142:577.
27 Little D, Campbell S. Ultrasound evaluation of intrauterine growth retardation. *Radiol Clin North Am* 1982;20:335.
28 Weiner CP, Williamson RA. Evaluation of severe retardation using cordocentesis: hematologic and metabolic alterations by etiology. *Obstet Gynecol* 1989;73:225.
29 Meschia G. Supply of oxygen to the fetus. *J Reprod Med* 1979;23:160.
30 Evans MI, Mukherjee AB, Schulman JD. Animal model of intrauterine growth retardation. *Obstet Gynecol Surv* 1983;38: 183.
31 Harbander S, Rutherford SE. Classification of intrauterine growth retardation. *Semin Perinatol* 1988;38:183.
32 Shabbagha RE. Intrauterine growth retardation. In: Sabbagha RE, ed. *Diagnostic ultrasound*. Hagerstown, MD: Harper & Row; 1980:112.
33 Anderson HF, Johnson TRB, Flora JD, et al. Gestational age assessment. II. Prediction from combined clinical observation. *Am J Obstet Gynecol* 1981;140:770.
34 Callen PW. Ultrasonography in obstetrics and gynecology. Philadelphia: W.B. Saunders; 1983:21.
35 Hobbins JC, Winsberg F, Berkowitz RL. *Ultrasonography in obstetrics and gynecology*, 3rd edn. Baltimore, MD: Williams & Wilkins; 1983:203.
36 Romero R, Jeanty P. The detection of fetal growth disorders. *Semin Ultrasound* 1984;5:130.
37 Campbell S, Thoms A. Ultrasound measurements of the fetal head to abdomen circumference ratio in the assessment of growth retardation. *Br J Obstet Gynaecol* 1977;84:165.
38 Geirsson RT, Persson PH. Diagnosis of intrauterine growth retardation using ultrasound. *Clin Obstet Gynaecol* 1982;11: 457.
39 Seeds JW. Impaired fetal growth: ultrasonic evaluation and clinical management. *Obstet Gynecol* 1984;63:577.
40 Arias F. The diagnosis and management of intrauterine growth retardation. *Obstet Gynecol* 1977;49:293.
41 Sabbagha RE. Intrauterine growth retardation: antenatal diagnosis by ultrasound. *Obstet Gynecol* 1978;52:252.
42 Queenan JT, Kubarych SF, Cook LN, et al. Diagnostic ultrasound for detection of intrauterine growth retardation. *Am J Obstet Gynecol* 1976;124:865.
43 Kurjak A, Kirkinen P, Latin V. Biometric and dynamic ultrasound assessment of small-for-dates infants: report of 260 cases. *Obstet Gynecol* 1980;56:281.
44 Campbell S, Dewhurst C. Diagnosis of small-for-date fetus by serial ultrasound cephalometry. *Lancet* 1971;ii:1002.
45 Deter RL, Harrist RB, Hadlock FP, et al. The use of ultrasound in the detection of intrauterine growth retardation. A review. *J Clin Ultrasound* 1982;10:9.
46 Shool JS, Woo D, Bubin JM, et al. Intrauterine growth retardation risk detection for fetuses of unknown gestational age. *Am J Obstet Gynecol* 1982;144:709.
47 Fescina RH, Martell M, Martinez G, et al. Small for dates: evaluation of different diagnostic methods. *Acta Obstet Gynecol Scand* 1987;66:221.
48 Rosendahl H, Kivinen S. Routine ultrasound screening for early detection of small for gestational age fetuses. *Obstet Gynecol* 1988;71:518.
49 Warsof SL, Cooper DJ, Little D, et al. Routine ultrasound screening for antenatal detection of intrauterine growth retardation. *Obstet Gynecol* 1986;67:33.
50 Goldstein I, Reece EA, Pilu G, et al. Cerebellar measurements with ultrasonography in the evaluation of fetal growth and development. *Am J Obstet Gynecol* 1987;156:1065.
51 Reece EA, Goldstein I, Pilu G, et al. Fetal cerebellar growth unaffected by intrauterine growth retardation: a new parameter for prenatal diagnosis. *Am J Obstet Gynecol* 1987;157:632.
52 Duchatel F, Mennesson B, Berseneff H, et al. Antenatal echographic measurement of the fetal cerebellum. Significance in the evaluation of fetal development. *J Gynecol Obstet Biol Reprod (Paris)* 1989;18:879.
53 Campbell WA, Narci D, Vintzileos AM, et al. Transverse cerebellar diameter/abdominal circumference ratio throughout pregnancy: a gestational age-independent method to assess fetal growth. *Obstet Gynecol* 1991;77:893.
54 Hill LM, Gyzick D, Rivello D, et al. The transverse cerebellar diameter cannot be used to assess gestational age in the small for gestational age fetus. *Obstet Gynecol* 1990;75:329.
55 Campbell S, Wilkin D. Ultrasonic measurement of fetal abdomen circumference in the estimation of fetal weight. *Br J Obstet Gynaecol* 1975:82;689.
56 Geirsson RT, Patel NB, Christie AD. Efficiency of intrauterine

volume, fetal abdominal area and biparietal diameter measurements with ultrasound in screening for small-for-dates babies. *Br J Obstet Gynaecol* 1985;92:929.

57 Geirsson RT, Patel NB, Christie AD. Efficiency of intrauterine volume, fetal abdominal area and biparietal diameter measurements with ultrasound in screening for small-for-dates babies in a high risk obstetric population. *Br J Obstet Gynaecol* 1985;92:936.

58 Wittman BK, Robinson HP, Aitchison T, et al. The value of diagnostic ultrasound as a screening test for intrauterine growth retardation: comparison of nine parameters. *Am J Obstet Gynecol* 1979;134:30.

59 Jeanty P, Coussaert E, Contraine F. Normal growth of the abdominal perimeter. *Am J Perinatol* 1984;1:129.

60 O'Brien GD, Queenan JR. Ultrasound fetal femur length in relation to intrauterine growth retardation. *Am J Obstet Gynecol* 1982;144:34.

61 Gohari P, Berkowitz RL, Hobbins JC. Prediction of intrauterine growth retardation by determination of total intrauterine volume. *Am J Obstet Gynecol* 1977;127:255.

62 Manning FA, Hill LM, Platt LD. Qualitative amniotic fluid volume determination by ultrasonic antepartum detection of intrauterine growth retardation. *Am J Obstet Gynecol* 1981;139:254.

63 Philipson EH, Sokol RJ, Williams T. Oligohydramnios: clinical association and predictive value for intrauterine growth retardation. *Am J Obstet Gynecol* 1983;146:271.

64 Grannum PA, Berkowitz RL, Hobbins JC. The ultrasonic changes in the maturing placenta and their relationship to fetal pulmonic maturity. *Am J Obstet Gynecol* 1979;133:915.

65 Petrucha R, Platt LD. Relationship of placenta grade to gestational age. *Am J Obstet Gynecol* 1982;144:733.

66 Grannum PA, Hobbins JC. The placenta. *Radiol Clin North Am* 1982;20:353.

67 Kazzi GM, Gross TL, Sokol RJ, et al. Detection of intrauterine growth retardation: a new use of sonographic placental grading. *Am J Obstet Gynecol* 1983;145:733.

68 Deter RL, Hadlock FP, Harrist RB. Evaluation of normal fetal growth and the detection of intrauterine growth retardation. In: Callen PW, ed. *Ultrasonography in obstetrics and gynecology.* Philadelphia: W.B. Saunders; 1983:113.

69 Hadlock FP, Deter RL, Harrist RB. A date-independent predictor of intrauterine growth retardation: femur length/abdominal circumference ratio. *Am J Roentgenol* 1983;141:979.

70 Benson CB, Doubilet PM, Saltzman DH, et al. FLqAC ratio: poor predictor of intrauterine growth retardation. *Invest Radiol* 1985;20:727.

71 Stocker J, Maward R, Deleon A, et al. Ultrasonic cephalometry. Its use in estimating fetal weight. *Obstet Gynecol* 1975;45:278.

72 Sampson MB, Thomason JL, Kelly SL, et al. Prediction of intrauterine fetal weight using real-time ultrasound. *Am J Obstet Gynecol* 1982;142:554.

73 Eik-Nes SH, Grottum P. Estimation of fetal weight by ultrasound measurement. I. Development of a new formula. *Acta Obstet Gynecol Scand* 1982;61:299.

74 Shepard MJ, Richards VA, Verkowitz RL, et al. An evaluation of two equations for predicting fetal weight by ultrasound. *Am J Obstet Gynecol* 1982;142:47.

75 Deter RL, Harrist RB, Hadlock FP, et al. Evaluation of three methods of obtaining fetal weight estimates using dynamic image ultrasound. *J Clin Ultrasound* 1981;9:421.

76 Hadlock FP, Harrist RB, Sharman RS, et al. Estimation of fetal weight with the use of head, body and femur measurements: a prospective study. *Am J Obstet Gynecol* 1985;151:333.

77 Warsof SL, Gohar P, Berkowitz RL, et al. The estimation of fetal weight by computer-assisted analysis. *Am J Obstet Gynecol* 1977;128:881.

78 Ott WJ, Doyle S. Ultrasonic diagnosis of altered fetal growth by use of a normal ultrasonic fetal weight curve. *Obstet Gynecol* 1984;63:201.

79 Hadlock FP, Deter RL, Carpenter RJ, et al. Estimating fetal age: effect of head shape on BPD. *Am J Roentgenol* 1981;137:83.

80 Divon MY, Chamberlain PF, Sipos L, et al. Underestimation of fetal weight in premature rupture of membranes. *J Ultrasound Med* 1984;3:529.

81 Weiner CP, Sabbagha RE, Vaisrub N, et al. Ultrasonic fetal weight prediction: the role of head circumference and femur length. *Obstet Gynecol* 1985;65:812.

82 Ferrazzi E, Bellotti M, Vegni C, et al. Umbilical flow waveforms versus fetal biophysical profile in hypertensive pregnancies. *Eur J Obstet Gynecol Reprod Biol* 1989;33:199.

83 Fleischer A, Schulman H, Farmakides G, et al. Umbilical artery velocity waveforms and intrauterine growth retardation. *Am J Obstet Gynecol* 1985;151:502.

84 Arduini D, Rizzo G. Doppler studies of deteriorating growth-retarded fetuses. *Curr Opin Obstet Gynecol* 1993;5:195.

85 Kingdom JC, Burrell SJ, Kaufmann P. Pathology and clinical implications of abnormal umbilical artery Doppler waveforms. *Ultrasound Obstet Gynecol* 1997;9:271.

86 Karsdorp VH, van Vugt JM, van Geijn HP, et al. Clinical significance of absent or reversed end diastolic velocity waveforms in umbilical artery. *Lancet* 1994;344:1664.

87 Pardi G, Cetin I, Marconi AM, et al. Diagnostic value of blood sampling in fetuses with growth retardation. *N Engl J Med* 1993;328:692.

88 Divon MY, Hsu HW. Maternal and fetal blood flow velocity waveforms in intrauterine growth retardation. *Clin Obstet Gynecol* 1992;35:156.

89 Ott WJ. Intrauterine growth restriction and Doppler ultrasonography. *J Ultrasound Med* 2000;19:661.

90 Alfirevic Z, Neilson JP. Doppler ultrasonography in high-risk pregnancies: systemic review with meta-analysis. *Am J Obstet Gynecol* 1995;172:179.

91 Hecker K, Campbell S, Doyle P, et al. Assessment of fetal compromise by Doppler ultrasound investigation of the fetal circulation: arterial, intracardiac and venous blood flow velocity studies. *Circulation* 1995;91:129.

92 Chien PF, Arnott N, Gordon A. How useful is uterine artery Doppler flow velocimetry in the prediction of pre-eclampsia, intrauterine growth retardation and perinatal death? An overview. *Br J Obstet Gynecol* 2000;107:196.

93 Kingdom JC, Burrell SJ, Kaufmann P. Pathology and clinical implications of abnormal umbilical artery Doppler waveforms. *Ultrasound Obstet Gynecol* 1997;9:271.

94 Farine D, Kelly EN, Ryan G, et al. Absent and reversed umbilical artery end-diastolic velocity. In: Copel JA, Reed KL, eds. *Doppler ultrasound in obstetrics and gynecology*, 1st edn. New York: Raven Press; 1995:187.

95 Veille JC, Hanson R, Tatum K. Longitudinal quantitation of middle cerebral artery blood flow in normal human fetuses. *Am J Obstet Gynecol* 1993;169:1393.

96 Mari G, Deter RL. Middle cerebral artery flow velocity waveforms in normal and small-for-gestational-age fetuses. *Am J Obstet Gynecol* 1992;166:1262.

97 Gramellini D, Folli MC, Raboni S, et al. Cerebral-umbilical Doppler ratio as a predictor of adverse perinatal outcome. *Obstet Gynecol* 1992;79:416.

98 Arduini D, Rizzo G. Prediction of fetal outcome in small for GA fetuses: comparison of Doppler measurements obtained from different fetal vessels. *J Perinat Med* 1992;20:29.

99 Rizzo G, Arduini D, Romanini C. Inferior vena cava flow velocity waveforms in appropriate- and small- for-gestational-age fetuses. *Am J Obstet Gynecol* 1992;166:1271.

100 Rizzo G, Arduini D. Fetal cardiac function in intrauterine growth retardation. *Am J Obstet Gynecol* 1991;165:876.

101 Makikallio K, Vuolteenaho O, Jouppila P, et al. Ultrasonographic and biochemical markers of human fetal cardiac dysfunction in placental insufficiency. *Circulation* 2002;105:2058.

102 Baschat AA, Gembruch U, Reiss I, et al. Relationship between arterial and venous Doppler and perinatal outcome in fetal growth restriction. *Ultrasound Obstet Gynecol* 2000;16: 407.

103 Sack RA. The large infant: a study of maternal, obstetric, fetal and newborn characteristics, including a long-term pediatric follow-up. *Am J Obstet Gynecol* 1969;104:195.

104 Nelson JH, Rovner IW, Barter RH. The large baby. *South Med J* 1958;51:23.

105 Posner AC, Friedman S, Posner LB. The large fetus: a study of 547 cases. *Obstet Gynecol* 1955;5:268.

106 Parks DG, Ziel HK. Macrosomia: a proposed indication for primary cesarean section. *Obstet Gynecol* 1983;61:715.

107 Boyd ME, Usher RH, McLean FH. Fetal macrosomia: prediction, risks, proposed management. *Obstet Gynecol* 1983;61:715.

108 Miller JM, Brown HL, Khawli OF, et al. Ultrasonographic identification of the macrosomic fetus. *Am J Obstet Gynecol* 1988;159:1110.

109 Elliott JP, Garite TJ, Freeman RK, et al. Ultrasonic prediction of fetal macrosomia in diabetic patients. *Obstet Gynecol* 1982;60:159.

110 Tamura RK, Sabbagha RE, Depp R, et al. Diabetic macrosomia: accuracy of third trimester ultrasound. *Obstet Gynecol* 1986;67:828.

30 Three- and four-dimensional ultrasound and magnetic resonance imaging in pregnancy

Teresita L. Angtuaco

Tremendous innovations in technology have propelled the field of medicine into a new dimension not imaginable 20 years ago. Ultrasound remains the mainstay of prenatal imaging, and the refinement in both hardware and software has led to the demonstration of fetal anatomy in exquisite detail beyond the imagination of ultrasound pioneers many years ago. Yet, in spite of the vast improvements in our ability to visualize the fetus, technology has not stopped evolving with regard to fetal imaging. Of all the new developments in technology applicable to obstetric imaging, three-dimensional/four-dimensional (3D/4D) ultrasound and magnetic resonance imaging (MRI) have benefited the most from the computer revolution. New horizons have been opened by the 3D/4D capabilities of ultrasound, and MRI is fast becoming an acceptable method in fetal diagnosis.[1–4] In most medical centers, ultrasound is performed as the initial examination, and MRI is performed as a complementary problem-solving tool. When both are performed to delineate a fetal anomaly, the MRI examination is often interpreted in conjunction with an ultrasound examination done just prior to the MRI study. As this practice becomes more and more widely accepted, it is becoming imperative that those who deal in prenatal diagnosis become familiar with these tools, as they increasingly gain acceptance as part of the routine armamentarium in fetal imaging.

Three-dimensional (3D) and four-dimensional (4D) ultrasound

Technique

Three-dimensional ultrasound provides a method of storing complete sets of volume data in a computer memory so that they can be accessed to reconstruct any desired image plane. To accomplish this, four steps have to be taken: data acquisition, 3D visualization, volume/image processing, and storage of images.[5] The acquisition of images in state-of-the-art machines uses internal integrated systems that are built into the ultrasound system. This calls for specialized 3D transducers that perform high-precision automated volume acquisition with the touch of a button. The transducer element is automatically swept in a fan-shaped pattern at a specified angle. After signal processing and quantification, the acquired planes are stored digitally at correlative sites in an electronic volume memory. Once stored, the acquisition planes are retrieved from the volume memory and displayed as multiplanar sections. This is usually accomplished by simultaneous display on the monitor of the three standard orthogonal planes (coronal, axial, and sagittal) (Fig. 30.1). As one plane is rotated or shifted, the changes are simultaneously displayed in the other two planes. This simultaneous display has the distinct advantage of allowing the anatomy in question to be viewed in several planes, thus making the diagnosis of an anomaly more certain. It is a well-known phenomenon in ultrasound that artifacts of scanning can produce suspicious images that can suggest anomalies where there are none (Fig. 30.2). When processing the images in three planes, the distinction between real findings and artifacts becomes obvious. In instances when volumetric determinations become necessary, the ability to determine the largest dimension of an object in all three planes results in more accurate volume calculations.

Four-dimensional imaging is a relatively recent addition to the tools of fetal imaging. It is 3D ultrasound with a dynamic display of rendered images rapidly updated over time (real-time 3D). Because of rapid acquisition rates, it is possible to capture all the acquired volumes sequentially. This results in the ability to document entire sequences of fetal movement, which can be stored with digital image quality. These volumes can then be retrieved sequentially from memory similar to cine loops in 2D ultrasound. With this technique, it is possible to view specific 3D movement phases and obtain remarkable "snapshot movements" (Fig. 30.3). These 3D surface images can therefore be demonstrated as separate images on the monitor or as animated displays on cine loops. Thus, digital video clips of fetal movements can be stored and shown repeatedly as isolated "images" without the need for video tapes, which used to be the mainstay of data storage.

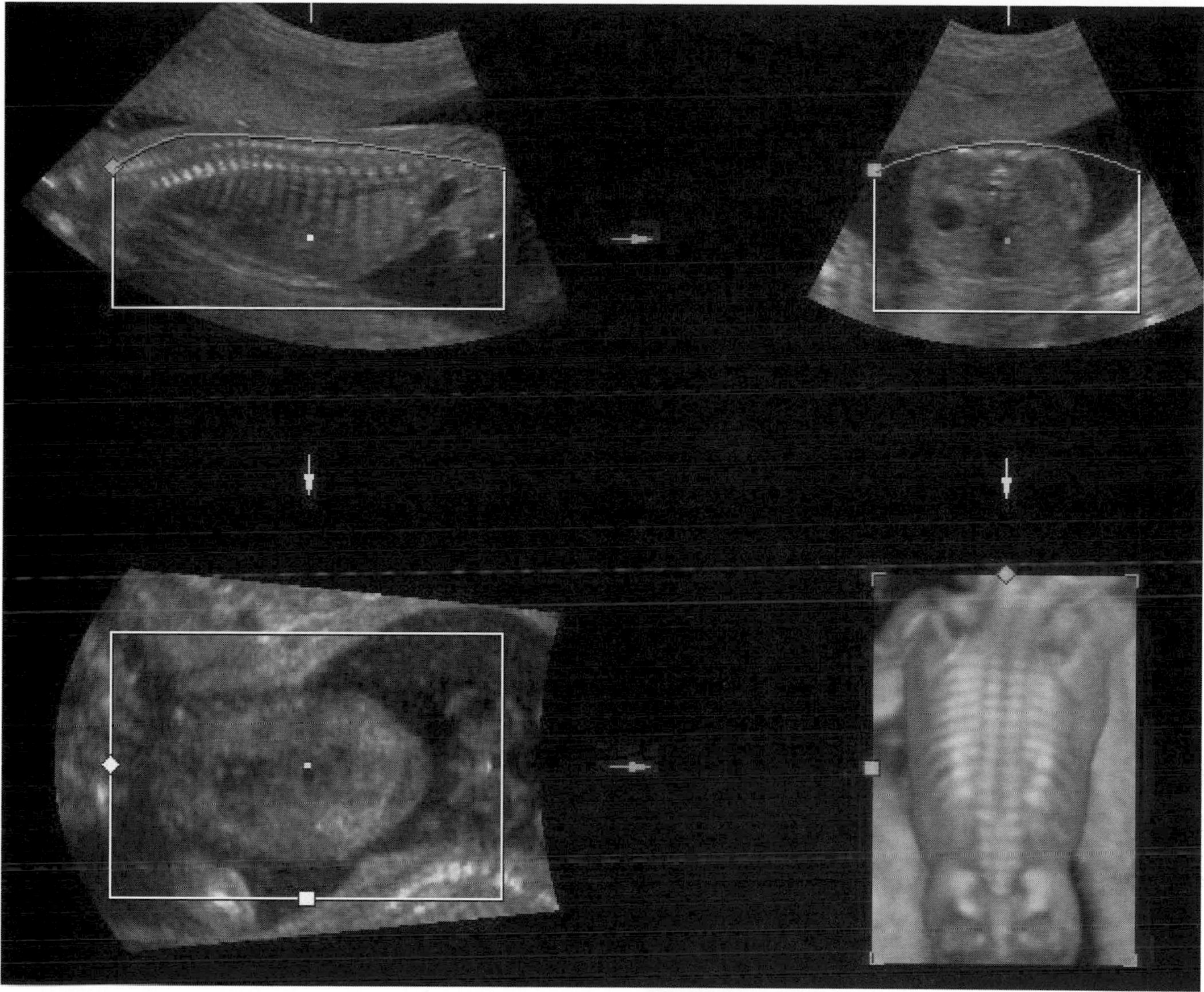

Figure 30.1 The fetal spine is shown in three orthogonal planes as well as a 3D-rendered coronal view. Upper left image, sagittal; lower left, coronal; upper right, axial.

Clinical impact

The advent of 3D ultrasound has taken away some of the "mystique" held by ultrasound over the years. For a very long time, only the sonologists and sonographers could recognize structures on the screen, leaving the patient and other nonexperts in ultrasound to wonder how anyone could make "head or tail" out of "weather maps" and come up with a determination regarding the presence or absence of fetal anomalies. Now, both the patient and the accompanying family and friends can actually relate to what the sonographer is seeing[6] (Fig. 30.4). This sudden familiarity is partly the reason behind the explosion of businesses offering ultrasound examinations for entertainment. Although an argument can be made for 3D ultrasound facilitating the "bonding experience," the Food and Drug Administration and the American Institute of Ultrasound in Medicine have jointly issued a statement discouraging the practice of performing 3D ultrasound solely for entertainment purposes.

Detection of fetal anomalies

When 3D ultrasound was first introduced, there was much anticipation of perceived improvements in the delineation of complex anomalies such as facial and limb deformities (Fig. 30.5). There have been several reports in the literature showing the feasibility and benefit of 3D ultrasound in demonstrating anomalies of the face and extremities[7–11] (Fig. 30.6). In addition, its use in the skull and brain has been explored, but with limited success[12,13] (Fig. 30.7). The fetal spine is among those structures more frequently imaged on 3D ultrasound because the three orthogonal planes of imaging can often follow the curvature of the spine even when the fetus is in a suboptimal lie[14,15] (Fig. 30.8). In the face, there is

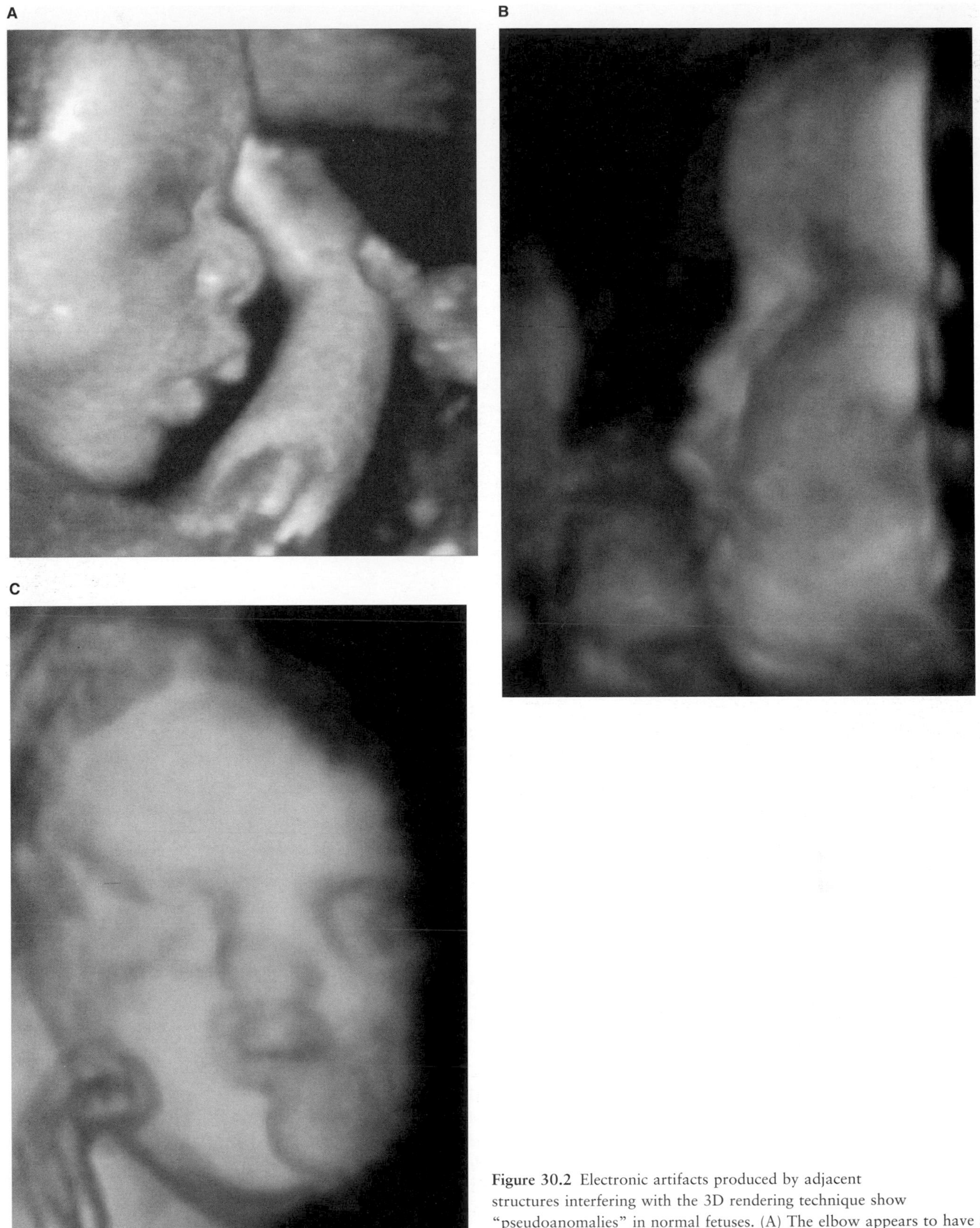

Figure 30.2 Electronic artifacts produced by adjacent structures interfering with the 3D rendering technique show "pseudoanomalies" in normal fetuses. (A) The elbow appears to have a soft tissue defect. (B, sagittal) and (C, coronal): The fetus appears to have a mass on the left chin, which extends anteriorly.

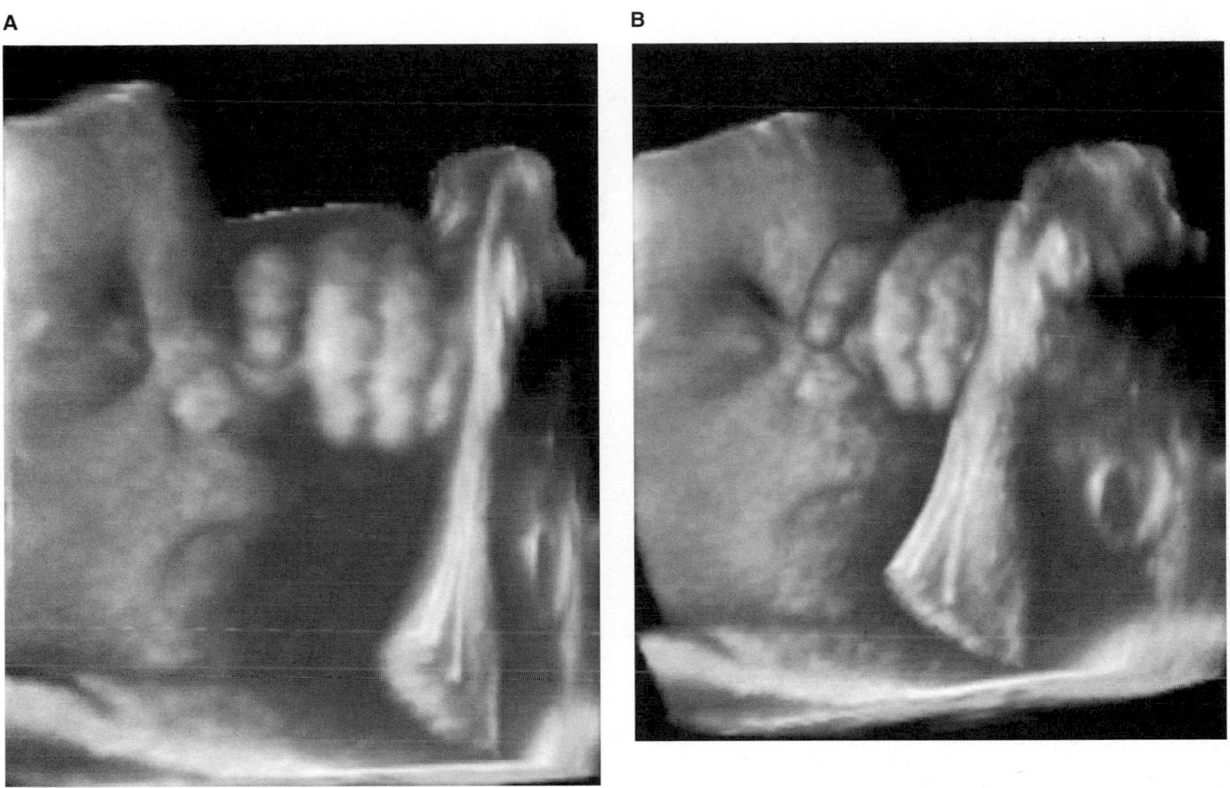

Figure 30.3 Serial 3D images obtained from a 4D volume slab of a fetus who appeared to be scratching its nose.

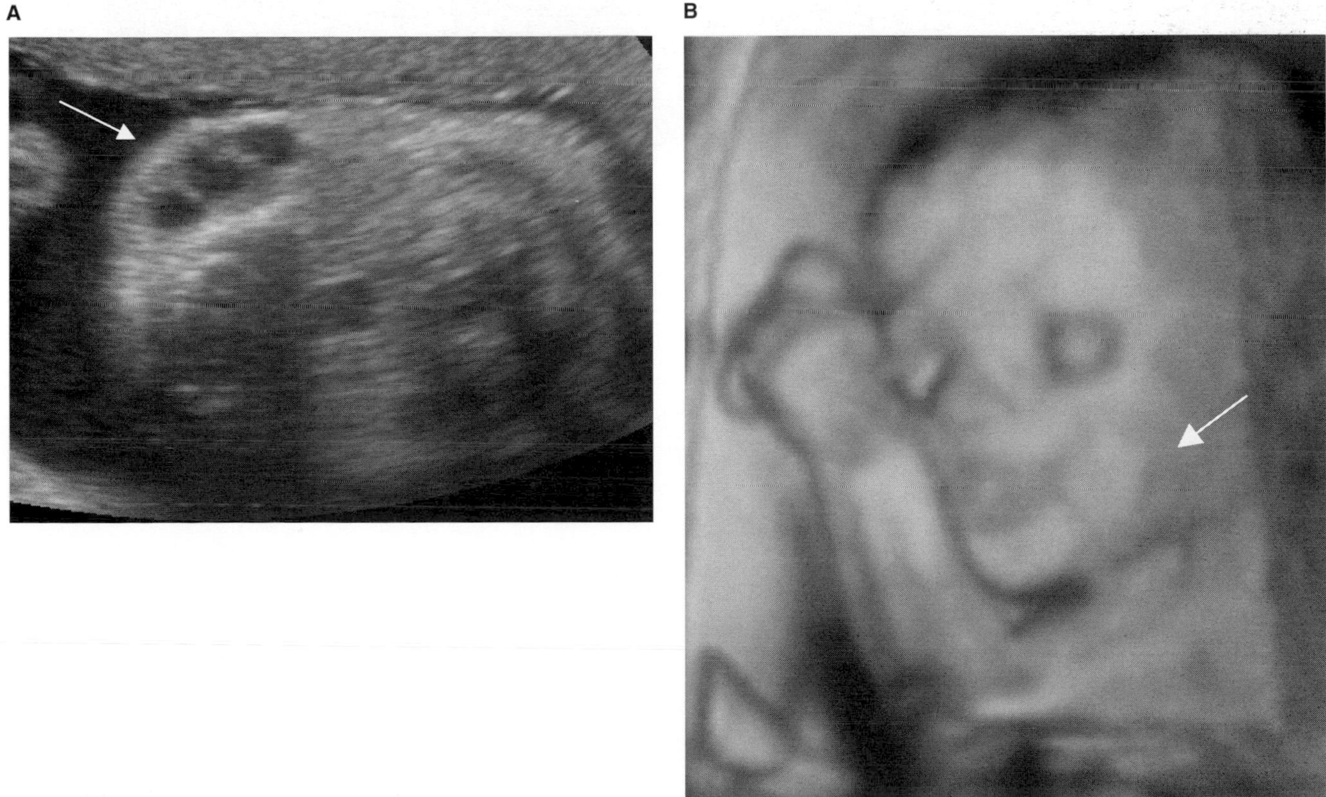

Figure 30.4 Facial cysts. Cystic masses (arrow) suspected to be in the fetal neck on a 2D image (A) are well localized on the 3D-rendered image (B) as cysts in the cheek (arrow), highly suggestive of lymphangiomas.

A

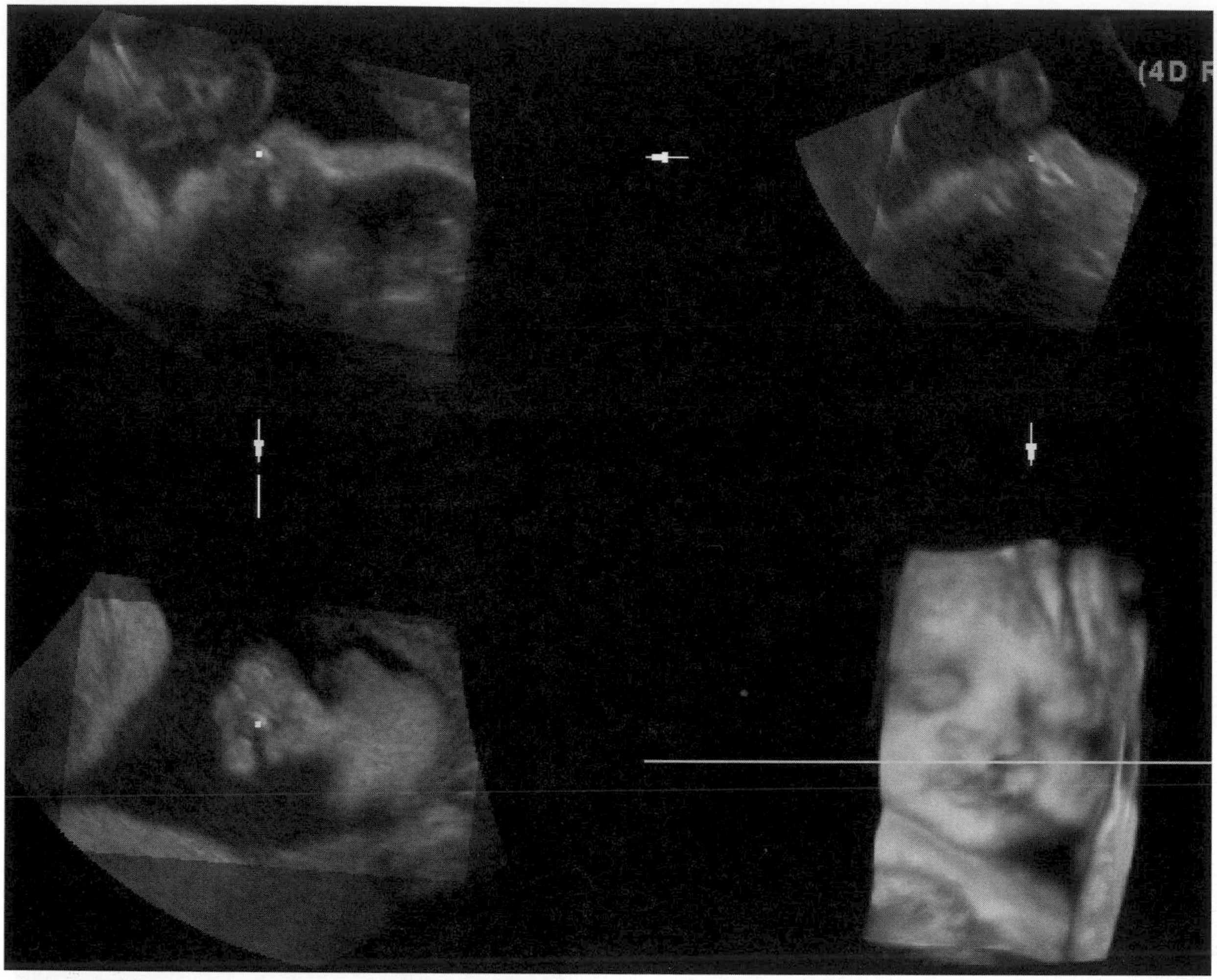

B

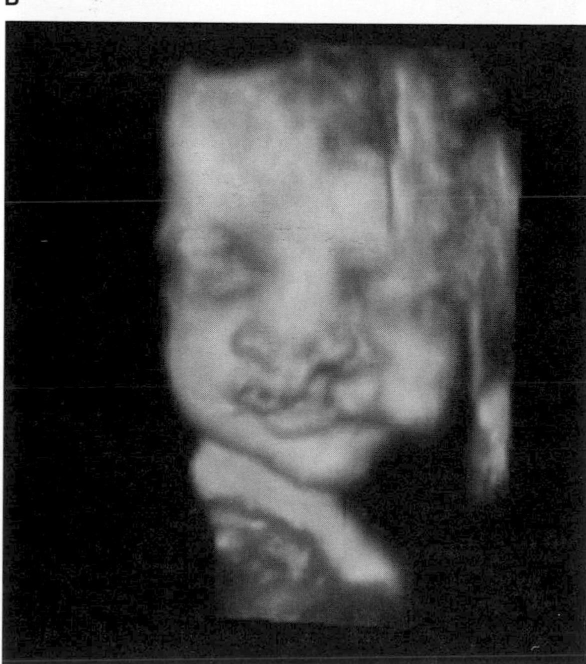

Figure 30.5 Unilateral cleft lip. 3D rendering (B) of the defect in the upper lip was guided by precise localization of the abnormality in three orthogonal planes (A).

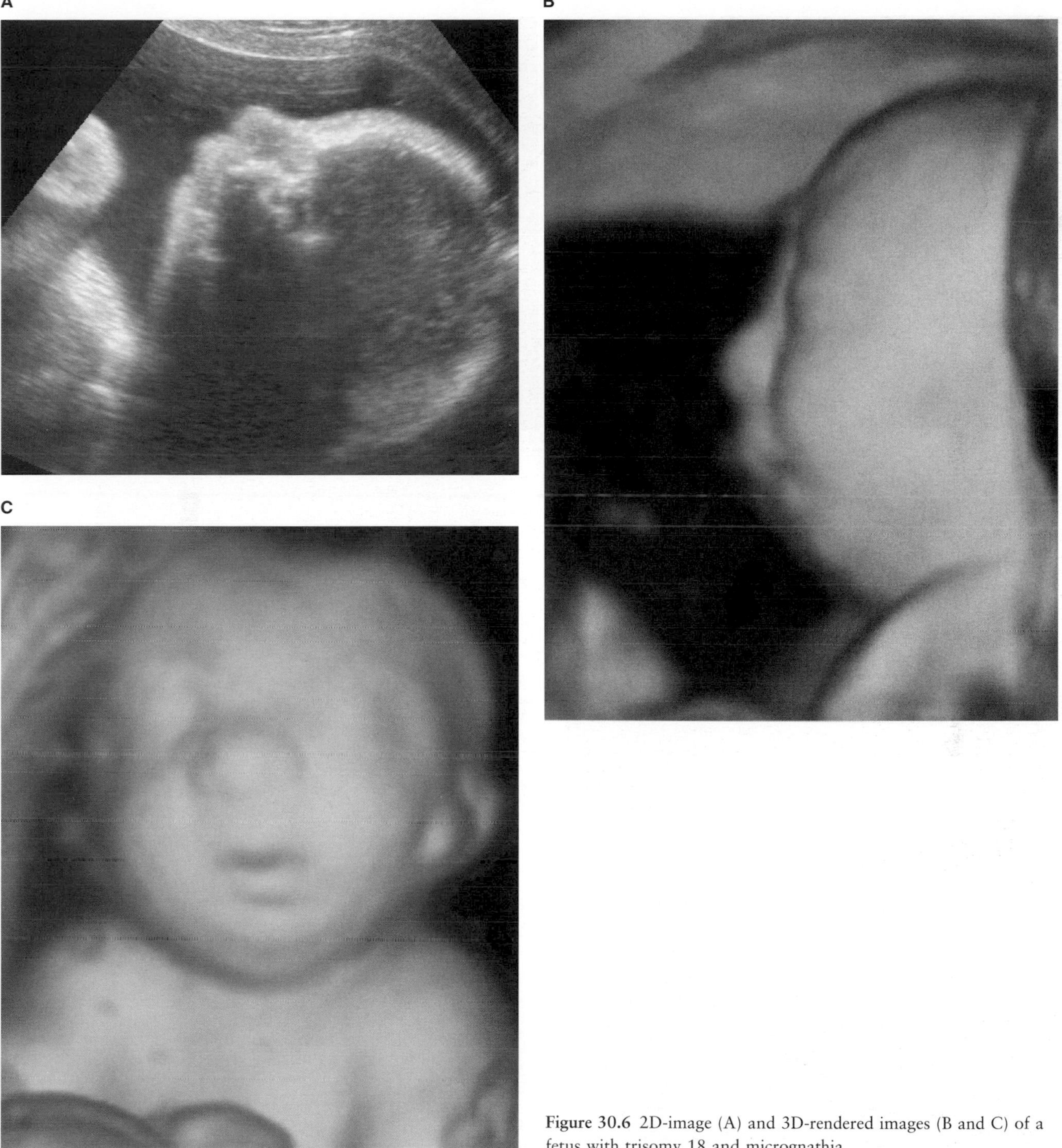

Figure 30.6 2D-image (A) and 3D-rendered images (B and C) of a fetus with trisomy 18 and micrognathia.

undoubtedly a distinct advantage in being able to see the extent of a complex midline anomaly, which may have a limited view on regular 2D images (Fig. 30.9). In a rotated and contorted limb, the confusing orientation of the whole extremity can be easier to appreciate on 3D ultrasound[16–20] (Fig. 30.10). In the past, this could only be appreciated on direct scanning as the mind processes the hundreds of real-time frames generated during the actual examination. With 3D surface rendering, the finding becomes obvious and easily documented by the sonographer when the sonologist is not physically present during the examination, as is often the case. However, as in any new advancement in imaging, many problems remain to be solved before 3D imaging of can fulfill its potential in producing these results in a constant, reproducible manner. Among these are oligohydramnios, shadowing from adjacent fetal parts, deep position of the head

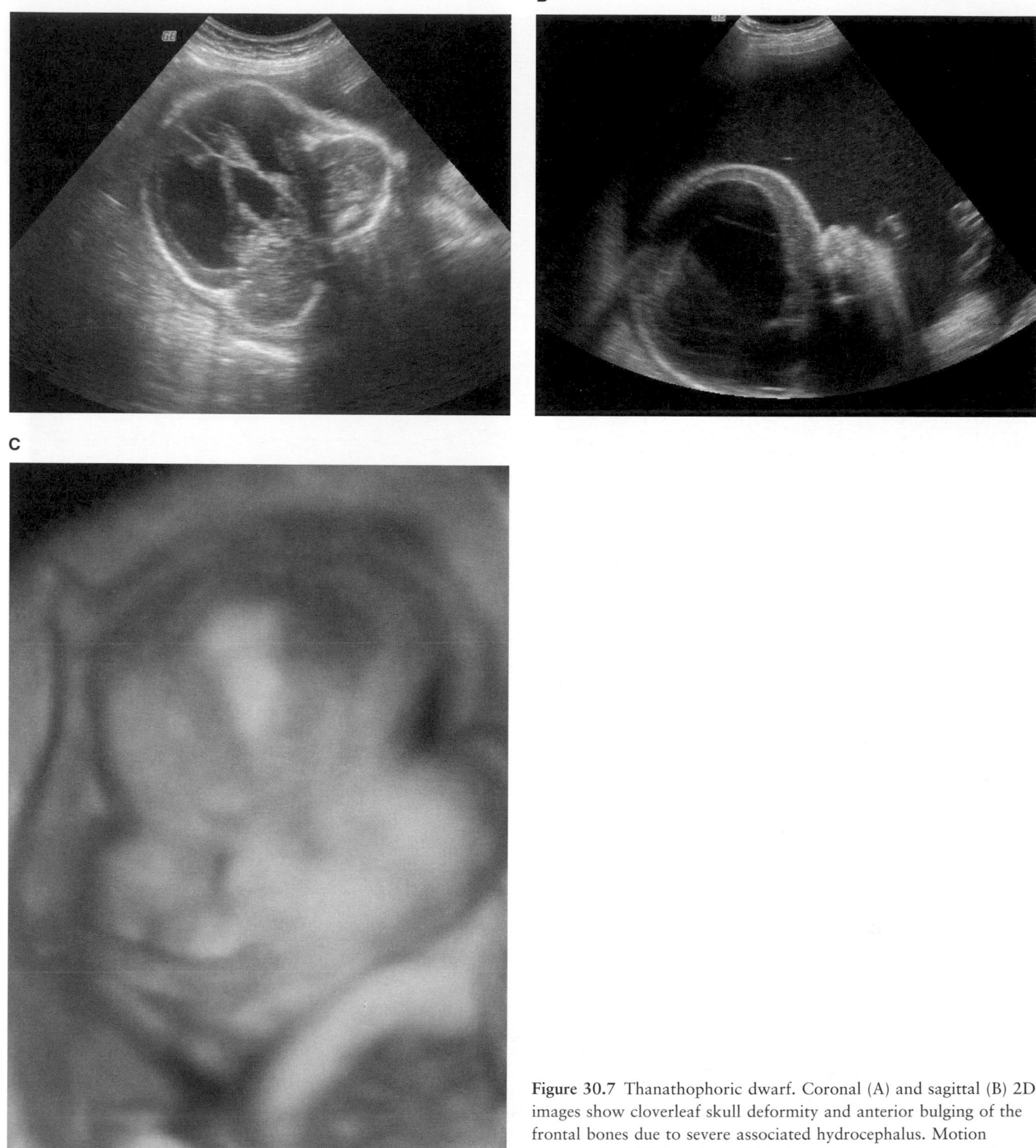

Figure 30.7 Thanathophoric dwarf. Coronal (A) and sagittal (B) 2D images show cloverleaf skull deformity and anterior bulging of the frontal bones due to severe associated hydrocephalus. Motion compromised 3D imaging, which showed the same findings (C).

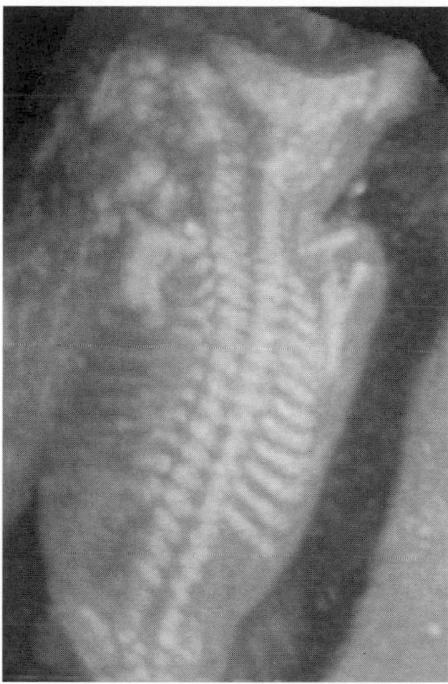

Figure 30.8 The fetal spine. Volume data are acquired and 3D-rendered as a surface image or reconstructed to display a series of 2D images.

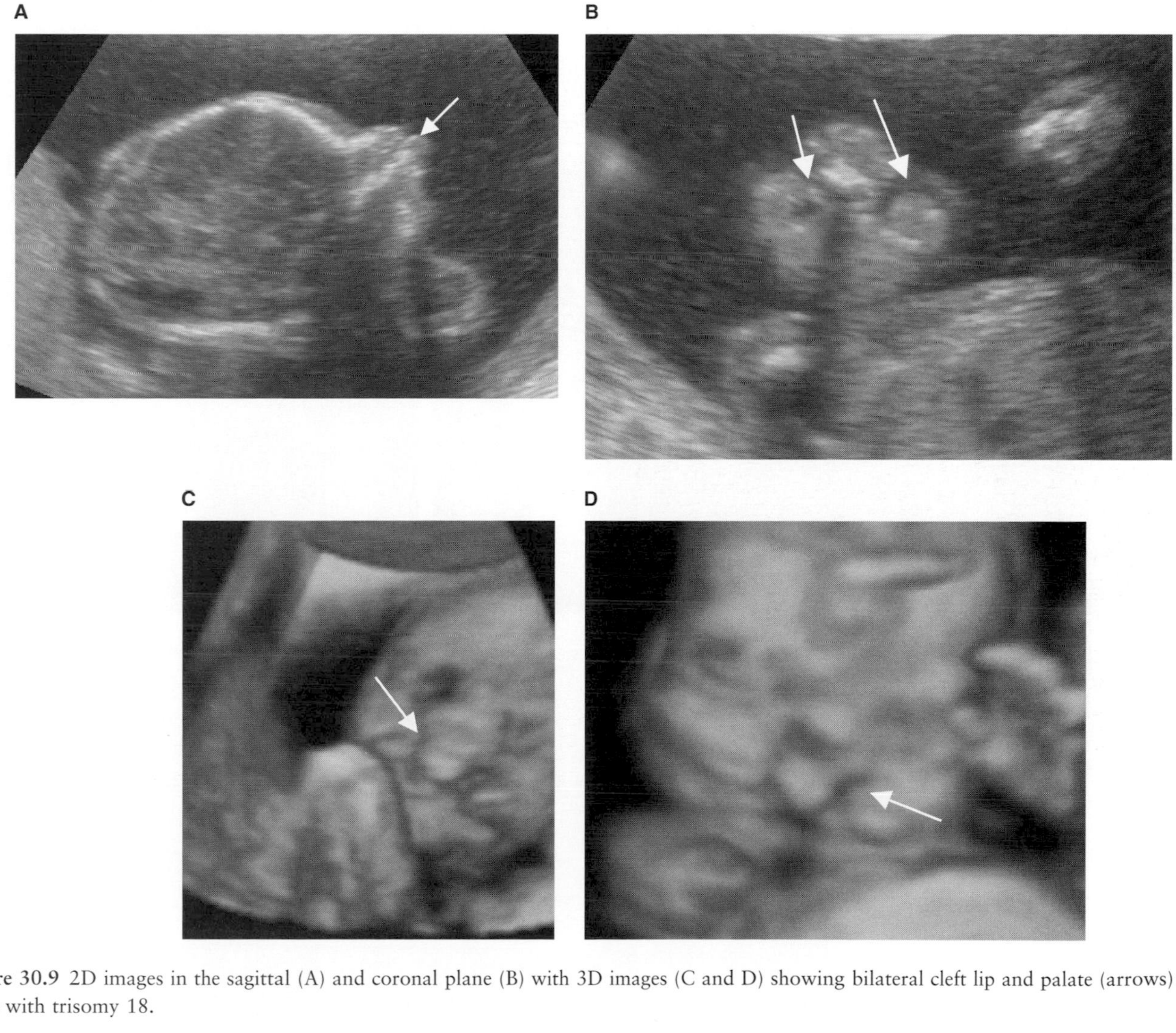

A

B

C

D

Figure 30.9 2D images in the sagittal (A) and coronal plane (B) with 3D images (C and D) showing bilateral cleft lip and palate (arrows) in a fetus with trisomy 18.

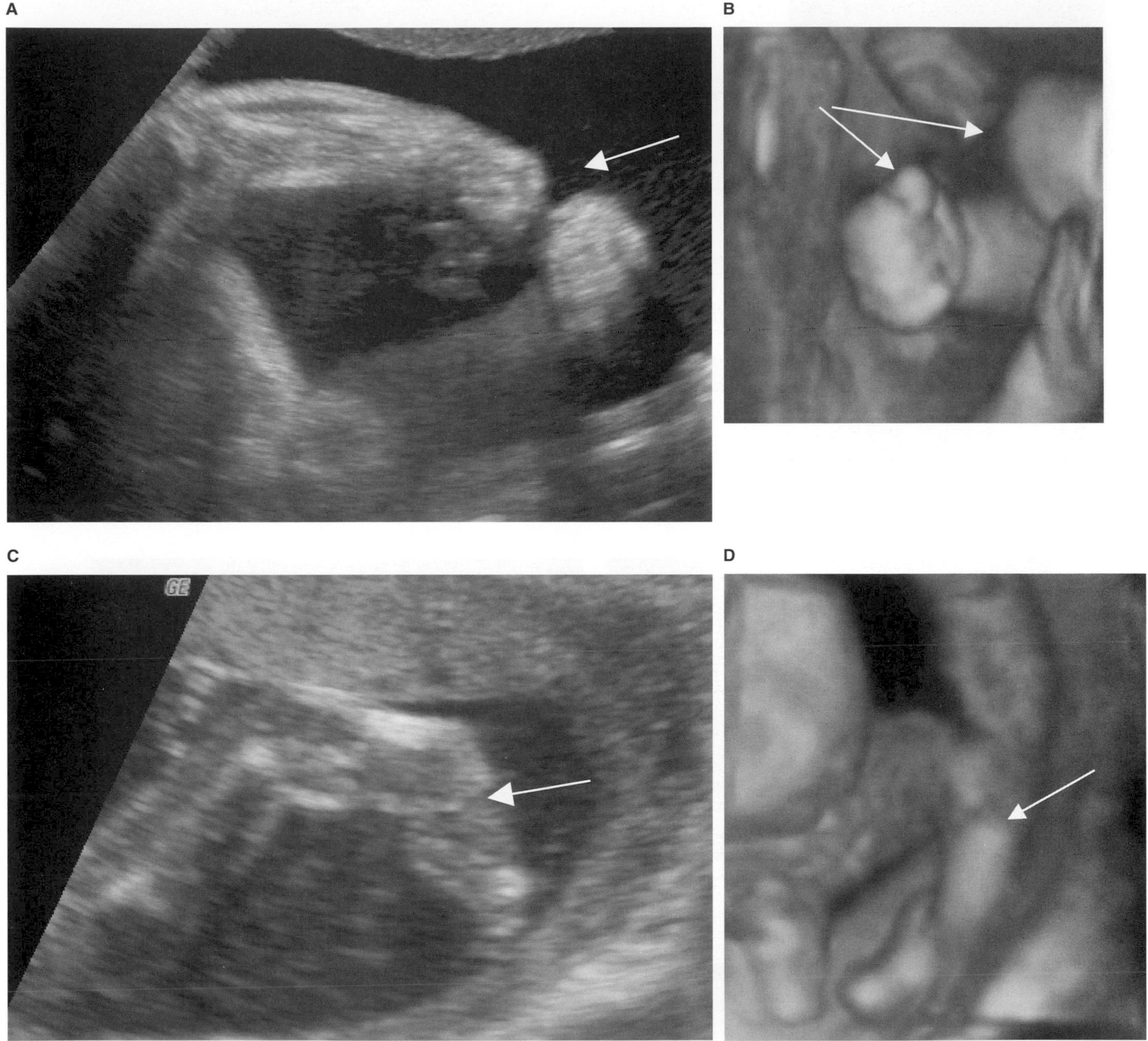

Figure 30.10 Extremities. 2D and 3D rendering of persistent clenched fists (A and B, respectively) and malpositioned lower leg (C and D, respectively) (arrows).

in the pelvis, very early gestation, and maternal body habitus. In oligohydramnios, the anatomy of interest could very easily be obscured by the adjacent placenta or uterine wall owing to the inability of the images to demonstrate a true plane of separation between these structures. Although it is possible to electronically "cut away" certain structures with an "electronic scalpel" and still obtain a 3D image on these occasions, it often leaves a suboptimal image (Fig. 30.11). This emphasizes the fact that the quality of 3D rendering is critically dependent upon the quality of the 2D image.[21] Similarly, an early gestational age tends to provide less prominent features for fetal imaging. The earlier the gestational age, the higher the chances of fetal motion, which can create motion artifacts. This can lead to images that simulate fetal defects. Also, the low resolution of the features of an embryo or fetus in the first trimester makes the rendered image suboptimal. In spite of these setbacks, a number of publications have documented the feasibility of performing 3D ultrasound in the first trimester, not only to demonstrate known embryologic events but also to diagnose anomalies resulting from faulty fetal development[22–26] (Fig. 30.12). As the fetus ages, surface rendering

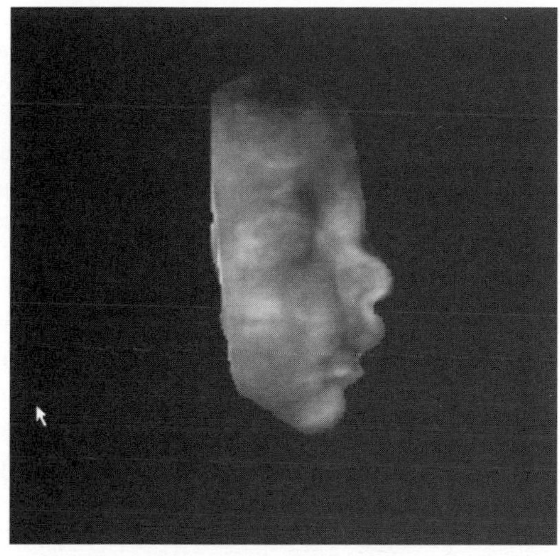

Figure 30.11 A close-up of a fetal profile using the "electronic scalpel" to eliminate other parts of the image.

A

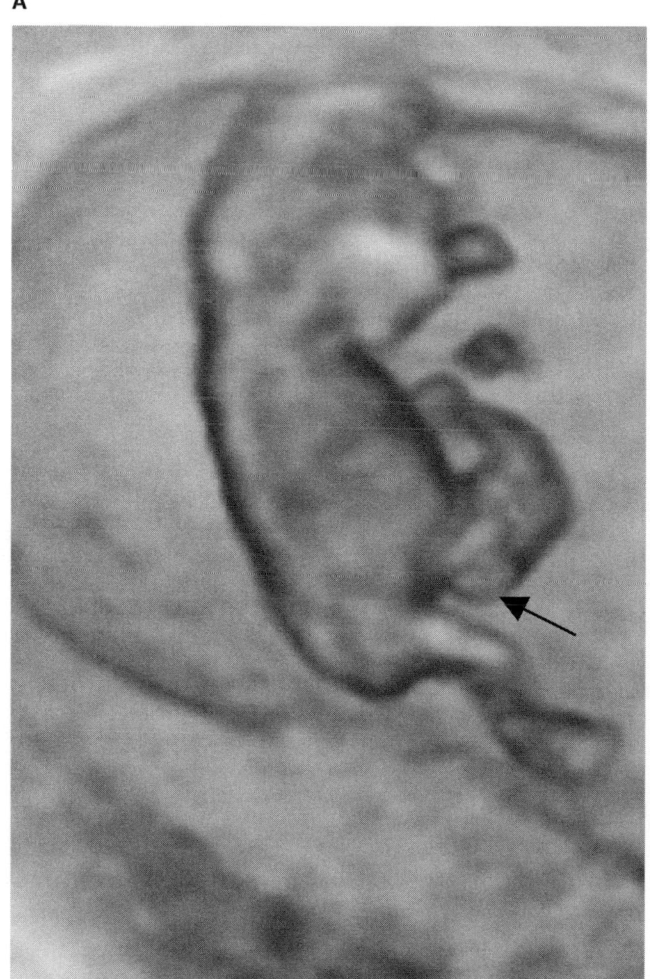

B

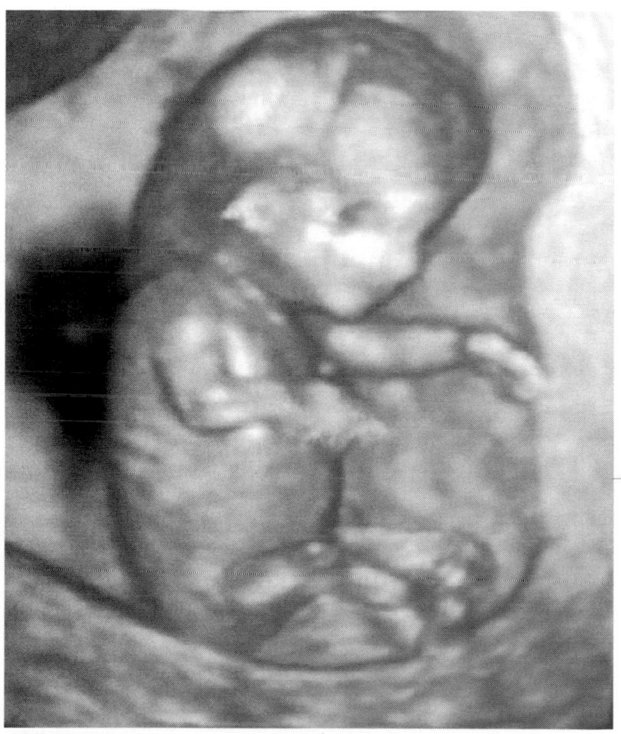

Figure 30.12 First-trimester 3D ultrasound. At 8 weeks (A), physiologic bowel herniation is seen at the cord insertion (arrow), which disappears by 12 weeks (B).

becomes less and less of a problem, and 3D ultrasound images obtained late in the third trimester become more impressive. It is in this scenario that 3D ultrasound has been employed in the chest[27–29] and the abdomen[30–32] (Figs 30.13 and 30.14). Although the results have been promising, these applications need to be validated by future studies that can convincingly show an improvement in visualization of the abnormalities on 3D ultrasound.

Detection of fetal cardiac anomalies has become possible with the development of the STIC technique (spatiotemporal image correlation) (Fig. 30.15). This allows the performance of 4D fetal echocardiography in B-mode without the use of external triggering devices.[33,34] Data acquired in one cardiac cycle are rearranged by correlation of their temporal and spatial domain. This can then be processed offline in a cine loop. This triplanar demonstration of the heart has allowed the assessment of both the cardiac chambers and the great vessels (Fig. 30.16). The possibility of reslicing the heart in all three dimensions and viewing these in different degrees of rotation has made possible the diagnosis of previously difficult anomalies.[35,36] The latest experience of cardiac 4D imaging has shown the detection of anomalies such as ventricular septal defects, tricuspid atresia, transposition of the great vessels, pulmonary atresia, and interruption of the inferior vena cava with azygous venous return. Although this experience is currently limited to a few referral centers, it is promising in that it provides another dimension in diagnosing complex cardiac defects that are typically difficult to see on conventional 2D ultrasound.[37–39] Faster computer processing has allowed this innovation to happen, but any further significant advances in 4D ultrasound depend upon the implementation of faster computer processing for imaging and the development of active matrix array transducers with further enhanced capabilities over those of the current machines.

Comparison of 3D/4D ultrasound over 2D ultrasound

The advantages of 3D ultrasound over conventional 2D ultrasound lie in its ability to store and retrieve complete volumes of data, its multiplanar display, surface rendering, and 4D display of fetal movements.[5] Because of its ability to store and retrieve volumes of data, the examiner can navigate precisely through fetal anatomy in three orthogonal planes simultaneously. Digital storage of complete sets of volumes allows us to manipulate the data even in the absence of the patient. This is a distinct advantage for sonologists and sonographers as it enables them to scrutinize equivocal findings in an unhurried fashion. This has tremendous implications in terms of time saved in actual scanning time, thus increasing patient turnover in a busy service. Consultations with peers and referring physicians can be conducted at mutually convenient times, and the need for additional images does not necessarily require return clinic visits. Retrospective analysis of the stored volume data is possible years later as the digital volume is stored without data loss. The same data can be copied and viewed by many examiners independently or used for training purposes. The multiplanar display allows for visualization of the anatomy in planes not possible during conventional 2D imaging, identification of the precise location of the imaged anatomic plane, and collection of more accurate volumetric measurements. Surface rendering allows the examiner a more vivid depiction of the fetal structures from various angles, increased confidence in the diagnosis of complex malformations, and the exclusion of anomalies in otherwise equivocal studies. For the parents, it is claimed to enhance the parental bonding experience owing to a more photorealistic depiction of fetal structures, better appreciation of any anomaly, and more reassurance in excluding fetal anomalies. In the acute clinical setting where an anomaly is discovered for the first time, the ability to display images that are easily recognized by the patient and her relatives becomes invaluable for counseling purposes.

Among the disadvantages of 3D ultrasound are: larger probes, motion artifacts (Fig. 30.17), production of iatrogenic structural defects by faulty electronic settings, the possibility of orientation problems in the stored volume, and the inability to perform surface rendering in the presence of oligohydramnios. Among these, only the problems related to oligohydramnios remain difficult to resolve (Fig. 30.18). The others should improve with experience and rapidly advancing technology. Another challenge facing any attempts at making 3D/4D ultrasound routine in obstetric imaging is the need for tremendous storage capacity for the acquired data. Each volume set can require 3–18 MB of memory depending upon the area of interest, and this could tax an overburdened common archiving device. With the widespread use of picture archiving and communication systems (PACS) workstations, this problem can only escalate with time as more and more people learn how to manipulate stored data. However, it is hoped that, as media storage becomes less and less expensive, this will not prove to be an impediment to a very promising diagnostic tool.

Magnetic resonance imaging (MRI)

General considerations

The applications of MRI in clinical medicine have spanned the whole human anatomy from head to foot. Over the past 10 years, there has been an increasing number of medical centers around the world embracing MRI as a primary diagnostic test. In obstetrics however, its applications are predominantly complementary to ultrasound and mainly as a problem-solving tool when ultrasound is inadequate for diagnosis.[40–42] Its use has been limited to the late second and third trimesters of pregnancy, mainly because of the uncertainty that bioeffects may eventually be proven in the fetus.[43] To date, no untoward incidents or fetal sequelae have been reported.[44,45] However, it is customary to obtain informed consent prior to

A

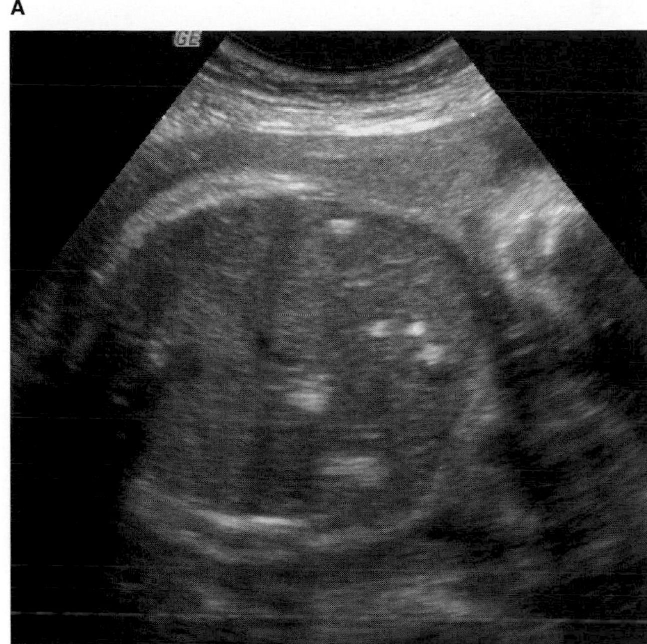

Figure 30.13 Liver calcifications. 2D image (A) shows multiple intrahepatic calcifications in a fetus suspected to have cytomegalovirus (CMV) infection. The 3D attempt at imaging the calcifications (B) did not add any further information.

B

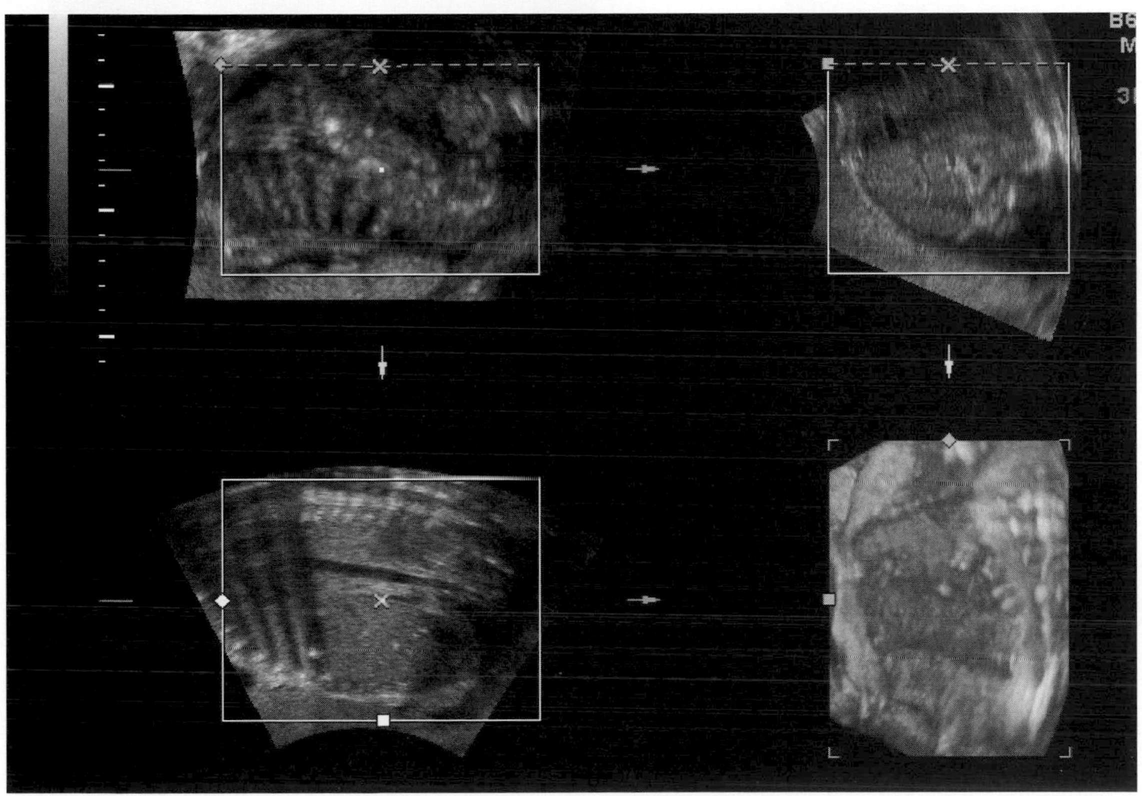

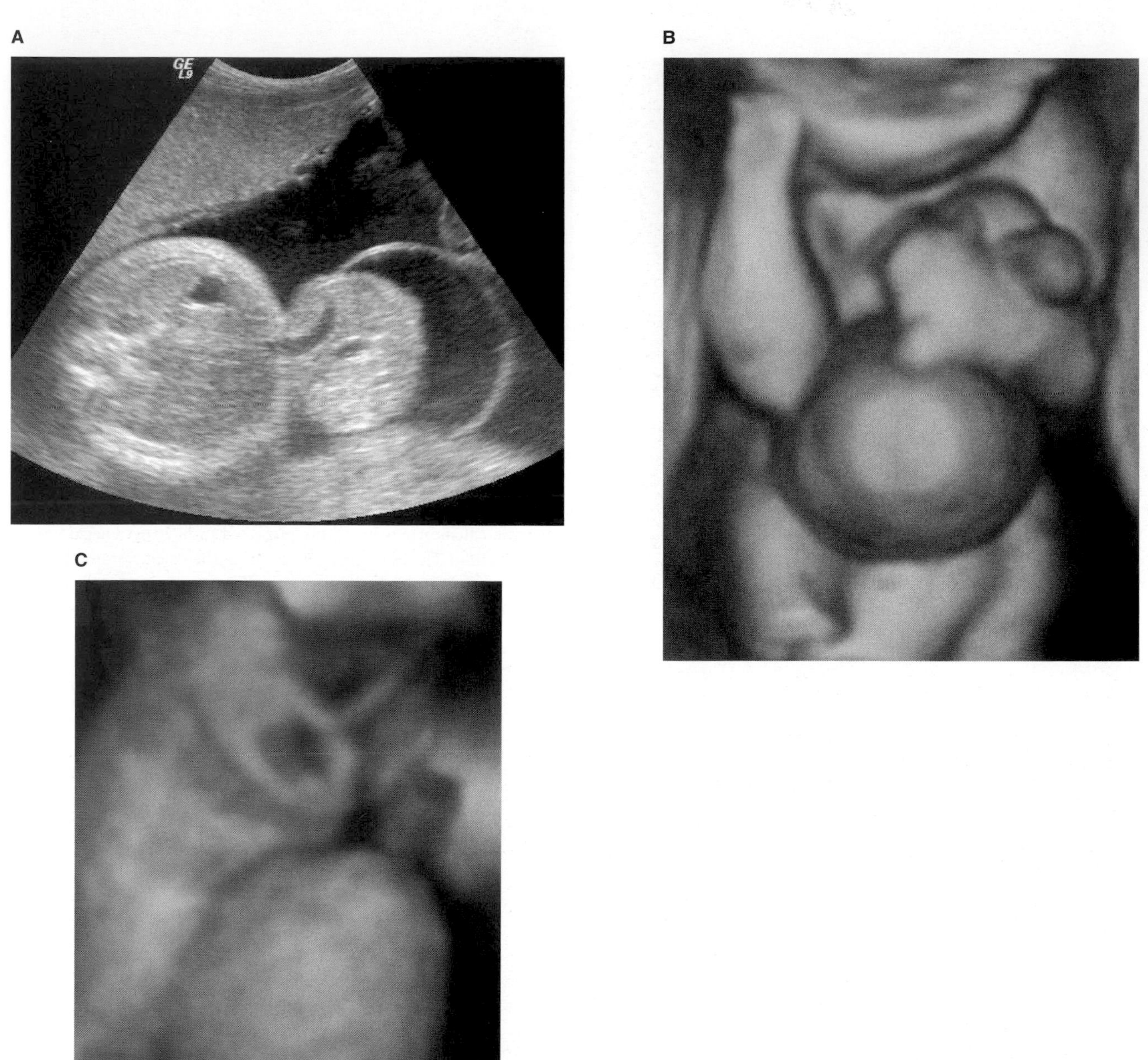

Figure 30.14 Omphalocele. The classic appearance of the herniated liver outside the abdomen is seen on a 2D axial images (A) and 3D rendering in the coronal (B) and sagittal (C) planes.

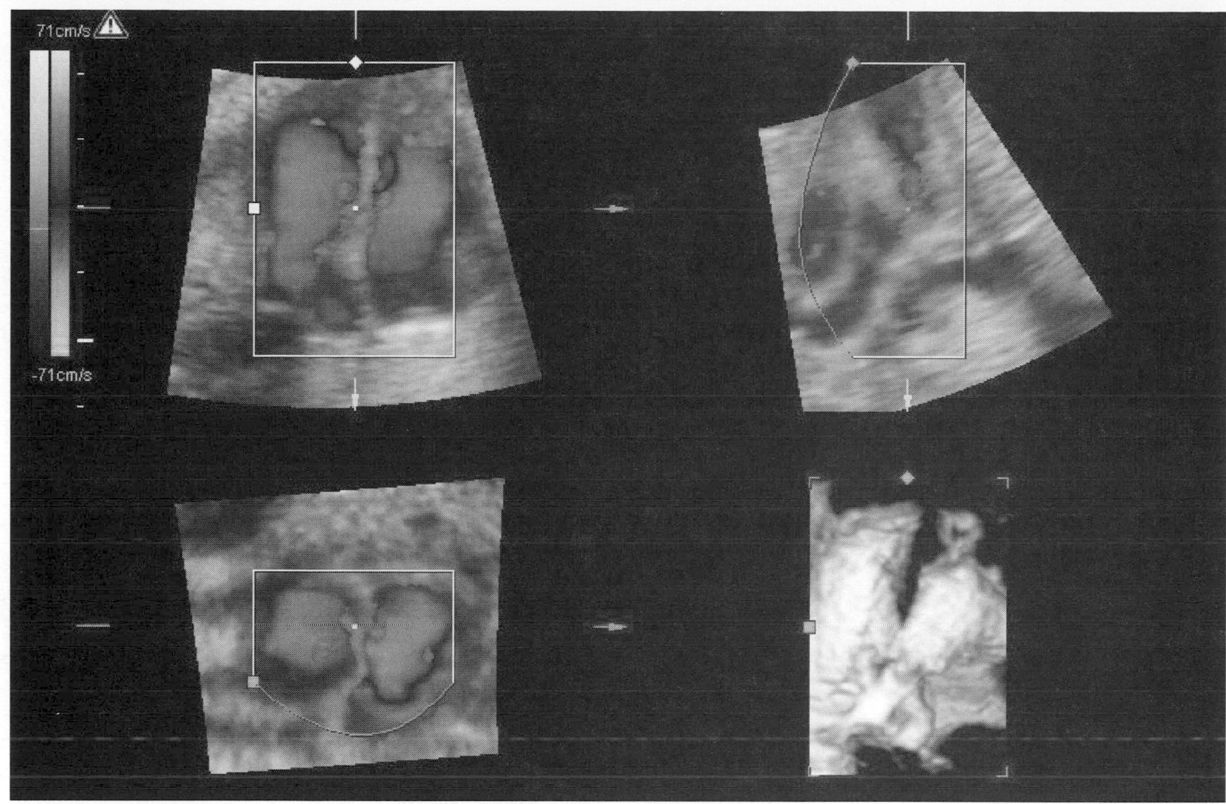

Figure 30.15 Normal heart. Color Doppler with 3D imaging of the heart shows an intact interventricular septum.

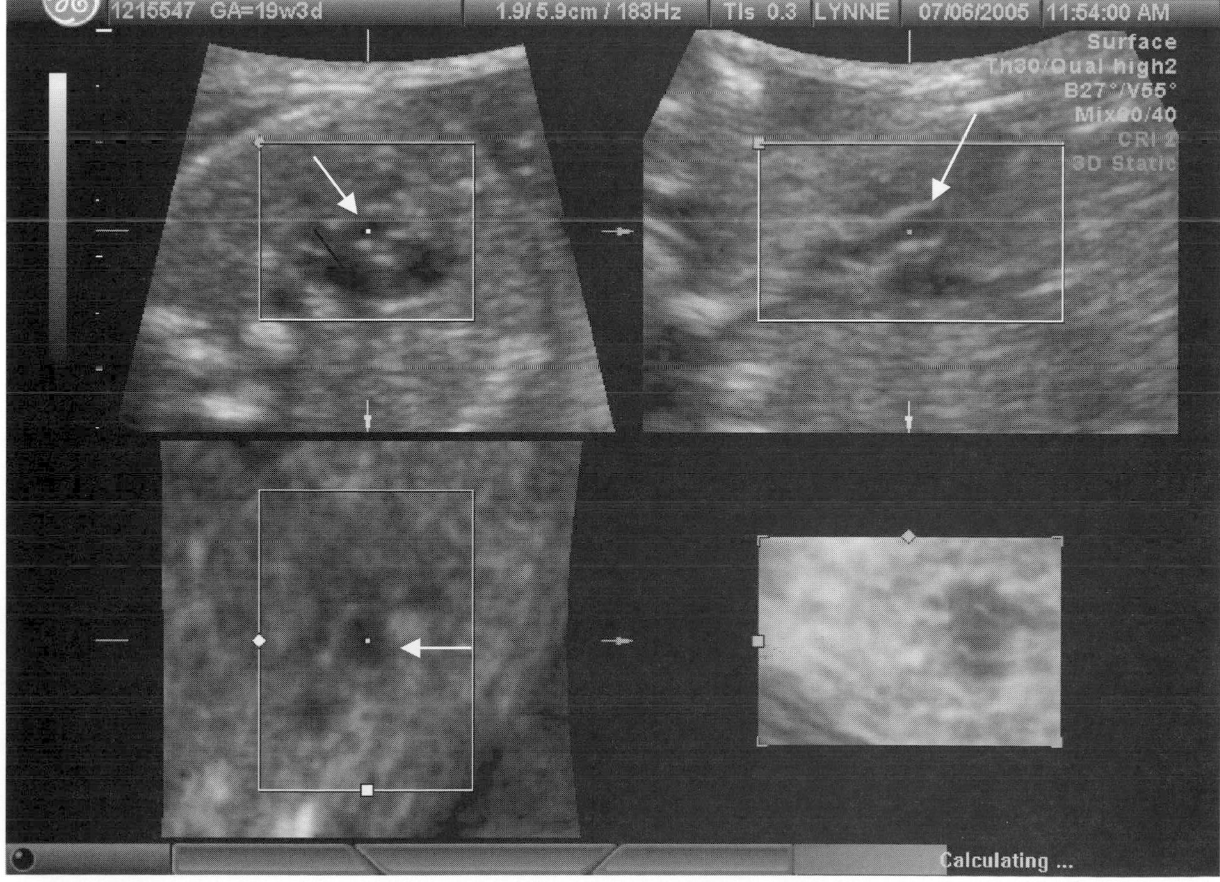

Figure 30.16 3D image of the heart showing the left ventricular outflow tract in three orthogonal planes.

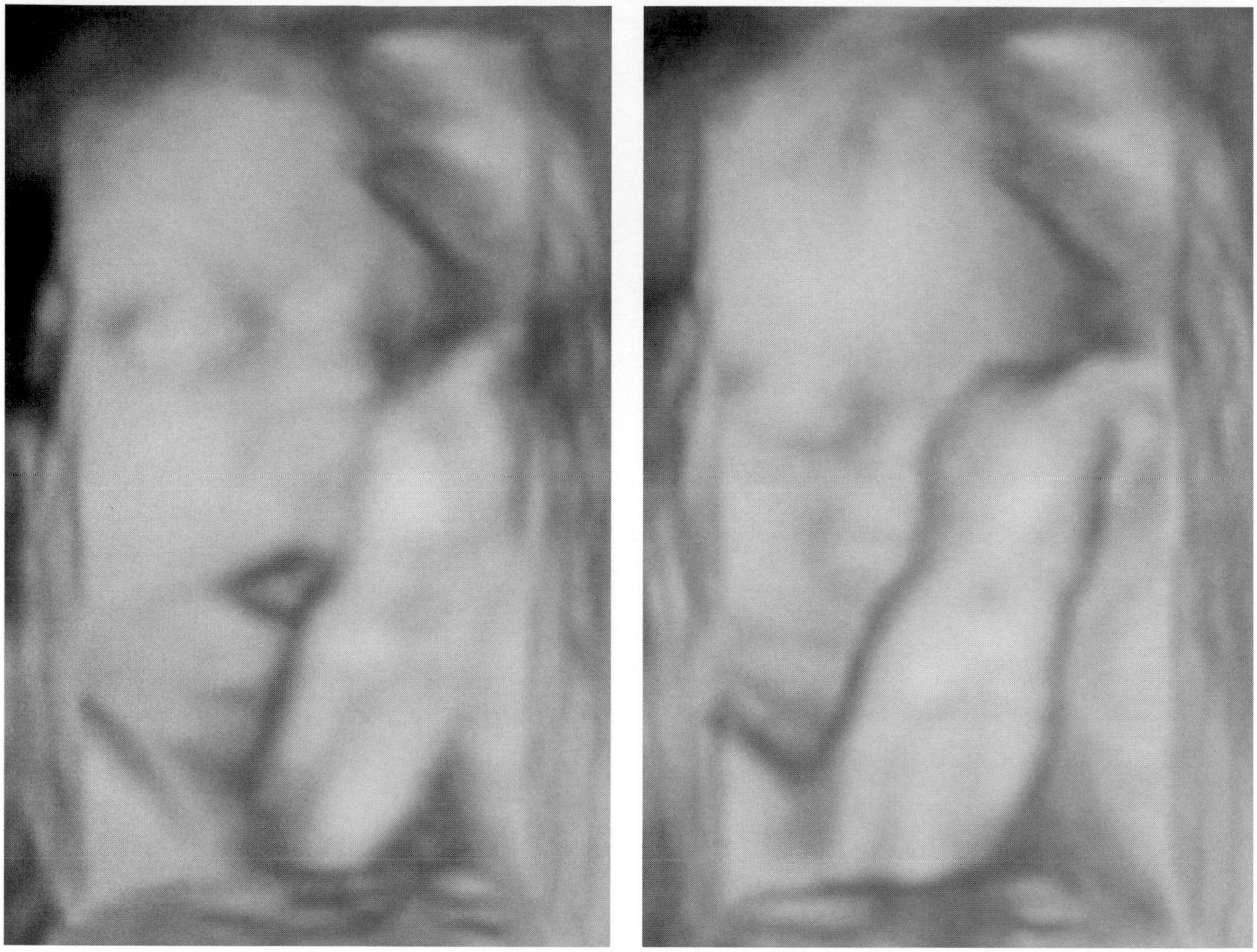

Figure 30.17 Serial images (A and B) from a 4D volume acquisition are rendered suboptimal by motion artifacts.

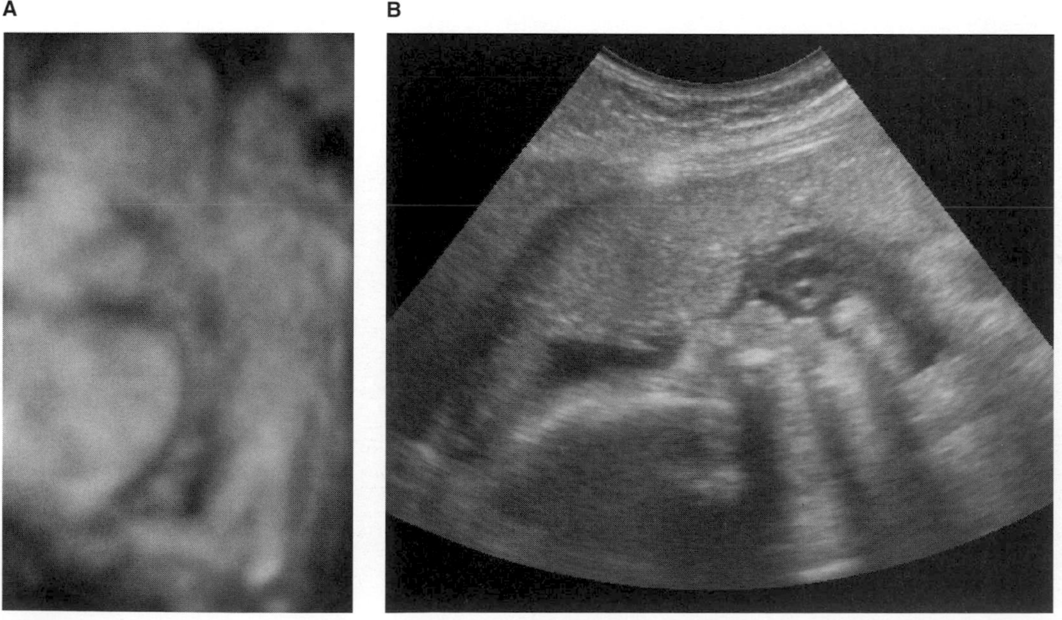

Figure 30.18 Oligohydramnios. The combination of decreased fluid in front of the fetal face and the resulting crowding of the upper extremities resulted in the inability to obtain a good image of the fetal profile. (A) Three-dimensional image; (B) two-dimensional image.

the examination so that the patient is aware of the nonroutine nature of the examination and its potential for causing unforeseen bioeffects in the future. It is best to reassure the patient that there is no conclusive evidence supporting the direct relationship between short-tem exposure to electromagnetic fields and any hazard to the developing fetus and that there are no documented ill-effects to either the mother or the fetus. In instances where MRI is indicated, it is always important to emphasize that the potential benefits obtained from the scan may outweigh any potential risks that exist.

MRI technique

It is suggested that patients be placed feet first into the magnet to minimize any possibility of claustrophobia. A pillow is placed under the knees for comfort, and the patient is scanned in the supine position. However, those who cannot tolerate this position for prolonged periods are scanned on their side.[46] It is important to monitor the examination as changes in fetal position can lead to alterations in any preplanned protocol.[47] It is routine to use the set of images from one sequence to decide on the next series of images. It is also best to correlate the images obtained on MRI with an ultrasound study preferably done immediately before the MRI or within a few days of the examination. This will tremendously facilitate the interpretation of the MRI examination and direct the conduct of the remainder of the study. The imaging sequences used in MRI vary depending upon the manufacturer-specific recommendations. The most popular is the half-Fourier single-shot turbo spin echo sequence that gives T2-weighted images of sufficient anatomic detail for both maternal and fetal structures[48,49] (Figs 30.19 and 30.20). This sequence comes under two proprietary technical names, HASTE (Half-Fourier Acquisition Single Shot Turbo Spin Echo) and SSFSE (Single Shot Fast Spin Echo). Another technique is the T1-weighted imaging sequence usually using gradient echo techniques (Fig. 30.21). This technique results in superb anatomic images that can be obtained in short periods of time that even allow for breath-holding sequences.[50] This becomes valuable especially in cases where there is suspected hemorrhage or fatty masses.

Excessive motion artifacts generated by the fetus early in pregnancy have likewise limited the early acceptance of MRI in fetal diagnosis (Fig. 30.22). In the early days of fetal MRI imaging, it was necessary to immobilize the fetus with an intramuscular dose of pancuronium because of the long imaging times.[51] This required percutaneous introduction of the drug into the fetal muscle (usually the thigh). The associated complications were similar to those of amniocentesis, compounded by the danger of inadvertently administering the drug partially to the mother, thus causing some respiratory problems. With current technological advances, whole imaging sequences can now be performed in seconds instead of the minutes that it used to take. This has eliminated the need for pancuronium and its potential complications. In occasional circumstances in which fetal motion compromises the study, diazepam or meperidine may be given to the mother to help lessen fetal motion artifacts. Another question raised about MRI was the possibility of using contrast agents such as gadolinium to enhance visualization of fetal organs. This has not been advocated in pregnancy, not only because gadolinium is known to cross the placental barrier, but also because it has not been needed in making the diagnosis of fetal abnormalities.

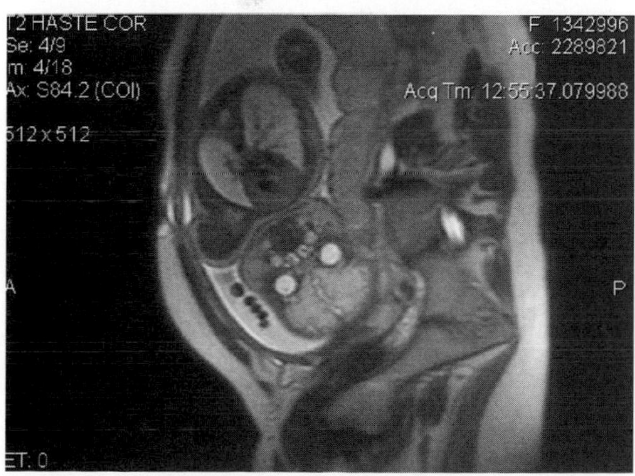

Figure 30.19 Sagittal MRI showing the fetal head and chest using the HASTE sequence of MRI data acquisition.

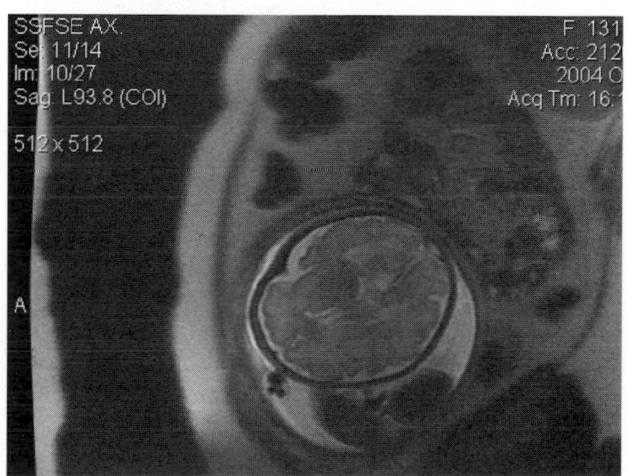

Figure 30.20 SSFSE sequence. A sagittal view of the maternal abdomen shows a normal axial image of the fetal brain surrounded by high-signal amniotic fluid.

Fetal anomalies

There is a potential for misdiagnosis on ultrasound in spite of experienced specialists (Figs 30.23 and 30.24). This is especially true when technical problems exist owing to maternal body habitus, suboptimal fetal lie, or oligohydramnios. What may seem like a simple diagnosis may actually be more complex and therefore need to be delineated prenatally for counseling purposes.[52,53] It is in circumstances such as these that the majority of fetal MRI studies are done, as a complement to a complete obstetric ultrasound that has already been performed. Often, an abnormality seen on ultrasound needs to be confirmed with certainty prior to the more invasive procedures necessary to correct the defect. This is especially true when specialists have been consulted prenatally to perform immediate neonatal intervention.[54] Examples are fetal abnormalities that may necessitate immediate invasive procedures at delivery because of airway obstruction. Entities such as lung masses or epignathus may benefit from an *ex utero* intrapartum treatment (EXIT) procedure in which the fetus is partially delivered and the airway is secured prior to clamping of the cord (Fig. 30.25). In these instances, it is critical to know the precise location and extent of the tumor so that management planning can be facilitated at the time of delivery.

The strength of MRI has been proven in the diagnoses of central nervous system (CNS) abnormalities where ultrasound may be inadequate[55–69]. However, there are instances when the etiology of the abnormality cannot be determined, even with better definition of anatomic structures on the MRI images. (Fig. 30.26). In brain anomalies associated with ventriculomegaly, the decision to shunt sometimes hinges on very subtle findings such as the presence or absence of a cerebral mantle in the high convexities (Fig. 30.27). This becomes crucial in the differentiation of hydrocephaly from hydranencephaly when the cerebral mantle is so compressed as to be almost invisible on ultrasound (Fig. 30.28). Similarly, the level of obstruction can be clearly defined on MRI, whereas it may only be determined on ultrasound by the process of exclusion (Fig. 30.29). Another example would be unilateral hydrocephalus due to an obstructing suprasellar arachnoid cyst. On ultrasound, the wall separating the body of the lateral ventricle from the cyst may not be obvious, and rare entities such as unilateral obstruction of the foramen of Monro may be entertained. MRI can clearly show the delineation between the dilated lateral ventricle and the large arachnoid cyst (Fig. 30.30). Other associated anomalies (such as agenesis of the corpus callosum) become clear on MRI. Future trends in diagnosis are geared toward earlier diagnosis of intracranial processes before they can produce detectable changes on ultrasound. One such possibility is the demonstration of subependymal tubers in tuberous sclerosis, which have been demonstrated as early as 21 weeks by MRI but not on ultrasound.[70]

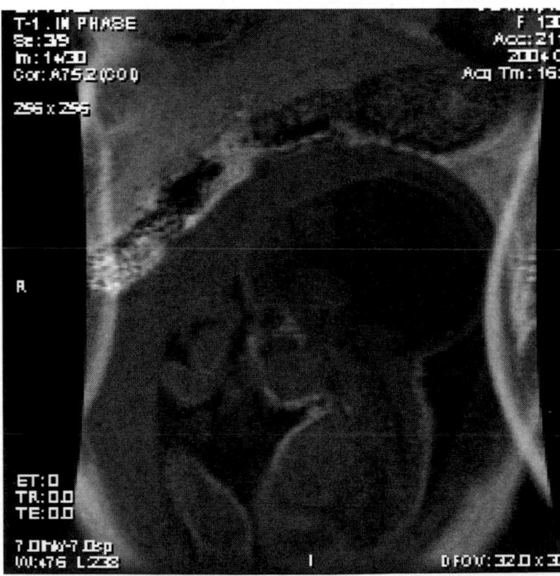

Figure 30.21 T1-weighted sagittal image of the fetus is distinguished by the low signal in the surrounding amniotic fluid and the high-intensity signal in the fetal and maternal subcutaneous fat.

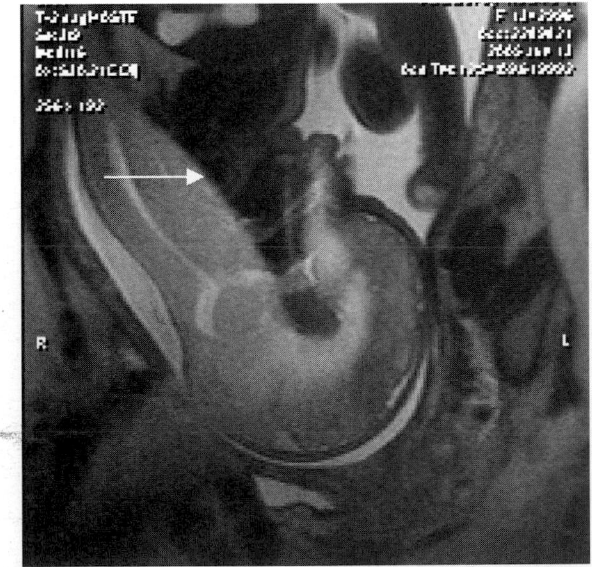

Figure 30.22 Fetal motion artifact has produced low-signal bands (arrow) in the middle of the fetal face, making the image uninterpretable.

The utility of MRI in other areas of the body has not been as successful as in the head or spine.[71–74] To a large extent, this is because of the many potential artifacts that can compromise imaging of the remainder of the fetus. Maternal bulk motion can be minimized by breath-holding techniques (Fig. 30.31). Fluid motion secondary to fetal respiration, urination, or swallowing can mimic masses, which can only be seen on a few images. This is usually not consistently imaged on multiple sequences. Many other technical artifacts are known to compromise the image such as aliasing, radiofrequency interference, susceptibility artifacts, and partial volume artifacts (Fig. 30.32). However, in spite of these, the indications for MRI of the fetal chest and abdomen are increasing.[75–81] These range from genitourinary abnormalities to unusual gastrointestinal abnormalities and a range of case reports in which MRI contributed significantly in making a diagnosis.[82–87]

Nonfetal complications of pregnancy

Nonfetal abnormalities can also be diagnosed with confidence on MRI whereas ultrasound can be doubtful.[88–90] At times, this could be crucial if an invasive procedure becomes indicated prior to term. A case in point would be the diagnosis of an abdominal pregnancy (Fig. 30.33). As this hinges on the demonstration of an empty uterus separate from the fetus, it is imperative that this be documented on prenatal ultrasound. A uterine leiomyoma can easily mimic the empty uterus, and MRI easily differentiates between the two entities (Fig. 30.34). A large adnexal mass may be difficult to demonstrate and characterize on ultrasound, not only because of its size but also because of its position. A large teratoma, for instance, can mimic a demised twin on account of its heterogeneous contents (Fig. 30.35). MRI can be definitive in characterizing these masses from their typical features and tissue content. Specifically, the identification of fat within the mass clinches the diagnosis (Fig. 30.36). In the case of uterine anomalies, the ultrasound picture can be very confusing. A uterus didelphys with a normal pregnancy in one of the uterine cavities can be associated with hematometra when the other cavity is obstructed (Fig. 30.37). A unicornuate uterus can be a difficult diagnosis even with MRI. In these cases, the abnormal orientation of the pregnancy can be a clue to the uterine anomaly (Fig. 30.38).

Clinical considerations

A significant factor driving the need for prenatal MRI is the level of comfort that the specialist has regarding ultrasound. Most neurosurgeons, who use MRI on almost every adult patient prior to intervention, sometimes require prenatal MRI before the initial consultation. This is increasingly true in spite of some excellent anatomical delineation that may already have been provided by the ultrasound examination. Similarly, with patients becoming more involved in management decisions regarding their pregnancy, the Internet has become their

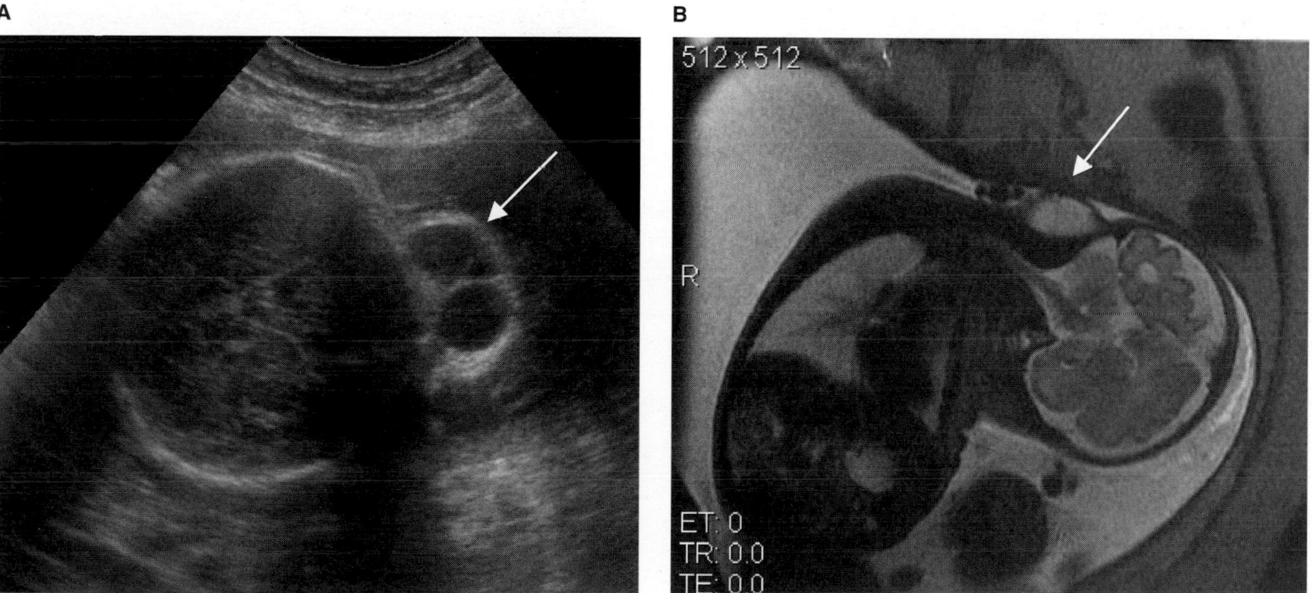

Figure 30.23 Cystic hygroma. 2D image of the fetal brain (A) suggested a mass arising from the occiput (arrow), perhaps a cephalocele. MRI (B) clearly shows that the cystic mass is in the neck (arrow), with no connection to the intracranial structure.

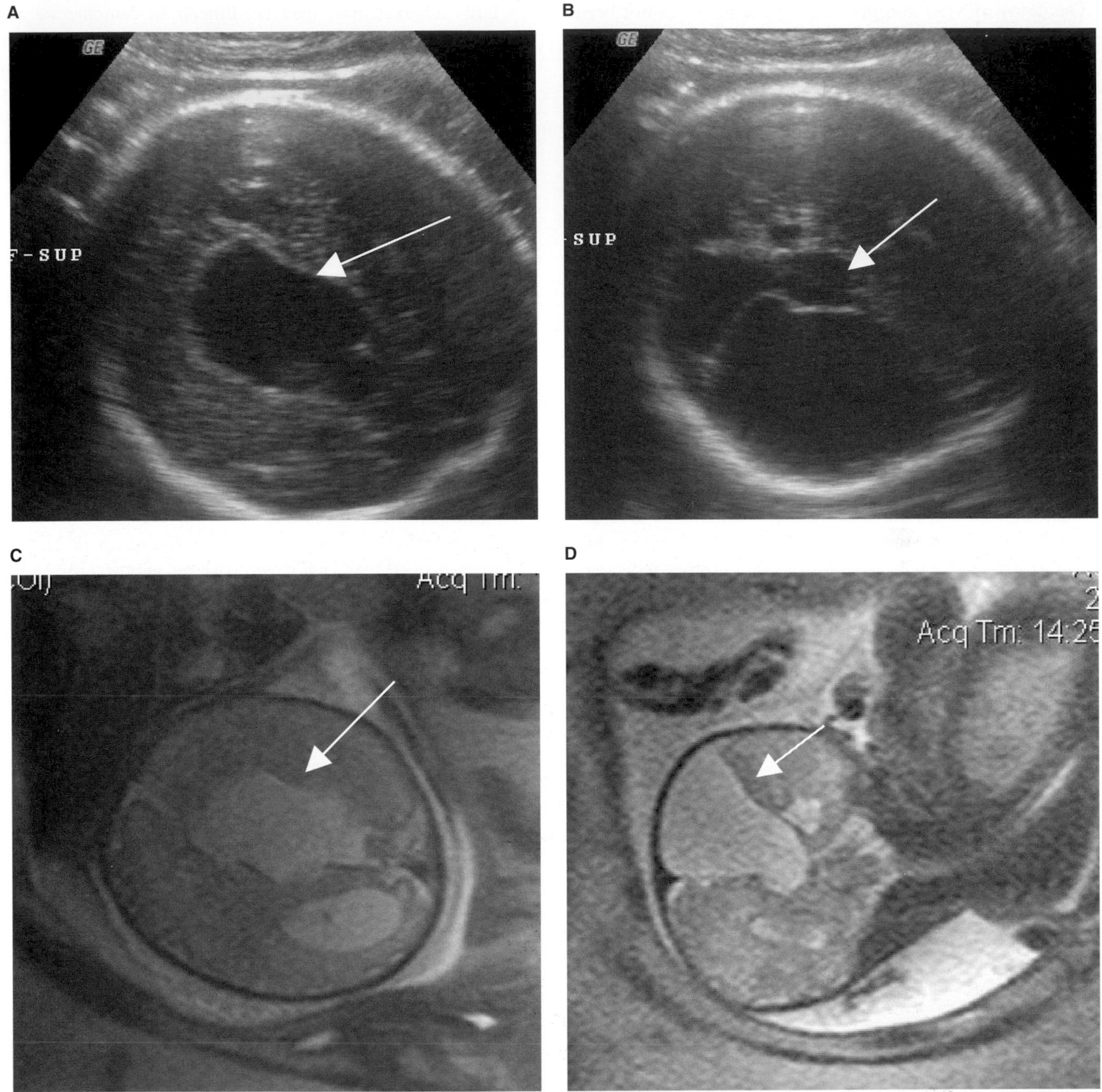

Figure 30.24 Suprasellar arachnoid cyst. A septated fluid collection (arrow) was seen on ultrasound (A and B) that extended to the parietal convexity. MRI (C–E) showed this to be a huge suprasellar cyst (arrow) that replaced part of the parietal cerebral cortex.

E

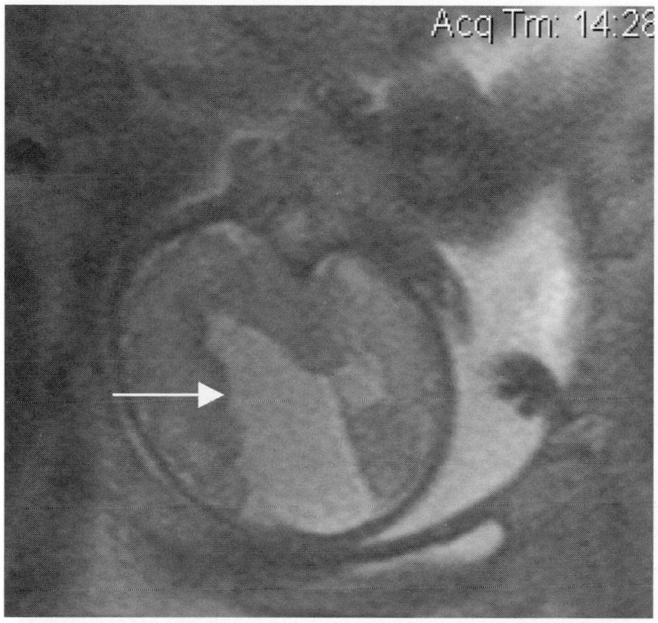

Acq Tm: 14:28

Figure 30.24 *Continued*

A

B

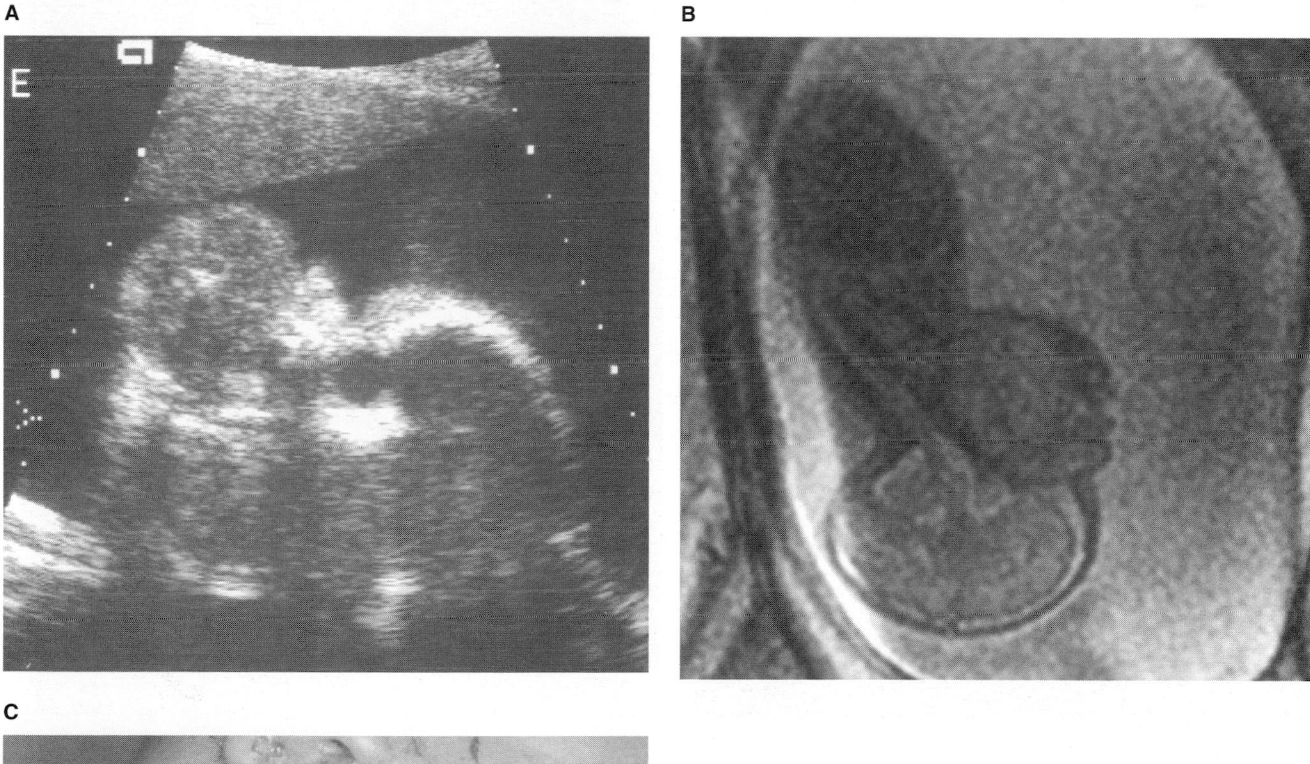

C

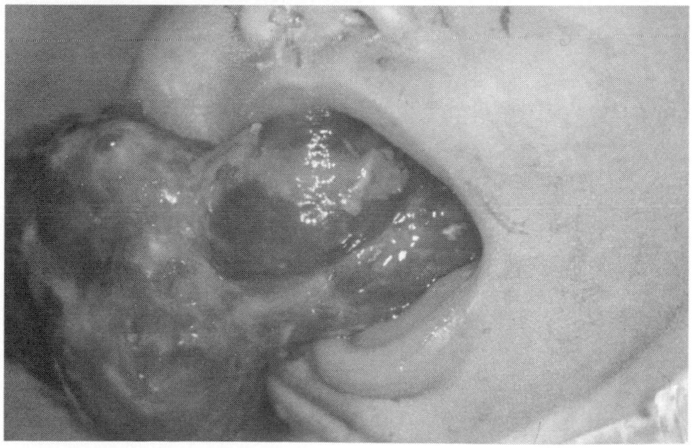

Figure 30.25 Epignathus. A large teratoma is seen protruding outside the oral cavity on ultrasound (A). MRI image (B) shows no intracranial extension. An EXIT procedure allowed maintenance of the airway during delivery (C).

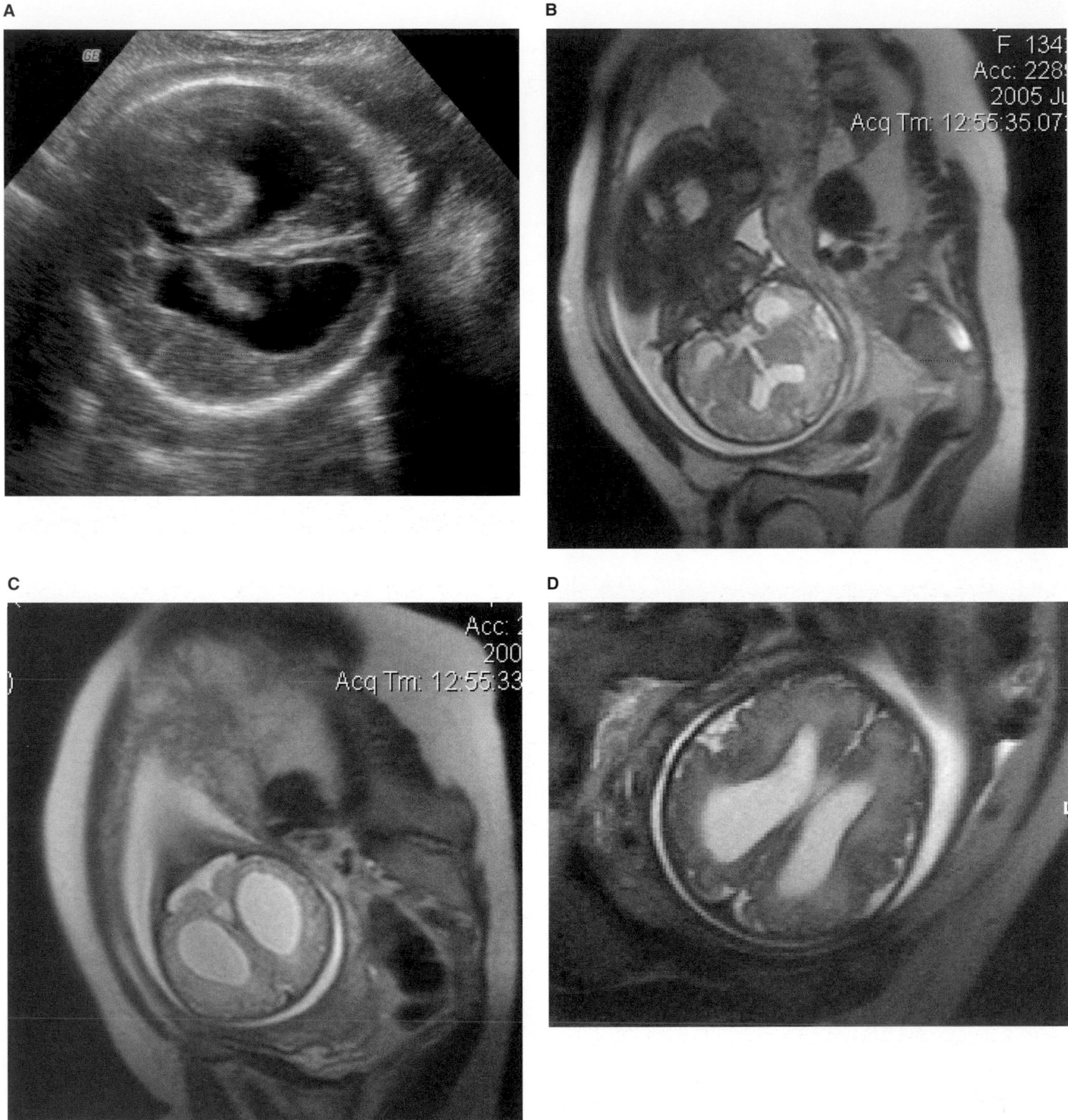

Figure 30.26 Moderate hydrocephalus. Both ultrasound (A) and MRI (B–D) failed to demonstrate an anatomical reason for the symmetric ventriculomegaly.

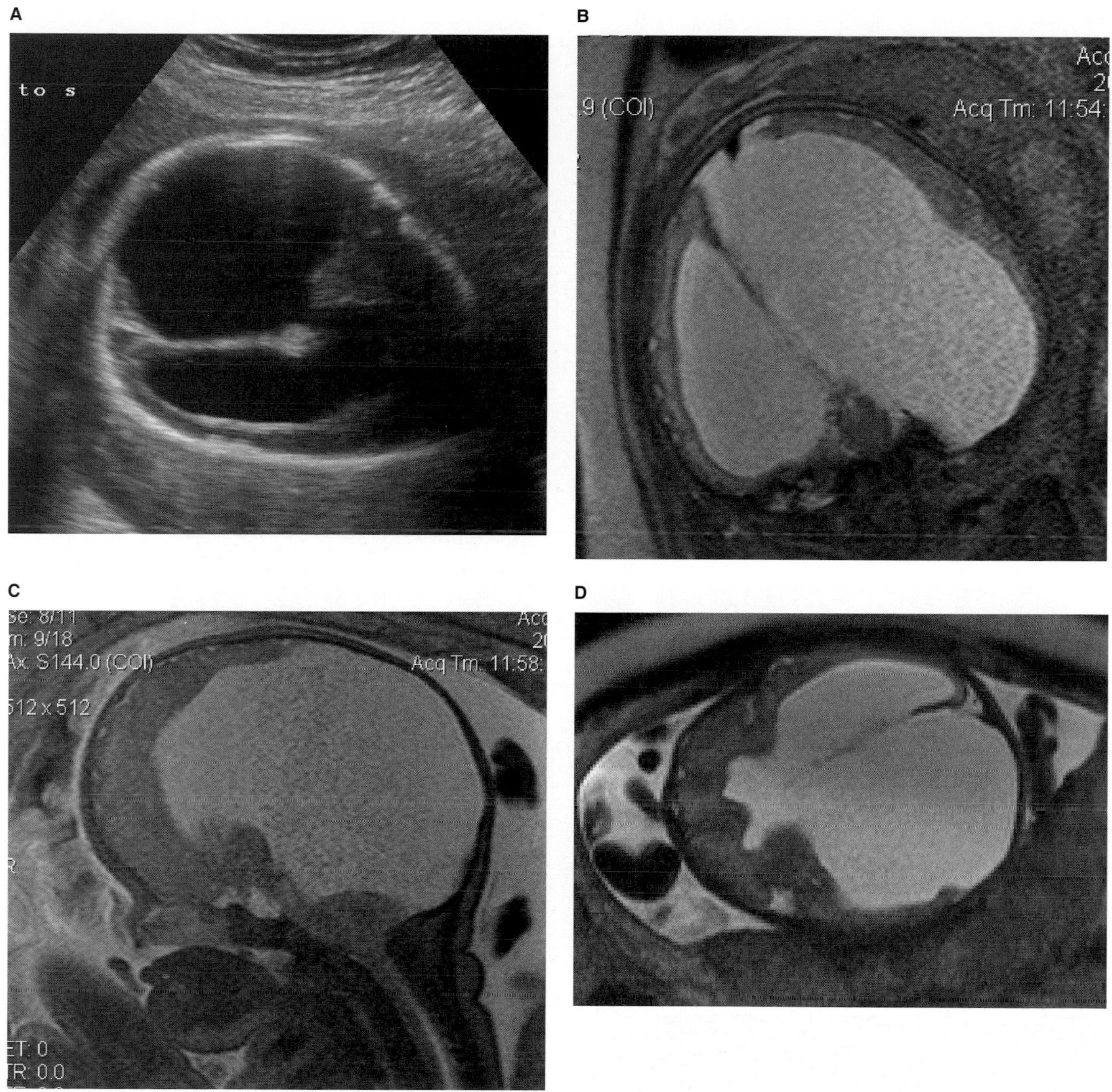

Figure 30.27 Asymmetric hydrocephalus. The ultrasound examination (A) did not find an etiology. MRI showed absence of cerebral cortex in the occipital region especially on the left. This is well demonstrated on coronal (B), sagittal (C), and axial (D) views.

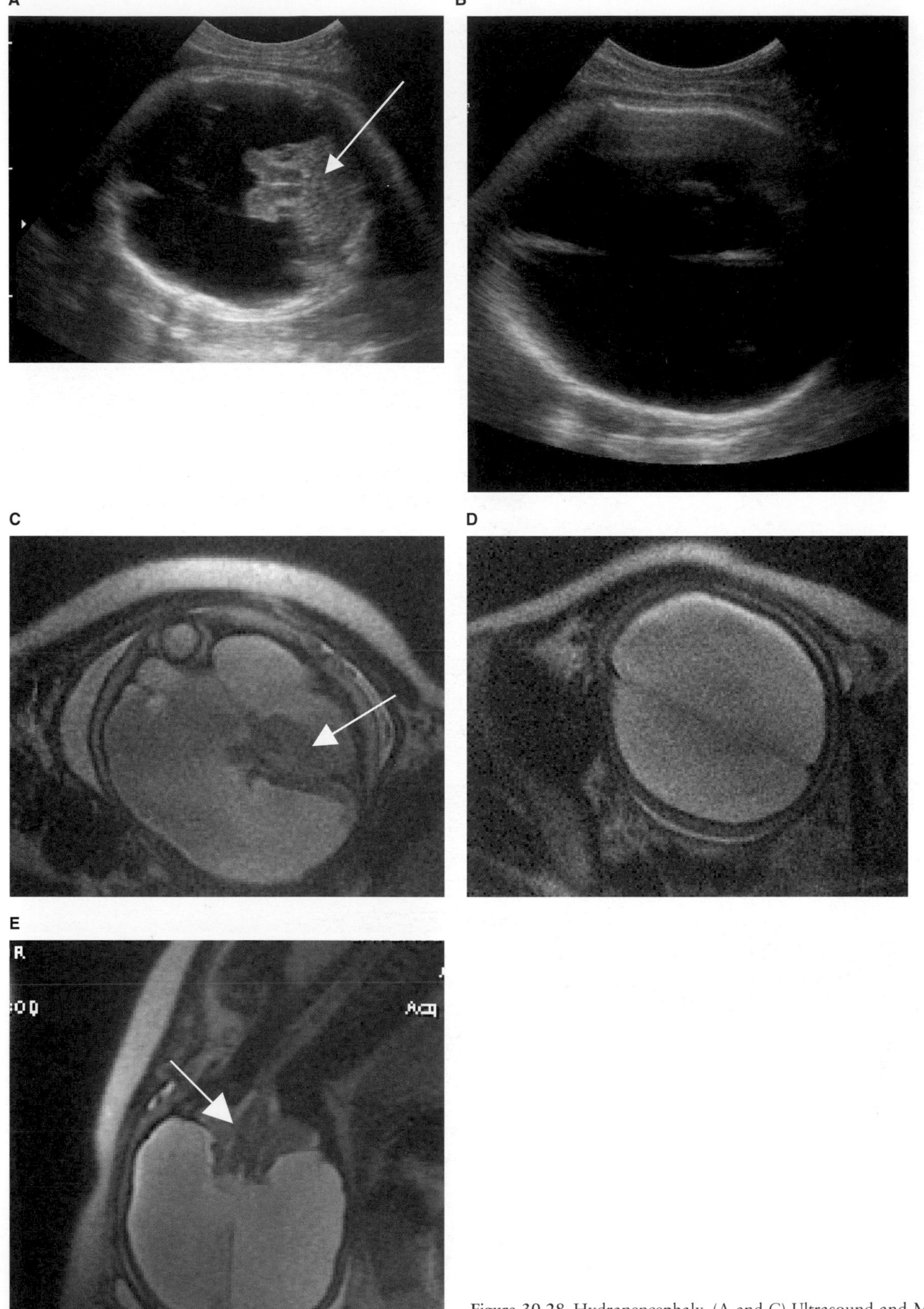

Figure 30.28 Hydranencephaly. (A and C) Ultrasound and MRI showed preservation of the midbrain and posterior fossa (arrow). (B and C) These images show nonvisualization of the cerebral cortex superiorly.

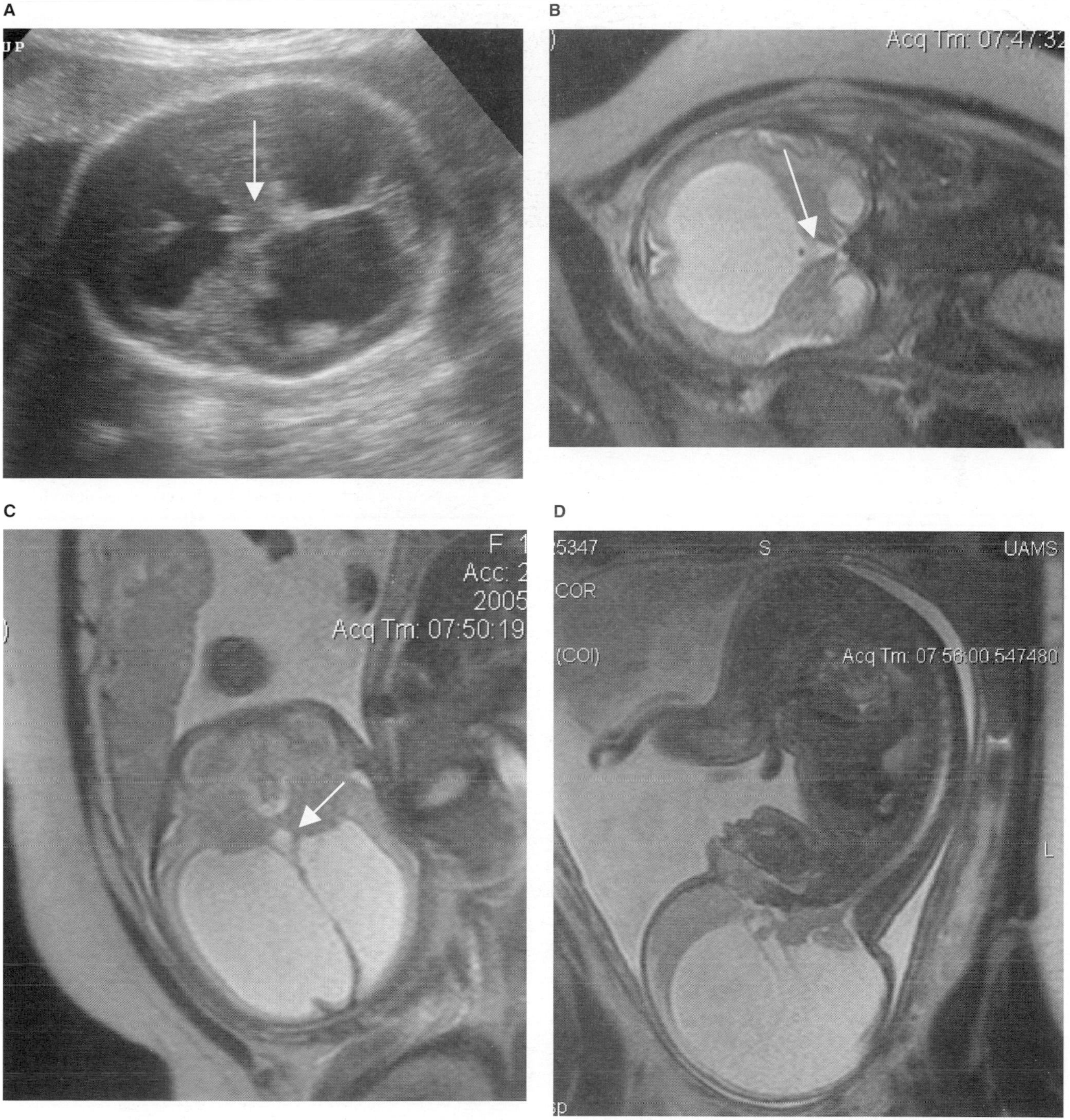

Figure 30.29 Aqueductal stenosis. Both ultrasound (A) and MRI (B and C) images show massive hydrocephalus with enlargement of the third ventricle (arrow). The cerebral mantle is very thin but preserved in all of the images.

A

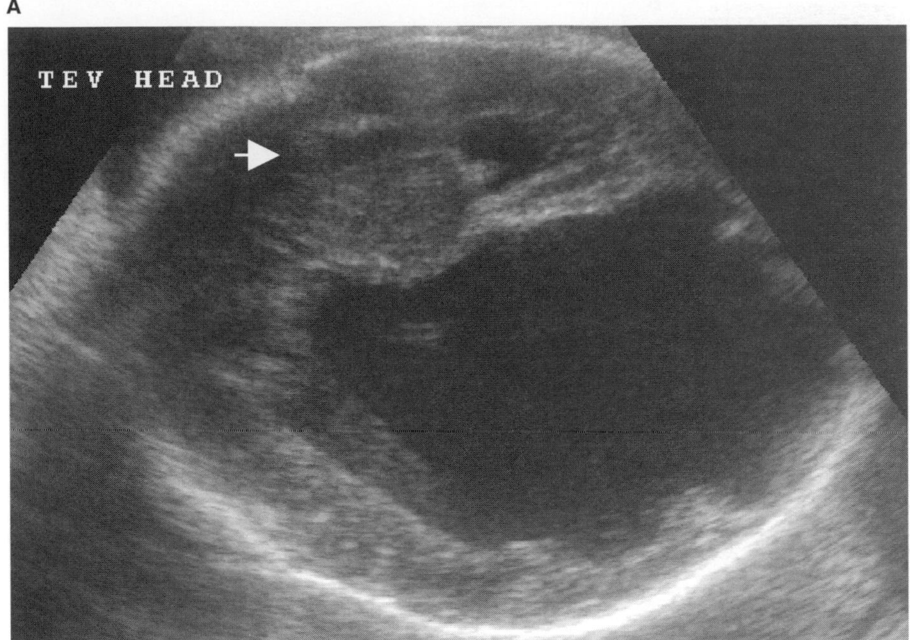

Figure 30.30 Agenesis of the corpus callosum with an interhemispheric cyst. The ultrasound image (A) suggested unilateral hydrocephalus. MRI (B–E) showed that the lateral ventricle (long arrow) is separate from the large interhemispheric cyst that has occupied the majority of the left side of the brain. There is no corpus callosum identified on MRI. The parallel orientation of the frontal horn (short arrow) and its wide separation from the midline is consistent with this diagnosis on both ultrasound and MRI.

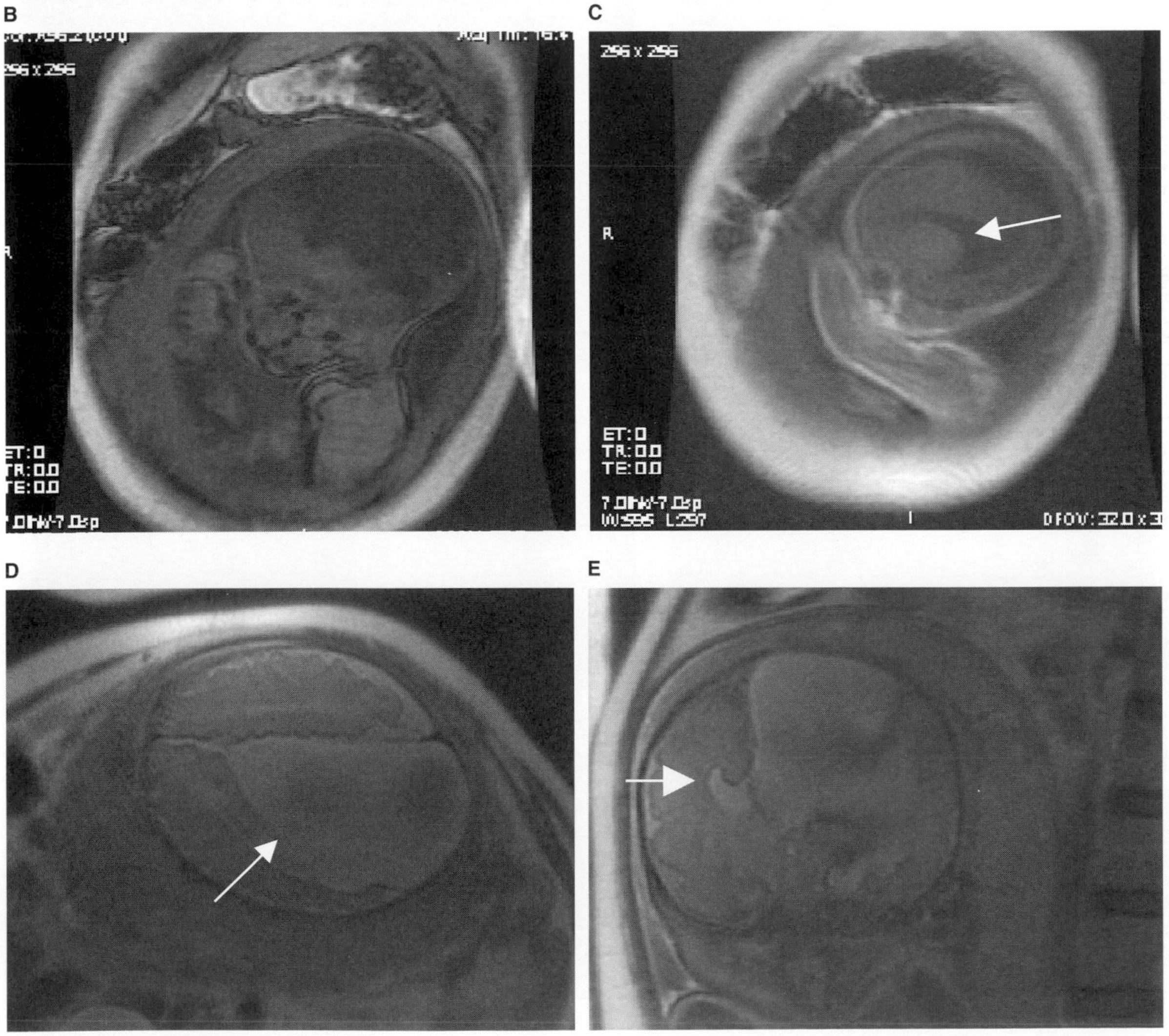

B

C

D

E

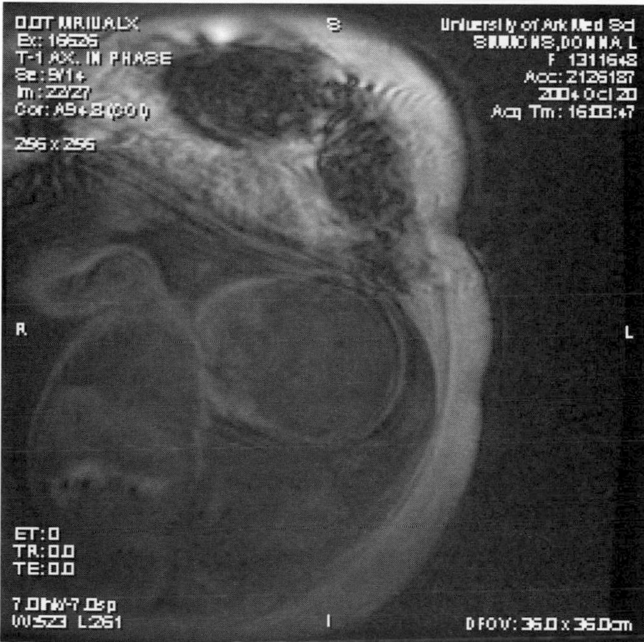

Figure 30.31 Maternal breathing motion has degraded MRI resolution of fetal anatomy.

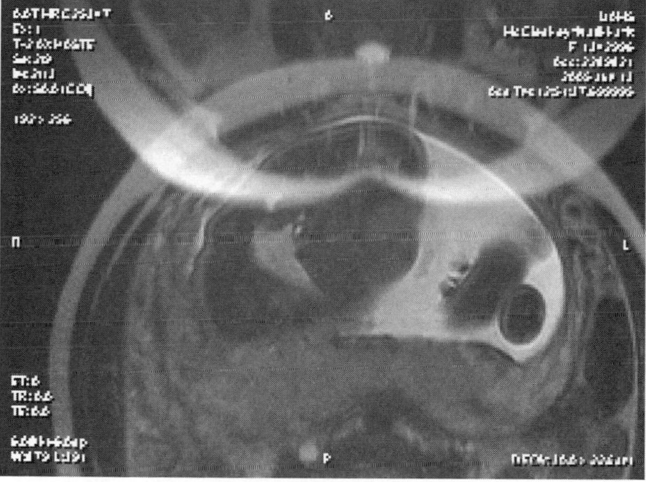

Figure 30.32 Inappropriate field of view settings can create wrap artifacts that superimpose on the region of interest.

most powerful resource. The numerous publications regarding the merits of prenatal MRI have often been brought up by patients during consultation. The obstetrician therefore becomes a gatekeeper in the determination of the need for MRI under a variety of instances.

In complicated cases, the MRI examination should be interpreted in consultation with a multispecialty team. The perspectives of a maternal–fetal medicine specialist, radiologist, or pediatrician can complement one another in a complex case and provide the best set of differential diagnoses. In CNS anomalies, for instance, neuroradiologists can provide a wider range of possible diagnoses than those who do not deal with these cases on an everyday basis. As always, the ultrasound findings need to come into play in the performance and interpretation of any MRI examination. In many instances, the findings on ultrasound determine the best planes to start an MRI examination. Frequent references to the ultrasound study can clarify any confusion brought about by fetal change in position or artifacts of scanning. In most instances, the MRI study is tailored to the area of concern on ultrasound. If the abnormality is within the brain, MRI of the fetal chest and abdomen are de-emphasized, and the planes of imaging are centered on those that will best demonstrate the brain abnormality. This focus will not only decrease the time required to keep the mother in the magnet, but will also simplify an examination that could otherwise not only take time but also produce hundreds of images for interpretation. When these factors are taken into consideration, the power of ultrasound and MRI together can increase the accuracy of diagnosis by several degrees of magnitude.

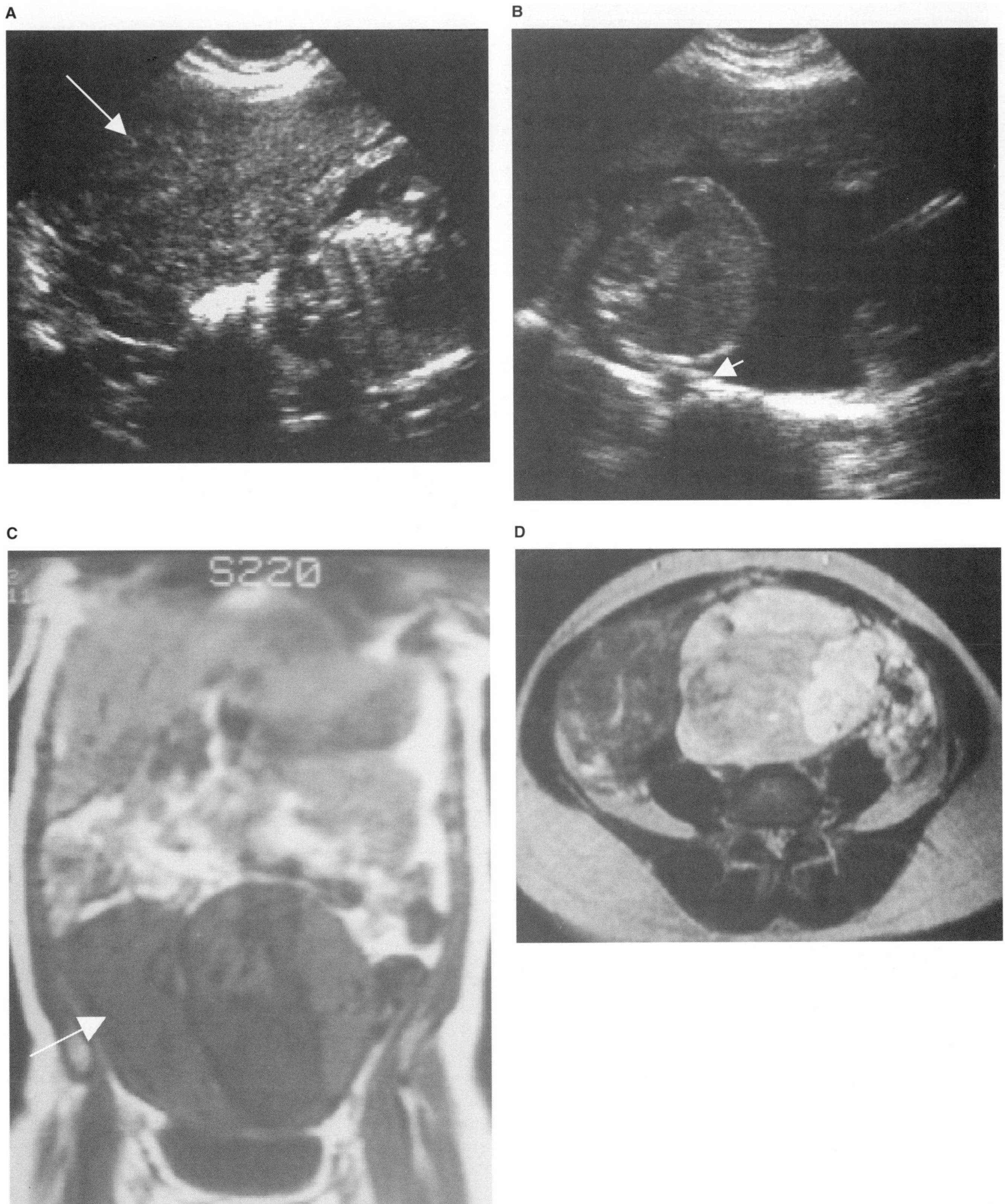

Figure 30.33 Abdominal pregnancy. Ultrasound images show the empty uterus (long arrow) anterior to the fetus (A). There is no myometrium posterior to the fetus separating the body from the common iliac artery (short arrow) (B). MRI confirmation images (C) and (D) show the uterus (long arrow) separate from the fetus on the coronal T1-weighted image (C). T2-weighted axial image (D) shows the typical high signal arising from the endometrium.

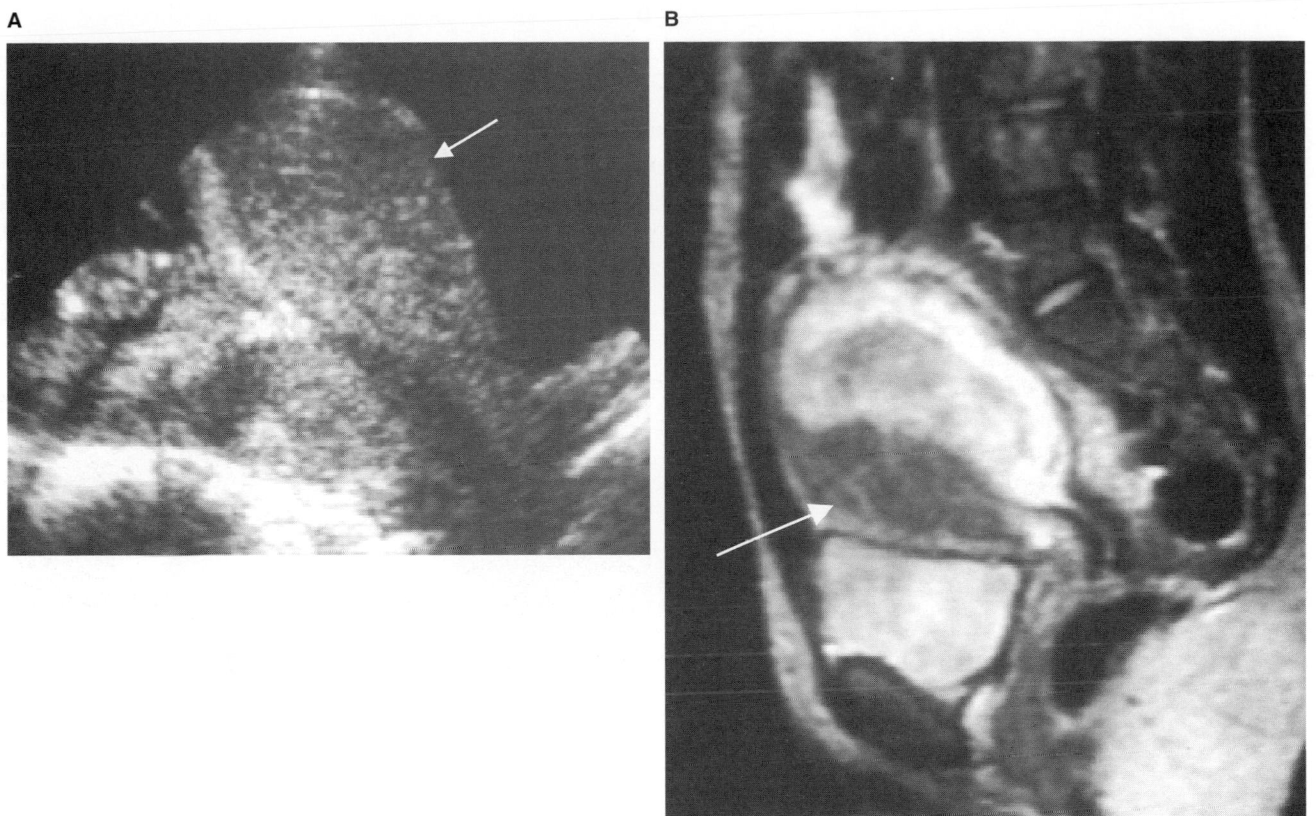

Figure 30.34 Uterine leiomyoma. An anterior myoma (arrow) raised the suspicion of an empty uterus in an abdominal pregnancy in ultrasound (A). MRI showed the normal gestational sac and the anterior myoma (B).

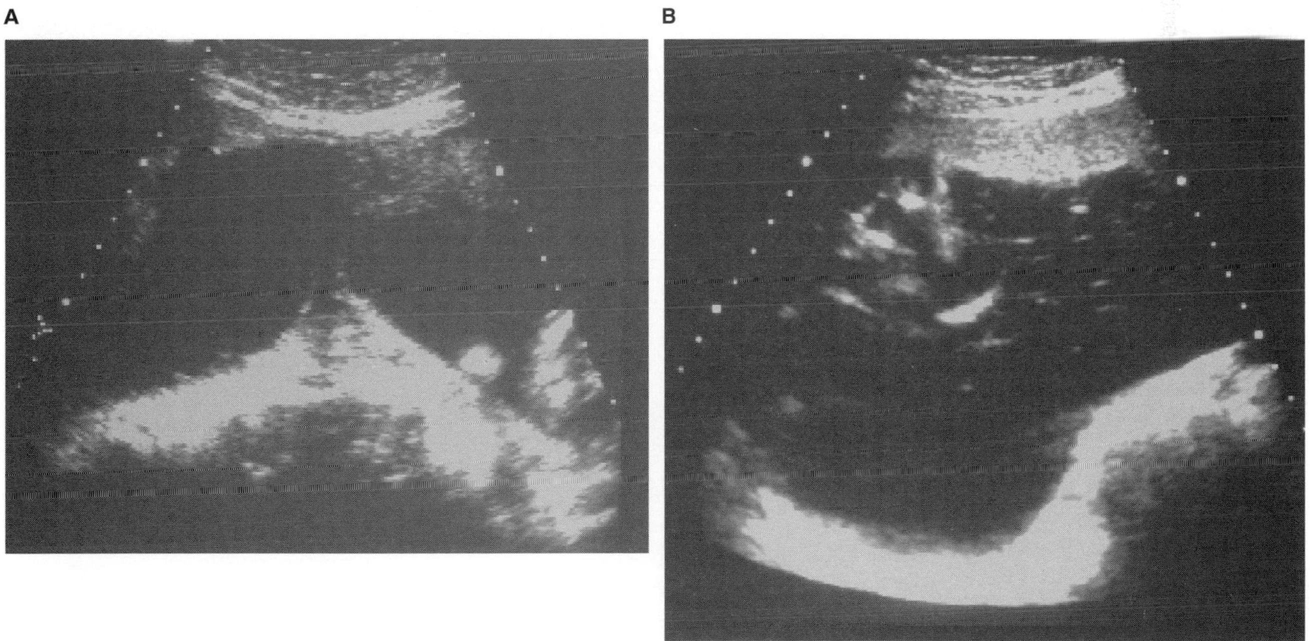

Figure 30.35 Teratoma. A large teratoma was mistaken for a demised twin on ultrasound (A and B). MRI shows a typical fat signal on T1-weighted image (C) and high-signal fluid component on T2-weighted image (D).

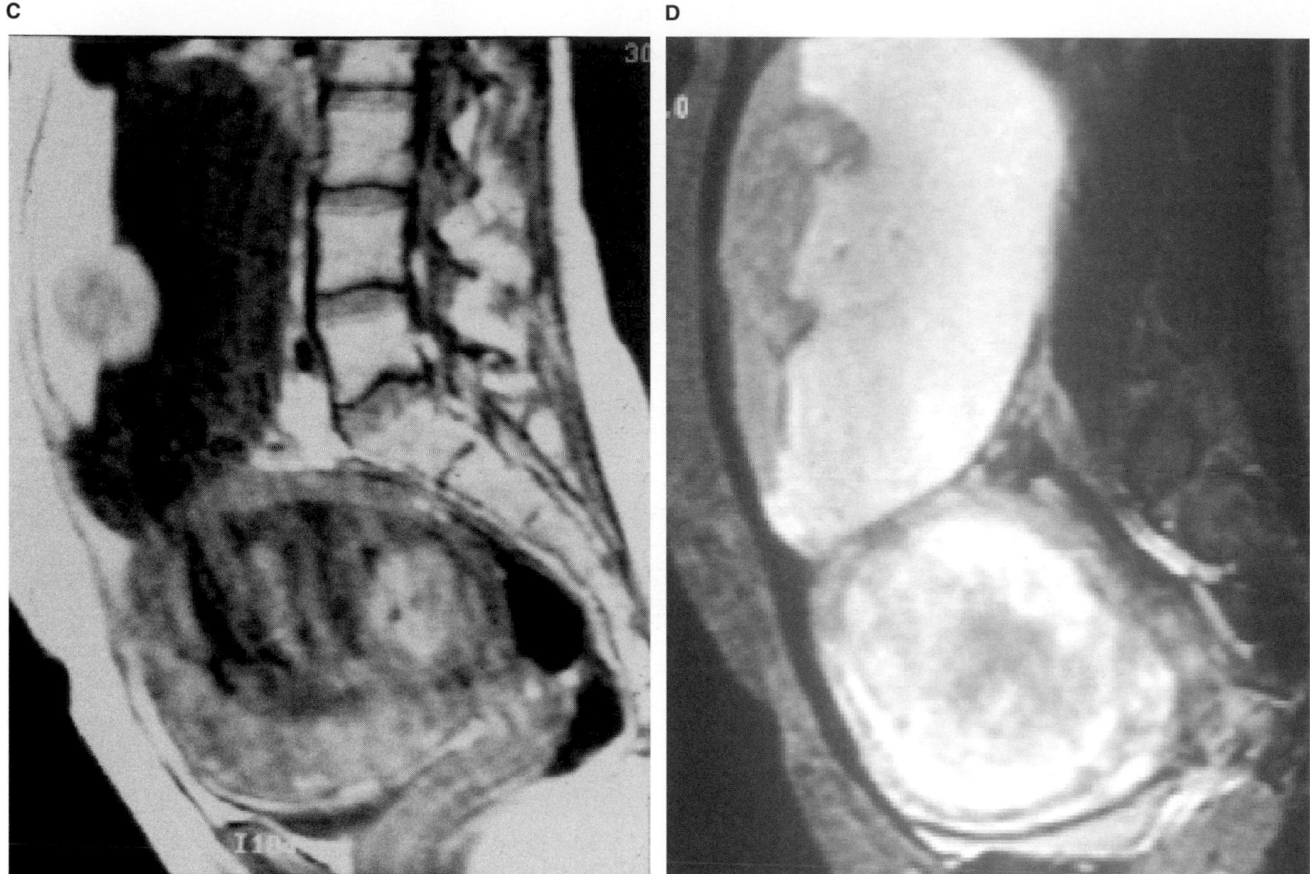

Figure 30.35 *Continued*

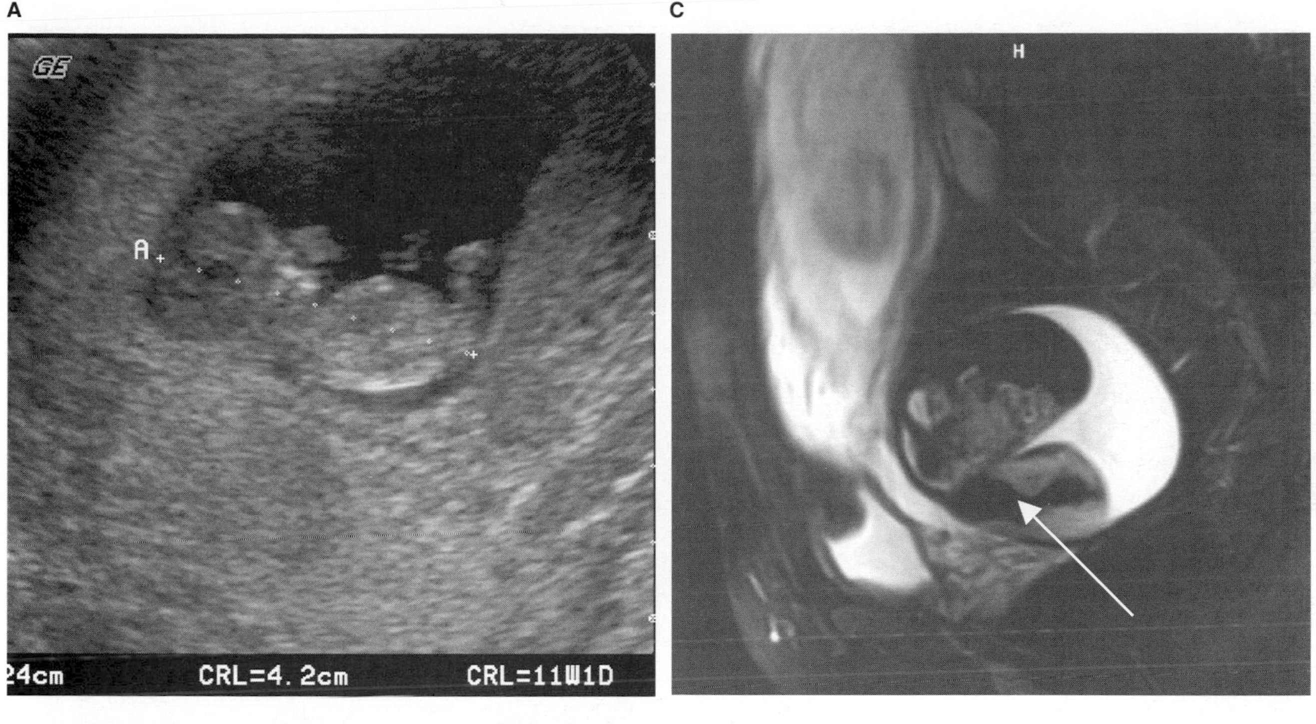

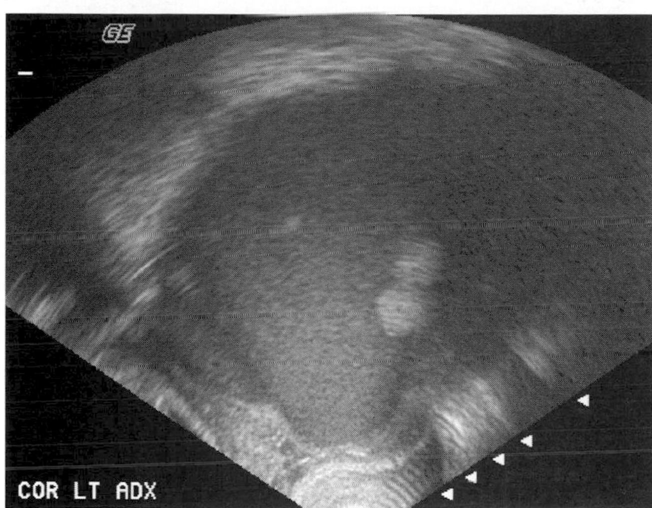

Figure 30.36 Teratoma. A mass associated with a first-trimester gestation showed typical MRI characteristics: on fat suppression, the fat-containing elements (arrow) decrease in signal relative to the fluid component (C). (A) The normal first-trimester fetus with a crown–rump length measurement corresponding to 11 weeks' gestation. (B) An endovaginal image of the dermoid showing better the cystic and solid components. Note the non-layering debris in the mass corresponding to a mixture of liquid and fat.

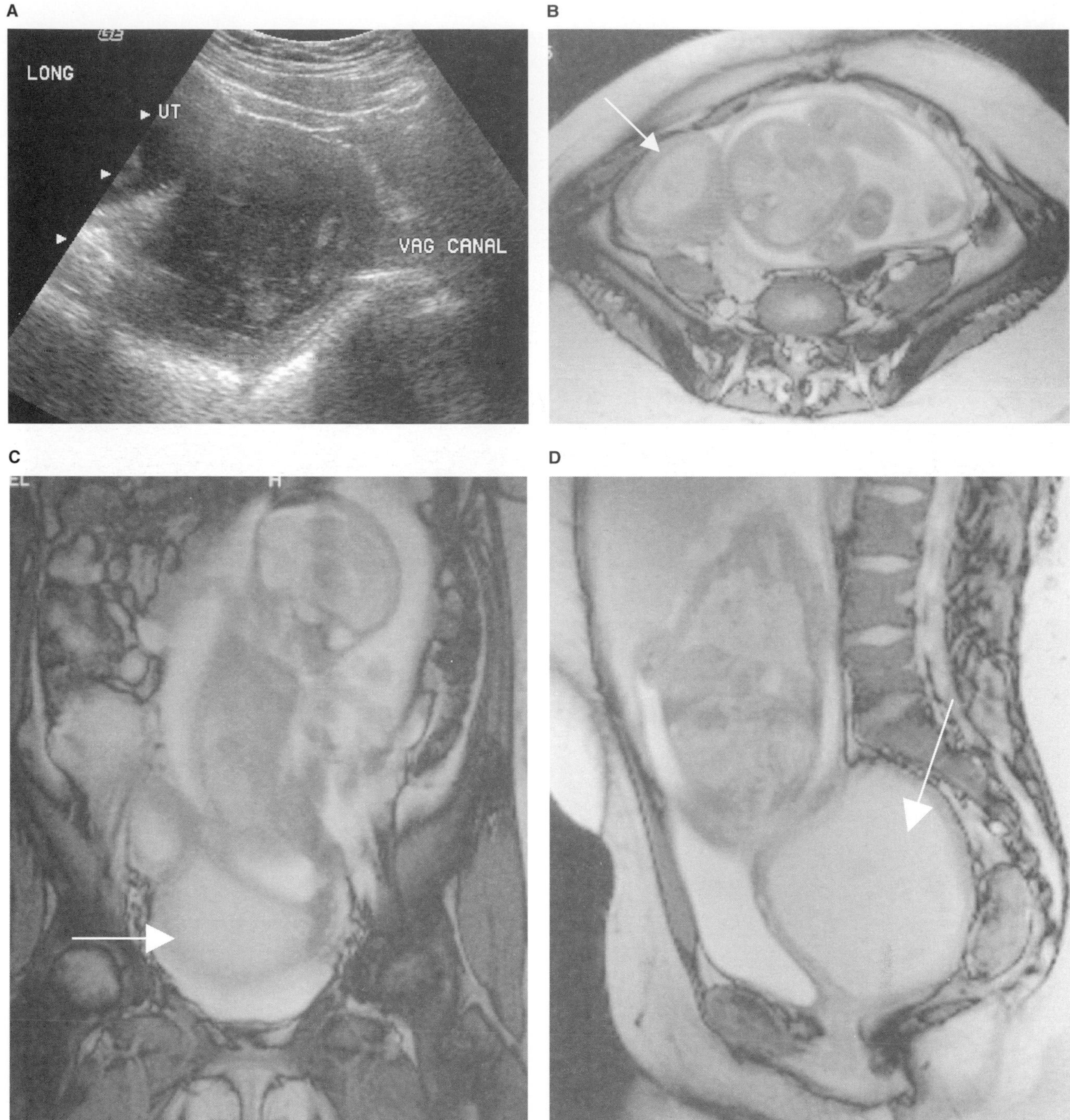

Figure 30.37 MRI images of uterus didelphys with normal pregnancy in the left uterine cavity and hematometra in the obstructed right uterine cavity (arrow) (B–D). This presented on ultrasound as a vaginal mass with heterogeneous echoes (A).

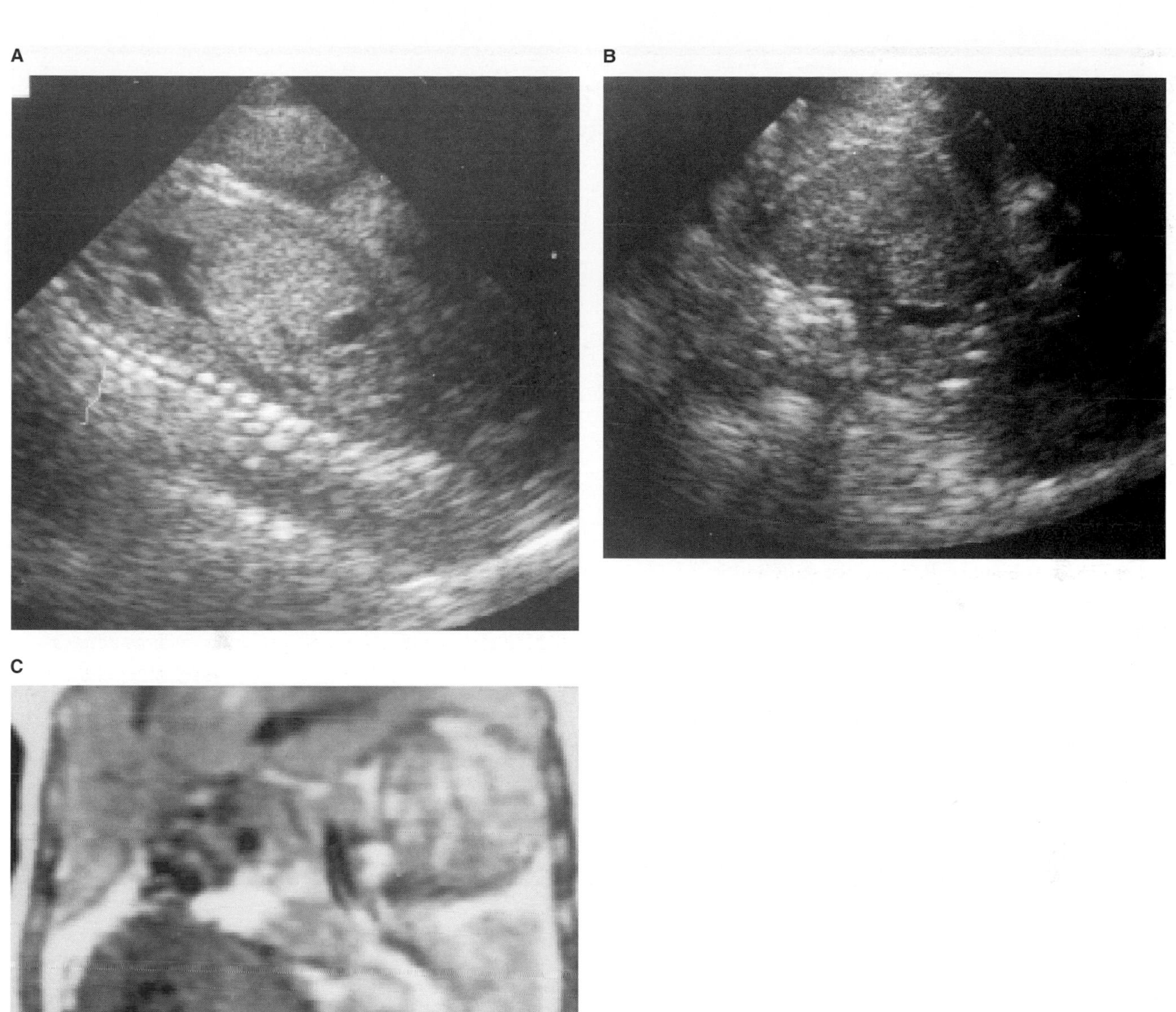

Figure 30.38 Unicornuate uterus. Severe oligohydramnios was seen on ultrasound (A and B) limiting fetal evaluation. MRI (C) shows the pregnancy in the unicornuate uterus, which was only diagnosed at Cesarean section.

Key points

1 Prenatal diagnosis expertise requires familiarity with 3D/4D ultrasound and MRI to remain at the cutting edge of technology.

2 3D ultrasound provides data storage that can be accessed to reconstruct any desired image plane.

3 Stored volumetric data can be reviewed by multiple examiners long after the examination has ended.

4 Digital storage of data allows for consultation among specialists at different locations.

5 4D ultrasound is 3D ultrasound with dynamic display of rendered images in real time.

6 The use of 3D/4D ultrasound solely for entertainment purposes is not a prudent use of medical technology and is discouraged.

7 3D/4D ultrasound has been promoted as a technique that enhances bonding between the fetus and its parents.

8 Detection of fetal anomalies with the use of 3D ultrasound has been proven useful in the demonstration of complex facial anomalies.

9 Complicated limb abnormalities are clearly shown on 3D imaging.

10 The application of 3D/4D ultrasound in the abdomen has seen limited use at this time.

11 Electronic artifacts can be generated by motion, oligohydramnios, and faulty electronic settings.

12 MRI applications in obstetrics have been proven in the second half of pregnancy, but have limited use in the first trimester.

13 Rapid scanning sequences available in modern MRI equipment have obviated the use of paralyzing agents for the fetus.

14 Artifacts can be generated on MRI images by both fetal motion and maternal motion.

15 The use of MRI should always be correlated with a recently performed ultrasound examination to facilitate the performance of the examination and the diagnosis of fetal abnormalities.

16 The greatest application of MRI in the fetus to date has been in the CNS, with increasing applications in the chest and abdomen.

17 Abnormalities detected but not conclusive on ultrasound should be pursued with an MRI examination.

18 Nonfetal complications of pregnancy such as adnexal masses and uterine anomalies are best evaluated with MRI.

19 The diagnosis of complicated fetal anomalies should be approached by a multidisciplinary team to maximize the diagnostic power of the examination.

20 The combination of ultrasound and MRI increases the accuracy of fetal diagnosis more than either modality alone.

References

1 Michailidis GD, Economides DL, Schild RL. The role of three-dimensional ultrasound in obstetrics. *Curr Opin Obstet Gynecol* 2001;13:207.

2 Kurjak A, Kupesic S, Kos M. Three-dimensional sonography for assessment of morphology and vascularization of the fetus and placenta. *J Soc Gynecol Invest* 2002;9:186.

3 Lee W, Kalache KD, Chaiworapongsa T, et al. Three-dimensional power Doppler ultrasonography during pregnancy. *J Ultrasound Med* 2003;22:91.

4 Dyson RL, Pretorius DH, Budorick NE, et al. Three-dimensional ultrasound in the evaluation of fetal anomalies. *Ultrasound Obstet Gynecol* 2000;16:321.

5 Merz E. 3-D Ultrasound in prenatal diagnosis. In: *Ultrasound in obstetrics and gynecology*, 2nd edn. New York: Thieme; 2005: 515–528.

6 Kurjak A, Hafner T, Kos M, et al. Three-dimensional sonography in prenatal diagnosis: a luxury or a necessity? *J Perinat Med* 2000;28:194.

7 Yanagihara T, Hata T. Three-dimensional sonographic visualization of fetal skeleton in the second trimester pregnancy. *Gynecol Obstet Invest* 2000;49:12.

8 Steiner H, Spitzer D, Weiss-Wichert PH, et al. Three-dimensional ultrasound in prenatal diagnosis of skeletal dysplasia. *Prenat Diagn* 1995;15:373.

9 Ploeckinger-Ulm B, Ulm MR, Lee A, et al. Antenatal depiction of fetal digits with three-dimensional ultrasonography. *Am J Obstet Gynecol* 1996;175:571.

10 Megier P, Esperandieu O, Martin JG, Desroches A. Three-dimensional ultrasound in the diagnosis of left upper limb amelia and right upper limb deficiency at 10 weeks gestation. *Ultrasound Obstet Gynecol* 2002;20:303.

11 Krakow D, Williams J, III, Poehl M, et al. Use of three-dimensional ultrasound imaging in the diagnosis of prenatal-onset skeletal dysplasia. *Ultrasound Obstet Gynecol* 2003;21:467.

12 Timor-Tritsch IE, Monteagudo A, Mayberry P. Three-dimensional ultrasound of the fetal brain: the three horn view. *Ultrasound Obstet Gynecol* 2000;16:302.

13 Pretorius DH, Nelson TR. Prenatal visualization of cranial sutures and fontanelles with three-dimensional ultrasonography. *J Ultrasound Med* 1994;13:871.

14 Schild RL, Wallny T, Fimmers R, Hansmann M. The size of the fetal thoracolumbar spine: a three-dimensional ultrasound study. *Ultrasound Obstet Gynecol* 2000;16:468.

15 Lee W, Chaiworapongsa T, Romero R, et al. A diagnostic approach for the evaluation of spina bifida by three-dimensional ultrasound. *J Ultrasound Med* 2002;21:619.

16 Lee W, McNie B, Chaiworapongsa T, et al. Three-dimensional

ultrasonographic presentation of micrognathia. *J Ultrasound Med* 2002;21:775.

17 Johnson DD, Pretorius DH, Budorick NE, et al. Fetal lip and primary palate: three-dimensional versus two-dimensional US. *Radiology* 2000;217:236.

18 Chmait R, Pretorius D, Jones M, et al. Prenatal evaluation of facial clefts with two-dimensional and adjunctive three-dimensional ultrasonography: a prospective trial. *Am J Obstet Gynecol* 2002;187:946.

19 Carlson DE. The ultrasound evaluation of cleft lip and palate – a clear winner for 3D. *Ultrasound Obstet Gynecol* 2000;16:299.

20 Benacerraf BR, Spiro R, Mitchell AG. Using three-dimensional ultrasound to detect craniosynostosis in a fetus with Pfeiffer syndrome. *Ultrasound Obstet Gynecol* 2000;16:391.

21 Xu HX, Zang QP, Lu MD, Xiao XT. Comparison of two-dimensional and three-dimensional sonography in evaluating fetal malformations. *J Clin Ultrasound* 2002;30:515.

22 Paul C, Krampl E, Skentou C, et al. Measurement of fetal nuchal translucency thickness by three-dimensional ultrasound. *Ultrasound Obstet Gynecol* 2001;18:481.

23 Kupesic S, Hafner T, Bjelos D. Events from ovulation to implantation studied by three-dimensional ultrasound. *J Perinat Med* 2002;30:84.

24 Hsu TY, Chang SY, Ou CY, et al. First trimester diagnosis of holoprosencephaly and cyclopia with triploidy by transvaginal three-dimensional ultrasonography. *Eur J Obstet Gynecol Reprod Biol* 2001;96:235.

25 Anandakumar C, Nurruddin Badruddin M, Chua TM, et al. First-trimester prenatal diagnosis of omphalocele using three-dimensional ultrasonography. *Ultrasound Obstet Gynecol* 2002; 20:635.

26 Benoit B, Hafner T, Kurjak A, et al. Three-dimensional sonoembryology. *J Perinat Med* 2002;30:63.

27 Osada H, Iitsuka Y, Masuda K, et al. Application of lung volume measurement by three-dimensional ultrasonography for clinical assessment of fetal lung development. *J Ultrasound Med* 2002;21:841.

28 Kalache KD, Espinoza J, Chaiworapongsa T, et al. Three-dimensional ultrasound fetal lung volume measurement: a systematic study comparing the multiplanar method with the rotational (VOCAL) technique. *Ultrasound Obstet Gynecol* 2003;21: 111.

29 Hubbard AM, Adzick NS, Crombleholme TM, et al. Congenital chest lesions: diagnosis and characterization with prenatal MR imaging. *Radiology* 1999;212:43.

30 Schild RL, Plath H, Hofstaetter C, Hansmann M. Diagnosis of a fetal mesoblastic nephroma by 3D-ultrasound. *Ultrasound Obstet Gynecol* 2000;15:533.

31 Cafici D, Iglesias A. Prenatal diagnosis of severe hypospadias with two- and three-dimensional sonography. *J Ultrasound Med* 2002;21:1423.

32 Chen CP, Shih JC, Tzen CY, Wang W. Three-dimensional ultrasound in the evaluation of complex anomalies associated with fetal ventral midline defects. *Ultrasound Obstet Gynecol* 2002;19: 102.

33 Goncalves LF, Lee W, Chaiworapongsa T, et al. Four-dimensional ultrasonography of the fetal heart with spatiotemporal image correlation. *Am J Obstet Gynecol* 2003;189:1792.

34 Goncalves LF, Romero R, Espinoza J, et al. Four-dimensional ultrasonography of the fetal heart using color Doppler spatiotemporal image correlation. *J Ultrasound Med* 2004;23:473.

35 Nelson TR, Pretorius DH, Sklansky M, Hagen-Ansert S. Three-dimensional echocardiographic evaluation of fetal heart anatomy and function: acquisition, analysis, and display. *J Ultrasound Med* 1996;15:1.

36 Zosmer N, Jurkovic D, Jauniaux E, et al. Selection and identification of standard cardiac views from three-dimensional volume scans of the fetal thorax. *J Ultrasound Med* 1996;15:25.

37 Bega G, Kuhlman K, Lev-Toaff A, et al. Application of three-dimensional ultrasonography in the evaluation of the fetal heart. *J Ultrasound Med* 2001;20:307.

38 Meyer-Wittkopf M, Rappe N, Sierra F, et al. Three-dimensional (3-D) ultrasonography for obtaining the four and five-chamber view: comparison with cross-sectional (2-D) fetal sonographic screening. *Ultrasound Obstet Gynecol* 2000;15:397.

39 Leventhal M, Pretorius DH, Sklansky MS, et al. Three-dimensional ultrasonography of normal fetal heart: comparison with two-dimensional imaging. *J Ultrasound Med* 1998:17:341.

40 Michel SC, Rake A, Treiber K, et al. MR obstetric pelvimetry: effect of birthing position on pelvic bony dimensions. *Am J Roentgenol* 2002;179:1063.

41 Nagayama M, Watanabe Y, Okumura A, et al. Fast MR imaging in obstetrics. *Radiographics* 2002;22:563.

42 Tamsel S, Ozbek SS, Sener RN, et al. MR imaging of fetal abnormalities. *Comput Med Imaging Graph* 2004;28:141.

43 Borowska-Matwiejczuk K, Lemancewicz A, Tarasow E, et al. Assessment of fetal distress based on magnetic resonance examinations: preliminary report. *Acad Radiol* 2003;10:1274.

44 Baker PN, Johnson IR, Harvey PR, et al. A three-year follow-up of children imaged in utero using echo planar magnetic resonance. *Am J Obstet Gynecol* 1994;170:32.

45 Kanal E, Gillen J, Evans JA, et al. Survey of reproductive health among female MR workers. *Radiology* 1993;187:395.

46 Levine D, Smith AS, McKenzie C. Tips and tricks of fetal MR imaging. *Radiol Clin North Am* 2003;41:729.

47 Ertl-Wagner B, Lienemann A, Strauss A, Reiser MF. Fetal magnetic resonance imaging: indications, technique, anatomical considerations, and a review of fetal abnormalities. *Eur Radiol* 2002;12:1931.

48 Levine D, Barnes PD, Robertson RR, et al. Fast MRI of fetal central nervous system abnormalities. *Radiology* 2003;229:51.

49 Peng SS, Shih JC, Liu HM, et al. Ultrafast fetal MR images of intracranial teratoma. *J Comput Assist Tomogr* 1999;23:318.

50 Glastonbury CM, Kennedy AM. Ultrafast MRI of the fetus. *Aust Radiol* 2002;46:22.

51 Angtuaco TL, Shah HR, Mattison DR, Quirk JG. Magnetic resonance imaging in high-risk obstetric patients: a valuable complement to ultrasound. *Radiographics* 1992;12:91.

52 Coakley FV, Hricak H, Filly FA, et al. Complex fetal disorders: effect of MR imaging on management – preliminary clinical experience. *Radiology* 1999;213:691.

53 Spielmann AL, Freed KS, Spritzer CE. MRI of conjoined twins illustrating advances in fetal imaging. *J Comput Assist Tomogr* 2001;25:88.

54 Coakley FV. Role of magnetic resonance imaging in fetal surgery. *Topics Magn Reson Imag* 2001;12:39.

55 Baldoli C, Righini A, Parazzini C, et al. Demonstration of acute ischemic lesions in the fetal brain by diffusion magnetic resonance imaging. *Ann Neurol* 2002;52:243.

56 Bargallo N, Peurto B, De Juan C, et al. Hereditary subependymal heterotopia associated with mega cisterna magna: antenatal diagnosis with magnetic resonance imaging. *Ultrasound Obstet Gynecol* 2002;20:86.

57 Claude I, Daire JL, Sebag G. Fetal brain MRI: segmentation and biometric analysis of the posterior fossa. *IEEE Trans Biomed Eng* 2004;51:617.

58 de Laveaucoupet J, Audibert F, Guis F, et al. Fetal magnetic resonance imaging (MRI) of ischemic brain injury. *Prenat Diagn* 2001;21:729.
59 Falkai P, Schneider-Axmann T, Honer WG, et al. Influence of genetic loading, obstetric complications, and premorbid adjustment on brain morphology in schizophrenia: a MRI study. *Eur Arch Psychiatry Clin Neurosci* 2003;253:92.
60 Garel C, Chantrel E, Elmaleh M, et al. Fetal MRI: normal gestational landmarks for cerebral biometry, gyration and myelination. *Childs Nerv Syst* 2003;19:422.
61 Girard N, Gire C, Sigaudy S, et al. MR imaging of acquired fetal brain disorders. *Childs Nerv Syst* 2003;19:490.
62 Golja AM, Estroff JA, Robertson RL. Fetal imaging of central nervous system abnormalities. *Neuroimag Clin North Am* 2004;14:293.
63 Guo WY, Wong TT. Screening of fetal CNS anomalies by MR imaging. *Childs Nerv Syst* 2003;19:410.
64 Kojima K, Suzuki Y, Seki K, et al. Prenatal diagnosis of lissencephaly (type II) by ultrasound and fast magnetic resonance imaging. *Fetal Diagn Ther* 2002;17:34.
65 Malinger G, Lev D, Lerman-Sagie T. Fetal central nervous system: MR imaging versus dedicated US – need for prospective, blind, comparative studies. *Radiology* 2004;232:306.
66 Merzoug V, Ferey S, Andre Ch, et al. Magnetic resonance imaging of the fetal brain. *J Neuroradiol* 2002;29:76.
67 Patel TR, Bannister CM, Thorne J. A study of prenatal ultrasound and postnatal magnetic imaging in the diagnosis of central nervous system abnormalities. *Eur J Pediatr Surg* 2003;13(Suppl. 1): 218.
68 Twickler DM, Magee KP, Caire J, et al. Second-opinion magnetic resonance imaging for suspected fetal central nervous system abnormalities. *Am J Obstet Gynecol* 2003;188:492.
69 Whitby EH, Paley NM, Sprigg A, et al. Comparison of ultrasound and magnetic resonance imaging in 100 singleton pregnancies with suspected brain abnormalities. *Br J Obstet Gynaecol* 2004;111: 784.
70 Levine D, Barnes P, Korf B, Edelman R. Tuberous sclerosis: second trimester diagnosis of subependymal tubers with fast MRI. *Am J Roentgenol* 2000;175:1067.
71 Ghi T, Tani G, Savelli L, et al. Prenatal imaging of facial clefts by magnetic resonance imaging with emphasis on the posterior palate. *Prenat Diagn* 2003;23:970.
72 Aronson OS, Hernanz-Schulman M, Bruner JP, et al. Myelomeningocele: prenatal evaluation – comparison between transabdominal US and MR imaging. *Radiology* 2003;227: 839.
73 Avni FE, Guibaud L, Robert Y, et al. MR imaging of fetal sacrococcygeal teratoma: diagnosis and assessment. *Am J Roentgenol* 2002;178:179.
74 Jeffrey JE, Campbell DM, Golden MH, et al. Antenatal factors in the development of the lumbar vertebral canal: a magnetic resonance imaging study. *Spine* 2003;28:1418.
75 Duncan KR, Gowland PA, Freeman A, et al. The changes in magnetic resonance properties of the fetal lungs: a first result and a potential tool for the non-invasive in utero demonstration of fetal lung maturation. *Br J Obstet Gynaecol* 1999;106:122.
76 Hubbard AM, Adzick NS, Crombleholme TM, et al. Congenital chest lesions: diagnosis and characterization with prenatal MR imaging. *Radiology* 1999:212:43.
77 Langer JC, Hussain H, Khan A, et al. Prenatal diagnosis of esophageal atresia using sonography and magnetic resonance imaging. *J Pediatr Surg* 2001;36:804.
78 Levine D, Barnewolt CE, Mehta TS, et al. Fetal thoracic abnormalities: magnetic resonance imaging. *Radiology* 2003;228:379.
79 Liu X, Ashtari M, Leonidas JC, Chan Y. Magnetic resonance imaging of the fetus in congenital intrathoracic disorders: preliminary observations. *Pediatr Radiol* 2001;31:435.
80 Sabogal JC, Becker E, Bega G, et al. Reproducibility of fetal lung volume measurements with 3-dimensional ultrasonography. *J Ultrasound Med* 2004;23:347.
81 Shinmoto H, Kuribayashi S. MRI of fetal abdominal abnormalities. *Abdom Imaging* 2003;28:877.
82 Cassart M, Massez A, Metens T, et al. Complementary role of MRI after sonography in assessing bilateral urinary tract anomalies in the fetus. *Am J Roentgenol* 2004;182:689.
83 Claire JT, Ramus RM, Magee KP, et al. MRI of fetal genitourinary anomalies. *Am J Roentgenol* 2003;181:1381.
84 Granata C, Dell'Acqua A, Lituania M, et al. Gastric duplication cyst: appearance on prenatal US and MRI. *Pediatr Radiol* 2003:33:148.
85 Martin C, Darnell A, Duran C, et al. Magnetic resonance imaging of the intrauterine fetal genitourinary tract: normal anatomy and pathology. *Abdom Imaging* 2004;29:286.
86 Matsuoka S, Takeuchi K, Yamanaka Y, et al. Comparison of magnetic resonance imaging and ultrasonography in the prenatal diagnosis of congenital thoracic abnormalities. *Fetal Diagn Ther* 2003;18:447.
87 Rohrer SE, Nugent CE, Mukherji SK. Fetal MR imaging of lymphatic malformation in a twin gestation. *Am J Roentgenol* 2003;181:286.
88 Kawamotoa S, Ogawa F, Tanaka J, et al. Chorioangioma: antenatal diagnosis with fast MR imaging. *Magn Reson Imag* 2000;18:911.
89 Verswijvel G, Grieten M, Gyselaers W, et al. MRI in the assessment of pregnancy related intrauterine bleeding: a valuable adjunct to ultrasound? *JBR-BTR J Belge Radiol* 2002;85:189.
90 Angtuaco TL. Sonography of non-fetal complications in pregnancy. *Contemp Diagn Radiol* 2002;25:1.

31 Doppler ultrasonography and fetal well-being

Brian J. Trudinger

Doppler ultrasound has provided a noninvasive clinical tool to assess blood flow in pregnancy in the circulations, previously precluded from direct study because of risk to the fetus from invasive procedures. The desire of obstetricians to measure blood flow, particularly to the placenta, has been achieved. Diagnoses such as "placental insufficiency" were created to express a hypothetical reduction in blood flow almost without any actual basis. The scope of Doppler studies has now extended from the placenta to many fetal vascular beds and a great variety of disorders of pregnancy. The information obtained from such studies has expanded our knowledge of the physiology of pregnancy and the pathophysiology of a variety of disorders, and provided a diagnostic tool for evaluation of the welfare of the fetus.

Doppler instrumentation

Doppler equipment used in obstetric practice ranges from the simplest fetal heart detectors through the fetal heart rate (FHR) monitors to the most sophisticated high-level ultrasound imaging systems. Common to all is the incorporation of the Doppler effect. When there is movement between a wave source and a reflecting target, there is a change in frequency of the reflected wave relative to the transmitted wave, and that change in frequency is proportional to movement velocity. The Doppler equation is:

$$F_D = F_1 - F_0 = (-2v\cos\theta \times F_0)/c$$

where F_0 is the transmitted frequency, F_1 the received frequency, c the velocity of sound in tissue, v the velocity of movement, and θ the angle between the ultrasound beam and the direction of flow. When an ultrasound beam strikes a blood vessel, the moving column of red blood cells scatters and reflects the ultrasound beam with a new frequency. The change in frequency or Doppler frequency shift (incident frequency minus reflected frequency) is proportional to the velocity of the red blood cell scatterers or blood flow velocity because the other terms are constants in the Doppler equation. This change in frequency may be displayed and used to calculate blood flow.

The ultrasound transducer of the Doppler used for flow studies can act as both the emitting source of the ultrasound beam and the receiver of the reflected signal. In continuous wave systems, there are separate crystals for each role, usually mounted side by side, whereas in a pulsed system, the single crystal emits an ultrasound pulse and then functions as a receiver. Activation of the crystal causes the conversion of electrical energy to an ultrasound beam during emission, and the returning ultrasound signal reverses this process. The weak returning signals are amplified and fed to the Doppler shift detector, which filters out unwanted frequencies (including the original ultrasound frequency) so that the Doppler frequency shift remains. This information is nondirectional. To separate the Doppler signals produced by flow toward and away from the transducer (forward and reverse flow), phase domain processing is commonly used. This requires two detectors with their reference inputs differing in phase by 90°. The filtered output signals are referred to as quadrature Doppler shift signals. Two types of Doppler systems are in use – continuous wave and pulsed. They differ in a number of ways. Continuous wave systems are continuously emitting from one crystal and receiving through another. They are relatively simple, cheap, and portable. The reflected echoes from any moving structure within the ultrasound beam are detected, so that there is no spatial resolution. Positioning the transducer and line of sight of the ultrasound beam is readily done. This system is used in simple fetal heart detectors. In the pulsed system, a short burst of the ultrasound wave is transmitted, and the crystal then acts as a receiver. A range gate circuit allows recording only at a specified time after the pulse emission, so the Doppler shift detected originates from a fixed depth. This type of processing may be referred to as setting the sample volume to a known depth. These Doppler velocimeters may exist as stand-alone items, but are now commonly built into ultrasound imaging systems. Integration with an imaging facility provides the ability to steer the ultrasound beam and, for pulsed Doppler systems, to locate the sample volume precisely over the vessel to be studied. In addition, the dimensions of the vessel under study may be measured.

The chosen frequency of the ultrasound beam is a compromise based on a number of considerations.[1] In general, the highest frequency producing a reliable signal is used. The depth of penetration (tissue attenuation) is inversely proportional to the square of the frequency. The degree of scattering is proportional to the fourth power of the frequency. The higher the transmitting frequency, the greater the Doppler frequency shift. With pulsed Doppler systems, there must be sufficient time to characterize the Doppler shift frequency before the next pulse is emitted. The laws of signal processing state that any Doppler signal with a frequency greater than the "Nyquist limit" (equal to half the pulse repetition rate) will be grossly distorted, suffering "frequency aliasing" and so appearing with quite different frequencies.

With medical equipment and vascular studies, the Doppler shift frequency usually falls in the audible range; therefore, the simplest display of the Doppler frequency shift is an audio signal. The method of choice is spectral analysis. If the vessel is totally insonated, the frequency spectrum represents all the different velocities across its lumen. The process of spectral analysis is carried out by a spectrum analyzer and is therefore also subject to the possibility of frequency aliasing if too fast a sampling rate is required. Equipment usually carries out the spectral analysis sufficiently quickly (less than 10 ms/spectrum) so that it is available in real time. It is also possible to display the frequency and direction of blood flow by color coding superimposed on the real-time ultrasound two-dimensional image ("color flow mapping"). This facility is particularly useful for locating vessels containing blood flow and determining the direction of flow of blood within a vessel. If the power of the frequency-shifted signals is displayed (rather than the frequency), then a power flow image is obtained. This facility is also a feature of ultrasound imaging systems now. Power imaging does not provide directional information.

Because blood flow velocity is directly proportional to the Doppler frequency shift, the information made available to the clinician by the Doppler instrumentation is a blood flow velocity waveform (FVW). The envelope of this wave is the maximum flow velocity. Beneath this is a frequency distribution, representing the various velocities of blood flow in the vessel under study. Both instantaneous and temporal mean flow velocities can be determined from this. If the angle between the ultrasound beam and the vessel is known, then the absolute velocity can be calculated. This requires the use of pulsed Doppler systems. Volume blood flow may be determined as the product of mean velocity and vessel area.

The blood flow velocity waveform

Blood flow is pulsatile. With each contraction of the heart, a pressure pulse or wave propagates down the aorta and its branches with an initial wave speed of 5 m/s. This creates a time-varying pressure gradient between neighboring points along the arterial tree. Blood flows ahead of this pressure gradient from high to low pressure. The blood flow is also pulsatile – the FVW. Doppler ultrasound systems record this FVW. Early in systole, the pressure and flow waveforms are in phase, but this breaks down later in systole because of the arrival of waves reflected from points of branching along the arterial tree and the periphery. The FVW travels more slowly than the pressure wave, and its amplitude decreases as it moves away from the heart. In the ascending aorta, following the opening of the aortic valve, blood flow velocity increases to a peak and then falls. After closure of the aortic valve, the blood is close to stationary for the remainder of the cardiac cycle.

The pressure and flow waveforms are influenced by cardiac contraction, the physical properties of the arterial walls and the blood within, and outflow impedance from the arterial tree. Traditionally, blood flow is described in terms of pressure and flow. Resistance has been defined as the ratio of mean pressure difference (or pressure head) across a vascular bed to mean flow through it. Resistance may also be conceptualized as how difficult it is to force blood through the circulation or the energy dissipation required for blood flow.[2] It is an artificial concept insofar as blood flow is not steady but pulsatile. Changes in resistance in clinical physiology are more often than not due to changes in the caliber of small blood vessels, but resistance is not necessarily only an index of arteriolar caliber. It also depends on the dispensability of the arterial walls (and transmural pressure) and blood viscosity.[3] The term impedance is introduced to take into consideration the pulsatile nature of blood flow, being the ratio of pulsatile pressure to pulsatile flow.[4] A consequence of pulsatile blood flow in comparison with steady flow is the requirement for more energy to move a given volume of blood, and much of this extra energy is used to distend the large arteries. The mean term resistance depends much more on arteriolar caliber than on large artery distention. Various indices derived from the FVW pattern have been defined to assess "resistance." They would appear to depend most on the size of the peripheral vascular bed.

When a blood vessel is interrogated with an ultrasound beam, not one but a spectrum of Doppler frequencies is found. This corresponds to all the different velocities across the flowing stream of blood. Each point across the vessel may be represented by a velocity vector, and a line through the tips of these vectors creates the velocity profile (Fig. 31.1). The variations in velocity result from the nonviscous and inhomogeneous nature of blood. The velocity profile also varies through the cardiac cycle and, in some circumstances, flow may not always be forward or in the same direction. Color flow mapping may demonstrate this.

If the lumen of the blood vessel has been totally insonated, all this information is available in the Doppler FVW. In order to recreate the exact velocity profile, it would be necessary to

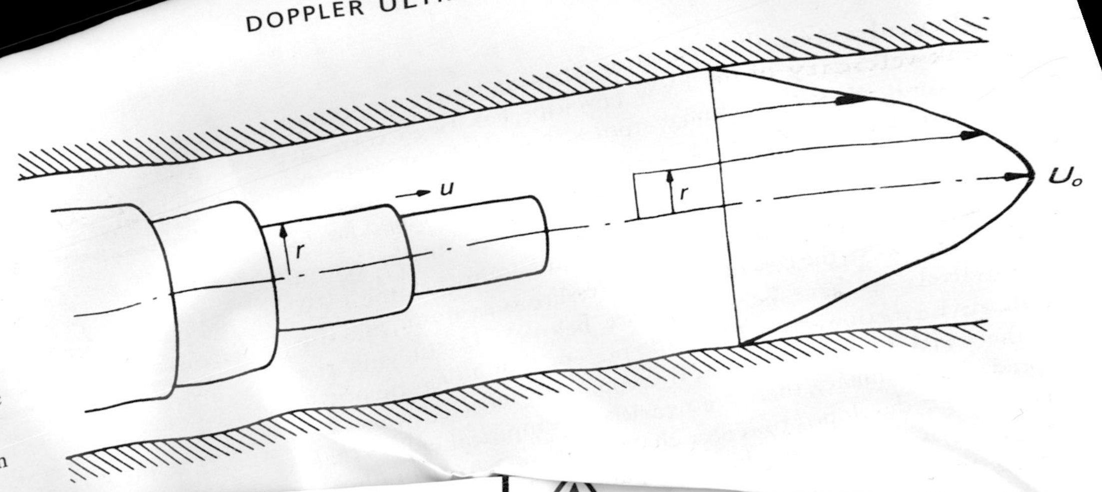

Figure 31.1 The blood flow velocity profile across a vessel. U_0, center line velocity; u, velocity at radial position r (modified from ref. 3, p. 47).

across the vessel. If the vessel is uniformly insonated, the mean Doppler frequency shift is proportional to the mean velocity, and this fact is used in the calculation of volume flow.[5] In a [illegible] with an established flow, the "boundary layer" is [illegible] laminar [illegible] increasing with distance [illegible] In the central stream, because there is movement is "en masse" and inertia is more important. If the disturbances of local geometry are ignored, then in large arterial vessels, inertial forces dominate blood flow, whereas in small vessels, viscous forces are more important. Reynold's number expresses the relative importance of these two forces.[3]

The Doppler FVW has been analyzed in a variety of different ways. In clinical applications, inferences about the cardiovascular system are made using empirical indices. The connection between an empirical index and a physiological variable may be based on a statistical association or evidence from an experimental model. In many situations, only the maximum velocity waveform (or the waveform envelope) is used. This is the easiest waveform to locate and is relatively error free. It does ignore all the information about the velocity profile contained within the frequency spectrum. The problems of analysis of the maximum mean and first moment of the velocity waveform in the fetal circulation have been reviewed.[6,7] The shape of the waveform envelope can be considered a characteristic of the vascular site. Waveforms recorded from arteries supplying low-impedance vascular beds (e.g., internal carotid, umbilical, and uterine artery in pregnancy) exhibit relatively high forward velocities throughout diastole. A triphasic waveform shape, where there is a period of reverse flow in diastole, is characteristic of sites with high distal impedance. The peripheral impedance, vessel wall elasticity, the degree and geometry of any proximal stenoses, and the condition of the upstream pump all affect the waveform. All these factors are important, all can be affected in the disease state being investigated, and none can be independently eliminated or controlled in clinical practice. Even in normal, presumably healthy subjects, blood flow patterns at a site with complicated geometry such as the carotid bifurcation are very complex.

The fetal circulation is uniquely suited to Doppler waveform analysis by simple empirical indices. This is because of the absence of degenerative arterial disease. The umbilical circulation was the first to be studied, and the indices used for this fetal circulation have been directed toward assessing downstream resistance. Three are in common usage (Fig. 31.2). All of these are highly correlated. Coefficients in excess of 0.9 have been demonstrated when the indices are compared.[6,8] This means that the indices are all providing the same information about the same physiological variables. Choice of index, then, is a matter of convenience relative to the investigational task. The systolic:diastolic ratio is easiest to calculate. Abnormally high values, when there is little or no diastolic value, tend to infinity and become meaningless. The pulsatility index has a precise mathematical definition. It requires determination of the mean velocity, and this is usually an inaccurate estimate. The resistance index (Pourcelot ratio) is the only one normally distributed and has the advantage that the maximum value attainable is one. It has an extra arithmetic step in comparison with the systolic–diastolic ratio. All these indices, when used to interpret the maximum velocity waveform, should be seen as simple descriptors of the waveform pattern. They are not precisely estimatable quantities. There is an inherent systematic error of 10–20% in their calculation.[8] The same indices have been used to assess vasodilation in the

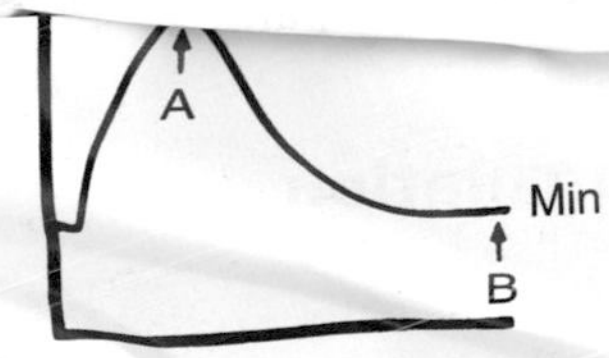

Pulsatility index $= \dfrac{A - B}{\text{Mean}}$

Pourcelot ratio $= \dfrac{A - B}{A}$

Systolic–diastolic ratio $= A/B$

Figure 31.2 The three indices of downstream resistance in common clinical use for the analysis of arterial flow velocity waveforms.

cerebral circulation (brain-sparing effect) in fetal compromise. The peak velocity of the FVW envelope has been correlated with volume flow[9] in animal studies, and this parameter has been used as an index in the cerebral circulation. In fetal anemia (e.g., rhesus alloimmunization), cerebral blood flow is increased. It has also been used in the aorta. In the central fetal veins (inferior vena cava and ductus venosus), the FVW pattern reflects the central venous pressure waveform, and different indices have been used (see below). In studying the maternal uterine artery FVW, the presence of a dicrotic notch at the end of systole, which is created by reflected waves, is noted. In summary, there are a variety of empirical indices that have been developed to reflect changes in the pattern of blood flow, which are the result of the pathophysiology of the disorder under study.

The umbilical circulation

The umbilical cord, linking the fetus and placenta, is long and suspended in amniotic fluid, and so is ideal for Doppler studies. The two umbilical arteries travel along this without branching or changes in lumen diameter. The radius of curvature of the loops of cord is large in comparison with the diameter of the umbilical arteries, and so is unlikely to significantly influence flow patterns. However, this spiraling course means that it is not possible to image a sufficient length of artery or vein to permit determination of the angle between the ultrasound beam and vessel, and so it is not possible to make Doppler volume flow measurements. Studies of the umbilical artery FVW using the indices of resistance have been carried out to assess the downstream vascular bed – the fetal placenta. The umbilical arteries can be readily studied with simple continuous wave Doppler ultrasound systems. They have been studied extensively, and these studies have been subjected to much critical appraisal.

Normal pregnancy

Blood flow through the umbilical circulation increases throughout pregnancy and represents some 40% of the combined ventricular output of the fetus.[10] The actual flow in the fetal lamb has been measured at 180–200 mL/min/kg fetus;[11] in human pregnancy, it is less, 100–110 mL/min/kg fetus.[12,13] The umbilical placental vascular bed is not innervated, and indeed is refractory to such circulating vasoconstrictors as epinephrine and norepinephrine.[11] Blood flow to the placenta appears to be the result of the balance between resistance to other fetal vascular beds and the placenta.[10] Almost certainly, there are local controls of placental blood flow that regulate the perfusion to keep a balance between the fetal and maternal placental flows.[14] It has been pointed out that the fetus does not need to regulate umbilical blood flow finely, because it has the capacity to vary tissue oxygen extraction ratios and, consequently, oxygen uptake.[15] The fetus requires oxygenated blood from the placenta for distribution to the fetal tissues, where uptake and delivery may be regulated.

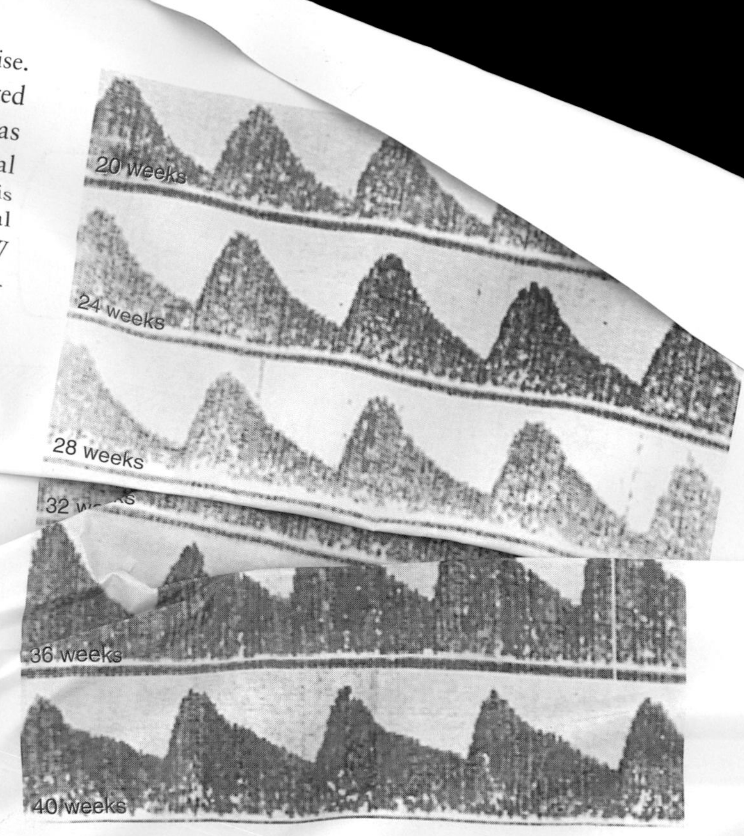

Figure 31.3 The changing form of the umbilical artery FVW recorded from one patient at varying periods of gestation.

The umbilical circulation is a low-resistance vascular bed, which is reflected in the pattern of the umbilical artery FVW (Fig. 31.3). Throughout pregnancy, the increase in umbilical blood flow is achieved by a decrease in resistance rather than an increase in driving pressure, although this also occurs in the last part of pregnancy.[11]

Gestational age is an important influence in determining the normality of the umbilical FVW (Fig. 31.3). The indices of resistance decrease as the placenta grows and expands its vascular bed. In early pregnancy, diastolic flow velocities may be absent. The range of variation in waveform pattern is much greater in early pregnancy. This is clearly apparent in the normal ranges of the various indices of resistance used to describe the umbilical waveform pattern (Fig. 31.4).

There has been debate about the influence of fetal heart rate (FHR) on the umbilical FVW. Two careful studies observed a weak relationship between FHR and waveform index over the physiological range of heart rates.[6,16] Others have reported

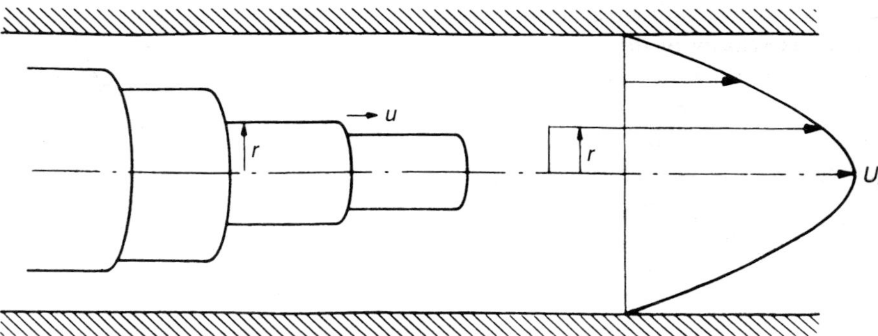

Figure 31.1 The blood flow velocity profile across a vessel. U_0, center line velocity; u, velocity at radial position r (modified from ref. 3, p. 47).

use a pulsed Doppler system and sample from each point across the vessel. If the vessel is uniformly insonated, the mean Doppler frequency shift is proportional to the mean velocity, and this fact is used in the calculation of volume flow.[5] In a blood vessel with an established flow, the "boundary layer" is the region of flow in which velocity is increasing with distance from the wall. Here, viscosity is important, because there is shear between adjacent flow lamina. In the central stream, the movement is "en masse" and inertia is more important. If the disturbances of local geometry are ignored, then in large arterial vessels, inertial forces dominate blood flow, whereas in small vessels, viscous forces are more important. Reynold's number expresses the relative importance of these two forces.[3]

The Doppler FVW has been analyzed in a variety of different ways. In clinical applications, inferences about the cardiovascular system are made using empirical indices. The connection between an empirical index and a physiological variable may be based on a statistical association or evidence from an experimental model. In many situations, only the maximum velocity waveform (or the waveform envelope) is used. This is the easiest waveform to locate and is relatively error free. It does ignore all the information about the velocity profile contained within the frequency spectrum. The problems of analysis of the maximum mean and first moment of the velocity waveform in the fetal circulation have been reviewed.[6,7] The shape of the waveform envelope can be considered a characteristic of the vascular site. Waveforms recorded from arteries supplying low-impedance vascular beds (e.g., internal carotid, umbilical, and uterine artery in pregnancy) exhibit relatively high forward velocities throughout diastole. A triphasic waveform shape, where there is a period of reverse flow in diastole, is characteristic of sites with high distal impedance. The peripheral impedance, vessel wall elasticity, the degree and geometry of any proximal stenoses, and the condition of the upstream pump all affect the waveform. All these factors are important, all can be affected in the disease state being investigated, and none can be independently eliminated or controlled in clinical practice. Even in normal, presumably healthy subjects, blood flow patterns at a site with complicated geometry such as the carotid bifurcation are very complex.

The fetal circulation is uniquely suited to Doppler waveform

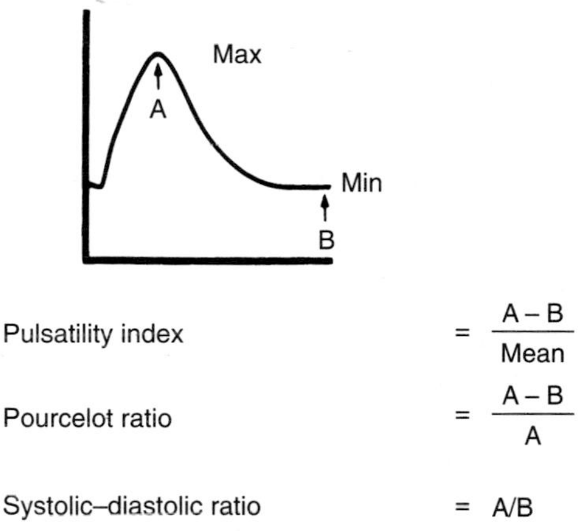

$$\text{Pulsatility index} = \frac{A - B}{\text{Mean}}$$

$$\text{Pourcelot ratio} = \frac{A - B}{A}$$

$$\text{Systolic–diastolic ratio} = A/B$$

Figure 31.2 The three indices of downstream resistance in common clinical use for the analysis of arterial flow velocity waveforms.

analysis by simple empirical indices. This is because of the absence of degenerative arterial disease. The umbilical circulation was the first to be studied, and the indices used for this fetal circulation have been directed toward assessing downstream resistance. Three are in common usage (Fig. 31.2). All of these are highly correlated. Coefficients in excess of 0.9 have been demonstrated when the indices are compared.[6,8] This means that the indices are all providing the same information about the same physiological variables. Choice of index, then, is a matter of convenience relative to the investigational task. The systolic:diastolic ratio is easiest to calculate. Abnormally high values, when there is little or no diastolic value, tend to infinity and become meaningless. The pulsatility index has a precise mathematical definition. It requires determination of the mean velocity, and this is usually an inaccurate estimate. The resistance index (Pourcelot ratio) is the only one normally distributed and has the advantage that the maximum value attainable is one. It has an extra arithmetic step in comparison with the systolic–diastolic ratio. All these indices, when used to interpret the maximum velocity waveform, should be seen as simple descriptors of the waveform pattern. They are not precisely estimatable quantities. There is an inherent systematic error of 10–20% in their calculation.[8] The same indices have been used to assess vasodilation in the cerebral circulation (brain-sparing effect) in fetal compromise. The peak velocity of the FVW envelope has been correlated with volume flow[9] in animal studies, and this parameter has been used as an index in the cerebral circulation. In fetal anemia (e.g., rhesus alloimmunization), cerebral blood flow is increased. It has also been used in the aorta. In the central fetal veins (inferior vena cava and ductus venosus), the FVW pattern reflects the central venous pressure waveform, and different indices have been used (see below). In studying the maternal uterine artery FVW, the presence of a dicrotic notch at the end of systole, which is created by reflected waves, is noted. In summary, there are a variety of empirical indices that have been developed to reflect changes in the pattern of blood flow, which are the result of the pathophysiology of the disorder under study.

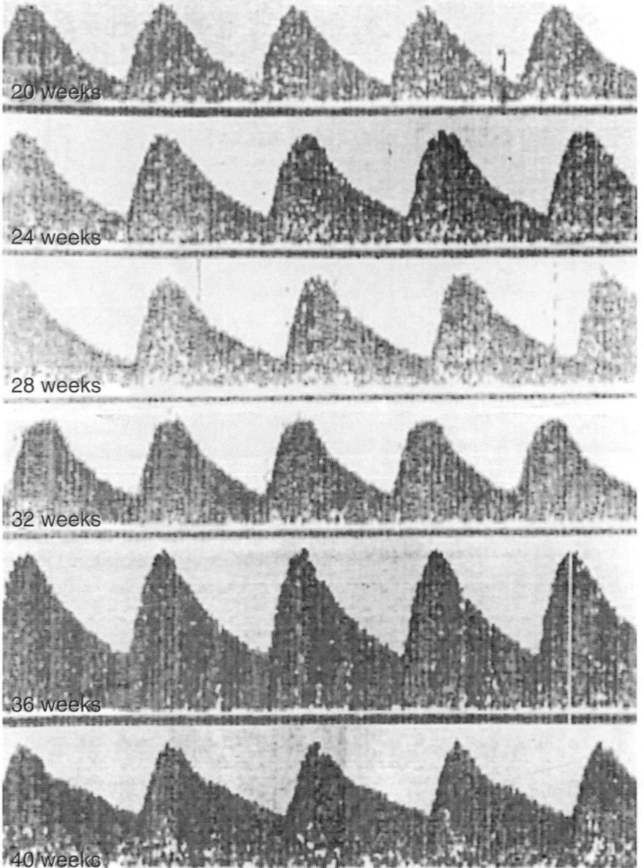

Figure 31.3 The changing form of the umbilical artery FVW recorded from one patient at varying periods of gestation.

The umbilical circulation

The umbilical cord, linking the fetus and placenta, is long and suspended in amniotic fluid, and so is ideal for Doppler studies. The two umbilical arteries travel along this without branching or changes in lumen diameter. The radius of curvature of the loops of cord is large in comparison with the diameter of the umbilical arteries, and so is unlikely to significantly influence flow patterns. However, this spiraling course means that it is not possible to image a sufficient length of artery or vein to permit determination of the angle between the ultrasound beam and vessel, and so it is not possible to make Doppler volume flow measurements. Studies of the umbilical artery FVW using the indices of resistance have been carried out to assess the downstream vascular bed – the fetal placenta. The umbilical arteries can be readily studied with simple continuous wave Doppler ultrasound systems. They have been studied extensively, and these studies have been subjected to much critical appraisal.

Normal pregnancy

Blood flow through the umbilical circulation increases throughout pregnancy and represents some 40% of the combined ventricular output of the fetus.[10] The actual flow in the fetal lamb has been measured at 180–200 mL/min/kg fetus;[11] in human pregnancy, it is less, 100–110 mL/min/kg fetus.[12,13] The umbilical placental vascular bed is not innervated, and indeed is refractory to such circulating vasoconstrictors as epinephrine and norepinephrine.[11] Blood flow to the placenta appears to be the result of the balance between resistance to other fetal vascular beds and the placenta.[10] Almost certainly, there are local controls of placental blood flow that regulate the perfusion to keep a balance between the fetal and maternal placental flows.[14] It has been pointed out that the fetus does not need to regulate umbilical blood flow finely, because it has the capacity to vary tissue oxygen extraction ratios and, consequently, oxygen uptake.[15] The fetus requires oxygenated blood from the placenta for distribution to the fetal tissues, where uptake and delivery may be regulated.

The umbilical circulation is a low-resistance vascular bed, which is reflected in the pattern of the umbilical artery FVW (Fig. 31.3). Throughout pregnancy, the increase in umbilical blood flow is achieved by a decrease in resistance rather than an increase in driving pressure, although this also occurs in the last part of pregnancy.[11]

Gestational age is an important influence in determining the normality of the umbilical FVW (Fig. 31.3). The indices of resistance decrease as the placenta grows and expands its vascular bed. In early pregnancy, diastolic flow velocities may be absent. The range of variation in waveform pattern is much greater in early pregnancy. This is clearly apparent in the normal ranges of the various indices of resistance used to describe the umbilical waveform pattern (Fig. 31.4).

There has been debate about the influence of fetal heart rate (FHR) on the umbilical FVW. Two careful studies observed a weak relationship between FHR and waveform index over the physiological range of heart rates.[6,16] Others have reported

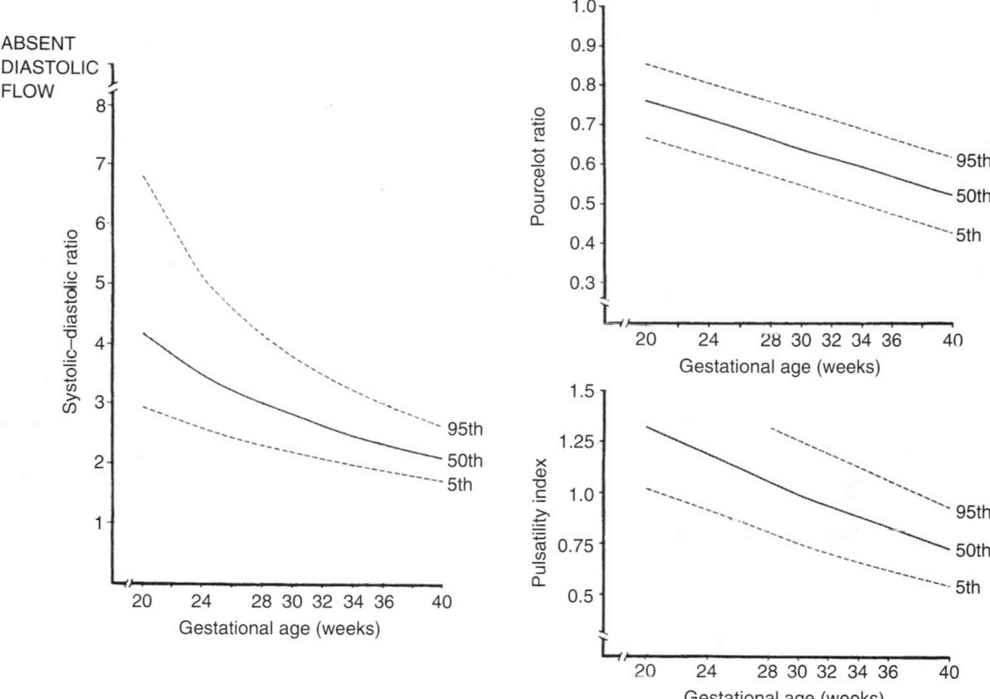

Figure 31.4 The normal range of values for the umbilical artery downstream resistance indices (from ref. 8).

strong associations, but included values outside the normal range, especially below 100 beats per minute (b.p.m.). Over the normal range of FHR, the correction suggested is less than the systematic error present in calculation of the various indices and very small in comparison with the difference between normal and abnormal waveform patterns. The suggestion that a correction factor is necessary is based in part on the assumption that the decay in the diastolic component of the maximum velocity is passive. This assumption is unfounded.

Fetal breathing movements do alter the FVW. During "inspiration," both peak systolic and least diastolic values are decreased, so that the systolic:diastolic ratio is increased (Fig. 31.5). It is interesting to speculate on the reason for this change. During inspiration, more of the right ventricular output has been directed through the pulmonary circulation and less bypasses this through the ductus arteriosus to the aorta and umbilical circulation. This implies that fetal breathing is associated with opening of the fetal pulmonary circulation.

Behavioral states do not influence the FVW pattern or indices of resistance in the umbilical circulation. This is in contrast to the aortic waveform.[17] Such an observation is not unexpected, because the aortic waveform is influenced by flow to various fetal organs under autonomic control, whereas the placenta is not so regulated.

There has been debate about variations in the umbilical FVW along the length of the cord. Close to the fetus, a higher value may be obtained for the systolic:diastolic ratio.[18] There is a transition from the typical aortic to umbilical waveform. At the placental end, the resistance indices have been reported

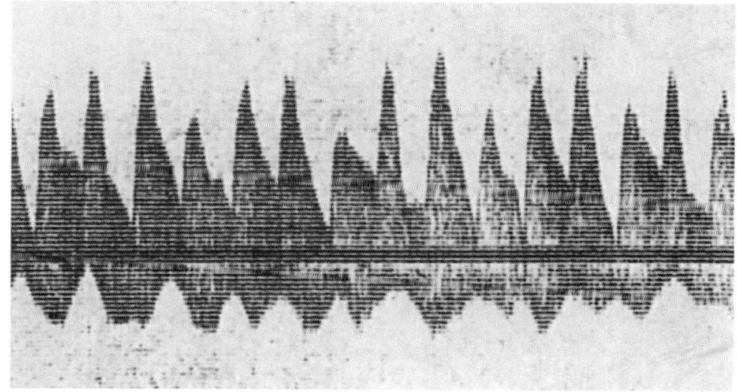

Figure 31.5 The influence of fetal breathing movements on the FVW of the umbilical artery (upper trace) and umbilical vein (lower trace).

to be lower than the values recorded from free-floating loops of cord. This difference is very small in comparison with differences between normal and abnormal pregnancy.

In recording the umbilical FVW, it is necessary to review a sequence of 10–20 cycles to confirm that variations due to fetal activity are absent. Ideally, at least five waveforms should be measured and averaged. To minimize errors, the measured waveforms should be those displaying the maximum obtainable peak systolic and least diastolic flow velocities. This requires that the angle between the ultrasound beam and the vessel is small, and an ideal image can be sought by small movements of the transducer. Simultaneous display of flow in the umbilical artery and vein allows confirmation of the origin of the signal from the umbilical cord by the characteristic pattern, and eliminates the possibility of superimposition of signals from the vein and artery, giving a false value for the diastolic velocity.

Experimental studies of the umbilical circulation relevant to FVW interpretation

The placental vasculature has been modeled as a lumped electrical circuit equivalent,[19,20] an approach widely used in other circulations. Thompson and Stevens[19] developed a computer-based model recreating the branching structure of the villus tree with each arterial vessel represented by a resistor and a capacitor in parallel. The validity of this approach was confirmed by substituting physiologically realistic values for vessel size, resistance, capacitance, and pressure, and demonstrating that calculated and clinically measured umbilical flow were similar. Using this model, it can be shown that the pulsatility index (PI) of the FVW is proportional to the pulsatility of the pressure waveform and the resistance of the umbilical placental villus vascular tree.[21]

Assuming a diffuse vascular pathology, it can be shown that the FVW index of resistance increases as the fraction (q) of terminal arterial vessels obliterated increases. This increase is not linear (Fig. 31.6). It is not until some 50–60% of the vessels have been obliterated that the PI is increased beyond the "normal range." Thereafter, it rises rapidly. It highlights the presence of extensive disease before Doppler detection is possible, and emphasizes the reserve capacity of the placenta. The model also showed a difference between the response of a large and a small placental vascular bed to superimposed vascular obliteration. The same fraction of obliteration (q) produced a much greater increase in PI when the placenta was small. It follows from this prediction that a large, late third-trimester placental vascular bed can accommodate a considerably greater degree of obliteration with minimal change in resistance index in comparison with a smaller, second-trimester placenta. This parallels clinical reports indicating

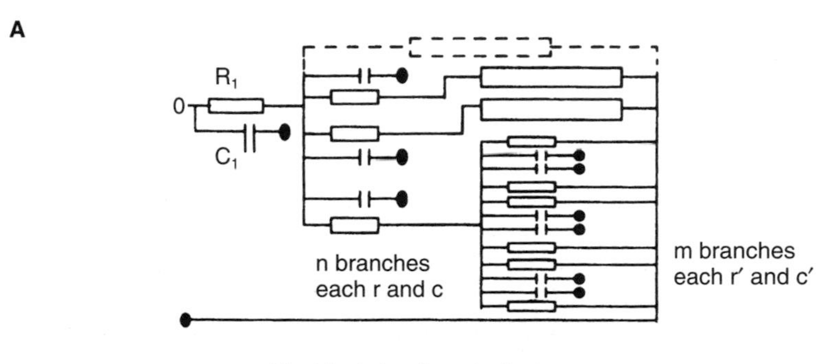

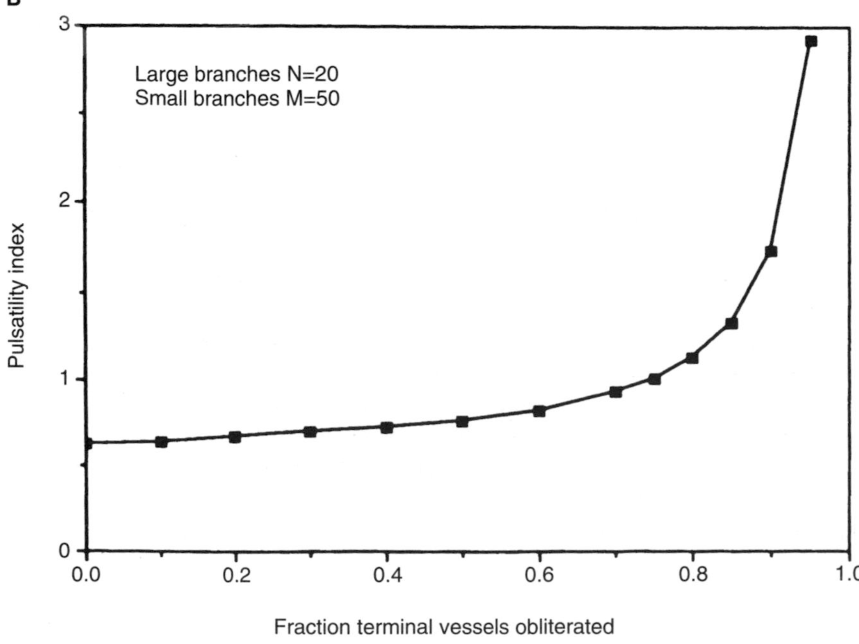

Figure 31.6 Using a mathematical model of the umbilical circulation, based on a lumped electrical circuit equivalent (A) [r = resistance, c = capacitance, of individual proximal branches (n) or distal branches (m)], the change in the umbilical artery pulsatility index was calculated in the presence of an increasing fraction (q) of the umbilical placental vascular bed (B). N is the total number of large (n) branches each having M small (m) branches chosen to be representative of a placenta at 30 weeks (from ref. 21, with permission).

that Doppler studies have a low sensitivity in predicting fetal compromise in postdate pregnancies.[22,23] Doppler umbilical studies are a far more sensitive test for the detection of placental vascular pathology earlier in pregnancy.

This model also demonstrated that variations in blood pressure will alter the PI, but this variation is small.[21] Over the physiological range of blood pressures, the very high values of PI seen in fetal compromise could not be obtained by variations in blood pressure. The PI was demonstrated independent of heart rate over the range 100–180 b.p.m. The effect of a fetal response (by increase in blood pressure) following placental vascular bed obliteration was examined using this mathematical model. If terminal vessels in the placenta were obliterated, the placental resistance increased, as did the PI, while umbilical volume flow decreased. However, a small, physiologically realistic increase in systolic pressure was sufficient to maintain umbilical flow until approximately 80% of the terminal arterial vessels were obliterated. Beyond this point, the pressure increase required was unrealistic (outside the physiological range).

The umbilical circulation in the fetal lamb has been studied with Doppler ultrasound. In ovine pregnancy, it is possible to demonstrate the same decrease in the FVW indices of resistance seen in human pregnancy.[24] The Doppler indices have been demonstrated to be a measure of resistance in the umbilical circulation in the fetal lamb. Embolization of the umbilical cotyledon circulation with microspheres was carried out to increase the resistance of the peripheral vascular bed.[25,26] This caused a rise in the umbilical systolic:diastolic ratio and a rise in calculated vascular resistance.

Pathophysiology of abnormal umbilical Doppler FVW

In normal pregnancy, placental growth continues throughout, as demonstrated by the progressive increase in the weight of the placenta. The overall increase in placental size is associated with an increase in the number of tertiary stem villi and, therefore, total small arterial channels. The continuing expansion of the umbilical placental vascular tree matches the decreasing vascular resistance measured directly in fetal lambs.[11] The decrease in the umbilical artery FVW indices of resistance seen in normal pregnancy is consistent with this. The abnormal umbilical Doppler FVW is characterized by a change in the opposite direction, with decreasing diastolic flow velocities relative to the systolic peak and, in extreme cases, by absence or even reversal of blood flow in diastole. This is a high resistance pattern and contrasts with the normal FVW discussed and illustrated above.

A histological study to correlate the umbilical artery FVW pattern with the "resistance" vessels in the umbilical placental vascular tree has been carried out.[27] Because the major drop in arterial pressure across the umbilical placental vascular bed occurs in the small arteries and arterioles of the tertiary villi, these are the "resistance" vessels. When these placental vessels were examined after delivery in pregnancies classified according to whether the antenatal umbilical Doppler studies were normal or abnormal, significant differences were found. The modal tertiary villus small arterial vessel count was significantly less in the group with the abnormal umbilical artery FVW (1–2 arteries/high-power field) in comparison with the normal group (7–8 arteries/field). This work has been confirmed by others.[28,29] Change in the walls of these resistance vessels was also recognized.[30] This placental lesion of vascular sclerosis, with obliteration of the small muscular arteries of the tertiary stem villi, could be expected to cause an increase in flow resistance in the umbilical placenta. This lesion in the fetal placenta could best be described as "umbilical placental insufficiency."

Placental pathologists have recently focused attention on vascular changes in the umbilical placental circulation. It is noteworthy that this has followed the Doppler definition of a changing vascular resistance in the fetal placenta. A large group of severe placental fetal vascular lesions (fetal thrombotic vasculopathy, chronic villitis with obliterative fetal vasculopathy, chorioamnionitis with severe vasculitis, and meconium-associated fetal vascular necrosis) have been identified and associated with neurological impairment.[31,32] Avascular villi are a common feature. However, it does not appear that the chronic inflammatory or vaso-occlusive histological patterns are specific.[33]

Studies of the fetal circulation and endothelium of the vessels of the placental villi have shed light on the pathogenic pathway. The umbilical artery Doppler high-resistance FVW pattern is associated with fetal platelet activation[34] and consumption.[35] The endothelium is activated,[36] and this is a likely cause. There is proinflammatory cytokine [interleukin (IL)-6 and IL-8] production by the endothelium.[37] These findings link the inflammatory change and thrombosis. The cause of this remains uncertain. The similarity of this to atherosclerosis in later life has been noted.[36] Fetuses with these findings also have an atherogenic lipoprotein profile.[38]

Clinical correlates of abnormal umbilical Doppler FVW in high-risk pregnancy

The abnormal umbilical artery Doppler FVW is characterized by a pattern of reduced, absent, or even reversed diastolic flow velocities relative to the systolic peak velocity (Fig. 31.7). In this situation, the indices of resistance are increased. A review of the normal ranges for these measures (see Fig. 31.4) illustrates the importance of knowledge of gestational age before an index is called abnormal. Before 18 weeks, absent diastolic flow may be seen in normal pregnancies. Particularly in early pregnancy, serial studies are necessary to determine whether the normal growth of the placental vascular tree is occurring, because the normal range is wide.

Before considering the clinical correlates of the abnormal

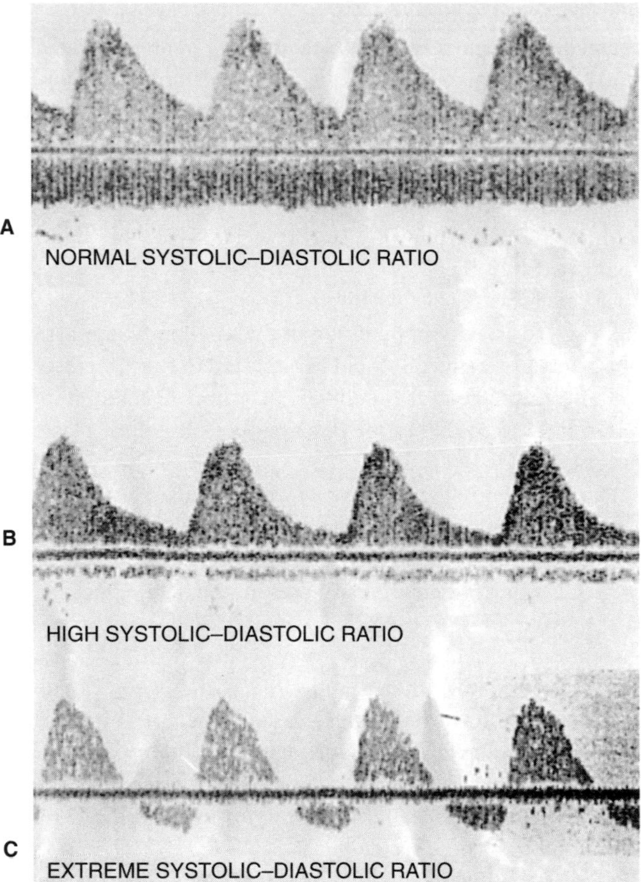

Figure 31.7 Examples of (A) a normal umbilical artery waveform, (B) a waveform in which the systolic:diastolic ratio is high, and (C) an extremely abnormal waveform, in which the diastolic flow velocities are reversed.

umbilical FVW, it is worth restating that analyzing the umbilical artery FVW with the various indices of resistance does not indicate a fetal condition, but rather the presence of a vascular lesion in the placenta – umbilical placental insufficiency. It is believed that this Doppler-defined umbilical placental insufficiency precedes the fetal deprivation. The fetal effects consequent upon this vascular lesion are the clinical correlates. Poor fetal outcome, particularly in terms of the birth of an infant small for gestational age (SGA), is the major clinical association reported. This has been the consistent finding in many reports of the results of Doppler studies in high-risk pregnancy.[39–41] However, what matters most to the obstetrician is not the recognition of the small fetus, but rather the fetus at risk of death *in utero*, distress in labor, and neonatal morbidity. Evidence that umbilical artery Doppler gives this information is provided by reviewing the results of a large study from a single laboratory[42] and collected studies from several centers.[43] The most abnormal studies (highest systolic:diastolic ratio group) had the greatest incidence of fetal growth failure, as indexed by the percentile birthweight. Both fetal and neonatal deaths were highest in this group.

Table 31.1 Results of the last study before delivery in the group of 53 SGA fetuses.

	Umbilical artery waveforms	
	Normal	Abnormal
Number of fetuses	19	34
Mean gestational age at delivery (weeks)	37.6	34.6
Admission to neonatal intensive care	3	23
Neonatal deaths	0	7

Data from ref. 46.

There has been considerable discussion about the group of patients that show an umbilical FVW pattern with absent diastolic flow velocities. Statements about the poor pregnancy outcome of this group and the need for delivery appear in the literature. It has been suggested that this constitutes a watershed for fetal risk. The outcome of patients with this finding has been reviewed in published reports.[44] In a collected review of 785 cases, there was an 84% incidence of birthweight less than the 10th percentile. Morbidity and mortality were high in this group. Careful anatomical ultrasound study is warranted as there is a 5–10% incidence of major anomalies including aneuploidy.[44] Absent diastolic flow is a part of the spectrum of FVW change from normal to extremely abnormal. It is not a level at which fetal morbidity starts to appear. It is the opinion of the author that absent end-diastolic flow velocities should not be the reason for delivery. Rather, it recognizes a severe vascular lesion in the placenta. Specific evidence of fetal effect should be sought as delivery may be warranted. Absent diastolic flow may be a feature of normal pregnancy before 18 weeks. This finding may occasionally result from error of technique. The greater incidence of hypoxemia in this group of fetuses is not surprising, but a number have normal gas tensions.[45] Caesarean delivery is usual.

Among a group of SGA fetuses, an abnormal Doppler umbilical study predicted those who were more likely to require early delivery and neonatal intensive care and those with the highest mortality (Table 31.1).[46]

The trend of umbilical Doppler results proved a very useful measure of neonatal morbidity in those patients with serial studies. This was analyzed among 794 high-risk pregnancies with three or more umbilical Doppler studies available.[42] A decreasing systolic:diastolic ratio was associated with a good outcome, even if the values were outside the normal range (Table 31.2). Such a result suggests continuing placental growth. This trend in serial studies will identify the single false-positive result. Serial studies are also helpful in determining the response to therapy.

Table 31.2 Pregnancy outcome in relation to trend in serial umbilical artery flow studies.

Outcome parameter	Pattern of serial Doppler studies		
	Normal	Abnormal/improving	Abnormal/deteriorating
Total number of cases	567	117	110
Gestational age at delivery	38.5	37.5*	34.5†
Birthweight (mean g)	3164	2708†	1906†
Percentile birthweight (mean)	43.8	26.5†	12.4†
Small for gestational age (< 10th percentile): number (%)	97 (17%)	47 (40%)†	78 (71%)†
Admission to NICU: number (%)	101 (18%)	27 (23%)†	65 (59%)†
Duration of stay in NICU (mean days)	6.1	11.1	34†
Perinatal mortality:			
Number	7	2	7
Rate per 1000	12.3	17.1	63.6†

Data from ref. 42.

NICU, neonatal intensive care unit.

Results shown are the number of patients in each grouping unless otherwise stated. The level of significance of results different from the normal Doppler study group is shown: $*P < 0.001$; $\dagger P < 0.0001$.

Umbilical Doppler FVW and specific pregnancy complications

Hypertensive disease of pregnancy

A high resistance pattern in the umbilical artery Doppler FVW is not present in all cases of pregnancy hypertension. It does appear that it predicts fetal mortality and morbidity.[47,48] It is not related to the severity or duration of the hypertension.

Diabetes mellitus

Umbilical artery FVWs have also been used in the management of diabetic pregnancies.[49,50] Umbilical artery resistance indices are not different from those found in nondiabetic pregnancy. Glycemic control does not appear to affect these indices. The expected relationship between abnormal umbilical artery FVWs and both antenatal fetal compromise and birthweight has been noted.[50] However, in diabetic pregnancy, abnormal nonstress FHR monitoring and biophysical profile have been noted in the presence of a normal umbilical artery FVW. Fetal death has also been reported. Two cases drawn from the author's experience provide further understanding of this problem. Illustrated in Fig. 31.8 is the development of a high-resistance pattern in the umbilical artery FVW in a macrosomic fetus. Diabetic control had been poor and, earlier in pregnancy, fetal growth was excessive. Late in pregnancy, growth was restricted as vascular pathology developed in the placenta. In Fig. 31.9 is the FHR tracing of a mother admitted with hyperglycemia and ketoacidosis in whom the umbilical Doppler result was normal. Good control was re-established, and the FHR tracing became normal. It is likely that many of the cases of unexpected fetal deterioration or demise in diabetes relate to swings in glycemic control, and this is not predicted by the umbilical artery FVW.

Multiple pregnancy

Premature labor, preeclampsia, and fetal growth restriction all contribute to high perinatal mortality and morbidity rates in twin pregnancies. Doppler umbilical studies are especially useful. Care with assignment of umbilical cord recording to the correct fetus is necessary.[51]

The great value of Doppler studies in twin pregnancy management lies in the early recognition of the fetus at risk. Two groups of twin pregnancy problems should be distinguished. In dizygotic twins, discordancy of fetal growth may occur, and this is typically associated with a high-resistance pattern in the umbilical artery Doppler in the small fetus. Such a finding then warrants close fetal surveillance. A recent randomized controlled trial showed no benefit from the use of Doppler[52] when all other fetal surveillance tests were available. Unexplained fetal deaths were reduced however. In contrast to this, an old study of historical data collected soon after the introduction of Doppler[53] into obstetrics showed benefits. Perinatal mortality and, in particular, fetal deaths were significantly reduced. The perinatal mortality was reduced from 58/1000 to 18/1000 ($P < 0.05$). This suggested that a program of intensive fetal surveillance improves outcome.

A consistent Doppler picture in the case of twin–twin transfusion syndrome has been disputed. Discordance in ultrasound measures of fetal size, cord diameter, amniotic fluid volume, and the urinary bladder between the members of the twin pair form the basis of grading.[54] The finding of absent or reversed end-diastolic flow velocities in the umbilical artery FVW indicates a poor prognosis, and this is a consistent observation in several published studies.[55] Interestingly, this finding may be intermittent. This is a subject of much controversy. Recent research has also focused on the possibility that it is pressure rather than volume overload that is the key factor in pathogenesis.[56]

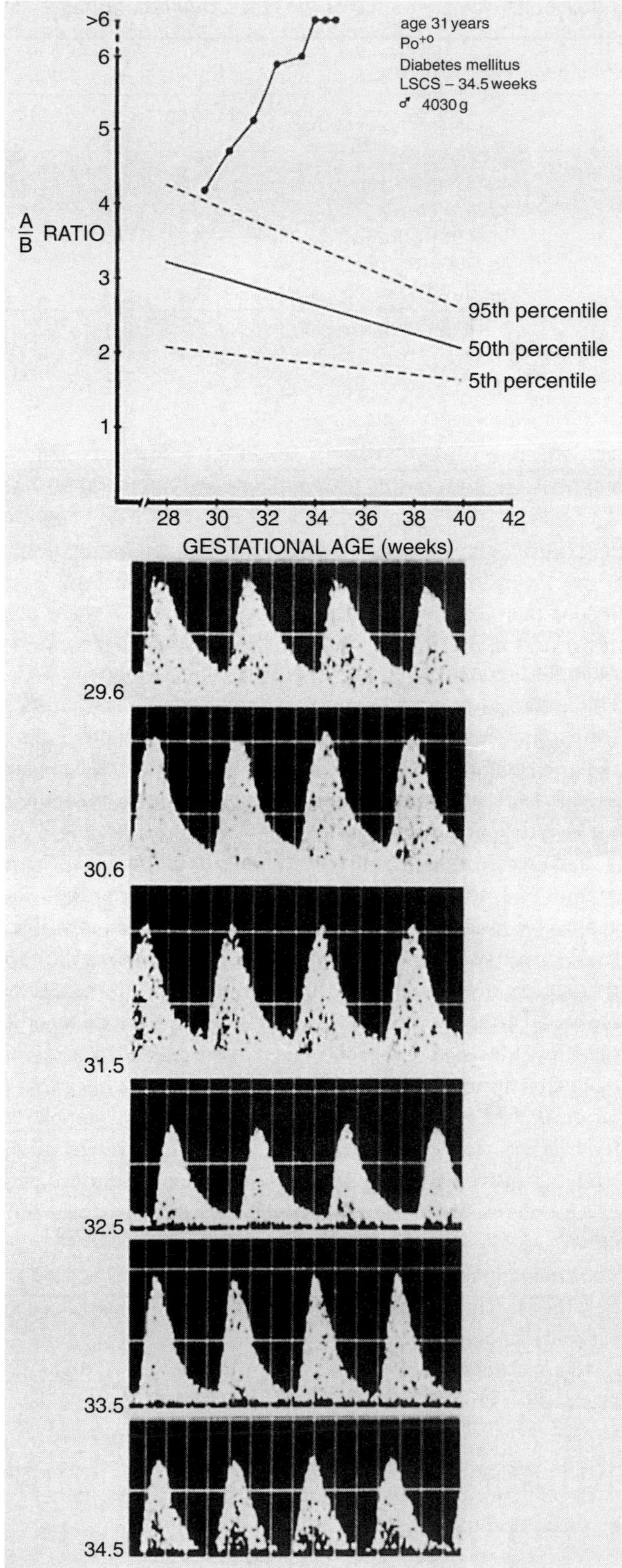

Figure 31.8 Sequential studies of the umbilical artery FVW in one patient with poorly controlled diabetes mellitus. Although the fetus was large, there was evidence of ultrasound fetal growth failure at the end of the pregnancy (from ref. 39).

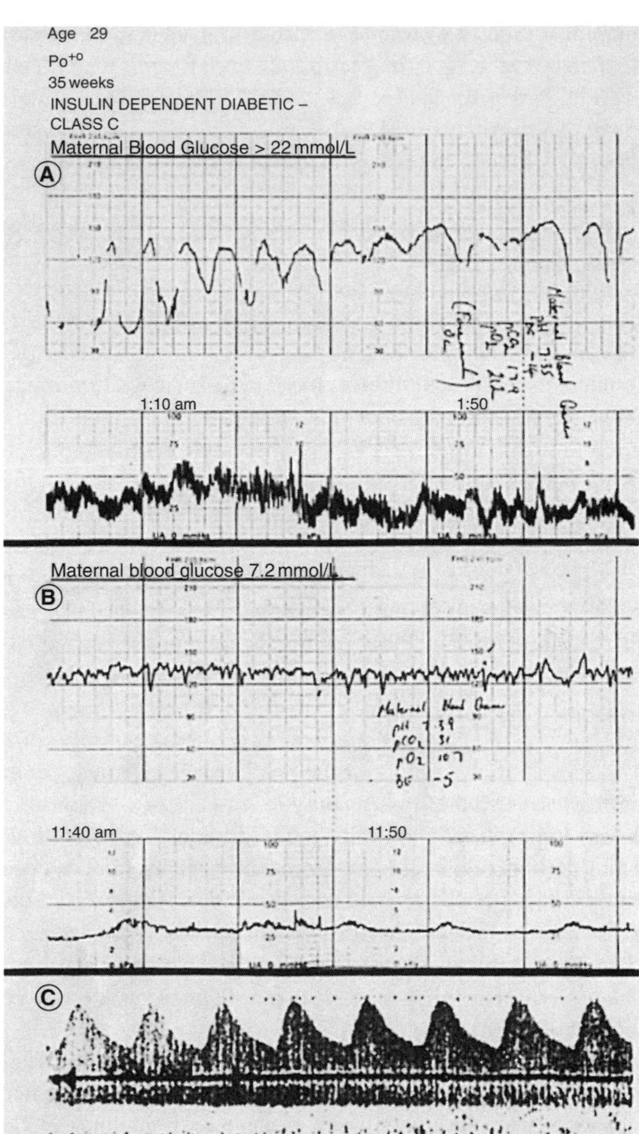

Figure 31.9 In one diabetic mother, with an episode of hyperglycemia and acidosis, the FHR monitoring trace was abnormal (A), although the umbilical artery Doppler FVW appeared normal (C). After correction for the metabolic problem, the FHR monitoring was normal (B).

Doppler studies have also been reported to be useful in fetal assessment of triplet pregnancies.[57] In triplet pregnancy, umbilical artery FVW studies may also be used to delineate those pregnancies requiring more intensive fetal surveillance.

Maternal thrombophilia

A high incidence of both early and late pregnancy fetal wastage and maternal hypertension and placental hemorrhage is seen in a variety of prothrombotic states collectively referred to as maternal thrombophilia. The antiphospholipid syndrome with or without systemic lupus erythematosus (SLE) or other autoimmune phenomena is the best known of these. However, also included are mothers with Factor V Leiden, hyperhomocysteinemia, protein S, protein C, or antithrombin (AT) III deficiency, or prothrombin mutations. Fetal deterioration is predicted by the development of an abnormal umbilical artery waveform, and these studies have aided the management of such pregnancies as this is a common sequelae. Frequent studies, at least weekly in the third trimester, are recommended because fetal demise may occur over a short time. Many of these are hereditary conditions, and there has been recent attention paid to the presence of the prothrombotic state of the fetus. This could be expected because thrombosis is a component of the umbilical placental pathology. Adverse long-term neurological outcome has also been related to fetal thrombophilia.

Major fetal anomaly

Major fetal anomaly is not consistently associated with an abnormal umbilical artery waveform, although such a finding is more common in this group.[58] The systolic–diastolic ratio has been reported to be high in fetuses with trisomy 13, 18, and 21.[58,59] Care should be taken before extrapolating these findings to a total population, because the reported cases studied by Doppler had come to the attention of the clinician before the Doppler study, and the reported findings may be the result of this selection bias. An incidence of abnormal karyotype of 16% has been reported in a series of profoundly growth-restricted fetuses confirmed by ultrasound scan (abdominal circumference less than the third percentile). Most of these fetuses had an abnormal Doppler study.[60]

Postdate pregnancy

It appears that the Doppler studies of the umbilical artery FVW do not predict fetal compromise in postdate pregnancy.[22,23] This may be due to the fact that the mechanism of fetal demise in this group differs from that operating before term. However, as noted above, mathematical modeling of the placental vascular tree has shown that the larger the placental size, the greater the fraction of the vascular tree that needs to be obliterated to cause a detectable increase in the systolic:diastolic ratio.[21] This, combined with a greater susceptibility of the mature fetus to the effects of hypoxemia, could account for the poor predictive value of the Doppler study. Doppler umbilical study as a method of surveillance is not recommended for postdate pregnancies.

The relationship of umbilical Doppler to fetal welfare tests

Tests of fetal welfare exist to identify the potentially compromised fetus (sometimes termed the "at-risk" fetus) and to quantitate fetal condition. The recognition of imminent fetal demise (i.e., the fetus in a terminal state) may be too late to prevent damage or loss of potential. It has been stated above that the umbilical Doppler study recognizes a vascular pathology in the fetal placenta that may lead to a fetal effect. Evaluation of umbilical Doppler studies against other fetal tests supports the fact that the umbilical studies better predict the potentially compromised pregnancy.

Antenatal nonstressed FHR monitoring is widely used in fetal surveillance protocols for high-risk pregnancy. Several comparative studies have demonstrated a greater sensitivity (the proportion of abnormal outcomes identified by the test) of umbilical Doppler in comparison with nonstressed FHR monitoring in recognizing the SGA fetus and a similar sensitivity in predicting adverse outcome.[61,62] The association of an abnormal nonstress FHR test with an abnormal Doppler study selects a group with a very high risk of morbidity. In a randomized trial, the umbilical Doppler was shown to allow antenatal monitoring and obstetric intervention to be aimed more precisely.[63]

The relationship between umbilical Doppler and ultrasonic estimation of fetal size has been examined.[64,65] Sonographic biometry is a more sensitive technique for identifying the small fetus. In a study of 179 fetuses identified by ultrasound measurements of having a small abdominal circumference, an abnormal umbilical Doppler result was shown to predict the need for preterm delivery and the risk of fetal distress in labor.[66] The authors of that study raised the question "is intrauterine growth retardation with normal umbilical artery blood flow a benign condition?" A Swedish study of all small fetuses identified from a total obstetric population, screened for ultrasound weight estimation at 32 weeks, reported operative delivery for fetal distress to be more likely in the group also exhibiting an abnormal Doppler study.[67,68] Serial umbilical Doppler studies in the genetically small, low growth potential fetus which is growing should reveal the normal decrease in systolic:diastolic ratio as the placenta grows even if the placenta is small and the initial Doppler index of resistance is high.

Because fetal compromise is not confined to the SGA fetus, larger fetuses in whom growth has stopped may also be identified by umbilical Doppler, although the ultrasonic measurements of fetal size are not small. Serial ultrasound measurements could be expected to reveal the growth failure in these fetuses, but this requires a delay of at least 2 weeks.[65]

The biophysical profile has not been widely compared with umbilical Doppler studies.

Screening of all pregnancies by umbilical Doppler studies

The possible use of umbilical Doppler studies to screen all pregnancies or low-risk pregnancy has been investigated by several groups. Results have been disappointing. The largest patient group examined was 2097, and these patients were seen at 28, 34, and 38 weeks.[69] There was a significant association between abnormal Doppler results and low percentile birthweight, but the authors suggested from receiver operating curves that this lacked sufficient sensitivity for clinical usage. The most important result was the presence of an

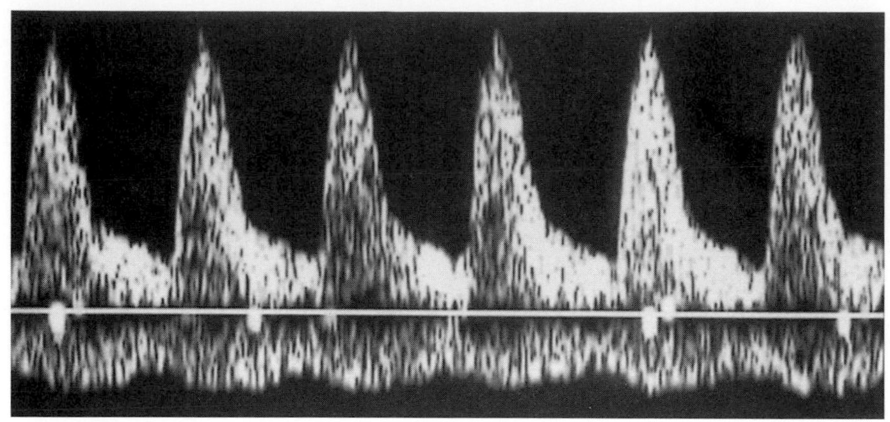

Figure 31.10 The FVW recorded from the umbilical vein to show venous pulsations. This may be seen normally in early pregnancy. In late pregnancy, it is a feature associated with high umbilical placental flow resistance.

abnormal waveform in all three of the unexplained stillbirths and one of two fetal deaths associated with placental abruption. This was emphasized in correspondence subsequent to the original report.[70] Other studies of smaller numbers from unselected low-risk pregnancy groups reported poor prediction of SGA infants and adverse perinatal outcomes.[71] The statistical power of these reports was low, because adverse outcome is infrequent in an unselected pregnancy population.

Fetal umbilical vein studies

The umbilical vein in the cord is readily imaged and a FVW recorded. Pulsations in the umbilical vein (Fig. 31.10) have been described in association with fetal compromise and fetal growth restriction.[72] They have been associated with the most profound fetal compromise. Two possible mechanisms have been advanced to explain the occurrence of this phenomenon. In fetal compromise with placental insufficiency, there is obliteration and so reduction in small arterial channels in the placenta. This results in a decrease in capacitance in the umbilical placental vascular bed so that compliance (its inverse) is changed. In this circumstance, arterial pulsation can be transmitted through to the venous circulation. This is predicted by placental model studies.[20] The alternative explanation is the retrograde transmission of the giant A waves backwards along the venous system. The validity of this observation has been challenged as pulsations may be seen in normal pregnancy.[73]

Doppler ultrasound measurement of volume flow in the umbilical circulation is possible by recording from the umbilical vein as it traverses the fetal liver.[5] The dimensions of the vessel need to be measured at the same time, and flow calculated as the product of average velocity and of vessel lumen. In normal pregnancy, flow in the umbilical vein increases with gestation. Flow per unit of fetal weight is relatively constant at 110 mL/min/kg fetus.[12]

Studies in high-risk pregnancy suggested that a reduced umbilical vein volume flow was associated with growth restriction, but only 40% of fetuses with a low flow had a birthweight below the 10th percentile.[74] The relationship between umbilical artery FVW and umbilical vein volume flow measurements has been examined.[75] The FVW was more sensitive and recognized more SGA fetuses. It had a higher predictive value and similar specificity. The ratio of umbilical vein flow to aortic flow was also measured in this series. In the normal fetuses, this was 39%; in those fetuses with an abnormal umbilical artery FVW systolic:diastolic ratio, it was 25%. This result suggests that the fetus is able to maintain umbilical placental circulation at least initially by an increase in cardiac output. The same observation has been made in experimental growth restriction in fetal lambs.[76] Thus, there is experimental and clinical evidence to suggest that the umbilical artery FVW will detect the compromised fetus earlier than volume flow measurements. A high umbilical vein volume flow has been seen in association with fetal hydrops associated with fetal anemia.[77]

The high umbilical vein volume flow has been reduced in rhesus isoimmunization by fetal transfusion.

The application of measures of umbilical vein volume flow to obstetric practice has been limited by the need for a detailed technique, measurement errors, and complex equipment.

Fetal arterial Doppler studies

Within the fetal body, arterial flow in the aortic and cerebral circulations has been most studied in the vascular trees, although reports of FVW in the renal, splanchnic, and external iliac arteries have been made.[78] Blood flow has been recorded from the fetal coronary arteries.[79]

Fetal aorta

Recordings from the fetal aorta (Fig. 31.11) are readily achieved using the duplex of a Doppler system integrated with real-time imaging.[80,81] The shape of the flow waveform varies along the aorta and, for reproducibility, most studies have concentrated on the midthoracic aorta, which is free of large branches. The fetal aortic blood FVW has been analyzed using

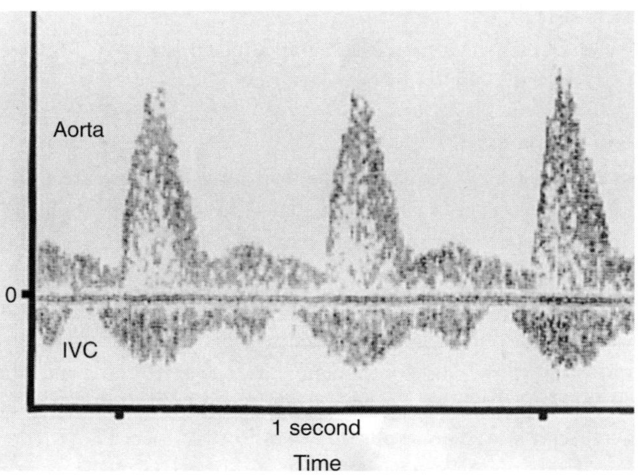

Figure 31.11 The normal FVW recorded from the aorta and inferior vena cava (IVC) in the lower thorax in the third trimester.

the same indices of downstream resistance as used for the umbilical circulation. Volume blood flow has been calculated from mean blood flow velocity and vessel area, but the pulsatile nature of the flow means that measuring diameter from a single frozen image has an error estimated to be 6%.

Normal pregnancy

The PI of the maximum velocity waveform in the thoracic aorta (1.68 ± 0.28) does not change with gestation[82] in the second half of pregnancy. Forward flow velocities are present throughout diastole. This index is significantly affected by changes in FHR. Within the normal FHR range, there is a small negative correlation with the PI. This index is also affected by behavioral state.[17] These observations are not surprising, because 60% of aortic blood is distributed to nonplacental fetal vascular beds in which the vasomotor tone will be regulated according to fetal behavioral and metabolic states. However, the variation due to FHR is small in comparison with the differences between normal and compromised pregnancy. The same influence of FHR and behavioral state has been reported in the growth-restricted fetus.[83] Fetal breathing movements affect the aortic flow waveform, and studies should be carried out during fetal apnea to ensure reproducible results.

Volume blood flow measurement in the fetal descending thoracic aorta increases with gestation up to 36–37 weeks, when a plateau is attained, whereas flow per unit fetal weight decreases during the third trimester.[84]

High-risk pregnancy

Studies of aortic FVW have been used to assess fetal condition in the presence of growth restriction and/or an abnormal fetal heart rate monitoring. Two approaches have been taken to analysis in this situation. Downstream resistance has been assessed by measuring the PI,[74,75,85] and the waveform pattern classified by the presence or absence of forward flow velocities in diastole.[76] Both methods predict perinatal morbidity and fetal growth restriction. Two factors are likely explanations for this. As so much of the blood flow down the aorta is directed to the placenta, the increase in downstream flow resistance in the placenta will dominate. In addition, an increase in resistance as part of the redistribution of blood flow away from the viscera and carcass to vital cerebral, coronary, and adrenal circulations will effect the aortic resistance. It has been reported that the ratio of the PI of the descending thoracic aorta and the middle cerebral artery (MCA) is the best Doppler predictor of fetal acidosis.[77] Fetuses that display absence of diastolic flow velocities in the fetal aorta have been shown to have more developmental disability at age 7 years in comparison with normal.[86]

A second approach to analysis of the aortic FVW has focused on the measurement of the peak mean velocity of the aortic waveform. Correlation with hypoxemia, hypercarbia, hyperlactemia, and acidemia, as determined from fetal blood obtained at cordocentesis,[87] has been demonstrated. These endpoints were used to compare the various methods of analysis of the FVW from aortic, cerebral, and umbilical fetal circulations. Again, the peak mean velocity of the aortic waveform was the most sensitive.[77] In fetal lamb studies, direct measurements of volume flow and the FVW from the fetal aorta have shown a strong correlation between peak and mean velocity of the aortic FVW and volume flow.[9] The correlation between the aortic FVW and blood gas analysis can therefore be explained by appreciating that those fetuses with abnormal blood gas results had depressed myocardial function and ventricular output. Many growth-restricted infants do not show these changes in blood gas analysis. They are present when the fetus is severely compromised. This highlights the different information that is provided by different Doppler studies. There is a distinction between the prediction of risk of fetal compromise and the identification of severe compromise.

Fetal cerebral circulation

The fetal intracranial arteries are readily visualized using a combined B-mode imaging ultrasound system and pulsed Doppler. The recording of FVWs from the fetal internal carotid artery and the individual arteries of the human fetal cerebral circulation spreading out from the circle of Willis is easily achieved. The internal carotid artery is best located at the level of its bifurcation into the middle and anterior cerebral artery.[88] This particular point can be readily identified on a transverse cross-section of the fetal cerebrum. The standard plane for measuring the biparietal diameter, which includes the thalamus and the cavum of the septum pellucidum, is visualized. The MCA can be seen pulsating at the level of the insula. If the transducer is now moved in a parallel fashion toward the base of the skull, a plane is reached that demonstrates a heart-shaped cross-section of the brain stem with the anterior

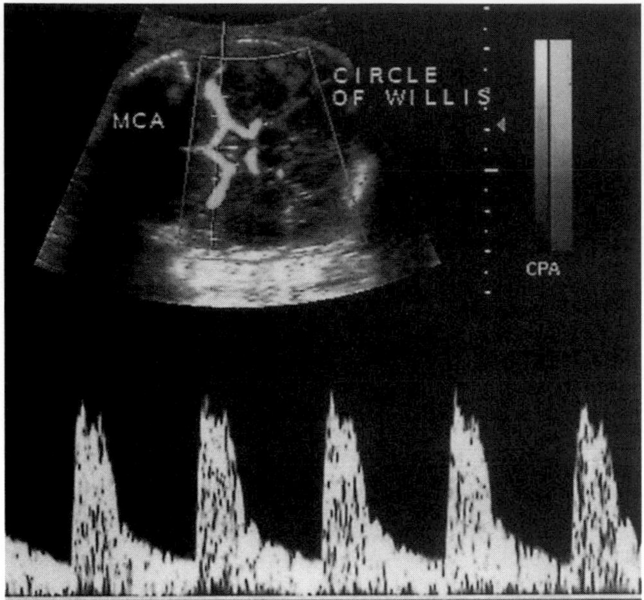

Figure 31.12 Color flow imaging of the circle of Willis of the fetal cerebral circulation. The FVW from the MCA is shown at the bottom.

lobes representing the cerebral peduncles. Anterior to this heart-shaped structure, on either side of the midline, is an oblique cross-section of the internal carotid artery as it divides into its middle and anterior cerebral branches. The MCA has become the standard vessel to image for recording cerebral FVWs. It sweeps out laterally from the internal carotid bifurcation, and a good straight length is usually seen in the transverse plane. It is usually possible to place the transducer so that the line of sight and sampling box is along this length of the vessel. The cosine θ term in the Doppler equation is then 1, and the maximum and peak velocity of the FVW do not need angle correction. Studies from right and left arteries yield similar FVWs, and only one needs to be recorded. Color Doppler imaging facilitates vessel identification (Fig. 31.12).

Normal pregnancy

The waveform of the fetal internal carotid and MCA is not unlike the umbilical artery in shape with forward flow through diastole. The indices of resistance have a higher value than those of the umbilical artery in normal pregnancy. With advancing gestation through the third trimester, this waveform reveals a small decrease in resistance. A normal range for the PI of the fetal internal carotid and MCA FVW has been reported.[89] In the third trimester, a value below 1.1 for the PI at 34 weeks (systolic–diastolic ratio below 2.5, resistance index above 0.67) is regarded as low – less than the fifth percentile value. Fetal breathing movements can cause fluctuations in the FVW which can be seen. Behavioral state also effects the FVW.[15] For clinical studies, the fetus should be inactive and apneic. Monitoring of the cerebral artery FVW waveform during labor[90] has not developed.

High-risk pregnancy

Intrauterine fetal growth restriction may be associated with a fetal cerebral artery FVW PI that is lower than normal.[91–93] Only some growth-restricted fetuses with a high-resistance pattern on umbilical artery Doppler show this low MCA PI. When a normal fetal MCA FVW was associated with a high-resistance umbilical FVW, it was suggested that normal cerebral blood flow was continuing. Later, when fetal condition deteriorates, cerebral vasodilation occurs, and there is an increase in flow. The cerebral FVW shows a lower PI. Whether this effect is adaptive to maintain cerebral oxygen supply or consequent to the occurrence of fetal hypoxia and hypercarbia is not known at present. Studies of the MCA indices of resistance have been related to the results of fetal blood sampling in SGA fetuses.[94] It was shown that the maximum reduction in PI was associated with a fetal PO_2 two to four standard deviations below the mean. In the most extreme cases with an oxygen deficit greater than this, the PI has been observed to rise, and it was suggested that this indicated developing brain edema.[95] The term "centralization of flow" was introduced to describe the situation with a low cerebral flow resistance. The suggested explanation was the redistribution of cardiac output to maintain blood flow to vital organs by the profoundly compromised fetus. Others have used the term "brain sparing" to describe this preservation of brain blood flow. The finding in the cerebral circulation is in contrast to the aorta.

Although the MCA indices of resistance are low in association with fetal compromise, the values overlap with the lower part of the normal range in many small fetuses. To improve discrimination and recognize a deteriorating situation, it has been suggested that the ratio of cerebral to umbilical index of resistance be used to identify the fetuses in whom the placental insufficiency is associated with altered cerebral blood flow. This ratio has been evaluated.[96] A group of fetuses with severe neonatal morbidity can be identified by a ratio of less than 1.0.

Fetal anemia, rhesus alloimmunization

The measurement of maximum velocity in the MCA FVW has become the standard method for assessment of fetal anemia in rhesus alloimmunization. It has obvious advantages over invasive testing. It can, of course, be used in any circumstance in which fetal anemia may occur, e.g., parvovirus infection, hemoglobinopathy. A detailed account is provided in Chapter 49.

Other fetal arterial circulations

In the fetal external iliac and femoral arteries, the resistance index was found to increase with gestation.[97] In fetal growth restriction, there was a small increase in the resistance index.

In the fetal brachial artery, the PI in the right and left arms was seen to be similar in normal pregnancy. In association with severe growth retardation and abnormal umbilical Doppler, the PI in the left arm was higher.[98]

Blood flow in the arteries of the fetal abdomen has been studied in normal and compromised fetuses. SGA fetuses have been identified as having decreased resistance in the splenic artery.[99]

Renal artery PI is reportedly increased in growth-restricted fetuses.[100]

In the coronary circulation, vasodilation has been reported in association with profound fetal compromise.[79] This has been referred to as the "heart-sparing effect." The coronary arteries can be imaged at an earlier gestation in profound fetal growth restriction, and this is a likely sign of dilation as a result of the circulatory redistribution to maintain this vital vascular bed. The FVW pattern is of low resistance in comparison with normal.

These studies in other vascular beds are not part of current clinical management protocols, but provide insight into pathophysiology and are an investigational tool.

Fetal venous Doppler studies

The studies of FVWs in fetal vessels have extended from the arterial circulation to the great veins. The ductus venosus, the inferior vena cava, and the umbilical vein have been the subject of most studies. The FVWs in the central fetal veins are influenced in form by the central venous pressure, and this in turn is a reflection of cardiac function. The form of the flow velocity wave is best understood by reviewing the shape of the central venous pressure waveform (Fig. 31.13). Four waves are identified on this. The A crest is associated with atrial contraction. The X trough occurs with atrial relaxation in early systole. The V crest is the result of rising central venous and atrial pressure as forward blood flow is obstructed while the atrioventricular valves are closed during ventricular systole. The Y trough begins as soon as the atrioventricular valves open at the end of isovolumetric ventricular relaxation. The pulsatile changes in the inferior vena cava reflect the same events of the cardiac cycle and are illustrated (Fig. 31.14). To understand the origin and interpretation of the changes in venous FVW pattern seen with fetal compromise, it is important to remember the differences in blood flow through the heart before and after birth. In the fetus, the pulmonary circulation is small, and systemic venous return passes to the left heart through the foremen ovale as well as through the right heart. Blood returning from the placenta is predominantly directed to the left heart. Ventricular outflow from the right heart enters the systemic circulation through the ductus arteriosus. Conceptually, there exists a combined ventricular output directed into the systemic circulation so that the afterload for both ventricles is systemic vascular resistance. However, blood from the left ventricle is directed to the head and upper body, whereas from the right, it is directed to the lower body and placenta. As 40% of the combined ventricular output is directed to the placenta, this is a major determinant of right ventricular afterload. Already in this chapter, changes in the arterial circulation in fetal growth restriction have been discussed. These have a profound effect on afterload, preload, and cardiac contractility. Umbilical placental resistance is high, so that a high right ventricular afterload is present. Resistance in the cerebral circulation is low, reducing the left ventricle afterload in the most compromised fetus. As the fetus becomes significantly hypoxemic, contractility and output from the heart fall. These are major changes in fetal cardiovascular hemodynamics and explain why venous Doppler has become widely incorporated in management protocols to define fetal condition.

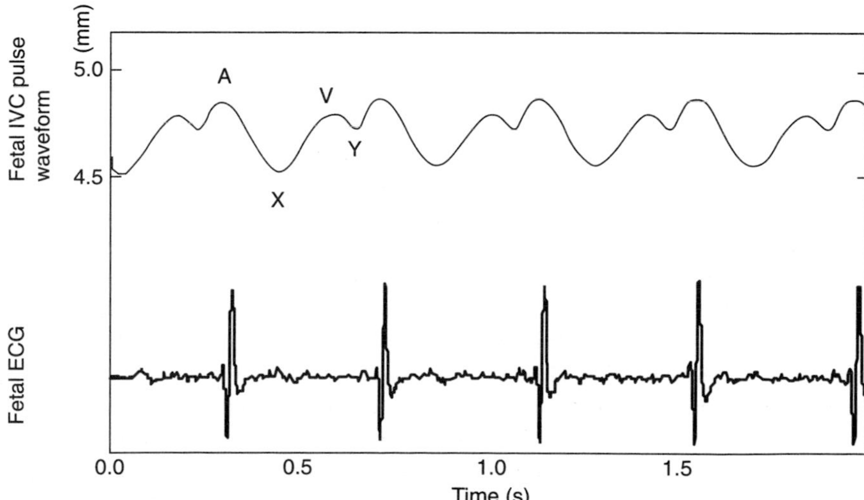

Figure 31.13 A fetal central venous pressure waveform with the "A", "X", "V", and "Y" components marked (see text) to show the associated events of the cardiac cycle (reprinted from ref. 107, with permission). ECG, electrocardiogram; IVC, inferior vena cava.

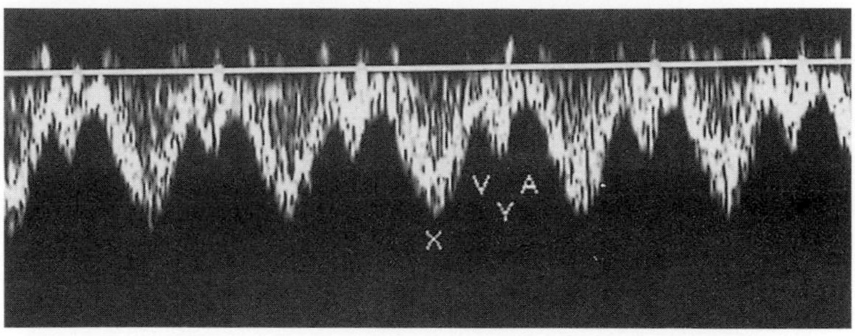

Figure 31.14 The FVW recorded from the fetal inferior vena cava in normal pregnancy at 34 weeks. The component A, X, V, and Y waves (see text) are shown.

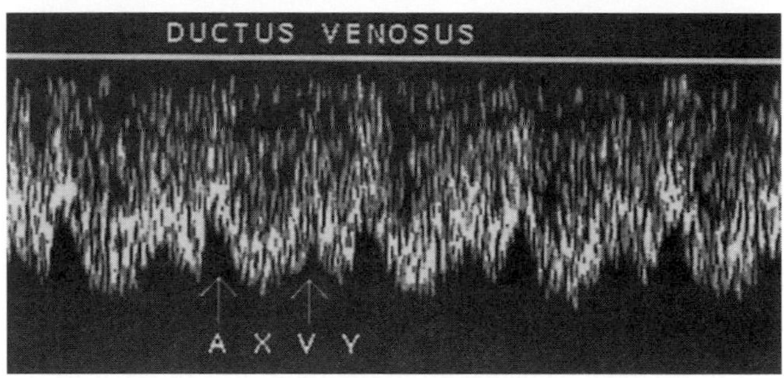

Figure 31.15 The FVW recorded from the fetal ductus venosus in normal pregnancy at 35 weeks. The component A, X, V, and Y waves (see text) are shown.

Fetal ductus venosus and inferior vena cava

The umbilical vein returns blood from the placenta. After entering the fetal abdomen, it is directed to the porta hepatis and into the liver. It is directed initially upwards and backwards and, at the point where it joins the portal vein to the right, it divides so that a thicker walled ductus venosus continues upwards to the sinus venosus entry to the right atrium. Although here the ductus venosus and inferior vena cava are a single sinus in open fetal lamb surgery, it is fascinating to see the two streams separately distinguished by differing color consequent upon the different degrees of oxygenation. This anatomy is relevant to the imaging of these vessels. The ductus venosus can be identified in a transverse plane directed upwards and backwards to include the region at which the umbilical vein joins the portal sinus. The inferior vena cava is best seen in a sagittal plane, which includes the region where it enters the right atrium. The ductus venosus may also be seen in this plane, but hepatic veins can confuse. The FVW patterns are, however, quite distinct, and the color Doppler imaging demonstrates the higher flow velocities[101] in the ductus venosus. A peak systolic velocity of 80 cm/s may be seen in the ductus venosus waveform in the third trimester of pregnancy in contrast to the inferior vena cava peak of 40 cm/s. Fetal breathing movements especially and fetal state affect these waveform patterns, and recordings should be made during quiet sleep.[102]

A large number of parameters have been calculated from the Doppler flow waveform of the inferior vena cava (Fig. 31.14) and ductus venous (Fig. 31.15). These figures should be contrasted with the central venous pressure wave (Fig. 31.13) as a different set of symbols has been used in fetal medicine. The "A" wave of atrial contraction is identified as the trough "A" because pressure and flow are inversely related. However, the "S" and "D" peaks in the FVW correspond to the "X" and "Y" troughs on the central venous pressure wave. This allows the events of the cardiac cycle to be timed. In two recent comprehensive studies,[103,104] these parameters (Fig. 31.16) have been related to fetal blood gas status and especially fetal hypoxemia. Normal ranges were reported for all parameters.[103] Among a group of growth-restricted fetuses (ultrasound estimate of weight less than the 5th percentile), all indices were abnormal. Fetal hypoxemia was associated with an increase in the percentage time of the cardiac period when there was reverse flow present and an increase in the preload index of the inferior vena cava.[105] For the ductus venosus, the systolic to atrial contraction peak velocity ratio and preload index were increased.[101] The dominant feature in growth-restricted fetuses was a reduction in the velocities during atrial contraction. Some workers have found better associations between fetal condition and parameters derived from the ductus venosus. Others prefer inferior vena cava parameters. The ductus venosus is the most widely used because of its unique pattern. The inferior vena cava FVW is very similar to the hepatic vein FVW, and this makes vessel identification more problematic. The underlying hemodynamic disturbance affecting both great veins is likely to be an increase in right ventricular end-diastolic pressure consequent to an increase in right ventricular afterload and reduction in cardiac contractility. Both of these are a consequence of the placental lesion (defined by the umbilical Doppler study).

In fetal anemia attributable to rhesus alloimmunization, a change in the waveform with an increase in the "S" peak and a decrease in the "A" trough has been noted. This is consistent with an increase in cardiac output and end-venous return.[106]

Recently, a technique to record the fetal central venous pressure waveform has been described.[107] Studies in normal and growth-restricted pregnancy demonstrate changes consistent with high right ventricular afterload (giant A waves) and, at a later stage, depressed myocardial function. Doppler FVWs of the central fetal vein are used as a surrogate for the central

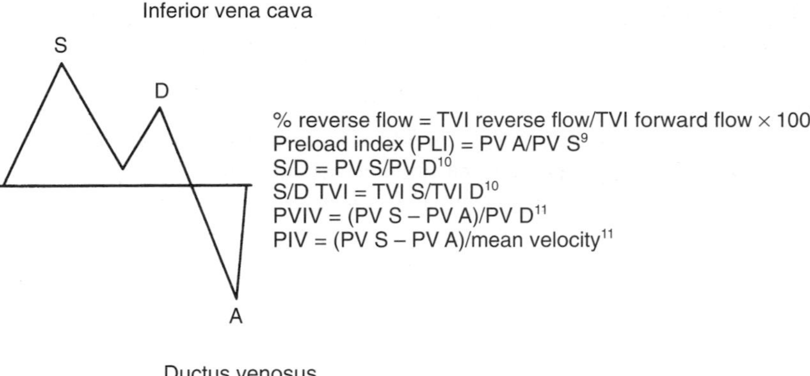

Inferior vena cava
S
D
A
% reverse flow = TVI reverse flow/TVI forward flow × 100[6]
Preload index (PLI) = PV A/PV S[9]
S/D = PV S/PV D[10]
S/D TVI = TVI S/TVI D[10]
PVIV = (PV S – PV A)/PV D[11]
PIV = (PV S – PV A)/mean velocity[11]

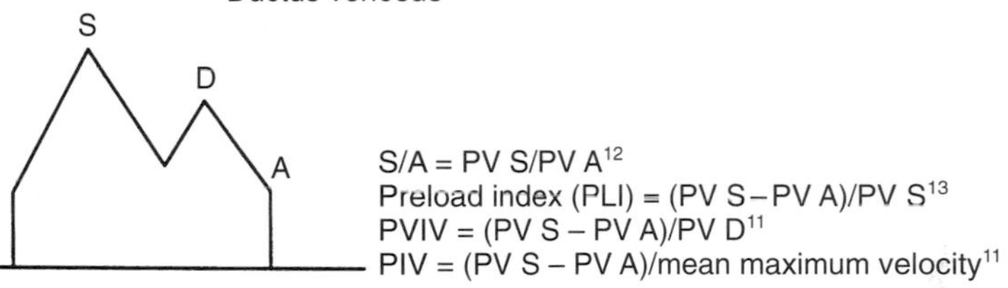

Ductus venosus
S
D
A
S/A = PV S/PV A[12]
Preload index (PLI) = (PV S – PV A)/PV S[13]
PVIV = (PV S – PV A)/PV D[11]
PIV = (PV S – PV A)/mean maximum velocity[11]

Figure 31.16 Various indices have been used to assess the FVWs from the fetal inferior vena cava and ductus venosus. This diagram shows these indices. The S and D peaks correspond to the X and Y troughs on the central venous pressure waveform (from ref. 103).

venous pressure wave to reflect changes in cardiac function, and these studies confirm such changes.

Fetal pulmonary veins

The pulmonary veins entering the left atrium are readily imaged with power Doppler or color flow mapping. The FVW is similar to the ductus venosus.[108] The hope that an alteration in pattern would identify pulmonary hypoplasia has not been achieved.[109]

Clinical strategies in Doppler and fetal compromise

The approach of the obstetrician to fetal compromise progresses through a sequence of steps, which can be summarized as:

1 Recognition of high-risk pregnancy on the basis of clinical history and examination, supported by the ancillary aids of maternal–fetal movement counting and fundal height measurement. (Is it a high-risk pregnancy?)

2 Confirmation of fetal risk by identifying the placental vascular lesion with Doppler ultrasound studies of the umbilical artery FVW. (Is there a placental pathology threatening the fetus?)

3 Determination of the extent to which the fetus is affected using the direct fetal assessments of biophysical profile, ultrasound growth, and FHR monitoring and direct fetal Doppler studies. This is relevant to the timing of delivery. (How sick is the fetus?)

4 Therapy aimed at improving the intrauterine environment by treating mother or fetus, and delivery if the risks to the fetus of intrauterine death or damage exceed that of delivery.

Included in this approach is the use of Doppler studies at two points. Umbilical Doppler studies are interposed between the clinical identification of the high-risk pregnancy and full fetal surveillance testing to quantitate the degree to which the fetus is affected. Umbilical Doppler is a doorway test confirming the potential for fetal compromise and so leading to intensive fetal testing. Direct fetal Doppler assessments are then used to quantify how sick the fetus is. These will be discussed.

The use of umbilical artery Doppler assumes that the placental vascular lesion identified by umbilical Doppler underlies all fetal compromise. Although this is common in the "chronic" situation, it is not always the case. Acute fetal deterioration (e.g., abruption) is not recognized. Fetal anemia, whether due to isoimmunization or other causes such as feto-maternal hemorrhage, is also not identified. However, chronic "placental insufficiency" is operating in the majority of cases, and these are identified. The one-quarter to one-third of SGA infants with normal umbilical Doppler studies have a good outcome (see above) and include cases of low growth potential where the growth velocity of the small fetus is normal and there is no placental constraint.[42] The concept of identification of umbilical placental insufficiency by umbilical Doppler studies also implies that the various clinical situations in which this is present operate through a final, common pathological pathway. This is recognized by the abnormal umbilical FVW.

The above scheme involves the use of the Doppler umbilical waveform study as a discriminator or doorway test to determine which fetuses are truly at risk and in need of intensive fetal surveillance. The relationship of the various direct fetal assessments to the umbilical FVW has been described above.

It cannot be stated too frequently that the Doppler umbilical artery waveform provides a guide to the presence of a placental pathology that is important in terms of the equation:

$$\text{placental lesion} \rightarrow \text{fetal effect}$$

It is not a direct fetal test and should not in itself be used as a measure of fetal condition, but rather as an indication of the need for detailed assessment of fetal welfare.

The use of umbilical Doppler in clinical practice has been evaluated by several randomized controlled trials. Indeed, umbilical Doppler studies have been subjected to more rigorous and extensive assessment than any previous test of fetal health or fetoplacental function. Meta-analysis[109] has established that women with high-fetal-risk pregnancies should have access to Doppler studies of the umbilical artery FVW. Meta-analysis of the umbilical Doppler trials demonstrated a reduction in the odds of a perinatal death by 38% (odds ratio 0.62, 95% confidence interval 0.45–0.85) (Fig. 31.17). This result was significant at the 1% level when umbilical studies were available to influence management. In the Doppler group, there was a significant reduction in the number of antenatal admissions, inductions of labor, and Cesarean section for fetal distress. The reviewers[110] noted that the results were consistent across all trials. The author[111] in the first published trial claimed that monitoring with umbilical Doppler led to more selective and appropriate elective delivery.

Direct fetal Doppler is increasingly used to quantify fetal condition and so determine the time of delivery. In the circumstance of fetal compromise, delivery is the definitive treatment. This is effected when the prospects for survival are better than the risk of remaining *in utero*. In late pregnancy, this is not so critical as delivery usually results in good fetal outcome. The clinical challenge at this gestational age lies in the identification of the potential for adverse outcome. At earlier gestations, this problem is not so simple. There are risks to the fetus from both prematurity and from continuing in the uterus in a situation of inadequate supply of oxygen and nutrients. It is the aim of management to prolong the pregnancy for as long as possible and deliver when there is a belief that fetal damage is occurring. Testing to define fetal condition is necessary. Of the nonDoppler flow tests, FHR monitoring relates to higher central nervous system (CNS) control of cardioregulation and biophysical profile to CNS behavior determination. Both therefore imply a CNS effect. Fetal Doppler adds new dimensions to testing. Cerebral Doppler defines the redistribution of cardiac output. Central venous Doppler defines changes in cardiac loading and contractility. There has been a search for evidence that they better predict the risk of fetal damage and, in particular, long-term neurological handicaps. There have been several recent studies aimed at defining longitudinally the sequence of change in these tests.[112–114] Unfortunately, a uniform pattern has not been documented, and it remains uncertain whether changes in cerebral or venous Doppler, FHR, or biophysical profile should guide the timing of delivery.[115] One randomized trial questioned the benefit of this precise definition using such testing and outcomes were comparable among early and late delivery groups.[116] More evaluation is needed, particularly with long-term neurological performance as an endpoint.

Doppler umbilical studies have also been used to guide specific therapies aimed at reversing the placental lesion. The demonstrated placental vascular obliteration[27] and fetal platelet consumption[35] suggested a role for thromboxane activity in the fetal placenta. It was the rationale for the

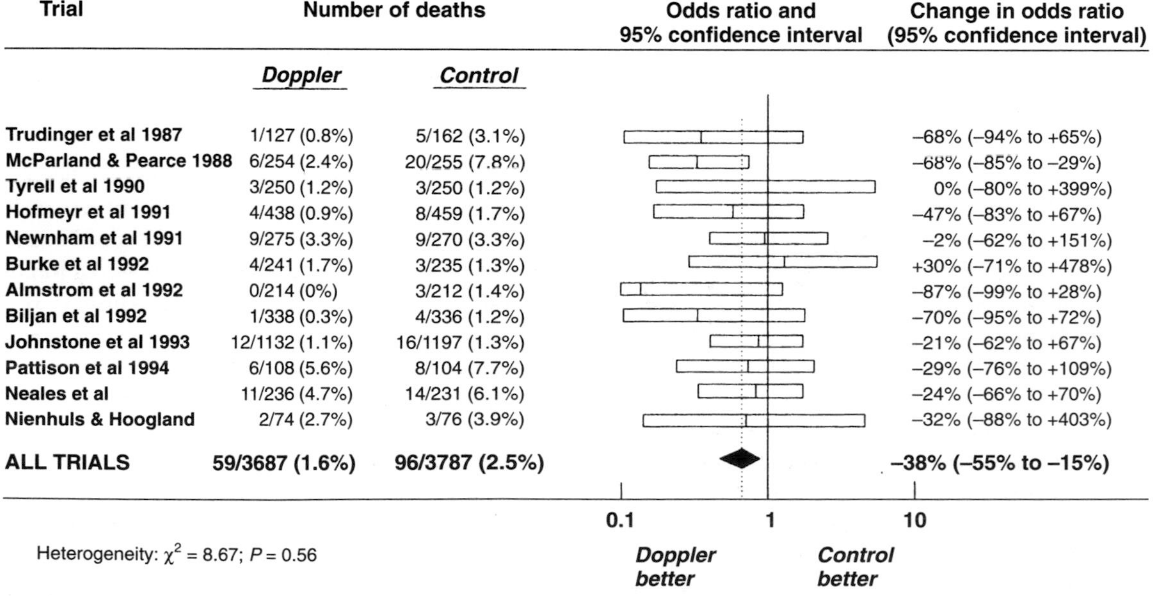

Trial
Number of deaths
Odds ratio and 95% confidence interval
Change in odds ratio (95% confidence interval)
Doppler
Control
Trudinger et al 1987 1/127 (0.8%) 5/162 (3.1%) −68% (−94% to +65%)
McParland & Pearce 1988 6/254 (2.4%) 20/255 (7.8%) −68% (−85% to −29%)
Tyrell et al 1990 3/250 (1.2%) 3/250 (1.2%) 0% (−80% to +399%)
Hofmeyr et al 1991 4/438 (0.9%) 8/459 (1.7%) −47% (−83% to +67%)
Newnham et al 1991 9/275 (3.3%) 9/270 (3.3%) −2% (−62% to +151%)
Burke et al 1992 4/241 (1.7%) 3/235 (1.3%) +30% (−71% to +478%)
Almstrom et al 1992 0/214 (0%) 3/212 (1.4%) −87% (−99% to +28%)
Biljan et al 1992 1/338 (0.3%) 4/336 (1.2%) −70% (−95% to +72%)
Johnstone et al 1993 12/1132 (1.1%) 16/1197 (1.3%) −21% (−62% to +67%)
Pattison et al 1994 6/108 (5.6%) 8/104 (7.7%) −29% (−76% to +109%)
Neales et al 11/236 (4.7%) 14/231 (6.1%) −24% (−66% to +70%)
Nienhuls & Hoogland 2/74 (2.7%) 3/76 (3.9%) −32% (−88% to +403%)
ALL TRIALS 59/3687 (1.6%) 96/3787 (2.5%) −38% (−55% to −15%)
0.1
1
10
Heterogeneity: $\chi^2 = 8.67$; $P = 0.56$
Doppler better
Control better

Figure 31.17 Meta-analysis of 12 randomized controlled trials demonstrated a significant benefit in reducing the number of fetal and neonatal deaths associated with the use of umbilical Doppler (from ref. 110).

A

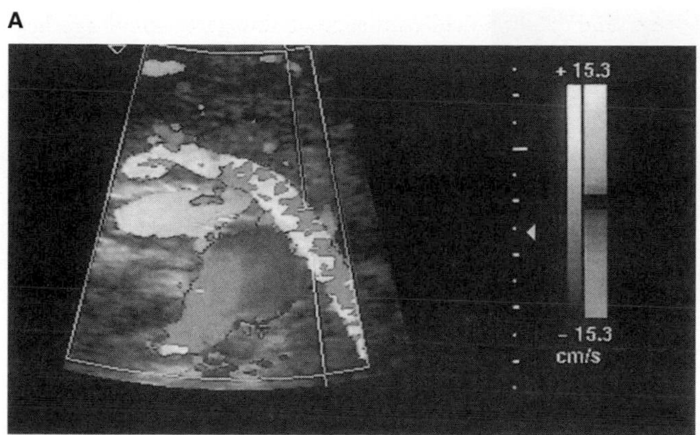

B

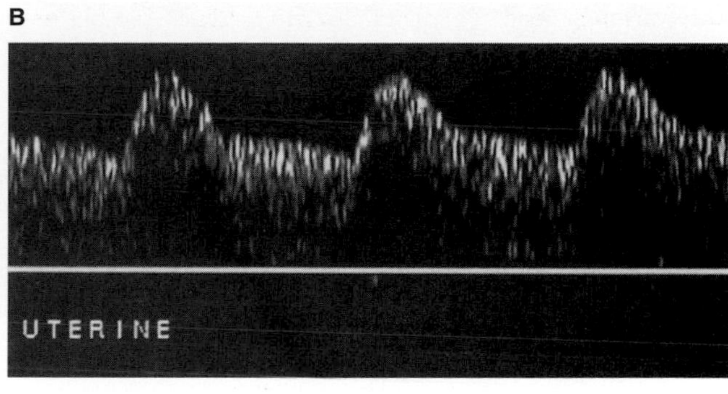

Figure 31.18 The uterine artery can be seen appearing to cross the external iliac vessels in this color Doppler mapping superimposed on a B-mode ultrasound image (A). The FVW in (B) is a normal uterine artery pattern with high diastolic flow velocities.

evaluation of low-dose aspirin as a therapy.[117] In a randomized clinical trial, soluble aspirin (150 mg/day) was administered to mothers with pregnancies identified by an umbilical artery waveform systolic:diastolic ratio above the 95th percentile. The treated pregnancies yielded infants with a 25% greater birthweight. There was an increase in head circumference. The placentas from the treated pregnancies showed the same proportional increase in size. This improvement was not seen in pregnancies in which the umbilical Doppler study was extremely abnormal, with absent diastolic flow velocities. Low-dose aspirin may provide a means of treatment of placental insufficiency if the Doppler diagnosis can be made early and before marked fetal effect. This study has not been repeated. The disappointing results obtained in using aspirin to prevent preeclampsia in large unselected groups have been allowed to overshadow the benefits demonstrated in small, highly selected studies.

Maternal uterine circulation

Both pulsed[118] and continuous wave[119] ultrasound have been used to record FVWs from the uterine circulation. The early problems of vessel identification in the study of uteroplacental circulation with continuous wave Doppler systems were overcome by the introduction of color Doppler and power Doppler imaging, which permit more precise localization of the uterine artery and its radial, arcuate, and spiral branches.[120] Color Doppler systems enable the main uterine artery to be studied[121] and identified, usually in the supracervical region after it is seen to cross the iliac veins (Fig. 31.18). The signal recorded from the side of placental implantation may have a lower resistance pattern in comparison with the nonplacental side.[122]

The same indices of downstream resistance that are described in the assessment of umbilical artery FVWs are used to assess FVWs of uteroplacental arteries. High diastolic flow velocities indicate low downstream resistance. Attention has also been focused on the presence or absence of an early diastolic "notch," which has been attributed to an increased downstream resistance.[47] The explanation for this is speculative. The distance between the main uterine artery and the vascular bed it feeds is short in comparison with the umbilical artery in the long umbilical cord. Reflected waves have little influence on the shape of the umbilical waveform, and no dicrotic notch is seen. In the uterine circulation, reflected waves from a high-resistance periphery can be expected (Fig. 31.19). The subjective yes–no present–absent use of a notch to identify a high-resistance pattern has been shown to be reproducible.[123]

Normal pregnancy

The process of trophoblast invasion of the spiral arteries of the decidual and inner third of the myometrium occurs during the first 20 weeks of gestation. Endovascular trophoblasts replace the endothelium of the spiral arteries in the placental bed, and the trophoblasts infiltrate into the musculoelastic coat. It is widely believed that this lowers the resistance to blood flow in the uterine artery branches opening into the intervillous space. A decrease in resistance in uterine artery branches causes higher end-diastolic flow velocities, and this can be detected in early pregnancy. This invasion extends from the decidua to the intramyometrial portion of the spiral arteries during the first half of pregnancy. After 20 weeks of gestation, there is little change in the waveform of the uteroplacental arteries throughout the remainder of the pregnancy. A pattern of low pulsatility and high end-diastolic velocity relative to peak systolic velocity is seen (Fig. 31.19).[119] After 20 weeks, the uterine artery S/D ratio is less than 2.0,[119] and the PI less than 1.5[121] in normal pregnancy. The early diastolic "notch" of the uteroplacental FVW has been reported in normal pregnancy until approximately 26 weeks' gestation. However, on the side of the uterus of the placental bed, it has been reported to be rarely found after 20 weeks' gestation.[121] The evidence linking the trophoblast invasion to the changing

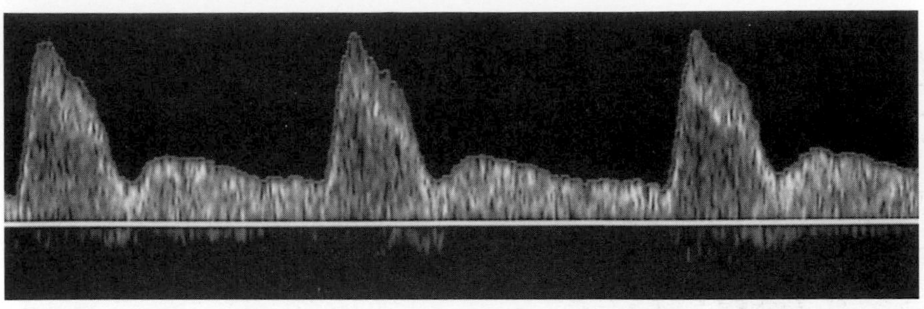

Figure 31.19 A uterine artery FVW from a pregnancy with preeclampsia. A dicrotic notch is present. Diastolic flow velocities are low. This is a high-resistance uterine artery pattern.

FVW pattern is the temporal relationship of these two processes. There has been much debate about the occurrence of intervillous blood flow in the first trimester as a result of Doppler studies. The inability to image intervillous flow until 10–12 weeks[124] is in conflict with the observation of a low-resistance flow pattern in the spiral arteries from very early in pregnancy,[125,126] and is probably attributable to limitations of the equipment.

High-risk pregnancy

Both severe fetal growth restriction and maternal hypertension may be associated with uteroplacental waveforms demonstrating a high systolic–diastolic ratio (Fig. 31.19). Among patients with pregnancies complicated by hypertension or intrauterine growth restriction, there were two patterns of results: those with FVWs similar to the normal population and those who had evidence of a high impedance to flow.[118] In this second group, there was a higher incidence of proteinuric hypertension, the time of delivery was significantly shorter, and the birthweight ratio of the infants (actual birthweight/mean birthweight for gestational age corrected for sex and parity) was lower. In women with hypertensive disorders of pregnancy of varying degrees, patients with an abnormal uterine waveform may be identified. This group has a significantly higher maternal uric acid level, shorter gestational period, higher Cesarean section rate for fetal distress, and lower infant birthweight than the patients with normal waveforms. Furthermore, in the pathologic group, there was a significantly higher incidence of SGA babies and a significant increase in stillbirths.[47] Whether the reduction in uteroplacental circulation is the cause or effect of pregnancy hypertension remains an open question. Others have not been able to demonstrate consistently abnormal studies in hypertension of pregnancy.[127]

Screening normal pregnancy

Based on the hypothesis that trophoblast invasion of the spiral arteries causes the change in the uterine waveforms during the first half of pregnancy, and that this invasion is less developed in pregnancy hypertension, uterine waveform studies have also been evaluated for screening in early pregnancy.[128] The test demonstrated a high sensitivity for prediction of preeclampsia and fetal growth restriction, but there was a high false-positive rate. The results of one study from a well-regarded center are illustrative of this.[129] From 1326 pregnancies, 214 women were identified at 19–21 weeks. Abnormal Doppler findings were still present in 110 of these women at 24 weeks. Three-quarters (77%) of the cases of preeclampsia and one-third of the SGA babies (32%) were found in this group of 110. The predictive value of 31% and 38% from the 24-week result appears good, but the denominator for this calculation should be the number identified at 19–21 weeks. This would halve the positive predictive value. Comment has been made that an incidence of 44 cases of proteinuric pregnancy hypertension out of 1326 pregnancies is high, suggesting that this was a high-risk population of low socioeconomic status. The performance of uterine Doppler in a truly low-risk population is debated. No adequate randomized controlled trials are available to settle this issue at the present time. A recent authoritative review[130] concluded that screening was not effective. This assessment was based on a collective total of 13 000 pregnancies screened. The authors noted a sixfold greater risk of preeclampsia if the Doppler findings were abnormal; however, the sensitivity in the reported studies was 20–60%, and the positive predictive value was 6-40%.

Relationship of umbilical and uterine flow studies

Study of umbilical and uterine waveforms allows classification into four groups, depending on whether these waveforms are normal or abnormal.[46,131,132] The two subgroups characterized by normal umbilical waveforms exhibit little fetal morbidity, irrespective of whether the uterine waveforms are normal or not. If the umbilical waveforms are abnormal, fetal morbidity is present. In patients with a normal uterine artery pattern, it has been suggested that the primary defect is on the fetal side of the placenta. Although the uterine waveform is normal, indicating normal resistance in that branch of the uterine artery, the total uterine flow may be low if the size of the uteroplacental bed (and number of branches of the uterine artery feeding it) is not extensive. In patients with both abnormal umbilical and uterine waveforms, disease may exist in the maternal uteroplacental vascular bed, and it is this that produces the constraint of the fetal–placental circulation. This result has been confirmed by others.[127,128]

Early pregnancy uterine flow studies

The advent of color Doppler ultrasound leading to precise vessel identification has permitted studies of the early first-trimester changes in the uterine artery FVWs. The waveform pattern and the various indices of resistance decrease between 6 and 16 weeks of gestation.[124] In early pregnancy failure (missed abortion, anembryonic pregnancy), there was no difference in these indices of resistance.[133] This finding is interesting as it suggests that early pregnancy failure does not result from failure of visualization.

Key points

1. The difference in frequency between incident and reflected waves produced when an ultrasound beam strikes a moving column of blood is proportional to the velocity of the blood flow. This is the Doppler principle.
2. The flow velocity waveform (FVW) is the collection of frequency differences produced by insonnating a vessel over a time base. The maximum velocity or envelope is the most widely used feature of this waveform in Doppler clinical studies, and a variety of empirical indices have been used to describe the waveform pattern; some reflect physiological hemodynamic quantities such as resistance and volume flow.
3. Blood flow in the umbilical artery in the umbilical cord can be recorded using Doppler ultrasound equipment.
4. Throughout pregnancy, there is a progressive decrease in resistance to blood flow to the placenta in the umbilical arteries as the placenta grows, and this is reflected by the changing pattern of the umbilical artery FVW.
5. Mathematical modeling studies confirm that in excess of 50% of small arteries and arterioles (resistance vessels) need to be obliterated before the umbilical artery Doppler FVW shows an abnormal (high-resistance) pattern.
6. Correlation studies of umbilical artery FVW pattern and placental villous histology confirm vascular disease with loss of small arterial channels in fetal villi when a high-resistance pattern is present.
7. The high-resistance pattern of the umbilical artery FVW is characterized by reduced, absent, or reversed diastolic flow relative to the systolic peak velocity.
8. The presence of a high-resistance pattern in the umbilical artery FVW is associated with an increased risk of intrauterine growth restriction, fetal distress *in utero*, fetal distress in labor, and need for early delivery.
9. Some 60–70% of small-for-gestional-age (SGA) fetuses have a high-resistance umbilical FVW.
10. In dizygotic twin pregnancy with discordant growth, a high-resistance pattern FVW is seen with a small fetus.
11. The use of umbilical artery Doppler FVWs to study high-risk pregnancy has been shown by meta-analysis of randomized controlled trials to be associated with a 32% reduction in perinatal mortality.
12. Volume flow in the umbilical circulation may remain normal when the FVW pattern is one of high resistance, presumably because there is an increase in fetal blood pressure, at least in the early phases.
13. FVW patterns can be recorded from the fetal aorta. The peak velocity of maximum or mean aortic FVW correlates with the degree of fetal hypoxemia and reflects depressed ventricular output.
14. FVW patterns can be recorded from the cerebral arteries. In the middle cerebral artery FVW, a pattern of low resistance predicts fetal hypoxemia.
15. In fetal anemia, the peak velocity of the middle cerebral artery FVW can be used as an index of the degree of anemia and requirement for fetal intravascular transfusion.
16. Changes in the FVWs from the central fetal veins (ductus venous, inferior vena cava) are produced in fetal compromise by a high central venous pressure, in turn reflecting changes in afterload, cardiac outflow, and ventricular end-diastolic pressure.
17. Retardation of flow velocity in the ductus venous waveform at the time of atrial systole indicates developing fetal hypoxemia. A variety of indices measure this.
18. The uterine artery FVW shows a low-resistance pattern in normal pregnancy from 8 weeks onwards.
19. A high-resistance pattern in the uterine artery FVW is signaled by low diastolic flow velocities and the appearance of an early diastolic notch. This predicts pregnancy at risk of preeclampsia and fetal growth restriction.
20. Abnormality in the umbilical artery FVW signals developing placental vascular pathology, which may lead to fetal hypoxemia and acidosis. Changes in the fetal aortic, middle cerebral artery, and ductus venous waveforms correlate with the degree of fetal hypoxemia and fetal condition. The information from Doppler studies of different fetal vessels is complementary.

References

1 Gill RW. Doppler ultrasound: physical aspects. *Semin Perinatol* 1987;11:292.

2 Milnor WR. Pulsatile blood flow. *N Engl J Med* 1972;187: 27.

3 Caro CG, Pedley TJ, Schroter CW, Seed WA. *The mechanics of the circulation*. London: Oxford University Press, 1978.

4 O'Rourke MF. Vascular impedance in studies of arterial and cardiac function. *Physiol Rev* 1982;62:571.

5 Gill RW. Pulsed Doppler with B-mode imaging for quantitative blood flow measurement. *Ultrasound Med Biol* 1979;5:223.

6 Thompson RS, Trudinger BJ, Cook CM. A comparison of Doppler ultrasound waveform indices in the umbilical artery. I: indices derived from the maximum velocity waveform. *Ultrasound Med Biol* 1986;12:835.

7 Thompson RS, Trudinger BJ, Cook CM. A comparison of Doppler ultrasound waveform indices in the umbilical artery. II: indices derived from the mean velocity and first moment waveforms. *Ultrasound Med Biol* 1986;12:845.

8 Thompson RS, Trudinger BJ, Cook CM. Doppler ultrasound waveform indices. AB ratio pulsatility index and Pourcelot ratio. *Br J Obstet Gynaecol* 1988;95:581.

9 Thompson RS, Trudinger BT, Reed VD, Turner AJ. Aortic Doppler velocity measurements and cardiac function in the fetal lamb. *Ultrasound Med Biol* 1994;20:893.

10 Rudolph AM, Heymann MA. Circulatory changes during growth in the fetal lamb. *Circ Res* 1970;26:289.

11 Dawes GS (ed.). The umbilical circulation. In: *Fetal neonatal physiology*. Chicago, IL: Year Book Medical Publishers; 1968:66.

12 Eik-Nes SH, Brubakk AO, Ulstein MK. Measurement of human fetal blood flow. *Br Med J* 1980;280:283.

13 Gill RW, Trudinger BJ, Garrett WJ, et al. Fetal umbilical venous flow measured in utero by pulsed Doppler and B-mode ultrasound. I: normal pregnancy. *Am J Obstet Gynecol* 1981;139: 720.

14 Rankin JHG, McLaughlin MK. The regulation of placental blood flows. *J Dev Physiol* 1979;1:3.

15 Itskovitz J, LaGamma EF, Rudolph AM. The effect of reducing umbilical blood flow on fetal oxygenation. *Am J Obstet Gynecol* 1983;145:813.

16 van Eyck J, Wladimiroff JW, Winjngaard JAGW, et al. The blood flow velocity waveform in the fetal internal carotid and umbilical artery: its relationship to fetal behavioural states in normal pregnancy at 37–38 weeks of gestation. *Br J Obstet Gynaecol* 1987;94:736.

17 van Eyck J, Wladimiroff JW, Noordam MJ, et al. The blood flow velocity waveform in the fetal descending aorta: its relationship to fetal behavioural state in normal pregnancy at 37–38 weeks. *Early Hum Dev* 1985;12:137.

18 Mehalex KE, Rosenberg J, Berkowitz GS, et al. Umbilical and uterine artery flow velocity waveforms effect of the sampling site on Doppler ratios. *J Ultrasound Med* 1989;8:171.

19 Thompson RS, Stevens RJ. A mathematical model for interpretation of Doppler velocity waveform indices. *Med Biol Eng Comput* 1989;27:269.

20 Surat DR, Adamson SL. Downstream determinants of pulsatility of the mean velocity waveform in the umbilical artery as predicted by a computer model. *Ultrasound Med Biol* 1996;22: 707.

21 Thompson RS, Trudinger BJ. Doppler waveform pulsatility index and resistance, pressure and flow in the umbilical placental circulation: an investigation using a mathematical model. *Ultrasound Med Biol* 1990;16:449.

22 Guidetti DA, Diven MY, Cavalieri RL, et al. Fetal umbilical artery flow velocimetry in postdate pregnancies. *Am J Obstet Gynecol* 1987;1157:1521.

23 Farmakides G, Schulman H, Winter D, et al. Prenatal surveillance using non-stress testing and Doppler velocimetry. *Obstet Gynecol* 1988;71:184.

24 Giles WB, Trudinger BJ, Stevens D, et al. Umbilical artery flow velocity waveform analysis in normal ovine pregnancy and after carunculectomy. *J Dev Physiol* 1989;11:135.

25 Trudinger BJ, Stevens D, Connelly A, et al. Umbilical artery flow velocity waveforms and placental resistance: the effects of embolization on the umbilical circulation. *Am J Obstet Gynecol* 1987;157:1443.

26 Morrow RJ, Adamson SL, Bull SB, Ritchie JWK. Effect of placental embolization on the umbilical arterial velocity waveform in fetal sheep. *Am J Obstet Gynecol* 1989;161:1056.

27 Giles WB, Trudinger BJ, Baird P. Fetal umbilical artery flow velocity waveforms and placental resistance: pathological correlation. *Br J Obstet Gynaecol* 1985;92:31.

28 McCowan LM, Mullen BM, Ritchie K. Umbilical artery flow velocity waveforms and the placental vascular bed. *Am J Obstet Gynecol* 1987;157:900.

29 Bracero LA, Beneck D, Kirshenbaum N, et al. Doppler velocimetry and placental disease. *Am J Obstet Gynecol* 1989;161:388.

30 Fok R, Parlova Z, Benirschke K, Paul R. The correlation of arterial lesions with umbilical artery Doppler velocimetry in the placentas of small for date pregnancies. *Obstet Gynecol* 1990;75: 578.

31 Redline RW, Ariel I, Baergen RN, et al. Fetal vascular obstructive lesions: nosology and reproducibility of placental reaction patterns. *Pediatr Dev Pathol* 2004;7:443.

32 Redline RW. Severe fetal placental vascular lesions in term infants with neurologic impairment. *Am J Obstet Gynecol* 2005;192: 452.

33 Moussa HA, Alfirevic Z. Do placental lesions reflect thrombophilia state in women with adverse pregnancy outcome? *Hum Reprod* 2000;15:1830.

34 Trudinger B, Song J, Wu Z, Wang J. Placental insufficiency is characterized by platelet activation in the fetus. *Obstet Gynecol* 2003;101:975.

35 Wilcox GR, Trudinger BJ, Cook CM, et al. Reduced fetal platelet counts in pregnancies with abnormal Doppler umbilical flow waveforms. *Obstet Gynecol* 1989;75:639.

36 Wang X, Athayde N, Trudinger B. Microvascular endothelial cell activation is present in umbilical placental microcirculation of fetal placental disease. *Am J Obstet Gynecol* 2004;190:596.

37 Wang X, Athayde N, Trudinger B. A proinflammatory cytokine response is present in the fetal placenta in placental insufficiency. *Am J Obstet Gynecol* 2003;189:1445.

38 Wang J, Trudinger B. Is an atherogenic lipoprotein profile in the fetus a prerequisite for placental vascular disease? *Br J Obstet Gynaecol* 2000;107:508.

39 Trudinger BJ, Giles WB, Cook CM, et al. Fetal umbilical artery flow velocity waveforms and placental resistance: clinical significance. *Br J Obstet Gynaecol* 1985;92:23.

40 Schulman H, Fleischer A, Stern W, et al. Umbilical velocity wave ratios in human pregnancy. *Am J Obstet Gynecol* 1984;148:986.

41 Reuwer PJHM, Bruinse HW, Stoutenbeek P, Haspels AA. Doppler assessment of the feto-placental circulation in normal and growth retarded fetuses. *Eur J Obstet Gynaecol Reprod Biol* 1984;18:199.

42 Trudinger BJ, Cook CM, Giles WB, et al. Fetal umbilical artery velocity waveforms and subsequent neonatal outcome. *Br J Obstet Gynaecol* 1991;98:378.

43 Karsdorp VH, van Vugt JM, van Geijn HP, et al. Clinical significance of absent or reversed end-diastolic velocity waveforms in umbilical artery. *Lancet* 1994;344:1664.

44 Farrine D, Kelly EN, Ryan G, et al. Absent and reversed umbilical artery end diastolic velocity in Doppler ultrasound. In: Copel J, Reed K, eds. *Obstetrician and gynaecology*. New York: Raven Press; 1995:187–198.

45 Nicholaides KH, Bilardo CM, Soothill PW, Campbell S. Absence of end diastolic frequencies in umbilical artery: a sign of fetal hypoxia and acidosis. *Br Med J* 1988;297:1026.

46 Trudinger BJ, Giles WB, Cook CM. Flow velocity waveforms in the maternal uteroplacental and fetal umbilical placental circulation. *Am J Obstet Gynecol* 1985;92:155.

47 Fleischer A, Schulman H, Farmakides G, et al. Uterine artery Doppler velocimetry in pregnant women with hypertension. *Am J Obstet Gynecol* 1986;154:807.

48 Trudinger BJ, Cook CM. Doppler umbilical and uterine flow waveforms in severe pregnancy hypertension. *Br J Obstet Gynaecol* 1990;97:142.

49 Landon MB, Gabbe SG, Bruner JP, Ludmir J. Doppler umbilical artery velocimetry in pregnancy complicated by insulin-dependent diabetes mellitus. *Obstet Gynecol* 1989;73:961.

50 Johnstone FD, Steel JH, Haddad NG, et al. Doppler umbilical artery flow velocity waveforms in diabetic pregnancy *Br J Obstet Gynaecol* 1992;99:135.

51 Giles WB, Trudinger BJ, Cook CM. Fetal umbilical artery flow velocity time waveforms in twin pregnancies. *Br J Obstet Gynaecol* 1985;92:490.

52 Giles WB, Trudinger BJ, Cook CM, Connelly A. Umbilical artery flow velocity waveforms and twin pregnancy outcome. *Obstet Gynecol* 1988;72:894.

53 Giles WB, Bisits A, O'Callaghan S, Gill A: DAMP Study Group. The Doppler assessment in multiple pregnancy randomized controlled trial of ultrasound biometry versus umbilical artery Doppler ultrasound and biometry in twin pregnancy. *Br J Obstet Gynaecol* 2003;110:593.

54 Quintero RA, Morales WJ, Allen MH, et al. Staging of twin–twin transfusion syndrome. *J Perinatol* 1999;19:550.

55 Quintero RA. Twin–twin transfusion syndrome. *Clin Perinatol* 2003;30:591.

56 Raboisson MJ, Fouron JC, Lamoureux J, et al. Early intertwin differences in myocardial performance during the twin-to-twin transfusion syndrome. *Circulation* 2004;110:3043.

57 Giles WB, Trudinger BJ, Cook CM, Connelly A. Umbilical artery waveforms in triplet pregnancy. *Obstet Gynecol* 1990;75:813.

58 Trudinger BJ, Cook CM. Umbilical and uterine artery flow velocity waveforms in pregnancy associated with major fetal abnormality. *Br J Obstet Gynaecol* 1985;92:666.

59 Rochelson B, Kaplan C, Guzman E, et al. A quantitative analysis of placental vasculature in the third-trimester fetus with autosomal trisomy. *Obstet Gynecol* 1990;75:59.

60 Campbell S. The detection of intrauterine growth retardation. In: Sharp F, Fraser RB, Milner RDG, eds. *Fetal growth*. London: Springer-Verlag; 1989:255.

61 Trudinger BJ, Cook CM, Jones L, Giles WB. A comparison of fetal heart rate monitoring and umbilical artery waveforms in the recognition of fetal compromise. *Br J Obstet Gynaecol* 1986;93:171.

62 Farmakides G, Schulman H, Winter D, et al. Prenatal surveillance using non-stress testing and Doppler velocimetry. *Obstet Gynecol* 1988;71:184.

63 Almstrom H, Axelsson O, Cnattingius S, et al. Comparison of umbilical artery velocimetry and cardiotocography for surveillance of small for gestational age fetuses. *Lancet* 1992;340:936.

64 Chambers SE, Hoskins PR, Haddad NG, et al. A comparison of fetal abdominal circumference measurements and Doppler ultrasound in the prediction of small-for-dates babies and fetal compromise. *Br J Obstet Gynaecol* 1989;96:803.

65 Chang TC, Robson SC, Spencer JAD, Gallivan S. Identification of fetal growth retardation: comparison of Doppler waveform indices and serial ultrasound measurements of abdominal circumference and fetal weight. *Obstet Gynecol* 1993;82:230.

66 Burke G, Stuart B, Crowley P, et al. Is intrauterine growth retardation with normal umbilical artery blood flow a benign condition? *Br Med J* 1990;300:1044.

67 Laurin J, Marsal K, Persson P-H, et al. Ultrasound measurement of fetal blood flow in predicting fetal outcome. *Br J Obstet Gynaecol* 1987;94:940.

68 Marsal K, Persson P. Ultrasonic measurement of fetal blood velocity waveform as a secondary diagnostic test in screening for intrauterine growth retardation. *J Clin Ultrasound* 1988;16:239.

69 Beattie RB, Dornan JC. Antenatal screening for intrauterine growth retardation with umbilical artery Doppler ultrasonography. *Br Med J* 1989;298:631.

70 Martin DH, Antenatal screening with umbilical artery Doppler ultrasonography. *Br Med J* 1989;298:1097.

71 Hanretty KP, Primrose MH, Neilson JP, Whittle MJ. Pregnancy screening by Doppler uteroplacental and umbilical artery waveforms. *Br J Obstet Gynaecol* 1989;96:1163.

72 Indik JH, Chen V, Reed KL. Association of umbilical venous with inferior vena cava blood flow velocities. *Obstet Gynecol* 1991;77:551.

73 Van Splunder P, Huisman TWA, Stijnen T, et al. Presence of pulsations and reproducibility of waveform recording in the umbilical and left portal vein in normal pregnancies. *Ultrasound Obstet Gynecol* 1994;4:49.

74 Griffin D, Bilardo K, Masini L, et al. Doppler blood flow waveforms in the descending thoracic aorta of the human fetus. *Br J Obstet Gynaecol* 1984;91:997.

75 Jouppila P, Kirkinen P. Increased vascular resistance in the descending aorta of the human fetus in hypoxia. *Br J Obstet Gynaecol* 1984;91:853.

76 Tonge HM, Wladimiroff JW, Noordam MH, van Kooten C. Blood flow velocity waveforms in the descending fetal aorta: comparison between normal and growth retarded pregnancies. *Obstet Gynecol* 1986;17:851.

77 Bilardo CM, Nicolaides KH, Campbell S. Doppler measurements of fetal and uteroplacental circulations: relationship with umbilical venous blood gases measured at cordocentesis. *Am J Obstet Gynecol* 1990;162:115.

78 Vyas S, Nicolaides KH, Campbell S. Renal artery flow velocity waveforms in normal and hypoxemic fetuses. *Am J Obstet Gynecol* 1989;161:168.

79 Baschat AA, Gembruch U, Reiss I, et al. Demonstration of fetal coronary blood flow by Doppler ultrasound in relation to arterial and venous flow velocity waveforms and perinatal outcome: the "heart sparing effect". *Ultrasound Obstet Gynecol* 1997;9:162.

80 Marsal K, Laurin J, Lindblad A, Lingman G. Blood flow in the fetal descending aorta. *Semin Perinatol* 1987;11:322.

81 Marsal K, Eik-Nes SH, Lindblad A, Lingman G. Blood flow in

the fetal descending aorta, intrinsic factors affecting fetal blood flow in fetal breathing movements and cardiac arrhythmia. *Ultrasound Med Biol* 1984;10:339.

82 Lingman G, Marsal K. Fetal central blood circulation in the third trimester of normal pregnancy. A longitudinal study. II: aortic blood velocity waveform. *Early Hum Dev* 1986;13:151.

83 van Eyck J, Wladimiroff JW, Noordam MJ, et al. The blood flow velocity waveform in the fetal descending aorta: its relationship to behavioural state in the growth retarded fetus at 37–38 weeks of gestation. *Early Hum Dev* 1986;14:99.

84 Lingman G, Marsal K. Fetal central blood circulation in the third trimester of normal pregnancy. A longitudinal study. I: aortic and umbilical blood flow. *Early Hum Dev* 1986;13:137.

85 Laurin J, Lingman G, Marsal K, Persson RH. Fetal blood flow in pregnancies complicated by intrauterine growth retardation. *Obstet Gynecol* 1987;69:895.

86 Ley D, Laurin J, Bjerre I, et al. Abnormal fetal aortic velocity waveform and minor neurological dysfunction at 7 years of age. *Ultrasound Obstet Gynecol* 1996;8:152.

87 Soothill PW, Nicolaides KH, Bilardo CM, Campbell S. Relation of fetal hypoxia in growth retardation to mean blood velocity in the fetal aorta. *Lancet* 1986;2:1118.

88 Wladimiroff JW, van Bel F. Fetal and neonatal cerebral blood flow. *Semin Perinatol* 1987;11:335.

89 van den Winjngaard JAGW, Groenenberg IAL, Wladimiroff JW, Hop WCJ. Cerebral Doppler ultrasound of the human fetus. *Br J Obstet Gynaecol* 1989;96:845.

90 Woo JSK, Liang ST, Lo RLS, Chan FY. Middle cerebral artery Doppler flow velocity waveforms. *Obstet Gynecol* 1987;70:613.

91 Kirkener P, Muller R, Huch R, Huch A. Blood flow velocity waveforms in human fetal intracranial arteries. *Obstet Gynecol* 1987;70:617.

92 Arbeille PH, Roncin A, Berson M, et al. Exploration of the fetal cerebral blood flow by duplex Doppler–linear array system in normal and pathological pregnancies. *Ultrasound Med Biol* 1987;13:329.

93 Waldimiroff JW, Tonge HM, Stewart PA. Doppler ultrasound assessment of cerebral blood flow in the human fetus. *Br J Obstet Gynaecol* 1986;93:471.

94 Vyas S, Nicolaides KH, Bower S, Campbell S, Middle cerebral artery flow velocity waveform in fetal hypoxaemia. *Br J Obstet Gynaecol* 1990;97:797.

95 Sepulveda W, Shennan AH, Peek MJ. Reverse end diastolic flow in the middle cerebral artery: an agonal pattern in the human fetus. *Am J Obstet Gynecol* 1996;174:1645.

96 Arias F. Accuracy of the middle cerebral to umbilical artery resistance index ratio in the production of neonatal outcome in patients at high risk for fetal and neonatal complications. *Am J Obstet Gynecol* 1994;171:1541.

97 Mari G. Arterial blood flow velocity waveforms of the pelvis and lower extremities in normal and growth retarded fetuses. *Am J Obstet Gynecol* 1991;165:143.

98 Sepulveda W, Bower S, Nicolidis P, et al. Discordant blood from velocity waveform in left and right brachial arteries in growth retarded fetuses. *Obstet Gynecol* 1995:86:734.

99 Abu Hamed A, Mari G, Bogdan D, Evans AT. Doppler color velocimetry of the splenic artery in the human fetus: is it a marker of chronic hypoxia. *Am J Obstet Gynecol* 1995;172: 820.

100 Arduini D, Rizzo G. Fetal renal artery velocity waveforms and amniotic fluid volume in growth retarded and post term fetuses. *Obstet Gynecol* 1991;77:370.

101 Kiserud T, Eik-Nes S, Blaas H, Hellevik LR. Ultrasonographic velocimetry of the fetal ductus venosus. *Lancet* 1991;338: 1412.

102 Huisman TW, Brezinka C, Stewart PA, et al. Ductus venosus flow velocity waveforms in relation to fetal behavioural states. *Br J Obstet Gynaecol* 1994;101:220.

103 Rizzo G, Capponi A, Talone PE, et al. Doppler indices from inferior vena cava and ductus venosus in predicting pH and oxygen tension in umbilical blood at cordocentesis in growth retarded fetuses. *Ultrasound Obstet Gynecol* 1996;7:401.

104 Hecher K, Snijders R, Campbell S, Nicolaides S. Fetal venous, intracardiac and arterial blood flow in intrauterine growth retardation. Relationship with blood gases. *Am J Obstet Gynecol* 1995;173:10.

105 Rizzo G, Capponi A, Arduini D, Romanini C. The value of fetal arterial cardiac and venous flow in predicting pH and blood gases in umbilical blood at cordocentesis in growth retarded fetuses. *Br J Obstet Gynecol* 1995;102:963.

106 Opekes D, Vandenbussche FP, Van Bel F, et al. Fetal ductus venosus blood flow velocities before and after transfusion in red cell alloimmunized pregnancies. *Obstet Gynecol* 1993;82:237.

107 Mori A, Trudinger BJ, Mori R, et al. The fetal central venous pressure waveform in normal pregnancy and in umbilical placental insufficiency. *Am J Obstet Gynecol* 1995;172:51.

108 Laudy JA, Huisman TW, de Ridder MA, et al. Normal fetal pulmonary venous blood flow. *Ultrasound Obstet Gynecol* 1995;6:277.

109 Laudy JA, Gaillard JL, van den Anker JN, et al. Doppler ultrasound imaging: a new technique to detect lung hypoplasia before birth? *Ultrasound Obstet Gynecol* 1996;7:189.

110 Alfirevic Z, Neilson JP. Doppler ultrasonography in high risk pregnancies: systematic review with meta-analysis. *Am J Obstet Gynecol* 1995;172:1379.

111 Trudinger BJ, Cook CM. Umbilical artery flow velocity waveform in high risk pregnancy: randomized controlled trial. *Lancet* 1987;1:188.

112 Hecher K, Bilardo CM, Stigter RH, et al. Monitoring of fetuses with intrauterine growth restriction: a longitudinal study. *Ultrasound Obstet Gynecol* 2001;18:564.

113 Baschat AA, Gembruch U, Harman CR. The sequence of changes in Doppler and biophysical parameters as severe fetal growth restriction worsens. *Ultrasound Obstet Gynecol* 2001;18: 571.

114 Ferrazzi E, Bozzo M, Rigano S, et al. Temporal sequence of abnormal Doppler changes in the peripheral and central circulatory systems of the severely growth restricted fetus. *Ultrasound Obstet Gynecol* 2002;19:140.

115 Romero R, Kalache KD, Kadar N. Timing the delivery of the preterm severely growth restricted fetus: venous Doppler, cardiotocography or biophysical profile? *Ultrasound Obstet Gynecol* 2002;19:118.

116 Thornton JG, Hornbuckle J, Vail A, et al. The GRIT study group. Infant wellbeing at 2 years of age in the Growth Restriction Intervention Trial (GRIT) : multicentred randomized controlled trial. *Lancet* 2004;364:513.

117 Trudinger BJ, Cook CM, Thompson RS, et al. Low dose aspirin therapy improves fetal weight in umbilical placental insufficiency. *Am J Obstet Gynecol* 1988;159:681.

118 Campbell S, Diaz-Recasens J, Griffin DR, et al. New Doppler technique for assessing uteroplacental blood flow. *Lancet* 1983;1:675.

119 Trudinger BJ, Giles WB, Cook CM. Uteroplacental blood flow velocity time waveforms in normal and complicated pregnancy. *Br J Obstet Gynaecol* 1985;92:39.

120 Campbell S, Vyas S, Beweley S. Doppler uteroplacental waveforms. *Lancet* 1988;1:1287.
121 Cohen-Overbeek T, Pearce JM, Campbell S. The antenatal assessment of utero-placental and feto-placental blood flow using Doppler ultrasound. *Ultrasound Med Biol* 1985;11:329.
122 Chambers SE, Johnstone FD, Muir BB, et al. The effects of placental site on the arcuate artery flow velocity waveform. *J Ultrasound Med* 1988;7:671.
123 Farrell T, Chien PD, Mires GJ. The reliability of detection of an early diastolic notch with uterine artery Doppler velocimetry. *Br J Obstet Gynaecol* 1998;105:1308.
124 Jauniaux E, Jurkovic D, Campbell S. In vivo investigation of the anatomy and the physiology on early human placental circulations. *Ultrasound Obstet Gynecol* 1991;1:435.
125 Dickey RP, Hower JF. Ultrasonographic features of uterine blood flow during the first 16 weeks of pregnancy. *Hum Reprod* 1995;10:2448.
126 Valentin L, Sladkevicius P, Laurini R, et al. Uteroplacental and luteal circulation in normal first trimester pregnancies: Doppler ultrasonographic and morphologic study. *Am J Obstet Gynecol* 1996;174:768.
127 Hanretty KP, Whittle M, Rubin PC. Doppler uteroplacental waveforms in pregnancy induced hypertension: a reappraisal. *Lancet* 1988;1:850.
128 Bower S, Schucter K, Campbell S. Doppler ultrasound screening as part of routine antenatal screening: prediction of preeclampsia and intrauterine growth retardation. *Br J Obstet Gynaecol* 1993:989.
129 Harrington K, Cooper D, Lees C, et al. Doppler ultrasound of the uterine arteries: the importance of bilateral matching in the prediction of preeclampsia, placental abruption on delivery of a small for gestational age baby. *Ultrasound Obstet Gynecol* 1996;7:182.
130 Sibai B, Dekker G, Kupferminc M. Pre-eclampsia. *Lancet* 2005;365:785.
131 Schulman H. The clinical implications of Doppler ultrasound examination of the uterine and umbilical arteries. *Am J Obstet Gynecol* 1987;136:889.
132 Gudmundsson S, Marsal K. Ultrasound Doppler evaluation of uteroplacental and fetoplacental circulation in pre-eclampsia. *Arch Gynecol Obstet* 1988;243:199.
133 Stabile I, Grudzinskas J, Campbell S. Doppler ultrasonographic evaluation of abnormal pregnancies in the first trimester. *J Clin Ultrasound* 1990;18:497.

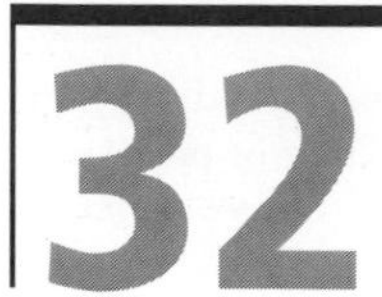

Antepartum and intrapartum surveillance of the fetus and the amniotic fluid

Lami Yeo, Michael G. Ross, and Anthony M. Vintzileos

Introduction

The challenge of assessing the intrauterine fetus as a patient lies in the inability to perform a truly direct examination. Instead, one must rely on current indirect modalities such as dynamic, high-resolution ultrasonography, fetal heart rate (FHR) monitoring via the nonstress test (NST) and contraction stress test (CST), and vibroacoustic stimulation (VAS), to name some examples. Fortunately, technological and scientific advances over the years have permitted more specific examinations of the fetus and its behavior. It is clear that one of the most important goals of perinatal medicine is to recognize fetal disease states, optimize fetal outcome, and prevent perinatal mortality. Therefore, surveillance of the fetus during the antepartum and intrapartum periods is an important component of this process, which has the intent of detecting fetal asphyxia so that appropriate and timely interventions can be made. It is also clear that, because fetal compromise has a diverse etiology, forms of testing must be able to survey both acute fetal asphyxia and more chronic disease states. In the past, both the method and the frequency of antepartum testing have been arbitrary and generalized. However, it is apparent that tailoring testing to each disease-specific state is not only practical, but also more appropriate. Surveillance of the amniotic fluid volume (AFV) is also crucial, as fluid disorders may not only represent but also lead to fetal disease states. By utilizing the information from fetal surveillance, conservative management may be possible and may allow continued maturation *in utero*, while reducing the potential of neonatal prematurity complications. This chapter will discuss the current techniques available to survey the fetus and amniotic fluid during both antepartum and intrapartum periods.

Antepartum surveillance techniques (fetus and amniotic fluid)

Currently, there are multiple maternal and fetal indications to perform antepartum surveillance (Table 32.1), although these are not absolute. The common basis for selecting these patients are those who are at increased risk of perinatal mortality, uteroplacental insufficiency, and fetal asphyxia. Many surveillance methods rely on natural fetal behavior. While the mechanisms controlling sleep and activity cycles in the fetus are not well understood, it is imperative that knowledge of this behavior is available to appropriately interpret FHR monitoring and fetal biophysical profile (BPP) activities. In the near-term fetus, there are four behavioral states (occurring repeatedly and stable over time) that have been described: quiet sleep, active sleep, quiet awake, and active awake.[1] Quiet sleep is characterized by absent eye or breathing movements, infrequent startle-type body movements, reduced FHR variability, and no accelerations. Active sleep is characterized by frequent gross body movements, rapid eye movements, breathing, normal FHR variability, and accelerations. The fetus predominantly spends its time in either a quiet or an active sleep state.[2]

Fetal movement monitoring

This method of surveillance (also known as "fetal kick counts") by the mother is advantageous because it lacks contraindications, is simple, inexpensive, noninvasive, and understandable to patients. In general, because the presence of good fetal movement is a sign of fetal well-being and an indirect measure of normal fetal acid–base status, it is a viable modality. However, a decrease in fetal movements often (but not invariably) precedes fetal death, in some cases by several days.[3] Around 16–18 weeks' gestation, most women become cognizant of fetal activity, and this perception appears to be at its maximum by 28–32 weeks.[4] However, awareness of fetal movements will vary from patient to patient, and is also affected by other maternal, fetal, and uterine factors (Table 32.2). In general, patients perceive about 80% of ultrasonographically visualized fetal movements.[5]

While several protocols have been utilized, neither the ideal duration for counting movements nor the optimal number of movements has been defined. Accordingly, there are many reported techniques that are acceptable, all of which rely on

Table 32.1 Selected indications for antepartum surveillance (fetus and amniotic fluid).

Indications
Diabetes mellitus
Hypertensive disorders (chronic hypertension, preeclampsia)
Renal disease
Collagen vascular disorders
Maternal thyrotoxicosis
Severe anemia or maternal hemoglobinopathies
Isoimmunization
Prior unexplained fetal demise
Third-trimester vaginal bleeding
Premature rupture of membranes
Maternal perception of decreased fetal movements
Postdate pregnancy (>41 weeks)
Elevated maternal serum AFP (normal amniotic fluid AFP)
Abnormal or irregular fetal heart rate on auscultation
Selected fetal anomalies (e.g., gastroschisis)
Multiple gestation
Intrauterine growth restriction
Amniotic fluid abnormalities (oligohydramnios or polyhydramnios)

AFP, alpha-fetoprotein.

Table 32.2 Fetal movement monitoring.

Factors influencing maternally perceived fetal movements
Maternal
Activity
Obesity
Ingestion of medications or drugs that depress (e.g., methadone) or increase (e.g., cocaine) fetal movements
Fetal
Behavioral states
Gestational age
Congenital anomalies (e.g., neuromuscular disorders, fetal akinesia syndrome)
Duration of fetal movements
Uterine
Placental location
Amniotic fluid volume

maternal compliance. A popular approach is to have the patient lie on her left side and count distinct fetal movements.[6] Counting 10 movements in a period of up to 2 h is felt to be reassuring. If the count is nonreassuring or decreased, further assessment is recommended (such as NST with AFV assessment or BPP), and the physician should be contacted immediately.

The relationship between decreased fetal activity and poor perinatal outcome has been well established.[7,8] Leader et al.[8] found that, among high-risk pregnancies, 15% perceived an inactive fetus; among these, 46% had a poor perinatal outcome (stillbirths or poor neonatal condition at birth). Rayburn[7] examined high-risk patients and found that patients with inactive fetuses were more likely to have a stillborn or do poorly during labor and the immediate neonatal period (abnormal labor FHR patterns, Cesarean for fetal distress, 5-min Apgar scores ≤ 6). In addition, in the inactive group, the incidence of severe fetal growth restriction was almost 10 times higher than that of the active group, and the overall risk of stillbirth was 35% (versus 0.6% in the active group).

While fetal movement monitoring is beneficial in high-risk pregnancies, it may also be useful in low-risk populations in reducing fetal mortality. In one large prospective study, during a 7-month control period (patients were not advised in formal fetal movement assessment), the fetal mortality rate was 8.7/1000 births.[6] However, in a subsequent study period, when a fetal movement screening program was instituted, this rate dropped to 2.1/1000 births. It should be noted that there was a 13% increase in the number of NSTs performed for "decreased fetal movement," and the intervention rate for fetal distress was 2.6 times higher (versus control subjects).

Contraction stress test (CST)

Designed to detect uteroplacental insufficiency before fetal compromise, this test is based on the response of the FHR to uterine contractions. It relies on the premise that fetal oxygenation will be transiently worsened by contractions. In the suboptimally oxygenated fetus, the resultant intermittent worsening in oxygenation will, in turn, lead to the FHR pattern of late decelerations.[9]

Lying in a lateral recumbent position, the patient has an external fetal monitor record both the FHR and uterine contractions simultaneously for a 20- to 30-min interval. If the patient is spontaneously contracting, and the frequency is ≥ 3 contractions/10 min, and the duration of each contraction is ≥ 45 s, then uterine stimulation is not required. However, if these criteria are not met, then either nipple stimulation or exogenous oxytocin can be used to elicit contractions. Once adequate contractions are achieved, the oxytocin infusion is discontinued. The CST should be avoided when there is a contraindication to labor. Examples include prior myomectomy or classical Cesarean section scar, placenta previa or placental abruption, premature rupture of membranes (PROM), current preterm labor, multiple gestations, and incompetent cervix.

Freeman's criteria (Table 32.3) are used by most to interpret CST results.[10] The most common result is a negative CST, which indicates adequate fetal oxygenation in the presence of contractions.[10–12] It has also been consistently associated with a good fetal outcome. One group reviewed data from their institution along with the literature, and found that the incidence of antepartum fetal death (within 1 week of a negative CST) was 0.2–0.7%.[11] Lagrew and colleagues[13] evaluated antepartum test results in 614 diabetic women. Only one

Table 32.3 Interpretation of the contraction stress test.

Interpretation	Criteria
Nonreactive	No acceleration of at least 15 b.p.m. in amplitude or of 15-s duration during test
Reactive	Any acceleration ≥ 15 b.p.m. for ≥ 15 s during test
Negative	No late deceleration, with at least three contractions/10 min
Positive	Consistent, persistent late decelerations, regardless of contraction frequency, in the absence of uterine hyperstimulation
Equivocal:	
Suspicious	Nonpersistent (< 50% of the contractions) late decelerations
Hyperstimulation	FHR deceleration in the presence of uterine contractions exceeding five/10 min or lasting ≥ 90 s
Unsatisfactory	Insufficient FHR tracing or inability to achieve appropriate uterine contractions

FHR, fetal heart rate; b.p.m., beats per minute.

patient had an intrauterine demise within 1 week of a negative CST. Thus, the literature suggests that there is a low incidence (< 1%) of antepartum fetal death within 1 week of testing. However, this test will not predict acute fetal compromise unrelated to placental insufficiency, such as cord prolapse. In addition, the fetal deaths that have been reported after a negative CST are often attributed to abruption, congenital malformations, and poor glucose control in diabetic women.[11] Fetal outcome is controversial when a negative, nonreactive CST is seen. Druzin et al.[14] have reported an increased likelihood of fetal death. Others have not found an increase in perinatal mortality or in low Apgar scores in this group; however, 12% of these fetuses had congenital anomalies.[15] Also, 18% of the mothers were on sedatives and 45% were hypertensive. Thus, it has been recommended that investigation into possible causes of nonreactivity (prematurity, medications, congenital anomalies) should be done, along with repeat testing within 24 h.[12]

In general, a positive CST implies uteroplacental insufficiency and has been associated with adverse perinatal outcome and an increased incidence of intrauterine demise.[10] However, an important drawback is the high incidence of false-positive CSTs. In fact, the false-positive rate has been reported to be > 50%, depending on which perinatal outcome is defined.[16] This may lead to intervention, which can be significant for the preterm fetus. The most ominous FHR pattern seen in this testing is when the CST is positive and nonreactive. In fact, the corrected perinatal mortality rate has been found to be as high as 17% in this group; nonreassuring FHR patterns have been found to occur during labor, and up to 25% of the cases demonstrate fetal growth restriction.[10,17] Thus, this type of CST result usually necessitates delivery, and Cesarean section should be considered. Another possible occurrence is the positive, reactive CST. Devoe[18] found that, in those with positive CSTs but accelerations, there were lower rates of perinatal mortality, intrapartum fetal distress, low 5-min Apgar scores, primary Cesarean sections, and neonatal morbidity (versus positive, nonreactive CSTs). Another group found that 70% of patients with a positive CST (and accelerations) could tolerate labor without distress.[17] Having this finding does not require abdominal delivery, and labor induction is acceptable. In addition, if the fetus is preterm, further alternative testing is a reasonable option.[12]

Varying results have been reported with the suspicious CST.[19,20] A retrospective evaluation of CST results found that 2.3% were suspicious; 26% of these went on to have a positive CST or subsequent perinatal death.[19] Conversely, Staisch and colleagues[20] performed 435 CSTs on 217 high-risk patients. A suspicious CST occurred in 24% of patients, and they found no association between this finding and neonatal morbidity or mortality. Thus, it is recommended that patients with a suspicious CST should have a repeat CST within 24 h or be evaluated with another form of antepartum testing. Equivocal tests resulting from uterine hyperstimulation or an inability to obtain a satisfactory FHR tracing should also be followed up similarly. Various causes of unsatisfactory CSTs include obesity, excessive fetal activity, and polyhydramnios.

Nonstress test (NST)

This testing modality is based on the premise that the heart rate of the fetus that is not acidemic or neurologically depressed will temporarily accelerate with fetal movement. FHR reactivity is felt to be a good indicator of normal fetal autonomic function and well-being; it depends on normal neurological development and normal integration of the central nervous system (CNS) control of FHR. In contrast, loss of reactivity is most commonly associated with a sleep cycle (an important point to remember), but can result from any cause of CNS depression (including fetal acidemia). The purpose of the NST is to identify both normal fetuses (who can remain *in utero*) and those with asphyxia/hypoxia (so that timely intervention can improve outcome). Fortunately, the NST (compared with the CST) has the advantages of time, easier interpretability, and lack of contraindications.[21]

The FHR is monitored with a Doppler ultrasound transducer, while a tocodynamometer may be used to record uterine contractions, if any. Fetal activity is also recorded with the results displayed on the strip; however, the patient does not need to document fetal movement for the test to be interpreted. Less than 1% of NSTs provide unsatisfactory results owing to inadequate recording of the FHR tracing.[22] Technical difficulties that may be encountered include obesity, fetal hiccups, excessive fetal activity, and polyhydramnios.[16]

The tracing is categorized as reactive (normal) or nonreactive. While various definitions of reactivity have been used, the most common is ≥ 2 FHR accelerations [which peak, but do not necessarily remain, at least 15 beats per minute (b.p.m.) in amplitude above the baseline, and last 15 s from baseline to baseline] within a 10- or 20-min period, with or without fetal movement.[23] It may be necessary to continue the tracing for 40 min to account for variations in the fetal sleep–wake cycle, because it may take this long for a healthy term fetus to display two FHR accelerations.[24] If, after 40 min (from the start of testing), the criteria are still not met, the test is considered nonreactive. On initial testing, almost 85% of high-risk patients show a reactive NST, and the remaining 15% are nonreactive.[22] Other factors (besides fetal hypoxia, asphyxia, behavioral states, gestational age) can lead to a nonreactive NST, such as depressants (narcotics, phenobarbital), beta-blockers (propranolol), and smoking (decreased NST reactivity).[25–27] It is also important to realize that variable decelerations can be observed in up to 50% of NSTs.[28] If they are not repetitive and brief (< 30 s), they likely indicate neither fetal compromise nor the need for obstetric intervention. However, repetitive variable decelerations (at least three in 20 min) even if mild, have been associated with an increased risk of Cesarean section for a nonreassuring intrapartum FHR pattern.[29]

Routine NST interpretation does not take gestational age into account; however, this is an important consideration, as preterm fetuses are less likely to have FHR accelerations in association with fetal movements. Navot et al.[30] found a linear increase in the incidence of FHR accelerations in association with fetal movements, from 20% (25 weeks) to 65% (40 weeks). The amplitude of accelerations also appears to be related to gestational age, as accelerations of > 15 b.p.m. are responsible for only 20% of the total number of accelerations at early gestations (24–26 weeks).[31] Gagnon et al.[32] described the normal maturation of the FHR pattern from 26 weeks to term: decrease in basal FHR, increase in amplitude of accelerations, and increase in long-term variability. All these changes evolved by 30 weeks, and no further significant changes developed later until term. As the gestational age increases, a higher percentage of reactive NSTs is found.[33] For instance, the percentage of reactive NSTs was 16.7%, 65.6%, 90.5%, and 94.4% at 23–27, 28–32, 33–37, and 38–42 weeks respectively.[33] This also implies that the lower the gestational age, the higher the percentage of nonreactive NSTs. This concept should be kept in mind, as fetuses may undergo antepartum surveillance at < 32 weeks. Preterm fetuses may also normally exhibit decelerations between 20 and 30 weeks.[34] They become less common as the gestation advances, and are more frequent at < 30 weeks. However, while it is clear that gestational age should always be considered when interpreting NSTs, nonreassuring FHR patterns in the preterm fetus should not be automatically and improperly attributed to prematurity.

Lavery[35] reviewed perinatal mortality among patients in whom the NST was the main method of fetal assessment. In nine separate studies (7759 patients), a gross perinatal mortality of 12.5/1000 was found. The predictive value of a negative NST (normal outcome associated with a reactive NST) is very high. The reactive NST predicts good perinatal outcome in about 95% of cases.[36] Accordingly, false-negative NSTs are infrequent. Within 1 week of a reactive NST, the perinatal mortality rate is about 3–5/1000.[10,22] In addition, Devoe[37] found that, compared with nonreactive tests, patients with reactive NSTs were less likely (5% versus 22%) to experience perinatal morbidity (intrapartum fetal distress, low Apgar scores, neonatal complications, intrauterine growth restriction). Barss et al.[38] found the antepartum stillbirth rate (within 7 days of a reactive test) was 2.7/1000 and 2.8/1000 for the general high-risk population and postdate pregnancies respectively. For the two groups, the mean interval between a reactive test and stillbirth was 3.8 and 3.5 days. Accordingly, some have recommended that increasing the testing frequency to twice per week could prevent some of these fetal deaths. Boehm et al.[39] found a reduction in the stillbirth rate in a high-risk population (6.1/1000 to 1.9/1000) when the NST frequency was increased from weekly to twice a week. In a review of 1000 patients with diabetes or fetal growth restriction, one group suggested that weekly testing was not effective, and that twice-weekly testing should be established.[40] However, the American College of Obstetricians and Gynecologists (ACOG) states that NSTs are typically repeated at weekly intervals (although certain high-risk conditions may warrant twice-weekly testing).[9]

While there is excellent specificity with a reactive NST, the predictive value of a positive test is low (in most large studies, it is < 40%).[41] The false-positive rate of a nonreactive NST is also very high. A literature review found false-positive rates of 57–100% for perinatal mortality, and 44–92% with softer outcome measures of perinatal morbidity.[16] Therefore, given this fact, when a nonreactive NST is seen, one can either extend the time of the NST or proceed with other forms of testing (such as the BPP). Studies have shown that a reactive FHR (even after a prolonged NST) may still be consistent with good fetal outcome. However, persistent absence of reactivity (without an obvious cause such as medication, prematurity, congenital anomalies) may be associated with fetal compromise in most cases. Devoe et al.[42] found that all tracings that became reactive did so by the end of 70 min. Those fetuses that remained nonreactive (after 90 min) had 67% and 93.3% perinatal mortality and morbidity rates respectively.

In summary, while a reactive NST is usually associated with good outcomes, most fetuses who do not show accelerations during an NST are also not compromised. We believe that, if the NST is used for fetal surveillance, once per week testing may not offer the most optimal outcome; one may consider the use of biweekly testing. As will be discussed later, indication-specific testing with a more individualized approach may be more appropriate.

Vibroacoustic stimulation (VAS)

Because the majority of nonreactive NSTs occur in healthy fetuses in a physiologically normal sleep state, some have tried to improve NST efficacy by "stimulating" the fetus, in the hope of distinguishing normal fetal sleep from asphyxia. This method may elicit FHR accelerations by utilizing an artificial larynx (positioned on the maternal abdomen over the fetal vertex) with a stimulus of 1–2 s being applied. This may be repeated up to three times (at 1-min intervals) for progressively longer durations (of up to 3 s) to elicit accelerations. The normal fetal response to VAS includes not only FHR accelerations, but also increases in long-term FHR variability and gross body movements. VAS has been conclusively demonstrated to be effective in achieving fetal arousal, is reasonably safe, and improves the efficiency of antepartum FHR testing. Utilizing this on the nonacidemic fetus may elicit accelerations that appear to be valid in predicting fetal well-being. It offers the advantage of safely reducing testing time, without compromising detection of the acidemic fetus.[43] While VAS produces increases in intrauterine sound, and although these sound pressure levels are elevated, they are thought to be safe and harmless to the fetus.

Trudinger and Boylan[44] found that using VAS with NST (versus NST alone) had a higher sensitivity in detecting abnormal outcomes (66% versus 39%). Those fetuses with an abnormal response (who remained nonreactive after VAS) demonstrated increased rates of intrapartum fetal distress, fetal growth restriction, and low Apgar scores.[44] Gestational age appears to affect the FHR response to VAS, with a maturational response as gestation advances. Gagnon et al.[45] found that in 26- to 28-week fetuses, the maximum amplitude of the first acceleration was lower, and in 75% of these fetuses, was < 15 b.p.m. In contrast, after 36 weeks, all the initial accelerations were > 15 b.p.m. Another study evaluated FHR responses to VAS in fetuses < 36 weeks and ≥ 36 weeks.[46] Baseline changes in FHR, as well as tachycardia in response to VAS, were common findings in both groups. Baseline changes in FHRs of ≥ 10 b.p.m. were observed in 46% and 70% of preterm and term fetuses respectively. Unusual FHR patterns (including prolonged tachycardia) were seen after VAS in some preterm fetuses. The authors cautioned that these unusual FHR patterns must be properly recognized to adequately interpret the FHR tracings in response to VAS.

In summary, VAS is an effective technique to improve the efficiency of antepartum FHR testing. It may decrease the time needed to perform NSTs, as well as the number of false-positive results. This is accomplished without changing the predictive reliability of a reactive NST.

Biophysical profile (BPP)

The BPP is performed using real-time ultrasonography to assess multiple fetal biophysical activities, as well as AFV. The observation is continued until either normal activity is seen or 30 consecutive minutes of scanning have elapsed. The BPP is unique in that it assesses both acute (FHR reactivity, fetal breathing movements, fetal movements, fetal tone) and chronic markers (AFV) of fetal condition. An understanding of the fetal biophysical response to hypoxemia and acidemia is essential to interpret the BPP score. The fetus will respond to central hypoxemia/acidemia by altering its movement, tone, breathing, and heart rate pattern. The corollary is also true that, in the presence of normal biophysical activities, CNS tissue is functional and is not significantly hypoxic.

Manning et al.[47] introduced the BPP score in 1980. It provides an estimate of the risk of fetal death in the immediate future, with the risk being low when a normal score is present. Scoring systems assign a numeric value (usually 0 or 2) to each of the biophysical components (Table 32.4). An advantage of the BPP is that observations of fetal movement and breathing (or their absence) are unequivocal, and there are no interobserver discrepancies in interpretation which, in contrast, exist with the NST. Fetal hiccups are interpreted as a variant of normal fetal breathing. Presently, the rate and pattern of the breathing movements are not considered clinically significant, except in extreme cases. Notably, each BPP

Table 32.4 Biophysical profile scoring: technique and interpretation.

Biophysical variable	Normal (score = 2)	Abnormal (score = 0)
Fetal breathing movements	≥ 1 episode of ≥ 30 s in 30 min	Absent or no episode of ≥ 30 s in 30 min
Gross body movements	≥ 3 discrete body limb movements in 30 min (episodes of active continuous movement considered)	≤ 2 episodes of body limb movements in 30 min as single movement
Fetal tone	≥ 1 episode of active extension with return to flexion of fetal limb(s) or trunk Opening and closing of hand considered normal tone	Either slow extension with return to partial flexion movement of limb in full extension or absent fetal movement
Reactive fetal heart rate	≥ 2 episodes of acceleration of ≥ 15 b.p.m. and of ≥ 15 s associated with fetal movement in 20 min	< 2 episodes of acceleration of fetal heart rate or acceleration of < 15 b.p.m. in 20 min
Qualitative amniotic fluid volume	≥ 1 pocket of fluid measuring 2 cm in vertical axis	Either no pockets or largest pocket < 2 cm in vertical axis

b.p.m., beats per minute.

parameter reflects a normally functioning area of the CNS, evolves *in utero* at predictable gestational ages, and is based on fetal neurophysiology. Vintzileos et al.[48] proposed the gradual hypoxia concept, which states that the biophysical activities developed last *in utero* are also the first to become abnormal in the presence of fetal acidemia or infection. At about 7.5 weeks, the CNS center controlling fetal tone is the first to develop, followed by development of body movement at 8.5–9.5 weeks. The center controlling regular breathing movements develops after 20–21 weeks, and the center controlling FHR reactivity functions by the end of the second/beginning of the third trimester. Therefore, in accordance with the gradual hypoxia concept, early stages of compromise are revealed by abnormalities in FHR reactivity and breathing, while movement and tone are not abolished until much later stages of compromise.

Absence of a particular activity may be due to diurnal variation, maternal drugs, short-term periodicity, acute fetal asphyxia, or fetal infection. The sequential loss of BPP variables serves as a marker of the degree of placental dysfunction. A BPP score of 8 or more is considered reassuring. In fact, if all four sonographic components are normal, the NST may be omitted without compromising the validity of the test results.[49] When the score is < 8, however, analyzing which individual components of the BPP are abnormal can assist in determining true fetal status and minimize false-positive examinations. The BPP score should also be interpreted within the overall clinical context. In general, a score of 6 is considered equivocal, and a score of ≤ 4 is abnormal. In the mature fetus, a BPP of 6/10 may indicate compromise and may be an indication for delivery; however, in the immature fetus, repeat testing or use of Doppler velocimetry may be in order before intervention is recommended. Also, regardless of the total score, in the presence of oligohydramnios (largest vertical pocket of AFV ≤ 2 cm), further evaluation is warranted.[50] Manning believes that oligohydramnios (in the presence of a normal fetus, functioning renal tissue, intact membranes) is always considered an indication for induction, despite the presence of normal FHR reactivity, breathing, movement, and tone. He bases this approach on an extensive review of the relationship between ultrasound-defined oligohydramnios and perinatal mortality,[51] and a subsequent prospective study indicating that intervention for oligohydramnios can improve perinatal outcome.[52] However, more recent data would advocate the use of Doppler velocimetry (umbilical artery, middle cerebral artery, ductus venosus) to assist in management.

The data strongly suggest that the application of BPP to the high-risk pregnant population results in a dramatic improvement in perinatal mortality rates. The corrected perinatal mortality rate for two large series (16 804 high-risk referred patients) was 2.2/1000.[53,54] Manning et al.[53] contrasted perinatal mortality among 12 620 high-risk tested patients with 65 979 nontested historical control subjects. The control population (the majority were low risk) yielded a gross perinatal mortality rate of 14.3/1000 (versus 7.37/1000 in the tested population) for a decrease in mortality of 48.5%. In this study, the corrected stillbirth rate among tested patients was 1.18/1000 (versus 6.35/1000 among historical control subjects), a decrease of 81%. A normal BPP conveys a low risk of stillbirth; the false-negative rate of the BPP (fetal death within 1 week of a last normal test result) ranges from 0.645 to 7.000 per 1000.[53,55] Figure 32.1 shows an inverse and exponential relationship (highly significant correlation) between last BPP score and perinatal mortality. There is also a strong relationship between the last BPP score and perinatal morbidity variables.[54,56] Figure 32.2 shows a highly significant inverse linear correlation between last BPP score and perinatal morbidity (fetal distress, admission to neonatal intensive care unit, intrauterine growth restriction, 5-min Apgar score ≤ 7, and cord pH < 7.20). Combinations of these variables also showed the same highly significant inverse linear correlation with BPP score. The interval of BPP testing frequency (1–2/week) is arbitrary, however, and is often a matter of individual judgment, training, preferences, and experience.

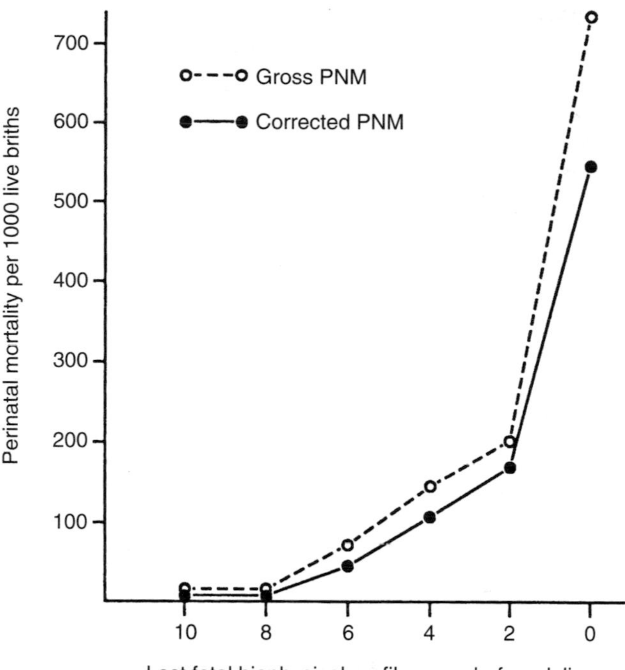

Figure 32.1 The relationship between perinatal mortality (either total or corrected for major anomaly) and the last biophysical profile scoring result. This relationship is exponential, yielding a highly significant inverse correlation using log 10 conversion. PNM, perinatal mortality.

Vintzileos et al.[57] examined the relationship between BPP components and cord pH in 124 patients undergoing Cesarean birth (prior to labor onset). An umbilical arterial pH of < 7.20 was used to define fetal acidemia. At pH < 7.20, inhibition of fetal breathing and FHR nonreactivity occurred; however, a pH < 7.10 was needed before movements and tone

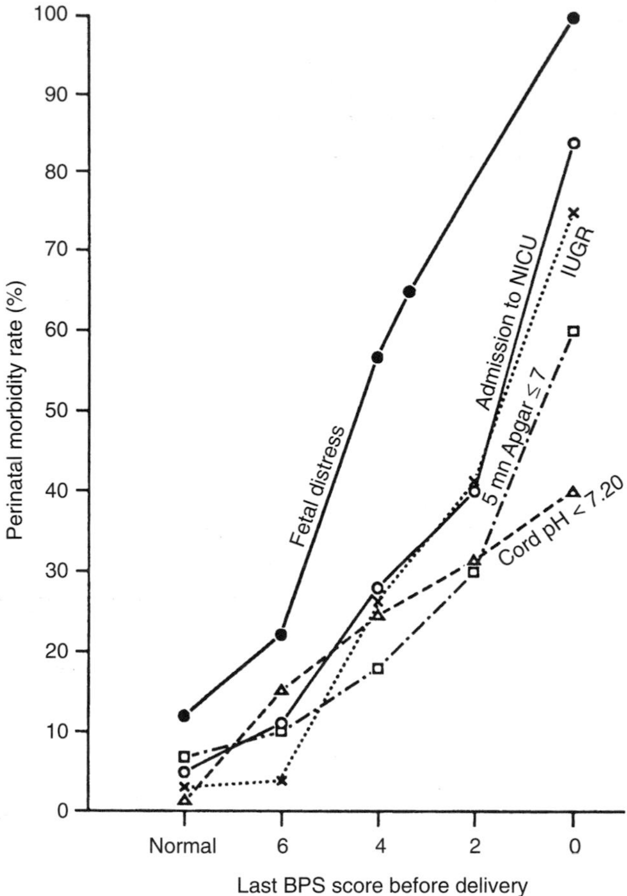

Figure 32.2 The relationship between last biophysical test score before delivery and individual perinatal morbidity variables: presence of fetal distress, admission to neonatal intensive care unit (NICU), intrauterine growth restriction (IUGR), 5-min Apgar score ≤ 7, and umbilical vein pH < 7.20, either alone or in any combination. BPS, biophysical profile score.

were abolished. Importantly, none of the fetuses with a reactive NST, or breathing, or both, had a pH < 7.20. By analyzing the individual components of the BPP (versus score), the sensitivity, specificity, positive and negative predictive values in predicting fetal acidemia were 100%, 92%, 71%, and 100% respectively. Vintzileos and colleagues[58] later examined the relationship between the absence of fetal biophysical activities and umbilical artery blood gas values (pH, Po_2, Pco_2, HCO_3, and base excess levels), thus confirming the gradual hypoxia concept.

The modified BPP is composed of the NST (an acute indicator of fetal acid–base status) and AFV (indicator of chronic uteroplacental function). It is used by many centers as a primary mode of surveillance. The amniotic fluid index (AFI) is the sum of measurements (cm) of the deepest cord-free amniotic fluid pocket in each of the maternal abdominal quadrants. Because an AFI > 5 cm is generally considered to be an adequate volume,[59] a normal modified BPP exists when the NST is reactive and the AFI is > 5 cm.[9] An abnormal test occurs if either the NST is nonreactive or the AFI is 5 cm or less. The advantage of using this modality is that the perinatal morbidity/mortality using this scheme compares favorably with previous studies (which use the entire BPP). Figure 32.3 shows our suggested protocol for the modified BPP. By using this protocol in 17211 tests, we had only four deaths of normal fetuses, for a false-negative rate of 0.02%.[60] Another study compared the outcomes of high-risk patients whose last antepartum assessment was a negative CST or negative modified BPP.[61] The incidence of adverse perinatal outcome (after reassuring testing) was significantly less in those managed by the modified BPP than in the CST group (5.1% versus 7.0%).

The BPP has also been useful as a method of assessing fetal well-being and predicting the development of infectious complications in patients with PROM. Vintzileos et al.[62] examined the effect of PROM on the biophysical components. They found that, in PROM patients (without intrauterine infection), there is an increased likelihood of FHR reactivity and oligohydramnios throughout gestation, adequate fetal breathing is decreased, and the other BPP components are not affected. A review of the literature found that, in most studies, a strong correlation was found between abnormal BPP assessment and the development of infectious outcome (maternal or neonatal) in patients with PROM.[63] The authors concluded that correlation between an abnormal BPP and infectious outcome is dependent on time. For instance, the relationship between an abnormal BPP and infection (neonatal, as well as intra-amniotic, as diagnosed by amniocentesis) exists only if the BPP is performed within 24 h of delivery. In contrast, no correlation exists between an abnormal BPP and infectious outcome if the test is performed > 24 h before delivery. It is also vital to remember that the development of maternal clinical chorioamnionitis alone (without neonatal infection) or invasion of the intra-amniotic cavity with *Mycoplasma* species are two conditions that are not necessarily associated with an abnormal BPP. Frequent NSTs or BPPs in patients with preterm PROM are helpful in distinguishing the healthy fetuses that can safely remain *in utero* from those that are either already infected or at high risk of developing neonatal infection.

Amniotic fluid volume (AFV) assessment

Amniotic fluid (AF) is essential to pregnancy, providing a compartment for normal development, growth, and movement of the fetus. AFV is a chronic marker of fetal well-being, and a normal AFV also protects the fetus from cord compression during fetal activity or uterine contractions. This volume changes during pregnancy (Fig. 32.4); at 22 weeks, the average AFV is 630 mL, and this increases to 770 mL at 28 weeks.[64] Between 29 and 37 weeks, there is little change in volume, which averages 800 mL. Beyond 39 weeks, AFV decreases sharply (averaging 515 mL at 41 weeks). Once a patient becomes postdate, there is a 33% decline in AFV per week,

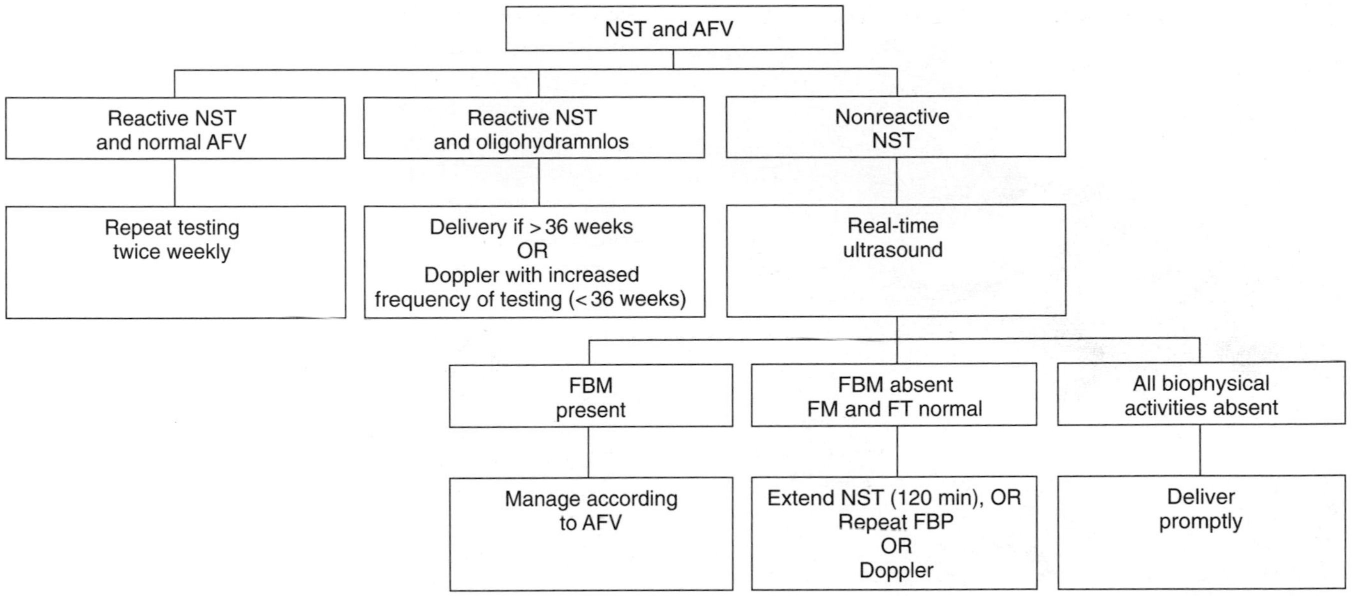

Figure 32.3 Suggested protocol for the modified fetal biophysical profile. AFV, amniotic fluid volume; FBM, fetal breathing movements; FBP, fetal biophysical profile; FM, fetal movements; FT, fetal tone; NST, nonstress test.

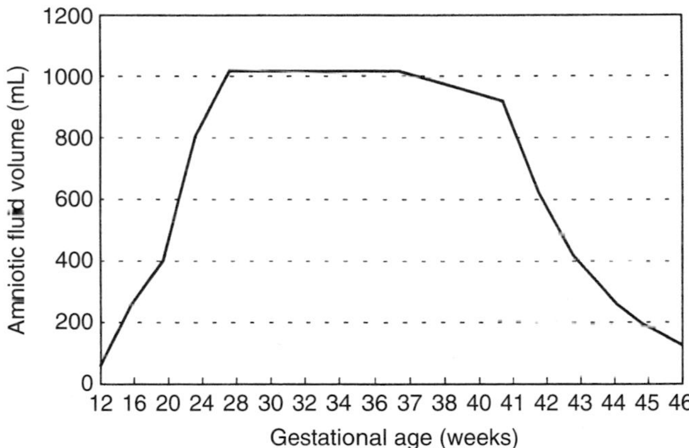

Figure 32.4 Mean amniotic fluid volume (AFV) changes during pregnancy.

consistent with clinical observations of an increased incidence of oligohydramnios in post-term gestations.[65]

During embryogenesis, little is known about AF dynamics. With advancing gestational age, the AF composition changes. In the second half of pregnancy, the main sources of AF include fetal urine excretion (especially) and fluid secreted by the fetal lung. However, unlike the role of the kidneys, the fetal lung does not play a role in regulating fetal body fluid homeostasis. Fetal urine production rates appear to be in the range of nearly 1 L/day near term. The primary pathways for fluid removal are fetal swallowing (mainly) and intramembranous absorption into fetal blood perfusing the fetal surface of the placenta. Thus, under pathologic conditions, fetal modulation of sites of fluid secretion (urine and lung liquid) and resorption (swallowing and intramembranous flow) contributes to the marked AFV changes seen. For example, increases in fetal blood volume (twin–twin transfusion) likely increase urine flow and induce polyhydramnios in the recipient twin. Alternatively, absent fetal swallowing due to gastrointestinal obstruction (e.g., esophageal atresia) or neurological deficits may also cause polyhydramnios. Placental dysfunction may result in decreased fetal renal perfusion, leading to oligohydramnios.

While a variety of techniques have been developed in the past to assess AFV, one of the initial methods involved vertically measuring a single (largest) AF pocket. Chamberlain et al.[51] developed the "2-cm rule". By using a 2-cm vertical pocket, they could reliably predict which fetuses were at risk of intrauterine growth restriction, oligohydramnios, and perinatal mortality; patients having pockets of > 2 cm were considered to have a normal AFV and were at low risk of these complications. One of the most common methods utilized today is the AFI, which was first described in 1987.[66] With the uterus "divided" into four quadrants (linea nigra and umbilicus divide the uterus into right/left halves and upper/lower halves respectively), the vertical diameter of the largest pocket in each quadrant (umbilical cord free) is measured. The summation of all four quadrant numbers equals the AFI (in cm) (Fig. 32.5). In low-risk pregnancies, the mean AFI was 16.2 ± 5.3 cm. Notably, the mean AFI is relatively stable from 24 weeks through term. Phelan et al.[66,67] also established definitions for oligohydramnios (AFI $\leq$ 5 cm) and polyhydramnios (AFI > 25 cm). In comparing the various techniques that have been described, some believe the AFI appears to be superior to the determinations of single vertical pockets.[51,59] It has been demonstrated that the AFI is not only simple and easy to perform, but is also reproducible and

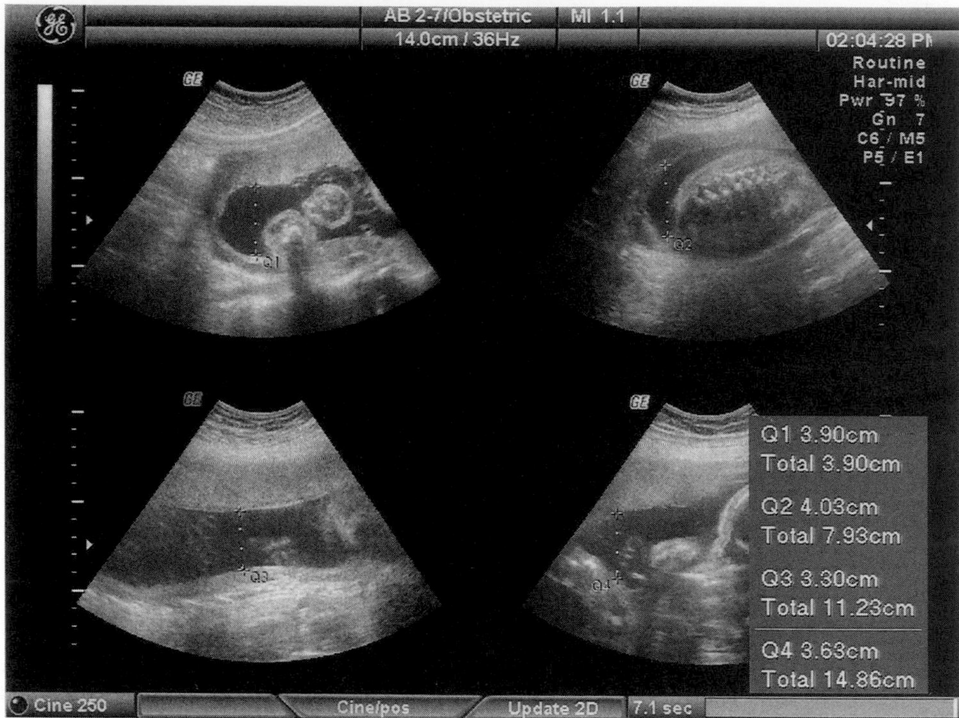

Figure 32.5 Prenatal ultrasound of 30-week fetus depicting vertical measurements (cm) of the amniotic fluid in all four quadrants (Q1–Q4) of the maternal abdomen, comprising the amniotic fluid index (14.86 cm in this case).

without substantial interobserver and intraobserver differences, which is important.[68] In addition, the AFI definitions of oligohydramnios and polyhydramnios are highly correlated with fetal outcome. Several limitations exist, however, with the AFI technique. First, prior to 20 weeks, a four-quadrant assessment may not be feasible. Second, a composite AFI does not provide quantitative information relative to each fetus in a twin pregnancy. Finally, the AFI does not correlate with actual AFV throughout gestation.

A recent study found that, during antepartum surveillance, measurement of the single deepest pocket (versus AFI) was associated with a significantly lower rate of suspected oligohydramnios (10% versus 17% respectively).[69] Another study found that the AFI offered no advantage in detecting adverse outcomes (compared with the single deepest pocket) when performed with the BPP.[70] In fact, they found that the AFI may cause more interventions by labeling twice as many at-risk pregnancies as having oligohydramnios (than with the single deepest pocket technique).

Preterm PROM affects 6% of all patients and is responsible for 30% of preterm deliveries. Early sonographic evaluation of AFV in patients admitted with preterm PROM is useful in counseling patients as to the chances of early delivery. While not absolute, patients with a normal AFV are four times more likely to be undelivered (after 1 week) than those with reduced fluid.[71] Vintzileos et al.[71] also showed that a normal AFV is associated with a significantly lower rate of Cesarean section, Apgar scores < 7 (1 and 5 min), and perinatal mortality. Assessment of AF either on admission or later can also serve as a predictor of amnionitis.[72,73] In patients with preterm PROM, Vintzileos et al.[72,73] showed that a low AFV or nonreactive FHR pattern is associated with a 67% probability of intrauterine infection, which is six or seven times higher than in patients with normal test results.

Table 32.5 Potential complications associated with polyhydramnios.

Complications
Premature labor
Placental abruption
Puerperal hemorrhage
Perinatal mortality
Maternal respiratory difficulties

The frequency at which AFI evaluations should be repeated in the antepartum period is not well established. Most recommend that follow-up examinations should be tailored individually and, in general, if the AFI is normal, fluid checks can be repeated weekly. However, with marginal or decreased fluid, or in a postdate pregnancy, a shorter test interval should be considered.

Polyhydramnios (pathologic accumulation of AF), which is defined as an AFI > 25 cm, occurs in 0.2–1.6% of the general population.[74] It is associated with increased maternal and perinatal morbidity and mortality (Table 32.5).[67–75] The causes of polyhydramnios depend on its severity. For instance, Hill et al.[74] found the cause to be apparent in only 17% of patients with mild polyhydramnios (idiopathic in the remaining 83%), but in 91% of those with moderate or severe polyhydramnios.

When the cause of polyhydramnios can be found, the diagnosis usually falls into the following categories:[67] fetal malformations and genetic disorders, diabetes, rhesus (Rh) sensitization, and congenital infections. Fetal swallowing impairment may also result in excess AFV. Once polyhydramnios is diagnosed, a targeted and detailed ultrasound should be performed to examine for fetal abnormalities and movement disorders (e.g., gastroschisis, duodenal atresia, anencephaly). In the absence of a sonographic abnormality, the patient evaluation may include (but not require) screening tests for maternal diabetes, Rh sensitization, and hemoglobinopathies. If a cause is diagnosed, when possible, it should be treated.

In some cases, it may be beneficial to attempt to reduce the risk of obstetric complications with AFV reduction. Techniques that have been used are amniocentesis and maternal administration of prostaglandin synthetase inhibitors (indomethacin), which reduce fetal urine flow.[76] However, because of continuous production of AF, repeated amniocenteses may be required, which is associated with both maternal and fetal risks. In addition, indomethacin must be administered carefully, as it is associated with potential fetal side-effects (oligohydramnios, premature closure of the ductus arteriosus, and increased incidence of neonatal necrotizing enterocolitis and renal compromise). While patients are on indomethacin, the AFV and, perhaps, fetal ductal flow should be monitored frequently.

Oligohydramnios (reduced AFV) occurs in 5.5–37.8% of pregnancies,[59,77] and is significant because of its known association with adverse pregnancy outcome (Table 32.6), such as umbilical cord occlusion, fetal distress in labor, meconium aspiration, operative deliveries, and stillbirth.[77] Some clinical conditions commonly associated with oligohydramnios include intrauterine growth restriction, urinary tract malformations, postdate pregnancies, and ruptured membranes. Decreased fluid may also be a sign of placental insufficiency. Evaluation of oligohydramnios should include a targeted sonogram, which may be difficult owing to the reduced AFV. Generally, second-trimester oligohydramnios is associated with a poor fetal prognosis. For instance, it may impair lung development with resulting neonatal morbidity/mortality.[78] Mercer and Brown[79] found that, of 34 pregnancies with second-trimester oligohydramnios (without PROM), 27% had fetal congenital malformations, 32% of fetuses died *in utero*, and 18% had an entirely normal outcome. However, second-trimester oligohydramnios should not be considered hopeless for patients with either intact or ruptured membranes. As third-trimester oligohydramnios has an increased risk of FHR decelerations and nonreactivity, ultrasound must often be complemented by FHR monitoring. It is important to remember, however, that, regardless of NST results, oligohydramnios in the third trimester (unrelated to PROM) should alert one to the potential for fetal compromise, and these patients should be considered for delivery.

Table 32.6 Potential consequences of oligohydramnios.

Consequences
Umbilical cord compression
Meconium-stained amniotic fluid
Fetal demise
Deformation syndrome
Pulmonary hypoplasia
Maternal or neonatal infection

Condition-specific antepartum fetal testing

Evidence-based observations have shown that there are different pathophysiologic processes that can place the fetus at risk; thus, the efficacy of the various fetal tests depends on the underlying pathophysiologic condition.[80] It also follows that no one test is ideal for all high-risk fetuses. Therefore, multiple parameter assessment or combinations of different tests may often be the optimal fetal strategy, depending on the testing indication. The most recent information in fetal testing reveals that, in order to improve accuracy, condition-specific fetal testing should be utilized. By using this method (at Robert Wood Johnson Medical School) in 12 766 high-risk fetuses, the number of fetal deaths was reduced to 1/3191 (four fetal deaths), which is three times lower than the number of fetal deaths that are seen when the same biophysical assessment tests are applied regardless of the underlying pathophysiologic process (1/1300).[61,80–82] The pathophysiologic processes that can lead to fetal death/damage include decreased utero-placental blood flow, decreased gas exchange at the trophoblastic membrane level, metabolic processes, fetal sepsis, fetal anemia, fetal heart failure, and umbilical cord accidents.[80] Table 32.7 shows the various pathophysiologic processes, examples of maternal/fetal conditions, and the specific surveillance tests that may be the most appropriate.

Intrapartum fetal surveillance techniques

Fetal heart rate (FHR) monitoring

The main surveillance technique for intrapartum fetal evaluation is FHR monitoring, which can be performed either intermittently or continuously. Intermittent FHR monitoring can be performed by either manual counting of the FHR (using a hand-held Doppler ultrasound on the abdomen or DeLee stethoscope) or using a continuous electronic FHR monitor intermittently (recorded on a tracing). In low-risk patients, it is recommended that the FHR should be determined at least every hour, every 30 min, and every 15 min in the latent phase, active phase, and second stages of labor respectively.[83] The FHR is generally monitored and recorded during a contraction, and for 30 s afterward. However, there are no studies

Table 32.7 Condition-specific antepartum fetal testing.

Pathophysiologic condition	Maternal/fetal condition	*Appropriate test(s)
Metabolic abnormalities	Type 1 diabetes	NST, CST, BPP, Doppler in class F–R diabetes, maternal blood glucose (goal is normal)
Decreased uteroplacental blood flow	Hypertensive disorders Collagen, renal, vascular disease Most cases IUGR (< 32–34 weeks)	NST, CST, BPP, AF assessment, Doppler, EFW by US (growth rate)
Decreased gas exchange	Postdate pregnancy Some cases IUGR (> 32–34 weeks)	NST, CST, BPP, AF assessment, first-trimester US (accurate dating), EFW by US
Fetal sepsis	PROM Intra-amniotic infection Maternal fever, primary subclinical intra-amniotic infection	NST, BPP, AF assessment, amniocentesis (rule out infection)
Fetal anemia	Fetomaternal hemorrhage Erythroblastosis fetalis Parvovirus B19 infection	NST (if hydrops present), CST (if hydrops present), BPP (if hydrops present), MCA peak systolic velocity, US to rule out hydrops, fetal liver length, cordocentesis, amniocentesis (> 28 weeks)
Fetal heart failure	Cardiac arrhythmia Nonimmune hydrops Chorioangioma placenta Aneurysm of the vein of Galen	NST or CST (if hydrops present/arrhythmia absent), BPP, Doppler (venous circulation), US to rule out hydrops, continuous FHR monitoring (determine time spent in sinus rhythm), M-mode echo (rule out arrhythmias)
Umbilical cord accident	Umbilical cord entanglement (monoamniotic twins) Velamentous cord insertion/funic presentation Noncoiled umbilical cord Oligohydramnios	Frequent NST, umbilical artery Doppler, color Doppler on US (verify diagnosis)

AF, amniotic fluid; BPP, biophysical profile; CST, contraction stress test; EFW, estimated fetal weight; FHR, fetal heart rate; IUGR, intrauterine growth restriction; MCA, middle cerebral artery; NST, nonstress test; PROM, premature rupture of membranes; US, ultrasound.

*Specific surveillance tests that may be the most appropriate and are suggested guidelines.

providing data on the optimal intervals for monitoring low-risk patients. In high-risk patients, it is recommended that the FHR be determined every 30 min, 15 min, and 5 min during the latent phase, active phase, and second stages of labor respectively.

Continuous electronic FHR monitoring (EFM) determines the FHR on a beat-to-beat basis and displays data continuously. It can be performed either externally or internally. External monitoring is noninvasive, and can be used in every patient by placing a Doppler transducer on the abdomen (overlying the fetal heart); however, signal loss can be a significant problem. In addition, the true beat-to-beat variability of the FHR can be assessed only from a fetal electrocardiogram by determining the R–R interval. This is accomplished via internal monitoring and direct FHR evaluation. Internal FHR monitoring requires ruptured membranes, and the cervix to be dilated ≥ 1–2 cm. A spiral electrode is applied to the presenting fetal part (either vertex or breech). Signal loss is reduced, and maternal obesity, fetal, and maternal movements should not alter the signal quality. An essential adjuvant component to FHR monitoring is uterine contraction monitoring, which can be accomplished via an external tocodynamometer (most commonly) on the maternal abdomen. While uterine frequency and duration of contractions are measured with reasonable accuracy, the strength/amplitude of the contractions cannot be determined using this modality. In contrast, another method involves insertion of an intrauterine pressure catheter, which requires cervical dilation and ruptured membranes. With this internal technique, the strength, amplitude, duration, and frequency of contractions can be assessed.

The interpretation of FHR patterns should incorporate knowledge of gestational age, maternal condition, medications, and other factors that could influence FHR components. In 1997, the National Institute of Child Health and Human Development (NICHHD) Research Planning Workshop developed standardized definitions for electronic FHR patterns and recommendations for interpreting them.[84] These definitions are found in Table 32.8. The workshop did not make a distinction between short-term variability (or beat-to-beat variability or R–R wave period differences in the electrocardiogram) and long-term variability, because they felt that, in actual practice, they are visually determined as a unit. Thus, the definition of variability was based visually on the amplitude of the complexes, with exclusion of the regular, smooth

Table 32.8 Fetal heart rate patterns.

Fetal heart rate pattern	Definition	Comments
Baseline FHR	Approximate mean FHR rounded to increments of 5 b.p.m. during a 10-min segment (excluding periodic/episodic changes, periods of marked FHR variability, segments of the baseline that differ by > 25 b.p.m.)	In any 10-min window, the minimum baseline duration must be ≥ 2 min, or the baseline for that period is indeterminate [one may then need to refer to the previous 10-min segment(s) for determination of the baseline]
Bradycardia	Baseline FHR < 110 b.p.m.	
Tachycardia	Baseline FHR > 160 b.p.m.	
Baseline FHR variability	Fluctuations in the baseline FHR of ≥ 2 cycles/min	Fluctuations are irregular in amplitude and frequency; visually quantitated as the amplitude of the peak-to-trough (b.p.m.)
Absent FHR variability	Amplitude range undetectable	
Minimal FHR variability	Amplitude range > undetectable and ≤ 5 b.p.m.	
Moderate FHR variability	Amplitude range 6–25 b.p.m.	
Marked FHR variability	Amplitude range > 25 b.p.m.	
Acceleration	Visually apparent abrupt increase (onset of acceleration to peak in < 30 s) in FHR above baseline. Increase is calculated from most recently determined portion of the baseline	Acme is ≥ 15 b.p.m. above baseline, and acceleration lasts ≥ 15 s and < 2 min from onset to return to baseline. Before 32 weeks, defined as acme ≥ 10 b.p.m. above baseline and duration ≥ 10 s
Prolonged acceleration	Duration ≥ 2 min and < 10 min	Acceleration of ≥ 10 min is a baseline change
Early deceleration	Visually apparent gradual (onset of deceleration to nadir ≥ 30 s) decrease and return to baseline FHR associated with UC	Decrease is calculated from most recently determined portion of baseline. Deceleration is coincident in timing, with nadir occurring at the same time as peak of contraction
Variable deceleration	Visually apparent abrupt decrease (onset of deceleration to beginning of nadir < 30 s) in FHR below baseline	Decrease is calculated from most recently determined portion of baseline. Decrease in FHR below baseline is ≥ 15 b.p.m., lasting ≥ 15 s and < 2 min from onset to return to baseline
Late deceleration	Visually apparent gradual (onset of deceleration to nadir ≥ 30 s) decrease and return to baseline FHR associated with UC	Decrease is calculated from most recently determined portion of baseline. Deceleration is delayed in timing, with nadir occurring after peak of contraction
Prolonged deceleration	Visually apparent decrease in FHR below baseline	Decrease is calculated from most recently determined portion of baseline. Decrease from baseline is ≥ 15 b.p.m., lasting ≥ 2 min, but < 10 min from onset to return to baseline. Prolonged deceleration of ≥ 10 min is a baseline change
Sinusoidal pattern	Smooth, sine wave-like pattern of regular frequency and amplitude	Excluded in the definition of FHR variability

Adapted from ref. 84.

b.p.m., beats per minute; FHR, fetal heart rate; UC, uterine contractions.

sinusoidal pattern. The workshop also stated that the individual components of the FHR patterns that were defined do not occur alone and generally evolve over time. Therefore, they felt that a full description of a FHR tracing requires a qualitative and quantitative description of: baseline rate, baseline FHR variability, presence of accelerations, periodic or episodic decelerations, and changes or trends in FHR patterns over time.[84]

While the baseline FHR normally ranges from 110 to 160 b.p.m. across all gestational ages, rates as low as 90 b.p.m. or as high as 180 b.p.m. are common in healthy fetuses. Such rates are not necessarily abnormal if they are transient and the other FHR parameters are normal. As gestation advances, there is a gradual slowing of the mean baseline FHR, from 160 b.p.m. (15 weeks) to 140 b.p.m. (term).[85] Fetal tachycardia has been associated with maternal fever, maternal thyrotoxicosis, atropine, excessive fetal movement, fetal infection, and tachyarrhythmias. Although fetal tachycardia can be associated with compromise, it is not usually associated with acidemia in the setting of normal FHR variability and absence of decelerations.[86] Fetal bradycardia can be seen with maternal hypotension or hypothermia, $MgSO_4$ toxicity,[35] and congenital heart block. Periodic FHR patterns are those associated with uterine contractions, while episodic patterns are those not associated with uterine contractions. Normal FHR variability is generally described as the most reliable indicator of fetal well-being, as it reflects intact integration of the CNS and cardiovascular systems. It is associated with fetal well-being despite the concomitant presence of FHR decelerations.[86–88] Various causes of decreased variability include fetal asphyxia, fetal behavioral states, gestational age, narcotics, and fetal anomalies.[35] During labor, extended periods of decreased FHR variability (up to 45 min) can normally be seen.[89] A clinical rule of thumb is that FHR decelerations reflect the nature of the insult to the fetus, while FHR variability reflects the fetal ability to tolerate the insult. If decreased variability is associated with baseline FHR changes, or is seen with recurrent decelerations, the likelihood of fetal compromise increases.[86–88]

The presence of FHR accelerations during labor is a sign of fetal well-being and indicates a well-oxygenated fetus.[90] Four types of decelerations are seen intrapartum, and they are classified as early, variable, late, or prolonged, based on their temporal relationship with contractions, as well as their configuration. The workshop stated that any deceleration is quantitated by the depth of the nadir in b.p.m. below the baseline (excluding transient spikes or electronic artifacts), and the duration is quantitated in minutes and seconds from the beginning to the end of the deceleration.[84] Accelerations are quantitated similarly. Decelerations are defined as recurrent if they occur with ≥ 50% of uterine contractions in any 20-min segment. Early decelerations are thought to be secondary to an increase in vagal tone due to fetal head compression during the contraction. These decelerations are innocuous, are not associated with fetal hypoxemia or acidemia,[86,91] can be observed throughout labor (but are seen most often at cervical dilations of 4–8 cm),[92] and no corrective measures are indicated. Variable decelerations are the most common decelerations seen in labor, are most often seen during the second stage, and indicate umbilical cord compression. Variable decelerations have been graded by some as mild, moderate, and severe based on the duration of the deceleration and the level to which the FHR drops.[91] Mild variable decelerations (in the presence of a normal FHR and variability) are usually of minimal clinical significance. However, prolonged and deep variable decelerations may result in a transient respiratory acidemia. If decelerations are severe, repetitive, and accompanied by decreased variability or changes in FHR baseline, fetal acidemia may be developing.[86,88] Late decelerations are caused by fetal hypoxia, which is often due to decreased intervillous exchange between mother and fetus (decreased placental perfusion). In advanced stages of fetal acidemia, late decelerations can also be a result of direct myocardial depression. For this pattern to become significant clinically, they must be repetitive. Although decelerations with larger amplitudes may be associated with lower fetal pH, shallow, repetitive, late decelerations with diminished FHR variability are nonreassuring, and there is a high likelihood of fetal acidemia.[88,92] Clinical situations in which late decelerations are seen include excessive uterine activity, placental abruption, and maternal hypotension. Prolonged decelerations may occur spontaneously, or be related to prolapsed cord, excessive uterine activity, maternal hypotension, or fetal manipulation. A sinusoidal FHR differs from variability in that it has a smooth, sine wave-like pattern of regular frequency and amplitude, and is excluded in the definition of FHR variability.[84] It may be nonreassuring in that it has been associated with severe fetal anemia. A transient "sinusoid-like" pattern may also be seen after maternal administration of some narcotic analgesics.[93] However, in this setting, it does not indicate fetal compromise.

Figure 32.6 shows a suggested protocol for managing nonreassuring FHR tracings or fetal heart decelerations in labor. The use of this should aid in detecting the acidemic fetus requiring delivery, and should limit the number of unnecessary interventions for suspected (but not proven) fetal distress. Conservative measures for resuscitation include discontinuation of oxytocin (if used), altering maternal position (left or right lateral, knee–chest), administering O_2, correcting maternal hypotension if present, amnioinfusion (if variable decelerations), tocolysis (if no contraindications), and performing a vaginal examination to rule out cord prolapse.

Introduced in the 1960s with the aim of detecting intrapartum fetal asphyxia and improving neonatal outcomes, EFM is now the main screening method for intrapartum fetal assessment in most developed countries, but has been disappointing on account of its subjective nature, frequency of falsely nonreassuring patterns, and persistent questions regarding efficacy.[94] Also, the widespread use of EFM does not appear to have reduced cerebral palsy.[95] Nonreassuring patterns occur in about 15% of labors.[96] Its diagnostic accuracy in predicting fetal compromise (positive predictive value) is not as good as its accuracy in confirming fetal well-being. Early randomized controlled trials (RCTs) in the 1970s and 1980s comparing intermittent auscultation with continuous monitoring failed to show a consistent improvement in neonatal outcome, despite the associated increase in operative deliveries with continuous EFM.[97–100] However, many of these early trials suffered from limitations, such as small sample sizes and low overall perinatal mortality rates in the studied populations. The Dublin trial had more than 6000 patients enrolled in each study arm.[98] The only significant difference found was a twofold higher rate of neonatal seizures and abnormal neurologic examinations in the intermittent auscultation group. However, crossover from one group to the other and the exclusion of many high-risk patients may have obscured any advantages of EFM over auscultation. In 1993, Vintzileos et al.[101] conducted a RCT that evaluated intermittent auscultation versus continuous EFM as the primary (and only) surveillance method, and included both low-risk and high-risk patients. No crossover was allowed from one group to the other. This study found a significant reduction in perinatal mortality secondary to hypoxia in those patients managed with continuous EFM. In addition, they found that EFM was superior to intermittent auscultation in detecting fetal acidemia at birth.[102] Our group performed a meta-analysis on the RCTs of monitoring

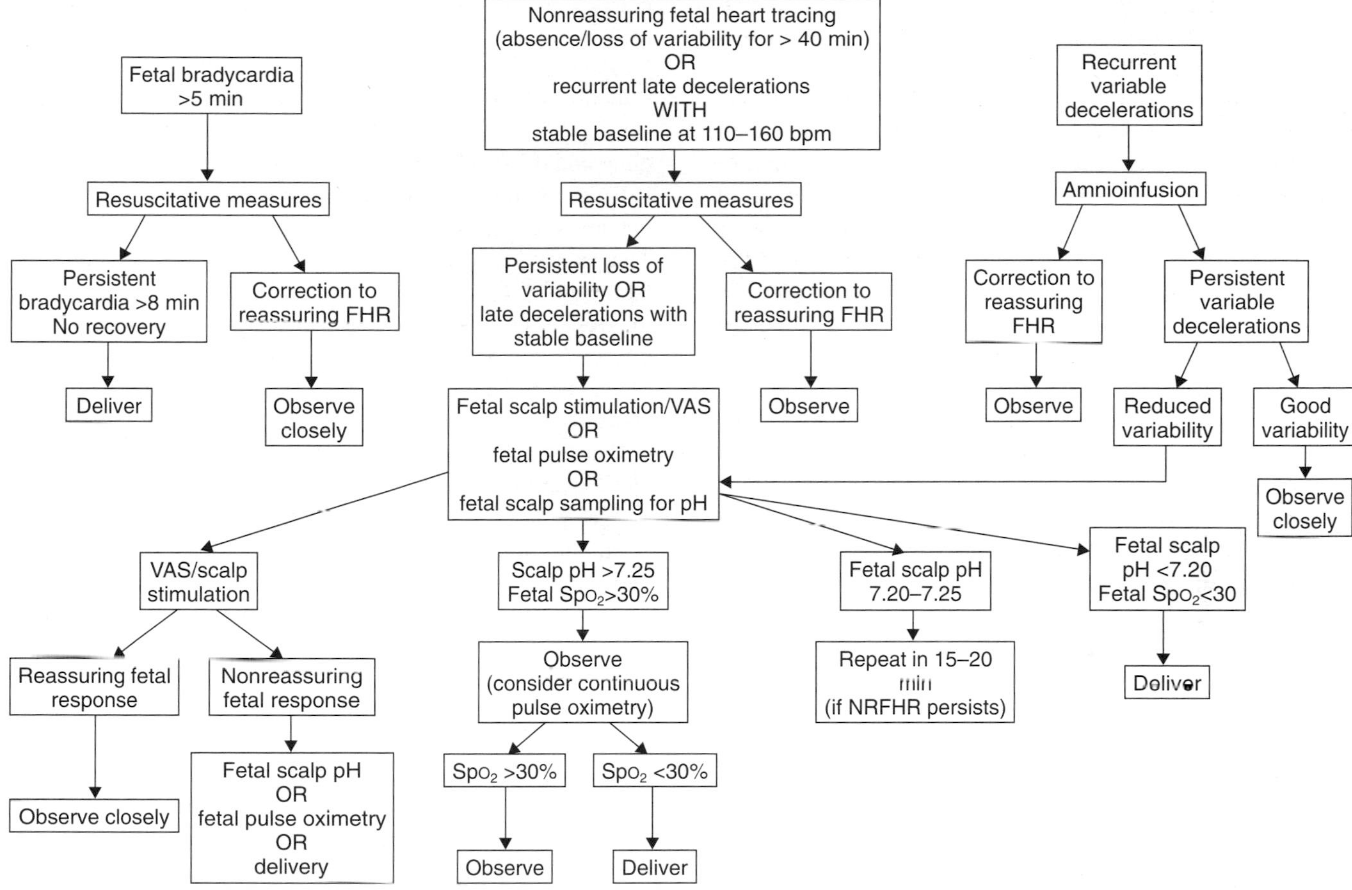

Figure 32.6 Management of nonreassuring fetal heart tracing or fetal heart decelerations in labor. FHR, fetal heart rate; NRFHR, nonreassuring fetal heart rate; SpO_2, arterial oxygen saturation; VAS, vibroacoustic stimulation (from Apuzzio JJ, Vintzileos AM, Iffy L, eds. *Operative obstetrics*, 3rd edn. Abingdon, United Kingdom: Taylor & Francis, 2005, with permission).

techniques.[103] Although perinatal mortality was no different with the two techniques (continuous versus intermittent), there was a significant reduction (about 40%) in perinatal deaths due to hypoxia in the continuous EFM group. Patients monitored electronically had overall higher rates of Cesarean and operative vaginal deliveries, as well as operative interventions for fetal distress. A recent Cochrane review[104] of nine RCTs concluded that the only clinically significant benefit from the use of routine continuous EFM (versus intermittent auscultation) was the reduction in neonatal seizures [relative risk (RR) 0.51, 95% confidence interval (CI) 0.32–0.82], with an increase in Cesarean and operative vaginal deliveries. There were no significant differences in 1-min Apgar scores below 4 or 7, and the rates of neonatal intensive care unit admissions, perinatal deaths, or cerebral palsy. Thus, although it appears that EFM is associated with reductions in neonatal seizures and perinatal deaths due to hypoxia, the price is a small (but significant) increase in operative deliveries.

Fetal acid–base evaluation

While EFM is mostly satisfactory, there is a clear need for an adjunctive method of intrapartum fetal surveillance when concerns arise about the EFM pattern. Fetal scalp capillary blood sampling was developed in the 1960s and is complementary to the FHR, by evaluating fetal acid–base status during labor. It has been used to improve the positive predictive value of FHR tracings. Figure 32.6 depicts a suggested protocol for managing nonreassuring FHR tracings or fetal heart decelerations in labor, incorporating scalp pH, fetal pulse oximetry, or fetal stimulation techniques. During labor, fetal acidemia may be secondary to impaired maternal–fetal exchange in the intervillous space. In acute umbilical cord compression, rapid CO_2 accumulation leads to a respiratory acidemia. Metabolic acidemia can occur secondary to lactic acid accumulation when the anaerobic pathway of energy production is used. If sufficient hypoxemia and acidemia develop and persist, significant fetal morbidity/mortality may result. A scalp pH ≥ 7.25 has been considered normal for a fetus during the intrapartum period.[105] A range of 7.20–7.24 indicates pre-acidemia, while values ≤ 7.19 indicate fetal acidemia. However, it is understood that pH values associated with pathologic fetal acidemia may be significantly lower than this. It is not common to find significant neonatal morbidity until the umbilical artery pH is < 7.10, and this cutoff may be as low as 7.00.[106,107] RCTs have shown that Cesarean delivery rates for fetal distress are lower in patients managed with EFM and intermittent scalp sampling.[98,108] Thacker et al. reported recently that the addition of fetal scalp blood sampling to standard EFM reduced the odds for Cesarean section, although the odds were still increased compared with intermittent auscultation of the fetal heart.[104] Intermittent fetal scalp blood sampling is now rarely utilized in the United States.[109]

Umbilical cord acid–base values are often obtained at the time of delivery, and are used to establish an objective measure of fetal status at the time of birth. Normal values for arterial and venous blood samples have been described.[110] Although umbilical artery blood gases are preferable to venous blood, sampling of both provides information on the fetal and utero-placental circulations respectively. It is also important to remember that, as fetal pH values normally fall during labor, abnormal cutoff values for defining acidemia at delivery are influenced by the presence or absence of labor. Values for defining the various types of acidemia at birth (labor versus no labor) have been described.[110] Nearly 80% of infants classified as depressed (1- or 5-min Apgar score < 7) have normal umbilical cord pH values.[111]

Recently, Ross and Gala[112] described how base excess values (versus umbilical cord pH values) have a significantly greater usefulness, because base excess does not change significantly with respiratory acidosis and demonstrates a linear correlation with the degree of metabolic acidosis. Umbilical artery base excess is the most direct measure of fetal metabolic acidosis, and threshold levels of base excess (–12 mmol/L) have been associated with an increased risk of neonatal neurological injury.[112] Through an interpolation of fetal base excess values throughout the course of labor, this approach can provide a framework for the assessment of FHR tracings during labor and, potentially, the timing of hypoxic/ischemic injury.[112]

Fetal stimulation techniques

Fetal scalp sampling has limitations and cannot be used in all patients. Equipment for pH analysis and skilled personnel to perform this technique may not be available. For these reasons, other methods of evaluating a nonreassuring FHR pattern have been proposed, such as fetal scalp stimulation and VAS. Clark et al.[113,114] evaluated FHR responses to scalp sampling, and correlated these FHR responses with fetal scalp blood pH. Evoked FHR accelerations of 15 b.p.m. (lasting 15 s) were associated with a scalp pH of ≥ 7.20 in all cases; there were no cases of a FHR acceleration response to the scalp puncture when the pH was < 7.20.[113] However, although acceleration presence indicated fetal well-being, a lack of response occurred in several normal, nonacidemic fetuses. A subsequent study showed that the need for scalp blood sampling could be reduced by 50% in the setting of an evoked FHR acceleration secondary to scalp stimulation.[114] Concerning, however, was that there was a false-negative rate of 60%. Thus, while evoked accelerations (15 b.p.m. for 15 s) indicate fetal well-being and imply a normal acid–base status, a lack of accelerations does not always predict fetal compromise. Others have used less stringent criteria (acceleration of 10 b.p.m. for at least 10 s) to define fetal response to scalp stimulation to try to decrease the need for scalp blood sampling.[115]

VAS has been used intrapartum to evoke FHR accelerations and thus identify the well fetus. Many studies have compared VAS responses with fetal acid–base determinations.[116–120] In evaluating 64 patients with abnormal intrapartum FHR patterns, all fetuses demonstrating a reactive response to VAS had a pH ≥ 7.25.[116] Of 34 fetuses not showing a response, half had a scalp pH of < 7.25. Another study evaluated 188 patients with scalp stimulation and VAS.[117] No patients demonstrated accelerations when scalp pH values were < 7.20. Bartelsmeyer et al.[118] suggested that VAS could predict fetal acidemia and differentiate between respiratory and metabolic acidemia. Patients with fetal scalp blood base deficits of > 10 mEq/L did not show a response of FHR accelerations after VAS; although five fetuses did show an acceleration with a scalp pH of < 7.20, all had base deficits of < 10 mEq/L. A meta-analysis evaluating the intrapartum assessment of fetal well-being with VAS found a fivefold increase in the risk of acidemia (scalp pH < 7.20) in laboring patients who did not respond with accelerations of 15 b.p.m. for 15 s after VAS.[121] Table 32.9 shows that, when data from studies using VAS[117–120] and studies evaluating scalp stimulation[113,114,117] are pooled and compared, the overall efficacy for predicting a scalp pH < 7.20 is similar, regardless of the method of stimulation. Although scalp and acoustic stimulation techniques are simple to perform, they are limited by falsely nonreassuring results.[122] Interestingly, one study has shown that the fetal response to VAS decreased as

Table 32.9 Efficacy of intrapartum fetal stimulation for prediction of a scalp pH of < 7.20.

	VAS (*n* = 405)	Scalp stimulation* (*n* = 488)
Sensitivity	83% (29/35)	98% (43/44)
Specificity	65% (241/370)	67% (298/444)
Positive predictive value	18% (29/158)	23% (43/189)
Negative predictive value	98% (241/247)	99% (298/299)

VAS, vibroacoustic stimulation.

*Scalp stimulation includes scalp puncture, digital pressure, and scalp pinch.

cervical dilation advanced.[123] Analgesia with low doses of nalbuphine has not been found to alter the fetal response to VAS in normal laboring patients.[124]

In summary, FHR acceleration as a response to fetal stimulation indicates a nonacidemic fetus, and thus scalp blood sampling may be omitted. In our opinion, using VAS or scalp stimulation may reduce the need for scalp pH analysis when FHR tracings are equivocal/nonreassuring. These fetal stimulation techniques are noninvasive, are not technically difficult, can be performed earlier in labor, and can be done when scalp pH sampling is not feasible. If the fetus responds normally to either VAS or scalp stimulation, significant acute fetal acidemia has been ruled out, and thus a scalp pH may be unnecessary.

Fetal pulse oximetry (FPO)

Recently, a new technology with practical potential has emerged, namely FPO. This emerged in the late 1980s, and is a tool that continuously and directly measures the fetal arterial O_2 saturation during the labor process, with the intent of improving the accuracy of evaluating fetal well-being in labor. It is generally reserved for use when a nonreassuring FHR has been recorded, to assist in identifying those hypoxemic fetuses who may benefit from further intervention, and as an adjunct to (not a replacement for) FHR monitoring. The hope is to decrease the Cesarean rate for fetal distress when fetal O_2 saturation is normal. A variety of sensors have been studied; some are placed during a vaginal examination to attach to the top of the fetal head by suction,[125] and others lie against the fetal temple or cheek.[126] The sensor remains *in situ*, and FPO values are recorded for approximately 81% of the monitoring time. Fetal acidemia is rare when the fetal arterial O_2 saturation is continually > 30% (critical threshold). Thus, FPO values ≥ 30% are considered reassuring (even when the EFM is nonreassuring), whereas values < 30% warrant consideration of interventions, such as maternal position change or urgent Cesarean delivery.[127] FHR abnormalities associated with normal scalp blood analysis and normal Apgar scores at delivery have been demonstrated in association with stable arterial O_2 saturation patterns.[128] It is currently recommended for singleton pregnancies only. An ominous EFM pattern has been defined as prolonged deceleration below 70 b.p.m. for at least 7 min. In 2003, the US Food and Drug Administration guidelines expanded the EFM patterns considered to be ominous, requiring prompt delivery despite reassuring FPO readings. They re-emphasized that FPO is meant as an adjunct to (not a replacement for) EFM, and that no technology is 100% predictive of the fetal acid–base condition.

In the 1990s, a large volume of data regarding the feasibility, physiology, and clinical application of FPO were published.[128–131] The only RCT published to date is an American multicenter study, which specifically defined mild to moderately nonreassuring EFM tracings.[132] They compared a group monitored using EFM alone with one monitored using both EFM and FPO. While the Cesarean rate for nonreassuring EFM was reduced by more than 50% in the EFM FPO group (without adversely affecting maternal or fetal/neonatal outcome), the overall Cesarean rate was unchanged between both control and test groups, because of an unanticipated increased incidence of Cesarean sections for dystocia (19%) in the EFM FPO group (versus 9% in control group). A higher proportion of those with nonreassuring variable decelerations were delivered by Cesarean section for dystocia in the oximetry group. The authors suggested that the nonreassuring EFM may indicate an underlying risk of dystocia.[132] Thus, the failure to reduce the overall Cesarean rate led many to question whether there was any clear benefit to FPO, despite the improved prediction of fetal condition/outcome using FPO. A follow-up prospective cohort study in 2004[133] was done to further elucidate the increased Cesarean rate for dystocia seen in the American RCT. Women whose fetuses demonstrated persistent, progressive, and moderately–severely nonreassuring EFM were more likely to have a Cesarean for dystocia, and had a significantly higher rate of persistent occipitoposterior position of the fetus, than those with intermittent, mildly nonreassuring EFM, despite adequate fetal oxygenation status, as measured by FPO. They concluded that nonreassuring EFM patterns predict Cesarean delivery for dystocia among nulliparous patients with normally oxygenated fetuses. In 2001, the American College of Obstetricians and Gynecologists (ACOG) released an opinion on FPO, with concerns about signal registration time, possible false-negative readings, and lack of proven cost–benefit.[134] They could not endorse the adoption of the FPO into clinical practice, and there has since been a reversal in enthusiasm for the FPO technology.[135] The NICHD MFM Units Network is currently conducting a RCT involving 10 000 nulliparous women in labor.[135] Subjects will be randomized to FPO with information available to the clinician (open device arm) or FPO with information masked to the clinician (blinded device arm). The primary outcome will be the impact of FPO as an adjunct to EFM on the Cesarean delivery rate. It is thought that future research should: (1) determine whether other mechanisms of intrapartum fetal brain injury besides hypoxemia (e.g., infection, ischemia) could escape surveillance by FPO; (2) establish the long-term outcomes of children monitored with FPO (compared with standard methods); and (3) establish whether there is a way to use FPO effectively in the setting of labor dystocia and a nonreassuring FHR pattern, to allow safe vaginal delivery.[135]

Fetal electrocardiogram (ECG) ST segment automated analysis (STAN)

Because animal and human studies have shown that fetal hypoxemia during labor can alter the shape of the fetal ECG waveform (notably the elevation or depression of the ST segment), technical systems have been developed to monitor the fetal ECG during labor, as an adjunct to continuous EFM with the aim of improving fetal outcome and minimizing unnecessary obstetric interference.[136] The fetal ECG ST segment automated analysis (STAN) analyzes the repolarization segment of the ECG (ST) waveform, which is altered by intramyocardial potassium release, resulting from metabolic acidemia.[137] A recent Cochrane review[136] of two RCTs assessing the use of fetal ECG as an adjunct to continuous EFM during labor found that using ST waveform analysis was associated with fewer babies with severe metabolic acidosis at birth (cord pH < 7.05 and base deficit > 12 mmol/L). This was achieved along with fewer fetal scalp samples during labor and fewer operative deliveries. Their conclusion was to restrict fetal ST waveform analysis to those fetuses demonstrating disquieting features on cardiotocography. However, in a study looking at the ability of EFM plus fetal ECG STAN monitoring to predict metabolic acidemia (umbilical cord artery pH < 7.15 and base deficit ≥ 12 mmol/L) at birth, they found a poor positive predictive value (8%) and a sensitivity of 43%.[138] Another Cochrane review[139] of the addition of fetal ECG monitoring reported a nonsignificant trend toward reducing the overall Cesarean rate, when compared with EFM only. Ross et al.[140] found that adding fetal ECG STAN to standard FHR monitoring improved FHR tracing interpretation and improved observer consistency in both the decision for and the timing of obstetric interventions, and that it may reduce the number of unneeded obstetric interventions when fetal compromise is absent.

In conclusion, there are currently a wide variety of techniques to survey the fetus and amniotic fluid during the antepartum and intrapartum periods. By utilizing the information from surveillance, fetal outcomes can hopefully be optimized and perinatal mortality prevented.

Key points

1 Both antepartum and intrapartum surveillance of the fetus have the intent of detecting fetal compromise (acidemia and/or infection), so that appropriate and timely interventions can be made. As fetal compromise has a diverse etiology, forms of testing must be able to survey both acute fetal status and more chronic disease states.

2 Fetal movement monitoring ("fetal kick counts") by the mother is an advantageous form of surveillance because it lacks contraindications, is simple, inexpensive, noninvasive, and understandable to patients. The relationship between decreased fetal activity and poor perinatal outcome has been well established.

3 A negative contraction stress test indicates fetal ability to tolerate uterine contractions. In general, however, a positive test implies potential uteroplacental insufficiency and has been associated with adverse perinatal outcome and an increased incidence of intrauterine demise.

4 Fetal heart rate (FHR) reactivity is a good indicator of normal fetal autonomic function and well-being; it depends on normal neurologic development and normal integration of the central nervous system control of FHR.

5 Preterm fetuses are less likely to have FHR accelerations in association with fetal movements.

6 The predictive value of a negative nonstress test (NST) (normal outcome associated with a reactive NST) is very high. The reactive NST predicts good perinatal outcome in about 95% of cases. The false-positive rate of a nonreactive NST is also very high.

7 The normal fetal response to vibroacoustic stimulation (VAS) includes not only FHR accelerations, but also increases in long-term FHR variability and gross body movements.

8 VAS has been conclusively demonstrated to be effective in achieving fetal arousal, is reasonably safe, and improves the efficiency of antepartum FHR testing. Utilizing VAS on the nonacidemic fetus may elicit accelerations that appear to be valid in predicting fetal well-being. It also offers the advantage of safely reducing testing time, without compromising detection of the acidemic fetus.

9 The biophysical profile (BPP) is unique in that it assesses both acute (FHR reactivity, fetal breathing movements, fetal movements, fetal tone) and chronic (amniotic fluid volume) markers of fetal condition.

10 The "gradual hypoxia concept" implies that the biophysical activities developed last *in utero* are also the first to become abnormal in the presence of fetal acidemia or infection. In accordance with this concept, early stages of fetal compromise are manifested by abnormalities in FHR reactivity and breathing, while movement and tone are generally not abolished until much later stages of compromise.

11 In the second half of pregnancy, the main sources of amniotic fluid include fetal urine excretion (especially) and fluid secreted by the fetal lung. However, unlike the role of the kidneys, the fetal lung does not play a role in regulating fetal body fluid homeostasis.

12 Polyhydramnios (pathologic accumulation of amniotic fluid), which is defined as an amniotic fluid index > 25 cm, occurs in 0.2–1.6% of the general population. When the cause of polyhydramnios can be found, the diagnosis usually falls into the following categories: fetal malformations and genetic disorders, diabetes, Rh sensitization, and congenital infections. Fetal swallowing impairment may also result in excess amniotic fluid volume.

13 Oligohydramnios (reduced amniotic fluid volume) occurs in 5.5–37.8% of pregnancies and is significant

because of its known association with adverse pregnancy outcome, such as umbilical cord occlusion, fetal distress in labor, meconium aspiration, operative deliveries, and stillbirth.

14 The pathophysiologic processes that can lead to fetal death/damage include decreased uteroplacental blood flow, decreased gas exchange at the trophoblastic membrane level, metabolic processes, fetal sepsis, fetal anemia, fetal heart failure, and umbilical cord accidents. Multiple parameter assessment or combinations of different tests may often be the optimal fetal strategy, depending on the testing indication. In order to improve accuracy, condition-specific fetal testing should be utilized.

15 The interpretation of FHR patterns should incorporate knowledge of gestational age, maternal condition, medications, and other factors that could influence FHR components.

16 In 1997, the National Institute of Child Health and Human Development Research Planning Workshop developed standardized definitions for electronic FHR patterns and recommendations for interpreting them.

17 The diagnostic accuracy of electronic FHR monitoring in predicting fetal compromise (positive predictive value) is not as good as its accuracy in confirming fetal well-being.

18 Other methods of evaluating an unreassuring FHR pattern have been proposed, such as fetal scalp stimulation and VAS. FHR acceleration as a response to fetal stimulation indicates a nonacidemic fetus, and thus scalp blood sampling may be omitted. Using VAS or scalp stimulation may reduce the need for scalp pH when FHR tracings are equivocal/nonreassuring.

19 Fetal pulse oximetry will reduce the Cesarean rate for nonreassuring electronic FHR monitoring patterns but, as currently used, will not decrease the overall Cesarean rate.

20 Technical systems have been developed to monitor the fetal electrocardiogram (ECG) during labor, as an adjunct to continuous electronic FHR monitoring, with the aim of improving fetal outcome and minimizing unnecessary obstetric interference. Some have found that, by adding fetal ECG ST segment automated analysis (STAN) to standard FHR monitoring, this has improved FHR tracing interpretation and improved observer consistency in both the decision for and the timing of obstetric interventions, and may reduce the number of unneeded obstetric interventions when fetal compromise is absent.

References

1 Nijhuis JG, Prechtl HFR, Martin CB, Bots RSGM. Are there behavioral states in the human fetus? *Early Hum Dev* 1982;6:177.

2 Van Woerdan EE, Van Geijn. Heart-rate patterns and fetal movements. In: Nijhuis JG, ed. *Fetal behavior: developmental and perinatal aspects*. New York: Oxford University Press; 1992:41.

3 Pearson JF, Weaver JB. Fetal activity and fetal wellbeing: an evaluation. *Br Med J* 1976;1:1305.

4 Rayburn WF. Clinical implications from monitoring fetal activity. *Am J Obstet Gynecol* 1982;144:967.

5 Rayburn WF. Clinical significance of perceptible fetal motion. *Am J Obstet Gynecol* 1980;138:210.

6 Moore TR, Piacquadio K. A prospective evaluation of fetal movement screening to reduce the incidence of antepartum fetal death. *Am J Obstet Gynecol* 1989;160:1075.

7 Rayburn WF. Antepartum fetal assessment: monitoring fetal activity. *Clin Perinatol* 1982;9:231.

8 Leader LR, Baillie P, VanSchalkwyk DJ. Fetal movements and fetal outcome: a prospective study. *Obstet Gynecol* 1981;57:431.

9 ACOG Practice Bulletin, no. 9. Antepartum fetal surveillance. Washington: American College of Obstetricians and Gynecologists; 1999;911.

10 Freeman RK, Anderson G, Dorchester W. A prospective multi-institutional study of antepartum fetal heart rate monitoring: risk of perinatal mortality and morbidity according to antepartum fetal heart rate test results. *Am J Obstet Gynecol* 1982;143:771.

11 Evertson LR, Gauthier RJ, Collea JV. Fetal demise following negative contraction stress tests. *Obstet Gynecol* 1978;51:671–673.

12 Lagrew DC. The contraction stress test. *Clin Obstet Gynecol* 1995;38:11.

13 Lagrew DC, Pircon RA, Towers CV, et al. Antepartum fetal surveillance in patients with diabetes: when to start? *Am J Obstet Gynecol* 1993;168:1820.

14 Druzin ML, Gratacos J, Paul RH. Antepartum fetal heart rate testing: predictive reliability of "normal" tests in the prevention of antepartum death. *Am J Obstet Gynecol* 1980;137:746.

15 Grundy H, Freeman RK, Lederman S, Dorchester W. Nonreactive contraction stress test: clinical significance. *Obstet Gynecol* 1984;64:337.

16 Thacker SB, Berkelman RL. Assessing the diagnostic accuracy and efficacy of selected antepartum fetal surveillance techniques. *Obstet Gynecol Surv* 1986;41:121.

17 Bissonnette JM, Johnson K, Toomey C. The role of a trial of labor with a positive contraction stress test. *Am J Obstet Gynecol* 1979;135:292.

18 Devoe LD. Clinical features of the reactive positive contraction stress test. *Obstet Gynecol* 1984;63:523.

19 Garite TJ, Freeman RK, Hochleutner I, Linzey EM. Oxytocin challenge test: achieving the desired goals. *Obstet Gynecol* 1978;51:614.

20 Staisch KJ, Westlake JR, Bashore RA. Blind oxytocin challenge test and perinatal outcome. *Am J Obstet Gynecol* 1980;138:399.

21 Keegan KA, Jr, Paul RH, Broussard PM, et al. Antepartum fetal heart rate testing. V. The nonstress test: an outpatient approach. *Am J Obstet Gynecol* 1980;136:81.

22 Phelan JP. The nonstress test: a review of 3000 tests. *Am J Obstet Gynecol* 1981;139:7.

23 Evertson LR, Gauthier RJ, Schifrin BS, Paul RH. Antepartum fetal heart rate testing. I. Evolution of the nonstress test. *Am J Obstet Gynecol* 1979;133:29.
24 Patrick J, Carmichael L, Chess L, Staples C. Accelerations of the human fetal heart rate at 38 to 40 weeks' gestational age. *Am J Obstet Gynecol* 1984;148:35.
25 Keegan KA, Paul RH, Broussard PM, et al. Antepartum fetal heart testing. III: The effect of phenobarbital on the nonstress test. *Am J Obstet Gynecol* 1979;133:579.
26 Margulis E, Binder D, Cohen AW. The effect of propanolol on the nonstress test. *Am J Obstet Gynecol* 1984;148:340.
27 Phelan JP. Diminished fetal reactivity with smoking. *Am J Obstet Gynecol* 1980;136:230.
28 Meis PJ, Ureda JR, Swain M, et al. Variable decelerations during nonstress tests are not a sign of fetal compromise. *Am J Obstet Gynecol* 1986;154:586.
29 Anyaegbunam A, Brustman L, Divon M, Langer O. The significance of antepartum variable decelerations. *Am J Obstet Gynecol* 1986;155:707.
30 Navot D, Yaffe H, Sadovsky E. The ratio of fetal heart rate accelerations to fetal movements according to gestational age. *Am J Obstet Gynecol* 1984;149:92.
31 Natale R, Nasello C, Turliuk R. The relationship between movements and accelerations in fetal heart rate at twenty-four to thirty-two weeks' gestation. *Am J Obstet Gynecol* 1984;148: 591.
32 Gagnon R, Campbell K, Hunse C, Patrick J. Patterns of human fetal heart rate accelerations from 26 weeks to term. *Am J Obstet Gynecol* 1987;157:743.
33 Smith CV, Phelan JP, Paul RH. A prospective analysis of the influence of gestational age on the baseline fetal heart rate and reactivity in a low-risk population. *Am J Obstet Gynecol* 1985;153:780.
34 Sorokin Y, Dierker LJ, Pillay SK, et al. The association between fetal heart rate patterns and fetal movements in pregnancies between 20 and 30 weeks' gestation. *Am J Obstet Gynecol* 1982;143:243.
35 Lavery JP. Nonstress fetal heart rate testing. *Clin Obstet Gynecol* 1982;25:689.
36 Devoe LD, Castillo RA, Sherline DM. The nonstress test as a diagnostic test: a critical reappraisal. *Am J Obstet Gynecol* 1985;152:1047.
37 Devoe LD. Clinical implications of prospective antepartum fetal heart rate testing. *Am J Obstet Gynecol* 1980;137:983.
38 Barss VA, Frigoletto FD, Diamond F. Stillbirth after nonstress testing. *Obstet Gynecol* 1985;65:541.
39 Boehm FH, Salyer S, Shah DM, Vaughn WK. Improved outcome of twice weekly nonstress testing. *Obstet Gynecol* 1986;67: 566.
40 Barrett JM, Salyer SL, Boehm FH. The nonstress test: an evaluation of 1000 patients. *Am J Obstet Gynecol* 1981;141: 153.
41 Devoe LD. The nonstress test. *Obstet Gynecol Clin North Am* 1990;17:111.
42 Devoe LD, McKenzie J, Searle NS, Sherline DM. Clinical sequelae of the extended nonstress test. *Am J Obstet Gynecol* 1985;151:1074.
43 Smith CV, Phelan JP, Platt LD, et al. Fetal acoustic stimulation testing. II. A randomized clinical comparison with the nonstress test. *Am J Obstet Gynecol* 1986;155:131.
44 Trudinger BJ, Boylan P. Antepartum fetal heart rate monitoring: value of sound stimulation. *Obstet Gynecol* 1980;55:265.
45 Gagnon R, Hunse C, Patrick J. Fetal responses to vibratory acoustic stimulation: influence of basal heart rate. *Am J Obstet Gynecol* 1988;159:835.
46 Thomas RL, Johnson TRB, Besinger RE, et al. Preterm and term fetal cardiac and movement responses to vibratory acoustic stimulation. *Am J Obstet Gynecol* 1989;161:141.
47 Manning FA, Platt LD, Sipos L. Antepartum fetal evaluation: development of a fetal biophysical profile. *Am J Obstet Gynecol* 1980;136:787.
48 Vintzileos AM, Campbell WA, Ingardia CJ, Nochimson DJ. The fetal biophysical profile and its predictive value. *Obstet Gynecol* 1983;62:271.
49 Manning FA, Morrison I, Lange IR, et al. Fetal biophysical profile scoring: selective use of the nonstress test. *Am J Obstet Gynecol* 1987;156:709.
50 Manning FA, Harman CR, Morrison I, et al. Fetal assessment based on fetal biophysical profile scoring. IV. An analysis of perinatal morbidity and mortality. *Am J Obstet Gynecol* 1990;162: 703.
51 Chamberlain PF, Manning FA, Morrison I, et al. Ultrasound evaluation of amniotic fluid volume. I. The relationship of marginal and decreased amniotic fluid volumes to perinatal outcome. *Am J Obstet Gynecol* 1984;150:245.
52 Bastide A, Manning FA, Harman CR, et al. Ultrasound evaluation of amniotic fluid: outcome of pregnancies with severe oligohydramnios. *Am J Obstet Gynecol* 1986;154:895.
53 Manning FA, Morrison I, Lange IR, et al. Fetal assessment based upon fetal biophysical profile scoring: experience in 12620 referred high risk pregnancies. I. Perinatal mortality by frequency and etiology. *Am J Obstet Gynecol* 1985;151;343.
54 Baskett TF, Allen AC, Gray JH, et al. Fetal biophysical profile and perinatal death. *Obstet Gynecol* 1987;70:357.
55 Platt LD, Eglinton GS, Sipos L, et al. Further experience with the fetal biophysical profile. *Obstet Gynecol* 1983;61:480.
56 Manning FA, Harman CR, Morrison I, et al. Fetal assessment based on fetal biophysical profile scoring. IV. An analysis of perinatal morbidity and mortality. *Am J Obstet Gynecol* 1990;162: 703.
57 Vintzileos AM, Gaffney SE, Salinger LM, et al. The relationship between fetal biophysical profile and cord pH in patients undergoing cesarean section before the onset of labor. *Obstet Gynecol* 1987;70:196.
58 Vintzileos AM, Fleming AD, Scorza WE, et al. Relationship between fetal biophysical activities and umbilical cord blood gases. *Am J Obstet Gynecol* 1991;165:707.
59 Rutherford SE, Phelan JP, Smith CV, Jacobs N. The four-quadrant assessment of amniotic fluid volume: an adjunct to antepartum fetal heart rate testing. *Obstet Gynecol* 1987;70: 353.
60 Vintzileos AM, Knuppel RA. Multiple parameter biophysical testing in the prediction of fetal acid-base status. *Clin Perinatol* 1994;21:823.
61 Nageotte MP, Towers CV, Tamerou A, et al. The value of a negative antepartum test: contraction stress test and modified biophysical profile. *Obstet Gynecol* 1994;84:231.
62 Vintzileos AM, Feinstein SJ, Lodeiro JG, et al. Fetal biophysical profile and the effect of premature rupture of the membranes. *Obstet Gynecol* 1986;67:818.
63 Hanley ML, Vintzileos AM. Biophysical testing in premature rupture of the membranes. *Semin Perinatol* 1996;20: 418.
64 Brace RA, Wolf EJ. Normal amniotic fluid volume changes throughout pregnancy. *Am J Obstet Gynecol* 1989;161:382.
65 Queenan JT, Thompson W, Whitfield CR, Shah SI. Amniotic fluid

volumes in normal pregnancies. *Am J Obstet Gynecol* 1972; 114:34.

66 Phelan JP, Smith CV, Broussard P, Small M. Amniotic fluid volume assessment with the four quadrant technique at 36–42 weeks' gestation. *J Reprod Med* 1987;32:540.

67 Phelan JP, Martin GI. Polyhydramnios: fetal and neonatal implications. *Clin Perinatol* 1989;16:987.

68 Rutherford SE, Smith CV, Phelan JP, et al. The four quadrant assessment of amniotic fluid volume: interobserver and intraobserver variation. *J Reprod Med* 1987;32:597.

69 Chauhan SP, Doherty DD, Magann EF, et al. Amniotic fluid index vs. single deepest pocket technique during modified biophysical profile: a randomized clinical trial. *Am J Obstet Gynecol* 2004;191:661.

70 Magann EF, Doherty DA, Field K, et al. Biophysical profile with amniotic fluid volume assessments. *Obstet Gynecol* 2004;104: 5.

71 Vintzileos AM, Campbell WA, Nochimson DJ, Weinbaum PJ. Degree of oligohydramnios and pregnancy outcome in patients with premature rupture of the membranes. *Obstet Gynecol* 1985;66:162.

72 Vintzileos AM, Campbell WA, Nochimson DM, et al. Qualitative amniotic fluid volume versus amniocentesis in predicting infection in preterm premature rupture of the membranes. *Obstet Gynecol* 1986;67:579.

73 Vintzileos AM, Campbell WA, Nochimson DJ, Weinbaum PJ. The use of the nonstress test in patents with premature rupture of the membranes. *Am J Obstet Gynecol* 1986;1515:149.

74 Hill L, Breckle R, Thomas ML, Fries JK. Polyhydramnios: ultrasonically detected prevalence and neonatal outcome. *Obstet Gynecol* 1987;69:21.

75 Phelan JP, Park YW, Ahn MO, Rutherford SE. Polyhydramnios and perinatal outcome. *J Perinatol* 1990;4:347.

76 Kirson B, Mari G, Moise KJ. Indomethacin therapy in the treatment of symptomatic polyhydramnios. *Obstet Gynecol* 1990; 75:202.

77 Mercer LJ, Brown LG, Petres RE, Messer RH. A survey of pregnancies complicated by decreased amniotic fluid. *Am J Obstet Gynecol* 1984;149:355.

78 King JC, Mitzner W, Butterfield AB, Queenan JT. Effect of oligohydramnios on fetal lung development. *Am J Obstet Gynecol* 1986;154:823.

79 Mercer LJ, Brown LG. Fetal outcome with oligohydramnios in the second trimester. *Obstet Gynecol* 1986;67:840.

80 Kontopoulos EV, Vintzileos AM. Condition-specific antepartum fetal testing. *Am J Obstet Gynecol* 2004;191:1546.

81 Miller DA, Rabello YA, Paul RH. The modified biophysical profile: antepartum testing in the 1990s. *Am J Obstet Gynecol* 1996;174:812.

82 Dayal AK, Manning FA, Berck DJ, et al. Fetal death after normal biophysical profile score: an eighteen-year experience. *Am J Obstet Gynecol* 1999;181:1231.

83 ACOG Technical Bulletin, no. 207. Fetal heart rate patterns: monitoring, interpretation, and management. Washington: American College of Obstetricians and Gynecologists; 1995: 454.

84 National Institute of Child Health and Human Development Research Planning Workshop. Electronic fetal heart rate monitoring: research guidelines for interpretation. *Am J Obstet Gynecol* 1997;17:1385.

85 Schifferli P, Cadeyro-Barcia R. Effects of atropine and beta adrenergic drugs on the heart rate of the human fetus. In: Boreus L, ed. *Fetal pharmacology*. New York: Raven Press; 1973:259.

86 Beard RW, Knight CA, Roberts GM. The significance of the changes in the continuous fetal heart rate in the first stage of labor. *J Obstet Gynaecol Br Commonw* 1971;78:865.

87 Martin CB. Physiology and clinical use of fetal heart rate variability. *Clin Perinatol* 1982;9:339.

88 Paul RH, Suidan AK, Yeh SY, et al. Clinical fetal monitoring. VII. The evaluation and significance of intrapartum baseline FHR variability. *Am J Obstet Gynecol* 1975;123:206.

89 Petrikovsky BM, Vintzileos AM, Nochimson DJ. Heart rate cyclicity during labor in healthy term fetuses. *Am J Perinatol* 1989;6:289.

90 Krebs HB, Petres RE, Dunn LJ, Smith PJ. Intrapartum fetal heart rate monitoring. VI. Prognostic significance of accelerations. *Am J Obstet Gynecol* 1982;142:297.

91 Kubli FW, Hon EH, Khazin AF, Takemura H. Observations on heart rate and pH in the human fetus during labor. *Am J Obstet Gynecol* 1969;104:1190.

92 Hon EH. The electronic evaluation of the fetal heart rate. Preliminary report. *Am J Obstet Gynecol* 1958;75:1215.

93 Angel JL, Knuppel R, Lake M. Sinusoidal fetal heart rate patterns associated with intravenous butorphanol administration: a case report. *Am J Obstet Gynecol* 1984;149:465.

94 Freeman RK. Problems with intrapartum fetal heart rate monitoring interpretation and patient management. *Obstet Gynecol* 2002;100:813.

95 Clark SL, Hankins GD. Temporal and demographic trends in cerebral palsy – fact and fiction. *Am J Obstet Gynecol* 2003;188: 628.

96 Umstad MP. The predictive value of abnormal fetal heart rate patterns in early labour. *Aust NZ J Obstet Gynaecol* 1993;33: 145.

97 Haverkamp AD, Thompson HE, McFee JG, Cetrulo C. The evaluation of continuous fetal heart rate monitoring in high-risk pregnancy. *Am J Obstet Gynecol* 1976;125:310.

98 MacDonald D, Grant A, Sheridan-Pereira M, et al. The Dublin randomized controlled trial of intrapartum fetal heart rate monitoring. *Am J Obstet Gynecol* 1985;152:524.

99 Kelso IM, Parsons RJ, Lawrence GF, et al. An assessment of continuous fetal heart rate monitoring in labor. A randomized clinical trial. *Am J Obstet Gynecol* 1978;131:526.

100 Wood C, Renou P, Oats J, et al. A controlled trial of fetal heart rate monitoring in a low-risk obstetric population. *Am J Obstet Gynecol* 1981;141:527.

101 Vintzileos AM, Antsaklis A, Varvarigos I, et al. A randomized trial of intrapartum electronic fetal heart rate monitoring versus intermittent auscultation. *Obstet Gynecol* 1993;81:899.

102 Vintzileos AM, Nochimson DJ, Antsaklis A, et al. Comparison of intrapartum electronic fetal heart rate monitoring versus intermittent auscultation in detecting fetal acidemia at birth. *Am J Obstet Gynecol* 1995;173:1021.

103 Vintzileos AM, Nochimson DJ, Guzman ER, et al. Intrapartum electronic fetal heart rate monitoring versus intermittent auscultation: a metaanalysis. *Obstet Gynecol* 1995;85:149.

104 Thacker SB, Stroup D, Chang M. Continuous electronic heart rate monitoring for fetal assessment during labor (Cochrane Review). *The Cochrane Library* Issue 4, 2004.

105 Beard RW. Fetal blood sampling. *Br J Hosp Med* 1970;3: 523.

106 Goldaber KG, Gilstrap LC, Leveno KJ, et al. Pathologic fetal acidemia. *Obstet Gynecol* 1991;78:1103.

107 Winkler CL, Hauth JC, Tucker M, et al. Neonatal complications at term as related to the degrees of umbilical artery acidemia. *Am J Obstet Gynecol* 1991;164:637.

108 Haverkamp AD, Orleans M, Langendoerfer S, et al. A controlled trial of the differential effects of intrapartum fetal monitoring. *Am J Obstet Gynecol* 1979;134:339.
109 Goodwin TM, Milner-Masterson L, Paul RH. Elimination of fetal scalp blood sampling on a large clinical service. *Obstet Gynecol* 1994;83:971.
110 Vintzileos AM, Egan JFX, Campbell WA, et al. Asphyxia at birth as determined by cord blood pH measurements in preterm and term gestations: correlation with neonatal outcomes. *J Matern Fetal Med* 1992;1:7.
111 Thorp JA, Sampson JE, Parisi VM, Creasy RK. Routine umbilical cord blood gas determinations? *Am J Obstet Gynecol* 1989;161:600.
112 Ross MG, Gala R. Use of umbilical artery base excess: algorithm for the timing of hypoxic injury. *Am J Obstet Gynecol* 2002;187: 1.
113 Clark SL, Gimovsky ML, Miller FC. Fetal heart rate response to scalp blood sampling. *Am J Obstet Gynecol* 1982;144: 706.
114 Clark SL, Gimovsky ML, Miller FC. The scalp stimulation test: a clinical alternative to fetal scalp blood sampling. *Am J Obstet Gynecol* 1984;148:274.
115 Elimian A, Figueroa R, Tejani N. Intrapartum assessment of fetal well-being: a comparison of scalp stimulation with scalp blood pH sampling. *Obstet Gynecol* 1997;89:373.
116 Smith CV, Nguyen HN, Phelan JP, Paul RH. Intrapartum assessment of fetal well-being: a comparison of fetal acoustic stimulation with acid base determinations. *Am J Obstet Gynecol* 1986;155:726.
117 Edersheim TG, Hutson JM, Druzin ML, Kogut EA. Fetal heart rate response to vibratory acoustic stimulation predicts fetal pH in labor. *Am J Obstet Gynecol* 1987;157:1557.
118 Bartelsmeyer JA, Sadovsky Y, Fleming B, Petrie RH. Utilization of fetal heart rate acceleration following vibroacoustic stimulation in labor to predict fetal acidemia and base deficit levels. *J Matern Fetal Med* 1995;4:120.
119 Ingemarsson I, Arulkumaran S. Reactive fetal heart rate response to vibroacoustic stimulation in fetuses with low scalp blood pH. *Br J Obstet Gynaecol* 1989;96:562.
120 Polzin GB, Blakemore KJ, Petrie RH, Amon E. Fetal vibroacoustic stimulation: magnitude and duration of fetal heart rate accelerations as a marker of fetal health. *Obstet Gynecol* 1988;72:621.
121 Benito CW, Vintzileos AM, Ananth CV. Intrapartum assessment of fetal acidosis by vibroacoustic stimulation: a meta-analysis (abstract 489). Proceedings of the Society of Perinatal Obstetricians, 17th Annual Meeting, Anaheim, CA, 1997.
122 Porter TF, Clark SL. Vibroacoustic and scalp stimulation. *Obstet Gynecol Clin North Am* 1999;26:657.
123 Richards DS, Cefalo RC, Thorpe JM, et al. Determinants of fetal heart rate response to vibroacoustic stimulation in labor. *Obstet Gynecol* 1988;71:535.
124 Poehlmann S, Pinette M, Stubblefield P. Effect of labor analgesia with nalbuphine hydrochloride on fetal response to vibroacoustic stimulation. *J Reprod Med* 1995;40;707.
125 Arikan GM, Scholz HS, Haeusler MCH, et al. Low fetal oxygen saturation at birth and acidosis. *Obstet Gynecol* 2000;95: 565.
126 Mallinckrodt Inc. *OxiFirst ™ fetal oxygen saturation monitoring system. Operator's manual. N-400 fetal pulse oximeter.* Pleasanton, CA: Mallinckrodt Inc., 2000.
127 Seelbach-Gobel B, Heupel M, Kuhnert M, Butterwegge M. The prediction of fetal acidoses by means of intrapartum fetal pulse oximetry. *Am J Obstet Gynecol* 1999;180:73.
128 Dildy GA, Clark SL, Loucks CA. Intrapartum fetal pulse oximetry: past, present, and future. *Am J Obstet Gynecol* 1996;175: 1.
129 Luttkus A, Fengler TW, Friedman W, Dudenhausen JW. Continuous monitoring of fetal oxygen saturation by pulse oximetry. *Obstet Gynecol* 1995;85:183.
130 Yam J, Chua S, Arulkumaran S. Intrapartum fetal pulse oximetry. Part 1. Principles and technical issues. *Obstet Gynecol Surv* 2000;55:163.
131 Yam J, Chua S, Arulkumarann S. Intrapartum fetal pulse oximetry. Part 2. Clinical application. *Obstet Gynecol Surv* 2000;55: 173.
132 Garite TJ, Dildy GA, McNamara H, et al. A multicenter controlled trial of fetal pulse oximetry in the intrapartum management of nonreassuring fetal heart rate patterns. *Am J Obstet Gynecol* 2000;183:1049.
133 Porreco RP, Boehm FH, Dildy GA, et al. Dystocia in nulliparous patients monitored with fetal pulse oximetry. *Am J Obstet Gynecol* 2004;190;113.
134 ACOG Committee Opinion, no. 258. Fetal pulse oximetry. *Obstet Gynecol* 2001;98:523.
135 Dildy GA. Fetal pulse oximetry: a critical appraisal. *Best Pract Res Clin Obstet Gynaecol* 2004;18:477.
136 Neilson JP. Fetal electrocardiogram (ECG) for fetal monitoring during labour. *Cochrane Database Syst Rev* 2003;2 CD000116.
137 Luttkus AK, Stupin JH, Callsen TA, Dudenhausen JW. Feasibility of simultaneous application of fetal electrocardiography and fetal pulse oximetry. *Acta Obstet Gynecol Scand* 2003;82: 443.
138 Dervaitis KL, Poole M, Schmidt G, et al. ST segment analysis of the fetal electrocardiogram plus electronic fetal heart rate monitoring in labor and its relationship to umbilical cord arterial blood gases. *Am J Obstet Gynecol* 2004;191:879.
139 Neilson JP. Fetal electrocardiogram (ECG) for fetal monitoring during labour (Cochrane Review). *The Cochrane Library*, 2004.
140 Ross MG, Devoe LD, Rosen KG. ST-segment analysis of the fetal electrocardiogram improves fetal heart rate tracing interpretation and clinical decision making. *J Matern Fetal Neonatal Med* 2004;15:181.

Part VIII

Fetal Therapy

33 The fetus at surgery

Robert H. Ball and Michael R. Harrison

The indications for fetal surgical interventions have expanded since the field was founded over two decades ago. Similarly, the total number of procedures performed, the centers at which they are performed, and the number of physicians performing them have increased. Nevertheless, overall, these procedures remain very limited when compared with the number of pregnancies and even the number of fetuses with malformations.

Over the last decade, technological advances have allowed a transition toward less invasive procedures. Initial fetal surgical procedures pioneered by one of the authors (MRH), at the University College of San Francisco, depended on maternal laparotomy and hysterotomy. This approach evolved into laparotomy and uterine endoscopy and, most recently, into percutaneous procedures using devices with diameters of 3 mm or less. Our experience suggests that the less invasive approaches are associated with a less complicated postoperative recovery for the mothers, but do not entirely eliminate morbidity.[1]

Open fetal surgery (hysterotomy)

The human experience with open fetal surgery is now quite extensive, both from our own center and others,[1–3] and is primarily associated with the large numbers of fetal spina bifida repairs (Fig. 33.1). We currently reserve maternal laparotomy/hysterotomy procedures for repair of spina bifida, resection of sacrococcygeal teratoma and other tumors, and lobectomy for cystic adenomatoid malformation (CCAM).

We have recently reviewed our experience at UCSF with maternal hysterotomy[1] (Table 33.1). Eighty-seven hysterotomies were performed between 1989 and 2003. There were significant immediate postoperative complications. In the early experience, pulmonary edema related to multiple tocolytic use, particularly nitroglycerin, and aggressive fluid management was a significant problem.[4] Thirteen percent of women required transfusion for intraoperative blood loss. Pregnancy outcomes were also significantly affected with a premature rupture of membrane (PROM) rate of 52%, 33% having preterm labor refractory to maximal tocolytic management leading to delivery. The mean time from hysterotomy to delivery was 4.9 weeks (range 0–16 weeks). The mean gestational age at the time of delivery was 30.1 weeks (range 21.6–36.7 weeks). Others[5,6] have had similar experiences with respect to an increased risk of preterm delivery following hysterotomy. Most of the morbidity associated with hysterotomy has decreased with experience. Significant pulmonary edema or blood loss is rare, and the mean gestational age at the time of delivery for repair of myelomeningocele (MMC) is now around 34 weeks.

The practical aspects of hysterotomy and postoperative management have evolved since the initial years of experience. Lengthy discussions regarding the risks, benefits, and alternatives of the procedure are important, including the experimental nature of the surgery. The risks to the mother are similar to any major abdominal surgery, although in this case there is no direct physical benefit to her. In addition, there are the risks associated with aggressive tocolytic therapy and bedrest in a hypercoagulable state. The risks to the fetus are primarily vascular instability and hypoperfusion intraoperatively, leading to injury or death, and prematurity due to postoperative complications. The risks to the pregnancy are primarily preterm labor and PROM and preterm delivery. Infectious complications are rare, except when premature rupture leads to prolonged latency. An important additional discussion point is that all subsequent deliveries, including the index pregnancy, must be by Cesarean section. Data regarding future fertility are reassuring, with no increased incidence of infertility in the UCSF experience in those patients attempting pregnancy.[7] Experience from the Children's Hospital of Pennsylvania suggests a concerning risk of uterine rupture in subsequent pregnancies that may be as high as 18%, which would be considerably higher than the risk after previous low transverse Cesarean section (1% or less) or classical Cesarean section (5–10%). Another potential risk in subsequent pregnancies is placenta accreta. The reason for this is that the site of a hysterotomy performed in the second trimester is never in the same area as a Cesarean section entry. There is an

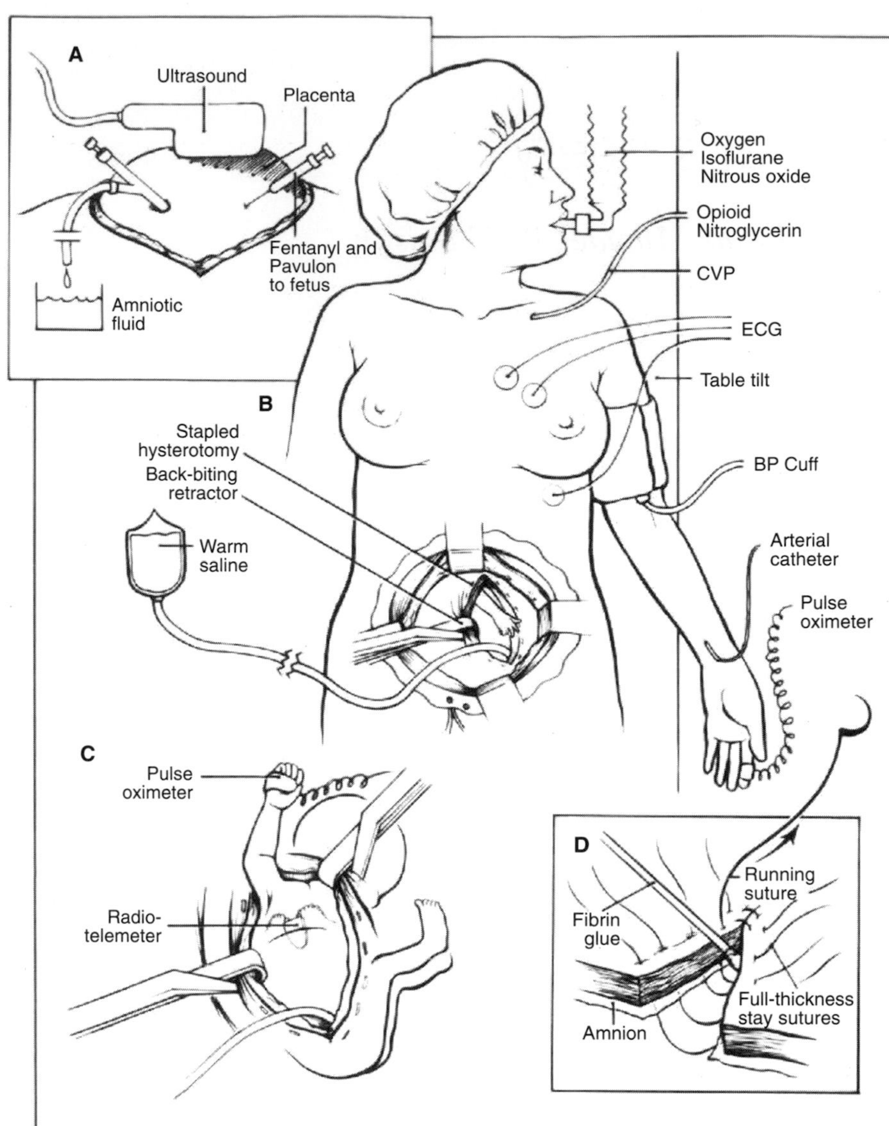

Figure 33.1 Summary of open fetal surgery techniques. (A) The uterus is exposed through a low, transverse abdominal incision. Ultrasonography is used to localize the placenta, inject the fetus with narcotic and muscle relaxant, and aspirate amniotic fluid. (B) The uterus is opened with staples that provide hemostasis and seal the membranes. Warm saline solution is continuously infused around the fetus. Maternal anesthesia, tocolysis, and monitoring are shown. BP, blood pressure; CVP, central venous pressure; ECG, electrocardiogram. (C) Absorbable staples and back-biting clamps facilitate hysterotomy exposure of the pertinent fetal part. A miniaturized pulse oximeter records pulse rate and oxygen saturation intraoperatively. A radiotelemeter monitors fetal electrocardiogram and amniotic pressure during and after the operation. (D) After fetal repair, the uterine incision is closed with absorbable sutures and fibrin glue. Amniotic fluid is restored with warm lactated Ringer's solution.

Table 33.1 Maternal morbidity and mortality for 178 interventions at UCSF with postoperative continuing pregnancy and divided into operative subgroups.

Postoperative result	Open hysterotomy	Endoscopy FETENDO/ Lap-FETENDO	Percutaneous FIGS/ Lap-FIGS	All interventions
Patients with postoperative continuing pregnancy	79	68	31	178
Gestational age at surgery (weeks)	25.1	24.5	21.1	24.2
Range (weeks)	17.6–30.4	17.9–32.1	17.0–26.6	17.0–32.1
Gestational age at delivery (weeks)	30.1	30.4	32.7	30.7
Range (weeks)	21.6–36.7	19.6–39.3	21.7–40.4	19.6–40.4
Interval surgery to delivery (weeks)	4.9	6.0	11.6	6.5
Range (weeks)	0–16	0–19	0.3–21.4	0–21.4
Pulmonary edema	22/79 (27.8%)	17/68 (25.0%)	0/31 (0.0%)	39/178 (21.9%)
Bleeding requiring blood transfusion	11/87 (12.6%)	2/69 (2.9%)	0/31 (0.0%)	13/187 (7.0%)
Preterm labor leading to delivery	26/79 (32.9%)	18/68 (26.5%)	4/31 (12.9%)	48/178 (27.0%)
Premature rupture of membranes (PROM)	41/79 (51.9%)	30/68 (44.1%)	8/31 (25.8%)	79/178 (44.4%)
Chorioamnionitis	7/79 (8.9%)	1/68 (1.5%)	0/31 (0.0%)	8/178 (4.5%)

FIGS, fetal intervention guided by sonography.

Table 33.2 Fetal conditions that may benefit from treatment before birth.

Fetal condition	Effect on development (rationale for treatment)	Result without treatment	Recommended treatment
Life-threatening defects			
Urinary obstruction (urethral valves)	Hydronephrosis Lung hypoplasia	→Renal failure →Pulmonary failure	Percutaneous vesicoamniotic shunt Fetoscopic ablation of valves Open vesicostomy
Cystic adenomatoid malformation	Lung hypoplasia–hydrops	→Hydrops, death	Open pulmonary lobectomy Ablation (laser/RFA) Steroids
Congenital diaphragmatic hernia	Lung hypoplasia	→Pulmonary failure	Open complete repair Temporary tracheal occlusion Tracheal clip (open and fetoscopic) Fetoscopic balloon (percutaneous/reversible)
Sacrococcygeal teratoma	High-output failure	→Hydrops, death	Open resection of tumor Vascular occlusion (alcohol/RFA) RFA
Twin–twin transfusion syndrome	Donor–recipient steal through placenta	→Fetal hydrops, death, neurologic damage to survivor	Fetoscopic laser ablation of placental vessels (NIH trial) Amnioreduction (NIH trial) Selective reduction (NIH trial)
Acardiac/anomalous twin (TRAP)	Vascular steal Embolization	→Death/damage to surviving twin	Selective reduction Cord occlusion/division RFA
Aqueductal stenosis	Hydrocephalus	→Brain damage	Ventriculoamniotic shunt
Valvular obstruction	Hypoplastic heart	→Heart failure	Balloon valvuloplasty
Congenital high airway obstruction (CHAOS)	Overdistention by lung fluid	→Hydrops, death	Fetoscopic tracheostomy *Ex utero* intrapartum treatment (EXIT)
Cervical teratoma	Airway obstruction High-output failure	→Hydrops, death	Open resection EXIT Vascular occlusion (alcohol/RFA)
Nonlife-threatening defects			
Myelomeningocle	Spinal cord damage	→Paralysis, neurogenic bladder/bowel, hydrocephalus	Open repair (NIH trial) Fetoscopic coverage
Gastroschisis	Bowel damage	→Malnutrition/ short bowel	Serial amnio-exchange
Cleft lip and palate	Facial defect	→Persistent deformity	Fetoscopic repair* Open repair
Metabolic and cellular defects			
Stem cell–enzyme defects	Hemoglobinopathy Immunodeficiency Storage diseases	→Anemia, hydrops →Infection/death →Retardation/death	Fetal stem cell transplant Fetal gene therapy*
Predictable organ	Agenesis/hypoplasia heart/lung/kidney	→Neonatal heart/lung/ kidney failure	Induce tolerance for postnatal organ transplant* Tissue engineering*

NIH, National Institutes of Health; RFA, radiofrequency ablation.

*Not yet attempted in human fetuses.

increased risk of placenta accreta in any case in which implantation is in an area of uterine scarring. Multiple incisions will increase the likelihood of implantation in such an area. To our knowledge, there has not been a case of accreta in a fetal surgical patient of ours in a subsequent pregnancy.

Indications for open fetal surgery (Table 33.2)

Myelomeningocele (MMC)

Currently, the most common indication for hysterotomy-based fetal intervention in our center is for MMCs. This is a devastating birth defect with sequelae that affect both the central and peripheral nervous systems. A change in cerebrospinal fluid (CSF) dynamics results in the Chiari II malformation and hydrocephalus. The abnormally exposed spinal cord results in lifelong lower extremity neurologic deficiency, fecal and urinary incontinence, sexual dysfunction, and skeletal deformities. This defect carries enormous personal, familial, and societal costs, as the near normal lifespan of the affected child is characterized by hospitalization, multiple operations, disability, and institutionalization. Although it has been assumed that the spinal cord itself is intrinsically malformed in children with this defect, recent work suggests that the neurologic impairment after birth may be due to exposure and trauma to the spinal cord *in utero*, and that covering the exposed cord may prevent the development of the Chiari malformation.[8]

Since 1997, more than 200 fetuses have had *in utero* closure of MMC by open fetal surgery. Preliminary clinical evidence suggests that this procedure reduces the incidence of shunt-dependent hydrocephalus and restores the cerebellum and brainstem to a more normal configuration. However, clinical results of fetal surgery for MMC are based on comparisons with historical control subjects, examine only efficacy and not safety, and lack long-term follow-up.

Cystic adenomatoid malformation (CCAM)

CCAM leading to hydrops is another indication for hysterotomy. Although CCAM often presents as a benign pulmonary mass in infants and children, some fetuses with large lesions die *in utero* or at birth from hydrops and pulmonary hypoplasia.[9] The pathophysiology of hydrops and the feasibility of resecting the fetal lung have been studied in animals.[9,10] Experience in managing more than 200 cases suggests that most lesions can be successfully treated after birth, and that some lesions resolve before birth.[11] Although only a few fetuses with very large lesions develop hydrops before 26 weeks of gestation, these lesions may progress rapidly, and the fetuses may die *in utero*. Careful sonographic surveillance of large lesions is necessary to detect the first signs of hydrops, because fetuses who develop hydrops can be treated successfully by emergency resection of the abnormal lobe *in utero*. Fetal pulmonary lobectomy has proved to be surprisingly simple and quite successful at two large fetal surgery centers. For lesions with single, large cysts, thoracoamniotic shunting has also been successful.[12] Percutaneous ablation techniques are being investigated. We have seen regression of very large lesions with hydrops after maternal steroid treatment.

Sacrococcygeal teratoma (SCT)

Hysterotomy is the most common fetal surgical approach to treat fetuses in a critical condition with large SCTs. Most neonates with SCT survive, and malignant invasion is unusual. However, the prognosis of patients with SCT diagnosed prenatally (by sonogram or elevated alpha-fetoprotein levels) is less favorable. There is a subset of fetuses (fewer than 20%) with large tumors who develop hydrops from high-output failure secondary to extremely high blood flow through the tumor. Because hydrops progresses very rapidly to fetal death, frequent sonographic follow-up is mandatory. Attempts to interrupt the vascular steal by sonographically guided or fetoscopic techniques have not yet been successful. Excision of the tumor reverses the pathophysiology if it is performed before the mirror syndrome (maternal preeclampsia) develops in the mother. Attempts to interrupt the vascular steal by ablating blood flow to the tumor by alcohol injection or embolization have not generally been successful. Hysterotomies in these cases may involve quite large incisions due to the large size of the masses.

Fetoscopic surgery (FETENDO)

With advances in technology and familiarity with endoscopic techniques, application of this technique to fetal surgery was natural. Common sense would suggest that the smaller the incision in the uterus, the lower the risk of subsequent pregnancy complications. At UCSF, endoscopic approaches were first applied to pregnancies complicated by diaphragmatic hernia, urinary tract obstruction, and twin-to-twin transfusion (Lap-FETENDO).

The initial pioneering approach involved maternal minilaparotomies, with direct exposure of the uterus. Ultrasound is used to determine the point of entry and the laparotomy site, depending on placental location and fetal lie. Once the uterus has been exposed, stay sutures are placed, and a 3- to 5-mm step trocar is advanced into the amniotic cavity under direct ultrasound visualization. Initially, several trocars were required for *in utero* dissections, placement of staples, etc. Later, many procedures could be performed through a single trocar using an endoscope with an operating channel. Initial caution regarding this approach led to similar perioperative management as in hysterotomy cases. This included general anesthesia, use of multiple tocolytics, and prolonged hospitalization. One important difference, even initially, was that patients could labor following FETENDO procedures. Since that time, endoscopic procedures have become less invasive with very small instruments passed through 3-mm ports.

Percutaneous FETENDO

Currently, we rarely use the more invasive Lap-FETENDO and have since progressed toward a completely percutaneous approach using a smaller 2 mm endoscope with an operating channel (Micro-FETENDO). We have used this technique for balloon tracheal occlusions, fetal cystoscopies, and for laser ablation in monochorionic twin gestations complicated by severe twin-to-twin transfusion. We anticipate that, based on our early experience and that of others[12] with percutaneous microendoscopy, the risk profile will be similar to that of percutaneous sonoguided procedures (see Fetal intervention guided by sonography). The perioperative management is very different. Patients are treated with prophylactic indomethacin and antibiotics. As uterine relaxation from inhalational agents is not required, we generally use spinal anesthesia. Ultrasound is again critical for safe uterine access to determine the best entry point. This is based on fetal position, placental location, membrane position in multiple gestations, and uterine vascularity. Postoperative tocolytic therapy is usually based on contraction activity. A 24–48 h, a course of indomethacin or nifedipine is often all that is required. In cases in which there are significant postoperative changes in uterine size, such as with interventions for twin–twin transfusion syndrome (TTTS), prophylactic intravenous magnesium sulfate may be helpful.

Indications for fetoscopic surgery (FETENDO)

(Table 33.2)

Congenital diaphragmatic hernia (CDH)

The fundamental problem in babies born with a CDH is pulmonary hypoplasia. Research in experimental animal models and later in human patients over two decades has aimed to improve growth of the hypoplastic lungs before they are needed for gas exchange at birth. Anatomic repair of the hernia by open hysterotomy proved feasible, but did not decrease mortality and was abandoned. Fetal tracheal occlusion was developed as an alternative strategy to promote fetal lung growth by preventing normal egress of lung fluid. Occlusion of the fetal trachea was shown to stimulate fetal lung growth in a variety of animal models. Techniques to achieve reversible fetal tracheal occlusion were explored in animal models and then applied clinically, evolving from external metal clips placed on the trachea by open hysterotomy or fetoscopic neck dissection, to internal tracheal occlusion with a detachable silicone balloon placed by fetal bronchoscopy through a single 5-mm uterine port, as described above.

Our initial experience suggested that fetal endoscopic tracheal occlusion improved survival in human fetuses with severe CDH[13,14]. To evaluate this novel therapy, we conducted a randomized, controlled trial comparing tracheal occlusion with standard care. Survival with fetal endoscopic tracheal occlusion (73%) met expectations (predicted 75%) and appeared to be better than that of historic control subjects (37%), but proved no better than that of concurrent randomized control subjects. The higher than expected survival in the standard care group may be because the study design mandated that patients in both treatment groups be delivered, resuscitated, and intensively managed in a unit experienced in caring for critically ill newborns with pulmonary hypoplasia. Attempts to improve outcome for severe CDH by treatments either before or after birth have proved to be double-edged swords. Intensive care after birth has improved survival, but has increased long-term sequelae in survivors, and is expensive.

Our ability to accurately diagnose and assess the severity of CDH before birth has improved dramatically. Fetuses with CDH who have associated anomalies do poorly, whereas fetuses with isolated CDH, no liver herniation, and a lung:head ratio (LHR) above 1.4 have an excellent prognosis (100% in our experience). In this study, fetuses with a LHR between 0.9 and 1.4 had a chance of survival of > 80% when delivered at a tertiary care center. The small number of fetuses with a LHR below 0.9 had a poor prognosis in both treatment groups, and should be the focus of further studies.[15]

Twin–twin transfusion syndrome (TTTS)

TTTS was one of the first entities to be treated endoscopically at UCSF. It is a complication of monochorionic multiple gestations resulting from an imbalance in blood flow through vascular communications. It is the most common serious complication of monochorionic twin gestations, affecting between 4% and 35% of monochorionic twin pregnancies, or approximately 0.1–0.9/1000 births each year in the USA. Yet, despite the relatively low incidence, TTTS disproportionately accounts for 17% of all perinatal mortality associated with twin gestations.[16] Standard therapy has been limited to serial amnioreduction, which appears to improve the overall outcome, but has little impact on the more severe end of the spectrum in TTTS. In addition, survivors of TTTS treated by serial amnioreduction have an 18–26% incidence of significant neurologic and cardiac morbidity. Selective fetoscopic laser photocoagulation of chorioangiopagus has emerged as an alternative treatment strategy with at least comparable, if not superior, survival to serial amnioreduction, as demonstrated in a randomized trial in Europe.[17]

Urinary tract obstruction

As a group at UCSF, we are particularly enthusiastic about the potential of fetal intervention in bladder outlet obstruction by percutaneous fetal cystoscopy. Fetal urethral obstruction produces pulmonary hypoplasia and renal dysplasia, and these often fatal consequences can be ameliorated by urinary tract decompression before birth. The natural history of untreated fetal urinary tract obstruction is well documented, and selection criteria based on fetal urine electrolyte and β_2-microglobulin levels and the sonographic appearance of fetal kidneys have proved reliable.[17–21] Of all fetuses with urinary tract dilation, as many as 90% do not require intervention. However, fetuses with bilateral hydronephrosis and bladder distention due to urethral obstruction who subsequently develop oligohydramnios require treatment. Depending on the gestational age, the fetus can be delivered early for postnatal decompression. Alternatively, the bladder can be decompressed *in utero* by a catheter Harrison vesicoamniotic shunt placed percutaneously under sonographic guidance,[22] by fetoscopic vesicostomy[23,24] or, more recently, by fetocystoscopic ablation of urethral valves.[25] Treatment with shunting has been relatively disappointing, as shunts often migrate or do not remain patent. Even when adequately decompressed, the obstructed bladder may not cycle correctly, resulting in a severe bladder dysfunction requiring surgery after birth. We have now developed a percutaneous fetal cystoscopic technique to disrupt posterior urethral valves through a single 3-mm port.

Fetal intervention guided by sonography (FIGS)

The first fetal procedure, developed in the early 1980s, was percutaneous sonographically guided placement of the Harrison fetal bladder catheter shunt. Many other catheter shunt procedures have been developed and described.[26] More recently, we have developed percutaneous sonographically guided radiofrequency ablation (RFA) procedures for management of anomalous multiple gestations. All these procedures we now group as "fetal intervention guided by sonography" or "FIGS". Very complicated procedures may still require laparotomy (Lap-FIGS).

Percutaneous or Micro-FIGS is used to sample or drain fetal blood, urine, and fluid collection, to sample fetal tissue, to place catheter shunts in the fetal bladder, chest, abdomen, or ventricles, and to do RFA. The most common indication at UCSF is RFA for acardiac twins/TRAP sequence or monochorionic twins for selective reduction. Other operators have used bipolar coagulation or umbilical cord ligation for similar indications. Compared with the 17-gauge RFA needles that we use, these techniques are more invasive, using at least 3-mm trocars. Additionally, the length of the cord or its position may preclude use of these instruments. The perioperative management of these patients is similar to that of the current Micro-FETENDO patients. The procedures are performed under spinal anesthesia, with prophylactic antibiotics and indomethacin. Postoperative tocolysis is rarely necessary, and patients are frequently discharged within hours of the procedure. Ultrasound is critical for both the planning and the execution of the procedure (Fig. 33.2).

There are a few complicated FIGS procedures that may

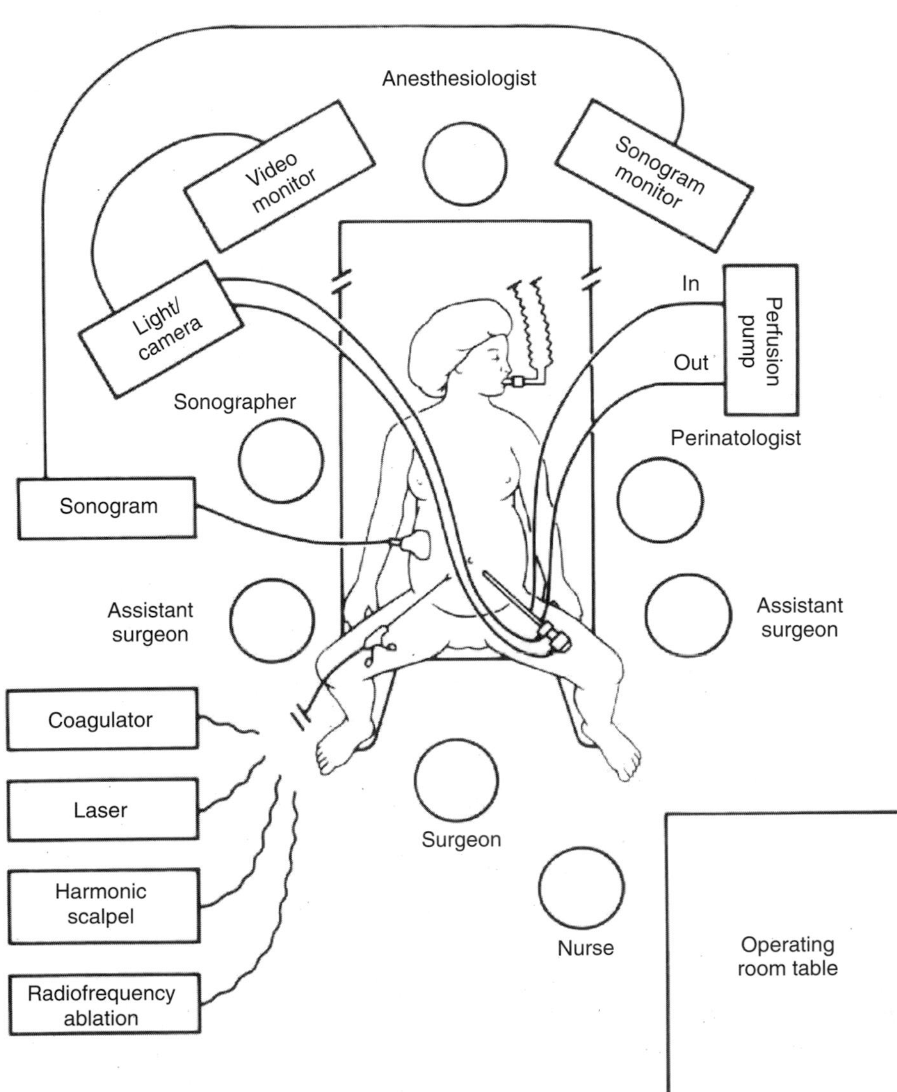

Figure 33.2 Drawing of the operating room setup. Note that there are two monitors at the head of the table: one for the fetoscopic picture and the other for the real-time ultrasound image.

require maternal laparotomy to allow fetal positioning and sonography directly on the uterus (Lap-FIGS). A few simple structural cardiac defects that interfere with development may benefit from prenatal correction. For example, if obstruction of blood flow across the pulmonary or aortic valve interferes with development of the ventricles or pulmonary or systemic vasculature, relief of the anatomic obstruction may allow normal development with an improved outcome. Similarly, congenital aortic stenosis may lead to hypoplastic left heart syndrome. Stenotic aortic valves have been dilated by a balloon catheter placed using both FIGS and Lap-FIGS with some promising results.[26] The procedure is technically difficult. Several centers are developing experimental techniques to correct fetal heart defects.[27]

In summary, fetal surgery has evolved considerably since its birth at UCSF two decades ago. The indications remain quite limited, but have the potential to expand numerically as patients and providers become increasingly informed. Recent advances in the development of less invasive fetal endoscopic (FETENDO) and sonography-guided techniques (FIGS) have extended the indications for fetal intervention.

Key points

1. The field of open fetal surgery was created at UCSF in the early 1980s.
2. Only a tiny fraction of fetal malformations are considered candidates for fetal surgery.
3. Generally, candidate malformations are ones that would be progressive and lethal *in utero* and which, if successfully treated, would lead to a near-normal outcome.
4. Fetal surgery is obviously maternal–fetal surgery, as the access to the fetus is through the mother.
5. There are three approaches to access for the procedures: open hysterotomy, FETENDO and FIGS.
6. Open hysterotomy involves maternal laparotomy under general anesthesia, and at least a 5- to 10-cm uterine incision.
7. Postoperative management includes maximal multiple tocolytic management and decreased activity for the remainder of the pregnancy.
8. Following open hysterotomy, delivery in the index as well as all subsequent pregnancies must be by Cesarean section.
9. FETENDO involves the use of small endoscopes, either percutaneously or at minilaparotomy.
10. Postoperative management is less challenging because suppression of contractions is less critical.
11. FIGS-IT involves even smaller diameter instruments, and patients often require prophylactic preoperative tocolytics only.
12. All fetal surgical procedures significantly increase the risk of premature rupture of membranes and premature delivery.
13. Currently, the most common procedure performed at open hysterotomy is fetal meningomyelocele repair.
14. There is some evidence that fetal repair reduces the rate of shunt placement. This is currently being studied in an NIH-funded randomized trial.
15. Hysterotomy is used to access the fetus for resection of chest masses and congenital tumors that have led to hydrops.
16. FETENDO is used for placement of intratracheal balloons to create lung growth in cases of congenital diaphragmatic hernia, treatment of the placental surface vessels leading to twin–twin transfusion syndrome, for releasing amniotic bands, and to perform fetal cystoscopy and anterograde disruption of posterior urethral valves.
17. FIGS-IT is used for ablation of vascular communications in acardiac twins (TRAP sequence), shunt placements, and fetal blood sampling and intrauterine transfusions.
18. All fetal surgical procedures depend on ultrasound and fetal magnetic resonance imaging for identification of the fetal malformation and determining the need for surgical intervention.
19. Fetal surgery of any sort requires a multidisciplinary team of experts, as it is as important to know when not to do a procedure as it is to know when to do it.
20. Maternal safety always has to be of paramount importance.

References

1 Golombeck K, Ball RH, Lee H, et al. Maternal morbidity after maternal–fetal surgery. *Am J Obstet Gynecol* 2006;194:834–839.

2 Bruner JP, Tulipan N, Reed G, et al. Intrauterine repair of spina bifida: preoperative predictors of shunt-dependent hydrocephalus. *Am J Obstet Gynecol* 2004;190:1305–1312.

3 Johnson MP, Sutton LN, Rintoul N, et al. Fetal myelomeningocele repair: short-term clinical outcomes. *Am J Obstet Gynecol* 2003;189:482–487.

4 DiFederico EM, Burlingame JM, Kilpatrick SJ, et al. Pulmonary edema in obstetric patients is rapidly resolved except in the presence of infection or of nitroglycerin tocolysis after open fetal surgery. *Am J Obstet Gynecol* 1998;179:925–933.

5 Wilson RD, Johnson MP, Crombleholme TM, et al. Chorioamni-

otic membrane separation following open fetal surgery: pregnancy outcome. *Fetal Diagn Ther* 2003;18:314–320.

6 Bruner JP, Tulipan NB, Richards WO, et al. In utero repair of myelomeningocele: a comparison of endoscopy and hysterotomy. *Fetal Diagn Ther* 2000;15:83–88.

7 Farrell JA, Albanese CT, Jennings RW, et al. Maternal fertility is not affected by fetal surgery. *Fetal Diagn Ther* 1999;14:190–192.

8 Bouchard S, Davey MG, Rintoul NE, et al. Correction of hindbrain herniation and anatomy of the vermis after in utero repair of myelomeningocele in sheep. *J Pediatr Surg* 2003;38:451–458.

9 Adzick NS, Harrison MR, Glick PL, et al. Fetal cystic adenomatoid malformation: prenatal diagnosis and natural history. *J Pediatr Surg* 1985;20:483–488.

10 Adzick NS, Hu LM, Davies P, et al. Compensatory lung growth after pneumonectomy in the fetus. *Surg Forum* 1986;37:648–649.

11 MacGillivray TE, Harrison MR, Goldstein RB, Adzick NS. Disappearing fetal lung lesions. *J Pediatr Surg* 1993;28:1321–1324.

12 Blott M, Nicolaides KH, Greenough A. Postnatal respiratory function after chronic drainage of fetal pulmonary cyst. *Am J Obstet Gynecol* 1988;159:858–865.

13 Harrison MR, Adzick NS, Flake AW, et al. Correction of congenital diaphragmatic hernia in utero VIII: Response of the hypoplastic lung to tracheal occlusion. *J Pediatr Surg* 1996;31:1339–1348.

14 Skarsgard ED, Meuli M, VanderWall KJ, et al. Fetal endoscopic tracheal occlusion ('Fetendo-PLUG') for congenital diaphragmatic hernia. *J Pediatr Surg* 1996;31:1335–1338.

15 Lipshutz GS, Albanese CT, Feldstein VA, et al. Prospective analysis of lung-to-head ratio predicts survival for patients with prenatally diagnosed congenital diaphragmatic hernia. *J Pediatr Surg* 1997;32:1634–1636.

16 Quintero RA. Twin–twin transfusion syndrome. *Clin Perinatol* 2003;30:591–600.

17 Senat MV, Deprest J, Boulvain M, et al. Endoscopic laser surgery versus serial amnioreduction for severe twin-to-twin transfusion syndrome. *N Engl J Med* 2004;351:136–144.

18 Adzick NS, Harrison MR, Glick PL, Flake AW. Fetal urinary tract obstruction: experimental pathophysiology. *Semin Perinatol* 1985;9:79–90.

19 Crombleholme TM, Harrison MR, Golbus MS, et al. Fetal intervention in obstructive uropathy: prognostic indicators and efficacy of intervention. *Am J Obstet Gynecol* 1990;162:1239–1244.

20 Manning FA, Harrison MR, Rodeck C. Catheter shunts for fetal hydronephrosis and hydrocephalus. Report of the International Fetal Surgery Registry. *N Engl J Med* 1986;315:336–334.

21 Nicolaides KH, Cheng HH, Snijders RJ, Moniz CF. Fetal urine biochemistry in the assessment of obstructive uropathy. *Am J Obstet Gynecol* 1992;166:932–937.

22 Johnson MP, Bukowski TP, Reitleman C, et al. In utero surgical treatment of fetal obstructive uropathy: a new comprehensive approach to identify appropriate candidates for vesicoamniotic shunt therapy. *Am J Obstet Gynecol* 1994;170:1770–1776.

23 Crombleholme TM, Harrison MR, Langer JC, et al. Early experience with open fetal surgery for congenital hydronephrosis. *J Pediatr Surg* 1988;23:1114–1121.

24 MacMahon RA, Renou PM, Shekelton PA, Paterson PJ. In-utero cystostomy. *Lancet* 1992;340:123.

25 Wilson RD, Baxter JK, Johnson MP, et al. Thoracoamniotic shunts: fetal treatment of pleural effusions and congenital cystic adenomatoid malformations. *Fetal Diagn Ther* 2004;19:413–420.

26 Allan LD, Maxwell D, Tynan M. Progressive obstructive lesions of the heart: an opportunity for fetal therapy. *Fetal Therapy* 1991;6:173–176.

27 Hanley FL. Fetal cardiac surgery. *Adv Cardiac Surg* 1994;5:47–74.

34 Fetal medical treatment

Mark I. Evans, Yuval Yaron, Charles S. Kleinman, and Alan W. Flake

Over the past three decades, numerous methods for the diagnosis of structural and physiologic fetal abnormalities have been devoloped.[1,2] When severe or lethal, pregnancy termination is viewed by many as reasonable. In countries that permit its availability and in cultures in which the fetus does not have more rights than the mother, a variable portion of patients chose this option.[3,4] With more moderate fetal anomalies, obstetric care can sometimes be modified to optimize outcomes and prevent secondary complications. In some instances, prenatal therapy of the underlying problem has emerged. In general, structural malformations are more logically approached with surgery, while metabolic disorders may benefit from pharmacologic or genetic therapies.[2]

The role of fetal therapy is still misunderstood, even four decades since the first transfusions by Lilley. If something can be treated safely postnatally, then there is generally no justification for prenatal intervention. However, profound and irreparable damage occurs for many conditions before birth, making fetal intervention the best or sometimes the only way to ameliorate the damage (Table 34.1). Fetal therapy has evolved using three major approaches: surgery, pharmacologic therapy, and stem cell/gene therapy. Other chapters will discuss the surgical approaches.

Pharmocologic therapies

Neural tube defects

Neural tube defects (NTDs) result from abnormal closure of the neural tube, which normally occurs between the third and fourth week of gestation. The etiology is complex and includes genetic and environmental factors. Historical data in humans suggest increased NTD frequencies in populations with poor dietary histories or with intestinal bypasses. Analysis of recurrence patterns within families and of twin–twin concordance data provides evidence of a genetic influence in nonsyndromal cases. However, factors such as socioeconomic status, geographic area, occupational expoşure, and maternal use of antiepileptic drugs are also associated with variations in the incidence of NTDs.[5] Smithells et al.[6] suggested that vitamin supplementation containing 0.36 mg of folate could reduce the frequency of NTD recurrence by sevenfold.[5–7] In 1991, a randomized, double-blinded trial designed by the MRC Vitamin Study Research Group demonstrated that preconceptual folate reduces the risk of recurrence in high-risk patients.[8] Subsequently, it was shown that preparations containing folate and other vitamins also reduce the occurrence of first-time NTDs.[8] In response to these findings, guidelines were issued calling for the consumption of 4.0 mg/day folic acid by women with a previous child affected with a NTD, for at least 1 month prior to conception through the first 3 months of pregnancy. In addition, 0.4 mg/day folic acid is recommended to all women planning a pregnancy, to be taken preconceptually. The data on NTD recurrence prevention are now very well established, and have become routine for high-risk cases. Since January 1998, the United States Food and Drug Administration mandated the supplementation of breads and grains with folic acid. NTD birth prevalence during the years 1990–1999, evaluated by assessing birth certificate reports before and after mandatory fortification, decreased by 19%.[9] Recently, Evans et al.[10] have shown a nearly 30% drop in high maternal serum alpha-fetoprotein (MSAFP) values in the United States when comparing 2000 values with 1997 values, before the introduction of folic acid supplementation.

Folate plays a central part in embryonic and fetal development because of its role in nucleic acid synthesis, which is mandatory for the widespread cell division that takes place during embryogenesis. Folate deficiency can occur because of low dietary folate intake or because of increased metabolic requirements, as seen in particular genetic alternations such as polymorphism of the thermolabile enzyme methyltetrahydrofolate reductase (MTHFR). However, evidence regarding its role in NTDs is unsupported, except in certain populations, suggesting that these variants are not large contributors to the etiology of NTDs.[11,12] Additional candidate genes other than MTHFR may be responsible for an increased risk of NTDs.[13] Methionine synthase (MTR) polymorphism is associated with an increased risk of NTDs that is not influenced by maternal preconception folic acid intake at doses of 0.4 mg/day.[14] Other candidate genes include the mitochondrial membrane transporter gene UCP2.[52] Despite previous studies suggesting that zinc deficiency plays a role in the etiology of NTDs,[16,17] further studies found that this observation was inconclusive.[18,19] Because methionine deficiency may be involved in NTDs, it may be beneficial in NTD risk reduction.[20] In conclusion, preconception folic acid intake, either as a sole vitamin or as part of multivitamin supplementation, reduces the risk of recurrence and first-time NTDs.

The traditional dogma that the pathogenesis of meningomyelocele was secondary to an abnormally developed spinal cord, which did not, in turn, engender the proper development of the bony spinal column, may not be the whole story. It is possible that the primary defect is in the bony spinal column, which exposes a presumptively undamaged spinal cord. The cord is then damaged by the toxic affects of amniotic fluid, trauma from the uterine environment, and repeated contact with the uterine wall. Thus came the rationale for attempts to cover and protect the spinal cord *in utero*, to minimize the sequelae.[21]

Table 34.1 Upper threshold values for selecting fetuses that might benefit from prenatal intervention.

Sodium	< 100 mg/dL
Chloride	< 90 mg/dL
Osmolality	< 190 mOsm/L
Calcium	< 8 mg/dL
β2-microglobulin	< 6 mg/L
Total protein	< 40 mg/dL

Endocrine disorders

Adrenal disorders: congenital adrenal hyperplasia

Congenital adrenal hyperplasia (CAH) is actually a group of autosomal recessive metabolic disorders, characterized by enzymatic defects in the steroidogenetic pathway.[22] A compensatory increase in adrenocorticotrophic hormone (ACTH) secretion leads to overproduction of the steroid precursors in the adrenal cortex, resulting in adrenal hyperplasia. Excess precursors are often converted to androgens, which may result in virilization of female fetuses. The phenotype is determined by the severity of the cortisol deficiency and the nature of the steroid precursors, which accumulate proximal to the enzymatic block. The most common abnormality, responsible for > 90% of patients with CAH, is caused by a deficiency in the 21-hydroxylase (21-OH) enzyme. Other, less common causes of CAH include deficiencies in 11β-hydroxylase and 17α-hydroxylase. Reduced 21-OH activity results in the accumulation of 17-hydroxyprogesterone (17-OHP) because of its decreased conversion to 11-deoxycorticosterone. Excess 17-OHP is then converted via androstenedione to androgens, the levels of which can increase by as much as several hundredfold (Fig. 34.1). Excess androgens produce virilization of the undifferentiated female external genitalia, which may vary from mild clitoral hypertrophy to the complete formation of a phallus and scrotum. In contrast, genital development in male fetuses is normal. The excess androgens cause postnatal virilization in both genders and may manifest in precocious puberty.[22] A severe enzyme deficiency or even a complete block of enzymatic activity produces the "classical" form of CAH. Two-thirds to three-quarters of cases have salt loss that may be life-threatening.

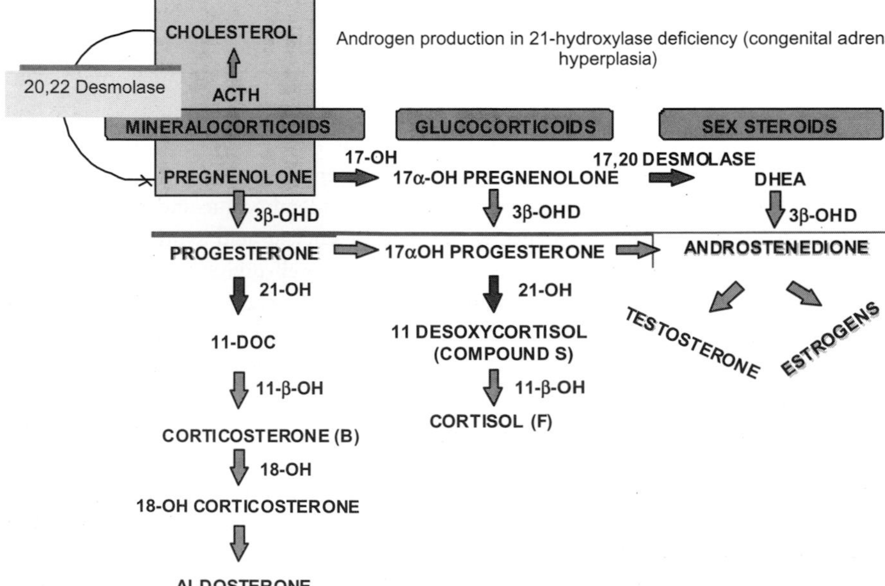

Figure 34.1 Steroidogenic pathway. Pathway of conversion from cholesterol to cortisol is vulnerable to enzymatic errors. Blockage at 21-hydroxylase (21-OH) leads to overproduction of 17-hydroxyprogesterone, which ultimately leads to excess androgens that produce masculinization of the external genitalia.

The classical form is easy to recognize in female newborns but may be overlooked in males, who may appear with severe dehydration and even demise. In the late 1970s and early 1980s, diagnosis of CAH could be made on amniocentesis by the finding of elevated levels of 17-OHP in the supernatant. In the 1980s, with the development of chorionic villus sampling (CVS), linkage-based molecular diagnosis became available in the first trimester, as the gene for 21-OH was found to be linked to the human leukocyte antigen (HLA) complex on chromosome 6.[23] The gene for 21-OH (*CYP21B*) was later mapped, allowing direct mutation analysis in informative families.[24]

We have known for two decades that the fetal adrenal gland can be pharmacologically suppressed by maternal replacement doses of dexamethasone.[25] Suppression can prevent masculinization of affected female fetuses in couples who are carriers of classical CAH. Evans et al.[25] were the first to administer dexamethasone to a carrier mother beginning at 10 weeks of gestation in an attempt to prevent masculinization. Differentiation of the external genitalia begins at about 7 weeks of gestation. Thus, for a carrier couple, pharmacologic therapy has to be initiated prior to diagnosis. Direct DNA diagnosis or linkage studies are then performed by CVS in the first trimester, and therapy is continued only if the fetus is found to be an affected female. Detailed inclusion criteria for treatment have been issued by the European Society for Pediatric Endocrinology and Wilkins Pediatric Endocrine Society.[26] Hundreds of fetuses have been successfully treated resulting in prevention or amelioration of masculinization.[26–28]

Hyperthyroidism

Neonatal hyperthyroidism is rare with an incidence of 1:4000 to 1:40 000 live births.[29] Fetal thyrotoxic goiter is usually secondary to maternal autoimmune disease, most commonly Graves' disease or Hashimoto's thyroiditis. As many as 12% of infants of mothers with a known history of Graves' disease are affected with neonatal thyrotoxicosis, which can occur even if the mother is euthyroid.[30] The underlying mechanism is the transplacental passage of maternal IgG antibodies. The antibodies, known as TSAb (or TSI), are predominantly directed against the thyroid-stimulating hormone (TSH) receptor. Often, fetal goiter is diagnosed on ultrasound in patients with elevated thyroid-stimulating antibodies. In some cases, fetal goiters are incidentally detected on routine ultrasonography. Others may be discovered in patients referred for a scan because of polyhydramnios. Untreated fetal hyperthyroidism may be associated with a mortality rate of 12–25% due to high-output cardiac failure.[30]

Once the diagnosis of fetal hyperthyroidism is confirmed, fetal treatment should be initiated. Authors have attempted to treat fetal hyperthyroidism with maternally administered antithyroid drugs. Porreco and Bloch[31] have reported maternal treatment of fetal thyrotoxicosis with PTU, which had a good outcome. The initial dose used was 100 mg p.o. three times a day, which was later decreased to 50 mg p.o. three times a day. A favorable outcome was shown using maternal methimazole to treat fetal hyperthyroidism in a patient who could not tolerate PTU.[32] Hatjis[32] also treated fetal goiterous hyperthyroidism with a maternal dose of 300 mg of PTU. This patient however, required supplemental synthroid to remain euthyroid. There was good fetal outcome in this case as well.

Hypothyroidism

Congenital hypothyroidism is relatively rare, affecting about 1:3000 to 1:4000 infants.[33] About 85% of cases are the result of thyroid dysgenesis, a heterogeneous group of developmental defects characterized by inadequate amounts of thyroid tissue. Congenital hypothyroidism is only rarely associated with errors of thyroid hormone synthesis, TSH insensitivity, or absence of the pituitary gland. Fetal hypothyroidism may not necessarily manifest in a goiter before birth, as maternal thyroid hormones may cross the placenta. Congenital hypothyroidism presenting with a goiter is found in only about 10–15% of cases.[34]

Fetal goiterous hypothyroidism usually follows maternal exposure to thyrostatic agents such as propylthiouracil (PTU), radioactive ^{131}I or iodide exposure used to treat maternal hyperthyroidism.[35] Maternal ingestion of amiodarone or lithium may also cause hypothyroidism in the fetus. Finally, fetal hypothyroidism may follow transplacental passage of maternal blocking antibodies (known as TBIAb or TBII). Rarely, it may be due to rare defects in fetal thyroid hormone biosynthesis.[29]

An enlarged fetal goiter may cause esophageal obstruction and polyhydramnios, leading to preterm delivery or premature rupture of membranes. Rarely, a goiter may even lead to high-output heart failure.[35] A large fetal goiter can also cause extension of the fetal neck, leading to dystocia. The effects of the fetal hypothyroidism itself may be devastating. Without treatment, postnatal growth delay and severe mental retardation may ensue. Even with immediate diagnosis and treatment at birth, long-term follow-up of children with congenital hypothyroidism has demonstrated that they have lower scores on perceptual–motor, visuospatial, and language tests.[36]

Inborn errors of metabolism

Methylmalonic acidemia

The methylmalonic acidemias (MMA) are a group of autosomal recessive enzyme deficiency diseases. Some cases are caused by mutations in the gene encoding methylmalonyl-coenzyme A mutase. Others are secondary to a defect that reduces the biosynthesis of adenosylcobalamin from vitamin B12. The disease has a wide clinical spectrum ranging from benign to fatal, characterized by severe metabolic acidosis, developmental delay, and biochemical abnormalities that include methylmalonic aciduria, long-chain ketonuria, and intermittent hyperglycinemia. Neurologic abnormalities may result from diminution of myelin content and of ganglioside N-acetylneuraminic acid in the cerebrum.[37] Patients with defects in adenosylcobalamin biosynthesis may respond to administration of large doses of vitamin B12, which may enhance the amount of active holoenzyme (mutase apoenzyme plus adenosylcobalamin).

Ampola et al.[38] first attempted prenatal diagnosis and treatment of a vitamin B12-responsive variant of MMA. Their patient had previously had a child who died of severe MMA. It is not clear whether *in utero* treatment actually resulted in an improved outcome, but it is likely that correction of the biochemical abnormality in the fetus had some beneficial effect on fetal development. Indeed, in a cohort of eight children with MMA, Andersson et al.[39] described congenital malformations, probably caused by prenatally abnormal cyanocobalamin metabolism. Growth was significantly improved in most cases after initiation of therapy postnatally and, in one case, microcephaly resolved. However, developmental delay of variable severity was always present regardless of treatment onset. These data suggest that prenatal therapy of MMA may be effective and may perhaps ameliorate some of the prenatal effects. Evans et al.[40] have documented the changing dose requirements necessary over the course of pregnancy to maintain adequate levels of vitamin B12. They sequentially followed maternal plasma and urine levels in a prenatally treated pregnancy.

Multiple carboxylase deficiency

Biotin-responsive multiple carboxylase deficiency is an inborn error of metabolism caused by diminished activity of the mitochondrial biotin-dependent enzymes (pyruvate carboxylase, propionyl-coenzyme A carboxylase, and α-methylcrotonyl-coenzyme A carboxylase). The condition may arise from mutations in the holocarboxylase synthetase gene or the biotinidase gene.[41–45] Affected patients present with dermatitis, severe metabolic acidosis, and a characteristic pattern of organic acid excretion. Metabolism can be restored toward normal levels by biotin supplementation. Prenatal diagnosis is based on the demonstration of elevated levels of typical organic acids (3-hydroxyisovalerate, methylcitrate) in the amniotic fluid or in the chorionic villi. However, the existence of a mild form of holocarboxylase synthetase gene deficiency can complicate prenatal diagnosis as organic acid levels in amniotic fluid might be normal.[46] Therefore, prenatal diagnosis must be performed by enzyme assay of cultured fetal cells in biotin-restricted medium.

Roth et al.[47] treated a fetus whose two previous siblings died of multiple carboxylase deficiency. The mother was first seen at 34 weeks' gestation, and prenatal diagnosis was not performed. Oral administration of biotin was begun at a dose of 10 mg/day. There were no apparent untoward effects. Maternal urinary biotin excretion increased by 100-fold and nonidentical twins were delivered at term. Cord blood and urinary organic acid profiles were normal, and cord blood biotin concentrations were four to seven times greater than normal. The neonatal course for both twins was unremarkable. Other cases of such treatment have been reported.[46,48,49]

Smith–Lemli–Opitz syndrome

Smith–Lemli–Opitz syndrome (SLOS) is an autosomal recessive disorder characterized by multiple anomalies, dysmorphic features, growth and mental retardation. Males with SLOS have ambiguous genitalia.[50] The severe form is associated with a high rate of neonatal mortality.[51] The incidence of SLOS is estimated to be 1:20 000 to 1: 40 000 live births with an estimated carrier frequency of 1:70.[52,53] SLOS is caused by an inborn error of cholesterol biosynthesis due to a deficiency in the enzyme dehydrocholesterol-Δ^7 reductase, leading to reduced cholesterol levels and elevated 7- and 8-dehydrocholesterol levels (7-DHC and 8-DHC respectively) in all body fluids and tissues including amniotic fluid and chorionic villi.[52,54,55] The diagnosis is based on elevated levels of 7-DHC (100 to 1000 times the normal value). Clinical manifestations correlate with cholesterol levels. Prenatal diagnosis of SLOS has been available since 1994 by either amniocentesis or CVS.[56–58]

Since the identification of the cholesterol metabolic defect in SLOS, a treatment protocol to provide exogenous cholesterol has been attempted. This form of therapy has now been provided to many patients with SLOS for several years in many centers in the United States and internationally,[56–58] with the goal of raising cholesterol levels and decreasing the levels of the precursors, 7-DHC and 8-DHC. Treatment has been attempted antenatally in several affected fetuses. In cases in which treatment was started late in pregnancy, the results were inconclusive. Although few descriptions of fetal therapy for SLOS exist, the latest report of antenatal treatment comes from that same group of investigators.[62]

Galactosemia

Galactosemia is an autosomal recessive disorder caused by decreased activity of galactose-1-phosphate uridyltransferase (GALT). Clinical manifestations include cataracts, growth deficiency, and ovarian failure. Clinical symptoms appear in the neonatal period and can be largely ameliorated by elimination of galactose from the diet. Cellular damage in galactosemia is thought to be mediated by the accumulation of galactose-l-phosphate intracellularly and of galactitol in the lens. Several disease-causing mutations in the *GALT* gene have been reported in classical galactosemia.[63] Galactosemia can also be diagnosed prenatally by biochemical studies of cultured amniocytes and chorionic villi.

Even the early postnatal treatment of galactosemic individuals with a low galactose diet may not be sufficient to ensure normal development. Some have speculated that prenatal damage to galactosemic fetuses could contribute to subsequent abnormal neurologic development and to lens cataract formation. Furthermore, it has been recognized that female galactosemics, even when treated from birth with galactose deprivation, have a high frequency of primary or secondary amenorrhea because of ovarian failure. Oocytes are probably irreversibly damaged long before birth.[64,65] There may also be some subtle abnormalities of male gonadal function as well. Thus, galactose restriction during pregnancy may be beneficial in affected fetuses. In humans, ovarian meiosis begins at 12 weeks, and ovarian damage may occur prior to prenatal diagnosis. Thus, anticipatory treatment in pregnancies at risk of having a galactosemic fetus might be best initiated very early in gestation or even preconceptually. We are unaware of studies that adequately assess the impact of prenatal administration of a low-galactose diet to galactosemic infants. Nevertheless, prenatal galactose restriction is probably desirable in galactosemia and should be harmless.

In utero cardiac therapy

The ability to diagnose structural or functional heart disease prenatally has, predictably, led to a growth of interest in the potential for prenatal therapy. It is, of course, necessary to identify fetal conditions that, if left untreated, will result in fetal death, or compromised conditions that will render the neonate in a condition that will result in a lower likelihood of cure or functional survival than would be the case if the fetus were to undergo the proposed therapy. It is essential, of course, to consider the potential risks to both the mother and the fetus, whose states of well-being are inextricably interwoven.

Fetal antiarrhythmic therapy has evolved in a more invasive direction over the past decades, including injection of medication directly into the amniotic fluid, intramuscular administration of medication directly to the fetus, and direct, repetitive administration of intravenous medication through the fetal umbilical vein.[66–70]

Direct instrumentation of the fetal heart was initially attempted in an effort to institute "transcatheter" pacing of a moribund fetus with congenital complete heart block and hydrops fetalis.[71] Subsequently, there have been several reports of attempted catheter treatment of congenital cardiac malformations, with varied success. Several centers have investigated techniques for the institution of surface cooling and rewarming, and for the provision of cardiopulmonary bypass in fetal animal models.[72,73]

Fetal antiarrhythmic therapy

The fetus with tachycardia

The administration of antiarrhythmic therapy to the mothers of fetuses with sustained supraventricular tachycardia represented the first examples of successful prenatal cardiac therapy that were reported in the medical literature.

The most commonly encountered sustained fetal tachycardia, supraventricular tachycardia, is most frequently (90–95%) a result of electrical "re-entry" at the atrioventricular junction, usually by way of an accessory connection between the atrial and ventricular myocardium, and less frequently via the atrioventricular node itself.[66,67,74,75] Supraventricular tachycardia resulting from electrical macro re-entry circuits typically presents with a monotonous fetal heart rate of 240–260 beats per minute (b.p.m.), and is usually exquisitely sensitive to treatment with antiarrhythmic agents that alter conduction velocity and/or refractoriness of the atrioventricular node or accessory pathways. Such agents include digoxin, propranolol, flecainide, and sotalol, among others. Multiple publications have described treatment protocols for this arrhythmia. Our group has approached these patients in a conservative fashion, reserving treatment for fetuses that appear to have no reasonable alternative. The characteristics that identify such patients are the development of hydrops fetalis in the face of sustained arrhythmia, at a gestational age that is early enough to preclude safe delivery and postnatal treatment. In such cases, we begin therapy with medications that have a relatively broad therapeutic margin, with a low risk of proarrhythmia (unwanted precipitation or exacerbation of arrhythmia) in the fetus or pregnant woman.[76,77]

The fetus with bradycardia

The most important sustained bradyarrhythmia is congenital complete heart block. Such fetuses may develop hydrops fetalis, which may occur in the subgroup of fetuses with associated congenital heart disease. The association of clinical heart failure with congenital heart block, with or without congenital heart disease, represents an absolute indication for electrical pacemaker therapy in the neonate.[78]

Hydrops fetalis in the presence of complete heart block *in utero* is a dire finding. The association of hydrops fetalis, complete heart block, and complex congenital heart disease is almost invariably fatal, with or without fetal therapy.[79]

The initial report of the application of electrical pacemaker therapy for fetal congenital heart block involved a fetus presenting with congenital heart block in the absence of congenital heart disease.[80] This fetus, with heart block presumably arising on the basis of immune complex-mediated damage to fetal conduction tissue and myocardium, presented with severe bradycardia and hydrops fetalis. In desperation, the treating physicians placed a pacing catheter within the fetal heart via percutaneous puncture of the maternal abdomen, uterus, and fetal thorax and ventricular wall. Fetal ventricular capture was demonstrated, without clinical improvement in the fetus. Subsequent attempts to utilize similar techniques had similarly discouraging outcomes.

Copel et al.[81] reported a preliminary experience with the administration of absorbable corticosteroid to pregnant women whose fetuses have developed high-grade, second-degree or recent-onset, third-degree heart block in the presence of high maternal titers of anti-SS-A and/or anti-SS-B antibodies. In this small subgroup of patients, there was demonstrable improvement in atrioventricular conduction that was attributed to amelioration of the immune-mediated inflammatory response of the fetal atrioventricular conduction tissue. This report has spawned a multicenter study designed to evaluate the impact of maternally administered corticosteroid on echocardiographically estimated fetal atrioventricular conduction intervals in a population of fetuses whose mothers have high anti-SS-A or anti-SS-B antibodies.[82]

Medical treatment of congestive heart failure in the fetus

The medical literature is replete with anecdotal reports of the administration of digoxin to pregnant women whose fetuses have evidence of impaired cardiac pump function. These have included cases in which structural heart disease (e.g., aortic stenosis) is associated with ventricular dysfunction and hydrops fetalis, and in whom the initiation of digoxin therapy is temporally associated with improved ventricular shortening and resolution of hydrops fetalis, with subsequent postnatal salvage of the child.[83,84] We have had similar personal experiences with two fetuses with similar presentation of hydrops fetalis and aortic stenosis. In addition, we have witnessed a close temporal association between the initiation of maternally administered digoxin and improved ventricular shortening and resolution of hydrops fetalis in several fetal patients who were presumed to have viral myocarditis, with viruses such as adenovirus, parvovirus, and coxsackievirus. In these cases, fetomaternal infection with the virus has been confirmed by analysis of maternal and fetal blood and amniotic fluid using the polymerase chain reaction (PCR). In two fetuses who showed an initial improvement, with eventual neonatal demise, the adenoviral genome was detected by PCR analysis of the infant's myocardial tissue. We have also recently demonstrated improved myocardial shortening and improved right ventricular dP/dT (calculated from the tricuspid regurgitant flow waveform) in two fetuses with progressively dilating right ventricles,[85] progressive tricuspid regurgitation and abnormal inferior vena caval flow waveforms, in the face of large hemangiomas with significant arteriovenous shunting. The findings of cardiomegaly, tricuspid regurgitation, and abnormal venous Doppler in the vena cavae were quite similar to those described by Tulzer and colleagues[86] in justification of the invasive pulmonary balloon valvuloplasties of two fetuses with pulmonary stenosis/atresia. We have also recently employed digoxin to empirically treat a fetus with severe dilated cardiomyopathy and marked cardiomegaly, bilateral atrioventricular valve regurgitation, and abnormal venous pulsatility, and demonstrated a remarkable improvement in biventricular shortening, partial amelioration of atrioventricular valve regurgitation, and improved biventricular dP/dT. This fetus survived pregnancy and delivery, and ultimately underwent successful cardiac transplantation, only to be diagnosed with an electron transport defect that was not identifiable in the studies performed on skeletal muscle biopsy prior to transplant. The same enthusiasm that we have criticized in others has led us to prescribe empirical treatment, without having done our "homework" with regard to ascertaining the mechanism of action of digoxin in the fetus. On the other hand, this medication has been in use for over 200 years, and is still being administered largely on an "empiric" basis. While the popularity of this agent for the treatment of congestive heart failure waxes and wanes every few years, recent studies have suggested some rationale for its inclusion in the therapeutic arsenal. It is, however, unclear whether the salutary effects are related to Na^+/K^+ ATPase inhibition and enhanced calcium availability to the myofilaments, or whether alterations in catecholamine concentration/effect alter the neuroendocrine manifestations of congestive heart failure. The underlying rationale for its use remains "it works." While it is possible that some of the fetuses that we and others have observed to improve in the days following digoxin administration spontaneously recovered from the underlying pathology that caused circulatory failure, and digoxin administration was simply serendipitous, in the last case we cited above (with an electron transfer deficiency), at least, the underlying nature of the cardiomyopathy would not logically have undergone spontaneous improvement after having demonstrated severe biventricular dilated myopathy. In any event, the centuries of use of this medication, in gravid and nongravid women, convinced us that, if one monitors the mother and fetus carefully for evidence of contraindications to the administration of digoxin (ventricular pre-excitation, severe maternal hypokalemia), or for indications calling for modulation of digoxin dose [e.g., maternal renal failure or concomitant treatment with medications that alter digoxin clearance (e.g., quinidine, amiodarone)], at the very least, you are unlikely to harm either the mother or the fetus.

Interventional cardiac catheterization of the human fetus

Aortic balloon valvuloplasty

Motivated by a dismal postnatal outcome for fetuses diagnosed to have critical aortic stenosis prenatally, a group from Guy's Hospital in London embarked upon an innovative program for percutaneous cardiac catheterization and aortic balloon valvuloplasty of fetuses with this condition. The initial experience was unsuccessful, although the feasibility of percutaneous entry of the maternal abdomen, uterus, and fetal chest and left ventricle, with subsequent wire entry of the ascending aorta, passage of an angioplasty balloon catheter, and subsequent retrieval of the system,[87] was established. Ultimately, this group performed a total of four such procedures, and reported the first survivor.[88] These initial reports suggested that balloon valvuloplasty was feasible, but that the prognosis for the fetus was dependent upon the ability to relieve aortic stenosis and to prevent or reverse damage to the left ventricular myocardium. Despite the survival of a single patient, this group declared a moratorium on such procedures until a clearer appreciation of hemodynamics and improvement in catheter technology was in place.[89]

Follow-up studies from that same center, only a few years later, documented improved survival in neonates who had not undergone fetal intervention, undermining the rationale for the introduction of fetal intervention as an alternative approach to an otherwise "hopeless" condition.[90]

Almost a decade later, Kohl et al.[91] summarized the world experience with such techniques. This report included 12 fetuses, including the four cases from Guy's Hospital. At the time of this review, the child from the Guy's experience represented the sole survivor. The conclusion was that the high failure rate was related to the selection of severe cases for treatment, technical problems during the procedure, and high postnatal operative mortality among patients who survived pregnancy. The conclusion of this paper was: "Improved patient selection and technical modifications in interventional methods may hold promise to improve outcome in future cases." This, I believe, is problematic. If one reviews this report at arm's length, we are presented with a "world experience" that included eight attempts, at multiple centers, without a single success. In any other situation, the inability to duplicate the single success of the initial investigators would have cast a cloud of doubt over the technique, at least until a fundamental review of the technique and its indications had taken place! In this situation, the honest eagerness of the investigators to provide help for an unfortunate patient population, and their personal conviction that this technique "should" work, may have influenced their level of enthusiasm for a "therapy in search of an indication."

Pulmonary balloon valvuloplasty

A recent report in *The Lancet*, from Tulzer and colleagues,[86] from Linz, documents the performance of pulmonary balloon valvuloplasty in two fetuses with severe right ventricular outlet obstruction ("complete" or "almost complete" pulmonary atresia), right ventricular compromise, and "imminent" hydrops fetalis. Both fetuses survived and have biventricular circulatory systems. It remains to be seen whether such therapy is justified, and whether these fetuses survived "because of," rather than "in spite of" what was done for (to) them.

Prenatal hematopoietic stem cell (HSC) transplantation

The engraftment and clonal proliferation of a relatively small number of normal HSCs can sustain normal hematopoiesis for a lifetime. This observation provides the compelling rationale for bone marrow transplantation (BMT) and is now supported by thousands of long-term survivors of BMT who would otherwise have succumbed to lethal hematologic disease.[92–94] Realization of the full potential of BMT, however, continues to be limited by a critical shortage of immunologically compatible donor cells, the inability to control the recipient or donor immune response, and the requirement for recipient myeloablation to achieve engraftment. The price of HLA mismatch remains high: the greater the mismatch, the higher the incidence of graft failure, graft-versus-host disease (GVHD), and delayed immunologic reconstitution. Current methods of myeloablation have high morbidity and mortality rates. In combination, these problems remain prohibitive for most patients who might benefit from BMT. A theoretically attractive alternative, which can potentially address many of the limitations of BMT, is *in utero* transplantation of HSCs.[95] This approach is potentially applicable to any congenital hematopoietic disease that can be diagnosed prenatally and can be cured or improved by engraftment of normal HSCs.

Rationale for *in utero* transplantation

The rationale for *in utero* transplantation is to take advantage of the window of opportunity created by normal hematopoietic and immunologic ontogeny. There is a period, prior to population of the bone marrow and thymic processing of self-antigen, when the fetus should theoretically be receptive to engraftment of foreign HSCs without rejection and without the need for myeloablation. In the human fetus, the ideal window would appear to be prior to 14 weeks' gestation, before the release of differentiated T lymphocytes into the circulation and while the bone marrow is just beginning to develop sites for hematopoiesis.[95] It may certainly extend beyond that in immunodeficiency states, particularly when T-cell development is abnormal. During this time, presentation of foreign antigen by thymic dendritic cells should theoretically result in clonal deletion of reactive T cells during the negative selection phase of thymic processing. Recent advances in prenatal diagnosis have made possible the diagnosis of a large number of congenital hematologic diseases during the first trimester. Technical advances in fetal intervention make transplantation feasible by 12–14 weeks' gestation. The ontologic window of opportunity falls well within these diagnostic and technical constraints, making the application of this approach a realistic possibility.

Because of the unique fetal environment, prenatal HSC transplantation could theoretically avoid many of the current limitations of postnatal BMT. There would be no requirement for HLA matching, resulting in expansion of the donor pool. Transplanted cells would not be rejected, and space would be available in the bone marrow, eliminating the need for toxic immunosuppressive and myeloablative drugs. The mother's uterus may ultimately prove to be the ultimate sterile isolation chamber, eliminating the high risk and costly 2–4 months of isolation required after postnatal BMT prior to immunologic reconstitution. Finally, prenatal transplantation would pre-empt the clinical manifestations of the disease, avoiding the recurrent infections, multiple transfusions, growth delay, and other complications that cause immeasurable suffering for the patient and often compromise postnatal treatment.

Source of donor cells

Identifying the best source of donor cells may ultimately prove to be the most critical factor for the success of engraftment. The most obvious advantage of the use of fetal HSCs is the minimal number of mature T cells in fetal liver-derived populations prior to 14 weeks' gestation. This alleviates any concern about GVHD and avoids the necessity of T-cell depletion processes, which can negatively impact on potential engraftment.[95,96,] The disadvantages of the use of fetal or embryonic tissue relates to availability and quality control, as well as the perceived ethical issues of some groups regarding the use of fetal tissue. Perhaps a more important limitation to the use of fetal tissues is the limited quantity available, and the inability to obtain more cells for donor-specific, tolerance-based, postnatal strategies. At the present time, these issues remain prohibitive in the United States, limiting the investigation and use of potentially efficacious donor sources.

Diseases amenable to prenatal treatment

Generally speaking, any disease that can be diagnosed early in gestation, that is improved by BMT, and for which postnatal treatment is not entirely satisfactory is a target disease. Some diseases, however, are far more likely to benefit from prenatal transplantation than others. The list can be divided into three general categories: hemoglobinopathies, immunodeficiency disorders, and inborn errors of metabolism. Each of the diseases has unique considerations for treatment and, in fact, each disease may respond differently (Table 34.2). Issues such as availability of engraftment sites within the bone marrow at time of transplantation, and the capacity of a needed enzyme to cross the blood–brain barrier at a particular gestational age must be considered. Of particular relevance to the prenatal approach, in which experimental levels of engraftment have been relatively low, is the observation that, in many of the target diseases, engrafted normal cells would be predicted to have a significant survival advantage over diseased cells. This would have the clinical effect of amplification of the specific lineage with the survival advantage. In addition, even with minimal levels of engraftment, specific tolerance for donor antigen should be induced, allowing additional cells from the same donor to be given to the tolerant recipient after birth.[97,98]

Table 34.2 Potential candidates for *in utero* stem cell fetal therapy.

Hematopoietic disorders
Disorders affecting lymphocytes
SCID (sex linked)
SCID (adenosine deaminase deficiency)
Ommen syndrome
Agammaglobinemia
Bare lymphocyte syndrome
Disorders affecting granulocytes
Chronic granulomatous disease
Infantile agranulocytosis
Neutrophil membrane GP-180
Lazy leukocyte syndrome
Disorders affecting erythrocytes
Sickle-cell disease
α-Thalassemia
β-Thalassemia
Hereditary spherocytosis
Fanconi anemia
Mannosidosis
α-Mannosidosis
β-Thalassemia
Mucolipidoses
Gaucher's disease
Metachromatic leukodystrophy
Krabbe disease
Niemann–Pick disease
β-Glucuronidase deficiency
Fabry disease
Adrenal leukodystrophy
Mucopolysaccharidoses
MPS I (Hurler's disease)
MPS II (Hunter's disease)
MPS IIIB (Sanfilippo B syndrome)
MPS IV (Morquio syndrome)
MPS VI (Maroteaux–Lamy syndrome)

SCID, severe combined immunodeficiency.

Hemoglobinopathies

The sickle cell anemia and thalassemia syndromes make up the largest patient groups potentially treatable by prenatal stem cell transplantation.[99–102] Both groups can be diagnosed within the first trimester. Both have been cured by postnatal BMT, but BMT is not recommended routinely because of its prohibitive morbidity and mortality rates, and the relative success of modern medical management. In both diseases, the success of BMT is indirectly related to the morbidity of the disease, that is, the younger the patient, the fewer transfusions received, and the less organ compromise from iron overload, the better the results. In both disorders, there is a survival advantage for normal erythrocytes, which results in amplification of the level of bone marrow engraftment in the peripheral red cell compartment. Thus, patients with relatively low levels of mixed chimerism after postnatal BMT have demonstrated high levels of normal hemoglobin peripherally with partial or complete amelioration of their disease.[92,93] Experimentally, this has been shown to be the case after *in utero* transplantation as well, with relatively high levels of circulating donor-derived erythrocytes despite low levels of mixed chimerism in the bone marrow.[103] This observation, in combination with the observation that engraftment can be enhanced after birth using nonmyeloablative approaches in the tolerant recipient,[97,98] makes it likely that hemoglobinopathies will be successfully treated by *in utero* transplantation in the future.

Immunodeficiency diseases

These represent an extremely heterogeneous group of diseases, which differ in their likelihood of cure by their capacity to develop hematopoietic chimerism.[104,105] Once again, the most likely to benefit from even low levels of donor cell engraftment are those diseases in which a survival advantage exists for normal cells. The best example of this situation is severe combined immunodeficiency (SCID) syndrome. Several different molecular causes of SCID have been identified, with approximately two-thirds of cases being of X-linked recessive inheritance (X-SCID). The genetic basis of X-SCID has been defined[106] as a mutation of the gene encoding the common -γ chain (-γ c), which is a common component of several members of the cytokine receptor superfamily. Children affected with X-SCID have a block in thymic T-cell development and diminished T-cell response. B cells, although present in normal or even increased numbers, are dysfunctional, either secondary to the lack of helper T-cell function or an intrinsic defect in B-cell maturation. Clinical experience with HLA-matched sibling bone marrow, fetal liver, or thymus transplantation has generally been successful without myeloablative therapy, suggesting that the lymphoid progeny of relatively few engrafted normal HSCs have a selective growth advantage *in vivo* over genetically defective cells.[107] The competitive advantage of normal cell populations in X-SCID is best supported by the discovery of skewed X-inactivation in female carriers.[108] Only T cells containing the normal X chromosome were found to be present in the circulation of carriers. Other characterized mutations in cytokine receptor signaling pathways (i.e., Jak 3 or ZAP-70), or adenosine deaminase deficiency, resulting in SCID, should also be favorable candidate diseases for *in utero* HSC transplantation. Based on the available clinical and experimental evidence, it is likely that any member of this group of disorders can be treated effectively by *in utero* HSC transplantation, using established protocols, with results comparable to the reported results for X-SCID. Ideally, clinical trials of *in utero* treatment for SCID would be established, and the results compared with early postnatal transplantation protocols, to determine whether there is a biologic advantage favoring *in utero* therapy. Unfortunately, such trials may not be possible because of the rarity of these diseases and the perception that postnatal therapy is adequate.[108] Unfortunately, other diseases such as chronic granulomatous disease would not be expected to provide a competitive advantage for donor cells. Nevertheless, in all these conditions, even a partial engraftment and expression of normal cell phenotype might at least partially ameliorate the clinical manifestations of the disease, and should result in donor-specific tolerance for later transplantation. If higher levels of engraftment are needed, further HSC transplants from the same donor could be performed after birth without fear of rejection.

Flake et al.[109] reported the successful treatment of a fetus with X-linked SCID in a family in which a previously afflicted child died at 7 months of age. Diagnosis by CVS at 12 weeks in the second pregnancy showed another affected male. For this couple, abortion was not an option. After lengthy informed consent, paternal bone marrow was harvested, T cells depleted, and enriched stem-cell populations injected intraperitoneally into the fetus beginning at about 16 weeks of gestation. Subsequent injections were performed at 17 and 18 weeks. The child presently shows a split chimerism with all of his T cells being derived from his father's and the majority of B cells being his own. He has achieved normal developmental milestones, and has had no serious infections through 10 years of age.[110] Additional cases have now been reported by Porta et al.[111] and Westgren et al.[112] with similarly favorable results.

Inborn errors of metabolism

An even more heterogeneous group of diseases, inborn errors of metabolism, can be caused by a deficiency in a specific lysosomal hydrolase, which results in the accumulation of substrates such as mucopolysaccharide, glycogen, or sphingolipid.[113] Depending on the specific enzyme abnormality and the compounds that accumulate, certain patterns of tissue damage and organ failure occur. These include central nervous system (CNS) deterioration, growth failure, dysostosis multiplex and joint abnormalities, hepatosplenomegaly, myocardial or cardiac disease, upper airway obstruction, pulmonary infiltration, corneal clouding, and hearing loss. The potential efficacy of prenatal HSC transplantation for the treatment of these diseases must be considered on an individual disease basis. The purpose of BMT in these diseases is to provide HSC-derived mononuclear cells that can repopulate various organs in the body, including the liver (Kupffer cells), skin (Langerhans cells), lung (alveolar macrophages), spleen (macrophages), lymph nodes, tonsils, and the brain (microglia).[114] Patients whose conditions have been corrected by postnatal BMT, such as Gaucher's disease or Maroteaux–Lamy syndrome (minimal CNS involvement), are certainly reasonable candidates for prenatal treatment. In many cases, postnatal BMT has corrected the peripheral manifestations of the disease and has arrested the neurologic deterioration. However, postnatal BMT has not reversed neurologic injury that is present in such disorders as metachromatic leukodystrophy and Hurler's disease.[115,116] In these cases, the neurologic injury may begin well before birth. Postnatal maturation of the blood–brain barrier restricts access to the CNS of transplanted cells or the deficient enzyme. Thus, a compelling rationale exists for prenatal therapy of these diseases. The primary unanswered question is whether donor HSC-derived microglial elements would populate the CNS, providing the necessary metabolic correction inside the blood–brain barrier. Based on experimental results with *in utero* HSC transplantation alone for these disorders, it is likely that a combination of *in utero* HSC transplantation and CNS-directed cellular or gene therapy will be needed to correct CNS manifestations of these diseases.[117]

To summarize, the only definitively successful transplants to date have been for SCID syndrome. All others have either failed to take or were afflicted with GVHD. Despite only limited evidence of clinical efficacy, interest in the field continues to gain momentum. Parallel advances in prenatal screening, molecular diagnosis, and the Human Genome Project make it highly likely that opportunities for the application of this approach will increase. However, at this point in the evolution of *in utero* HSC transplantation, there are more questions than answers. Widespread clinical application is premature, based on the extremely limited clinical success that has been achieved. The biology of each disease is unique, and expectations of success or failure can only be based on sound clinical investigation guided by experimental work in relevant animal models. The barriers to prenatal engraftment need to be investigated and understood prior to further clinical efforts in diseases in which host cell competition is prohibitive. Clinical centers should be associated with an active research effort to solve the remaining problems with this potentially promising clinical approach. In the near future, advances in our understanding of stem cell biology in the context of the prenatal microenvironment may allow *in utero* stem cell transplantation to achieve its full potential.

Conclusion

There are an increasing number of congenital and genetic abnormalities for which *in utero* treatment is possible and, in some cases, now relatively routine. Advances in therapies have progressed at different paces for different disorders, but there is great hope and enthusiasm that progress will continue to expand the number of disorders for which therapy can be effective.[118]

Key points

1. Prenatal diagnosis of fetal abnormalities has been developing over the last 30 years.
2. When congenital abnormalities are detected, couples should have the option of continuing, terminating (when legal) or, in selected cases, attempting prenatal therapeutic procedures.
3. Structural abnormalities are best approached surgically, and metabolic ones pharmacologically or genetically.
4. Neural tube defects (NTDs) are a multifactorial genetic disorder with a wide variation in incidence among racial and ethnic groups.
5. The neural tube normally closes within 30 days of conception.
6. The recurrence incidence of NTDs can be reduced from about 3–5%, depending upon the ethnic group, to about 1% with the use of 4.0 mg of preconceptual folic acid.
7. Since 1998, the United States FDA has mandated the supplementation of breads and grains with folic acid.
8. The primary incidence of NTDs has been reduced by about 30% in the United States from about 1:700 in the Caucasian population, 1:1000 in the African population, and 1:1200 in the Asian population.
9. Congenital adrenal hyperplasia, an autosomal recessive condition, is the most common cause of female hermaphroditism.
10. 21-Hydroxylase deficiency produces a salt-losing, glucocorticoid and mineralocorticoid deficiency, which can be life-threatening in the nursery if unrecognized.
11. Prenatal therapy by pharmacologic suppression of the fetal adrenal gland has been performed for over 20 years through the use of maternally administered dexamethasone, which "turns off" the fetal adrenal gland and is the model for the first prevention of a birth defect.
12. Such babies still have the biochemical abnormality, which requires medication, but are spared from the anatomic masculinization of the external genitalia.
13. Fetal hyperthyroidism can produce high-output cardiac failure and can be treated.
14. Fetal hypothyroidism can produce classic "cretinism" and can be treated with intra-amniotic fluid thyroxine.
15. Methylmalonic aciduria and multiple carboxylase deficiency are biochemical defects that have neonatal consequences; they can be treated *in utero*, but it is unclear how much prenatal amelioration helps.
16. Smith–Lemli–Opitz syndrome can be treated with cholesterol, but the data to show any efficacy are still lacking. Galactosemia can produce rapid depletion of ovarian follicles in female fetuses. No one has yet tried to reverse the process.
17. Fetal cardiac arrhythmias can be diagnosed by their specific type. The implications vary tremendously by type.

18 *In utero* treatment of such arrhythmias has to be tailored to the specific diagnosis, but correction is commonly feasible and lowers perinatal morbidity and mortality in appropriate cases.

19 Valvoplasties have been performed in a very limited number of cases with conflicting interpretations of their success.

20 Genetic therapies using stem cells have been attempted for immunodeficiency disorders and inborn errors of metabolism. To date, only the treatment of immunodeficiency disorders has had any success. New methods are needed to improve the receptivity of the fetus to stem cell transplants.

References

1 Evans MI, ed. *Reproductive risks and prenatal diagnosis.* Norwalk, CT: Appleton & Lange Publishing, 1992.

2 Harrison MR, Evans MI, Adzick NS, Holzgrove W. *The unborn patient.* Philadelphia, PA: W.B. Saunders, 2000.

3 Pryde PG, Odgers AE, Isada NB, et al. Determinants of parental decision to abort (DTA) or continue for non-aneuploid ultrasound detected abnormalities. *Obstet Gynecol* 1992;80:52–56.

4 Evans MI, Sobecki MA, Krivchenia EL, et al. Parental decisions to terminate/continue following abnormal cytogenetic prenatal diagnosis: "What" is still more important than "when". *Am J Med Genet* 1996;61:353–355.

5 Lemire RJ. Neural tube defects. *JAMA* 1988;259:558–562.

6 Smithells RW, Sheppard S, Schorah CJ, et al. Possible prevention of neural tube defects by preconceptual vitamin supplementation. *Lancet* 1980;1:399–340.

7 Frey L, Hauser WA. Epidemiology of neural tube defects. *Epilepsia* 2003;44(Suppl. 3):4–13.

8 MRC Vitamin Study Research Group. Prevention of neural tube defects: results of the MRC vitamin study. *Lancet* 1991;338: 132–137.

9 Honein MA, Paulozzi LJ, Mathews TJ, et al. Impact of folic acid fortification of the US food supply on the occurrence of neural tube defects. *JAMA* 2001;285:2981–2986.

10 Evans MI, Llurba E, Landsberger EJ, et al. Impact of folic acid supplementation in the United States: markedly diminished high maternal serum AFPs. *Obstet Gynecol* 2004;103:474–479.

11 Parle-McDermott A, Mills JL, Kirke PN, et al. Analysis of MTHFR 1298A→C and 677 C→T polymorphisms as risk factors for neural tube defects. *J Hum Genet* 2003;48:190–193.

12 Finnell RH, Shaw GM, Lammer EJ, Volcik KA. Does prenatal screening for 5,10-methylenetetrahydrofolate reductase (MTHFR) mutations in high-risk neural tube defect pregnancies make sense? *Genet Test* 2002;6:47–52.

13 Rampersaud E, Melvin EC, Siegel D, et al. Updated investigations of the role of methylenetetrahydrofolate reductase in human neural tube defects. *Clin Genet* 2003;63:210–214.

14 Zhu H, Wicker NJ, Shaw GM, et al. Homocysteine remethylation enzyme polymorphisms and increased risks for neural tube defects. *Mol Genet Metab* 2003;78:216–221.

15 Volocik KA, Shaw GM, Zhu H, et al. Risk factors for neural tube defects: associations between uncoupling protein 2 polymorphisms and spina bifida. *Birth Defects Res Part A Clin Mol Teratol* 2003;67:158–161.

16 Sever LE. Zinc deficiency in man. *Lancet* 1973;I:887.

17 McMichael AJ, Dreosti IE, Gibson GT. A prospective study of serial maternal serum zinc levels and pregnancy outcome. *Early Hum Dev* 1982;7:59–69.

18 Stoll C, Dott B, Alembik Y, Koehl C. Maternal trace elements, vitamin B12, vitamin A, folic acid, and fetal malformations. *Rep Toxicol* 1999;13:53–57.

19 Hambidge M, Hackshaw A, Wald N. Neural tube defects and serum zinc. *Br J Obstet Gynaecol* 1993;100:746–749.

20 Shoob HD, Sargent RG, Thompson SJ, et al. Dietary methionine is involved in the etiology of neural defect-affected pregnancies in humans. *J Nutr* 2001;131:2653–2658.

21 Meuli M, Meuli-Simmen C, Hutchins GM, et al. In utero surgery rescues neurological function at birth in sheep with spina bifida. *Nature Med* 1995;1:342–346.

22 MacLaughlin DT, Donahoe PK. Sex determination and differentiation. *N Engl J Med* 2004;350:323–324.

23 Dupont B, Oberfield SE, Smithwick EM, et al. Close genetic linkage between HLA and congenital adrenal hyperplasia (21-hydroxylase deficiency). *Lancet* 1977;2:1309–1312.

24 White PC, Grossberger D, Onufer BJ, et al. Two genes encoding steroid 21-hydroxylase are located near the genes encoding the fourth component of complement in man. *Proc Natl Acad Sci USA* 1985;82:1089–1093.

25 Evans MI, Chrousos GP, Mann DL, et al. Pharmacologic suppression of the fetal adrenal gland in utero: attempted prevention of abnormal external genital masculinization in suspected congenital adrenal hyperplasia. *JAMA* 1985;253:1015.

26 Forrest M, David M. Prenatal treatment of congenital adrenal hyperplasia due to 21-hydroxylase deficiency. 7th International Congress of Endocrinology, Abstract y11, Quebec, Canada, 1984.

27 New MI, Carlson A, Obeid J, et al. Prenatal diagnosis for congenital adrenal hyperplasia in 532 pregnancies. *Clin Endocrinol Metab* 2001;86:5651–5657.

28 Clayton PE, Miller WL, Oberfield SE, et al. ESPE/LWPES CAH Working Group. Consensus statement on 21-hydroxylase deficiency from the European Society for Paediatric Endocrinology and the Lawson Wilkins Pediatric Endocrine Society. *Horm Res* 2002;58:188–195.

29 Fisher DA, Klein AH. Thyroid development and disorders of thyroid function in the newborn. *N Engl J Med* 1981;304: 702–712.

30 Bruinse HW, Vermeulen-Meiners C, Wit JM. Fetal treatment for thyrotoxicosis in non-thyrotoxic pregnant women. *Fetal Ther* 1988;3:152–157.

31 Porreco RP, Bloch CA. Fetal blood sampling in the management of intrauterine thyrotoxicosis. *Obstet Gynecol* 1990;76: 509–512.

32 Hatjis CG. Diagnosis and successful treatment of fetal goitrous hyperthyroidism caused by maternal Graves' disease. *Obstet Gynecol* 1993;81:837–839.

33 Fisher DA. Neonatal thyroid disease of women with autoimmune thyroid disease. *Thyroid Today* 1986;9:1–7.

34 Volumenie JL, Polak M, Guibourdenche J, et al. Management of

fetal thyroid goitres: a report of 11 cases in a single perinatal unit. *Prenat Diagn* 2000;20:799.

35 Morine M, Takeda T, Minekawa R, et al. Antenatal diagnosis and treatment of a case of fetal goitrous hypothyroidism associated with high-output cardiac failure. *Ultrasound Obstet Gynecol* 2002;19:506–509.

36 Rovet J, Ehrlich R, Sorbara D. Intellectual outcome in children with fetal hypothyroidism. *J Pediatr* 1987;110:700–704.

37 Brusque A, Rotta L, Pettenuzzo LF, et al. Chronic postnatal administration of methylmalonic acid provokes a decrease of myelin content and ganglioside N-acetylneuraminic acid concentration in cerebrum of young rats. *Braz J Med Biol Res* 2001;34:227–231.

38 Ampola MG, Mahoney MI, Nakamura E, et al. Prenatal therapy of a patient with vitamin B responsive methylmalonic acidemia. *N Engl J Med* 1975;293:313–317.

39 Andersson HC, Marble M, Shapira E. Long term outcome in treated combined methylmalonic acidemia and homocysteinemia. *Genet Med* 1999;1:146–150.

40 Evans MI, Duquette DA, Rinaldo P, et al. Modulation of B12 dosage and response in fetal treatment of methylmalonic aciduria (MMA); titration of treatment dose to serum and urine MMA. *Fetal Diagn Ther* 1997;12:21–23.

41 Leon Del Rio A, Leclerc D, Gravel RA. Isolation of a cDNA encoding human holocarboxylase synthetase by functional complementation of a biotin auxotroph of *E. coli*. *Proc Natl Acad Sci USA* 1995;92:4626–4630.

42 Suzuki Y, Akoi Y, Ishida Y, et al. Isolation and characterization of mutations in the holocarboxylase synthetase cDNA. *Nature Genet* 1994;8:122–128.

43 Aoki Y, Suzuki Y, Sakamoto O, et al. Molecular analysis of holocarboxylase synthetase deficiency: a missense mutation and a single base deletion are predominant in Japanese patients. *Biochim Biophys Acta* 1995;1272:168–174.

44 Dupuis L, Leon-Del-Rio A, Leclerc D, et al. Clustering of mutations in the biotin-binding region of holocarboxylase synthetase in biotin responsive multiple carboxylase deficiency. *Hum Mol Genet* 1996;5:1011–1016.

45 Pompponio RJ, Hymes J, Reynolds TR, et al. Mutation in the human biotinidase gene that cause profound biotinidase deficiency in symptomatic children: molecular, biochemical, and clinical analysis. *Pediatr Res* 1997;42:840–848.

46 Suormala T, Fowler B, Jakobs C, et al. Late onset holocarboxylase synthetase deficiency: pre- and post-natal diagnosis and evaluation of effectiveness of antenatal biotin therapy. *Eur J Pediatr* 1998;157:570–575.

47 Roth KS, Yang W, Allen L, et al. Prenatal administration of biotin: biotin responsive multiple carboxylase deficiency. *Pediatr Res* 1982;16:126–129.

48 Packman S, Cowan MJ, Golbus MS, et al. Prenatal treatment of biotin responsive multiple carboxylase deficiency. *Lancet* 1982;1:1435–1438.

49 Thuy LP, Jurecki E, Nemzer L, et al. Prenatal diagnosis of holocarboxylase synthetase deficiency by assay of the enzyme in chorionic villus material followed by prenatal treatment. *Clin Chim Acta* 1999;284:59–68.

50 Smith DW, Lemli L, Opitz JM. A newly recognized syndrome of multiple congenital anomalies. *J Pediatr* 1964;64:210–217.

51 Curry CJR, Carey JC, Holland JS. Smith–Lemli–Opitz syndrome–type II: multiple congenital anomalies with male pseudohermaphroditism and frequent early lethality. *Am J Med Genet* 1987;26:45–57.

52 Opitz JM. RSH-SLO ("Smith–Lemli–Opitz") syndrome: historical, genetic, and development considerations. *Am J Med Genet* 1994;50:344–346.

53 Kelley RI. A new face for an old syndrome. *Am J Med Genet* 1997;65:251–256.

54 Kelley RI. Diagnosis of Smith–Lemli–Opitz syndrome by gas chromatography/mass spectrometry of 7-dehydrocholesterol in plasma, amniotic fluid and cultured skin fibroblasts. *Clin Chim Acta* 1995;236:45–58.

55 Waterham HR, Wijburg FA, Hennekam RCM, et al. Smith–Lemli–Opitz is caused by mutations in the 7-dehydrocholesterol reductase gene. *Am J Hum Genet* 1998;63:329–338.

56 Johnson JA, Aughton DJ, Comstock CH, et al. Prenatal diagnosis of Smith–Lemli–Opitz syndrome, type II. *Am J Med Genet* 1994;49:240–243.

57 Hobbins JC, Jones OW, Gottesfeld MD, Persutte W. Transvaginal ultrasonography and transabdominal embryoscopy in the first-trimester diagnosis of Smith-Lemli-Opitz syndrome, type II. *Am J Obstet Gynecol* 1994;171:546–549.

58 Sharp P, Haan E, Fletcher JM, et al. First trimester diagnosis of Smith–Lemli–Opitz syndrome. *Prenat Diagn* 1997;17:355–361.

59 Irons M, Elias E, Tint GS, et al. Abnormal cholesterol metabolism in the Smith–Lemli–Opitz syndrome: report of clinical and biochemical findings in 4 patients and treatment in 1 patient. *Am J Med Genet* 1994;50:347–352.

60 Irons M, Elias ER, Abuelo D, et al. Treatment of Smith–Lemli–Opitz syndrome: results of a multicenter trial. *Am J Med Genet* 1997;68:311–314.

61 Nowaczyk MJM, Whelan DT, Heshka TW, Hill R. Smith–Lemli–Opitz syndrome: a treatable inherited error of metabolism causing mental retardation. *Can Med Assoc J* 1999;161:165–170.

62 Irons MR, Nores J, Stewart TL, et al. Antenatal therapy of Smith–Lemli–Opitz syndrome. *Fetal Diagn Ther* 1999;14:133–137.

63 Elsas LJ. Prenatal diagnosis of galactose-1-phosphate uridyltransferase (GALT) deficient galactosemia. *Prenat Diagn* 2001;21:302–303.

64 Chen YT, Mattis'on DR, Feigenbaum L, et al. Reduction in oocyte number following prenatal exposure to a high galactose diet. *Science* 1981;314:1146–1147.

65 Bandyopadhyay S, Chakrabarti J, Banerjee S, et al. Prenatal exposure to high galactose adversely affects initial gonadal pool of germ cells in rats. *Hum Reprod* 2003;18:276–282.

66 Kleinman CS, Donnerstein RL, DeVore GR, et al. Fetal echocardiography for evaluation of in utero congestive heart failure: a technique for study of nonimmune fetal hydrops. *N Engl J Med* 1982;306:568–575.

67 Kleinman CS, Copel JA, Nehgme RA. The fetus with cardiac arrhythmia. In: Harrison MR, Evans MI, Adzick NS, Holzgreve W, eds. *The unborn patient: the art and science of fetal therapy*. Philadelphia, PA: W.B. Saunders; 2001:417–441.

68 Weiner CP, Thompson MIB. Direct treatment of fetal supraventricular tachycardia after failed transplacental therapy. *Am J Obstet Gynecol* 1988;158:570–573.

69 Hansmann M, Gembruch U, Bald RK, et al. Fetal tachyarrhythmias: transplacental and direct treatment of the fetus. A report of 60 cases. *Ultrasound Obstet Gynecol* 1991;1:162–167.

70 Younis JS, Granat M. Insufficient transplacental digoxin transfer in severe hydrops fetalis. *Am J Obstet Gynecol* 1987;157:1268–1269.

71 Simpson PC, Trudinger BJ, Walker A, Baird PJ. The intrauterine

treatment of fetal cardiac failure in a twin pregnancy with an acardiac, acephalic monster. *Am J Obstet Gynecol* 1983;147: 842–844.

72 Slate RK, Stevens MB, Verrier ED, et al. Intrauterine repair of pulmonary stenosis in fetal sheep. *Surg Forum* 1985;36:246–247.

73 Turley K, Vlahakes GI, Harrison MR, et al. Intrauterine cardiothoracic surgery: the fetal lamb model. *Ann Thorac Surg* 1982;34:422–426.

74 Gillette PC. The mechanisms of supraventricular tachycardia in children. *Circulation* 1980;54:133–139.

75 Naheed ZJ, Strasburger JF, Deal BJ, et al. Fetal tachycardia: mechanisms and predictors of hydrops fetalis. *J Am Coll Cardiol* 1996;27:1736–1740.

76 Morganroth J. Risk factors for the development of proarrhythmic events. *Am J Cardiol* 1987;59:32E–37E.

77 Wellens JHH, Durrer D. Effect of digitalis on atrioventricular conduction and circus movement tachycardia in patients with the Wolff–Parkinson–White syndrome. *Circulation* 1973;47:1229–1236.

78 Michaelsson M, Engle MA. Congenital complete heart block: an international study of the natural history. *Cardiovasc Clin* 1972;4:85–101.

79 Anandakumar C, Biswas A, Chew SS, et al. Direct fetal therapy for hydrops secondary to congenital atrioventricular heart block. *Obstet Gynecol* 1996;87:835–837.

80 Carpenter RJ, Strasburger JF, Garson A, Jr, et al. Fetal ventricular pacing for hydrops secondary to complete atrioventricular block. *J Am Coll Cardiol* 1986;8:1434–1436.

81 Copel JA, Buyon JP, Kleinman CS. Successful in utero therapy of fetal heart block. *Am J Obstet Gynecol* 1995;173:1384–1390.

82 Harris JP, Alexson CG, Manning JA, Thompson HO. Medical therapy for the hydropic fetus with congenital complete atrioventricular block. *Am J Perinatol* 1993;10:217–219.

83 Bitar FF, Byrum CJ, Kveselis DA, et al. In utero management of hydrops fetalis caused by critical aortic stenosis. *Am J Perinatol* 1997;14:389–391.

84 Schmider A, Henrich W, Dahnert I, Dudenhausen JW. Prenatal therapy of non-immunologic hydrops fetalis caused by severe aortic stenosis. *Ultrasound Obstet Gynecol* 2000;16:275–278.

85 Kleinman CS, Donnerstein RL. Ultrasonic assessment of cardiac function in the intact human fetus. *J Am Coll Cardiol* 1985;5(Suppl. 1):84S–94S.

86 Yagel S, Weissman A, Rotstein Z, et al. Congenital heart defects. natural course and in utero development. *Circulation* 1997;96: 550–555.

87 Maxwell D, Allan L, Tynan MJ. Balloon dilatation of the aortic valve in the fetus. A report of two cases. *Br Heart J* 1991;65: 256–261.

88 Allan LD, Maxwell DJ, Carminati, Tynan MJ. Survival after fetal aortic balloon valvoplasty. *Ultrasound Obstet Gynecol* 1995;5: 90–91.

89 Kohl T, Szabo X, Suda K, et al. Fetoscopic and open transumbilical fetal cardiac catheterization in sheep. Potential approaches for human fetal cardiac intervention. *Circulation* 1997;95:1048–1053.

90 Simpson JM, Sharland GK. Natural history and outcome of aortic stenosis diagnosed prenatally. *Heart* 1997;77:205–210.

91 Kohl T, Sharland G, Chaoui R, et al. World experience of percutaneous ultrasound-guided balloon valvuloplasty in human fetuses with severe aortic valve obstruction. *J Am Coll Cardiol* 2000;15:1230–1233.

92 Lucarelli G, Clift RA, Galimberti M, et al. Bone marrow transplantation in adult thalassemic patients. *Blood* 1999;93:1164–1167.

93 Walters MC, Patience M, Leisenring W, et al. Bone marrow transplantation for sickle cell disease. *N Engl J Med* 1996;335: 369–376.

94 Walters MC, Storb R, Patience M, et al. Impact of bone marrow transplantation for symptomatic sickle cell disease: an interim report. Multicenter investigation of bone marrow transplantation for sickle cell disease. *Blood* 2000;95:1918–2466.

95 Flake AW, Zanjani ED. In utero hematopoietic stem cell transplantation: ontogenic opportunities and biologic barriers. *Blood* 1999;94:2179–2191.

96 Touraine JL, Raudrant D, Laplace S. Transplantation of hematopoietic cells from the fetal liver to treat patients with congenital disease postnatally or prenatally. *Transplant Proc* 1997;29:712–713.

97 Hayashi S, Peranteau WH, Shaaban AF, Flake AW. Complete allogeneic hematopoietic chimerism achieved by a combined strategy of in utero hematopoietic stem cell transplantation and postnatal donor lymphocyte infusion. *Blood* 2002;100:804–812.

98 Peranteau WF, Hayashi S, Hsieh M, et al. High level allogeneic chimerism achieved by prenatal tolerance induction and postnatal non-myeloablative bone marrow transplantation. *Blood* 2002;100:2225–2234.

99 Flake AW, Zanjani ED. In utero hematopoietic stem cell transplantation. A status report. *JAMA* 1997;278:932–937.

100 Hayward A, Ambruso D, Battaglia F, et al. Microchimerism and tolerance following intrauterine transplantation and transfusion for alpha-thalassemia-1. *Fetal Diagn Ther* 1998;13:8–14.

101 Westgren M, Ringden O, Eik Nes S, et al. Lack of evidence of permanent engraftment after in utero fetal stem cell transplantation in congenital hemoglobinopathies. *Transplantation* 1996;61:1176–1179.

102 Touraine JL, Raudrant D, Royo C, et al. In utero transplantation of hematopoietic stem cells in humans. *Transplant Proc* 1991;23:1706–1708.

103 Hayashi S, Abdulmalik O, Peranteau WH, et al. Mixed chimerism following in utero hematopoietic stem cell transplantation in murine models of hemoglobinopathy. *Exp Hematol* 2003;31:176–184.

104 Flake AW. Stem cell and genetic therapies for the fetus. *Semin Pediatr Surg* 2003;12:202–208.

105 Shields LE, Lindton BIM, Andrews RG, Westgren M. Fetal hematopoietic stem cell transplantation. a challenge for the twenty-first century. *J Hematother Stem Cell Res* 2002;11:617–631.

106 Noguchi M, Yi H, Rosenblatt HM, et al. Interleukin-2 receptor gamma chain mutation results in X-linked severe combined immunodeficiency in humans. *Cell* 1993;73:17–157.

107 Slavin S, Naparstek E, Ziegler M, Lewin A. Clinical application of intrauterine bone marrow transplantation for treatment of genetic diseases–feasibility studies. *Bone Marrow Transplant* 1992;9:189–190.

108 Buckley RH, Schiff SE, Schiff RI, et al. Hematopoietic stem-cell transplantation for the treatment of severe combined immunodeficiency. *N Engl J Med* 1999;340:508–516.

109 Flake AW, Roncarolo MG, Puck JM, et al. Treatment of X-linked severe combined immunodeficiency by in utero transplantation of paternal bone marrow. *N Engl J Med* 1996;335:1806–1810.

110 Flake AW, Zanjani ED. Treatment of severe combined immunodeficiency syndrome. *N Engl J Med* 1999;341:291–292.

111 Pirovano S, Notarangelo LD, Malacarne F, et al. Reconstitution of T-cell compartment after in utero stem cell transplantation: analysis of T-cell repertoire and thymic output. *Haematologica* 2004;89:450–461.
112 Westgren M, Ringden O, Bartmann P, et al. Prenatal T-cell reconstitution after in utero transplantation with fetal liver cells in a patient with X-linked severe combined immunodeficiency. *Am J Obstet Gynecol* 2002;187:475–482.
113 Moses S. Pathophysiology and dietary treatment of the glycogen storage diseases. *J Pediatr Gastr Nutr* 1990;11:155–174.
114 Kaye E. Therapeutic approaches to lysosomal storage diseases. *Curr Opin Pediatr* 1995;7:650–654.
115 Imaizumi M, Gushi K, Kurobane I, et al. Long-term effects of bone marrow transplantation for inborn errors of metabolism: a study of four patients with lysosomal storage diseases. *Acta Paediatr Japon* 1994;36:30–36.
116 Krivit W, Lockman L, Watkins P, et al. The future for treatment by bone marrow transplantation for adrenoleukodystrophy, metachromatic leukodystrophy, globoid cell leukodystrophy and Hurler syndrome. *J Inher Metabol Dis* 1995;18:398–412.
117 Westlake V, Jolly R, Jones B, et al. Hematopoietic cell transplantation in fetal lambs with ceroid-lipofuscinosis. *Am J Med Genet* 1995;57:365–368.
118 Tulipan N, Hermanz-Schulman M, Bruner JP. Reduced hindbrain herniation after intrauterine myelomeningocele repair. A report of four cases. *Pediatr Neurosurg* 1998;29:274–278.

Part IX

Maternal biological adaptations to pregnancy

35 Maternal biological, biomechanical, and biochemical changes in pregnancy

Edward K.S. Chien and Helen Feltovich

Pregnancy induces changes in all maternal physiologic systems to accommodate the developing fetus. A thorough understanding of normal adaptations is important in identifying pathologic changes that may adversely affect both fetus and mother. In this chapter, we focus on general maternal physiologic changes, as well as specific changes within the uterus, in order to understand how these changes protect the fetomaternal environment and ultimately allow normal delivery.

Cardiovascular system

Profound cardiovascular changes are required throughout gestation to meet fetal oxygen and nutritional requirements as well as to meet the increased demands of maternal organ systems (Fig. 35.1). Many of these can be detected in the first trimester, such as changes in heart rate, cardiac output, vascular tone, and blood pressure.

The maternal heart is displaced by the growing uterus and increases in mass, which may lead to misinterpretation of both the electrocardiogram (ECG) and the chest radiograph (as depicted in Fig. 35.2).[1] Left axis deviation due to diaphragmatic elevation is approximately 15°, although deviation up to 28° has been described. ECG changes include low-voltage QRS complexes, flattened or inverted T waves in anterior chest leads and lead III, as well as ST segment depression in chest and limb leads.[1] Conduction abnormalities resulting from pregnancy are uncommon, although extrasystoles of atrial and ventricular origin are more frequent in pregnancy.

Auscultation of the heart reflects the change in its position (Fig. 35.3).[2,3] Splitting of the first heart sound, due to closure of the mitral valve prior to the tricuspid valve, is commonly heard. The second heart sound (closure of the aortic and pulmonary valves) typically does not change. Between the first and second heart sounds, it is common to detect systolic ejection murmurs because of increased cardiac output. The third heart sound (diastolic filling) can often be heard during mid- to late pregnancy when end-diastolic volume peaks.

Blood pressure is followed closely during pregnancy and undergoes a series of changes (Fig. 35.1).[4] The mean arterial pressure decreases gradually over the first half of gestation, with a nadir at approximately 20 weeks.[5] A greater decrease in diastolic (average 10–20 mmHg) versus systolic (average 5–10 mmHg) pressure is observed in the first half of gestation, whereas in the second half of gestation, greater elevations are seen in systolic versus diastolic pressures. Vascular tone is altered during pregnancy, leading to the decline in systemic blood pressure.[6] Venous compliance increases as a result of a number of circulating factors, leading to an increase in venous capacitance and stasis.[7] Blood pressure during pregnancy is dependent on maternal position; both systolic and diastolic blood pressures are elevated an average of 10 mmHg in the sitting compared with the lateral recumbent position.[8]

Pregnancy leads to redistribution and a 30–50% increase in cardiac output (heart rate × stroke volume) to accommodate increased demand by all maternal organ systems, particularly the pregnant uterus, which at term requires a fifth of the total cardiac output (500–800 mL/min) (Fig. 35.1).[9–11] The increase in cardiac output is secondary to changes in both heart rate and stroke volume, and can be detected as early as the 5th week of gestation.[9] Most investigators have demonstrated that cardiac output peaks around the 32nd week of gestation, although some have suggested that it continues to rise to term; however, this may represent technical differences in measurements.[12] During the late second and third trimesters, venacaval compression secondary to maternal supine positioning can decrease venous return, reducing cardiac output by 25–30%.[13,14] For this reason, the supine position is not recommended.

Respiratory system

The pulmonary system must also adapt to the increased oxygen and ventilatory demands placed upon it by pregnancy. Oxygen consumption undergoes a 15–20% increase by the end of gestation (Fig. 35.4).[15,16] This increased requirement for oxygen is compensated for by an increase in ventilation.[17] The

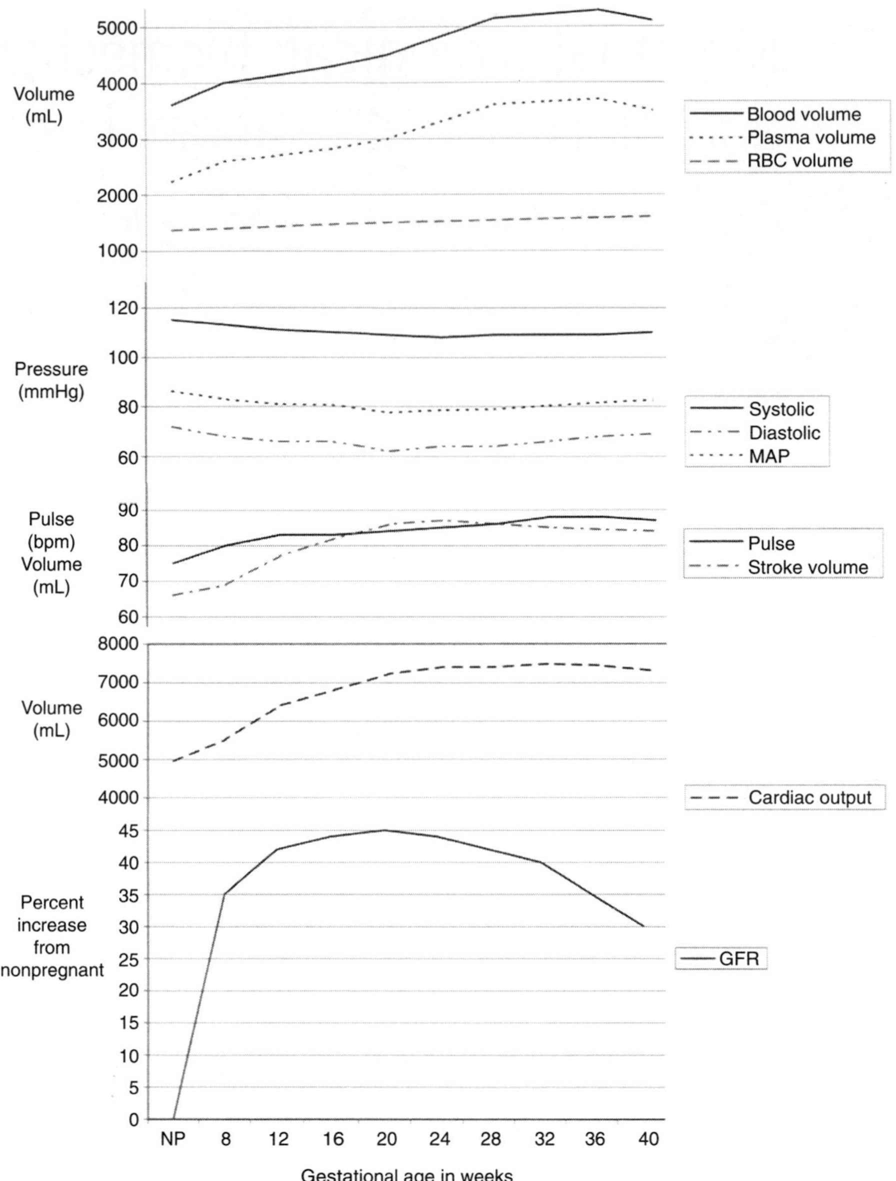

Figure 35.1 The body makes a number of physiologic adjustments throughout pregnancy, which can be detected as early as 5 weeks from the last menstrual period. Systems with easily measurable changes include the cardiovascular, hematologic, and renal systems. To accommodate the increased cardiovascular demands, blood volume progressively increases with advancing gestation. The blood volume is determined by both red cell mass and plasma volume. Plasma volume increases occur during the first trimester and continue to late in the third trimester. The red cell mass increases at a slower rate, leading to a dilutional anemia, which usually reaches its nadir around 28 weeks of gestation. Blood pressure also falls owing to decreased peripheral vascular resistance, reaching a nadir around 20 weeks. A decrease in both systolic and diastolic pressure is observed. From mid-gestation to term, blood pressure rises to near nonpregnant levels. Cardiac output, which is determined by both pulse and stroke volume, increases progressively throughout gestation. Cardiac output is believed to peak around 32 weeks, although some studies suggest a gradual increase to term. Early increases in cardiac output are mainly due to increases in heart rate, but increases in stroke volume contribute a greater proportion later in pregnancy. Glomerular filtration increases with the increase in cardiac output. The marked increase in glomerular filtration rate (GFR) is primarily due to an increase in effective renal plasma flow. The increase in effective renal plasma flow results from an increase in perfusion and decreased renal vascular resistance. MAP, mean arterial pressure; NP, nonpregnant; RBC, red blood cell.

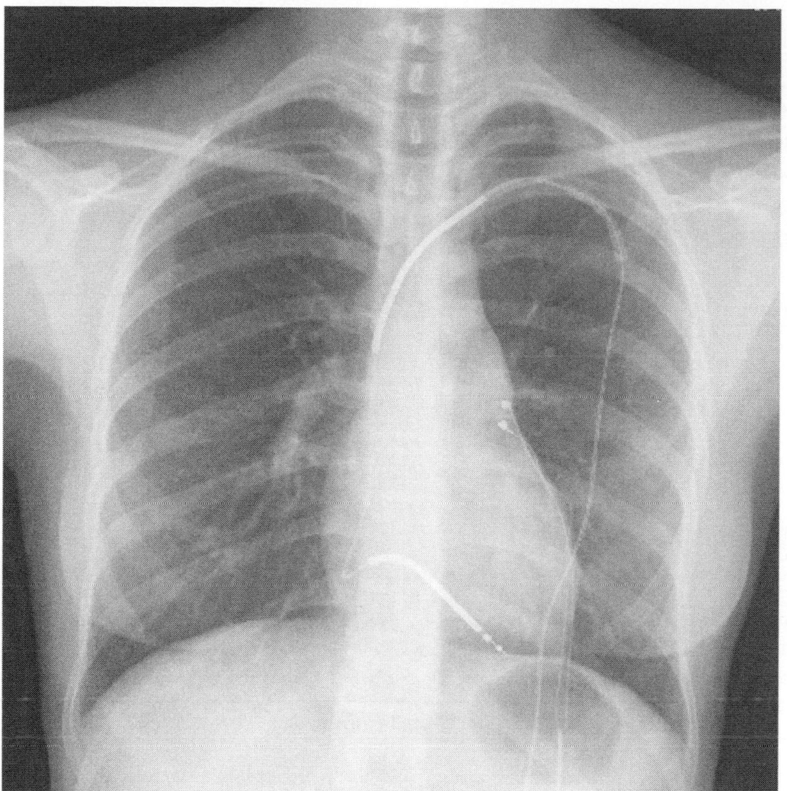

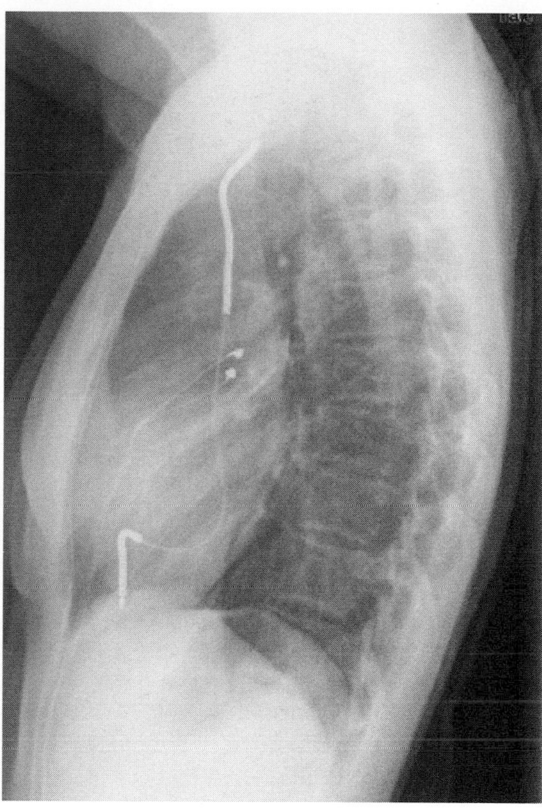

Figure 35.2 Anatomic changes in the pulmonary and cardiovascular systems are well demonstrated on chest radiography. The heart is rotated forward and deviated upward during pregnancy owing to diaphragmatic elevation, resulting in apical displacement into the fifth intercostal space. This rotation may falsely suggest right atrial enlargement on lateral views of the chest. It also causes increased prominence of the left cardiac border, giving the impression of cardiac hypertrophy. Together, these changes cause the cardiac volume to increase by approximately 12%. The chest dimensions are also altered. The diaphragm is elevated by 4 cm, which leads to flattening of the subcostal angle from 68° to 103°. This potential decrease in lung volume is compensated by a 2-cm increase in chest diameter, which allows maintenance of vital capacity.

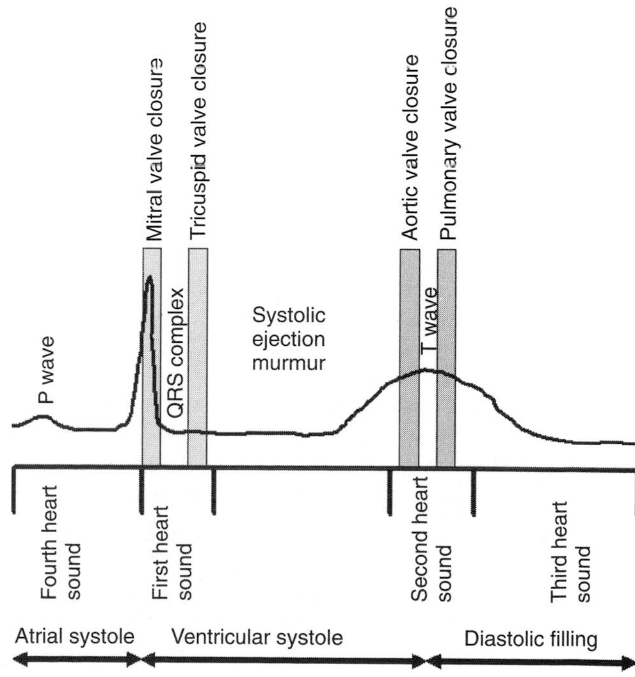

Figure 35.3 Identification of additional heart sounds on auscultation of the maternal heart is common. These include splitting of the first heart sound and systolic ejection murmurs. Splitting of the first heart sound is due to closure of the tricuspid valve after the mitral valve. Delayed closure results from an increase in blood volume and extended filling of the left ventricle. Flow murmurs detected between the first and second heart sounds are also common owing to increased blood flow. The electrical changes associated with the cardiac cycle and heart sounds are also depicted. Atrial and ventricular systole are depicted below the heart sounds as well as diastolic filling periods.

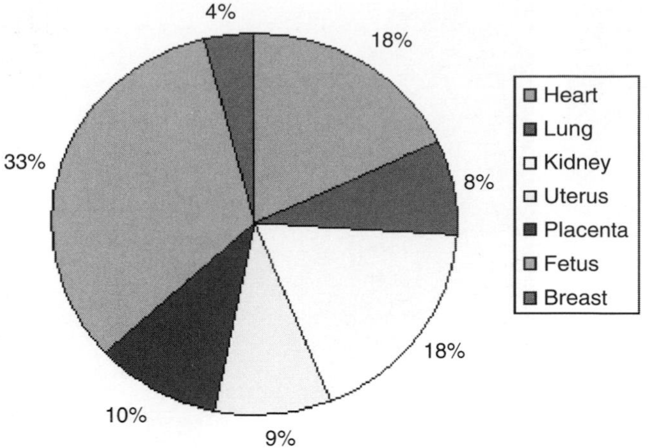

Figure 35.4 Oxygen consumption increases progressively by 15–20% over the course of pregnancy. The increase in oxygen consumption is due mainly to increased cardiac, pulmonary, renal, and reproductive system demands. The reproductive system accounts for over half of the required increase. The cardiovascular and renal systems require a similar increase in oxygen consumption, although the increase in the renal system is seen early in pregnancy and remains constant throughout gestation. The increase in oxygen consumption parallels the increase in cardiac output.

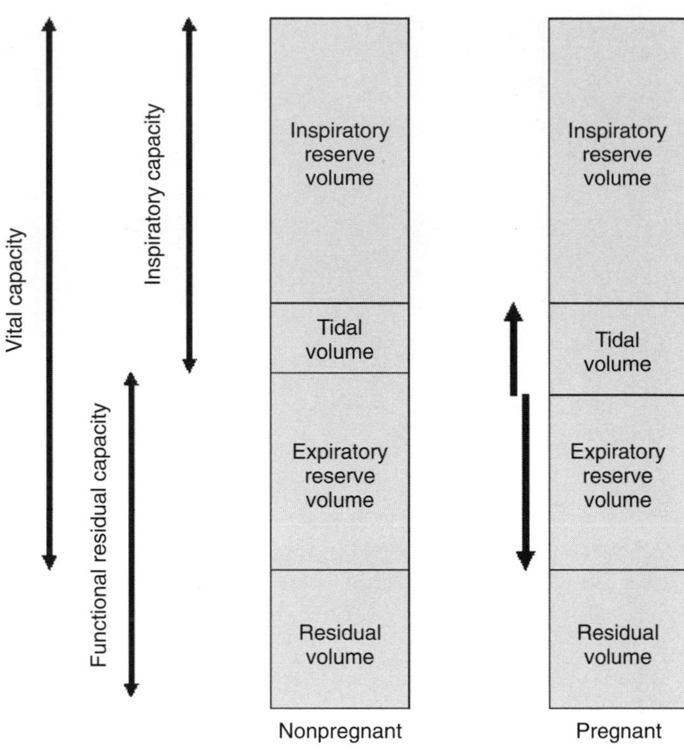

Figure 35.5 The increase in oxygen requirement is accommodated by an increase in tidal volume without an increase in respiratory rate. This increase in tidal volume is at the expense of the end-expiratory reserve volume. The inspiratory reserve volume and the vital capacity remain constant. The forced expiratory volume in 1 s (FEV_1) and forced vital capacity (FVC) remain unchanged during pregnancy.

respiratory system, although adaptable, is also remarkably susceptible to failure in the event of injury to other physiologic systems.

The increased ventilatory requirements are met by anatomic, ventilatory, and biochemical mechanisms (minute ventilation = tidal volume × respiratory rate). Increased ventilation is due to increased tidal volume (Fig. 35.5);[18,19] respiratory rate does not change during pregnancy. Maternal hyperventilation leads to changes in normal blood gas parameters (Table 35.1).[20] Beginning early in the first trimester, tidal volume increases by 40% (500 mL to 700 mL) due to direct stimulation of the central respiratory control center by progesterone.[18,19] This increase in tidal volume comes at the expense of functional residual capacity (the volume remaining in the lungs at forced end expiration) (Fig. 35.5).[18,21,22] The vital capacity does not change, nor do a number of spirometric parameters.[23] Anatomic changes are demonstrated in Figure 35.2.

Table 35.1 Arterial blood gas values in pregnancy.

	pH	Po_2 (mmHg)	Pco_2 (mmHg)	HCO_2 (mEq/L)	Sao_2 (%)
Nonpregnant	7.40	98	40	22–26	98
Pregnant	7.44	101	28	18–22	98

Increased ventilation leads to alterations in normal blood gas values in pregnancy. The Po_2 is elevated from the normal nonpregnant value of 98 to 101 mmHg in pregnancy, and Pco_2 falls from 40 to 28 mmHg. The renal system compensates for the decline in Pco_2 by increasing bicarbonate (HCO_2) secretion to 18–22 mEq/L. These changes result in slightly higher average pH values (7.44 vs. 7.40). This pH alteration also permits increased oxygen delivery by shifting the oxygen dissociation curve, which allows for enhanced oxygen release into tissue where oxygen is being consumed.

Hematologic system

Pregnancy affects all components of the hematologic system, and includes changes in plasma volume and red blood cell volume, the immunologic system, and coagulation components.

Both plasma volume and red blood cell volume increase over the course of gestation, together contributing to a 20–40% increase in blood volume during pregnancy (Fig. 35.1).[24,25] Plasma volume expands as early as 6 weeks and continues through 32 weeks of gestation, leading to an increase of 40–50% in singleton pregnancies, and more with multiple gestations.[26] Red blood cell volume only increases by 20–30% over gestation, which leads to a fall in hemoglobin concentration often referred to as the physiologic anemia of pregnancy.[24]

Platelet quantity generally remains unchanged throughout

Table 35.2 Coagulation components and test values in pregnancy.

Component or test	Change	Nonpregnant	Pregnant (relative change compared with nonpregnant values)
PT	None	11–12 s	No change
PTT	None	24–36 s	No change
Bleeding time	None	1–5 min	No change
Platelet count	None	$150–400 \times 10^3/mm^3$	No change
Fibrinogen	Increase	200 mg/dL	50–100%
Factor IIc	Increase	20 mg/dL	10–20%
Factor Vc	None	100 U/dL	No change
Factor VIIc	Increase	100 IU/dL	30–50%
Factor VIIIc	Increase	100 IU/dL	100%
Factor IXc	None	100 IU/dL	No change
Factor Xc	Increase	100 IU/dL	20–60%
Factor XIc	Decrease	100 U/dL	20–30%
Factor XIIc	Increase	100 IU/dL	40%
vW An	Increase	100 IU/dL	100–300%
Protein C	None	100%	No change
Protein S	Decrease	100%	50%
Antithrombin III	None	100%	No change

vW An, von Willebrand antigen.

gestation, although up to 10% of women will have a decrease in total platelets due to increased turnover.[27,28] Although pregnancy does not appear to change the platelet's lifespan, studies suggest that pregnancy is associated with increased platelet activation, which may contribute to increased turnover and gestational thrombocytopenia.[28]

Altered levels of coagulation components, together with increased venous stasis, create a hypercoagulable state during pregnancy. The alterations in coagulation components are complex with both increases and decreases in specific components (Table 35.2).[29,30] These alterations make identification of coagulation disorders difficult, although tests of coagulation such as prothrombin time (PT), partial thromboplastin time (PTT), and bleeding time are unchanged by pregnancy. By 6 weeks' postpartum, most coagulation factors have returned to prepregnant values, although the timing varies by component.

Maternal immunologic adaptation to pregnancy is poorly understood. Pregnancy requires the recognition and acceptance of the fetus, which is considered a semi-allograft because it expresses antigens of both maternal and paternal origin. Studies suggest that local immunity within the uterus is altered to permit the development of the fetoplacental unit. A subset of T cells (helper T cells) is believed to be important in the recognition of the fetal allograft and local immune suppression.[31–34]

Other immune system changes include an increase in the white blood cell count (WBC) (Table 35.3), even in the absence of an acute infection.[31] This increase is due primarily to an increase in granulocytes belonging to the innate immune response that is mediated by neutrophils, macrophages, monocytes, and natural killer cells. These cell types reside locally in tissues and are recruited in response to local challenges. Changes in the adaptive immune response can be subdivided into cellular and humoral responses mediated by T and B lymphocytes.[32] Total lymphocyte counts remain unchanged during pregnancy, but alterations in lymphocyte populations do occur.

Table 35.3 Change in WBC populations.

Component	Change in pregnancy
WBC	Increase
Granulocytes	Increase
Lymphocytes	No change
Monocytes	No change
Total T cells	Decrease
B cells	No change
T-helper cells	Decrease
T-suppressor cells	No change

Urinary tract system

Pregnancy produces both anatomic and functional changes in the urinary tract. Renal abnormalities are associated with an increased risk of preterm delivery.[35] The renal system increases in size during pregnancy. The dimensions of the kidneys increase with the increase in glomerular filtration rate (GFR). These changes resolve during the postpartum period. Dilation of the collecting system can often be seen and is more common on the right than on the left side. Ureteral dilation is commonly seen above the pelvic brim, but can be observed all the way down to the level of trigone, thought to be secondary to hormonal effects on smooth muscle tone. The pregnant uterus may contribute to intermittent obstruction of the ureters, especially at the level of the pelvic brim. Standard tests to assess renal function are often inaccurate in the pregnant state because of anatomic changes in the renal system.[36] Thus, accepted normal values of renal function outside of pregnancy may suggest intrinsic renal disease in pregnancy.

The kidney becomes hypertrophied during pregnancy, then returns to normal in the postpartum period. Hormonal changes likely contribute to the alterations in renal anatomy and function,[37] as well as to increases in renal parenchyma and the collecting system.[38,39] Dilation of renal calices and ureters is observed as early as the first trimester, often more on the right side compared with the left. Mechanical obstruction of the ureters by the expanding uterus is believed to be responsible for some of the anatomic changes.[40] Radiologic studies indicate that ureteral dilation occurs mainly above the pelvic brim, suggesting compression against the bony pelvis. This intermittent obstruction and increased stasis produces inaccurate results of renal function using spot collections and increases the risk of lower urinary tract infections.

Increases in the GFR (Fig. 35.1) and effective renal plasma flow (ERPF) occur early in the first trimester;[41,42] GFR increases by 30–50% while ERPF increases by 50–80%. These increases peak by the end of the first trimester and persist throughout gestation. Measurements of plasma solutes are altered by the increased GFR.[43] Normal serum creatinine declines by 0.1–0.2 mg/dL and blood urea nitrogen decreases by more than 10 mg/dL. Glycosuria during pregnancy is common, and may be normal due to increased solute filter load and decreased tubular resorption.[44,45] Decreased uric acid levels result more from increased filtration load than decreased tubular resorption.[46] The physiologic hyperventilation of pregnancy reduces $P\text{CO}_2$ and therefore serum bicarbonate levels, which decreases the body's buffering capacity, increasing its susceptibility to acidosis.

Plasma osmolality decreases during pregnancy,[47] beginning after conception and reaching a nadir by the end of the first trimester. This is due largely to a decrease in serum sodium and, to a lesser extent, to a fall in blood urea nitrogen. The change in osmotic threshold is attributed to alterations in vasopressin metabolism.[48] Vasopressin secretion is not suppressed at normal osmotic thresholds, which leads to fluid retention. The increased secretion is balanced partly by placental vasopressinase, an enzyme that degrades vasopressin.

The body's volume sensor response is unaltered during pregnancy, while the alterations in osmolality and AVP metabolism produce a relative state of hypervolemia. Thus, pregnancy is associated with relative activation of the renin–angiotensin–aldosterone system.[48] This activation is thought to contribute to the retention of sodium as well as an increase in total body water. Pregnancy is associated with a 6- to 8-L increase in total body water, two-thirds of which is stored extracellularly.

Table 35.4 Change in liver function tests during pregnancy.

	Change
Total bilirubin	None
Alkaline phosphatase	Increase
Alanine aminotransferase	None
Aspartate aminotransferase	None
γ-Glutamyl transferase	Increase
Albumin	Decrease
Cholesterol	Increase
Triglycerides	Increase
Binding globulins	Increase
Lactate dehydrogenase	Increase
Fibrinogen	Increase

Gastrointestinal system

Gastrointestinal complaints are common in pregnancy. Symptomatic complaints such as nausea and vomiting, while common, may represent conditions with significant morbidity and mortality. However, many of the symptoms are pregnancy limited, resolving spontaneously after delivery.

Anatomic changes occur throughout the alimentary system and affect physiological function. Gastroesophageal reflux is a common complaint that is related to decreased pyloric sphincter tone resulting from smooth muscle relaxation and increased intra-abdominal pressure from the expanding uterus.[49,50] Gastric emptying times are elevated by 50% with pregnancy,[51,52] and delayed emptying contributes to symptomatic complaints.

Biochemical and physiologic parameters in the biliary system are affected by pregnancy, although no anatomic changes occur.[53] Gallbladder size is unchanged, while motility is diminished because of decreased smooth muscle activity, similar to that occurring in the intestine. The liver does not change in size, although parameters of liver function may be altered (Table 35.4). Increased alkaline phosphatase occurs secondary to increased placental production.[54] In contrast, aspartate aminotransferase (AST) and alanine aminotransferase (ALT) may be elevated in normal pregnancy.[55] Albumin production is unchanged, but plasma levels are often decreased on account of plasma volume expansion.[56] Pregnancy has major effects on the lipid profile, with significant elevations of both triglycerides and cholesterol.[57] Increases in binding globulins alter normal total circulating hormone levels.

The exocrine pancreas is less well studied than the endocrine pancreas. Its secretory response does not appear to be altered, although animal studies suggest that pregnancy increases the basal secretion of digestive enzymes.[58] Amylase and lipase levels are unaffected by pregnancy.

Endocrine system

Multiple anatomic and functional changes occur throughout pregnancy within the endocrine system. A thorough understanding of these changes is key to interpreting laboratory results during pregnancy.

Euglycemia in pregnancy is important. The fetus requires adequate maternal glucose, but hyperglycemia is associated with birth defects and fetal macrosomia.[59] Pregnancy changes carbohydrate metabolism, causing fasting hypoglycemia, postprandial hyperglycemia, and hyperinsulinemia.[60] The normal response to a carbohydrate challenge in pregnancy is a twofold or greater increase in stimulated insulin release compared with the nonpregnant state.[60]

Basal glucose levels in pregnancy, particularly during the first trimester, are lowered by approximately 10%.[61] Placental secretion of counter-regulatory hormones causes decreased peripheral insulin sensitivity. Unlike glucose, insulin and other protein hormones do not cross the placenta, although insulin probably does affect nutrient transport and availability to the fetus.

An increase in anterior pituitary size during pregnancy, primarily because of an increase in the number of prolactin-secreting cells, has been described.[62] In contrast to the increased number of lactotrophs, growth hormone-secreting cells decrease in number along with the number of gonadotropin-secreting cells. No changes in thyrotropic or adrenocorticotropin-secreting cells have been identified. Increased pituitary size seems to correlate with increased levels of circulating hormones. During pregnancy, prolactin levels are up to 10 times higher than in the nonpregnant state.[63] Elevations of both corticotropin-releasing hormone (CRH) and adrenocorticotrophic hormone (ACTH) occur during delivery.[64] Gonadotropin releasing hormone (GnRH), follicle-stimulating hormone (FSH), and luteinizing hormone (LH) levels are suppressed in pregnancy.

Thyroid hormone metabolism is altered during pregnancy.[65,66] The thyroid gland does not normally change in size. Iodine absorption during pregnancy is improved, although excretion is also increased owing to enhanced GFR. Thyroxine (T_4) is bound by thyroid-binding globulin (85%) and thyroxine-binding prealbumin (15%). Less than 1% of T_4 circulates in the unbound, active form. The increased production of estrogens during pregnancy stimulates an increase in T_4-binding proteins (over twofold), leading to elevated levels of total T_4. Free T_4 levels remain in the normal range, but have been shown to fluctuate.

T_4 production and release is regulated by thyrotropin (TSH), which in turn is under the direct control of thyrotropin-releasing hormone (TRH). TRH is produced in the hypothalamus, released from the pituitary gland, and inhibited via direct feedback by T_4. Elevated levels of human chorionic gonadotropin (hCG) during the first and early second trimesters stimulate the release and production of T_4, which feeds back on the pituitary to decrease the secretion of TSH. This may cause a transient low TSH level. Triiodothyronine (T_3), produced by both the thyroid and peripheral conversion of T_4, is also metabolically active. Two of the three enzymes responsible for converting T_4 to metabolically active T_3 or to inactive reverse T_3 are expressed in the placenta, causing elevated local and peripheral levels of these hormones.

The maternal adrenal cortex plays a significant metabolic role through the production of mineralocorticoids, glucocorticoids, and sex steroids.[64] Aldosterone (mineralocorticoid) is regulated mainly by the renin–angiotensin system. Cortisol (glucocorticoid) levels are elevated during pregnancy. Cortical secretion is normally regulated by hypothalamic CRH and pituitary ACTH. The latter normally feeds back to inhibit CRH production, thereby decreasing cortisol release. In pregnancy, the placenta and fetal membranes both produce CRH, particularly in the third trimester, which circumvents the normal regulatory loop, leading to elevations in circulating cortisol.

Pregnancy requires enhanced absorption of calcium to meet fetal demands. This demand is met by increased synthesis of vitamin D and by physiological hyperparathyroidism.[67,68] Vitamin D is synthesized by the skin and activated by hydroxylation in the kidneys and placenta. Activated vitamin D increases calcium membrane channel activity, which increases transplacental transport to the fetus. Physiological hyperparathyroidism is due to both parathyroid hormone (PTH) and parathyroid hormone-related peptide (PTHrp).[69] PTH levels decline over gestation, but this is compensated for by placental production of PTHrp, which has amino acid homology to PTH and is thus able to stimulate PTH receptors. PTHrp mediates placental calcium transport more than increased synthesis of activated vitamin D.

Reproductive system

Of all maternal physiologic systems, the reproductive system undergoes the most dramatic changes during pregnancy. The uterus can be divided into three functional components, all of which must adapt to the developing fetus: the cervix, the endometrium (decidua), and the myometrium.

Cervix

The cervix performs two opposite functions during pregnancy: it maintains the fetus *in utero* and then dilates with the onset of labor. Cervical biomechanics and biochemistry are less well understood than that of the myometrium, although greater attention has been paid to the cervix in the past decade, since the recognition that early cervical shortening often precedes the increased uterine activity associated with preterm delivery.[70]

The cervix is composed of a cellular component and an extracellular matrix.[71] The latter is composed of many different macromolecules, including collagen (primarily types I and

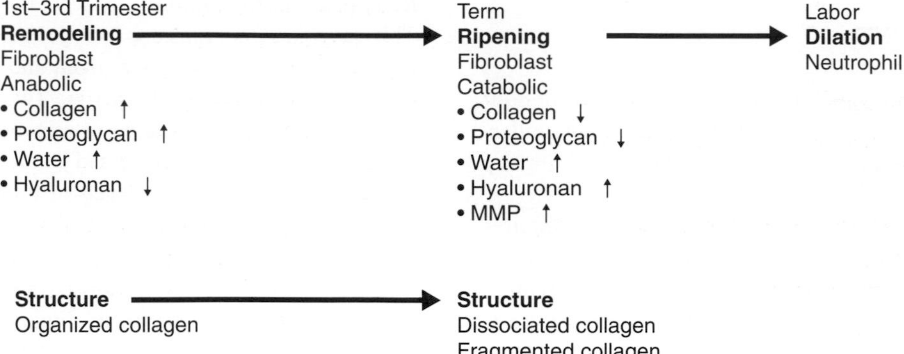

Figure 35.6 The cervix remodels during pregnancy in order to perform its two main functions. The first phase is an anabolic process, which involves an increased production of both collagen and proteoglycans. The increase in cervical size is associated with an increase in water content. The production of hyaluronan is diminished during this phase of remodeling. Imaging of cervical collagen demonstrates a packed and organized structure. As term approaches, the concentration of both collagen and proteoglycans is diminished, which may be due to either decreased production or increased degradation, which are catabolic processes. Increased expression of degradative enzymes has been described including members of the MMP (matrix metalloproteinase) family. Cervical ripening is associated with dissociation and fragmentation of collagen fibers. The degradative enzymes are thought to be produced from fibroblasts prior to the onset of labor and from infiltrating neutrophils with the onset of labor.

III), proteoglycans (decorin and biglycan), glycosaminoglycans (dermatan sulfate, chondroitin sulfate, and heparin sulfate), and the nonsulfated, nonprotein-bound glycosaminoglycan hyaluronate.[72] Throughout gestation, but particularly in the second half of pregnancy, cervical mass increases due to the influence of estrogen, progesterone, and relaxin.[73] The increase in mass results from increases in both the cellular and the extracellular components. Increases in collagen, proteoglycans, glycosaminoglycans, and water have been measured. Smooth muscle cells undergo both hyperplasia and hypertrophy.[74]

Cervical changes during pregnancy can be divided into remodeling and ripening phases (Fig. 35.6).[72] Remodeling is an anabolic process regulated by the hormonal milieu of pregnancy. During this phase, collagen, proteoglycans, and glycosaminoglycans are deposited into the extracellular matrix. An increased deposition of hyaluronate leads to an influx of water that is associated with cervical softening. The alterations in the proportion of collagen, proteoglycans, and glycosaminoglycans are believed to contribute to the progressive decline in cervical tensile strength, as is a gradual decrease in collagen fibril length.[75]

The ripening phase is believed to be a catabolic process in which the extracellular matrix components are degraded.[72] Unlike remodeling, which is affected by steroid hormones, ripening involves release of proteases that degrade collagen and other extracellular matrix components. Elevated levels of prostaglandins, seen with both term and preterm labor, can stimulate the release of extracellular proteases. Marked collagen fragmentation, believed to be important to cervical dilation, occurs during the active phase of labor.[76] Ripening is thought to be an inflammatory process, and is accelerated by infiltration of leukocytes and release of proinflammatory cytokines.[77] Leukocytes such as neutrophils are a rich source of proteases that may contribute to the degradative process. Proinflammatory cytokines such as tumor necrosis factor (TNF)-alpha or interleukin (IL)-8, which induce an inflammatory infiltrate, can induce cervical ripening.[77,78]

Regulation of this process is poorly understood, although a number of pharmacologic and mechanical methods artificially reproduce these changes. For instance, administration of prostaglandin E_2 induces structural changes in the cervix similar to those seen with physiologic ripening.[76]

Progesterone also plays a role in cervical remodeling, but has not been well studied. Progesterone receptor antagonists such as mifepristone (RU-486) also decrease cervical resistance.[79] This is used for cervical ripening in the first and second trimesters. In humans, circulating progesterone levels do not decrease prior to or at the onset of labor; however, a shift in expression of progesterone receptors (from predominantly the B isoform to the A isoform) occurs within the uterus,[80]

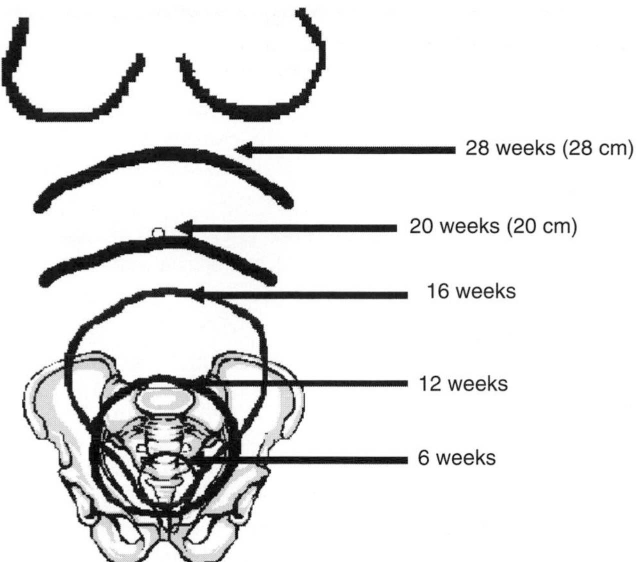

Figure 35.7 The uterus undergoes marked changes during pregnancy, from an organ weighing approximately 60 g to one weighing approximately 1000 g at term. The uterus progressively increases in size from the size of a small pear at 6 weeks, completely filling the pelvis at 12 weeks to reaching the xiphoid at term. The uterus at 16 weeks is midway between the umbilicus and the symphisis pubis, and at the umbilicus at 20 weeks. From 20 weeks until term, fundal height in centimeters, as measured from the symphisis to the top of the uterine fundus, corresponds roughly to the gestational age from the last menstrual period.

possibly simulating progesterone withdrawal, which is seen in other species.

Endometrium (decidua)

The decidua has been poorly studied during pregnancy. It is clear that it plays an important role in anchoring the placenta, is metabolically active, and is critical to the early establishment and continued maintenance of pregnancy. It is infiltrated by maternal leukocytes, which assist in pregnancy maintenance by regulating immune responses. The decidua produces a number of different hormones, including prolactin, relaxin, CRH, and prostaglandin dehydrogenase (prostaglandin-inactivating enzyme).[81]

Myometrium

The myometrium, like the cervix, undergoes marked changes in size during pregnancy, increasing from approximately 60 g in early pregnancy to 1000 g at term.[82] This is primarily due to hypertrophy rather than hyperplasia of smooth muscle. Myometrial cells increase in size from 50–90 μm to 500–800 μm in length. The increase in size appears to be dependent on the presence of both estrogen and progesterone. The uterus remains a pelvic organ until approximately 12 weeks. At this point, the uterus becomes spherical compared with its nonpregnant pear-like shape. The myometrium becomes soft to palpation, probably due to the increase in amniotic fluid within the uterine cavity. The uterus continues to increase in size, reaching the level of the umbilicus at approximately 20 weeks of gestation. A measurement of fundal height (distance from the symphisis pubis to the top of the uterine fundus) in centimeters roughly corresponds to gestational age from this point until term (Fig. 35.7).[83] At term, fundal heights may decline as the fetal head becomes engaged within the maternal pelvis.

To accommodate the increased uterine size as well as the developing fetus, blood flow increases throughout gestation to approximately 500 mL/min by term.[84,85] It is unclear what mechanism is responsible for the increase in uterine blood flow, but it is thought to be secondary to an increase in production of placental hormones. The uterine vessels increase in both diameter and length to accommodate the increase in blood flow. An increase in vasodilating substances such as prostaglandins and nitric oxide within the uterine circulation is believed to contribute to the decrease in vascular tone and increase in uterine blood flow.[86] In addition, the uterine vasculature becomes less responsive to vasoactive substances such as angiotensin.

Although the myometrium readily contracts when stimulated in pregnancy, spontaneous uterine contractions are relatively infrequent, occurring up to two or three times per hour during normal gestation.[87] These uterine contractions are usually appreciated during the third trimester, if not earlier, and are referred to as "Braxton–Hicks" contractions. Low-amplitude irregular bursts of electrical activity can be detected using electromyography and correlate with uterine contractions.[88]

As term approaches, spontaneous activity increases gradually, particularly during the late third trimester. In addition, the uterus becomes significantly more responsive to stimulatory agents. This increase in uterine activity is believed to be due to increased electrical coupling of myometrial cells.[89] Coupling occurs because of channels between cells produced by connexin proteins. These proteins provide low-resistance channels for the passage of ions such as calcium. Animal studies have demonstrated a correlation between increased levels of connexin proteins and increased uterine electrical activity. An increase in a number of other proteins associated with contractile activity has been described in parallel with connexin proteins.[90] This group of proteins, which is necessary for force production, is often referred to as contractile-associated proteins.

In summary, a comprehensive understanding of normal maternal physiologic adaptations to pregnancy is paramount to diagnosing pathologic changes associated with disease states during gestation.

Key points

1. Pregnancy-associated cardiovascular changes seen as early as the first trimester include increases in heart rate and cardiac output, and decreases in vascular tone and blood pressure.
2. Displacement of the maternal heart by the expanding uterus results in predictable chest radiograph and ECG changes.
3. Cardiac output peaks at approximately 32 weeks' gestation owing to increases in both heart rate and stroke volume.
4. Systolic ejection murmurs are common during pregnancy owing to increased cardiac output.
5. Systemic blood pressure normally declines until around 20 weeks' gestation, then gradually increases, but should remain equal to or below nonpregnant values throughout pregnancy.
6. Pulmonary changes in the first trimester include an increase in tidal volume and, therefore, minute ventilation.
7. Respiratory rate does not change during pregnancy.
8. Maternal hyperventilation leads to a slight metabolic alkalosis, with an increase in pH, decrease in PCO_2, decrease in bicarbonate, and an increase in PO_2.
9. Because spirometric parameters should not change during pregnancy, this can be used to evaluate for obstructive and restrictive airway disease.
10. Pregnancy often causes a "physiologic anemia" because plasma volume increases to a greater extent than red blood cell volume.
11. Pregnancy typically does not affect platelet count, although up to 10% of the population may become thrombocytopenic, believed to be secondary to increased platelet activation and consumption.
12. Bleeding time, PT, and PTT are not altered during pregnancy despite marked changes in different coagulation components.
13. An elevated WBC count may be normal during pregnancy because of an increase in circulating granulocytes.
14. The kidney and renal collecting system may increase in size during pregnancy, potentially causing urinary stasis, which may contribute to lower and upper tract infections.
15. The GFR increases during pregnancy and is associated with increased (nonpathologic) glucosuria and decreases in serum creatinine and blood urea nitrogen.
16. The osmotic threshold is altered during pregnancy, reflected by a decrease in plasma osmolality and an increase in fluid retention.
17. Decreased plasma osmolality during pregnancy is reflected by decreases in serum albumin, serum sodium, and blood urea nitrogen.
18. Gastric emptying is delayed during pregnancy, and contributes to benign gastrointestinal complaints as well as an increased risk of aspiration from anesthesia.
19. Diminished esophageal sphincter tone during pregnancy increases the incidence of gastroesophageal reflux.
20. Pregnancy alters some parameters of liver function, including alkaline phosphatase and lipid profile.
21. Decreased TSH and increased total thyroxine may be seen in pregnancy, although free thyroxine levels should not be altered.
22. Cervical remodeling mainly occurs during the second half of pregnancy.
23. Cervical ripening, which decreases tensile strength, is associated with changes in collagen, proteoglycan, and glycosaminoglycan composition.
24. The uterus grows mainly because of uterine myocyte hypertrophy, although hyperplasia also occurs.
25. Blood flow to the uterus consumes approximately 20% of the total cardiac output at term.
26. Increase in uterine activity at term involves expression of contractile-associated proteins and increased electrical coupling.

References

1 Hollander AG, Crawford JH. Roentgenologic and electrocardiographic changes in the normal heart during pregnancy. *Am Heart J* 1943;26:364.

2 Cutforth R, MacDonald CB. Heart sounds and murmurs in pregnancy. *Am Heart J* 1966;71:741–747.

3 Proctor H. Alteration of the cardiac physical examination in normal pregnancy. *Clin Obstet Gynecol* 1975;18:51–63.

4 MacGillivray I, R.G., Rowe B. Blood pressure survey in pregnancy. *Clin Sci* 1969;37:395–407.

5 Wilson M, Morganti AA, Zervoudakis I, et al. Blood pressure, the renin-aldosterone system and sex steroids throughout normal pregnancy. *Am J Med* 1980;68:97–104.

6 Duvekot JJ, Peeters LL. Maternal cardiovascular hemodynamic adaptation to pregnancy. *Obstet Gynecol Surv* 1994; 49(Suppl.):S1–14.

7 Fawer R, Dettling A, Weihs D, et al. Effect of the menstrual cycle, oral contraception and pregnancy on forearm blood flow, venous distensibility and clotting factors. *Eur J Clin Pharmacol* 1978;13:251–257.

8 Schwarz R. Das Verhalten des Kreislaufs in der normalen Schwangershaft. *Arch Gynäkol* 1964;199:549.

9 Robson SC, Hunter S, Boys RJ, Dunlop W. Serial study of factors influencing changes in cardiac output during human pregnancy. *Am J Physiol* 1989;256:H1060–1065.

10 Robson SC, Dunlop W, Moore M, Hunter S. Combined Doppler and echocardiographic measurement of cardiac output: theory and application in pregnancy. *Br J Obstet Gynaecol* 1987;94:1014–1027.

11 Lee W, Rokey R, Cotton DB. Noninvasive maternal stroke volume and cardiac output determinations by pulsed Doppler echocardiography. *Am J Obstet Gynecol* 1988;158:505–510.

12 Metcalf J, Ueland K. Maternal cardiovascular adjustments to pregnancy. *Prog Cardiovasc Dis* 1974;16:363–374.

13 Kerr MG. The mechanical effects of the gravid uterus in late pregnancy. *J Obstet Gynaecol Br Commonw* 1965;72:513–529.

14 Quilligan EJ, Tyler C. Postural effects on the cardiovascular status in pregnancy: a comparison of the lateral and supine postures. *Am J Obstet Gynecol* 1959;78:465–471.

15 Emerson K, Jr, Saxena BN, Poindexter EL. Caloric cost of normal pregnancy. *Obstet Gynecol* 1972;40:786–794.

16 Pernoll ML, Metcalfe J, Schlenker TL, et al. Oxygen consumption at rest and during exercise in pregnancy. *Respir Physiol* 1975;25:285–293.

17 Milne JA. The respiratory response to pregnancy. *Postgrad Med J* 1979;55:318–324.

18 Cugell DW, Frank NR, Gaensler EA, Badger TL. Pulmonary function in pregnancy. I. Serial observations in normal women. *Am Rev Tuberc* 1953;67:568–597.

19 Lehmann V, Fabel H. [Investigations of respiratory function in pregnancy. II. Ventilation, mechanics of respiration and diffusion-capacity (author's transl)]. *Z Geburtshilfe Perinatol* 1973;177:397–410.

20 Awe RJ, Nicotra MB, Newsom TD, Viles R. Arterial oxygenation and alveolar–arterial gradients in term pregnancy. *Obstet Gynecol* 1979;53:182–186.

21 Baldwin GR, Moorthi DS, Whelton JA, MacDonnell KF. New lung functions and pregnancy. *Am J Obstet Gynecol* 1977;127:235–239.

22 Gilroy RJ, Mangura BT, Lavietes MH. Rib cage and abdominal volume displacements during breathing in pregnancy. *Am Rev Respir Dis* 1988;137:668–672.

23 Weinberger SE, Weiss ST, Cohen WR, et al. Pregnancy and the lung. *Am Rev Respir Dis* 1980;121:559–581.

24 Pritchard JA. Changes in the blood volume during pregnancy and delivery. *Anesthesiology* 1965;26:393–399.

25 Lund CJ, Donovan JC. Blood volume during pregnancy. Significance of plasma and red cell volumes. *Am J Obstet Gynecol* 1967;98:394–403.

26 Rovinsky JJ, Jaffin H. Cardiovascular hemodynamics in pregnancy. I. Blood and plasma volumes in multiple pregnancy. *Am J Obstet Gynecol* 1965;93:1–15.

27 Fay RA, Hughes AO, Farron NT. Platelets in pregnancy: hyperdestruction in pregnancy. *Obstet Gynecol* 1983;61:238–240.

28 Schwartz KA. Gestational thrombocytopenia and immune thrombocytopenias in pregnancy. *Hematol Oncol Clin North Am* 2000;14:1101–1116.

29 Clark P. Changes of hemostasis variables during pregnancy. *Semin Vasc Med* 2003;3:13–24.

30 Djelmis J, Ivanisevic M, Kurjak A, Mayer D. Hemostatic problems before, during and after delivery. *J Perinat Med* 2001;29:241–246.

31 Gall SA. Maternal adjustments in the immune system in normal pregnancy. *Clin Obstet Gynecol* 1983;26:521–536.

32 Weetman AP. The immunology of pregnancy. *Thyroid* 1999;9:643–646.

33 Szekeres-Bartho J. Immunological relationship between the mother and the fetus. *Int Rev Immunol* 2002;21:471–495.

34 Laird SM, Tuckerman EM, Cork BA, et al. A review of immune cells and molecules in women with recurrent miscarriage. *Hum Reprod Update* 2003;9:163–174.

35 Cunningham FG, Cox SM, Harstad TW, et al. Chronic renal disease and pregnancy outcome. *Am J Obstet Gynecol* 1990;163:453–459.

36 Lindheimer MD, Davidson M. Renal disorders. In: Barron L, Lindheimer MD, eds. *Medical disorders during pregnancy*. Chicago: Mosby; 1991:42–72.

37 Marchant DJ. Effects of pregnancy and progestational agents on the urinary tract. *Am J Obstet Gynecol* 1972;112:487–501.

38 Rasmussen PE, Nielsen FR. Hydronephrosis during pregnancy: a literature survey. *Eur J Obstet Gynecol Reprod Biol* 1988;27:249–259.

39 Schulman A, Herlinger H. Urinary tract dilatation in pregnancy. *Br J Radiol* 1975;48:638–645.

40 Fried AM, Woodring JH, Thompson DJ. Hydronephrosis of pregnancy: a prospective sequential study of the course of dilatation. *J Ultrasound Med* 1983;2:255–259.

41 Baylis C. Impact of pregnancy on underlying renal disease. *Adv Ren Replace Ther* 2003;10:31–39.

42 Baylis C. Glomerular filtration rate in normal and abnormal pregnancies. *Semin Nephrol* 1999;19:133–139.

43 Dunlop W, Davison JM. Renal haemodynamics and tubular function in human pregnancy. *Baillieres Clin Obstet Gynaecol* 1987;1:769–787.

44 Bishop JH, Green R. Effects of pregnancy on glucose reabsorption by the proximal convoluted tubule in the rat. *J Physiol* 1981;319:271–285.

45 Davison JM, Lovedale C. The excretion of glucose during normal pregnancy and after delivery. *J Obstet Gynaecol Br Commonw* 1974;81:30–34.

46 Dunlop W, Davison JM. The effect of normal pregnancy upon the renal handling of uric acid. *Br J Obstet Gynaecol* 1977;84:13–21.

47 Davison JM, Vallotton MB, Lindheimer MD. Plasma osmolality and urinary concentration and dilution during and after pregnancy: evidence that lateral recumbency inhibits maximal urinary concentrating ability. *Br J Obstet Gynaecol* 1981;88:472–479.

48 Davison JM. Edema in pregnancy. *Kidney Int* 1997;59(Suppl.):S90–96.

49 Nagler R, Spiro HM. Heartburn in pregnancy. *Am J Dig Dis* 1962;7:648–655.

50 Olans LB, Wolf JL. Gastroesophageal reflux in pregnancy. *Gastrointest Endosc Clin North Am* 1994;4:699–712.

51 Simpson KH, Stakes AF, Miller M. Pregnancy delays paracetamol absorption and gastric emptying in patients undergoing surgery. *Br J Anaesth* 1988;60:24–27.

52 Lawson M, Kern F, Jr, Everson GT. Gastrointestinal transit time in human pregnancy: prolongation in the second and third trimesters followed by postpartum normalization. *Gastroenterology* 1985;89:996–999.

53 Combes B, Shibata H, Adams R, et al. Alterations in sulfobromophthalein sodium-removal mechanisms from blood during normal pregnancy. *J Clin Invest* 1963;42:1431–1442.

54 Kaplan MM. Alkaline phosphatase. *N Engl J Med* 1972;286:200–202.

55 Cerutti R, Ferrari S, Grella P. Behaviour of serum enzymes in pregnancy. *Clin Exp Obstet Gynecol* 1976;3:22.

56 Honger PE. Albumin metabolism in normal pregnancy. *Scand J Clin Lab Invest* 1968;21:3–9.
57 Herrera E. Lipid metabolism in pregnancy and its consequences in the fetus and newborn. *Endocrine* 2002;19:43–55.
58 O'Sullivan GM, Bullingham RE. The assessment of gastric acidity and antacid effect in pregnant women by a non-invasive radiotelemetry technique. *Br J Obstet Gynaecol* 1984;91: 973–978.
59 Reece EA, Sivan E, Francis G, Homko CJ. Pregnancy outcomes among women with and without diabetic microvascular disease (White's classes B to FR) versus non-diabetic controls. *Am J Perinatol* 1998;15:549–555.
60 Phelps RL, Metzger BE, Freinkel N. Carbohydrate metabolism in pregnancy. XVII. Diurnal profiles of plasma glucose, insulin, free fatty acids, triglycerides, cholesterol, and individual amino acids in late normal pregnancy. *Am J Obstet Gynecol* 1981;140: 730–736.
61 Lind T, Billewicz WZ, Brown G. A serial study of changes occurring in the oral glucose tolerance test during pregnancy. *J Obstet Gynaecol Br Commonw* 1973;80:1033–1039.
62 Goluboff LG, Ezrin C. Effect of pregnancy on the somatotroph and the prolactin cell of the human adenohypophysis. *J Clin Endocrinol Metab* 1969;29:1533–1538.
63 Rigg LA, Lein A, Yen SS. Pattern of increase in circulating prolactin levels during human gestation. *Am J Obstet Gynecol* 1977;129:454–456.
64 Mastorakos G, Ilias I. Maternal and fetal hypothalamic–pituitary–adrenal axes during pregnancy and postpartum. *Ann NY Acad Sci* 2003;997:136–149.
65 Glinoer D. What happens to the normal thyroid during pregnancy? *Thyroid* 1999;9:631–635.
66 Fantz CR, Dagogo-Jack S, Ladenson JH, Gronowski AM. Thyroid function during pregnancy. *Clin Chem* 1999;45:2250–2258.
67 Steichen JJ, Tsang RC, Gratton TL, et al. Vitamin D homeostasis in the perinatal period: 1,25-dihydroxyvitamin D in maternal, cord, and neonatal blood. *N Engl J Med* 1980;302:315–319.
68 Kumar R, Cohen WR, Epstein FH. Vitamin D and calcium hormones in pregnancy. *N Engl J Med* 1980;302:1143–1145.
69 Rouffet J, Barlet JP. [Parathyroid hormone related peptide (PTHrP) and bone metabolism]. *Arch Physiol Biochem* 1995;103: 3–13.
70 Welsh A, Nicolaides K. Cervical screening for preterm delivery. *Curr Opin Obstet Gynecol* 2002;14:195–202.
71 Uldbjerg N, Ulmsten U. The physiology of cervical ripening and cervical dilatation and the effect of abortifacient drugs. *Baillieres Clin Obstet Gynaecol* 1990;4:263–282.
72 Winkler M, Rath W. Changes in the cervical extracellular matrix during pregnancy and parturition. *J Perinat Med* 1999;27:45–60.
73 Too CK, Kong JK, Greenwood FC, Bryant-Greenwood GD. The effect of oestrogen and relaxin on uterine and cervical enzymes: collagenase, proteoglycanase and beta-glycuronidase. *Acta Endocrinol (Copenh)* 1986;111:394–403.
74 Winn RJ, Baker MD, Merle CA, Sherwood OD. Individual and combined effects of relaxin, estrogen, and progesterone in ovariectomized gilts. II. Effects on mammary development. *Endocrinology* 1994;135:1250–1255.
75 Yu SY, Tozzi CA, Barbiarz J, Leppert PC. Collagen changes in rat cervix in pregnancy – polarized light microscopic and electron microscopic studies. *Proc Soc Exp Biol Med* 1995;209:360–368.
76 Rath W, Osmers R, Adelmann-Grill BC, et al. Biochemical changes in human cervical connective tissue after intracervical application of prostaglandin E2. *Prostaglandins* 1993;45:375–384.
77 Osmers RG, Blaser J, Kuhn W, Tschesche H. Interleukin-8 synthesis and the onset of labor. *Obstet Gynecol* 1995;86:223–229.
78 Watari M, Watari H, DiSanto ME, et al. Pro-inflammatory cytokines induce expression of matrix-metabolizing enzymes in human cervical smooth muscle cells. *Am J Pathol* 1999;154:1755–1762.
79 Gupta JK, Johnson N. Should we use prostaglandins, tents or progesterone antagonists for cervical ripening before first trimester abortion? *Contraception* 1992;46:489–497.
80 Brown AG, Leite RS, Strauss JF, III. Mechanisms underlying "functional" progesterone withdrawal at parturition. *Ann NY Acad Sci* 2004;1034:36–49.
81 Johnson RF, Mitchell CM, Clifton V, et al. Regulation of 15-hydroxyprostaglandin dehydrogenase (PGDH) gene activity, messenger ribonucleic acid processing, and protein abundance in the human chorion in late gestation and labor. *J Clin Endocrinol Metab* 2004;89:5639–5648.
82 Reynolds S. *Physiology of the uterus*. New York: Hafner Publishing, 1965.
83 Jimenez JM, Tyson JE, Reisch JS. Clinical measures of gestational age in normal pregnancies. *Obstet Gynecol* 1983;61:438–443.
84 Metcalfe J, Romney SL, Ramsey LH, et al. Estimation of uterine blood flow in normal human pregnancy at term. *J Clin Invest* 1955;34:1632–1638.
85 Rekonen A, Luotola H, Pitkanen M, et al. Measurement of intervillous and myometrial blood flow by an intravenous 133Xe method. *Br J Obstet Gynaecol* 1976;83:723–728.
86 Carbillon L, Uzan M, Uzan S. Pregnancy, vascular tone, and maternal hemodynamics: a crucial adaptation. *Obstet Gynecol Surv* 2000;55:574–581.
87 Moore TR, Iams JD, Creasy RK, et al. Diurnal and gestational patterns of uterine activity in normal human pregnancy. The Uterine Activity in Pregnancy Working Group. *Obstet Gynecol* 1994;83:517–523.
88 Maul H, Maner WL, Saade GR. The physiology of uterine contractions. *Clin Perinatol* 2003;30:665–676.
89 Lye SJ, Ou CW, Teoh TG, et al. The molecular basis of labour and tocolysis. *Fetal Maternal Med Rev* 1998;10:121–136.
90 Chow L, Lye SJ. Expression of the gap junction protein connexin-43 is increased in the human myometrium toward term and with the onset of labor. *Am J Obstet Gynecol* 1994;170:788–795.

36 Maternal nutrition

Barbara Luke

Nutrition in maternity has experienced a renaissance in recent years, with increasing evidence linking alterations in both fetal growth and maternal health with subsequent metabolic and vascular disease.[1–8] For the developing fetus, altered nutrition *in utero* may result in developmental adaptations that permanently change structure, physiology, and metabolism, favoring fetal survival, but with metabolic and vascular disease consequences in adulthood. For the mother, pregnancy complications such as gestational diabetes, preeclampsia, intrauterine growth restriction, and preterm delivery, and subsequent metabolic and vascular disease may share common underlying disease mechanisms. Maternal nutrition, therefore, plays a central role in the immediate and long-term health of the mother and her child. This chapter presents an overview of current knowledge in this area. The *Guidelines for perinatal care* (5th edn, 2002)[9] acknowledge that nutrition counseling is an integral component of perinatal care, and that it is most effectively accomplished by referral to a nutritionist or registered dietitian. Their recommendations, which are issued jointly by the American Academy of Pediatrics and the American College of Obstetricians and Gynecologists, cover preconception care, nutrition in pregnancy, postpartum guidelines, and neonatal nutrition.

Diet during pregnancy

Both the quality and the quantity of the diet during pregnancy critically influence the health of the mother and her unborn child.[10] Energy and nutrient requirements increase during pregnancy to insure appropriate maternal adaptation to pregnancy and optimal fetal growth. In singleton pregnancies, the daily caloric requirement is approximately 27–30 kcal/kg maternal prepregnancy weight during the first trimester, and 30 kcal/kg maternal prepregnancy weight plus 200–300 kcal during the second and third trimesters. In underweight women, these caloric prescriptions would need to be adjusted upward. The recommended caloric distribution of macronutrients during pregnancy is the same as for all healthy adults: 20% of kcal from protein, 30–35% of kcal from fat, and the remainder (45–50% of kcal) from carbohydrates. A summary of recommended dietary allowances (RDAs) and dietary reference intakes from the Food and Nutrition Board, the Institute of Medicine (IOM), is given in Table 36.1.

Use of vitamin–mineral supplements

Ideally, pregnant women should get the level and range of required nutrients through a balanced diet. However, in order to insure the adequate intake of prenatal vitamins, it is recommended that all pregnant women take prenatal vitamins daily throughout the course of pregnancy. Recent national dietary surveys indicate that adult women fail to meet the RDAs for five nutrients: calcium, magnesium, zinc, and vitamins E and B_6.[11] In addition, prenatal use of vitamin–mineral supplements among low-income women has been shown to reduce the risks of preterm delivery and low birthweight, particularly if initiated during the first trimester.[12] Data from national surveys indicate that the majority of Americans, including half to two-thirds of women of childbearing age, take some form of vitamin–mineral supplements.[13–15] Vitamin–mineral supplement use is more common among women than men, among individuals with one or more health problems, and among older individuals.[13]

Supplementation in excess of twice the RDA (see Table 36.1) should be avoided, because of the potential for birth defects. The fat-soluble vitamins, particularly vitamins A and D, are the most potentially toxic during pregnancy. The pediatric and obstetric literature includes case reports of kidney malformations in children whose mothers took between 40 000 and 50 000 IU of vitamin A during pregnancy. Even at lower doses, excessive amounts of vitamin A may cause subtle damage to the developing nervous system, resulting in serious behavioral and learning disabilities in later life. The margin of safety for vitamin D is smaller than for any other. Birth defects of the heart, particularly aortic stenosis, have been reported in both humans and experimental animals with

Table 36.1 Summary of recommended dietary allowances and dietary reference intakes for nonpregnant, pregnant, and lactating women aged 1–50 years.

Nutrient	Nonpregnant 19–30 years	Nonpregnant 31–50 years	Pregnancy	Lactation (first 6 months)	Food sources
Folate	400 mcg	400 mcg	600 mcg	500 mcg	Liver, green leafy vegetables, enriched cereals, oranges
Thiamin	1.1 mg	1.1 mg	1.4 mg	1.5 mg	Meats, poultry, pork, beans, enriched cereals and breads
Riboflavin	1.1 mg	1.1 mg	1.4 mg	1.6 mg	Dairy products, meats, liver, eggs, enriched cereals
Niacin	14 mg	14 mg	18 mg	17 mg	Meats, poultry, fish, nuts, legumes, enriched cereals
Vitamin A	800 mcg	800 mcg	800 mcg	1300 mcg	Dark green, yellow, or orange fruits and vegetables, liver
Vitamin B6	1.3 mg	1.3 mg	1.9 mg	2.0 mg	Meats, liver, poultry, fish, nuts, legumes, enriched cereals
Vitamin B12	2.4 mcg	2.4 mcg	2.6 mcg	2.8 mcg	Meats, liver, poultry, eggs, fish, dairy products
Vitamin C	60 mg	60 mg	70 mg	95 mg	Citrus fruits, tomatoes, green leafy vegetables
Vitamin D*	5 mcg	5 mcg	5 mcg	5 mcg	Fortified dairy products
Vitamin E	8 mg α-TE	8 mg α-TE	10 mg α-TE	12 mg α-TE	Vegetable oils, seeds, and cereal grains
Calcium	1000 mg	1000 mg	1000 mg	1000 mg	Dairy products, salmon
Iron	15 mg	15 mg	30 mg	15 mg	Meats, liver, eggs, enriched and whole grains
Magnesium	310 mg	320 mg	350 mg	310 mg	Whole grains, legumes, nuts, green vegetables
Phosphorus	700 mg	700 mg	700 mg	700 mg	Meats, poultry, eggs, pork, fish, dairy products
Zinc	12 mg	12 mg	15 mg	19 mg	Meats, pork, seafood, eggs, legumes
Energy	2200 kcal	2200 kcal	2500 kcal	2700 kcal	Proteins, fats, and carbohydrates
Protein	50 g	50 g	60 g	65 g	Meats, poultry, eggs, fish, and dairy products

Adapted from the National Academy of Sciences, Food and Nutrition Board. Recommended Dietary Allowances, 10th edn, 1989; and Dietary Reference Intakes, 1998.

*As cholecalciferol, 1 mcg = 40 IU of vitamin D.

doses as low as 4000 IU, which is 10 times the RDA during pregnancy.

Maternal iron status

There are no absolute requirements for routine dietary supplementation, with the possible exception of iron. In instances in which inadequacies cannot be remedied through diet, or if a woman has unique nutritional requirements, such as multiple gestation, diagnoses of hemoglobinopathies or seizure disorders, or other circumstances, daily supplementation may be the most reasonable alternative. The IOM 1990 report[16] recommended daily iron supplementation with 30 mg/day during the second and third trimesters, as prophylaxis for iron deficiency. The treatment of iron-deficiency anemia requires daily doses of 60–120 mg of elemental iron, to be taken between meals or at bedtime to facilitate absorption. Iron should not be taken as part of a vitamin–mineral supplement, on account of inhibition by other minerals, as well as poor iron release.[17] To minimize their side-effects, iron supplements should be taken with a nondairy snack.

Iron-deficiency anemia is significantly associated with low birthweight (LBW), preterm delivery, and inadequate maternal weight gain. In a study of adolescent and young gravidas, iron-deficiency anemia (based on the Centers for Disease Control criteria of hemoglobin values < 11.0 g/dL for the first and third trimesters and < 10.5 g/dL for the second trimester) was significantly associated with inadequate maternal weight gain [adjusted odds ratio (AOR) 2.67, 95% confidence interval (CI) 1.13 to 6.30], preterm delivery (AOR 2.66, 95% CI 1.15 to 6.17), and LBW (AOR 3.10, 95% CI 1.16 to 4.39).[18] Iron-deficiency anemia during the second trimester of pregnancy has also been significantly associated with preterm delivery (AOR 4.3, 95% CI 1.2 to 15.5), particularly among black women (AOR 1.9, 95% CI 1.5 to 2.3).[19]

Iron-deficiency anemia, as measured at 16–18 weeks (second trimester) and at 25–32 weeks (third trimester), is significantly associated with preterm delivery, with increased risks with ORs ranging from 2.7 to 4.3 and 1.8 to 3.5, respectively, depending on the age and racial composition of the study populations.[18–21] Serum ferritin levels, which are elevated in the presence of infection and lowered with iron deficiency, have also been linked to prematurity. Extremes of maternal serum ferritin, measured early in the second trimester (15–17 weeks), as well as elevated levels at 24, 26, or 28 weeks have been associated with preterm birth.[22–26] Recently, it has been shown that, when elevated third-trimester serum ferritin levels show a failure to decline, they are significantly associated with preterm and very preterm birth (AOR 8.77, 95% CI 3.9 to 19.7 and AOR 3.81, 95% CI 1.93 to 7.52 respectively), with iron-deficiency anemia and poor maternal nutritional status underlying the relationship.[26]

Iron status during pregnancy has also been linked to fetal programming and the development of chronic disease. Low maternal hemoglobin is strongly related to the development of a large placenta and high placental–birthweight ratio, which is seen as predictive of long-term programming of hypertension and cardiovascular disease. Severe maternal iron-deficiency anemia leads to placental adaptive hypertrophy, a fall in the cortisol metabolizing system, and increased susceptibility to hypertension in later life. Because the iron demands of pregnancy may exceed 1 g, with nearly half this amount in the red cell mass increase in blood volume, the maternal preconceptional and early pregnancy iron status is extremely important.

Mineral intake and supplementation

In addition to being the nutrients most often lacking in women's diets, calcium, magnesium, and zinc have been identified as having the most potential for reducing pregnancy complications and improving outcomes.[11,27–29] A recent review by the World Health Organization concluded that these nutrients "be rigorously evaluated as these . . . substances may have effects on both impaired fetal growth and preterm delivery."[27]

Calcium

During pregnancy, there is an increased physiologic demand for calcium such that a full-term infant accretes about 30 g, primarily in the third trimester, when there is active ossification of the fetal skeleton. Prenatal diets low in calcium have been associated with increased blood pressure because of heightened smooth muscle reactivity, resulting in an increased risk of pregnancy-induced hypertension and preterm delivery. Nearly all calcium supplementation trials have been shown to lower blood pressure levels.[30–35]

Results of calcium supplementation trials among high-risk women have been promising, with significant reductions in preterm deliveries among teenagers (7.4% versus 21.1%, $P < 0.007$) and significantly longer mean gestations among women with very low dietary calcium intakes (37.4 versus 39.2 weeks, $P < 0.01$).[30,31,34] Other studies have shown inconsistent results in lowering the rates of pregnancy-induced hypertension, or no effect on preterm delivery and small for gestational age births.[32,35] Calcium supplementation trials among high-risk women (teenagers in Baltimore and women with very low calcium intakes in Quito, Ecuador) were promising in decreasing the rate of preterm delivery. Among teenagers (aged 16 years) in Baltimore, with similar overall dietary calcium intakes, the calcium-supplemented group had a lower incidence of preterm delivery than the placebo group (7.4% versus 21.1%, $P < 0.007$).[30] Life-table analysis demonstrated an overall shift to a higher gestational age in the calcium-supplemented group. In Ecuador, length of gestation was increased from 37.4 to 39.2 weeks for the calcium-supplemented group versus the placebo group.[31,34] On the other hand, a large calcium supplementation trial of over 1000 adult women from Argentina showed a decrease in pregnancy-induced hypertension, but no effect on preterm delivery,[32] and a recent multicenter trial of calcium supplementation in the United States with more than 4500 adult women showed no difference in pregnancy-induced hypertension, preterm deliveries, or small for gestational age births.[35] The ability of supplemental calcium to decrease the risk of preterm delivery may be confined to high-risk populations where there is either a severe dietary restriction of calcium or, as in the case of adolescents and multiple pregnancy, an increased demand for this nutrient.

Prenatal calcium supplementation may have more far-reaching effects, beyond pregnancy. Belizàn et al.[36] evaluated blood pressure in 7-year-old children whose mothers had received calcium supplementation during pregnancy. They reported significantly lower systolic blood pressure and lower risk of high systolic blood pressure [relative risk (RR) 0.59, 95% CI 0.39 to 0.90], particularly among children in the highest quartile of body mass index [BMI, weight/(height)^2], (RR 0.43, 95% CI 0.26 to 0.71).

Magnesium

Magnesium supplementation trials have also reported inconsistent results.[37–39] These inconsistencies may have been due to differences in study design, study populations, and the concurrent use of other medications such as β-sympathomimetic agents.[39] Recent studies have demonstrated that magnesium is not only effective as therapy for and prophylaxis against eclampsia, but is safe and potentially beneficial for the neonate.[40,41] In a case–control study examining the risk of cerebral palsy in premature infants exposed to magnesium *in utero*, Nelson and Grether[42] reported a protective effect (OR 0.14, 95% CI 0.05 to 0.51), regardless of whether the magnesium had been given for preeclampsia or as treatment for preterm labor. In a population-based cohort study of prenatal magnesium exposure among children who had very LBW, Schendel et al.[43] also reported a protective effect against cerebral palsy (OR 0.11, 95% CI 0.02 to 0.81), and possibly against mental retardation (OR 0.30, 95% CI 0.07 to 1.29). Recent analyses indicate that reduced long-term morbidity with prenatal magnesium exposure is unlikely because of selective mortality of vulnerable infants.[44] Magnesium therapy, as prenatal supplementation or as therapy for preeclampsia or preterm labor, may play a neuroprotective role.

Maternal zinc status

During pregnancy, plasma zinc concentrations decline by 20–30% compared with nonpregnant values, reflecting the transfer of zinc from mother to fetus and the normal expansion of the maternal plasma volume. Plasma zinc concentrations and available zinc intakes are significantly correlated, with zinc supplementation increasing maternal plasma levels.[45] Using plasma zinc as an indicator of zinc status, Neggers et al.[45] found a positive correlation between duration of gestation and zinc concentration at entry to prenatal care. A recent randomized trial of zinc supplementation of women with plasma zinc levels below the median showed that zinc supplementation resulted in an increase in gestation duration by approximately 0.5 weeks and an increase in birthweight.[46] Plasma zinc levels in the lowest quartiles are associated with significantly greater frequency of maternal complications, including infection.[47,48] Maternal zinc nutriture, as a composite index of zinc measured from maternal whole blood, hair, and colostrum, has been shown to be related to the risk of premature rupture of membranes (PROM).[48] Women with PROM were found to have significantly lower levels of zinc compared with women who gave birth at term.

Scholl et al.[49] evaluated the association between dietary zinc intake and pregnancy outcome in a cohort of 818 low-income, mostly minority women in Camden, NJ, USA. A low zinc intake during pregnancy (< 6 mg/day or < 40% of the RDA for pregnancy) was associated with an increased incidence of iron-deficiency anemia at entry to care, a lower use of prenatal supplements during pregnancy, and a higher incidence of inadequate weight gain during pregnancy. Even after adjusting for other confounding variables (e.g., energy intake, maternal age, ethnicity, cigarette smoking), a low dietary intake of zinc was associated with a twofold increase in the risk of LBW (AOR 2.10, 95% CI 1.19 to 3.67), a nearly twofold increase in preterm delivery (AOR 1.86, 95% CI 1.11 to 3.09), and a threefold increased risk of early preterm birth (< 33 weeks' gestation) (AOR 3.46, 95% CI 1.04 to 11.47). In addition, there was a joint effect of iron-deficiency anemia at entry to care and a low zinc intake during pregnancy. When both were present, there was a fivefold increased risk of preterm delivery (AOR 5.44, 95% CI 1.58 to 18.79).

Although maternal zinc nutriture has been significantly related to length of gestation, infection, and risk of premature rupture of membranes,[45,47,48] clinical trials of zinc supplementation have yielded equivocal results.[50,51] A clinical trial that randomly supplemented only women with plasma zinc levels below the median reported an increase in length of gestation of approximately 0.5 weeks ($P = 0.06$), and an increase in birthweight, about half of which was explained by the longer duration of gestation.[46] Consistent with prior results, effects were increased for nonobese women (pregravid BMI < 26.0). Studies of prenatal zinc supplementation have reported an improvement in fetal neurobehavioral development.[52]

Maternal pregravid weight and gestational weight gain

The factors most strongly correlated with both length of gestation and birthweight are maternal height, pregravid or early pregnancy body weight, maternal fat deposition, and gestational weight gain. Although each factor independently influences birthweight and length of gestation, their effects are neither equal nor additive. The landmark studies in this area are from the Collaborative Perinatal Project, which was conducted between 1959 and 1964.[53–56] Based on term singleton pregnancies, these studies demonstrated that: (1) a progressive increase in weight gain was paralleled by an increase in mean birthweight and a decline in the incidence of LBW; (2) increasing pregravid weight diminishes the effect of weight gain on birthweight; (3) there is an inverse relationship between weight gain and perinatal mortality, with gains up to 30 pounds (13.6 kg); and (4) higher gestational weight gains are related to higher birthweights and better growth and development during the first postnatal year. As a result of these and subsequent studies, in 1990, the IOM issued pregravid BMI-specific weight gain guidelines for singleton pregnancies (Table 36.2).[16] Many investigators have subsequently confirmed these

Table 36.2 Institute of Medicine (IOM) categories of pregravid body mass index (BMI) and suggested weight gain ranges for singleton pregnancies.

Weight status	BMI range (kg/m^2)	Total gain at 40 weeks	Weight gain at trimester 1	Rate of gain at trimesters 2 and 3
Underweight	< 19.8 kg/m^2	12.5–18.0 kg (28–40 lb)	2.3 kg (5.1 lb)	0.49 kg/week (1 lb/week)
Normal weight	19.8–26.0 kg/m^2	11.5–16.0 kg (25–35 lb)	1.6 kg 0.44 kg/week (3.5 lb)	(1 lb/week)
Overweight	26.1–29.0 kg/m^2	7.0–11.5 kg (15–25 lb)	0.9 kg 0.30 kg/week (2.0 lb)	(0.5–0.75 lb/week)
Obese	> 29.0 kg/m^2	≥ 6.8 kg (≥ 15 lb)	No recommendation	

associations, including the link between low prepregnancy weight and both prematurity and intrauterine growth retardation (IUGR), with reported increased risks ranging from 1.7 to 3.0, depending on the study population.[57] The population-attributable risk for early preterm birth (< 32 weeks) with low prepregnancy weight is as much as 31–43%, depending on race and ethnicity.[58] Low maternal weight gain has also been significantly associated with both IUGR and preterm birth, with reported risks with ORs in the range of 2.1–4.3.[16,59–63] Significant interaction has also been documented between low pregravid weight and low weight gain on the risk of preterm birth (AOR 5.63, 95% CI 2.35 to 13.8).[61]

Pattern of weight gain

Although cumulative or total weight gain is an important predictor of birthweight, the pattern of weight gain and rates of gain also play significant roles in modifying birthweight and predicting preterm delivery.[64,65] Hediger et al.[64] demonstrated that both early gains (before 24 weeks' gestation) and later weight gains (after 24 weeks) have independent effects on the outcome of singleton births. In a multiracial sample of 1790 teenagers from Camden County, NJ, USA, early inadequate weight gain (< 4.3 kg by 24 weeks) was associated with an increased risk of small for gestational age outcomes (SGA, < 10th percentile for gestation) (AOR 2.08, 95% CI 1.31 to 3.30).[64] Even if there were compensatory gains after 24 weeks, bringing the cumulative total gain up to levels deemed adequate, the risk of an SGA birth was still increased (AOR 1.88, 95% CI 1.08 to 3.27). This strongly suggests that early weight gains, which presumably reflect gains in maternal nutrient stores, are important in enhancing fetal growth, whether by serving as a nutrient reserve later in pregnancy or as a marker for adequate placental growth and development. In these studies, preterm delivery (< 37 weeks) was relatively unaffected by early inadequate weight gain, but was increased with late inadequate weight gain (< 400 g/week). Again, this occurred even when the total pregnancy weight gain never fell below the targets set in clinical standards (AOR 1.69, 95% CI 1.12 to 2.55).[64]

Changes in maternal body fat

A substantial portion of gestational weight gain is maternal body fat, which, when measured as the triceps skinfold thickness or mid-upper arm circumference (MUAC), increases in the first two trimesters and decreases in the third, reflecting the early accretion of maternal body fat and the subsequent utilization in late gestation to meet increasing energy needs. The components of maternal weight gain, particularly changes in body fat, may be more important determinants of pregnancy outcome than absolute weight gain. Prior studies of well-nourished women, based on deuterium oxide and underwater weighing[66–69] as well as anthropometric measures,[70–72] have reported a pattern of small gains in maternal body fat early in pregnancy, rapid accumulation between 20 and 30 weeks' gestation, and a leveling off between 30 weeks and delivery. A consistent finding in studies with diverse ethnic and racial groups is the correlation between triceps skinfold or MUAC measures during the second trimester and birthweight, with the loss of upper arm fat or the failure to accrue maternal fat during the second trimester associated with poor fetal growth and subsequent lower birthweights.[70–74]

Examining the components of weight gain in pregnancy, Hediger et al.[75] demonstrated that, for teenagers and adults whose pregravid weights were above the 25th percentile for age, the loss of subcutaneous fat (> 6.4 cm^2) from 28 weeks through 4–6 weeks postpartum (measured at the mid-upper arm) was associated with a higher birthweight (+ 144 g, $P < 0.01$). At the same time, there appeared to be a mobilization of fat stores; there was an increase in arm muscle area. However, when pregravid weight was below the 25th percentile for age, a loss of upper arm fat was associated instead with a lower birthweight (–339 g, $P < 0.01$), suggesting that the nutrient stores of these women may have been relatively depleted. Continued weight gain and increases in upper arm fat area (> 5 cm^2), accompanied by a loss of upper arm muscle, was also associated with a lower birthweight (–123 g, $P < 0.02$). Thus, a change in upper arm fat is a significant predictor of variation in infant birthweight, and serial monitoring by arm anthropometry, as well as maternal weight, may help to determine risk for IUGR.

Postpartum weight retention

Gestational weight gain is the single most important factor influencing postpartum weight retention, a finding consistent throughout the medical literature. The challenge with pregnancy weight gain is to have an optimal balance. That is, sufficient gain for good fetal growth, but low enough to avoid postpartum weight retention. Li et al.[76] have shown that each kilogram of maternal weight gain in the second and third trimester was associated with significant increases in birthweight of 62 g ($P < 0.001$) and 26 g ($P < 0.05$) respectively. Each kilogram of maternal weight gain during midpregnancy (but not late pregnancy) was also associated with significant increases in birth length of 0.24 cm ($P < 0.01$) and head circumference of 0.14 cm ($P < 0.001$). Brown et al.[77] reported that each kilogram of maternal weight gain in the first and second trimesters significantly increased birthweight by 31 g ($P < 0.0007$) and 26 g ($P < 0.0007$), but maternal gain in the third trimester had a minimal and nonsignificant effect (7 g, $P = 0.40$). These researchers also reported that, per kilogram of maternal weight gain in the first trimester, newborn ponderal index (in kg/m^3) increased by 0.21 units ($P < 0.0003$) and, per kilogram maternal gain in the third trimester, newborn ponderal index increased by 0.12 units ($P < 0.03$), but not by maternal gain in the second trimester. Newborn birthweight was 211 g lower ($P < 0.006$) and ponderal index 1.2 units lower ($P < 0.02$) with maternal weight loss in the first trimester.

Likewise, Strauss and Dietz,[78] in their analyses of the National Collaborative Perinatal Project (NCPP) and the Child Health and Development Study (CHDS), reported that maternal weight gain < 0.3 kg/week in the second or third trimester was associated with increased risks for IUGR. Low maternal gain in the second and third trimesters was associated with relative risks of IUGR of 1.8 (95% CI 1.3 to 2.6) and 1.7 (95% CI 1.3 to 2.3), respectively, in the NCPP cohort and 2.6 (95% CI 1.6 to 4.1) and 2.5 (95% CI 1.7 to 3.8), respectively, in the CHDS cohort. To and Cheung[79] have shown that women who gain weight excessively after mid-pregnancy retained more weight postpartum, and their weight gain had less of an effect on the birthweight of their infants than women who had gained weight earlier in pregnancy but who did not gain weight excessively in late pregnancy. Kac et al.,[80] in their study of 405 Brazilian women aged 18–45 years, reported that women with the highest gestational weight gain and with baseline body fat ≥ 30% had the highest likelihood of developing maternal obesity. They reported that 35% of each kilogram of weight gained during pregnancy was retained at 9 months postpartum, even after adjustment for age, prepregnancy BMI, body fat at baseline, and years since first parturition. In their study of healthy, nonsmoking, white women in Canada, Muscati et al.[81] reported that a pregnancy weight gain of 12 kg was associated with 2.5 kg postpartum weight retention, and that total pregnancy weight gain was more strongly associated with postpartum weight retention than infant birthweight.

Multiple pregnancy

In 2002, in the United States, there were 132 535 infants of multiple births, the highest number ever recorded in the history of the vital statistics system.[82] The incidence of twin births has increased by 65% since 1980 and by 38% since 1990, while the triplet and higher order multiple rate increased an average of 13% per year between 1980 and 1998, and is currently 5% lower than the 1998 peak.[82] An estimated one-fourth of this rise is due solely to older maternal age, which is associated with a higher natural frequency of multiple births.[83,84] It is likely that the single most important factor in the rising multiple birth rate is fertility-enhancing therapies: fertility drugs, artificial insemination, and assisted reproductive technology (ART). Recent analyses by the CDC estimated that ART has contributed 39–43% of the increase in triplet and higher order multiple births in the US since 1996, and about 40% was due to ovulation-inducing drugs.[85,86] The twin and triplet and higher rates for ART patients are estimated to be 14-fold and 54-fold higher, respectively, than for the United States as a whole.[86] It is estimated that ART accounted for more than 40% of all triplet births in 2000, double the proportion of triplet and higher order births that were estimated to have been conceived using ART in 1990.[85] By 2000, it is estimated that only about two-thirds of twins and one-fifth of triplet and other higher order multiples were conceived spontaneously.[87] Infants of multiple births are disproportionately represented among the LBW (< 2500 g), very LBW (< 1500 g), preterm (< 37 weeks) and very preterm (< 32 weeks) infant populations (Table 36.3). Specialized prenatal care has been shown to reduce adverse outcomes in these high-risk pregnancies, including targeted diet therapy (Table 36.4) and BMI-specific weight gain recommendations (Table 36.5).[88]

Conclusions

Technological advances during the twentieth century will continue to push back the limits of viability. In future decades, the nutrition–fertility link will be expanded at the opposite end of the spectrum, and nutrition *in utero* will emerge as a powerful tool with which to augment growth, development, and vitality. Careful evaluation and aggressive therapy will help to ensure the most positive outcomes during gestation as a foundation for childhood health.

Table 36.3 Birthweight and gestation by plurality, USA, 2002.

Plurality	Singletons	Twins	Triplets	Quadruplets	Quintuplets
Number	3 889 191	125 134	6898	434	69
Percent very preterm (< 32 weeks)	1.6%	11.9%	36.1%	59.9%	78.3%
Percent preterm (< 37 weeks)	10.4%	58.2%	92.4%	96.8%	91.3%
Mean gestational age (weeks, SD)	38.8 (2.5)	35.3 (3.7)	32.2 (3.8)	29.9 (4.0)	28.5 (4.7)
Percent very low birthweight (< 1500 g)	1.1%	10.2%	34.5%	61.1%	83.8%
Percent low birthweight (< 2500 g)	6.1%	55.4%	94.4%	98.8%	94.1%
Mean birthweight (g, SD)	3332 (573)	2347 (645)	1687 (561)	1309 (522)	1105 (777)

Adapted from ref. 82.

Table 36.4 BMI-specific dietary recommendations for twin gestations.

BMI group BMI range	Underweight < 19.8	Normal 19.8–26.0	Overweight 26.1–29.0	Obese > 29.0
Calories	4000	3500	3250	3000
Protein (20% of calories)	200g	175g	163g	150g
Carbohydrate (40% of calories)	400g	350g	325g	300g
Fat (40% of calories)	178g	156g	144g	133g
Exchanges (servings) per day				
Dairy	10	8	8	8
Grains	12	10	8	8
Meat and meat equivalents	10	10	8	6
Eggs	2	2	2	2
Vegetables	5	4	4	4
Fruits	8	7	6	6
Fats and oils	7	6	5	5

Adapted from ref. 29.

Table 36.5 Optimal rates of maternal weight gain and cumulative gain by pregravid BMI status.

Pregravid BMI	Rates of weight gain (lbs/week)			Cumulative weight gain (lbs)		
	0–20 weeks	20–28 weeks	28 weeks to delivery	to 20 weeks	to 28 weeks	to 36–38 weeks
Underweight (BMI < 19.8)	1.25–1.75	1.50–1.75	1.25	25–35	37–49	50–62
Normal weight (BMI 19.8–26.0)	1.00–1.50	1.25–1.75	1.00	20–30	30–44	40–54
Overweight(BMI 26.1–29.0)	1.00–1.25	1.00–1.50	1.00	20–25	28–37	38–47
Obese (BMI > 29.0)	0.75–1.0	0.75–1.25	0.75	15–20	21–30	29–38

Adapted from ref. 88.

Results are from models controlling for diabetes and gestational diabetes, preeclampsia, smoking during pregnancy, parity, placental membranes, and fetal growth before 20 weeks.

BMI, body mass index.

Key points

1 Altered nutrition *in utero* may result in fetal developmental adaptations that permanently alter structure, physiology, and metabolism, and may manifest as chronic disease in adulthood.

2 Pregnancy complications and subsequent metabolic and vascular disease may share common underlying disease mechanisms.

3 Supplementation in excess of twice the recommended dietary allowance during pregnancy should be avoided, because of the potential for birth defects.

4 Iron should not be taken as part of a vitamin–mineral supplement, because of inhibition by other minerals as well as poor iron release.

5 Low maternal hemoglobin is strongly related to the development of a large placenta and high placental–birthweight ratio, which is seen as predictive of long-term programming of hypertension and cardiovascular disease.

6 Severe maternal iron-deficiency anemia leads to placental adaptive hypertrophy, a fall in the cortisol metabolizing system, and increased susceptibility to hypertension in later life.

7 Calcium is actively transferred to the fetus during pregnancy, and diets low in calcium have been associated with increased maternal blood pressure.

8 The ability of supplemental calcium to decrease the risk of preterm delivery may be confined to high-risk populations in which there is either a severe dietary

restriction of calcium or, as in the case of adolescents and multiple pregnancy, an increased demand for this nutrient.

9 Magnesium is neuroprotective and is an effective therapeutic agent for preterm labor.

10 Zinc is actively transferred to the fetus during pregnancy, with low maternal intakes and levels significantly associated with complications, including infections.

11 Many investigators have confirmed the associations between low prepregnancy weight and both prematurity and intrauterine growth retardation.

12 The population-attributable risk for early preterm birth (< 32 weeks) with low prepregnancy weight is as much as 31–43%, depending on race and ethnicity.

13 Although cumulative or total weight gain is an important predictor of birthweight, the pattern of weight gain and rates of gain also play significant roles in modifying birthweight and predicting preterm delivery.

14 The components of maternal weight gain, particularly changes in body fat, may be more important determinants of pregnancy outcome than absolute weight gain.

15 Gestational weight gain is the single most important factor influencing postpartum weight retention.

16 Maternal weight gain in the third trimester has less effect on fetal growth and more effect on retained maternal weight postpartum.

17 Maternal weight loss in the first trimester is associated with significantly lower subsequent birthweights.

18 Multiple births in the United States are at their all-time high.

19 Infants of multiple births are disproportionately represented among the low birthweight and premature infant populations.

20 Targeted diet therapy, BMI-specific weight gain goals, and specialized prenatal care have all been shown to improve outcomes in multiple pregnancies.

References

1 Lucas A, Fewtrell MA, Cole TJ. Fetal origins of adult disease: the hypothesis revisited. *Br Med J* 1999; 319:245–249.

2 Petry CJ, Hales CN. Long-term effects on offspring of intrauterine exposure to deficits in nutrition. *Hum Reprod Update* 2000;6:578–586.

3 Godfrey KM, Barker DJP. Fetal nutrition and adult disease. *Am J Clin Nutr* 2000;71(Suppl.):1344S–1352S.

4 Phenekos C. Influence of fetal body weight on metabolic complications in adult life: review of the evidence. *J Pediatr Endocrinol Metab* 2001;14:1361–1363.

5 Sattar N, Greer IA. Pregnancy complications and maternal cardiovascular risk: opportunities for intervention and screening? *Br Med J* 2002;325:157–169.

6 Wu G, Bazer FW, Cudd TA, et al. Maternal nutrition and fetal development. *J Nutr* 2004;134:2169–2172.

7 Bateson P, Barker D, Clutton-Brock T, et al. Developmental plasticity and human health. *Nature* 2004;430:419–21.

8 Gluckman PD, Hanson MA. Living with the past: evolution, development, and patterns of disease. *Science* 2004;305:1733–1736.

9 American Academy of Pediatrics and the American College of Obstetricians and Gynecologists. *Guidelines for perinatal care*, 5th edn. Elk Grove, IL: American Academy of Pediatrics, 2002.

10 Lagiou P, Tamimi RM, Mucci LA, et al. Diet during pregnancy in relation to maternal weight gain and birth size. *Eur J Clin Nutr* 2004;58:231–237.

11 Enns CW, Goldman JD, Cook A. Trends in food and nutrient intakes by adults: NFCS 1977–78, CSFII 1989–91, and CSFII 1994–95. *Fam Econ Nutr Rev* 1997;10:2–15.

12 Scholl TO, Hediger ML, Bendich A, et al. Use of multivitamin/mineral prenatal supplements: influence on the outcome of pregnancy. *Am J Epidemiol* 1997;146:134–141.

13 Bender MM, Levy AS, Schucker RE, et al. Trends in prevalence and magnitude of vitamin and mineral supplement usage and correlation with health status. *J Am Diet Assoc* 1992;92:1096–1101.

14 Block G, Cox C, Madans J, et al. Vitamin supplement use by demographic characteristics. *Am J Epidemiol* 1988;127:297–309.

15 Koplan JP, Annest JL, Layde PM, et al. Nutrient intake and supplementation in the United States (NHANES II). *Am J Public Health* 1986;76:287–289.

16 Subcommittee on Nutritional Status and Weight Gain During Pregnancy, Committee on Nutritional Status During Pregnancy and Lactation, Institute of Medicine. *Nutrition during pregnancy*. Washington, DC: National Academy Press, 1990.

17 Seligman PA, Caskey JH, Frazier JL, et al. Measurements of iron absorption from prenatal multivitamin–mineral supplements. *Obstet Gynecol* 1983;61:356–362.

18 Scholl TO, Hediger ML, Fischer RL, et al. Anemia vs iron deficiency: increased risk of preterm delivery. *Am J Clin Nutr* 1992;55:985–988.

19 Klebanoff MA, Shiono PH, Selby JV, et al. Anemia and spontaneous preterm birth. *Am J Obstet Gynecol* 1991;164:59–63.

20 Siega-Riz A, Adair LS, Hobel CJ. Maternal hematologic changes during pregnancy and the effect of iron status on preterm delivery in a West Los Angeles population. *Am J Perinatol* 1998;15:515–522.

21 Mitchell MC, Lerner E. Maternal hematologic measures and pregnancy outcome. *J Am Diet Assoc* 1992;92:484–486.

22 Holzman C, Katnik R, Jetton J, et al. Do maternal serum ferritin levels have a role in predicting preterm delivery? *Am J Epidemiol* 1996;143:S73 (Abstract).

23 Tamura T, Goldenberg RL, Johnston KE, et al. Serum ferritin: a predictor of early spontaneous preterm delivery. *Obstet Gynecol* 1996;87:360–365.

24 Goldenberg RL, Tamura T, DuBard M, et al. Plasma ferritin and pregnancy outcome. *Am J Obstet Gynecol* 1996;175:1356–1359.

25 Goldenberg RL, Mercer BM, Miodovnik M, et al. Plasma ferritin, premature rupture of membranes, and pregnancy outcome. *Am J Obstet Gynecol* 1998;179:1599–1604.

26 Scholl TO. High third-trimester ferritin concentration: associations with very preterm delivery, infection, and maternal nutritional status. *Obstet Gynecol* 1998;92:161–166.

27 Gülmezoglu AM, de Onis M, Villar J. Effectiveness of interventions to prevent or treat impaired fetal growth. *Obstet Gynecol Surv* 1997;6:139–149.

28 Ramakrishnan U, Manjrekar R, Rivera J, et al. Micronutrients and pregnancy outcome: a review of the literature. *Nutr Res* 1998;19:103–159.

29 Luke B, Brown MB, Misiunas R, et al. Specialized prenatal care and maternal and infant outcomes in twin pregnancy. *Am J Obstet Gynecol* 2003;189:934–938.

30 Villar J, Repke JT. Calcium supplementation during pregnancy may reduce preterm delivery in high-risk populations. *Am J Obstet Gynecol* 1990;163:1124–1131.

31 López-Jaramillo P, Narváez M, Weigel RM, et al. Calcium supplementation reduces the risk of pregnancy-induced hypertension in an Andes population. *Br J Obstet Gynaecol* 1989;96:648–655.

32 López-Jaramillo P, Narváez M, Felix C, et al. Dietary calcium supplementation and prevention of pregnancy hypertension. *Lancet* 1990;335:293.

33 Repke JT, Villar J. Pregnancy-induced hypertension and low birth weight: the role of calcium. *Am J Clin Nutr* 1991;272:237–241S.

34 Belizàn JM, Villar J, Gonzalez L, et al. Calcium supplementation to prevent hypertensive disorders of pregnancy. *N Engl J Med* 1991;325:1399–1405.

35 Levine RJ, Hauth JC, Curet LB, et al. Trial of calcium to prevent preeclampsia. *N Engl J Med* 1997;337:69–76.

36 Belizàn JM, Vilar J, Bergel E, et al. Long term effect of calcium supplementation during pregnancy on the blood pressure of offspring: follow up of a randomized controlled trial. *Br Med J* 1997;315:281–285.

37 Sibai BM, Villar MA, Bray E. Magnesium supplementation during pregnancy: a double-blind randomized controlled clinical trial. *Am J Obstet Gynecol* 1989;161:115–119.

38 Conradt A, Weidinger H, Algayer H. On the role of magnesium in fetal hypotrophy, pregnancy-induced hypertension and preeclampsia. *Mag Bull* 1984;6:68–76.

39 Spätling L, Spätling G. Magnesium supplementation in pregnancy. A double-blind study. *Br J Obstet Gynaecol* 1988;95:120–125.

40 Lucas MJ, Leveno KJ, Cunningham FG. A comparison of magnesium sulfate with phenytoin for the prevention of eclampsia. *N Engl J Med* 1995;333:201–205.

41 The Eclampsia Trial Collaborative Group. Which anticonvulsant for women with eclampsia? Evidence from the Collaborative Eclampsia Trial. *Lancet* 1995;345:1455–1463.

42 Nelson KB, Grether JK. Can magnesium sulfate reduce the risk of cerebral palsy in very low birthweight infants? *Pediatrics* 1995;95:263–269.

43 Schendel DE, Berg CJ, Yeargin-Allsopp M, et al. Prenatal magnesium sulfate exposure and the risk for cerebral palsy or mental retardation among very low-birth-weight children aged 3 to 5 years. *JAMA* 1996;276:1805–1810.

44 Grether JK, Hoogstrate J, Selvin S, et al. Magnesium sulfate tocolysis and risk of neonatal death. *Am J Obstet Gynecol* 1998;178:1–6.

45 Neggers YH, Cutter GR, Acton RT, et al. A positive association between maternal serum zinc concentration and birth weight. *Am J Clin Nutr* 1990;51:678–684.

46 Goldenberg RL, Tamura T, Neggers Y, et al. The effect of zinc supplementation on pregnancy outcome. *JAMA* 1995;274:463–468.

47 Mukherjee MD, Sandstead HH, Ratnaparkhi MV, et al. Maternal zinc, iron, folic acid, and protein nutriture and outcome of human pregnancy. *Am J Clin Nutr* 1984;40:496–507.

48 Sikorski R, Juszkiewicz T, Paszkowski T. Zinc status in women with premature rupture of membranes at term. *Obstet Gynecol* 1990;76:675–677.

49 Scholl TO, Hediger ML, Schall JI, et al. Low zinc intake during pregnancy: its association with preterm and very preterm delivery. *Am J Epidemiol* 1993;137:1115–1124.

50 Hunt IF, Murphy NJ, Lleaver AE, et al. Zinc supplementation during pregnancy: Effects on selected blood constituents and on progress and outcome in low-income women of Mexican descent. *Am J Clin Nutr* 1984;40:508–521.

51 Cherry FF, Sandstead HH, Rojas P, et al. Adolescent pregnancy: associations among body weight, zinc nutriture, and pregnancy outcome. *Am J Clin Nutr* 1989;50:945–954.

52 Merialdi M, Caufield LE, Zavaleta N, et al. Adding zinc to prenatal iron and folate tablets improves fetal neurobehavioral development. *Am J Obstet Gynecol* 1998;180:483–490.

53 Eastman NJ, Jackson E. Weight relationships in pregnancy: the bearing of maternal weight gain and pre-pregnancy weight on birthweight in full term pregnancies. *Obstet Gynecol Surv* 1968;23:1003–1025.

54 Niswander KR, Singer J, Westphal M, et al. Weight gain during pregnancy and prepregnancy weight: association with birth weight of term gestations. *Obstet Gynecol* 1969;33:482–491.

55 Niswander K, Jackson E. Physical characteristics of the gravida and their association with birth weight and perinatal death. *Am J Obstet Gynecol* 1974;119:306–313.

56 Singer JE, Westphal M, Niswander K. Relationship of weight gain during pregnancy to birth weight and infant growth and development in the first year of life. *Obstet Gynecol* 1968;31: 417–423.

57 World Health Organization. Maternal anthropometry and pregnancy outcomes: a WHO collaborative project. *Bull WHO* 1995;73(Suppl.).

58 Goldenberg RL, Iams JD, Mercer BM, et al. The preterm prediction study: the value of new vs standard risk factors in predicting early and spontaneous preterm births. *Am J Public Health* 1998;88:233–238.

59 Abrams B, Newman V, Key T, et al. Maternal weight gain and preterm delivery. *Obstet Gynecol* 1989;74:577–583.

60 Abrams B, Newman V. Small-for-gestational-age birth: maternal predictors and comparison with risk factors of spontaneous preterm delivery in the same cohort. *Am J Obstet Gynecol* 1991;164:785–790.

61 Spinillo A, Capuzzo E, Piazzi G, et al. Risk for spontaneous preterm delivery by combined body mass index and gestational weight gain patterns. *Acta Obstet Gynecol Scand* 1998;77:32–36.

62 Virji SK, Cottington E. Risk factors associated with preterm deliveries among racial groups in a national sample of married mothers. *Am J Perinatol* 1991;8:347353.

63 Berkowitz GS. Clinical and obstetric risk factors for preterm delivery. *Mt Sinai J Med* 1985;52:239–247.

64 Hediger ML, Scholl TO, Salmon RW. Early weight gain in pregnant adolescents and fetal outcome. *Am J Hum Biol* 1989;1: 665–672.

65 Hediger ML, Scholl TO, Belsky DH, et al. Patterns of weight gain in adolescent pregnancy: effects on birth weight and preterm delivery. *Obstet Gynecol* 1989;74:6–12.

66 Pipe NGG, Smith T, Halliday D, et al. Changes in fat, fat-free mass and body water in human normal pregnancy. *Br J Obstet Gynaecol* 1979;86:929–940.

67 Hytten FE, Thomson AM, Taggart N. Total body water in normal pregnancy. *J Obstet Gynaecol Br Commonwlth* 1966;73:553–561.
68 Seitchik J, Alper C, Szutka A. Changes in body composition during pregnancy. *Ann NY Acad Sci* 1963;110:821–829.
69 Van Raaij JMA, Schonk CM, Vermaat-Miedema SH, et al. Body fat mass and basal metabolic rate in Dutch women before, during, and after pregnancy: a reappraisal of energy cost of pregnancy. *Am J Clin Nutr* 1989;49:765–772.
70 Villar J, Cogswell M, Kestler E, et al. Effect of fat and fat-free mass deposition during pregnancy on birthweight. *Am J Obstet Gynecol* 1992;167:1344–1352.
71 Viegas OAC, Cole TJ, Wharton BA. Impaired fat deposition in pregnancy: an indicator for nutritional intervention. *Am J Clin Nutr* 1987;45:23–28.
72 Neggers Y, Goldenberg RL, Cliver SP, et al. Usefulness of various maternal skinfold measurements for predicting newborn birth weight. *J Am Diet Assoc* 1992;92:1393–1394.
73 Bissenden JG, Scott PH, King J, et al. Anthropometric and biochemical changes during pregnancy in Asian and European mothers having well grown babies. *Br J Obstet Gynaecol* 1981;88:992–998.
74 Bissenden JG, Scott PH, King J, et al. Anthropometric and biochemical changes during pregnancy in Asian and European mothers having light for gestational age babies. *Br J Obstet Gynaecol* 1981;88:999–1008.
75 Hediger ML, Scholl TO, Schall JI, et al. Changes in maternal upper arm fat stores are predictors of variation in infant birth weight. *J Nutr* 1994;124:24–30.
76 Li R, Haas JD, Habicht J-P. Timing of the influence of maternal nutritional status during pregnancy on fetal growth. *Am J Hum Biol* 1998;10:529–539.
77 Brown JE, Murtaugh MA, Jacobs DR, et al. Variation in newborn size according to pregnancy weight change by trimester. *Am J Clin Nutr* 2002;76:205–209.
78 Strauss RS, Dietz WH. Low maternal weight gain in the second or third trimester increases the risk for intrauterine growth retardation. *J Nutr* 1999;129:988–993.
79 To WW, Cheung W. The relationship between weight gain in pregnancy, birth weight and postpartum weight retention. *Aust NZ J Obstet Gynaecol* 1998;38:176–179.
80 Kac G, Benício MHDA, Velásquez-Meléndez G, et al. Gestational weight gain and prepregnancy weight influence postpartum weight retention in a cohort of Brazilian women. *J Nutr* 2004;134: 661–666.
81 Muscati SK, Gray-Donald K, Koski KG. Timing of weight gain during pregnancy: promoting fetal growth and minimizing maternal weight retention. *Int J Obes* 1996;20:526–532.
82 Martin JA, Hamilton BE, Sutton PD, et al. *Final data for 2002. National Vital Statistics Reports*, vol. 52, no. 10, December 17, 2003.
83 Jewell SE, Yip R. Increasing trends in plural births in the United States. *Obstet Gynecol* 1995;85:229–232.
84 Lynch A, McDuffie R, Murphy J, et al. Assisted reproductive interventions and multiple birth. *Obstet Gynecol* 2001;97:195–200.
85 MMWR. Contribution of assisted reproductive technology and ovulation-inducing drugs to triplet and higher-order multiple births – United States, 1980–1997. *Morbidity Mortality Weekly Rep* 2000;49:535–538.
86 Reynolds MA, Schieve LA, Martin JA, et al. Trends in multiple births conceived using assisted reproductive technology, United States, 1997–2000. *Pediatrics* 2003;111:1159–1162.
87 Wright VC, Schieve, LA, Reynolds MA, et al. Assisted Reproductive Technology Surveillance – United States, 2000. In: *Surveillance summaries*, August 29, 2003. *Morbidity Mortality Weekly Rep* 2003;52(SS-9):1–16.
88 Luke B, Hediger ML, Nugent C, et al. Body mass index-specific weight gains associated with optimal birthweights in twin pregnancies. *J Reprod Med* 2003;48:217–224.

Part X

Maternal Diseases Complicating Pregnancy

37 Trauma, shock, and critical care obstetrics

Erin A.S. Clark, Gary A. Dildy, and Steven L. Clark

Definition of shock

Shock is a condition in which circulation fails to meet the nutritional needs of the cell and remove metabolic wastes.[1] This may result from cardiac dysfunction, hypovolemia (relative or absolute), maldistribution of flow, or intravascular obstruction (Table 37.1). When the circulating blood volume is less than the capacity of its vascular bed, hypotension with diminished tissue perfusion results, leading to cellular hypoxia and, ultimately, cell death.[2] Depending on the duration and severity of the insult, irreversible organ damage or even death may ensue.

Incidence of shock in the obstetric population

The actual incidence of shock in obstetric patients is unclear. However, by extrapolating mortality data, we can obtain an indication of the relative incidence of shock severe enough to result in the death of the patient. A steady decline in maternal mortality has been noted since 1915, when national vital statistics in the United States were first recorded (Fig. 37.1). Recent statistics for the United States suggest that overall maternal mortality was 11.5 maternal deaths per 100 000 live births during 1991–97.[3] The pregnancy-related maternal mortality ratio was threefold greater among black women than in white women[4] (Table 37.2). The National Health Promotion and Disease Prevention objectives of the *Healthy People 2010* indicators specifies a goal of no more than 3.3 maternal deaths per 100 000 live births in the United States.[5] This objective remains elusive. The chief cause of a pregnancy-related maternal death depends on whether the pregnancy results in a liveborn, stillbirth, ectopic pregnancy, abortion, or molar gestation (Table 37.3). For the period 1987–1990, hemorrhage was recorded in 28.8% of all deaths, leading to an overall pregnancy-related mortality ratio (PRMR) for hemorrhage of 2.6 per 100 000 live births, followed by embolism-related deaths (1.8), and hypertensive diseases (1.6). Among live births, hypertensive diseases were the most frequent cause of death (23.8%). Among stillbirths and ectopic pregnancies, the chief cause of death was hemorrhage (27.2 and 94.9% respectively). Infections were the leading cause of abortion-related deaths (49.4%).

Tracking maternal deaths is helpful, but may not give the best indication of the incidence of shock and critical illness in the obstetric population as the majority of such cases do not result in maternal death. Unlike mortality, which is a definable endpoint, shock and critical illness in pregnancy are difficult to define and, therefore, difficult to measure and study precisely. Furthermore, maternal mortality data collection is well established in many places, but specific surveillance systems that record severe complications of pregnancy not associated with maternal mortality are rare. An examination of cases admitted to intensive care units (ICUs) has provided insight into the incidence and etiology of shock and critical illness in the obstetric population, although nearly two-thirds of maternal deaths may occur in women who never reach an ICU.[7] In 2004, Ananth and Smulian[8] reviewed 22 studies involving 1 550 723 deliveries and found that 0.07–0.88% of deliveries resulted in admission to an ICU. Reported maternal mortality for critically ill obstetric patients admitted to an ICU was 5.0%. Hypertensive diseases and obstetric hemorrhage were responsible for over 50% of the primary admitting diagnoses, and specific organ system dysfunction was responsible for the majority of the remaining admissions.

General supportive measures

Initial treatment

Several important initial steps should be performed when the diagnosis of shock is made in the obstetric patient. Placement of two large-bore intravenous lines, preferably 16-gauge, for rapid expansion of intravascular volume is the first step. One liter of crystalloid solution should be infused over the first 15 min while other measures are taken. An indwelling bladder

Table 37.1 Classification scheme for shock.

Type	Physiologic derangement	Examples
Cardiogenic	Diminished cardiac function	Cardiomyopathy, myocardial infarction
Hypovolemic	Decreased intravascular volume	Hemorrhage, dehydration
Distributive	Inappropriate distribution of perfusion	Septic shock, neurogenic shock
Obstructive	Intravascular obstruction	Pulmonary embolus

Table 37.2 Number of pregnancy-related deaths and pregnancy-related mortality ratios (PRMRs)* among Hispanic, Asian/Pacific Islander, American Indian/Alaska Native, non-Hispanic black (black), and non-Hispanic white (white) women, by age group, United States, 1991–1997.[4]

Age group (years)	Hispanic		Asian/ Pacific Islander		American Indian/ Alaska Native		Black		White		Total	
	No.	PRMR	No.	PRMR	No.	PRMR	No.	PRMR	No.	PRMR	No.	PRMR
< 20	45	5.5	–†		–†		160	16.0	96	5.8	**306**	**8.5**
20–29	200	7.4	43	8.4	16	11.0‡	590	25.0	35	6.0	**1384**	**9.3**
30–34	125	16.0	28	8.7	–†		260	38.8	330	7.4	**749**	**11.9**
35–39	82	26.0	34	22.7	–†		202	70.8	226	12.3	**549**	**21.1**
> 39	31	48.2	14	42.4§	–†		80	151.2	79	25.5	**205**	**44.3**
Total	**483**	**10.3**	**121**	**11.3**	**31**	**12.2**	**1292**	**29.6**	**1266**	**7.3**	**3193**	**11.5**
RR§		1.4		1.6		1.7		4.0		(ref)		
95% CI**		(1.3–1.6)		(1.3–1.9)		(1.2–2.4)		(3.8–4.4)				

* Per 100 000 live births.

† Fewer than seven pregnancy-related deaths; considered unreliable (relative standard error [RSE] => 38%).

‡ Point estimates based on 7–19 deaths are highly variable (RSE = 23–38%).

§ Relative ratio of PRMR for each racial/ethnic group divided by PRMR for white women.

** Confidence interval.

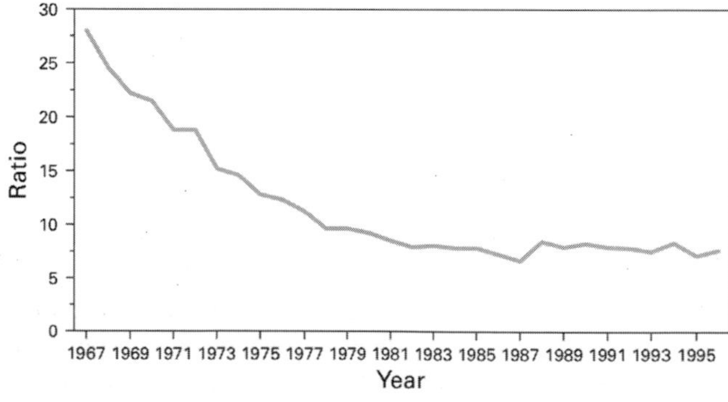

Figure 37.1 Maternal mortality ratio, by year, United States, 1967–1996.[4]

catheter is placed for hourly determination of urine output. An arterial line allows continuous measurement of systemic blood pressure, as well as easy access for laboratory investigations. Oxygen should be administered via a face mask at 8–10 L/min, and the inspired oxygen concentration adjusted according to arterial blood gas results. Inability to maintain an adequate tidal volume, poor arterial oxygenation, and airway obstruction may require endotracheal intubation with positive pressure ventilation. Initial laboratory investigation should include blood type and cross-match, complete blood count, platelets, fibrinogen, electrolytes, blood urea nitrogen, creatinine, and arterial blood gas. Urine should be sent for analysis and microscopic evaluation. When the patient is stabilized, cultures from blood, urine, sputum, amniotic fluid, endometrial cavity, and stool are taken, as indicated, if sepsis is suspected.

Volume replacement

Whether to give crystalloid or colloid solutions for initial treatment is controversial.[9] Rackow and colleagues[10] showed that two to four times as much 0.9% saline was required to reach the same hemodynamic endpoints as 6% hetastarch and 5% albumin. Colloid osmotic pressure rose when albumin and hetastarch were administered and fell when saline was given. Resuscitation with normal saline resulted in a higher incidence of pulmonary edema, probably related to the fall in colloid osmotic pressure. Standard dextran, with a molecular weight averaging 75 000, may initiate intravascular coagulation. Low-molecular-weight dextran, with a molecular weight aver-

Table 37.3 Percentage of pregnancy-related deaths by outcome of pregnancy and cause of death, percentage of all outcomes of pregnancy, and PRMR,* United States, 1987–1990.[6]

	Outcome of pregnancy (% distribution)							All outcomes	
Cause of death	Live birth	Stillbirth	Ectopic	Abortion†	Molar‡	Undelivered	Unknown	Percentage	PRMR
Hemorrhage	21.1	27.2	94.9	18.5	16.7	15.7	20.1	28.8	2.6
Embolism	23.4	10.7	1.3	11.1	0.0	35.2	21.1	19.9	1.8
Pregnancy-induced hypertension	23.8	26.2	0.0	1.2	0.0	4.6	16.3	17.6	1.6
Infection	12.1	19.4	1.3	49.4	0.0	13.0	9.0	13.1	1.2
Cardiomyopathy	6.1	2.9	0.0	0.0	0.0	2.8	13.9	5.7	0.5
Anesthesia complications	2.7	0.0	1.9	8.6	0.0	1.8	1.0	2.5	0.2
Other/unknown	11.1	13.6	0.6	11.1	83.3	27.5	19.3	12.8	1.2
Total§	**100.0**	**100.0**	**100.0**	**100.0**	**100.0**	**100.0**	**100.0**	**100.0**	9.2

* Pregnancy-related deaths per 100 000 live births.

† Includes spontaneous and induced abortions.

‡ Also known as gestational trophoblastic neoplasia.

§ Percentages may not add to 100.0 due to rounding.

aging 40 000, carries a smaller risk of initiating disseminated intravascular coagulopathy (DIC), but also has less tendency to pull fluid into the intravascular space.[11] A 1984 American College of Obstetricians and Gynecologists technical bulletin titled *Hemorrhagic Shock* recommends avoidance of dextran because of its anticoagulant effect and risk of anaphylaxis.[12] Owing to its expense and tendency to extravasate into the interstitium, albumin is also probably not a colloid of first choice. Given these objections, hetastarch may be a better choice of colloid if initial crystalloid therapy does not result in the desired clinical improvement. In a meta-analysis of several randomized controlled trials, there was no evidence that colloids achieve a superior clinical outcome when compared with crystalloid therapy.[13] Crystalloids are therefore reasonable and cost-effective first-line therapy for volume resuscitation. When severe, correction of metabolic acidosis may be aided by adding sodium bicarbonate to intravenous fluids. Lactated solutions should be avoided because aerobic metabolism is required for the conversion of lactate to bicarbonate.[2,14]

Blood component therapy

In the case of hemorrhagic hypovolemic shock and DIC, blood component therapy is often indicated. Which components should be used is determined largely by laboratory parameters. An obvious exception is profuse hemorrhagic shock, for which immediate blood components, specifically packed red blood cells, are indicated. It must be remembered that the degree of hemorrhage is often underestimated by as much as 50%.[15]

Packed red blood cells are administered through an 18-gauge or larger intravenous line in order to increase blood volume and oxygen-carrying capacity to the tissues. The term *massive blood replacement* is used when the total blood volume of the patient is replaced over a 24-hour period.[15] In those patients who have been typed and screened for antibodies, the risks of abbreviating the major cross-match in an urgent transfusion (after the "immediate spin" phase of the cross-match) are low and are often outweighed by the risk of hemorrhagic shock.[16]

The use of fresh frozen plasma (FFP) requires specific indications: replacement of isolated or combined factor deficiencies, reversal of warfarin effect in patients actively bleeding or requiring emergency surgery, antithrombin III deficiency, immunodeficiencies, thrombotic thrombocytopenia purpura, and massive blood transfusion in cases in which factor deficiencies are presumed to be the sole or principal derangement.[17,18] Besides containing the components of the coagulation, fibrinolytic, and complement systems, FFP also contains proteins that maintain oncotic pressure and modulate immunity. Because of risks, including disease transmission, anaphylactoid reactions, alloimmunization, and volume overload, alternative therapy with crystalloids is encouraged for volume replacement. Pathologic hemorrhage in the patient receiving massive transfusion is usually due to thrombocytopenia rather than depletion of coagulation factors. Empiric administration of FFP should therefore be allowed only in those patients in whom factor deficiencies are presumed to be the sole or principal derangement.[17] In massively transfused patients, there is no evidence to support prophylactic transfusion of FFP after transfusion of a certain number of units of packed red blood cells unless coagulation factor defects have been documented.[19] The most useful tests for predicting abnormal bleeding and guiding therapy in massively transfused trauma patients are the platelet count and fibrinogen level.[20] Normal hemostasis requires no more than 30% of normal values of clotting factors. Bleeding would therefore not be expected until the prothrombin time (PT) and activated partial thromboplastin time (aPTT) have exceeded 1.5 times their reference values.[21]

Thrombocytopenia may be secondary to a dilutional effect or to consumption of platelets. Adults have a limited mobile platelet pool and a limited ability to increase production acutely.[22] Moreover, platelets in refrigerated blood quickly become nonviable.[23] Platelet transfusion should be considered when the platelet count falls to less than 10 000/μL, or to less than 35 000/μL in preparation for a surgical procedure or in the face of active bleeding. Minimization of blood product transfusion can be effected by correcting thrombocytopenia and specific coagulation factor defects.[15] In trauma patients, platelets are usually required after a patient receives more than 20 units of blood in a 12-hour period.[23] However, in obstetric patients who experience thrombocytopenia secondary to other causes (e.g., preeclampsia), platelet transfusion may be indicated much earlier in the course of treatment.

Cryoprecipitate should be administered instead of FFP when the calculated coagulation factor deficit based on blood fibrinogen levels suggests that FFP will result in inadequate replacement or in volume overload (Fig. 37.2). Table 37.4 demonstrates the therapeutic contents per volume of each blood product.[24]

Pharmacologic agents

If adequate intravascular volume replacement is not successful in supporting blood pressure (i.e., mean arterial pressure ≥65 mmHg) and other reversible causes of shock are not found (e.g., cardiac arrhythmia, tension pneumothorax), an advanced stage of shock should be suspected. In order to ensure tissue perfusion in these refractory cases, cardiac performance should be enhanced through the use of inotropic agents (Table 37.5). Dopamine is considered a first-line inotropic agent. Dopamine is an endogenous catecholamine, structurally similar to norepinephrine and epinephrine. Dopamine increases myocardial contractility and heart rate via beta-adrenergic receptors and releases norepinephrine from myocardial storage sites. Its action on blood vessels is dose dependent, resulting in vasodilation of renal, mesenteric, coronary, and intracerebral vessels via dopamine receptors, and vasoconstriction of all vascular beds in higher doses via alpha-adrenergic receptors.[26] Dopamine should be started at 2–5 μg/kg/min and titrated to the desired clinical parameters.[26] Although there is considerable variance, generally, doses between 2 and 5 μg/kg/min result in vasodilation of renal and mesenteric vasculature via β2 and dopaminergic receptors, whereas doses between 5 and 10 μg/kg/min tend to result in

Table 37.4 Summary chart of blood components.

Component	Content	Indications for use	Amount of active substance per unit	Volume (mL)
Red blood cells	Red blood cells, some plasma, some white blood cells and platelets their degradation products	Increase red blood cell mass for symptomatic anemia	200 mL packed red blood cell mass	250–350
Leukocyte-poor red blood cells	Red blood cells, some plasma, few white blood cells	Prevent febrile reactions due to leukocyte antibodies, and increase red blood cells mass	185 mL packed red blood cell mass	200–250
Frozen–thawed washed red blood cells	Red blood cells, no plasma, minimal white blood cells and platelets	Increase red blood cell mass; prevent sensitization to HLAs; prevent febrile or anaphylactic reactions to white blood cells, platelets, and proteins (IgA); provide rate blood cells	170–190 mL packed red blood cells	300
Platelet concentrations	Platelets, few white blood cells, some plasma	Bleeding due to thrombocytopenia or thrombocytopathia	At least 5.5×10^{10} platelets	30–50
Fresh frozen plasma	Plasma, all coagulation factors, no platelets	Treatment of coagulation disorders	0.7–1.0 U factors II, V–VI, VIII–XIII, 500 mg fibrinogen	220–250
Cryoprecipitate	Fibrinogen, factor VIII, factor XIII, von Willebrand's factor	Factor VIII deficiency (hemophilia A) von Willebrand's disease; factor XIII deficiency; fibrinogen deficiency	80 U factor VIII; 200 mg fibrinogen	20–25
Albumin				
5%	Albumin	Plasma volume expansion	12.5 g	250
25%			12.5 g	50

Source: modified from ref. 24.

Blood volume (mL) = weight (kg) × 70 mL/kg

Plasma volume (mL) = Blood volume (mL) × (1.0 − hematocrit)

Fibrinogen requirement (mg) = [Desired fibrinogen level (mg/dL) − initial fibrinogen level (mg/dL)] × plasma volume (mL) × 0.01 dL/mL

1 unit cryoprecipitate (22.5 mL) contains 200 mg fibrinogen
1 unit FFP (225 mL) contains 400 mg fibrinogen

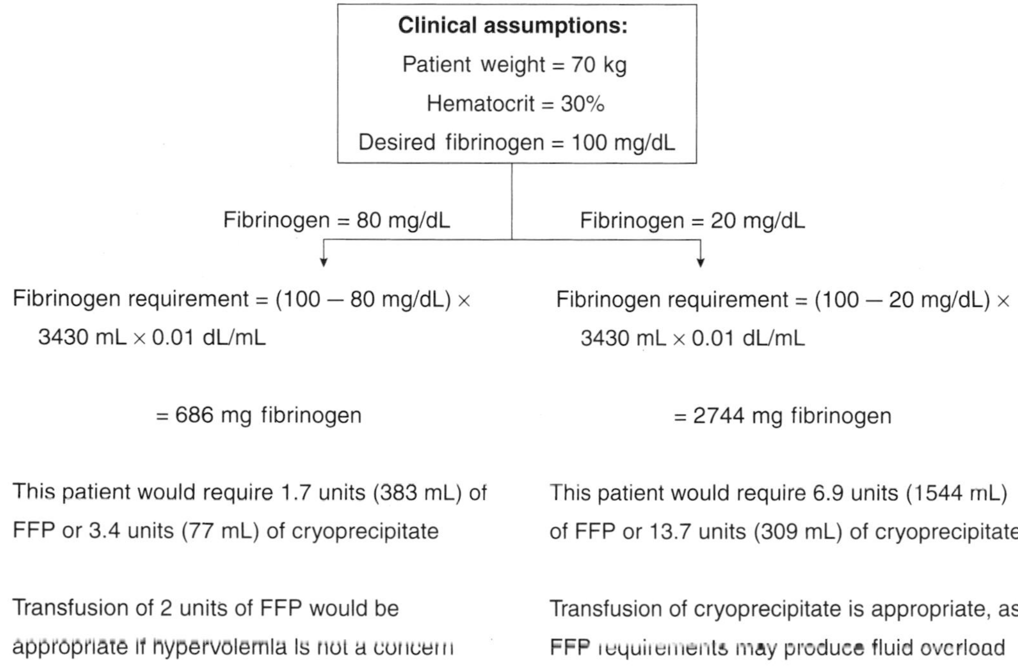

Clinical assumptions:
Patient weight = 70 kg
Hematocrit = 30%
Desired fibrinogen = 100 mg/dL
Fibrinogen = 80 mg/dL
Fibrinogen = 20 mg/dL
Fibrinogen requirement = (100 − 80 mg/dL) × 3430 mL × 0.01 dL/mL
= 686 mg fibrinogen
This patient would require 1.7 units (383 mL) of FFP or 3.4 units (77 mL) of cryoprecipitate
Transfusion of 2 units of FFP would be appropriate if hypervolemia is not a concern
Fibrinogen requirement = (100 − 20 mg/dL) × 3430 mL × 0.01 dL/mL
= 2744 mg fibrinogen
This patient would require 6.9 units (1544 mL) of FFP or 13.7 units (309 mL) of cryoprecipitate
Transfusion of cryoprecipitate is appropriate, as FFP requirements may produce fluid overload

Figure 37.2 Calculation of fibrinogen requirements for obstetric hemorrhage. FFP, fresh frozen plasma.

Table 37.5 Inotropic agents.

Inotropic agent	Mechanism of action	Dosage
Dopamine	Dopaminergic (0.5–5.0 μg/kg/min) vasodilation of renal and mesenteric vasculature; β_1-adrenergic (5.0–10.0 μg/kg/min) increased myocardial contractility SV, CO; alpha-adrenergic (15–20 μg/kg/min) increased general vasoconstriction	2–5 μg/kg/min and titrate to BP and CO
Dobutamine	Myocardial β_1-receptor stimulant increased CO, minimal tachycardia	2–10 μg/kg/min
Isoproterenol	β-adrenergic receptors increased contractility and heart rate, but ventricular ectopy, tachycardia, vasodilation	1–20 μg/min
Digoxin	Improved contractility of myocardium	0.5 mg IV push and 0.25 mg q4h × 2, then 0.25–0.37 mg/day

BP, blood pressure; CO, cardiac output; SV, stroke volume.

Source: modified from ref. 25.

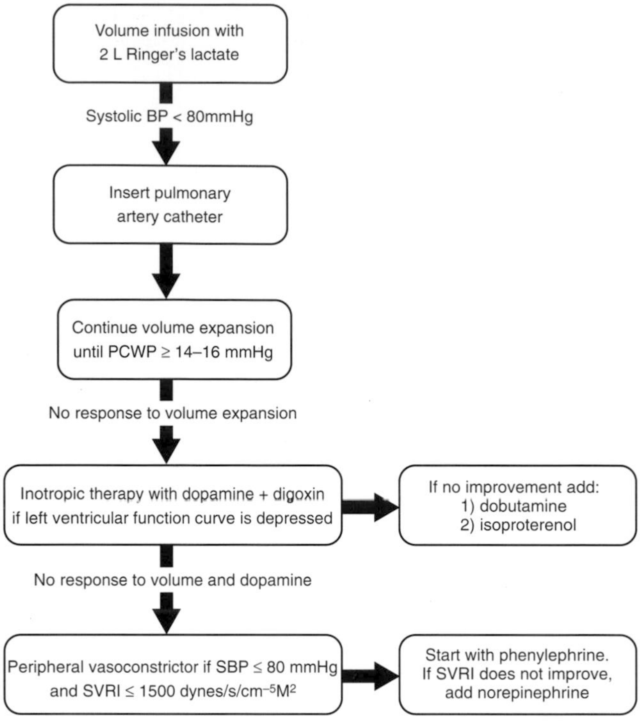

Figure 37.3 Hemodynamic algorithm for obstetric septic shock. BP, blood pressure; PCWP, pulmonary catheter wedge pressure; SBP, systolic blood pressure; SVRI, systemic vascular resistance index (reprinted from ref. 25, with permission).

increased myocardial contractility and cardiac output via β1 receptors.[27] Doses of more than 20 μg/kg/min result in generalized vasoconstriction via alpha-adrenergic receptors. High-dose dopamine has been demonstrated to decrease uterine blood flow in healthy and hypotensive pregnant sheep.[28,29] This should be kept in mind when administering dopamine during pregnancy.

If satisfactory hemodynamic performance is not achieved and the patient is not profoundly hypotensive, dobutamine may be added to the dopamine regimen at 2.5–10 μg/kg/min (Fig. 37.3). Dobutamine increases cardiac output with minimal tachycardia by acting as a myocardial beta-receptor stimulant. Unfortunately, it may also reduce afterload and lower systemic blood pressure, and must be used with caution in severe hypotension. If dobutamine does not provide adequate improvement, isoproterenol, a beta-adrenergic agonist, may be added. Increased heart rate and contractility are achieved at the risk of ventricular ectopy, excessive tachycardia, and peripheral vasodilation. Although rarely used in acute hypotension, other inotropic agents, such as digoxin and amrinone, may also be used to improve myocardial contractility.[30] Digoxin is usually administered with continuous electrocardiographic monitoring by giving an initial bolus of 0.5 mg by intravenous push, followed by 0.25-mg doses every 4 hours for a total loading dose of 1.0 mg. The maintenance dosage in pregnant patients is usually at least 0.25–0.37 mg/day, depending on plasma levels.[25,31] Amrinone, an inotropic agent with vasodilatory activity, is indicated for the short-term management of cardiac failure.[30] A bolus of 0.75 mg/kg over 2–3 min is given, and an infusion of 5–10 μg/kg/min should follow. Vasodilation may be undesirable, particularly in distributive shock, and agents producing vasodilation should only be used with caution.

Table 37.6 Vasopressor agents.

Vasopressor agent	Mechanism of action	Dosage
Phenylephrine (Neo-synephrine)	Alpha-adrenergic increased systemic vascular resistance	1–5 μg/kg/min
Norepinephrine (Levophed)	Mixed adrenergic alpha and beta generalized vasoconstriction increased systemic vascular resistance	1–4 μg/min

Source: modified from ref. 25.

When blood pressure does not respond to inotropic therapy, a peripheral vasoconstrictor should be considered to maintain appropriate vascular tone (Table 37.6). Phenylephrine, an alpha-adrenergic agonist, may be initiated at 1–5 μg/kg/min. Norepinephrine, a mixed alpha- and beta-agonist with powerful vasoconstrictive properties, may be added to provide generalized vasoconstriction and increased systemic vascular resistance. This agent is used in situations in which blood pressure is dangerously low (mean arterial pressure < 60 mmHg) despite other therapy, because perfusion to vital organs, such as the kidneys and lungs, may be reduced by the vasoconstriction. Although vasoconstrictors are commonly used, there are few data to suggest they improve outcome.[31,32]

Particular caution must be exercised with the use of these agents in gravid patients. Only correction of maternal hypovolemia will maintain placental perfusion and prevent fetal compromise. Although vasopressors may temporarily correct hypotension, they do so at the expense of uteroplacental perfusion, as the uterine spiral arterioles are especially sensitive to these agents. Vasopressors should therefore be used in the treatment of obstetric hemorrhagic shock only when essential for maternal survival.

In hypovolemic shock, vasopressors or inotropic agents are rarely indicated and should not be given until the intravascular volume has been adequately replaced.

Hemodynamic monitoring

The pulmonary artery catheter was introduced in 1970 for the determination of pressures in the right side of the heart and pulmonary capillary wedge pressure.[33] The pulmonary artery catheter provides direct measurement of central venous pressure, pulmonary artery systolic and diastolic pressure, and

Table 37.7 Hemodynamic indices in nonpregnant and normal third-trimester pregnant women measured by pulmonary artery catheter.

Parameter	Normal nonpregnant (n = 10)* mean ± SD	Normal third trimester (n = 10)* mean ± SD	Severe preeclampsia (n = 45)† mean ± SD	Amniotic fluid embolism (n = 15)‡ mean ± SD
Cardiac output (L/min)	4.3 ± 0.9	6.2 ± 1.0	7.5 ± 0.2	–
Heart rate (beats per minute)	71 ± 10	83 ± 10	95 ± 2	–
Systemic vascular resistance (dyne/m/s^{-5})	1,530 ± 520	1.210 ± 266	1,496 ± 64	–
Pulmonary vascular resistance (dyne/cm/s^{-5})	119 ± 47	78 ± 22	70 ± 5	176 ± 72
Colloid osmotic pressure (mm Hg)	20.8 ± 1.0	18.0 ± 1.5	19.0 ± 0.5	–
Mean arterial pressure (mm Hg)	86 ± 8	90 ± 6	138 ± 3	–
Pulmonary capillary wedge pressure (mm Hg)	6.3 ± 2.1	7.5 ± 1.8	10 ± 1	18.9 ± 9.2
Central venous pressure (mm Hg)	3.7 ± 2.6	3.6 ± 2.5	4 ± 1	–
Left ventricular stroke work index (g/m/m^{-2})	41 ± 8	48 ± 6	81 ± 2	26 ± 19
Mean pulmonary artery pressure (mm Hg)	11.9 ± 2.0	12.5 ± 2.0	17 ± 1	26.2 ± 15.7

Source: data from refs 34–36, and unpublished data from the National Amniotic Fluid Embolism Registry.

SD, standard deviation; SEM, standard error of the mean.

Observations in pathophysiologic states (severe preeclampsia and amniotic fluid embolism) are shown for comparison.

*Data from ref. 34.

†Data from ref. 35.

‡Data from ref. 36.

pulmonary capillary wedge pressure, whereas thermodilution techniques and physiologic equations allow derivation of cardiac output, systemic vascular resistance, and other hemodynamic parameters. Normal values during pregnancy have been published[34,35] and are summarized in Table 37.7. In select cases, placement of a pulmonary artery catheter should be considered to aid in assessing cardiac function and hemodynamic status. Several prospective trials have demonstrated the benefits of pulmonary catheterization in selected critically ill patients. These benefits may include a reduction in morbidity and mortality in complicated surgical patients and in patients in shock. This technique, however, is not without its critics.[38] A nonrandomized observational study demonstrated increased mortality and cost associated with pulmonary artery catheterization.[39] In contrast, a recent randomized controlled trial (n = 201) of the pulmonary artery catheter in critically ill patients by Rhodes et al.[40] concluded that its use is not associated with increased mortality.

Some pathophysiologic conditions secondary to, or in association with, the pregnant state may be diagnosed and treated appropriately with the Swan–Ganz catheter. The differentiation between pulmonary edema secondary to high pulmonary capillary wedge pressure versus low pulmonary capillary wedge pressure can be determined with the pulmonary artery catheter. Kirshon and Cotton[30] found that the development of hydrostatic pulmonary edema may occur at lower pulmonary capillary wedge pressures during pregnancy secondary to a lower colloid osmotic pressure. Numerous studies have documented the frequent discrepancy between measurements of central venous pressure and pulmonary capillary wedge pressure during pregnancy.[37,41–43] Central venous pressure would be misleading in these circumstances, and so central venous monitoring is seldom indicated in obstetric critical care. Potential clinical indications for use of the pulmonary artery catheter in obstetric patients are summarized in Table 37.8. One simple but clinically helpful use for the Swan–Ganz catheter is to guide volume resuscitation through use of the volume challenge (Fig. 37.4).

Table 37.8 Indications for pulmonary artery catheterization during pregnancy.

1. Massive blood loss with large transfusion requirements, particularly in the face of oliguria or pulmonary edema
2. Septic shock, especially when accompanied by hypotension or oliguria, required volume resuscitation or vasopressor therapy
3. Cardiac failure or pulmonary edema of uncertain etiology
4. Severe pregnancy-induced hypertension complicated by pulmonary edema, oliguria unresponsive to initial fluid challenge, or severe hypertension refractory to conventional therapy (hydralazine)
5. Labor and delivery in patients with significant cardiovascular disease (New York Heart Association functional class III and IV patients)
6. Intraoperative cardiovascular decompensation (e.g., pulmonary hypertension with shunting secondary to amniotic fluid embolism)
7. During peripartum period in patients with severe preeclampsia and structural cardiac defects
8. Thyroid storm with evidence of high output failure
9. Diabetic ketoacidosis with severe hypovolemia and oliguria

Source: Date from refs. 35, 44, 45, 369, and 442.

On insertion of the Swan–Ganz catheter, advancement to

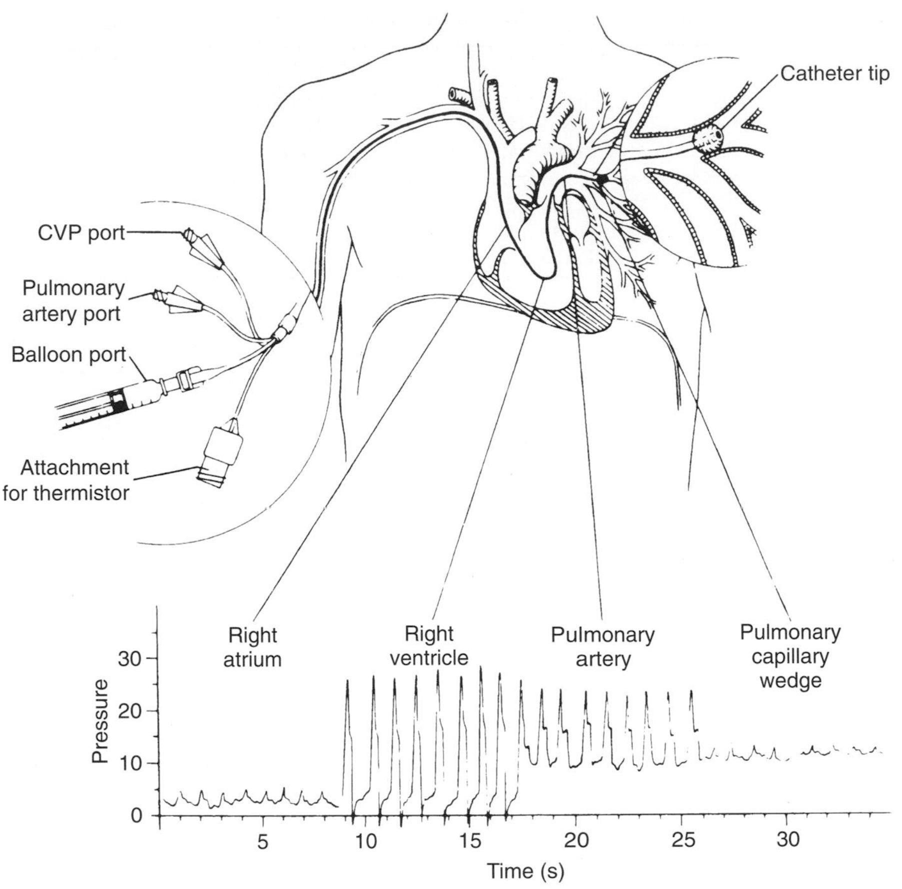

Figure 37.4 Swan–Ganz catheter placement. Swan–Ganz catheter depicting central venous pressure (CVP) port, pulmonary artery and balloon port, and attachment for thermistor. During advancement through the right side of the heart, characteristic pressure tracings are recorded from the right atrial, right ventricular, pulmonary artery, and pulmonary capillary wedge positions (reprinted from ref. 46, with permission).

Table 37.9 Hemodynamic and ventilatory parameters.

	Nonpregnant	Pregnant
Central venous pressure (mm Hg)	1–7	Unchanged
Pulmonary capillary wedge pressure (mm Hg)	6–12	Unchanged
Mean pulmonary artery pressure (mm Hg)	9–16	Unchanged
Systemic vascular resistance (dyne/cm/s^{-5})	800–1,200	Decreased 25%
Pulmonary vascular resistance (dyne/cm/s^{-5})	20–120	Decreased 25%
Cardiac output (L/min)	4–7	Increased 30–45%
Arterial P_{O_2} (mm Hg)	90–95	104–108
Arterial P_{CO_2} (mm Hg)	38–40	27–32
Arterial pH	7.35–7.40	7.40–7.45
Oxygen consumption (mL/min)	173–311	249–331

Source: from ref. 30, with permission.

the right side of the heart demonstrates characteristic pressure tracings through the right atrium, right ventricle, pulmonary artery, and pulmonary capillary wedge positions (Fig. 37.5). From these waveforms, specific hemodynamic and ventilatory parameters can be determined (Table 37.9). Cardiac output may then be used to construct a ventricular function curve (Fig. 37.6). Hemodynamic subsets of ventricular function can be evaluated by plotting stroke index against left ventricular filling pressure (Fig. 37.7). A knowledge of pulmonary capillary wedge pressure, pulmonary artery diastolic-wedge gradient, and the arteriovenous oxygen difference makes it possible to ascertain the precise etiology of cardiopulmonary compromise (Fig. 37.8).

After placement of the Swan–Ganz catheter, a chest radiograph should be obtained to rule out pneumothorax and to confirm the catheter's position. Most complications encountered in patients undergoing pulmonary artery catheterization are a result of obtaining central venous access. These compli-

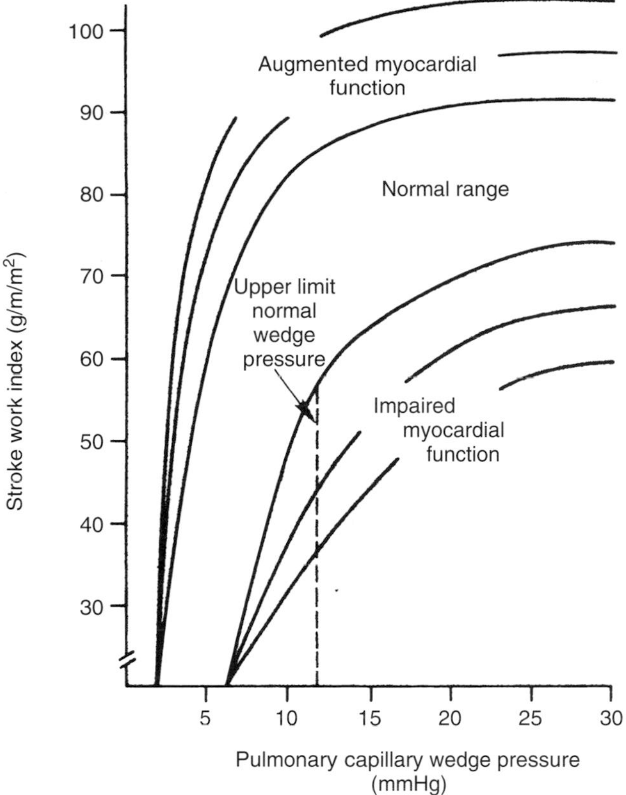

Figure 37.5 Normal ventricular function curve. (reprinted from ref. 36, with permission).

cations, which include pneumothorax and insertion site infection, occur in 1–5% of patients undergoing the procedure.[47–49] Potential complications of pulmonary artery catheterization include air embolism, thromboembolism, pulmonary infarction, catheter-related sepsis, direct trauma to the heart or vessels, Horner's syndrome and catheter intrapment.[50–55] These complications are uncommon and occur in 1% or fewer patients.

Development of accurate noninvasive methods of central hemodynamic assessment would help to minimize risks associated with invasive techniques. Such methods generally focus on sonographic or bioimpedance techniques to estimate cardiac output and have been described in both pregnant and nonpregnant patients.[31,56–59] Techniques to investigate noninvasive central pressure determination are also continuing.[60] For now, invasive techniques remain the standard for ongoing management of critically ill obstetric patients.

Electronic fetal heart rate monitoring

During the development of shock in the pregnant patient, redistribution of maternal cardiac output to vital organs such as the brain and heart may occur at the expense of the uteroplacental fetal unit. In the pregnant patient, fetal hypoxia may lead to changes in the heart rate pattern before the mother becomes overtly hypotensive.[61] In the absence of abnormal changes in the fetal heart rate pattern, significant maternal shock is unlikely.[61] Consequently, fetal heart rate is a clinically useful window to endorgan perfusion, and continuous electronic fetal heart rate monitoring with appropriate interpretation may be an important adjunct in the care of the critically ill pregnant patient.

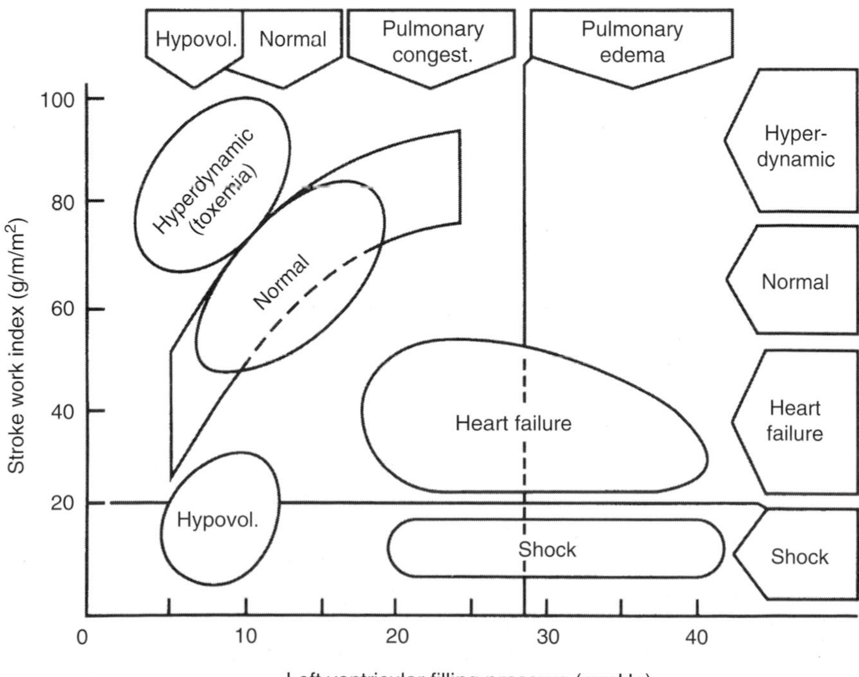

Figure 37.6 Hemodynamic subsets of ventricular function. Congest., congestion; Hypovol., hypovolemic (reprinted from ref. 36, with permission).

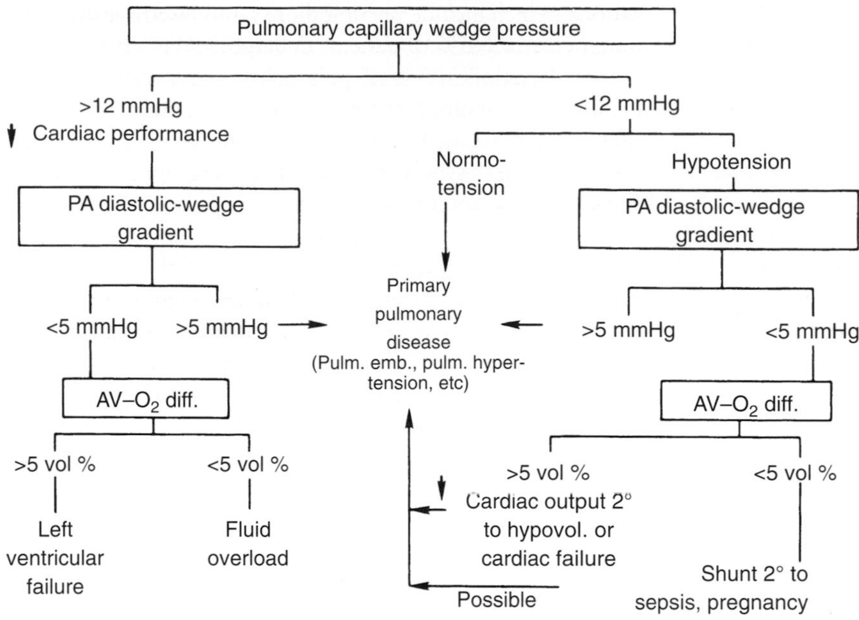

Figure 37.7 Flow diagram for interpretation of Swan–Ganz catheter. AV O_2 diff., arteriovenous oxygen difference; emb., embolism; hypovol., hypovolemia; PA, pulmonary artery; pulm., pulmonary; ventr., ventricular (reprinted from ref. 36, with permission).

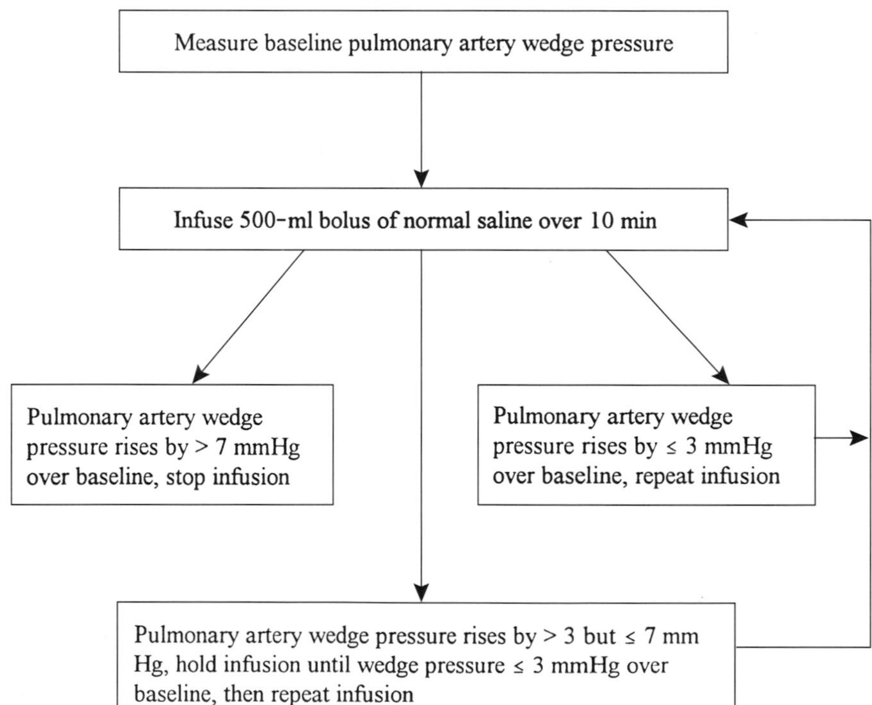

Figure 37.8 Pulmonary artery catheter-guided volume challenge.

The appropriate duration of electronic fetal monitoring after trauma has been the subject of investigation. The occurrence of adverse outcomes including abruptio placentae is not always predictable on the basis of injury severity.[62] Williams et al.[63] and Pearlman et al.[64] studied pregnant trauma patients with electronic fetal monitoring. No cases of placental abruption were seen in the absence of uterine contractions or if contractions occurred at a frequency of less than one every 10 min after 4 hours of monitoring. In patients with more frequent contractions, nearly 20% had placental abruptions. If complications do not occur after 4 hours of monitoring, an outcome similar to uninjured control subjects may be expected.[64] If uterine contractions, uterine tenderness, vaginal bleeding, rupture of membranes, nonreassuring fetal heart rate, or serious maternal injury are present, further monitoring and evaluation are indicated. Current evidence suggests that a period of continuous fetal monitoring is prudent in most cases of trauma during pregnancy of more than 22–24 weeks' gestation. In patients without signs or symptoms of abruption, a period of 2–6 hours of monitoring will suffice.[60] Prolonged monitoring is indicated in clinically unstable patients. In cases of hemodynamic instability, the maternal condition should be stabilized before delivery is considered for persistent evidence of fetal distress. The fetus may recover as maternal hypoxia, acidosis, and hypotension are corrected. Serial evaluations of fetal status and *in utero* resuscitation are generally preferable to the emergency delivery of a depressed infant from a hemodynamically unstable mother.

Surgical therapy

Surgical therapy may be an integral part of managing obstetric patients in hemorrhagic shock. Uterine bleeding can occur in the antepartum, intrapartum, and postpartum periods, and requires prompt evaluation and management. As in the case of uterine rupture, definitive surgical therapy may need to be initiated prior to stabilization. With postpartum hemorrhage resulting from uterine atony, surgical therapy may be required if the conventional treatments of uterine compression and pharmacologic therapies have been unsuccessful. Uterine artery ligation, initially described by Waters,[66] is performed by grasping the uterine wall and broad ligament and passing a single no. 1 chromic catgut suture anteroposteriorly through the lower uterine segment. The ascending uterine vessels are encompassed, and the suture is exited through the avascular area at the base of the broad ligament.[67] The fundus compression suture as described by B-Lynch[68] has also been reported to abate uterine hemorrhage in many cases.

If hemorrhage persists after these measures, the hemodynamic stability of the patient should determine whether one proceeds with a hypogastric artery ligation or hysterectomy. Hypogastric artery ligation should likely be reserved for stable patients of low parity who strongly desire further childbearing, as hypogastric artery ligation has been associated with a high complication rate and a low success rate in obtaining control of uterine hemorrhage. The ligation should be performed distal to the posterior division of the hypogastric artery. Hysterectomy is clearly indicated for profound intractable hemorrhage if the patient is unstable or not desirous of future childbearing.[69]

Transcatheter arterial embolization

Advances in interventional radiology have produced alternatives to the surgical management of obstetric hemorrhage. Arterial embolization with gel foam, coils, and glue have been reported to successfully control massive bleeding.[70,71] Vascular access is usually via the femoral or axillary artery, and diagnostic localization is performed with an intra-aortic injection of radiopaque dye below the renal arteries.[72] Once the site of hemorrhage is identified, selective catheterization is performed, and the vessel embolized. If catheterization of the bleeding artery is unsuccessful, embolization is attempted at or near the distal end of the anterior division of the internal iliac artery.[72] In patients with prior hypogastric artery ligation, collateral arteries may be identified, selectively catheterized, and embolized. However, embolization appears to be easier if performed before arterial ligation. Complications due to the procedure may include tissue ischemia (e.g., buttock claudication), guidewire perforation of an arterial blood vessel, and "postembolization syndrome."[73] Gelfoam appears to be the embolizing agent of choice in most obstetric series.[72–75] Prophylactic arterial catheterization for selective embolization has been proposed in cases at high risk for obstetric hemorrhage requiring surgical intervention.[73,76] Techniques for achieving medical and surgical hemostasis in patients with postpartum bleeding have been discussed more comprehensively by Dildy.[77]

Military antishock trousers

Military antishock trousers may be useful in controlling intra-abdominal and pelvic hemorrhage and in stabilizing pelvic and lower extremity fractures. In the pregnant shock victim, the abdominal compartment is not inflated, as uterine compression against the inferior vena cava may decrease venous return, thus reducing cardiac output and worsening the hemodynamic condition.[78] Although widely accepted recommendations for use during pregnancy have not been delineated, obstetric and gynecologic applications of the gravity suit have been proposed.[79]

Pelvic pressure pack

After hysterectomy for severe obstetric hemorrhage, diffuse bleeding may persist from pelvic surgical sites due to associated coagulopathy. The use of a transvaginal pressure pack was first reported by Logothetopulos in 1926[79] to tamponade diffuse venous bleeding. Others have since described a similar approach.[80,82] Hallak and colleagues[82] used a mushroom-shaped pack, created from a sterile plastic bag filled with gauze, placed transabdominally in the pelvis, with the stalk exiting the vagina. Traction on the stalk produces pressure on the pelvic floor, which tamponades low-pressure venous bleeding and controls hemorrhage. The pack is removed either transabdominally or transvaginally once the patient is hemodynamically and hematologically stable.

Cardiopulmonary resuscitation

If cardiac or pulmonary arrest occurs in the pregnant woman, cardiopulmonary resuscitation is initiated in the same fashion as for nonpregnant victims.[83] Technical variations specific for pregnancy include lateral uterine displacement to improve venous return and cardiac output, and perimortem Cesarean section if resuscitation is not successful within 4 min of the initial event.[84]

Perimortem Cesarean section

Postmortem Cesarean delivery has been described for centuries as an attempt to save the life of the unborn child.[84,85] Katz and colleagues[84] stress that the chance of fetal survival after perimortem Cesarean section is improved if maternal death is sudden. The timing of the operation is also important, and they have suggested that Cesarean delivery should be initiated within 4 min, and the baby delivered within 5 min of maternal cardiac arrest. The longest documented time interval from maternal death to delivery with fetal survival is 25 min,[86] although this remains disputed. In a series of patients who underwent cardiac arrest in association with amniotic fluid embolism, if delivery occurred within 15 min, most fetuses survived neurologically intact. However, even poor neonatal outcomes have been encountered with delivery within 5 min of maternal cardiac arrest.[87] Given the critical nature of time, perimortem Cesarean section should not be delayed to obtain an obstetric ultrasound; the physician should assess fundal height to confirm a potentially viable gestational age before making the abdominal incision.[88] In cases of moribund patients suffering from chronic disease, preparation for perimortem Cesarean section should be planned well in advance.

Case reports have indicated an increased success rate of delivering live infants, which may be related to both changing causes of maternal death and improved neonatal resuscitation. Most important, fetal outcome is related to fetal gestational age and the amount of time that has elapsed between maternal death and delivery.[89] However, underreporting of unsuccessful cases may prohibit an establishment of the actual success rate.

Katz and colleagues[84] have concluded that there is minimal legal risk for the physician in performing a perimortem section. The benefits include a chance for infant survival and improved maternal cardiopulmonary resuscitation. Removal of the placenta at the time of delivery is encouraged, as postoperative placental expulsion has been known to occur.[85–89]

Controversial and experimental modalities

Corticosteroids

Historically, the most controversial modality in the treatment of septic shock has been the use of high-dose steroids. Theoretic benefits include stabilization of lysosomal membranes, inhibition of complement-induced inflammatory changes, and attenuation of the effects of cytokines and other inflammatory mediators.[90] Numerous animal model studies and a few human studies have produced widely conflicting results. Human clinical studies have been criticized for flaws in study design and nonstandardization of regimens.[91] In 1984, Sprung et al.[92] demonstrated in a prospective, randomized study of 56 patients that corticosteroids may improve outcome if administered early in septic shock. Although short-term improvement was noted, mortality rates were not altered, and more than 25% of patients treated with steroids developed superinfections. Hoffman et al.[93] reported in 1984 that the mortality of patients with severe typhoid fever could be decreased by treatment with corticosteroids. In contrast, in 1987, the Methylprednisolone Severe Sepsis Study Group published data from a prospective, randomized, double-blind, placebo-controlled trial of 382 patients, concluding that the use of high-dose corticosteroids provided no benefit in the treatment of septic shock. Furthermore, they reported an increased mortality secondary to infections.[91] Additionally, potential side-effects from the administration of corticosteroids include gastrointestinal bleeding, hyperglycemia, and superinfection.[90,94] Currently, there is insufficient evidence to recommend the use of corticosteroids for septic shock, and their use should be reserved for patients with documented adrenal insufficiency.

Naloxone

Naloxone, an opiate antagonist, has been studied in animals[95] and humans[96–98] for the reversal of opiate-induced hypotension in endotoxic shock. The rationale for use of naloxone is that the endogenous opiate beta-endorphin is stored with adrenocorticotropic hormone, and both seem to be released simultaneously under physical stress.[98,99] Studies using the rat endotoxic shock model have suggested that naloxone both prophylactically blocks and rapidly reverses endotoxin-induced hypotension, which appears to be partially mediated by endogenous opiates.[100] Naloxone has been shown to inhibit the production of tumor necrosis factor-alpha induced by lipopolysaccharide.[101] Canine studies demonstrated improved cardiovascular parameters and survival in animals treated with naloxone in endotoxic shock.[102–104] Data published so far on humans have been controversial. Roberts and colleagues[97] suggest that earlier studies found no positive effects secondary to short observation periods.[96,105] Their data suggested that the continuous intravenous infusion of naloxone resulted in decreased inotrope and vasopressor requirements in patients with septic shock. Positive hemodynamic effects (decreased heart rate with increased stroke volume) were observed more than 4 hours after an initial naloxone bolus, and no side-effects were identified. A meta-analysis showed naloxone therapy to be associated with statistically significant hemodynamic improvement, but the case fatality rate was not decreased.[106] Further controlled clinical studies are required before the general use of naloxone for endotoxic shock can be recommended. It should be noted that the treatment of patients who are receiving opiates for chronic pain relief with naloxone can precipitate opiate withdrawal and even cardiovascular collapse.[100]

Nonsteroidal anti-inflammatory drugs

Prostaglandins are suspected to play a central role in septic shock, particularly in controlling regional blood flow distribution. Nonsteroidal anti-inflammatory drugs (NSAIDs) are thought to protect against the many deleterious effects of the prostaglandins on the cardiovascular, pulmonary, and coagulation systems during endotoxic shock. Increased production and decreased degradation of prostaglandins in severe sepsis has been demonstrated.[107] These alterations may be associated with endotoxin-induced pulmonary vascular changes.[108] Prostaglandin synthetase inhibitors have been used to blunt this pathophysiologic response in sheep.[109] Similar beneficial effects have been observed in other organ systems when experimental animals were pretreated with prostaglandin synthetase inhibitors prior to endotoxin exposure.[110–112] Current data regarding the effects of NSAIDs on humans are lacking, and future clinical investigation in humans appears to be warranted before routine clinical use.

Immunotherapy

Preliminary immunotherapy studies have shown that antibodies specifically directed against endotoxin or inflammatory mediators reduce mortality in animal models and human septic shock patients.[113] Clinical trials, however, have produced inconsistent results. Anti-lipopolysaccharide (anti-LPS) immunoglobulin has been found to bind to LPS from a wide range of Gram-negative bacteria.[114] Anti-LPS IgG has been administered to obstetric patients in septic shock with reductions in morbidity and mortality.[115] Control patients demonstrated a mortality of 47.4% (9 of 19), compared with a mortality of 7.1% (1 of 14) in the treated group. Ziegler and colleagues[116] treated bacteremic patients with human antiserum to a mutant *Escherichia coli* during the onset of the illness and observed a significant reduction in deaths from Gram-negative bacteremia and septic shock. Despite some promising studies, clinical success with antiendotoxin and anticytokine therapies has been less than hoped for,[117–121] and these agents are still of questionable benefit in the therapy of septic shock. Circulating natural inhibitors of proinflammatory cytokines have been described and, in animal models, these inhibitors have been shown to decrease mortality in endotoxic shock. The effect of these natural inhibitors on the clinical course of sepsis is being investigated. The presence of these inhibitors may explain the inconsistent results observed with the exogenous administration of inflammatory mediators in clinical trials.[122]

Anticoagulants

Activation of the coagulation system and depletion of endogenous anticoagulants have been found in patients with severe sepsis and septic shock. Diffuse microthrombus formation may induce organ dysfunction and lead to excess mortality in this situation. It has been hypothesized that antithrombin III may provide protection from multiorgan failure and improve survival in critically ill patients. However, studies using antithrombin III replacement in septic shock have shown no survival benefit. A double-blind, placebo-controlled, multicenter phase 3 trial of antithrombin III replacement showed no survival benefit and was associated with a significant increase in the risk for hemorrhagic complications in patients receiving antithrombin III in combination with heparin.[123] Recombinant activated protein C has also been studied. Bernard et al.[124] showed a significant reduction in mortality with the administration of recombinant activated protein C in septic shock. Unfortunately, an increased risk of bleeding was also noted, including two fatal intracranial hemorrhages. The authors calculated a rate of one serious bleeding event for every 66 patients treated and a 28-day survival benefit for one patient out of every 16 treated.

Specific etiologies and their management: hypovolemic shock

Hypovolemia may result from hemorrhage or solely from loss of intravascular fluids. The causes of hemorrhage in obstetrics are numerous, with the most common cause of postpartum hemorrhage being uterine atony followed by obstetric trauma.[15] Hemorrhage is still the leading cause of pregnancy-related mortality in the United States.[4] Pritchard[125] showed that the average amount of blood volume expansion during pregnancy is approximately 1500 mL. The average amount of blood lost during a vaginal delivery and elective repeat Cesarean section is 500 mL and 1000 mL respectively. No physiologic compromise should be encountered so long as the volume of blood lost at delivery does not exceed the amount added during pregnancy. When this balance is exceeded, hypovolemia results in decreased venous return and reduced cardiac output. The diagnosis of shock is most often made by the presence of hypotension, oliguria, acidosis, and collapse in the late stage, when therapy is frequently ineffective. Early in the course of massive hemorrhage, there are decreases in mean arterial pressure (MAP), cardiac output (CO), central venous pressure (CVP), and pulmonary capillary wedge pressure (PCWP), stroke volume and work, mixed venous oxygen saturation, and oxygen consumption. Increases are seen in systemic vascular resistance (SVR) and arteriovenous oxygen content differences, which serve to improve tissue oxygenation in the face of reduced blood flow. Catecholamine release causes a generalized increase in venular tone, resulting in an autotransfusion effect. These changes are accompanied by compensatory increases in heart rate, SVR, pulmonary vascular resistance, and myocardial contractility. Redistribution of CO and blood volume occurs via selective arteriolar constriction mediated by the central nervous system and adrenomedullary stress response. This results in diminished perfusion to the skin, kidneys, gut, and uterus and

Table 37.10 Uterotonic agents for uterine atony.

Agent	Administration route	Dose	Comments
Oxytocin (Pitocin)	Intravenous	10–40 U in 1000 mL of LR or NS	Not to exceed 100 mU/min
Methylergonovine (Methergine)	Intramuscular	0.2 mg q6h	Avoid in hypertensive patients
15-methyl $PGF_{2\alpha}$ (Hemabate)	Intramuscular or intramyometrial	0.25 mg q15–60 min	Side effects include arterial O_2 desaturation, bronchospasm, hypertension
Dinoprostone (Prostin E_2)	Per rectum	20-mg suppository	Use with caution in hypotensive patient because of vasodilation; if available, $PGF_{2\alpha}$ is preferable

LR, lactated Ringer's solution; NS, normal saline; $PGF_{2\alpha}$, prostaglandin F_2 alpha.

Source: modified from ref. 128.

maintenance of blood flow to the heart, brain, and adrenal glands. In the pregnant patient, this redistribution may result in fetal hypoxia and distress. This will likely occur before the mother becomes overtly hypotensive. Regardless of the maternal MAP, significant maternal shock is unlikely in the absence of fetal distress.[61] Three vital organs in addition to the placenta are especially susceptible to damage in the setting of hypotension due to hemorrhagic shock. These organs are the anterior pituitary gland, the kidneys, and the lungs. Sheehan and Murdoch[126] first described the syndrome of hypopituitarism secondary to postpartum hemorrhage and subsequent hypotension. This condition is now a rare obstetric complication. Hypovolemia leading to reduced renal perfusion can result in acute tubular necrosis. Severe hemorrhage may also precipitate ARDS.

Treatment of hemorrhagic shock involves correcting the initiating process as well as instituting general supportive measures, as previously discussed. When hemorrhage is suspected, the clinician should: (1) estimate actual blood loss and prehemorrhage blood volume as accurately as possible; (2) consider factors affecting the patient's ability to tolerate blood loss; (3) seek clinical evidence of hypovolemia and shock; (4) identify and correct the source of blood loss; (5) restore blood volume and oxygen carrying capacity; and (6) attempt to prevent further blood loss.[127] If medical therapy is unsuccessful, surgical procedures such as uterine artery ligation, internal iliac artery ligation, and emergency hysterectomy may be required. Other modalities, such as percutaneous transcatheter hypogastric artery embolization, may have their place in certain situations, but are not without their own risks. Response to therapy is reflected by hemodynamic parameters and laboratory values. Blood products should be administered after identifying the underlying disorder by laboratory indices.

Uterine atony

Uterine atony is the most common cause of primary postpartum hemorrhage, accounting for 80% of all cases. Diagnosis is made after delivery of the placenta when excessive bleeding is noted per vagina, and the uterine fundus is boggy. Examination of the birth canal reveals no lacerations that may account for bleeding. The uterine cavity should be explored to rule out retained placenta, retained blood clots, and disruption of the uterine wall. Initial management includes bimanual fundal massage and administration of uterotonic agents (Table 37.10).

Oxytocin (Pitocin, Syntocinon) is administered intravenously or via intramyometrial injection. Given intravenously, it has an almost immediate onset of action. The usual dose is 20–40 units/L of crystalloid. It has approximately 5% of the antidiuretic effect of vasopressin and, if given in large volumes of electrolyte-free solution, can cause water overload.

Methylergonovine maleate (Methergine) acts via stimulation of α-adrenergic myometrial receptors. The dose is 0.2 mg intravenously or via intramyometrial injection and may be repeated after 2–4 hours if necessary. Vasoconstriction is a side-effect, and contraindications include patients with heart disease, hypertension (including preeclampsia/eclampsia), and peripheral vascular disease.

Prostaglandin derivatives have been shown to be effective in treating postpartum uterine atony where other modalities have failed. Prostaglandin F2α results in contraction of smooth muscle cells.[127,129] Carboprost/hemabate (15-methyl prostaglandin F2α) is an established second-line treatment for postpartum hemorrhage unresponsive to oxytocic agents. It is available in single-dose vials of 0.25 mg to be given intramuscularly. Small case series have reported an efficacy of 85% or more in refractory postpartum hemorrhage.[130,131] The largest case series to date involved a multicenter surveillance study of 237 patients with postpartum hemorrhage refractory to oxytocin, which found that 15-methyl prostaglandin F2α was effective in 88% of patients.[132] Takagi and associates[133] showed that intramyometrial injection of prostaglandin F2α was superior to intravenous or intramuscular administration. The intramyometrial route of administration may be preferred to peripheral intramuscular injection, especially in patients who are in shock with compromised circulation. Side-effects include bronchospasm, nausea, vomiting, and diarrhea. There are case reports of hypotension and intrapulmonary shunting with arterial oxygen desaturation. This medication is therefore contraindicated in patients with cyanotic cardiac or pulmonary disease.

Misoprostol is a synthetic analog of prostaglandin E1 and can be given orally, vaginally, or rectally. An international multicenter randomized trial reported that oral misoprostol is less successful than parenteral oxytocin administration as prophylaxis for postpartum hemorrhage.[134] However, two small case series have reported good responses in postpartum hemorrhage refractory to oxytocin and syntometrine (oxytocin and ergometrine) with rectal doses of 600–1000 μg.[135,136] A single-blinded randomized trial of misoprostol 800 mg rectally versus syntometrine intramuscularly plus oxytocin by intravenous infusion found that misoprostol resulted in cessation of bleeding within 20 min in 30/32 cases (93%) compared with 21/32 (66%).[137] There was no difference in need for blood transfusion. The advantages of misoprostol include low cost and ease of administration. If hemorrhage persists despite medical therapy, surgical intervention is mandated.

Placenta accreta, increta, and percreta

Placenta accreta occurs when Nitabuch's membrane is deficient and trophoblastic tissue attaches directly to the deciduas basalis or myometrium. If the trophoblast invades the myometrium or penetrates adjacent structures, placenta increta or placenta percreta exist. In a study of 40 cases of such placental abnormalities, the relative proportions of accreta, increta, and percreta were 78%, 17%, and 5% respectively.[138] When the placenta detaches, areas of adherence prevent the normal mechanism of myometrial contraction and compression of vascular channels from occurring, resulting in hemorrhage. Clinical studies reveal an increasing trend in incidence, perhaps secondary to better case reporting and increasing rates of Cesarean section. Read and colleagues[139] state that the hallmark of placenta accreta is multiparity. The most common associated factors were placenta previa and previous Cesarean sections. A linear increase in risk of placenta accreta in patients with placenta previa and previous uterine scars has been demonstrated.[140] It has been noted that patients presenting with placenta previa and an unscarred uterus have a 5% risk of having placenta accreta. The risk of placenta accreta increased to 24% in patients with a placenta previa and one previous Cesarean section. Those patients with placenta previa and four previous Cesarean sections experienced a 67% incidence of placenta accreta.[140]

Treatment generally involves hysterectomy; however, conservative management may be appropriate in certain cases. McHattie's 1972[141] review of the literature showed a maternal mortality of 41.9% with conservative management and a maternal mortality of 6.5% with hysterectomy. In a review of patients treated between 1977 and 1983, no maternal deaths were observed in the 28% of those patients treated with conservative methods.[140] Individualized treatment and conservative procedures, such as curettage, local repair, and uterine artery ligation, may be appropriate in selected patients. When future fertility is desired and the placental site is not bleeding, conservative management has been advocated leaving the placenta *in situ*.[142] Methotrexate chemotherapy has also been used to enhance destruction of placental tissue;[143] however, cumulative experience is limited, and this approach may not always be successful.[144]

Placental invasion into extrauterine structures, such as the bladder (requiring bladder resection and massive transfusion) has been reported.[145–148] According to Thorp's[142] review of the English language literature, the maternal mortality of placenta percreta with bladder involvement is 9.5% (2 in 21). Antenatal detection by color Doppler ultrasound or magnetic resonance imaging has afforded predelivery preparation in some cases.[142,148,149]

Uterine rupture

Uterine rupture may occur in an unscarred uterus or at the site of a previous Cesarean section or gynecologic surgery. The overall rate varies from 2 to 8 per 10 000 deliveries.[150] The most common clinical sign in labor is the sudden onset of fetal decelerations, reported in 81% of cases.[150] Abdominal pain, cessation of contractions, and recession of the presenting part are less common. Bleeding may be intraperitoneal and into the broad ligament rather than revealed vaginally, and profound shock may occur before rupture is suspected. Uterine rupture should be considered in every obstetric patient with undiagnosed hemorrhagic shock. Rupture of an unscarred uterus is frequently related to obstetric intervention. This includes the excessive use of uterotonic drugs for induction or augmentation of labor, mid-forceps delivery, or breech extraction with internal podalic version.[151] Prolonged labor in the presence of malpresentation or cephalopelvic disproportion also predisposes to uterine rupture. External trauma and grand multiparity are also risk factors. The overall risk of uterine rupture for women attempting a trial of labor following low transverse Cesarean section is 0.5–1%, but higher if the trial of labor is unsuccessful.[152] A previous classical Cesarean section has a risk of rupture of 3–6%; this becomes 12% if a trial of labor takes place. Use of uterotonic drugs has been associated with an increased risk of rupture in the presence of a Cesarean section scar. Prostaglandin agents used for labor induction or cervical ripening have been associated with an even higher risk.[153] Management options include surgical repair and hysterectomy. Many authors consider hysterectomy to be the procedure of choice.[151,154] Repair may be considered when technically feasible, especially in cases of desired fertility. In these cases, planned Cesarean section should be performed as soon as fetal lung maturity can be confirmed. Repair may also be considered in cases where successful control of hemorrhage can be attained in hemodynamically unstable patients in order to avoid risking further blood loss.

Nonobstetric trauma

The incidence of accidental injury during pregnancy is estimated to be 6–7%.[89] An increased incidence of minor trauma has been observed as pregnancy progresses.[155] In most cases, injury is minimal and is not associated with a significant increase in perinatal mortality.[151,156] Major trauma, however, may place the mother and infant at severe risk.

The initial management of a pregnant woman who has sustained severe or major trauma is essentially the same as that of a nonpregnant person.[157] Crosby[158] has described in detail the initial evaluation of the gravid trauma patient. Maternal stabilization often leads to fetal stabilization, and delivery of the fetus before stabilization of the mother may worsen the mother's condition and result in the delivery of a premature fetus. Electronic fetal monitoring during maternal evaluation provides information regarding fetal and maternal well-being because deteriorating maternal cardiovascular status may be reflected early via fetal distress.[159] Signs of fetal well-being reflect maternal cardiovascular stability.

Blunt trauma

Causes of blunt abdominal trauma include motor vehicle accidents, pedestrian accidents, falls, and assaults. A recent large retrospective study revealed motor vehicle accidents to be the leading cause of fetal death related to maternal trauma.[159] In these accidents, the most common cause of fetal death is maternal death.[160] Among maternal survivors, premature separation of the placenta was the most frequent cause of fetal death. Fetal injuries, usually skull fractures and intracranial hemorrhage, tend to occur later in gestation because of a reduced amniotic fluid–fetus ratio, fixation of the fetal head in the bony pelvis, and placement of the fetal body outside the bony pelvis.[161] Expulsion from the vehicle and maternal head trauma are associated with poor maternal and fetal outcomes. Automobile passenger restraining systems have been shown to improve maternal and fetal outcomes. Crosby and Costiloe[162] noted a 33% mortality in unrestrained gravid automobile accident victims compared with a 5% mortality when two-point restraints (traditional lap belt) were used. In a more recent study of gravid accident victims using three-point restraint belts, it was noted that proper use of seat belts was the best predictor of maternal and fetal outcomes.[163]

The severity and mechanism of injury may not correlate directly with the incidence or severity of fetomaternal hemorrhage. Relatively minor blunt abdominal trauma may result in abruption. Up to 40% of severe blunt abdominal trauma is associated with placental abruption, but a 2.6% rate of abruption is seen with relatively minor abdominal trauma.[62,164–166] Uterine rupture is a relatively infrequent result of blunt traumatic injury during pregnancy. The incidence increases with advancing gestation and severity of force. Most traumatic uterine ruptures involve the uterine fundus or posterior aspect of the uterus.[161] Patients with a history of prior Cesarean delivery may be at increased risk.

Evaluation of the pregnant trauma patient is similar to evaluation of the nonpregnant patient with a few exceptions. The presence of the gravid uterus may alter the patterns of injury observed. Bowel injury is less frequent,[167] but hepatic and splenic injury appears to be more frequent.[168] Abdominal ultrasound is an important diagnostic tool in the identification of intraperitoneal fluid collections secondary to hemorrhage and has been demonstrated to have similar sensitivity and specificity as in nonpregnant trauma patients. Computed tomography (CT) scans may add additional diagnostic information. Exploratory laparotomy is indicated in pregnant patients who are hemodynamically unstable, have evidence of viscus perforation, infection, or fetal distress at a viable gestation. Diagnostic peritoneal lavage may be useful in less severe cases and is as useful in pregnancy as in nonpregnant abdominal trauma patients.[156] An open technique should be performed (analogous to open laparoscopy) in pregnant patients to help the catheter to avoid the gravid uterus. It should be noted that, because of changes in maternal physiology and pregnancy-related anatomic alterations, pregnant patients with significant abdominal injuries may not have significant abdominal signs or symptoms at presentation. Maternal hypotension (systolic pressure < 90 mmHg) and tachycardia may represent late findings. Diagnosis may be significantly delayed and result in a higher risk of pregnancy loss.[169] The presence of rib or pelvic fractures should increase the suspicion for other abdominal and pelvic injuries. Pelvic fractures are usually associated with motor vehicle accidents, and serious complications are related to urologic and vascular damage. Retroperitoneal hemorrhage may be massive. Less than 10% of patients with pelvic fractures require subsequent Cesarean section secondary to pelvic deformity or instability.[170]

Providers should have a high index of suspicion for physical abuse during pregnancy. Blunt abdominal trauma and other injuries, especially to the face, neck, breasts, and proximal extremities, may occur as a result of physical abuse.

Penetrating trauma

As the uterus expands during pregnancy, the bowel is compartmentalized into the upper abdomen and, therefore, the gravid uterus becomes the most frequently injured organ in cases of penetrating abdominal trauma.[158] Because of the physical forces involved, gunshot wounds carry a substantially higher mortality than stab wounds. Gunshot wounds are the most common type of penetrating injury during pregnancy.[171] A review by Buchsbaum[171] indicated a lower than expected maternal mortality in association with gunshot wounds to the uterus, as reflected by no reported deaths between 1912 and 1979. Fetal mortality, however, was high. An 89% incidence of fetal injury and a 66% perinatal mortality were noted in this series. Reported data from stab wounds are similar in that fetal mortality was high (42%) and maternal mortality was not seen.[172] Prematurity contributes significantly to perinatal mortality.

Traditional management of gunshot wounds to the

abdomen has included exploratory laparotomy to determine the extent of visceral injury.[171,173] Patients in whom the projectile or object enters anteriorly and below the level of the uterine fundus often do not have maternal visceral involvement.[174] Most authors recommend abdominal exploration for all extrauterine intra-abdominal gunshot wounds and most intrauterine wounds. Some authors suggest an individualized approach to intrauterine injures, and that selective laparotomy may be considered in gravidas with stable vital signs, when the missile entry site is anterior and subfundal, and when imaging studies indicate that the missile has not crossed the posterior uterine wall.[175–177] Posterior abdominal wounds, upper abdominal wounds, uterine location of the projectile, and fetal or maternal compromise are not optimal for expectant management.[176] Surgical exploration of all pregnant intra-abdominal gunshot wounds is generally advocated.[178]

Stab wounds require surgical repair in approximately one-half of reported cases.[179] Small bowel involvement is more frequent with upper abdominal stab wounds in pregnancy.[174,180] Because of the propensity of small intestinal injury and the potentially lethal effect of diaphragmatic rupture with herniation of intra-abdominal organs, exploration of upper abdominal stab wounds during pregnancy is recommended. As with gunshot wounds, if the wound is confined to the lower abdomen, the uterus usually sustains most injuries, whereas other viscera are spared.

Cesarean section is indicated for fetal distress at a viable gestational age. Exploratory laparotomy is not a reason to perform a Cesarean section if another indication does not exist. If direct uterine perforation is noted in the presence of a viable pregnancy, abdominal delivery is probably warranted. Maternal indications for delivery include severely compromised maternal cardiovascular status and obstruction of the operating field by the gravid uterus that limits surgical exposure of damaged vital structures. Fetal indications for delivery include fetal hemorrhage and distress and intra-amniotic infection. Such factors as suspected fetal injury and fetal distress must be balanced against those of fetal maturity. Even if labor has begun, some authors believe that vaginal delivery after exploratory laparotomy is preferable to hysterotomy.[159] However, if significant uterine injury involves the active uterine segment, Cesarean section is the preferred route of delivery to avoid uterine rupture in labor.

Burns

Approximately 2.2 million people each year in the United States suffer burns significant enough to present for medical treatment.[181] Most burns are minor, defined as superficial or partial-thickness injuries covering less than 10% of the total body surface. Major burns are partial-thickness or full-thickness injuries covering more than 10% of the total body surface. Major burns may be further classified as moderate (10–19% total body burn), severe (20–39% total body burn), or critical (40% or greater total body burn).[182] The first step in the management of the pregnant burn patient is to determine the depth of the burn and the percentage of body surface involved. The more severe the maternal burn, the higher the maternal and perinatal mortality.[182,183] With a burned total body surface area greater than or equal to 60%, the rate of maternal and fetal mortality was 100%, whereas a burned total body surface area of 40–59% was associated with 50% maternal and fetal mortality.[184] Pregnancy alone does not appear to alter maternal survival; however, with serious maternal burns, the fetal death rate is high.

Early complications of burns include severe hypovolemia secondary to fluid and electrolyte shifts resulting from vascular damage.[185] Hypovolemia, hypotension, and shock are prevented by aggressive fluid and electrolyte replacement.[183] Electrolytes must be monitored carefully as sodium and potassium values may fluctuate widely.[182] Hypoxemia may occur in conjunction with hypovolemia or secondary to upper and lower respiratory damage as a result of inhalation of noxious fumes. Oxygenation warrants close monitoring, and supplemental oxygen should be administered as required, occasionally via endotracheal intubation.

Later complications of burns include wound infection and sepsis. Hospital-acquired resistant organisms may complicate therapeutic management. Septicemia and pneumonia are reported to contribute to nearly one-half of all deaths in burn patients.[181] Abdominal scarring can also be problematic. Rai and Jackson[186] reported no increase in difficulties during labor or Cesarean section from severe abdominal scarring secondary to burns. Adverse effects of previous abdominal burn scars on subsequent pregnancies have been reported to include scar pain, occasional scar tissue breakdown, and uterine displacement.[186,187]

Because experience with pregnant burn patients is limited, few specific treatment guidelines beyond electrolyte and fluid replacement, adequate ventilatory support, and antibiotic therapy have been proposed. The route and timing of delivery should likely be based on obstetric indications, although assessment of fetal well-being in the burn patient may be difficult. The ability to determine fetal status with ultrasound or fetal monitoring will depend on the size and location of the burn. Because of such monitoring difficulties and the direct relationship between the size of the burn and perinatal outcome, some practitioners[184,188] have recommended immediate Cesarean delivery in any pregnant burn patient with a fetus of potentially viable age and a burn that involves 50% or more of the maternal body surface area. Early delivery of third-trimester pregnancies is an alternative option.[178]

Specific etiologies and their management: distributive shock

Causes of distributive shock include neurogenic, anaphylactic, and septic shock. Neurogenic shock in obstetrics may accompany conduction anesthesia, central nervous system trauma and puerperal uterine inversion. Uterorelaxant agents used for uterine inversion are listed in Table 37.11. Anaphylactic and septic shock will be discussed in detail.

Anaphylactic shock

Anaphylactic reactions are rare events, but may be fatal in as many as 10% of cases (Table 37.12).[189] Antibiotics, NSAIDs, oxytocin, anesthetic agents, blood products, colloid solutions, and latex exposures are some of the more common causes of anaphylaxis in pregnancy. Few reports exist in the current obstetric literature regarding this subject. Anaphylaxis is a series of events that occur in a sensitized individual on subsequent exposure to a specific antigen. It refers to an IgE-mediated, type I hypersensitivity response, produced by antigen-stimulated mast cell mediator release. The result may range from a localized response to a life-threatening systemic reaction with subsequent hypotension, cardiovascular collapse, and multiorgan system failure (Table 37.13). An anaphylactoid reaction may be clinically indistinguishable, and involves similar mediators, but does not require IgE antibody or previous exposure to the inciting substance. Exposure to the triggering agent results in release of primary mediators, such as histamine, prostaglandins, leukotrienes, eosinophil chemotactic factor of anaphylaxis, neutrophil chemotactic factor, and platelet-activating factor. These initiate release of

Table 37.11 Uterorelaxant agents for uterine inversion.

$MgSO_4$	2 g i.v. over 5–10 min
Terbutaline	0.125–0.250 mg IVP*
Nitroglycerin	100 μg IVP*
Halothane	≥ 2% general endotracheal

IVP, intravenous push.

*May exacerbate hypotension.

Source: reprinted from ref. 128, with permission.

Table 37.12 Clinical spectrum of anaphylactic reactions.

Mild	Moderate	Severe
Local erythema and itching	Dizziness	Hypotension, cyanosis
Pruritus and urticaria	Generalized skin reactions	Angioedema
Coryza	Hoarseness	Stridor and wheezes
Nausea/vomiting	Swelling of lips and tongue	Cardiac arrhythmias
Diarrhea	Tachypnea	Syncope and seizures
Conjunctiva suffusion	Tachycardia	Altered mental status
Anxiety	Increasing respiratory distress and anxiety	Shock, cardiopulmonary arrest

Source: reprinted from ref. 189, with permission.

Table 37.13 Specific organ failure in multisystem organ failure.

Organ	Pathophysiology	Result
Lung	Increased permeability and ventilation-perfusion mismatch; decreased metabolism of vasoactive substances; antimicrobial dysfunction and impaired lung defenses	Decreased compliance and hypoxemia; hemodynamic instability; nosocomial pneumonia
Liver synthesis	Early increase; late decrease; decreased lgA production; decreased bile salts	Acute-phase protein synthesis and hypermetabolism; jaundice and coagulopathy; increased gastrointestinal tract bacteria; increased gastrointestinal tract endotoxin
Immunologic	Kupffer's cell activation; decreased fibronectin and decreased phagocytosis	Hepatocyte depression and peripheral catabolism; bacteremia, endotoxemia, and microvascular emboli
Kidney	Hypovolemia, redistribution of renal blood flow, and nephrotoxic drugs	Azotemia with or without oliguria
Gastrointestinal tract	Decreased IgA and use of antibiotics and antacids; mucosal atrophy and increased permeability	Increased luminal bacteria and endotoxin; leaks bacteria and endotoxin, stress bleeding
Heart	Circulating myocardial depressant factor	Decreased ejection fraction
Central nervous system	Circulating false neurotransmitters; endogenous opioid-mimetics	Altered mental status; hemodynamic stability

Source: reprinted from ref. 190, with permission.

the secondary mediators via the complement, intrinsic coagulation, fibrinolytic, and kallikrein–kinin enzyme systems. Multiple products, such as leukotrienes, prostaglandins, vasoactive amines, and oxygen radicals, are then released from white blood cells, platelets, and eosinophils.[189]

Early recognition and treatment of anaphylactic reactions is essential. Risk factors, including a prior history of anaphylaxis, should be noted carefully at admission. The clinical presentation of anaphylactic and anaphylactoid reactions has been reviewed.[191] Hypotension and tachycardia are universal, and rhythm and conduction disturbances are frequently seen. The first priority is removal of the offending antigen, if possible. Further management in severe cases includes ventilation, oxygenation, and external cardiac massage, which, in general, is followed by the subcutaneous administration of epinephrine in 0.2-mg increments every 20 min up to a total dose of 1.0 mg.[192] In obstetric patients, ephedrine, 25–50 mg by intravenous push, has been recommended for treatment of hypotension because other vasoactive agents carry detrimental uteroplacental effects. However, failure to achieve rapid clinical response with ephedrine should be followed by the use of other, more potent agents, such as epinephrine or dopamine. A trial of terbutaline may also be an acceptable alternative treatment in cases of mild anaphylaxis or asthma but, in cases of life-threatening reactions, epinephrine should be used. Other drugs, such as corticosteroids, aminophylline, and antihistamines, have been recommended to enhance clinical response.[189,193] Hydrocortisone (100 mg), or its equivalent, should be administered every 6 hours. If wheezing is unresponsive to epinephrine, aminophylline (5–6 mg/kg) may be given over 20 min, followed by a maintenance dose of 0.9 mg/kg/hour. Aggressive fluid replacement is required. In severe cases of anaphylactic shock, colloid volume expanders may be required, because crystalloids have been observed to be ineffective in volume replacement.[192,193]

Septic shock

Septic shock is characterized by hypotension and inadequate tissue perfusion resulting from overwhelming sepsis.[194] Septic shock is rare in obstetrics, yet it remains one of the most frequent causes of maternal mortality in the United States.[195] Even with optimal care, the mortality rate from septic shock remains 40–50% in most series.[196] Many infections may result in septic shock in obstetric patients, but endometritis, chorioamnionitis, and pyelonephritis are the most common causes. Before legalization of abortion, septic shock resulting from criminal abortion was common.[197,198] Other infections that may develop in obstetric patients include pneumonia, appendicitis, septic abortion, toxic shock syndrome, septic pelvic thrombophlebitis, and endocarditis. Significant risk factors for septic shock include prolonged rupture of membranes, retained products of conception, and instrumentation of the genitourinary tract.[25]

Although genitourinary and other infections are common among obstetric patients, septic shock is an infrequent event. The incidence of septic shock in bacteremic obstetric and gynecologic patients is estimated to be 0–12%.[199–201] Physiologic changes in pregnancy may result in higher pulmonary morbidity in septic pregnant patients. Pregnancy decreases the gradient between colloid oncotic pressure and PCWP.[35] This results in an increased propensity for pulmonary edema in the setting of infection.

Mortality from septic shock in the general population is reported to be as high as 40–90%, as opposed to less than 3% in obstetric and gynecologic patients.[2,199,201,202] This may be explained by the relative good health and youth of obstetric patients, prompt vigorous treatment, and infrequency of underlying disease processes.[201] Obstetric infections are usually caused by organisms normally found in the genital tract and thus are often polymicrobial.[203–205] Common organisms include *E. coli*, *Klebsiella–Enterobacter*, *Pseudomonas*, and *Serratia*.[206] Most cases of bacterial infection complicated by shock are caused by Gram-negative enteric organisms.[207] Lee and colleagues[25] found that 80% of cases of septic shock during pregnancy developed during the postpartum period.

Septic shock has classically been described in three phases that correlate with progressive physiologic derangement: early (warm) shock, late (cold) shock, and secondary (irreversible) shock.[14,206] Flushed warm skin, fever, chills, diaphoresis, and tachycardia are manifest in the early phase. Pulse pressure and urine output remain stable. The late phase is characterized by cool and clammy skin, a decrease in body temperature, and diminished mental status. Hypotension, tachycardia, and oliguria develop. Myocardial depression becomes a prominent feature of severe septic shock, with marked reductions in cardiac output and SVR.[208] This phase is reversible with treatment. If medical intervention is not begun and cellular hypoxia and anaerobic metabolism continue, the irreversible phase of septic shock develops. Metabolic acidosis, anuria, respiratory distress, cardiac distress, DIC, and coma are ominous signs.

Cultures should be obtained in all patients from the urine, blood, and, if possible, the amniotic fluid or the endometrium. Other specific sources (e.g., stool, wound, and sputum) are cultured as indicated, and lumbar puncture should be considered in patients with altered mental status.[94] Chest radiography should be obtained to rule out infiltrates, evidence of pulmonary edema, and acute respiratory distress syndrome. Abdominal radiography should be considered to rule out free air under the diaphragm or a foreign body in some clinical circumstances.[14]

Treatment of septic shock requires general supportive measures, including restoration of intravascular volume and inotropic support (see section on general supportive measures). Lee and colleagues[194] recommend that acute stabilization of obstetric patients with septic shock be performed in the following sequence: (1) volume repletion and hemostasis; (2) inotropic therapy with dopamine on the basis of left ventricular function curves; and (3) addition of peripheral vasoconstrictors (phenylephrine first, then norepinephrine) to maintain vascular afterload. Considerable fluid resuscitation is often necessary secondary to profound vasodilation, increased capillary permeability, and extravasation of fluid into the extravascular space. Blood pressure, heart rate, urine output, and hematocrit may be used to initially guide resuscitation, but a PA catheter may ultimately be the best means of guiding optimal fluid and inotrope management in critically ill patients with septic shock and/or multiorgan system dysfunction.[33,209,210] Adequate oxygenation is essential. Antibiotic therapy for sepsis should be tailored directly to the suspected source and guided by information obtained by Gram's stain. Empiric therapy in the obstetric patient should include broad coverage for aerobic and anaerobic Gram-negative and Gram-positive bacteria.

Failure of the patient to respond promptly to simple volume resuscitation warrants transfer to an intensive care setting.[211] If response to treatment is not satisfactory, close examination for abscessed or necrotic tissue must be carried out and surgical intervention considered.[209] Timely drainage of abscesses and debridement of necrotic tissue, sometimes via hysterectomy, are required for clinical improvement.

Specific etiologies and their management: cardiogenic shock

Most etiologies of cardiogenic shock are described elsewhere in the text. In this chapter, cardiac compression and electric shock will be discussed.

Cardiac compression

Tension pneumothorax, pericardial tamponade, and rupture of the diaphragm with herniation of the abdominal contents into the thoracic cavity may cause significant cardiac compression resulting in decreased venous return and decreased cardiac output.

Placement of a chest tube alleviates compression secondary to a tension pneumothorax. Pericardiocentesis relieves the high intrapericardial pressure produced by cardiac tamponade. Diaphragmatic rupture with herniation of abdominal viscera is a surgical emergency.[212] Maternal death secondary to constrictive pericarditis occurring after thoracic radiotherapy has been reported.[214]

Electric shock

Reports of electrical injury during pregnancy are relatively few in the medical literature. The electric shock threshold for a mild sensation is 1 mA, for local muscular tetany 10 mA, and for ventricular fibrillation about 100 mA.[214] The fetus appears to be more susceptible to the adverse effects of electric shock, as the hyperemic gravid uterus, amniotic fluid, and fetal skin are all excellent conductors of electricity.[215] In a series of 15 cases of electric shock in pregnancy, there were no maternal deaths, 11 fetal deaths, and only one normal fetal outcome.[215] The path of the current appears to be an important factor, as accidental shocks have a hand-to-foot (including the uterus) passage of current. Intentional therapeutic shock (electroconvulsive therapy and DC cardioversion) does not include the uterus in the current path, and published reports would suggest its safety during pregnancy. Fatovich[215] recommends immediate obstetric evaluation with fetal monitoring and ultrasound in any pregnant victim of electric shock. Maternal cardiac monitoring after electric shock with single-phase alternating current at household voltage may not be necessary if the patient is asymptomatic and has had a normal electrocardiographic result on presentation.[212]

Specific etiologies and their management: obstructive shock

Obstruction of the pulmonary vessels may result in pulmonary hypertension, right-sided heart failure, cardiogenic shock, and death. Pulmonary embolism is one of the leading causes of maternal death in the United States and is discussed elsewhere in this text.

Key points

1. Maternal mortality in the United States is steadily declining, and recent statistics for the United States suggest an overall maternal mortality of 11.5 maternal deaths per 100 000 live births.
2. Hemorrhage is the leading cause of pregnancy-related mortality, followed by embolism-related deaths and hypertensive diseases.
3. Shock in the obstetric patient includes hypovolemic, distributive, cardiogenic, and obstructive etiologies.
4. Initial supportive measures in the treatment of shock include volume resuscitation, blood component replacement, ensuring adequate oxygenation, and supporting blood pressure with pharmacologic agents if indicated.
5. Crystalloids are first-line therapy for volume resuscitation.
6. Blood component replacement should be guided by clinical evaluation and by laboratory parameters. FFP

and platelets should be transfused only if factor or platelet deficiencies are presumed to be the principal derangement.

7 If intravascular volume replacement is not successful in supporting blood pressure and other reversible causes of shock are not found, inotropic agents may be necessary. When blood pressure does not respond to inotropic therapy, use of a peripheral vasoconstrictor should be considered.

8 In hypovolemic shock, vasopressors or inotropic agents are rarely indicated and should not be given until intravascular volume has been adequately replaced.

9 Use of a pulmonary artery catheter to assess cardiac function and hemodynamic status may be helpful in select critically ill patients.

10 Electronic fetal heart rate monitoring in the critically ill pregnant patient yields clinically useful information about endorgan perfusion. Fetal hypoxia may lead to changes in the heart rate pattern before the mother becomes overtly hypotensive. In the absence of abnormal changes in the fetal heart rate pattern, significant maternal shock is unlikely.

11 In cases of hemodynamic instability, the maternal condition should be stabilized before delivery is considered for persistent fetal distress. Fetal recovery will likely occur as maternal hypoxia, acidosis, and hypotension are corrected.

12 Perimortem Cesarean section should be initiated within 4 min of cardiac arrest with a goal of delivery of the fetus within 5 min of the initial event.

13 Average blood loss during a vaginal delivery and elective Cesarean section is 500 mL and 1000 mL respectively. No physiologic compromise should be encountered so long as the volume lost at delivery does not exceed this amount.

14 Management of hemorrhage includes: estimation of blood loss; consideration of factors affecting the patient's ability to tolerate blood loss; evaluation for possible hypovolemia and shock; identification of the source of blood loss; restoration of blood volume and oxygen-carrying capacity; and an attempt to prevent further blood loss.

15 Uterine atony is the most common cause of postpartum hemorrhage.

16 The severity and mechanism of blunt traumatic injury during pregnancy does not directly correlate with the incidence or severity of fetomaternal hemorrhage. Relatively minor trauma may result in abruption. A high suspicion for abruption after traumatic injuries is crucial, and a period of continuous fetal monitoring is prudent in most cases of trauma during pregnancy of viable gestational age.

17 The gravid uterus is the most frequently injured organ in cases of penetrating abdominal trauma during pregnancy. In these cases, fetal mortality is high.

18 Infection is a leading cause of morbidity and mortality in the obstetric population, and common causes include endometritis, chorioamnionitis, and pyelonephritis. Treatment of septic shock requires general supportive measures and broad-spectrum antibiotic coverage.

19 If a patient in septic shock fails to improve with supportive measures and broad-spectrum antibiotics, a close examination for abscessed or necrotic tissue must be performed and surgical intervention considered.

20 Clinical assessment of preexisting risk factors for the development of obstetric complications and advance preparation may decrease fetomaternal morbidity and mortality in the event of maternal cardiovascular collapse and shock.

References

1 Holcroft JW, Blaisdell FW. Shock: causes and management of circulatory collapse. In: Sabiston DC, ed. *Textbook of surgery*, 13th edn. Philadelphia, PA: W.B. Saunders; 1986:38.

2 Cavanagh D, Knuppel RA, Shepherd JH, et al. Septic shock and the obstetrician/gynecologist. *South Med J* 1982;75: 809.

3 Morbidity and Mortality Weekly Report. Maternal Mortality – United States, 1982–1996. US Department of Health and Human Services. *Morbidity Mortality Weekly Rep* 1998;47:705.

4 Morbidity and Mortality Weekly Report. Pregnancy-related deaths among Hispanic, Asian/Pacific Islander, and American Indian/Alaska Native Women – United States, 1991–1997. US Department of Health and Human Services. *Morbidity Mortality Weekly Rep* 2001;50:361.

5 National Center for Health Statistics. *Healthy people 2000 review, 1992*. Hyattsville, MD: US Department of Health and Human Services, Public Health Service, CDC, 1993.

6 Morbidity and Mortality Weekly Report. Pregnancy-related surveillance – United States, 1987–1990. US Department of Health and Human Services. *Morbidity Mortality Weekly Rep* 1997; 46:17.

7 Hazelgrove JF, Price C, Pappachan GD. Multicenter study of obstetric admissions to 14 intensive care units in southern England. *Crit Care Med* 2001;29:770.

8 Ananth CV, Smulian JC. Epidemiology of critical illness and outcomes in pregnancy. In: Dildy GA, Belfort MA, Saade GR, et al., eds. *Critical care obstetrics*, 4th edn. Maldon: Blackwell Science; 2004:3.

9 Kirshon B, Cotton DB. Fluid replacement in the obstetric patient. In: Sciarra JJ, ed. *Gynecology and obstetrics*, Vol. 3. Hagerstown, MD: Harper & Row; 1989:1.

10 Rackow EC, Falk JL, Fein IA, et al. Fluid resuscitation in circulatory shock: a comparison of the cardiorespiratory effects of albumin, hetastarch, and saline solutions in patients with hypovolemic and septic shock. *Crit Care Med* 1983;11:839.

11 Hardaway RM. Coagulation disorders and hemorrhagic shock in the parturient. *Int Anesthesiol Clin* 1968;6:743.

12 American College of Obstetricians and Gynecologists. Hemorrhagic shock. *Tech Bull* 1984;82.

13 Velanovich V. Crystalloid versus colloid fluid resuscitation: a meta-analysis of mortality. *Surgery* 1989;105(1):65.
14 Cavanagh D. Septic shock in a pregnant or recently pregnant woman. *Postgrad Med* 1977;62:62.
15 Hayashi RH. Hemorrhagic shock in obstetrics. *Clin Perinatol* 1986;13:755.
16 Oberman HA, Barnes BA, Friedman BA. The risk of abbreviating the major crossmatch in urgent or massive transfusion. *Transfusion* 1978;18:137.
17 Consensus Conference. Fresh-frozen plasma. Indications and risks. *JAMA* 1985;253:551.
18 Oberman HA. Uses and abuses of fresh frozen plasma. In: Garratty A, ed. *Current concepts in transfusion therapy*. Arlington, VA: American Association of Blood Banks; 1985:109.
19 Mannucci PM, Federici AB, Sirchia G. Hemostasis testing during massive blood replacement: a study of 172 cases. *Vox Sang* 1982;42:113.
20 Counts RB, Haisch C, Simon TL, et al. Hemostasis in massively transfused trauma patients. *Ann Surg* 1979;190:91.
21 Reiss RF. Hemostatic defects in massive transfusion: rapid diagnosis and management. *Am J Crit Care* 2000;9:158.
22 Shulman NR, Watkins SP, Itscoits SB, et al. Evidence that the spleen retains the youngest and hemostatically most effective platelets. *Trans Assoc Am Phys* 1968;81:302.
23 Murphy S, Gardner FH. Platelet preservation: effect of storage temperature on maintenance of platelet viability – deleterious effect of refrigerated storage. *N Engl J Med* 1969;280:1094.
24 Borucki DT, ed. *Blood component therapy: a physician's handbook*, 3rd edn. Washington, DC: American Association of Blood Banks; 1981:25.
25 Lee W, Clark SL, Cotton DB, et al. Septic shock during pregnancy. *Am J Obstet Gynecol* 1988;159:410.
26 Goldberg LI. Dopamine: clinical uses of an endogenous catecholamine. *N Engl J Med* 1974;291:707.
27 Abboud FM. Shock. In: Wyngaarden JB, Smith LH, eds. *Cecil textbook of medicine*, 17th edn. Philadelphia, PA: W.B. Saunders; 1985:211.
28 Callender K, Levinson G, Shnider SM, et al. Dopamine administration in the normotensive pregnant ewe. *Obstet Gynecol* 1978;51:586–589.
29 Rolbin SH, Levinson G, Shnider SM, et al. Dopamine treatment of spinal hypotension decreases uterine blood flow in the pregnant ewe. *Anesthesiology* 1979;51:37–40.
30 Kirshon B, Cotton DB. Invasive hemodynamic monitoring in the obstetric patient. *Clin Obstet Gynecol* 1987;30:579.
31 Lee W, Rokey R, Cotton DB. Noninvasive maternal stroke volume and cardiac output determinations by pulsed Doppler echocardiography. *Am J Obstet Gynecol* 1988;158:505.
32 Ruiz C, Weil MH, Carlson R. Treatment of circulatory shock with dopamine. *JAMA* 1979;242:165.
33 Swan HJC, Ganz W, Forrester J, et al. Catheterization of the heart in man with use of a flow-directed balloon-tipped catheter. *N Engl J Med* 1970;283:447.
34 Clark SL, Cotton DB, Gonik B, et al. Central hemodynamic alterations in amniotic fluid embolism. *Am J Obstet Gynecol* 1988;158:1124.
35 Clark SL, Cotton DB, Lee W, et al. Central hemodynamic assessment of normal term pregnancy. *Am J Obstet Gynecol* 1989;161:1439.
36 Cotton DB, Benedetti TJ. Use of the Swan-Ganz catheter in obstetrics and gynecology. *Obstet Gynecol* 1980;56:641.
37 Benedetti TJ, Cotton DB, Read JC, et al. Hemodynamic observations in severe preeclampsia with a flow-directed pulmonary artery catheter. *Am J Obstet Gynecol* 1980;136:465.
38 Cruz K, Franklin C. The pulmonary artery catheter: uses and controversies. *Crit Care Clin* 2001;17(2):271.
39 Connors AF, Jr, Speroff T, Dawson NV, et al. The effectiveness of right-heart catheterization in the initial care of critically ill patients. *JAMA* 1996;18:889.
40 Rhodes A, Cusack RJ, Newman PJ, et al. A randomized, controlled trial of the pulmonary artery catheter in critically ill patients. *Intens Care Med* 2002;28(3):256.
41 Cotton DB, Gonik B, Dorman K, et al. Cardiovascular alterations in severe pregnancy induced hypertension: relationship of central venous pressure to pulmonary capillary wedge pressure. *Am J Obstet Gynecol* 1985;151:762.
42 Clark SL, Cotton DB. Clinical opinion: clinical indications for pulmonary artery catheterization in the patient with severe preeclampsia. *Am J Obstet Gynecol* 1988;158:453.
43 Bolte AC, Dekker GA, vanEyck J, et al. Lack of agreement between central venous pressure and pulmonary capillary wedge pressure in preeclampsia. *Hypertens Pregnancy* 2000;19(3): 261.
44 Clark SL, Horenstein JM, Phelan JP, et al. Experience with the pulmonary artery catheter in obstetrics and gynecology. *Am J Obstet Gynecol* 1985;152:374.
45 Nolan TE, Wakefield ML, Devoe LD. Invasive hemodynamic monitoring in obstetrics. A critical review of its indications, benefits, complications, and alternatives. *Chest* 1992;101:1429.
46 Gibson RS, Kistner JR. In: Suratt PM, Gibson RS, eds. *Manual of medical procedures*. St Louis, MI: C.V. Mosby; 1982:59.
47 Patel C, Laboy V, Venus B, et al. Acute complications of pulmonary artery catheter insertion in critically ill patients. *Crit Care Med* 1986;14:195.
48 Scott WL. Complications associated with central venous catheters. A survey. *Chest* 1988;91:1221.
49 Gilbert WM, Towner DR, Field NT, et al. The safety and utility of pulmonary artery catheterization in severe preeclampsia and eclampsia. *Am J Obstet Gynecol* 2000;182(6):1397.
50 Lanigan C, Cornwell E. Pulmonary artery catheter entrapment. *Anaesthesia* 1991;46:600.
51 Vaswani S, Garvin L, Matuschak GM. Postganglionic Horner's syndrome after insertion of a pulmonary artery catheter through the internal jugular vein. *Crit Care Med* 1991;19: 1215.
52 Yellin LB, Filler JJ, Barnette RE. Nominal hemoptysis heralds pseudoaneurysm induced by a pulmonary artery catheter. *Anesthesiology* 1991;74:370.
53 Manager D, Connell GR, Lessin JL. Catheter induced pulmonary artery haemorrhage resulting from a pneumothorax. *Can J Anaesth* 1993;40:1069.
54 Bernardin G, Milhaud D, Roger PM, et al. Swan–Ganz catheter related pulmonary valve infective endocarditis: a case report. *Intens Care Med* 1994;20:142.
55 Soding PF, Klinck JR, Kong A, et al. Infective endocarditis of the pulmonary valve following pulmonary artery catheterization. *Intens Care Med* 1994;20:222.
56 Easterling T, Watts D, Schmucker B, et al., Measurement of cardiac output during pregnancy: validation of Doppler technique and clinical observations in preeclampsia. *Obstet Gynecol* 1987;69:845.
57 Belfort MA, Rokey R, Saade GR, et al. Rapid echocardiographic assessment of left and right heart hemodynamics in critically ill obstetric patients. *Am J Obstet Gynecol* 1991;171:884.

58 Clark SL, Southwick J, Pivarnik JM, et al. A comparison of cardiac index in normal term pregnancy using thoracic electrical bioimpedance and oxygen extraction (Fick) technique. *Obstet Gynecol* 1994;83:669.
59 Weiss S, Calloway E, Cairo J, et al. Comparison of cardiac output measurements by thermodilution and thoracic electrical bioimpedance in critically ill vs. noncritically ill patients. *Am J Emerg Med* 1995;13:626.
60 Ensing G, Seward J, Darragh R, et al. Feasibility of generating hemodynamic pressure curves from noninvasive Doppler echocardiographic signals. *J Am Coll Cardiol* 1994;23:434.
61 Clark SL. Shock in the pregnant patient. *Semin Perinatol* 1990;14:52.
62 Fries MH, Hankins GDV. Motor vehicle accident associated with minimal maternal trauma, but subsequent fetal demise. *Ann Emerg Med* 1989;18:301.
63 Williams JK, McClain L, Rosemursy AS, et al. Evaluation of blunt abdominal trauma in the third trimester of pregnancy. *Obstet Gynecol* 1990;75:33.
64 Pearlman MD, Tintinalli JE, Lorenz RP. A prospective controlled study of outcome after trauma during pregnancy. *Am J Obstet Gynecol* 1990;162:1502.
65 American College of Obstetricians and Gynecologists. Obstetric aspects of trauma management. *Tech Bull* 1998;251.
66 Waters EG. Surgical management of postpartum hemorrhage with particular reference to ligation of uterine arteries. *Am J Obstet Gynecol* 1952;64:1143.
67 O'Leary JL, O'Leary JA. Uterine artery ligation in the control of intractable postpartum hemorrhage. *Am J Obstet Gynecol* 1966;94:920.
68 B-Lynch C, Coker A, Lawal AH, et al. The B-Lynch surgical technique for the control of massive postpartum hemorrhage: an alternative to hysterectomy? *Br J Obstet Gynecol* 1997;104: 372.
69 Clark SL, Yeh S-Y, Phelan JP, et al. Emergency hysterectomy for the control of obstetric hemorrhage. *Obstet Gynecol* 1984;64: 376.
70 Smith DC, Wyatt JF. Embolization of the hypogastric arteries in the control of massive vaginal hemorrhage. *Obstet Gynecol* 1977;49:317.
71 Walker WJ. Case report: successful internal iliac artery embolization with glue in a case of massive obstetric hemorrhage. *Clin Radiol* 1996;51:442.
72 Greenwood LH, Glickman MG, Schwartz PE, et al. Obstetric and nonmalignant gynecologic bleeding: treatment with angiographic embolization. *Radiology* 1987;164:155.
73 Alvarez M, Lockwood CJ, Ghidini A, et al. Prophylactic and emergent arterial catheterization for selective embolization in obstetric hemorrhage. *Am J Perinatol* 1992;9:441.
74 Yamashita Y, Takahashi M, Ito M, et al. Transcatheter arterial embolization in the management of postpartum hemorrhage due to genital tract injury. *Obstet Gynecol* 1991;77: 160.
75 Gilbert WM, Moore TR, Resnik R, et al. Angiographic embolization in the management of hemorrhage complications of pregnancy. *Am J Obstet Gynecol* 1992;166:493.
76 Mitty HA, Sterling KM, Alvarez M, et al. Obstetric hemorrhage: prophylactic and emergency arterial catheterization and embolotherapy. *Radiology* 1993;188:183.
77 Dildy GA. Postpartum hemorrhage: new management options. *Clin Obstet Gynecol* 2002;45(2):330.
78 Pearlman MD, Tintinalli JE. Evaluation and treatment of the gravida and fetus following trauma during pregnancy. *Obstet Gynecol Clin North Am* 1991;18:371.
79 Gunning JE. For controlling intractable hemorrhage: the gravity suit. *Contemp Obstet Gynecol* 1983;22:23.
80 Logothetopulos K. Eine absolute sichere Blutstillungsmethode bei vaginalen und abdominalen gynakologischen Operationen. *Zentralbl Gynakol* 1926;50:3202.
81 Robie GF, Morgan MA, Payne GG, et al. Logothetopulos pack for the management of uncontrollable postpartum hemorrhage. *Am J Perinatol* 1990;7:327.
82 Hallak M, Dildy GA, Hurley TJ, et al. Transvaginal pressure back for life-threatening pelvic hemorrhage secondary to placenta accreta. *Obstet Gynecol* 1991;78:938.
83 Dildy GA, Clark SL. Cardiac arrest during pregnancy. *Obstet Gynecol* Clin 1995;22:303.
84 Katz VL, Dotters DJ, Droegemueller W. Perimortem cesarean delivery. *Obstet Gynecol* 1986;68:571.
85 Weber CE. Postmortem cesarean section: review of the literature and case reports. *Am J Obstet Gynecol* 1971;110:158.
86 Buchsbaum HJ. Traumatic injury in pregnancy. In: Barber HRK, Garber EA, eds. *Surgical disease in pregnancy*. Philadelphia, PA: W.B. Saunders; 1974:184.
87 Clark SL, Hankins GD, Dudley DA, et al. Amniotic fluid embolism: analysis of the national registry. *Am J Obstet Gynecol* 1995;172:1158.
88 Morris JA, Rosenbower TJ, Jurkovich GJ, et al. Infant survival after cesarean section for trauma. *Ann Surg* 1996;223:481.
89 Patterson RM. Trauma in pregnancy. *Clin Obstet Gynecol* 1984;27:32.
90 Schein RMH, Long WM, Sprung CL. Controversies in the management of sepsis and septic shock: corticosteroids, naloxone and non-steroidal anti-inflammatory agents. In: Sibbald WJ, Sprung CL, eds. *Perspectives on sepsis and septic shock*. Fullerton, CA: Society of Critical Care Medicine; 1986:339.
91 Bone RC, Fisher CJ, Clemmer TP, et al. A controlled clinical trial of high-dose methylprednisolone in the treatment of severe sepsis and septic shock. *N Engl J Med* 1987;317:653.
92 Sprung CL, Caralis PV, Marcial EH, et al. The effects of high-dose corticosteroids in patients with septic shock. A prospective, controlled study. *N Engl J Med* 1984;311:1137.
93 Hoffman SL, Punjabi NH, Kumula S, et al. Reduction of mortality in chloramphenicol treated severe typhoid fever by high-dose dexamethasone. *N Engl J Med* 1984;310:82.
94 Rackow EC. Clinical definition of sepsis and septic shock. In: Sibbald WJ, Sprung CL, eds. *Perspectives on sepsis and septic shock*. Fullerton, CA: The Society of Critical Care Medicine; 1986:1.
95 Holaday JW, Faden AI. Naloxone reversal of endotoxin hypotension suggests role of endorphins in shock. *Nature* 1978;275:450.
96 Bonnet F, Bilaine J. Lhoste F, et al. Naloxone therapy of human septic shock. *Crit Care Med* 1985;13:972.
97 Roberts DE, Dobson KE, Hall KW, et al. Effects of prolonged naloxone infusion in septic shock. *Lancet* 1988;2:699.
98 Guillemin R, Vargo T, Rossier J, et al. Beta-endorphin and adrenocorticotropin are secreted concomitantly by the pituitary gland. *Science* 1977;197:1367.
99 Rossier J, French ED, Rivier C, et al. Foot-shock induced stress increases beta-endorphin levels in blood but not brain. *Nature* 1977;270:618.
100 Holaday JW, Faden AI. Naloxone treatment in shock. *Lancet* 1981;ii:201.
101 Greeneltch KM, Haudenschild CC, Keegan AD, et al. The opioid

antagonist naltrexone blocks acute endotoxic shock by inhibiting tumor necrosis factor-alpha production. *Brain Behav Immun* 2004;18(5):476.

102 Thijs LG, Balk E, Tuynman HARE, et al. Effects of naloxone on hemodynamics, oxygen transport, and metabolic variables in canine endotoxin shock. *Circ Shock* 1983;10:147.

103 Reynolds DG, Gurll NJ, Vargish T, et al. Blockade of opiate receptors with naloxone improves survival and cardiac performance in canine endotoxic shock. *Circ Shock* 1980;7:39.

104 Raymond RM, Harkema JM, Stoffs WV, et al. Effects of naloxone therapy on hemodynamics and metabolism following a superlethal dosage of *Escherichia coli* endotoxin in dogs. *Surg Gynecol Obstet* 1981;152:159.

105 DeMaria A, Heffernan JJ, Grindlinger GA, et al. Naloxone versus placebo in treatment of septic shock. *Lancet* 1985;i: 1363.

106 Boeuf B, Gauvin F, Guerguerian AM, et al. Therapy of shock with naloxone: a meta-analysis. *Crit Care Med* 1998;26(11): 1910.

107 Oettinger WK, Walter GO, Jensen UM, et al. Endogenous prostaglandin F2-alpha in the hyperdynamic state of severe sepsis in man. *Br J Surg* 1983;70:237.

108 Vada P. Elevated plasma phospholipase A2 levels: correlation with the hemodynamic and pulmonary changes in gram-negative septic shock. *J Lab Clin Med* 1984;104:873.

109 Cefalo RC, Lewis PE, O'Brien WF, et al. The role of prostaglandins in endotoxemia: comparisons in response in the nonpregnant, maternal, and fetal model. *Am J Obstet Gynecol* 1980;137:53.

110 O'Brien WF, Cefalo RC, Lewis PE, et al. The role of prostaglandins in endotoxemia and comparisons in response in the nonpregnant, maternal, and fetal models. II. Alterations in prostaglandin physiology in the nonpregnant, pregnant, and fetal experimental animal. *Am J Obstet Gynecol* 1981;139:535.

111 Rao PS, Cavanagh D, Gaston LW. Endotoxic shock in the primate: effects of aspirin and dipyridamole administration. *Am J Obstet Gynecol* 1981;140:914.

112 Makabali GL, Mandal AK, Morris JA. An assessment of the participatory role of prostaglandins and serotonin in the pathophysiology of endotoxic shock. *Am J Obstet Gynecol* 1983;145:439.

113 Beutler B, Milsark IW, Cerami AC. Passive immunization against cachectin/tumor necrosis factor protects mice from lethal effect of endotoxin. *Science* 1985;229:869.

114 Badsha N, Vorster B, Gaffin SL. Properties of human LPS specific gamma-globulin. *Circ Shock* 1983;10:248.

115 Lachman E, Pitsoe SB, Gaffin SL. Antilipopolysaccharide immunotherapy in management of septic shock of obstetric and gynaecologic origin. *Lancet* 1984;1:981.

116 Ziegler EJ, McCutchan JA, Fierer J, et al. Treatment of gram-negative bacteremia and shock with human antiserum to a mutant *Escherichia coli. N Engl J Med* 1982;307:1225.

117 Greenman RL, Schein RMH, Martin MA, et al. A controlled clinical trial of E5 murine monoclonal IgM antibody to endotoxin in the treatment of gram-negative sepsis. *JAMA* 1991;266: 1097.

118 Wenzel RP. Monoclonal antibodies and the treatment of gram-negative bacteremia and shock. *N Engl J Med* 1991; 324:486.

119 Ziegler EJ, Fisher CJ, Jr, Sprung CL, et al. Treatment of gram-negative bacteremia and septic shock with HA-1A human monoclonal antibody against endotoxin. *N Engl J Med* 1991;324: 429.

120 Warren HS, Danner RL, Munford RS. Anti-endotoxin monoclonal antibodies. *N Engl J Med* 1992;326:1153.

121 Natanson C, Hoffman WD, Suffredini AF, et al. Selected treatment strategies for shock based on proposed mechanisms of pathogenesis. *Ann Intern Med* 1994:120:771.

122 Goldie AS, Fearon KDH, Ross JA, et al. Natural cytokine antagonists and endogenous antiendotoxin core antibodies in sepsis syndrome. *JAMA* 1995;274:172.

123 Warren BL, Eid A, Siger P, et al. KyberSept Trial Study Group. Caring for the critically ill patients. High-dose antithrombin III in severe sepsis: a randomized controlled trial. *JAMA* 2001; 286;1869.

124 Bernard GR, Vincent JL, Laterre PF, et al. Efficacy and safety of recombinant human activated protein C for severe sepsis. *N Engl J Med* 2001;344:699.

125 Pritchard JA. Changes in the blood volume during pregnancy and delivery. *Anesthesiology* 1965;26:393.

126 Sheehan HL, Murdoch R. Postpartum necrosis of the anterior pituitary: pathologic and clinical aspects. *Br J Obstet Gynaecol* 1938;45:456.

127 Lowe TW. Hypovolemia due to hemorrhage. *Clin Obstet Gynecol* 1990;33:454.

128 Dildy GA, Clark SL. Acute puerperal uterine inversion. *Contemp Obstet Gynecol* 1993;38:13.

129 Dollery C, ed. *Therapeutic drugs*, 2nd edn. Edinburgh: Churchill Livingstone, 1999.

130 Toppozada M, El-Bossaty M, El-Rahman HA, et al. Control of intractable atonic postpartum hemorrhage by 5-methyl prostaglandin F2α. *Obstet Gynecol* 1981;58:327.

131 Hayashi RH, Castillo MS, Noah ML. Management of severe postpartum hemorrhage with a prostaglandin F2α analogue. *Obstet Gynecol* 1984;63:806.

132 Oleen MA, Mariano JP. Controlling refractory atonic postpartum haemorrhage with Hemabate sterile solution. *Am J Obstet Gynecol* 1990;162:205.

133 Takagi S, Yoshida T, Togo Y, et al. The effects of intramyometrial injection of prostaglandin F2α on severe postpartum hemorrhage. *Prostaglandins* 1976;12:565.

134 Gulmezoglu AM, Villar J, Ngoc NT, et al. WHO multicentre randomized trial of misoprostol in the management of the third stage of labour. *Lancet* 2001;358:689–695.

135 O'Brien P, El-Refaey H, Gordon A, et al. Rectally administered misoprostol for the treatment of postpartum haemorrhage unresponsive to oxytocin and ergometrine: a descriptive study. *Obstet Gynecol* 1998;92:212.

136 Abdel-Aleem H, El-Nashar I, Abdel-Aleem A. Management of severe postpartum hemorrhage with misoprostol. *Int J Gynecol Obstet* 2001;72:75.

137 Lokugamage AU, Sullivan KR, Niculescu I, et al. A randomized study comparing rectally administered misoprostol versus syntometrine combined with an oxytocin infusion for the cessation of primary postpartum hemorrhage. *Acta Obstet Gynecol Scand* 2001;80:835.

138 Breen JL, Neubecker R, Gregori CA, et al. Placenta accreta, increta, and percreta: survey of 40 cases. *Obstet Gynecol* 1977;49:43.

139 Read JA, Cotton DB, Miller FC. Placenta accreta: changing clinical aspects and outcome. *Obstet Gynecol* 1980;56: 31.

140 Clark SL, Koonings PP, Phelan JP. Placenta previa/accreta and prior cesarean section. *Obstet Gynecol* 1985;66:89.

141 McHattie TJ. Placenta previa accreta. *Obstet Gynecol* 1972;40: 795.

142 Gibb DM, Soothill PW, Ward KJ. Conservative management of placenta accreta. *Br J Obstet Gynaecol* 1994;101:79.
143 Legro RS, Price FV, Hill LM, et al. Nonsurgical management of placenta percreta: a case report. *Obstet Gynecol* 1994;83:847.
144 Jaffe, R, DuBeshter B, Sherer DM, et al. Failure of methotrexate treatment for term placenta percreta. *Am J Obstet Gynecol* 1994;171:558.
145 Aho AJ, Pulkkinen MO, Vaha-Eskeli K. Acute urinary bladder tamponade with hypovolemic shock due to placenta percreta with bladder invasion. Case report. *Scand J Urol Nephrol* 1985;19:157.
146 Cox SM, Carpenter RJ, Cotton DB. Placenta percreta: ultrasound diagnosis and conservative surgical management. *Obstet Gynecol* 1988;71:454.
147 Bakri YN, Sundin T, Mansi M, et al. Placenta percreta with bladder invasion: report of three cases. *Am J Perinatol* 1993;10:468.
148 Thorp JM, Councell RB, Sandredge DA, et al. Antepartum diagnosis of placenta previa percreta by magnetic resonance imaging. *Obstet Gynecol* 1992;80:506.
149 Bakri YN, Rifai A, Legarth J. Placenta previa-percreta: magnetic resonance imaging findings and methotrexate therapy after hysterectomy. *Am J Obstet Gynecol* 1993;169:213.
150 Phelan JP. Uterine rupture. *Clin Obstet Gynecol* 1990;33:432.
151 Plaunche WC, von Almen W, Muller R. Catastrophic uterine rupture. *Obstet Gynecol* 1984;64:792.
152 McMahon MJ. Vaginal birth after cesarean. *Clin Obstet Gynecol* 1998;2:369.
153 Lydon-Rochelle M, Holt VL, Easterling TR, et al. Risk of uterine rupture during labor among women with a prior cesarean delivery. *N Engl J Med* 2001;345:3.
154 Eden RD, Parker RT, Gall SA. Rupture of the pregnant uterus: a 53-year review. *Obstet Gynecol* 1986;68:671.
155 Fort AT, Harlin RS. Pregnancy outcome after noncatastrophic maternal trauma during pregnancy. *Obstet Gynecol* 1970;35:912.
156 Rothenberger DA, Quattlebaum FW, Zabel J, et al. Diagnostic peritoneal lavage for blunt trauma in pregnant women. *Am J Obstet Gynecol* 1977;129:479.
157 Jacobson M, Mitchell R. Trauma to the abdomen in pregnancy. *S Afr J Surg* 1983;21:71.
158 Crosby WM. Trauma during pregnancy: maternal and fetal injury. *Obstet Gynecol Surv* 1974:29:683.
159 Crosby WM. Traumatic injuries during pregnancy. *Clin Obstet Gynecol* 1983:26:902.
160 Weiss HB, Songer TJ, Fabio A. Fetal deaths related to maternal injury. *JAMA* 2001;286:1863.
161 Kimball IM. Maternal fetal trauma. *Semin Pediatr Surg* 2001;10(1):32.
162 Crosby WM, Costiloe JP. Safety of lap-belt restraint for pregnant victims of automobile collisions. *N Engl J Med* 1971;284:632.
163 Pearlman MD, Klinich KD, Schneider LW, et al. A comprehensive program to improve safety for pregnant women and fetuses in motor vehicle crashes: a preliminary report. *Am J Obstet Gynecol* 2000;182:1554.
164 Agran PF, Dunkle DE, Winn DG, et al. Fetal death in motor vehicle accidents. *Ann Emerg Med* 1987;16:1355.
165 Lane PL. Traumatic fetal deaths. *J Emerg Med* 1989;7:433–435.
166 Hankins GD, Barth WH, Satin AJ. Critical care medicine and the obstetric patient. In: Ayers SM, Grenuik A, Holbrook PR, et al, eds. *Textbook of critical care*, 3rd edn. Philadelphia, PA: W.B. Saunders; 1995:50.
167 Goodwin TM, Breen MT. Pregnancy outcome and fetomaternal hemorrhage after noncatastrophic trauma. *Am J Obstet Gynecol* 1990;162:665.
168 Sparkman RS. Rupture of the spleen in pregnancy: a report of two cases and review of the literature. *Am J Obstet Gynecol* 1958;76:587.
169 Baerga VY, Zietlow S, Scott P, et al. Trauma in pregnancy. *Mayo Clinic Proc* 2000;75(12):1243.
170 Eastman NJ. Editorial comment. *Obstet Gynecol* Surv 1958;13:69.
171 Buchsbaum HJ. Diagnosis and management of abdominal gunshot wounds during pregnancy. *J Trauma* 1975;15:425.
172 Sakala EP, Kost DD. Management of stab wounds to the pregnant uterus. A case report and review of the literature. *Obstet Gynecol Surv* 1988;43:319.
173 Kobak AJ, Hurwitz CH. Gunshot wounds of the pregnant uterus: review of the literature and two case reports. *Obstet Gynecol* 1954;4:383.
174 Stone IK. Trauma in the obstetric patient. *Obstet Gynecol Clin North Am* 1999;26:459.
175 Del Rossi AJ, ed. Blunt thoracic trauma. *Trauma Quarterly* 1990;6(3):1.
176 Awwad JT, Azar GB, Seoud MA, et al. High-velocity penetrating wounds of the gravid uterus: review of 16 years of civil war. *Obstet Gynecol* 1994;83:259.
177 Kuhlmann RS, Cruikshank DP. Maternal trauma during pregnancy. *Clin Obstet Gynecol* 1994;37:274.
178 Grubb DK. Non-surgical management of penetrating uterine trauma in pregnancy – a case report. *Am J Obstet Gynecol* 1992;166:583.
179 Buchsbaum HJ. Penetrating injury of the abdomen. In: Buchsbaum HJ, ed. *Trauma in pregnancy*. Philadelphia, PA: W.B. Saunders; 1979:82.
180 Cunningham FG, Gant N, Leveno KJ, et al. Maternal adaptations to pregnancy. In: *Williams obstetrics*, 21st edn. Norwalk, CT: Appleton and Lange; 2001:167.
181 Feller I, Archambeault C. *Nursing the burned patient*. Ann Arbor, MI: National Institute for Burn Medicine, 1975.
182 Smith BK, Rayburn WF, Feller I. Burns and pregnancy. *Clin Perinatol* 1983;10:383.
183 Guo SS, Greenspoon JS, Kahn AM. Management of burn injuries during pregnancy. *Burns* 2001;27:394.
184 Polko LE, McMahon MJ. Burns in pregnancy. *Obstet Gynecol* Surv 1998;53:50.
185 Rayburn W, Smith B, Feller I, et al. Major burns during pregnancy: effects on fetal well-being. *Obstet Gynecol* 1984;63:392.
186 Rai YS, Jackson D. Childbearing in relation to the scarred abdominal wall from burns. *Burns* 1974;1:167.
187 Webb JC, Baack BR, Osler TM, et al. A pregnancy complicated by mature abdominal burn scarring and its surgical solution: a case report. *J Burn Care Rehabil* 1995;16:276.
188 Matthews RN. Obstetric implications of burns in pregnancy. *Br J Obstet Gynaecol* 1982;89:603.
189 Carlson RW, Bowles AL, Haupt MT. Anaphylactic, anaphylactoid, and related forms of shock. *Crit Care Clin* 1986;2:347.
190 DeCamp MM, Demling RH. Posttraumatic multisystem organ failure. *JAMA* 1988;260:530.
191 Moneret-Vautrin DA, Laxenaire MC. Anaphylactic and anaphylactoid reactions. Clinical presentation. *Clin Rev Allergy* 1991;91:249.
192 Smith BE. Anesthetic emergencies. *Clin Obstet Gynecol* 1985;28:391.

193 Fisher M. Anaphylaxis. *Semin Respir Med* 1982;3:257.
194 Lee W, Cotton DB, Hankins GDV, et al. Management of septic shock complicating pregnancy. *Obstet Gynecol Clin North Am* 1989;16:431.
195 Gibbs CE, Locke WE. Maternal deaths in Texas, 1969 to 1973. *Am J Obstet Gynecol* 1976;126:687.
196 Brun-Buisson C, Doyon F, Carlet J, et al. Incidence, risk factors, and outcome of severe sepsis and septic shock in adults. A multicenter prospective study in intensive care units. *JAMA* 1995;274:968.
197 Gordon M, Horowitz A. Septic shock in obstetrics and gynecology. *Postgrad Med* 1969;46:144.
198 Stubblefield PG, Grimes DA. Septic abortion. *N Engl J Med* 1994;331:310.
199 Ledger WJ, Norman M, Gee C, et al. Bacteremia on an obstetric–gynecologic service. *Am J Obstet Gynecol* 1975;121: 205.
200 Monif GRG, Baer H. Polymicrobial bacteremia in obstetric patients. *Obstet Gynecol* 1976;48:167.
201 Blanco JD, Gibbs RS, Castaneda YS. Bacteremia in obstetrics: clinical course. *Obstet Gynecol* 1981;58:621.
202 Weinstein MP, Murphy JR, Reller LB, et al. The clinical significance of positive blood cultures: a comparative analysis of 500 episodes of bacteremia and fungemia in adults. II. Clinical observations, with special reference to factors influencing prognosis. *Rev Infect Dis* 1983;5:54.
203 Duff P. Pathophysiology and management of septic shock. *J Reprod Med* 1980;24:109.
204 Gibbs RS, Blanco JD, St Clair PF, et al. Quantitative bacteriology of amniotic fluid from women with clinical intraamniotic infection at term. *J Infect Dis* 1982;145:1.
205 Gonik B. Septic shock in obstetrics. *Clin Perinatol* 1986;13:741.
206 Knuppel RA, Rao PS, Cavanagh D. Septic shock in obstetrics. *Clin Obstet Gynecol* 1984;27:3.
207 Weil M. Current understanding of mechanisms and treatment of circulatory shock caused by bacterial infections. *Ann Clin Res* 1977; 9:181.
208 Parker MM, Parillo JE. Septic shock: hemodynamics and pathogenesis. *JAMA* 1983;250:3324.
209 Shippy CR, Appel PL, Shoemaker WC. Reliability of clinical monitoring to assess blood volume in critically ill patients. *Crit Care Med* 1984;12:107.
210 Shoemaker WC, Kram HB, Appel PL, et al. The efficacy of central venous and pulmonary artery catheters and therapy based upon them in reducing mortality and morbidity. *Arch Surg* 1990;125:1332.
211 Hawkins DF. Management and treatment of obstetric bacteraemic shock. *J Clin Pathol* 1980;33:895.
212 Dudley AG, Teaford H, Gatewood TS, Jr. Delayed traumatic rupture of the diaphragm in pregnancy. *Obstet Gynecol* 1979;53:25S.
213 Gray SF, Muers MF, Scott JS. Maternal death from constrictive pericarditis 15 years after radiotherapy. Case report. *Br J Obstet Gynaecol* 1988;95:518.
214 Fatovich DM, Lee KY. Household electric shocks: who should be monitored? *Med J Aust* 1991;155:301.
215 Fatovich DM. Electric shock in pregnancy. *J Emerg Med* 1993;11:175.

38 Hypertensive diseases in pregnancy

Frederick U. Eruo and Baha M. Sibai

Approximately 10% of pregnancies are complicated by hypertension. The incidence varies according to the population studied and the criteria used for diagnosis. Preeclampsia accounts for 70% of hypertension in pregnancy, and chronic hypertension accounts for most of the remaining 30%. The quoted figures may be underestimated as the incidence of hypertension is said to have increased by about 40–50% in the past 10 years.[1,2] This increase is probably due to the increase in obesity in the United States,[3] delay of pregnancy until later in life (advanced maternal age), and increased rate of multifetal pregnancy.[4]

Patients with hypertension in pregnancy have higher incidence of eclampsia, abruptio placentae, preterm delivery (very often iatrogenic preterm delivery due to obstetric intervention secondary to hypertension or its complications), disseminated intravascular coagulation (DIC), hemorrhage, pulmonary edema, renal insufficiency, stroke, and death. Apart from being the most common medical complication of pregnancy, hypertensive disorders are associated with significant maternal, fetal, and neonatal morbidity and mortality.[5,6] African–American women have a fourfold increase in mortality.[7] Mortality rate is also increased for women over 35 years of age.[8]

Blood pressure measurement

The American College of Obstetricians and Gynecologists (ACOG) defines hypertension in pregnancy as either a systolic blood pressure of ≥ 140 mmHg or a diastolic blood pressure ≥ 90 mmHg observed on two occasions at least 6 hours apart.[9] Blood pressure is measured with the patient in the sitting position with an appropriately sized blood pressure cuff. The measurement of blood pressure is subject to many inaccuracies. Potential sources of error in blood pressure measurement include faulty equipment, observer bias, improper technique, cuff size, and position of the arm during blood pressure measurement.[10,11]

Direct intra-arterial blood pressure measurement is the gold standard for blood pressure monitoring and is the preferred method for critically ill patients. However, in clinical practice, the indirect (auscultatory) method is the more convenient and widely accepted technique in use. Of the indirect methods, the use of a mercury sphygmomanometer is the gold standard in clinical practice. An aneroid sphygmomanometer may be used, but it needs to be validated every 6 months for accuracy.[12]

There is controversy regarding the use of Korotkoff phase 4 (muffling of sound) versus phase 5 (disappearance of sound) to measure the diastolic blood pressure. Korotkoff phase 4 measures approximately 5–10 mmHg higher than phase 5 if using the auscultatory technique, or up to 20 mmHg difference if compared with intra-arterial measurement.[13] It has been suggested that both phases should be measured, but that the phase 5 reading should be used for diagnosis and clinical trials.[14]

Classification of hypertensive disorders in pregnancy

Numerous attempts have been made to classify hypertensive disorders of pregnancy. However, it is often difficult to differentiate between preeclampsia (hypertension with proteinuria diagnosed after 20 weeks of gestation), gestational hypertension (elevated blood pressures without symptoms or proteinuria after 20 weeks of gestation), chronic hypertension (elevated blood pressure prior to conception or prior to 20 weeks of gestation), and chronic hypertension with superimposed preeclampsia. The normal second-trimester fall in blood pressure may conceal the presence of underlying chronic hypertension and, unless the patient presents in the first trimester or has a well-documented history of chronic hypertension, accurate classification is very difficult. It is classified as:

- preeclampsia (mild preeclampsia, severe preeclampsia, eclampsia, HELLP syndrome);
- gestational hypertension;

- chronic hypertension;
- chronic hypertension with superimposed preeclampsia.

Preeclampsia

The preeclampsia group includes mild preeclampsia, severe preeclampsia, eclampsia, and HELLP syndrome (hemolysis, elevated liver enzymes, and low platelets). Preeclampsia is the presence of proteinuria with elevated blood pressure (after 20 weeks' gestation) measured on two occasions at least 6 hours apart within 7 days. Mild preeclampsia is systolic blood pressure (BP) > 140 mmHg or diastolic BP > 90 mmHg with proteinuria (Table 38.1). Severe preeclampsia is proteinuria with systolic BP ≥ 160 mmHg or diastolic BP ≥ 110 mmHg or the presence of cerebral or visual disturbances (Table 38.2). Other features of preeclampsia include headache, visual disturbance, persistent visual changes, right upper quadrant pain, epigastric pain, nausea, and vomiting. Some of these features are indicative of severe preeclampsia rather than mild preeclampsia.

Protein excretion in the urine increases in normal pregnancy from approximately 5 mg/100 mL in the first and second trimesters to 15 mg/100 mL in the third trimester. These low levels are not detected by the dipstick technique. Significant proteinuria is defined as > 0.3 g in a 24-hour urine collection or 0.1 g/L (> 2+ on the dipstick), in at least two random samples collected 6 or more hours apart.

There is still confusion in the world literature regarding the true definition of preeclampsia despite the above diagnostic criteria.[15] This is further complicated by problems with urinary protein estimation. The concentration of urinary protein is highly variable, especially if estimated with the dipstick technique. It is influenced by several factors, including contamination with vaginal secretions, blood, or bacteria; urine specific gravity and pH; exercise; and posture.[16]

Reported incidence of preeclampsia ranges from 2% to 7% depending on the diagnostic criteria and the population studied. It is principally a disease of primigravidas and rarely presents before 20 weeks' gestation. Early presentation is more likely to be associated with unrecognized renal disease.[17]

Several factors have been identified as predisposing to the development of preeclampsia. Risk factors for the development of preeclampsia include diabetes (particularly poorly controlled pregestational diabetes mellitus), obesity, nulliparity or primiparity, extremes of age (more common in teenagers and women with advanced maternal age, i.e., ≥ 35 years old), renal insufficiency or chronic renal disease, preexisting hypertension, personal history of preeclampsia, family history of preeclampsia, molar pregnancy, multifetal gestation, thrombophilia, and fetal hydrops. The risk factors may be present prior to conception (Table 38.3) or may appear during pregnancy (Table 38.4).[18]

Table 38.1 Criteria for the diagnosis of mild preeclampsia.

Systolic BP ≥ 140 mmHg or diastolic BP ≥ 90 mmHg on two occasions 6 hours apart after 20 weeks of gestation in a woman known not to have chronic hypertension prior to the pregnancy
Proteinuria ≥ 0.3 g in a 24-hour urine collection or 2+ proteinuria on qualitative examination or urinalysis
Edema and excessive weight gain may be present in preeclampsia but are no longer necessary for the diagnosis of preeclampsia

Table 38.2 Criteria for the diagnosis of severe preeclampsia.

- Systolic BP ≥ 160 mmHg on two occasions 6 hours apart
- Diastolic BP ≥ 110 mmHg on two occasions 6 hours apart
- Proteinuria ≥ 5 g in a 24-hour urine collection
- Oliguria of ≤ 500 mL in 24 hours
- Cerebral or visual disturbances
- Epigastric pain/right upper quadrant pain
- Pulmonary edema
- Abnormal liver function tests: aspartate aminotransferase (AST) or alanine aminotransferase (ALT) more than twice the upper limit for the laboratory
- Thrombocytopenia (platelet count < 100 000/mm^3)

Eclampsia

Eclampsia is the occurrence of seizures or coma (not attributable to any other cause) in a woman with preeclampsia. Antepartum eclampsia occurs in approximately 75% of cases, with the remaining 25% of cases occurring postpartum. Eclampsia rarely occurs before 20 weeks' gestation.[19] Late postpartum eclampsia is defined as that beginning more than 48 hours postpartum but less than 4 weeks after delivery.[20] In one study, late postpartum eclampsia constituted 56% of postpartum eclampsia and 16% of all cases of eclampsia.[20]

Table 38.3 Preconception risk factors for preeclampsia.

Preconception risk factors for preeclampsia	Frequency of occurrence
Previous preeclampsia	20–30%
Previous preeclampsia at ≤ 28 weeks	50%
Chronic hypertension	15–25%
Severe hypertension	40%
Renal disease	25%
Pregestational diabetes mellitus	20%
Class B/C diabetes	10–15%
Class F/R diabetes	35%
Thrombophilia	10–40%
Obesity/insulin resistance	10–15%
Age > 35 years	10–20%
Family history or preeclampsia	10–15%
Nulliparity/primiparity	6–7%

Courtesy of Sibai.[18]

Table 38.4 Pregnancy-related risk factors for preeclampsia. (magnitude of risk depends on the number of factors)

Unexplained midtrimester elevations in serum AFP, hCG, inhibin A	Twice normal
Abnormal uterine artery Doppler velocimetry	10–30%
Hydrops/hydropic degeneration of placenta	0–30%
Multifetal gestation (depends on the number of fetuses and maternal age)	10–20%
Partner who fathered preeclampsia in another woman	10%
Gestational diabetes mellitus	8–10%
Limited sperm exposure (teenage pregnancy)	8–10%
Nulliparity/primiparity	6–7%
Donor insemination, oocyte donation	Limited data
Unexplained persistent proteinuria or hematuria	Limited data
Unexplained fetal growth restriction	Unknown

Courtesy of Sibai.[18]

The reported incidence of eclampsia varies between 0.5% and 0.2% of all deliveries. Eclampsia is associated with multi-organ dysfunction. Factors determining the degree of dysfunction include a delay in the treatment of preeclampsia and the presence of complicating obstetric and medical factors. Eclampsia is associated with a wide spectrum of signs and symptoms, ranging from extreme hypertension, hyperreflexia, proteinuria, and generalized edema to isolated mild hypertension. Some cases present without warning signs or symptoms. A small proportion of cases will occur despite normal blood pressure, but such cases will show other features of preeclampsia (proteinuria, elevated liver enzymes, etc.).[17] Laboratory findings also vary. Serum uric acid and creatinine are usually elevated, and creatinine clearance is reduced. Hemoconcentration, reflected by an increased hematocrit and reduced plasma volume, is common as liver enzymes are found in 11–74% of eclamptic patients. HELLP syndrome complicates approximately 10% of eclampsia and usually occurs in longstanding disease and in patients with medical complications.

Why some women with symptoms of preeclampsia develop convulsions or coma while others do not is unknown. Several mechanisms have been suggested as predisposing factors to the development of eclampsia:

- cerebral vasospasm;
- cerebral hemorrhage;
- cerebral ischemia;
- cerebral edema;
- hypertensive encephalopathy;
- metabolic encephalopathy.

Most women with eclamptic seizures have an abnormal electroencephalogram.[21] However, electroencephalographic changes are almost always transient and resolve completely. The neurologic and cerebrovascular changes of eclampsia serve as a model for hypertensive encephalopathy, with the occipital and parietal zones most vulnerable. The similar pathogenetic events of forced vasodilation and altered cerebral autoregulation seen in hypertensive encephalopathy may be operative in eclampsia. However, an additional factor, such as endothelial cell dysfunction, seems to be present in eclampsia. Although routine neuroimaging studies are not advocated for all women with eclampsia, focal neurologic deficits or prolonged coma (atypical eclampsia) require prompt investigation.

Table 38.5 Criteria for the diagnosis of HELLP syndrome.*

Hemolysis
Abnormal peripheral blood smear (burr cells, schistocytes)
Elevated bilirubin ≥ 1.2 mg/dL
Increased LDH of more than twice the upper limit of normal for the laboratory
Elevated liver enzymes
Elevated ALT or AST ≥ twice the upper limit of normal for the laboratory
Increased LDH more than twice the upper limit of normal for the laboratory
Low platelet count (< 100 000/mm^3)

*Requires at least two of the abnormalities listed.

LDH, lactate dehydrogenase; ALT, alanine aminotransferase; AST, aspartate aminotransferase.

HELLP syndrome

Hemolysis, elevated liver enzymes, and low platelet counts have been recognized as complications of preeclampsia or eclampsia for many years.[22–24] The criteria for the diagnosis of HELLP syndrome (Table 38.5) include: (1) hemolysis: abnormal peripheral blood smear, total bilirubin exceeding 1.2 mg/dL, lactic dehydrogenase (LDH) > 600 U/L; (2) elevated liver enzymes: serum aspartate aminotransferase (AST) > 70 U/L, elevated alanine aminotransferase (ALT) and LDH > 600 U/L: and (3) low platelet count: < 100 000/μL.

The reported incidence of HELLP syndrome in preeclampsia ranges from 2% to 12%, which reflects different diagnostic criteria.[25] In the series reported by Sibai,[26] women with HELLP syndrome may present with a variety of signs and symptoms, none of which is diagnostic and all of which may be found in women with severe preeclampsia or eclampsia without HELLP syndrome. Nausea, vomiting, and epigastric pain are the most common symptoms.[25–27] Right upper quadrant or epigastric pain is thought to result from obstructed blood flow in the hepatic sinusoids, which are blocked by intravascular fibrin deposition and capsular distention.

About 15–50% of cases have mild hypertension, about 12–18% have no hypertension, and 13% of cases have no proteinuria.[28] As a result, patients are often misdiagnosed as having various medical and surgical disorders, including appendicitis, gastroenteritis, glomerulonephritis, pyelonephritis, viral hepatitis, or even acute fatty liver of pregnancy (AFLP).

Pathogenesis of preeclampsia

A familial factor has been established in the pathogenesis of preeclampsia.[29] However, the exact mode of inheritance and the interactions between maternal and fetal genotype have not been elucidated.[30]

There is evidence that abnormal placental angiogenesis occurs in pregnancies complicated by preeclampsia.[31] There are reduced serum levels of vascular endothelial growth factor (VEGF) and placental growth factor (PIGF) in women with preeclampsia,[32,33] coupled with altered expression of angiogenesis-related proteins.[34] According to Myatt,[35] hypoxia may affect trophoblast invasion and alter villous angiogenesis, leading to a poorly developed fetoplacental vasculature with abnormal reactivity.

An imbalance of prostaglandin metabolism has been implicated in the pathophysiology of preeclampsia.[36,37] The renin–angiotensin–aldosterone system (RAAS) plays an important role in the control of vascular tone and blood pressure. Angiotensin-converting enzyme (ACE) activity, ACE protein expression, and ACE mRNA expression are higher in preeclamptic placentas than in placentas from uncomplicated pregnancies.[38]

Gestational hypertension

Mild gestational hypertension is defined as systolic BP ≥ 140 mmHg or diastolic BP ≥ 90 mmHg (without proteinuria) measured on two occasions at least 6 hours apart and no more than 7 days apart after 20 weeks of gestation.[39] It is usually mild hypertension, late in onset, often occurs close to term, and occurs intrapartum or within 24 hours of delivery. It often resolves within 10 days of the postpartum period without treatment.

Severe gestational hypertension is defined as sustained systolic BP ≥ 160 mmHg and/or diastolic BP ≥ 110 mmHg measured at least 6 hours apart with no proteinuria.[40] Women with severe gestational hypertension have higher maternal and perinatal morbidities than those with mild gestational hypertension.[40,41] Women with mild gestational hypertension may progress to severe gestational hypertension or preeclampsia. The rate of progression from gestational hypertension to preeclampsia is dependent on the gestational age at the time of diagnosis; the rate reaches 50% when gestational hypertension develops before 30 weeks of gestation.[42]

Latent or transient hypertension was described in the last edition of this text as hypertension occurring antepartum, in labor, or in the first 24 hours postpartum without generalized edema or proteinuria and with a return to normotension within 10 days of delivery. Latent or transient hypertension is gestational hypertension in the intrapartum period but becomes transient hypertension (a retrospective diagnosis) if blood pressure returns to a normal value and no proteinuria is identified 12 weeks postpartum.[43] If proteinuria occurs before 12 weeks' gestation, then the diagnosis will be gestational hypertension with progression to postpartum preeclampsia. If high blood pressure alone persists beyond 12 weeks of the postpartum period, then the patient has chronic hypertension.

Chronic hypertension

Chronic hypertension (CHTN) is diagnosed if there is persistent elevation of blood pressure to at least 140/90 mmHg on two occasions more than 24 hours apart prior to conception, prior to 20 weeks of gestation, or beyond 12 weeks postpartum. Other factors that may suggest the presence of chronic hypertension include the following:

- retinal changes on fundoscopic examination;
- radiologic and electrocardiographic evidence of cardiac enlargement;
- compromised renal function or associated renal disease;
- multiparity with a previous history of hypertensive pregnancies.

It may be difficult to be certain of a diagnosis of chronic hypertension because of significant changes in blood pressure that occur during midpregnancy. Women with mild chronic hypertension show greater decreases in their blood pressure during pregnancy than do normotensive women.[44]

Chronic hypertension occurs in 1–5% of pregnancies. The most common etiology of chronic hypertension is essential or primary hypertension, contributing 90% of CHTN cases, while secondary hypertension accounts for the rest.[17] Causes of chronic hypertension (Table 38.6) include renal diseases (glomerulonephritis, polycystic kidneys, renal artery stenosis, or renovascular disease), systemic lupus erythematosus, polyarteritis nodosa, endocrine disorders (hyperaldosteronism, pheochromocytoma, diabetes mellitus), and coarctation of the aorta.[45] Most of the secondary causes require specific treatment in addition to antihypertensive therapy. Early diagnosis is important because, if untreated, many of these disorders

Table 38.6 Etiology of chronic hypertension.

Renal factors	Acute and chronic glomerulonephritis Acute and chronic pyelonephritis Polycystic renal disease Renovascular disease
Collagen disease with renal involvement	Lupus erythematosus Periarteritis nodosa Scleroderma
Endocrine factors	Diabetes with vascular involvement Thyrotoxicosis Aldosterone-producing tumors Pheochromocytoma
Vascular system	Coarctation of the aorta

are associated with significant maternal/fetal morbidity and mortality.

In pheochromocytoma, there is increased production of epinephrine and norepinephrine by adrenal tumors or extra-adrenal catecholamine-producing tumors. There is excessive stimulation of adrenergic receptors causing peripheral vasoconstriction and a rise in blood pressure. Diagnosis is based on clinical presentation (high blood pressure not responding to conventional antihypertensives; hypertensive crisis with paroxysmal features and palpitation) and the presence of excess urinary catecholamines or products of catecholamine breakdown [vanylmandelic acid (VMA), etc.].

Maternal renal artery duplex sonography may be used for initial screening in renovascular disease.[45] Definitive diagnosis requires more invasive procedures (isotopic renography and plasma renin levels after administration of oral captopril challenge), which are reserved for nonpregnant patients as such tests may have adverse effects on the fetus.

Chronic hypertension in pregnancy may be subclassified into mild hypertension (diastolic BP $\geq$ 90 to < 110 mmHg or systolic BP $\geq$ 140 to < 180 mmHg) or severe hypertension (diastolic BP $\geq$ 110 mmHg or systolic BP $\geq$ 180 mmHg). For the purpose of clinical management, chronic hypertension in pregnancy may also be divided into a low-risk group (hypertension with no endorgan damage or associated significant comorbidities) or a high-risk CHTN group (hypertension with endorgan damage or associated morbidities). These subdivisions are discussed in detail under the management of chronic hypertension in pregnancy.

Chronic hypertension with superimposed preeclampsia

Chronic hypertension may be complicated by superimposed preeclampsia (or eclampsia), which is diagnosed when there is an exacerbation of hypertension and development of proteinuria that was not present earlier in the pregnancy. Approximately 15–30% of chronic hypertensive women develop superimposed preeclampsia. Conditions for the diagnosis of superimposed preeclampsia on pre-existing chronic hypertension include:

- sudden exacerbation of blood pressure in a woman with previously well-controlled hypertension on antihypertensives;
- new-onset proteinuria ($\geq$ 0.5 g protein in 24-hour urine collection) in a woman with chronic hypertension but no proteinuria prior to 20 weeks' gestation;
- worsening proteinuria in a woman with chronic hypertension and proteinuria prior to 20 weeks' gestation;
- new-onset elevated AST or ALT;
- new-onset thrombocytopenia with a platelet count less than 100 000/mm^3;
- new-onset symptoms of severe preeclampsia (persistent headache, right upper quadrant pain, epigastric pain, scotomata, nausea, and vomiting).

Management of hypertension in pregnancy

Management of preeclampsia

The most effective therapy for preeclampsia is delivery of the fetus and placenta. In pregnancies at or near term in which the cervix is favorable, labor should be induced. There is no need for antihypertensive medication unless the blood pressure is in the severe preeclampsia range. Mild preeclampsia prior to term may be monitored in the hospital or at home with daily fetal kick/movement counts, twice-weekly nonstress tests, and amniotic fluid assessment.

Indications for hospitalization and/or delivery of a patient with mild preeclampsia include:

- worsening maternal or fetal parameters;
- a favorable cervix at term;
- spontaneous rupture of membranes.

Conservative management of mild or severe preeclampsia beyond term is not beneficial to the fetus because uteroplacental blood flow may be suboptimal. After 37 weeks' gestation, labor should be induced as soon as the cervix is favorable.

Severe preeclampsia warrants hospitalization, administration of magnesium sulfate for seizure prophylaxis while antihypertensive medication is instituted for diastolic BP $\geq$ 110 mmHg or systolic BP $\geq$ 160 mmHg, and delivery of the fetus (except where conservative management is indicated as discussed below). The therapeutic objective for treatment of severe hypertension is to prevent maternal cerebrovascular accidents and congestive heart failure without compromising cerebral perfusion or jeopardizing uteroplacental blood flow. Profound and rapid reduction in blood pressure may compromise the uteroplacental circulation; therefore, continuous fetal monitoring should be employed. Therapeutic goals include reduction of blood pressure to a level compatible with a decreased risk of cerebrovascular accidents and maintenance of cerebral autoregulation. Accordingly, the goal of initial antihypertensive therapy is to limit the reduction in mean arterial pressure to 20–25% or to a diastolic blood pressure of 100 mmHg.[46]

Parenteral or oral antihypertensive agents (labetalol, hydralazine, nifedipine, sodium nitroprusside, etc.) are used for acute reduction of blood pressure in women with severe preeclampsia or eclampsia. Oral medications are also used for maintenance or chronic therapy (Table 38.7). The choice of agents is dependent on the stage in pregnancy (antepartum, intrapartum, or postpartum), the side-effect profile of the agent in question, the presence of other medical problems (renal insufficiency, diabetes mellitus, pulmonary edema, myocardial ischemia, etc.), and, if postpartum, whether the woman is breastfeeding or not. The different agents used are discussed later under antihypertensive agents.

Table 38.7 Antihypertensive medication in pregnancy.

Class	Medication	Dose	
		Starting dose	Maximum dose
Common drugs for chronic therapy of hypertension			
Central alpha-2 agonist	Methyldopa	250 mg p.o. tid	2 g/day
Calcium channel blocker	Nifedipine	10 mg p.o. qid	120 mg p.o. qid
Alpha- and beta-blocker	Labetalol	100 mg p.o. tid	1200 mg/day
Common drugs for acute therapy of severe hypertension			
Arteriolar dilator	Hydralazine	5–10 mg i.v. every 15–30 min	
Calcium channel blocker	Nifedipine	10–20 mg p.o. every 30 min	
Alpha- and beta-blocker	Labetalol	5–10 mg i.v. per dose, cumulative to 40–80 mg over 20 min (maximum dose is 300 mg)	
Arterial and venous dilator	Nitroprusside	0.2–0.5 μg/kg/min	

Table 38.8 Guidelines for expectant management of severe preeclampsia remote from term.

Management plan	Clinical findings
Expedited delivery (within 72 h)	One or more of the following: Uncontrolled severe hypertension* Eclampsia Platelet count of < 100 000 cells/mL AST or ALT more than twice upper limit of normal with epigastric pain or right upper quadrant tenderness Pulmonary edema Compromised renal function† Persistent severe headache or visual changes
Expectant management	One or more of the following: Controlled hypertension Urinary protein > 5000 mg/24 h Oliguria (< 0.5 mL/kg/h) that resolves with routine fluid and food intake AST or ALT more than twice upper limit of normal epigastric pain or right upper quadrant tenderness

ALT, alanine aminotransferase; AST, aspartate aminotransferase.

*Blood pressure persistently ≥ 160 mmHg systolic or ≥ 110 mmHg diastolic despite maximum recommended doses of two antihypertensive medications.

†Persistent oliguria (< 0.5 mL/kg/h) or rise in serum creatinine of 1 mg/dL over baseline values.

Reproduced from ref. 47.

Conservative or expectant management of severe preeclampsia

Severe preeclampsia or superimposed preeclampsia developing early in pregnancy presents an obstetric dilemma. Delivery is the ultimate cure for maternal disease. However, delivery of infants before 34 weeks of gestation with immature lungs is associated with significant neonatal morbidity and mortality. Therefore, expectant or conservative management of the pregnant woman with severe preeclampsia remote from term (Table 38.8) is a feasible alternative to immediate delivery.[47]

After admission, all women are observed in the labor and delivery unit for 12–24 hours to determine their eligibility for conservative management. Intravenous magnesium sulfate therapy is administered for seizure prophylaxis, glucocorticoid therapy is given for fetal lung maturation, antihypertensive drug therapy is administered as indicated, and baseline laboratory studies (complete blood count with platelets, serum levels of creatinine, uric acid, total bilirubin, AST, and LDH, and 24-hour urine collection for total protein and creatinine clearance) are obtained. Fetal testing includes a baseline ultrasound examination and biophysical profile.

Once the woman and the fetus are judged to be suitable candidates for expectant management, the magnesium sulfate therapy is discontinued, and the patient is managed on the antepartum ward/floor. Blood pressure is measured every 4–6 hours, platelets every day, and serum AST and ALT every other day. Oral antihypertensive therapy is administered as needed to maintain blood pressure in the range 130–150 mmHg over 80–100 mmHg. Fetal biophysical profiles are obtained daily and ultrasound estimates of fetal weight biweekly. Hospitalization is continued until delivery.

Conservative management in severe preeclampsia at 28–32 weeks of gestation has been shown to prolong pregnancy by an average of 15.4 days (range 4–36 days), to reduce the incidence of admission to the neonatal intensive care unit, and to reduce length of stay in the unit.[48] Expectant management of severe preeclampsia is beneficial in a select group of women and should be practiced at tertiary care centers or at facilities that have the services of a specialist obstetrician with experience in managing such high-risk patients. Prompt delivery is indicated for the presence of imminent eclampsia, multiorgan dysfunction, fetal distress, or severe preeclampsia developing after 34 weeks of gestation. Mode of delivery is based on obstetric indications.

Management of HELLP syndrome

Delivery is the definitive therapy for HELLP syndrome beyond 34 weeks' gestation or with evidence of fetal lung maturity or fetal or maternal jeopardy. Without laboratory evidence of DIC, steroid therapy may be given to promote fetal lung maturity at gestational age under 34 weeks. During this period of conservative management, maternal and fetal conditions must be continuously assessed.

HELLP syndrome is not an indication for immediate Cesarean delivery. Guidelines similar to those described above for women with severe preeclampsia should be followed. The use of pudendal block or epidural anesthesia is contra-indicated because of the bleeding risk. General anesthesia is the method of choice for Cesarean delivery.

Platelet transfusion is indicated either before or after vaginal delivery if the woman is bleeding and the platelet count is less than 20 000/mL. Repeated platelet transfusions are not necessary because consumption is rapid and the effect is transient. Platelet transfusion should be considered before Cesarean delivery if the platelet count is less than 40 000/mL. Six to ten units of platelets can be administered just before tracheal intubation. Generalized oozing from the operative site is common. The bladder flap should be left open, and a subfascial drain should be used for 24–48 hours postpartum to minimize the risk of hematoma formation. The wound may be left open from the level of the fascia, or a subcutaneous drain may be placed and the skin closed. Open wounds are usually closed within 48–72 hours.

After delivery, the woman with HELLP syndrome should be monitored closely in an intensive care facility (labor and delivery recovery unit or medical/surgical intensive care unit) for at least 48 hours. Most women show evidence of resolution of the disease process within 48 hours postpartum. Some (especially those with DIC) may demonstrate delayed resolution or even deterioration. These women are at risk for the development of pulmonary edema from transfusion of blood products, fluid mobilization, and compromised renal function.

HELLP syndrome may also develop in the postpartum period. The time of onset in the postpartum group ranges from a few hours to 6 days, with the majority developing HELLP syndrome within 48 hours postpartum. Postpartum management is similar to that in the antepartum woman with HELLP syndrome, including the need for antiseizure prophylaxis. Steroids (dexamethasone or betamethasone) have been suggested in a few studies to improve the hematological parameters and, possibly, the clinical outcome of HELLP syndrome.[49,50] However, the use of steroids in HELLP syndrome is considered experimental.

Women with delayed resolution of HELLP syndrome (including persistent severe thrombocytopenia) represent a management dilemma. Exchange plasmapheresis with fresh-frozen plasma (FFP) has been advocated.[51,52] Early initiation of plasmapheresis may result in unnecessary treatment because the majority of these women have spontaneous resolution of their disease.

Women presenting with shoulder pain, shock, or evidence of massive ascites or pleural effusions should have imaging studies of the liver to rule out the presence of subcapsular hematoma of the liver. A ruptured subcapsular liver hematoma resulting in shock is a surgical emergency requiring an acute multidisciplinary approach. Resuscitation should consist of massive transfusion of blood products, correction of coagulopathy with FFP and platelets, and immediate laparotomy. Options at laparotomy include any combination of the following: packing, drainage, surgical ligation of the hepatic artery, embolization of the hepatic artery to the involved liver segment, resection of the involved hepatic segment, and liver transplantation, if indicated.[53]

Management of eclampsia

The protocol used to manage eclampsia is outlined in Table 38.9. Magnesium sulfate therapy is discussed in detail under antiseizure medications. Once convulsions have been abolished, arterial blood gas measurements and a chest radiograph should be obtained to insure adequate maternal oxygenation and exclude aspiration. Hypoxemia and acidemia should be corrected and maternal hypertension treated.

The fetal heart rate and uterine activity must be closely monitored. Fetal bradycardia is a common finding during an

Table 38.9 Sibai's protocol for the management of eclampsia.

Convulsions are controlled or prevented with a loading dose of 6 g magnesium sulfate in 100 mL of 5% dextrose in Ringer's lactated solution, given over 15 min, followed by a maintenance dose of 2 g/h. The dose is adjusted according to patellar reflexes and urine output in the previous 4-h period
Induction or delivery is initiated within 4 h after maternal stabilization
Magnesium sulfate is continued for 24 h after delivery or, if postpartum, 24 h after the last convulsion. In some cases, the infusion may be continued for a longer period
Diuretics, plasma volume expanders, and invasive hemodynamic monitoring used only if clinically indicated

eclamptic seizure,[54] but the rate usually returns to normal once convulsions cease. If bradycardia persists or the uterus is hypertonic, placental abruption should be suspected and evaluated as appropriate. After stabilization of the maternal condition, steps should be taken to deliver the fetus, which is the definitive treatment for eclampsia. The mode of delivery is dependent on the usual obstetric indications. Hemodynamic monitoring with Swan–Ganz catheters is rarely necessary and should be based on the usual indications.[55]

Management of gestational hypertension

Mild gestational hypertension is managed essentially as mild preeclampsia as detailed above, whereas women with severe gestational hypertension are managed as if they had severe preeclampsia. Women with severe gestational hypertension have a higher rate of maternal and perinatal morbidities than those who have mild gestational hypertension or normotensive women.[40,56,57] The rates of abruptio placentae, small for gestational age (SGA) babies, and iatrogenic preterm deliveries are similar to those in women with severe preeclampsia. Women with gestational hypertension have higher birthweight at delivery, higher rates of induction of labor for maternal reasons, and higher rates of Cesarean delivery than normotensive women.[58] To all intents and purposes, severe gestational hypertension should be managed just like severe preeclampsia.

Management of CHTN and CHTN with superimposed preeclampsia

Management of secondary hypertension is that of the underlying disease. However, most patients with chronic hypertension have essential hypertension, and the discussion that follows is directed toward this group of patients. The presence of chronic hypertension in pregnancy increases maternal and perinatal morbidity and mortality.[59] Most of the morbidity and mortality is related to the development of superimposed preeclampsia and abruptio placentae. Maternal and fetal risks can be reduced by proper antepartum surveillance (Table 38.10).

Preconception counseling in women with chronic hypertension provides an opportunity to:

- determine the severity of hypertension and identify any endorgan damage;
- implement prepregnancy lifestyle changes (exercise, weight loss, reduction in sodium intake, etc.) necessary for adequate blood pressure control;
- establish baseline laboratory data that will help in the future diagnosis of superimposed preeclampsia;
- discuss the potential side-effects of antihypertensive drugs.

Laboratory investigation should include the following:

- electrocardiogram (ECG);
- urinalysis, culture, and sensitivity;
- 24-hour urine collection for total protein and creatinine clearance;
- biochemistry: renal panel (in particular creatinine level), uric acid, lactate dehydrogenase, liver function test;
- hematology: full or complete blood count, prothrombin time (PT), partial thromboplastin time (PTT);
- optional tests (depending on the clinical evaluation/judgment): antinuclear antibody (ANA), VMA and catecholamines, anticardiolipin antibodies (ACA), etc.

Uncomplicated CHTN in pregnancy is labeled low-risk CHTN, whereas the high-risk group (Table 38.11) includes patients with renal disease, diabetes mellitus, etc. The discussion of management focuses on the control of blood pressure and the assessment of fetal and maternal well-being. Most women are seen by a nutritionist and given dietary advice. Daily sodium intake should be restricted to 2 g. The harmful effects of smoking, stress, and caffeine on maternal blood pressure and fetal well-being are emphasized, and frequent rest periods are encouraged.

Table 38.10 Evaluation of pregnancy complicated by chronic hypertension.

Name:	Date of birth:
Parity: G . . . P . . . :	LMP:
Gestational age:	EDD or EDC:

Ultrasound:
- First trimester ultrasound [for correct dating and nuchal translucence (NT) measurement]:
- Fetal biometry/anatomy ultrasound (at 18–20 weeks):
- Follow-up growth ultrasound at 4-weekly intervals starting in late second trimester

Fetal testing starting in late second or early third trimester (for patients with renal insufficiency):
- Twice-weekly testing or BPP
- Nonstress test (NST) if there is poor growth
- NST and Doppler studies if IUGR (< 10%)

Renal evaluation: 24-h urine protein and creatinine clearance, electrolytes, urea, and creatinine levels

ECG: (cardiology consultation if ECG is abnormal)

Cardiac echocardiography:

Comments/comorbid conditions:

Table 38.11 High-risk chronic hypertension in pregnancy.

Maternal age greater than 40 years (may consider age ≥ 35 years)
Duration of hypertension more than 15 years
Blood pressure exceeding 160 over 110 mmHg early in pregnancy
Diabetes mellitus (classes B–F)
Cardiomyopathy
Renal disease
Connective tissue disorders
Consider morbid obesity (weight ≥ 300 lb)

Women are seen every 2–3 weeks until 34 weeks and then weekly until delivery. At each visit, systolic and diastolic blood pressure should be recorded and the urine tested for the presence of glucose and protein. Evaluation of maternal status includes serial measurements of hematocrit, serum creatinine, and 24-hour urinary excretion of protein. Prompt hospitalization is indicated if there is an exacerbation of hypertension, development of pyelonephritis, or significant proteinuria. An elevation of uric acid > 6 mg/dL may be an early warning sign of superimposed preeclampsia.

Fetal evaluation includes serial growth scans and antepartum fetal heart rate testing from the early third trimester. For those considered high risk, nonstress testing (NST) may commence as early as 28 weeks. Daily fetal movement counts and weekly or biweekly biophysical profiles (BPP) or NSTs are generally employed.

Antihypertensive therapy is restricted to women with severe hypertension. Low-risk pregnancy is allowed to continue to 40–41 weeks' gestation with close monitoring. High-risk pregnancies and women receiving antihypertensive drugs are delivered at or before 40 weeks' gestation.

The outcome in women with chronic hypertension is closely related to the development of superimposed preeclampsia. Sibai and Anderson[60] studied 44 pregnant women with severe hypertension in the first trimester. Fifty-two percent developed superimposed preeclampsia.

Women with severe chronic hypertension in early pregnancy or underlying renal disease require early referral for antenatal care, intensive fetal and maternal monitoring as described earlier, and delivery in a tertiary care center. Antihypertensive therapy is indicated and should maintain systolic blood pressure between 140 and 150 mmHg and diastolic pressure between 90 and 100 mmHg. Persistent blood pressure levels below these ranges in women who have previously been very hypertensive may jeopardize placental perfusion.

Antiseizure medications in preeclampsia

Parenteral magnesium sulfate ($MgSO_4$) has become the drug of choice for therapy and prophylaxis of eclampsia (Magpie trial[61]). Magnesium causes relaxation of smooth muscle by competing with calcium for entry into cells at the time of cellular depolarization, but its exact mechanism of action in the control of eclamptic seizures is unknown. Central nervous system depression and suppression of neuronal activity are postulated as mechanisms. Additional theories about the efficacy of magnesium sulfate therapy for seizure prophylaxis include its role as a cerebral vasodilator (particularly acting on the smaller diameter vessels). The potential for magnesium to relieve cerebral ischemia through its antagonism of calcium-dependent arterial constriction may explain its antiseizure activity. Conversely, once widespread cerebral vasoconstriction has occurred in severe preeclampsia, the resultant cerebral ischemia could lower the threshold for seizure activity in those affected areas.[62]

Table 38.12 Clinical findings associated with increasing maternal serum levels of magnesium.

Serum magnesium level (mg/dL)	Clinical findings
1.5–2.5	Normal level
4–8	Therapeutic range for seizure prophylaxis
9–12	Loss of patellar reflex
15–17	Muscular paralysis, respiratory arrest
30–35	Cardiac arrest

Most eclamptic convulsions resolve in 60–90 seconds. After the convulsion has ended, an initial intravenous 6-g loading dose of magnesium sulfate should be given over 15–20 min. If another convulsion occurs after the initial loading dose, an additional intravenous bolus of 2 g may be given over 3–5 min. Approximately 10–15% of women have a second convulsion after receiving the loading dose of magnesium sulfate; most women remain free of seizures after the additional 2-g bolus. Maintenance infusion of 2 g/h magnesium sulfate is then begun. Serum magnesium levels may be followed to guide maintenance infusion therapy of magnesium sulfate if there is renal dysfunction. The initial level may be obtained 4 h after the loading dose.

Clinical findings associated with elevated serum magnesium levels will help in monitoring therapy (Table 38.12). The first sign of magnesium toxicity is loss of patellar reflexes (10–12 mg/dL). Other early signs and symptoms of magnesium toxicity include nausea, feeling of warmth, flushing, slurred speech, and somnolence (9–12 mg/dL). Magnesium toxicity should also be considered in women who do not regain consciousness after an eclamptic seizure.

Serum magnesium levels may also be used for monitoring evidence of drug toxicity. Magnesium is excreted by the kidneys; renal dysfunction may result in toxicity. The following guidelines may help to prevent magnesium toxicity:

- monitor hourly urine output;
- evaluate deep tendon reflexes hourly;
- monitor respiratory rate;
- monitor serum magnesium levels regularly.

If magnesium toxicity is suspected, the magnesium infusion should be discontinued, supplemental oxygen administered, and a serum magnesium level obtained. Pharmacologic treatment of magnesium toxicity includes administration of 10 mL of 10% calcium gluconate (1 g in total) as a slow intravenous push. Calcium competitively and briefly inhibits magnesium at the neuromuscular junction. Symptoms of magnesium toxicity may recur if the magnesium level remains elevated. Respiratory arrest secondary to magnesium toxicity requires intubation and assisted ventilation.[63]

Magnesium sulfate may inhibit uterine contraction, causing uterine atony. Magnesium sulfate therapy appears to prolong bleeding time,[64,65] to increase blood loss at delivery,[66] and to be associated with increased postpartum hemorrhage.[67]

Magnesium sulfate may also decrease beat-to-beat variability of the fetal heart rate,[68] and signs of neonatal hypermagnesemia have been reported after only 24 hours of intravenous therapy.[69]

Women who have recurrent convulsions while receiving therapeutic maintenance magnesium sulfate may be given a short-acting barbiturate, such as sodium amobarbital, in a dose up to 250 mg intravenously over 3–5 min.

Antihypertensive therapy

Treatment of severe hypertension is associated with a reduction in maternal morbidity and mortality.[70] Antihypertensive therapy does not prevent preeclampsia or abruptio placentae, neither does it improve perinatal outcome.[71,72]

Central-acting agents (methyldopa, clonidine)

Methyldopa acts by stimulating central alpha-2 receptors. It may also be an alpha-2 blocker acting by a false neurotransmitter effect. The drug is given orally in a loading dose of 1 g followed by maintenance therapy of 1–2 g daily in four divided doses. Peak plasma levels occur within 2 h of an oral dose, and the fall in blood pressure is maximal 4 h after tablet ingestion. Side-effects include drowsiness and a dry mouth. Hepatitis, hemolytic anemia, and a positive Coombs' test have been reported in association with long-term use. Differentiating cholestatic jaundice or abnormal LFT due to methyldopa from elevated liver enzymes resulting from severe preeclampsia might be difficult.

Until recently, methyldopa was the most frequently used antihypertensive agent in pregnancy, probably because of its safety profile. It is no longer the first-line agent because it has a slow onset of action and is not as efficacious as other available antihypertensive agents. In breastfeeding mothers with hypertension requiring medication, when there is difficulty with the choice of antihypertensive agents, methyldopa may be an option.

Clonidine is a powerful alpha-2 adrenergic central stimulant. The usual oral dose in pregnancy is 0.1 (morning) and 0.3 mg/day (bedtime), increasing incrementally to a maximum of 1.2 mg daily. Rebound hypertension has been reported after abrupt cessation of the drug. The safety of clonidine in pregnancy appears to be well established;[73] however, it is more likely to be used as a second- or third-line agent. Also, it is a useful alternative in breastfeeding mothers.

Alpha- and beta-blocking agents

Labetalol is a combined alpha- and beta-adrenoceptor blocker. It is probably the most commonly used antihypertensive agent in pregnancy. Parenteral labetalol has a rapid onset of action. The initial intravenous dose is 20 mg with subsequent escalating doses every 20 min (40, 80, 80, and 80 mg) until either a desired effect or a maximum dose of 300 mg is reached. Oral labetalol may also be used for long-term therapy: an initial oral dose of 300 mg daily may be increased to a maximum daily dose of 1200 mg. Side-effects of labetalol therapy include scalp tingling, tremulousness, and headache. Avoid the use of labetalol in women with second-degree heart block.

Other beta blockers (metoprolol, atenolol, oxprenolol) have been studied in pregnancy. Exercise caution with the use of these drugs because of reports of intrauterine growth restriction with the use of atenolol in the first trimester, but not later in pregnancy.[74] Metoprolol is sometimes used as a last resort in the management of hypertension not responding to other common antihypertensive agents.

Doxazosin, an alpha-blocker, has no role in the management of hypertension in pregnancy. Its role in the nonpregnant population seems to be under scrutiny.[75]

Diuretics

Thiazide diuretics are commonly used to treat hypertension in the nonpregnant population, but their role in pregnancy is highly controversial. Although preeclampsia and eclampsia patients may have edema and appear to be fluid overloaded, they are very frequently intravascularly depleted. Sibai et al.[76] observed a marked reduction in volume in pregnant women treated with diuretics compared with a control group receiving no medication. Although this effect was reversed after discontinuing the diuretic therapy, plasma volume depletion is associated with a poor perinatal outcome. Consequently, most doctors avoid diuretics in pregnant preeclampsia patients for fear of depleting the intravascular volume. Whereas that may be a concern in the intrapartum period, there is no reason not to use it in the postpartum period, especially if there is pulmonary edema or evidence of fluid overload.

In the postpartum period, there is pooling of fluid from the periphery and the uterus into the circulation, thus increasing the intravascular fluid volume; therefore, the use of diuretics is acceptable. Hopefully, more people will start using diuretics as first-line antihypertensive agents in the postpartum period.

Thiazide diuretics may cause hyperglycemia, thus adversely affecting the control of hyperglycemia in diabetic patients, but this side-effect is unlikely to have a huge impact on outcome when diuretics are used for only a short period. Other side-effects include hyponatremia, hyperuricemia, acute pancreatitis, and fetal thrombocytopenia.

Loop diuretics are useful in patients with signs of fluid overload or pulmonary edema. Prolonged use of loop diuretics may lead to hypokalemia. Therefore, the serum potassium level should be checked if the woman is receiving a loop diuretic for more than a couple of days.

Hydralazine

Hydralazine is a potent vasodilator that acts directly on smooth muscle. It is administered as an intravenous bolus injection. After intravenous administration, the hypotensive effects develop gradually over 15–30 min. The usual bolus dose is 5–10 mg to be repeated every 20–30 min as needed. Maternal side-effects include headache, facial flushing, tachycardia, palpitations, nausea, and vomiting. Mabie et al.[77] reported fetal distress secondary to hypotension from overtreatment in two of six cases. Chronic administration may be associated with a maternal lupus syndrome and neonatal thrombocytopenia. Oral hydralazine is a weak antihypertensive when used alone and is usually combined with methyldopa or a diuretic.

Sodium nitroprusside

Sodium nitroprusside is a potent arterial and venous dilator used for emergent therapy of patients with hypertensive crisis. It is given as a continuous intravenous infusion because of its immediate onset of action and short duration of action (1–10 min). It is metabolized by the liver and excreted by the kidneys. The initial infusion dose in gravid women should be 0.2 μg/kg/min rather than the usual dose of 0.5 μg/kg/minute, as is standard in nonpregnant patients. This drug should be reserved for hypertensive emergencies because of concerns about thiocyanate toxicity in the neonate.

Calcium channel blockers (CCB)

Calcium channel blockers (CCB) have a very good safety profile in pregnancy and have been used successfully to manage hypertension in pregnancy. They may have a renoprotective effect that might be useful in patients with renal insufficiency. Nifedipine is used extensively in obstetric practice for both blood pressure control and preterm labor with no obvious teratogenic effects documented.[78,79]

Nifedipine is available orally in both short-acting and extended-release forms. It may improve uteroplacental blood flow and has a tocolytic effect on the uterus. In addition to oral therapy for chronic hypertension in pregnancy, nifedipine may be used for emergent reduction of severe hypertension. The use of sublingual nifedipine in the past for rapid reduction in blood pressure posed significant risks to the mother and fetus; hence, the sublingual route is contraindicated. Exercise caution when using nifedipine in patients on magnesium sulfate as they may have a synergistic action leading to severe hypotension. The maximum daily dose for nifedipine is 120 mg. Common side-effects include headache, flushing, tachycardia, and fatigue.

Although less often used, other CCBs (verapamil and diltiazem) may be used for blood pressure control in patients with cardiac disease. Additional experience with verapamil use in pregnancy is available because of its use in treating arrhythmias in pregnancy.

Angiotensin-converting enzyme (ACE) inhibitors

The chronic use of ACE inhibitors in pregnancy is associated with fetal renal insufficiency/renal failure, fetal growth retardation, oligohydramnios, cranial anomalies, severe fetal hypotension, and death, especially in the second and third trimesters.[80,81] Postpartum use of ACE inhibitors is indicated for women with diabetic nephropathy and peripartum cardiomyopathy. Women are advised to stop ACE inhibitors prior to conception; however, if exposed to ACE inhibitors in the first trimester, the medication may be stopped without significant damage to the fetus.[82,83] In summary, ACE inhibitors are contraindicated in pregnancy but may be useful in the postpartum period.

Anesthesia and hypertensive disorders of pregnancy

Exaggerated hemodynamic response

Sudden increase in blood pressure may occur in general anesthesia during either intubation or extubation, leading to a cerebrovascular event. An increase in arterial blood pressure accompanies laryngoscopy performed with or without tracheal intubation. Therefore, blood pressure should be reduced prior to intubation or extubation. This hypertensive response is prevented with a short-acting antihypertensive agent, such as nitroglycerin, sodium nitroprusside, or labetalol.[84,85] Esmolol, a pure β-receptor antagonist with a rapid onset of action, is a popular agent for blunting the hypertensive response to tracheal intubation in nonpregnant patients. Unfortunately, it crosses the placenta and causes severe fetal bradycardia; hence, it is not recommended in pregnant patients but may be used in postpartum preeclampsia.[86]

Decreased sympathetic activity due to regional anesthesia leads to dilatation of the capacitance vessels that cause hypotension. Adequate intravascular volume repletion (fluid preloading) performed before initiating regional anesthesia avoids this relative hypovolemia. Management of volume status varies according to the severity of the patient's disease. Hypotension can also occur with intravenous administration of antihypertensive medication. This effect is more pronounced if the mother has been in a supine position for a long period; hence, the need to have the patient in a "tilted" position to avoid compression of the vena cava by the uterus.

Difficulty with intubation

Preeclamptic women may have pharyngeal and laryngeal edema rendering intubation and ventilation difficult. A laryngeal mask airway (LMA) may be a useful alternative in cases of difficult airway management and should be anticipated in severe preeclampsia.[87]

Magnesium sulfate interaction with neuromuscular blocking agents

Magnesium decreases the release of acetylcholine from the presynaptic portion of the myometrial junction as well as decreasing the sensitivity of the motor endplate to the effects of acetylcholine. Women receiving magnesium sulfate are more sensitive to the depolarizing and nondepolarizing neuromuscular blocking agents; therefore, the dose of muscle relaxant must be adjusted accordingly.[84,88] This neuromuscular transmission defect correlates with increased serum magnesium levels and decreased serum calcium levels.

Bleeding problems

Decreased platelet count and function occur in up to 18% of women with preeclampsia.[84] Epidural anesthesia is safe for women with platelet counts ≥ 100 000/μL in the peripartum period.[89–91] The rate of fall in platelet count is equally important because a rapid fall in platelet count may be indicative of severe disease. Estimation of bleeding time is no longer deemed necessary as a routine test in severe preeclampsia. It is, however, important to check other indicators of coagulopathy, including prothrombin time (PT), partial thromboplastin time (PTT), and international normalized ratio (INR), especially if there are clinical signs of coagulopathy. If an epidural catheter is already in place, then the platelet count should be checked before removal of the epidural catheter.

Postpartum hemorrhage secondary to uterine atony may be due to magnesium sulfate (a tocolytic agent) and/or anesthetic agents (especially the inhalational agents) used in general anesthesia. Platelet dysfunction or thrombocytopenia, as in HELLP syndrome, will increase the risk of bleeding. Ramanathan et al.[92] showed that platelet dysfunction is related to the severity of preeclampsia.

Regional anesthesia is now established as the preferred mode of anesthesia for preeclampsia patients as long as there is no contraindication to regional anesthesia such as coagulopathy. Regional anesthesia is the anesthetic of choice in most women with preeclampsia or eclampsia, for some of the following reasons. Epidural analgesia reduces maternal plasma catecholamine levels in laboring women. This may benefit preeclamptic women who are already exhibiting increased vascular reactivity to circulating catecholamines. Compromised intervillous blood flow in preeclamptic women may be improved by lumbar epidural analgesia. In turn, lumbar epidural analgesia may improve uteroplacental perfusion by reversal of uterine arterial vasospasm.[84]

Prediction and prevention of preeclampsia

Preeclampsia discussion often evokes emotions and controversies, whether it is the etiology, diagnosis, pathogenesis, prediction, prevention, or treatment. Is magnesium sulfate indicated in the management of mild preeclampsia? What is the role of aspirin in the management of preeclampsia? Any role for antioxidants, placental growth factors, etc. in the evaluation of a woman with preeclampsia?

Prediction of preeclampsia

Over 100 clinical, biophysical, and biochemical tests have been recommended to predict or identify women at risk for future development of preeclampsia.[93–96] The results of the combined data and lack of agreement between serial tests suggest that none of these clinical tests is reliable for use as a screening test.

Numerous biomarkers have been proposed for the prediction of women who are destined to develop preeclampsia. The markers may indicate placental dysfunction,[96,97] endothelial and coagulation activation,[98,99] and systemic inflammation.[43,97] Many of these markers suffer from poor specificity and predictive values and, therefore, are not used in routine clinical practice.

Doppler ultrasound in the second trimester may show abnormal uterine artery velocity waveforms characterized by a high resistance index or by the presence of an early diastolic notch (unilateral or bilateral notch). The presence of these Doppler findings in the second trimester increases the rate of preeclampsia with a 20–60% sensitivity and a 6–40% positive predictive value.[100–102] A review by Chien et al.,[103] which included 27 studies with nearly 13 000 patients, claimed that uterine artery Doppler assessment had limited value as a screening tool for preeclampsia.

Prevention of preeclampsia

Magnesium sulfate for the prevention of eclampsia

Magnesium sulfate is now established as the drug of choice for the prevention of eclampsia, having been shown to be superior to placebo or no treatment in the prevention of convulsions in women with severe preeclampsia.[61,67,104–106] These trials demonstrated that magnesium sulfate prophylaxis, compared with placebo (two trials with a total of 10 795 women), nimodipine (one trial with 1750 women), and no treatment (one trial with 228 women) in the management of severe preeclampsia, is associated with a significantly lower rate of eclampsia. One of the largest trials to date enrolled 10 141 women with preeclampsia in 33 countries (mainly developing countries).[61] Most of the enrolled patients had severe disease by current United States standards; half of them received antihypertensives prior to randomization; 75% had antihypertensives following randomization. Among the enrolled women, the rate of eclampsia was significantly lower in those assigned to magnesium sulfate. However, of the 1560 women enrolled in the Western world, the rate of eclampsia was 0.5% in the magnesium group versus 0.8% in the placebo group, which was not significant [relative risk (RR) 0.67 within a 95% confidence interval].[61]

Two randomized placebo-controlled trials evaluated the efficacy and safety of magnesium sulfate in the management of mild preeclampsia. One study had 135 women[67] and the other had 222 women,[107] which revealed that magnesium sulfate does not affect the duration of labor, nor does it affect the rate of Cesarean section. Both trials lacked sufficient power to clarify the role of magnesium sulfate in the prevention of convulsions in mild preeclampsia.[108]

Aspirin

Several studies of aspirin for the prevention of preeclampsia have been performed. Hauth et al.[109] showed that the incidence of preeclampsia was significantly lower in the aspirin-treated group; however, there were no differences in gestational age at delivery, neonatal birthweight, or frequency of fetal growth restriction or preterm delivery. A subsequent study by Sibai et al.[110] showed a reduction in the incidence of preeclampsia by 26% in the aspirin-treated women. However, a significantly higher incidence of abruptio placentae was identified in women receiving aspirin. The CLASP trial,[111] a multinational, randomized trial involving 9364 women and using low-dose aspirin (60 mg), failed to identify a difference in the incidence of preeclampsia, intrauterine growth restriction, abruptio placentae, or perinatal deaths. The aspirin-treated group did, however, have a lower incidence of preterm delivery. A meta-analysis suggested that low dose aspirin improved pregnancy outcome in women with persistent elevations in uterine Doppler resistance index at both 18 and 24 weeks of gestation.[117] Other studies, however, did not show aspirin administration to prevent subsequent development of preeclampsia.[100,102] It thus appears that our hope for low-dose aspirin therapy as an effective prophylaxis for preeclampsia has not materialized, yet.

Oral supplementation with magnesium, zinc, calcium, vitamin C, vitamin E, etc.

Although the early reports of calcium supplementation for the prevention of and reduction in the severity of preeclampsia appeared promising, the results have not been convincing.[113–117] Zinc supplementation[118] and oral magnesium supplementation[119] studies did not show any change in the rate of preeclampsia. Fish oil supplementation showed no significant change in the incidence of preeclampsia.[120] Although Chappell et al.[121] showed improvement in the biochemical indices of preeclampsia after the administration of antioxidants, recent studies indicate that some antioxidants may not necessarily improve the clinical outcome in preeclampsia. Meanwhile, the role of calcium, vitamin E, vitamin C, and other antioxidants remains unclear.[122,123]

Prospects for the future

Maternal morbidity and mortality related to preeclampsia are principally associated with eclampsia and HELLP syndrome. Fetal morbidity and mortality are associated mainly with second-trimester severe preeclampsia and preterm delivery. Greater understanding of the pathophysiology of preeclampsia is the key to improving both fetal and maternal outcomes. In the present state of knowledge, women with severe disease should be referred to a tertiary center with the experience and facilities to manage maternal complications and provide intensive care for a preterm infant. In the future, it may be possible to identify factors that clearly distinguish between pregnant women at low risk of developing hypertensive complications and those at high risk. This would allow for appropriate antenatal care and maternal–fetal monitoring.

Key points

1 Hypertension is the most common medical complication of pregnancy, being present in 8–10% of pregnancies.

2 Mild preeclampsia is systolic blood pressure (BP) ≥ 140 mmHg or diastolic BP ≥ 90 mmHg observed on two occasions at least 6 hours apart with proteinuria.

3 Severe preeclampsia is proteinuria with systolic BP ≥ 160 mmHg or diastolic BP ≥ 110 mmHg or the presence of cerebral or visual disturbances. Other features of severe preeclampsia include persistent headache, persistent visual changes (scotomata), right upper quadrant pain, epigastric pain, nausea, and vomiting.

4 Preeclampsia accounts for 70% of hypertension in pregnancy, and chronic hypertension (CHTN) accounts for most of the remaining 30%.

5 Most women with eclamptic seizures have an abnormal electroencephalogram. However, electroencephalographic changes are almost always transient and resolve completely.

6 The outcome in women with CHTN is closely related to the development of superimposed preeclampsia and abruptio placentae.

7 Patients with hypertension in pregnancy have an increased incidence of eclampsia, abruptio placentae, preterm delivery (mainly iatrogenic preterm delivery due to obstetric intervention secondary to hypertension or its complications), disseminated intravascular coagulation (DIC), hemorrhage, renal insufficiency, pulmonary edema, stroke, and death.

8 Hypertension in pregnancy increases perinatal morbidity and mortality including preterm delivery/prematurity and intrauterine growth retardation (IUGR).

9 Treatment of severe hypertension is associated with a reduction in maternal morbidity and mortality, but does not prevent preeclampsia or abruptio placentae; neither does it improve perinatal outcome.

10 The most effective therapy for preeclampsia is delivery of the fetus and placenta.

11 No clinically useful and universally accepted predictive or screening test has been identified for preeclampsia.

12 Preconception counseling is very important in the management of patients with CHTN. It is important to establish the etiology and severity of hypertension, to identify endorgan damage, and to achieve adequate blood pressure control prior to conception.

13 Calcium channel blockers (diltiazem, nifedipine, etc.) are helpful in patients with CHTN and diabetes mellitus because of their renoprotective effect.

14 Angiotensin-converting enzyme (ACE) inhibitors may cause fetal renal insufficiency, oligohydramnios, growth restriction, cranial anomalies, and severe fetal hypotension especially in the second and third trimesters. The ACE inhibitors are contraindicated in pregnancy but may be used in diabetic patients in the postpartum period if they are not breastfeeding.

15 Hypertension and diabetes mellitus are both systemic diseases with significant impact on the micro- and macrocirculation leading to nephropathy, retinopathy, cardiac disease, etc. This underscores the need for aggressive control of blood pressure in such women.

References

1 Roberts JM, Pearson GD, Cutler JA, et al. for the National Heart Lung and Blood Institute. Summary of the NHLBI Working Group on Research on Hypertension During Pregnancy. *Hypertens Pregnancy* 2003;22(2):109–127.

2 Labarthe D, Ayala C. Nondrug interventions in hypertension prevention and control. *Cardiol Clin* 2002;20(2):249–263.

3 Wyatt HR. The prevalence of obesity. *Prim Care* 2003:30(2): 267–279.

4 Sibai BM, Dekker G, Kupferminc M. Preeclampsia—an update on its causation, diagnosis, prevention and management. *Lancet* 2005;365:785–799.

5 Koonin LM, Mackay AP, Berg CJ, et al. Pregnancy-related mortality surveillance, United States, 1987–1990. *Morbidity Mortality Weekly Rep CDC Surveill Summ* 1997;46(4):17–36.

6 Confidential Enquiry into Maternal and Child Health. *Why mothers die 2000–2002: Improving care for mothers, babies and children*. The Sixth Report of the Confidential Enquiries into Maternal Deaths in the United Kingdom. London: Royal College of Obstetrics and Gynaecology Press, 2004.

7 Berg CJ. Pregnancy-related mortality in the United States, 1991–1997. *Obstet Gynecol* 2003;101(2):289–296.

8 Callaghan WM. Pregnancy-related mortality among women aged 35 years and older, United States, 1991–1997. *Obstet Gynecol* 2003;102(5 Pt a):1015–1021.

9 American College of Obstetricians and Gynecologists. *Hypertension in pregnancy*. Technical Bulletin No. 219. Washington, DC: ACOG, 1996.

10 Sibai BM. Pitfall in the diagnosis and management of preeclampsia. *Am J Obstet Gynecol* 1988;159:1–5.

11 Karnath B. Review of clinical signs: sources of error in blood pressure measurement. *Hosp Phys* 2002;38(3):33–37.

12 Canzanello VJ, Jensen PL, Schwarts GL. Are aneroid sphygmomanometers accurate in hospital and clinic settings? *Arch Intern Med* 2001;161:729–731.

13 Neufeld PD, Johnson DL. Observer error in blood pressure measurement. *Can Med Assoc J* 1986;135:633–637.

14 National Institute of Health (NIH): National Heart, Lung, and Blood Institute. *National High Blood Pressure Education Program: working group report on high blood pressure in pregnancy*. NIH Publication No. 00-3029, 2000.

15 Chappell L, Pulton L, Halligan A, et al. Lack of consistency in research papers over the definition of preeclampsia. *Br J Obstet Gynaecol* 1999;106:983–985.

16 Henry CS, Biedermann SA, Campbell MF, et al. Spectrum of hypertensive emergencies in pregnancy. *Crit Care Clin* 2004; 20(4):697–712.

17 Sibai BM. Diagnosis, prevention, and management of eclampsia. *Obstet Gynecol* 2005;102(2):402–410.

18 Sibai BM. Best practices for diagnosis and management of preeclampsia. Part 1 of 3. Preeclampsia: 3 preemptive tactics. *Obstet Gynecol Manage* 2005;17(2):20–32.

19 Sibai BM, Abdella TH, Taylor HA. Eclampsia in the first half of pregnancy. A report of three cases and review of the literature. *J Reprod Med* 1982;27:706.

20 Lubarsky SL, Barton JR, Friedman SA, et al. Late postpartum eclampsia revisited. *Obstet Gynecol* 1994;83:502–505.

21 Sibai BM, Spinnato JA, Watson DL, et al. Eclampsia IV. Neurological findings and future outcome. *Am J Obstet Gynecol* 1985; 152:184.

22 Chesley LC. Disseminated intravascular coagulation. In: Chesley LC, ed. *Hypertensive disorders in pregnancy*. New York: Appleton-Century-Crofts; 1978:88.

23 Goodlin RC. Beware the great imitator-severe preeclampsia. *Contemp Obstet Gynecol* 1982;20:215.

24 Weinstein L. Syndrome of hemolysis, elevated liver enzymes, and

low platelet count: a severe consequence of hypertension in pregnancy. *Am J Obstet Gynecol* 1982;142:159–167.

25 Sibai BM, Taslimi MM, El-Nazer A, et al. Maternal–perinatal outcome associated with the syndrome of hemolysis, elevated liver enzymes, and low platelets in severe preeclampsia–eclampsia. *Am J Obstet Gynecol* 1986;155:501.

26 Sibai BM. The HELLP syndrome (hemolysis, elevated liver enzymes, and low platelets). Much ado about nothing? *Am J Obstet Gynecol* 1990;162:311–316.

27 Weinstein L. Preeclampsia/eclampsia with hemolysis, elevated liver enzymes, and thrombocytopenia. *Obstet Gynecol* 1985;66: 657–660.

28 Sibai BM. Diagnosis, controversies, and management of the syndrome of hemolysis, elevated liver enzymes, and low platelet count. *Obstet Gynecol* 2004;103(5 Pt 1):981–991.

29 Dawson LM, Parfrey PS, Hefferton D, et al. Familial risk of preeclampsia in Newfoundland: A population-based study. *J Am Soc Nephrol* 2002;13(7):1901–1906.

30 Bernard N, Giguere Y. Genetics of preeclampsia: what are the challenges? *J Obstet Gynaecol Can* 2003;25(7):578–585.

31 Taylor RN, et al. Longitudinal serum concentrations of placental growth factor: evidence for abnormal placental angiogenesis in pathologic pregnancies. *Am J Obstet Gynecol* 2003;188(1): 177–182.

32 Levine JL, Maynard SE, Qian C, et al. Circulating angiogenic factors and the risk of preeclampsia. *N Engl J Med* 2004; 350:672–683.

33 Torry DS, Wang HS, Wang TH, et al. Preeclampsia is associated with reduced serum levels of placental growth factor. *Am J Obstet Gynecol* 1998;179(6 Pt 1):1539–1544.

34 Wolf M, et al. Preeclampsia and future cardiovascular disease: potential role of altered angiogenesis and insulin resistance. *J Clin Endocrinol Metab* 2004;89(12):6239–6243.

35 Myatt L. Role of placenta in preeclampsia. *Endocrine* 2002;19(1):103–111.

36 Walsh SW. Preeclampsia: an imbalance in placental prostacyclin and thromboxane production. *Am J Obstet Gynecol* 1985;152: 335.

37 Francois H, Athirakul K, Mao L, et al. Role for thromboxane receptors in angiotensin-II-induced hypertension. *Hypertension* 2004;43:364.

38 Ito M, et al. Possible activation of the renin–angiotensin system in the feto-placental unit in preeclampsia. *J Clin Endocrinol Metab* 2002;87(4):1871–1877.

39 American College of Obstetricians and Gynecologists. *Chronic hypertension in pregnancy*. ACOG Practice Bulletin no.29. Washington, DC: ACOG, 2001.

40 Buchbinder A, Sibai BM, Caritis S, et al. Adverse perinatal outcomes are significantly higher in severe gestational hypertension than in mild preeclampsia. *Am J Obstet Gynecol* 2002;186:66–71.

41 Sibai BM, Gordon T, Thom E, et al. Risk factors for preeclampsia in healthy nulliparous women: a prospective multicenter study. The National Institutes of Child Health and Human Development Network of Maternal and Fetal Medicine Units. *Am J Obstet Gynecol* 1995;172:642–648.

42 Barton JR, O'Brien JM, Bergauer NK, et al. Mild gestational hypertension remote from term: progression and outcome. *Am J Obstet Gynecol* 2001;184:979–983.

43 Report of the National High Blood Pressure Education Program Working Group on High Blood Pressure in Pregnancy. *Am J Obstet Gynecol* 2000;183(1):S1–S22.

44 Sibai BM, Abdella TN, Anderson GD. Pregnancy outcome in 211 patients with mild chronic hypertension. *Obstet Gynecol* 1983;61:571.

45 Kaplan NM. Systemic hypertension: mechanisms and diagnosis. In: Braunwald E, Zipes DP, Libby P, eds. *Heart disease: a textbook of cardiovascular medicine*, 6th edn. Philadelphia: W.B. Saunders; 2001:941–971.

46 Calhoun DA, Oparil S. Treatment of hypertensive crisis. *N Engl J Med* 1990;323:1177–1183.

47 Schiff E, Friedman SA, Sibai BM. Conservative management of severe preeclampsia remote from term. *Obstet Gynecol* 1994;84: 626–630.

48 Sibai BM, Mercer BM, Schiff E, et al. Aggressive versus expectant management of severe preeclampsia at 28 to 32 weeks gestation: a randomized controlled trial. *Am J Obstet Gynecol* 1994;174:818–822.

49 Isler CM, Magann EF, Rinehart BK, et al. Dexamethasone compared with betamethasone for glucocorticoid treatment of postpartum HELLP syndrome. *Int J Gynecol Obstet* 2003;80:291–297.

50 Crane JM, Tabarsi B, Hutchens D. The maternal benefits of corticosteroids with HELLP (hemolysis, elevated liver enzymes, low platelet count) syndrome. *J Obstet Gynaecol Can* 2003; 8:650–655.

51 Schwartz ML. Possible role for exchange plasmapheresis with fresh frozen plasma for maternal indications in selected cases of preeclampsia and eclampsia. *Obstet Gynecol* 1986;68:136–139.

52 Martin JN, Jr, Files JC, Black PG, et al. Plasma exchange for preeclampsia 1. Postpartum use for persistently severe preeclampsia-eclampsia with HELLP syndrome. *Am J Obstet Gynecol* 1990;162:126–137.

53 Wicke C, Pereira PL, Neeser E. Subcapsular liver hematoma in HELLP syndrome: Evaluation of diagnostic and therapeutic options—a unicenter study. *Am J Obstet Gynecol* 2004;190(1): 106–112.

54 Paul RH, Koh KS, Bernstein SG. Changes in fetal heart rate—uterine contraction patterns associated with eclampsia. *Am J Obstet Gynecol* 1978;130:165.

55 Hankins GDV, Wendel GD, Cunningham FG, et al. Longitudinal evaluation of hemodynamic changes in eclampsia. *Am J Obstet Gynecol* 1984;150:506.

56 Hauth JC, Ewell MG, Levine RI, et al. Pregnancy outcomes in healthy nulliparous women who subsequently developed hypertension. *Obstet Gynecol* 2000;95:24–28.

57 Knuist M, Bonsel GJ, Zondervan HA, et al. Intensification of fetal and maternal surveillance in pregnant women with hypertensive disorders. *Int J Gynecol Obstet* 1998;61:127.

58 Sibai BM. Diagnosis and management of gestational hypertension and preeclampsia. *Obstet Gynecol* 2003;102(1):181–192.

59 Sibai BM, Lindheimer M, Hauth J, et al. Risk factors for preeclampsia, abruptio placentae, and adverse neonatal outcomes among women with chronic hypertension. National Institute of Child Health and Human Development Network of Maternal–Fetal Medicine Units. *N Engl J Med.* 1998;339(10): 667–671.

60 Sibai BM, Anderson GD. Pregnancy outcome of intensive therapy in severe hypertension in first trimester. *Obstet Gynecol* 1986;67:517.

61 Magpie Trial Collaboration Group. Do women with pre-eclampsia, and their babies, benefit from magnesium sulphate? The Magpie Trial: a randomized placebo-controlled trial. *Lancet* 2002;359(9321):1877–1890.

62 Belfort MA, Moise KJ. Effect of magnesium sulfate on maternal

brain blood flow in preeclampsia: a randomized, placebo-controlled study. *Am J Obstet Gynecol* 1992;167:661–666.

63 Bohman VR, Cotton DB. Supralethal magnesium with patient survival. *Obstet Gynecol* 1990;76:984–986.

64 Fuentes A, Rojas A, Porter KB, et al. The effect of magnesium sulfate on bleeding time in pregnancy. *Am J Obstet Gynecol* 1995;173:1246–1249.

65 Kynezl-Leisure M, Cibils LA. Increased bleeding time after magnesium sulfate infusion. *Am J Obstet Gynecol* 1996;175:1293–1294.

66 Friedman SA, Lim K, Baker CA, et al. Phenytoin versus magnesium sulfate in preeclampsia: a pilot study. *Am J Perinatol* 1993;10:233–238.

67 Witlin AG, Friedman SA, Sibai BM. The effect of magnesium sulfate therapy on the duration of labor in women with mild preeclampsia at term: a randomized, double-blind, placebo-controlled trial. *Am J Obstet Gynecol* 1997;176:623–627.

68 Stallworth JC, Yeh SY, Petrie RH. The effect of magnesium sulfate on fetal heart rate variability and uterine activity. *Am J Obstet Gynecol* 1981;140:702.

69 Duley L, Gulmezoglu AM, Henderson-Smart DJ. Magnesium sulphate and other anticonvulsants for women with pre-eclampsia. *Cochrane Database Syst Rev* Jan 1 2003(2): CD000025.

70 Livingston JC, Sibai BM. Chronic hypertension in pregnancy. *Obstet Gynecol Clin North Am* 2001;28(3):447–463.

71 Sibai BM, Anderson GD. Pregnancy outcome of intensive therapy in severe hypertension in first trimester. *Obstet Gynecol* 1986;67:517–522.

72 McCowan LM, Buist RG, North FA, et al. Perinatal morbidity in chronic hypertension. *Br J Obstet Gynaecol* 1996;103: 123–129.

73 Horvath JS, Phippard A, Korda A, et al. Clonidine hydrochloride: a safe and effective antihypertensive agent in pregnancy. *Obstet Gynecol* 1985;66:634.

74 Rubin PC, Butters L, et al. Placebo-controlled trial of atenolol in treatment of pregnancy associated hypertension. *Lancet* 1983;I: 431–434.

75 Davis BR, Cutler JA, Furberg CD, et al. ALLHAT Collaborative Research Group. Relationship of antihypertensive treatment regimens and change in blood pressure to risk for heart failure in hypertensive patients randomly assigned to doxazosin or chlorthalidone: further analyses from the Antihypertensive and Lipid-Lowering Treatment to prevent Heart Attack Trial. *Ann Intern Med* 2002;137(5 Pt 1):313–320.

76 Sibai BM, Abdella TN, Anderson, GD, et al. Plasma volume findings in pregnant women with mild hypertension. *Am J Obstet Gynecol* 1983;145:539.

77 Mabie WC, Gonzalez AR, Sibai BM, et al. A comparative trial of labetalol and hydralazine in the acute management of severe hypertension complicating pregnancy. *Obstet Gynecol* 1987;70: 328–333.

78 Sibai BM, Barton JR, Akl S, et al. A randomized prospective comparison of nifedipine and bed rest versus bed rest alone, in the management of preeclampsia remote from term. *Am J Obstet Gynecol* 1992;167:879–884.

79 Magee LA, Schick B, Donnenfeld AF, et al. The safety of calcium channel blockers in human pregnancy: a prospective, multicenter cohort study. *Am J Obstet Gynecol* 1996;174:823–828.

80 Leguizamon G, Reece EA. Effect of medical therapy on progressive nephropathy: influence of pregnancy, diabetes and hypertension. *J Matern Fetal Med* 2000;9:70–78.

81 Rosa FW, Bosco LA, Graham CF, et al. Neonatal anuria with maternal angiotensin converting enzyme inhibitor. *Obstet Gynecol* 1989;74:371–374.

82 How HY, Sibai BM. Use of angiotensin-converting enzyme inhibitors in patients with diabetic nephropathy. *J Matern Fetal Neonatal Med* 2002;12(6):402–407.

83 Lip GYH, Churchill D, Beevers M, et al. Angiotensin-converting enzyme inhibitors in early pregnancy. *Lancet* 1997;350:1446.

84 Chadwick HS, Easterling T. Anesthetic concerns in the patient with preeclampsia. *Semin Perinatol* 1991;15:397–409.

85 Birnbach DJ, Browne IM. Anesthesia for obstetrics. In: Miller RD, ed. *Miller's anesthesia*, 6th edn. New York: Churchill Livingstone, 2005.

86 Ramanathan J, Bennett K. Pre-eclampsia: fluids, drugs, and anesthetic management. *Anesthesiol Clin North Am* 2003;21(1): 145–163.

87 Keller C, Brimacombe J, Lirk P, et al. Failed obstetric tracheal intubation and postoperative respiratory support with the ProSeal laryngeal mask airway. *Anesth Analg* 2004;98(5):1467–1470.

88 Ramanathan J, Sibai BM, Pillai R, et al. Neuromuscular transmission studies in preeclamptic women receiving magnesium sulfate. *Am J Obstet Gynecol* 1988;158:40–46.

89 Rolbin SH, Abbott K, Musclow E, et al. Epidural anesthesia in pregnant patients with low platelet counts. *Obstet Gynecol* 1988;71:918–920.

90 Rasmus KT, Rottman RL, Kotelko DM, et al. Unrecognized thrombocytopenia and regional anesthesia in parturients: a retrospective review. *Obstet Gynecol* 1989;73:943–946.

91 Wallace DH, Leveno KJ, Cunningham FG, et al. Randomized comparison of general and regional anesthesia for cesarean delivery in pregnancies complicated by severe preeclampsia. *Obstet Gynecol* 1995;86:193–199.

92 Ramanathan J, Sibai BM, Vu T, et al. Correlation between bleeding times and platelet counts in women with preeclampsia undergoing cesarean delivery. *Anesthesiology* 1989;71:188–191.

93 Friedman SA, Lindheimer MD. Prediction and differential diagnosis. In: Lindheimer MD, Roberts JM, Cunningham GF, eds. *Chesley's hypertensive disorders in pregnancy*. Stamford, CT: Appleton & Lange; 1999:201.

94 August P, Helseth G, Cook F, et al. A prediction model for superimposed preeclampsia in women with chronic hypertension during pregnancy. *Am J Obstet Gynecol* 2004;191:1666–1672.

95 Conde-Agudelo A, Villar J, Linheimer M. World Health Organization systematic review of screening tests for preeclampsia. *Obstet Gynecol* 2004;104:1367–1391.

96 Tjoa ML, Qwdejans CBM, Van Vugt JMG, et al. Markers for presymptomatic prediction of preeclampsia and intrauterine growth restriction. *Hypertens Pregnancy* 2004;23:171–189.

97 Sargent IL, Germain SJ, Sacks GP, et al. Trophoblast deportation and the maternal inflammatory response in preeclampsia. *J Reprod Immunol* 2003;59:153–160.

98 Savidou MD, Hingorani AD, Tsikas D, et al. Endothelial dysfunction and raised plasma concentrations of asymmetric dimethylarginine in pregnant women who subsequently develop pre-eclampsia. *Lancet* 2003;361:1151–1157.

99 Wang Y, Gu Y, Zhang Y, et al. Evidence of endothelial dysfunction in preeclampsia: decreased endothelial nitric oxide synthase expression is associated with increased cell permeability in endothelial cells from preeclampsia. *Am J Obstet Gynecol* 2004;190:817–824.

100 Yu CKH, Papageorghiou AT, Parra M, et al. Randomized controlled trial using low-dose aspirin in the prevention of pre-eclampsia in women with abnormal uterine artery Doppler at 23

weeks' gestation. *Ultrasound Obstet Gynecol* 2003;22:233–239.

101 Yu CKH, Papageorghiou AT, Boli A, et al. Screening for pre-eclampsia and fetal growth restriction in twin pregnancies at 23 weeks of gestation by transvaginal uterine artery Doppler ultrasound. *Obstet Gynecol* 2002;20:535–540.

102 Subtil D, Goeusse P, Houfflin-Debarge V, et al. Essai Regional Aspirine Mere-Enfant (ERASME) Collaborative Group. Randomized comparison of uterine artery Doppler and aspirin (100 mg) with placebo in nulliparous women: The Essai Regional Aspirine Mere-Enfant study (Part 2). *Br J Obstet Gynaecol* 2003;110:485–491.

103 Chien PE, Arnott N, Gordon A, et al. How useful is uterine artery Doppler flow velocimetry in the prediction of pre-eclampsia, intra-uterine growth retardation and perinatal death? An overview. *Br J Obstet Gynaecol* 2000;107:196–208.

104 Coetzee EJ, Dommisse J, Anthony J. A randomized controlled trial of intravenous magnesium sulfate versus placebo in the management of women with severe preeclampsia. *Br J Obstet Gynaecol* 1998;105:300–303.

105 Moodley J, Moodley VV. Prophylactic anticonvulsant therapy in hypertensive crises of pregnancy—the need for a large, randomized trial. *Hypertens Pregnancy* 1994;13:245–252.

106 Belfort MA, Anthony J, Saade GR, et al. for the Nimodipine Study Group. A comparison of magnesium sulfate and nimodipine for the prevention of eclampsia. *N Engl J Med* 2003;348:304–311.

107 Livingston JC, Livingston LW, Ramsey R, et al. Magnesium sulfate in women with mild preeclampsia: a randomized, double blinded, placebo-controlled trial. *Obstet Gynecol* 2003;101:217–220.

108 Sibai BM. Magnesium sulfate prophylaxis in preeclampsia. Lessons learned from recent trials. *Am J Obstet Gynecol* 2004;190:1520–1526.

109 Hauth JC, Goldenberg RL, Parker CR Jr, et al. Low-dose aspirin therapy to prevent preeclampsia. *Am J Obstet Gynecol* 1993;168:1083–1091(discussion 1091–1093)

110 Sibai BM, Caritis SN, Thom E, et al. Prevention of preeclampsia with low-dose aspirin in healthy, nulliparous pregnant women. *N Engl J Med* 1993;329:1213–1218.

111 CLASP (Collaborative Low-dose Aspirin Study in Pregnancy) Group. CLASP: a randomized trial of low-dose aspirin for the prevention and treatment of pre-eclampsia among 9364 pregnant women. *Lancet* 1994;343:619–629.

112 Coomarasamy A, Papaioannou S, Gee H, et al. Aspirin for the prevention of preeclampsia in women with abnormal uterine artery Doppler: a meta-analysis. *Obstet Gynecol* 2001;98:861–866.

113 Levine RL. Calcium for preeclampsia prevention (CPEP): a double-blind, placebo-controlled trial in healthy nulliparas. *Am J Obstet Gynecol* 1997;176:S2.

114 Sibai BM, Dekker G, Kupferminc M. Pre-eclampsia. *Lancet* 2005;365:785.

115 Sibai BM. Prevention of preeclampsia: a big disappointment. *Am J Obstet Gynecol* 1998;179:1275–1278.

116 Atallah AN, Hofmeyr GJ, Duley L. Calcium supplementation during pregnancy for preventing hypertensive disorders and related problems (Cochrane Review). In: *The Cochrane Library*, Issue 1, 2003. Oxford: Update Software.

117 Levine RJ, Hauth JC, Curet LB, et al. Trial of calcium to prevent preeclampsia. *N Engl J Med* 1997;337;69.

118 Mohamed K, James DK, Golding J, et al. Zinc supplementation during pregnancy: a double-blind randomized controlled trial. *Br Med J* 1989;299:826.

119 Sibai BM, Villar MA, Bray E. Magnesium supplementation during pregnancy: a double-blind randomized controlled clinical trial. *Am J Obstet Gynecol* 1989;161:115.

120 Olsen SF, Secheer NJ, Tabor A, et al. Randomized clinical trials of fish oil supplementation in high risk pregnancies. Fish Oil Trials in Pregnancy (FOTIP) Team. *Br J Obstet Gynaecol* 2000;107(3):382–395.

121 Chappell LC, Seed PT, Kelly FJ, et al. Vitamin C and E supplementation in women at risk of preeclampsia is associated with changes in indices of oxidative stress and placental function. *Am J Obstet Gynecol* 2002;187(3):777–784.

122 Dekker G, Sibai B. Primary, secondary, and tertiary prevention of pre-eclampsia. *Lancet*. 2001;357(9251):209–215.

123 Beazley D, Ahokas R, Livingston J, et al. Vitamin C and E supplementation in women at high risk for preeclampsia: a double-blind, placebo-controlled trial. *Am J Obstet Gynecol* 2005;192:520–521.

39 Cardiac diseases in pregnancy

Kjersti Aagaard-Tillery and Steven L. Clark

Pregnancy causes significant alterations in the maternal cardiovascular system. The pregnant patient with normal cardiac function accommodates these physiologic changes without difficulty. In the presence of cardiac disease, however, pregnancy may be extremely hazardous, resulting in decompensation and even death. Despite advances in the diagnosis and treatment of maternal cardiovascular disease, such conditions continue to account for 10–25% of maternal deaths.[1–3] Given an observed increasing prevalence of pregnancies among women with cardiac disease, currently estimated to range between 0.1% and 4%, the need for obstetricians to be well versed in proper counseling and management of these conditions is paramount.[4] This chapter focuses on the interaction between structural cardiac disease and pregnancy, with an emphasis on the means of achieving optimal maternal and perinatal outcomes.

Counseling the pregnant cardiac patient

The Criteria Committee of the New York Heart Association (NYHA) has recommended a classification of cardiac disease based on clinical function (classes I–IV). Although such a classification is useful in discussing the pregnant cardiac patient, up to 40% of patients developing congestive heart failure and pulmonary edema during pregnancy are functional class I before pregnancy. In one review, the majority of maternal deaths during pregnancy occurred in patients who were initially class I or II.[5] In general, however, women who begin pregnancy as functional class I or II have a better outcome than those initially in class III or IV.[6,7] Counseling the pregnant cardiac patient regarding her prognosis for successful pregnancy is further complicated by recent advances in medical and surgical therapy, fetal surveillance, and neonatal care. Such advances render invalid many older estimates of maternal mortality and fetal wastage.

Table 39.1 represents a synthesis of maternal risk estimates for various types of cardiac disease initially developed by Clark et al.[8] in 1987. Counseling of the pregnant cardiac patient, as well as general management approaches, were based on this classification. Category I included conditions that, with proper management, were associated with negligible maternal mortality (less than 1%). Cardiac lesions in category II traditionally carried a 5–15% risk of maternal mortality. Patients with cardiac lesions in group III were, and probably remain, subject to a mortality risk exceeding 25%. In all but exceptional cases, this risk is unacceptable, and it is our continued belief that prevention or interruption of pregnancy is generally recommended.

While our initial classification schema has proven useful in grossly predicting mortality risk in the past, a review of more recent data from the United States and Europe suggests the need to selectively revise these estimates; this is summarized in Table 39.2. In some of these current studies, it may generally be said that maternal mortality is almost exclusively seen in patients with pulmonary hypertension, endocarditis, coronary artery disease, cardiomyopathy, and sudden arrhythmia.[1–3,9–33] deSwiet,[1] reporting on maternal mortality from heart disease in the United Kingdom between 1997 and 1999, found that all deaths could be accounted for from the following entities: puerperal cardiomyopathy (20%), myocardial infarction (14%), aortic dissection (14%), cardiomyopathy and myocarditis (14%), primary pulmonary hypertension (9%), secondary pulmonary hypertension (11%), endocarditis (9%), and dysrhythmia (3%). These authors attribute the changing pattern of heart disease in recent decades to a dramatic reduction in rheumatic heart disease. In support of this hypothesis, a review of maternal mortality in Utah from 1982 to 1994 revealed 13 cardiac deaths, four from pulmonary hypertension (31%), four secondary to cardiomyopathy (31%), two from coronary artery disease (15%), and three (23%) from sudden arrhythmia.[3] This is not to imply that the relative risk categories outlined in Table 39.1 are not still valid with respect to the likelihood of maternal complications or that interruption of pregnancy or cardiac surgery before term may not be necessary. The possibility of fetal morbidity and mortality, especially in cases of cyanotic heart disease, also cannot be overlooked. However, it would appear that, with

Table 39.1 Maternal risk associated with pregnancy, by general categorization.

Group	Cardiovascular disorder
Group I: Minimal risk of complications (< 1%)	Atrial septal defect
	Ventricular septal defect
	Patent ductus arteriosus
	Pulmonic or tricuspid disease
	Corrected tetralogy of Fallot
	Bioprosthetic valve
	Mitral stenosis, NYHA classes I and II
	Marfan syndrome with normal aorta*
Group II: Moderate risk of complications (5–15%)	Mitral stenosis with atrial fibrillation
	Artificial valve
	Mitral stenosis, NYHA classes III and IV
	Aortic stenosis
	Coarctation of aorta, uncomplicated
	Uncorrected tetralogy of Fallot
	Previous myocardial infarction
Group III: Major risk of complications or death (> 25%)	Pulmonary hypertension
	Coarctation of the aorta, complicated
	Marfan syndrome with aortic involvement

*Normal aorta, defined as aortic root diameter < 4 cm and no evidence of dissection.

NYHA, New York Heart Association.

appropriate obstetric care, the presence or absence of the above secondary complications or cardiomyopathy appears to play a much more important role in determining ultimate maternal outcome than the primary structural nature of the cardiac lesion itself.[8] Indeed, the most recent recommendations from the American Heart Association and the American College of Cardiology regarding classification of maternal and fetal risk during pregnancy on the basis of the type of valvular abnormality and NYHA functional class (Table 39.3) note that the absolute risk conferred on a given women by pregnancy is modified by additional clinical factors.[34,35]

Congenital cardiac disease

The relative frequency of congenital as opposed to acquired heart disease is changing.[5,36] With the wide introduction of efficacious penicillin therapy for rheumatic fever, sequelent valvular stenosis is relatively uncommon in the United States. Concomitant advances in heart–lung bypass have enabled the surgical correction of many previously fatal congenital cardiac lesions. Thus, patients with congenital cardiac disease now account for the vast majority of pregnant women with heart disease. In a review in 1954, the ratio of rheumatic to congenital heart disease seen during pregnancy was 16:1; the current ratio approximates 1:1.5.[5,34–37] In the following discussion of specific cardiac lesions, no attempt is made to duplicate existing comprehensive texts regarding physical

Table 39.2 Summary of current revised maternal mortality risks associated with selected cardiovascular disorders.

Group	Cardiovascular disorder	Maternal mortality (%)
Group I: Minimal risk of complications	Atrial septal defect	< 1
	Ventricular septal defect, without pulmonary hypertension	< 1
	Patent ductus arteriosus	< 1
	Pulmonic or tricuspid disease	0–0.5
	Corrected tetralogy of Fallot	0.05–1
	Bioprosthetic valve	1
	Mitral stenosis, NYHA classes I and II	0–1.6
	Marfan syndrome with normal aorta*	0–1.1
Group II: Moderate risk of complications	Mitral stenosis with atrial fibrillation	12–17
	Mechanical valve	1–4
	Mitral stenosis, NYHA classes III and IV	5–7
	Aortic stenosis	2–18
	Coarctation of aorta, uncomplicated	2–5
	Uncorrected tetralogy of Fallot	12–15
	Previous myocardial infarction, remote	2–15
Group III: Major risk of complications or death	Primary pulmonary hypertension	35–50
	Coarctation of the aorta, complicated	> 25
	Marfan syndrome with aortic involvement	50
	Previous myocardial infarction, within 2 weeks of delivery	50

The maternal mortality rates represent a compilation from available and identified references.[1–4,8–33] As such, they represent varying degrees of disorder severity, a spectrum of patient ages and ethnic background, and additional associated risk factors. They must thus be regarded as generalizable approximations.

*Normal aorta, defined as aortic root diameter < 4 cm and no evidence of dissection.

Table 39.3 Valvular heart lesions stratified by maternal and fetal risk derived from ACC/AHA Guidelines.[35]

Maternal risk	Lesion	Description
Low maternal and fetal risk	Asymptomatic aortic stenosis	Low mean outflow gradient (< 50 mmHg) Normal LV systolic function (EF > 50%)
	Aortic regurgitation, NYHA I or II	Normal LV systolic function (EF > 50%)
	Mild/moderate mitral stenosis	Mitral valve area > 1.5 cm^2 Low gradient (< 5 mmHg) Absence of severe pulmonary hypertension (severe pulmonary hypertension defined as pulmonary pressure > 75% of systemic pressures)
	Mitral regurgitation, NYHA I or II	Normal LV systolic function (EF > 50%)
	Mitral valve prolapse	Absence of mitral regurgitation OR Mild/moderate mitral regurgitation with normal LV systolic function (EF > 50%)
High maternal and fetal risk	Severe aortic stenosis	Valve area <1.5 cm^2
	Aortic regurgitation, NYHA III or IV	Symptomatic per NYHA criteria
	Aortic regurgitation in Marfan syndrome	
	Mitral stenosis, NYHA II, III, or IV	Symptomatic per NYHA criteria
	Mitral regurgitation, NYHA III or IV	Symptomatic per NYHA criteria
	Aortic and/or mitral valve disease, with severe pulmonary hypertension	Resultant severe pulmonary hypertension (severe pulmonary hypertension defined as pulmonary pressure > 75% of systemic pressures)
	Aortic and/or mitral valve disease, with left ventricular systolic dysfunction	Abnormal LV systolic function (EF < 40%)
	Maternal cyanosis	

NYHA, New York Heart Association classification. By functional status, NYHA I is asymptomatic; NYHA II is symptoms with greater than normal activity; NYHA III is symptoms with normal activity; NYHA IV is symptoms at rest.

LV, left ventricular; EF, ejection fraction.

diagnostic, electrocardiographic, and radiographic findings of specific cardiac lesions. (For a comprehensive discussion of diagnostic findings, see Braunwald E, ed. *Heart disease. A textbook of cardiovascular medicine*, 6th edn. Philadelphia: W.B. Saunders, 2001.) Instead, the discussion here focuses on aspects of congenital cardiac disease that are unique to pregnancy. We preface our discussion regarding congenital cardiac lesions with the longstanding acknowledgment that patients at risk of developing right-to-left shunts with increased pulmonary hypertension are at highest risk for unacceptably high maternal and fetal morbidity and mortality; surgical correction prior to the development of increased pulmonary vascular resistance and pulmonary hypertension (Eisenmenger's syndrome) is the greatest single contributor to improved outcomes observed over the preceding four decades.

Atrial sepal defect

Atrial septal defect (ASD) is the most common congenital lesion seen during pregnancy and is generally asymptomatic.[38–42] As a result of the disproportionate number of women with ostium secundum defects being asymptomatic until the reproductive years, it is not unheard of to have women present with a sentinel ASD diagnosis in pregnancy.[43] The two significant potential complications seen with ASD are arrhythmias and ventricular failure.

As a result of pregnancy-associated increases in atrial volume, biatrial enlargement and resultant supraventricular dysrhythmias are occasionally encountered. In general, although atrial arrhythmias are not uncommon in patients with ASD, their onset generally occurs after the fourth decade of life. Thus, such arrhythmias are unlikely to be encountered in the majority of pregnant woman. That said, in patients with ASD, atrial fibrillation is the most common arrhythmia encountered; however, supraventricular tachycardia and atrial flutter also may occur.[44] Initial therapy is with digoxin; less commonly, propranolol, quinidine, or cardioversion may be necessary.

The hypervolemia and increased cardiac output associated with pregnancy accentuates the left-to-right shunt through the ASD, and thus a significant burden is imposed on the right ventricle. Although this additional burden is tolerated well by most patients, congestive failure and death have been reported with ASD.[45–47] Thus, peripartum management centers on avoiding vascular resistance changes that increase the degree

Table 39.4 Antibiotic prophylaxis for the prevention of bacterial endocarditis.

Cardiac lesion	Prophylaxis for uncomplicated delivery	Prophylaxis for suspected bacteremia (i.e., chorioamnionitis)
Negligible risk category		
Functional heart murmurs	Not recommended	Not recommended
Mitral valve prolapse without regurgitation	Not recommended	Not recommended
Previous rheumatic fever without valve dysfunction	Not recommended	Not recommended
Previous Kawasaki disease without valve dysfunction	Not recommended	Not recommended
Cardiac pacemakers and implanted defibrillators	Not recommended	Not recommended
Prior coronary bypass graft surgery	Not recommended	Not recommended
Moderate-risk category		
Acquired valve dysfunction (rheumatic fever)	Not recommended	Recommended
Congenital cardiac malformations EXCEPT: repaired ASD, VSD, or PDA, or isolated secundum ASD	Not recommended	Recommended
Hypertrophic cardiomyopathy	Not recommended	Recommended
Mitral valve prolapse with regurgitation or thickened leaflets	Not recommended	Recommended
High-risk category		
Prosthetic cardiac valves	Optional	Recommended
Prior bacterial endocarditis	Optional	Recommended
Complex cyanotic congenital cardiac malformations	Optional	Recommended
Surgically constructed systemic pulmonary shunts/conduits	Optional	Recommended

Adapted from ACOG Practice Bulletin No. 47 Prophylactic Antibiotics in Labor and Delivery, October 2003. These recommendations are based on ACC/AHA guidelines,[35] which specifically discourage endocarditis prophylaxis for "routine" vaginal or Cesarean delivery. Given a possible increased risk of endocarditis with complicated deliveries such as retained placenta,[48] alongside recommendations to give antibiotics before or within 30 min of starting a "complicated" procedure, the decision to hold or administer subacute bacterial endocarditis (SBE) prophylaxis is not necessarily straightforward.[35] Thus, many obstetricians may elect to administer prophylactic antibiotics to cover unpredictable complicated deliveries.

of the shunt. In contrast to the high-pressure/high-flow state seen with ventricular septal defect (VSD) and patent ductus arteriosus (PDA), ASD is characterized by high pulmonary blood flow associated with normal pulmonary artery pressures. Because pulmonary artery pressures are low, pulmonary hypertension is unusual. The majority of patients with ASD tolerate pregnancy, labor, and delivery without complication. Neilson and colleagues[45] reported 70 pregnancies in 24 patients with ASD; all patients had an uncomplicated ante- and intrapartum course. During labor, placement of the patient in the lateral recumbent position, avoidance of fluid overload, oxygen administration, and pain relief with epidural anesthesia, as well judicious use of prophylaxis against bacterial endocarditis, are the most important considerations (Tables 39.4 and 39.5).

Ventricular septal defect

VSD may occur as an isolated lesion or in conjunction with other congenital cardiac anomalies, including tetralogy of Fallot, transposition of the great vessels, and coarctation of the aorta. The size of the septal defect is the most important determinant of clinical prognosis during pregnancy. Small defects are tolerated well, whereas larger defects are associated more frequently with congestive heart failure, arrhythmias, or the development of pulmonary hypertension. In addition, a large VSD is often associated with some degree of aortic regurgitation, which then modifies the risk of congestive failure. Pregnancy, labor, and delivery are tolerated well by patients with uncomplicated VSD. Schaefer and colleagues[46] compiled a series of 141 pregnancies in 56 women with VSD. The only two maternal deaths were in women whose VSD was complicated by pulmonary hypertension (Eisenmenger's syndrome). Although very rarely indicated, successful primary closure of a large VSD during pregnancy has been reported.[47,49] Because of the significance of unrecognized Eisenmenger's syndrome, careful measurements of pulmonary artery pressures are mandatory in any patient in whom persistent VSD is suspected or in whom the status of a previous repair is uncertain.[50,51] In general, invasive hemodynamic monitoring is unnecessary. Management considerations for patients with uncomplicated VSD are similar to those outlined for ASD.

Patent ductus arteriosus

Although PDA is one of the most common congenital cardiac anomalies, its almost universal detection and closure in the newborn period make it uncommon during pregnancy.[52,53] As with uncomplicated ASD and VSD, most patients are asymptomatic, and PDA is generally well tolerated during pregnancy,

Table 39.5 Endocarditis prophylaxis regimens for genitourinary/gastrointestinal procedures.[35]

Patient group	Agent	Dosage*
High risk	Ampicillin plus gentamicin	Load: Ampicillin 2 g i.v./i.m. Gentamicin 1.5 mg/kg i.v. to a maximum of 120 mg 6 h later: Ampicillin 1 g i.v./i.m. or amoxicillin 1 g p.o.
Ampicillin-allergic high risk	Vancomycin plus gentamicin	Load: Vancomycin 1 g i.v. over 1–2 h Gentamicin 1.5 mg/kg i.v. to a maximum of 120 mg 6 h later: Ampicillin 1 g i.v./i.m. or amoxicillin 1 g p.o.
Moderate risk	Amoxicillin or ampicillin	Amoxicillin 2 g p.o. 1 h before procedure or ampicillin 2 g i.v./i.m.
Ampicillin-allergic moderate risk	Vancomycin plus gentamicin	Load: Vancomycin 1 g i.v. over 1–2 h

*With respect to i.v.- or i.m.-administered ampicillin, gentamicin, or vancomycin, complete infusion within 30 min of starting the procedure.[35]

labor, and delivery. As with a large VSD, however, the high-pressure/high-flow, left-to-right shunt associated with a large, uncorrected PDA can lead to pulmonary hypertension. In such cases, the prognosis unacceptably worsens. In one study of 18 pregnant women who died of congenital heart disease, three had PDA; however, all these patients had secondary severe pulmonary hypertension.[47] Management considerations for patients with uncomplicated PDA, without pulmonary hypertension, are similar to those outlined under ASD.

Eisenmenger's syndrome and pulmonary hypertension

Eisenmenger's syndrome develops when, in the presence of congenital left-to-right shunt, progressive pulmonary hypertension leads to shunt reversal or bidirectional shunting as a result of chronically increased pulmonary vascular blood flow with accompanying pulmonary vascular resistance exceeding systemic vascular resistance. Although this syndrome may rarely occur with ASD, VSD, or PDA, the low-pressure and high-flow shunt seen as ASD is far less likely to result in pulmonary hypertension and shunt reversal than is the condition of high-pressure and high-flow symptoms seen with VSD and PDA. Regardless of the etiology, pulmonary hypertension carries a guarded prognosis during pregnancy, although there are published reports suggesting that the greatest risk may be seen in women with Eisenmenger's syndrome.[54,55] After Eisenmenger's pathophysiology is established, the pulmonary hypertension is permanent, and surgical correction of the defect is unhelpful and may increase mortality.[33,59]

During the antepartum period, the decreased systemic vascular resistance associated with pregnancy increases both the likelihood as well as the degree of right-to-left shunting. Pulmonary perfusion decreases, with systemic hypotension resulting in hypoxemia with subsequent maternal then fetal deterioration. The peripartum development of systemic hypotension leads to decreased right ventricular filling pressures; in the concomitant presence of a fixed cardiac output state (e.g., pulmonary hypertension), such decreased right heart pressures may be insufficient to perfuse the pulmonary arterial bed, leading to a sudden and profound hypoxemia and death. While there may exist any number of inciting events resulting in systemic hypotension in pregnancy, it most frequently results from hemorrhage or complications of conduction anesthesia.[53–61] Thus, avoidance of systemic hypotension is the principal clinical concern in the intrapartum management of patients with pulmonary hypertension of any etiology. This fact is underscored by the longstanding knowledge that the greatest maternal risk occurs in the peripartum period, and most deaths occur between 2 and 9 days postpartum. The precise pathophysiology of such decompensation is unclear, and it is uncertain what, if any, therapeutic maneuvers prevent or ameliorate such deterioration.

Maternal mortality in the presence of Eisenmenger's syndrome ranges from 30% to 60%.[27,52,59] In their classic review of the subject, Gleicher and colleagues[55] reported a 39% mortality associated with vaginal delivery and a 75% mortality associated with Cesarean section. These authors' original observations still stand; a more recent review looking at mortality from 1978 to 1996 fails to demonstrate significant improvement in maternal mortality.[61] Eisenmenger's syndrome associated with VSD appears to carry a higher mortality risk than that associated with PDA or ASD. In addition to the previously discussed problems associated with hemorrhage and hypovolemia, thromboembolic phenomena have been associated with up to 43% of all maternal deaths in Eisenmenger's syndrome.[55] Pitts and colleagues[58] reported increased mortality associated with prophylactic peripartum heparinization. However, other authors have reported that the use of heparin therapy (with bedrest and supplemental oxygen) may modestly positively influence maternal and fetal outcomes; there are no large trials supporting these findings to date.[59] Sudden delayed postpartum death, occurring 4–6 weeks after delivery, has also been reported.[55,60] Such deaths may involve a rebound worsening of pulmonary hypertension associated with the loss of pregnancy-associated hormones, or thromboembolic events.

Because of the high mortality associated with continuing pregnancy,[27] pregnancy termination ought to be presented to the patient as the preferred management of choice for the woman with pulmonary hypertension of any etiology. Pregnancy termination in either the first or the second trimester has long been considered the safer alternative over allowing the pregnancy to progress to term.[62] Dilation and curettage in the first trimester or dilation and evacuation in the second trimester is the method of choice. Hypertonic saline and F-series prostaglandins (prostaglandin $F_2\alpha$) are contraindicated, although the careful use of E-series prostaglandins is probably appropriate as long as systemic hypotension is avoided.

For the patient with a continuing gestation, management centers on avoiding increases in pulmonary vascular resistance, maintaining right ventricular preload, left ventricular afterload, and right ventricular contractility. Thus, factors that increase pulmonary vascular resistance ought to be avoided. In general terms, sympathetic agonists (epinephrine and norepinephrine) and conditions resulting in hypoxia or hypercarbia are associated with a poor outcome. Thus, the mainstays of therapy and management continue to be inpatient care in a tertiary care center with experienced providers, with continuous administration of oxygen, use of pulmonary vasodilators, avoidance of hypotension and anemia, and limited use of operative deliveries.[8,63–68]

With respect to pulmonary vasodilators, recent success with inhaled nitric oxide (iNO) alongside prostacyclin and its analogs has been observed.[63–68] Administration of iNO via facemask or nasal cannula has been shown to be effective when estimated final alveolar concentrations of 5–40 p.p.m. are reached; great care is taken to avoid accumulation of toxic nitrogen dioxide with the use of continuous monitoring of tidal iNO concentrations using electrochemical monitors (similar to those found in neonatal intensive care unit settings). Given a risk of both maternal and fetal methemoglobinemia, it is also recommended that concentrations should be measured hourly during administration with a goal of < 5 g/dL; in the fetus, postnatal monitoring through the first 48 hours of life is also recommended.[66–68] High concentrations of methemoglobin can be treated with methylene blue at 2 mg/kg i.v.[63] Prostacylin, a naturally occurring prostaglandin (PGI_2), is a potent vasodilator and inhibitor of platelet aggregation. Infusions of 1–10 ng/kg/min effectively reduce pulmonary vascular resistance, but at the risk of decreasing right ventricular preload. However, its synthetic analog (iloprost) has a minimal effect on systemic vascular resistance, and has been used successfully to reduce pulmonary artery pressures either alone or in combination with iNO.[64–68] When administered with nebulizers, the systemic effect is minimized; iloprost is administered diluted in 0.9% NaCl (20 μg/2 mL up to six times daily), and prostacylin at 60 μg/h.[64,65]

In cyanotic heart disease of any etiology, fetal outcome correlates well with maternal hematocrit; successful pregnancy is unlikely with an initial hemoglobin > 20 g/dL.[69,70] Thus, we recommend judicious iron therapy and packed red blood cell transfusion to maintain a hematocrit above 24–30 g%.[8] Maternal P_aO_2 should be maintained with exogenous oxygen at a level of 70 mmHg or higher.[67–69] In addition, third-trimester fetal surveillance with antepartum testing is necessitated as at least 30% of the fetuses are growth restricted,[55,70] and pregnancy interruption due to fetal deterioration is common.[70]

The issue of pulmonary artery catheterization is controversial. Among some patients with moderate to severe pulmonary hypertension from interatrial shunts, a pulmonary artery catheter will provide useful information.[8,60] However, we share the concern of other authors that, among those with interventricular shunts, catheter placement is associated with a high rate of complications, including arrythmias, embolization, and pulmonary artery rupture.[66] In instances in which pulmonary artery catheterization may be of benefit, simultaneous cardiac imaging with ultrasound may be helpful in catheter placement. If the possibility of right-to-left shunting exists, balloon inflation with carbon dioxide is preferable to that with air in an effort to avoid systemic air embolus associated with the rare occurrence of balloon rupture.

In consideration of catheter placement, it is of note that, during labor, uterine contractions are associated with a decrease in the ratio of pulmonary to systemic blood flow.[71–73] Pulmonary artery catheterization and serial arterial blood gas determinations thus theoretically allow the clinician to detect and treat early changes in cardiac output, pulmonary artery pressure, and shunt fraction. As point of reference, central hemodynamic assessment references are provided in Table 39.6.[6] We have used a fiberoptic pulmonary artery catheter in conjunction with an oximeter to detect early changes in mixed venous oxygen saturation during the successful intrapartum management of patients with pulmonary hypertension. Because the primary concern in such patients is the avoidance of hypotension, any attempt at preload reduction (i.e., diuresis) must be undertaken with great caution, even in the face of initial fluid overload. We prefer to manage such patients on

Table 39.6 Reference values with central hemodynamic assessment.

Parameter	Nonpregnant	Pregnant
Cardiac output (L/min)	4.3	6.2
Heart rate (b.p.m.)	71	83
Pulmonary vascular resistance (dyne/cm/s[5])	119	78
Systemic vascular resistance (dyne/cm/s[5])	1530	1210
Colloid oncotic pressure (mmHg)	21	18
Mean arterial pressure (mmHg)	86	90
Pulmonary capillary wedge pressure (mmHg)	6.3	7.5
Central venous pressure (mmHg)	3.7	3.6

Values are derived from 10 selected patients at 36–38 weeks' gestation, and again at 11–13 weeks postpartum with arterial lines and Swan–Ganz catheters to characterize central hemodynamic values of pregnancy.[6]

the "wet" side (wedge pressure range of 16–18 mmHg), maintaining a preload margin of safety against unexpected blood loss with an a priori acknowledged risk of pulmonary edema. Because of the increased risk of significant blood loss and hypotension associated with operative delivery, Cesarean section should be reserved for standard obstetric indications. Similarly, midforceps delivery is not warranted to shorten the second stage, but should be reserved for obstetric indications only.

If surgery is necessary, meticulous attention to hemostasis and surgical technique with an experienced surgical team minimizes the risk of blood loss, hypotension, and death in these patients. Despite expert management, a substantial risk of maternal mortality remains during labor and delivery. Laparoscopic tubal ligation under local anesthesia has also been described in a group of women with various types of cyanotic cardiac disease.[74]

Anesthesia for patients with pulmonary hypertension is controversial. Theoretically, conduction anesthesia, with its accompanying risk of hypotension, should be avoided. Regional techniques for both vaginal (epidural) and Cesarean (spinal) delivery have been described, and successfully used.[63–68,72–74] To summarize this expanding volume of data, with the concomitant use of systemic vasoconstrictors (ephedrine) and pulmonary vasodilators (iNO and prostacylin analogs), the use of epidural or intrathecal morphine sulfate will be theoretically devoid of any overt effect on systemic blood pressure and thus represents one reasonable approach to the anesthetic management of these difficult patients.

Coarctation of the aorta

Coarctation of the aorta accounts for approximately 9% of all congenital cardiac disease.[75] The most common site of coarctation is the origin of the left subclavian artery. Associated anomalies of the aorta and left heart, including VSD and PDA, are common, as are intracranial aneurysms in the circle of Willis.[76] Coarctation is usually asymptomatic. Its presence is suggested by hypertension confined to the upper extremities, although Goodwin[76] cites data suggesting a generalized increase in peripheral resistance throughout the body. Resting cardiac output may be increased, but increased left atrial pressure with exercise suggests occult left ventricular dysfunction. Aneurysms may also develop below the coarctation, or involve the intercostal arteries, and may lead to rupture. In addition, ruptures without prior aneurysm formation have been reported.[75,76]

More than 400 patients with coarctation have been reported during pregnancy, with maternal mortality ranging from none to 17%.[46,75,76] Half the fatalities occur during the first pregnancy. In a review of 200 pregnant women with coarctation of the aorta before 1940, Mendelson[77] reported 14 maternal deaths and recommended routine abortion and sterilization of these patients.[77] Deaths in this series were from aortic dissection and rupture, congestive heart failure, cerebrovascular accidents, and bacterial endocarditis. Six of the 14 deaths occurred in women with associated lesions. In contrast to this historical dismal prognosis, an initial series by Deal and Wooley[75] in 1973 reported 83 pregnancies in 23 women with uncomplicated coarctation of the aorta. All were NYHA class I or II before pregnancy. In these women, there were no maternal deaths or permanent cardiovascular complications. In a recent series, these findings were confirmed, which suggest that patients with coarctation of the aorta uncomplicated by aneurysmal dilation or associated cardiac lesions who enter pregnancy as class I or II have a good prognosis and a minimal risk of complications or death.[21,22] Even if uncorrected, uncomplicated coarctation carries with it a risk of maternal mortality of only 3–4%.[22] In the presence of aortic or intervertebral aneurysm, known aneurysm of the circle of Willis, or associated cardiac lesions, however, the risk of death may approach 15%; therefore, pregnancy termination must be strongly considered.[8]

Tetralogy of Fallot

Tetralogy of Fallot encompasses the cyanotic complex of VSD, overriding aorta, right ventricular hypertrophy, and pulmonary stenosis. Most cases of tetralogy of Fallot are corrected during infancy or childhood; the vast majority of women may be assumed to have undergone repair in order to survive to reproductive age. Several published reports attest to the relatively good outcome of pregnancy in patients with corrected tetralogy of Fallot.[7,78–81] In a review of 55 pregnancies in 46 patients, there were no maternal deaths among nine patients with correction before pregnancy. However, in patients with an uncorrected lesion, maternal mortality ranges from 4% to 15%, with a 30% fetal mortality as a result of hypoxia.[7,80] In patients with uncorrected VSD, the decline in systematic vascular resistance that accompanies pregnancy can lead to worsening of the right- to-left shunt.[7] This condition can be aggravated further by systemic hypotension as a result of peripartum blood loss. A poor prognosis has been related to prepregnancy hematocrit exceeding 65%, history of syncope or congestive failure, electrocardiographic evidence of right ventricular strain, cardiomegaly, right ventricular pressure in excess of 120 mmHg, and peripheral oxygen saturation of less than 80%.

Pulmonic stenosis

Pulmonic stenosis is a common congenital defect. Although obstruction can be valvular, supravalvular, or subvalvular, the degree of obstruction, rather than its site, is the principal determinant of clinical performance. A transvalvular pressure gradient exceeding 80 mmHg is considered severe and mandates surgical correction.[8] A compilation (totaling 106 pregnancies) of three series of patients with pulmonic stenosis revealed no maternal deaths.[45–47] With severe stenosis, right heart failure can occur; fortunately, this is usually less severe clinically than the left heart failure associated with mitral or aortic valve lesions. Pulmonic stenosis in association with cyanotic congenital lesions has a worse prognosis.

Ebstein's anomaly

Ebstein's anomaly accounts for a rare 1% of all congenital cardiac disease.[82–86] This anomaly consists of apical displacement of the tricuspid valve with secondary tricuspid regurgitation and enlargement of both right atrium and ventricle. In a review of 111 pregnancies in 44 women, no serious maternal complications were noted. Seventy-six percent of pregnancies ended in live births, although there was a 6% incidence of congenital heart disease in the offspring of these women.[86]

Acquired cardiac lesions

By way of introduction, it is often helpful to keep a number of commonly accepted considerations regarding acquired valvular lesions in mind. First, regurgitant lesions are generally better tolerated in pregnancy than stenotic lesions due to pregnancy-associated systemic vascular resistance improving forward flow, and thus limiting the effects of regurgitation (assuming an absence of left ventricular dysfunction). However, in stenotic lesions, increased cardiac output and tachycardia result in an elevation in left atrial pressure (i.e., mitral stenosis) and thus increased incidence of atrial fibrillation and high-output cardiac failure. Second, maternal and fetal risks of acquired cardiac lesions in pregnancy generally vary with the functional classification at pregnancy onset and term. Thus, the common collective wisdom is that women with functional class I or II heart disease have a favorable prognosis in pregnancy (with the notable exception of mitral stenosis; Table 39.3). Moreover, patients who reach term as class I or II usually tolerate properly managed labor without invasive monitoring. Third, because of increasing cardiovascular demand in the high-output state, functional status will deteriorate during pregnancy among functional class II, III, and IV patients.[5–7] This is evidenced by the fact that nearly half of all women with acquired valvular lesions will first develop heart failure and pulmonary edema in their third trimester of pregnancy.[1–3,5]

Acquired valvular lesions are commonly rheumatic in origin, although endocarditis secondary to intravenous drug use ought to be considered as an underlying etiology of acquired right heart lesions. During pregnancy, maternal morbidity and mortality with rheumatic lesions results from congestive failure or arrhythmias with a final common sequelae of pulmonary edema, embolic event, or fatal dysrhythmia. Indeed, pulmonary edema is the leading cause of death in rheumatic heart disease patients during pregnancy.[1,4–6] Szekely and colleagues[5] found the risk of pulmonary edema in pregnant patients with rheumatic heart disease to rise with increasing age and with increasing length of gestation. The onset of atrial fibrillation during pregnancy carries with it a higher risk of right and left ventricular failure (63%) than fibrillation with onset before gestation. In addition, the risk of systemic embolization after the onset of atrial fibrillation during pregnancy may exceed that associated with onset in the nonpregnant state.[5] In counseling the patient with severe rheumatic cardiac disease on the advisability of initiating or continuing pregnancy, the physician must also consider the long-term prognosis of the underlying disease. For up to 44 years, Chesley[87] followed 134 women who had functionally severe rheumatic heart disease and who had completed pregnancy. He reported a mortality of 6.3% per year but concluded that, in patients who survived the gestation, maternal life expectancy was not shortened by pregnancy. These data would therefore suggest that, in the absence of an acute morbid event, pregnancy has no long-term sequelae for patients who survive the pregnancy.[62,87]

Pulmonic and tricuspid lesions

Physiologic valvular regurgitation is common during pregnancy, especially with right-sided valves, and the degree of regurgitation progresses as pregnancy advances.[88] Isolated right-sided valvular lesions of rheumatic origin are uncommon; however, such lesions are seen with increased frequency in intravenous drug abusers, in whom they are secondary to valvular endocarditis. For the reasons reviewed above, pregnancy-associated hypervolemia is far less likely to be symptomatic with right-sided lesions than with those involving the mitral or aortic valves. In a review of 77 maternal cardiac deaths, Hibbard[47] reported none associated with isolated right-sided lesions. In several recent reviews, congestive heart failure has been noted to occur in less than 2% of women with pulmonic stenosis.[87–89] A successful pregnancy has been reported after Fontan repair of congenital tricuspid atresia.[89] Even after complete tricuspid valvectomy for endocarditis, subsequent pregnancy, labor, and delivery are generally well tolerated. Given the propensity toward pulmonary edema in the puerperium,[91] cautious fluid administration is the mainstay of labor and delivery management in patients with right-sided lesions.[87–91] In general, invasive hemodynamic monitoring during labor and delivery is not necessary.

Mitral stenosis

Mitral stenosis is the most common rheumatic valvular lesion encountered during pregnancy.[59] It can occur as an isolated lesion or in conjunction with aortic or right-sided lesions. Severe mitral stenosis (valve area < $1.5\,cm^2$) carries a maternal mortality approximated at 5%.[11] Secondary to a severe stenosis, ventricular diastolic filling obstruction yields elevated left atrial pressure with a relatively fixed cardiac output. Marked increases in cardiac output accompany normal pregnancy, labor, and delivery. When the pregnant patient is unable to accommodate volume fluctuations, right-sided heart failure results in pulmonary edema.

The ability to accommodate an increased cardiac output in patients with mitral stenosis depends largely on two factors.[59] First, these patients depend on adequate diastolic filling time. However, in instances of stenotic mitral lesions, a rapid and dramatic fall in cardiac output and blood pressure in response to tachycardia will compromise this tenuous filling time. Given that an increase in heart rate of approximately 10 b.p.m. is common in normal pregnancy, labor, and delivery, consideration ought to be given to oral beta-blocker therapy for any patient with severe mitral stenosis who enters labor with even a mild tachycardia. Control of acute-onset tachycardia with an intravenous beta-blocking agent may be employed at the following dosages: propranolol 1 mg i.v. every 2 min; metoprolol 5 mg i.v. over 5 min, repeated in 10 min; esmolol drip at 500 μg/kg i.v. over 1 min with an infusion rate of 50–200 μg/kg/min; or labetalol 20–40 mg i.v. followed by 20–80 mg i.v. every 10 min to a maximum dose of 180 mg.

A second important consideration in patients with mitral stenosis centers on left ventricular preload. In the presence of mitral stenosis, pulmonary capillary wedge pressure fails to accurately reflect left ventricular filling pressures. Such patients often require high-normal or elevated pulmonary capillary wedge pressure to maintain adequate ventricular filling pressure and cardiac output. Any preload manipulation (i.e., diuresis) must therefore be undertaken with extreme caution and careful attention to the maintenance of cardiac output. However, it has long been recognized that potentially dangerous intrapartum fluctuations in cardiac output can be minimized by using epidural anesthesia;[92] however, the most hazardous time for these women appears to be the immediate postpartum period. Such patients often enter the postpartum period already operating at maximum cardiac output and cannot accommodate the volume shifts that follow delivery. In our series of patients with severe mitral stenosis, we found that a postpartum rise in wedge pressure of up to 16 mmHg could be expected in the immediate postpartum period.[60] Because frank pulmonary edema generally does not occur with wedge pressures of less than 28–30 mmHg,[93] it follows that the optimal predelivery wedge pressure for such patients is 14 mmHg or lower, as indicated by pulmonary artery catheterization.[60] Such a preload may be approached by cautious intrapartum diuresis with careful attention to the maintenance of adequate cardiac output (Table 39.6). Active diuresis is not always necessary in patients who enter with evidence of only mild fluid overload. In such patients, simple fluid restriction alongside sensible and insensible fluid losses endogenous to labor can result in a significant fall in wedge pressure before delivery.

In a patient with hemodynamically significant mitral stenosis, many of the same management considerations apply as those previously discussed under the section dealing with Eisenmenger's syndrome and pulmonary hypertension. Bedrest with the administration of oxygen and pulmonary vasodilators to maintain the therapeutic goal of a $P\text{O}_2$ of greater than 70 mmHg are essential. As previously discussed, pulmonary artery catheterization allows the hemodynamic condition to be optimized before the stress of labor. Because pulmonary edema is the major concern in these patients, we recommend incremental diuresis be carried out to approach a wedge pressure of 12–14 mmHg. Such manipulation, however, must be performed with careful attention to maintaining cardiac output; patients with mitral stenosis cannot necessarily tolerate a normal wedge pressure. Thus, wedge pressures of 20 mmHg or more may be necessary to maintain cardiac output and blood pressure.[8,60] If the pulse rises to more than 100 b.p.m., we recommend the administration of a beta-blocking agent (note the above discussion regarding dosing) to avoid tachycardia and subsequent falls in cardiac output.

Previous recommendations for delivery in patients with cardiac disease have included the liberal use of midforceps to shorten the second stage of labor. In cases of severe disease, Cesarean section with general anesthesia has also been advocated as the preferred mode of delivery. With the aggressive and attentive management scheme presented, we have found that spontaneous vaginal delivery is generally safe and preferable, even in patients with severe disease and pulmonary hypertension.

Mitral insufficiency

Hemodynamically significant mitral insufficiency is usually rheumatic in origin and most commonly occurs in conjunction with other valvular lesions. Fortunately, this lesion is tolerated well during pregnancy, and heart failure is unusual. However, these patients are at risk for the development of atrial enlargement and fibrillation. Given an observed increased risk of developing atrial fibrillation in pregnancy,[4,5–8] some authors have recommended prophylactic digitalization during pregnancy for patients with significant mitral insufficiency.[94] That said, the current mainstay of therapy among nonpregnant patients is rate control with anticoagulation;[95] by extrapolation, we would recommend therapeutic interventions with beta-blocking agents and thromboembolic prophylaxis as outlined previously. In Hibbard's review[47] of 28 maternal deaths associated with rheumatic valvular lesions, no patient died with complications of mitral insufficiency unless there was coexisting mitral stenosis.

Congenital mitral valve prolapse is much more common during pregnancy than rheumatic mitral insufficiency and can occur in up to 17% of young healthy women. This condition is generally asymptomatic.[4–9] The midsystolic click and murmur associated with congenital mitral valve prolapse are characteristic. However, the intensity of this murmur, as well as that associated with rheumatic mitral insufficiency, may decrease during pregnancy because of decreased systemic vascular resistance.[96] In the largest reported series to date, outcomes of 42 pregnancies from 25 women demonstrated only a single instance of heart failure, which occurred in the context of severe preeclampsia being managed with intravenous betamimetic therapy and glucocorticoids.[97]

Aortic stenosis

Aortic stenosis is commonly congenital in origin, secondary to a bicuspid aortic valve, and thus represents 5% of all congenital cardiac anomalies.[99,101] In several recent series of pregnancies in women with cardiac disease, no maternal deaths due to aortic stenosis were observed.[1–5,99–101] In contrast to mitral valve stenosis, aortic stenosis generally does not become hemodynamically significant until the orifice has diminished to one-third or less of normal. Indeed, severe aortic stenosis is defined as a peak gradient > 50 mmHg with a valve area < 1 cm^2.[98–102] Given that the major problem experienced by patients with valvular aortic stenosis is maintenance of cardiac output, the relative hypervolemia associated with gestation enables such patients generally to tolerate pregnancy well. This is evidenced by a series of five patients with congenital aortic stenosis demonstrating relatively uncomplicated pregnancies, albeit balloon valvuloplasty was necessary in one case.[98,99] With severe disease, however, a fixed cardiac output limits adequate coronary artery or cerebral perfusion under conditions of physical exertion. Inadequate cardiac perfusion subsequently results in angina, myocardial infarction, syncope, or sudden death. Thus, among patients with severe aortic stenosis, limitation of physical activity may be necessary.

Consistent with these recommendations is the longstanding observation that delivery and pregnancy termination are the intervals in pregnancy with the greatest risk for inadequate cardiac perfusion.[4,5,7,98–102] The maintenance of cardiac output is crucial: any factor leading to diminished venous return results in an increase in the valvular gradient with subsequent diminished cardiac output. Indeed, patients with shunt gradients exceeding 100 mmHg are at greatest risk of hemodynamic decompensation. As such, management considerations for the patient with aortic stenosis are similar to those in women with pulmonary hypertension. Of note, because hypovolemia is of greater concern than pulmonary edema, the wedge pressure should be maintained in the range 14–18 mmHg in order to provide a margin of safety against unexpected peripartum blood loss. Hypotension resulting from blood loss, ganglionic blockade from epidural anesthesia, or supine vena caval occlusion by the pregnant uterus may result in sudden death. Pregnancy termination in the midtrimester may be especially hazardous in this regard and has been reported to carry a mortality of up to 40%.[98] Thus, women who have severe stenosis or symptoms are advised to undergo repair prior to attempting pregnancy in an effort to substantially reduce pregnancy-associated morbidity and mortality.[100–102] That said, there are reports of women with severe aortic stenosis having undergone successful balloon valvoplasty in pregnancy.[103] In contrast, open valve replacement is associated with a 30% fetal mortality risk.[104]

The cardiovascular status of patients with aortic stenosis is occasionally complicated by the frequent coexistence of ischemic heart disease. In these instances, death associated with aortic stenosis may occur secondary to myocardial infarction rather than as a direct complication of the valvular lesion itself.[88,99]

Aortic insufficiency

Aortic insufficiency is most commonly rheumatic in origin and, as such, is associated almost invariably with mitral valve disease. The aortic insufficiency is generally tolerated well during pregnancy because the increased heart rate seen with advancing gestation decreases time for regurgitant flow during diastole. In Hibbard's series[47] of 28 maternal rheumatic cardiac deaths, only one was associated with aortic insufficiency in the absence of concurrent mitral stenosis. If symptomatic, patients respond favorably to diuretics and vasodilators; epidural anesthesia is thus appropriate and reduces the risk of left ventricular failure at delivery.[33,34]

Peripartum cardiomyopathy

Peripartum cardiomyopathy is defined as cardiomyopathy developing in the last month of pregnancy or the first 6 months postpartum in women without previous cardiac disease and after exclusion of other causes of cardiac failure, as shown in Table 39.7.[32,105–107] It is therefore a diagnosis of exclusion that should not be made without a concerted effort to identify valvular, metabolic, infectious, or toxic causes of cardiomyopathy.[108] Much of the current controversy surrounding this condition is the result of many older reports in which these causes of cardiomyopathy were not investigated adequately. Other peripartum complications, such as amniotic fluid embolism, severe preeclampsia, and corticosteroid- or

Table 39.7 Clinical parameters defining peripartum cardiomyopathy.

Parameter	Echocardiographic parameters
Cardiac failure in last month of pregnancy, or within 5 months of delivery No prior history of cardiac disease Absence of clearly identifiable etiology	
Echocardiographic findings of left ventricular dysfunction	EF < 45% and/or M-mode fractional shortening of < 30% End-diastolic dimension > 2.72 cm/m^2

Echocardiographic parameters as described by Hibbard et al.[32]

sympathomimetic-induced pulmonary edema, must also be considered before making the diagnosis of peripartum cardiomyopathy.[108] However, prior to concluding a definitive etiologic role for beta-agonists, it must be considered that sympathomimetic agents may unmask rather than induce an underlying peripartum cardiomyopathy.[109] To date, there remains no definitive proven association between tocolytic therapy and peripartum cardiomyopathy.

The incidence of peripartum cardiomyopathy is estimated at between 1 in 1500 and 1 in 4000 deliveries in the United States.[29–31,110] An incidence as high as 1% has been suggested in women from certain African tribes.[110] However, idiopathic heart failure in these women may be primarily a result of unusual culturally mandated peripartum customs involving excessive sodium intake, as such, and may represent simple fluid overload.[110] In the United States, the peak incidence of peripartum cardiomyopathy occurs in the first postpartum month and appears most frequently among older, multiparous, black females.[105,108,110] Other suggested risk factors include twinning and pregnancy-induced hypertension.[28–31,108–111] In some cases, a familial recurrence pattern has been reported.

The condition is manifest clinically by increasing fatigue, dyspnea, and peripheral or pulmonary edema. As most women in the last trimester of pregnancy manifest these conditions, suspicion for a cardiomyopathy should arise with paroxysmal nocturnal dyspnea, chest pain, nocturnal cough, new regurgitant murmurs, pulmonary crackles, and hepatomegaly.[94] Physical examination reveals classic evidence of congestive heart failure, including elevated jugular venous pressure, rales, and an S3 gallop. Cardiomegaly and pulmonary edema are found on chest radiograph, and the electrocardiogram often demonstrates left ventricular and atrial dilation and diminished ventricular performance, with the reported observance of inverted T waves, Q waves, and nonspecific ST segment changes. In addition, up to 50% of patients with peripartum cardiomyopathy may manifest evidence of pulmonary or systemic embolic phenomena. The diagnosis rests on the echocardiographic finding of new left ventricular systolic dysfunction during a limited period around parturition (Table 39.7).[32] Overall mortality ranges from 25% to 50%.[29–31,108–111]

The histologic picture of peripartum cardiomyopathy involves nonspecific cellular hypertrophy, degeneration, fibrosis, and increased lipid deposition. Although some reports have documented the presence of a diffuse myocarditis, the common collective wisdom suggests that peripartum cardiomyopathy may represent a type of myocarditis arising from an infectious (viral), autoimmune, or idiopathic process.[106,108,111] Its existence as a distinct entity is supported primarily by epidemiologic evidence suggesting that 80% of cases of idiopathic cardiomyopathy in women of childbearing age occur in the peripartum period.[112] Such an epidemiologic distribution could also be attributed to an exacerbation of underlying subclinical cardiac disease related to the hemodynamic changes accompanying normal pregnancy.[29,31] However, as such changes are maximal in the third trimester of pregnancy and return to normal within a few weeks postpartum, such a pattern does not explain the peak incidence of peripartum cardiomyopathy occurring, in most reports, during the second month postpartum. Nevertheless, the diagnosis of peripartum cardiomyopathy remains primarily a diagnosis of exclusion and cannot be made until underlying conditions, including chronic hypertension, valvular disease, and viral myocarditis, have been excluded.

Therapy includes digoxin (dosed to achieve a serum level of 1–2 ng/dL), diuretics (furosemide 20–40 mg orally daily), fluid and sodium restriction (2 L/day and 4 mg/day, maximum, respectively), and prolonged bedrest.[28–33,105–111] In refractory cases or with clear evidence of systolic dysfunction, we employ concomitant afterload reduction with vasodilators (25–100 mg of oral q.i.d. hydralazine being the drug of choice peripartum, with either long-acting nitroglycerin or 5–10 mg of oral daily amlodipine as second-line agents) or use epidural regional analgesia approximating delivery. In general, because of the adverse effects of negative ionotropic agents, other calcium channel blockers ought to be avoided. In recent years, angiotensin-converting enzyme inhibitors (enalapril 5–20 mg oral twice daily) have been the mainstay of treatment postpartum; breastfeeding women should be counseled accordingly. Early endomyocardial biopsy to identify a subgroup of patients who have a histologic picture of inflammatory myocarditis and who may be responsive to immunosuppressive therapy has been suggested.[113] It is of note that patients with poor cardiac function (EF < 40%) are at increased risk of thromboembolism; we recommend anticoagulation with unfractionated heparin (5000–7500 units s.c.) or low-molecular-weight enoxaparin (40 mg s.c. daily) during pregnancy, and consideration of warfarin in the postpartum interval.

When peripartum cardiomyopathy occurs in the last trimester of pregnancy, delivery is indicated. The mode of delivery should be based on obstetric indications. Indeed, the advantages of vaginal delivery over Cesarean section are evident: minimal blood loss, greater hemodynamic stability, and decreased pulmonary and thromboembolic complications. In addition, regional epidural analgesia has the distinct advantage of reducing both preload and afterload, as well as minimizing fluctuations in cardiac output associated with labor.[94] In instances of obstetrically indicated Cesarean delivery, we and others[94] recommend careful monitoring of fluid balance with central monitoring in an effort to clearly define and monitor the central venous pressure.

A notable feature of peripartum cardiomyopathy is its tendency to recur with subsequent pregnancies. Several reports have suggested that the prognosis for future pregnancies is related to heart size. Patients whose cardiac size returned to normal within 6–12 months had an 11–14% mortality in subsequent pregnancies; patients with persistent cardiomegaly had a 40–80% mortality.[28–31] Recently, persistent decreased contractile reserve has been demonstrated in women who have recovered from peripartum cardiomyopathy.[30,107] Thus, pregnancy is contraindicated in all patients with persistent cardiomegaly accompanying left ventricular dysfunction; the 11–14% risk of maternal mortality with subsequent pregnancy seen in patients with normal heart size would seem, in most cases, to be unacceptable as well.

Idiopathic hypertrophic subaortic stenosis

Idiopathic hypertrophic subaortic stenosis (IHSS) or hypertrophic cardiomyopathy (HCM) is an autosomal dominant condition with variable penetrance, generally characterized by left ventricular hypertrophy with reduced left ventricular size and compliance. IHSS manifests clinically in the second or third decade of life; thus, its sentinel presentation is likely to occur during pregnancy. Detailed physical and echocardiographic diagnostic criteria have been described elsewhere.[113,114] IHSS is unique among the hypertrophies in that the left ventricular hypertrophy involves the septum to a greater extent than the free wall, resulting in obstruction to left ventricular outflow and secondary mitral regurgitation, the two principal hemodynamic concerns of the clinician.[113–116] Although the increased blood volume associated with normal pregnancy should enhance left ventricular filling and improve hemodynamic performance, this positive effect of pregnancy is countereffected by the fall in arterial pressure and vena caval obstruction common in the last trimester of pregnancy. In addition, tachycardia resulting from pain in labor and Valsalva with active maternal efforts in the second stage of labor diminish left ventricular filling and aggravate the relative outflow obstruction. Thus, it may be generally surmised that reduction of preload and afterload in IHSS patients results in an increase in the outflow gradient with a concomitant reduction in left ventricular filling. As such, regional analgesia is relatively contraindicated, although reports of its use are observed.[115]

The keys to successful management of the peripartum period in patients with IHSS involve avoidance of hypotension (resulting from conduction anesthesia or blood loss), control of tachycardia, conduction of labor in the left lateral recumbent position, and avoidance of maternal Valsalva with the use of forceps or vacuum. As with most other cardiac diseases, Cesarean section of IHSS patients should be reserved for obstetric indications only.

Despite the potential theoretical risks, maternal and fetal outcome in IHSS patients is generally good. In a report of 54 pregnancies in 23 patients with IHSS, no maternal or neonatal deaths occurred.[114] Although beta-blocking agents were once used routinely in patients with IHSS, they are currently reserved for patients with angina, recurrent supraventricular tachycardia, or occasional beta-blocker-responsive arrhythmias. In these patients, we recommend antibiotic prophylaxis against subacute bacterial endocarditis.

Marfan syndrome

Marfan syndrome is an autosomal dominant disorder resulting from multiple lineage-specific mutations in the fibrillin gene on chromosome 15; the weakness results in skeletal, ocular, and cardiovascular abnormalities. Among the cardiovascular manifestations, mitral valve prolapse, mitral regurgitation, aortic insufficiency, and aortic root dilation with a marked propensity toward aortic root dissection are common. The most common cause of death among women under 40 years of age with Marfan syndrome is an aortic complication, and 50% of aortic aneurysm ruptures in these women occur during pregnancy.[77] Rupture of splenic artery aneurysms also occurs more frequently during pregnancy.[77] In addition, 60% of patients with Marfan syndrome have associated mitral or aortic regurgitation.[117] Thus, patients are followed prior to and during pregnancy for aortic root diameter, as it may predict the risk of aortic dissection or rupture. Generally, the longstanding recommendation for replacement of the ascending aorta in asymptomatic patients is recommended when the root diameter exceeds 5.5 cm.[117]

Although some authors believe that pregnancy is contraindicated in any woman with documented Marfan syndrome, prognosis is best individualized and should be based on echocardiographic and computed tomography (CT) assessment of aortic root diameter and postvalvular dilation.[23–25,117] It is important to note that enlargement of the aortic root is not demonstrable by chest radiograph until dilation has become pronounced.[117] Women with an abnormal aortic valve or aortic dilation may have up to a 50% pregnancy-associated mortality; women without these changes and with an aortic root diameter of less than 40 mm have a mortality of less than 5%.[23–25] Even in patients meeting these echocardiographic criteria, however, special attention must be given to signs or symptoms of aortic dissection because even serial echocardiographic assessment is not invariably predictive of complications.[118–120] In counseling women with Marfan syndrome, the genetics of this condition and the shortened maternal lifespan must be considered, in addition to the immediate maternal risk.[23–25]

Gestational management hinges on aggressive control of hypertension with beta-blocker therapy; utilization of labetalol (an alpha- and beta-antagonist) has the added advantage of controlling mean arterial blood pressure in a rapid fashion, alongside its ability to decrease pulsatile pressure on the aorta.[119] In instances of aortic root dilation approximating 5 cm, we and others[33,120] would recommend Cesarean delivery to minimize episodic hypertension that may precipitate aortic root dissection. If Cesarean section is performed, retention sutures should be used because of generalized connective tissue weakness.

It is worthy of mention that type IV Ehlers–Danlos syndrome similarly bears an equivalent risk of aortic root dissection and should be managed accordingly.[120]

Myocardial infarction

Coronary artery disease is uncommon in women of reproductive age; therefore, myocardial infarction in conjunction with pregnancy is rare and occurs in less that 1:10 000 pregnancies.[121] In a review of 68 reported cases, myocardial infarction during pregnancy was associated with a 35% mortality rate.[122] Only 13% of patients were known to have had coronary artery disease before pregnancy. Two-thirds of the women suffered infarction in the third trimester; mortality for these women was 45%, compared with 23% in those suffering infarction in the first or second trimesters. Thus, it appears that the increased hemodynamic burden imposed on the maternal cardiovascular system in late pregnancy may unmask latent coronary artery disease in some women and worsen the prognosis for patients suffering infarction.[27] Fetuses from surviving women appear to have an increased risk of spontaneous abortion and unexplained stillbirth.

Women with class H diabetes mellitus face risks beyond those imposed by their cardiac disease alone. Although successful pregnancy outcome may occur, maternal and fetal risks are considerable. Such considerations, as well as the anticipated shortened lifespan of these patients, make special counseling of such women of major importance.[124]

In the largest series published to date, Roth and Elkayam[123] reviewed 125 cases of myocardial infarction during pregnancy or within 3 months of delivery; 78 occurred antepartum, 17 peripartum, and 30 postpartum. Among these cases, 43% were attributed to coronary atherosclerosis, with coronary thrombus without atherosclerosis in 21%, coronary artery dissection in 16%, and acute or coronary aneurysm in 4%. Maternal mortality in this series was 21%, and fetal mortality was 13%. Mode of delivery was not associated with maternal mortality.

Antepartum care of women with prior myocardial infarction centers on efforts to minimize myocardial oxygen demands. Diagnostic radionuclide cardiac imaging during pregnancy results in a fetal dose of no more than 0.8 rad and thus does not carry the potential for teratogenesis.[62] If cardiac catheterization becomes necessary, the simultaneous use of contrast echocardiography may reduce the need for cineangiography and thus reduce radiation exposure to the fetus.[125] In women with angina, nitrates have been used without adverse fetal effects. Delivery within 2 weeks of infarction is associated with increased mortality; therefore, if possible, attempts should be made to allow adequate convalescence before delivery. If the cervix is favorable, cautious induction under controlled circumstances after a period of hemodynamic stabilization is optimal. Labor in the lateral recumbent position, the administration of oxygen, pain relief with epidural anesthesia, and shortening of the second stage to reduce myocardial oxygen demands with assisted vaginal delivery are important management considerations; Cesarean delivery is reserved for obstetric indications. Having six or more pregnancies has been associated with a small but significant increase in the risk of subsequent coronary artery disease.[126]

Anticoagulation

Anticoagulation in the patient with an artificial heart valve or atrial fibrillation during pregnancy is controversial and has been the focus of many recent and comprehensive reviews.[127–131] The key issue involves the lack of consensus on an ideal agent for anticoagulation during pregnancy.

Warfarin (coumadin) is relatively contraindicated at all stages of gestation because of its association with fetal warfarin syndrome (warfarin embryopathy, characterized by nasal hypoplasia and stippled epiphyses) in weeks 6–12, and because of its theoretical relationship to fetal intracranial hemorrhage and secondary brain scarring at later stages. In addition, there are reports suggesting that central nervous system and ocular abnormalities may be associated with warfarin exposure during the second and third trimesters.[127–131] Several studies have suggested that the presumed risk of warfarin embryopathy beyond the first trimester has been overstated; one deficiency in these studies is a lack of detailed neonatal neurologic evaluation and follow-up.[132] Thus, although the risk of embryopathy when warfarin derivatives are taken between weeks 6 and 9 is historically estimated to be between 8% and 30%, recent reports suggest an anomaly rate of 3.9% of all pregnancies and 7.4% of live births,[128] with prospective studies supporting a rate of 10.2%;[131] the frequency of intracranial hemorrhage in fetuses whose mothers receive warfarin after the first trimester is unknown. Several series from outside the United States have reported on the use of warfarin in pregnant patients with prosthetic valves, and demonstrated a 2% incidence of embryopathy.[135] Thus, while one can debate the precise risk of embryopathy based on prospective or retrospective acquired data, this risk unequivocally exists.

Balancing the fetal risks with warfarin therapy are the maternal risks with heparin and low-molecular-weight heparin therapy. In sum of a large body of data, there are now multiple series comparing maternal thromboembolic events in patients receiving unfractionated heparin, which demonstrate a two- to fourfold increased risk of treatment failure with maternal mortality from thrombosed valves.[127–131] However, as noted by Nassar et al.,[132] the risk of valve thrombosis relies on many factors, including type, number, and position of the valve with higher risk in mitral valves, arrythmias, previous thrombosis, and adequacy of anticoagulation. In addition, it is suggested that bileaflet valves (St Jude valves) may actually have a lowered thrombogenic potential, albeit one study did not support such findings.[136]

Reported and hypothesized treatment failures with unfractionated heparin led both cardiologists and obstetricians to employ low-molecular-weight heparin (LMWH) for prosthetic valve prophylaxis. However, this too is fraught with

Table 39.8 Treatment approaches for women with mechanical heart valves.

Approach	Dosing regimen	Therapeutic parameters
Adjusted-dose unfractionated heparin throughout pregnancy	Adjusted dosage s.c. every 12h	Maintain midinterval aPTT at a minimum of twice control OR anti-factor Xa heparin level of 0.3U/ml
Adjusted-dose LMWH throughout pregnancy	Adjusted dosage s.c. every 12h	Maintain peak anti-factor Xa heparin levels (4h post injection) > 0.8U/mL
Heparin or LMWH in adjusted dose (as above) through the 12th week of gestation, then warfarin until 36 weeks, followed by reinitiation of adjusted-dose heparin or LMWH (as above)	As above, with warfarin after 12 weeks daily	Target INR 2.5–3.5 with warfarin therapy Otherwise as above

INR, international normalized ratio; aPTT, activated partial thromboplastin time.

controversy and limitations. Both the Food and Drug Administration (FDA) and the American College of Obstetricians and Gynecologists (ACOG) warn against the use of enoxaparin and other LMWHs during pregnancy, citing risk of thrombosis.[138] Understandably, many clinicians were thereafter frustrated with the elimination of potentially acceptable therapeutic options. This frustration prompted a flurry of reports, most notably the Report and Recommendations of the Anticoagulation in Prosthetic Valves and Pregnancy Consensus Report (APPCR) Panel and Scientific Roundtable.[127] This panel of experts ultimately came to the consensus opinion that "There is a substantial body of published, peer-reviewed, trial- and cohort study-based evidence, institutional data sets, and expert clinical experience/opinion to support safe and effective use of enoxaparin for anticoagulation management of non-pregnant patients with prosthetic mechanical heart valves. There are insufficient data to reliably predict, compare clinical outcomes, or to confirm the safety or effectiveness of enoxaparin, UFH, or warfarin in pregnant patients with mechanical heart valves. In light of the predicatable, published, and problematic aspects encountered with each of the aforementioned anticoagulants currently available in the armamentarium for pregnant patients with mechanical valves, the Panel felt strongly that while concerns about efficacy and safety were justified for all agents (i.e., warfarin, heparin, and LMWH [enoxaparin]), the available literature and index cases did not support selective, asymmetrical warning language in the case of enoxaparin."[127]

In essence, a choice between fetal and maternal risks must be made, and neither choice is considered ideal. That said, two approaches may be termed "acceptable."[127–131,139] One involves substitution of heparin or enoxaparin for warfarin from the time pregnancy is diagnosed until 12 weeks' gestation, followed by warfarin until 32 weeks, at which time heparin or enoxaparin is reinstituted until delivery. The second approach involves using adjusted-dose subcutaneous heparin or enoxaparin throughout pregnancy. We recommend dosage regimens as outlined in Table 39.8, with acknowledgment of the paucity of data supporting these recommendations. Given the controversies outlined above, with their ensuing medicolegal implications, the patient must be involved in this choice and thoroughly informed of the risks and benefits of either approach.

Patients with bioprosthetic or xenograft valves are not usually treated with anticoagulants during pregnancy. This fact makes the bioprosthetic valve the ideal choice of prosthesis for young women of childbearing age.[139] Patients with a bioprosthetic valve who are in atrial fibrillation or have evidence of thromboembolism, however, should be anticoagulated and rate controlled accordingly.[95]

Cardiovascular surgery

There are numerous reports of cardiovascular surgery during pregnancy, most of which are favorable; they include successful correction of most types of congenital and acquired cardiac disease (as reviewed above). Early reports of closed mitral valve commissurotomy during pregnancy were also favorable and indicated a maternal death rate of 1–2% and perinatal loss in the region of 10%.[4,8] This procedure has been replaced by open valvuloplasty with equally good results.

Initial reports of cardiopulmonary bypass during pregnancy were not nearly as favorable, indicating a fetal wastage of up to 33%.[140,141] Initiation of cardiopulmonary bypass is generally followed by fetal bradycardia, which may be correctable by high flow rates.[142] With the use of continuous electronic fetal heart rate monitoring, flow rate can be adjusted to avoid or correct fetal hypoperfusion and bradycardia, thus reducing fetal mortality to less than 10%. High-flow/high-pressure normothermic perfusion and continuous electronic fetal heart rate monitoring appear to be optimal for the fetus.[8] Maternal mortality is highly dependent on the specific nature of the procedure being performed and does not appear to be increased significantly by pregnancy. Successful pregnancy after heart transplantation has been reported. Principles of counseling and management for these complex patients have been summarized previously.[8]

Key points

1 Normal physiologic changes of pregnancy may mimic cardiac disease.

2 Despite (1), suspected cardiovascular abnormalities must be worked up aggressively in pregnancy.

3 Most maternal deaths in developed countries due to cardiac disease are secondary to cardiomyopathy, ischemic heart disease, endocarditis, pulmonary hypertension, and arrythmia.

4 Women with cardiac disease should seek preconception counseling.

5 Women with pulmonary hypertension, complicated or unrepaired aortic coarctation, and Marfan syndrome with a dilated aortic root should be counseled toward pregnancy termination.

6 Women with ischemic cardiac disease or prior peripartum cardiomyopathy should also be encouraged to consider pregnancy termination.

7 No method of anticoagulation is ideal or risk free in patients with mechanical valves during pregnancy.

8 Any woman with suspected pulmonary hypertension must have a definitive diagnosis as soon as possible, usually via right heart catheterization.

9 With the exception of conditions listed in (5) and (6) above, prepregnancy NYHA classification is prognostic of how the woman will tolerate pregnancy.

10 In women with cyanotic heart disease, fetal deterioration is a very common cause of early delivery.

11 Most valvular insufficiency is tolerated well during pregnancy.

12 In patients with significant mitral stenosis, the risks of pulmonary edema due to peripartum volume shifts must be weighed against the risks of falling cardiac output if active diuresis is considered during labor.

13 Patients with pulmonary hypertension incur intrapartum risk primarily from conditions resulting in hypovolemia or reduced venous return to the heart.

14 Patients with obstructive congenital cardiac disease have up to a 10% risk of a cardiac defect in their fetus.

15 The postpartum period is the time of greatest risk of pulmonary edema in women with mitral stenosis.

16 The major hemodynamic considerations complicating pregnancy in women with heart disease are increased intravascular volume, decreased systemic vascular resistance, increased tendency for pathologic clot formation, and hemodynamic fluctuations during the peripartum period.

17 The need for endocarditis prophylaxis during uncomplicated vaginal delivery in women with structural heart disease is controversial, but is recommended by many authorities.

18 Even in most forms of severe cardiac disease, forceps or vacuum delivery should be reserved for standard obstetric indications.

19 With proper management, many women with cardiac disease can expect successful pregnancy.

20 Management of significant cardiac disease in pregnancy should be a team effort, involving obstetrics, cardiology, maternal–fetal medicine, and anesthesia specialists.

References

1 deSwiet M. Cardiac disease. In: Lewis G, Drife J, eds. *Why mothers die 1997–1999. The confidential enquiries into maternal deaths in the United Kingdom*. London: Royal College of Obstetricians and Gynaecologists; 2001: 153.

2 Chang J, Elam-Evans LD, Berg CJ, et al. Pregnancy related mortality surveillance, United States, 1991–1999. *Morbidity Mortality Weekly Rep* 2003;52:1.

3 Jacob S, Bloebaum L, Shah G, et al. Maternal mortality in Utah. *Obstet Gynecol* 1998;91:187.

4 McFaul PB, Dornan JC, Lamki H, et al. Pregnancy complicated by maternal heart disease: a review of 519 women. *Br J Obstet Gynaecol* 1988;95:861.

5 Szekely P, Turner R, Snaith L. Pregnancy and the changing pattern of rheumatic heart disease. *Br Heart J* 1973;35: 1293.

6 Clark SL, Cotton DB, Lee W, et al. Central hemodynamic assessment of normal term pregnancy. *Am J Obstet Gynecol* 1989;161: 1439.

7 Shime J, Mocarski EJM, Hastings D, et al. Congenital heart disease in pregnancy: short- and long-term implications. *Am J Obstet Gynecol* 1987;156:313.

8 Clark SL. Structural cardiac disease in pregnancy. In: Clark SL, Cotton DB, Phelan JP, eds. *Critical care obstetrics*, 3rd edn. Boston: Blackwell Scientific, 1997.

9 Avila WS, Rossi EG, Ramires JA, et al. Pregnancy in patients with heart disease: experience with 1,000 cases. *Clin Cardiol* 2003;26:135.

10 Ullery JC. Management of pregnancy complicated by heart disease. *Am J Obstet Gynecol* 1954;67:834.

11 Siu SC, Sermer M, Colman JM, et al. Prospective multicenter study of pregnancy outcomes in women with heart disease. *Circulation* 2001;104:515.

12 Ramsey PS, Ramin KD, Ramin SM. Cardiac disease in pregnancy. *Am J Perinatol* 2001;18:245.

13 Sawhney H, Aggarwal N, Suri V, et al. Maternal and perinatal outcome in rheumatic heart disease. *Int J Gynaecol Obstet* 2003;80:9.

14 Silversides CK, Colman JM, Sermer M, et al. Cardiac risk in pregnant women with rheumatic mitral stenosis. *Am J Cardiol* 2003;91:1382.

15 vanCoeverden de Groot HA. Maternal mortality in Cape Town, 1978–83. *S Afr Med J* 1986;69:797.

16 Schoon MF, Bam RH, Wolmarans L. Cardiac disease during pregnancy – a Free State perspective on maternal morbidity and mortality. *S Afr Med J* 1997;87:19.

17 Naidoo DP, Desai DK, Moodley J. Maternal deaths due to preexisting cardiac disease. *Cardiovasc J S Afr* 2002;13:17.

18 Murphy DJ, Charlett P. Cohort study of near-miss maternal mortality and subsequent reproductive outcome. *Eur J Obstet Gynecol Reprod Biol* 2002;102:173.

19 Loverro G, Pansini V, Greco P, et al. Indications and outcome for intensive care unit admission during puerperium. *Arch Gynecol Obstet* 2001;265:195.

20 Hameed A, Karaalp IS, Tummala PP, et al. The effect of valvular heart disease on maternal and fetal outcome of pregnancy. *J Am Coll Cardiol* 2001;37:893.

21 Goodwin J. Pregnancy and coarctation of the aorta. *Lancet* 1958;1:16.

22 Beauchesne LM, Connolly HM, Ammash NM, et al. Coarctation of the aorta: outcome of pregnancy. *J Am Coll Cardiol* 2001;38:1728.

23 Lipscomb KJ, Smith JC, Clarke B, et al. Outcome of pregnancy in women with Marfan's syndrome. *Br J Obstet Gynecol* 1997; 104:201.

24 Murdoch JL, Walker BA, Halpern BL, et al. Life expectancy and causes of death in the Marfan syndrome. *N Engl J Med* 1972;286:804.

25 Rossiter JP, Repke JT, Morales AJ, et al. A prospective longitudinal evaluation of pregnancy in the Marfan syndrome. *Am J Obstet Gynecol* 1995;173:1599.

26 Nienaber CA, Eagle KA. Aortic dissection: new frontiers in diagnosis and management. Part I: from etiology to diagnostic strategies. *Circulation* 2003;108:628.

27 Avila WS, Grinberg M, Snitcowsky R, et al. Maternal and fetal outcomes in pregnant women with Eisenmenger's syndrome. *Eur Heart J* 1995;16:460.

28 Weiss BM, Zemp L, Seifert B, et al. Outcome of pulmonary vascular disease in pregnancy: a systematic review from 1978–1996. *J Am Coll Cardiol* 1998;31:1650.

29 Sutton MS, Cole P, Plappert M, et al. Effects of subsequent pregnancy on left ventricular function in peripartum cardiomyopathy. *Am Heart J* 1991;121:1776.

30 Elkayam U, Tummala PP, Rao K, et al. Maternal and fetal outcomes of subsequent pregnancies in women with peripartum cardiomyopathy. *N Engl J Med* 2001;344:1567.

31 Witlin AG, Mabie WC, Sibai BM. Peripartum cardiomyopathy: an ominous diagnosis. *Am J Obstet Gynecol* 1997;176:182.

32 Hibbard JU, Lindheimer M, Lang RM. A modified definition for peripartum cardiomyopathy and prognosis based on echocardiography. *Obstet Gynecol* 1999;94:311.

33 Klein LL, Galan HL. Cardiac disease in pregnancy. *Obstet Gynecol Clin North Am* 2004;31:429.

34 Reimold SC, Rutherford JD. Valvular heart disease in pregnancy. *N Engl J Med* 2003;349:52.

35 ACC/AHA Guidelines for the Management of Patients with Valvular Heart Disease: a Report of the American College of Cardiology/American Heart Association Task Force on Practice Guidelines (Committee on Management of Patients with Valvular Heart Disease). *J Am Coll Cardiol* 1998;32: 1486.

36 Sommerville J. Grown-up congenital heart disease: medical demands look back, look forward 2000. *Thorac Cardiovasc Surg* 2001;49:21.

37 Siu SC, Colman JM, Sorenson S, et al. Adverse neonatal and cardiac outcomes are more common in pregnant women with cardiac disease. *Circulation* 2002;105:2179.

38 Ullery JC. Management of pregnancy complicated by heart disease. *Am J Obstet Gynecol* 1954;67:834.

39 Rush RW, Verjans M, Spraklen FH. Incidence of heart disease in pregnancy. *S Afr Med J* 1979:55:808.

40 Etheridge MJ, Pepperell RJ. Heart disease and pregnancy at the Royal Women's Hospital. *Med J Aust* 1971;2:277.

41 Stayer SA, Andropoulos DB, Russel IA. Anesthetic management of the adult patient with congenital heart disease. *Anesthesiol Clin North Am* 2003;21:653.

42 Perloff JK. Congenital heart disease and pregnancy. *Clin Cardiol* 1994;17:579.

43 Mishra M, Chambers JB, Jackson G. Murmurs in pregnancy: an audit of echocardiography. *Br Med J* 1992;304: 1413.

44 Ellison CR, Sloss CJ. Electrocardiographic features of congenital heart disease in the adult. In: Roberts WC, ed. *Congenital heart disease in adults*. Philadelphia: F.A. Davis Co.; 1979:119.

45 Neilson G, Galea EG, Blunt A. Congenital heart disease and pregnancy. *Med J Aust* 1970;30:1086.

46 Schaefer G, Arditi LI, Solomon HA, et al. Congenital heart disease and pregnancy. *Clin Obstet Gynecol* 1968;11:1048.

47 Hibbard LT. Maternal mortality due to cardiac disease. *Clin Obstet Gynecol* 1975;18:27.

48 Sugrue D, Blake S, Troy P, et al. Antibiotic prophylaxis against infective endocarditis after a normal delivery—is it necessary? *Br Heart J* 1980;44:499.

49 Zitnick RS, Brandenburg RO, Sheldon R, et al. Pregnancy and open heart surgery. *Circulation* 1969;39:157.

50 Gilman DH. Cesarean section in undiagnosed Eisenmenger's syndrome. Report of a patient with a fatal outcome. *Anesthesia* 1991;46:371.

51 Jackson GM, Dildy GA, Varner MW, et al., Severe pulmonary hypertension in pregnancy following successful repair of ventricular septal defect in childhood. *Obstet Gynecol* 1993;82(S): 680.

52 Szekely P, Julian DG. Heart disease and pregnancy. *Curr Problems Cardiol* 1979;4:1.

53 Knapp RC, Arditi LI. Pregnancy complicated by patent ductus arteriosus with reversal of flow. *NY J Med* 1967;67:573.

54 Tahir H. Pulmonary hypertension, cardiac disease and pregnancy. *Obstet Gynecol* 1995;51:109.

55 Gleicher N, Midwall J, Hochberger D, et al. Eisenmenger's syndrome and pregnancy. *Obstet Gynecol Surv* 1979;34: 721.

56 Pirlo A, Herren AL. Eisenmenger's syndrome and pregnancy. *Anesth Rev* 1979;6:9.

57 Sinnenberg RJ. Pulmonary hypertension in pregnancy. *South Med J* 1980;73:1529.

58 Pitts JA, Crosby WM, Basta LL. Eisenmenger's syndrome in pregnancy. Does heparin prophylaxis improve the maternal mortality rate. *Am Heart J* 1977;93:321.

59 Avila WS, Grinber M, Snitcowsky R, et al. Maternal and fetal outcome in pregnant women with Eisenmenger's syndrome. *Eur Heart J* 1995;15:460.

60 Clark SL, Phelan JP, Greenspoon J, et al. Labor and delivery in the presence of mitral stenosis: central hemodynamic observations. *Am J Obstet Gynecol* 1985;152:984.

61 Weiss BM, Semp L, Seigert B, et al. Outcome of pulmonary vascular disease in pregnancy: a systematic overview from 1978–1996. *J Am Coll Cardiol* 1998;31:1650.

62 Elkayam V, Gleicher N. Cardiac problems in pregnancy. I. Maternal aspects: the approach to the pregnant patient with heart disease. *JAMA* 1984;251:2838.

63 Lust KM, Boots RJ, Dooris M, et al. Management of labor in Eisenmenger's syndrome with inhaled nitric oxide. *Am J Obstet Gynecol* 1999;181:419.

64 Lam GK, Stafford RE, Thorp J, et al. Inhaled nitric oxide for primary pulmonary hypertension in pregnancy. *Obstet Gynecol* 2001;98:895.

65 Monnery L, Nanson J, Charlton G. Primary pulmonary hypertension in pregnancy: a role for the novel vasodilators. *Br J Anaesth* 2001;87:295.

66 Stewart R, Tuazon D, Olson G, et al. Pregnancy and primary pulmonary hypertension: successful outcome with epoprostenol therapy. *Chest* 2001;119:973.

67 Weiss BM, Maggiorini M, Jenni R, et al. Pregnant patient with primary pulmonary hypertension: inhaled pulmonary vasodilators and epidural anesthesia for cesarean delivery. *Anesthesiology* 2000;92:1191.

68 Rout CC. Anasthesia and analgesia for the critically ill parturient. *Best Pract Res Clin Obstet Gynecol* 2001;15:507.

69 Sobrevilla LA, Cassinelli MT, Carcelen A, et al. Human fetal and maternal oxygen tension and acid–base status during delivery at high altitude. *Am J Obstet Gynecol* 1971;111:1111.

70 Prestbitero P, Somerville J, Stone S. Pregnancy in cyanotic congenital heart disease. Outcome of mother and fetus. *Circulation* 1994;89:2673.

71 Penning S, Robinson KD, Major CA, et al. A comparison of echocardiography and pulmonary artery catheterization for evaluation of pulmonary artery pressures in pregnant patients with suspected pulmonary hypertension. *Am J Obstet Gynecol* 2001;184:1568.

72 Weiss BM, Hess OM. Pulmonary vascular disease and pregnancy: current controversies, management strategies, and perspective. *Eur Heart J* 2000;21:104.

73 Penning S, Thomas N, Atwal D, et al. Cardiopulmonary bypass support for emergency cesarean delivery in a patient with severe pulmonary hypertension. *Am J Obstet Gynecol* 2001;184:225.

74 Snabes MC, Poindexter AN. Laparoscopic tubal sterilization with local anesthesia in women with cyanotic heart disease. *Obstet Gynecol* 1991;78:437.

75 Deal K, Wooley CF. Coarctation of the aorta and pregnancy. *Int Med* 1973;78:706.

76 Goodwin JF. Pregnancy and coarctation of the aorta. *Clin Obstet Gynecol* 1961;4:645.

77 Mendelson CL. Pregnancy and coarctation of the aorta. *Am J Obstet Gynecol* 1940;39:1014.

78 Zuber M, Gautschi N, Oechslin E, et al. Outcome of pregnancy in women with congenital shunt lesions. *Heart* 1999;81:271.

79 Jacoby WJ. Pregnancy with tetralogy and pentalogy of Fallot. *Cardiology* 1964;14:866.

80 Meyer EC, Tulsky AS, Sigman P, et al. Pregnancy in the presence of tetralogy of Fallot. *Am J Cardiol* 1964;14:874.

81 Loh TF, Tan NC. Fallot's tetralogy and pregnancy: a report of successful pregnancy after complete correction. *Med J Aust* 1975;2:141.

82 Simon A, Sadovsky E, Aboulatia Y, et al. Fetal activity in pregnancy complicated by rheumatic heart disease. *J Perinat Med* 1986;14:331.

83 Waikman LA, Skorton DJ, Varner MW, et al. Ebstein's anomaly in pregnancy. *Am J Cardiol* 1984;53:357.

84 Connoly JE, Brown JM, Radford DJ. Pregnancy outcome with Ebstein's anomaly. *Br Heart J* 1991;66:368.

85 Whittemore R, Hobbins JC, Engle MA. Pregnancy and its outcome in women with and without surgical correction of congenital heart disease. *Am J Cardiol* 1982:50:641.

86 Connoly HM, Warnes CA. Ebstein's anomaly: outcome of pregnancy. *J Am Coll Cardiol* 1994;23:1194.

87 Chesley LC. Severe rheumatic heart disease and pregnancy: the ultimate prognosis. *Am J Obstet Gynecol* 1980;126:552.

88 Gei AF, Hankins GD. Cardiac discase and pregnancy. *Obstet Gynecol Clin North Am* 2001;28:465.

89 Campos O, Andrade JL, Bocanegra J, et al. Physiologic multivalvular regurgitation during pregnancy: a longitudinal doppler echocardiographic study. *Int J Cardiol* 1993;40:265.

90 Hess DB, Hess LW, Heath BJ, et al. Pregnancy after Fontan repair of tricuspid atresia. *South Med J* 1991;84:532.

91 Robson SC, Hunter S, Boys RJ, et al. Serial study of factors influencing changes in cardiac output during human pregnancy. *Am J Physiol* 1989;256:H1060.

92 Ueland K, Akamatsu TH, Eng M, et al. Maternal cardiovascular dynamics. VI. Cesarean section under epidural anesthesia with epinephrine. *Am J Obstet Gynecol* 1972;114:775.

93 Forester JS, Swan HJC. Acute myocardial infarction: a physiologic basis for therapy. *Crit Care Med* 1974:2:283.

94 Ray P, Murphy GJ, Shutt LE. Recognition and management of maternal cardiac disease in pregnancy. *Br J Anaesth* 2004;93: 428.

95 The AFFIRM Investigators. Survival of patients presenting with atrial fibrillation in the Atrial Fibrillation Follow-Up Investigation of Rhythm Management (AFFIRM) study. *N Engl J Med* 2002;347:1825.

96 Haas JM. The effect of pregnancy on the midsystolic click murmur of the prolapsing posterior leaflet of the mitral valve. *Am Heart J* 1976;92:407.

97 Rayburn WF, Fontana ME. Mitral valve prolapse and pregnancy. *Am J Obstet Gynecol* 1981;141:9.

98 Arias F, Pineda J. Aortic stenosis and pregnancy. *J Reprod Med* 1978;20:229.

99 Ramin SM, Maberry MC, Gilstrap LC. Congenital heart disease. *Clin Obstet Gynecol* 1989;32:41.

100 Carabello BA. Evaluation and management of patients with aortic stenosis. *Circulation* 2002;105:1746.

101 Sullivan HJ. Valvular heart surgery during pregnancy. *Surg Clin North Am* 1995;75:59.

102 Silversides CK, Colman MF, Sermer M, et al. Early and intermediate term outcomes of pregnancy with congenital aortic stenosis. *Am J Cardiol* 2003;91:1386.

103 Presbitero P, Prever S, Bursca A. Interventional cardiology in pregnancy. *Eur Heart J* 1996;17:182.

104 Chambers CE, Clark SL. Cardiac surgery during pregnancy. *Clin Obstet Gynecol* 1994;37:316.

105 Demakis JG, Rahtimoola SH, Sutton GC, et al. Natural course of peripartum cardiomyopathy. *Circulation* 1971;44: 1053.

106 Brown CS Bertolet BD. Peripartum cardiomyopathy: a comprehensive review. *Am J Obstet Gynecol* 1998;178:409.

107 deSouza J L, de Carvalho, Frimm C, et al. Left ventricular function after a new pregnancy in patients with peripartum cardiomyopathy. *J Card Fail* 2001;7:30..

108 Felker GM, Thompson RE, Hare JM, et al. Underlying causes and long term survival in patients with initially unexplained cardiomyopathy. *N Engl J Med* 2000;342:1077.

109 Blickstein I, Zale Y, Katz Z, et al. Ritodrine-induced pulmonary edema unmasking underlying peripartum cardiomyopathy. *Am J Obstet Gynecol* 1988;159:332.

110 Seftel H, Susser M. Maternity and myocardial failure in African women. *Br Heart J* 1961;23:43.

111 Cunningham FG, Pritchard JA, Hankins GDV, et al. Peripartum heart failure: idiopathic cardiomyopathy or compounding cardiovascular events? *Obstet Gynecol* 1986;67:157.

112 Witlin AG, Mable SC, Sibai BM. Peripartum cardiomyopathy: an ominous diagnosis. *Am J Obstet Gynecol* 1997;176:182.

113 Kolibash AJ, Ruiz DE, Lewis RP. Idiopathic hypertophic subaortic stenosis in pregnancy. *Ann Intern Med* 1975;82:791.

114 Oakley GDG, McGarry K, Limb DG, et al. Management of pregnancy in patients with hypertrophic cardiomyopathy. *Br Med J* 1979;1:1749.

115 Autore C, Brauneis S, Apponi F, et al. Epidural anesthesia for cesarean section in patients with hypertrophic cardiomyopathy: a report of 3 cases. *Anesthesiology* 1999;90:1205.

116 Autore C, Conte MR, Piccininno M, et al. Risk associated with pregnancy in hypertrophic cardiomyopathy. *J Am Coll Cardiol* 2002;40:1864.

117 Pyretz RE, McKusick VA. The Marfan syndrome: diagnosis and management. *N Engl J Med* 1979;300:772.

118 Rosenblum NG, Grossman AR, Gabbe SG, et al. Failure of serial echocardiographic studies to predict aortic dissection in a pregnant patient with Marfan's syndrome. *Am J Obstet Gynecol* 1983;146:470.

119 Slater EE, DeSanctis RW. Dissection of the aorta. *Med Clin North Am* 1979;63:141.

120 Nienaber CA, Eagle KA. Aortic dissection: New frontiers in diagnosis and management. Part I: from etiology to diagnostic strategy. *Circulation* 2003;108:628.

121 Thilen U, Olsson SB. Pregnancy and heart disease: a review. *Eur J Obstet Gynecol Reprod Biol* 1997;75:43.

122 Hankins GDV, Wendel GD, Leveno KJ, et al. Myocardial infarction during pregnancy: a review. *Obstet Gynecol* 1985;65:139.

123 Roth A, Elkayam U. Acute myocardial infarction associated with pregnancy. *Ann Intern Med* 1996;125:751.

124 Bast MJ, Rigg LA. Class H diabetes and pregnancy. *Obstet Gynecol* 1985;66:5.

125 Elkayam U, Kawanishi D, Reid CL, et al. Contrast echocardiography to reduce ionizing radiation associated with cardiac catheterization during pregnancy. *Am J Cardiol* 1983;52:213.

126 Ness RB, Harris T, Cobb J, et al. Number of pregnancies and the subsequent risk of cardiovascular disease. *N Engl J Med* 1993;328:1528.

127 APPCR Panel and Scientific Roundtable. Anticoagulation and enoxaparin use in patients with prosthetic heart valves and/or pregnancy. *Clin Cardiol Consensus Rep* 2002;3(9).

128 Hung L, Rahimtoola SH. Prosthetic heart valves and pregnancy. *Circulation* 2003;107:1240.

129 Rowan JA, McCowan LME, Raudkivi PJ, et al. Enoxaparin treatment in women with mechanical heart valves during pregnancy. *Am J Obstet Gynecol* 2001;185:633.

130 Meschengieser SS, Fondevila CG, Santarelli MT, et al. Anticoagulation in pregnant women with mechanical heart valve prostheses. *Br Heart J* 1999;82:23.

131 Chan W, Anand S, Ginsberg J. Anticoagulation of pregnant women with mechanical heart valves: a systematic review of the literature. *Arch Intern Med* 2000;160:191.

132 Nassar AH, Hobeika EM, Hasan M, et al. Pregnancy outcome in women with prosthetic heart valves. *Am J Obstet Gynecol* 2004;191:1009.

133 Golby AJ, Bush EC, DeRook FA. Failure of high dose heparin to prevent recurrent cardioembolic strokes in a pregnant patient with a mechanical heart valve. *Neurology* 1992;42:2204.

134 Salazar E, Isaguirre R, Verdejo J, et al. Failure of subcutaneous heparin to prevent thromboembolic events in pregnant patients with mechanical cardiac valve prosthesis. *Cardiology* 1996;27:1698.

135 Vitale N, DeFeo M, DeSanto LS, et al. Dose dependent fetal complications of warfarin in pregnant women with mechanical heart valves. *J Am Coll Cardiol* 1999;33:1637.

136 Sadler L, McCowna L, White H, et al. Pregnancy outcomes and cardiac complications in women with mechanical, bioprosthetic, and homograft valves. *Br J Obstet Gynaecol* 2000;107:245.

137 Lev-Ran O, Kramer A, Gurevitch J, et al. Low-molecular weight heparin for prosthetic heart valves: treatment failure. *Ann Thoracic Surg* 2000;69:264.

138 ACOG. Safety of lovenox in pregnancy. *ACOG Comm Opin* 2002;276.

139 Ginsberg JS, Chan WS, Bates SM, et al. Anticoagulation of pregnant women with mechanical heart valves. *Arch Intern Med* 2003;163:694.

140 Ueland K. Cardiovascular surgery and the OB patient. *Contemp Obstet Gynecol* 1984;10:117.

141 Koh KS, Friesen RM, Livingstone RA, et al. Fetal and maternal cardiac surgery with cardiopulmonary shunt. *Heart* 1975;112:1102.

142 Chambers CE, Clark SL. Cardiac surgery during pregnancy. *Obstet Gynecol* 1994;37:316.

40 Maternal pulmonary disorders complicating pregnancy

Steven L. Clark and Calla Holmgren

Pregnant women are afflicted by the same respiratory ailments as nonpregnant women, but these conditions are complicated by the physiologic alterations of pregnancy. Certain lung diseases, such as asthma, are common in women of childbearing age and may often be seen in pregnant women. However, asthma and other pulmonary diseases may first manifest during pregnancy or change their course during gestation. In this chapter, we first review diagnostic techniques for lung disease, including history and physical examination, pulmonary function tests, arterial blood gases, and radiographic tests. We then summarize the physiologic alterations of the respiratory system during pregnancy. Specific respiratory illnesses are discussed, including those found in women with chronic disease as well as those found in women who were previously normal.

Diagnostic techniques

History and physical examination

Most common respiratory disorders lead to symptoms such as shortness of breath, exercise intolerance, cough, sputum production, wheezing, chest tightness, fever, chills, night sweats, or hemoptysis. A careful history should elicit information about medications, smoking history, and prior respiratory illness. Physical examination should be carried out with particular attention to the duration of the expiratory phase, the use of accessory muscles, and the presence of rales, rhonchi, wheezes, pleural rubs, signs of pleural effusions, consolidation, and chest wall abnormalities. Taken together, these aspects of the history and physical examination provide the necessary database for the care of patients with pulmonary disease during pregnancy. If the patient has been pregnant in the past, the presence of respiratory symptoms during the previous pregnancy should be noted and compared with the patient's usual respiratory symptoms when not pregnant.

Dyspnea is the most common respiratory complaint during pregnancy, with as many as 60–70% of previously normal women having this symptom at some time during pregnancy. The complaint usually begins in the first or second trimester but is most prevalent at term.[1] It is not usually due to underlying lung disease, but appears to result from the subjective perception of hyperventilation that normally accompanies pregnancy. With increased progesterone levels in pregnancy, the volume of air taken into the lungs with each breath (tidal volume) increases, giving a sensation of hyperventilation. This occurs despite a lack of change in breathing frequency. As the woman acclimatizes to this new sensation, her perception of dyspnea is reduced, and dyspnea stabilizes as the pregnancy progresses. Maximum dyspnea seems to correlate with the time of lowest arterial carbon dioxide tension, which suggests a potential role for hypocarbia in mediating this symptom.

Arterial blood gases

Arterial blood sampling provides valuable data about maternal oxygenation and acid–base status. Because of the well-documented risks of fetal hypoxia with decreasing maternal oxygenation, arterial blood gas data should be obtained when any serious acute respiratory complaint is present. Interpretation of acid–base abnormalities is greatly aided by reference to base nomograms, such as the one shown in Figure 40.1.[2] In a normal pregnant female, arterial blood gas measurements usually show a compensated respiratory alkalosis due to maternal hyperventilation.

The pH generally ranges from 7.40 to 7.47, and the partial pressure of arterial carbon dioxide is 25–32 mmHg.[3–6] The partial pressure of arterial oxygen (P_aO_2) may be as high as 106 mmHg in early pregnancy, decreasing during pregnancy but remaining at 100 mmHg, or slightly higher, at term. In patients at moderate altitude, partial pressure of oxygen (PO_2) values are lower, averaging 88 mmHg.[6] The measured arterial O_2 tension represents the partial pressure of O_2 dissolved in blood, but is only an indirect reflection of the blood's O_2 content. Calculating the O_2 content of blood requires a knowledge of the amount of O_2 dissolved in the blood, the maximum amount of O_2 able to be carried per gram of hemoglobin, the

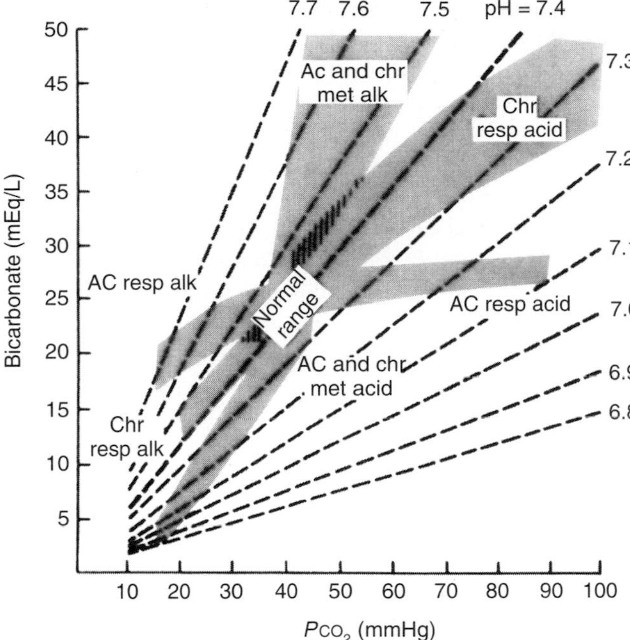

Figure 40.1 Nomogram showing bands for uncomplicated respiratory or metabolic acid–base disturbances in intact subjects. Each "confidence" band represents the mean ± standard deviation for the compensatory response of normal subjects or patients to a given primary disorder. Ac, acute; acid, acidosis; alk, alkalosis; chr, chronic; met, metabolic; resp, respiratory. (Modified from Arbus.) (Reprinted from ref. 2, with permission.)

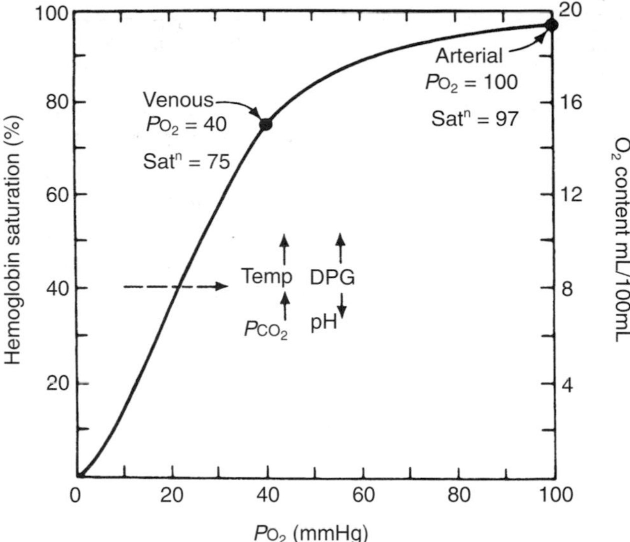

Figure 40.2 Anchor points of the oxygen dissociation curve. The curve is shifted to the right by an increase in temperature, $P\text{CO}_2$ and 2,3-DPG and a fall in the pH. The oxygen content scale is based on a hemoglobin concentration of 14.5 g per 100 mL. (Reprinted from ref. 7, with permission.)

hemoglobin concentration, and the O_2 saturation of hemoglobin.

O_2 content = [(hemoglobin [Hb] (g/dL) × 1.39 mL O_2/g Hb) × (O_2 saturation)] + [(0.003 mL O_2/100 ml of blood) × P_aO_2 (mmHg)]

As the equation shows, 1 g of fully saturated Hb can combine with 1.39 mL of O_2. Because normal blood has approximately 15 g of Hb per 100 mL, the maximal O_2-carrying capacity is usually approximately 20.8 mL of O_2 per 100 mL of blood. The O_2 saturation of Hb is usually taken from the oxyhemoglobin dissociation curve (Fig. 40.2)[7] and is affected by such variables as pH, partial pressure of carbon dioxide ($P\text{CO}_2$), temperature, and the amount of 2,3-diphosphoglycerate (DPG) present. The amount of dissolved O_2 is calculated by applying Henry's law, which states that the amount of dissolved gas is proportional to its partial pressure. For each 1 mmHg of partial pressure of O_2, 0.003 mL of O_2 is dissolved per 100 mL of blood (0.003 mL O_2 per 100 mL of blood). Thus, the dissolved O_2 content of arterial blood with a P_aO_2 of 100 mmHg is 0.3 mL of O_2 per 100 mL of blood.

The adequacy of alveolar gas exchange depends on the matching of ventilation and blood perfusion within various regions of the lung. Mismatching of ventilation and perfusion is responsible for most of the defective gas exchange in pulmonary diseases. The adequacy of alveolar gas exchange can be assessed by calculating the alveolar–arterial O_2 tension gradient and, if the alveolar O_2 tension (P_AO_2) greatly exceeds the P_aO_2, then alveolar gas exchange is abnormal. Ideal P_aO_2 is calculated as follows:

$$P_aO_2 = F_IO_2 \times (PB - 47) - P_aCO_2/0.8$$

F_IO_2 = fractional percentage of inspired O_2; PB = barometric pressure; 47 = water vapor pressure; P_aCO_2 = arterial blood tension of carbon dioxide; 0.8 = respiratory quotient.

This equation states that a patient's P_aO_2 equals the tension of O_2 in inspired air minus the amount of O_2 taken up in the lung in exchange for carbon dioxide. This latter exchange relationship, the respiratory quotient, is equal to 0.8 of the volume of carbon dioxide released in exchange for every volume of O_2 delivered. P_aO_2, obtained from blood gas measurement is subtracted from P_AO_2 to obtain a measure of the (A–a) O_2 gradient.

In the nonpregnant patient, the (A–a) O_2 gradient varies with age, but a prediction formula for the expected range of normal is not applicable during pregnancy. In one study, the mean (A–a) O_2 gradient in normal pregnant women in the supine position during the third trimester was 20 mmHg, whereas in the sitting position it decreased to 14.3 mmHg.[8] In another study of normal obstetric patients, P_aO_2 increased by 13 mmHg when changing from a supine to a sitting position, and arterial $P\text{CO}_2$ decreased by 2 mmHg, leading to a net decrease in the (A–a) O_2 gradient of 10 mmHg.[9] The increased gradient noted in the supine position may be the result of decreased cardiac output attributable to decreased venous return from compression of the inferior vena cava by the uterus.[8,10]

On the other hand, a more recent study performed at moderate altitude showed no effect of position or oxygenation in normal pregnant women.[5]

Because most acute lung diseases are accompanied by an increased (A–a) O_2 gradient, the gradient should be assessed with the pregnant patient in the upright position and should be considered abnormal if it exceeds 25 mmHg. Blood gas analysis should be accompanied by calculation of the gradient because, given the usual decreased $P\text{CO}_2$ of pregnancy, on casual observation, a "normal" $P_a\text{CO}_2$ can be seen even with an abnormally increased (A–a) O_2 gradient.

Pulmonary function tests

Normal respiratory physiology is altered in pregnancy, and these changes must be considered when evaluating tests of lung function. In the terminology of pulmonary function testing (Table 40.1), a volume is a single discrete component of the lung. Four such volumes exist: tidal volume (TV), residual volume (RV), inspiratory reserve volume (IRV), and expiratory reserve volume (ERV). The term capacity refers to a sum of volumes. Except for RV, each of the volumes defined can be recorded and measured by simple spirometry. RV, the volume of gas remaining in the thorax at the end of a maximal exhalation, can be measured only by indirect methods (e.g., helium dilution, nitrogen washout, or body plethysmography). The enlarging fetus and the increased concentration of circulating hormones during pregnancy account for the changes in pulmonary function seen with gestation. The hyperventilation of pregnancy is characterized by an increased depth of breathing (TV increases from 450 to 600 mL) rather than a higher respiratory rate.[11] Minute ventilation is increased in excess of the rise in O_2 consumption associated with pregnancy and is thought to be due to a progesterone-mediated increase in sensitivity to carbon dioxide. In one study, at term, minute ventilation was 48% higher than normal, whereas oxygen consumption increased by only 21%.[12] Vital capacity generally remains unchanged because there is an increase in inspiratory capacity but a decrease in ERV. In the second half of pregnancy, a slight reduction in functional residual capacity (FRC) (18%), RV, and total lung capacity (TLC) occurs, caused by compression of the resting lung by the elevated intra-abdominal pressure secondary to uterine enlargement.[13] Typical pulmonary volumes and capacities and the modifications caused by pregnancy are shown schematically in Figure 40.3. In women with a moderate deficiency of serum protease inhibitor, forced expiratory volume (FEV), forced vital capacity (FVC), and other tests of pulmonary function increase with increasing numbers of children.[14]

Abnormal spirometry is usually classified as fitting a pattern of either obstruction or restriction. Normal spirometric lung values are within 20% of a predicted normal, which is based on a patient's age, sex, height, and weight. Flow rates are preserved in both large and small airways during a normal pregnancy.

A restrictive pattern is present when TLC is less than 80% of the predicted normal. With restrictive disease, air flow rate, expressed by volume of air expired in 1 s from maximum inspiration (FEV) as a percentage of FVC (FEV_1 per FVC), can be increased to more than 85%. Restrictive ventilatory defects are caused by skeletal, neuromuscular, pleural, interstitial, and alveolar diseases that lead to a reduction in lung volume or chest wall expansion. Sarcoidosis and chest wall deformity are the most common restrictive lung diseases seen in women of childbearing age.

An obstructive pattern is present when the FEV/FVC ratio is less than 75% and FEV is less than 80% of the predicted value, indicating a reduction in air flow rates. Lung volumes

Table 40.1 Pulmonary parameters.

Lung volumes	Description
Tidal volume (TV)	The volume of air inhaled or exhaled with each normal breath
Residual volume (RV)	The volume of air remaining in the lungs after a vital capacity maneuver
Inspiratory reserve volume (IRV)	The maximal additional volume of gas that can be inhaled after a tidal breath is inhaled
Expiratory reserve volume (ERV)	The maximal volume of gas that can be exhaled after a tidal breath is exhaled
Total lung capacity (TLC)	The volume of air in the lungs at maximal inspiration
Vital capacity (VC)	The maximum amount of air that can be exhaled after a maximal inspiration to TLC
Inspiratory capacity (IC)	The maximal volume of gas that can be inspired from the resting expiratory level
Functional residual capacity (FRC)	The volume of air remaining in the lungs after a tidal volume exhalation
Forced vital capacity (FVC)	The volume of air exhaled during a rapid forced expiration starting at full inspiration
Other measurements made by spirometry	
Forced expiratory volume in 1 s (FEV)	The volume of air expelled in 1 s during a forced expiration starting at full inspiration
Minute ventilation (MV)	The amount of air exhaled per minute, measured under resting conditions
Peak expiratory flow rate (PEFR)	The peak rate (L/min) of a forceful expiration of a vital capacity

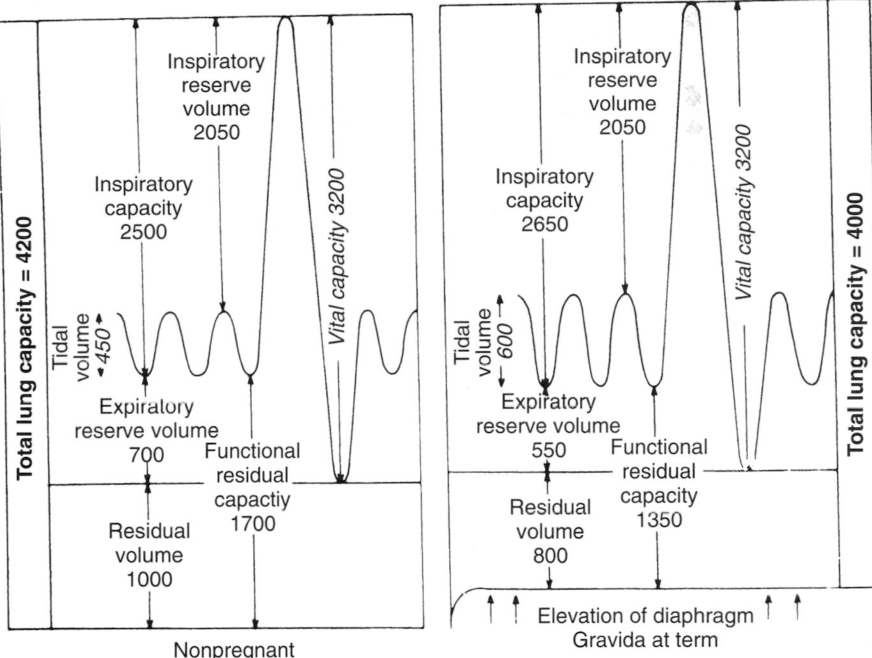

Figure 40.3 Alterations in pulmonary volumes and capacities associated with pregnancy. (Reprinted from ref. 11, with permission.)

may be normal, or they may be increased if air is trapped as a result of early airway closure. Asthma is the most common obstructive airway disease encountered in pregnancy.[15] Other obstructive lung diseases include cystic fibrosis, bronchiectasis, and emphysema. The diffusing capacity of the lung, which reflects the amount of O_2 that can be taken up by the pulmonary capillary blood, is either unchanged or increased during pregnancy. Diffusing capacity has been reported to be most elevated in the first trimester[16,17] as a result of the increase in capillary blood volume that accompanies pregnancy. Diffusing capacity may also be increased in asthmatic patients because relative pulmonary hypertension, secondary to hypoxemia, results in redistribution of pulmonary blood flow to the upper lobes, where alveoli have higher ventilation–perfusion ratios.[18]

When a patient with known lung disease seeks advice about the risks of pregnancy, pulmonary function studies should be obtained. These studies combined with other clinical data can be used to make an objective assessment of the patient's risks during pregnancy. However, no strict guidelines can be given as to the level of pulmonary function that will prohibit a safe pregnancy. A patient with a vital capacity less than 1 L generally has significant difficulties. If the FEV exceeds 1 L in a woman with obstructive disease, she does not ordinarily experience dyspnea at rest, even at term. Resting ventilation during pregnancy increases less in patients with lung disease than in normal subjects.[19] Although patients with obstructive lung disease vary widely in their tolerance of pregnancy, most women with restrictive disease tolerate pregnancy well. Studies in patients with lung disease resulting from lung resection have shown the potential for normal pregnancy and fetal development. Indeed, even intrapartum lung resection has been carried out when necessary without adverse outcome.[20] In view of these data, women with respiratory disease that is unlikely to worsen during pregnancy, an FEV of greater than 1 L, and no dyspnea at rest can generally undertake pregnancy safely.

When a pregnant patient must undergo general anesthesia and serious lung disease is suspected, ideally, pulmonary function should be assessed. Postoperative respiratory complications of atelectasis, inadequate secretion clearance, infection, and respiratory failure are more likely to occur when the FEV is less than 2 L. A higher FEV is required to undergo uncomplicated surgery than is needed to tolerate pregnancy alone because of an expected reduction in lung function in the immediate postoperative period. Both spinal and epidural anesthesia impair cough effectiveness as well as most other respiratory variables during pregnancy.[21]

Radiographic testing

Radiologic evaluation is a cornerstone of pulmonary medicine. Chest radiography performed on a pregnant patient may expose the fetus to 8–36 mrad.[22,23] Chest fluoroscopy exposes the fetus to approximately 70 mrad, an estimate that varies depending on the operator, shielding, and reason for fluoroscopy.[22] Technetium-99m, a radionuclide frequently used in lung scanning, has a short half-life (6 h), is rapidly excreted, emits no beta rays, and is attached to macroaggregates of human albumin with a particle size of approximately 20 μm, which does not cross the placenta. Fetal radiation exposure has been estimated to range between 500 mrad and 1 rad,[22] and thus poses no hazard to the developing fetus. If at any time during pregnancy, the health of the mother or fetus would be compromised by failure to perform a radiologic examination, the examination should be performed, and every care should be taken to shield the fetus from scatter radiation and from the direct beam when appropriate. Although available data are not conclusive, both epidemiologic and laboratory studies indicate that some levels of radiographic exposure can be harmful to the developing human. Irradiation *in utero* may increase the risk of childhood leukemia and other malignancies by 40–50%.[22,24] Experimental studies show that doses as low as 5 rad can kill the early embryo, cause neural and skeletal malformations, and impair several aspects of behavior, including learning ability and emotional response to varied stimuli.[23] Obvious malformations are particularly associated with irradiation during the period of major organogenesis, which extends from approximately week 2 through week 9 after conception.[25] Taking into account the greatest oncogenic risk, the overall risk of any adverse effect from exposure to 1 rad is estimated to be 0.1%,[26] a risk that is thousands of times smaller than the risks of spontaneous abortion, malformation, or genetic disease.[22] Fetal exposure to less than 5 rad is considered insufficient reason to recommend termination of a desired pregnancy.[23,25,26]

When chest radiographs are performed in the pregnant patient, normal findings differ from those seen in nonpregnant women of childbearing age. The diaphragm may be elevated 4 cm at term, but there is a compensatory increase in anteroposterior diameter. The subcostal angle increases from 68.5° to 103.5° from early to late pregnancy.[27] Also, lung markings may be increased, giving a false impression of mild congestive heart failure. Hughson and colleagues reported that pleural effusions frequently occurred in the first 24 h after delivery[28] and that, in the absence of symptoms or signs of illness, no intervention was necessary. A subsequent prospective ultrasound study of 50 women within 1–45 h of delivery found only one patient with a pleural effusion, a patient who was also in pulmonary edema.[29] The results of this study suggest that postpartum pleural effusions may not be a normal occurrence.

Maternal–fetal oxygen exchange

Fetal O_2 delivery depends on maternal respiratory function, hemoglobin concentration, and cardiac output. During pregnancy, plasma volume increases by 30 mL/kg (from 40 to 70 mL/kg), and red cell volume increases from 25 mL/kg to 30 mL/kg.[30] As a result, even though erythrocyte mass is increased, there is a decrease in hemoglobin concentration to a value as low as 10.5–11.0 g/dL. Maternal cardiac output, however, is enhanced by 30–40% early in the second trimester because of an increase in stroke volume, left ventricular compliance, and heart rate, along with a reduced systemic vascular resistance (Table 40.2).[31] The net result of these physiologic changes is to ensure a high rate of O_2 delivery to the gravid uterus.

Table 40.2 Hemodynamic alterations in pregnancy.

Plasma volume	++
Red cell volume	+
Hemoglobin	–
Hematocrit	–
Stroke volume	+
Left ventricular compliance	+
Heart rate	+
Systemic vascular resistance	–
Cardiac output	+++

+++, greatly increased; ++, increased; +, slightly increased; –, slightly decreased; –, decreased.

In a woman with no pulmonary disease who is breathing room air, arterial blood typically has a P_aO_2 of 91 mmHg and a $P\text{CO}_2$ of 36 mmHg. In the fetal umbilical vein, a simultaneous blood gas typically shows a $P\text{O}_2$ of 32 mmHg and a $P\text{CO}_2$ of 50 mmHg. The same woman breathing 100% O_2 would raise her P_aO_2 to 583 mmHg, and the $P\text{O}_2$ of the umbilical vein would increase from 32 to 40 mmHg, thereby illustrating a large shunt effect.[32] Experimental data in sheep demonstrate that the O_2 tension in the fetal umbilical vein is always less than that in the uterine arteries at all levels of maternal oxygenation.[32] Increases in the concentration of inspired O_2 result in the expected rise in O_2 tension in the maternal arteries, but not in large increases in the O_2 tension of the fetal umbilical veins. The fetus is sensitive to large shifts in O_2 delivery caused by a fall in cardiac output. With complete interruption of O_2 supply to the umbilical vein, the fetus has only a limited O_2 reserve. In the normoxic fetus, the effects of maternal administration of nasal cannula or standard mask O_2 on fetal O_2 saturation are negligible.[33,34]

Blood pH is an important determinant of uterine blood flow, and the finding of an acute, uncompensated respiratory alkalosis in a pregnant female signals possible compromise of fetal oxygenation. In one study of women at term, hyperventilation during inspiration of room air was associated with an increase in maternal O_2 tension from 91 to 100 mmHg, but fetal scalp O_2 tension fell from 25 to 19 mmHg because of a reduction in maternal carbon dioxide tension from 25 to 19 mmHg. Maternal inhalation of 95% O_2 and 5% carbon dioxide restored the fetal O_2 tension to a normal level.[35] These data and studies in sheep have suggested that maternal alkalosis can result in decreased fetal O_2 tension because of reduced uterine blood flow due to hypocarbia-induced vasoconstriction of uterine arteries. This effect occurs because of the mechanical effects of hyperventilation causing decreased maternal venous return and because of a shift in the maternal oxyhemoglobin dissociation curve to the left, thereby impairing O_2 transfer to the fetus. In the studies by Wulf and colleagues, fetal O_2 delivery was compromised when maternal pH exceeded 7.6 and $P\text{CO}_2$ was 15 mmHg.[32]

Asthma

Approximately 1–4% of pregnancies are complicated by bronchial asthma.[15] During the past decade, the prevalence, morbidity, and mortality of asthma have all increased. In about 0.05–2% of cases, asthma presents as a life-threatening event. In general, data suggest that the severity of asthma during pregnancy improves in about one-third of women, remains stable in one-third and worsens in one-third of patients. In addition, there appears to be a tendency for the course of asthma to be similar in subsequent pregnancies.[35] The working group on Asthma and Pregnancy of the National Institutes of Health concluded that undertreatment, principally because of unfounded fears of fetal effects of medication, is the major problem in asthma management during pregnancy in the United States.[36,37]

Traditionally, asthma treatment relied on symptomatic therapy with bronchodilators. This reflected the view of asthma as an intermittent illness that is primarily a bronchospastic event. However, recent pathophysiologic insights have defined more clearly the dominant role of chronic airway inflammation in bronchial hyperreactivity and exacerbations of reversible airway obstruction. Thus, asthma is now viewed as a chronic process characterized by acute exacerbations. Control of inflammation should minimize or eliminate the acute exacerbations and dramatically decrease morbidity and mortality from the illness.

Pathogenesis

Asthma is a lung disease involving airway obstruction that is partially or completely reversible and involves both airway inflammation and airway hyperresponsiveness to a variety of stimuli, including environmental irritants, viral respiratory infections, cold air, and exercise.[15] Several mechanisms have been proposed to explain airway hyperresponsiveness in asthma, including airway inflammation, abnormalities in bronchial epithelial integrity, alterations in autonomic neural control of airways, changes in intrinsic bronchial smooth muscle function, alterations in the volume and composition of the airway liquid lining layer, defects in control of bronchial blood flow, and abnormal airway geometry.[15] Airway inflammation is thought to be a key factor in airway hyperresponsiveness, even in individuals with mild asthma. Cellular infiltrates of eosinophils, neutrophils, lymphocytes, mast cells, and macrophages are present. During an asthmatic attack, the release of inflammatory mediators leads to migration and activation of more inflammatory cells, destruction of the epithelial cell layer integrity, abnormalities of autonomic neural control of airway tone, changes in mucociliary function, and increased airway smooth muscle responsiveness.[15] Desquamation of epithelial cells and alteration in their barrier function as a consequence of the airway inflammatory process can lead to increased permeability to inhaled allergens and other provoking agents, impaired mucociliary clearance, impaired metabolism of peptide hormones, impaired regulation of the bronchial fluid lining layer, and increased response to cholinergic stimulation.[15] Although airway smooth muscle is clearly hypertrophic in asthma, it does not show increased constriction to pharmacologic stimulation. However, there may be impaired relaxation characteristics of the airway smooth muscle *in vivo*. Narrowing of the airway lumen may also occur through the development of bronchial mucosal edema, inflammatory cellular infiltrates, excess mucus and fluid, and smooth muscle hypertrophy or constriction. This narrowing may contribute to airway hyperresponsiveness.[15]

Exacerbations of asthma manifest as acute or subacute episodes of progressively worsening shortness of breath, cough, wheezing, or chest tightness. Exacerbations are characterized by decreases in expiratory air flow and an increase in FRC, leading to increased work in breathing, use of accessory muscles of respiration, hypoxemia because of mismatching of ventilation and perfusion, hypercapnia due to respiratory muscle failure, increases in pulmonary vascular resistance, and the development of negative pleural pressures associated with lung hyperinflation manifested by pulsus paradoxus.[15] In an acute asthma exacerbation, maternal P_aO_2 falls. Because the fetus operates on the steep portion of the O_2 dissociation curve (normal fetal venous P_aO_2 is close to 33 mmHg), decreases in maternal P_aO_2 below 60–70 mmHg result in a rapid and profound decrease in fetal O_2 saturation and fetal hypoxia. Careful monitoring of the fetal heart rate is essential in the late second or third trimester in a clinically unstable or marginally hypoxic mother.[15]

Effects on pregnancy

Two large epidemiologic studies have clearly defined the potential adverse effects of maternal asthma on pregnancy and the infant. One study described pregnancy outcomes in 381 women with asthma compared with a control population of 112 530 pregnant women with no medical illness.[38] There was a statistically significant increase in preterm births and low birthweights, decreased mean birthweight, and increased neonatal mortality in the pregnancies of women with asthma compared with control pregnancies. These investigators also found a statistically significant increase in hyperemesis gravidarum, vaginal hemorrhage, preeclampsia, and induced and complicated labors in the women with asthma compared with normal control subjects. No increased incidence of congenital malformations was found. Another study compared pregnancy outcomes between 277 women with asthma and the entire cohort population of 30 861 women.[39] A statistically significant increase in perinatal mortality was found in the pregnancies of women with asthma compared with the control women. Subsequent studies have reported increases in low birthweight infants, chronic hypertension, and preeclampsia in the pregnancies of women with asthma compared with those of women without asthma.[40–42]

The mechanism(s) of the potential adverse effects of asthma on pregnancy and the infant have not been fully defined. However, good asthma control is perhaps the most important factor in improving maternal and fetal outcomes.[37] Acute exacerbations of asthma are associated with maternal hypoxia as well as hypocapnia and alkalosis, factors that may further impair fetal oxygenation.[37] Relative hypoxia in high-altitude pregnancies is associated with lower infant birthweight, and chronic hypoxia seen in women with cyanotic heart disease is associated with both fetal growth restriction and prematurity.[15] Lower mean birthweights occur in infants whose mothers are hospitalized for asthma during pregnancy compared with infants whose mothers did not require emergency therapy for asthma.[15] In addition, diminished pulmonary function is associated with decreased birthweight and asymmetric growth restriction in infants of asthmatic mothers.[15]

Another recent study suggests that asthma morbidity during pregnancy is related to the original severity classification of mild, moderate, or severe based on the 1993 National Asthma Education Program Working Group on Asthma recommendations.[42] In this investigation, 1793 patients with asthma were evaluated throughout pregnancy. Exacerbations during pregnancy occurred in 12.6% of patients initially classified as mild, in 25.7% of patients classified as moderate, and in 51.9% of patients classified as severe. Although the course of asthma may change during pregnancy, with up to 30% of patients manifesting an increasing severity classification during pregnancy,[42] experience in a previous pregnancy often predicts the course of asthma in a subsequent gestation. The condition of women with severe asthma before pregnancy is more likely to deteriorate during pregnancy. The variable effect of pregnancy on the course of asthma appears to be more than random fluctuations in the natural history of the disease because the changes generally revert to the prepregnancy level of severity within 3 months postpartum.[15,43]

Effective management of asthma in pregnant women relies on four components:

1 patient education;
2 avoidance or control of environmental precipitating factors;
3 objective assessment of maternal lung function and fetal well-being;
4 pharmacologic therapy.[15,37]

Patient education is an invaluable component of treating asthma during pregnancy. The key educational messages are that none of the drugs commonly prescribed for asthma during pregnancy is associated with significant teratogenic effects and that control of maternal symptoms (and thus fetal hypoxia) is vital to fetal and maternal well-being. This awareness often improves compliance with therapeutic recommendations and enhances fetal oxygenation in pregnant women who are justifiably concerned about the potential adverse effects of drugs taken during pregnancy. Other educational components are the nature of the disease, specifically identification of triggers, and proper utilization of medications prescribed for asthma. Written guidelines may be necessary for some patients.

Known environmental precipitants of asthma attacks should be eliminated. Cigarette smoke, either primary or secondary, is perhaps the most common of such agents. Animal dander is also highly allergenic; sensitive individuals should remove pets from their environments. An alternative strategy involves the use of 3% tannic acid shampoo to render such dander less allergenic. Mites are ubiquitous in most mattresses and in household dust, and mite feces is one of the most potent environmental allergens known. Thus, the patient's mattress should be enclosed in an airtight cover, and she should wear a mask or leave the house for 1 h after cleaning, vacuuming, or dusting (preferably performed by someone else!). Household filters in the heating and cooling systems should be changed regularly. When specific allergens have been identified, immunotherapy may be considered and is safe during pregnancy. Other common asthma triggers to avoid include sulfite food additives, aspirin, and beta-blockers.[37]

Another preventive measure to be considered in women with a history of asthma is influenza vaccination. Since 1998, the American College of Obstetricians and Gynecologists and the Centers for Disease Control (CDC) have recommended influenza vaccination for all pregnant women who will be in the second and third trimester during influenza season. It is also recommended at all stages of pregnancy for women with chronic medical conditions such as asthma.[44] One population-based study by Hartert et al. in 2003 found that, after evaluating eight influenza seasons, those patients with asthma accounted for half of all respiratory-related hospitalizations.[45] With women in later stages of pregnancy being at increased risk of serious influenza-related maternal morbidity, particularly with underlying respiratory disease, patients with asthma should be strongly encouraged to be vaccinated.

Objective measurements of lung volumes or flow rates are essential for assessing and monitoring the severity of asthma in order to recommend appropriate therapy and to identify asthma attacks early in their course. This practice allows treatment even before the patient becomes overtly symptomatic. Such measures are desirable because both patient and physician perceptions of asthma severity are often insensitive or inaccurate.[44] Furthermore, objective measures of lung function differentiate asthma from other causes of dyspnea during pregnancy. The single best measure of pulmonary function for assessing the severity of asthma is the FEV. However, the peak expiratory flow rate (PEFR) correlates well with FEV and can be measured reliably with inexpensive, portable peak flowmeters. Because PEFR reflects only large airway function, its measurement may not be sufficient to diagnose or fully evaluate the severity of asthma. Nevertheless, patient PEFR monitoring at home is valuable for giving insight into the course of asthma throughout the day. Such monitoring is important for assessing circadian variation in pulmonary function (an indication of airway hyperresponsiveness), detecting early signs of deterioration (often before symptoms appear), and assessing response to therapy (Table 40.3).[15,37]

In general, pregnant women with moderate to severe asthma should make daily PEFR measurements at home with a peak flowmeter. Ideally, the measurements should be made and recorded twice a day, in the morning on rising and approximately 12 h later. These records should be brought to each prenatal visit. Predicted values of PEFR are in the range 380–550 ml^3/min for women, and these values do not change during pregnancy. Rather than use the predicted value, however, it is often better to establish a personal best PEFR for each patient after a period of monitoring when the asthma is well controlled. This is most easily performed by administering a "burst" of corticosteroids (such as prednisone, 40 mg p.o., tapering over the course of 1 week). Recommendations for adjustments in asthma therapy may then be based on deviations from this personal best level.

Table 40.3 Status asthmaticus: warning signs of fatal attack.

Previous or recurrent episodes of status asthmaticus, especially previous intubation
FVC <1.0 L; FEV_1 <0.5 L; PEFR <100 L/min
Little or no response to bronchodilator therapy at 1 h (ΔFEV_1 of <400 mL; ΔPEFR of <60 mL/min)
Altered consciousness
Unequivocal central cyanosis; arterial Po_2 of <50 mmHg
Pco_2 of >45 mmHg
Pulsus paradoxus
Echocardiographic abnormalities
Presence of pneumothorax or pneumomediastinum

FEV_1, forced expiratory volume in 1 second; FVC, forced vital capacity; PEFR, peak expiratory flow rate.

Reprinted from Summer WR. Status asthmaticus. *Chest* 1985;87[Suppl]:895, with permission.

Early sonography provides a benchmark for progressive fetal growth. Sequential sonographic evaluations of fetal growth are indicated in the second and third trimesters if asthma is moderate or severe or if fetal growth restriction is suspected. Antepartum fetal surveillance in the third trimester should be used as needed to ensure fetal well-being. Daily maternal assessment of fetal activity in the late third trimester should be encouraged.[15,37]

Because asthma is an airway disease, inhalation therapy is generally preferable to systemic treatment. Aerosolized medications deliver the drug directly to the airways, minimizing systemic side-effects. Inhaled β_2-agonists, by themselves, are usually sufficient therapy for mild, intermittent asthma (Table 40.4).[37] If symptoms disappear and pulmonary function normalizes with inhaled β_2-agonists, they can be used indefinitely as needed. However, their use on a daily basis, or even more often than three times a week, usually indicates a need for anti-inflammatory therapy.[15,37] The category of moderate asthma includes patients who, before treatment, have symptoms that are not controlled or that are poorly regulated by episodic administration of a β_2-agonist. Some patients have frequent (more than three times a week) symptomatic exacerbations of asthma. Others do not have acute exacerbations and can regulate symptoms by modulating their lifestyle, even though

Table 40.4 Drugs and dosages for asthma and associated conditions preferred for use during pregnancy.

Drug class	Specific drug	Dosage
Anti-inflammatory	Cromolyn sodium	2 puffs q.i.d. (inhalation)
		2 sprays in each nostril b.i.d.–q.i.d. (intranasal for nasal symptoms)
	Beclomethasone	2–5 puffs b.i.d.–q.i.d. (inhalation)
		2 sprays in each nostril b.i.d.–q.i.d. (intranasal for allergic rhinitis)
	Prednisone	Burst for active symptoms: 40 mg/day, single or divided dose for 1 week, then taper for 1 week. If prolonged course is required, single morning dose on alternate days may minimize adverse effects
Bronchodilator	Inhaled β_2-agonist	2 puffs every 4 h as needed
	Theophylline	Oral: Dose to reach serum concentration level of 8–12 mg/mL
Antihistamine	Chlorpheniramine	4 mg by mouth up to q.i.d.
		8–12 mg sustained-release b.i.d.
	Tripelennamine	25–50 mg by mouth up to q.i.d.
		100 mg sustained-release b.i.d.
Decongestant	Pseudoephedrine	60 mg by mouth up to q.i.d.
		120 mg sustained-release b.i.d.
	Oxymetazoline	Intranasal spray or drops up to 5 days for rhinosinusitis
Cough	Guaifenesin	10 mL by mouth q.i.d.
	Dextromethorphan	
Antibiotics	Amoxicillin	3 weeks therapy for sinusitis

This table presents drugs and suggested dosages for the home management of asthma and associated conditions. Drugs and dosages for the treatment of exacerbations in the emergency department or hospital are presented in the full report of the working group.

From ref. 37, with permission.

their pulmonary function (FEV or PEFR) is 60–80% of the predicted range.[15,37]

Inhaled anti-inflammatory agents are the primary therapy for moderate asthma. Choices include cromolyn sodium or inhaled corticosteroids, which provide effective asthma control with minimal side-effects at recommended doses. However, suppression of symptoms and PEFR improvement are often not maximal until 2–4 weeks of treatment. A spacer, used to bypass the oropharynx during the administration of aerosolized medication, should be considered not only to reduce oropharyngeal candidiasis but also to improve respiratory tract penetration and reduce systemic effects. A short tapering course of oral corticosteroids is indicated when asthma is not controlled by a combination of bronchodilators, cromolyn sodium, and inhaled corticosteroids. Such deterioration of asthma may be characterized by a reduction in PEFR of 20% or more from normal values that fails to respond to inhaled bronchodilators, by greater intolerance of exercise, or by the development of nocturnal symptoms. At the end of this course, oral corticosteroids can be stopped; if asthma symptoms do not recur and pulmonary functions remain normal, no additional oral steroid therapy is necessary. However, if this burst of prednisone does not control symptoms, is effective for less than 10 days, or must be repeated frequently, the patient has severe asthma and needs additional therapy.[15,37]

Leukotriene modifiers, such as montelukast (Singulair) and zafirlukast (Accolate), are available for the treatment of asthma. The cysteinyl leukotrienes (LTC4, LTD4, and LTE4) are produced by way of arachidonic acid metabolism and are released by mast cells and eosinophils. They then bind to leukotriene receptors in the human airway, causing airway edema, smooth muscle contraction, and altered cellular activity. Leukotriene modifiers bind to these leukotriene receptors, inhibiting the actions of leukotriene at the level of the mast cell and eosinophil. These medications are pregnancy category B and may be continued during pregnancy.[37]

Sustained release theophylline or a long-acting oral agonist once a day in the evening may be helpful for the patient with primarily nocturnal symptoms. Otherwise, oral theophylline is generally not used in current clinical practice. Asthma not controlled on maximal doses of bronchodilators and inhaled anti-inflammatory agents is classified as severe, and these patients may also need oral corticosteroids on a routine basis. Although the prolonged use of high doses of oral corticosteroids may be associated with increased risk of gestational diabetes and maternal adrenal insufficiency, use of these agents is justified in women with chronic severe asthma to avoid potentially fatal attacks.

Several risk factors for fatal asthma have been identified, and these include the following:

- a history of intubation for asthma;
- two or more hospitalizations for asthma within 1 year;
- three or more emergency room visits for asthma within 1 month;
- recent withdrawal from systemic corticosteroids;
- history of syncope or seizure associated with an asthmatic attack;
- previous admission to a hospital intensive care unit for asthma;
- coexisting psychiatric disease or psychosocial problems.

Individuals with one or more of these risk factors require especially intensive patient education, close monitoring, and prompt treatment of exacerbations.[48]

For symptomatic exacerbations with PEFR above 80% of baseline, the patient administers two puffs of a β_2-agonist inhaler every 20 min for up to 1 h if needed. If the response is good (PEFR of more than 70%), two puffs every 3–4 h are given for 6–12 h. If the response is not good (PEFR of less than 70%), the patient must begin or increase a dose of inhaled or systemic corticosteroids. If the PEFR is less than 50% of baseline, the patient is instructed to seek immediate medical attention. It is important to emphasize to patients that they should not delay seeking medical help if an asthma exacerbation is severe, if therapy does not give rapid improvement, if sustained improvement is not achieved, or if there is further deterioration.[37]

The emergency management of acute, severe asthma in pregnancy involves several initial steps:

1 Administer O_2 to maintain a P_aO_2 as near normal as possible but at least above 60 mmHg or O_2 of at least 95%.

2 Perform baseline arterial blood gases, continuous pulse oximetry, and intensive fetal monitoring for late second- or third-trimester fetuses.

3 Obtain baseline pulmonary function tests (FEV or PEFR).

4 Administer an inhaled β-agonist, such as albuterol, 2.5 mg in 2–3 mL of diluent with a pressure-driven nebulizer, every 20 min for up to three doses. Alternately, terbutaline sulfate, 0.25 mg, is administered subcutaneously every 20–30 min for up to three doses.

Further management is based on clinical response and improvements in pulmonary function testing. If these maneuvers improve the PEFR to more than 70% of baseline, the patient may be discharged, often with a short course of oral corticosteroids. For a PEFR that is 40–70% of baseline, the β-agonist therapy is continued (at intervals as frequent as every hour in patients without heart disease) and methylprednisolone, 80 mg every 6 h, is initiated. If the initial response results in a PEFR less than 40% of baseline, the patient should be admitted to hospital. A PEFR of less than 25% or $P\text{CO}_2$ of more than 35 mmHg suggests imminent respiratory failure. The patient should be admitted to an intensive care unit, where intravenous aminophylline may be added and nebulized beta-agonist therapy intensified. Intubation may be necessary if deterioration continues[15,37,43] (see Table 40.3).

Other obstructive lung disorders

Severe emphysema due to α_1-antitrypsin deficiency and cystic fibrosis (CF) can occur in women of childbearing age. Care of these patients is primarily supportive, with attention to the physiologic parameters of lung function and oxygenation discussed earlier. As noted, the effect of pregnancy on these diseases and the effect of these diseases on fetal outcome are more variable than with restrictive lung disorders. This is true primarily because pulmonary function can deteriorate rapidly as a result of the respiratory infections that frequently complicate these diseases.

A National Institutes of Health study followed 129 pregnancies in CF patients and found only 86 viable infants, leading the investigators to conclude that CF patients have greatly increased fetal wastage.[49] In the study, there were six spontaneous abortions, 25 therapeutic abortions, and 11 perinatal deaths. Ten of the perinatal deaths occurred in infants born at less than 37 weeks' gestation. Premature labor occurred in 26 of the 129 pregnancies, and infant mortality was 18% within 24 months of delivery.

The authors recommended that pregnancy be avoided unless the potential CF mother was clinically healthy. Published studies relate the severity of maternal disease at the onset of pregnancy more than the effects of CF on pregnancy to outcomes.[50,51] Factors such as pancreatic insufficiency, nutritional status, and low Taussig score were predictors of poor prognosis in pregnancy. Any woman with pulmonary hypertension should not undertake pregnancy.[50] A reasonable set of guidelines is to advise against pregnancy in any CF patient with a vital capacity (VC) of less than 50% of predicted, hypoxemia, pulmonary hypertension, or pancreatic insufficiency. The absence of pancreatic insufficiency may identify a subgroup more able to tolerate pregnancy.[52] A recent study showed that women with CF, after adjusting for demographic differences, who became pregnant did not have worse survival.[53]

Bronchial drainage, antibiotic therapy, prophylactic immunization (including annual influenza vaccine administration), and optimal nutritional and psychosocial care are essential components in the care of the CF patient contemplating pregnancy. Respiratory infections may be responsible for increased fetal and maternal mortality during pregnancy. Although the use of continuous antibiotic prophylaxis is controversial, therapy for acute exacerbations accompanied by a change in sputum character is effective.[54] Therapy is often given intravenously with antibiotics directed against *Pseudomonas aeruginosa* and *Staphylococcus aureus*, which commonly infect CF patients. Antibiotic therapy can be guided further by the results of sputum cultures. Most pregnant women with CF can successfully breastfeed, maintaining their own weight and supporting the growth of a healthy infant.[55]

Patients with α_1-antitrypsin deficiency or bronchiectasis are managed using the same principles. All should be regarded as high-risk patients, and serial spirometries and blood gas analyses are indicated.

Aspiration of stomach contents

The aspiration of low-pH liquid stomach contents into the tracheobronchial tree, with subsequent chemical pneumonitis, was first described in women undergoing labor and delivery. This syndrome is most likely to develop if aspirated material has a pH of less than 2.5, but some reports suggest that some degree of respiratory dysfunction can occur even if the pH of the aspirate is higher.[56,57] Other syndromes that can result from aspiration are bronchial obstruction by an aspirated foreign body and bacterial pneumonia from aspiration of oropharyngeal bacteria. Foreign body aspiration is managed by bronchoscopic removal, whereas aspiration pneumonia is treated with antibiotics, chosen on the basis of whether the event occurred out of hospital, shortly after admission, or during a prolonged hospitalization.[58]

In the pregnant patient, the acid aspiration syndrome is encountered more frequently and can lead to maternal mortality.[59] The pregnant woman is vulnerable to this problem because increased circulating progesterone levels tend to relax the esophageal sphincter and because the gravid uterus can compress the stomach and elevate intragastric pressure. Labor itself delays gastric emptying and, in one study, 55% of intrapartum patients had more than 40 mL of liquid gastric juice and 42% had a pH of less than 2.5.[60] Forceful abdominal manipulation and obtundation during anesthesia also add to the risk of aspiration.

In aspiration pneumonitis, there is generally a delay of at least 6–8 h before the first appearance of signs and symptoms such as bronchospasm, tachycardia, hypotension, tachypnea, cyanosis, and frothy pink sputum. Treatment of acid aspiration is supportive with O_2 and mechanical ventilation if needed. If aspiration is observed, endotracheal suctioning should be performed, but saline lavage is not indicated and may even serve to spread the acid to uninvolved areas. Bronchodilators may be used to control bronchospasm, and the prophylactic use of broad-spectrum antibiotics should be considered. Corticosteroids have been used in the treatment of witnessed gastric aspiration, but are of unproven benefit.

Prophylaxis of aspiration should always be undertaken in the pregnant patient undergoing surgery, with antacids given during labor to raise the gastric pH to more than 2.5 and thus reduce the chance of a dangerous aspiration. One study found that the risk of serious aspiration of gastric fluid with a pH of more than 2.5 could be reduced with the use of 30 mL of antacid given every 3 h after the onset of labor.[61] Gibbus and colleagues have demonstrated that adverse pulmonary reactions may result from aspirating antacid particles; thus, the use of nonparticulate agents is preferred.[62] Recently, various combinations of oral nonparticulate antacids and H_2-receptor blockers have been advocated as a convenient prophylactic regimen for patients about to undergo elective or emergency Cesarean section, but no particular combination appears to be clearly superior.[62] Additional prophylactic measures include limiting oral intake to essential medications once labor has started, nasogastric evacuation of a distended stomach, selection of regional anesthesia when possible, use of a cuffed endotracheal tube, and use of cricoid pressure during intubation.

Bacterial pneumonia

Pneumonia of all etiologies is a relatively common cause of maternal mortality. It has been reported in 0.1–0.84% of all pregnancies, with a mortality rate of 3.5–8.6%,[63] although antibiotics and modern obstetric care have improved the prognosis.[64] *Streptococcus pneumoniae* is the most common infectious agent implicated in antepartum pneumonia, and other common bacterial pathogens include *Mycoplasma pneumoniae* and *Haemophilus influenzae*.[64] *Legionella pneumoniae* and *Listeria monocytogenes* have rarely been reported to cause respiratory failure in pregnancy.[65–67]

Pneumococcal pneumonia classically begins with the abrupt onset of shaking chills, fever, pleuritic chest pain, cough productive of purulent sputum, and shortness of breath. The physical examination often shows signs of consolidation, such as dullness to percussion, tactile fremitus, and egobronchophony. A chest radiograph usually reveals evidence of lobar consolidation, but bronchopneumonia may also occur. Laboratory examination may reveal a polymorphonuclear leukocytosis in the range of 12 000–25 000 cells/mL, but a normal white blood cell count can also be seen, especially in patients with overwhelming infection and bacteremia. A sputum specimen for culture and Gram's stain should generally be obtained and may demonstrate Gram-positive encapsulated cocci in pairs and short chains. Blood cultures are positive in approximately 20–30% of patients and should be collected before the administration of antibiotics.

Although penicillin U has long been considered the antibiotic of choice, recent evidence suggests that penicillin nonsusceptibility is found in nearly 40% of strains of *Streptococcus pneumoniae* causing disease in adults.[68,69] Given this, any gravid patient thought to have bacterial pneumonia should be admitted to the hospital and started on a third-generation cephalosporin and a macrolide (e.g., azithromycin) until sputum culture reveals the causal organism and sensitivities. Once established, antibiotic treatment can be tailored to the responsible organism. This will typically lead to defervescence within 48 h. Once the patient is afebrile for 48 h, parenteral antibiotic therapy can be discontinued and oral cephalosporin continued for 10–14 days.[69]

Mycobacterium pneumoniae produces symptoms similar to a viral infection, with a flu-like syndrome, interstitial infiltrates, and alveolar filling. Small pleural effusions are common, and approximately 50% of affected patients have cold agglutinins in their serum. Because tetracycline is relatively contraindicated in pregnancy, erythromycin is the drug of choice. *Haemophilus influenzae* pneumonia may have a gradual rather than an abrupt onset and may be clinically indistinguishable from *S. pneumoniae*. It is infrequently seen in young adults unless the patient has a history of chronic obstructive lung disease or is an alcoholic. Sputum Gram's stain usually shows abundant neutrophils and pleomorphic coccobacillary Gram-negative organisms. The chest radiograph may show either bronchial or lobar consolidation, and pleural effusions are common. Again, because the occurrence of ampicillin resistance may be significant,[70] the patient should be managed as stated above with susceptibility testing performed on all culture isolates and antibiotic therapy tailored appropriately.

Influenza

Although the exact mortality rate from influenza during pregnancy is not known, during the 1918 influenza epidemic, maternal mortality with the illness varied from 30% to 50%.[71,73] In one study from the 1957 epidemic, pregnancy increased mortality ninefold in the 20- to 29-year age group.[73] In a review of all deaths due to influenza from 1957 through 1960, 1–11% occurred in pregnant patients.[73] These deaths were concentrated late in the third trimester and early puerperium and were more likely to occur with increased maternal age. In more recent studies, 39–60% of asymptomatic pregnant women had serologic evidence of recent influenza infection, and up to 35% of pregnant symptomatic women had no serologic evidence of recent influenza infection.[71,74,75] Because earlier studies were based on the clinical diagnosis of influenza, the conclusion that pregnancy predisposes to infection or to an enhanced severity of illness is controversial.[71]

Influenza usually begins abruptly with systemic symptoms, such as headache, fever, chills, myalgia, and malaise accompanied by an upper respiratory illness. In an uncomplicated case, complaints of a sore throat and cough may persist for a week or more. Physical findings may be minimal, but reddened engorgement of the mucous membranes and a postnasal discharge can be seen along with mild cervical adenopathy. The chest examination may be normal but can reveal rhonchi, wheezes, and scattered rales. Occasionally, the disease can progress rapidly to fulminant cardiopulmonary failure, or it can be complicated by secondary bacterial or mixed viral–bacterial pneumonia involving *Streptococcus*, *Staphylococcus*, or *H. influenzae*.

Amantadine, an oral antiviral agent active against influenza A, can be used therapeutically and prevents 70–90% of experimentally produced and natural infections. It is not effective in treating infections due to influenza B. If used within 48 h of the onset of symptoms, amantadine shortens the duration of the illness by up to 50%, reduces fever, and hastens the resumption of normal activities.[76,77] If given concomitantly with an influenza vaccine, it can protect the patient for the 2–3 weeks necessary for immunity to develop during exposure to an epidemic. Other antivirals, such as zanamivir and osteltamivir, may reduce the duration of uncomplicated influenza A and B. No clinical study has been conducted regarding the safety or efficacy of any of these antiviral medications during pregnancy. Because safety during pregnancy has not been adequately established, the Committee on Obstetric Practice recommends that these medications be used only if the practitioner thinks the "potential benefits justify the potential risks."[76]

Although influenza virus can cross the placenta, it has not been isolated from fetal blood,[71] and transplacental passage does not appear to cause congenital defects. Fetal abnormalities, such as circulatory defects, central nervous system malformations, cleft lip, and childhood cancer, have been attributed to influenza, but most investigators have concluded that no influenza-induced congenital syndrome exists.[71,78] Influenza vaccine may be administered appropriately in pregnant women in any trimester with standard indications for such immunization. Because increased mortality from infections usually occurs late in pregnancy, vaccination can often be delayed until the middle of the second trimester if necessary.[79]

Viral pneumonia

Other life-threatening viral pneumonias can develop in the pregnant patient, including varicella pneumonia, which may accompany chickenpox and can range from a mild to a rapidly fatal illness. In pregnancy, varicella is rare; however, if pneumonia develops, mortality is high, ranging from 30% to 40% in some series.[80–82] Varicella pneumonia has been associated with an increased incidence of premature labor.[82] The pneumonia can be completely asymptomatic but, in its severe form, it is accompanied by tachypnea, high fever, cough, dyspnea, and pleuritic chest pain. The chest examination may be unimpressive and correlates poorly with the severity of the pneumonia, but the chest radiograph usually shows extensive bilateral, peribronchial, fluffy, nodular infiltrates, which are more prominent when the skin eruption is maximal.[82] In severe cases, rapid pulmonary deterioration requiring intubation can occur within a matter of hours. Maternal varicella infection in any trimester of pregnancy can be associated with infrequent, but possibly lethal, congenital anomalies. If the maternal infection occurs within 5 days of delivery, the infant is at risk of fatal disseminated infection. Given the high mortality rate associated with varicella pneumonia occurring in pregnancy and the lack of demonstrated human fetal toxicity, it is recommended that any gravid patient with varicella pneumonia be admitted to the hospital for parenteral therapy with acyclovir. The dose is 500 mg/m^2 every 8 h and should be continued until symptoms of the illness resolve.[83,84] An important consideration of varicella pneumonia during pregnancy is the issue of prevention. Patients considering pregnancy should be questioned regarding their history of varicella and, if unsure, titers should be drawn to confirm immunity. If the patient is not immune, then the varicella vaccine can be given prior to pregnancy. If the patient is not immune, but exposed to varicella peripartum, many authors have recommended administration of varicella zoster immune globulin.[85]

Fungal pneumonia

Cryptococcus neoformans, *Blastomyces dermatitidis*, and *Sporothrix schenckii* have rarely been reported as causing serious respiratory infection in pregnancy. The clinical course and outcome are generally the same in pregnant and nonpregnant patients.[86] It has been estimated that coccidioidomycosis occurs in less than 1 in every 1000 pregnancies.[87] However, infection in pregnancy, particularly during the second and third trimesters, increases the rate of disseminated infection from 0.2% to more than 20%.[87] It has been suggested that 17β-estradiol has a stimulatory effect on the fungus and may be responsible for the increased risk of dissemination associated with pregnancy.[88] Maternal mortality rate from disseminated coccidioidomycosis approaches 100%, a rate approximately twice that seen in nonpregnant patients,[87] and dissemination is associated with increased fetal prematurity and mortality.[87]

Symptomatic pulmonary coccidioidomycosis manifests as cough, fever, chest pain, malaise, and occasionally hypersensitivity reactions. Chest radiography may show an infiltrate, hilar adenopathy, or pleural effusions. The peripheral blood count may show eosinophilia. The diagnosis is made by serologic testing and by culture and wet smear examination of sputum, urine, and pus. Dissemination should be suspected in the setting of rapidly progressive respiratory failure with a clinical picture similar to miliary tuberculosis.[65]

Amphotericin B has been used to treat cryptococcoses, blastomycosis, and disseminated coccidioidomycosis in pregnancy.[86,87] It crosses the placenta and can be found in both amniotic fluid and fetal blood. Although use in pregnancy has not been well studied, normal, full-term infants have been born to patients who received amphotericin B in the first trimester.[88] Its use is associated with anemia; thus, serial hematocrits must be followed.

Pneumocystis carinii pneumonia

Pneumocystis carinii pneumonia is the most common opportunistic infection affecting the lungs of patients with acquired immunodeficiency syndrome (AIDS).[89–92] It can be confused with atypical mycobacterial infection, cryptococcoses, and histoplasmosis. Clinically, *P. carinii* pneumonia manifests with fever, dyspnea, and nonproductive cough, which may have an insidious onset followed by a rapid progressive deterioration. Arterial blood gases usually demonstrate hypoxemia with an increased alveolar–arterial gradient and respiratory alkalosis, and the chest radiograph classically shows bilateral diffuse infiltrates beginning in the perihilar regions and lower lung fields that progress to involve the entire parenchyma. Diagnosis is made by specific staining of sputum, bronchial aspirates, or material obtained by bronchoscopically performed bronchoalveolar lavage or biopsy.

There are several case reports of *P. carinii* pneumonia (PCP) complicating pregnancy[90–92] and evidence to suggest that PCP has a more aggressive course during pregnancy, with increased morbidity and mortality. Because of the current level of asymptomatic human immunodeficiency virus (HIV) infection and because women of childbearing age represent a significant portion of some of the groups at risk for AIDS, the number of infected mothers will continue to increase. In one published case series of 22 pregnant women with PCP, 60% of these patients required mechanical ventilation and 11 patients died of pneumonia. These patients were treated with a variety of regimens, but the treatment of choice in pregnant women with AIDS and *P carinii* pneumonia is trimethoprim–sulfamethoxazole (SXT).[92] Concomitant use of steroids is controversial. Studies of *in utero* exposure to SXT failed to show an increase in prematurity, hyperbilirubinemia, or kernicterus.[93] Patients should be monitored for drug toxicity, such as rash, fever, neutropenia, thrombocytopenia, and hepatitis. Nausea and vomiting may occur and can exacerbate hyperemesis gravidarum. Pentamidine is an alternative therapy, but its use has not been studied in pregnancy.

In patients who cannot tolerate trimethoprim–sulfamethoxazole, pentamidine may be required because of the life-threatening risk of withholding treatment from the mother.[94] If pentamidine is used, the mother should be closely monitored for hypoglycemia. Aerosolized pentamidine, because of poor systemic absorption and decreased systemic side-effects, has been advocated as safe, effective prophylaxis for *P. carinii* pneumonia.[95] Treatment of even mild cases of *P. carinii* pneumonia with aerosolized pentamidine may be effective, but some investigators have discouraged this therapy because of a concern about treatment failure.[96] Pyrimethamine–sulfadoxine has been used as prophylaxis, and no fetal malformations have been associated with its use. However, because it is a folate antagonist, it should be used cautiously. Prophylaxis against PCP with trimethoprim–sulfamethoxazole is known to be very effective, with rates of prevention of 90–95%.[96] Given this, in pregnant patients with known HIV-positive status, prophylaxis should be strongly considered.

Amniotic fluid embolism

Amniotic fluid embolism (AFE) is a devastating, pregnancy-specific condition in which both maternal and fetal death is the most probable outcome.[97] It is one of the principal causes of maternal death in developed countries. In a high percentage of survivors, profound neurologic impairment is seen. Although an immunologic basis for this syndrome (similar to anaphylaxis) has been postulated and discussed for decades, a recent report from the national AFE registry provided direct support for the anaphylactoid nature of this condition, based on marked clinical similarities between a large series of patients with AFE and patients with both septic and anaphylactic shock.[97]

Clinically, AFE manifests by the sudden development of hypoxia, hypotension, or cardiac arrest and disseminated intravascular coagulation (DIC). All components of the full AFE syndrome are not invariably present. AFE occurs as fetal tissue enters the maternal circulation and incites the reaction described above, probably via the release of various endogenous mediators. This most commonly occurs during labor but, in susceptible maternal–infant pairs, it has clinical onset at the time of Cesarean section with roughly the same frequency as the Cesarean rate in the general population.[97]

Table 40.5 Signs and symptoms found in patients with amniotic fluid embolism.

Sign or symptom	No. of patients	%
Hypotension	43	100
Fetal distress*	30	100
Pulmonary edema or adult respiratory distress syndrome	28	93
Cardiopulmonary arrest	40	87
Cyanosis	38	83
Coagulopathy	38	83
Dyspnea	22	49
Seizure	22	48
Atony	11	23
Bronchospasm	7	15
Transient hypertension	5	11
Cough	3	7
Headache	3	7
Chest pain	1	2

*In undelivered fetuses.

From ref. 89, with permission.

In the past, a pattern of hypertonic uterine contractions was implicated in the genesis of AFE.[98] This theory has been clearly rejected on statistical, clinical, and theoretical grounds.[98,99] Uterine hypertonicity, similar to that seen with eclamptic seizures, is a response to hypoxia and stress-induced norepinephrine release, and is an early manifestation of impending hemodynamic collapse.[100] Fetal bradycardia commonly precedes maternal physiologic manifestations. Commonly observed clinical signs and symptoms are outlined in Table 40.5.[97]

There is currently no way to predict or prevent AFE. Treatment of the mother is supportive and involves the administration of O_2 in response to clinical hypoxia, preload and inotropic support of falling blood pressure, and blood component replacement for DIC with clinical hemorrhage. With the development of lethal cardiac dysrhythmia, standard basic and advanced cardiac life support protocols should be instituted.

In the presence of maternal cardiac arrest, maternal survival without profound neurologic impairment is rarely achieved.[97] However, a clear relationship exists between arrest-to-delivery interval and neonatal outcome (Table 40.6).[97] Thus, expeditious perimortem Cesarean section should be initiated on the diagnosis of maternal cardiac arrest, regardless of its etiology, assuming the gestation has advanced to the point of fetal via-

Table 40.6 Cardiac arrest-to-delivery interval and neonatal outcome in amniotic fluid embolism.

Interval (minutes)	Survival (no. of subjects)	Intact survival (no. of subjects)
< 5	3/3	2/3 (67%)
5–15	3/3	2/3 (67%)
16–25	2/5	2/5 (40%)
26–35	3/4	1/4 (25%)
36–54	0/1	0/1 (0%)

bility.[97] When maternal hemodynamic or respiratory instability exists short of frank arrest, the situation becomes far more complex, and valid generalizations about fetal intervention are not possible.

The diagnosis of AFE is a clinical one based on physiologic manifestations and must be made after the exclusion of other conditions, such as myocardial infarction and pulmonary thromboembolism. The presence of a consumptive coagulopathy, although not required for the diagnosis of AFE, supports its diagnosis because acute consumptive coagulopathy in obstetrics is limited to AFE and placental abruption.[97,98,101] Further, because placental abruption provides a classic opportunity for admixture of placental thromboplastin and other tissue of fetal origin with the maternal circulation, these two entities commonly occur together, with clinical manifestations depending on the maternal response to the fetal tissue.[102] Because some fetal debris is commonly found in the maternal circulation, the presence or absence of histologic pulmonary findings is not sufficient by itself to make the diagnosis of AFE, nor does its absence rule this syndrome out in the presence of appropriate clinical manifestations.[98,99]

Venous air embolism

Venous air embolism may account for as many as 1% of maternal deaths,[65] with risk factors being the performance of surgery, intravenous infusions, and central venous catheter placement. However, because the venous sinuses of the uterus are particularly susceptible to the entry of air during pregnancy, air embolism can occur during normal labor, delivery of a placenta previa, criminal abortions using air, orogenital sex,[103] and insufflation of the vagina during gynecologic procedures.[103,104] Maternal mortality associated with a clinically significant event exceeds 90% in untreated cases.[105] The severity of a venous air embolism depends on the amount and rate of air entry. Small amounts of venous air are clinically undetectable, but accidental bolus injections of 100–300 mL^3 of air have been reported to be fatal.[103] However, there are reports of patients surviving infusions of up to 1600 mL^3.[105,106]

Embolization of a large bolus of venous air to the right ventricle results in mechanical obstruction to the forward flow of blood in the pulmonary artery outflow tract.[107] In addition, the pumping action of the right ventricle acting on blood and air may produce platelet damage and fibrin formation, resulting in fibrin emboli that lodge in the pulmonary vascular bed. Maldistribution of pulmonary blood flow may result in ischemia or hyperperfusion, with the hyperperfused areas being susceptible to developing interstitial and alveolar edema. Areas that are initially ischemic may also become abnormally permeable once perfusion is restored.[107] In animal models, the permeability pulmonary edema after venous air embolism has been related to leukocyte production and the release of toxic O_2 metabolites.[108] Paradoxical embolization can occur if there is an atrial septal defect, resulting in arterial ischemia or occlusion.[109]

The patient initially presents with a feeling of faintness, dizziness, fear of impending doom, dyspnea, cough, diaphoresis, and substernal chest pain.

Physical examination may reveal a state of altered consciousness, cyanosis, tachypnea, wheezing, tachycardia, hypotension, elevated jugular venous pressure, gallop rhythm, and an evanescent "mill wheel" or "waterwheel" murmur heard over the precordium.[65,109] Paradoxical embolism may be evidenced by bubbles in the retinal arterioles, marble-like skin (air in superficial dermal vessels), and possibly stroke or myocardial infarction.[109] A blood gas test characteristically reveals hypoxemia, and there may be an associated metabolic acidosis. Chest radiography may occasionally demonstrate air in the right side of the heart or the main pulmonary artery, and the electrocardiogram may show signs of right heart strain, ischemia, or arrhythmia.[65,109] Therapy must be instituted promptly, and the patient should be placed in the left lateral decubitus position to minimize obstruction to the right ventricular outflow tract.

Administration of 100% O_2 promotes removal of nitrogen from the air bubble and results in more rapid absorption of the embolus. Nitrous oxide is highly soluble and, in a patient receiving general anesthesia, it should be discontinued because it can increase the size of the air embolus.[106] In the presence of cardiovascular collapse, closed chest compression and aspiration of air from the right side of the heart via venous catheterization or transthoracic puncture have been suggested, although actual improved survival of pregnant women so treated has not been demonstrated. Hyperbaric O_2 may be useful in the setting of cerebral venous air embolism, and anticoagulation has been suggested to minimize the formation of fibrin microemboli.[106,107] Mechanical ventilation may be necessary to treat permeability pulmonary edema.

Adult respiratory distress syndrome

Adult respiratory distress syndrome (ARDS) is the final common pathway of pathophysiologic changes occurring in the lungs as a consequence of a variety of acute bodily insults that reach the lung directly or via the vasculature (Table 40.7).

Table 40.7 Causes of adult respiratory distress syndrome in pregnant women.

Abruptio placentae
Air embolism
Amniotic fluid embolism
Aspiration
Bacterial pneumonia
Blood transfusion
Carcinomatosis
Dead fetus syndrome
Diabetic ketoacidosis
Drugs (narcotics, barbiturates)
Fat embolism
Fractures
Fungal and *Pneumocystis carinii* pneumonia
Head trauma
Inhaled toxin
Intra-abdominal abscess
Lung contusion
Nonthoracic trauma
Pancreatitis
Preeclampsia, eclampsia
Seizure
Septic abortion
Septicemia
Shock
Tocolytic therapy with sympathomimetics and glucocorticoids
Tuberculosis
Uremia

Clinically, patients present with marked respiratory distress, tachypnea, hypoxemia refractory to O_2 therapy, "stiff' noncompliant lungs that require high pressures to achieve inflation, and diffuse bilateral interstitial and alveolar infiltrates on chest radiograph.[110] The central pathophysiologic event in ARDS is injury to the alveolar–capillary membrane, either directly or via mediators delivered by the pulmonary vasculature, which results in increased vascular permeability and noncardiogenic pulmonary edema. Severe hypoxemia results from both increased shunting of unoxygenated blood and impaired ventilation and perfusion matching in the alveoli, with an arterial PO_2 of typically less than 50–60 mmHg despite an inspired O_2 concentration of 60% or more.[111] To make the diagnosis of ARDS, chronic pulmonary disease and left heart failure (cardiogenic pulmonary edema) must be excluded, and an appropriate precipitating event should be present. Right heart catheterization is often required to demonstrate that the pulmonary capillary hydrostatic pressure is not elevated,[112] but the data thus obtained should be assessed in the light of the expected decrease in colloid oncotic pressure during pregnancy and in the immediate postpartum period.[113] Mortality in patients with ARDS continues to exceed 50%, a figure that has remained fairly constant over the last 20 years.[114]

In the pregnant patient, ARDS can be associated with many of the factors that complicate pregnancy and delivery, including septicemia, AFE, aspiration of stomach contents, eclampsia, septic abortion, venous air embolism, abruptio placentae, blood transfusion (with white blood cell agglutination in the pulmonary circulation), dead fetus syndrome (with DIC), drug overdose (narcotics, barbiturates, aspirin), fat embolism (after long bone fracture), hemorrhagic shock, seizures, and overwhelming pneumonia. The incidence of ARDS in pregnancy is unknown but, in one general hospital respiratory care unit, 9.5% of all patients carried this diagnosis, and it is estimated that more than 150 000 cases occur annually in the United States.[115]

Pathophysiology

Except in cases of direct damage to the alveolar–capillary membrane (e.g., via inhaled toxins, aspiration, invasive organisms), the specific mechanisms that initiate lung injury in ARDS are generally incompletely understood. Multiple humoral and cellular mediators contribute to the intense inflammatory response that characterizes ARDS. These mediators include polymorphonuclear leukocytes, alveolar macrophages, platelets, free fatty acids, arachidonic acid metabolites (prostaglandins, leukotrienes, thromboxane A), fibrin-derived peptides, and tumor necrosis factor.[111,116–119] Initial injury to the alveolar–capillary membrane results in increased endothelial cell permeability and noncardiogenic pulmonary edema.[111,120,121] This capillary leak is the earliest finding in ARDS and results in the accumulation of protein-rich fluid in the extravascular space of the lung, initially in the interstitium and later in the alveolar sacs. Alveolar type I epithelial cells are injured, the alveolar basement membrane is denuded, and the alveolar space fills with red blood cells, leukocytes, macrophages, and cell debris. Damage to the epithelium results in the loss of surfactant and alveolar collapse. Early hyaline membranes composed of protein, fibrin, and cellular debris can be seen.[122]

Morphologically, epithelial cell injury is more obvious than endothelial cell injury, which may indicate a greater reparative capacity of the endothelial cells.[122] After 24–96 h, the early exudative phase of injury is followed by a cellular proliferative phase, with repopulation of the alveolar basement membrane by alveolar type 2 cells. The hyaline membrane begins to organize, and morphologic evidence of endothelial injury is more obvious.[122] This phase is present from the third to the 10th day and is followed by a fibrotic proliferative phase as the hyaline membranes undergo fibrosis.

Clinical presentation

Clinically, the patient with ARDS of any etiology may go through four clinical stages:

1 injury;
2 apparent stability;
3 respiratory insufficiency;
4 terminal stage.

The initial injury may occur without outward clinical signs and usually lasts for 6 h or more. Next, the patient develops dyspnea associated with rapid shallow breathing and a persistent cough. Approximately 12–24 h after injury, the chest radiograph may begin to show bilateral infiltrates that coalesce into a diffuse haze, representing perivascular fluid accumulation, interstitial edema, and alveolar edema. As the disease progresses, mechanical ventilation is usually required because the pulmonary edema and localized atelectasis have resulted in ventilation–perfusion mismatching and an increased alveolar–arterial O_2 gradient that is resistant to high inspired O_2 concentrations.[111] Other physiologic derangements include an increase in physiologic dead space, frequently exceeding 60% of each breath and resulting in significant carbon dioxide retention, despite the presence of a very high minute ventilation. Narrowing and obstruction of the pulmonary vessels, primarily caused by edema fluid, results in "stiff" lungs and is often associated with a high pulmonary arterial pressure despite a low or normal capillary hydrostatic pressure.

Therapy

Corticosteroids, in doses up to several grams of methylprednisolone over 24 h, have been widely used in the treatment of full-blown ARDS without good evidence that they are effective.[123] However, although corticosteroids have not been shown to be effective in treating "early ARDS," there is some evidence to suggest that their use in the management of "late ARDS" is useful. The ARDS Net group recently completed enrollment in a randomized, double-blind trial comparing corticosteroid with placebo treatment in severe, late ARDS, a study which suggested the usefulness of corticosteroids. The use of corticosteroids and mineralocorticoids to treat patients who are in shock that might be caused by or accompanied by adrenal insufficiency is warranted. Surfactant, a complex substance containing phospholipids and apoproteins, is used to treat RDS in premature infants, but there are some data to suggest that, when instilled by way of bronchoscopy, it may be useful in the treatment of ARDS.[124,125] Efforts to identify pharmacologic agents effective in enhancing lung repair or blocking mediators of lung injury in ARDS have been largely unsuccessful. Nonsteroidal anti-inflammatory drugs, such as ibuprofen, meclofenamate, and indomethacin, have been studied *in vitro* and in animals and have shown some promise.[126,127]

The care of a patient with ARDS is primarily supportive, with the mainstays of therapy being supplemental O_2 and the application of positive end-expiratory pressure (PEEP). Despite the lack of any clear evidence that its use improves mortality rates, PEEP is almost universally employed because it improves oxygenation and can reduce O_2 needs below potentially toxic concentrations.[128] The early application of PEEP (prophylactic PEEP) cannot prevent the development of ARDS.[129]

Reversible causes of ARDS, such as occult intra-abdominal or pelvic abscesses, should be sought because early surgical intervention and antimicrobial therapy may be life-saving. Patients with abruptio placentae, dead fetus syndrome, and septic abortion often have accompanying DIC. These patients should undergo delivery of the fetus or evacuation of the uterus as soon as the coagulopathy has been addressed and the patient is surgically stable.

Mechanical ventilation

Ventilator therapy should be instituted when refractory hypoxemia is present and should be considered at the earliest recognition of ARDS-related symptoms to ensure fetal well-being. With correction of hypoxemia and respiratory alkalosis, fetal O_2 delivery can often be maintained at an adequate level. Pregnant patients with ARDS should be placed in the left lateral decubitus position, with the right buttock and hip elevated approximately 15°, or with the uterus manually displaced to the left, to maximize venous return. Continuous external fetal heart monitoring should be instituted when appropriate, and pulse oximetry can permit continuous monitoring of arterial oxygenation. Periodic blood gas determinations should be obtained to check acid–base status.

When indicated, volume-cycled mechanical ventilation is begun, using 100% O_2, at a respiratory rate of 10–12 breaths/min. Traditionally, a TV of 10–15 mL/kg was utilized, but a National Institutes of Health (NIH)-sponsored ARDS Net trial compared the outcomes of 861 patients with ARDS at a TV of 6 versus 12 mL/kg. They found an overall 22% reduction in mortality rate, more ventilator-free days, and more organ failure-free days in the low tidal volume group.[129] The maternal pH should be maintained in the normal pregnancy range of 7.4 to 7.47, with an arterial CO_2 between 25 and 32 mmHg. Under normobaric conditions, the F_IO_2, initially set at 1.0, can be continued for up to 24 h without the threat of pulmonary O_2 toxicity.[128] An F_IO_2 of 0.5 can be administered indefinitely without adverse sequelae. In ARDS, the increased work of breathing caused by noncompliant lungs and the increased airway resistance caused by bronchial edema and possibly bronchospasm can be relieved using the continuous mandatory ventilation mode of mechanical ventilation, which allows the respiratory muscles to rest completely, thereby reducing O_2 consumption. Use of the continuous mandatory ventilation mode may require sedation or paralysis to maximize ventilation and minimize patient O_2 requirements and discomfort. Should a vaginal delivery of the fetus be contemplated while the patient is intubated, withdrawal of sedation and a change of respirator mode to intermittent mandatory ventilation is probably warranted to allow the patient to assist in the delivery effort.[130]

If the maternal arterial O_2 saturation cannot be maintained at or above 90%, with an F_IO_2 of 0.6 or less, then PEEP should be added. PEEP recruits atelectatic areas for gas exchange that would otherwise collapse during expiration and which are difficult to expand due to the loss of surfactant and structural derangements. The result is an increase in systemic arterial O_2 tension and in the lung's FRC and compliance.[131–133] The use of PEEP is not without pitfalls, however, as it can overdistend alveoli, thereby decreasing compliance and increasing the risk of pneumothorax. The most important adverse effect is to decrease cardiac output by impeding venous return to the right side of the heart, particularly when the blood volume is low.[134] Application of PEEP is accomplished by titrating upward from levels of 5 cmH_2O and checking P_aO_2 15–30 min later. By following serial arterial blood gases or using a pulse oximeter, PEEP can be increased until either the required F_IO_2 is less than 0.6 or cardiac output declines. Generally, levels of more than 15 cmH_2O are not required, but values as high as 20 cmH_2O may occasionally be necessary to provide an appreciable increase in arterial O_2. Applying PEEP at high levels may lead to retention of excessive lung water. If PEEP is then decreased, this lung water can flood alveoli and lead to a deterioration in gas exchange, which is not easily reversible by simply raising levels of PEEP.[135] This problem can be avoided by starting PEEP at low levels and then gradually increasing as needed.[129]

An optimal PEEP has been defined as a level that increases oxygenation without significantly reducing cardiac output and, consequently, O_2 delivery. Studies have shown that this level correlates with maximal pulmonary compliance.[134] Use of a pulmonary artery catheter permits the calculation of maximal pulmonary compliance or "best PEEP" by direct sampling of the mixed venous O_2 saturation (S_vO_2) and measuring the cardiac output by the thermodilution method. The S_vO_2 reflects the balance between tissue O_2 delivery and tissue O_2 utilization and declines with inadequate tissue perfusion. The normal average value for S_vO_2 is 73%, with saturations of less than 60% considered low. Because of the altered pulmonary capillary permeability inherent in ARDS, an increase in pulmonary capillary blood pressure that would be well tolerated by a healthy individual may cause life-threatening pulmonary edema in a patient with ARDS. Therefore, the ultimate goal of fluid management in ARDS is to maintain adequate maternal and fetal tissue O_2 delivery while keeping pulmonary microvascular pressures as low as possible, a task made easier with the use of a pulmonary artery catheter to measure pulmonary capillary wedge pressure and cardiac output serially. Units of packed red cells are given to patients who are anemic and who would benefit from the increased O_2-carrying capacity provided by blood transfusion.

Therapy of ARDS in the pregnant patient is complicated because a cardiac output sufficient to supply maternal needs may not be adequate for placental perfusion. Additionally, vasopressor drugs often used to increase cardiac output may have deleterious effects on uterine blood flow. Given the lack of available information on the effects of hemodynamic and pharmacologic manipulation on uterine blood flow in the critically ill patient, it seems prudent to lower intravascular volume only to a level tolerated by the circulation and to avoid excessive pharmacologic manipulation. External fetal heart rate monitoring is a useful adjunct in assessing fetal O_2 delivery.[130]

After the initiation of therapy for ARDS, the patient may begin to show signs of improvement, with less impairment of gas exchange and increases in lung compliance and S_vO_2. If the F_IO_2 can be reduced to less than 0.5 and PEEP can be reduced to 5 cmH_2O, consideration should be given to weaning the patient from mechanical ventilation. Most patients who are successfully weaned require supplemental O_2 for several days or more after mechanical ventilation is discontinued.

Complications

Therapy of ARDS requires knowledge not only of the disease process and its management but also of associated complications. Table 40.8 lists complications resulting from intubation

Table 40.8 Complications associated with adult respiratory distress syndrome.

Pulmonary
Pulmonary emboli
Pulmonary barotrauma
Pulmonary fibrosis
Pulmonary complications of ventilatory and monitoring procedures
Mechanical ventilation
Right main stem intubation
Alveolar hypoventilation
Swan–Ganz catheterization
Pulmonary infarction
Pulmonary hemorrhage
Gastrointestinal
Gastrointestinal hemorrhage
Ileus
Gastric distention
Pneumoperitoneum
Renal
Renal failure
Fluid retention
Cardiac
Arrhythmia
Hypotension
Low cardiac output
Infection
Sepsis
Nosocomial pneumonia
Hematologic
Anemia
Thrombocytopenia
Disseminated intravascular coagulation
Other
Hepatic
Endocrine
Neurologic
Psychiatric

From ref. 100, with permission.

and mechanical ventilation and emphasizes that this severe disease can involve many organ systems in addition to the lungs. Two specific complications, pulmonary barotrauma and infection, merit special attention.

Pulmonary barotrauma is common. In one series of ARDS patients, 38% of the group was found to have pneumomediastinum or pneumothorax.[136] Pneumothorax may cause further deterioration in gas exchange, and tension pneumothorax may produce life-threatening pulmonary and cardiovascular deterioration. Factors that have been implicated as predisposing to these complications include high inflation pressures resulting from poor lung compliance, large TVs, and high levels of PEEP. Approximately two-thirds of all critically ill patients have respiratory tract colonization with Gram-negative bacteria, and Brodie and colleagues found concurrent pneumonia in a majority of patients with ARDS.[137] Intravenous catheters, endotracheal tubes, bladder catheters, and intra-arterial cannulae can all be sources of infection. Respiratory assistance devices and medical personnel are other potential sources of infection.[138,139]

Infection can be both an important etiologic factor in ARDS and a secondary complication that increases mortality. Ashbaugh and Petty,[140] in a retrospective review of 51 patients with ARDS, reported a mortality of 70% in patients who acquired respiratory infection, in contrast to a fatality rate of 40% in patients without respiratory tract infection. Seidenfeld et al.[141] found a mortality of more than 70% in ARDS patients with infection, whereas mortality was only 20% when patients were free from infection.

Pneumonia in the setting of ARDS is notoriously difficult to diagnose. In one study, although 58% of patients with ARDS had histologic evidence of pneumonia,[126] 36% of these cases were not clinically detected, and 20% of those without pneumonia were incorrectly given this diagnosis. Fever, leukocytosis, and focal infiltrates may be present in ARDS patients, independent of the presence of pneumonia. The relatively recent development of the bronchoscopically directed, protected specimen brush may help to make this diagnosis in complicated patients.[142]

In addition to pneumonia, other infections may complicate the course of ARDS. Nasotracheal and large nasogastric tubes predispose to bacterial sinusitis by blocking ventilation and drainage of the sinuses. Sinus infections are particularly likely to occur in patients who have underlying disorders of the nasal passages and in those who have sustained either facial trauma or trauma due to instrumentation. Parenteral empiric antibiotics should cover both Gram-positive and nosocomial Gram-negative organisms, and patients may benefit from a topical nasal decongestant. Other complications of ARDS include airway trauma from translaryngeal intubation[143] and persistent pulmonary function abnormalities (both small airways disease and reduced diffusion).[144,145]

Key points

1 Normal respiratory physiology is altered in pregnancy, and these changes must be considered when evaluating tests of lung function.

2 When a patient with known lung disease seeks advice about the risks of pregnancy, pulmonary function studies should be obtained.

3 If at any time during pregnancy, the health of the mother or fetus would be compromised by failure to perform a radiologic examination, the examination should be performed and every care should be taken to shield the fetus from scatter radiation and from the direct beam when appropriate.

4 Chest radiographs performed in the pregnant patient have normal findings that differ from those seen in nonpregnant women of childbearing age. The diaphragm may be elevated 4 cm at term, but there is a compensatory increase in anteroposterior diameter. The subcostal angle increases from 68.5° to 103.5° from early to late pregnancy. Lung markings may be increased, giving a false impression of mild congestive heart failure.

5 Because the fetus operates on the steep portion of the O_2 dissociation curve (normal fetal venous P_aO_2 is close to 33 mmHg), decreases in maternal P_aO_2 below 60–70 mmHg during an acute asthma exacerbation can result in rapid and profound decrease in fetal O_2 saturation and fetal hypoxia.

6 Good asthma control is perhaps the most important factor in improving maternal and fetal outcomes.

7 Effective management of asthma in pregnant women relies on four components: patient education, avoidance or control of environmental precipitating factors, objective assessment of maternal lung function and fetal well-being, and pharmacologic therapy.

8 It is reasonable to advise any patient with cystic fibrosis against pregnancy if there is evidence of a VC of less than 50% of predicted or of hypoxemia, pulmonary hypertension, or pancreatic insufficiency. The absence of pancreatic insufficiency may identify a subgroup more able to tolerate pregnancy.

9 Bronchial drainage, antibiotic therapy, prophylactic immunization (including annual influenza vaccine administration), and optimal nutritional and psychosocial care are essential components in the care of the CF patient contemplating pregnancy.

10 In aspiration pneumonitis, there is generally a delay of at least 6–8 hours before the first appearance of signs and symptoms such as bronchospasm, tachycardia, hypotension, tachypnea, cyanosis, and frothy pink sputum.

11 Prophylaxis of aspiration should always be undertaken in the pregnant patient undergoing surgery and during labor to raise the gastric pH to more than 2.5 and thus reduce the chance of a dangerous aspiration.

12 *Streptococcus pneumoniae* is the most common infectious agent implicated in antepartum pneumonia, but other common bacterial pathogens include *Mycoplasma pneumoniae* and *Haemophilus influenzae.*

13 Gravid patients thought to have bacterial pneumonia should be admitted to hospital and started on a third-generation cephalosporin and a macrolide.

14 Influenza vaccine may be appropriately administered in pregnant women in any trimester.

15 Amantadine, an oral antiviral agent active against influenza A, can be used therapeutically and prevents 70–90% of infections.

16 Given the high mortality rate associated with varicella pneumonia occurring in pregnancy, it is recommended that any gravid patient with varicella pneumonia be admitted to the hospital for parenteral therapy with acyclovir.

17 *Pneumocystis carinii* pneumonia (PCP) is the most common opportunistic infection affecting the lungs of patients with acquired immunodeficiency syndrome (AIDS) and prophylaxis against PCP with trimethoprim–sulfamethoxazole is known to be very effective, with rates of prevention of 90–95%.

18 Amniotic fluid embolism (AFE) is a devastating, pregnancy-specific condition in which both maternal and fetal death is the most probable outcome.

19 The diagnosis of AFE is clinical, based on physiologic manifestations, and is made after exclusion of other conditions, such as myocardial infarction and pulmonary thromboembolism.

20 Clinically, the patient with ARDS of any etiology may go through four clinical stages: injury, apparent stability, respiratory insufficiency, terminal stage.

21 The care of a patient with ARDS is primarily supportive, with the mainstays of therapy being supplemental O_2 and the application of positive end-expiratory pressure (PEEP).

References

1 Milne JA, Howie AD, et al. Dyspnoea during normal pregnancy. *Br J Obstet Gynaecol* 1978;85(4):260–263.

2 Levinsky NG. Acidosis and alkalosis. In: Braunwald E, Isselbacher KJ, Wilson JD et al., eds. 11th edn. New York: McGraw-Hill; 1994:253.

3 Lim VS, Katz AI, et al. Acid–base regulation in pregnancy. *Am J Physiol* 1976;231(6):1764–1769.

4 Templeton A, Kelman GR. Maternal blood-gases, PAo2–Pao2, physiological shunt and VD/VT in normal pregnancy. *Br J Anaesth* 1976;48(10):1001–1004.

5 Hankins GD, Harvey CJ, et al. The effects of maternal position and cardiac output on intrapulmonary shunt in normal third-trimester pregnancy. *Obstet Gynecol* 1996;88(3):327–330.

6 Hankins GD, Clark SL, et al. Third-trimester arterial blood gas and acid base values in normal pregnancy at moderate altitude. *Obstet Gynecol* 1996; 88(3):347–350.

7 West JB. *Pulmonary pathology – the essentials*, 3rd edn. Baltimore: Williams & Wilkins, 1987.

8 Awe RJ, Nicotra MB, et al. Arterial oxygenation and alveolar-arterial gradients in term pregnancy. *Obstet Gynecol* 1979; 53(2):182–186.

9 Ang CK, Tan TH, et al. Postural influence on maternal capillary oxygen and carbon dioxide tension. *Br Med J* 1969;4(677): 201–203.

10 Lees MM, Scott DB, et al. The circulatory effects of recumbent postural change in late pregnancy. *Clin Sci* 1967;32(3):453–465.

11 Leontic EA. Respiratory disease in pregnancy. *Med Clin North Am* 1977;61(1):111–128.

12 Milne JA, Mills RJ, et al. The effect of human pregnancy on the pulmonary transfer factor for carbon monoxide as measured by the single-breath method. *Clin Sci Mol Med* 1977;53(3): 271–276.

13 Milne JA. The respiratory response to pregnancy. *Postgrad Med J* 1979;55(643):318–324.

14 Horne SL, Chen Y, et al. Risk factors for reduced pulmonary function in women. A possible relationship between Pi phenotype, number of children, and pulmonary function. *Chest* 1992;102(1):158–163.

15 Clark SL. Asthma in pregnancy. National Asthma Education Program Working Group on Asthma and Pregnancy. National Institutes of Health, National Heart, Lung and Blood Institute. *Obstet Gynecol* 1993;82(6):1036–1040.

16 Greenberger PA. Asthma in pregnancy. *Clin Perinatol* 1985;12(3):571–584.

17 Hung CT, Pelosi M, et al. Blood gas measurements in the kyphoscoliotic gravida and her fetus: Report of a case. *Am J Obstet Gynecol* 1975;121(2):287–289.

18 Gaensler EA, Patton WE, et al. Pulmonary function in pregnancy. III. Serial observations in patients with pulmonary insufficiency. *Am Rev Tuberc* 1953;67(6):779–797.

19 Weinberger SE, Weiss ST, et al. Pregnancy and the lung. *Am Rev Respir Dis* 1980;121(3):559–581.

20 Laros KD. The postpneumonectomy mother. Pregnancy, delivery and motherhood in 80 patients followed through more than 20 years after surgery. *Respiration* 1980;39(4):185–187.

21 Harrop-Griffiths AW, Ravalia A, et al. Regional anaesthesia and cough effectiveness. A study in patients undergoing caesarean section. *Anaesthesia* 1991;46(1):11–13.

22 Amatuzzi R. Hazards to the human fetus from ionizing radiation at diagnostic dose levels: review of the literature. *Perinatology-Neonatology* 1980;4(6):23.

23 Committee on the Biological Effects of Ionizing Radiations. Division of Medical Sciences, Assembly of Life Sciences, National

Research Council. *Somatic effects: effects other than cancer. The effects on populations of exposure to low levels of ionizing radiation*. Washington, DC: National Academy Press; 1980:477.
24 Swartz HM, Reichling BA. Hazards of radiation exposure for pregnant women. *JAMA* 1978;239(18):1907–1908.
25 Brent RL. The effects of embryonic and fetal exposure to X-ray, microwaves, and ultrasound. *Clin Obstet Gynecol* 1983;26(2): 484–510.
26 Mole RH. Radiation effects on pre-natal development and their radiological significance. *Br J Radiol* 1979;52(614):89–101.
27 Thompson KJ, Cohen ME. Studies on the circulation in pregnancy. II: Vital capacity observations in normal pregnant women. *Surg Gynecol Obstet* 1938;66:591.
28 Hughson WG, Friedman PJ, et al. Postpartum pleural effusion: a common radiologic finding. *Ann Intern Med* 1982;97(6): 856–858.
29 Udeshi UL, McHugo JM, et al. Postpartum pleural effusion. *Br J Obstet Gynaecol* 1988;95(9):894–897.
30 Cheek TG, Gutsche BB. Maternal physiologic alterations during pregnancy. In: Shnider SH, Levinson G, eds. *Anesthesia for obstetrics*. Baltimore: Williams & Wilkins; 1984:3.
31 Clark SL, Cotton DB, et al. Central hemodynamic assessment of normal term pregnancy. *Am J Obstet Gynecol* 1989;161(6 Pt 1):1439–1442.
32 Wulf KH, Kunzel W, Lehmann V. Clinical aspects of gas exchange. In: Longo LD, Bartels H, eds. *Respiratory gas exchange and blood flow in the placenta*. Bethesda, MD: Public Health Service; 1972:505.
33 Dildy GA, Clark SL, et al. Intrapartum fetal pulse oximetry: the effects of maternal hyperoxia on fetal arterial oxygen saturation. *Am J Obstet Gynecol* 1994;171(4):1120–1124.
34 Weinstein AM, Dubin BD, et al. Asthma and pregnancy. *JAMA* 1979;241(11):1161–1165.
35 Weinberger M. Salmeterol for the treatment of asthma. *Ann Allergy Asthma Immunol* 1995;75(3):209–211.
36 Barth W. Asthma in pregnancy. In: Clark SL, Cotton DB, Hankins GDV, Phenlan J, eds. *Critical care obstetrics*, 3rd edn. Malden, MA: Blackwell Science, 1997.
37 Working Group on Asthma and Pregnancy. *Management of asthma during pregnancy*. National Institutes of Health Publication No. 93-3279A, 1993.
38 Schatz M, Harden K, et al. The course of asthma during pregnancy, post partum, and with successive pregnancies: a prospective analysis. *J Allergy Clin Immunol* 1988;81(3):509–517.
39 Gordon M, Niswander KR, et al. Fetal morbidity following potentially anoxigenic obstetric conditions. VII. Bronchial asthma. *Am J Obstet Gynecol* 1970;106(3):421–429.
40 Fitzsimons R, Greenberger PA, et al. Outcome of pregnancy in women requiring corticosteroids for severe asthma. *J Allergy Clin Immunol* 1986;78(2):349–353.
41 Greenberger PA, Patterson R. The outcome of pregnancy complicated by severe asthma. *Allergy Proc* 1988;9(5):539–543.
42 Schatz M, Dombrowski MP, et al. Asthma morbidity during pregnancy can be predicted by severity classification. *J Allergy Clin Immunol* 2003;112(2):283–288.
43 Barth BA. Acute severe asthma in pregnancy. In: Clark SL, Cotton DB, Hankins GDV, Phenlan JP, eds. *Critical care obstetrics*, 3rd edn. Malden, MA: Blackwell Science, 1997.
44 Bridges CB, Fukuda K, et al. Prevention and control of influenza. Recommendations of the Advisory Committee on Immunization Practices (ACIP). *MMWR Recomm Rep* 2002;51(RR-3):1–31.
45 Hartert TV, Neuzil KM, et al. Maternal morbidity and perinatal outcomes among pregnant women with respiratory hospitalizations during influenza season. *Am J Obstet Gynecol* 2003;189(6):1705–1712.
46 McFadden ER Jr, Kiser R, et al. Acute bronchial asthma. Relations between clinical and physiologic manifestations. *N Engl J Med* 1973;288(5):221–225.
47 Gardner MO, Doyle NM. Asthma in pregnancy. *Obstet Gynecol Clin North Am* 2004;31(2):385–413.
48 Miller TP, Greenberger PA, et al. The diagnosis of potentially fatal asthma in hospitalized adults. Patient characteristics and increased severity of asthma. *Chest* 1992;102(2):515–518.
49 Cohen LF, di Sant'Agnese PA, et al. Cystic fibrosis and pregnancy. A national survey. *Lancet* 1980;2(8199):842–844.
50 Huang NN. Special features, survival rate and prognostic factors in young adults with cystic fibrosis. *Am J Med* 1987;82:871.
51 Pittard WB 3rd, Sorensen RU, et al. Pregnancy outcome in mothers with cystic fibrosis: normal neonatal immune responses. *South Med J* 1987;80(3):344–346.
52 Corky CWB, Newth CJL, Corey M, Levison H. Pregnancy in cystic fibrosis: a better prognosis in patients with pancreatic function. *Am J Obstet Gynecol* 1981;140:737.
53 Kulich M, Rosenfeld M, et al. Improved survival among young patients with cystic fibrosis. *J Pediatr* 2003;142(6):631–636.
54 Hyatt AC, Chipps BE, et al. A double-blind controlled trial of anti-Pseudomonas chemotherapy of acute respiratory exacerbations in patients with cystic fibrosis. *J Pediatr* 1981;99(2): 307–314.
55 Michael SH, Mueller DH Impact of lactation on women with cystic fibrosis and their infants: a review of a few cases. *J Am Diet Assoc* 1994;51:452.
56 Bond VK, Stoelting RK, et al. Pulmonary aspiration syndrome after inhalation of gastric fluid containing antacids. *Anesthesiology* 1979;51(5):452–453.
57 Schwartz DJ, Wynne JW, et al. The pulmonary consequences of aspiration of gastric contents at pH values greater than 2.5. *Am Rev Respir Dis* 1980;121(1):119–126.
58 Bartlett JG, Gorbach SL. The triple threat of aspiration pneumonia. *Chest* 1975;68(4):560–566.
59 Baggish MS, Hopper S. Aspiration as a cause of maternal death. *Obstet Gynecol* 1979;53:182.
60 Roberts RB, Shirley MA. The obstetrician's role in reducing the risk of aspiration pneumonitis. With particular reference to the use of oral antacids. *Am J Obstet Gynecol* 1976;124(6): 611–617.
61 Gibbs CP, Schwartz DJ, et al. Antacid pulmonary aspiration in the dog. *Anesthesiology* 1979;51(5):380–385.
62 Sweeney B, Wright I. The use of antacids as a prophylaxis against Mendelson's syndrome in the United Kingdom. A survey. *Anesthesia* 1986;41(4):419–422.
63 Hopwood HG Jr. Pneumonia in pregnancy. *Obstet Gynecol* 1965;25:875–879.
64 Benedetti TJ, Valle R, et al. Antepartum pneumonia in pregnancy. *Am J Obstet Gynecol* 1982;144(4):413–417.
65 Hollingsworth HM, Pratter MR, Irwin RS. Acute respiratory failure in pregnancy. *J Intensive Care Med* 1989;4:11.
66 Boucher M, Yonekura ML, et al. Adult respiratory distress syndrome: a rare manifestation of *Listeria monocytogenes* infection in pregnancy. *Am J Obstet Gynecol* 1984;149(6):686–688.
67 Soper DE, Melone PJ, et al. Legionnaire disease complicating pregnancy. *Obstet Gynecol* 1986;67(3 Suppl):10S–12S.
68 Whitney CG, Farley MM, et al. Increasing prevalence of

multidrug-resistant *Streptococcus pneumoniae* in the United States. *N Engl J Med* 2000;343(26):1917–1924.
69 Jacobs MR. *Streptococcus pneumoniae*: epidemiology and patterns of resistance. *Am J Med* 2004;117 Suppl 3A:3S–15S.
70 Schwartz RH, Goldenberg RI, et al. The increasing prevalence of bacteremic ampicillin-resistant *Haemophilus influenzae* infections in a community hospital. *Pediatr Infect Dis* 1982;1(4): 242–244.
71 Korones SB. Uncommon virus infections of the mother, fetus, and newborn: influenza, mumps and measles. *Clin Perinatol* 1988;15(2):259–272.
72 MacKenzie JS, Houghton M. Influenza infections during pregnancy: association with congenital malformations and with subsequent neoplasms in children, and potential hazards of live virus vaccines. *Bacteriol Rev* 1974;38(4):356–370.
73 Eickhoff TC, Sherman IL, et al. Observations on excess mortality associated with epidemic influenza. *JAMA* 1961;176: 776–82.
74 Walker WM, McKee AM. Asian influenza in pregnancy; relationship to fetal anomalies. *Obstet Gynecol* 1959;13(4):394–398.
75 Wilson MG, Stein AM. Teratogenic effects of Asian influenza. *JAMA* 1971;216:1022.
76 Influenza vaccination and treatment during pregnancy. *ACOG Committee Opinion No. 305* 2004:1125–1126.
77 Mostow SR. Prevention, management, and control of influenza. Role of amantadine. *Am J Med* 1987;82(6A):35–41.
78 Kirshon B, Faro S, et al. Favorable outcome after treatment with amantadine and ribavirin in a pregnancy complicated by influenza pneumonia. A case report. *J Reprod Med* 1988;33(4):399–401.
79 Coffey VP, Jessop WJ. Congenital abnormalities. *Ir J Med Sci* 1955;6(349):30–48.
80 Schoenbaum SC, Weinstein L. Respiratory infection in pregnancy. *Clin Obstet Gynecol* 1979;22(2):293–300.
81 Fleisher G, Henry W, et al. Life-threatening complications of varicella. *Am J Dis Child* 1981;135(10):896–899.
82 Harris RE, Rhoades ER. Varicella pneumonia complicating pregnancy. Report of a case and review of literature. *Obstet Gynecol* 1965;25:734–740.
83 Hockberger RS, Rothstein RJ. Varicella pneumonia in adults: a spectrum of disease. *Ann Emerg Med* 1986;15(8):931–934.
84 Smego RA Jr, Asperilla MO. Use of acyclovir for varicella pneumonia during pregnancy. *Obstet Gynecol* 1991;78(6): 1112–1116.
85 Hankins GD, Gilstrap 3rd LC, et al. Acyclovir treatment of varicella pneumonia in pregnancy. *Crit Care Med* 1987; 15(4):336–337.
86 DeNicola LK, Hanshaw JB. Congenital and neonatal varicella. *J Pediatr* 1979;94(1):175–176.
87 Catanzaro A. Pulmonary mycosis in pregnant women. *Chest* 1984;86(3 Suppl):14S–18S.
88 Harris RE. Coccidioidomycosis complicating pregnancy. Report of 3 cases and review of the literature. *Obstet Gynecol* 1966;28(3):401–405.
89 US Department of Health and Human Services Clinical Practice Guidelines. *Evaluation and management of early HIV infection*. Publication No. 94-0572. Washington, DC: US Department of Health and Human Services, 1994.
90 Jensen LP, O'Sullivan MJ, et al. Acquired immunodeficiency (AIDS) in pregnancy. *Am J Obstet Gynecol* 1984;148(8): 1145–1146.
91 Minkoff H, deRegt RH, et al. *Pneumocystis carinii* pneumonia associated with acquired immunodeficiency syndrome in pregnancy: a report of three maternal deaths. *Obstet Gynecol* 1986;67(2):284–287.
92 Ahmad H, Mehta NJ, et al. *Pneumocystis carinii* pneumonia in pregnancy. *Chest* 2001;120(2):666–671.
93 Baskin CG, Law S, et al. Sulfadiazine rheumatic fever prophylaxis during pregnancy: does it increase the risk of kernicterus in the newborn? *Cardiology* 1980;65(4):222–225.
94 Feinkind L, Minkoff HL. HIV in pregnancy. *Clin Perinatol* 1988;15(2):189–202.
95 Armstrong D, Bernard E. Aerosol pentamidine. *Ann Intern Med* 1988;109(11):852–854.
96 Palella FJ Jr, Delaney KM, et al. Declining morbidity and mortality among patients with advanced human immunodeficiency virus infection. HIV Outpatient Study Investigators. *N Engl J Med* 1998;338(13):853–860.
97 Clark SL, Hankins GD, et al. Amniotic fluid embolism: analysis of the national registry. *Am J Obstet Gynecol* 1995;172(4 Pt 1):1158–1167; discussion 1167–1169.
98 Clark SL. New concepts of amniotic fluid embolism: a review. *Obstet Gynecol Surv* 1990;45:360–368.
99 ACOG. Amniotic fluid embolus in prologue. In: *Obstetrics*, 3rd edn. Washington, DC: American College of Obstetricians and Gynecologists, 1993.
100 Paul RH, Koh KS, et al. Changes in fetal heart rate-uterine contraction patterns associated with eclampsia. *Am J Obstet Gynecol* 1978;130(2):165–169.
101 Porter TF, Clark SL, Dildy GA, et al. Isolated disseminated intravascular coagulation in amniotic fluid embolism. *Am J Obstet Gynecol* 1996;174: 486.
102 Clark SL, Pavlova Z, et al. Squamous cells in the maternal pulmonary circulation. *Am J Obstet Gynecol* 1986;154(1): 104–106.
103 Fyke FE 3rd, Kazmier FJ, et al. Venous air embolism. Life-threatening complication of orogenital sex during pregnancy. *Am J Med* 1985;78(2):333–336.
104 Baker B, Brooks PG. Air emboli risked with laparoscopy and hysteroscopy. *Obstet Gynecol News* 1996;31:19.
105 Gottlieb JD, Ericsson JA, et al. Venous air embolism: a review. *Anesth Analg* 1965;44(6):773–779.
106 O'Quinn RJ, Lakshminarayan S. Venous air embolism. *Arch Intern Med* 1982;142:2173.
107 Fowler MJ Jr, Thomas CE, et al. Diffuse cerebral air embolism treated with hyperbaric oxygen: a case report. *J Neuroimaging* 2005;15(1):92–96.
108 Ence TJ, Gong H Jr. Adult respiratory distress syndrome after venous air embolism. *Am Rev Respir Dis* 1979;119(6):1033–1037.
109 Clark MC, Flick MR. Permeability pulmonary edema caused by venous air embolism. *Am Rev Respir Dis* 1984;129(4):633–635.
110 Petty TL, Ashbaugh DG. The adult respiratory distress syndrome. Clinical features, factors influencing prognosis and principles of management. *Chest* 1971;60(3):233–239.
111 Balk R, Bone RC. The adult respiratory distress syndrome. *Med Clin North Am* 1983;67(3):685–700.
112 Hansen-Flaschen J, Fishman AP. Adult respiratory distress syndrome: clinical features and pathogenesis. In: Fishman AP, ed. *Pulmonary diseases and disorders*, 2nd edn. New York: McGraw-Hill; 1988:2201.
113 Berkowitz RL. The Swan–Ganz catheter and colloid osmotic pressure determinations. In: Berkowitz RL, ed. *Critical care of the obstetric patient*. New York: Churchill Livingstone; 1983:1.
114 Maunder RJ. Clinical prediction of the adult respiratory distress syndrome. *Clin Chest Med* 1985;6(3):413–426.

115 Mabie WC, Barton JR, et al. Adult respiratory distress syndrome in pregnancy. *Am J Obstet Gynecol* 1992;167(4 Pt 1):950–957.

116 Andreadis N, Petty TL. Adult respiratory distress syndrome: problems and progress. *Am Rev Respir Dis* 1985;132(6):1344–1346.

117 Rinaldo JE, Rogers RM. Adult respiratory-distress syndrome: changing concepts of lung injury and repair. *N Engl J Med* 1982;306(15):900–909.

118 Bernard GR. N-acetylcysteine in experimental and clinical acute lung injury. *Am J Med* 1991;91(3C):54S–59S.

119 Bernard GR, Reines HD, Halvshka RV, et al. Prostacyclin and thromboxane A2 formation is increased in human sepsis syndrome: effects of cyclooxygenase inhibitors. *Am Rev Respir Dis* 1991;144: 1095.

120 Snapper JR. Lung mechanics in pulmonary edema. *Clin Chest Med* 1985;6(3):393–412.

121 Verghese GM, Ware LB, et al. Alveolar epithelial fluid transport and the resolution of clinically severe hydrostatic pulmonary edema. *J Appl Physiol* 1999;87(4):1301–1312.

122 Bachofen M, Weibel ER. Structural alterations of lung parenchyma in the adult respiratory distress syndrome. *Clin Chest Med* 1982;3(1):35–56.

123 Flick MR, Murray JF. High-dose corticosteroid therapy in the adult respiratory distress syndrome. *JAMA* 1984;251(8):1054–1056.

124 Walmrath D, Gunther A, et al. 1996; Bronchoscopic surfactant administration in patients with severe adult respiratory distress syndrome and sepsis. *Am J Respir Crit Care Med* 154(1):57–62.

125 Wiswell TE, Smith RM, et al. Bronchopulmonary segmental lavage with Surfaxin (KL(4)-surfactant) for acute respiratory distress syndrome. *Am J Respir Crit Care Med* 1999;160(4):1188–1195.

126 Bernard GR, Brigham KL. Pulmonary edema. Pathophysiologic mechanisms and new approaches to therapy. *Chest* 1986;89(4):594–600.

127 Bernard GR, Artigas A, et al. Report of the American–European consensus conference on ARDS: definitions, mechanisms, relevant outcomes and clinical trial coordination. The Consensus Committee. *Intensive Care Med* 1994;20(3):225–232.

128 Winter PM, Smith G. The toxicity of oxygen. *Anesthesiology* 1972;37(2):210–241.

129 Brower RG, Lanken PN, et al. Higher versus lower positive end-expiratory pressures in patients with the acute respiratory distress syndrome. *N Engl J Med* 2004;351(4):327–336.

130 Sosin D, Krasnow J, et al. Successful spontaneous vaginal delivery during mechanical ventilatory support for the adult respiratory distress syndrome. *Obstet Gynecol* 1986;68(3 Suppl):19S–23S.

131 Demling RH. Current concepts on the adult respiratory distress syndrome. *Circ Shock* 1990;30(4):297–309.

132 Mason B, Hankins GDV. Adult respiratory distress syndrome. In: Clark SL, Hankins GDV, Cotton DB, Phelan JP, eds. *Critical care obstetrics*, 3rd edn. Cambridge, MA: Blackwell Science, 1997.

133 VanHook JW, Witty J. Ventilation therapy. In: Clark SL, Hankins GDV, Cotton DB, Phelan JP, eds. *Critical care obstetrics*, 3rd edn. Cambridge, MA: Blackwell Science, 1997.

134 Suter PM, Fairley B, et al. Optimum end-expiratory airway pressure in patients with acute pulmonary failure. *N Engl J Med* 1975;292(6): 284–289.

135 Lynch JP, Mhyre JG, et al. Influence of cardiac output on intrapulmonary shunt. *J Appl Physiol* 1979;46(2):315–321.

136 de Latorre FJ, Tomasa A, et al. Incidence of pneumothorax and pneumomediastinum in patients with aspiration pneumonia requiring ventilatory support. *Chest* 1977;72(2):141–144.

137 Browdie DA, Deane R, et al. Adult respiratory distress syndrome (ARDS), sepsis, and extracorporeal membrane oxygenation (ECMO). *J Trauma* 1977;17(8):579–586.

138 Albert RK, Condie F. Hand-washing patterns in medical intensive-care units. *N Engl J Med* 1981;304(24):1465–1466.

139 Cross AS, Roup B. Role of respiratory assistance devices in endemic nosocomial pneumonia. *Am J Med* 1981;70(3):681–685.

140 Ashbaugh DG, Petty TL. Sepsis complicating the acute respiratory distress syndrome. *Surg Gynecol Obstet* 1972;135(6):865–869.

141 Seidenfeld JJ, Pohl DF, et al. Incidence, site, and outcome of infections in patients with the adult respiratory distress syndrome. *Am Rev Respir Dis* 1986;134(1):12–16.

142 Andrews CP, Coalson JJ, et al. Diagnosis of nosocomial bacterial pneumonia in acute, diffuse lung injury. *Chest* 1981;80(3):254–258.

143 Niederman MS, Fein AM. The interaction of infection and the adult respiratory distress syndrome. *Crit Care Clin* 1986;2(3):471–495.

144 Ingbar DH, Matthay RA. Pulmonary sequelae and lung repair in survivors of the adult respiratory distress syndrome. *Crit Care Clin* 1986;2(3):629–665.

145 Ghio AJ, Elliott CG, et al. Impairment after adult respiratory distress syndrome. An evaluation based on American Thoracic Society recommendations. *Am Rev Respir Dis* 1989;139(5):1158–1162.

41 Diabetes mellitus in pregnancy

Carol J. Homko, Zion J. Hagay, and E. Albert Reece

Diabetes mellitus is a heterogeneous disorder characterized by hyperglycemia, which is a result of relative or absolute insulin deficiency. It is estimated that diabetes mellitus affects approximately 4 million women of childbearing age in the United States.

Peel, in an excellent historic review of diabetes and pregnancy, noted that, before 1856, there were few reports of pregnancy-complicated diabetes.[1] At that time, diabetes was a disease with a dismal prognosis, and infertility was common in women with diabetes. The advent of insulin brought about a dramatic change in the overall outlook for diabetics and their reproductive potential. A dramatic fall in maternal mortality from 45% to just over 2% was observed shortly after the introduction of insulin in 1922.[2] A decline in perinatal mortality was achieved more gradually, however, and must be credited to a number of developments. Infant survival can be credited to a better understanding of metabolism in diabetic patients, a recognition of the need for stringent metabolic control to achieve glucose levels that are as close as possible to nondiabetic values to insure a better pregnancy outcome, the improvement in neonatal intensive care units, new techniques for fetal surveillance, and devices for self-monitoring blood glucose. In fact, perinatal mortality rates have been reduced remarkably, from approximately 15–20% in the 1960s to approximately 2–3% at present.[2–4] Furthermore, if mortality secondary to major congenital malformations is excluded, then perinatal mortality rates in well-controlled diabetics approximates that of nondiabetics. Unresolved problems remain, however, such as macrosomia and congenital anomalies.

At present, there is no doubt that the goal in treating diabetic patients is not only a reduction in perinatal mortality but also decreases in perinatal and maternal morbidity.

Classification

Diabetes during pregnancy is still generally classified using the original system proposed by Priscilla White almost 40 years ago.[5] White's classification relates the onset of diabetes, its duration, and the degree of vasculopathy to the outcome of pregnancy. Because there were differences and some confusion in the interpretation of class A diabetes, particularly when the patient required insulin for therapy, a revision made by Hare and White proposed that class A diabetes should include women known to have diabetes before pregnancy and who are treated with diet alone.[6] Thus, White's class A classification includes only patients with pregestational diabetes and defines gestational diabetes as a completely separate group.

Practically speaking, women with pregnancies complicated by diabetes mellitus may be separated into one of two groups:

1 Gestational diabetes: women with carbohydrate intolerance of variable severity, with onset or first recognition during the present pregnancy.

2 Pregestational diabetes: women known to have diabetes before pregnancy.

Table 41.1 presents the classifications that include these two groups.[7]

Epidemiology and etiology

Significant advances in the understanding of genetic features of diabetes mellitus have been achieved in the last 20 years.[8] Because diabetes mellitus is a heterogeneous disorder rather than a single disease, the different types of diabetes should be distinguishable from each other. To improve differentiation of the various forms of diabetes, the National Diabetes Data Group (NDDG) was updated in 1997 by the Expert Committee on The Diagnosis and Classification of Diabetes Mellitus (see Table 41.2).[9]

Ninety percent of all pregnant diabetic patients have gestational diabetes mellitus (GDM), whereas type 1 (insulin-dependent diabetes) and type 2 (noninsulin-dependent diabetes) account for the remaining 10%.[10] The clinical distinction between the ketosis-prone type 1 and the nonketosis-prone type 2 has been recognized by clinicians for many years, but the two types were thought to represent differences in the expression of a single disease.[11] Twenty years ago, it was discovered that type 1 is a human leukocyte antigen (HLA)-linked disorder, whereas type 2 is not, and thus they are two different diseases genetically.[12–14] In general, type 1 and type 2 can be distinguished from each other using clinical criteria or islet cell antibody (ICA) studies (Table 41.3).

Type 1 accounts for 6–10% of all cases of diabetes in the

Table 41.1 Classification of diabetes in pregnancy.

Pregestational diabetes:

Class	Age of onset (years)	Duration (years)	Vascular disease	Therapy
A	Any	Any	No	Diet only
B	> 20	< 10	No	Insulin
C	10–19	10–19	No	Insulin
D	Before 10	> 20	Benign retinopathy	Insulin
F	Any	Any	Nephropathy	Insulin
R	Any	Any	Proliferative retinopathy	Insulin
H	Any	Any	Heart disease	Insulin

Gestational diabetes:

Class	Fasting glucose level		Postprandial glucose level
A-1	< 105 mg/dL	*and*	< 120 mg/dL
A-2	> 105 mg/dL	*and/or*	> 120 mg/dL

Based on the American College of Obstetricians and Gynecologists (ACOG), Technical Bulletin no. 92 (Chicago), May 1986, with modifications.

Table 41.2 Classification of glucose intolerance.

	Nomenclature	Old name(s)
Type I	Type 1 diabetes	Insulin-dependent diabetes Juvenile-onset diabetes
Type II	Type 2 diabetes	Noninsulin-dependent diabetes Maturity-onset diabetes
Type III	Other specific types	Secondary diabetes
Type IV	Gestational diabetes mellitus	

From ref. 9.

general population.[15,16] It has an increased prevalence rate in white people but is rare in certain ethnic groups (e.g., Japanese, Chinese, and Eskimos).[17,18] The prevalence of type 1 in Europe and the United States is estimated to be in the range of 0.1–0.4% in various age groups younger than age 30 years.[19]

In contrast, type 2 is the most common form of diabetes observed in the general population. It has a peak incidence at age 65 years, with 80% of cases appearing after age 40 years.[18,19] However, in recent years, type 2 diabetes has been steadily increasing among younger individuals and, as a result, in many parts of the world, including the United States, the number of pregnancies complicated by type 2 diabetes is actually exceeding those with type 1 diabetes. A study of diabetes prevalence in the United States found that, while the overall prevalence of type 2 diabetes increased by 33% from 1990 to 1998, the prevalence in individuals aged 30–39 years increased by 70%.[5,20] In 1994, type 2 diabetes accounted for approximately a third of all cases of diabetes in teenagers and as many as half of all new cases of diabetes in certain populations.[21]

Genetics of type 1 diabetes mellitus

In the past few years, it has become increasingly clear that autoimmunity plays a key role in type 1 diabetes.[22–24] It is currently believed that type 1 diabetes mellitus is actually a slow process in which insulin-secreting cells are gradually destroyed, leading to islet cell failure and hyperglycemia.

The exact mechanism of the inheritance of type 1 diabetes is not known. Formerly, it was suggested that the risk of inheriting diabetes in offspring with one affected parent was in the range of 1–6%.[25–27] Based on recent information,[28] it has become clear that type 1 diabetes is transmitted less frequently to the offspring of diabetic mothers (1%) than to children of diabetic fathers (6%). This preferential paternal transmission rate may be related to greater transfer of DR_4 alleles to the offspring of DR_4 fathers than to the offspring of DR_4 mothers.[29] Family studies have shown that the estimated risk of type 1 diabetes in offspring in a family with one affected sibling but unaffected parents is 5–6%.[30,31]

Genetics of type 2 diabetes mellitus

There are clear genetic and immunologic differences between type 1 and type 2 diabetes. Type 2 diabetes is not linked to HLA, and no specific genetic markers have been found. Furthermore, type 2 diabetes does not seem to be an autoimmune

Table 41.3 Predominant characteristics of type 1 and type 2 diabetes.

Characteristic	Type 1	Type 2
Prevalence	0.1–0.5%	5–10%*
Weight at onset	Nonobese	Often obese
Age at onset	Usually young, < 30 years	Usually older, > 40 years
Seasonal variations	Yes	No
Insulin level	Low or absent	Variable
Ketosis	Most often	Unusual
MHC gene associations	HLA-DR_4, HLA-DR_3, HLA-DQ	No
Twin studies	30–50% concordance	80–100% concordance
Anti-islet cell antibodies	Positive in 70% of individuals with new type 1	No

MHC, major histocompatibility complex.

*Prevalence in Western countries.

or endocrine disease. Currently available information indicates that type 2 diabetes occurs when there is both impaired insulin secretion and insulin antagonism.[32]

For relatives of individuals with type 2 diabetes, the empiric risk of developing the disease is much higher than it is for relatives of type 1 diabetics (Table 41.4). The risk of transmitting type 2 diabetes to first-degree relatives is almost 15%, and as many as 30% have impaired glucose tolerance.[16] When both parents have type 2 diabetes, the chance of developing the disease is much higher, reaching 60–75%.[19]

Genetics of gestational diabetes mellitus

Historically, GDM was believed to be a variant of type 2 diabetes; however, available data now support the concept that GDM is a heterogeneous disorder representing, at least in part, patients who are destined to develop either type 1 or type 2 diabetes in later life.[33,34] The exact percentage difference of each subgroup is unknown, but it appears that most GDM cases represent a preclinical state of type 2 diabetes. Immunologic studies have shown that as many as 30% of GDM patients may have circulating ICAs,[35] and anti-ICAs have been found in many patients with pretype 1 diabetes.[36–39] Furthermore, it has been shown that GDM patients who were ICA positive had a higher prevalence of HLA-DR_3 or -DR_4 than those who were ICA negative. More than half the patients who were ICA positive developed type 1 diabetes within an 11-year period after the diagnosis of GDM.

Metabolic changes in normal and diabetic pregnancies

Insulin secretion and insulin resistance in normal pregnancy

Insulin is the major hormonal signal regulating metabolic responses to feeding and tissue use of carbohydrates; it is also the major glucose-lowering hormone. It is produced by the B cells of the pancreas and is secreted into the hepatic portal circulation, from which it reaches and acts on the liver and other peripheral tissues (i.e., muscle and fat). Insulin suppresses endogenous glucose production by inhibiting hepatic glycogenolysis and gluconeogenesis. On the other hand, it stimulates glucose uptake and fuel storage of glycogen and triglyceride in the liver, muscle, and adipose tissue (Table 41.5).[40]

Table 41.4 Empiric risk for offspring of parents with type 1 and type 2 diabetes developing diabetes.

Affected parent(s)	Empiric risk estimate of offspring
Type 1 diabetes	
Mother	1%
Father	6%
Parents unaffected, sibling affected	Overall 5–6% No. of haplotypes shared: 1 haplotype = 5% 2 haplotypes = 13% No haplotypes = 2%
Both parents affected	33%
Type 2 diabetes	
MODY	50%
Obese	7%
Nonobese	15%
Both parents affected	60–75%

MODY, maturity-onset diabetes of youth.

During pregnancy, fasting values of insulin rise from roughly 5 mU/L to approximately 8 mU/L until term (Fig. 41.1).[41,42] The increase in insulin release in response to a glucose load becomes pronounced by the third trimester.[41,43–45] Data show that the release of insulin in response to a challenge with oral or intravenous glucose in the last trimester of

Table 41.5 Summary of the metabolic effects of insulin.

Target tissue	Enhances glucose and amino acid uptake Increases glycogen synthesis Converts glucose into fatty acids Inhibits glyconeogenesis
Muscle	Enhances glucose and amino acid uptake Increases glycogen synthesis
Adipose tissue	Increases glucose and amino acid transport Increases fatty acid synthesis Inhibits release of fatty acids from fat stores "Fat-sparing effect" is enhanced by glucose utilization in many tissues
Central nervous system	Has little or no effect on uptake or metabolism of glucose
All tissues	Increases protein synthesis Inhibits protein catabolism

From ref. 40.

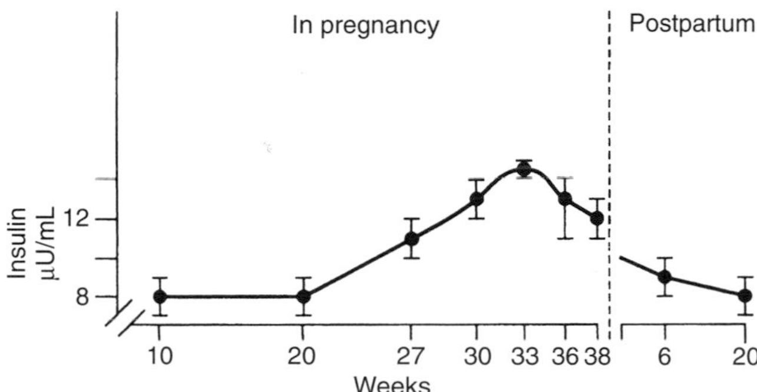

Figure 41.1 Plasma insulin in normal pregnancy and postpartum after overnight fast. Basal insulin levels are increased in the last half of pregnancy. (Modified from ref. 71.)

pregnancy is approximately 1.5–2.5 times greater than it is in nonpregnant women.[43,46]. In the first trimester of pregnancy, insulin action is enhanced by estrogen and progesterone; thus, an increase in peripheral glucose use leads to lower fasting plasma glucose levels,[47] a decrease that may explain the clinical observation of increased episodes of hypoglycemia experienced by pregnant diabetic patients in early pregnancy.

Late pregnancy is characterized by accelerated growth of the fetoplacental unit, rising plasma concentrations of several diabetogenic hormones including human placental lactogen and estrogens, and increasing insulin resistance. Several investigators[48–50] have demonstrated increased first- and second-phase insulin release during late gestation as well as increased plasma insulin/glucose ratios. Buchanan and colleagues,[49] using the minimal model technique, found that peripheral insulin sensitivity was reduced to approximately one-third of normal during late gestation. Similar findings have been reported by Catalano et al.[48] and Ryan et al.,[50] both using the euglycemic–hyperinsulinemic clamp technique. They reported decreases of 50% and 33%, respectively, in insulin-stimulated glucose uptake, indicating peripheral insulin resistance during the third trimester of pregnancy. In another publication, Catalano et al.[51] observed a 30% increase in basal hepatic glucose output despite elevated basal serum insulin levels, suggesting hepatic insulin resistance. Our own investigations,[52,53] in overweight women using the insulin clamp technique, have demonstrated a 40% reduction in insulin-stimulated glucose uptake during the third trimester of pregnancy compared with the postpartum period. In addition, we found that, after 2 h of hyperinsulinemia, endogenous glucose production was significantly less inhibited during the third trimester when compared with either the second trimester or the nonpregnant state. Thus, there appears to be general agreement that the second half of pregnancy is associated with increasing insulin resistance in the periphery (muscle and, in obese women, also at the hepatic level).

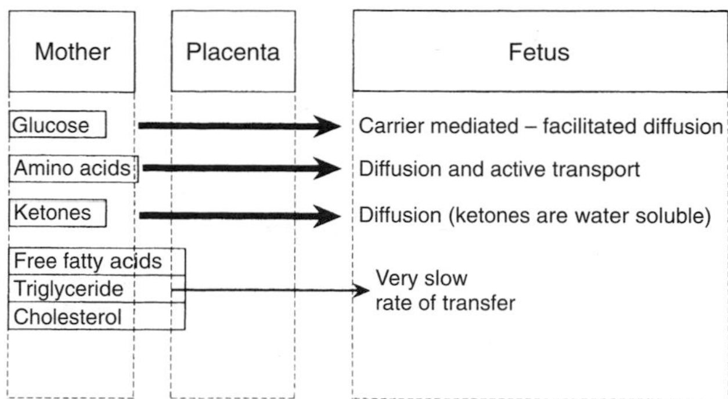

Figure 41.2 Transplacental transfer of maternal fuels to the fetus (for details, see text).

Placental transfer of nutrients

The placenta is a complex organ that has an important function in the transfer of gases and nutrients between mother and fetus. Fetal growth is controlled by various factors and depends on the uptake of nutrients and oxygen by the placenta and on their transfer to the fetus. The availability of nutrients to the fetus depends principally on the maternal metabolic state. Placental transfer of the principal nutrients is discussed briefly here (Fig. 41.2).

Glucose

Experimental studies have provided evidence that the process of transplacental glucose transfer involves a carrier-mediated active transport system.[54,55] In this process of facilitated diffusion, the net result is that fetal blood glucose levels are 15–20% lower than maternal levels. It is believed that this difference in blood glucose levels between maternal and fetal blood is a result of placental use of glucose. It has been shown that the placenta contains insulin receptors, but their role is not yet clear.[56] The fetus seems to be protected from very high maternal glucose levels. In fact, it has been found that the placental transport system of glucose is saturated when maternal glucose levels are maintained up to approximately 250 mg/dL. It is not possible to increase fetal plasma glucose levels above this threshold.[57,58]

Amino acids

Placental transfer of amino acids is an active process. Amino acids are transferred against a concentration gradient; in the fetus, amino acid levels are three to four times higher than those in the maternal blood. However, the concentration of amino acids in the placenta is higher than that in either fetal or maternal blood.[59]

Metabolism in the diabetic pregnancy

Islet cells function completely differently in type 1 than in type 2 diabetes. It is therefore unsurprising that there is a difference in insulin secretion between the two forms of diabetes. C peptide, which is the connecting peptide between the A and B chains of insulin, was found to be higher in pregnant women with type 2 diabetes than in normal control subjects. However, C-peptide release in type 2 diabetes was lower after meals.[60] This may indicate impaired effectiveness of insulin in target tissues and pancreatic B-cell dysfunction in patients with type 2 diabetes.

In type 1 diabetes, C-peptide levels were found to be very low or almost undetectable, which may indicate no residual B-cell function.[61] It has also been shown that, in patients with type 1 diabetes, the increase in insulin requirement is almost 40%, whereas in type 2 it can be much higher, reaching as high as 100%.[62] For several years, it has been known that maternal fuel levels other than that of glucose can be abnormal in diabetic pregnant patients. Metzger and colleagues[63] have shown that plasma triglyceride levels are elevated in obese pregnant patients with GDM and type 2 diabetes. Skryten and colleagues[64] reported higher than normal plasma triglyceride concentrations in pregnant patients with type 1 diabetes during the third trimester. However, this has not been confirmed in more recent studies.[64]

Metzger et al.[63] reported that plasma free fatty acid (FFA) levels tend to be higher in patients with gestational diabetes than in normal pregnant patients. Furthermore, FFA levels were also found to be elevated in pregnant patients with type 1 diabetes. A correlation between these concentrations and neonatal birthweight was reported.[65] In yet another study, high-density lipopolysaccharide (HDL) cholesterol concentrations were found to be low in type 2 diabetes and not significantly changed in women with type 1 diabetes compared with nondiabetic pregnant control subjects.[66]

In summary, the metabolic disturbances in diabetic pregnant patients are expressed in increased concentrations of circulating metabolic fuels, including carbohydrate, protein, and fat. This increased circulating maternal level can be transferred to the fetus and may contribute to the development of fetal macrosomia.[64,67]

Gestational diabetes mellitus

Definition and incidence

GDM is defined as carbohydrate intolerance of variable severity with onset or first recognition during the present pregnancy.[68] This means that the glucose intolerance may have antedated the pregnancy but was not recognized by the patient or physician. The incidence of GDM varies in different study populations and is estimated to occur in 3–5% of pregnant women.[69] The likelihood of developing gestational diabetes is significantly increased among certain subgroups, and these include women with a family history of type 2 diabetes, advancing maternal age, obesity, and nonwhite ethnicity.

Screening for gestational diabetes

In the United States, screening for gestational diabetes mellitus consists of a 50-g oral glucose load, followed 1 h later by a plasma glucose determination. The screen is performed without regard to the time of day or interval since the last meal. It is recommended that screening be carried out at 24–28 weeks' gestation in average-risk women not known to have diabetes mellitus. Women deemed to be a high risk for GDM should be tested as soon as possible. This approach is endorsed by the American College of Obstetricians and Gynecologists (ACOG),[7] the Expert Committee on the Diagnosis and Classification of Diabetes Mellitus,[9] and the Fourth International Workshop Conference on Gestational Diabetes Mellitus.[68]

However, there is a lack of agreement among clinicians and experts as to whether screening should be selective or universal. This controversy is apparent from the varying recommendations from different but related professional organizations. The ACOG[7] recommended selective screening in 1986 but made no definite recommendations in 1994. The American Diabetes Association recommended universal screening until 1997.[70] At that time, the Fourth International Workshop Conference on GDM[68] took a stand that there appears to be a low-risk group in whom screening may not be cost-effective. They defined low-risk women as those possessing all of the following characteristics: < 25 years of age, of normal weight, without a history of abnormal glucose metabolism or poor obstetric outcome, and with no first-degree relative with diabetes.

A value of plasma venous glucose between 130 and 140 mg/dL has been recommended as a threshold to indicate the need for a full diagnostic oral glucose tolerance test (OGTT). Lowering the threshold to 130 mg/dL increases the sensitivity of the test but increases the number of diagnostic tests performed and, therefore, increases the cost per case diagnosed. When the plasma glucose screening test results are

Table 41.6 Incidence of a positive glucose tolerance test among 96 gravidas with 50-g, 1-h screening test values > 134 mg/dL (plasma, glucose oxidase).

Screening test result (mg/dL)	Incidence of gestational diabetes (%)
135–144	14.6
145–154	17.4
155–164	28.6
165–174	20.0
175–184	50.0
> 185	100.0

From ref. 73.

Table 41.7 Oral glucose tolerance test (100-g) values for the diagnosis of gestational diabetes (mg/dL).

	O'Sullivan (ref. 71)	NDDG (ref. 72)	Carpenter and Coustan (ref. 73)
Fasting	90	105	95
1-h	165	190	180
2-h	145	165	155
3-h	125	145	140

> 185 mg/dL, patients are gestational diabetics and no further testing is required (Table 41.6).

Diagnosis

The diagnosis of GDM is, in most cases, based on an abnormal result of an OGTT during pregnancy. A minority of cases are diagnosed on the basis of high fasting glucose levels during pregnancy, in which case the OGTT does not have to be performed. The OGTT is administered under standard conditions: 100 g of glucose is given orally in at least 400 mL of water after an overnight fast of 8–14 h. The patient should have at least 3 days of unrestricted diet with more than 150 g of carbohydrates and should be at rest during the study. Diagnosis requires that at least two of four glucose levels of the OGTT meet or exceed the upper limits of normal values. The normal upper limit was determined by O'Sullivan and Mahan as two standard deviations (SD) above the mean for each of four glucose values of 752 pregnant patients undergoing 100-g OGTT.[27] Their criteria for the OGTT in pregnancy are the most widely used in the United States. O'Sullivan and Mahan studied whole blood using the Somogyi–Nelson method, which has been shown to identify other saccharides in addition to glucose.[71] The NDDG[72] has modified O'Sullivan's data for plasma values by increasing whole blood values by 15% because plasma glucose values are approximately 15% higher than those in whole blood.

Further modifications of O'Sullivan's criteria were proposed by Carpenter and Coustan, who took into consideration not only the change in the medium tested (whole blood versus plasma), as had been done by the NDDG, but also the changes in methodology.[73] Currently, the most widely used methods of glucose measurement in plasma are the glucose oxidase, or hexokinase, assay. These new methodologies are more specific for glucose and have been shown to result in approximately 5-mg/dL lower values than the less specific Somogyi–Nelson method. Thus, the criteria of Carpenter and Coustan for oral glucose tolerance testing are stricter.[73] Whole blood and plasma glucose criteria of the OGTT used for the diagnosis of GDM are presented in Table 41.7.

Long-term maternal outcome of gestational diabetes

Several investigators have shown that patients with GDM are at increased risk of developing diabetes years after pregnancy.[74] O'Sullivan et al.,[75] in a long-term study of the outcome of women with GDM, has shown the development of overt diabetes at 20 years after pregnancy to be as high as 20%, and 50% had impaired glucose tolerance.

It is recommended, therefore, that women with GDM be followed postpartum to detect diabetes early in its course. They should be evaluated at the first postpartum visit by a fasting plasma glucose test and by a 2-h OGTT (30, 90, and 120 min) using a 75-g glucose load. The criteria of the NDDG[72] for the diagnosis of diabetes mellitus in nonpregnant adults include a fasting plasma glucose level of more than 140 mg/dL on more than one occasion, or a 75-g, 2-h OGTT in which the 2-h value and at least one other value are more than 200 mg/dL. The criteria for the diagnosis of impaired glucose tolerance are the following: fasting plasma glucose below 140 mg/dL, a 2-h value between 140 and 200 mg/dL, and at least one other value of 200 mg/dL or more.

Pregestational diabetes mellitus

Congenital anomalies in infants of diabetic mothers

The frequency of major congenital anomalies among infants of diabetic mothers has been estimated at 6–10%, which represents a two- to fivefold increase over the frequency observed in the general population.[76] Congenital malformations in fetuses of diabetic patients are now responsible for approximately 40% of all perinatal deaths, replacing respiratory distress syndrome (RDS) as the leading cause of infant death.[77] These malformations usually involve multiple organ systems (Table 41.8), with cardiac anomalies being the most common, followed by central nervous system and skeletal malformations.[78]

Table 41.8 Congenital anomalies of infants of diabetic mothers.

Skeletal and central nervous system
Caudal regression syndrome
Neural tube defects excluding anencephaly
Anencephaly with or without herniation of neural elements
Microcephaly
Cardiac
Transposition of the great vessels with or without ventricular septal defects
Ventricular septal defects
Coarctation of the aorta with or without ventricular septal defects or patent ductus arteriosus
Atrial septal defects
Cardiomegaly
Renal
Hydronephrosis
Renal agenesis
Ureteral duplication
Gastrointestinal
Duodenal atresia
Anorectal atresia
Small left colon syndrome
Other
Single umbilical artery

From ref. 141.

Pathogenesis of diabetes-associated congenital anomalies

Both clinical and experimental studies agree that diabetes-associated birth defects occur after disruption of developmental processes during organogenesis and are associated with abnormal metabolism, which is thought to be related mostly to hyperglycemia.[79,80] *In vivo* studies in which rats were made diabetic by streptozotocin or alloxan therapy resulted in fetal anomalies.[81,82] These studies suggest a cause and effect relationship between altered glucose metabolism and congenital anomalies; however, the target site of action remains unknown. Studies in our laboratory at Yale on diabetes-related teratogenesis focused on the mechanism and possible target site of action.[82,83] Using the *in vitro* rodent conceptus culture system, we conducted studies of glucose-induced embryopathy. In all cases of embryopathy, concomitant characteristic yolk sac changes were observed in both gross and microscopic examinations. These findings support our hypothesis that the yolk sac is the primary target site for the adverse metabolic effect of diabetes and that embryonic malformations occur as a secondary phenomenon to the primary yolk sac damage. Factors other than hyperglycemia have been implicated in diabetes-associated birth defects, including ketone bodies, hypoglycemia, low levels of trace metals, and somatomedin-inhibiting factors.[84,85]

A correlation between maternal oxygen free radicals produced in excess in patients with diabetes mellitus and the induction of fetal anomalies has been suggested in the past few years. *In vitro* studies demonstrated that the addition of oxygen free radical-scavenging enzymes to culture medium protects embryos against glucose-induced maldevelopment and growth impairment. More recently, Hagay et al.[85] demonstrated the role of oxygen free radicals in the genesis of diabetic embryopathy *in vivo* in an animal model. Mice used in this study produced elevated levels of copper or zinc superoxide dismutase (SOD), a key enzyme in the metabolism of free oxygen radicals. This enzyme was found to elicit a protective effect against diabetes-associated embryopathy. Although this finding has yet to be verified in humans, it provides important information for designing interventions effective in the prevention of diabetic embryopathy.

Prevention of fetal anomalies

Clinical studies suggest that euglycemia during organogenesis is critical in the prevention of congenital anomalies.[86] Several investigators have recruited diabetic women before pregnancy and attempted to place them under tight glycemic control before conception.[86–90] These studies are summarized in Table 41.9.

Periconceptional care

Management of the pregnant diabetic woman is a complex task that ideally begins before conception. Prepregnancy clinics for diabetics were initiated in Edinburgh in 1976. In such clinics, physicians have the opportunity to explain to the patient and her partner the practice of diabetes care during pregnancy, in particular the need for stringent glycemic control. At the initial visit, the patient's general medical status is assessed, and signs of retinopathy, nephropathy, hypertension, and ischemic heart disease are looked for. The patient undergoes ophthalmologic evaluation, electrocardiography, and kidney function tests.[91] Optimization of blood glucose control should be achieved before a woman is advised to become pregnant. It is generally recommended that women achieve a glycosylated hemoglobin level that is less than 1% above the upper limit of normal. Women should receive appropriate contraceptive therapy while preparing for pregnancy. For women who are not already following an intensive diabetes regimen, an extensive period of education and the institution of self blood glucose monitoring is also necessary.

Diabetes management during pregnancy

Diabetes during pregnancy has been associated with increased perinatal mortality, an increased rate of Cesarean sections, significant risk of macrosomia, and other neonatal morbidities, including serious birth trauma, hypoglycemia, hypocalcemia, polycythemia, and hyperbilirubinemia.[92,93] Management is therefore directed toward reducing perinatal mortality and morbidity, a goal that may be achieved by maintaining close surveillance of the mother and fetus and stringent glucose control.

Table 41.9 Summary of selected clinical studies using a program of preconceptional metabolic control to prevent diabetes-associated birth defects.

Investigator (year)	No. of patients	Malformation rate (%)	Glucose control achieved	No. of patients	Malformation rate (%)	Glucose control achieved
	Control group			*Study group*		
Pedersen et al. (1979)	284	14.1	Inadequate	363	7.4	Improved
Miller et al. (1981)	58	22.4	$HbA_{1c} > 8.5\%$	58	3.4	$HbA_{1c} \leq 8.5\%$
Fuhrmann et al. (1983)	292	7.5	Mean daily plasma glucose ≥ 110 mg/dL in 88.3% of patients	128	0.8	Mean daily plasma glucose ≥110 mg/dL in 20.7% of patients
Steel (1988)	65	9.2	–	78	3.9	–
Goldman et al. (1986)	31	9.6	MBG = 163 ± 10.2 mg/dL $HbA_{1c} = 10.42 \pm 0.47\%$	44	0	MBG = 110 ± 6.5 mg/dL $HbA_{1c} = 7.39 \pm 0.34\%$
Kitzmiller et al. (1986)	53	15.1	$HbA_{1c} < 9.0\%$ in 47% of patients	46	2.2	$HbA_{1c} < 9.0\%$ in 87% of patients
Mills et al. (1988)	279	9.0	–	397	4.9	–
Damm et al. (1989)	61	8.2	Mean HbA_{1c} 7.3 ± 1.5%	193	1.0	Mean HbA_{1c} 7.1 ± 1.2%
Steel et al. (1990)	143	10.4		96	1.4	
Kitzmiller et al. (1991)	110	25	$HbA_{1c} > 10.6\%$	84	1.7	$HbA_{1c} < 7.9\%$
Wilhoite et al. (1993)	123	6.5	–	62	1.6	–

HbA_{1c}, hemoglobin A_{1c}; MBG, mean blood glucose.

From Reece EA, Friedman AM, Copel J, Kleinman CS. Prenatal diagnosis and management of deviant fetal growth and congenital malformations. In: *Diabetes mellitus in pregnancy*, 2nd edn. New York: Churchill Livingstone, 1995.

Diet

Diet therapy is considered a standard treatment for diabetes mellitus. The goals of diet therapy are to provide adequate maternal and fetal nutrition, appropriate gestational weight gain, and to minimize glucose excursions. For women with pregestational diabetes, guidelines suggest that diet composition be based on an individualized nutrition assessment.[94] In GDM, it is generally accepted that carbohydrate levels should not exceed 40–45% of total calories. Restricted saturated fats and cholesterol and increased dietary fiber are suggested. Most patients are instructed on how to maintain a diet that consists of three meals and one to three snacks, the last snack usually being taken at bedtime. The bedtime snack should be composed of complex carbohydrates with proteins to maintain adequate blood glucose levels during the night, thereby avoiding nocturnal hypoglycemia.

Patient weight gains are assessed at each visit to the clinic, and caloric intake is adjusted accordingly. The aim is to prevent weight reduction and its associated ketogenic risk while ensuring optimal weight gain. It is desirable to increase weight by 2–4 lb (0.9–1.7 kg) in the first trimester and 0.5–1.0 lb (200–450 g) per week thereafter until term. A total weight gain of 22–30 lb (10–13 kg) during normal and diabetic pregnancy is recommended.[95]

It is generally agreed that pregnancy is not the time for weight reduction; however, excessive weight gain should be firmly discouraged. Dietary advice to the obese pregnant diabetic patient is a matter of controversy. Several authors have indicated that caloric restriction in obese pregnant patients is contraindicated.[95] However, there are data to show that modest caloric restriction (25–30 kcal/day), especially for the morbidly obese patient, is not associated with ketonuria or elevated plasma ketone concentrations.[96,97]

Insulin administration

Insulin is the only pharmacological therapy currently recommended to treat diabetes during pregnancy. The goal of insulin therapy is to achieve blood glucose levels that are nearly identical to those observed in healthy pregnant women. Therefore, multiple injections of insulin are usually required in women with pre-existing diabetes. Human insulin is the least immunogenic of all insulins and is exclusively recommended in pregnancy. The rapid-acting insulin analogs with peak hypoglycemic action 1–2 h after injection offer the potential for

Table 41.10 General guidelines for insulin administration.

Regimen no.	Prebreakfast insulin	Prelunch insulin	Predinner insulin	Bedtime insulin	Comments
I. Two-injection scheme	NPH + regular or rapid-acting analog; 2:1	–	NPH + regular or rapid-acting analog	–	Give two-thirds of the total dose as prebreakfast dose and one-third as predinner dose Disadvantage: predinner NPH may cause nocturnal hypoglycemia (1–3 AM) and may not be effective in controlling the early morning glucose level
II. Three-injection scheme	NPH + regular or rapid-acting analog; 2:1	–	Regular or rapid-acting analog	NPH	This regimen may be more effective than regimen I. By changing the administration of NPH to bedtime, nocturnal hypoglycemia may be prevented and early morning glucose control may be achieved
III. Four-injection scheme	NPH + regular or rapid-acting analog	Regular or rapid-acting analog	Regular or rapid-acting analog	NPH	This is the most effective regimen. We use it as an alternative to regimen II. Here the dose of insulin given at bedtime replaces basal daily insulin requirements. This regimen (with a rapid-acting analog) works especially well for patients with morning sickness or erratic schedules

NPH, neutral protamine Hagedorn.

improved postprandial glucose control. Studies support their safety during pregnancy and ability to improve blood glucose control. Insulin requirements may change dramatically throughout the various stages of gestation. In the first trimester, the maternal insulin requirement is approximately 0.7 U/kg of body weight/day.[98] This is increased in the third trimester to 1.0 U/kg/day. There are several different approaches to insulin administration, as outlined in Table 41.10. We prefer to use the three-injection scheme, which permits better control of the fasting blood glucose levels while minimizing the risk of middle-of-the-night hypoglycemia.[99]

In addition, continuous subcutaneous insulin infusion pumps have also been shown to be effective during pregnancy. Insulin therapy delivered by a subcutaneous infusion pump more closely resembles that of physiologic insulin release. Insulin pumps deliver a continuous basal rate of insulin infusion with pulse-dose increments before meals. Published studies have demonstrated that comparable glucose control and pregnancy outcomes can be achieved by both conventional insulin therapy and pump therapy.[100,101] However, Gabbe[102] reported that HbA1c levels were significantly lower 1 year after delivery in women who elected to remain on pump therapy after delivery compared with women who had continued to use conventional insulin treatment. Therapy guidelines for converting patients to pump therapy are provided in Table 41.11.

Insulin therapy should be initiated in all women with GDM who fail to maintain euglycemia with diet. We start women on a daily insulin dose of 20 U of neutral protamine Hagedorn (NPH) and 10 U of regular insulin daily. Insulin doses are adjusted according to blood glucose levels, and an evening injection is added if fasting hyperglycemia persists. Some investigators have advocated the use of prophylactic insulin in GDM to reduce the risk of macrosomia. However, the advantages of this therapy must be weighed against the disadvantages of no treatment.

Table 41.11 Guidelines for insulin schedule for patients converting to pump therapy.

Use the same total daily dose of insulin that the patient received with conventional therapy
Fifty percent of the daily insulin dose is given as a constant basal rate
The remaining 50% is divided into three doses, each administered as a bolus before each meal:
20% before breakfast
15% before lunch
15% before dinner

Although the current data demonstrate a relationship between metabolic control and neonatal complications, maternal glycemia may not be the sole parameter of optimal control. In women with gestational diabetes, Buchanan and colleagues[103,104] have suggested the use of fetal ultrasound to identify pregnancies at risk of fetal macrosomia and related morbidity. They have found that a fetal abdominal circumference < 75th percentile for gestational age obtained in the late second trimester or early third trimester can distinguish pregnancies at low risk from those at high risk of producing large for gestational age (LGA) infants. Their data suggest that maternal glucose concentrations alone may not accurately predict which fetuses are at high risk of excessive fetal growth and support the use of fetal criteria to direct metabolic therapies in GDM.

Self-monitoring of blood glucose

Self blood glucose monitoring has become the mainstay of management for pregnancies complicated by diabetes mellitus. A variety of small, battery-powered blood glucose reflectance meters are currently available for home use. Accurate readings depend on performing the test correctly; however, most of the newest models are less technique dependent. Some models are extremely sophisticated, having memories that permit the storage of results with the day and time they were collected, whereas others can even be downloaded onto a personal computer. All women should be seen by a qualified nurse educator for an individualized assessment to insure that her technique is accurate. Ongoing education is also important to help the woman make necessary changes to her treatment plan to maintain euglycemia throughout gestation.

Although it has been shown that, in general, self-monitored blood glucose levels correlate very well with automated laboratories, reports have shown that sometimes patients falsely report blood glucose levels both during and outside pregnancy. These findings are worrisome as accurate information is essential for optimal management of the pregnancy complicated by diabetes. Therefore, verified blood glucose determinations (i.e., the utilization of blood glucose meters with memory) are recommended to enhance the reliability and accuracy of self-monitored blood glucose results.

Blood glucose measurements should be obtained at least four times a day (fasting and 1–2 h after meals) in women with gestational diabetes and five to seven times a day in women with pre-existing diabetes. In addition to this regular monitoring, patients should also test whenever they feel symptoms of either hyperglycemia or hypoglycemia. Detailed record keeping is useful to help identify glucose patterns. Daily urine ketone testing should be performed to insure early identification of the development of starvation ketosis or ketoacidosis. Ketone testing should also be performed any time the blood glucose level exceeds 200 mg/dL, during illness, or when the patient is unable to eat.

Blood glucose levels are measured in both fasted and postprandial states. A recent randomized controlled trial compared the efficacy of preprandial and postprandial glucose determinations in reducing the incidence of neonatal macrosomia and other complications in women with gestational diabetes.[105] Women requiring insulin treatment were randomly assigned to have their diabetes managed according to the results of preprandial self blood glucose monitoring or postprandial monitoring, which was performed 1 h after meals. Both groups had similar success in achieving blood glucose targets and demonstrated similar degrees of adherence to the monitoring schedule. Nevertheless, the women in the postprandial monitoring group received significantly more insulin and achieved a greater decrease in glycoslyated hemoglobin values during treatment than those in the preprandial monitoring group. In addition, there was significantly less macrosomia and neonatal hypoglycemia among the offspring of the mothers in the postprandial monitoring group. These data suggest that adjustment of insulin therapy according to the results of postprandial blood glucose values improves glycemic control and pregnancy outcomes. Previous studies in pregnant women with pregestational diabetes have also found that postprandial blood glucose levels are better predictors of fetal macrosomia than are fasting blood glucose levels.[106,107]

In conclusion, the target ranges for blood glucose during pregnancy should be based on maternal plasma glucose levels in normal pregnancy. The logical approach is to achieve as near normal glucose levels as possible without undue severe hypoglycemia. Current recommendations are that whole blood glucose levels should not exceed 95 mg/dL in the fasted state and 120 mg/dL after meals.

Oral agents

Traditionally, insulin therapy has been considered the gold standard for management because of its efficacy in achieving tight glucose control and the fact that it does not cross the placenta. As GDM and type 2 diabetes are characterized by insulin resistance and relatively decreased insulin secretion, treatment with oral hypoglycemic agents that target these defects is of potential interest. However, because of concerns regarding transplacental passage and, therefore, the possibility of fetal teratogenesis and prolonged neonatal hypoglycemia, these agents are not currently recommended in pregnancy.

There are no randomized controlled trials on which to draw conclusions regarding the teratogenicity of these oral agents. However, most retrospective studies and the published clinical experience have not demonstrated an increased risk of malformed infants among women treated with oral hypoglycemic agents.[108–110] Rather, the data indicate that the increased risk of major congenital anomalies appears to be related to maternal glycemic control during the periconceptual period. These studies and currently available data on the use of both metformin and sulfonylureas in pregnancy have also failed to demonstrate an increased risk of neonatal hypoglycemia and other neonatal morbidities. To date, there has only been one randomized controlled trial to test the effectiveness and safety of sulfonylurea therapy (glyburide) in the management of women with GDM.[111] Both the insulin- and the glyburide-treated women were able to achieve satisfactory glucose control and had similar perinatal outcomes. Glyburide was not detected in the cord serum of any infant in the glyburide group.

In summary, based on the currently available data, it would appear that glyburide could be safely and effectively utilized in the management of GDM. More intensive investigation regarding the safety and feasibility of oral agents in pregnancies complicated by type 2 diabetes is necessary.

Antepartum assessment

Maternal assessment

Ophthalmologic and renal function tests, including creatinine clearance and total urinary protein excretion, are performed in each trimester or more often, if indicated. In patients with vasculopathy, an electrocardiogram is performed at the initial visit and repeated, if clinically indicated. In patients in White's class H, the electrocardiogram is performed routinely in each trimester. The echocardiogram is performed at enrollment and repeated in the pregnancy, depending on the initial findings. It is extremely important to detect early signs of pregnancy-induced hypertension; therefore, an assessment of blood pressure and the signs of proteinuria and edema formation is essential. It is estimated that approximately 25% of all diabetics develop preeclampsia during pregnancy. The highest incidence is seen among patients with vasculopathy.[112] In many cases, differentiation between pregnancy-induced hypertension and chronic hypertension is very difficult. In patients with diabetic nephropathy, the diagnosis of preeclampsia may be challenging. We have used a number of factors as adjunctive clues: acute increase in blood pressure, the elevation of fibrin split products, liver function test abnormality, or thrombocytopenia. Most helpful is the increase in fibrin split products as a reasonably sensitive marker of underlying consumptive coagulopathy. We recognize that this is less than ideal but, at the present time, it is the best diagnostic aid available.

Fetal surveillance

All pregnancies complicated by diabetes require extra assessment. The use of ultrasonography provides essential information about the fetus. A first-trimester scan is used to date the pregnancy and to establish viability and fluid volume status. A second-trimester scan is repeated at 18–20 weeks' gestation to rule out fetal anomalies. Subsequent ultrasound evaluations are then performed at 4- to 6-week intervals to assess fluid volume and fetal growth. Because diabetic patients are at risk of growth aberrations (intrauterine growth restriction and macrosomia), this frequency is recommended to identify states of altered growth.

Fetal macrosomia

Macrosomia, arbitrarily defined as fetal weight in excess of 4000g, or a birthweight above the 90th percentile for gestational age, occurs in approximately 10% of all pregnancies. Almost 30% of all diabetics deliver infants weighing more than 4000g.[113] Gabbe and colleagues[114] reported an incidence of macrosomia of 20% and 25% in GDM and type 1 patients respectively.

Fetal macrosomia is thought to be related to maternal hyperglycemia which induces fetal hyperglycemia and hyperinsulinemia. Fetal hyperinsulinemia results in enhanced glycogen synthesis, lipogenesis, increased protein synthesis and, thus, fetal organomegaly and fat deposition.

Macrosomic fetuses have higher rates of perinatal morbidity and mortality, a result caused mainly by the traumatic delivery. These fetuses are at increased risk of severe fetal asphyxia due to head and neck birth trauma. Shoulder dystocia is common in macrosomic fetuses; therefore, infants of diabetics experience more shoulder dystocia than those of nondiabetics. Disproportional growth of the body compared with the head is believed to be the cause of shoulder dystocia. Acker and associates[115] reported the incidence of shoulder dystocia in nondiabetic offspring weighing 4000–4499g as 10% and in those weighing 4500g or more as 22%. Among the offspring of diabetics, the incidence is much higher, and in infants with birthweights of 4000–4499g and 4500g or more, the incidence doubles, reaching 23.1% and 50% respectively.

It has been suggested that Cesarean section should be employed to deliver diabetic mothers of babies of 4000g or more.[115] In our institutions, primary Cesarean section is performed if the estimated fetal weight is 4500g or more. In cases of estimated fetal weight of 4000–4500g, the mode of delivery is determined individually for each patient and is based on the clinical assessment of the pelvis and the past history (e.g., birthweight of previous babies). In such cases, midpelvic instrumental delivery should be avoided as much as possible.

Antepartum fetal testing

In pregnant diabetic patients, stillbirth occurs with increased frequency, particularly in the third trimester.[116] Therefore, a program of fetal monitoring should be initiated, usually at 32–33 weeks. Currently, in most medical centers, outpatient protocols for antepartum fetal surveillance include either once- or twice-weekly nonstress tests (NSTs), once-weekly oxytocin challenge tests (OCTs), or biophysical profiles.[117] Which is the best test remains controversial because controlled, prospective randomized studies comparing the various methods of antepartum fetal assessment are lacking. Many investigators have concluded that the NST is simple, inexpensive, and reasonably reliable. Therefore, the NST is most widely used for pregnancies complicated by diabetes mellitus.[117,118]

Gabbe and colleagues[114] observed no intrauterine fetal death within 1 week of a negative contraction stress test (CST) in 211 metabolically well-controlled type 1 patients. This observation suggests that a negative CST in metabolically controlled patients predicts fetal survival for 1 week. The high incidence of false-positive CSTs (50%) and the potential unnecessary intervention as a result of these false-positive findings are major disadvantages.

The biophysical profile has been shown to have a lower false-abnormal test rate than either the CST or NST.[119] Golde and Plan[117] have demonstrated that a biophysical score of 8 is reliable in predicting good fetal outcome in diabetics, which is comparable to the reliability of reactive NSTs.

Sadovsky[120] has shown that maternal evaluation of fetal movements has a very low false-negative rate and that patients with decreased fetal movements of less than 10 in 12 h may show severe fetal compromise. Therefore, further testing is necessary in cases of decreased fetal movements. Maternal assessment of fetal activity seems to be not only a practical approach toward evaluation of fetal condition but a simple, inexpensive, and valuable screening technique. Patients with diabetes are instructed to count fetal movements, beginning as early as 28–29 weeks of gestation, and to report any decrease in fetal movements so that further testing can be initiated if necessary.

A large body of evidence shows that maternal glucose control is the most important factor in improved perinatal mortality and morbidity rates. Therefore, any method of fetal surveillance is ineffective unless strict control of maternal diabetes is maintained.[117] In fact, the need for elective intervention resulting from abnormal antepartum fetal testing in diabetics in good metabolic control is very low compared with patients in poor metabolic control.[121] Several investigators reported an intervention rate of 1–5%, based on abnormal fetal testing in pregnant type 1 patients.[122–124] In one report, no intervention for abnormal fetal testing was required in 82 type 1 patients.[125] Drury and colleagues[124] have shown that, when strict maternal metabolic control is achieved, antepartum fetal testing can be used less frequently and that, despite limited use of antepartum testing, the perinatal mortality was low, approaching 3%.

In summary, in recent years, management protocols using strict metabolic control consistent with various techniques of antepartum surveillance have allowed more diabetic patients to deliver at term and to achieve good fetal outcome similar to that of the general obstetric population.

Timing and mode of delivery

In recent years, there has been a significant change in the attitude of obstetricians and perinatologists toward the mode and timing of delivery of type 1 and type 2 pregnant patients. It is now recognized worldwide that, if the pregnant diabetic patient and her fetus are under stringent metabolic control and antepartum surveillance, delivery may be safely delayed in most cases until term or the onset of spontaneous labor.[114,126]

Management during labor and delivery

During labor and delivery, it is necessary to maintain maternal euglycemia to avoid neonatal hypoglycemia. Induced maternal hyperglycemia during labor in diabetics is associated with neonatal hypoglycemia.[127,128] Soler and associates[127] have demonstrated that mean glucose levels of more than 90 mg/dL during labor are associated with higher rates of neonatal episodes of hypoglycemia. Therefore, the goal should be to maintain glucose levels of 70–90 mg/dL during labor.

Caloric and insulin requirements in diabetic patients during labor have been studied extensively.[129] Investigators have documented a decrease in insulin requirement, particularly in the first stage of labor, with constant glucose requirement during this time. Jovanovic and Peterson,[129] using an artificial pancreas (Biostator) for 12 type 1 patients during labor, have demonstrated the lack of insulin requirement during the first stage of labor, despite a constant and continuous glucose infusion rate of 2.5 mg/kg/min. In another study by Golde and colleagues,[130] 48% of type 1 patients undergoing induction of labor required no insulin therapy.

Therefore, in patients undergoing induction of labor, the morning insulin doses should be withheld and glucose levels determined once every hour with a home glucose meter. In well-controlled patients, 1 U of insulin/h and 3–6 g of glucose/h are usually required to maintain a glucose level of 70–90 mg/dL. If the initial glucose level is between 80 and 120 mg/dL, 10 U of regular insulin can be added to 1000 mL of 5% dextrose in 0.5% normal saline or 5% dextrose 5% and Ringer's lactate, and administered at an infusion rate of 125 mL/h. If initial glucose levels are less than 70 mg/dL, it is recommended that, initially, 5% dextrose in water without insulin at a rate of 100–120 mL/h be given throughout labor.

If the patient presents in spontaneous labor and has already taken her morning intermediate-acting insulin, additional insulin may not be required throughout labor and delivery, but a continuous glucose infusion will be necessary (125 mL/h of 5% dextrose in water).

When an elective Cesarean section is planned for a diabetic patient, the procedure should be scheduled early in the morning, when glucose levels are usually in the normal range because of the action of the intermediate-acting insulin dose given the night before. Infusion without glucose is preferred (i.e., normal saline), and glucose levels are monitored frequently. If the patient is under regional anesthesia, it is easier to detect signs of hypoglycemia.

After delivery, a dramatic decrease in the insulin requirement is almost the rule because of a significant decrease in the level of placental hormones that have anti-insulin action. At this time, there is no need for stringent glucose control, and glucose levels of less than 200 mg/dL are satisfactory. In the first few days after delivery, it is preferable to give regular insulin subcutaneously before each meal on the basis of plasma glucose levels. After the patient is able to eat regular meals, she may receive one-half of the prepregnancy dosage of insulin, usually divided into two daily injections.

Maternal complications

Diabetic women have a markedly higher risk of a number of pregnancy complications. Because of a paucity of data on maternal complications during diabetic pregnancy, the exact relative risk for each complication is not known. Complications that have been reported to be more frequent in diabetic pregnancy include spontaneous abortion, preterm labor, pyelonephritis, polyhydramnios, and hypertensive disorders. Also directly related to metabolic control are hypoglycemia and diabetic ketoacidosis (DKA). These complications, together with the vascular alterations and the higher Cesarean section rate, contribute to the higher maternal morbidity and mortality among diabetic pregnant patients.

Maternal mortality

The advent of insulin in 1922 and its widespread introduction in 1935 brought about a dramatic fall in the maternal mortality rate from 45% to just over 2%.[2] Together with improved medical and obstetric care, the maternal mortality rate has decreased to as low as 0.5%.[131] More recently, a mortality rate of 0.11% was reported among 2584 pregnant diabetic patients.[132] Causes or events related to maternal death among diabetics include acute myocardial infarction during Cesarean section,[133] sepsis, hemorrhage, ketoacidosis, hypoglycemia, and anesthetic and hypertensive complications.[131] Maternal mortality seems to be highest (approaching 65%) among patients with coronary artery disease.[134]

Diabetic ketoacidosis

In recent years, the incidence of DKA during pregnancy has decreased significantly. Cousins,[132] in a review of a large number of studies, found an incidence of 9.3% of DKA among 1508 diabetics. Ketoacidosis has been reported to occur in pregnant diabetic patients more rapidly and at lower blood glucose levels than in nonpregnant patients. It may be precipitated by stress, infection (e.g., urinary tract), or omission of insulin because of patient neglect. The use of beta-sympathomimetic agents in pregnant diabetics may induce DKA.[135]

Omission of insulin or insulin deficiency in type 1 pregnant patients results in hyperglycemia and glucosuria. Osmotic diuresis results in urinary potassium, sodium, and water losses. Hyperglycemia is aggravated because, as a consequence of hypovolemia, there is an increase in the secretion of glucagon and catecholamines.[136,137] Lipolysis consequent to insulin deficiency leads to increased hepatic oxidation of fatty acids, with the formation of ketone bodies (acetone, β-hydroxybutyrate, and acetoacetate), which leads to the production of metabolic acidosis (Fig. 41.3).

The following are some general guidelines for the treatment of DKA:

1 Insert two intravenous lines; obtain blood to assess levels of glucose, serum electrolytes and ketones, and arterial blood gases; and administer oxygen by face mask. Frequently assess the clinical status and follow urinary output. Repeat blood and urinary testing often.

2 Patients with DKA require simultaneous correction of fluid and electrolyte imbalance and treatment of hyperglycemia and acidosis.

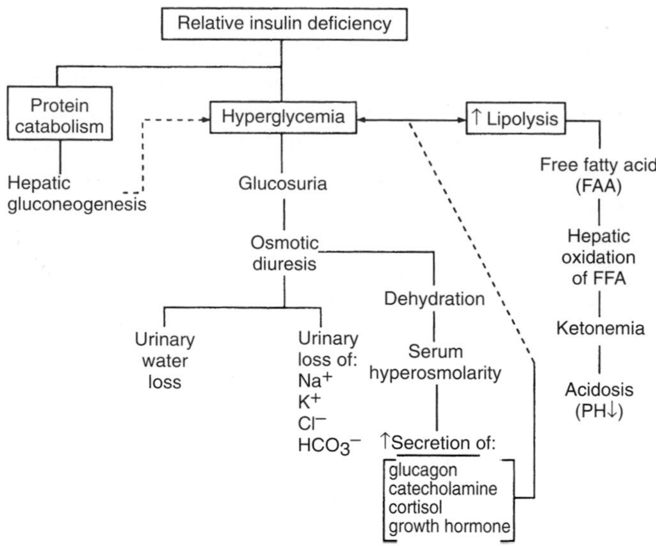

Figure 41.3 Metabolic alterations in diabetic ketoacidosis.

- Replacement of fluid. The average fluid deficit is 3–5 L. It is therefore necessary to administer 1000–2000 mL of isotonic saline rapidly during the first hour. If hypernatremia is present, 0.45% sodium chloride is preferred. After the first hour, 300–500 mL/h is given, depending on hemodynamic status. Normal saline is given to hypotensive patients in larger amounts. In these cases, a central line may be necessary.
- Insulin therapy. Administer an initial bolus of 10–20 U of regular insulin intravenously. Follow this with a constant infusion of approximately 10 U/h (Add 50 U of regular insulin per 500 mL of normal saline.) Larger doses of constant regular insulin infusion of 12–20 U/h may be required if acidosis does not begin to respond within 3 h or if plasma glucose level does not fall by 30%.
- Glucose administration. To reduce the risk of hypoglycemia and cerebral edema, change the intravenous solution to 5% dextrose when the plasma glucose level reaches 200–250 mg/dL, and simultaneously decrease the rate of the insulin infusion.
- Potassium administration. Hyperkalemia is usually present on administration. At this point, potassium administration is not required and, in fact, may be dangerous or even lethal because hyperkalemia may rapidly reach cardiotoxic levels. Potassium administration is usually started after 3–4 h of insulin therapy, when potassium begins to fall to normal or low levels. It is given by adding 40 mEq of potassium chloride per 1000 mL of normal saline at a rate of 10–20 mEq/h, as needed. It should be stressed that, when potassium is administered, it is given with extreme caution, and that potassium and urinary output are monitored carefully.
- Bicarbonate administration. Add 44 mEq of sodium bicarbonate to 1 L of 0.45% saline and administer intra-

venously only if arterial pH is less than 7.1 or serum bicarbonate is less than 5 mEq. If the pH is less than 7, the sodium bicarbonate dose should be doubled (88 mEq). Bicarbonate administration should be terminated if arterial pH has been corrected to 7.2. Alkali administration in DKA is still controversial because this therapy might aggravate tissue hypoxia.

Hypoglycemia

The goal of very stringent glycemic control during diabetic pregnancy places the patient at increased risk for hypoglycemic episodes. Coustan and associates[101] observed a high frequency of both symptomatic and biochemical hypoglycemia. Forty-five percent of type 1 patients treated with multiple daily insulin injections had severe hypoglycemia requiring hospitalization or emergency room care.

Pyelonephritis

Pedersen[138] reported a 6% incidence of pyelonephritis in diabetic pregnant patients, including it as one of the "prognostic bad signs of pregnancy" because it is associated with higher perinatal mortality and morbidity. Cousins[132] reported an incidence of pyelonephritis of 2.2% among 356 class B and C diabetics, and 4.9% among 264 class D, F, and R diabetics in an extensive literature review. In no study, however, was a nondiabetic control group used for comparison. It appears that, in recent years, there has been a reduction in the frequency of pyelonephritis in diabetic pregnancy.[139] However, this reduction has not been confirmed statistically.[132] Nevertheless, it is our practice to perform serial urine cultures at least once in each trimester of pregnancy and to treat asymptomatic bacteriuria vigorously in diabetic pregnant patients because, if left untreated, it may result in frank pyelonephritis.

Polyhydramnios

Polyhydramnios occurs commonly in diabetics, with a reported incidence that varies from 3% to 32%.[132] Although this condition can be associated with central nervous system and gastrointestinal abnormalities, in almost 90% of diabetics with polyhydramnios, no etiology can be found.[140]

The etiology of polyhydramnios in diabetics is not clear. Suggested mechanisms include increases in amniotic fluid osmolality caused by increases in glucose load, decreased fetal swallowing, high gastrointestinal tract obstruction, and fetal polyuria secondary to fetal hyperglycemia. Experimental work, however, has not provided strong evidence for any of these explanations.[141] Although the most likely reason for the higher fluid volume is increased fetal urine production in diabetics, this was not demonstrated by sequential estimation of bladder volume over time.[142]

Preterm labor

Earlier studies have found that the incidence of prematurity in diabetic pregnancies is three times higher than that in nondiabetics.[143] This high rate was attributed in part to the higher rate of iatrogenic preterm delivery. In a study by Miodovnik and colleagues,[144] the rate of spontaneous preterm labor was 31.1% in type 1 patients, a rate that is three to four times more than that reported in the general obstetric population. The authors found two factors to be significantly associated with premature labor: premature rupture of membranes and previous history of preterm labor and delivery. Furthermore, patients with poor glycemic control during the second trimester of pregnancy had increased rates of preterm delivery. Interestingly, polyhydramnios was not significantly associated with preterm labor in this study.

Magnesium sulfate is considered the drug of choice in diabetic patients with premature labor because it has no effect on diabetic control. In contrast, beta-sympathomimetic tocolytic agents or glucocorticosteroids have been reported to induce hyperglycemia and ketoacidosis.[139] Therefore, treatment with both medications in diabetics requires great caution, intensive monitoring of glucose levels, and treatment with intravenous insulin infusion as needed.

Spontaneous abortions

The rate of spontaneous abortion in pregestational pregnant diabetic patients varies considerably between reports, ranging from 6% to 29%.[145] Most studies are retrospective and do not have nondiabetic control groups for comparison. Kalter,[146] in an extensive literature review of the years 1950–1986, concluded that the incidence of spontaneous abortion in diabetic women is similar to that in nondiabetic women, approaching 10%. However, a prospective study reported from Cincinnati, Ohio, showed a significantly higher rate of spontaneous abortions among pregnant type 1 patients than among pregnant nondiabetic women (30% vs 15%).[147] Furthermore, the same group demonstrated in another study that the higher rate of spontaneous abortions in type 1 women was associated with poor glycemic control in the early postconceptional period, as reflected by high levels of HbA_{1c} early in pregnancy.[148] The latter findings were confirmed by the results of the Diabetes in Early Pregnancy Study.[106]

Diabetic retinopathy

Diabetic retinopathy is usually classified as background simple diabetic retinopathy and proliferative diabetic retinopathy. The characteristic lesions of diabetic retinopathy are presented in Table 41.12.

Microaneurysms alone are not usually associated with severe loss of vision but, when maculopathy is present with either macular edema or macular ischemia, serious loss of vision can occur. The most serious condition, however, is proliferative retinopathy, which carries a high risk of blindness. It is believed that background retinopathy represents an early stage of the disease: as it worsens, it leads to proliferative retinopathy, which, when developed, is usually associated with the characteristic lesions of background retinopathy.[149]

Table 41.12 Characteristic lesions of diabetic retinopathy.

Background diabetic retinopathy
Microaneurysms
Small vessel obstruction, soft exudates, intraretinal microvascular abnormalities
Venous abnormalities
Retinal hemorrhages
Hard exudates
Disk edema
Maculopathy
Proliferative diabetic retinopathy
Neovascularization
Fibrous deposition
Vitreous hemorrhage
Retinal detachment

Pregnancy and progression of diabetic retinopathy

Investigators have reported controversial findings on the role of pregnancy in the development and progression of diabetic retinopathy. Most recent reports have shown that, in some diabetic patients, pregnancy is associated with progression of diabetic retinopathy from minimal to marked deterioration of the retina.[150–153] However, many changes during pregnancy have proved to be reversible, and many patients have experienced regression of their lesion after delivery.

Tight metabolic control in pregnancy and diabetic retinopathy

Studies in nonpregnant type 1 patients investigated the effect of glycemic control on the progression of diabetic retinopathy.[154,155] These studies have shown that progression of diabetic retinopathy was significantly higher over an 8-month period compared with a control group with proper metabolic control.[154,155] After 2 years of follow-up, no statistical significance was found between the rates of progression of retinopathy in the two groups. The authors suggest that caution should be used and that one should avoid achieving good glycemic control too rapidly in type 1 patients with retinopathy and poor glycemic control.

Principal management of diabetic retinopathy in pregnant diabetics

Diabetic retinopathy occurring during pregnancy should be treated in essentially the same manner as in the nonpregnant state.[149] Laser treatment can be used safely during pregnancy, when indicated. It is recommended that diabetic patients undergo careful retinal examination before conception and be treated with laser photocoagulation before pregnancy, if necessary. It is our practice to perform ophthalmoscopy every trimester in pregnant type 1 patients and even more frequently in patients with documented retinopathy before pregnancy.

The preferred mode of delivery in patients with active proliferative retinopathy remains controversial. In the past, the performance of Cesarean section was suggested to avoid the Valsalva maneuver and the risk of vitreous hemorrhage.[156–158] Today, however, most investigators do not recommend Cesarean delivery in patients with active neovascularization because it has been found that vitreous hemorrhages during childbirth are extremely rare.[158] Furthermore, there are no data to show any advantage of Cesarean section over vaginal delivery in patients with proliferative retinopathy.

Diabetic nephropathy

Diabetic nephropathy is a disease that develops slowly and appears on average 17 years after the onset of type 1 diabetes. Background retinopathy complicates almost all these pregnancies, and proliferative retinopathy affects approximately 35–65% of patients.[159,160]

The prevalence of diabetic nephropathy in type 1 pregnant patients is estimated at 6%.[138] Five evolutionary stages of nephropathy in diabetics have been described for type 1 diabetes:[161]

1 early hypertrophy or hyperfunction;
2 glomerular lesions without clinical disease;
3 incipient nephropathy characterized by microproteinuria;
4 overt nephropathy characterized by macroproteinuria;
5 endstage diabetic renal disease.

In type 1 diabetes, renal insufficiency eventually occurs in all patients who exhibit macroproteinuria, whereas in type 2 diabetes, deterioration occurs in only 10% of cases.[162] A diagnosis of diabetic nephropathy in pregnancy is made if there is persistent proteinuria of more than 300 mg/day in the first half of pregnancy in the absence of urinary tract infection.[160]

Several studies examining fetal outcome and maternal risks in women with diabetic nephropathy suggest that most patients have an increase in proteinuria during the course of pregnancy.[159,163] Reece and colleagues[160] reported an increase in third-trimester proteinuria that exceeded 3.0 g/day in 70% of the pregnancies studied. Kitzmiller and colleagues[159] also found increasing proteinuria in the third trimester, with almost 60% exceeding 6.0 g/day in the third trimester.

Acute worsening of hypertension is very common in patients with diabetic nephropathy and occurs in almost 60% of cases. In the report by Reece and colleagues,[160] hypertension during pregnancy developed in 32% of women who began pregnancy with normal blood pressure levels. However, after delivery, changes in renal function, proteinuria, and hypertension returned to values observed in the first trimester. Based on a 9-year follow-up study, the long-term maternal course was judged to be consistent with the expected course of diabetic nephropathy in nonpregnant women.

Many investigators have shown that the likelihood of a successful fetal and neonatal outcome in patients with diabetic nephropathy is comparable to that of type 1 patients without overt renal disease.[105,109] Fetal survival has been reported to exceed 90% when contemporary methods of fetal and maternal care are applied.[159,160,163] Perinatal mortality and morbidity in patients with diabetic nephropathy may be attributed to the higher incidence of early delivery (31%), a higher incidence of low birthweight infants (21%),[159] and an increased incidence of fetal distress and preeclampsia. Therefore, pregnant patients with diabetic nephropathy require an intensive program of maternal and fetal evaluation, adequate bedrest during pregnancy, assessment of renal function and retinal status at regular intervals, blood pressure monitoring, and treatment of hypertension, when required, using methyldopa, arteriolar vasodilator, or beta-blockers. In patients on antihypertensive medications before pregnancy, the same regimen is continued during pregnancy (with the exception of diuretics and ace inhibitors, which should be discontinued). A modest sodium restriction (1500 mg of Na) in all patients with significant proteinuria (> 500 mg/dL) is suggested to reduce the rate of edema formation.

Morbidity of the infant of the diabetic mother

In the last decade the perinatal morbidity rate in pregnancies complicated by diabetes mellitus has been remarkably reduced. However, severe neonatal morbidity in infants of diabetic mothers is still a problem that may affect even infants delivered at term.[164,165] The following sections briefly discuss the most common neonatal morbidities.

Hypoglycemia

Hypoglycemia is diagnosed when plasma glucose levels are less than 35 mg/dL and 25 mg/dL in term and preterm infants respectively. Infants of diabetic mothers in unsatisfactory glycemic control often develop hypoglycemia during the first few hours of life. The reported incidence ranges from 25% to 40% of infants of diabetic mothers. Poor glycemic control during pregnancy and high maternal plasma glucose levels at the time of delivery increase the risk of occurrence, particularly if the patients have been delivered by Cesarean section.[166]

Because prolonged and severe hypoglycemia may be associated with neurologic sequelae, initiation of treatment is advised in all neonates of diabetic mothers with plasma glucose levels of less than 40 mg/dL. The most efficient means of therapy for hypoglycemia is continuous dextrose infusion at a rate of 4–6 mg/kg/min. The use of a bolus of a hypertonic glucose infusion should be avoided to prevent later rebound hypoglycemia.[167] Occasionally, hypoglycemia may persist beyond the second day of life and may require the use of glucocorticoids.[168,169]

Hypocalcemia and hypomagnesemia

There is a significant increase in the incidence of hypocalcemia and hypomagnesemia in infants of diabetic mothers.[170,171] The incidence of neonatal hypocalcemia, defined as calcium levels at or below 7 mg/dL, has been reported to approach 20% in a group of infants with a mean gestational age at delivery of 38 ± 0.2 weeks.[172] Serum calcium levels in infants of diabetic mothers are lowest on the second to third days of life. The etiology of hypocalcemia in neonates of diabetic mothers is not yet clear, but some evidence shows that it is associated with "relative" neonatal hypoparathyroidism.[173] It has also been postulated that magnesium deficiency may contribute to hypoparathyroidism and hypocalcemia in infants of diabetic mothers.[167]

Polycythemia

Polycythemia is diagnosed when the venous hematocrit exceeds 65%. This condition has been reported to affect one-third of neonates of diabetic mothers in the first few hours of life.[174] The mechanism responsible for polycythemia in these babies may be related to chronic intrauterine hypoxia that leads to an increase in erythropoietin and a consequent increase in red blood cell production.

Usually, polycythemia is associated with hyperviscosity of the blood, which may impede the velocity of blood flow and increase the risk of microthrombus formation in multiple organs.[175,176] Kidneys, adrenals, and lungs are the most commonly affected organs. Clinically, infants with polycythemia appear plethoric. Some of these infants have convulsions, respiratory distress, tachycardia, congestive heart failure, and hyperbilirubinemia. The treatment of polycythemia consists of partial exchange transfusion with a volume expander (e.g., plasma) to reduce the hematocrit to approximately 55%.[177]

Respiratory distress syndrome (RDS)

RDS was considered a common neonatal morbidity in the infants of diabetic mothers in the past. However, the incidence has dramatically decreased with the initiation of strict glycemic control. Factors contributing to the development of RDS in these infants are preterm deliveries, delayed fetal lung maturation, and a high rate of elective Cesarean section.

In poorly controlled diabetic patients, the reason for the increased risk of RDS seems to be related to the inhibitory effect of high fetal insulin levels on surfactant phospholipid synthesis and secretion and possibly to decreased prolactin levels.[178,179]

Hyperbilirubinemia

Infants of diabetic mothers have a higher incidence of hyperbilirubinemia than do infants of nondiabetic mothers matched for gestational age.[180] The mechanism of this increased risk of jaundice is not clear. Early treatment of polycythemia may further reduce the risk of hyperbilirubinemia.

Cardiomyopathy

Infants of diabetic mothers have a higher risk of hypertrophic types of cardiomyopathy and congestive heart failure.[181] The incidence of cardiomyopathy in neonates of diabetic mothers is not known. According to one study, 10% of infants of diabetic mothers may have evidence of myocardial and septal hypertrophy. The characteristic findings in echocardiography are generalized myocardial hypertrophy with disproportionate hypertrophy of the interventricular septum. Infants of diabetic mothers with severe cardiomyopathy may develop left ventricular outflow tract obstruction with reduced cardiac output and congestive heart failure.[182,183] The natural history of cardiomyopathy in infants of diabetic mothers is different from other types of cardiomyopathy in that there is a complete regression of hypertrophic changes to normal after several months.[181,184] Several studies have demonstrated a strong correlation between the risk of cardiomyopathy in infants of diabetic mothers and poor maternal diabetic control.[182,185,186]

Conclusion

The diagnosis of diabetes mellitus during pregnancy has certain implications for the well-being of both the mother and the fetus. Advances in medical and obstetric care have dramatically improved the outlook for women with diabetes and their offspring. However, both mother and child remain at increased risk for a number of complications. Research indicates that the majority of these complications are associated with hyperglycemia. The achievement and maintenance of euglycemia has therefore become the major focus of management.

Key points

1 Diabetes mellitus is a heterogeneous disorder characterized by hyperglycemia. It is estimated that diabetes mellitus affects approximately 4 million women of childbearing age in the United States.

2 Diabetes mellitus is generally classified into the following categories: type 1, type 2, and GDM. The prevalences of type 1, type 2, and GDM are all increasing.

3 The development of insulin resistance during late pregnancy is a normal physiologic adaptation that shifts maternal energy metabolism from carbohydrate to lipid oxidation and thus spares glucose for the growing fetus.

4 Screening for gestational diabetes mellitus consists of a 50-g oral glucose load, followed 1 h later by a plasma glucose determination. The screen is performed without regard to the time of day or interval since the last meal.

5 This screening should be carried out at 24–28 weeks' gestation in average-risk women not known to have diabetes mellitus.

6 Current research studies indicate that optimization of blood glucose control in the periconceptual period can dramatically reduce the rate of congenital malformations in the offspring of women with diabetes.

7 All diabetic women of childbearing age should be counseled regarding the importance of preconception care and planning of their pregnancies.

8 Women with diabetes and their offspring are at greater risk of a number of pregnancy-related complications.

9 Strict blood glucose control prior to conception and throughout gestation can reduce and/or eliminate the excess risk for both mother and baby.

10 The achievement of euglycemia requires frequent daily self blood glucose determinations in both the fasted and the postprandial states.

11 Subcutaneous insulin pump therapy can be a safe and effective means of glucose control in pregnant women with diabetes.

12 The introduction of new rapid-acting insulin analogs has expanded our options for the treatment of diabetes during pregnancy.

13 Serial ultrasound measurements need to be performed during pregnancy to identify infants at risk of excessive fetal growth.

14 Most clinicians institute some form of antenatal surveillance based on diabetes classification, existence of comorbidities, and degree of glycemic control.

15 Hypertensive complications are more common in women with diabetes than in their nondiabetic counterparts.

16 Diabetic ketoacidosis is one of the most significant complications in pregnancy and requires both timely and aggressive treatment.

17 Pregnancy *per se* is an independent risk factor that accelerates retinopathy.

18 Macrosomic fetuses have higher rates of morbidity and mortality, a result caused mainly by traumatic delivery.

19 Euglycemia should be maintained during labor and delivery to reduce the risk of neonatal hypoglycemia.

References

1 Peel J. A historical review of diabetes and pregnancy. *J Obstet Gynaecol Br Commonw* 1972;79:385.

2 Reece EA, Gabbe SG. The history of diabetes mellitus in women. In: Reece EA, Coustan DR, Gabbe SG, eds. *Diabetes in women.* Philadelphia, PA: Lippincott Williams & Wilkins; 2004:6–7.

3 Evers IM, deValk HW, Visser GH. Risk of complications of pregnancy in women with type 1 diabetes: nationwide prospective study in the Netherlands. *Br Med J* 2004;328:915.

4 Dunne R, Brydon P, Smith K, Gee H. Pregnancy in women with Type 2 diabetes: 12 years outcome data 1990–2002. *Diabetic Med* 2003;20:734.

5 White P. Pregnancy complicating diabetes. *Am J Med* 1949;7:609.

6 Hare JW, White P. Gestational diabetes and the White classification. *Diabetes Care* 1980;3:394.

7 ACOG Technical Bulletin. Diabetes and pregnancy. No. 200, December 1994 (replaces No. 92, May 1986). Committee on Technical Bulletins of the American College of Obstetricians and Gynecologists. *Int J Gynaecol Obstet* 1995;480:331.

8 Hitman GA. Progress with the genetics of insulin-dependent diabetes mellitus. *Clin Endocrinol* 1986;25:463.

9 Report of the Expert Committee on the Diagnosis and Classification of Diabetes Mellitus. *Diabetes Care* 1997;7:1183.

10 Freinkel N. Gestational diabetes 1979: philosophical and practical aspects of a major health problem. *Diabetes Care* 1980; 3:399.

11 Barnett AH, ed. *Immunogenetics of insulin-dependent diabetes.* Lancaster: MTP Press; 1987:11.

12 Singal DP, Blajchman MA. Histocompatibility (L-A) antigens, lymphocytotoxic antibodies and tissue antibodies in patients with diabetes mellitus. *Diabetes* 1973;22:429.

13 Nerup J, Platz P, Anderson OO, et al. ALA-antigens and diabetes mellitus. *Lancet* 1974;ii:864.

14 Cudworth AG, Woodrow JC. HLA system and diabetes mellitus. *Diabetes* 1975;24:245.

15 Rotter N, Rimoin DL. The genetics of diabetes. *Hosp Pract* 1987;22:79.

16 Ekoe JM. *Diabetes mellitus. Aspects of world-wide epidemiology of diabetes mellitus and its long-term complications.* Amsterdam: Elsevier; 1988:34.

17 Zinunet P, Taylor RR, Whitehouse S. Prevalence rates of impaired glucose tolerance and diabetes mellitus in various Pacific populations according to the new WHO criteria. *WHO Bull* 1982;60:279.

18 Zimmet P, Taft P. The high prevalence of diabetes mellitus in Nauru, a Central Pacific Island. *Adv Metab Disord* 1978;9:225.

19 Thompson G, Robinson WP, Kuhner MK, et al. Genetic heterogeneity, modes of inheritance, and risk estimates for a joint study of Caucasians with insulin-dependent diabetes mellitus. *Hum Genet* 1988;43:799.

20 Mokdad AH, Ford ES, Bowman BA, et al. Diabetes trends in the US: 1990–1998. *Diabetes Care* 2000;23:1278.

21 Pinhas-Hamiel O, Standiford D, Hamiel D, et al. The type 2 family: a setting for development and treatment of adolescent type 2 diabetes mellitus. *Arch Pediatr Adolesc Med* 1999;153:1063.

22 Eisenbarth BS. Type I diabetes mellitus. A chronic autoimmune disease. *N Engl J Med* 1986;314:1360.

23 Todd IA, Bell N, McDevitt HO. A molecular basis for genetic susceptibility to type I (insulin dependent) diabetes: analysis of the HLA-DR association. *Diabetologia* 1984;24:224.

24 Ridgway WM, Fathman CO. The association of MHC with autoimmune diseases: understanding the pathogenesis of autoimmune diabetes. *Clin Immunopathol* 1998;86:3.

25 Dorman IS. Molecular epidemiology of insulin-dependent diabetes mellitus. *Epidemiol Rev* 1997;19:91.

26 Kobberling I, Bruggeboes B. Prevalence of diabetes among children of insulin-dependent diabetic mothers. *Diabetologia* 1980;18:459.

27 Wagener DK, Sacks JM, Laporte RE, et al. The Pittsburgh study of insulin-dependent diabetes mellitus: risk for diabetes among relatives of IDDM. *Diabetes* 1982;31:136.

28 Warram IH, Krolewski AS, Gottlieb MS, et al. Differences in risk of insulin-dependent diabetes in offspring of diabetic mothers and diabetic fathers. *N Engl J Med* 1984;311:149.

29 Vadheim CM, Rotter N, Maclaren NK, et al. Preferential transmission of diabetic alleles within the HLA gene complex. *N Engl J Med* 1986;315:1314.

30 Gamble DR. An epidemiological study of childhood diabetes affecting two or more siblings. *Diabetologia* 1980;19:341.

31 Tillil H, Kobberling I. Age-corrected empirical genetic risk estimates for first-degree relatives of IDDM patients. *Diabetes* 1987;36:93.

32 Cahill F, Jr. Heterogeneity in type II diabetes (editorial). *West J Med* 1985;142:240.

33 Permutt MA, Andreone T, Chirgwin I, et al. The genetics of type I and type II diabetes: analysis by recombinant DNA methodology. *Adv Exp Med Biol* 1985;189:89.

34 Ober C, Wason CJ, Andrew K, et al. Restriction fragment length polymorphisms of the insulin gene hypervariable region in gestational onset diabetes mellitus. *Am J Obstet Gynecol* 1987;157: 1364.

35 Ginsberg-Fellner F, Mark EM, Nechemias C, et al. Islet cell antibodies in gestational diabetics. *Lancet* 1980;ii:362.

36 Freinkel N, Metzger BE. Gestational diabetes: problems in classification and implications for long-range prognosis. In: Vranic M, Hollenberg CH, Steiner A, eds. *Comparison of type I and type II diabetes. Similarities and dissimilarities in etiology, pathogenesis, and complications.* New York. Plenum, 1985:47.

37 Vardi P, Dib SA, Tuttlemen M, et al. Competitive insulin autoantibody assay. Prospective evaluation of subjects at high risk for development of type I diabetes mellitus. *Diabetes* 1987;36: 1286.

38 Ginsberg-Fellner F, Witt ME, Franklin BH, et al. Triad of markers for identifying children at high risk of developing insulin-dependent diabetes mellitus. *JAMA* 1985;254:1469.

39 Pettit DL, Aleck KA, Baird HR, et al. Congenital susceptibility to NIDDM. Role of intrauterine environment. *Diabetes* 1988;37:622.

40 Brumfield C, Huddleston JF. The management of diabetic ketoacidosis in pregnancy. *Clin Obstet Gynecol* 1984;27:50.

41 Lind T, Billewicz WZ, Brown G. A serial study of changes occurring in the oral glucose tolerance test during pregnancy. *J Obstet Gynaecol Br Commonw* 1973;80:1033.

42 Kuhl C, Hoist II. Plasma glucagon and insulin:glucagon ratio in gestational diabetes. *Diabetes* 1976;25:16.

43 Spellacy WN, Goetz FC. Plasma insulin in normal late pregnancy. *N Engl J Med* 1963;268:988.

44 Kalkhoff R, Schalch DS, Walker JL, et al. Diabetogenic factors associated with pregnancy. *Trans Assoc Am Phys* 1964;77:270.

45 Bleicher SI, O'Sullivan JB, Freinkel N. Carbohydrate metabolism in pregnancy. V. The interrelations of glucose, insulin, and free fatty acids in late pregnancy and postpartum. *N Engl J Med* 1964;271:866.

46 Kuhl C. Glucose metabolism during and after pregnancy in normal and gestational diabetic women. I. Influence of normal pregnancy on serum glucose and insulin concentration during basal fasting conditions and after a challenge with glucose. *Acta Endocrinol* 1975;79:709.
47 Kalkhoff RK, Kissebah AH, Kim H-I. Carbohydrate and lipid metabolism during normal pregnancy: relationship to gestational hormone action. *Semin Perinatol* 1978;12:291.
48 Catalano PM, Tyzbir ED, Roman NM, et al. Longitudinal changes in insulin resistance in non-obese pregnant woman. *Am J Obstet Gynecol* 1991;165:1667.
49 Buchanan TA, Metzger BE, Freinkel N et al. Insulin sensitivity and B-cell responsiveness to glucose during late pregnancy in lean and moderately obese women with normal glucose tolerance or mild gestational diabetes. *Am J Obstet Gynecol* 1990;162: 1008.
50 Ryan EA, O'Sullivan MJ, Skyler JS. Insulin action during pregnancy: studies with the euglycemic clamp technique. *Diabetes* 1985;34:380.
51 Catalano PM, Tyzbir ED, Wolfe RR, et al. Carbohydrate metabolism during pregnancy in control subjects and women with gestational diabetes. *Am J Physiol* 1993;264:E60.
52 Sivan E, Chen XC, Homko CJ, et al. A longitudinal study of carbohydrate metabolism in healthy, obese pregnant women. *Diabetes Care* 1997;20:1470–1475.
53 Homko CJ, Sivan E, Reece EA, Boden G. Fuel metabolism during pregnancy. *Semin Reprod Endocrinol* 1999;17:119.
54 Rice PA, Rourke JE, Nesbitt REL. Some characteristics of the glucose transport. *Gynecol Invest* 1976;7:213.
55 Johnson LW, Smith CH. Monosaccharide transport across microvillous membrane of human placenta. *Am J Physiol* 1980;2387:160.
56 Battaglia FC, Meschia G. *An introduction to fetal physiology*. New York: Academic Press, 1986.
57 Cordero L, Yea SY, Grunt JA, et al. Hypertonic glucose infusion during labor. Maternal-fetal blood glucose relationships. *Am J Obstet Gynecol* 1970;107:295.
58 Oakley NW, Beard RW, Turner RC. Effect of sustained maternal hyperglycaemia on the fetus in normal and diabetic pregnancies. *Br Med J* 1972;1:466.
59 Young M. Techniques for studying placental metabolism and transfer. In: Beaconsfield P, Billee C, eds. *Placenta, a neglected experimental animal.* Oxford: Pergamon Press; 1979:96.
60 Hollingsworth DR. Alterations of maternal metabolism in normal and diabetic pregnancies. Differences in insulin-dependent, non-insulin-dependent and gestational diabetes. *Am J Obstet Gynecol* 1983;146:417.
61 Lewis SB, Wallin JD, Kuzuya H, et al. Circadian variation of serum glucose, C-peptide immunoreactivity and free insulin in normal and insulin treated diabetic pregnant patients. *Diabetologia* 1976;12:343.
62 Knopp R, Montes A, Childs M, et al. Metabolic adjustments in normal and diabetic pregnancy. *Clin Obstet Gynecol* 1980;24: 21.
63 Metzger BE, Phelps RL, Freinkel N, et al. Effects of gestational diabetes on diurnal profiles of plasma glucose, lipids, and individual amino acids. *Diabetes Care* 1980;3:402.
64 Skryten A, Johnson G, Samisoe G, et al. Studies in diabetic pregnancy. I. Serum lipids. *Acta Obstet Gynecol Scand* 1976;55:211.
65 Knopp RH, Chapman M, Bergelin R, et al. Relationships of lipoprotein lipids to mild fasting hyperglycemia and diabetes in pregnancy. *Diabetes Care* 1980;3:416.
66 Molsted-Pedersen L, Wagner L, Klege G, et al. Aspects of carbohydrate metabolism in newborn infants of diabetic mothers. IV. Neonatal changes in plasma free fatty acid concentration. *Acta Endocrinol* 1972;71:338.
67 Szabo AJ, Opperman W, Hanover B, et al. Fetal adipose tissue development: relationship to maternal free fatty acid levels. In: Camerini-Davalos RA, Cole HS, eds. *Early diabetes in early life.* New York: Academic Press, 1975.
68 Metzger BE, Coustan DR. Summary and recommendations of the Fourth International Workshop Conference on Gestational Diabetes Mellitus. *Diabetes Care* 1998;21(Suppl. 2): B161.
69 Sepe SJ, Connell FA, Geiss LS, et al. Gestational diabetes. Incidence, maternal characteristics, and perinatal outcome. *Diabetes* 1985;34(Suppl. 2):13.
70 Metzger BE, the Organizing Committee. Summary and recommendations of the Third International Workshop-Conference on Gestational Diabetes Mellitus. *Diabetes* 1991:40(Suppl. 2): 197.
71 O'Sullivan JB, Mahan CM. Criteria for the oral glucose tolerance test in pregnancy. *Diabetes* 1964;13:278.
72 National Diabetes Data Group. Classification and diagnosis of diabetes mellitus and other categories of glucose intolerance. *Diabetes* 1979;28:1039.
73 Carpenter MW, Coustan DR. Criteria for screening tests for gestational diabetes. *Am J Obstet Gynecol* 1982;144:768.
74 Stowers JM, Sutherland HW, Kerridge DF. Long-range implications for the mother. The Aberdeen experience. *Diabetes* 1985;34(Suppl. 2):106.
75 O'Sullivan JB, Charles D, Mahan CM, et al. Gestational diabetes and perinatal mortality rate. *Am J Obstet Gynecol* 1973;116: 901.
76 Reece EA, Gabrielli S, Abdalla M. The prevention of diabetes-associated birth defects. *Semin Perinatol* 1988;12:292.
77 Mills JL. Malformations in infants of diabetic mothers. *Teratology* 1982;25:385.
78 Kucera J. Rate and type of congenital anomalies among offspring of diabetic women. *J Reprod Med* 1971;7:61.
79 Goldman AS, Baker L, Piddington R, et al. Hyperglycemia-induced teratogenesis is mediated by a functional deficiency of arachidonic acid. *Proc Natl Acad Sci USA* 1985;82:8277.
80 Pinter E, Reece EA, Leranth C, et al. Arachidonic acid prevents hyperglycemia-associated yolk sac damage and embryopathy. *Am J Obstet Gynecol* 1986;155:691.
81 Mintz DH, Chez RA, Hutchinson DL. Subhuman primate pregnancy complicated by streptozotocin-induced diabetes mellitus. *J Clin Invest* 1972;51:837.
82 Pinter E, Reece EA, Leranth C, et al. Yolk sac failure in embryopathy due to hyperglycemia. Ultrastructural analysis of yolk sac differentiation of rat conceptuses under hyperglycemic culture conditions. *Teratology* 1986;33:363.
83 Pinter E, Reece EA, Leranth C, et al. Ultrastructural analysis of malformations of the embryonic neural axis induced by in vitro hyperglycemic culture conditions. Fifth Annual Scientific Meeting of the Society of Perinatal Obstetricians (Abstract), 1985.
84 Eriksson UI, Borg LAH. Protection by free oxygen radicals scavenging enzymes against glucose induced embryonic malformations in vitro. *Diabetologia* 1991;34:325.
85 Hagay, Z, Weiss Y, Zusman I, et al. Prevention of diabetes-associated embryopathy by overexpression of the free radical scavenger copper zinc superoxide dismutase in transgenic mouse embryos. *Am J Obstet Gynecol* 1995;173:1036.

86 Reece EA, Homko CJ. Why do diabetic women deliver malformed infants? *Obstet Gynecol Clin* 2000;43:32.
87 Pedersen JF, Pedersen-Molsted L. Congenital malformations: the possible role of diabetes care outside pregnancy. Ciba Foundation Symposium, 1979:265.
88 Mills JL, Knopp RH, Simpson JL, et al. Lack of relation of increased malformation rates in infants of diabetic mothers to glycemic control during organogenesis. *N Engl J Med* 1988; 318:671.
89 Fuhrmann K, Risker H, Semmler K, et al. Prevention of congenital malformations in infants of insulin-dependent diabetic mothers. *Diabetes Care* 1983;6:219.
90 Reece EA, Eriksson UJ. The pathogenesis of diabetes-associated congenital malformations. *Obstet Gynecol Clin North Am* 1996;23:29.
91 Steel JM, Johnstone FD, Smith AF, et al. Five years' experience of a "pre-pregnancy" clinic for insulin-dependent diabetics. *Br Med J* 1982;285:353.
92 Reece EA, Homko CJ. Infant of the diabetic mother. *Semin Perinatol* 1994;18:459.
93 Weintrob N, Karp M, Hod M. Short and long-range complications in offspring of diabetic mothers. *J Diabetes Complic* 1996;10:294.
94 American Diabetes Association. Principles of nutrition and dietary recommendations for individuals with diabetes mellitus. *Diabetes Care* 1979;2:520.
95 Pitken RM. Nutritional influences during pregnancy. *Med Clin North Am* 1977;61:3.
96 Coetzee EJ, Jackson WP, Berman PA. Ketonuria in pregnancy, with special reference to calorie-restricted food intake in obese diabetics. *Diabetes* 1980;29:177.
97 Kay RM, Grobin W, Track NS. Diets rich in natural fiber improve carbohydrate tolerance in maturity-onset, non-insulin-dependent diabetics. *Diabetologia* 1981;20:18.
98 Jovanovic L, Peterson CM. Optimal insulin delivery for the pregnant diabetic patient. *Diabetes Care* 1982;5(Suppl. 2):24.
99 Homko CJ, Reece EA. Ambulatory management of the pregnant woman with diabetes. *Obstet Gynecol Clin North Am* 1998;41: 584.
100 Rudolf MCI, Coustan DR, Sherwin RS, et al. Efficacy of the insulin pump in the home treatment of pregnant diabetics. *Diabetes* 1981;30:891.
101 Coustan DR, Reece RA, Sherwin R, et al. A randomized clinical trial of insulin pump vs. intensive conventional therapy in diabetic pregnancies. *JAMA* 1986;255:631.
102 Gabbe SG. New concepts and applications in the use of the insulin pump during pregnancy. *J Matern–Fetal Med* 2000;9: 42.
103 Buchanan TA, Kjos SL, Montoror MN, et al. Use of fetal ultrasound to select metabolic therapy for pregnancies complicated by mild gestational diabetes. *Diabetes Care* 1994;17: 275.
104 Kjos SL, Schaefer-Graf U, Sardesi S, et al. A randomized controlled trial using glycemic plus fetal ultrasound parameters versus glycemic parameters to determine insulin therapy in gestational diabetes with fasting hyperglycemia. *Diabetes Care* 2001;24:1904.
105 deVeciana M, Major CA, Morgan MA, et al. Postprandial versus preprandial blood glucose monitoring in women with gestational diabetes requiring insulin therapy. *N Engl J Med* 1995;333: 1237.
106 Jovanovic-Peterson CM, Reed GF, Metzger BE, et al. Maternal postprandial glucose levels and infant birth weight. The Diabetes in Early Pregnancy Study. *Am J Obstet Gynecol* 1991;164: 103.
107 Combs CA, Gunderson E, Kitzmiller JL, et al. Relationship of fetal macrosomia to maternal postprandial glucose control during pregnancy. *Diabetes Care* 1992;15:1251.
108 Towner D, Kjos S, Leung B, et al. Congenital malformations in pregnancies complicated by NIDDM. *Diabetes Care* 1995;18: 1446.
109 Piacquadio K, Hollingsworth DR, Murphy H. Effects of in-utero exposure to oral hypoglycemic drugs. *Lancet* 1991;383: 866.
110 Homko CJ, Sivan E, Reece EA. Is there a role for oral antihyperglycemics in gestational diabetes and type 2 diabetes during pregnancy? *Treat Endocrinol* 2004;3:133.
111 Langer O, Conway DL, Berkus MD, et al. A comparison of glyburide and insulin in women with gestational diabetes mellitus. *N Engl J Med* 2000;343:1134.
112 Simonson DC. Etiology and prevalence of hypertension in diabetic patients. *Diabetes Care* 1988;11:821.
113 Elliot JP, Garite TL, Freeman RK, et al. Ultrasonic prediction of fetal macrosomia in diabetic patients. *Obstet Gynecol* 1982;60: 159.
114 Gabbe SG, Mestman JH, Freeman RK, et al. Management and outcome of class A diabetes mellitus. *Am J Obstet Gynecol* 1977;127:465.
115 Acker D, Sachs BP, Friedman EA. Risk factors for shoulder dystocia. *Obstet Gynecol* 1985;66:762.
116 North AF, Mazumdar S, Logrillo VM. Birth weight, gestational age, and perinatal death in 5,471 infants of diabetic mothers. *J Pediatr* 1977;90:444.
117 Golde S, Plan L. Antepartum testing in diabetes. *Clin Obstet Gynecol* 1985;28:516.
118 Phelan JP. The nonstress test: a review of 3000 tests. *Am J Obstet Gynecol* 1981;139:7.
119 Manning FA, Morrison I, Lange IR, et al. Fetal assessment based on fetal biophysical profile scoring: experience in 12,260 referred high-risk pregnancies. *Am J Obstet Gynecol* 1985;151:343.
120 Sadovsky E. Fetal movements and fetal health. *Semin Perinatol* 1981;5:131.
121 Adashi EY, Pinto H, Tyson JE. Impact of maternal euglycemia on fetal outcome in diabetic pregnancy. *Am J Obstet Gynecol* 1979;133:268.
122 Golde SH, Montoro M, Good-Anderson B, et al. The role of NST, fetal biophysical profile and CST in the outpatient management of insulin-requiring diabetic pregnancies. *Am J Obstet Gynecol* 1984;148:269.
123 Teramo K, Ammala P, Ylinen K, et al. Pathologic fetal heart rate associated with poor metabolic control in diabetic pregnancies. *Obstet Gynecol* 1983;61:559.
124 Drury MI, Stronge IM, Foley ME, et al. Pregnancy in the diabetic patient: timing and mode of delivery. *Obstet Gynecol* 1983;62:279.
125 Jovanovic R, Jovanovic L. Obstetric management when normoglycemia is maintained in diabetic pregnant women with vascular compromise. *Am J Obstet Gynecol* 1984;149:617.
126 Coustan DR. Delivery: timing, mode and management. In: Reece EA, Coustan DR, eds. *Diabetes mellitus in pregnancy.* Edinburgh: Churchill Livingstone; 1988:525.
127 Soler NG, Soler SM, Malins IM. Neonatal morbidity among infants of diabetic mothers. *Diabetes Care* 1978;1:340.
128 Grylack U, Chu SS, Scanlon JW. Use of intravenous fluids before cesarean section: effect on perinatal glucose insulin and sodium hemostasis. *Obstet Gynecol* 1984;63:654.

129 Jovanovic L, Peterson CM. Insulin and glucose requirements during the first stage of labor in insulin-dependent diabetic women. *Am J Med* 1983;75:605.
130 Golde SH, Good-Anderson B, Montoro M, et al. Insulin requirements during labor: a reappraisal. *Am J Obstet Gynecol* 1982; 144:556.
131 Gabbe S, Mestman J, Hibbard L. Maternal mortality in diabetes mellitus. An 18 year survey. *Obstet Gynecol* 1976;48:549.
132 Cousins L. Pregnancy complications among diabetic women: review 1965–1985. *Obstet Gynecol Surv* 1987;42:140.
133 Olofsson P, Liedholm H, Sartor A, et al. Diabetes and pregnancy. A 21-year Swedish material. *Acta Obstet Gynecol Scand* 1984;122:3.
134 Reece EA, Egan JFX, Coustan DR, et al. Coronary artery disease in diabetic pregnancies. *Am J Obstet Gynecol* 1986;154:150.
135 Thomas D, Gill B, Brown P, et al. Salbutamol-induced diabetic ketoacidosis. *Br Med J* 1977;2:438.
136 Kitzmiller JL. Diabetes ketoacidosis and pregnancy. *Contemp Obstet Gynecol* 1982;20:141.
137 Schade DS, Eaton RP. The pathogenesis of diabetes ketoacidosis: a reappraisal. *Diabetes Care* 1979;2:296.
138 Pedersen J. *The pregnant diabetic and her newborn*, 2nd edn. Copenhagen: Munksgaard, 1977.
139 Diamond M, Vaughn W, Salyer S. Efficacy of outpatient management of insulin-dependent diabetic pregnancies. *J Perinatol* 1985;5:2.
140 Lufkin G, Nelson R, Hill L, et al. An analysis of diabetic pregnancies at Mayo Clinic, 1950–79. *Diabetes Care* 1984;7:539.
141 Reece EA, Hobbins IC. Diabetes embryopathy, pathogenesis, prenatal diagnosis and prevention. *Obstet Gynecol Surv* 1986;41:325.
142 Wladirniroff JW, Barentsen R, Wallenburg HCS, et al. Fetal urine production in a case of diabetes associated with polyhydramnios. *Obstet Gynecol* 1975;46:100.
143 Molsted-Pedersen L. Preterm labour and perinatal mortality in diabetic pregnancy: obstetric considerations. In: Sutherland HW, Stowers JM, eds. *Carbohydrate metabolism in pregnancy and the newborn*. Berlin: Springer-Verlag; 1979:392.
144 Miodovnik M, Mimouni F, Siddiqi TA, et al. High spontaneous premature labor rate in insulin-dependent diabetic (IDD) pregnant women: an association with poor glycemic control. Scientific Abstracts of the Seventh Annual Meeting of the Society for Perinatal Obstetrics, Lake Buena Vista, Florida, February 5–7, 1987.
145 Miodovnik M, Mimouni F, Siddiqi TA, et al. Periconceptional metabolic status and risk for spontaneous abortion in insulin-dependent diabetic pregnancies. *Am J Perinatol* 1988;5:368.
146 Kalter H. Diabetes and spontaneous abortion: an historical review. *Am J Obstet Gynecol* 1987;156:1243.
147 Miodovnik M, Lavin JP, Knowles HC, et al. Spontaneous abortion among insulin-dependent diabetic women. *Am J Obstet Gynecol* 1984;150:372.
148 Miodovnik M, Skillman C, Holroyde JC, et al. Elevated maternal hemoglobin Al in early pregnancy and spontaneous abortion among insulin-dependent diabetic women. *Am J Obstet Gynecol* 1985;153:439.
149 Puklin J. Diabetic retinopathy. In: Reece EA, Coustan D, eds. *Diabetes mellitus in pregnancy.* Edinburgh: Churchill Livingstone, 1988.
150 Klein R, Klein BEK, Moss SE, et al. Effect of pregnancy on progression of diabetic retinopathy. *Diabetes Care* 1990;13:34.
151 Laatikainen L, Teramo K, Hieta-Heikurainen H, et al. A controlled study of the influence of continuous subcutaneous insulin infusion treatment on diabetic retinopathy during pregnancy. *Acta Med Scand* 1987;221:367.
152 Price JH, Hadden DR, Archer DB, et al. Diabetic retinopathy in pregnancy. *Br J Obstet Gynaecol* 1984;91:11.
153 Serup L. Influence of pregnancy on diabetic retinopathy. *Acta Endocrinol (Copenh)* 1986;277:122.
154 Kroc Collaborative Study Group. The Kroc study patients at 2 years: a report on further retinal changes. *Diabetes* 1985; 34(Suppl. 1):39A.
155 Lauritzen T, Frost-Larsen K, Larsen HW, et al. Two year experience with continuous subcutaneous insulin infusion in relation to retinopathy and neuropathy. *Diabetes* 1985;34(Suppl. 3):74.
156 Kitzmiller IL, Aiello LM, Kaldany A, et al. Diabetic vascular disease complicating pregnancy. *Clin Obstet Gynecol* 1981;24: 107.
157 Elman K, Welch RA, Frank RN, et al. Diabetic retinopathy in pregnancy: a review. *Obstet Gynecol* 1990;75:119.
158 Sunness JS. The pregnant woman's eye. *Surv Ophthalmol* 1988;32:219.
159 Kitzmiller IL, Brown ER, Phillippe N, et al. Diabetic nephropathy and perinatal outcome. *Am J Obstet Gynecol* 1981;141:741.
160 Reece EA, Coustan DR, Hayslen JP, et al. Diabetic nephropathy: pregnancy performance and fetomaternal outcome. *Am J Obstet Gynecol* 1988;159:56.
161 Mogensen CE. Renal function changes in diabetes. *Diabetes* 1976;25:871.
162 Deckert T, Andersen AR, Christiansen JS, et al. Course of diabetic nephropathy. Factors related to development. *Acta Endocrinol* 1981;97:242.
163 Redman CWG. Controlled trials of treatment of hypertension during pregnancy. *Obstet Gynecol Surv* 1982;37:523.
164 Landon MB, Gabbe SG, Piana R, et al. Neonatal morbidity in pregnancy complicated by diabetes mellitus: predictive value of maternal glycemic profiles. *Am J Obstet Gynecol* 1987;156: 1089.
165 Kitzmiller JL, Younger MD, Tabatabaii A, et al. Diabetic pregnancy and perinatal morbidity. *Am J Obstet Gynecol* 1978;131:560.
166 Hertel I, Kiihl C. Metabolic adaptations during the neonatal period in infants of diabetic mothers. *Acta Endocrinol (Copenh)* 1986;277:136.
167 Tsang RC, Ballard I, Colleen B. The infant of the diabetic mother: today and tomorrow. *Clin Obstet Gynecol* 1981;24:125.
168 Haworth JC, Dilling LA, Vidyasagar D. Hypoglycemia in infants of diabetic mothers. Effect of epinephrine therapy. *J Pediatr* 1973;82:94.
169 Wu PYK, Modanlou H, Karelitz M. Effect of glucagon on blood glucose homeostasis in infants of diabetic mothers. *Acta Paediatr Scand* 1975;64:441.
170 Tsang RC, Kleinman L, Sutherland JM, et al. Hypocalcemia in infants of diabetic mothers: studies in Ca, P and Mg metabolism and in parahormone responsiveness. *J Pediatr* 1972;80: 384.
171 Tsang RC, Strub R, Steichen H, et al. Hypomagnesemia in infants of diabetic mothers. Perinatal studies. *J Pediatr* 1976;89:115.
172 Fallucca F, Gargiulo P, Troili F, et al. Amniotic fluid insulin, C-peptide concentrations, and fetal morbidity in infants of diabetic mothers. *Am J Obstet Gynecol* 1985;153:534.
173 Noaguchi A, Eren M, Tsang RC. Parathyroid hormone in hypocalcemic and normocalcemic infants of diabetic mothers. *J Pediatr* 1980;97:112.
174 Gamsu HR. Neonatal morbidity in infants of diabetic women. *J R Soc Med* 1978;71:211.

175 Nichols MM, Laharopoulos P. Thrombosis of superior mesenteric artery in a newborn infant. *Am J Dis Child* 1969;117: 599.
176 Oh W. Neonatal outcome and care. In: Reece EA, Coustan DR, eds. *Diabetes mellitus in pregnancy.* Edinburgh: Churchill Livingstone; 1988:547.
177 Nogee L, McMahan M, Witsett JA. Hyaline membrane disease and surfactant protein, SAP-35, in diabetes in pregnancy. *Am J Perinatol* 1988;5:374.
178 Bourbon JR, Farrell PM. Fetal lung development in the diabetic pregnancy. *Pediatr Res* 1985;19:253.
179 Saltzman DH, Barbieri RL, Frigoletto FD. Decreased fetal cord prolactin concentration in diabetic pregnancy. *Am J Obstet Gynecol* 1986;154:1035.
180 Taylor PM, Wofson JH, Bright NH, et al. Hyperbilirubinemia in infants of diabetic mothers. *Biol Neonate* 1963;5:289.
181 Breitweser JA, Meyer RA, Sperling MA, et al. Cardiac septal hypertrophy in hyperinsulinemic infants. *J Pediatr* 1980;96:535.
182 Mace S, Hirschfeld SS, Riggs T, et al. Echocardiographic abnormalities in infants of diabetic mothers. *J Pediatr* 1979;95:1013.
183 Gutgesell HP, Speer ME, Rosenburg HS. Characterization of the cardiomyopathy in infants of diabetic mothers. *Circulation* 1980;61:441.
184 Leslie J, Shen SC, Strauss L. Hypertrophic cardiomyopathy in a mid trimester fetus born to a diabetic mother. *J Pediatr* 1982;100:631.
185 Way GL, Wolfe RR, Eshaghpour E, et al. The natural history of hypertrophic cardiomyopathy in infants of diabetic mothers. *J Pediatr* 1979;95:1020.
186 Reller MD, Tsang RC, Meyer RA, et al. Relationship of prospective diabetes control in pregnancy to neonatal cardiorespiratory function. *J Pediatr* 1985;106:86.

42 Endocrine disorders in pregnancy

Fred H. Faas

In this chapter on endocrine disorders in pregnancy, changes in endocrine function that occur during normal pregnancy will be reviewed. Following this, those endocrine disorders whose diagnosis, course, or treatment are affected by pregnancy will be discussed. This chapter is intended to present a practical review of these issues and will emphasize the most common dilemmas facing the practicing clinician. The diagnostic and therapeutic areas of confusion or controversy will be reviewed in the greatest detail to provide the information necessary for decisions in patient management.

Endocrine changes associated with a normal pregnancy

There are a number of endocrine changes that occur during normal pregnancy. Although the mechanisms for these changes are not always understood, they presumably occur for the health of the mother and her developing offspring. The known mechanism(s) of these changes and the importance to the physician of understanding these changes will be reviewed. Some of these changes occur through the existing maternal endocrine system, and some occur as a result of effects of placental hormones on the maternal endocrine system. For additional information on this subject, see Chapters 5 and 9.

Pituitary

Lactotroph hyperplasia causes an increase in pituitary size in normal pregnancy, mainly due to estrogen stimulation of the pituitary lactotrophs. Prolactin levels rise progressively during pregnancy in preparation for lactation. Prolactin levels rise to 100–300 ng/mL by late pregnancy, levels in the range of those seen in pituitary prolactinomas in the nonpregnant patient[1,2] (see Fig. 42.1). The new diagnosis of a prolactinoma in a pregnant patient is not a common problem, as substantial prolactin elevations typically result in amenorrhea and infertility. However, it is important to be aware that prolactin levels are normally elevated during pregnancy to avoid confusion in diagnosis. For the management of patients during pregnancy with known pituitary prolactinomas prior to pregnancy, see the section in this chapter on Prolactinomas under Pituitary disorders.

Cortisol and adrenocorticotrophic hormone (ACTH) levels rise normally during pregnancy as a result of large rises in corticotropin-releasing hormone (CRH), derived from the fetal–placental unit[3–5] (see Table 42.1). CRH levels can be detected in maternal plasma at levels averaging at least 100 times those in nonpregnant plasma.[3] Estrogen-induced increases in cortisol-binding globulin increase total plasma cortisol without affecting plasma free cortisol. However, total and free plasma cortisol, ACTH and 24 h urine free cortisol all increase during normal pregnancy. Twenty-four-hour urine free cortisol levels average three times higher than those in the nonpregnant state.[3] Thus, pregnancy is a normal physiologic state of mild hypercortisolism, which on occasion has corresponding clinical features of mild hypercortisolism. Interestingly, it has been suggested that activation of the hypothalamic–pituitary–adrenal axis during pregnancy, resulting from the large rises in CRH derived from the fetal–placental unit, combined with the central suppression of maternal hypothalamic CRH secretion, might explain the increased vulnerability to affective disorders during the postpartum period.[6] A practical implication of these changes in the hypothalamic–pituitary–adrenal axis during and immediately after pregnancy is that diagnosis of Cushing syndrome, particularly the ACTH-dependent type, should be made with caution during this time period. Unless there is a profound clinical situation indicating severe Cushing syndrome, diagnostic evaluation is best deferred until after delivery.

Salt and water metabolism

The renin–aldosterone system is a major determinant of sodium balance in pregnancy, as in the nonpregnant state. Salt retention occurs during pregnancy accompanied by a rise in renin and aldosterone levels, producing a form of secondary

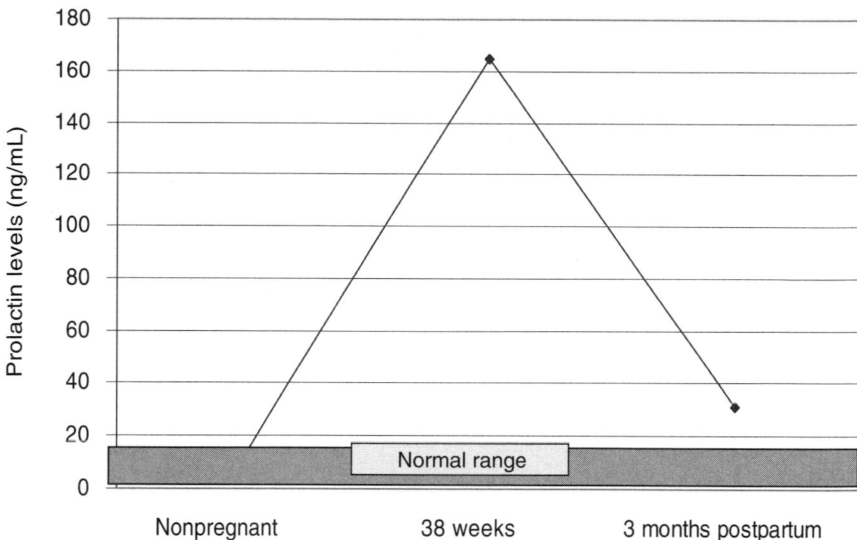

Figure 42.1 Changes in serum prolactin during pregnancy and in the postpartum period. Data shown in the figure were derived from the data from refs 1 and 2.

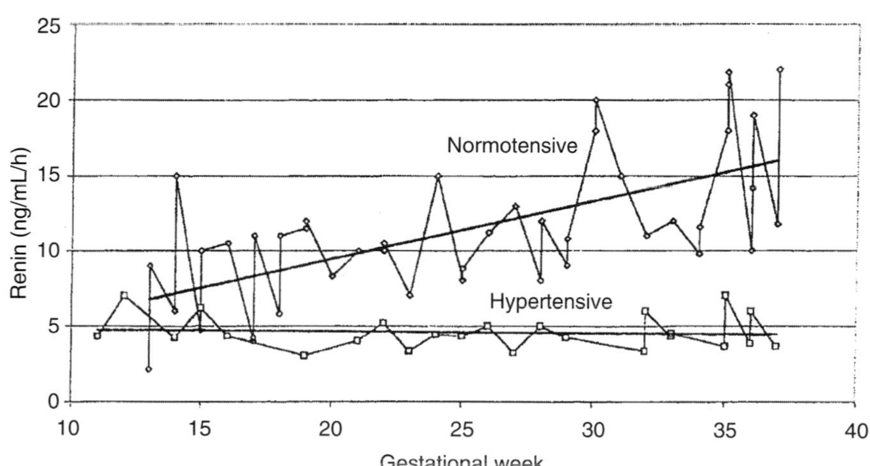

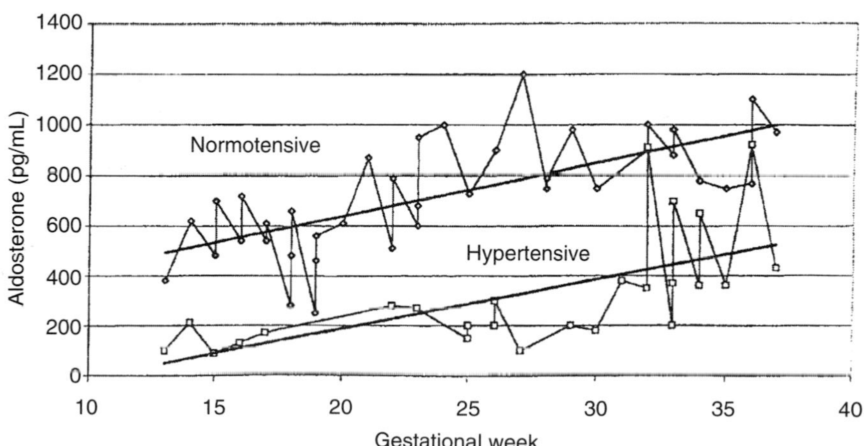

Figure 42.2 Plasma renin activity and aldosterone levels during pregnancy in normotensive and hypertensive women. Reprinted from ref. 7.

hyperaldosteronism. Renin and aldosterone levels may increase to three or four times the levels in the nonpregnant state[7] (see Fig. 42.2). Interestingly, in gestational hypertension, this effect is dampened. In general, unless there is an urgent clinical situation, diagnostic evaluation of hyperaldosteronism is better delayed until the postpartum period, although a very low renin activity level during pregnancy might suggest primary hyperaldosteronism.

Table 42.1 Mean concentrations of CRH, ACTH, cortisol, and urine free cortisol in pregnant and nonpregnant women.

Study group	CRH (pg/mL)	ACTH (pg/mL)	Serum cortisol (μg/dL)	Urine free cortisol (μg/24 h)
Nonpregnant	< 41	1.3 ± 0.4	9.2 ± 4.0	29 ± 1
21–24 weeks' gestation	158 ± 5	8.2 ± 1.8	15.4 ± 1.9	–
25–28 weeks' gestation	315 ± 50	11.4 ± 0.9	23.7 ± 3.1	–
29–32 weeks' gestation	705 ± 115	15.0 ± 0.9	31.9 ± 5.0	–
22–34 weeks' gestation	–	–	–	89 ± 14
33–36 weeks' gestation	2060 ± 490	16.4 ± 3.2	36.7 ± 5.4	–
37–40 weeks' gestation	4410 ± 893	13.2 ± 1.8	37.7 ± 4.0	–

Adapted from ref. 3.

In normal pregnancy, there is a decrease in plasma osmolality to a level of about 10 mOsmol/kg below normal.[8,9] This seems to result from a new steady-state setpoint caused by a decrease in the osmotic thresholds for both thirst and vasopressin suppression, similar to that seen in the syndrome of inappropriate antidiuretic hormone secretion (SIADH).

Calcium metabolism

A detailed discussion of changes in calcium and bone mineral metabolism occurring during pregnancy is beyond the scope of this chapter. One new area of interest related to calcium metabolism and pregnancy is the importance of parathyroid hormone-related peptide (PTHrp) in pregnancy. PTHrp, the protein responsible for causing humoral hypercalcemia of malignancy in many patients, has been found to be necessary for development of the fetal skeleton. In fact, in animal models, absence of PTHrp results in severe abnormalities and an incompletely developed fetal skeleton.[10] PTHrp is also instrumental in the transport of calcium in the lactating mammary gland.[11] The calcium receptor present in nonparathyroid tissues appears to be partially regulated by PTHrp. Increasing blood levels of PTHrp during pregnancy further suggest that it plays an important role during normal pregnancy. The practical implications of changes in PTHrp levels in normal pregnancy are unknown at this time.

There is an obvious need for increased available calcium in the mother for the developing fetal skeleton. Calcium homeostasis appears to be attained by more efficient intestinal calcium absorption and by renal calcium conservation during pregnancy and lactation.[12] Although total calcium levels may fall during pregnancy due to hemodilution, ionized calcium levels remain normal. It has been suggested that the increased calcium needed for infant growth during pregnancy and lactation may come in part from the maternal skeleton. Regarding the need for maternal dietary calcium during pregnancy, it has been the standard practice for many years to give pregnant women supplemental calcium with vitamin D, usually 400 IU of vitamin D daily. Serum 25(OH)vitamin D levels are considered the best measure of endogenous vitamin D status. Although 1,25(OH)vitamin D levels increase during pregnancy, 25(OH)vitamin D and parathyroid hormone levels are typically normal during pregnancy. It has been recognized in recent years that vitamin D deficiency is an increasingly common condition in healthy nonpregnant adults, particularly in dark-skinned people. There is evidence that severe vitamin D deficiency may cause rickets and affect fetal growth. A better understanding of vitamin D requirements and vitamin D levels in normal pregnant women taking usual amounts of dietary calcium and vitamin D is needed. Although the dose of dietary vitamin D necessary during pregnancy has not been determined scientifically, it may be as much as 1000 IU daily or more.[13,14] One concern is the possibility that increased intake of vitamin D in association with the hypercalciuria that often occurs in pregnancy may increase the frequency of kidney stones during pregnancy, although the dose of vitamin D necessary to elevate serum 25(OH)vitamin D levels and cause hypercalciuria is likely to be much higher than this (see the section on Vitamin D deficiency below).

Thyroid

Thyroid-binding globulin (TBG) levels increase during pregnancy as a result of increased estrogen levels, and lead to increases in total thyroxine (T_4) and total triiodothyroxine (T_3), but this increase in TBG does not affect free thyroid hormone or thyroid-stimulating hormone (TSH) levels. However, there is often a transient rise in free T_4 (although usually within the normal range) during the first trimester of pregnancy associated with a mild decrease in TSH due to the high circulating human chorionic gonadotropin (hCG) levels (see section below on hCG). This requires different normal ranges for TSH during each trimester of pregnancy. In some cases, these changes may be more pronounced and may be considered an abnormal change in thyroid function during pregnancy rather than "normal." This has been referred to as gestational transient thyrotoxicosis. This syndrome may also overlap with the transient thyrotoxicosis associated with hyperemesis gravidarum (see section below on Thyrotoxicosis). In addition to changes in thyroid hormone levels, an increase in thyroid size sometimes occurs during pregnancy, which may be related to a relative iodine deficiency (see section below on Goiter).

Placental/fetal hormones affecting the maternal endocrine system

These hormones are discussed in more detail in other sections of this book. Here, the emphasis will be on effects they may have on the maternal endocrine system.

Human chorionic gonadotropin

hCG is a glycoprotein, a unique gonadotropin produced by the syncytiotrophoblast of the placenta. It is an analog of luteinizing hormone (LH) with the same alpha subunit but a different beta subunit. Although its main function is maintenance of the corpus luteum, the fetal testis is a target organ for hCG. It is largely responsible for the early development of the fetal testis and for testosterone production prior to fetal LH control. The main effect of this hormone relevant to maternal endocrine function is the well-documented thyrotropic effect which, in cases of trophoblastic disease, can cause hyperthyroidism in the mother. Not only can hCG have a thyrotropic effect, but there is recent evidence that the hCG molecule from women with trophoblastic diseases displays enhanced thyrotropic activity compared with that from normal pregnant women.[15] This thyrotropic effect in normal women causes a mild lowering of TSH early in pregnancy, recognized by most laboratories, which report lower normal ranges of TSH during pregnancy. It is important that this be recognized and taken into consideration when considering the diagnosis of hyperthyroidism in the mother, another fairly common condition that is discussed in more detail below.

Thyrotropin-releasing hormone

Thyrotropin-releasing hormone (TRH) is produced by the placenta and enters the maternal and fetal circulation.[16,17] However it seems to be more important in fetal thyroid function than in maternal thyroid function.

Human chorionic somatomammotropin (human placental lactogen)

Human chorionic somatomammotropin, also known as human placental lactogen, is a polypeptide that has a structure very similar to that of human growth hormone. Its major function is to provide the nutritional needs of the fetus during pregnancy. The role of this hormone in pregnancy relates more to its metabolic properties than to its somatotropic or lactogenic effects.[17] Its major effect on the maternal endocrine system relates to its effect on carbohydrate and fat metabolism, playing a role in the shift of energy metabolism from carbohydrate to fat during pregnancy. Despite these effects, it probably does not play a major role in altering glucose and insulin levels during pregnancy.

Placental growth hormone

There is a placental growth hormone variant synthesized by the syncytiotrophoblast and secreted into the circulation during pregnancy, the levels of which relate to fetal growth.[17] This also results in increased insulin-like growth factor (IGF)-1 levels during pregnancy[18] (see Fig. 42.3). Although there is a specific antibody for measuring the placental growth hormone variant, some commercial growth hormone assays may measure this along with the maternal pituitary growth hormone. Thus, elevated growth hormone and IGF-1 levels may confuse the diagnostic evaluation of a patient with a possible growth hormone-secreting pituitary tumor during pregnancy.

Insulin-like growth factor

IGF-1 is a peptide that is important for fetal and placental growth during pregnancy.[18,19] It is bound by a family of binding proteins. IGFBP-1, IGFBP-4, and perhaps others are synthesized by the endometrium and placenta. They probably

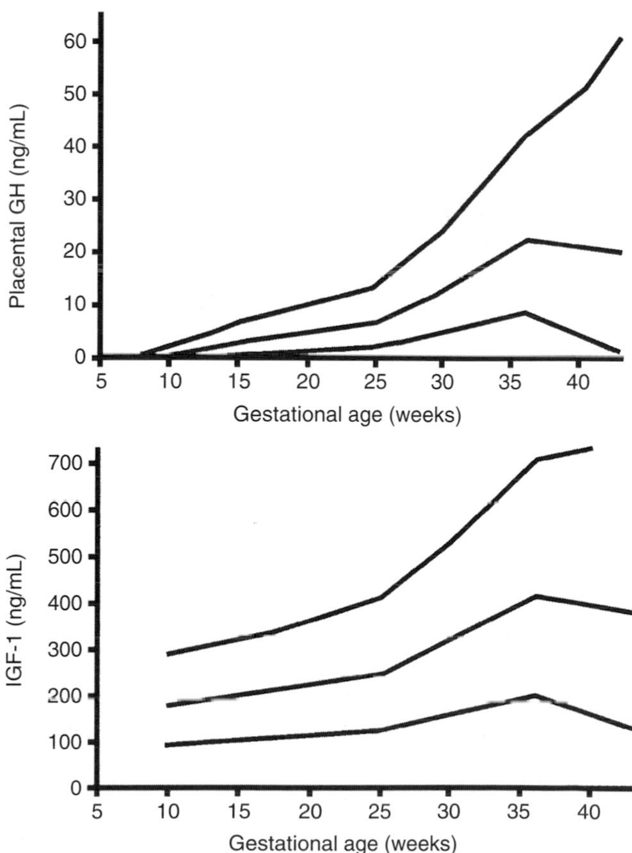

Figure 42.3 Placental growth hormone (GH) and IGF-1 levels during pregnancy. The lines shown represent the mean and 95% confidence interval. Reprinted with minor changes from ref. 18.

play an important part in the insulin–glucose homeostasis system during pregnancy (see Chapter 5).

Endocrine disorders of pregnancy

There are a variety of endocrine disorders which, when associated with pregnancy, have unique aspects of importance to the mother, newborn, or both that may alter the usual diagnostic or therapeutic strategies.[20] In some instances, the disease is more likely to occur or may be worsened by the pregnancy; in some, changes resulting from the pregnancy and/or the associated alterations in metabolism influence the diagnostic evaluation; and, in some, the treatment strategy of the endocrine disorder may require alterations to avoid detrimental effects on the fetus.

Thyroid disorders

Thyroid disorders in pregnancy are relatively common in the general population and are much more common than previously thought because of increased screening and the increased sensitivity of current diagnostic techniques. Overt hypothyroidism and hyperthyroidism have clearly been shown to have detrimental effects on the pregnancy and the fetus. It is more difficult to establish the risk to the fetus of untreated mild hypothyroidism or hyperthyroidism. Although there is no clear consensus on thyroid screening of all pregnant women,[21] thyroid disease is sufficiently common that all pregnant women should be screened with a serum TSH antibody. This is mainly to detect overt biochemical hypo- or hyperthyroidism that has been overlooked clinically. Some have recommended adding free T_4 and thyroid thrombopoietin (TPO) antibodies to the screen, but this should probably be reserved for patients with an abnormal TSH level or a family history of autoimmune thyroid disease. Several comprehensive reviews of thyroid disorders in pregnancy have been published.[20–25] This review of thyroid diseases during pregnancy will emphasize the practical management issues.

Goiter

Thyroid size has historically been said to increase in pregnancy. However, objective studies have shown that this only occurs in the presence of iodine insufficiency.[26] It seems that marginal iodine insufficiency is enough of a stimulus to cause thyroid enlargement during pregnancy, whereas a normal iodine intake is adequate to maintain normal thyroid size. Such an increase in thyroid size can be prevented by as little as 100 μg of supplemental dietary iodine daily, an amount easily consumed by simply using iodized salt.

Thyrotoxicosis

The term thyrotoxicosis is used for an increased metabolic state associated with excess thyroid hormone levels from any source. Hyperthyroidism is the term reserved for thyrotoxicosis due to thyroid gland hyperfunction, i.e., Graves' disease or toxic nodular goiter. Although both thyroid hyperfunction and hypofunction may be associated with infertility, these conditions are not uncommonly seen in pregnancy.

Thyrotoxicosis is the most frequent thyroid disorder in the pregnant patient and is the most difficult to evaluate and manage. Being certain that one is dealing with hyperthyroidism as the cause of thyrotoxicosis may be difficult as performing a radioactive iodine uptake is contraindicated in pregnancy. Silent thyroiditis (postpartum thyroiditis) may occur during late pregnancy and may cause transient thyrotoxicosis. This may be difficult to differentiate from Graves' hyperthyroidism, again, because a radioactive iodine uptake cannot be done. If the patient is sufficiently symptomatic and the diagnosis is not clear during pregnant, antithyroid drug therapy may be instituted, which will be beneficial for Graves' hyperthyroidism but not for the thyrotoxicosis due to silent thyroiditis. Painful subacute thyroiditis is no more likely to occur in the pregnant than in the nonpregnant state. This condition is recognized by the presence of an enlarged, painful, tender thyroid gland, sometimes with fever, and may be associated with transient thyrotoxicosis. It is generally self-limiting and resolves in a few weeks. Another potentially difficult differential diagnosis is the transient gestational thyrotoxicosis of hyperemesis gravidarum. In hyperemesis gravidarum, biochemical thyrotoxicosis is commonly seen. Such patients usually do not have supporting clinical features of thyrotoxicosis, and free T_4 and TSH generally return to normal by 15–20 weeks of gestation with free T_4 preceding TSH in the return to normal[27] (Fig. 42.4).

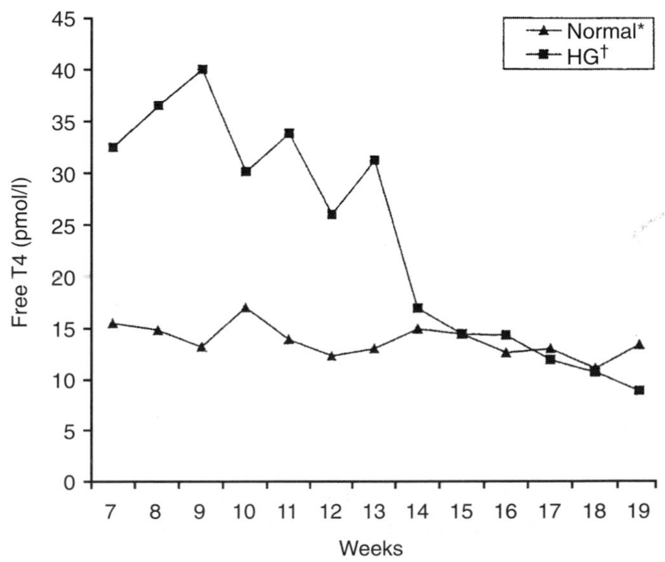

Figure 42.4 Mean free T_4 levels by gestation. *Mean free T_4 levels established in the normal population. †Mean free T_4 levels in women with hyperemesis gravidarum. Reprinted from ref. 27.

Even after hyperthyroidism is established as the probable cause of thyrotoxicosis, management is complicated by the fact that the antithyroid drugs propylthiouracil (PTU), methimazole (MMI), and carbimazole cross into the fetal circulation readily whereas thyroid hormone does so less readily. A unique study in patients with thyroid hormone resistance has shown that high maternal thyroid hormone levels *per se* are detrimental to the fetus.[28] Inadequate treatment of maternal hyperthyroidism is associated with prematurity, low birthweight infants, small for gestational age infants, and stillbirths. It is less certain whether there is an increase in congenital malformations. Uncontrolled maternal hyperthyroidism in the last trimester may result in transient central hypothyroidism in the newborn, presumably due to suppression of fetal TSH and impaired maturation of the fetal hypothalamic–pituitary–thyroid system.[29] Diagnosis requires a T_4 as well as a TSH determination in the newborn. The hypothyroidism may last for weeks to months and may require treatment of the infant. On the other hand, aggressive treatment of maternal thyrotoxicosis may cause fetal goiter, fetal hypothyroidism, and the associated consequences of either fetal loss or impaired intellectual development.

Radioactive iodine therapy is contraindicated in hyperthyroidism in the pregnant mother, although in the few reports in which this was done inadvertently, the results were for the most part not catastrophic.[30,31] The greatest risk appears to be if radioactive iodine is given late in the first trimester, at the time of fetal thyroid development and high sensitivity to radioactive iodine. Thus, surgical thyroidectomy or antithyroid drug therapy are the only two therapeutic options for hyperthyroidism in pregnancy. The main indication for surgical thyroidectomy is the hyperthyroid patient who cannot tolerate thionamide therapy or whose hyperthyroidism cannot be adequately controlled with thionamides. Thus, in the vast majority of patients, therapy with a thionamide, either PTU or MMI in the United States or carbimazole in Europe, has become the preferred therapy.

In view of the risks of untreated or undertreated hyperthyroidism as well as overtreatment of hyperthyroidism, one must always evaluate the risk/benefit ratio of treating maternal hyperthyroidism on a case by case basis. In the newly diagnosed hyperthyroid woman, beta-blockers such as propranolol are effective in controlling symptoms and signs of hyperthyroidism in a short period of time and appear to be safe. However, long-term treatment with beta-blockers, particularly during the third trimester is not recommended, as there have been reports of neonatal morbidity and mortality associated with such long-term use, although it is always difficult to know whether it is the beta-blocker therapy or the underlying condition that might be responsible for any fetal effects. In extremely severe maternal hyperthyroidism, short-term therapy with stable iodine may be helpful and appears to be safe. Chronic maternal iodine therapy may be associated with fetal goiter or hypothyroidism.

Even though there are no well-controlled studies of various treatment regimens using thionamides for hyperthyroidism in the pregnant mother, the standard treatment recommendation is to treat the mother with a thionamide. The dose should be sufficient to keep the free T4 level in the upper normal or mildly elevated range, which is usually accompanied by a low or suppressed TSH. This approach balances minimizing the risk of overt hyperthyroidism to fetal development and survival while at the same time avoiding the risk of excessive thionamide therapy, which may affect fetal thyroid development and function and fetal survival. PTU has traditionally been preferred over MMI because PTU was thought to cross the placenta less well and because of reports of cutis aplasia and other possible congenital abnormalities in the infant related to MMI therapy. However, a recent study has questioned the evidence for this advantage of PTU over the other thionamides and has emphasized the importance of individualization of the thionamide dose.[32] As such a large experience with successful outcomes has been developed using PTU, this continues to be the main antithyroid drug used by most endocrinologists treating hyperthyroidism in pregnancy. A pregnant woman who has hyperthyroidism should be monitored at 4- to 6-week intervals during the pregnancy.

As the third trimester approaches, one must be aware that hyperthyroidism in the mother frequently improves, allowing dose reduction or discontinuation of antithyroid drug therapy. There is evidence that improvement is associated with a decline in thyroid-stimulating antibodies and TSH-binding inhibitory immunoglobulins during pregnancy.[33] As symptomatic Graves' hyperthyroidism commonly recurs in the postpartum period, either continuation of low-dose antithyroid therapy during the third trimester or careful frequent monitoring during the postpartum period with reinstitution of antithyroid therapy as soon as biochemical hyperthyroidism recurs may prevent clinically symptomatic hyperthyroidism during this time.[34]

In addition, early in the third trimester is an appropriate time to measure TSH receptor-stimulating antibodies and/or thyroid-stimulating immunoglobulins in the mother.[35,36] These antibodies cross the placenta and can produce transient hyperthyroidism in the infant. It should be emphasized that all women with a history of Graves' disease, even if not hyperthyroid during the present pregnancy, may have these circulating antibodies and should have them measured early in the third trimester of the pregnancy. Transient hyperthyroidism in the infant occurs in about 17% of patients with high levels of thyroid-stimulating immunoglobulins,[36] and the risk relates to the antibody titer[36] (Fig. 42.5). TSH receptor-blocking antibodies may also be present, which can lead to transient fetal hypothyroidism. It is probably not necessary to measure blocking antibodies routinely, but one can obtain a TSH level in the newborn, as is done routinely. Several recent studies have demonstrated the value of ultrasonographic monitoring of fetal thyroid size during thionamide therapy, which might be an indicator of either fetal Graves' disease or fetal hypothyroidism.[37] In one study, umbilical blood sampling was done in patients with positive thyroid-

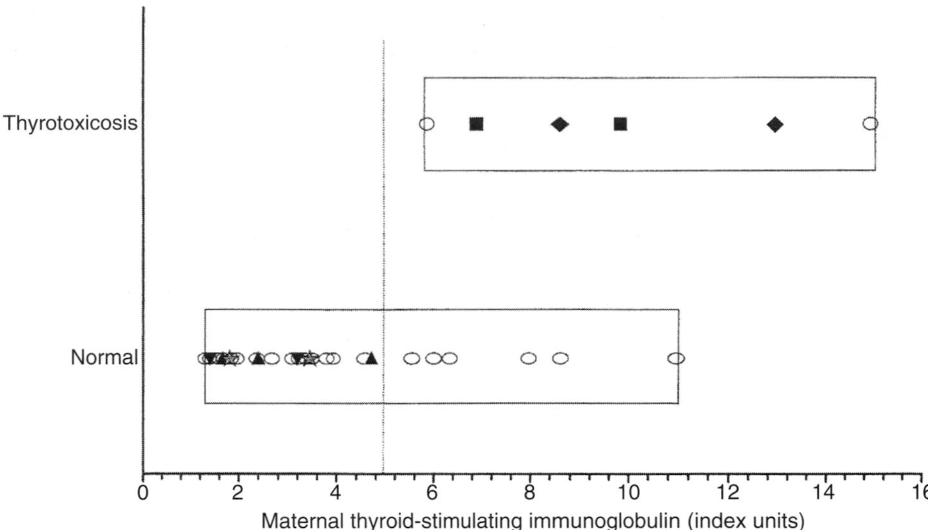

Figure 42.5 Maternal thyroid-stimulating immunoglobulin values and pregnancy outcomes in 35 pregnancies. There are 29 data points in the bar with normal outcomes. Solid figures of similar shape represent different pregnancies from the same mother. Reprinted from ref. 36.

stimulating or -blocking antibody levels for diagnosis of fetal hyperthyroidism or hypothyroidism, treated with maternal thionamide therapy in the former instance or T_4 injection into the amniotic sac in the latter case.[38] Whether such an aggressive approach is justifiable remains to be determined.

Regarding continued management during the postpartum period, an advantage of PTU over MMI is that it appears to be secreted in breast milk in lower concentrations. Daily doses of PTU of up to 600 mg have been shown to have no significant affect on the infant's thyroid hormone level.[22] Current evidence supports the view that breastfeeding with either of the thionamides appears to be safe for the infant. Thus, PTU can be continued or reinstituted during breastfeeding. In such a case, it would always be reasonable to check the infant's TSH levels after several months to be absolutely certain that fetal thyroid function has not been affected. Obtaining a radioactive iodine uptake and administering radioactive iodine therapy should be withheld until breastfeeding has been completed.

Hypothyroidism

Hypothyroidism is most commonly due to primary thyroid gland failure resulting from radioactive iodine treatment of hyperthyroidism, surgical thyroidectomy, or idiopathic primary hypothyroidism, often related to underlying Hashimoto's thyroiditis. Rarely, hypothyroidism may be due to underlying pituitary disease. This is unlikely as patients with pituitary hypothyroidism usually have pituitary hypogonadism and are unlikely to achieve a pregnancy. Primary hypothyroidism may be diagnosed prior to pregnancy or may be first diagnosed during pregnancy. Gestational hypothyroidism is linked to fetal cognitive development and an increased rate of fetal death. This relationship has been most clearly established for severe hypothyroidism and, as one might expect, less well established for mild hypothyroidism. Worldwide, iodine deficiency is a common cause of hypothyroidism and may be more common in Western societies than previously thought. It is readily preventable by small supplemental doses of dietary iodine.[39] There is an increasing consensus that clinical and subclinical maternal hypothyroidism requires early detection and treatment.[39] In addition to screening pregnant women with a TSH antibody for the presence of primary hypothyroidism, any woman on replacement L-thyroxine therapy should have their TSH and free T_4 levels monitored periodically during pregnancy as L-thyroxine requirements often increase during pregnancy. This has recently been carefully studied with the finding that the average increase in T_4 requirement in pregnant women is nearly 50% during the first half of pregnancy.[40] Therefore, because of the known importance of maternal thyroid function for normal fetal cognitive development, and the fact that increased T_4 requirements may occur as early as the fifth week of pregnancy, it has been recommended that treatment be initiated as soon as pregnancy is confirmed. Patients should be given about a 30% increase in their thyroid hormone dose and then be monitored and have their T_4 dose adjusted as necessary.[40]

Postpartum thyroid disease

In the postpartum period (up to 1 year postpartum), one must be sensitive to the possibility of silent thyroiditis (postpartum thyroiditis), generally manifest as transient thyrotoxicosis, sometimes followed by transient hypothyroidism.[41] This may easily be overlooked in the mother going through emotional changes following pregnancy and the many responsibilities in caring for a newborn. In the thyrotoxic phase, this can be confirmed by demonstrating high free T_4 and free T_3 levels with a suppressed TSH level. If the mother is not breastfeeding, a low radioactive iodine uptake may be helpful in making the diagnosis. This transient thyrotoxicosis may be followed by a transient phase of hypothyroidism in up to 40% of patients. Recovery of normal thyroid function usually occurs (Fig. 42.6),

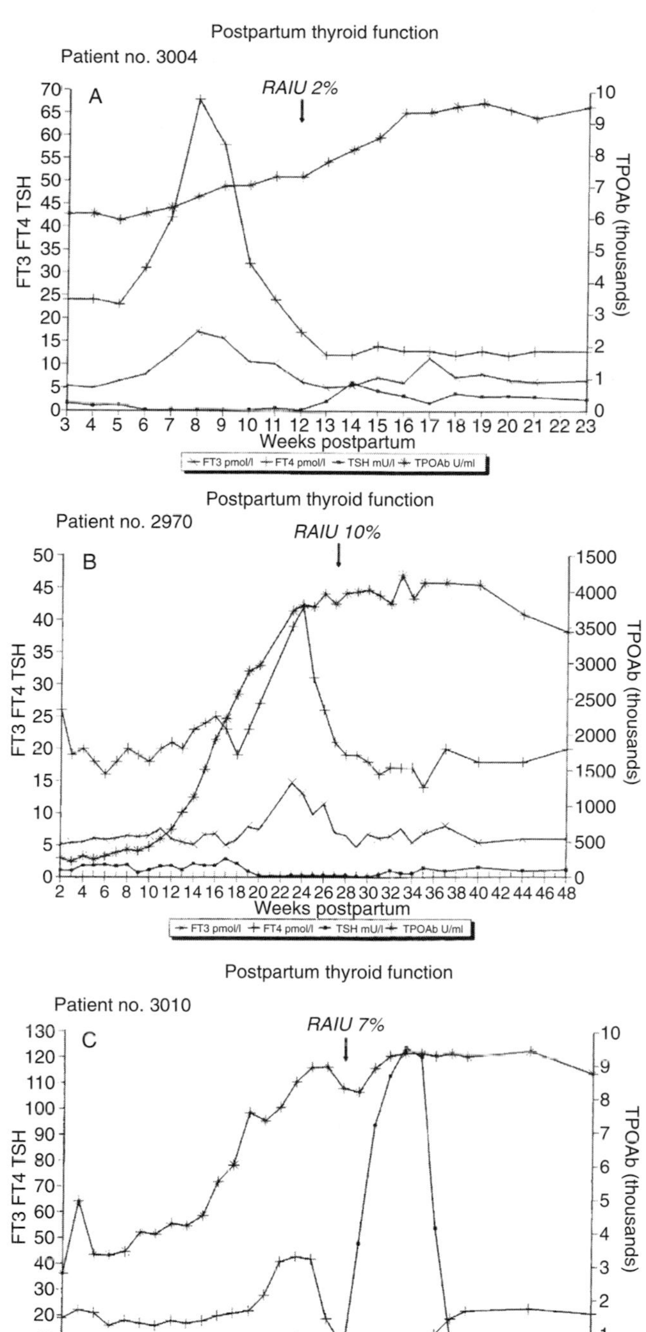

Figure 42.6 Clinical pattern of postpartum thyroid dysfunction in three women studied weekly for 30 weeks postpartum. FT3, free T_3; FT4, free T_4; RAIU, percent radioactive iodine uptake at 24 h; TPOAb, thyroid peroxidase antibodies. The top part of the figure shows hormone levels from a patient with transient hyperthyroidism developing 8–9 weeks postpartum; the middle part of the figure is from a patient with transient hyperthyroidism developing 22–24 weeks postpartum; and the lower part of the figure is from a patient developing modest transient hyperthyroidism followed by severe transient hypothyroidism. Note the significant rise in anti-TPO antibody. Reprinted from ref. 56.

although long-term follow-up of such patients indicates that permanent hypothyroidism is common.[42] Beta-blocker therapy is appropriate during the hyperthyroid phase for the symptomatic patient.

Fetal thyroid disease

Fetal primary hypothyroidism is now usually detected through fetal screening at birth. Transient fetal hyperthyroidism usually occurs in conjunction with maternal Graves' hyperthyroidism (see above). An excellent detailed review of this topic is available.[23]

Pituitary disorders

Prolactinoma

The pituitary gland normally enlarges during pregnancy owing to lactotroph hyperplasia.[43] The most common potentially serious therapeutic problem associated with pituitary gland disorders and pregnancy is the coexistence of a pituitary prolactin-producing tumor and pregnancy. This is being seen with increasing frequency, as the diagnosis of a prolactinoma is made during the evaluation of infertility in a woman with amenorrhea and galactorrhea. An elevated serum prolactin level leads to a pituitary magnetic resonance image (MRI), which demonstrates a pituitary tumor, most commonly a microadenoma (< 1 cm) but occasionally a macroadenoma (> 1 cm). Although this can be a gratifying situation in which infertility is very treatable, before therapy with a dopamine agonist such as bromocryptine or cabergoline, the physician should discuss the potential risks and benefits to the mother and fetus of a pregnancy resulting from dopamine-induced fertility. Such fertility is a result of lowering of the serum prolactin, with cessation of galactorrhea and resumption of menses. The physician is then faced with optimal management of this woman during her pregnancy. A large experience from a single center in patients with pregnancy and a coexisting prolactinoma has been published.[44]

If a microprolactinoma was known to be present before the pregnancy, there is a very small risk of significant tumor growth requiring therapy during the pregnancy. Although it appears that bromocryptine is likely to be safe when taken during pregnancy, it is recommended that it be stopped as soon as the pregnancy is recognized. In a recent review, only 1.4% of over 300 patients with microprolactinomas had symptomatic tumor enlargement defined by headaches and/or visual field disturbance, and none required surgery.[45] Any documented visual field disturbance or significant increase in headaches would indicate the need for a follow-up MRI during the pregnancy. Although some authors have indicated that there is no value in monitoring prolactin levels in such patients because of the normal rise in prolactin during pregnancy (Fig. 42.1), it would seem reasonable to monitor prolactin levels periodically. If a substantial rise in serum prolactin occurs beyond that expected from the pregnancy, a follow-up MRI of the pituitary might be considered even in the absence of increasing headaches or visual field disturbance.

In the occasional patient with a macroprolactinoma diagnosed prior to pregnancy, most endocrinologists would advise against any attempt at pregnancy until the tumor showed substantial regression following medical therapy or surgical resection. The problem with doing a surgical resection in such a patient is that there is a significant risk of postoperative hypogonadotropic hypogonadism, making it much more difficult for the woman to conceive. When a pregnancy occurs in a patient with a diagnosed macroprolactinoma, one must undertake frequent follow-up including regular visual field determinations by a neuro-ophthalmologist and a follow-up MRI during the pregnancy. The risk of significant symptomatic tumor enlargement during pregnancy is about 25%, and the risk seems to be greater in patients with no prior therapy compared with those with prior surgical or radiation therapy.[45] There is little information available on the incidence of tumor enlargement following first shrinkage of the tumor with dopamine agonist therapy followed by a pregnancy. In all patients with a present or prior macroprolactinoma, one must weigh up the advantages and disadvantages of discontinuing dopamine agonist therapy against those of continuing or initiating dopamine agonist therapy. The data available suggest that both bromocryptine and cabergoline are safe when given during pregnancy, although there are much less data available for use throughout pregnancy compared with use of these drugs only early in pregnancy. As there are more data available for bromocryptine than for cabergoline, when the decision is made to use dopamine agonist therapy, it is preferable to use bromocryptine. One helpful point in making this decision is the size of the tumor and the amount of suprasellar or lateral extension of the tumor. If the tumor is less than 2 cm and not overtly impinging on the optic apparatus, it would seem reasonable to discontinue the dopamine agonist therapy, as in a patient with a microprolactinoma, and observe carefully. On the other hand, for a large tumor or one that is pressing on the optic chiasm or invading the cavernous sinus, it would seem reasonable to continue dopamine agonist therapy throughout the pregnancy and follow carefully with visual field determinations and MRI. If the tumor enlarges substantially during pregnancy or visual field abnormalities occur, one must be prepared to undertake surgical decompression of the tumor.

Other pituitary tumors

Pituitary tumors other than prolactinomas have no particularly association with pregnancy, but may coexist with pregnancy. This includes secretory and nonsecretory pituitary tumors. Nonsecretory tumors are not commonly seen in pregnancy as the frequent hypopituitarism present in such patients makes pregnancy unlikely. Secretory pituitary tumors such as pituitary Cushing disease and acromegaly have occasionally been seen in pregnancy, although the frequently associated infertility makes this situation uncommon.[44–46] These diseases are not more likely to occur during pregnancy. However, they each have special diagnostic problems, and great caution should be exercised in making these diagnoses in a pregnant patient.

Regarding acromegaly, the placental growth hormone variant secreted into the circulation during pregnancy may not be distinguished from the normal adult growth hormone in clinical growth hormone assays and may give a falsely high serum growth hormone level. Maternal IGF-1 levels also normally rise during pregnancy[17] (Fig. 42.3). In the absence of unequivocal dramatic clinical features, the diagnosis of acromegaly or a growth hormone-secreting tumor should be delayed until the postpartum period. If a patient with known acromegaly becomes pregnant, there might be a greater problem with hypertension and diabetes than in the nonacromegalic patient. Therapeutically, as the potential fetal effects of octreotide during pregnancy have not been clearly established, and as bromocryptine is in general only modestly effective, such patients are probably best left untreated until the pregnancy is complete. The only major exception would be an increase in tumor size during pregnancy with pressure symptoms on the optic apparatus, making surgical therapy a consideration during the pregnancy.

Regarding Cushing syndrome of any type, particularly pituitary Cushing disease, once again it is best to delay biochemical evaluation until the postpartum period. This is because, as indicated above, urine free cortisol, plasma cortisol, and ACTH levels normally increase during pregnancy (Table 42.1), making diagnostic studies difficult to interpret, including dexamethasone suppressibility. The exception would be a patient with dramatic catabolic features of Cushing syndrome or a patient with ACTH-independent Cushing syndrome with a low ACTH due to an adrenal tumor. If profound pituitary Cushing disease is thought to be present, one should treat any resulting hypertension or diabetes, deferring definitive therapy until the postpartum period.

Hypopituitarism

Patients with partial hypopituitarism who become pregnant should simply be monitored carefully. If they require cortisol replacement due to ACTH deficiency, one might consider a slightly higher replacement dose of 30 mg of hydrocortisone daily in divided doses rather than the usual 15–20 mg daily as cortisol levels typically increase during normal pregnancy. Patients with diabetes insipidus may experience worsening of their condition during pregnancy related to increased clearance of arginine vasopressin by the increased levels of vasopressinase known to exist in pregnancy.[20] As desmopressin is resistant to vasopressinase, this is probably the preferred therapy in the rare case in which diabetes insipidus is present.

Lymphocytic hypophysitis

Lymphocytic hypophysitis is an uncommon inflammatory autoimmune disorder of unknown etiology occurring with increased frequency in the postpartum period or rarely in late pregnancy.[47,48] It usually presents with symptoms of a mass effect including headaches, visual field disturbances, and a sellar/suprasellar mass visualized on MRI. Anterior pituitary hormonal deficiencies and hyperprolactinemia occur in approximately half of such patients. Diabetes insipidus is frequently present. The main differential diagnosis is between an inflammatory mass and a pituitary macroadenoma. The other inflammatory disorders in the differential diagnosis include granulomatous diseases, most commonly sarcoidosis. The Tolusa–Hunt syndrome may also have similar MRI characteristics, but is usually differentiated clinically by the presence of orbital pain and cranial nerve palsies. There are certain MRI characteristics suggestive of an inflammatory process. If these MRI characteristics are present, the diagnosis is often made clinically without histological confirmation. The presence of diabetes insipidus is supportive of the diagnosis of an inflammatory etiology as this rarely occurs in patients with a pituitary adenoma. Although a female preponderance is described in patients diagnosed with lymphocytic hypophysitis, this depends on the definitions used and the institutional experience. In one center reporting 16 patients with primary hypophysitis, 13 of whom had histological verification of the diagnosis, half were male.[49] In this series, two had had a recent pregnancy and one occurred in late pregnancy. Lymphocytic hypophysitis often improves spontaneously or responds to glucocorticoid therapy, although persistent partial hypopituitarism is common. Surgical therapy may be required because of the mass effect, which at the same time provides tissue to document the diagnosis. If one discovers a new symptomatic pituitary mass during late pregnancy or in the postpartum period, particularly if associated with diabetes insipidus, the likelihood is that this is an inflammatory hypophysitis rather than a pituitary macroadenoma.

Sheehan syndrome

Although Sheehan syndrome does not occur during pregnancy, it is a complication of pregnancy. Sheehan syndrome is infarction of the pituitary gland postpartum, which was originally described as resulting from hypotension following massive bleeding at or around the time of delivery. Current information indicates that, although it still usually occurs following severe postpartum vaginal bleeding, it may occur in the absence of massive bleeding, presumably secondary to vasospasm, thrombosis, or vascular compression of the anterior pituitary. The enlarged pituitary gland of pregnancy may be more susceptible to such events. Typically, the key to diagnosis is the history of bleeding, the failure to lactate in the postpartum period, and failure of the resumption of menses. This syndrome may occasionally present similarly to pituitary apoplexy. Most commonly, it is insidious in its presentation and, although imaging may show an enlarged nonhemorrhagic pituitary gland if the patient presents early, more commonly imaging shows an empty sella by the time the diagnosis is made. The newer as well as the older aspects of this disease have been reviewed recently.[50] Any patient with an obstetric hemorrhage and prolonged hypotension following delivery should have hormonal evaluation of possible hypopituitarism and be treated with stress doses of steroids until cortisol levels measured prior to treatment are available. If the diagnosis is in question, the patient can gradually be tapered off steroids after clinical improvement and undergo formal testing with a metyrapone test as well as assessment of other pituitary endorgan hormones.

Adrenal gland disorders

Congenital adrenal hyperplasia

Although pregnancy in a woman with congenital adrenal hyperplasia is a matter that the obstetrician and endocrinologist do not deal with often, it presents some special issues, namely that of prenatal diagnosis and possible early therapeutic intervention.[51] The congenital adrenal hyperplasias are a group of disorders involving enzymatic defects of adrenal steroid biosynthesis usually inherited as a recessive trait. As more than 95% of such patients who achieve pregnancy will be those with the 21-hydroxylase deficiency, this is the only disorder reviewed here. 21-Hydroxylase deficiency may be either the salt-losing type or the classic virilizing type. Such patients are typically managed with glucocorticoids in doses adequate to maintain 17 hydroxyprogesterone, androstenedione, and testosterone levels in the normal or near normal range. Although fertility is often decreased in such patients, patients who are able to be well controlled biochemically and those with milder disease often menstruate regularly and are fertile. Monitoring the adequacy of steroid hormone therapy during pregnancy is complicated by the fact that 17-hydroxy-

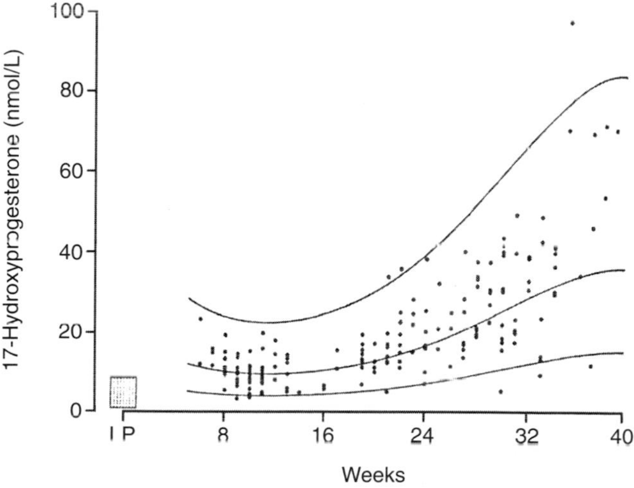

Figure 42.7 The luteal phase (LP) reference interval for 17-hydroxyprogesterone, 0.8–8.7 nmol/L, is shown in the shaded area at the left. Changes in maternal serum concentrations of 17-hydroxyprogesterone during pregnancy. Data are from 60 women who had hormone levels measured at three different times during the pregnancy. The solid lines correspond to the mean and central 95th percentile values. Reprinted from ref. 2.

progesterone levels rise substantially during normal pregnancy (Fig. 42.7). Total testosterone levels rise, but free testosterone levels are unchanged during gestation and may be used as a guide to the adequacy of steroid hormone suppression. Although many authors do not recommend a change in steroid hormone doses during pregnancy in such patients, in view of the normally increased cortisol levels during pregnancy, it would seem reasonable to treat such patients with slightly higher steroid doses, i.e., 30 mg of hydrocortisone daily in divided doses in contrast to the more usual 15–20 mg daily in adrenal insufficiency. There is insufficient data to provide much information on pregnancy outcomes in such patients.

Prenatal diagnosis of 21-hydroxylase deficiency in the fetus is now possible, raising possible therapeutic decisions and ethical concerns. A detailed discussion of these issues is beyond the scope of this chapter. However, such decisions must be made after detailed counseling of the parents by someone trained in genetic counseling, informing them of the potential risks of the procedure, the probability of the fetus being affected, and the risks and benefits of identifying an affected fetus.[51] Such counseling should take into consideration the parents' moral and religious values. Optimal treatment to prevent virilization in the affected female fetus requires administration of glucocorticoids, preferably dexamethasone, prior to the seventh week of gestation followed by chorionic villus sampling at 10 weeks.[52] If genotyping demonstrates that the fetus is a male or unaffected female, dexamethasone is tapered and discontinued over a 1-week period. Depending on the parents' genetics, the chances of the fetus being an affected female are fairly small. This results in the unnecessary exposure of the majority of fetuses to dexamethasone, which has an undetermined long-term effect. This issue is currently under intensive study.[52] An alternative approach is to evaluate the fetal perineum and adrenal glands by ultrasound as soon as possible and, if there appears to be an affected female fetus, therapy can be started at that time. Although this approach is probably much less effective than earlier treatment, it may have some benefit.[51]

Endocrine hypertension in pregnancy

As hypertension in pregnancy is extremely common, the most difficult decision is deciding when one should look for correctable causes of hypertension in the pregnant woman. This is a decision that must be individualized and must be made by the patient's obstetrician. A detailed review of the endocrine causes of hypertension in pregnancy is available.[53] Some of the most serious causes are discussed here in more detail.

Adrenal gland tumors

Although any adrenal gland tumor including benign secretory or nonsecretory tumors of the adrenal cortex, adrenal cortical carcinoma, or pheochromocytoma may occur or be diagnosed during pregnancy, there is nothing to indicate that these occur with an increased frequency in pregnancy. The main issue to consider is whether such disorders require any special diagnostic or therapeutic considerations because of the pregnancy. Other than the biochemical diagnostic studies used to diagnose an adrenal gland disorder, the only safe abdominal radiologic studies to identify such a lesion are an MRI or ultrasound. In a pregnant woman who is thought to have a benign nonsecretory tumor of the adrenal gland, a definitive diagnosis should be delayed until the postpartum period unless a very large tumor is present and an adrenal carcinoma is suspected. In such a case, intervention should be carried out with a laparoscopic adrenalectomy immediately unless the tumor is too large to approach by this technique. An androgen-secreting tumor is unlikely because of the usual associated infertility.

Primary hyperaldosteronism

In primary hyperaldosteronism, the primary diagnostic difficulty relates to the fact that aldosterone levels rise during normal pregnancy (Fig. 42.2). A suppressed renin level during pregnancy, which does not normally occur, is a clue that primary hyperaldosteronism might be present, but is insufficient to make the definitive diagnosis. Therefore, unless there is a pressing clinical situation, definitive diagnostic procedures should be delayed until the postpartum period. Spironolactone is contraindicated as medical therapy. Hypokalemia is best managed simply by potassium replacement. If the hypertension cannot be adequately controlled by other drugs that are acceptable during pregnancy, and if the diagnosis seems clear, consideration can be given to a laparoscopic adrenalectomy during the second trimester.

ACTH-independent Cushing syndrome

In Cushing syndrome resulting from a cortisol-producing adenoma, cortisol levels are of limited value for diagnosis as they normally rise substantially during pregnancy (Table 42.1). However, a suppressed ACTH level may be of value. As in primary hyperaldosteronism, most patients can simply be followed through their pregnancy without specific treatment, but with treatment of their hypertension. If they have evidence of severe Cushing syndrome with catabolic features, a laparascopic adrenalectomy may be performed during the second trimester.

Pheochromocytoma

Although the presence of a pheochromocytoma during pregnancy is rare, proper diagnosis and management is vital. The diagnosis of pheochromocytoma is usually not complicated by the presence of the pregnancy because urine catecholamines, metanephrines, and vanylmandelic acid (VMA) are generally normal in the pregnant patient who is not unduly stressed. The benefit of medical management in such a patient far outweighs the unknown possible risk to the fetus resulting from the use of appropriate pharmacotherapy. The patient should be treated with alpha blockade, using a drug such as phenoxybenzamine, and beta blockade as necessary. Timing of adrenalectomy for this condition in pregnancy is controversial. If the patient is relatively stable, it is probably best to delay resection of the pheochromocytoma until the fetus is viable. However, if any threat to the mother's health ensues, surgical therapy should be undertaken at that time.

Renovascular hypertension

Although renovascular hypertension is not a primary endocrine disorder, this may become a consideration in the pregnant women with accelerated hypertension. Although aldosterone and renin levels are of limited value because of the increases that occur in normal pregnancy (Fig. 42.2), and many of the usual diagnostic techniques such as nuclear medicine scans and angiography are contraindicated in pregnancy, ultrasound Doppler blood flow of the renal arteries and MRI may be helpful. Beta-blocker therapy is the preferred medical therapy. If possible, definitive therapy of renal artery stenosis with angioplasty or renal artery bypass should be delayed until the postpartum period.

A pregnant woman, recently seen at our institution and screened for renovascular hypertension with an ultrasound during the second trimester, was found to have a 6 × 8-cm adrenal tumor. Endocrine evaluation indicated that the tumor was secreting cortisol, as demonstrated by a very high 24-h urine free cortisol level of 1300 μg/24 h and a low plasma ACTH level of 7 pg/mL. It was possibly also secreting aldosterone, but this evaluation was complicated by the known increase in aldosterone levels during pregnancy. A decision was made for her to undergo an open adrenalectomy immediately because of the size of the tumor and uncontrolled hypertension. This was done near the end of the second trimester. The tumor was an adrenal carcinoma. Unfortunately, intrauterine death of the fetus occurred 1 month later at 27 weeks. The patient was followed for the next 3 years with no signs of anatomical or biochemical recurrence of her tumor and thus is one of the few patients likely cured of an adrenal carcinoma because of early diagnosis and immediate therapy.

Addison's disease

If a patient with Addison's disease becomes pregnant, management should be the same as in the nonpregnant state except that it may be best to use hydrocortisone doses at the higher end of usual replacement therapy such as 30 mg daily in divided doses rather than the 15–20 mg daily commonly used; this is because of the increase in urine and plasma cortisol levels seen during normal pregnancy. The dosage of mineralocorticoid therapy may also decrease during pregnancy because of the secondary hyperaldosteronism occurring with pregnancy.

Disorders of calcium metabolism

Vitamin D deficiency

As indicated above, vitamin D requirements during pregnancy have not been clearly established. Nutritional rickets may be more common than previously thought.[13] Even though 25(OH)vitamin D levels are typically normal during pregnancy, adequate vitamin D intake is likely important during pregnancy, and may be even more important in the postpartum period while the mother is nursing. A recent study has indicated that mothers taking 2000–4000 IU of supplemental vitamin D daily while nursing during the first few months after birth do not develop high serum levels of 25(OH)vitamin D. Furthermore, such doses are safe for both the mother and the infant and increase the infant's 25(OH)vitamin D levels to 25–30 ng/dL, ensuring an adequate nutritional status for both mother and infant.[14]

Hyperparathyroidism

Hyperparathyroidism, a common endocrine disorder, may occur coincidentally with pregnancy. As the mean age of patients with primary hyperparathyroidism is substantially older than the mean age of pregnancy, these two conditions do not coincide frequently. However, primary hyperparathyroidism in pregnancy has not been reported as frequently as one might expect. This may be due to masking of hypercalcemia by the physiologic hypoalbuminemia that occurs with pregnancy causing a lower than expected total calcium, although the ionized calcium level accurately reflects the hypercalcemia.

When primary hyperparathyroidism occurs with pregnancy, there may be more complications from the hyperparathyroidism than expected.[54] An increased incidence of maternal and fetal complications has been reported. Nephrolithiasis is reported to occur in hyperparathyroidism associated with pregnancy more frequently than in the nonpregnant state because of the hypercalciuria that occurs in pregnancy. Pancreatitis is also reported to be a more common complication during pregnancy than in the nonpregnant state. Regarding fetal complications, the most common fetal complication is neonatal hypocalcemia. This is presumably due to suppression of the fetal parathyroid glands by the maternal hypercalcemia. This can generally be managed successfully, although neonatal deaths have been reported.

Regarding management of the hyperparathyroidism, one must weigh up the risks of uncontrolled hyperparathyroidism against the benefits and risks of parathyroidectomy. Some have recommended that, if the total serum calcium is less than 12 mg/dL, attempts should be made at conservative management with hydration and decreasing calcium intake.[54] In patients whose calcium is greater than 12 mg/dL, parathyroidectomy should be considered. Intravenous pamidronate therapy may be safe, but there are significant concerns about potential effects on the fetus, and it should not be used unless there is life-threatening hypercalcemia. As surgical parathyroidectomy in large numbers of patients using current standard techniques with ultrasound-guided localization and intraoperative parathyroid hormone assays by an experienced parathyroid surgeon have only been published in recent years in the nonpregnant patient, this procedure will likely be shown to be safely used with increasing frequency in the pregnant patient undergoing surgery during pregnancy. The most important decision if surgery is contemplated is to identify an experienced parathyroid surgeon. Preoperative sestamibi parathyroid scans should probably not be done although they may be safe.

Hypoparathyroidism

Patients with idiopathic or surgical hypoparathyroidism who become pregnant should be managed just as if they were not pregnant with sufficient doses of calcitriol and calcium to keep the serum calcium in the low normal range.[55] As total calcium levels may be falsely low in pregnancy, monitoring the ionized calcium is probably preferable during pregnancy if a reliable ionized calcium assay is available.

Summary

In this chapter, the endocrine changes that occur during normal pregnancy have been reviewed, emphasizing the impact of these changes on the diagnosis and treatment of various endocrine disorders in pregnancy. Substantial increases in ACTH, cortisol, prolactin, renin, aldosterone, and IGF-1 occur during normal pregnancy. These changes complicate the diagnosis of Cushing syndrome, primary hyperaldosteronism, acromegaly, and pituitary prolactinoma. In addition, the diagnosis and treatment of common thyroid disorders occurring in pregnancy that present special problems have been reviewed as well as treatment of pregnant women with a pituitary prolactin-producing tumor. Other issues such as dealing with the pregnant woman with congenital adrenal hyperplasia have been discussed. It is hoped that this review will make the physician better able to diagnose and treat the pregnant woman with an endocrine disorder.

Key points

1. Lactrotroph hyperplasia causes pituitary size to increase during pregnancy, and prolactin levels may rise to values as high as > 10 times the upper limit of normal for the nonpregnant state.
2. Corticotropin-releasing hormone derived from the fetal–placental unit appears in the maternal circulation at very high levels, causing maternal increases in ACTH and true free cortisol levels.
3. Diagnosis of Cushing syndrome during pregnancy should be made with caution.
4. Plasma osmolality decreases by about 10 mOsm/kg, and renin and aldosterone levels increase three- to fourfold during normal pregnancy.
5. Diagnoses of abnormalities in salt and water metabolism, i.e., hyperaldosteronism, are complicated by the normal changes occurring during pregnancy.
6. Maternal vitamin D requirements during pregnancy and lactation may be greater than previously thought.
7. Normal pregnancy causes a mild lowering of TSH levels because of the thyrotropic effect of the high chorionic gonadotropin levels.
8. Pregnancy-adjusted normal ranges for TSH should be taken into consideration when diagnosing or managing disorders of thyroid function during pregnancy.
9. A placental growth hormone variant is secreted during normal pregnancy, which suppresses maternal pituitary growth hormone and increases maternal IGF-1 levels.
10. Diagnosis of growth hormone deficiency or excess during pregnancy must take into consideration the effects of secretion of the placental growth hormone variant.
11. As maternal hypothyroidism or hyperthyroidism may have adverse fetal effects, pregnant women should have their TSH level determined early in pregnancy.
12. Thyrotoxicosis during pregnancy due to Graves' hyperthyroidism may be difficult to distinguish from thyroiditis or hyperemesis gravidarum.
13. Hyperthyroidism during pregnancy should be treated with antithyroid drugs in doses sufficient to achieve adequate control of maternal hyperthyroidism without causing fetal hypothyroidism.
14. Pregnant women with present or past Graves' disease should be screened during the early part of the third trimester for TSH receptor antibodies to determine the fetal risk for neonatal thyrotoxicosis.
15. Pregnant women being treated with L-thyroxine for hypothyroidism should be monitored frequently during pregnancy as a 30–50% increase in L-thyroxine requirement is commonly seen.
16. Women with amenorrhea and galactorrhea may have a pituitary prolactin-producing tumor, and fertility can be restored by treatment with a dopamine agonist such as bromocryptine.
17. Patients with a microprolactinoma who become pregnant after taking a dopamine agonist should have the dopamine agonist stopped as soon as they learn of their pregnancy because the growth of the microprolactinoma during pregnancy is very small.

18 In the unusual patient with a macroprolactinoma who becomes pregnant, the therapeutic decision must be individualized, weighing up the risks and benefits of continuing dopamine agonist therapy against follow-up therapy.

19 The postpartum period, a time when the mother is dealing with the physical and emotional stresses of a new baby, is a time when thyroiditis commonly occurs, which may present as transient thyrotoxicosis or hypothyroidism.

20 Presentation with headaches and amenorrhea in the postpartum period should lead one to entertain the possible diagnoses of lymphocytic hypophysitis or Sheehan's syndrome.

21 Pregnancy in a woman with congenital adrenal hyperplasia presents special ethical issues regarding possible prenatal diagnosis and/or therapeutic intervention in a potentially affected infant.

References

1 Campino C, Torres C, Rioseco A, et al. Plasma prolactin/oestradiol ratio at 38 weeks gestation predicts the duration of lactational amenorrhoea. *Hum Reprod* 2001;16:2540.

2 O'Leary P, Boyne P, Flett P, et al. Longitudinal assessment of changes in reproductive hormones during normal pregnancy. *Clin Chem* 1991;37:667.

3 Goland R, Conwell I, Warren W, et al. Placental corticotrophin-releasing hormone and pituitary–adrenal function during pregnancy. *Neuroendocrinology* 1992;56:742.

4 Magiakou M, Mastorakos G, Rabin D, et al. The maternal hypothalamic–pituitary–adrenal axis in the third trimester of human pregnancy. *Clin Endocrinol* 1996;44:419.

5 Mastorakos G, Ilias I. Maternal and fetal hypothalamic–pituitary–adrenal axis during pregnancy and postpartum. *Ann NY Acad Sci* 2003;997:136.

6 Magiakouo M, Mastorakos G, Rabin D, et al. Hypothalamic corticotrophin-releasing hormone suppression during the postpartum period: implications for the increase in psychiatric manifestations at this time. *J Clin Endocrinol Metab* 1996;81:1912.

7 Elsheikh A, Creatsas G, Mastorakos G, et al. The renin–aldosterone system during normal and hypertensive pregnancy. *Arch Gynecol Obstet* 2001;264:182.

8 Lindheimer M, Davidson J. Osmoregulation, the secretion of arginine vasopressin and its metabolism during pregnancy. *Eur J Endocrinol* 1995;132:133.

9 van der Post J, van Buul B, van Heerikhuize J, et al. Vasopressin and oxytocin levels during normal pregnancy: effect of chronic dietary sodium restriction. *J Endocrinol* 1997;152:345

10 Miao D, He B, Karaplis A, et al. Parathyroid hormone is essential for normal fetal bone formation. *J Clin Invest* 2002;109:1173.

11 VanHouten J, Dann P, McGeoch G, et al. The calcium-sensing receptor regulates mammary gland parathyroid hormone-related protein production and calcium transport. *J Clin Invest* 2004;113:598.

12 Prentice A. Calcium in pregnancy and lactation. *Annu Rev Nutr* 2000;20:249.

13 Hollis B, Wagner C. Assessment of dietary vitamin D requirements during pregnancy and lactation. *Am J Clin Nutr* 2004;79:717.

14 Hollis B, Wagner C. Vitamin D requirements during lactation: high-dose maternal supplementation as therapy to prevent hypovitaminosis D for both the mother and nursing infant. *Am J Clin Nutr* 2004;80(Suppl.):1752S.

15 Kato K, Mostafa M, Mann K, et al. The human chorionic gonadotropin molecule from patients with trophoblastic diseases has a high thyrotropic activity but is less active in the ovary. *Gynecol Endocrinol* 2004;18:269.

16 Bajoria R, Babawale M. Ontogeny of endogenous secretion of immunoreactive-thyrotropin releasing hormone by the human placenta. *J Clin Endocrinol Metab* 1998;83:4148.

17 Reis F, Florio P, Cobellis L, et al. Human placenta as a source of neuroendocrine factors. *Biol Neonate* 2001;79:150.

18 Chellakooty M, Vangsgaard K, Larsen T, et al. A longitudinal study of intrauterine growth and the placental growth hormone (GH)-insulin-like growth factor I axis in maternal circulation: association between placental GH and fetal growth. *J Clin Endocrinol Metab* 2004;89:384.

19 Zhou R, Diehl D, Hoeflich A, et al. IGF-binding protein-4: biochemical characteristics and functional consequences. *J Endocrinol* 2003;178:177.

20 Nader S. Thyroid disease and other endocrine disorders in pregnancy. *Obstet Gynecol Clin North Am* 2004;31:257.

21 Gharib H, Tuttle R, Baskin J, et al. Consensus statement. Subclinical thyroid dysfunction: a joint statement on management from the American Association of Clinical Endocrinologists, the American Thyroid Association, and the Endocrine Society. *J Clin Endocrinol Metab* 2005;90:581.

22 Dallas J. Autoimmune thyroid disease and pregnancy: relevance for the child. *Autoimmunity* 2003;36:339.

23 Fisher D. Fetal thyroid function: diagnosis and management of fetal thyroid disorders. *Clin Obstet Gynecol* 1997;40:16.

24 Glinoer D. Management of hypo- and hyperthyroidism during pregnancy. *Growth Hormone IGF Res* 2003;13:S45.

25 Mestman J. Diagnosis and management of maternal and fetal thyroid disorders. *Curr Opin Obstet Gynecol* 1999;11:167.

26 Berghout A, Wiersinga W. Thyroid size and thyroid function during pregnancy: an analysis. *Eur J Endocrinol* 1998;138:536.

27 Tan J, Loh K, Yeo G, et al. Transient hyperthyroidism of hyperemesis gravidarum. *Br J Obstet Gynecol* 2002;109:683.

28 Anselmo J, Cao D, Karrison T, et al. Fetal loss associated with excess thyroid hormone exposure. *JAMA* 2004;292:691.

29 Kempers M, Tijn D, van Trotsenburg A, et al. Central congenital hypothyroidism due to gestational hyperthyroidism; detection where prevention failed. *J Clin Endocrinol Metab* 2003,88:5851.

30 Ayala C, Navarro E, Rodriguez J, et al. Conception after iodine-131 therapy for differentiated thyroid cancer. *Thyroid* 1998;8:1009.

31 Lin J, Wang H, Weng H, et al. Outcome of pregnancy after radioactive iodine treatment for well differentiated thyroid carcinomas. *J Endocrinol Invest* 1998;212:662.

32 Momotani N, Noh J, Ishikawa N, et al. Effects of propylthiouracil and methimazole on fetal thyroid status in mothers with Graves' hyperthyroidism. *J Clin Endocrinol Metab* 1997;82:3633.

33 Amino N, Izumi Y, Hidaka Y, et al. No increase of blocking type anti-thyrotropin receptor antibodies during pregnancy in patients with Graves' disease. *J Clin Endocrinol Metab* 2003;88:5871.
34 Nakagawa Y, Mori K, Hoshikawa S, et al. Postpartum recurrence of Graves' hyperthyroidism can be prevented by the continuation of antithyroid drugs during pregnancy. *Clin Endocrinol* 2002;57: 467.
35 Laurberg P, Nygaard B, Glinoer D, et al. Guidelines for TSH-receptor antibody measurements in pregnancy: results of an evidence-based symposium organized by the European Thyroid Association. *Eur J Endocrinol* 1998;139:584.
36 Peleg D, Cada S, Peleg A, et al. The relationship between maternal serum thyroid-stimulating immunoglobulin and fetal and neonatal thyrotoxicosis. *Obstet Gynecol* 2002;99:1040.
37 Cohen O, Pinhas-Hamiel O, Sivan E, et al. Serial in utero ultrasonographic measurements of the fetal thyroid: a new complementary tool in the management of maternal hyperthyroidism in pregnancy. *Prenatal Diagn* 2003;23:740.
38 Nachum Z, Rakover Y, Weiner E, et al. Graves' disease in pregnancy: prospective evaluation of a selective invasive treatment protocol. *Am J Obstet Gynecol* 2003;189:159.
39 de Escobar G, Obregon M, del Rey F. Role of thyroid hormone during early brain development. *Eur J Endocrinol* 2004;151:U25.
40 Alexander E, Marqusee E, Lawrence J, et al. Timing and magnitude of increases in levothyroxine requirements during pregnancy in women with hypothyroidism. *N Engl J Med* 2004;351:241.
41 Terry A, Hague W. Postpartum thyroiditis. *Semin Perinatol* 1998;22:497.
42 Lazarus J. Thyroid dysfunction: reproduction and postpartum thyroiditis. *Semin Reprod Med* 2002;20:381.
43 Chiodini I, Liuzzi A. PRL-secreting pituitary adenomas in pregnancy. *J Endocrinol Invest* 2003;26:96.
44 Bronstein M, Salgado L, de Castro Musolino N. Medical management of pituitary adenomas: the special case of management of the pregnant woman. *Pituitary* 2002;5:99.
45 Molitch M. Pituitary tumors and pregnancy. *Growth Hormone IGF Res* 2003;13:S38.
46 Lindsay J, Jonklass J, Oldfield E, et al. Cushing's syndrome during pregnancy: personal experience and review of the literature. *J Clin Endocrinol Metab* 2005;90:3077.
47 Cheung C, Ezzat S, Smyth H, et al. The spectrum and significance of primary hypophysitis. *J Clin Endocrinol Metab* 2001;86:1048.
48 Kidd D, Wilson P, Unwin B, et al. Lymphocytic hypophysitis presenting early in pregnancy. *J Neurol* 2003;250:1385.
49 Leung G, Lopes M, Thorner M, et al. Primary hypophysitis: a single-center experience in 16 cases. *J Neurosurg* 2004;101;262.
50 Kelestimur F. Sheehan's syndrome. *Pituitary* 2003;6:181.
51 Garner P. Congenital adrenal hyperplasia in pregnancy. *Semin Perinatol* 1998;22:446.
52 Lajic S, Nordenstrom A, Ritzen E, et al. Prenatal treatment of congenital adrenal hyperplasia. *Eur J Endocrinol* 2004;151:U63.
53 Keely E. Endocrine causes of hypertension in pregnancy – when to start looking for zebras. *Semin Perinatol* 1998;22:471.
54 Schnatz P, Curry S. Primary hyperparathyroidism in pregnancy: evidence-based management. *Obstet Gynecol Surv* 2002;57:365.
55 Callies F, Arlt W, Scholz H, et al. Management of hypoparathyroidism during pregnancy – report of twelve cases. *Eur J Endocrinol* 1998;139:284.
56 Lazarus J, Hall R, Othman S, et al. The clinical spectrum of postpartum thyroid disease. *Q J Med* 1996;89:429.

43 Gastrointestinal diseases complicating pregnancy

Washington Clark Hill and Alfred D. Fleming

Pregnancy can complicate almost any gastrointestinal disease. The pregnant woman may enter pregnancy with a gastrointestinal disorder, or it may develop during pregnancy. The physiologic effects of pregnancy may cause gastrointestinal disturbances such as nausea, vomiting, hyperemesis gravidarum, and esophageal reflux. Conversely, gastrointestinal disorders such as ruptured appendix, gallbladder, and inflammatory bowel disease may affect the course of pregnancy. New findings and diagnostic advances warrant revisiting key features of acute nonobstetric abdominal pain in pregnancy.[1] This chapter discusses the various gastrointestinal diseases complicating pregnancy and their effect on the fetus and mother.

Diseases within the gastrointestinal tract

Nausea, vomiting, and hyperemesis gravidarum

Nausea with or without vomiting is an especially common symptom during early pregnancy and the most common gastrointestinal complaint. It usually occurs during the first trimester of pregnancy and, by mid-second trimester, most women no longer complain of these symptoms. It occurs in approximately 60–80% of pregnancies. In its mildest form, it is referred to as morning sickness, which is unpleasant and distressing, both physically and psychologically, but requires no particular therapy. Approximately 1–2 per 1000 pregnant patients may experience some morning sickness throughout their entire pregnancy. It is unknown why some patients experience no morning sickness and others are bothered by it all the time.

The cause of nausea and vomiting during pregnancy is also unknown. The smooth muscles of the stomach do relax during pregnancy, and this physiologic change may play some role. The role of human chorionic gonadotropin (hCG) has been studied; however, a clear correlation between maternal serum hCG levels and the severity of morning sickness has not been demonstrated.[2] Patients with high levels of hCG, as in multiple gestation or hydatidiform moles, may or may not experience exaggerated nausea and vomiting throughout pregnancy.

The management of nausea and vomiting during pregnancy is primarily supportive. Therapeutic regimens include reassurance, physical and psychological support, frequent small meals, the avoidance of foods that are unpleasant or that may initiate symptoms, adequate hydration and fluid intake, and selective, occasional use of antiemetics. There is no ideal antiemetic currently available for the treatment of morning sickness. Until 1983, Bendectin was available; this drug was a combination of doxylamine succinate (10 mg) and pyridoxine (10 mg). Bendectin, which had been approved by the Food and Drug Administration (FDA) for the treatment of nausea and vomiting in pregnancy, was removed from the market by the pharmaceutical company in 1983, primarily because of litigation. There was no evidence that Bendectin was teratogenic.[3–7] When symptoms require treatment, both pyridoxine and doxylamine are still available over the counter as Unisom (25 mg). Several studies have shown that pyridoxine alone may be effective in treating patients with severe nausea and vomiting in the hospital or as an outpatient.[8,9] Antiemetic therapy should be used when supportive measures are not effective. Other antiemetics that have also been used successfully in the treatment of nausea and vomiting in pregnancy include the phenothiazines, trimethobenzamide, metoclopramide, and diphenhydramine.

Hyperemesis gravidarum is the abnormal condition of pregnancy associated with pernicious nausea and vomiting. Hyperemesis is both infrequent and uncommon. These patients experience persistent intractable nausea and vomiting associated with weight loss, fluid and electrolyte imbalance, ketonuria, and ketonemia. Electrolyte imbalance may include decreased sodium, potassium, and chloride, and metabolic alkalosis. The patient usually becomes clinically dehydrated and may even develop jaundice, hyperpyrexia, and peripheral neuritis. Recurrent hyperemesis gravidarum has caused recurrent first-trimester jaundice.[10] Wernicke's encephalopathy has even been reported in patients with hyperemesis gravidarum.[11] If the patient is not appropriately treated, there may be a failure of the mother and fetus to increase their weight. A patient with hyperemesis gravidarum who has abnormal electrolyte, renal, or liver test results should be promptly hospitalized for fluid management. Outpatient, hospital, or home therapy consisting of intravenous fluid hydration with pyridoxine, 100 mL/L, can be sufficient along with supportive care. The management of hyperemesis in the home can be both safe and efficacious.[12] Furthermore, successful therapy can be achieved at a significantly reduced cost. However, when the patient's condition does not improve, hospitalization with appropriate electrolyte, caloric, and fluid management is necessary, if not mandatory.

Refractory hyperemesis gravidarum has been successfully treated with corticosteroid therapy. Corticosteroids are effective in suppressing symptoms of intractable hyperemesis, decreasing the length of hospitalization, and allowing normal maternal nutrition. The exact mechanism of action of corticosteroids is unclear. It has been assumed that they act directly on a vomiting center in the brain. The safety of corticosteroid therapy early in pregnancy has been established by its use in other disorders. Corticosteroid therapy should be considered not as a first-line therapy but when: (1) all other causes of vomiting have been excluded; (2) vomiting has been prolonged and associated with dehydration; (3) the risks and benefits of the treatment have been clearly explained to the patient; and (4) intravenous fluid replacement and conventional antiemetics have failed. Studies have established the efficacy and safety of corticosteroid therapy for refractory hyperemesis. Methylprednisolone in tapering doses is the drug of choice. The use of droperidol and diphenhydramine in the management of hyperemesis gravidarum has been reported but is now used infrequently.[13] Levine and Esser[14] have reported the safe and effective use of first-trimester total parenteral nutrition in the management of hyperemesis gravidarum, which was initiated in the hospital and was continued in the patient's homes. Hsu and colleagues[15] have reported that enteral feeding via nasogastric tube seems to be effective as an alternative for relieving intractable nausea and vomiting and providing adequate nutrition support.

The role of psychosocial stressors, such as an undesired pregnancy, in the etiology of nausea, vomiting, and hyperemesis gravidarum has been only partially studied. It is believed that psychological factors contribute to excessive nausea and vomiting during pregnancy. Several studies have shown that these symptoms occur more frequently in women with undesired pregnancies or negative relationships with their mothers or partners.[15,16]

Although most patients with pernicious nausea and few patients with hyperemesis gravidarum have transient hyperthyroidism,[17] thyroid evaluation should be part of the workup of these patients. Whether the hyperthyroidism is a cause of hyperemesis or is present because of the condition is controversial and a difficult differential diagnosis. Whether or not antithyroid medication is necessary in the treatment of transient hyperthyroidism occurring in hyperemetic pregnancies has in the past been controversial. However, Goodwin and coworkers,[18] in the largest series of hyperemesis subjects studied prospectively with respect to thyroid function, show that hyperthyroidism in these patients is common, self-limited, and requires no therapy.

Most patients with hyperemesis gravidarum improve with appropriate medical therapy. Maternal mortality is rare, but has been reported when severe metabolic abnormalities go untreated, esophageal tears (Mallory–Weiss syndrome) occur, or hematemesis develops. Intrauterine fetal demise can also occur in severe cases. The association of nausea and vomiting in pregnancy with other pregnancy outcomes has been investigated by several authors. Women admitted on multiple occasions for hyperemesis had significantly lower birthweight infants.[19] Although nausea and vomiting in early pregnancy may be a bothersome and a common symptom, there is no consistent or significant effect from this gastrointestinal disorder on pregnancy outcome, good or bad.[20]

Oral cavity complications of pregnancy

Many pregnant women enter pregnancy with poor dental care. They may not have seen a dentist since their own childhood. Their teeth are in poor condition, and numerous cavities and gingivitis are present owing to poor dental hygiene. They should be urged to practice good oral hygiene and referred and encouraged to see a dentist because dental care is not prohibited during pregnancy. Pregnant women are no more susceptible to tooth decay than the nonpregnant patient. There is no agreement that normal pregnancy causes a decreased or increased incidence of caries. Rather, the worsening of dental caries during pregnancy is due to poor dental hygiene. This may not be true for the diabetic pregnancy where the prevalence of gingivitis is higher.[21]

The chemical and mineral composition of human teeth has not been shown to be changed by pregnancy or lactation. Pregnancy does not cause gingivitis; it is caused by bacteria.[22] The increase in gingival vascularity can result in accentuated gingival hyperplasia or enlargement, which is commonly referred to as pregnancy gingivitis. The incidence of this common oral condition during pregnancy is unknown, but it probably occurs in at least one-half of pregnant women. Once the hormonal changes of pregnancy decline, the exaggerated gingivitis due to pregnancy decreases. Pregnancy does not increase the amount of oral calculus present on the teeth. When oral hygiene is poor, calculus may, however, lead to mild, moderate, or severe gingivitis and other periodontal disease. Bleeding from the gingivae, a common complaint of pregnant women, due to pregnancy gingivitis, requires no treatment.[22] Gingivitis due to poor dentition and hygiene is treated by good cleaning of the teeth and by meticulous dental care. There is no basis for delaying dental care during pregnancy, and patients who require treatment should obtain it promptly. Prenatal care should, but frequently does not, include a good examination of the teeth by a dentist who may then consult with the obstetrician about the best treatment plan.

Pregnancy tumor is a granuloma that forms as a result of exaggerated gingival enlargement during pregnancy.[23] It appears as a localized enlargement of the hyperplastic gingivae or pedunculated growth. Pregnancy tumors are pyogenic granulomas because they result from nonspecific inflammatory gingivitis secondary to poor oral hygiene, associated with deposits of plaque and calculus on the teeth. The poor teeth and gums adjacent to these lesions are responsible for the local irritation resulting in the pregnancy tumor. These predisposing inflammatory factors, along with the hormonal effects of pregnancy on the gingival tissues, predispose to the development of pregnancy tumors. They occur in approximately 1–5% of pregnant women. The tumors are typically painless, pedunculated, lobulated, red owing to their vascularity, and soft with a smooth surface. Consultation with a dentist is indicated. The treatment for pregnancy tumor is complete surgical excision.[22] The adjacent teeth should be cleaned aggressively to remove debris, plaque, and calculus. If the tumor is not completely removed, it may recur, and recurrence during a future pregnancy is not uncommon.

The treatment of dental problems associated with pregnancy is rarely contraindicated and, when several guidelines are used, may be performed safely.[24] If the treatment is necessary but elective, it is best delayed until the second trimester, when there is the least risk of teratogenesis. Emergency treatment should be obtained whenever indicated. Fillings, extractions, and crowns can be safely performed during pregnancy. The supine hypotensive syndrome, which occurs most frequently during the third trimester, can be avoided by keeping the patient turned toward her side while she is in the dental chair.

Radiographs, which are often necessary to establish a proper dental diagnosis, may be taken safely during any stage of pregnancy. The maternal abdomen should be shielded with a lead apron. Using fast X-ray film, the exposure time is minimized. There is no harm to the fetus when dental radiographs are taken with the necessary precautions, good techniques, and today's modern equipment.[25] Dental procedures may cause pain. Efforts should be made by the dentist to reduce the pain and stress of the treatment. Although the dentist may be concerned, a local or topical anesthetic is usually recommended and is safe for both mother and fetus. The smallest amount necessary to achieve satisfactory anesthesia should be used. When incorporated with a vasoconstrictor such as epinephrine, the anesthetic's effect is prolonged, blood loss decreased, and the dosage of anesthesia is minimized. Lidocaine and mepivacaine combined with epinephrine have become the local anesthetics of choice for dental work during pregnancy. Low doses of intravenous medications may be used, but should be titrated to an acceptable level before administering the local anesthesia.[24] Inhalation or general anesthesia should be reserved for those patients who are hospitalized and require extensive dental surgery. The anesthesia should be administered by an anesthetist or anesthesiologist who is familiar with the risks of the procedure.[26] It is best, whenever possible, to avoid the use of an inhalational anesthetic for dental procedures during pregnancy. Laboring patients with oral jewelry should remove the hardware before receiving anesthesia for safety reasons.[27]

Most dental procedures require no antibiotics. When antibiotics are necessary, tetracycline should not be given to the pregnant woman.[28] Penicillin, frequently used by the dentist for treatment or prophylaxis therapy, is safe to use during pregnancy and would be the drug of choice.[28] There is now evidence that maternal periodontal disease and incident progression are significant contributors to obstetric risk for preterm delivery.[29]

Reflux esophagitis

The esophagus is a fibromuscular tube that connects the oral pharynx and the stomach. It is predominantly an interthoracic organ, although a small portion of the esophagus is located beneath the diaphragm. The function of the esophagus is to move food from the oral pharynx to the stomach. The esophagus also prevents or helps to prevent the movement of air from the oral pharynx to the stomach and the movement of food from the stomach into the oral pharynx, called gastroesophageal reflux. Peristalsis carries food into the stomach. At the distal end of the esophagus is the lower esophageal sphincter, consisting of circular muscle fibers approximately 2 cm in length. Normally, the lower esophageal sphincter is in a state of tonic contraction, thus preventing gastroesophageal reflux. Heartburn is really a symptom of reflux esophagitis. Heartburn is a common, bothersome complaint during pregnancy and occurs in as many as 70% of pregnant patients. A quarter of pregnant patients experience some degree of heartburn daily.[30] The symptoms of heartburn include burning and substernal discomfort radiating to the back of the neck. Heartburn is usually more severe after meals and is aggravated by recumbent positions. The pain is not limited to substernal discomfort, but may also be epigastric, between the shoulders or, rarely, generalized chest pain. Usually, the symptoms of reflux esophagitis occur in the last trimester, but they can occur at any time during pregnancy.[31] They subside after 36 weeks of gestation and improve, as expected, postpartum with the decrease in the size of the uterus.

The exact cause of heartburn and reflux esophagitis of pregnancy remains unknown and controversial.[30] It probably occurs as a result of some degree of gastroesophageal reflux favored by the decreased gastric emptying time during pregnancy and by the increased intra-abdominal pressure created by the enlarged uterus. The differential diagnosis of esophageal reflux includes cardiac symptoms, peptic ulcer disease, and hiatal hernia. Treatment of reflux esophagitis during pregnancy consists primarily of neutralizing the acid material that is being refluxed into the esophagus, thereby decreasing gastroesophageal reflux.[31,32] Symptomatic strategies include dietary modification. Foods and drinks such as chocolate, caffeine, peppermint, and alcohol may actually decrease the lower esophageal sphincter pressure. Fatty or spicy foods aggravate the symptoms and are to be avoided. The avoidance of recumbency, particularly immediately after eating a meal, is likewise to be avoided. Elevation of the head of the bed while reclining may provide symptomatic relief. A variety of antacids have been prescribed for heartburn. All these over-the-counter preparations neutralize gastric acid, which is responsible for the symptoms. In the nonpregnant patient, the lower esophageal sphincter pressure has been elevated with a variety of medications, including metoclopramide.[33] The use of this and similar drugs, although safe, should be avoided except in severe cases. The histamine H2 receptor antagonists and/or the proton pump inhibitors can also be prescribed for severe and persistent symptoms.[30] Prolonged esophageal reflux can result in complications such as peptic esophageal stricture, hemorrhagic esophagitis, gastrointestinal bleeding, and hemorrhage. Ulceration of the esophageal mucosa can also occur with significant bleeding. The symptoms of reflux esophagitis can be so severe or difficult to treat that esophagoscopy, parenteral hyperalimentation, and parenteral nutrition are necessary.[30] These procedures may be performed safely, when necessary, during pregnancy for this and other gastrointestinal diseases complicating pregnancy.

Peptic ulcer disease

An ulcer is a defect that occurs in the gastrointestinal mucosa and extends through the muscularis mucosa. The stomach, pylorus, or duodenum are the usual sites for ulcers. However, they may occur in the esophagus as a result of gastroesophageal reflux. Benign ulcers of the upper gastrointestinal tract are caused by a number of factors including the action of hydrochloric acid and pepsin on the gastrointestinal mucosa.[34,35] Because of the action of acid and pepsin, these defects are called peptic ulcers. Factors known to play a role in the development of peptic ulcer are infections of the stomach and nonsteroidal inflammatory drugs.[34] Ulcerations of the stomach affect both sexes equally and are less common than duodenal ulcer disease, which is twice as common in men as in women.[34] The development of peptic ulcer disease during pregnancy is uncommon and rare. Patients who have peptic ulcers before pregnancy frequently experience fewer symptoms during pregnancy and may even become totally asymptomatic. This is the primary reason why complications of ulcer disease, such as perforation, bleeding, and pyloric stenosis, are quite rare during pregnancy. The exact cause of the decrease in symptoms remains unknown. There was a recurrence in 50% of the patients by 3 months and in 75% of patients by 6 months after delivery. There are no conclusive studies regarding gastric acid secretion changes during pregnancy. Studies to date have shown conflicting data, with some showing no change and others a slight decrease in gastric acid secretion.[35]

The symptoms of peptic ulcer disease are quite similar to those of reflux esophagitis.[30] The diagnosis during pregnancy may therefore be delayed. The most common symptom of peptic ulcer disease is complaints of heartburn or dyspepsia. The patient may experience nausea and vomiting, which is a common complaint of pregnancy. She may also have anorexia, bloating, or epigastric pain and discomfort. Patients with duodenal ulcer disease more frequently have epigastric pain than those with gastric ulcers. There are no typical physical findings. When presenting to her obstetrician, the patient may already have taken antacids and found that they may have helped her symptoms. Peptic ulcer disease is diagnosed by the visualization of the ulcer by radiography or endoscopy. Although the upper gastrointestinal series is sometimes used to diagnose peptic ulcer disease in a nonpregnant patient, esophagoscopy when necessary should be used in the pregnant patient. This is usually not necessary except in the patient who has symptoms that do not respond to antacids. However, patients with persistent and serious gastrointestinal signs and symptoms from peptic ulcer disease or other disorders may require endoscopy during pregnancy. Gastrointestinal endoscopy, both esophagogastroduodenoscopy and colonoscopy, has been used safely in the diagnosis and treatment of pregnant patients. Not only may the procedure be useful, but it may be necessary in making an accurate and early diagnosis.[34]

Complications of peptic ulcer disease rarely occur during pregnancy, because in most cases the disease does not worsen. Complications that can occur include perforation, hemorrhage or other bleeding, pyloric stenosis, and gastrointestinal obstruction.[34] When serious complications occur, they should be managed as in the nonpregnant patient. By doing so, there is less maternal and fetal mortality. There is disagreement in the literature as to whether or not a Cesarean section should be performed at the time of an emergency gastric resection. The decision to perform a Cesarean section would depend on the gestational age of the fetus. The experience of most clinicians is not to perform an emergency Cesarean before the peptic ulcer surgery. Patients who have had previous peptic ulcer disease surgery are at no increased risk for complications during future pregnancies.[35]

Lewis and Weingold[7] have extensively reviewed the use of gastrointestinal drugs during pregnancy and lactation. The treatment of peptic ulcer disease consists primarily of the use of antacids, which are safe to use during pregnancy.[7,36] The usual recommended dose is 15–30 mL 1–3 h after meals and at bedtime. Antacids neutralize acid that has been secreted by the gastrointestinal lining. In most cases, antacids improve symptoms. A combination of magnesium trisilicate and aluminum hydroxide is found in most antacid preparations. Sodium bicarbonate should not be used as an antacid during pregnancy, because it can lead to the absorption of large amounts of sodium. Sucralfate is a mucosal-protective aluminum hydroxide salt that has been used in the nonpregnant patient to enhance mucosal defense. Some investigators have suggested that sucralfate forms a shield over the ulcer crater.

There has been no adverse fetal or maternal effect of this drug when used during pregnancy.[7,36]

Patients with peptic ulcer disease should avoid a diet of foods that cause discomfort. Some authorities suggest that milk, which is frequently included in the diet of the pregnant patient, stimulates acid secretion and should be taken in moderation. Other dietary modification is not necessary, although bedtime snacks are to be avoided. Smoking, which should be avoided in both pregnant and nonpregnant woman, and alcohol should certainly be eliminated from the diets of these patients. Patients who are smokers and have a previous history of peptic ulcer disease are at highest risk for ulcer disease during pregnancy.[34] Aspirin and the nonsteroidal and inflammatory drugs such as indomethacin, which is used for tocolysis, can produce gastric irritation and, with prolonged use, gastric and duodenal ulcers; their use should be avoided in patients with active or a history of peptic ulcer disease.[32,34]

Histamine H2 blockers such as cimetidine, famotidine, nizatidine, ranitidine, and others are second-line therapy for peptic ulcer disease. They do cross the placenta, but no teratogenic risk has been detected from their use during the first trimester.[30,35] H2 receptors are located on parietal cells of the gastrointestinal lining. Their stimulation results in the production of histamine. H2 receptor antagonists decrease the production of histamine. Histamine H2 blockers are a mainstay in the medical therapy of peptic ulcer disease. There are several concerns about the use of cimetidine during pregnancy. It is an antiandrogen and has produced gynecomastia and impotence in a small number of male animals and male users.[30,35] Its effect on the H2 receptors in the uterine myometrium has not been well studied, but no adverse effect on uterine activity has been reported. Cimetidine does cross the placenta. No teratogenicity has been linked to the use of cimetidine during pregnancy.[7,36] However, its use is and should be reserved for those patients who have symptoms refractory to antacid therapy. There are no data to support the discontinuation of cimetidine during pregnancy in patients prescribed it before conception.

Ranitidine, famotidine, and nizatidine are other H2 receptor antagonists that have been used for ulcer therapy during pregnancy without maternal or neonatal complications.[30,35] The newest antisecretory agents are the proton pump inhibitors omeprazole, lansoprazole, esomeprazole, pantoprazole, and rabeprazole. These drugs suppress gastric acid secretion by a direct inhibitory effect on the gastric parietal cell. They are potent agents that promote faster healing of peptic ulcers. The use of these drugs during pregnancy has been limited.[30,35] The use of proton pump inhibitors during pregnancy does not present a teratogenic risk when used in recommended doses. Increased maternal or fetal morbidity is not caused by peptic ulcer disease.

Acute intestinal obstruction

Intestinal obstruction is a serious complication of pregnancy that is occurring with increasing frequency. The incidence is approximately 1 in 2500 to 1 in 3500 pregnancies.[37] There has been an increasing incidence because of the increasing number of abdominal surgeries performed on women. Matthews and Mitchell[38] noted three time periods during pregnancy when obstruction is likely to occur: (1) during the fourth and fifth months, when the enlarging uterus is no longer a pelvic organ; (2) during the eighth and ninth months, when the fetal head descends into the pelvis; and (3) during the puerperium, when there is a marked change in the size of the uterus. Acute intestinal obstruction is most common in the third trimester, less common in the second, and least likely in the first trimester.[39,40]

The most common cause of intestinal obstruction in the pregnant and nonpregnant woman is adhesions.[37,39] More than half of intestinal obstructions are secondary to adhesions that are usually, but not always, due to prior abdominal surgery. Previous laparotomy for appendectomy or gynecologic surgery is the most frequent preceding operation.[37,40] Intussusception and hernias are less common causes of intestinal obstruction during pregnancy.[39]

Volvulus usually involves the sigmoid colon rather than the small intestine or cecum and is the second most common cause of intestinal obstruction during pregnancy.[40] Sigmoid volvulus is usually treated by surgery. Goldthorp[41] determined that 80% of intestinal obstruction cases caused by past appendectomy adhesions occurred during the first pregnancy after the operation. Spontaneous small bowel obstruction associated with a spontaneous triplet gestation has been reported by Ludmir and co-workers. Their patient had no predisposing factors, a delayed diagnosis, delivered preterm, and required surgery to alleviate the obstruction. The authors emphasized the importance of considering the diagnosis of intestinal obstruction when nausea, vomiting, and an overdistended abdomen occur during pregnancy.

The diagnosis of intestinal obstruction in pregnancy is not easy.[39,40,42] As with appendicitis, delay in diagnosis is not uncommon. This can result in perforated or strangulated bowel, preterm labor, and increased maternal and fetal mortality. The classic triad of presenting symptoms in intestinal obstruction is abdominal pain, vomiting, and constipation. All these are common symptoms during normal pregnancy. The physician must have a high index of suspicion for the presence of acute intestinal obstruction. Pain, although usually present, may be constant, colicky, mild, severe, diffuse, or localized. Preterm labor or increased uterine contractions may be present. Physical examination may or may not reveal guarding or rebound tenderness. Abdominal distention can easily be missed in late pregnancy because of the normally large uterus and abdomen. When present, it usually indicates large bowel rather than small bowel obstruction. Bowel sounds may be normal, absent, or high pitched with rushes. Physical examination, however, can be completely nondiagnostic. The white blood cell count is usually not helpful because it is normally elevated in pregnancy. If there is considerable delay in diagnosis and the patient is not appropriately treated, then third spacing of fluids occurs. This results in dehydration, electrolyte imbalance, hypotension, oliguria, fever, tachycardia and, eventually, shock and death.

Diagnosis, once expected clinically, can be made by limited radiographic studies showing bowel distention, intraluminal fluid levels, and decreased gas in the large bowel.[39,40] The concern of obtaining radiographic studies during pregnancy should be tempered by the increased maternal and fetal mortality associated with delayed or misdiagnosis. Radiographic or serial studies showing dilated, gas-filled loops of bowel with air–fluid levels is diagnostic.

Treatment of intestinal obstruction during pregnancy is the same as in the nonpregnant patient.[42,43] Exploratory laparotomy is the treatment of choice. Before surgery, close attention must be paid to correction of fluid and electrolyte imbalance, maintenance of adequate urinary output, administration of blood and blood products, and fetal monitoring. Antibiotics may be indicated. A vertical abdominal incision should be made to provide adequate exposure. Care should be taken by the operating surgeon to avoid manipulating, touching, or tugging on the pregnant uterus, because this could result in preterm labor. If labor occurs while the patient is in surgery, tocolysis should be initiated. The prophylactic use of tocolytic therapy before, during, or after surgery has not been proven and remains debatable.[37] When surgery occurs at term, a well-repaired abdominal incision will tolerate labor without difficulty. At the time of surgery, a Cesarean section should be performed only for obstetric reasons and not because the abdomen is open. Vaginal delivery can occur without difficulty following abdominal surgery. There do not appear to be many, if any, clinical indications for the use of a long intestinal tube rather than surgery to treat obstruction.

Maternal and fetal mortality from undiagnosed cases of intestinal obstruction have decreased over the years.[37,38] Because this is a disease of the third trimester, preterm labor and neonatal death can cause significant fetal mortality.[39] This should be reduced with early diagnosis and aggressive operative treatment. It is good, therefore, for the clinician to remember that an abdominal scar on a pregnant woman with abdominal pain should raise the suspicion of acute intestinal obstruction.[38,42]

Inflammatory bowel disease

The term inflammatory bowel disease refers to a group of idiopathic chronic inflammatory diseases of the intestinal tract.[44,45] The two most commonly seen during pregnancy are ulcerative colitis and Crohn's disease, also called regional enteritis. Both these disorders are not uncommon in women during their reproductive years and are frequently seen either before or during pregnancy.[34,44–48]

The pathologic features of these two diseases distinguish and differentiate them.[34,44] Ulcerative colitis is an inflammatory ulcerative pathologic process involving the mucosal lining of the colon and/or rectum. It is characteristically not transmural. A typical biopsy of ulcerative colitis lesions shows diffuse mucosal ulceration and a chronic inflammatory response consisting of polymorphonuclear cells, lymphocytes, and plasma cells. There may be abscesses of the mucosa. The mucosal lining is edematous and replaced by a chronic inflammatory infiltrate. As this chronic process continues over time, the bowel may become thickened. Areas of stricture, fibrosis, and stenosis develop. Intestinal obstruction and toxic dilation of the colon with resultant perforation can complicate ulcerative colitis.[49]

Crohn's disease, on the other hand, is an inflammatory disease that may involve any area of the gastrointestinal tract, but the distal small intestine, colon, and anal rectal regions are most often affected. The pathologic process is transmural, and the granulomatous enteritis involves all layers of the bowel, mesentery, and lymph nodes. The inflammatory process consists primarily of plasma cells and lymphocytes. The bowel that is affected is edematous, thickened, hyperemic and ulcerated. There may be adhesions of the involved portion with other loops of intestine. Intestinal obstruction, perforation, and fistula formation between loops of bowel can result. The nearby mesentery lymphadenopathy is present. The chronic inflammatory process is more granulomatous than in ulcerative colitis. Granulomas, multinucleated giant cells, and chronic ulcerations may be present. Skipped areas are common and characteristically found in removed bowel affected by regional enteritis. These are unaffected areas of the bowel located next to diseased areas.

These two disorders share a common cause, clinical findings, and management.[34,44] Ulcerative colitis and Crohn's disease may be so similar clinically that a specific diagnosis of the type of inflammatory disease present cannot be made. They can be characterized as chronic disorders that go through periods of quiescence and exacerbation, making differentiation even more difficult.

The effect of inflammatory bowel disease on fertility has been studied by several authors. Most reports show that ulcerative colitis does not affect or alter female fertility.[45,50] Numerous reports have shown and there is general agreement that fertility is decreased in patients with Crohn's disease.[45] This is probably due to the chronic pelvic adhesions that occur as a result of the inflammatory process. The activity of the disease process also affects fertility. Although it is decreased during exacerbations, there is also a decrease in fertility when the disease is quiescent. Improved and reduced fertility after the removal of intestine affected by regional enteritis has been reported.[45]

Ulcerative colitis and regional enteritis can affect pregnancy. The earliest and most extensive report is by Abramson et al.,[51] who reviewed the effect of ulcerative colitis on pregnancy. This report suggests that the best prognosis for pregnancy is in those patients who had inactive disease at the time of conception or whose active disease is limited to early pregnancy. In general, a good prognosis can be expected, and ulcerative colitis does not adversely affect fetal outcome. Brostrom[52] has suggested that pregnancy, if planned, should be encouraged when the patient is in remission, although the disease or its standard treatment does not seem to dangerously affect the patient, fetus, or the newborn infant. The more inactive the disease at the time of conception, the better the prognosis for a more favorable pregnancy outcome.[53]

The effect of Crohn's disease on pregnancy is similar. Numerous investigators have concluded that there is little or no decrease in the live birth rate.[45,48] Adverse pregnancy outcome, as reflected by prematurity, stillbirths, spontaneous abortion, or congenital anomalies, does not appear to be increased. The route of delivery may be affected by inflammatory bowel disease. Cesarean section has been recommended if severe perineal fistulas or scarring, which can occur as a complication of Crohn's disease, are present. Patients who have recently had a proctocolectomy to promote healing of perineal disease should also be delivered by Cesarean section. However, in a small study by Rogers and Katz[54] of 17 women whose pregnancies were complicated by Crohn's disease, the mode of delivery was not protective against worsening perineal disease. Active disease at the onset of pregnancy tends to remain active, and quiescent disease tends to remain quiescent.[54] Cesarean section is not indicated in patients simply because they have had successful restorative surgery for inflammatory bowel disease. However, the full clinical picture, including gestational and fetal age, should be assessed.[45]

The clinical manifestations of inflammatory bowel disease depend on the area of the gastrointestinal tract involved.[34,44] Some symptoms occur with both diseases or are more common with one or the other. Symptoms occurring with both these diseases may include soft stools, rectal bleeding, diarrhea, abdominal pain, weight loss, and urgency of defecation. Rectal bleeding is more common in ulcerative colitis. Abdominal pain, diarrhea, weight loss, fever, and rectal bleeding are the most frequent symptoms occurring in ulcerative colitis. The symptoms of Crohn's disease are most frequently episodic abdominal pain, fever, diarrhea, and weight loss. Perineal fistulas and scarring are more commonly present with regional enteritis and occur in one-third to one-half of the patients with this disease.

The clinical features and presentations of these two disorders can be quite similar, requiring sigmoidoscopy, colonoscopy, radiography, and histologic examination of a biopsy to tell the difference.[34,44] The endoscopic techniques are safe during pregnancy and have replaced radiography in making a diagnosis.[55,56] Extraintestinal manifestations of the inflammatory bowel diseases occur in both the pregnant and the nonpregnant patient.[34,44,47] These include nutritional and metabolic abnormalities, hematologic abnormalities, skin and mucous membrane lesions, arthritis, and eye and renal complications. Hepatic and biliary complications can also occur with the development of sclerosing cholangitis and gallstones. Systemic complications and manifestations have been reported to occur all over the body.[44] Local complications requiring surgical and gastroenterologic intervention can occur, depending on the severity of the disease. These complications include stricture, stenosis, bleeding, malignancy, abscess formation, perforation, fistulas, and perineal problems.

There is little evidence to suggest that pregnancy has an effect on inflammatory bowel disease. The clinical course of ulcerative colitis can be worsened when pregnancy occurs when the disease is active. The risk of exacerbation of ulcerative colitis in pregnant patients is approximately 50%, not dissimilar from that in the nonpregnant patient. One-third of patients who conceive while their colitis is inactive have an exacerbation during their pregnancy. The worst prognosis for the pregnant woman, according to Nielsen and colleagues,[57] occurs when the patient develops ulcerative colitis for the first time during pregnancy. The maternal mortality rate under those circumstances was 15%. Pregnancy should therefore be avoided if possible while the disease is active; one-third of pregnant patients experience worsening of their disease, and less than a half show remission or improvement. Pregnancy has little or no effect on Crohn's disease, and the overall maternal prognosis is good. When an exacerbation in inflammatory bowel disease occurs during pregnancy, it most frequently happens during the first trimester or the postpartum period.

Inflammatory bowel disease is treated by both medical and surgical measures during pregnancy. In general, the treatment is the same as in the nonpregnant patient,[34,44] with several special considerations.[34,44] The mainstay of medical therapy for both ulcerative colitis and Crohn's disease is the use of mesalamine preparations, sulfasalazine, and corticosteroids. Mesalamine is more efficacious in the treatment of ulcerative colitis than in regional enteritis. The corticosteroids most frequently used are prednisone, hydrocortisone, and prednisolone. Metronidazole, azathioprine, and 6-mercaptopurine have also been used in the medical therapy of inflammatory bowel disease. These three agents have possible teratogenic effects, and their use during pregnancy must be carefully evaluated and weighed against their expected benefit.[36,58] Metronidazole has been shown to be effective in the management of inflammatory bowel disease, particularly Crohn's disease for perineal fistula. Although efficacious, it should be used during pregnancy and postpartum only in severe and unusual cases because, although not teratogenic, its use is of concern.[7,36,58] Mesalamine is now the most commonly used drug in the treatment of inflammatory bowel disease and is safe to use during pregnancy (FDA risk category B; see Tables 43.1 and 43.2). It does not appear to pose a teratogenic risk when used at recommended doses. Azathioprine is also indicated for treatment and maintenance of remission of Crohn's disease, but is regarded as unsafe in pregnancy (category D). Remicade can be used in patients with Crohn's disease unresponsive to the above drugs. Although there are limited data for its use in pregnancy, it is a category B drug.[58,59]

Corticosteroid therapy has been used in both these diseases to suppress the inflammatory response present in the bowel.[34,44,47] It is also frequently used in treating exacerbations of Crohn's disease. Doses of prednisone range from 40 to 60 mg daily for a period of several weeks to a month. Some pregnant patients who have been unable to be weaned from corticosteroids may enter pregnancy on a low dose. The continuation of their medication or even the institution of corticosteroid therapy during pregnancy is not contraindicated.[7,58,59] The mother may experience the usual side-effects of corticosteroid therapy, but there are no adverse effects on the fetus from the use of corticosteroids during pregnancy. Breastfeeding is likewise not contraindicated in the mother on corticosteroid therapy.[58,59] None of the drugs used to treat inflammatory bowel diseases is associated with poor pregnancy outcome.[60]

Medical management should include nutritional assessment and treatment, as in any patient with a chronic disease.[34,44] Adequate calories should be provided to help prevent weight loss. Parenteral nutrition, sometimes required in the management of some of the other gastrointestinal complications of pregnancy, is infrequently needed in these patients. If medically necessary to provide adequate caloric intake, total parenteral nutrition may be used safely during pregnancy.[47,61] General therapeutic measures include antidiarrheal drugs such as codeine, opium, paregoric, and diphenoxylate with atropine (Lomotil). As in the treatment of hyperemesis gravidarum, the patient should have the opportunity to discuss the psychological factors of pregnancy or other aspects of her life, which may be playing a part in the precipitation of inflammatory bowel disease.

Inflammatory bowel disease may require surgical treatment of ulcerative colitis including total proctocolectomy with construction of an ileostomy or ileoanal pullthrough.[34,45] Indications for surgery include perforation (with or without abscess formation), massive bleeding, and carcinoma of the colon. Patients who develop toxic megacolon and do not respond to other therapy may also be candidates for this surgical therapy. The procedure should not be done during pregnancy, because the surgery would not only be difficult to perform as the pregnant uterus enlarges, but could also initiate preterm labor.[49] Patients with ulcerative colitis who have been treated with surgery before pregnancy have no increased risk during their pregnancy. Care of the ileostomy is not hampered by pregnancy. There is no evidence that the enlarging uterus interferes with the function of the ileostomy. Vaginal delivery is not contraindicated and should be encouraged. The performance of a Cesarean section for obstetric indications only is recommended, with draping of the ileostomy out of the surgical site.

Surgical therapy for Crohn's disease or regional enteritis is the same as for ulcerative colitis.[34,44] Intractability of symptoms is the most frequent indication for surgery. Perianal complications such as fistulas may also lead to total proctocolectomy with ileostomy or some other variation of this surgery. As with ulcerative colitis, there is a high recurrence rate of the disease with an internal anastomosis. Unlike ulcerative colitis, Crohn's disease is not cured by total proctocolectomy; there is a recurrence rate as high as 80% in 5 years. Surgery for both these disorders should be performed during pregnancy only after intensive medical therapy has failed.[45,62] The interested reader is referred to several other extensive and recent reviews of inflammatory bowel disease in pregnancy.[45–48]

Appendicitis

Appendicitis is the most common cause of an acute abdomen during pregnancy. The incidence during pregnancy has been reported to vary from 1 per 1000 to 1 per 2000 pregnancies, with an average incidence of 1 per 1500 deliveries. There appears to be no increased frequency during any particular trimester.[63] Appendicitis occurring postpartum is fortunately rare as it is particularly difficult to diagnose because peritonitis is a less prominent finding. During pregnancy, the usual symptoms and physical changes may delay the diagnosis or confuse the clinical picture of appendicitis. This delay in diagnosis can be further compounded by the commonly experienced nausea, vomiting, and abdominal discomfort of pregnancy and the displacement of the appendix upward by the enlarging uterus (Fig. 43.1). Additionally, the usual elevation in the white blood cell count during pregnancy and the elevated sedimentation rate may also delay the diagnosis. Unfortunately, pregnant women have a higher mortality rate

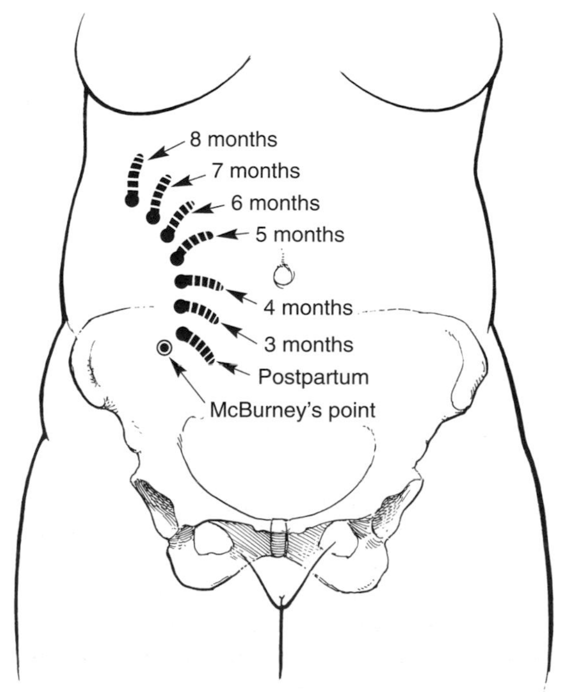

Figure 43.1 Change in the position of the appendix during pregnancy.

when they develop appendicitis. This is primarily because of procrastination in diagnosis and treatment, with resultant perforation of the appendix and peritonitis.[39,63] Therefore, in pregnancy the frequent association of appendicitis with peritonitis is caused by a delay in diagnosis.

The pregnant woman with appendicitis has symptoms and signs similar to those in the nonpregnant patient, but may not experience abdominal rigidity, rebound, or similar signs of peritonitis. Abdominal pain is present, but usually not at McBurney's point. This is because of the change in the position and direction of the appendix during pregnancy.[39,63,64] As pregnancy advances, the cecum is displaced toward the iliac crest, thus moving the appendix laterally, superiorly, and posteriorly. The abdominal pain of appendicitis is typically mild at onset. During pregnancy, it is even less severe. It may be intermittent or colicky, due to a fecalith within the appendix. The pain is followed within an hour or two by anorexia, nausea, and vomiting, symptoms frequently seen during a normal pregnancy. The temperature may be normal, or there may be a low-grade fever. An increasing left shift in the differential may be helpful in making the diagnosis. The urinalysis is usually not helpful other than in excluding the diagnosis of urinary tract infection.

To reduce both maternal and perinatal mortality associated with appendicitis during pregnancy, the diagnosis must be made promptly. These adverse sequelae are obviated by prompt operative exploration when appendicitis is suspected and prevention of appendiceal perforation. A delay in diagnosis appears to increase with gestational age.[39,63] The diagnosis must be suspected in the pregnant patient who experiences persistent right-sided abdominal pain and atypical gastrointestinal symptoms. The removal of a normal appendix may occur in half the cases and should not be criticized, because such an operation rate may be necessary to detect the case with minimal or unusual symptoms, thus decreasing fetal and maternal mortality.[39,63,65] An uncomplicated appendectomy does not increase the risk of preterm labor. However, the presence of peritonitis and a perforated appendix more frequently results in preterm labor and preterm birth. If in doubt, the appendix should be removed, especially during pregnancy.[42,65]

The differential diagnosis of appendicitis during pregnancy includes threatened abortion, ectopic pregnancy, pelvic inflammatory disease, pyelonephritis, placental accidents, twisted ovarian cyst, pancreatitis, gallbladder disease, degenerating fibroids, ruptured corpus luteum, chorioamnionitis, infracted omentum, and the difficult-to-diagnose "round ligament syndrome." Both computed tomography (CT) and magnetic resonance imaging (MRI) are helpful and safe during pregnancy in the diagnosis of acute appendicitis. The clinician or radiologist or emergency room physician should not hesitate to use them when they are indicated. The use of laparoscopy and graded compression sonography in the differential diagnosis of acute appendicitis in the nonpregnant patient may be helpful. Sonography can be helpful in the diagnosis of a postappendectomy abscess. The diagnosis of appendicitis in pregnancy must always be considered when a pregnant patient presents with abdominal pain. The most frequent condition misdiagnosed as appendicitis is pyelonephritis.

Appendectomy is the treatment of choice for appendicitis during pregnancy. It is the most frequent nonobstetric procedure performed during pregnancy. Laparoscopic appendectomy is now as safe as open surgery in pregnancy. It is becoming the standard of care for appendicitis and cholelithiasis management during pregnancy.[66] Some surgeons still suggest the use of a transverse muscle-splitting incision directly over the point of maximum tenderness. When necessary, this incision can be extended without much difficulty. During the operation, the uterus should be manipulated as little as possible. The left lateral position with uterine displacement should be used to minimize the chance of the development of supine hypotension. There is no need for drainage of the incision if the appendix is unruptured and the incision can be primarily closed. Antibiotics are indicated when the appendix is perforated or there is extensive inflammation. There are no data to indicate that tocolysis reduces the incidence of uterine contractions or preterm labor. The routine usage of such agents in these circumstances cannot be recommended. When the diagnosis is made in the third trimester, there are few, if any, indications for a simultaneous Cesarean delivery, except in the presence of obstetric indications. On occasion, a patient presents with appendicitis in labor. Vaginal delivery is not precluded, with minilaparotomy and appendectomy immediately postpartum. This scenario presumes the patient is not in acute distress from a possible perforation.

The complication rate with rupture of the appendix can be very high, including fetal loss and maternal morbidity. When the diagnosis is made promptly and procrastination in treatment does not occur, fetal loss is lowered.[42,63] Prophylactic appendectomy at the time of Cesarean section has been studied prospectively by Parsons and colleagues,[67] who found that this procedure does not add to the risk of elective Cesarean section. Nevertheless, most elective Cesarean sections performed today are not accompanied by an incidental appendectomy, even though they may be safe.

Pregnancy after operation for morbid obesity

Pregnant patients today are more obese than in the past. Over the past 30 years, patients who are morbidly obese have been undergoing a variety of surgical bypass operations to induce weight loss.[68] Seventy-five percent of these patients are women and therefore may be seen after their bypass pregnant. There are basically two types of bypass operations: the older jejunoileal and the more recently developed gastric techniques. The jejunoileal bypass results in weight loss by bypassing approximately 90% of the small bowel, which decreases the area of the bowel available for absorption of food.[68,69] In performing the jejunoileal shunt, an end-to-end or end-to-side anastomosis of the jejunum is accomplished.

A newer procedure, the gastric bypass, involves altering the stomach in some manner to produce a slower, as well as a physiologically better tolerated, weight loss. This can be accomplished by a variety of techniques.[68] The gastric procedures have less long-term morbidity and mortality, making the jejunoileal bypass operation now obsolete.[68]

Successful pregnancy after jejunoileal bypass continues to occur.[69] Knudsen and Kallen studied delivery of women who, before pregnancy, had undergone an intestinal bypass operation. The infants born to these women had an increased rate of low birthweight, short gestation, and also growth retardation. In their study, there was no distinct difference between these infants, whether they were conceived less than 24 months or more than 24 months after the operation. A previous report by Stenning et al.[70] had suggested that pregnancy not long after the procedure could result in fetal loss and a complicated maternal course.

Most pregnant women with a jejunoileal bypass tolerate pregnancy quite well. It has been recommended that they receive supplemental iron, folic acid, vitamin B12, and a prenatal vitamin–mineral preparation.[67] Pregnancy is not contraindicated after jejunoileal bypass,[71] but a 2-year interval before pregnancy is undertaken has been suggested so that the patient will not become pregnant during the highest phase of weight loss and to allow the weight loss to plateau. The longer the interval from surgery to pregnancy, the better the prognosis for both mother and newborn.[70] Pregnancies after gastric restrictive operations are usually well tolerated by both the mother and the fetus. However, complications reported have included severe maternal and fetal electrolyte imbalance, other nutritional deficiencies, and gastrointestinal hemorrhage during pregnancy.[72] Total parenteral nutrition may be necessary in some patients who have previously undergone a jejunoileal bypass when they have evidence of intrauterine growth retardation and inadequate absorption of nutrients.[72]

Because of long-term complications, including persistent electrolyte abnormalities, the jejunoileal bypass procedure is no longer performed. Gastric restrictive operations have now developed as the operations of choice for the patient who is morbidly obese.[68] These include gastroplasty, gastric stapling, and gastric bypass techniques. It has been recommended that a woman undergoing one of these procedures does not become pregnant for at least 1 year because, during that year, significant postoperative metabolic changes occur in the patient. Even after 1 year, severe iron deficiency anemia resulting from malabsorption can complicate pregnancy that occurs after gastric bypass surgery. Pregnancy after at least 1 year has for the most part been uncomplicated, and the patient may actually benefit from the weight loss that has occurred before conception.[68]

Constipation

A decrease in the frequency of stools, painful defecation, increased straining, or increased consistency of the stool is usually thought of as constipation. A patient may complain of being constipated if she experiences any of these symptoms, but a patient's perception of being constipated may differ considerably from that of her physician. Constipation is a common symptom of pregnancy, particularly in late pregnancy. Levy and coworkers[73] interviewed 1000 healthy postpartum women about their bowel habits before and during pregnancy. In 54.6%, there was no change in the bowel frequency during pregnancy. Increased frequency occurred in 34.4%, and only 11% experienced a decreased frequency. Five percent of the subjects actually reported diarrhea of 2–8 weeks' duration in the last trimester. Ninety percent of the women interviewed experienced either no change or an increase in bowel frequency during pregnancy, contrary to the generally accepted view that constipation is frequent in pregnancy. Why pregnancy may cause constipation remains unclear and unknown.

The prevention and treatment of constipation during pregnancy should consist mainly of nutrition counseling, increasing fluid intake, daily exercise, and dietary modification to increase the fiber content.[74,75] If these measures are unsuccessful, then mild laxatives, bulk-producing substances, and stool softeners may be used. These preparations should be used sparingly and are not usually necessary. Castor oil may initiate preterm uterine contractions and preterm labor and is not recommended. Laxatives most commonly recommended are the bulk-forming preparations containing fiber (e.g., Metamucil, Citrucel, and Konsyl) because no systemic absorption occurs. The use of excess laxatives by patients to induce labor should not be condoned. The stool softener dioctyl sulfosuccinate may be used to make the stool softer and able to be passed with less straining. No teratogenic effects have been reported from the use of these common laxatives, stool softeners, or bulk-forming preparations.[58,59] Lewis and Weingold[7] have suggested that they be used cautiously in the breastfeeding patient because they may be transmitted to the infant. Constipation may result in the development of hemorrhoids and, less commonly, rectal prolapse. These can usually be treated by topical ointments or sprays, stool softeners, sitz baths, and over-the-counter preparations such as Preparation H. When hemorrhoids develop during the puerperium after vigorous pushing, they may become thrombosed. Incision after local anesthesia may be necessary and beneficial. Rectal bleeding should be evaluated as in the nonpregnant patient.

Diarrhea

Diarrhea occurs during pregnancy at an incidence up to 34%. Although it is not a common occurrence, it may be due to drugs, malabsorption, osmotic diarrhea, food poisoning, and infections, particularly viral. When persistent, routine evaluation or consultation with a gastroenterologist is indicated;[75] evaluation is the same as in the nonpregnant patient and flexible sigmoidoscopy is safe. Most diarrhea that occurs during pregnancy is nonspecific and can be managed with a variety of nonsystemic and systemic medications. Nonsystemic medications are preferable and should be tried initially. These include kaolin with pectin (Kaopectate) and stool-bulking agents. These substances are not absorbed from the gastrointestinal tract and therefore can cause no systemic side-effects or cross the placenta. Systemic medications frequently prescribed include loperamide (Imodium), diphenoxylate atropine (Lomotil), and bismuth subsalicylate (Pepto-Bismol). All these systemic therapies have been used during pregnancy. No teratogenic effects have been demonstrated from their use.[58,59]

Diseases adjacent to the gastrointestinal tract

Gallbladder disease

Classically, the female patient with gallbladder disease has been described as "fair, fat, forty, and fertile."[39] Gallbladder disease is uncommon during pregnancy. It may present as cholelithiasis or acute cholecystitis.

Cholelithiasis

Pregnancy predisposes to gallstones, increasing the risk of cholesterol gallstone formation by causing incomplete emptying of the gallbladder, particularly in late pregnancy, leaving a large residual volume because of decreased gallbladder contractility. The decreased gallbladder motility is theorized to result from the high progesterone levels present in the second and third trimesters of pregnancy that stimulate progesterone receptors and decrease mobility. The risk of developing gallstone disease increases in association with increasing parity, particularly among younger women, and most stones develop during the second and third trimester.[39] Older women have a decreased risk of developing gallstones.

The exact incidence of cholelithiasis during pregnancy in female patients is unknown, because many gallstones are asymptomatic. It has been reported that 2.0–5.3% of asymptomatic women undergoing routine obstetric ultrasound examinations have cholelithiasis.[76] Consequently, approximately 0.05% of pregnant women will develop symptomatic cholelithiasis and 40% of these women will require surgery.[77] When asymptomatic gallstones are found incidentally during a prenatal ultrasound examination, no therapy is indicated. The authors advise the patient that she has cholelithiasis and to seek follow-up evaluation after her pregnancy. There is no evidence that asymptomatic gallstones become symptomatic at a higher or lower frequency during pregnancy. Gallstones create a problem by passing through or becoming impacted in the biliary tract, producing colic. It has been estimated that one-half of asymptomatic silent stones will cause a problem during a patient's life. The most common complication of cholelithiasis is choledocholithiasis. This occurs in approximately 15–25% of patients with gallstones. The incidence of choledocholithiasis and biliary colic does not appear to be affected by pregnancy. The presence of gallstones may also lead to the development of acute and chronic cholecystitis.

Biliary colic, which is due to choledocholithiasis, is a form of chronic cholecystitis in which the gallstones become impacted or pass through the biliary tract and is the most common symptom that gallstones produce during pregnancy. It affects 15% of patients with cholelithiasis.[34] The pain is due to the passage of the gallstones from the gallbladder into the cystic duct or the common bile duct. This produces a spasm of the gallbladder or the biliary duct involved. The pain is in the right upper quadrant and moderate to severe. It may be cramping or steady. The pain may come on abruptly, particularly after eating a fatty meal. It does not usually last more than a few hours. Although biliary colic is most frequently present in the right upper quadrant, it may also be epigastric, colicky, or steady in intensity. Unlike appendicitis, the pain of biliary colic is not altered in location or character. The patient may also experience nausea, vomiting, and, if cholangitis is present, fever. Jaundice may be present, although gallstones account for only 5% of the causes of jaundice during pregnancy. Depending on where the stone becomes impacted in the biliary tree, obstructive jaundice (common bile duct) or acute pancreatitis (ampulla of Vater) may occur. The symptoms of cholelithiasis may cease spontaneously once the stone is passed through the biliary tract or may persist, requiring surgical removal.

Laboratory diagnosis of gallstones in pregnancy is the same as in nonpregnant patients. The leukocyte count and differential may be normal or slightly elevated, depending on the degree of cholangitis. Hyperbilirubinemia and elevation in levels of aminotransferases [aspartate aminotranferase, AST (formerly called SGOT) and alanine aminotransferase, ALT (formerly called SGPT)] may be present. The serum alkaline phosphatase level is elevated by biliary obstruction. This is not helpful during pregnancy because elevated serum alkaline phosphatase is normal in the pregnant patient as a result of placental production. The presence of acute pancreatitis as a result of common duct stones may cause pancreatitis and elevated serum amylase and lipase levels.[34]

Real-time ultrasound has revolutionized the diagnosis of biliary tract disease during pregnancy. In a review, the maternal gallbladder was visualized in 97.4% of women who underwent gallbladder ultrasound as part of routine obstetric ultrasound screening.[76] An adequate view of the gallbladder could be visualized in 96% of patients within 2 min, suggesting that the gallbladder can be readily, quickly, and adequately visualized during pregnancy. While routine gallbladder sonography is not necessary, any symptomatic patients should be evaluated for gallbladder disease during pregnancy. Several other studies have also shown ultrasound to be 95–98% sensitive in diagnosing both solitary and multiple gallstones in the gallbladder or biliary tract.[77] The technique used in the pregnant and nonpregnant patient is the same and has been well described.[77] Ultrasonography, which has been used in all trimesters to identify gallstones, is completely safe during pregnancy and should be part of the evaluation of any pregnant woman with right upper quadrant pain.[77]

The treatment of cholelithiasis during pregnancy is the same as in the nonpregnant patient. Accurate diagnosis should be made as described previously. Therapy should be tailored to the patient's symptoms, physical examination, gestational age, duration of illness, and clinical condition. Asymptomatic gallstones do not require any therapy. Most patients who have silent gallstones never develop symptoms. Cholecystectomy is recommended for the patient with gallstones who has recurrent episodes of biliary colic, common bile duct gallstones, and gallstone pancreatitis.[39] Cholecystectomy is the second most frequent nonobstetric abdominal surgical procedure performed in pregnancy. Nonoperative therapy consisting of hospitalization, antibiotics, analgesia, nil by mouth, and nasogastric suction may be all that is necessary in patients who have mild illness. Patients with symptoms that do not improve with observation and medical therapy require prompt cholecystectomy. Many authors have demonstrated that a delay in surgery for biliary tract disease complications results in increased maternal and fetal morbidity and mortality.[39] Gallbladder rupture, an unusual complication, has also occurred during pregnancy.[78] In their review, Davis et al.[79] reported that only 40% of patients with symptomatic cholelithiasis responded to conservative medical management. Nineteen percent of their patients required readmission, and 45% who failed conservative management required surgery. Cholecystectomy, when indicated, can be performed by either the laparotomy or the more popular laparoscopic approach.[39] During pregnancy, it should be performed during the second trimester if possible when pregnancy outcome is best. Several additional recommendations should be kept in mind when a patient requires cholecystectomy in the second half of pregnancy:

- Tocolytic therapy may be necessary and should be instituted if preterm labor occurs.
- There are no data to support or condemn the use of prophylactic tocolysis around the time of surgery.
- Surgery should be delayed until after delivery if possible when symptoms arise in the third trimester, although laparoscopic cholecystectomy has been performed safely even at that time.[80]

The safety of laparoscopic cholecystectomy during pregnancy has been reviewed by several authors, and it is a safe procedure during pregnancy. The procedure has become the standard of care for treatment.[39]

Endoscopic management of biliary disease during pregnancy has been proposed.[81] Endoscopic retrograde cholangiopancreatography (ERCP) has been shown to decrease morbidity, mortality, and costs as a definitive treatment alternative for pancreaticobiliary disease in pregnancy. However, further clinical evaluation of this aggressive endoscopic intervention during pregnancy is necessary.[39]

Intraoperative cholangiography is a controversial method of treating biliary disease during pregnancy. Several authors propose that intraoperative cholangiography is probably safe in the second and third trimesters because of the small amount of radiation used during a period when organogenesis is complete.[77] Liberman and colleagues[82] advocate routine intraoperative cholangiography in all pregnant patients undergoing laparoscopic cholecystectomy because of the increased incidence of common bile duct stones. Some argue that intraoperative cholangiography should be used only when there is a question of choledocholithiasis on the basis of clinical, biochemical, or ultrasonic evidence.[77] Alternative methods of investigating the common bile duct during surgery without X-ray exposure include intraoperative ultrasonography, transcystic duct choledochoscopy, and endoscopic papillotomy performed under ultrasonographic guidance.[77] If there is high clinical suspicion for choledocholithiasis or cholangitis, preoperative ERCP should be attempted and has a high degree of success.

Acute cholecystitis

Acute cholecystitis is a rare gastrointestinal disorder during pregnancy. The incidence is not well known. Landers et al.,[83] investigating patients at two hospitals in San Francisco, reported an incidence of 1 per 1000 births. The rate of acute cholecystitis in pregnancy in their report is higher than the 6–20 per 100 000 expected from other series. Fewer pregnant women develop acute cholecystitis than appendicitis during pregnancy.

Acute cholecystitis and appendicitis must be included frequently in the differential diagnosis of the pregnant patient presenting with right upper quadrant pain. Acute pancreatitis must also be considered in the differential diagnosis and may coexist with acute cholecystitis. The incidence of acute cholecystitis does not change through all three trimesters.

The clinical manifestations of acute cholecystitis during pregnancy are the same as in the nonpregnant patient. An attack usually begins with abdominal pain, which may increase in severity. The pain is in the right upper quadrant or epigastrium, and a positive Murphy's sign (right upper quadrant tenderness that is increased with while taking a deep breath) is elicited. Between 70% and 80% of patients have had a previous episode of biliary colic, and a history of previous fatty food intolerance can usually be obtained. The pain may radiate to the back and be associated with low-grade fever, chills, nausea, vomiting, and anorexia. As with other intra-abdominal inflammation, peritoneal signs may be absent. The leukocyte count may be normal or mildly elevated. If gallstone pancreatitis is present, there is an elevation in the serum amylase. When common bile duct obstruction occurs, there will be hyperbilirubinemia and liver enzyme elevation. The evaluation of laboratory data is rarely diagnostic, but the use of ultrasound can be.

There is no evidence that the ultrasonographic appearance of the gallbladder changes during pregnancy. Gallstones within the gallbladder or biliary tract are easily seen with sonography and appear as an echodense area within the gallbladder or biliary tract. They usually cast a shadow and move with a change in position of the patient. The gallbladder wall may be thickened due to chronic cholecystitis, and the biliary ducts dilated due to an impacted stone. Conservative medical management is the mainstay of the treatment of the pregnant patient with acute cholecystitis. This consists of nasogastric suction when necessary, analgesia, intravenous hydration, and antibiotics. Most patients will respond to this medical management. Cholecystectomy should be reserved for those patients who have gallstone pancreatitis, jaundice, repeated attacks, or who fail medical management. When necessary, it should be performed during the second trimester. In the series by Landers et al.,[83] 84% of the patients were successfully treated conservatively. Favorable pregnancy outcomes occurred when those patients who failed conservative management had their cholecystectomy, preferably during the second trimester. Because conservative management of acute cholecystitis or cholelithiasis is not always successful during pregnancy, surgical therapy should be considered.[39] Surgery during the first trimester can result in spontaneous abortion.[39,83] As discussed in the previous section, laparoscopic cholecystectomy can be performed safely and effectively during pregnancy.[84] While the optimal time for laparoscopic surgery remains the second trimester of pregnancy, no increase in fetal loss has been shown when the procedure is performed in the first trimester.[84] Preterm labor remains a concern of laparoscopic cholecystectomy performed in the third trimester, but the incidence may be lower than with a laparotomy surgical approach.[79,84]

In a study performed by Affleck et al.,[85] 47 patients underwent laparoscopic cholecystectomy during pregnancy. The incidence of preterm delivery among these patients was 11.9%. Younger patient age was found to correlate with preterm delivery. In the same study, 15 laparoscopic cholecystectomies were performed during the third trimester, each without any adverse maternal or fetal outcomes. These outcomes suggest that laparoscopic cholecystectomy may be performed safely in all trimesters.

If preterm labor occurs as a result of performing a cholecystectomy, it should be treated with aggressive tocolysis. Maternal morbidity is not increased when cholecystectomy is performed during pregnancy. Fetal loss after cholecystectomy during pregnancy has been reported to occur most frequently during the first trimester.[86] When necessary (gallstone pancreatitis, worsened maternal condition with medical therapy, or complications), cholecystectomy should not be delayed because of pregnancy. Patients should be educated on the potential risks associated with laparoscopic surgery, including trocar injury to the uterus and fetus, effect of pneumoperitoneum on both mother and fetus, induction of preterm labor, decreased uterine blood flow, and increased fetal acidosis. The Society of American Gastrointestinal Endoscopic Surgeons (SAGES)[86] has adopted some guidelines to enhance operative safety in the pregnant patient including:

1 When possible, operative intervention should be deferred until the second trimester, when fetal risk is low.
2 Because pneumoperitoneum enhances lower extremity venous stasis already present in a gravid patient, and because pregnancy is a hypercoagulable state, pneumatic compression devices must be used.
3 Fetal and uterine status, as well as maternal endtidal carbon dioxide and arterial blood gases, should be monitored.
4 The uterus should be protected with a lead shield if intraoperative cholangiography is a possibility. Fluroscopy should be used selectively.
5 Given the enlarged gravid uterus, abdominal access should be attained using an open technique.
6 Dependent positioning should be used to shift the uterus off the inferior vena cava.
7 Pneumoperitoneum pressures should be minimized (8–12 mmHg) and not allowed to exceed 15 mmHg.
8 Obstetric consultation should be obtained preoperatively.

Pancreatitis

The exact incidence of acute pancreatitis during pregnancy has been difficult to determine. It is not common and has been reported to occur in 1 per 1000 to 1 per 12 000 pregnancies in an extensive review by Wilkinson.[87] Although acute pancreatitis may occur at any stage of gestation, it is a disease of late pregnancy, particularly the third trimester, or the early postpartum period.[88,89] Relapses of pancreatitis occur, with an average of two readmissions during the affected pregnancy. It is important to counsel pregnant patients about the relapsing nature of pancreatitis, occuring during the first trimester; however, a favorable prognosis for the pregnancy should be expected.[90] Pancreatitis can reoccur during the same, a subsequent pregnancy, or the puerperium.[91] When pancreatitis develops in women of less than 30 years of age, half of them are pregnant.[89]

Pregnancy probably predisposes a woman to the development not of pancreatitis but of cholelithiasis,[92] which is the most common cause of acute pancreatitis in the pregnant patient. Other factors that predispose to the development of acute pancreatitis during pregnancy include alcoholism, acute infections, abdominal surgery, abdominal trauma, pyelonephritis, tetracycline or thiazide use during pregnancy, and, rarely, pregnancy-induced hypertension.[31] Hyperlipidemia may be the second most common cause of pancreatitis during pregnancy after cholelithiasis.[93] Gestational diabetes in the presence of severe hyperlipidemia has also been reported as a cause of acute pancreatitis. However, biliary disease is at least present in, if not responsible for, 90% of pancreatitis in pregnancy.[88,89] The gallstone can block the ampulla of Vater, causing active pancreatic proteolytic enzymes to cause autodigestion. The most common predisposing factor in the nonpregnant patient is alcoholism.[34]

The clinical picture of acute pancreatitis is characteristic. The symptoms and signs include a rapid onset of constant, central mid-epigastric pain that may radiate to the chest and back and can be quite severe. In mild cases of pancreatitis, pain may be the only symptom that the patient experiences. Not infrequently, however, nausea and severe vomiting may occur alone or with pain. Low-grade fever and absent or decreased bowel sounds also aid in the diagnosis. The classic clinical presentation of a patient with pancreatitis is an individual rocking in the bed with her knees drawn up and trunk flexed in agony.[44] The pain may also radiate to the flanks or shoulders due to the development of peritoneal irritation. Other symptoms include tachycardia in response to the pain, hypotension, ascites, pleural effusion, hypotonic bowel sounds or ileus, tenderness over the epigastrium, and generalized peritonitis. An adynamic ileus may be demonstrated on radiographic examination. The severity of the clinical features depends on the severity of the pancreatitis and whether or not complications occur, such as pseudocyst or abscess formation.[34,94] Rarely is the white blood cell count above 30 000 cells per mL. It may even be within the range for normal pregnancy, 10 000–20 000 cells/mL. The serum amylase is the specific test used to diagnose pancreatitis and is usually elevated to more than 200 IU/mL. However, it is elevated in other conditions causing an acute abdomen, such as perforation of a peptic ulcer, cholecystitis, intestinal bowel obstruction, hepatic trauma, and ruptured ectopic pregnancy.[42] The increase occurs rather quickly after the onset of the illness, usually within 12–24 h, but values do not correlate with the severity of the disease. A serum amylase above 1000 IU/mL is almost always indicative of pancreatitis or an obstruction of the pancreatic duct.[91] Serum amylase has been reported to be both increased and unchanged in the normal pregnancy.[95,96] These mild changes result in fluctuations in the serum amylase, but not to the degree that would cause confusion in the diagnosis of acute pancreatitis.

Other abnormal laboratory data seen in acute pancreatitis include slight elevation of liver function test results, elevated serum lipase, hemoconcentration, hyperglycemia, hypocalcemia, and acidemia due to abnormal pancreatic function. Diagnostic ultrasound can be used to visualize the pancreas for the presence of pseudocyst or abscess.[34] At the same time, the gallbladder and biliary ducts can be visualized to rule out the presence of gallstones. The pancreas can also be evaluated during pregnancy by a CT scan. This procedure is safe to perform during pregnancy, because the dose of radiation given to the fetus is low.[32,58] As both ultrasound and CT demonstrate pancreatitis, failure to demonstrate enlargement of the pancreas in a case of suspected acute pancreatitis should institute a search for other causes of hyperamylasemia.

Treatment for acute pancreatitis is primarily nonoperative.[34,44] Management includes intravenous fluid hydration to correct hypovolemia and electrolyte imbalance, correction of hyperglycemia, enteric rest with nasogastric suction, broad-spectrum antibiotics, and adequate analgesia. Insulin may be necessary to reduce the blood sugar. Acute pancreatitis, when managed appropriately, usually subsides in 2–3 days. Cholecystectomy is reserved for the patient with recurrent attacks of pancreatitis due to gallstones.[42] Cholecystectomy in the midtrimester has been recommended because of the relapsing nature of gallstone pancreatitis. The risks of anesthesia and preterm labor are also lowest at that time. If pancreatitis during pregnancy is due to hyperlipidemia, hemodialysis, plasma exchange, immunospecific apheresis, and a combination of these have been used for the treatment.[97] Several reports suggest a maternal mortality rate as high as 20% in cases of acute pancreatitis secondary to hyperlipidemia during pregnancy. Because of peritoneal irritation, if the patient is in the second half of pregnancy, an attempt should be made to detect preterm labor early and to treat it once diagnosed. Magnesium sulfate would be the tocolytic drug of choice, because hyperglycemia could be worsened if the betamimetic drugs were used.[98] Theoretically, the prostaglandin antagonists may be effective, because animal experiments have shown an elevation of prostaglandin-like activity in the pancreatic venous drainage and peritoneal exudates with induced pancreatitis.[99] The clinician should be concerned about maintaining adequate volume replacement and electrolyte balance and should be vigilant for the appearance of complications in the patient who does not improve rapidly.

The most feared complications are hypocalcemia, pancreatic abscess, and pseudocyst formation, but they occur rarely during pregnancy or postpartum. Patients with necrotizing pancreatitis require hospitalization in an intensive care unit. They should receive treatment with intravenous fluids, antibiotics and, if necessary, surgical debridement.[100] Total parenteral nutrition can be used safely and effectively in the management of pancreatitis during pregnancy, when there is concern for the nutritional status of the mother or the development of intrauterine growth restriction.[88] Maternal mortality is low when diagnosis is made promptly and appropriate management is instituted. Pancreatitis is now a rare cause of maternal death unless the diagnosis is either delayed or missed entirely. The prognosis for the fetus is also good unless severe peritonitis occurs, which predisposes the patient to spontaneous abortion or preterm birth. Preterm labor occurs in 60% of patients when pancreatitis develops late in pregnancy. The mode of delivery is not affected by pancreatitis and, unless contraindicated for obstetric reasons, vaginal delivery is recommended.[88,91]

Effects on the fetus of drugs used in treating gastrointestinal diseases

Throughout this chapter, statements have been made about the teratogenic effect of drugs used in managing these conditions on the fetus. In 1979, the US FDA established a system of five categories to indicate the potential of systemically absorbed drugs to be teratogenic. These risk categories were defined as A, B, C, D, and X and are used by manufacturers to rate their

Table 43.1 Food and Drug Administration risk categories.

Category A	Controlled studies in women fail to demonstrate a risk to the fetus in the first trimester (and there is no evidence of a risk in later trimesters), and the possibility of fetal harm appears remote.
Category B	Either animal reproduction studies have not demonstrated a fetal risk but there are no controlled studies in pregnant women or animal reproduction studies have shown an adverse effect (other than a decrease in fertility) that was not confirmed in controlled studies in women in the first trimester (and there is no evidence of a risk in later trimesters).
Category C	Either studies in animals have revealed adverse effects on the fetus (teratogenic, embryocidal, or other) and there are no controlled studies in women or studies in women and animals are not available. Drugs should be given only if the potential benefit justifies the potential risk to the fetus.
Category D	There is positive evidence of human fetal risk, but the benefits from use in pregnant women may be acceptable despite the risk (e.g., if the drug is needed in a life-threatening situation or for a serious disease for which safer drugs cannot be used or are ineffective).
Category X	Studies in animals or human beings have demonstrated fetal abnormalities, or there is evidence of fetal risk based on human experience, or both, and the risk of the use of the drug in pregnant women clearly outweighs any possible benefit. The drug is contraindicated in women who are or may become pregnant.

products for use during pregnancy (Table 43.1).[101] This classification is currently under revision by the FDA. A review of data on teratology by the American College of Obstetricians and Gynecologists found none of the commonly used drugs in the treatment of gastrointestinal disease during pregnancy to be teratogenic.[102] Table 43.2 lists drugs frequently used in the treatment of gastrointestinal diseases during pregnancy with their FDA risk category.[58,59] The maternal condition, gestational age, treatment need, and benefit to the mother and risk to the fetus, especially of category C or X drugs, must be considered when these drugs are used during pregnancy.[58,59]

Table 43.2 Gastrointestinal drugs frequently used in the treatment of gastrointestinal disorders during pregnancy.

Drugs	FDA risk category (see Table 43.1)
Azathioprine	D
Cimetidine	B
Diazepam	D
Diphenoxylate	C
Doxylamine	B
Droperidol	C
Esomeprazole	B
Famotidine	B
Lansoprazole	B
Lidocaine	C
Loperamide	B
Meperidine	B
Mesalamine	B
Metoclyopramide	B
Misoprostol	X
Nizatidine	C
Olsalazine	C
Omeprazole	C
Pantoprazole	B
Prednisone	B
Prochlorperazine	C
Promethazine	C
Rabeprazole	B
Ranitidine	B
Sulcralfate	B
Tetracycline	D
Trimethobenzamide	C

Total parenteral nutrition in pregnancy

Pregnant patients unable to consume sufficient nutrients orally require an effective method of feeding. Alternative forms of nutrition are being used more frequently in obstetrics.[103] This may be particularly necessary to maintain maternal nutrition when a gastrointestinal disease complicates pregnancy, and can be given as enteral nutrition (tube feeding) or as total parenteral nutrition. Total parenteral nutrition, parenteral nutrition, hyperalimentation, intravenous hyperalimentation, and intravenous feedings are used synonymously and interchangeably to describe the various methods of providing all required nutrients intravenously.[104] Total parenteral nutrition, in order to meet basal, maintenance level of required nutrients, as well as the additional demands of growth and development of the patient and fetus, is hyperosmolar and requires jugular or subclavian venous catheterization.[105,106] Subclavian venous catheterization is now the preferred technique for long-term inpatient total parenteral nutrition.

Numerous authors have reported long-term total parenteral nutrition with good results in a variety of hospitalized or outpatient pregnant patients at significant risk for malnutrition and poor fetal outcome.[14,105–107] Patients at high risk for malnutrition during pregnancy may also benefit from total parenteral nutrition. Silberman and Eisenberg[104] discuss in detail, but succinctly, therapeutic nutrition in the hospitalized patient and principles applicable to the outpatient and pregnant patient.

Total parenteral nutrition can be complicated by death of the nonpregnant patient or by maternal and/or fetal death in the pregnant patient. Other complications include accidental pneumothorax or hemothorax, catheter infection, various metabolic disorders, glycosuria, hypoglycemia and, rarely, clinical sepsis.[104,108] New findings and diagnostic advances warrant revisiting key features of acute nonobstetric abdominal pain in pregnancy.[1] Wernicke–Korsakoff syndrome, with irreversible neurologic abnormalities, has occurred after institution of total parenteral nutrition and has been reported by various authors.[103,106]

There is general agreement that total parenteral nutrition does not cause preterm labor, small for gestational age infants, or fetal death. However, the disease process for which parenteral nutrition is being given may be the cause of this adverse perinatal outcome.[109] It has been demonstrated that enteral or total parenteral nutrition can be safely and effectively administered during pregnancy. A team of qualified, knowledgeable individuals who are familiar with the technique being used should explain it to the patient, obtain written consent, and manage the administration of the parenteral nutrition. Total parenteral nutrition should be administered in hospitals with an intensive care nursery, because many of the infants of the mothers who are receiving this therapy deliver preterm.[110–112]

Key points

1 Nausea with or without vomiting is an especially common symptom during early pregnancy and the most common gastrointestinal complaint. It usually occurs during the first trimester of pregnancy and, by mid-second trimester, most women no longer complain of these symptoms.

2 Hyperemesis gravidarum is the abnormal condition of pregnancy associated with pernicious nausea and vomiting. Hyperemesis is both infrequent and uncommon.

3 Refractory hyperemesis gravidarum has been successfully treated with corticosteroid therapy, which is effective in suppressing symptoms of intractable hyperemesis, decreasing the length of hospitalization, and allowing normal maternal nutrition.

4 The role of psychosocial stressors, such as undesired pregnancy, in the etiology of nausea, vomiting, and hyperemesis gravidarum has been only partially studied. It is believed that psychological factors contribute to excessive nausea and vomiting during pregnancy.

5 A few patients with hyperemesis gravidarum have transient hyperthyroidism, which in these patients is common, self-limited, and requires no therapy.

6 Many pregnant women enter pregnancy with poor dental care. Their teeth are in poor condition, and numerous cavities and gingivitis are present owing to poor dental hygiene.

7 Radiographs, which are often necessary to establish a proper dental diagnosis, may be safely taken during any stage of pregnancy. The maternal abdomen should be shielded with a lead apron.

8 Heartburn is really a symptom of reflux esophagitis that is a common, bothersome complaint during pregnancy and occurs in as many as 70% of pregnant patients.

9 Treatment of reflux esophagitis during pregnancy consists primarily of neutralizing the acid material that is being refluxed into the esophagus, thereby decreasing gastroesophageal reflux.

10 The development of peptic ulcer disease during pregnancy is uncommon and rare. Patients who have peptic ulcers before pregnancy frequently experience fewer symptoms during pregnancy and may even become totally asymptomatic.

11 Patients with peptic ulcer disease should avoid a diet of foods that cause discomfort. The H2 receptor antagonists and the proton pump inhibitors appear to be safe to use during pregnancy.

12 The most common cause of intestinal obstruction in the pregnant woman is adhesions.

13 The term inflammatory bowel disease refers to a group of idiopathic chronic inflammatory diseases of the intestinal tract. The two most commonly seen during pregnancy are ulcerative colitis and Crohn's disease.

14 There is little evidence to suggest that pregnancy has an effect on inflammatory bowel disease. Pregnancy has little or no effect on Crohn's disease and the overall maternal prognosis is good.

15 Appendicitis is the most common cause of an acute abdomen during pregnancy. The most frequent condition misdiagnosed as appendicitis is pyelonephritis.

16 Pregnant women have a higher mortality rate when they develop appendicitis. This is primarily due to procrastination in diagnosis and treatment, with resultant perforation of the appendix, peritonitis, and preterm labor.

17 Both computed axial tomography and magnetic resonance imaging are helpful and safe during pregnancy in the diagnosis of acute appendicitis and other gastrointestinal diseases of pregnancy. The emergency room physician, other clinicians, or radiologists should not hesitate to use them when they are indicated.

18 Gastric restrictive operations have now developed as the operation of choice for the patient who is morbidly obese. It has been recommended that a woman undergoing one of these procedures should not become pregnant for at least 1 year because, during that year,

significant postoperative metabolic changes occur in the patient.

19 The prevention and treatment of constipation during pregnancy should consist mainly of nutrition counseling, increasing fluid intake, daily exercise, and dietary modification to increase the fiber content.

20 Most diarrhea that occurs during pregnancy is nonspecific and can be managed with a variety of nonsystemic and systemic medications.

21 Pregnancy predisposes a woman to developing gallstones by decreasing gallbladder contractility and mobility. About 2–5.3% of asymptomatic women undergoing routine obstetrical ultrasound examinations have cholelithiasis for which no immediate treatment is required.

22 The gallbladder can be readily, quickly, and adequately visualized by ultrasound during pregnancy. Ultrasound has been shown to be 95–98% sensitive in diagnosing both solitary and multiple gallstones in the gallbladder or biliary tree.

23 Biliary colic occurs when gallstones become impacted or pass through the biliary tree, and it is the most common symptom that gallstones produce during pregnancy. Biliary colic typically presents with right upper quadrant pain that is epigastric, colicky, or steady in intensity accompanied by nausea, vomiting and, if cholangitis is present, fever.

24 Obstructive jaundice can occur when the gallstone becomes impacted in the common bile duct or ampulla of Vater causing acute pancreatitis.

25 Cholecystectomy should be reserved for the patient with gallstones who has recurrent episodes of biliary colic, common bile duct gallstones, and gallstone pancreatitis. Nonoperative therapy for a patient with gallstones includes hospitalization, analgesia, nil by mouth, and nasogastric suction.

26 When performed during the second trimester, cholecystectomy carries the most favorable pregnancy outcome.

27 The clinical manifestations of acute cholecystitis during pregnancy are right upper quadrant or epigastric pain that radiates to the back and can be associated with low-grade fever and chills. Nausea, vomiting, anorexia, and fatty food intolerance may accompany the pain.

28 Conservative medical management is the mainstay of treatment of acute cholecystitis during pregnancy.

29 Pancreatitis is uncommon during pregnancy and most typically develops in the third trimester. Treatment for acute pancreatitis is primarily nonoperative.

30 Factors that predispose to the development of acute pancreatitis during pregnancy include alcoholism, acute infections, abdominal surgery, abdominal trauma, pyelonephritis, tetracycline or thiazide use during pregnancy, pregnancy-induced hypertension, eclamptic seizures, hyperlipidemia, gestational diabetes, and hyperparathyroidism.

31 Cholelithiasis is the most common cause of acute pancreatitis during pregnancy. The symptoms and signs of acute pancreatitis during pregnancy include a rapid onset of constant, central mid-epigastric pain that may radiate to the chest and back and can be quite severe. A low-grade fever and absent or decreased bowel sounds may also be present.

32 Serum amylase level is usually elevated to more than 200 IU/mL in acute pancreatitis. A serum amylase level above 1000 IU/mL is almost always indicative of pancreatitis or an obstruction of the pancreatic duct.

33 Careful consideration should be made when prescribing drugs that fall under categories C, D, and X of the Food and Drug Administration's risk category classification, which is being revised.

34 Pregnant patients at high risk of malnutrition during pregnancy may benefit from total parenteral nutrition, which can be used safely during pregnancy.

References

1 Angelini DJ. Obstetric triage revisited. *J Midwifery Wom Health* 2003;48:111.

2 Soules MR. Nausea and vomiting of pregnancy: role of human chorionic gonadotropin and 17-hydroxyprogesterone. *Obstet Gynecol* 1980;55:696.

3 US Department of Health and Human Services. Indications for Bendectin narrowed. *FDA Drug Bull* 1981;11:1.

4 Cordero JF, Oakley GP, Greenberg F, et al. Is Bendectin a teratogen? *JAMA* 1981;245:2307.

5 Shapiro S, Heinonen OP, Siskind V, et al. Antenatal exposure to Benedictin in relation to congenital malformations, perinatal mortality rate, birth weight, intelligence quotient score. *Am J Obstet Gynecol* 1977;128:480.

6 Holmes LB. Teratogen update: Benedictin. *Teratology* 1983;27: 277.

7 Lewis JH, Weingold AB. The use of gastrointestinal drugs during pregnancy and lactation. *Am J Gastroenterol* 1985;80:912.

8 Sahakian V, Rouse D, Sipes S, et al. Vitamin B6 is effective therapy for nausea and vomiting of pregnancy: a randomized, double-blind placebo-controlled study. *Obstet Gynecol* 1991;78: 33.

9 Vutyavanich T, Wongtrangan S, Ruangrsi R. Pyridoxine for nausea and vomiting of pregnancy: a randomized, double-blind, placebo-controlled trial. *Am J Obstet Gynecol* 1995;173: 881.

10 Larrey D, Rueff B, Feldmann G, et al. Recurrent jaundice caused by recurrent hyperemesis gravidarum. *Gut* 1984;25: 1414.

11 Lavin PJM, Smith D, Kori SH, Elinburger C. Wernicke's encephalopathy: a predictable complication of hyperemesis gravidarum. *Obstet Gynecol* 1983;62(Suppl.):13.
12 Naef RW, III, Chauhan SP, Roach H, et al. Treatment for hyperemesis gravidarum in the home: an alternative to hospitalization. *J Perinatol* 1995;154:289.
13 Nageotte MP, Briggs GG, Towers CV, Asrat R. Droperidol and diphenhydramine in the management of hyperemesis gravidarum. *Am J Obstet Gynecol* 1996;174:1801.
14 Levine MG, Esser D. Total parenteral nutrition for the treatment of severe hyperemesis gravidarum: maternal effects and fetal outcome. *Obstet Gynecol* 1988;72:102.
15 Hsu JJ, Clark-Glena R, Nelson DK, Kim CH. Nasogastric enteral feeding in the management of hyperemesis gravidarum. *Obstet Gynecol* 1996;88:343.
16 Fitzgerald CM. Nausea and vomiting in pregnancy. *Br J Med Psychol* 1984;57:159.
17 Dozeman R, Kaiser FE, Cass O, Pries J. Hyperthyroidism appearing as hyperemesis gravidarum. *Arch Intern Med* 1983;143: 2202.
18 Goodwin TM, Montoro M, Mestman JH. Transient hyperthyroidism and hyperemesis gravidarum: clinical aspects. *Am J Obstet Gynecol* 1992;167:648.
19 Klebanoff MA, Koslowe PA, Kaslow R, Rhoads GG. Epidemiology of vomiting in early pregnancy. *Obstet Gynecol* 1985;66:612.
20 Eliakim R, Abulafio O, Sherer DM. Hyperemesis gravidarum: a current review. *Am J Perinatol* 2000;17:207.
21 Albrecht M, Banoczy J, Baranyi E, et al. Studies of dental and oral changes of pregnant diabetic women. *Acta Diabetol Lat* 1987;24:1.
22 Shafer WG, Hine MK, Levy BM. *A textbook of oral pathology*, 4th edn. Philadelphia, PA: W.B. Saunders, 1993.
23 Regezi JA, Sciubba JJ. *Oral pathology: clinical pathologic correlations*, 2nd edn. Philadelphia, PA: W.B. Saunders, 1993.
24 Carranza F. *Glickman's clinical periodontology*, 7th edn. Philadelphia, PA: W.B. Saunders, 1990.
25 Schwartz H, Reichling B. Hazards of radiation exposure for pregnant women. *JAMA* 1978;239:1907.
26 Levinson G, Shnider SM. *Anesthesia for obstetrics*. Baltimore, MD: Williams & Wilkins, 1993.
27 Kuczkowski KM, Benumof JL. Tongue piercing and obstetric anesthesia: is there cause for concern? *J Clin Anesth* 2002;14: 447.
28 Hamod KA, Khouzami VA. Antibiotics in pregnancy. In: Niebyl JR, ed. *Drug use in pregnancy*, 2nd edn. Philadelphia, PA: W.B. Saunders, 1993.
29 Offenbacher S, Lieff S, Boggess KA, et al. Maternal periodontitis and prematurity. *Am Periodontol* 2001;6:164.
30 Richter JE. Gastrocsophageal reflux disease during pregnancy. *Gastroenterol Clin North Am* 2003;32:235.
31 Scott LD, Abu-Hamda E. Gastrointestinal disease in pregnancy. In: Creasy RK, Resnik R, Iams J, eds. *Maternal–fetal medicine: principles and practice*, 5th edn. Philadelphia, PA: W.B. Saunders; 2004:1109.
32 Gastrointestinal disorders. In: Cunningham FG, Hauth JC, Leveno KJ, et al., eds. *Williams obstetrics*, 22nd edn. New York: McGraw Hill; 2005:1273.
33 Diav-Citrin O, Arron J, Shechtman S, et al. The safety of proton pump in pregnancy: a multicentre prospective controlled study. *Aliment Pharmacol Ther* 2005;21:269.
34 Feldman M, Friedman LS, Sleisinger MH. *Sleisenger and Fortran's gastrointestinal and liver disease*, 7th edn. Philadelphia, PA: W.B. Saunders, 2004.
35 Cappell MS. Gastric and duodenal ulcers during pregnancy. *Gastroenterol Clin North Am* 2003;32:263.
36 Williamson C. Drugs in pregnancy. Gastrointestinal disease. *Best Pract Res Clin Obstet Gynaecol* 2001;15:937.
37 Davis MR, Bohon CJ. Intestinal obstruction and pregnancy. *Clin Obstet Gynecol* 1983;26:832.
38 Matthews S, Mitchell PR. Intestinal obstruction in pregnancy. *J Obstet Gynaecol Br Emp* 1948;55:653.
39 Malangoni MA. Gastrointestinal surgery and pregnancy. *Gastroenterol Clin North Am* 2003;32:181.
40 Connolly MM, Unti JA, Nora PF. Bowel obstruction in pregnancy. *Surg Clin North Am* 1995;75:101.
41 Goldthorp WO. Intestinal obstruction during pregnancy and the puerperium. *Br J Clin Pract* 1966;20:367.
42 Ludmir J, Samuels P, Armson BA, Torosian MH. Spontaneous small bowel obstruction associated with a spontaneous gestation. A case report. *J Reprod Med* 1990;34:945.
43 Sharp HT. The acute abdomen during pregnancy. *Clin Obstet Gynecol* 2002;45:405.
44 Goldman L, Ausiello B, eds. *Cecil textbook of medicine*, 22nd edn. Philadelphia, PA: W.B. Saunders, 2004.
45 Kane S. Inflammatory bowel disease in pregnancy. *Gastroenterol Clin North Am* 2003;32:323.
46 Sorokin JJ, Levine SM. Pregnancy and inflammatory bowel disease in the pregnant woman. *Obstet Gynecol* 1983;62: 247.
47 Hanan IM, Kirsner JB. Inflammatory bowel disease in the pregnant woman. *Clin Perinatol* 1985;12:669.
48 Warsof SL. Medical and surgical treatment of inflammatory bowel disease in pregnancy. *Clin Obstet Gynecol* 1983;26: 822.
49 Becker IM. Pregnancy and toxic dilatation of the colon. *Am J Dig Dis* 1972;17:79.
50 Willoughby CP, Truelove SC. Ulcerative colitis and pregnancy. *Gut* 1980;21:469.
51 Abramson D, Jankelson IR, Milner LR. Pregnancy in idiopathic ulcerative colitis. *Am J Obstet Gynecol* 1951;6: 121.
52 Brostrom O. Prognosis in ulcerative colitis. *Med Clin North Am* 1990;74:201.
53 Bush MC, Patel S, Lapinksi RH, Stone JL. Perinatal outcomes in inflammatory bowel disease. *J Matern Fetal Neonatal Med* 2004;15:237.
54 Rogers RG, Katz VL. Course of Crohn's disease during pregnancy and its effects on pregnancy outcome: a retrospective review. *Am J Perinatol* 1995;12:262.
55 Cappell MS, Colon VJ, Sidhom OA. A study at 10 medical centers of the safety and efficacy of 48 flexible sigmoidoscopies and 8 colonoscopies during pregnancy with follow-up of fetal outcome and with comparison to control groups. *Dig Dis Sci* 1996;41:2353.
56 Cappell MS. The fetal safety and clinical efficacy of gastrointestinal endoscopy during pregnancy. *Gastroenterol Clin North Am* 2003;32:123.
57 Nielsen OH, Andreasson B, Bondesen S, et al. Pregnancy in Crohn's disease. *Scand J Gastroenterol* 1984;19:724.
58 Briggs GG, Freeman RK, Yaffee SJ, eds. *Drugs in pregnancy and lactation*, 7th edn. Philadelphia, PA: Lippincott, Williams and Wilkins, 2005.
59 Weiner CP, Buhimschi C, eds. *Drugs for pregnant and lactating women*. Philadelphia, PA: Churchill Livingstone, 2004.
60 Moskovitz DN, Bodian C, Chapman ML, et al. The effects on the fetus of medications used to treat pregnant inflammatory-

bowel disease patients. *Am J Gastroenterol* 2004;99: 656.
61 Folk JJ, Leslie-Brown HF, Nosovitch JT, et al. Hyperemesis gravidarum: outcomes and complications with and without total parenteral nutrition. *J Reprod Med* 2004;49:497.
62 Mogadam M, Korelitz BI, Ahmed SW, et al. The course of inflammatory bowel disease during pregnancy and postpartum. *Am J Gastroenterol* 1981;75:265.
63 Cappell MS, Friedel D. Abdominal pain during pregnancy. *Gastroenterol Clin North Am* 2003;32:1.
64 Baer JL, Reis RA, Arens RA. Appendicitis in pregnancy with changes in position and axis of the normal appendix in pregnancy. *JAMA* 1932;98:1359.
65 Viktrup L, Hee P. Appendicitis during pregnancy. *Am J Obstet Gynecol* 2001;185:259.
66 Rollins MD, Chan K-J, Price RR. Laparoscopy for appendicitis and cholelithiasis during pregnancy: a new standard of care. *Surg Endosc* 2004;18:237.
67 Parsons AK, Sauer MV, Parsons MT, et al. Appendectomy at cesarean section: a prospective study. *Obstet Gynecol* 1986;68: 479.
68 Zuidema G. *Shackelford's surgery of the alimentary tract*, 5th edn. Philadelphia, PA: W.B. Saunders, 2001
69 Knudsen LB, Kallen B. Intestinal bypass, operation and pregnancy outcome. *Acta Obstet Gynecol Scand* 1986;65: 831.
70 Stenning H, Campbell R, Brake I, et al. Pregnancy after jejunoileal shunt. *Med J Aust* 1977;1:781.
71 Woods JR, Brinkman CR. The jejunoileal bypass and pregnancy. *Obstet Gynecol Surv* 1978;33:697.
72 Weissman A, Hagay Z, Schachter M, Dreazen E. Severe maternal and fetal electrolyte imbalance in pregnancy after gastric surgery for morbid obesity. A case report. *J Reprod Med* 1995;40:813.
73 Levy N, Lenberg E, Sharf M. Bowel habit in pregnancy. *Digestion* 1971;4:216.
74 Brucker MC. Management of common minor discomforts in pregnancy. III: managing gastrointestinal problems in pregnancy. *J Nurse Midwifery* 1988;33:67.
75 Wald A. Constipation, diarrhea and symptomatic hemorrhoids during pregnancy. *Gastroenterol Clin North Am* 2003;32: 309.
76 Deutchman ME, Conner P, Hahn RG, Rodney WM. Maternal gallbladder assessment during obstetric ultrasound: results, significance, and technique. *J Fam Pract* 1994;39:33.
77 Graham G, Baxil L, Tharakan T. Laparoscopic cholecystectomy during pregnancy: a case series and review of the literature. *Obstet Gynecol Surv* 1998;53:566.
78 Petrozza JC, Mastrobattista JM, Monga M. Gallbladder perforation in pregnancy. *Am J Perinatol* 1995;12:339.
79 Davis A, Katz VL, Cox R. Gallbladder disease in pregnancy. *J Reprod Med* 1995;40:759.
80 Eichenberg BJ, Vanderlinden J, Miguel C, et al. Laparoscopic cholecystectomy in the third trimester of pregnancy. *Am Surg* 1996;62:874.
81 American Society for Gastrointestinal Endoscopy. Consensus statement: appropriate use of gastrointestinal endoscopy. *Gastrointest Endosc* 2000;52:831.
82 Liberman MA, Phillips EH, Carroll B, et al. Management of choledocholithiasis during pregnancy: a new protocol in the laparoscopic era. *J Laparoendosc Surg* 1995;5:399.
83 Landers D, Carmona R, Crombleholme W, Lim R. Acute cholecystitis in pregnancy. *Obstet Gynecol* 1987;69:131.
84 Barone JE, Beans S, Chen S, et al. Outcome study of cholecystectomy during pregnancy. *Am J Surv* 1999;177:232.
85 Affleck DG, Handrahan DL, Egger MJ, Price RR. The laparoscopic management of appendicitis and cholelithiasis during pregnancy. *Am J Surg* 199;178:523.
86 Patel SG, Veverka TJ. Laparoscopic cholecystectomy in pregnancy. *Curr Surg* 2002;59:74.
87 Wilkinson EJ. Acute pancreatitis in pregnancy: a review of 98 cases and a report of 8 new cases. *Obstet Gynecol Surv* 1973;28:281.
88 Ramin KD, Ramsey PS. Disease of the gallbladder and pancreas in pregnancy. *Obstet Gynecol Clin North Am* 2001;281: 571.
89 McKay AJ, O'Neill J, Imrie CW. Pancreatitis, pregnancy, and gallstones. *Br J Obstet Gynaecol* 1980;87:47.
90 Legro RS, Laider SA. First-trimester pancreatitis: maternal and neonatal outcome. *J Reprod Med* 1995;40:689.
91 Corlett RC, Mishell DR. Pancreatitis in pregnancy. *Am J Obstet Gynecol* 1972;113:281.
92 Cohen S. The sluggish gallbladder of pregnancy. *N Engl J Med* 1980;302:397.
93 Chen CP, Wang KG, Su TH, Yang YC. Acute pancreatitis in pregnancy. *Acta Obstet Gynecol Scand* 1995;74:607.
94 Winship D. Pancreatitis: pancreatic pseudocysts and their complications. *Gastroenterology* 1977;73:593.
95 Kaiser R, Berk JE, Fridhandler L, et al. Serum amylase changes during pregnancy. *Am J Obstet Gynecol* 1975;122:283.
96 Strickland DM, Hauth JC, Widish J, et al. Amylase and isoamylase activities in serum of pregnant women. *Obstet Gynecol* 1984;63:389.
97 Swoboda K, Derfler K, Koppensteiner R, et al. Extracorporeal lipid elimination for treatment of gestational hyperlipidemic pancreatitis. *Gastroenterology* 1993;104:1527.
98 Besinger RE, Niebyl JR. The safety and efficacy of tocolytic agents for the treatment of preterm labor. *Obstet Gynecol Surv* 1990;45:415.
99 Glazer G, Bennett A. Elevation of prostaglandin-like activity in the blood and peritoneal exudates of dogs with acute pancreatitis. *Br J Surg* 1974;61:922.
100 Gosnell FE, O'Neill BB, Harris HW. Necrotizing pancreatitis during pregnancy: a rare cause and review of the literature. *J Gastrointest Surg* 2001;5:371.
101 US Food and Drug Administration. Pregnancy labeling. *FDA Drug Bull* 1979;9:23.
102 ACOG. *Teratology*. ACOG Educational Bulletin 236. Washington, DC. ACOG, 1997.
103 Catanzarite VA, Argubright K, Mann BA, Brittain VL. Malnutrition during pregnancy? Consider parenteral feeding. *Contemp Obstet Gynecol* 1986;27:110.
104 Silberman H, Eisenberg D. *Parenteral and enteral nutrition for the hospitalized patient*, 2nd edn. Norwalk, CT: Appleton-Lange, 1989.
105 Hew LR, Deitel M. Total parenteral nutrition in gynecology and obstetrics. *Obstet Gynecol* 1980;55:464.
106 Seifer DB, Silberman H, Catanzarite VA, et al. Total parenteral nutrition in obstetrics. *JAMA* 1985;253:14.
107 Subramaniam R, Soh EB, Dhillon HK, Abidin HZ. Total parenteral nutrition (TPN) and steroid usage in the management of hyperemesis gravidarum. *Aust NZ J Obstet Gynaecol* 1998;38:339.
108 Nugent FW, Rajala M, O'Shea RA, et al. Total parenteral nutrition in pregnancy: conception to delivery. *J Parenter Enteral Nutr* 1987;11:424.

109 Greenspoon JS, Safarik RH, Hayashi JT, Rosen DJ. Parenteral nutrition during pregnancy. Lack of association with idiopathic preterm labor or preeclampsia. *J Reprod Med* 1994;39:87.
110 Landon MB, Gabbe SG, Mullen JL. Total parenteral nutrition during pregnancy. *Clin Perinatol* 1986;13:57.
111 Rayburn W, Wolk R, Mercer N, Roberts J. Parenteral nutrition in obstetrics and gynecology. *Obstet Gynecol Surv* 1986;41: 200.
112 Russo-Stieglitz K, Levine AB, Wagner BA, Armenti VT. Pregnancy outcome in patients requiring parenteral nutrition. *J Mat–Fetal Med* 1999;8:164.

44 Liver disease in pregnancy

Vivek Raj

Pregnancy is an altered but normal physiological state. Pregnancy causes alterations in the normal physiology of many organs, but its effect on the liver is minimal. Liver disease is uncommon in pregnancy, but its effect on the patient and the fetus can be severe, thus making it more challenging to manage. While any disease of the liver can affect the pregnant woman, there are some diseases that are unique to pregnancy, such as hemolysis, elevated liver function, and low platelets (HELLP) syndrome, acute fatty liver of pregnancy, etc. Some other diseases such as hepatitis E may take a more serious course in pregnant women compared with the general population. Because of the altered physiological state, some disorders are more likely to occur in pregnancy, e.g., Budd–Chiari syndrome, due to the hypercoagulable state (Table 44.1).

Normal pregnancy and liver

Pregnancy alters the normal hemodynamics of the body and causes certain biochemical and physical changes, which should be kept in mind when assessing clinical and biochemical parameters, as some of these can be similar to changes associated with liver disease.[1] Spider angiomata and palmer erythema are seen in pregnancy, as well as in liver disease patients. However, these changes are normal in pregnancy, can be seen in more than 50% of pregnant women, and disappear after delivery. There is no hepatosplenomegaly in pregnancy. Liver histology remains unchanged. Jaundice is not a normal physiological finding in pregnancy, and should prompt further investigation. Hemodynamic and biochemical changes in normal pregnancy are outlined in Table 44.2. Most biochemical tests used to assess liver injury or liver function are not altered in pregnancy. Therefore, increase in levels of aspartate aminotransferase (AST), alanine aminotransferase (ALT), serum bilirubin, and fasting serum bile acid concentration indicate liver disease, should be considered abnormal, just as in a non-pregnant woman, and should be investigated further.[2–4]

Liver diseases unique to pregnancy

Liver diseases unique to pregnancy include hyperemesis gravidarum, intrahepatic cholestasis of pregnancy (ICP), preeclampsia- and eclampsia-related liver diseases including HELLP syndrome, and acute fatty liver of pregnancy (AFLP). These present at different gestational periods, and this knowledge can be very helpful in suspecting and diagnosing these diseases (Table 44.3). Diseases that are not unique to pregnancy, such as viral hepatitis, drug hepatotoxicity, etc., can also occur in a pregnant woman and should be considered in the differential diagnosis of liver disease in a pregnant woman. Salient features of liver diseases unique to pregnancy are summarized later in the text (see Table 44.6).

Hyperemesis gravidarum

Hyperemesis gravidarum is characterized by severe nausea and vomiting during pregnancy. It can lead to dehydration and ketosis. It is more severe than the common morning sickness. While nausea and vomiting can be seen in up to 50% of pregnancies, hyperemesis gravidarum is seen in only 1–1.5% of all pregnancies.[5,6] It generally occurs in the first trimester of pregnancy, but can occur as late as the 20th week. Abnormal liver enzymes and mild hyperbilirubinemia can be seen in more than 50% of cases.[7,8]

Pathophysiology and pathology

The pathogenesis of hyperemesis gravidarum remains unclear. Liver involvement is secondary to the disorder itself and not the cause of the disorder. Gestational hormones that peak in early pregnancy may affect both liver and thyroid. Liver biopsy is not needed in most situations but, if performed, it is usually normal or may show centrilobular vacuolation, cell dropout, and rare bile plugs. There is usually no inflammation, and either no or minimal fat.[7,9]

Table 44.1 Liver diseases in pregnancy.

Liver diseases unique to pregnancy
Hyperemesis gravidarum
Intrahepatic cholestasis of pregnancy
Preeclampsia and liver disease including HELLP syndrome, hepatic infarction, hepatic hematoma, and rupture
Acute fatty liver of pregnancy
Common liver diseases occurring concurrently with pregnancy or exacerbated by pregnancy
Acute viral hepatitis: A, B, C, E, Herpes simplex
Drug hepatotoxicity
Biliary and pancreatic diseases
Budd–Chiari syndrome
Other diseases
Pregnancy in the presence of chronic liver disease
Cirrhosis and portal hypertension
Chronic hepatitis B
Chronic hepatitis C
Autoimmune hepatitis
Primary biliary cirrhosis
Focal nodular hyperplasia and hepatic adenoma
Liver transplantation

Table 44.2 Hemodynamic and biochemical changes in normal pregnancy.

Hemodynamic changes	
Plasma volume	↑ Between weeks 6 and 36 by 50%. ↓ After delivery
Red cell volume	↑ By about 20%. ↓ After delivery
Cardiac output	↑ Until second trimester. Normalizes by term
Systemic vascular resistance	↓ Due to systemic vasodilation and placental circulation
Absolute hepatic blood flow	Unchanged
Biochemical changes	
Serum albumin	↓ As pregnancy advances, due to hemodilution
ALP	↑ Mainly placental ALP
ALT	No change
AST	No change
Serum bilirubin	No change or mild ↓
Direct bilirubin	No change
Fasting total bile acid	No change
GGT	Mild ↓
Serum fibrinogen	↑
Prothrombin time/INR	No change

ALP, alkaline phosphatase; ALT, alanine aminotransferase; AST, aspartate aminotransferase; GGT, gamma-glutamyltransferase; INR, international normalized ratio.

Table 44.3 Onset of liver diseases unique to pregnancy by trimester.

Hyperemesis gravidarum	Early first trimester
Intrahepatic cholestasis of pregnancy	Anytime. Usually late second or third trimester
Preeclampsia	Late second or third trimester
HELLP syndrome	Third trimester. Sometimes postpartum
Acute fatty liver of pregnancy	Third trimester. Sometimes postpartum

Clinical and biochemical features

Patients usually present with intractable severe nausea and vomiting in the 4th to 10th week of gestation, but can present as late as the 20th week. Vomiting can be severe and lead to dehydration, malnutrition, and ketosis. It is more common in primiparous than in multiparous women. Usually, the patient has no other complaint such as abdominal pain or fever. When the liver is involved, there can be significant elevations of AST and ALT ranging from mild elevation to 500–1000 IU/L. Bilirubin elevation is usually mild and so is alkaline phosphatase (ALP; up to twice normal levels).[9,10]

Management, maternal and fetal outcome

Most patients respond to intravenous rehydration and bowel rest for a few days, followed by a high-carbohydrate, low-fat diet. The symptoms, as well as liver test abnormalities, usually resolve quickly with this treatment. Antiemetics such as ondansetron, phenargan, and droperidol are frequently needed for symptom control.[11,12] Corticosteroids may be useful in refractory cases.[13] Enteral nutrition via a gastric or duodenal feeding tube can be useful[14] and, rarely, parenteral nutrition may be needed. Symptoms usually resolve by late first or early second trimester. There is usually no impact on the child. Infants born to affected patients do not differ from those of normal patients in terms of birthweight, maturity at birth, or birth defects.[5,6] However, in patients with severe hyperemesis, the infant birthweight may be lower than normal.[15]

Intrahepatic cholestasis of pregnancy (ICP)

ICP is a benign cholestatic disorder that usually occurs during the second or third trimester of pregnancy and disappears shortly after delivery. It is characterized by pruritis, cholestatic liver test abnormalities, and occasionally jaundice. It is not a life-threatening disease, but can cause significant discomfort and affect maternal well-being.[16] It can sometimes be associated with an increased incidence of postpartum hemorrhage, probably as a result of vitamin K malabsorption. There is wide variation in its prevalence across the world, with low rates of 1–2 per 10 000 pregnancies in the United States, Asia, and Australia, and high rates up to 10–200 per 10 000 pregnancies in Europe.[17,18] Prevalence of 15.6% was reported from Chile,[19] although lower rates of 4–6.5% have been reported in more recent studies.[20,21] The reason for this is unclear. ICP can occur in primiparous or multiparous women, can recur in subsequent pregnancies, and is more common in multiple gestations.[18,22]

Pathophysiology and pathology

The exact cause of ICP is unknown. Genetic factors, hormonal exposure, and exogenous factors may all play a role in its pathogenesis.[23] Genetic factors may explain the wide geographical variation and high incidence in some ethnic groups such as Native Americans in Chile.[19] Premature truncation or missense mutation of the *MDR3* gene has been reported.[24] A role for estrogens has been strongly suggested. ICP occurs in the third trimester, when estrogen levels peak,[18,21,25] and occurs five times more commonly in multiple gestations, where estrogen levels are high.[26] Experimental cholestasis can be induced in nonpregnant women with a previous history of ICP by the administration of ethinylestradiol.[27,28] Abnormal progesterone metabolism may also be involved in the pathogenesis of ICP. In ICP patients, the levels of sulfated metabolites of progesterone are increased.[28] Oral administration of progesterone in the third trimester of pregnancy has been shown to increase serum bile acid concentration and serum ALT levels.[29] Progesterone should not be prescribed in pregnant women with a history of ICP, or in late pregnancy, and should be withdrawn if cholestasis occurs during pregnancy.[1,16] Exogenous factors may also be important in the pathogenesis of ICP, as suggested by a recurrence rate of 45–70%[30,31] in subsequent pregnancies, seasonal variation in incidence in many countries, and decreasing incidence in some high-prevalence countries such as Sweden[32] and Chile.[30] Liver biopsy is rarely necessary for diagnosis. Histopathology shows cholestasis, with bile plugs in hepatocytes and canaliculi, predominantly in the centrilobular region. There is no inflammation or necrosis, and portal tracts are unaffected (Fig. 44.1).[33]

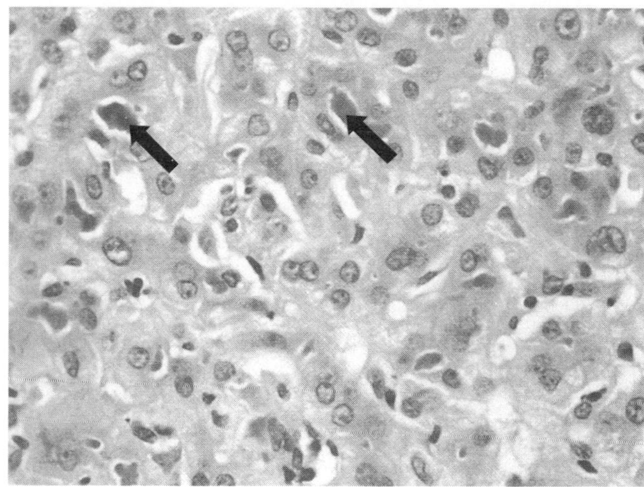

Figure 44.1 Liver biopsy showing cholestasis of pregnancy. Arrows point to bile plugs within canaliculi (bilirubinostasis). Note minimal accompanying inflammation (reprinted from Burt et al., with permission from Elsevier).

Clinical and biochemical features

The main symptom of ICP is pruritis, which can be very severe, uncomfortable, and difficult to tolerate. It can involve any part of the body, but usually involves the hands and feet, especially the palms and soles. It is often generalized and is usually worse at night, resulting in sleep deprivation and psychological distress.[26,34–36] Pruritis generally develops in the third trimester, but can occur as early as the sixth week.[31,37] Jaundice develops in only 10–15% of cases, is usually mild, with serum bilirubin less than six times the upper limit of normal, and resolves rapidly after delivery, within 1–40 days. Jaundice in the absence of pruritis is rare.[26,31,38] ALT and AST are elevated 2- to 10-fold above the upper limit of normal. ALT elevation is a sensitive test for ICP.[39] Viral hepatitis should be ruled out in all cases with elevated ALT and AST. Liver histology does not show any hepatocyte injury, and the cause of elevated liver transaminases is thought to be an increase in membrane permeability. Serum gamma-glutamyltransferase (GGT) is usually normal or mildly increased. Serum total bile acid (TBA) concentrations are increased. Increased serum cholic acid levels, or a ratio of cholic to chenodeoxycholic acid level of > 1 may be the earliest and most sensitive predictor of ICP, even before the onset of symptoms.[33] Measurement of serum TBA concentration is a useful diagnostic test for ICP, especially when the patient has pruritis but normal ALT and AST levels.[30] The serum bile acid and aminotransferase levels decrease rapidly after delivery and, as a rule, normalize in a few weeks. Prothrombin time is usually normal. It can sometimes be abnormal because of vitamin K deficiency, and should be checked before delivery and corrected with vitamin K, to avoid bleeding complications.

Maternal and fetal outcome

Severe pruritis can lead to fatigue and psychological distress for the mother. However, the overall maternal prognosis is good. There is a slight increase in the risk of postpartum hemorrhage due to vitamin K malabsorption, but this is easily corrected by administration of vitamin K prior to delivery. ICP does increase the risk for the fetus, with an increase in risk of prematurity, stillbirth, meconium-stained amniotic fluid, and abnormal fetal heart rate patterns.[21,40–43] The higher rate of multiple pregnancies in ICP may also contribute to high rates of prematurity.[31] Antenatal testing, amniocentesis, and early induction of labor, once fetal lung maturity is achieved, decrease fetal mortality rates.[22,44]

Medical and obstetric management

The aim of management is treatment of maternal symptoms and improvement of fetal outcome. Hydroxyzine, other antihistaminics, benzodiazepines, and tranquilizers are used to treat symptoms, but have limited success and do not improve biochemical parameters or fetal outcome. Low-dose phenobarbital (2–5 mg/kg) has been found to be effective in controlling pruritis in about 50% of patients in one study,[18] but not in others.[21] Cholestyramine (8–16 g/day) decreases ileal absorption and increases fecal excretion of bile acids by binding bile acids in the small bowel. It improves maternal symptoms to some extent, but does not improve biochemical parameters or fetal outcome.[21,45] In many studies, ursodeoxycholic acid (UDCA) has been effective. It is a naturally occurring bile acid, which modifies the bile acid pool composition by replacing lithocholic acid, which is mildly cytotoxic to hepatocyte membranes, and by decreasing the absorption of cholic and chenodeoxycholic acid. It relieved pruritis, improved liver blood test values, and prevented prematurity in most patients. No major side-effects have been reported in mother or baby, and it was not found to be teratogenic.[28,46–49] Fetal outcome improves if the condition is diagnosed early and managed actively, including fetal surveillance. It is difficult to decide the best time for delivery. Risk of prematurity and the risk of intrauterine death of the fetus have to be taken into account when deciding the best time to deliver. In patients with severe cholestasis, delivery should be considered after 36 weeks' gestation if the fetal lungs have matured, or as soon as possible thereafter.[21]

Preeclampsia and liver disease

Preeclampsia is a multisystem disorder of unknown etiology that presents in the late second or third trimester of pregnancy and is characterized by a triad of hypertension, proteinuria, and edema.[3] It complicates 3–5% of all pregnancies and is a major cause of maternal and fetal morbidity and mortality. The etiology and pathogenesis of preeclampsia are poorly understood. Genetic and immunological factors have been implicated,[50–52] as well as paternal or fetal factors.[53] The drop in systemic vascular resistance typically seen in normal pregnancy fails to occur, and the sensitivity of the vascular system to vasospasm is enhanced, resulting in poor perfusion of a variety of organs including the liver, causing ischemic injury. The spectrum of liver disease in preeclampsia ranges from subclinical involvement at one end of the spectrum to HELLP syndrome, hepatic infarction, and rupture of liver at the other end of the spectrum. Acute fatty liver of pregnancy is also associated with preeclampsia in about half the cases, but is a distinct syndrome. The commonest liver disorder seen in the presence of preeclampsia is HELLP syndrome. The exact mechanism for this is unknown.

HELLP syndrome

HELLP syndrome is defined as hemolysis, elevated liver test values and low platelets in a patient with preeclampsia. It affects approximately 0.1–0.6% of pregnancies, and 4–12% of patients with severe preeclampsia. The majority of cases (about 70%) occur in the third trimester, and the rest occur postpartum.[1]

Pathophysiology and pathology

The peripheral smear characteristically shows features of microangeopathic hemolytic anemia, with characteristic schistocytes and burr cells. Liver biopsy is not necessary for diagnosis and can be high risk given the possibility of hematoma and liver rupture seen in HELLP syndrome. Liver histology is characterized by periportal hemorrhage, and periportal and focal parenchymal necrosis, with hyaline deposits[54,55] (Fig. 44.2). There is fibrin deposition and microthrombi in sinusoids. Steatosis can be seen in some patients, but it is usually macrovesicular fat distribution throughout the liver lobule that distinguishes it from the microvesicular centrizonal fat distribution typical of acute fatty liver of pregnancy.[56] Rarely, hepatic infarction and rupture of the liver capsule from underlying bleeding can occur.

A

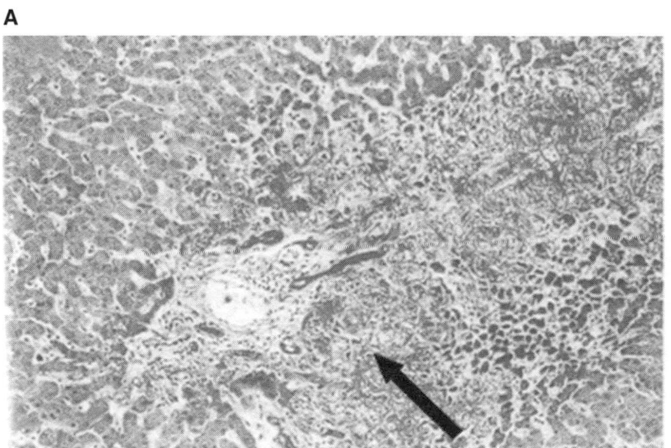

B

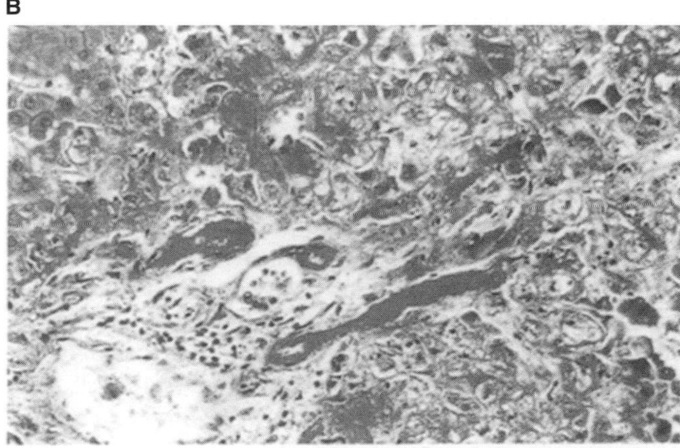

Figure 44.2 Liver in toxemia of pregnancy. (A) Area of periportal necrosis (arrow) with intrasinusoidal fibrin deposition. (B) Hepatic arterioles showing vacuolosis and intrasinusoidal fibrin deposition. Masson's trichrome stain (reprinted from Burt et al., with permission from Elsevier).

Clinical and biochemical features:

There is wide variation in the clinical presentation, varying from no symptoms other than mild abdominal pain to severe life-threatening illness. The typical presenting symptoms are right upper quadrant or epigastric pain (65–90% of patients), malaise (90%), nausea and vomiting (36–50%), and headache (31%). Although liver enzyme elevation is common, jaundice is seen in only 5% of patients.[57,58] Hypertension and proteinuria typical of preeclampsia are seen in the majority of patients. Hypertension can be absent in 15–20% of patients.[58,59] Physical examination reveals right upper quadrant tenderness (80%) and weight gain with edema (60%).[58] On laboratory testing, there is evidence of hemolytic anemia with a drop in hemoglobin, abnormal peripheral smear showing schistocytes and burr cells, and elevated serum lactate dehydrogenase (LDH). Liver enzymes are elevated modestly, but may sometimes be above 1000 IU/L. Usually, AST levels are higher than ALT levels. Platelet count is decreased below 100 000 cells/mm^3.[16] Coagulation studies including prothrombin time and fibrinogen levels are usually normal (Table 44.4).

Maternal and fetal outcome

The mortality rate for women with HELLP syndrome is 1–3%, although rates as high as 25% have been reported.[3,57] The most important causes of maternal morbidity and mortality are stroke, disseminated intravascular coagulation (DIC; 20% of patients), and spontaneous or postpartum hemorrhage. Other causes of morbidity and mortality include hypertension, eclampsia, pulmonary edema (6%), acute renal failure (7%), abruptio placentae (16%) and, rarely, hepatic rupture.[57] Perinatal mortality of infants is about 35% (range 10–60% in different series). Besides prematurity, infants born to mothers with HELLP are at increased risk of thrombocytopenia.[60,61]

Table 44.4 Diagnostic laboratory and pathological features of HELLP syndrome.

Hemolytic anemia
Decrease in Hb
Peripheral smear: schistocytes and burr cells
Total bilirubin > 1.2 mg/dL, mainly unconjugated
Lactate dehydrogenase > 600 U/L
Elevated liver enzymes
Serum AST > 70 U/L or > twice normal
AST > ALT
AST and ALT up to 1000 IU/L
Thrombocytopenia
Platelet count < 100 000/mL
Liver biopsy
Periportal hemorrhage and periportal or focal parenchymal necrosis with hyaline deposits. Fibrin microthrombi and fibrinogen deposits in sinusoids

ALT, alanine aminotransferase; AST, aspartate aminotransferase; Hb, hemoglobin.

The risk of recurrent HELLP in subsequent pregnancies is 3–27% according to different studies.[62,63]

Management

Management of HELLP and preeclampsia is supportive and may require intensive care unit (ICU) care. Delivery is the definitive treatment for HELLP, preeclampsia, and eclampsia.[3] The best timing for delivery is determined by the balance between fetal gestational age and lung maturity and the severity of HELLP and preeclampsia. If preeclampsia is severe or develops after the 36th week of gestation and the fetal lungs are likely to be mature, the baby should be delivered. If preeclampsia is seen in the early third trimester and is mild, then expectant management can be followed with close monitoring.[64] Corticosteroids have been shown to improve maternal platelet count and liver enzymes, and to promote fetal lung maturity, along with a trend toward improving fetal outcome.[61,65,66]

Hepatic infarction

Hepatic infarction is a severe but rare complication of preeclampsia, and may be considered an extension of HELLP syndrome.[67] Patients present with severe abdominal or chest pain and fever without an obvious source. White blood cell (WBC) count is elevated and aminotransferases may be very high, sometimes > 5000 U. In severe cases, patient may have acute liver failure due to massive liver damage, with encephalopathy, coagulopathy, and jaundice.[68] Abdominal computerized tomography (CT) scan or magnetic resonance imaging (MRI) are the imaging modalities of choice for seeing liver infarcts.[69] Management is mainly supportive. Fortunately, most patients recover completely, with no long-term sequelae.

Subcapsular hematoma and rupture of liver

These are rare but the most severe complications of preeclamptic liver involvement. When the rupture is contained within the capsule of the liver, the patient presents with severe right upper quadrant abdominal pain, but is hemodynamically stable.[70] Abdominal CT helps to make a definitive diagnosis. Management is supportive. Patients with hepatic rupture present with severe abdominal pain, shock, and hemoperitoneum. Mortality is very high. Most patients undergo emergency laparotomy with liver resection and packing.[71] Arterial embolization to control hemorrhage has also been suggested.[72] Liver transplant has been done in some cases.[73,74] Early diagnosis and prompt delivery are essential.[74,75]

Acute fatty liver of pregnancy (AFLP)

AFLP was first described by Sheehan in 1940.[76] It is a rare disease, occurring in the third trimester, and has a high mortality risk. It occurs in 1 in every 7000–14 000 deliveries and has a worldwide prevalence.[77,78] Women in their first pregnancy or women carrying more than one fetus are most often affected.[79,80] It occurs in the third trimester, although in some cases it may be diagnosed postpartum, even though the disease starts before delivery in all cases. Rare cases have been described occurring between 22 and 26 weeks.[81–83] Before 1980, both maternal and fetal mortality rates of 70–90% were reported,[77,84–87] but recent data show mortality rates of less than 20%,[88–90] mostly because of greater disease awareness, earlier diagnosis, and improved ICU care. Patients who survive have no long-term sequelae, and liver histology completely returns to normal.[78,85] Recurrence in subsequent pregnancies is rare.[3]

Pathophysiology and pathology

The etiology of AFLP is not known. It belongs to a group of liver diseases characterized by microvesicular steatosis and mitochondrial dysfunction. Other disorders in this group include Reye syndrome, drug hepatotoxicity with sodium valproate and tetracycline, and Jamaican vomiting sickness.[1] A genetic factor has been suggested, but no familial cases have been reported. Recently, a mutation (Glu474Gln mutation) in the long-chain 3-hydroxyacyl-coenzyme A dehydrogenase (LCHAD), a fatty acid β-oxidation enzyme, has been suggested.[86,87,91] Women with LCHAD deficiency do not always have liver disease. Liver disease occurs most often when severe fetal deficiency of the enzyme activity results in accumulation of metabolites in the fetus and fetal–maternal transfer.[92] Liver biopsy is the most definitive way to confirm diagnosis but, as it is invasive, the benefit and risk have to be assessed. It is definitely indicated after common illnesses such as viral hepatitis have been excluded, and there is doubt about the diagnosis of AFLP. The overall liver architecture is intact. There is microvesicular fatty infiltration of hepatocytes, which are swollen. Minute fatty droplets surround the central nucleus, giving a foamy appearance to the cytoplasm. The changes are most prominent in the pericentral zone and midzone (zones 2 and 3), and spare the periportal hepatocytes. Subtle inflammation and necrosis of hepatocytes may be present[93] (Fig. 44.3). Electron microscopy can confirm fat droplets in the cytoplasm and changes in mitochondrial morphology.[81]

A

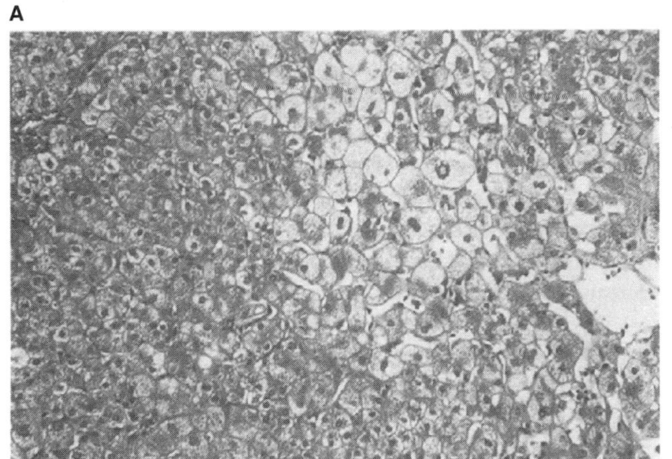

B

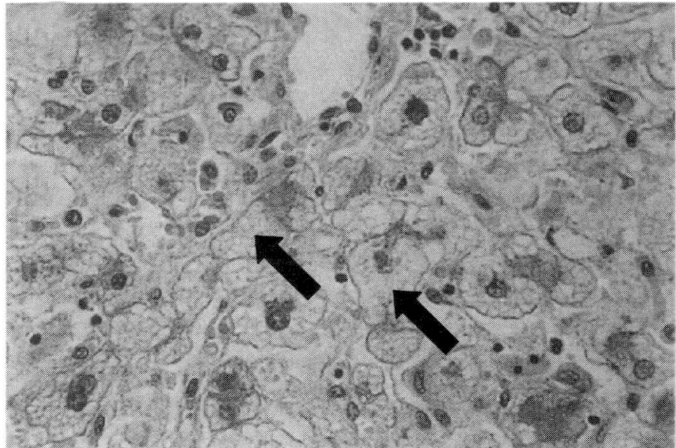

C

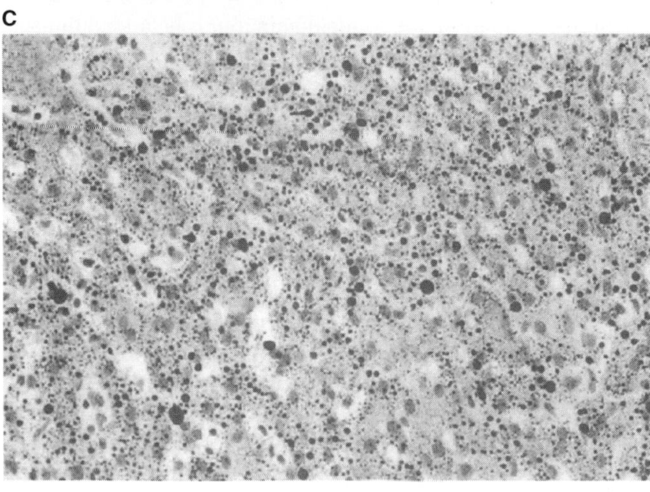

Figure 44.3 Acute fatty liver of pregnancy. (A) Microvesicular steatosis involving centrilobular (perivenular) zones, H&E. (B) High-power micrograph showing swollen hepatocytes and microvasicular fat accumulation (arrows), H&E, and (C) Oil red O stain (reprinted from ref. 134, with permission from Elsevier).

Table 44.5 Diagnostic clinical, laboratory, and pathological features of acute fatty liver of pregnancy.

Clinical
Acute-onset nausea, vomiting
Right upper quadrant or epigastric pain
Flu-like symptoms: malaise, anorexia, headache
Jaundice
Encephalopathy: somnolence, irritability, sleep alterations, asterexis, progressing to seizures and coma
Laboratory tests
Leukocytosis
Coagulation disorders: increased prothrombin time, decreased fibrinogen and clotting factors, thrombocytopenia, DIC
Elevated liver enzymes: AST, ALT (up to 1000 IU/L), bilirubin (up to 5–15 mg/dL), ALP
Hypoglycemia
Renal failure: elevated BUN and creatinine
Liver biopsy
Microvesicular steatosis with foamy appearance of cytoplasm. Mild inflammation and hepatocyte necrosis

ALP, alkaline phosphatase; ALT, alanine aminotransferase; AST, aspartate aminotransferase; BUN, blood urea nitrogen; DIC, disseminated intravascular coagulation.

Clinical and biochemical features (Table 44.5)

AFLP generally presents with acute onset of nausea and vomiting (70% of cases), right upper quadrant or epigastric abdominal pain (50–80%), or flu-like symptoms of malaise, headache, and anorexia.[78,81,90] Jaundice usually occurs 1–2 weeks after the onset of these systemic symptoms. Pruritis is rare.[81,89] About half the patients have preeclampsia. Physical examination is usually unremarkable except for jaundice. The liver edge may be palpable.

Leukocytosis is common. Coagulation disorders, including thrombocytopenia, decreased clotting factors, and DIC, are frequently seen. Liver enzymes are elevated with moderate increases in ALT and AST (usually < 1000 IU/L), increased ALP, and increased hyperbilirubinemia (usually between 5 and 15 mg/dL and mostly conjugated). Hypoglycemia and renal dysfunction can develop.[16,81,89] Radiological imaging studies (ultrasound, CT, MRI) can show fatty liver, but do not have any specific pattern on which to base a radiological diagnosis.[94]

Maternal and fetal outcome

Most patients improve 1–4 weeks postpartum, following spontaneous or induced delivery or Cesarean section. Rarely, the disease may worsen postpartum.[84,86,95,96] If untreated, AFLP typically progresses to fulminant hepatic failure with encephalopathy, coagulopathy, DIC, cerebral edema, renal failure, pancreatitis, gastrointestinal or uterine bleeding, seizures, coma, and death. Infection is a common complication.[81,89] As pointed out earlier, with better management, maternal and fetal mortality has decreased from 85% before 1980 to less than 20% in 2000.

Management

Timely diagnosis, intensive monitoring and management, and early delivery are the key to a successful outcome. There is no specific therapy. Prompt delivery is recommended to improve maternal and fetal outcomes. Severely affected patients (encephalopathy, coagulopathy, severe jaundice, etc.) should be monitored in the ICU.[84,86,95,97,98] Liver transplantation is a possible therapeutic option in postpartum patients who do not improve rapidly after delivery.[88,99]

Liver diseases occurring concurrently with pregnancy or exacerbated by pregnancy

Viral hepatitis in pregnancy

All the hepatotrophic viruses can affect a pregnant woman. A detailed discussion of viral hepatitis is beyond the scope of this book. A brief discussion of hepatitis A, B, C, E, and herpes simplex viral hepatitis, pertinent to pregnancy, follows. For detailed discussion, the reader is referred to a liver textbook.[1,100] Acute viral hepatitis is a systemic illness with fever, malaise, nausea, vomiting, anorexia, and fatigue at presentation, followed by jaundice. Aminotransferase concentrations are markedly elevated (> 500 IU/L and usually > 1000 IU/L).

Hepatitis A has the same course in pregnant women as in nonpregnant women.[101] Although intrauterine transmission to the fetus has been reported, it is rare. Maternal or fetal outcomes are not affected by hepatitis A. In cases of possible exposure, pooled serum immunoglobulin administration 3–6 months before to 2 weeks after exposure can attenuate or prevent the clinical symptoms. Hepatitis vaccine can be safely and successfully administered to a pregnant woman at high risk of exposure, such as when traveling to an endemic area or a healthcare worker at high risk.[102]

Hepatitis B is usually acquired by the parenteral route as in blood transfusion, intravenous drug use, or exposure to blood or sexual secretions from an infected patient. Its main relevance in pregnancy is the risk of vertical transmission to the child, who can then develop chronic hepatitis B. More than 95% of perinatal transmission occurs intrapartum. Risk of maternal–fetal transmission is 90% in hepatitis Be antigen (HBeAg)-positive mothers and 10–40% in HBeAg-negative mothers.[103,104] Therefore, antepartum hepatitis B surface antigen (HBsAg) testing is essential in pregnant women. Seronegative mothers can safely receive hepatitis B virus (HBV) vaccine. Infants born to HBsAg-positive mothers should receive human hepatitis B immune globulin (HBIG) at delivery, followed by HBV vaccine.[102] Active and passive immunization of the infant also decreases the risk of HBV transmitted by maternal milk in breastfed infants.[105] Lamivudine, a nucleoside analog therapy for hepatitis B, has also been used safely in the last 4 weeks of pregnancy to decrease the risk of vertical transmission.[106] Infants who acquire infection at birth have a high risk of developing chronic hepatitis B, as their immune system is immature. The infected infants may remain completely asymptomatic and have normal liver enzymes, despite active replication of hepatitis B.

Hepatitis C virus (HCV) infection during pregnancy does not interfere with normal pregnancy unless the patient has cirrhosis. Pregnancy does not alter the natural course of infection either.[16] The risk of vertical transmission of HCV from mother to fetus is up to 10% in women who are antibody positive but negative on polymerase chain reaction (PCR) analysis, and up to 33% in women who are positive for HCV RNA on PCR.[107] Risk of transmission is higher if the patient has a HCV viral load of more than 1 million copies/mL or is co-infected with human immunodeficiency virus (HIV).[108,109] Breastfeeding does not increase transmission risk.[110] Unlike hepatitis B, as yet, there is no vaccine and no known method for interrupting the transmission of the hepatitis C virus.

Hepatitis E virus (HEV) is notorious for its severe course and bad outcome in pregnant women. It occurs mainly in developing countries and is rare in the United States. HEV is a feco-orally transmitted infection, which is usually a mild and self-limited illness in nonpregnant patients, but commonly causes fulminant hepatic failure during pregnancy (up to 58%).[111] Mortality is 1.5% in the first trimester, 8.5% in the second, and 21% during the third trimester.[112] HEV infection in the third trimester is associated with higher fetal mortality.[112] Treatment is supportive.

Herpes simplex hepatitis

Similar to hepatitis E, herpes simplex follows a more severe course in pregnant women and can cause fulminant hepatitis in these women.[113,114] Patients usually present with a nonspecific viral syndrome including fever and upper respiratory symptoms. On laboratory tests, they are found to have markedly elevated transaminases and only mild elevation of bilirubin. Accompanying genital vesicular eruptions are common, and culture of these lesions can establish the diagnosis. In other cases, liver biopsy may be needed for diagnosis. It demonstrates classical intranuclear inclusions (Fig. 44.4). Immunocytochemistry may be needed to confirm the diagnosis. Patients can be treated successfully with acyclovir, and early delivery is not necessary.

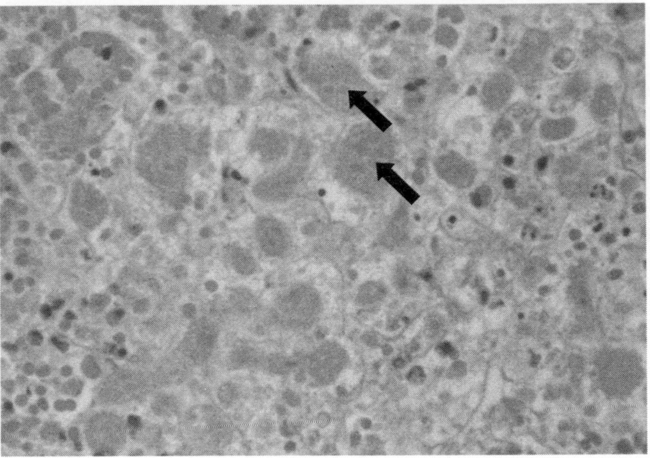

Figure 44.4 Herpes simplex hepatitis. High-power view showing zones of necrotic hepatocytes with intranuclear inclusions typical of Herpes simplex infection (arrows) (courtesy of Laura W. Lamps, Department of Pathology, University of Arkansas for Medical Sciences, Little Rock, AR, USA).

Hepatic vein thrombosis (Budd–Chiari syndrome)

Budd–Chiari syndrome is caused by hepatic vein thrombosis involving a large hepatic vein. It occurs most commonly in the setting of a hypercoagulable state. Both pregnancy and oral contraceptive therapy are associated with a hypercoagulable state,[115] and are associated with an increased incidence of Budd–Chiari syndrome. Reports from India suggest that it is more common in pregnant women, usually occurring after delivery.[1,116,117] In the Western literature, many reports have linked Budd–Chiari syndrome with underlying procoagulant disorders such as anticardiolipin antibody,[118,119] factor V Leiden mutation,[120] thrombotic thrombocytopenic purpura,[121] or myeloproliferative disorders such as polycythemia rubra vera.[122] Patients usually present soon after delivery with abdominal pain, rapid accumulation of ascites, and hepatomegaly. Liver function deteriorates rapidly. Prognosis is poor. Liver transplantation may be needed to save the patient,[120,123] but many patients can be managed successfully with supportive care, prompt delivery, and anticoagulation.[1]

Cholelithiasis

Gallbladder motility decreases during pregnancy, and the lithogenicity of bile increases, resulting in an increased incidence of gallstones.[124] About 2% of women develop gallstones during pregnancy, with multigravida at higher risk.[125] Most of the women remain asymptomatic. Sometimes, the patient presents with one of the complications of cholelithiasis such as biliary colic, acute cholecystitis, or acute gallstone pancreatitis. Most of these patients respond very well to conservative management but, if they remain symptomatic, then cholecystectomy may be necessary[126,127] and can be performed either laparoscopically or by the open route. Common bile duct stones can be managed with endoscopic retrograde cholangiopancreatography (ERCP) and sphincterotomy.[128]

Cirrhosis and portal hypertension

Chronic liver disease is associated with a decrease in fertility, with anovulation, amenorrhea, and premature menopause being more common in these patients. If a woman has cirrhosis and does get pregnant, she can usually sustain the pregnancy without major worsening of liver function.[129] However, progressive liver failure, ascites, and hepatic coma have been reported in a few patients who have cirrhosis and become pregnant.[129,130] There is an increased incidence of stillbirths and premature delivery.[129,131,132] On the other hand, in patients with noncirrhotic portal hypertension, fertility is not decreased.[133] However, worsening of portal hypertension with increased risk of variceal bleeding occurs, due to a marked increase in blood volume and azygous flow during pregnancy.[131–133]

For a summary of liver diseases in pregnancy, see Table 44.6.

Table 44.6 Salient features of liver diseases in pregnancy by trimester.

Trimester of onset	Liver condition	Main symptoms	Laboratory tests	Histology	Management
First	Hyperemesis gravidarum	Nausea, vomiting	↑ AST, ALT, ketosis	Central vacuolization	Intravenous hydration, bowel rest, antiemetics. TPN in severe cases
Second	Cholestasis of pregnancy	Pruritis, jaundice ±	↑ AST, ALT, total bile acids. Mild ↓ bilirubin	Cholestasis. No inflammation	Antihistaminics, phenobarbital, ursodeoxycholic acid. Early delivery ±
Third	HELLP syndrome	Abdominal pain, malaise, nausea, vomiting	Low platelets. ↑ AST, ALT, LDH. Hemolysis	Periportal hemorrhage, focal parenchymal necrosis	Supportive. Early delivery when possible
	Hepatic infarction	Severe abdominal or chest pain. Acute liver failure	↑ WBC, ↑↑ AST, ALT, ↑ bilirubin, coagulopathy. CT/MRI diagnostic	–	Supportive. May need ICU
	Hepatic rupture	Severe abdominal pain. Shock	Abdominal CT	–	Laparotomy. Prompt delivery
	Acute fatty liver of pregnancy	Nausea, vomiting, abdominal pain	↑ Prothrombin time, DIC. ↑ AST, ALT, bilirubin, ALP	Microvesicular fat in hepatocytes	Supportive care. Prompt delivery
Any	Viral hepatitis	Nausea, vomiting, jaundice	↑ AST, ALT, bilirubin. Hepatitis serology	Inflammation and hepatocyte necrosis	Supportive

ALP, alkaline phosphatase; ALT, alanine aminotransferase; AST, aspartate aminotransferase; CT, computerized tomography; DIC, disseminated intravascular coagulation; HELLP, hemolysis, elevated liver function, and low platelets; ICU, intensive care unit; LDH, lactate dehydrogenase; MRI, magnetic resonance imaging; TPN, total parenteral nutrition; WBC, white blood cells.

Key points

1. Most liver blood tests are not altered in pregnancy. Therefore, elevation of bilirubin, AST, ALT, or TBA concentration indicates liver disease and should be investigated.
2. Elevation of alkaline phosphatase in pregnancy is usually of placental origin and should not be considered abnormal unless associated with other liver test abnormalities or clinical features of liver disease.
3. Some liver diseases are seen only in pregnancy, e.g., intrahepatic cholestasis of pregnancy (ICP), hyperemesis gravidarum, HELLP syndrome, and acute fatty liver of pregnancy (AFLP). Gestational age can help significantly in differential diagnosis. For example: first trimester – hyperemesis gravidarum; second or third trimester – ICP; third trimester – HELLP syndrome or AFLP.
4. Common liver diseases such as viral hepatitis, drug hepatotoxicity, etc. can occur during pregnancy and should always be considered in the differential diagnosis.
5. Pregnancy in patients with advanced chronic liver disease is rare. Some patients with conditions such as autoimmune hepatitis, Wilson's disease, etc. may regain fertility after successful treatment and should continue their treatment during pregnancy. In patients with mild chronic liver disease such as hepatitis B or C, pregnancy is common.

6 Acute viral hepatitis E and Herpes simplex hepatitis can take a more severe course in pregnant patients, with higher mortality rates than in nonpregnant patients.

7 The incidence of some diseases such as cholelithiasis and Budd–Chiari syndrome is increased during pregnancy because of alterations in biliary physiology and the hypercoagulable state associated with pregnancy respectively.

8 Patients with hyperemesis gravidarum present with severe nausea and vomiting between the 4th and 10th weeks of gestation, far worse and more prolonged than common morning sickness, which can lead to dehydration and ketosis. AST and ALT can be mildly or significantly elevated (up to 500–1000 IU/L), but bilirubin elevation is mild. All symptoms and laboratory abnormalities usually resolve with conservative supportive management by the second trimester.

9 ICP is a benign cholestatic disorder that occurs during the second or third trimester, and resolves after delivery. It is characterized by pruritis, elevated serum TBA concentration, mild to moderate AST and ALT elevation and, in 10–15% of cases, mild elevation of bilirubin. It may have an adverse effect on the fetus, and early delivery after 36 weeks of gestation may have to be considered.

10 Preeclampsia is a multisystem disorder that occurs in 3–5% of pregnancies in the second or third trimester, and is characterized by hypertension, edema, and proteinuria. It can be associated with many liver disorders including HELLP syndrome, hepatic infarction, subcapsular hematoma, and hepatic rupture. The commonest of these is HELLP syndrome.

11 HELLP syndrome is characterized by hemolysis (drop in Hb, schistocytes and burr cells on peripheral smear, high LDH), elevated liver enzymes (elevated AST and ALT), and low platelets (< 100 000 cells/mm^3). Clinical symptoms can vary in severity and include abdominal pain, malaise, nausea, and vomiting. It can be associated with increased maternal and fetal mortality. Management is supportive. Delivery is the definitive treatment for HELLP and preeclampsia.

12 Hepatic infarction should be considered in a patient with preeclampsia presenting with severe abdominal pain and fever without an obvious source. WBC count is elevated, and liver enzymes can be very high (ALT, AST > 1000 IU/L). CT and MRI can establish the diagnosis. Management is supportive and most patients recover.

13 Hepatic rupture is a rare complication of preeclampsia, but should be considered in a patient presenting with severe right upper quadrant abdominal pain, shock, and hemoperitoneum. Emergency CT to confirm diagnosis, followed by urgent laparotomy with liver resection and packing should be done. Mortality is very high. Arterial embolization has been tried in some cases.

14 AFLP is a rare disorder, but has a very high mortality rate (20%, despite high-quality care). It occurs in the third trimester, and rarely postpartum. The histological hallmark is microvesicular steatosis with fatty droplets in hepatocyte cytoplasm, giving a foamy appearance.

15 Clinical symptoms of AFLP are nonspecific, including nausea, vomiting, abdominal pain, and malaise. AST and ALT are elevated (usually < 1000 IU/L), and bilirubin is elevated to 5–15 mg/dL. The patient can progress rapidly to fulminant liver failure with encephalopathy, coagulopathy, DIC, and cerebral edema. Other complications include hypoglycemia, renal failure, pancreatitis, gastrointestinal and uterine bleeding, and seizures. The patient can die of bleeding complications, hepatic coma, infection, or multisystem failure. Timely diagnosis, intensive monitoring, ICU care, and prompt delivery are key to a successful outcome. Most patients improve 1–4 weeks postpartum, with complete recovery of liver function and no long-term sequelae.

16 Hepatitis B is acquired by the parenteral route or via sexual secretions. It causes acute hepatitis with elevated liver enzymes, jaundice, and hyperbilirubinemia, severe malaise, anorexia and, infrequently, fulminant liver failure. If acquired in adulthood, about 90–95% of patients clear the infection spontaneously, 2–5% develop chronic active hepatitis B, and 2–5% become carriers. Persistence of HBsAg 6 months after exposure indicates chronicity. Anyone with HBsAg in the blood can be infectious, and the risk of transmission is much higher if there is active replication, indicated by the presence of HBeAg in the blood. If the infection is acquired in infancy, the risk of chronicity is about 90%, and the patient may have no symptoms and normal liver enzymes. This is thought to be due to the immature immune system of infants.

17 If the mother has hepatitis B, there is a high risk of vertical maternal–fetal transmission (90% in HBeAg-positive mothers and 10–40% in HBeAg-negative, HBsAg-positive mothers). Ninety-five percent of perinatal transmission occurs in the intrapartum period, and less than 5% is transplacental. Infants born to HBsAg-positive mothers should receive human hepatitis B immune globulin (HBIG) at delivery, followed by HBV vaccine, to decreases the risk of the child developing hepatitis B. All pregnant women should be tested for hepatitis B.

18 Hepatitis C is parenterally acquired (blood products, intravenous drug use, multiple sexual partners, etc.) and causes chronic hepatitis in 85% of those infected. Unlike hepatitis B, the spontaneous clearance rate for hepatitis C is only 15%. It progresses to cirrhosis in 20% of cases over a 20-year period. It does not interfere with normal pregnancy. The risk of transmission to the fetus is 10% in HCV antibody-positive but PCR-negative patients, and 33% in PCR-positive patients. As yet, there is no vaccine for

hepatitis C and no known method of interrupting transmission to the fetus.

19 Hepatitis E occurs mainly in developing countries and is rare in the United States. It is transmitted feco-orally and usually causes a self-limiting hepatitis but, in the setting of pregnancy, it takes a more severe course and causes fulminant hepatic failure, with high mortality.

20 Pregnancy causes a decrease in gallbladder motility and increased lithogenicity of bile, resulting in increased incidence of gallstones and a risk of complications of cholelithiasis, such as acute cholecystitis, gallstone colic, gallstone pancreatitis, etc.

21 Budd–Chiari syndrome is caused by hepatic vein thrombosis, and its incidence is increased in pregnancy owing to a physiological hypercoagulable state. Patients present with abdominal pain, rapid accumulation of ascites, and hepatomegaly. Prognosis is poor, with progression to liver failure. Management includes supportive care, prompt delivery, and anticoagulation.

References

1 Bacq Y, Riely CA. The liver in pregnancy. In: *Schiffs textbook of liver disease*, Vol. 2, 9th edn. Lippincott Williams and Wilkins, 2003:1435.

2 Bacq Y, Zarka O, Brechot JF, et al. Liver function tests in normal pregnancy: a prospective study of 103 pregnant women and 103 matched controls. *Hepatology* 1996;23:1030.

3 Knox TA, Olans LB. Liver disease in pregnancy. *N Engl J Med* 1996;335:569.

4 Lunzer M, Barnes P, Byth K, O'Halloran M. Serum bile acid concentrations during pregnancy and their relationship to obstetric cholestasis. *Gastroenterology* 1986;91:825.

5 Tsang IS, Katz VL, Wells SD. Maternal and fetal outcomes in hyperemesis gravidarum. *Int J Gynaecol Obstet* 1996;55: 231.

6 Hallak M, Tsalamandris K, Dombrowski MP, et al. Hyperemesis gravidarum. Effects on fetal outcome. *J Reprod Med* 1996;41:871.

7 Abell TL, Riely CA. Hyperemesis gravidarum. *Gastroenterol Clin North Am* 1992;21:835.

8 Wallstedt A, Riely CA, Shaver DEA. Prevalence and characteristics of liver dysfunction in hyperemesis gravidarum. *Clin Res* 1990;38:970A.

9 Adams RH, Gordon J, Combes B. Hyperemesis gravidarum. I. Evidence of hepatic dysfunction. *Obstet Gynecol* 1968;31:659.

10 Abell TL. Nausea and vomiting of pregnancy and the electrogastrogram: old disease, new technology. *Am J Gastroenterol* 1992;87:689.

11 Sullivan CA, Johnson CA, Roach H, et al. A pilot study of intravenous ondansetron for hyperemesis gravidarum. *Am J Obstet Gynecol* 1996;174:1565.

12 Nageotte MP, Briggs GG, Towers CV, Asrat T. Droperidol and diphenhydramine in the management of hyperemesis gravidarum. *Am J Obstet Gynecol* 1996;174:1801.

13 Safari HR, Fassett MJ, Souter IC, et al. The efficacy of methylprednisolone in the treatment of hyperemesis gravidarum: a randomized, double-blind, controlled study. *Am J Obstet Gynecol* 1998;179:921.

14 Hsu JJ, Clark-Glena R, Nelson DK, Kim CH. Nasogastric enteral feeding in the management of hyperemesis gravidarum. *Obstet Gynecol* 1996;88:343.

15 Gross S, Librach C, Cecutti A. Maternal weight loss associated with hyperemesis gravidarum: a predictor of fetal outcome. *Am J Obstet Gynecol* 1989;160:906.

16 Sandhu BS, Sanyal AJ. Pregnancy and liver disease. *Gastroenterol Clin North Am* 2003;32:407.

17 Davidson KM. Intrahepatic cholestasis of pregnancy. *Semin Perinatol* 1998;22:104.

18 Berg B, Helm G, Petersohn L, Tryding N. Cholestasis of pregnancy. Clinical and laboratory studies. *Acta Obstet Gynecol Scand* 1986;65:107.

19 Reyes H, Gonzalez MC, Ribalta J, et al. Prevalence of intrahepatic cholestasis of pregnancy in Chile. *Ann Intern Med* 1978; 88:487.

20 Ribalta J, Reyes H, Gonzalez MC, et al. S-adenosyl-L-methionine in the treatment of patients with intrahepatic cholestasis of pregnancy: a randomized, double-blind, placebo-controlled study with negative results. *Hepatology* 1991;13:1084.

21 Rioseco AJ, Ivankovic MB, Manzur A, et al. Intrahepatic cholestasis of pregnancy: a retrospective case–control study of perinatal outcome. *Am J Obstet Gynecol* 1994;170:890.

22 Palmer DG, Eads J. Intrahepatic cholestasis of pregnancy: a critical review. *J Perinat Neonatal Nurs* 2000;14:39.

23 Bacq Y. Intrahepatic cholestasis of pregnancy. *Clin Liver Dis* 1999;3:1.

24 Jacquemin E, De Vree JM, Cresteil D, et al. The wide spectrum of multidrug resistance 3 deficiency: from neonatal cholestasis to cirrhosis of adulthood. *Gastroenterology* 2001;120:1448.

25 Holzbach RT, Sivak DA, Braun WE. Familial recurrent intrahepatic cholestasis of pregnancy: a genetic study providing evidence for transmission of a sex-limited, dominant trait. *Gastroenterology* 1983;85:175.

26 Davies MH, Ngong JM, Yucesoy M, et al. The adverse influence of pregnancy upon sulphation: a clue to the pathogenesis of intrahepatic cholestasis of pregnancy? *J Hepatol* 1994;21: 1127.

27 Bacq Y. [Acute fatty liver in pregnancy]. *Gastroenterol Clin Biol* 1997;21:109.

28 Meng LJ, Reyes H, Axelson M, et al. Progesterone metabolites and bile acids in serum of patients with intrahepatic cholestasis of pregnancy: effect of ursodeoxycholic acid therapy. *Hepatology* 1997;26:1573.

29 Reyes H. Review: intrahepatic cholestasis. A puzzling disorder of pregnancy. *J Gastroenterol Hepatol* 1997;12:211.

30 Axten S. Obstetric cholestasis. *Mod Midwife* 1996;6:32.

31 Benifla JL, Dumont M, Levardon M, et al. [Effects of micronized natural progesterone on the liver during the third trimester of pregnancy]. *Contracept Fertil Sex* 1997;25:165.

32 Fagan EA. Intrahepatic cholestasis of pregnancy. *Clin Liver Dis* 1999;3:603.

33 Rolfes DB, Ishak KG. Liver disease in pregnancy. *Histopathology* 1986;10:555.

34 Brites D, Rodrigues CM. Elevated levels of bile acids in colostrum of patients with cholestasis of pregnancy are decreased

following ursodeoxycholic acid therapy (see comments). *J Hepatol* 1998;29:743.
35 Brites D, Rodrigues CM, Oliveira N, et al. Correction of maternal serum bile acid profile during ursodeoxycholic acid therapy in cholestasis of pregnancy. *J Hepatol* 1998;28:91.
36 Palma J, Reyes H, Ribalta J, et al. Ursodeoxycholic acid in the treatment of cholestasis of pregnancy: a randomized, double-blind study controlled with placebo. *J Hepatol* 1997;27:1022.
37 Drill VA. Benign cholestatic jaundice of pregnancy and benign cholestatic jaundice from oral contraceptives. *Am J Obstet Gynecol* 1974;119:165.
38 Svanborg A, Ohlsson S. Recurrent jaundice of pregnancy; a clinical study of twenty-two cases. *Am J Med* 1959;27:40.
39 Heikkinen J, Maentausta O, Ylostalo P, Janne O. Changes in serum bile acid concentrations during normal pregnancy, in patients with intrahepatic cholestasis of pregnancy and in pregnant women with itching. *Br J Obstet Gynaecol* 1981;88:240.
40 Reid R, Ivey KJ, Rencoret RH, Storey B. Fetal complications of obstetric cholestasis. *Br Med J* 1976;1:870.
41 Lammert F, Marschall HU, Glantz A, Matern S. Intrahepatic cholestasis of pregnancy: molecular pathogenesis, diagnosis and management. *J Hepatol* 2000;33:1012.
42 Reyes H, Simon FR. Intrahepatic cholestasis of pregnancy: an estrogen-related disease. *Semin Liver Dis* 1993;13:289.
43 Reyes H, Wegmann ME, Segovia N, et al. HLA in Chileans with intrahepatic cholestasis of pregnancy. *Hepatology* 1982;2:463.
44 Bergasa NV. The pruritus of cholestasis. *Semin Dermatol* 1995;14:302.
45 Sadler LC, Lane M, North R. Severe fetal intracranial haemorrhage during treatment with cholestyramine for intrahepatic cholestasis of pregnancy. *Br J Obstet Gynaecol* 1995;102:169.
46 Floreani A, Paternoster D, Grella V, et al. Ursodeoxycholic acid in intrahepatic cholestasis of pregnancy. *Br J Obstet Gynaecol* 1994;101:64.
47 Palma J, Reyes H, Ribalta J, et al. Effects of ursodeoxycholic acid in patients with intrahepatic cholestasis of pregnancy. *Hepatology* 1992;15:1043.
48 Floreani A, Paternoster D, Melis A, Grella PV. S-adenosylmethionine versus ursodeoxycholic acid in the treatment of intrahepatic cholestasis of pregnancy: preliminary results of a controlled trial. *Eur J Obstet Gynecol Reprod Biol* 1996;67:109.
49 Rodrigues CM, Marin JJ, Brites D. Bile acid patterns in meconium are influenced by cholestasis of pregnancy and not altered by ursodeoxycholic acid treatment. *Gut* 1999;45:446.
50 Arngrimsson R, Bjornsson S, Geirsson RT, et al. Genetic and familial predisposition to eclampsia and pre-eclampsia in a defined population. *Br J Obstet Gynaecol* 1990;97:762.
51 Grandone E, Margaglione M, Colaizzo D, et al. Factor V Leiden, C>T MTHFR polymorphism and genetic susceptibility to preeclampsia. *Thromb Haemost* 1997;77:1052.
52 Smith GN, Walker M, Tessier JL, Millar KG. Increased incidence of preeclampsia in women conceiving by intrauterine insemination with donor versus partner sperm for treatment of primary infertility. *Am J Obstet Gynecol* 1997;177:455.
53 Dekker GA, Sibai BM. The immunology of preeclampsia. *Semin Perinatol* 1999;23:24.
54 Aarnoudse JG, Houthoff HJ, Weits J, et al. A syndrome of liver damage and intravascular coagulation in the last trimester of normotensive pregnancy. A clinical and histopathological study. *Br J Obstet Gynaecol* 1986;93:145.
55 Hannah ME, Gonen R, Mocarski EJ, et al. Elevated liver enzymes and thrombocytopenia in the third trimester of pregnancy: an unusual case report and a review of the literature. *Am J Obstet Gynecol* 1989;161:322.
56 Barton JR, Riely CA, Adamec TA, et al. Hepatic histopathologic condition does not correlate with laboratory abnormalities in HELLP syndrome (hemolysis, elevated liver enzymes, and low platelet count). *Am J Obstet Gynecol* 1992;167:1538.
57 Sibai BM, Ramadan MK, Usta I, et al. Maternal morbidity and mortality in 442 pregnancies with hemolysis, elevated liver enzymes, and low platelets (HELLP syndrome). *Am J Obstet Gynecol* 1993;169:1000.
58 Sibai BM. The HELLP syndrome (hemolysis, elevated liver enzymes, and low platelets): much ado about nothing? *Am J Obstet Gynecol* 1990;162:311.
59 Chandran R, Serra-Serra V, Redman CW. Spontaneous resolution of pre-eclampsia-related thrombocytopenia. *Br J Obstet Gynaecol* 1992;99:887.
60 Sibai BM, Taslimi MM, el-Nazer A, et al. Maternal–perinatal outcome associated with the syndrome of hemolysis, elevated liver enzymes, and low platelets in severe preeclampsia–eclampsia. *Am J Obstet Gynecol* 1986;155:501.
61 Thiagarajah S, Bourgeois FJ, Harbert GM Jr, Caudle MR. Thrombocytopenia in preeclampsia: associated abnormalities and management principles. *Am J Obstet Gynecol* 1984;150:1.
62 Sibai BM, Ramadan MK, Chari RS, Friedman SA. Pregnancies complicated by HELLP syndrome (hemolysis, elevated liver enzymes, and low platelets): subsequent pregnancy outcome and long-term prognosis. *Am J Obstet Gynecol* 1995;172:125.
63 Sullivan CA, Magann EF, Perry KG, Jr, et al. The recurrence risk of the syndrome of hemolysis, elevated liver enzymes, and low platelets (HELLP) in subsequent gestations. *Am J Obstet Gynecol* 1994;171:940.
64 Barron WM. The syndrome of preeclampsia. *Gastroenterol Clin North Am* 1992;21:851.
65 Magann EF, Bass D, Chauhan SP, et al. Antepartum corticosteroids: disease stabilization in patients with the syndrome of hemolysis, elevated liver enzymes, and low platelets (HELLP). *Am J Obstet Gynecol* 1994;171:1148.
66 Magann EF, Perry KG, Jr, Meydrech EF, et al. Postpartum corticosteroids: accelerated recovery from the syndrome of hemolysis, elevated liver enzymes, and low platelets (HELLP). *Am J Obstet Gynecol* 1994;171:1154.
67 Krueger KJ, Hoffman BJ, Lee WM. Hepatic infarction associated with eclampsia. *Am J Gastroenterol* 1990;85:588.
68 Riely CA. Liver diseases in pregnancy. In: Reece AE, Hobbins JC, eds. *Medicine of the fetus and mother*, 2nd edn. Philadelphia, PA: Lippincott-Raven Publishers; 1999:1153.
69 Barton JR, Sibai BM. Hepatic imaging in HELLP syndrome (hemolysis, elevated liver enzymes, and low platelet count). *Am J Obstet Gynecol* 1996;174:1820.
70 Manas KJ, Welsh JD, Rankin RA, Miller DD. Hepatic hemorrhage without rupture in preeclampsia. *N Engl J Med* 1985;312:424.
71 Minuk GY, Lui RC, Kelly JK. Rupture of the liver associated with acute fatty liver of pregnancy. *Am J Gastroenterol* 1987;82:457.
72 Herbert WN, Brenner WE. Improving survival with liver rupture complicating pregnancy. *Am J Obstet Gynecol* 1982;142:530.
73 Strate T, Broering DC, Bloechle C, et al. Orthotopic liver transplantation for complicated HELLP syndrome. Case report and review of the literature. *Arch Gynecol Obstet* 2000;264:108.
74 Erhard J, Lange R, Niebel W, et al. Acute liver necrosis in the HELLP syndrome: successful outcome after orthotopic liver transplantation. A case report. *Transpl Int* 1993;6:179.

75 Hunter SK, Martin M, Benda JA, Zlatnik FJ. Liver transplant after massive spontaneous hepatic rupture in pregnancy complicated by preeclampsia. *Obstet Gynecol* 1995;85:819.
76 Sheehan HL. The pathology of acute yellow atrophy and delayed chloroform poisoning. *J Obstet Gynaecol Br Empire* 1940;47: 49.
77 Vigil-De Gracia P, Lavergne JA. Acute fatty liver of pregnancy. *Int J Gynaecol Obstet* 2001;72:193.
78 Riely CA. Acute fatty liver of pregnancy. *Semin Liver Dis* 1987;7:47.
79 Buytaert IM, Elewaut GP, Van Kets HE. Early occurrence of acute fatty liver in pregnancy. *Am J Gastroenterol* 1996;91:603.
80 Pereira SP, O'Donohue J, Wendon J, Williams R. Maternal and perinatal outcome in severe pregnancy-related liver disease. *Hepatology* 1997;26:1258.
81 Rolfes DB, Ishak KG. Acute fatty liver of pregnancy: a clinicopathologic study of 35 cases. *Hepatology* 1985;5:1149.
82 Monga M, Katz AR. Acute fatty liver in the second trimester. *Obstet Gynecol* 1999;93:811.
83 Riely C. Liver diseases of pregnancy. In: *Liver and biliary diseases*. Baltimore, MD: Williams and Wilkins; 1996:483.
84 Sheehan HL. Jaundice in pregnancy. *Am J Obstet Gynecol* 1961;81:427.
85 Riely CA, Latham PS, Romero R, Duffy TP. Acute fatty liver of pregnancy. A reassessment based on observations in nine patients. *Ann Intern Med* 1987;106:703.
86 Ibdah JA, Bennett MJ, Rinaldo P, Zhao Y, et al. A fetal fatty-acid oxidation disorder as a cause of liver disease in pregnant women. *N Engl J Med* 1999;340:1723.
87 Tyni T, Ekholm E, Pihko H. Pregnancy complications are frequent in long-chain 3-hydroxyacyl-coenzyme A dehydrogenase deficiency. *Am J Obstet Gynecol* 1998;178:603.
88 Ockner SA, Brunt EM, Cohn SM, et al. Fulminant hepatic failure caused by acute fatty liver of pregnancy treated by orthotopic liver transplantation. *Hepatology* 1990;11:59.
89 Kaplan MM. Acute fatty liver of pregnancy. *N Engl J Med* 1985;313:367.
90 Usta IM, Barton JR, Amon EA, et al. Acute fatty liver of pregnancy: an experience in the diagnosis and management of fourteen cases. *Am J Obstet Gynecol* 1994;171:1342.
91 Brackett JC, Sims HF, Rinaldo P, et al. Two alpha subunit donor splice site mutations cause human trifunctional protein deficiency. *J Clin Invest* 1995;95:2076.
92 Bernuau J, Degott C, Nouel O, et al. Non-fatal acute fatty liver of pregnancy. *Gut* 1983;24:340.
93 Bacq Y, Riely CA. Acute fatty liver of pregnancy: the hepatologist's view. *Gastroenterologist* 1993;1:257.
94 Moise KJ, Jr, Shah DM. Acute fatty liver of pregnancy: etiology of fetal distress and fetal wastage. *Obstet Gynecol* 1987;69:482.
95 Borum ML. Hepatobiliary diseases in women. *Med Clin North Am* 1998;82:51.
96 Campillo B, Bernuau J, Witz MO, et al. Ultrasonography in acute fatty liver of pregnancy. *Ann Intern Med* 1986;105:383.
97 Hou SH, Levin S, Ahola S, et al. Acute fatty liver of pregnancy. Survival with early cesarean section. *Dig Dis Sci* 1984;29:449.
98 Amon E, Allen SR, Petrie RH, Belew JE. Acute fatty liver of pregnancy associated with preeclampsia: management of hepatic failure with postpartum liver transplantation. *Am J Perinatol* 1991;8:278.
99 Johnston WG, Baskett TF. Obstetric cholestasis. A 14 year review. *Am J Obstet Gynecol* 1979;133:299.
100 Sherlock S, Dooley J. *Diseases of the liver and biliary system*. Blackwell Science, 2002.
101 Zhang RL, Zeng JS, Zhang HZ. Survey of 34 pregnant women with hepatitis A and their neonates. *Chin Med J (Engl)* 1990;103:552.
102 Reinus J, Leikin E. Viral hepatitis in pregnancy. *Clin Liver Dis* 1999;3:115.
103 McMahon BJ, Alward WL, Hall DB, et al. Acute hepatitis B virus infection: relation of age to the clinical expression of disease and subsequent development of the carrier state. *J Infect Dis* 1985;151:599.
104 Okada K, Kamiyama I, Inomata M, et al. e antigen and anti-e in the serum of asymptomatic carrier mothers as indicators of positive and negative transmission of hepatitis B virus to their infants. *N Engl J Med* 1976;294:746.
105 World Health Organization. Hepatitis B and breastfeeding. *J Int Assoc Physicians AIDS Care* 1998;4:20.
106 van Nunen AB, de Man RA, Heijtink RA, et al. Lamivudine in the last 4 weeks of pregnancy to prevent perinatal transmission in highly viremic chronic hepatitis B patients. *J Hepatol* 2000;32:1040.
107 Sabatino G, Ramenghi LA, di Marzio M, Pizzigallo E. Vertical transmission of hepatitis C virus: an epidemiological study on 2,980 pregnant women in Italy. *Eur J Epidemiol* 1996;12:443.
108 Giovannini M, Tagger A, Ribero ML, et al. Maternal–infant transmission of hepatitis C virus and HIV infections: a possible interaction. *Lancet* 1990;335:1166.
109 Ohto H, Terazawa S, Sasaki N, et al. Transmission of hepatitis C virus from mothers to infants. The Vertical Transmission of Hepatitis C Virus Collaborative Study Group. *N Engl J Med* 1994;330:744.
110 Lin HH, Kao JH, Hsu HY, et al. Absence of infection in breast-fed infants born to hepatitis C virus-infected mothers. *J Pediatr* 1995;126:589.
111 Jaiswal SP, Jain AK, Naik G, et al. Viral hepatitis during pregnancy. *Int J Gynaecol Obstet* 2001;72:103.
112 Tsega E, Hansson BG, Krawczynski K, Nordenfelt E. Acute sporadic viral hepatitis in Ethiopia: causes, risk factors, and effects on pregnancy. *Clin Infect Dis* 1992;14:961.
113 Klein NA, Mabie WC, Shaver DC, et al. Herpes simplex virus hepatitis in pregnancy. Two patients successfully treated with acyclovir. *Gastroenterology* 1991;100:239.
114 Yaziji H, Hill T, Pitman TC, et al. Gestational herpes simplex virus hepatitis. *South Med J* 1997;90:347.
115 Lowe GD, Drummond MM, Forbes CD, Barbenel JC. Increased blood viscosity in young women using oral contraceptives. *Am J Obstet Gynecol* 1980;137:840.
116 Khuroo MS, Datta DV. Budd–Chiari syndrome following pregnancy. Report of 16 cases, with roentgenologic, hemodynamic and histologic studies of the hepatic outflow tract. *Am J Med* 1980;68:113.
117 Covillo FV, Nyong AO, Axelrod JL. Budd–Chiari syndrome following pregnancy. *Mol Med* 1984;81:356.
118 Segal S, Shenhav S, Segal O, et al. Budd–Chiari syndrome complicating severe preeclampsia in a parturient with primary antiphospholipid syndrome. *Eur J Obstet Gynecol Reprod Biol* 1996;68:227.
119 Ouwendijk RJ, Koster JC, Wilson JH, et al. Budd–Chiari syndrome in a young patient with anticardiolipin antibodies: need for prolonged anticoagulant treatment. *Gut* 1994;35: 1004.
120 Fickert P, Ramschak H, Kenner L, et al. Acute Budd–Chiari syndrome with fulminant hepatic failure in a pregnant woman with factor V Leiden mutation. *Gastroenterology* 1996;111: 1670.

121 Hsu HW, Belfort MA, Vernino S, et al. Postpartum thrombotic thrombocytopenic purpura complicated by Budd–Chiari syndrome. *Obstet Gynecol* 1995;85:839.
122 Valla D. Obstruction of the hepatic veins. *Dig Dis* 1990;8:226.
123 Salha O, Campbell DJ, Pollard S. Budd–Chiari syndrome in pregnancy treated by caesarean section and liver transplant. *Br J Obstet Gynaecol* 1996;103:1254.
124 Everson GT. Gastrointestinal motility in pregnancy. *Gastroenterol Clin North Am* 1992;21:751.
125 Tsimoyiannis EC, Antoniou NC, Tsaboulas C, Papanikolaou N. Cholelithiasis during pregnancy and lactation. Prospective study. *Eur J Surg* 1994;160:627.
126 Amos JD, Schorr SJ, Norman PF, et al. Laparoscopic surgery during pregnancy. *Am J Surg* 1996;171:435.
127 Davis A, Katz VL, Cox R. Gallbladder disease in pregnancy. *J Reprod Med* 1995;40:759.
128 Jamidar PA, Beck GJ, Hoffman BJ, et al. Endoscopic retrograde cholangiopancreatography in pregnancy. *Am J Gastroenterol* 1995;90:1263.
129 Borhanmanesh F, Haghighi P. Pregnancy in patients with cirrhosis of the liver. *Obstet Gynecol* 1970;36:315.
130 Schweitzer IL, Peters RL. Pregnancy in hepatitis B antigen positive cirrhosis. *Obstet Gynecol* 1976;48:53S.
131 Cheng YS. Pregnancy in liver cirrhosis and/or portal hypertension. *Am J Obstet Gynecol* 1977;128:812.
132 Schreyer P, Caspi E, El-Hindi JM, Eshchar J. Cirrhosis – pregnancy and delivery: a review. *Obstet Gynecol Surv* 1982;37:304.
133 Kochhar R, Kumar S, Goel RC, et al. Pregnancy and its outcome in patients with noncirrhotic portal hypertension. *Dig Dis Sci* 1999;44:1356.
134 Burt A, Portman B, MacSween R. Liver pathology associated with diseases of other organs or systems. In: MacSween RNM, Burt AD, Portman BC, eds. *Pathology of the liver*, 4th edn. Churchill Livingstone; 2002:827.

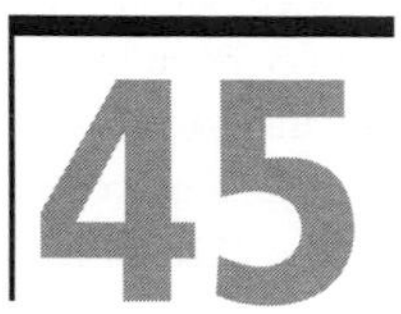

Pregnancy complicated by renal disorders

Michelle W. Krause and Sudhir V. Shah

Recent epidemiological studies indicate that chronic kidney disease (CKD) is common and affects 20 million Americans.[1] This, coupled with the evidence that the incidence of pregnancy in women with CKD is rising, makes it important to understand how pregnancy affects the kidney as well as how kidney disease affects both the mother and the fetus. In addition, women are susceptible to acute renal failure (ARF) with causes unique to pregnancy. Despite the advancement of medical technology in both obstetrics and neonatology, kidney disease in pregnancy is associated with significant maternal and fetal morbidity and mortality. In this chapter, we focus on the impact of the physiological changes of pregnancy in normal and in diseased kidneys as well as the importance of renal function on maternal and fetal outcomes.

Renal physiology and pregnancy

The marked decrease in the peripheral vascular resistance during pregnancy results in a reduction in blood pressure and significant changes in systemic and renal hemodynamics, including net retention of sodium and water, an increase in cardiac output, and an increase in the glomerular filtration rate (GFR) (Table 45.1).[2,3] These changes occur early in conception and are generally maintained throughout pregnancy. The increase in the GFR results in lower values for blood urea nitrogen (BUN) and creatinine. Thus, serum markers of renal function that are considered normal for non-pregnant women may signify underlying renal impairment in pregnancy.

Acute renal failure in pregnancy

Advancements in sterile technique and obstetric delivery have led to a dramatic decrease in ARF during pregnancy, now accounting for only 15% of ARF compared with 50% previously.[4,5] Traditionally, ARF is categorized into three distinct entities: prerenal ARF, intrinsic renal ARF, and postrenal ARF, based on the type of injury causing changes in renal function. Pregnant women are at risk for the same causes of ARF as in the general population; however, etiologies specific for pregnancy-related ARF are depicted in Figure 45.1. Prerenal ARF refers to conditions in which the kidney itself is normal, but in which there is a decrease in renal perfusion. In certain pregnancy states, such as hyperemesis gravidarum, severe vomiting with volume depletion may be a contributing cause of prerenal ARF. Additionally, septic abortions in the first trimester with alterations in renal perfusion have been associated with prerenal ARF. Causes of intrinsic renal ARF in pregnancy are generally more serious than the prerenal or postrenal disorders. Intrinsic renal ARF is characterized by tissue damage with loss of renal tubular function. The most common etiologies of intrinsic renal ARF are the hemolysis, elevated liver function, and low platelets (HELLP) syndrome, postpartum hemorrhage, and the preeclampsia/eclampsia syndrome. Uncommon conditions of intrinsic renal ARF in pregnancy are glomerulonephritis, abruptio placentae, cortical necrosis, and acute fatty liver of pregnancy.[5,6] Lastly, postrenal causes of ARF result from a blockage of urine flow beyond the kidney itself. In pregnancy, the gravid uterus may exert pressure on the ureters, resulting in mild to moderate hydronephrosis, but not typically renal failure.[7] In conditions of polyhydramnios in the third trimester, the enlarged uterus may compress the ureters causing obstructive ARF.[8] Nephrolithiasis may also result in postrenal ARF in pregnancy. Pregnancy alone does not cause an increased risk for the development of renal calculi compared with the general population, but they may be difficult to diagnose as the presentation of back pain and urinary symptoms may be identical to urinary infections or premature labor.

The evaluation of ARF in pregnancy consists of a detailed history and physical examination as well as evaluation of the urine, laboratory studies, and radiographic imaging of the kidneys and the collecting system to distinguish between prerenal ARF and intrinsic or postrenal ARF (Table 45.2). The majority of causes of ARF are prerenal, and the diagnosis is supported by a bland urine sediment, a low fractional excretion of sodium (FeNa), and a BUN to creatinine ratio > 20:1. Distinguishing between intrinsic ARF disorders such as preeclampsia or glomerulonephritis may be challenging in the pregnant patient, as both may present with hypertension, proteinuria, edema, and renal failure. The clinical history may support glomerulonephritis with symptoms and signs of systemic diseases such as arthritis and skin rashes in autoimmune disorders that are not common in preeclampsia. Additionally, there may be laboratory abnormalities such as a positive antinuclear antibody (ANA) test and hypocomplementemia in lupus nephritis or coexisting hepatitis C infection in membranoproliferative glomerulonephritis and cryoglobulinemia, whereas in preeclampsia, there are no associated serological abnormalities. Moreover, the urine sediment may have hematuria, pyuria, or casts in nonpreeclamptic intrinsic renal disorders. In rare instances, a renal biopsy may be performed to determine the underlying renal pathology if the clinical and laboratory evaluation is unable to distinguish between preeclampsia and intrinsic renal disease. On renal histology, there is swelling of glomerular cells in preeclampsia termed "endotheliosis" (Fig. 45.2), and there is no appreciable glomerular proliferation or immune complex deposition that is seen in some types of glomerulonephritis. Lastly, the diagnosis of postrenal ARF largely relies on radiographic imaging with ultrasonography of the kidneys and collecting system to assess for hydronephrosis, renal calculi, masses, or increased postvoid urinary residuals in the bladder.

The treatment of ARF is based on correcting the underlying etiology. An intravenous fluid challenge to correct volume depletion and impaired renal perfusion is warranted in a hospitalized setting with careful monitoring for signs of volume overload to distinguish between prerenal ARF and intrinsic renal ARF. The treatment of preeclampsia with renal dysfunction is delivery of the fetus, whereas some of the glomerular disorders can be managed with immunosuppressive therapy to prolong pregnancy for fetal viability. Failure of proteinuria and renal function to return to normal within 12 weeks postpartum suggests underlying glomerular pathology, and a referral to a nephrologist for evaluation and treatment is indicated. For postrenal ARF, polyhydramnios can be corrected by fluid aspiration with amniocentesis or, more

Table 45.1 Systemic and renal physiologic changes in pregnancy.

	Normal	Pregnancy
Blood pressure	120/80 mmHg	110/60 mmHg
Cardiac output	4–5 L/min	6–7 L/min
Plasma volume	2.5–3.0 L	3.75–4.5 L
Renal plasma flow	650 mL/min	975–1000 mL/min
Glomerular filtration rate	100 mL/min/1.73 m^2	140 mL/min/1.73 m^2
Blood urea nitrogen	8–10 mg/dL	5–8 mg/dL
Creatinine	1.0–1.2 mg/dL	0.4–0.8 mg/dL
Sodium	135–145 mEq/L	130–135 mEq/L
Hematocrit	36–46%	30–36%
Serum bicarbonate	22–30 mEq/L	18–22 mEq/L

Table 45.2 Evaluation of acute renal failure in pregnancy.

	Prerenal ARF	Intrinsic renal ARF	Postrenal ARF
BUN : Cr ratio	20 : 1	10–15 : 1	10–15 : 1
Urinalysis			
Urine sodium	< 20 mEq/L	> 40 mEq/L	> 40 mEq/L
Hematuria	–	±	±
Proteinuria	–	±	±
Volume	Low	Low or normal	Low
Osmolality	High	Low	Low/normal
FeNa	< 1%	> 1%	> 1%
Volume status	Low	Normal/high	Normal/high
Renal ultrasonography	Normal	Normal	Abnormal

Cr, creatinine.

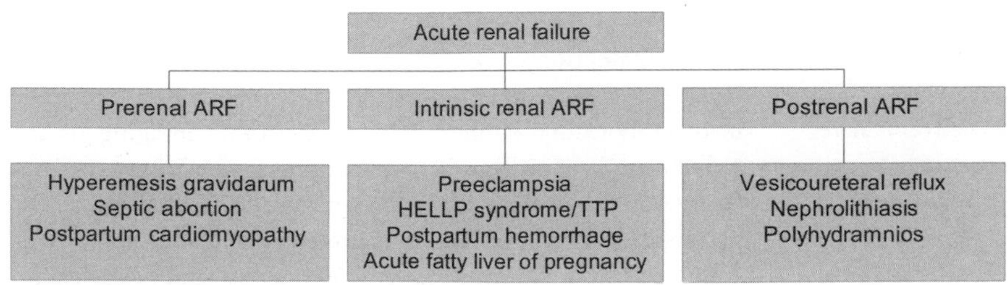

Figure 45.1 Etiologies of acute renal failure in pregnancy. TTP, thrombotic thrombocytopenic purpura.

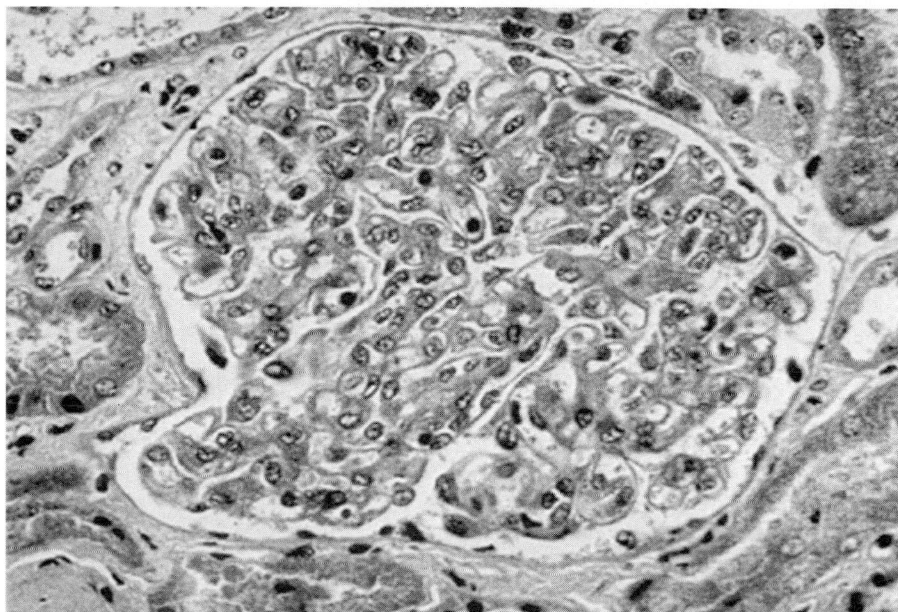

Figure 45.2 Renal pathological changes in preeclampsia. Light micrograph of a renal glomerulus in preeclampsia. "Endotheliosis" refers to swelling of the mesangial and endothelial cells with loss of the capillary lumen and absence of cellular proliferation.

Table 45.3 Maternal and fetal outcomes in women with normal pregnancy compared with those with pre-existing renal disease.

	Normal	Increased creatinine	Proteinuria < 500 mg/day	Proteinuria > 500 mg/day
Maternal outcomes				
Preeclampsia/eclampsia	5–8%	25%	42%	29–64%
Progressive renal failure	< 1%	15–30%	–	–
Endstage renal disease (1 year)	< 1%	6–45%	–	–
Fetal outcomes				
Intrauterine growth restriction	5%	33%	4%	23–45%
Prematurity	10%	33%	62%	45–91%

Data derived from refs 10–19 and 21.

rarely, placement of percutaneous nephrostomy tubes.[8] The treatment of nephrolithiasis is largely supportive as > 70% of stones will pass spontaneously. For those stones that do not pass, ureteral stents, percutaneous nephrostomy tubes, and ureteroscopy with stone removal are all safe methods that may be utilized during pregnancy.[9]

Renal replacement therapy in the form of dialysis is required in < 1% of all cases of ARF. Dialysis is indicated in pregnancy for hyperkalemia and metabolic acidosis that is not responding to medical therapy, volume overload, uremia, or the inability to maintain adequate nutrition.

Pregnancy and pre-existing renal disease

In contrast to ARF, which is characterized as a sudden change in renal function, chronic kidney disease (CKD) is defined as kidney damage for ≥ 3 months with structural or functional abnormalities of the kidney. Renal disease in pregnancy can be classified into those with CKD diagnosed prior to conception, CKD unknown prior to conception but discovered during the pregnancy and, thirdly, renal disease that develops during pregnancy. Regardless of the etiology of CKD, with the exception of lupus nephritis, the degree of renal impairment at the time of conception largely defines the risk and outcome for both the mother and the fetus (Table 45.3). In general, women with CKD have a fourfold increased risk of adverse maternal outcomes including preeclampsia, eclampsia, and abruptio placentae compared with women without renal disease. Similarly, there is a twofold increased risk of adverse fetal events including intrauterine growth restriction, low birthweight, prematurity, and neonatal death in women with renal disease compared with women without renal disease.[10]

Vesicoureteral reflux (VUR) is one of the most common causes of CKD in women during pregnancy. VUR results from urine flowing back from the bladder into the ureters causing chronic infections and scarring of the kidney with loss of renal function. The diagnosis may be missed prior to conception, as recurrent urinary tract infections may have been underappreciated, and no laboratory or urinary studies may have been performed before the first prenatal visit. As with other disorders of CKD, VUR has adverse maternal and fetal effects, especially when there is pre-existing chronic hypertension. It is estimated that 25% of women will have preeclampsia, 33% premature births, and 20% will have deterioration of renal function during pregnancy. Interestingly, there appears to be a genetic predisposition to VUR as almost half of infants born to mothers with urinary reflux will have abnormal micturating cystourethrography consistent with VUR.[11] Urinary tract infection is a common sequela in pregnant women with VUR, so surveillance and treatment for asymptomatic bacteriuria are recommended.[12]

Another common cause of CKD in pregnancy is diabetes mellitus. Individuals with diabetes mellitus may have normal proteinuria (< 30 mg/24 h), microalbuminuria (30–300 mg/24 h), or increased macroalbuminuria (> 300 mg/24 h) in addition to abnormal renal function defined by a GFR < 90 mL/min/1.73 m^2. Even with normal renal function and a lack of proteinuria, women with diabetes mellitus suffer from a higher risk of premature births and preeclampsia than the general population. Superimposed microalbuminuria and proteinuria have an additive risk. Some 62% of women with microalbuminuria experience preterm births, and 42% are diagnosed with preeclampsia, whereas the risks for preterm births and preeclampsia are 91% and 64%, respectively, in women with overt proteinuria.[13]

Nephrotic syndrome and glomerular disorders such as membranous glomerulonephritis, focal segmental glomerulosclerosis (FSGS), and immunoglobulin (Ig) A nephropathy are typically detected prior to conception, but may be diagnosed or develop *de novo* during pregnancy. As these disorders are relatively uncommon in the pregnant population, there is a paucity of data as to how best to manage these patients. Women with chronic proteinuria have successful pregnancies with > 90% resulting in live births; there is a worse outcome for those with > 500 mg of proteinuria in 24 h at the time of conception. These women have a high incidence of hypertension, and more than half will have increases in proteinuria throughout the duration of the pregnancy. There is also an associated 45% risk of premature births, a 25% risk of intrauterine growth restriction, and a 30% risk of preeclampsia. Interestingly, even with normal renal function at the start of pregnancy, a small proportion of women with chronic proteinuria will progress to endstage renal disease (ESRD) within 1 year of delivery.[14]

Women with CKD are at risk for progressive loss of renal function throughout gestation. In those women with a creatinine of < 1.5 mg/dL at the time of conception, there is an associated 15% decline in renal function during pregnancy, and an estimated 6% will progress to ESRD within 1 year. For those women with a creatinine of 1.5–2.9 mg/dL at the time of conception, there is an associated 30% decline in renal function during pregnancy, and an estimated 20% will progress to ESRD in 1 year. For those women with a creatinine of > 3.0 mg/dL at the time of conception, 45% will progress to ESRD in 1 year.[15,16] It is thought that the increased stress imposed on the kidney with pregnancy, uncontrolled hypertension, and urinary tract infections contribute to loss of renal function during pregnancy.

Systemic lupus erythematosus (SLE) deserves special mention, as pregnancy may be associated with worsening disease activity and a high rate of fetal loss. Disease flares are estimated to occur in about one-third of pregnancies in women with underlying SLE. Approximately 50% of these flares occur in the postpartum period, and one quarter will occur in the second trimester. Lupus flares have been linked to stopping immunosuppressive therapy, a history of active disease as defined by more than three flares prior to conception, as well as active disease at the time of conception.[17] Adverse fetal outcomes such as death, prematurity, and intrauterine growth restriction are higher in women with lupus and concomitant antiphospholipid antibody syndrome, hypocomplementemia, and hypertension.[18] The antiphospholipid antibody syndrome is of particular concern in pregnancy because of risks of recurrent miscarriage, intrauterine growth restriction, preeclampsia, preterm labor, and fetal death. Renal involvement of the antiphospholipid antibody syndrome has been described historically with thrombotic vascular events and cortical necrosis resulting in permanent renal failure. Recently, there have been cases of the antiphospholipid antibody syndrome associated with glomerular disorders such as membranous glomerulopathy, minimal change disease, and even pauci-immune glomerulonephritis.[19]

The treatment of CKD in pregnant women is primarily directed at control of blood pressure with antihypertensive agents that are considered safe in pregnancy (Table 45.4) and monitoring and treatment of asymptomatic bacteriuria and urinary tract infections angiotensin-coverting enzyme (ACE).

Table 45.4 Antihypertensive agents in pregnancy.

Central-acting adrenergic agents
Methyldopa 0.25–3.0 g/day
Clonidine 0.1–1.2 mg/day
Beta-adrenergic blocking agents
Atenolol 25–100 mg/day
Metoprolol 25–400 mg/day
Labetalol 200–2400 mg/day
Propranolol 40–240 mg/day
Calcium-channel blocking agents
Nifedipine 30–120 mg/day
Diltiazem 60–360 mg/day
Verapamil 80–480 mg/day
Vasodilators
Hydralazine 50–300 mg/day

Women taking angiotensin-converting enzyme (ACE) inhibitors in the first trimester of pregnancy have a nearly threefold risk of congenital fetal malformations than women not taking these agents and thus women should be counseled to discontinue these agents if trying to conceive or stop as soon as a pregnancy is recognized.[18] For women with diabetes, the goal hemoglobin A1c (HbA1c) should be less than 7%, and close involvement with a dietitian is necessary to avoid hyperglycemia that may contribute to macrosomia and polyhydramnios. For those women with underlying glomerular disorders, immunosuppressive agents such as cyclosporine and prednisone are safe in pregnancy and are useful in keeping renal disease in remission and treating disease flares activated by pregnancy. For those with the antiphospholipid antibody syndrome and renal failure, plasma exchange has been associated with improvement in renal function.[21] Lastly, delivery is recommended for women if there is rapid deterioration of renal function or if there is concern for superimposed preeclampsia or eclampsia.

Pregnancy in endstage renal disease

Pregnancy is a relatively uncommon phenomenon in women with ESRD on renal replacement therapy. In the mid-1990s, the conception rate for women of childbearing age on dialysis was 2.2%.[22] Other reports similarly estimate the conception rate at 0.3–1.5% each year.[23] There is no difference in maternal or fetal outcomes based on dialysis modality. Rather, because of the enlarging gravid uterus, most pregnant women with ESRD on peritoneal dialysis therapy will temporarily transfer to hemodialysis therapy for comfort in the second and third trimesters.[24] In recent years, with aggressive dialysis therapy and management of hypertension, approximately 50% of pregnancies in women with ESRD result in live births.[25] Most pregnancies will be complicated by intrauterine growth restriction, preeclampsia, and prematurity. In one study of pregnancies in women on renal replacement therapy, the average time to delivery was 30.5 weeks.[26]

The care of a pregnant dialysis patient is complex and begins with a dialysis prescription aimed at reducing the BUN to less than 45–50 mg/dL.[27] This translates into > 20 hours/week on hemodialysis, often over five or six treatments. The metabolic disturbances are also challenging for the pregnant dialysis patient. The target hemoglobin and hematocrit is 11–12 g/dL and 33–36%, respectively, with the use of erythropoietin. There needs to be judicious monitoring of calcium, phosphorous, and potassium as levels may decrease with the increase in weekly dialysis. In addition, the target bicarbonate level should also be maintained at 18–20 mEq/L to avoid ill-effects from metabolic acidosis. Hypertensive therapy should be continued using medications with a favorable safety profile in pregnancy (Table 45.4). Lastly, the dry weight of the patient needs to be watched carefully and on average increase by 0.5 kg/week after the first trimester to take into account the weight gain required for fetal growth.[24,28]

Pregnancies in renal transplant recipients are more successful than those in women with ESRD on renal replacement therapy. Generally, ovarian function and resumption of menstruation will occur within the first year after transplantation. For those women who wish to conceive, > 90% of pregnancies will result in live births after the first trimester.[29,30] Despite this, women with a renal transplant should still be considered at high risk with an increased incidence of prematurity in 45–60% of cases, intrauterine growth restriction in 20–30%, and 30% superimposed preeclampsia.[29,31] Although most nephrologists agree that pregnancy itself does not permanently alter renal allograft function or predispose to acute rejection of the renal transplant, one small study reported an increase in the serum creatinine of 0.5–0.7 mg/dL within 1 year of pregnancy in transplant patients compared with nonpregnant control subjects.[32] Ideally, it is recommended that women should wait until a year after their renal transplant to conceive when they are on a stable maintenance immunosuppressive regimen. Several immunosuppressive transplant medications have a documented safety profile in pregnancy, and these include prednisone, cyclosporine, and azathioprine.[33,34] Other immunosuppressive transplant medications such as mycophenolate mofetil and sirolimus are contraindicated in pregnancy because of an association with fetal malformations and should be stopped several weeks prior to conception.[35] There are limited data on the use of tacrolimus in pregnant transplant recipients, so most nephrologists favor a regimen utilizing prednisone, cyclosporine, and/or azathioprine. There is no contraindication for vaginal deliveries in renal transplant recipients. If Cesarean delivery is required, the obstetrician should have access to the operative history of the patient to avoid complications arising from the change in anatomy associated with the transplanted kidney and ureter in the pelvis.

Conclusions

Women with renal disease who plan to become pregnant need to make their wishes clear and have an open dialogue with their physicians as many medications such as ACE inhibitors, angiotensin receptor blocking medications, and certain immunosuppressive medications need to be discontinued prior to conception. Additionally, women with renal disease need to be informed of the increased risk for themselves as well as for the fetus of adverse outcomes. In the ESRD population, aggressive dialysis needs to be instituted early in pregnancy, as the risk of miscarriage is high in the first trimester. Special attention and interactions with nurses and dietitians may also be helpful in monitoring adequate nutritional intake, fetal development, blood pressure monitoring, and weight gain. Although this unique group of women with renal disease and pregnancy is challenging to manage from a medical perspective, successful outcomes can be achieved with careful monitoring of both the fetus and the mother.

Key points

1 Chronic kidney disease is common, and there is a high likelihood that obstetricians will manage women with chronic kidney disease during pregnancy.

2 Changes in peripheral vascular resistance and reductions in blood pressure during pregnancy result in significant alterations in renal and systemic hemodynamics.

3 Serum markers of renal function are lower in pregnancy and may confound the ability to diagnose pre-existing renal disease.

4 There are unique causes of acute renal failure that occur in pregnancy.

5 Certain types of renal disease can present with the same signs and symptoms as preeclampsia/eclampsia and may be difficult to distinguish clinically.

6 Dialysis is safe in pregnancy for acute renal failure when the kidney is unable to maintain fluid and metabolic homeostasis.

7 The degree of renal impairment in chronic kidney disease largely determines the outcome for both the mother and the fetus.

8 Women with pre-existing renal disease have an increased risk of preeclampsia/eclampsia, progressive renal failure, and abruptio placentae.

9 Infants born to women with pre-existing renal failure have an increased risk of intrauterine growth restriction, prematurity, and fetal death.

10 Women with renal disease and significant proteinuria have worse outcomes than those with microalbuminuria or without proteinuria.

11 Pregnancy in women with systemic lupus erythematosus can be associated with increased disease activity and fetal loss.

12 The antiphospholipid antibody syndrome is associated with thrombotic events and renal failure.

13 Blood pressure control with antihypertensive medications that are safe in pregnancy is required for the majority of women with chronic kidney disease.

14 Immunosuppressive medications can be maintained in pregnancy to keep underlying renal glomerular disorders in remission.

15 Pregnancy is uncommon in women with endstage renal disease.

16 An increase in the amount of dialysis and careful monitoring of blood pressure and volume status are needed for pregnant women on dialysis.

17 Pregnancy is safe in women with kidney transplants without an increased risk of rejection or loss of the graft.

18 Immunosuppression may need to be adjusted during pregnancy in women with kidney transplants.

19 Collaboration with nephrologists and obstetricians is necessary to manage pregnancy in women with kidney disease.

20 Referral for dietary counseling and serial monitoring of fetal development is warranted in women with kidney disease because of the unique requirements in this population.

References

1 K/DOQI Advisory Board Members. Clinical Practice Guidelines for Chronic Kidney Disease. Part 4. Definition and Classification of Stages of Chronic Kidney Disease. *Am J Kidney Dis* 2002;39:S46–S75.

2 Hytten FE, Leitch I. *The physiology of human pregnancy*, 2nd edn. Oxford, UK: Blackwell Scientific Publications, 1971.

3 Davison JM, Dunlop W. Renal hemodynamics in normal human pregnancy. *Kidney Int* 1980;18:152–161.

4 Merrill JP, Ober WB, Reid DE, Romney SL. Renal lesions and acute renal failure in pregnancy. *Am J Med* 1956;21:781–810.

5 Selcuk NY, Tonbul HZ, San A, Odabas AR. Changes in frequency and etiology of acute renal failure in pregnancy (1980–1997). *Ren Fail* 1998;20:513–517.

6 Selcuk NY, Odabas AR, Cetinkaya R, et al. Outcome of pregnancies with HELLP syndrome complicated by acute renal failure (1989–1999). *Ren Fail* 2000;22:319–327.

7 Fried AM. Hydronephrosis of pregnancy: ultrasonographic study and classification of asymptomatic women. *Am J Obstet Gynecol* 1979;135:1066–1070.

8 D'Elia FL, Brennan RE, Brownstein PK. Acute renal failure secondary to ureteral obstruction by a gravid uterus. *J Urol* 1982;128:803–804.

9 McAleer SJ, Loughlin KR. Nephrolithiasis in pregnancy. *Curr Opin Urol* 2004;14:123–127.

10 Fisher MJ, Lehnerz SD, Herbert JR, Parikh CR. Kidney disease is an independent risk factor for adverse fetal and maternal outcomes in pregnancy. *Am J Kidney Dis* 2004;43:415–423.

11 North RA, Taylor RS, Gunn TR. Pregnancy outcome in women with reflux nephropathy and the inheritance of vesicoureteric reflux. *Aust NZ J Obstet Gynaecol* 2000;40:280–285.

12 El-Khatib M, Packman DK, Becker GJ, Kincaid-Smith P. Pregnancy-related complications in women with reflux nephropathy. *Clin Nephrol* 1994;41:50–55.

13 Ekbom P, Damm P, Feldt-Rasmussen B, et al. Pregnancy outcome in type I diabetic women with microalbuminuria. *Diabetes Care* 2001;24:1739–1744.

14 Stettler RW, Cunningham FG. Natural history of chronic protein-

uria complicating pregnancy. *Am J Obstet Gynecol* 1992;167: 1219–1224.

15 Katz, AI, Lindheimer, MD. Does pregnancy aggravate primary glomerular disease? *Am J Kidney Dis* 1985;6:261–265.

16 Cunningham FG, Cox SM, Harstad TW, et al. Chronic renal disease and pregnancy outcome. *Am J Obstet Gynecol* 1990; 163:453.

17 Cortes-Hernandez J, Ordi-Ros J, Paredes F, et al. Clinical predictors of fetal and maternal outcome in systemic lupus erythematosus: a prospective study of 103 pregnancies. *Rheumatology* 2002;41:643–650.

18 Moroni G, Quaglini S, Banfi G, et al. Pregnancy in lupus nephritis. *Am J Kidney Dis* 2002;40:713–720.

19 Fakhouri F, Noel LH, Zuber J, et al. The expanding spectrum of renal diseases associated with the antiphospholipid syndrome. *Am J Kidney Dis* 2003;41:1205–1211.

20 Cooper WO, Hernandez-Diaz S, Arbogast PG, et al. Major congenital malformations after the first-trimester exposure to ACE inhibitors. *N Engl J Med* 2006;354:2443–2451.

21 Roberts G, Gordon MM, Porter D, et al. Acute renal failure complicating HELLP syndrome, SLE, and anti-phospholipid syndrome: successful outcome using plasma exchange therapy. *Lupus* 2003;12:251–257.

22 Okundaye I, Abrinko P, Hou S. Registry of pregnancy in dialysis patients. *Am J Kidney Dis* 1998;31:766–773.

23 Hou S. Pregnancy in chronic renal insufficiency and end stage renal disease. *Am J Kidney Dis* 1999;33:235–252.

24 Hou S. Pregnancy in dialysis patients: where do we go from here? *Semin Dial* 2003;16:376–378.

25 Hou SH. Frequency and outcome of pregnancy in women on dialysis. *Am J Kidney Dis* 1994;23:60–63.

26 Giatras I, Levy DP, Malone FD, et al. Pregnancy during dialysis: case report and management guidelines. *Nephrol Dial Transplant* 1998;13:3266.

27 Jungers P, Chauveau D. Pregnancy in renal disease. *Kidney Int* 1997;52:871.

28 Hou SH. Pregnancy in women on haemodialysis and peritoneal dialysis. *Baillieres Clin Obstet Gynaecol* 1994;8:481.

29 Holley JL, Reddy SS. Pregnancy in dialysis patients: a review of outcomes, complications, and management. *Semin Dial* 2003;16:384–388.

30 Hou S. Pregnancy in renal transplant recipients. *Adv Ren Replace Ther* 2003;10:40–47.

31 Davidson JM. Dialysis, transplantation, and pregnancy. *Am J Kidney Dis* 1991;17:127.

32 Thompson BC, Kingdon EJ, Tuck SM, et al. Pregnancy in renal transplant recipients: the Royal Free Hospital experience. *Q Med J* 2003;96:837–844.

33 Salmela KT, Kyllonen LE, Holmberg C, Gronhagen-Riska C. Impaired renal function after pregnancy in renal transplant recipients. *Transplantation* 1993;56:1372.

34 Bar Oz B, Hackman R, Einarson T, Koren G. Pregnancy outcome after cyclosporin therapy during pregnancy. *Transplantation* 2001;71:1051.

35 European Best Practice Guidelines (Part 2). *Nephrol Dial Transplant* 2002;17(Suppl. 4):50.

46 Neurological disorders in pregnancy

R. Lee Archer, Stacy A. Rudnicki, and Bashir S. Shihabuddin

Pregnancy predisposes to some serious neurological problems, such as eclampsia, cerebrovascular disorders, and benign intracranial hypertension, and to a number of disorders that are relatively benign, including carpal tunnel syndrome, meralgia paresthetica, and Bell's palsy. In addition, women of childbearing age can have other neurological problems that are not uncommon and often require special attention during pregnancy. These include epilepsy, migraine headaches, and autoimmune diseases such as multiple sclerosis, myasthenia gravis, and Guillain–Barré syndrome.

Headaches

Headaches are among the most common of human ills and can be a sign of many different neurological problems.[1–4] A flow diagram to guide management is presented in Fig. 46.1. If headaches during pregnancy have been present for years, are unchanged in character, and the neurological examination is normal, then further attention is rarely warranted,[1] except perhaps to modify medications to protect the fetus.[3]

Most tension headaches are manageable without daily medication but, in severe cases, preventative treatment with low doses of tricyclic antidepressants (e.g., imipramine 10–50 mg at bedtime) may be justified.[1] Migraine headaches are often improved during pregnancy, but still constitute a large share of the headaches seen. They are most often unilateral with a throbbing quality and may be accompanied by nausea, photophobia, and phonophobia.[7] When necessary, migraine preventative medications may be used, such as beta-blockers[3] (e.g., atenolol 50–100 mg daily) or tricyclic antidepressants but, in general, migraineurs are managed best with limited doses (10–20 per month) of analgesics. Combinations of caffeine, butalbital, and acetaminophen (with codeine when necessary) are particularly effective and safe. Patients who use analgesics on more than 3 days/week are predisposed to analgesic rebound headaches,[7] and the frequent use of opioid analgesics runs the risk of withdrawal problems in the newborn.

The new onset of headaches or a significant change in the character or frequency of headaches during pregnancy should always cause concern. Preeclampsia is frequently accompanied by headache,[16] and all gravidas with new-onset headache deserve careful observation for this disorder. Benign intracranial hypertension is more likely to occur during pregnancy and usually presents with a constant holocephalic headache and papilledema.[1] Blindness may result without treatment. Treatments include serial lumbar punctures (the mainstay), cautious control of weight gain, occasionally acetazolamide (a class C drug), and, very rarely, surgical procedures such as lumboperitoneal shunting or optic nerve sheath fenestration.[1] Regular ophthalmological follow-up with visual field determination is imperative to confirm stability, as the visual loss tends to occur peripherally and may not be noticed by the patient until it is advanced.

The presence of new problems with focal neurological signs, such as hemianesthesia or hemiparesis, with a headache should prompt further investigation as a rule. Confidence that the symptoms represent a migraine aura would be a notable exception. Magnetic resonance imaging (MRI) has never been known to cause fetal harm and is considered the imaging procedure of choice in neurological evaluations during pregnancy.[3,5,6] When a cerebrovascular insult is in the differential, consideration should be given to doing diffusion-weighted imaging, as well as magnetic resonance angiography and venography at the same sitting, as these will usually clarify the pathology and guide management.

The very sudden onset of a severe or even moderately severe headache should raise concern for the possibility of a subarachnoid hemorrhage (SAH). A computerized tomographic (CT) scan will discern the presence of blood more often than MRI, but even a normal CT scan will miss a SAH 5% of the time; a lumbar puncture is mandatory when this diagnosis is suspected (preferably after urgent imaging).[1] The risk of SAH increases around the time of delivery.[9] Causes include berry aneurysms and arteriovenous malformations. Immediate workup and treatment are mandatory with neurosurgical consultation to help determine the timing of arteriography, as the risk of a fatal subsequent bleed is high, and arteriography may cause a stroke by inducing vasospasm.[8]

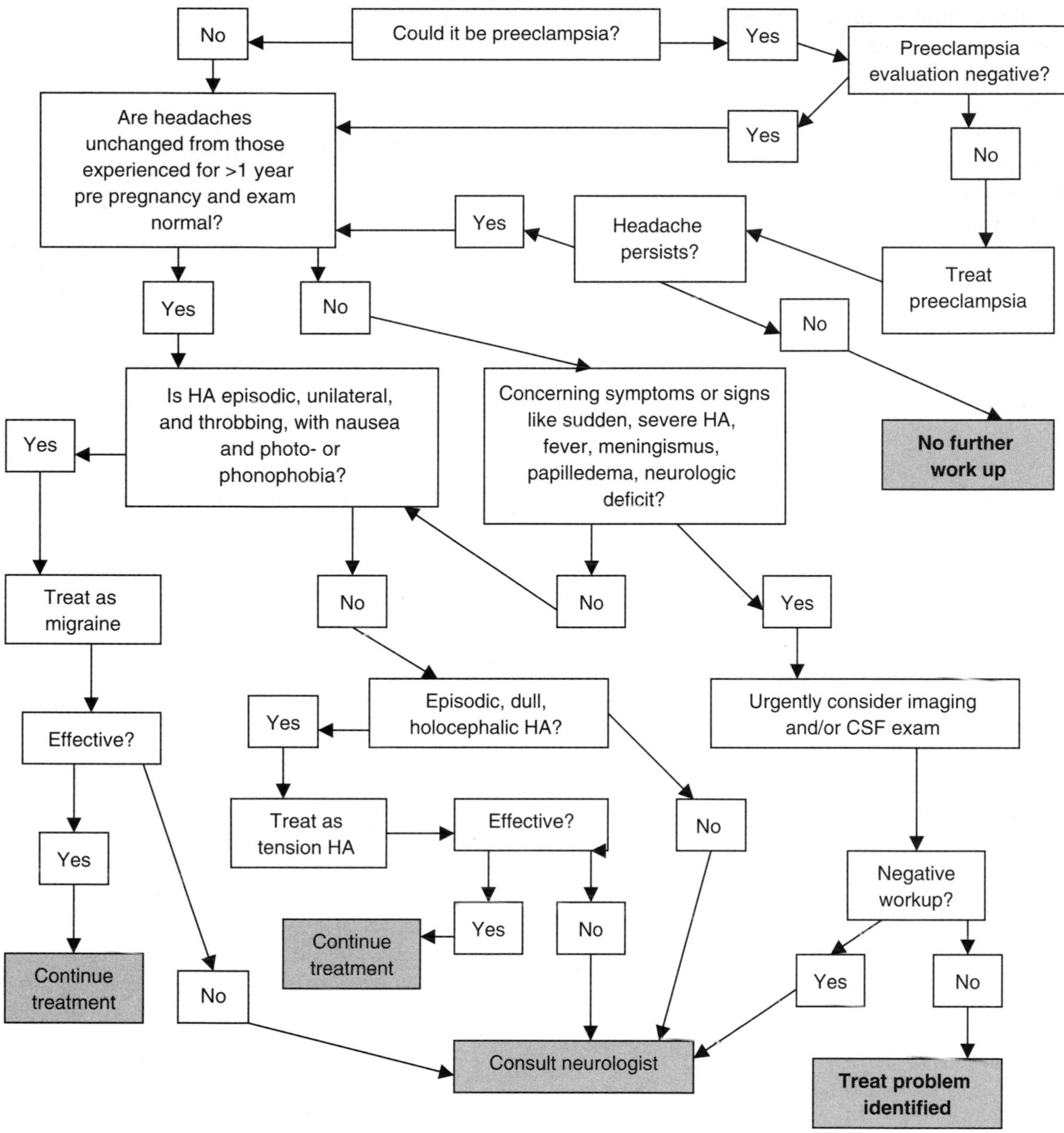

Figure 46.1 Flow diagram for headaches in pregnancy. CSF, cerebrospinal fluid; HA, headache.

Strokes

Strokes occur in 5–15 out of 100 000 pregnancies.[8] Urgent evaluation is indicated for the pregnant patient with stroke, just as in the general population.[10] Intracerebral hemorrhages generally present with profound hemiparesis and headache, sometimes progressing quickly to coma.[8] Treatment is primarily supportive, unless the size of the hemorrhage or bleeding into the ventricular system necessitates surgical intervention to relieve pressure on other parts of the brain.[8] Nonhemorrhagic strokes are either thrombotic or embolic. Thrombotic strokes may be arterial or venous. Venous sinus thrombosis is more common in the puerperium, and the new onset of headaches with any neurological symptoms or signs (such as headache with papilledema) during this period should cause concern for this possibility. Other cerebrovascular disorders associated with or more common during pregnancy include air or amniotic fluid embolism, embolic strokes caused by right-to-left shunts through a patent foramen ovale, hypercoagulable states (such as antiphospholipid syndrome), and metastatic choriocarcinoma.

Appropriate testing and treatment is evolving rapidly in this field, with clot retrieval devices recently becoming available and intra-arterial thrombolysis an option at many institutions, so management should involve neurological consultation. Anticoagulation with warfarin or heparin has been proven to be of benefit in atrial fibrillation and, in addition, many authorities recommend it with venous sinus thrombosis, hypercoagulable states, acute arterial dissection, and in the case of many other types of cardiac embolic strokes. Heparin (particularly low-molecular-weight heparin) is considered by most the anticoagulant of choice in pregnancy, because it does not cross the placenta and because warfarin is teratogenic in the first trimester.[8]

Multiple sclerosis

A diagnosis of multiple sclerosis does not contraindicate pregnancy, but the postpartum period is associated with an increased incidence of exacerbations,[11,14] and any neurological disability present (such as paraplegia) can certainly complicate management. None of the available treatments is approved for use during pregnancy, but anecdotal reports suggest that glatiramer acetate may be safe.[12,13] There are no known anesthetic contraindications.[12,15]

Focal neuropathies during pregnancy

Up to 62% of pregnant women have symptoms of carpal tunnel syndrome (which includes numbness and tingling in all fingers except the little one).[17] Wrist splints at night are beneficial, and steroid injections may be used when symptoms are severe. Spontaneous resolution following delivery is common.[18–20] Bell's palsy is three times more likely to occur in pregnancy. Onset is typically during the third trimester or puerperium.[21] It is associated with an increased risk of preeclampsia and hypertension.[23] Prognosis for recovery from an incomplete Bell's palsy is excellent but, for those with complete facial paralysis, pregnancy is associated with a worse prognosis.[24] Meralgia paresthetica (a neuropathy of the lateral femoral cutaneous nerve) causes numbness or burning pain in the lateral thigh. Symptoms generally resolve within a few months after delivery as weight is lost.[25] For patients who have significant pain, topical capsaicin may be beneficial.[26] Approximately 1% of postpartum women have leg numbness or weakness confirmed by neurological examination. The femoral and lateral femoral cutaneous nerves are commonly involved. The common fibular, sciatic, and obturator nerves, lumbosacral plexus, and lumbosacral roots are occasionally involved.[27] Injuries may be more common in small and/or nulliparous women, in those with a prolonged second stage of labor, when the fetus is large, or with midforceps rotation.[27–29] Recovery may take anywhere from a week to 18 months, with some patients having persistent problems.[27]

Peripheral neuropathy

Thiamine deficiency may occur with hyperemesis gravidarum, resulting in either a peripheral neuropathy or Wernicke's encephalopathy. Intravenous thiamine may reverse the encephalopathy, but the neuropathy, which may be severe, improves slowly and recovery may be incomplete.[30,31] Guillain–Barré syndrome may occur during pregnancy, but pregnant women do not appear to be at increased risk. Plasmapheresis for Guillain–Barré syndrome appears to be safe.[32]

Neuromuscular junction and muscle disorders

Women with myasthenia gravis (MG) may occasionally have their first symptoms during pregnancy. Exacerbations occur during pregnancy in 15–41% of myasthenics, and in an additional 16–30% during the puerperium. The latter is not influenced by mode of delivery.[35–37]

Because magnesium impairs neuromuscular transmission, it should be used very cautiously in treating preeclampsia and eclampsia in myasthenics.[38] Similarly, neuromuscular blocking agents should be avoided.[39] MG may cause fatigue during the second phase of labor, but the first stage is not affected as MG does not affect smooth muscle.

As weight gain increases during pregnancy, there may be increased ambulation difficulties in patients with muscular dystrophies and congenital myopathies.[40] Both increased incidences of preterm labor and a higher rate of Cesarean sections occur in women with myotonic dystrophy (the most common muscular dystrophy of adulthood).[41] Rarely, women with myotonic dystrophy may develop a cardiomyopathy with congestive heart failure during pregnancy.[42,43] Inflammatory myopathies (dermatomyositis and polymyositis) have rarely been reported during pregnancy, but there is a sense that increased fetal loss and premature labor are common, particularly when the diseases are active.[45,46]

Treatment of any of the autoimmune neurologic diseases should be done in conjunction with a neurologist, as the risks of immunosuppression in a pregnant patient must be carefully weighed against the risks of untreated disease. Prednisone is considered safe during pregnancy when needed for autoimmune diseases. Azathiaprine, a class D drug, may be the safest of the other immune suppressants.

Epilepsy

Although women with epilepsy have an increased risk of obstetric complications, worsening seizure control, and adverse neonatal outcomes, around 95% have an uncomplicated pregnancy course and give birth to normal offspring. These women, however, do have a higher rate of spontaneous and elective abortion than the general population and are more likely to undergo labor induction and Cesarean section procedures.[47–49]

Factors leading to increased seizure frequency during pregnancy include declining antiepileptic drug (AED) concentrations, noncompliance, stress, and sleep deprivation.[51,54,55] Serum AED concentrations start declining in the first trimester, reach a nadir near term, then return to preconception levels within 4–12 weeks postpartum if the dose is not altered.[56] Anticonvulsant levels should be checked every 1–3 months, and the goal should be to maintain prepregnancy levels. Anticonvulsant changes should be considered prior to pregnancy to optimize safety to the fetus and, in general, should not be done during pregnancy. Infants born to women with epilepsy are at increased risk of congenital malformations, cognitive impairment, and developmental delays. Contributing factors to these adverse outcomes are intrauterine AED exposure, folic acid deficiency, seizure control, seizure type, genetics, maternal health, smoking, and lower socioeconomic class.[57] The incidence of major congenital malformations in infants born to women with epilepsy is 4–8%, which represents a twofold increase over the incidence in the general population.[58] Phenytoin, carbamazepine, phenobarbital, primidone, and valproic acid (VPA) are associated with an increased risk of major malformations, especially for women on polytherapy and women exposed to high serum AED concentrations during the first trimester. This has been demonstrated most consistently with the use of VPA.[59,60] Therefore polytherapy and VPA should be avoided whenever possible. Adequate information regarding the safety of other, newer AEDs during pregnancy is not available yet, although lamotrigine looks promising. Kaplan[61] and Tomson and Battino.[62] have provided excellent reviews of AEDs and teratogenicity.

Folic acid deficiency is associated with the development of congenital malformations, mainly neural tube defects (NTDs). Folic acid levels decline during pregnancy, and the antifolate effect of some AEDs predisposes women with epilepsy to folic acid deficiency.[65] Folic acid supplementation of 0.4–4 mg daily, beginning 1 month before conception and continuing through pregnancy, reduces the incidence of NTDs by 50–70%. The higher dose of 4 mg daily is used in women who have a prior history of offspring with NTDs.[66] Infants born to women taking enzyme-inducing AEDs are also at greater risk of hemorrhagic complications because of the reduced activity of vitamin K-dependent clotting factors.[67] For this reason, women taking enzyme-inducing AEDs should be treated with oral vitamin K 10–20 mg daily during the last month of pregnancy. Infants should receive vitamin K 1 mg intramuscularly at birth and, if needed, fresh frozen plasma.

Key points

1. Azathioprine is possibly safe (FDA pregnancy class D).
2. Magnesium should be used judiciously in myasthenics, and neuromuscular blocking agents should be avoided as they can exacerbate MG symptoms.
3. Multiple sclerosis does not contraindicate pregnancy, but exacerbations are more frequent in the postpartum period.
4. Anticonvulsant level checks and necessary medication changes should be made at 1- to 3-month intervals during pregnancy in all women with epilepsy.
5. Oral vitamin K 20 mg supplementation should be given daily for women on enzyme-inducing anticonvulsants (e.g., phenytoin and carbamazepine) during the last month of pregnancy; newborns should be given vitamin K 1 mg intramuscularly and fresh frozen plasma if necessary.
6. Medication compliance, adequate rest, and stress reduction should be encouraged in all women with epilepsy.
7. The incidence of major congenital malformations is 4–8% for all women with epilepsy.
8. Strokes are more common during pregnancy.
9. Strokes should be treated urgently, as with any nonpregnant patient.
10. Unusual causes of stroke that are more common in pregnancy include: right-to-left shunt through a patent septal defect; air embolism; amniotic fluid embolism; venous sinus thromboses in the puerperium; choriocarcinoma; hypercoagulable states (e.g., antiphospholipid antibody syndrome)
11. MRI is the imaging method of choice (except when hemorrhage is suspected).

12 CT scans have a 5% chance of missing a SAH.

13 Sudden, severe headaches may herald the onset of a SAH (which occur more commonly during the third trimester).

14 A change in headache pattern during pregnancy should prompt concern as to the cause because many serious disorders, including preeclampsia, benign intracranial hypertension, cerebral venous sinus thrombosis, and subarachnoid hemorrhage, can present with a headache.

15 Concerning symptoms and signs that may accompany headache include: sudden onset of a severe headache, papilledema, fever, and focal neurological signs (such as hemiparesis and hemianesthesia).

16 Headaches that have been present for over a year before pregnancy and that have not changed in frequency or type, in someone with a normal neurological examination, do not require additional workup as a rule.

17 Benign intracranial hypertension presents with a constant holocephalic headache and papilledema; it may cause blindness if untreated.

18 Cerebral venous sinus thrombosis is more common in the puerperium.

19 Heparin is generally considered to be the anticoagulant of choice during pregnancy as warfarin is teratogenic in the first trimester and heparin does not cross the placenta.

20 Carpal tunnel syndrome symptoms occur in 62% of pregnant women, and wrist splints at night generally help. Spontaneous resolution after delivery is common.

21 Meralgia paresthetica causes a burning pain on the side of the thigh and typically improves spontaneously after pregnancy. It may improve with topical capsaicin.

22 Approximately 1% of women have postpartum leg weakness or numbness attributed to a focal neuropathy, the most common of which are the femoral and lateral femoral cutaneous nerves.

23 A thiamine deficiency neuropathy may be caused by hyperemesis gravidarum.

24 Treatment of any autoimmune neurological disease in pregnancy should involve a neurologist to assist in weighing the pros and cons of immune suppression.

25 Guillain–Barré syndrome can be safely treated with plasmapheresis during pregnancy.

26 Women with epilepsy on anticonvulsants should be on 0.4–4 mg of folic acid daily, the higher dose being used for women with previous infants affected by neural tube defects.

27 Polytherapy and valproic acid should be avoided in epileptic women during pregnancy, if feasible, as both increase the chances of birth defects.

28 Consideration for changing AEDs to benefit the fetus should be done before and generally not during the pregnancy course.

29 Prednisone is generally safe to use when necessary for autoimmune diseases during pregnancy.

30 The AED serum levels during pregnancy should be maintained at prepregnancy levels.

References

1 Martin SR, Foley RF. Approach to the pregnant patient with headache. *Clin Obstet Gynecol* 2005;48:2.

2 Marcus DA. Headache in pregnancy. *Curr Pain Headache Rep* 2003;7:288.

3 Silberstein SD. Headaches in pregnancy. *Neurol Clin* 2004;22:727.

4 Von Wald T, Walling AD. Headache during pregnancy. *Obstet Gynecol Surv* 2002;57:179.

5 Levine D, Barnes PD, Edleman RR. Obstetric MR imaging. *Radiology* 1999;211:609.

6 ACR standards. MRI safety and sedation. World Wide Web URL: http://www.acr.org. Accessed September 12, 2002.

7 Headache Classification Subcommittee of the International Headache Society. The International Classification of Headache Disorders, 2nd edn. *Cephalagia* 2004;24(Suppl. 2): 9.

8 Turan TN, Stern GJ. Stroke in pregnancy. *Neurol Clin* 2004;22:821.

9 Kittner SJ, Stern BJ, Feeser BR, et al. Pregnancy and the risk of stroke. *N Engl J Med* 1966;335:768.

10 Pathan M, Kittner SJ. Pregnancy and stroke. *Curr Neurol Neurosci Rep* 2003;3:27.

11 Vukusic S, Hutchinson M, Hours M, et al. Pregnancy in Multiple Sclerosis Group. Pregnancy and multiple sclerosis (the PRIMS study): clinical predictors of post-partum relapse. *Brain* 2004;127:1353.

12 Ferrero S, Pretta S, Ragni N. Multiple sclerosis: management

issues during pregnancy. *Eur J Obstet Gynecol Reprod Biol* 2004;115:3.
13 Hughes MD. Multiple sclerosis and pregnancy. *Neurol Clin* 2004;22:757.
14 Salemi G, Callari G, Gammino M, et al. The relapse rate of multiple sclerosis changes during pregnancy: a cohort study. *Acta Neurol Scand* 2004;110:23.
15 Bennett K. Pregnancy and multiple sclerosis. *Clin Obstet Gynecol* 2005;48:38.
16 Kaplan P. Neurologic aspects of eclampsia. *Neurol Clin* 2004;22:841.
17 Padua L, Aprile I, Caliandro P, et al. Italian Carpal Tunnel Syndrome Study Group. Carpal tunnel syndrome in pregnancy: multiperspective follow-up of untreated cases. *Neurology* 2002;59:1643.
18 Padua L, Aprile I, Caliandro P, et al. Italian Carpal Tunnel Syndrome Study Group. Symptoms and neurophysiological picture of carpal tunnel syndrome in pregnancy. *Clin Neurophysiol* 2001;112:1946.
19 Stolp-Smith KA, Pascoe MK, Ogburn PL. Carpal tunnel syndrome in pregnancy: frequency, severity, and prognosis. *Arch Phys Med Rehabil* 1998;79:1285.
20 Stahl S, Blumenfeld Z, Yarnitsky D. Carpal tunnel syndrome in pregnancy: indications for early surgery. *J Neurol Sci* 1996; 136:182.
21 Hilsinger RL, Jr, Adour KK, Doty HE. Idiopathic facial paralysis, pregnancy, and the menstrual cycle. *Ann Otol Rhinol Laryngol* 1975;84:433.
22 Shehata HA, Okosun H. Neurological disorders in pregnancy. *Curr Opin Obstet Gynecol* 2004;16:117.
23 Shmorgun D, Chan WS, Ray JG, Association between Bell's palsy in pregnancy and pre-eclampsia. *Q J Med* 2002;95:359.
24 Gillman GS, Schaitkin BM, May M, Klein SR. Bell's palsy in pregnancy: a study of recovery outcomes. *Otolaryngol Head Neck Surg* 2002;126:26.
25 Wiezer MJ, Franssen H, Rinkel GJ, Wokke JH. Meralgia paraesthetica: differential diagnosis and follow-up. *Muscle Nerve* 1996;19:522.
26 Puig L, Alegre M, de Moragas JM. Treatment of meralgia paraesthetica with topical capsaicin. *Dermatology* 1995;191:73.
27 Wong CA, Scavone BM, Dugan S, et al. Incidence of postpartum lumbosacral spine and lower extremity nerve injuries. *Obstet Gynecol* 2003;101:279.
28 Feasby TE, Burton SR, Hahn AF. Obstetrical lumbosacral plexus injury. *Muscle Nerve* 1992;15:937.
29 Katirji B, Wilbourn AJ, Scarberry SL, Preston DC. Intrapartum maternal lumbosacral plexopathy. *Muscle Nerve* 2002;26:340.
30 Nel JT, van Heyningen CF, van Eeden SF, et al. Thiamine deficiency induced gestational polyneuropathy and encephalopathy. A case report. *S Afr Med J* 1985;67:600.
31 Spruill SC, Kuller JA. Hyperemesis gravidarum complicated by Wernicke's encephalopathy. *Obstet Gynecol* 2002;99:875.
32 Clifton ER. Guillain–Barré syndrome, pregnancy, and plasmapheresis. *J Am Osteopath Assoc* 1992;92:1279.
33 McCombe P, McManis PG, Frith JA, et al. Chronic inflammatory demyelinating polyradiculoneuropathy associated with pregnancy. *Ann Neurol* 1987;21:102.
34 Drachman DB. Myasthenia gravis. *N Engl J Med* 1994;330:1797.
35 Djelmis J, Sastarko M, Mayer D, et al. Myasthenia gravis in pregnancy: report on 69 cases. *Eur J Obstet Gynecol Reprod Biol* 2002;104:21.
36 Plauche WC. Myasthenia gravis in mothers and their newborns. *Clin Obstet Gynecol* 1991;34:82.
37 Osserman KE. Pregnancy in myasthenia gravis and neonatal myasthenia gravis. *Am J Med* 1955;19:718.
38 Krendel DA. Hypermagnesemia and neuromuscular transmission. *Semin Neurol* 1990;10:42.
39 Dillon FX. Anesthesia issues in the perioperative management of myasthenia gravis. *Semin Neurol* 2004;24:83.
40 Rudnik-Schoneborn S, Glauner B, Rohrig D, Zerres K. Obstetric aspects in women with facioscapulohumeral muscular dystrophy, limb-girdle muscular dystrophy, and congenital myopathies. *Arch Neurol* 1997;54:888.
41 Rudnik-Schoneborn S, Zerres K. Outcome in pregnancies complicated by myotonic dystrophy: a study of 31 patients and review of the literature. *Eur J Obstet Gynecol Reprod Biol* 2004;114:44.
42 Fall LH, Young WW, Power JA, et al. Severe congestive heart failure and cardiomyopathy as a complication of myotonic dystrophy in pregnancy. *Obstet Gynecol* 1990;76:481.
43 Dodds TM, Haney MF, Appleton FM. Management of peripartum congestive heart failure using continuous arteriovenous hemofiltration in a patient with myotonic dystrophy. *Anesthesiology* 1991;75:907.
44 Dalakas MC, Hohlfeld R. Polymyositis and dermatomyositis. *Lancet* 2003;362:971.
45 Silva CA, Sultan SM, Isenberg DA. Pregnancy outcome in adult-onset idiopathic inflammatory myopathy. *Rheumatology* 2003;42: 1168.
46 Ishii N, Ono H, Kawaguchi T, Nakajima H. Dermatomyositis and pregnancy. Case report and review of the literature. *Dermatologica* 1991;183:146.
47 Tanganelli P, Regesta G. Epilepsy, pregnancy, and major birth anomalies: an Italian prospective, controlled study. *Neurology* 1992;42(Suppl. 5):89.
48 Sawhney H, Vasishta K, Suri V, et al. Pregnancy with epilepsy: a retrospective analysis. *Int J Gynaecol Obstet* 1996;54:17.
49 Yerby M, Koepsell T, Daling J. Pregnancy complications and outcomes in a cohort of women with epilepsy. *Epilepsia* 1985;26:631.
50 Devinsky O, Yerby MS. Women with epilepsy: reproduction and effects of pregnancy on epilepsy. *Neurol Clin* 1994;12:479.
51 Schmidt D, Canger R, Avanzini G, et al. Change of seizure frequency in epileptic woman. *J Neurol Neurosurg Psychiatry* 1983;46:751.
52 Teramo K, Hiilesmaa V, Bardy A, et al. Fetal heart rate during a maternal grand mal epileptic seizure. *J Perinat Med* 1979;7:3.
53 Yerby MS. Problems and management of the pregnant woman with epilepsy. *Epilepsia* 1987;28(Suppl. 3):S29.
54 Lander CM, Eadie MJ. Plasma antiepileptic drug concentrations during pregnancy. *Epilepsia* 1991;32:257.
55 Tomson T, Lindbom U, Ekqvist B, et al. Disposition of carbamazepine and phenytoin in pregnancy. *Epilepsia* 1994;35:131.
56 Yerby MS, Friel PN, McCormick K. Antiepileptic drug disposition during pregnancy. *Neurology* 1992;42(Suppl. 5):12.
57 Yerby MS. Pregnancy, teratogenesis and epilepsy. *Neurol Clin* 1994;12:749.
58 Leavitt AM, Yerby MS, Robinson N, et al. Epilepsy in pregnancy: developmental outcome of offspring at 12 months. *Neurology* 1992;42(Suppl. 5):141.
59 Canger R, Battino D, Canevini MP, et al. Malformations in offspring of women with epilepsy: a prospective study: *Epilepsia* 1999;40:1231.
60 Omtzigt JGC, Los FJ, Grobbee DE, et al. The risk of spina bifida aperta after first-trimester exposure to valproate in a prenatal cohort. *Neurology* 1992;42(Suppl. 5):119.
61 Kaplan P. Reproductive health and teratogenicity of antiepileptic drugs. *Neurology* 2004;63(Suppl. 4):13.

62 Tomson T, Battino D. Teratogenicity of antiepileptic drugs: state of the art review. *Curr Opin Neurol* 2005;18:135.
63 Kaneko S, Battino D, Andermann E, et al. Congenital malformations due to antiepileptic drugs. *Epilepsy Res* 1999;33:145.
64 Steeger-Theunissen RPM, Renier WO, Borm GF, et al. Factors influencing the risk of abnormal pregnancy outcome in epileptic women: a multi-centre prospective study. *Epilepsy Res* 1994;18:261.
65 Dansky LV, Andermann E, Rosenblatt D, et al. Anticonvulsants, folate levels, and pregnancy outcome: a prospective study. *Ann Neurol* 1987;21:176.
66 Yerby MS. Management issues for women with epilepsy: neural tube defects and folic acid supplementation. *Neurology* 2003;61(Suppl. 2):23.
67 Thorp JA, Gaston L, Caspers DR, et al. Current concepts and controversies in the use of vitamin K. *Drugs* 1995;49:376.

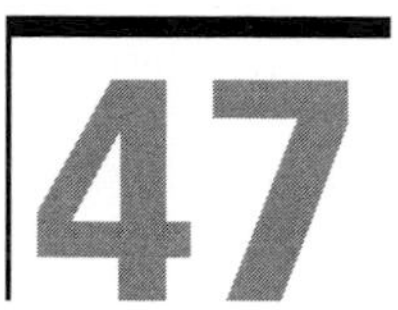

Thromboembolic disorders of pregnancy

Michael J. Paidas, Christian M. Pettker, and Charles J. Lockwood

Venous thromboembolism (VTE) poses significant maternal and fetal risks in pregnancy. It is estimated that VTE complicates 1 in 1000 pregnancies, but the precise frequency of thromboembolism is probably underestimated, given the reluctance to perform diagnostic tests in pregnancy secondary to fears of radiation exposure to the fetus. Pregnancy has been associated with a sixfold higher incidence of VTE compared with age-matched nonpregnant women, and pulmonary embolism remains a leading cause of maternal mortality.[1,2] In the USA, death from pulmonary embolism occurs in 2 in 100 000 deliveries and represents 11% of maternal deaths.[3] Postpartum deep venous thrombosis (DVT) is more common than antepartum DVT, with reported rates of 0.61 in 1000 and 0.13 in 1000 pregnancies respectively.[4] Timely diagnosis and treatment of DVT are essential as a quarter of patients with DVT develop pulmonary embolism, with a 15% mortality rate,[5] and two-thirds of these deaths occur within 30 min of the pulmonary embolism.[6] Institution of anticoagulation once the diagnosis of DVT has been made significantly reduces both the risk of pulmonary embolism (5%) and the mortality rate (< 1%).[7]

Pregnancy and the hemostatic system: clot formation, thrombin regulation, and fibrinolysis

Platelet plug formation: adhesion, activation, and aggregation

Following vascular disruption, platelets adhere to subendothelial collagen, mediated by von Willebrand factor "bridges" anchored at one end to subendothelial collagen and at the other to the platelet GPIb/IX/V receptor.[8] Platelets also adhere to other subendothelial extracellular matrix proteins. Adherent platelets are then activated, and increases in phospholipase C activity promote the synthesis of thromboxane and the phosphorylation of key platelet proteins that promote granule release, including α-granules containing von Willebrand factor, thrombospondin, platelet factor 4, fibrinogen, beta-thromboglobulin, and platelet-derived growth factor, as well as dense granules containing adenosine diphosphate and serotonin. Adenosine diphosphate induces a conformational change in the GPIIb/IIIa receptor on the platelet membrane, resulting in platelet aggregation via high-affinity fibrinogen formation and other proteins.[9]

Alpha-granule release also promotes exteriorization of platelet factor 4, a chemokine with potent heparin-neutralizing activity, as well as other procoagulant factors, leading to thrombin generation. Thrombin binds to type 1 and type 4 protease-activated receptors (PAR-1, -4) on the platelet membrane, serving as stimuli for platelet activation. Other factors, such as epinephrine and platelet activation factor, contribute to platelet activation. Platelet activation is limited by blood flow and agents elaborated by an intact endothelium, including prostacyclin, nitric oxide, and adenosine diphosphatase (ADPase) (Fig. 47.1).

Fibrin plug formation: the coagulation cascade

Tissue factor (TF), a cell membrane-bound glycoprotein, is ultimately responsible for the initiation of adequate hemostasis, as platelet activation alone cannot generate an effective hemostatic plug.[10] Intrauterine survival is not possible in the absence of TF, unlike the absence of either platelets or fibrinogen.[11] Tissue factor is expressed on the cell membranes of perivascular smooth muscle cells, fibroblasts, and tissue parenchymal cells; TF also circulates in the blood in very low concentrations as part of cell-derived microparticles or in a truncated soluble form.[11,12] These TF-bearing microparticles contribute to clotting by binding to platelets at sites of vascular injury through the interaction of P-selectin glycoprotein ligand-1 on microparticles with surface P-selectin on activated platelets.[13] In the presence of ionized calcium, perivascular cell- or platelet-bound TF comes into contact with plasma factor VII on negatively charged (anionic) cell membrane phospholipids (Fig. 47.1).

Factor VII has low intrinsic clotting activity, autoactivates after binding to TF, and/or can be activated by thrombin, as

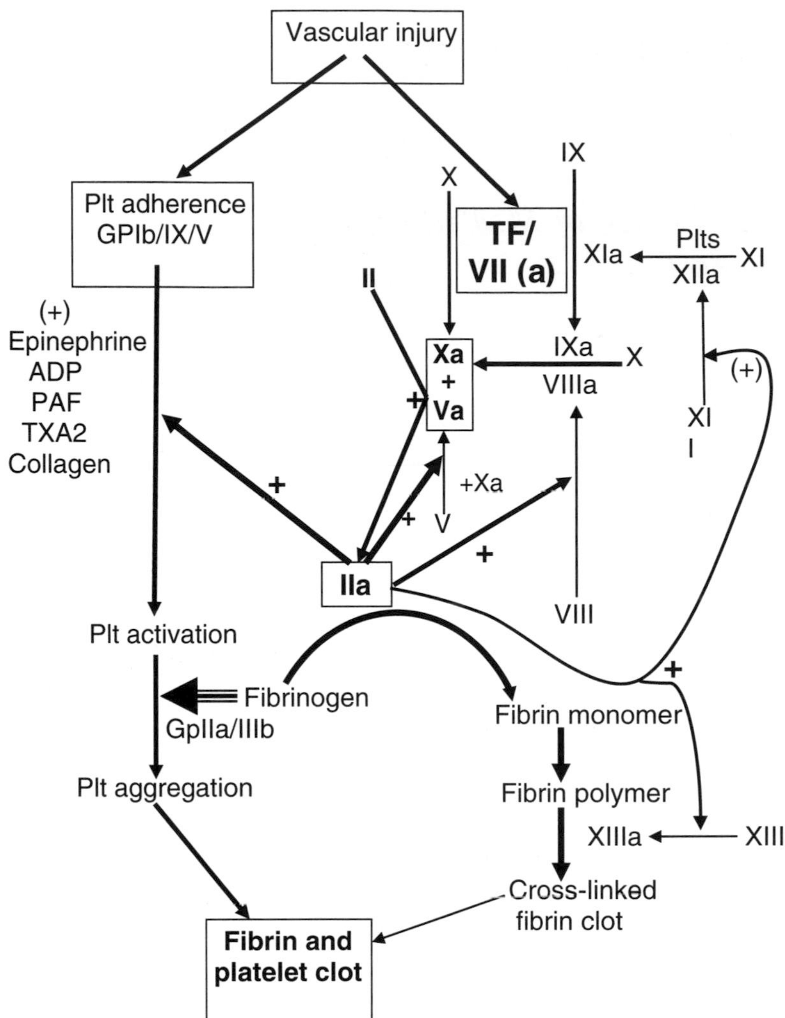

Figure 47.1 Activation of the clotting cascade leading to formation of a fibrin plug. Tissue factor initiates the extrinsic clotting cascade. Factor Xa complexes with its cofactor, factor Va, to convert prothrombin to thrombin. Thrombin cleaves fibrinogen to produce fibrin. A second pathway of thrombin generation is also available. See text for details.

well as factors IXa, Xa, or XIIa.10.[10,14] The complex of TF/factor VII(a) can either directly activate factor X (formerly known as the extrinsic pathway) or generate factor Xa by initially activating factor IX. Factor IX complexes with its cofactor, factor VIIIa, to activate factor X (formerly known as the intrinsic pathway). Once activated, factor Xa complexes with its cofactor, factor Va, to convert factor II (prothrombin) to factor IIa (thrombin). The cofactors, factors V and VIII, can each be activated by either thrombin or factor Xa (Fig. 47.1).

A second pathway of thrombin generation is available, which results from activation of factor XI by thrombin-activated factor XIIa, typically on the surface of activated platelets. Factor XII can be activated by the action of kallikrein and its cofactor, high-molecular-weight kininogen, and by plasmin. Factor IX activation can also occur via factor XIa.

Fibrinogen is cleaved by thrombin to produce fibrin. A stable hemostatic plug is created as fibrin monomers self-polymerize and are cross-linked by thrombin-activated factor XIIIa (Fig. 47.1). Thus, thrombin is the ultimate arbiter of clotting as it not only activates platelets and generates fibrin but, along with factor Xa, activates the crucial clotting cofactors, factors V and VIII, and mediates the aforementioned activation of factors VII, XII, and XIII (Fig. 47.1).

The anticoagulant system

The anticoagulant system provides balance in the hemostatic system to prevent excessive or inappropriate thrombin generation. The anticoagulant system consists of effector and inhibitor molecules (Fig. 47.2). The first inhibitory molecule is tissue factor pathway inhibitor (TFPI), which forms a complex with TF, factor VIIa, and factor Xa (the prothrombinase complex).[15] This block can be bypassed by the generation of factor XIa. Additionally, during the time period (10–15 s) before TFPI-mediated prothrombinase inhibition, a sufficient amount of factors Va, VIIIa, IXa, Xa, and thrombin can be generated to sustain clotting.

The protein C system plays a central role in regulating thrombin. Once thrombin is formed, it binds to thrombomodulin on the endothelial cell surface. A resultant conformational change permits thrombin to activate protein C when

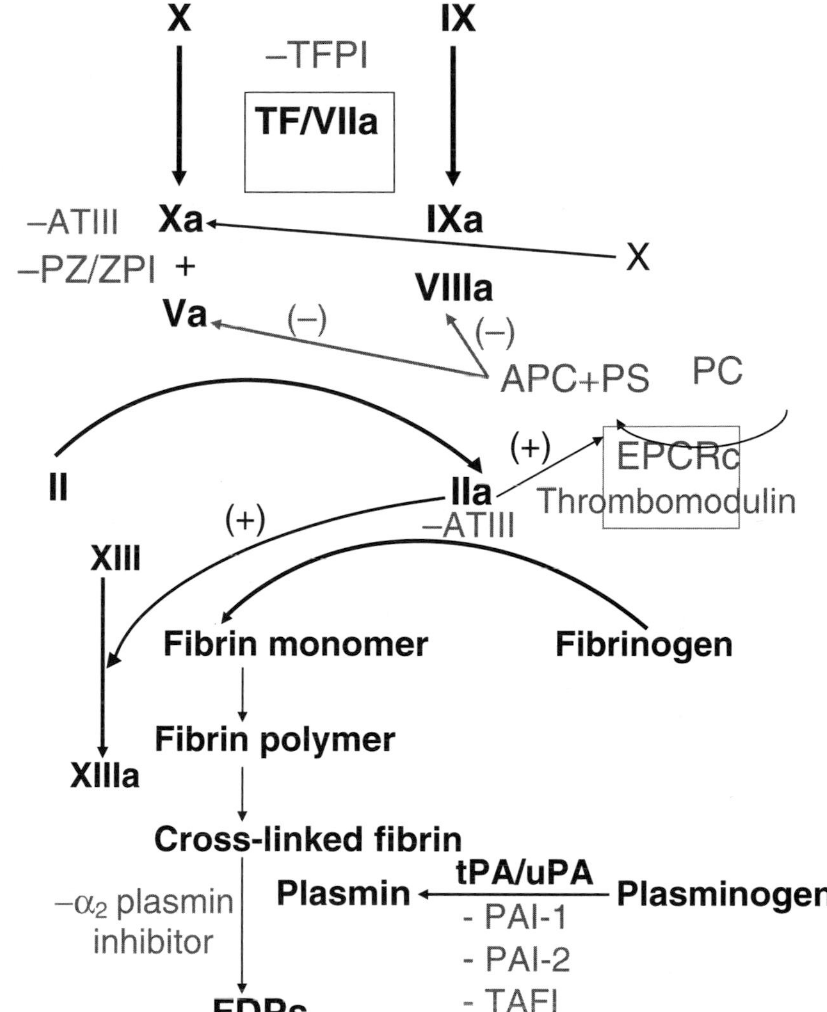

Figure 47.2 The anticoagulant and fibrinolytic systems. Key components of the anticoagulant system, which prevents excessive or inappropriate thrombin generation, consists of tissue factor pathway inhibitor, the protein C system, and antithrombin. The fibrinolytic system is critical for the prevention of thrombosis. Plasmin degrades fibrin, leading to the formation of fibrin degradation products. Plasmin is created by the proteolysis of plasminogen under proteolysis by urokinase-type plasminogen activator (uPA) or tissue-type plasminogen activator (tPA). Inhibitors of fibrinolysis include plasminogen activator inhibitor-1 (PAI-1), plasminogen activator inhibitor-2 (PAI-2), and thrombin-activatable fibrinolysis inhibitor (TAFI). See text for details.

bound to damaged endothelium or to the endothelial protein C receptor (EPCR). Activated protein C (APC) then binds to its cofactor, protein S (PS), to inactivate factors Va and VIIIa.[16] Factor Va acts as a second cofactor in APC-mediated factor VIIIa inactivation.

Protein Z (PZ) is a 62-kDa, vitamin K-dependent plasma protein that serves as a cofactor for a PZ-dependent protease inhibitor (ZPI) of factor Xa.[17,18] When ZPI is complexed to PZ, its inhibitory activity is enhanced 1000-fold.[19] The ZPI molecule also inhibits factor XIa in a PZ-independent process. PZ is critical for regulation of factor Xa activity along with TFPI.[19–21] PZ increases rapidly during the first months of life, followed by slow increases in childhood, with adult levels reached during puberty.[22,23] PZ deficiency influences the prothrombotic phenotype in factor V Leiden patients,[24] and low plasma PZ levels have been reported in patients with antiphospholipid antibodies.[25,26] There is also some evidence suggesting a role for PZ deficiency in a bleeding tendency.[27]

The most active inhibitor of both factor Xa and thrombin is antithrombin. Antithrombin binds either thrombin or factor Xa and vitronectin. A conformational change facilitates binding to heparin, which augments antithrombin's rate of thrombin inactivation 1000-fold.[28] A similar inhibitory mechanism is initiated by heparin cofactor II and α-2 macroglobulin.

Fibrinolysis

Fibrinolysis is also crucial to the prevention of thrombosis (Fig. 47.2). Plasmin degrades fibrin, leading to fibrin degradation products. Plasmin is created by the proteolysis of plasminogen via tissue-type plasminogen activator (tPA) embedded in fibrin. Endothelial cells produce a second plasminogen activator, urokinase-type plasminogen activator (uPA). There is also a series of inhibitors of fibrinolysis (Fig. 47.2). Plasmin is directly inhibited by α2-plasmin inhibitor, which can be bound to the fibrin clot to prevent premature fibrinolysis. Platelets and endothelial cells release type 1 plasminogen activator inhibitor (PAI-1) in response to thrombin binding to its PARs. The decidua is also a very rich source of

PAI-1, while the placenta is the chief source of PAI-2.[29] Thrombin-activatable fibrinolysis inhibitor (TAFI), activated by the thrombin–thrombomodulin complex, is a fourth fibrinolysis inhibitor.[30] The fibrinolytic system exerts anticoagulant effects. For example, fibrin degradation products inhibit thrombin action, a major source of hemorrhage in disseminated intravascular coagulation (DIC). In addition, PAI-1 bound to vitronectin and heparin directly inhibits thrombin and factor Xa activity.[31]

Risk factors for VTE

Clinical risk factors for VTE in pregnancy

Vascular stasis, hypercoagulability, and vascular trauma (Virchow's triad) remain the three prime antecedents to thrombosis. Clinical risk factors for VTE include pregnancy, obesity, surgery, infection, trauma, cancer, nephrotic syndrome, hyperviscosity syndromes, immobilization, congestive heart failure, estrogen-containing contraceptives and postmenopausal hormone therapy, prior VTE, and the presence of acquired and inherited thrombophilias. These conditions increase clotting potential through a variety of mechanisms including: increases in TF, clotting factors, and PAI-1; decreases in PS levels; increasing stasis; vascular injury. In women, pregnancy in thrombophilic patients and pregnancy in patients with a prior history of thromboembolism confer the highest risks of thromboembolism (Table 47.1).[32] Specific pregnancy-associated clinical risk factors can be stratified and are detailed in Table 47.2.[33–35]

Hemostatic changes in pregnancy

Substantial changes must occur in local decidual and systemic coagulation, anticoagulant, and fibrinolytic systems to meet the hemostatic challenges of pregnancy, including avoidance of hemorrhage at implantation, placentation, and the third stage of labor. Progesterone augments perivascular decidual cell TF and PAI-1 expression.[29,36] Transgenic TF knockout mice rescued by the expression of low levels of human TF have been found to have a 14% incidence of fatal postpartum hemorrhage, underscoring the importance of decidual TF.[37] Obstetric conditions associated with impaired decidualization (e.g., ectopic and Cesarean scar pregnancy, placenta previa and accreta) are associated with potential lethal hemorrhage in humans.

Pregnancy is associated with significant elevations of a number of clotting factors. Fibrinogen concentration is doubled, and 20–1000% increases in factors VII, VIII, IX, X, XII, and von Willebrand factor have been observed, with maximum levels reached at term.[38] Prothrombin and factor V levels remain unchanged, while levels of factors XIII and XI decline modestly. The net effect of these changes is to increase thrombin-generating potential. Coagulation activation markers in normal pregnancy are elevated, as evidenced by

Table 47.1 Risk of venous thromboembolic disease in women: a qualitative systematic review.[32]

Risk factor	Risk per 1000 women–years
Pregnancy	1.23
Puerperium	3.2
Pregnancy in thrombophilic patient	40
Pregnancy and history of VTE	110
Third-generation oral contraception	0.3
Postcoital pill	No risk
Hormone replacement	0.2–5.9
Tamoxifen	3.6–12
Raloxifene	9.5

Table 47.2 Pregnancy-associated clinical risk factors for venous thromboembolism (odds ratios with confidence intervals).[33–35]

	Lindqvist, 1999 (*n* = 603)	Danilenko-Dixon, 2001 (*n* = 90)	Anderson, 2003 (*n* = 1231)
Moderate-risk factors			
Age ≥ 35 years	1.3 (1–1.7)	–	2.0 (age > 40 years)
Parity (2)	1.5 (1.1–1.9)	1.1 (0.9–1.4)	–
(≥ 3)	2.4 (1.8–3.1)	–	–
Smoking	1.4 (1.1–1.9)	2.5 (1.3–4.7)	–
Multiple gestation	1.8 (1.1–3.0)	7 (0.4–135.5)	–
Preeclampsia	2.9 (2.1–3.9)	1 (0.14–7.1)	–
Varicose veins	–	2.4 (1.04–5.4)	4.5
Obesity	–	1.5 (0.7–3.2)	< 2
Cesarean section	3.6 (3.0–4.3)	–	–
Obstetric hemorrhage	–	9 (1.1–71.0)	–
High-risk factors	–	–	–
Spinal cord injury	–	–	> 10
Major abdominal surgery ≥ 30 min	–	–	> 10

Table 47.3 Coagulation parameters in pregnancy.

Variables (mean ± SD)	First trimester*	Second trimester*	Third trimester*	Normal range
Platelet (× 10^9/L)	275 ± 64	256 ± 49	244 ± 52	150–400
Fibrinogen (g/L)	3.7 ± 0.6	4.4 ± 1.2	5.4 ± 0.8	2.1–4.2
Prothrombin complex (%)	120 ± 27	140 ± 27	130 ± 27	70–30
Antithrombin (U/mL)	1.02 ± 0.10	1.07 ± 0.14	1.07 ± 0.11	0.85–1.25
Protein C (U/mL)	0.92 ± 0.13	1.06 ± 0.17	0.94 ± 0.2	0.68–1.25
Protein S, total (U/mL)	0.83 ± 0.11	0.73 ± 0.11	0.77 ± 0.10	0.70–1.70
Protein S, free (U/mL)	0.26 ± 0.07	0.17 ± 0.04	0.14 ± 0.04	0.20–0.50
Soluble fibrin (nmol/l)	9.2 ± 8.6	11.8 ± 7.7	13.4 ± 5.2	< 15
Thrombin–antithrombin (μg/L)	3.1 ± 1.4	5.9 ± 2.6	7.1 ± 2.4	< 2.7
D-Dimers (μg/L)	91 ± 24	128 ± 49	198 ± 59	< 80
Plasminogen activator inhibitor-1 (AU/mL)	7.4 ± 4.9	14.9 ± 5.2	37.8 ± 19.4	< 15
Plasminogen activator inhibitor-2 (μg/l)	31 ± 14	84 ± 16	160 ± 31	< 5
Cardiolipin antibodies positive	2/25	2/25	3/23	0
Protein Z (μg/mL)†	2.01 ± 0.76	1.47 ± 0.45	1.55 ± 0.48	–
Protein S, free antigen (%)†	–	38.9 ± 10.3	31.2 ± 7.4	–

Table modified from ref. 38 and †ref. 40.
*First trimester, weeks 12–15; second trimester, week 24; third trimester, week 35.
†First trimester, 0–14 weeks; second trimester, 14–27 weeks; third trimester, ≥ 27 weeks.

increased thrombin activity, increased soluble fibrin levels (9.2–13.4 nmol/L), increased thrombin–antithrombin (TAT) complexes (3.1–7.1 μg/L), and increased levels of fibrin D-dimer (91–198 μg/L).[39] Fifty percent of women had elevated TAT levels (11/22), and 36% of women had elevated levels of D-dimers (9/25) in the first trimester.

Significant changes in the natural anticoagulant and fibrinolytic systems occur in normal pregnancy. Protein S levels decrease significantly in normal pregnancy. Mean PS free antigen levels have been reported to be 38.9 ± 10.3% and 31.2 ± 7.4% in the second and third trimesters respectively.[40] In a follow-up study, free PS antigen levels in the first trimester were found to be 39% (SD 10.5), compared with the reference range in nonpregnancy of 88% (SD 19), $P < 0.05$.[41] The PS carrier molecule, complement 4B-binding protein, is increased in pregnancy, and is one explanation for the diminished PS levels in pregnancy. Studies on PZ levels in pregnancy are conflicting, with one group of investigators demonstrating lower levels as pregnancy progresses in a cross-sectional study,[40] while another group of investigators have demonstrated that PZ levels are increased by 20% ($P = 0.006$) from first trimester to delivery, followed by a 30% decrease ($P < 0.0001$) 6–12 weeks after delivery.[42] Levels of PAI-1 increase three- to fourfold during pregnancy; plasma PAI-2 values are low prior to pregnancy and reach concentrations of 160 μg/L at term. Table 47.3 summarizes the relevant pregnancy-associated changes in the hemostatic system.[43] The prothrombotic hemostatic changes are exacerbated by pregnancy-associated venous stasis in the lower extremities because of compression of the inferior vena cava and pelvic veins by the enlarging uterus, as well as a hormone-mediated increase in deep vein capacitance secondary to increased circulating levels of estrogen and the local production of prostacyclin and nitric oxide. In summary, the most significant pregnancy-related prothrombotic factors are listed in Table 47.4.

Table 47.4 Most significant prothrombotic changes in pregnancy.

Increased levels of procoagulants
Fibrinogen
Factor VIII
Diminished fibrinolysis
Decreased protein S
Resistance to activated protein C
Mechanical factors
Venous distension
Vessel injury
Compression of left iliac vein

Inherited thrombophilias

Inherited thrombophilias are a heterogeneous group of disorders associated with varying degrees of increased thrombotic risk. Until recently, these disorders consisted of deficiencies in PS, PC, and antithrombin. An association between a mutation in the factor V gene and increased thrombotic risk was first reported in 1994, termed the factor V Leiden mutation.[44] This relatively common mutation is present in 5% of American Caucasians, 1% of African–Americans, and 5–9% of Europeans, but is rare in Asian and African populations.[45,46] The factor V mutation is associated with resistance to APC and is inherited primarily in an autosomal-dominant fashion.[46,47] Heterozygosity is found in 20–40% of nonpregnant patients with thromboembolic disease, whereas homozygosity confers a > 100-fold risk of thromboembolic disease.[46] More recently, the prothrombin gene mutation (prothrombin G20210A) has been found to increase circulating prothrombin levels and, hence, the risk of both thrombosis and pregnancy complications.[46,48] In women with a history of VTE during pregnancy, prothrombin G20210A was found in 17% of patients compared with 1% of age-matched controls, and the factor V Leiden mutation was found in nearly 45% of patients.[49] However, a prospective study involving over 5000 patients designed to determine whether patients carrying the factor V Leiden mutation were at increased risk for venous thromboembolism compared with patients who were factor V Leiden negative did not find that factor V Leiden conferred an increased risk of thromboembolism.[50] Homozygosity for prothrombin G20210A confers an equivalent risk of VTE to that of factor V Leiden homozygosity.[46]

Other inherited thrombophilic mutations, including methylene tetrahydrafolate reductase (MTHFR) C667T and A1298C (often associated with hyperhomocysteinemia) and PAI gene mutations 4G/4G, 4G/5G, and 5G/5G, have been weakly associated, if at all, with thrombotic risk and pregnancy complications.[51–53] Table 47.5 summarizes the thromboembolic risks associated with the significant known thrombophilic mutations.[54–61] Heterozygous factor V Leiden is associated with a 0.2% risk of thromboembolism associated with pregnancy, while heterozygous prothrombin gene mutation is associated with a 0.5% risk. Compound heterozygous factor V Leiden and prothrombin gene mutations are associated with a 4.6% risk of thromboembolism.

Acquired thrombophilia

The well-characterized antiphospholipid antibody syndrome (APS) is defined by the combination of VTE, obstetric complications, and antiphospholipid antibodies (APA).[62] By definition APA-related thrombosis can occur in any tissue or organ except superficial veins, while accepted associated obstetric complications include at least one fetal death at or beyond the 10th week of gestation, or at least one premature birth at or before the 34th week, or at least three consecutive spontaneous abortions before the 10th week. All other causes of pregnancy morbidity must be excluded. APAs must be present on two or more occasions at least 6 weeks apart, and are immunoglobulins directed against proteins bound to negatively charged surfaces, usually anionic phospholipids.[63] Thus, APAs can be detected by screening for antibodies that:

- directly bind these protein epitopes (e.g., anti-β2-glycoprotein-1, prothrombin, annexin V, APC, PS, PZ, ZPI, high- and low-molecular-weight kininogens, tPA, factors VIIa and XII, the complement cascade constituents, C4 and CH, and oxidized low-density lipoprotein antibodies); or
- are bound to proteins present in an anionic phospholipid matrix (e.g., anticardiolipin and phosphatidylserine antibodies); or
- exert downstream effects on prothrombin activation in a phospholipid milieu (i.e., lupus anticoagulants).[64]

Venous thrombotic events associated with APA include DVT with or without acute pulmonary embolus, while the most common arterial events include cerebral vascular accidents and transient ischemic attacks. At least half of patients with APA have systemic lupus erythematosus. Anticardiolipin

Table 47.5 Inherited thrombophilias and their association with VTE.

Thrombophilia	Inheritance	Prevalence in European populations (from large cohort studies)	Prevalence in patients with VTE (range)	Relative risk or odds ratio (OR) of VTE [95% CI] (lifetime)	Reference
Factor V Leiden (FVL) (homozygous)	AD	0.07%*	< 1%*	80 [22–289]	54–56
FVL (heterozygous)	AD	5.3%	6.6–50%	2.7 [1.3–5.6]	54, 55
Prothrombin G20201A (PGM) (homozygous)	AD	0.02%*	< 1%	> 80-fold*	57
PGM (heterozygous)	AD	2.9%	7.5%	3.8 [3.0–4.9]	58
FVL/PGM (compound heterozygous)	AD	0.17%*	2.0%	20.0 [11.1–36.1]	58
Hyperhomocysteinemia	AR	5%	< 5%	3.3 [1.1–10.0]†	56, 59
Antithrombin deficiency (< 60% activity)	AD	0.2%	1–8%	17.5 [9.1–33.8]	56, 60
Protein S deficiency: Heerlen S460P mutation or free S antigen < 55%	AD	0.2%	3.1%	2.4 [0.8–7.9]	61
Protein C (< 60% activity)	AD	0.2%	3–5%	11.3 [5.7–22.3]	56, 60

AD, autosomal dominant; AR, autosomal recessive; CI, confidence interval.

*Calculated based on a Hardy–Weinberg equilibrium.

†OR adjusted for renal disease, folate, and B12 deficiency, while odds ratios are adjusted for these confounders.

antibodies were associated with an odds ratio (OR) of 2.17 (1.51–3.11; 14 studies) for any thrombosis, 2.50 (1.51–4.14) for DVT and APE, and 3.91 (1.14–13.38) for recurrent VTE.[65] Patients with systemic lupus erythematosus and lupus anticoagulants were at a sixfold greater risk of VTE compared with systemic lupus erythematosus patients without lupus anticoagulants, while systemic lupus erythematosus patients with anticardiolipin antibodies had a twofold greater risk of VTE compared with systemic lupus erythematosus patients without these antibodies. The lifetime prevalence of arterial or venous thrombosis in affected patients with antiphospholipid antibodies is about 30%, with an event rate of 1% per year.[64] These antibodies are present in up to 20% of individuals with VTE.[66] A review of 25 prospective, cohort and case–control studies involving more than 7000 patients observed an OR range for arterial and venous thromboses in patients with lupus anticoagulants of 8.65–10.84 and 4.09–16.2, respectively, and 1.0–18.0 and 1.0–2.51 for anticardiolipin antibodies.[64]

There is a 5% risk of VTE during pregnancy and the puerperium among patients with APA despite treatment.[67] Recurrence risks of up to 30% have been reported in APA-positive patients with a prior VTE; thus, long-term prophylaxis is required in these patients. A severe form of APS is termed catastrophic APS, or CAPS, which is defined as a potentially life-threatening variant with multiple vessel thromboses leading to multiorgan failure.[68] In the Euro-Phospholipid Project Group (13 countries included), DVT, thrombocytopenia, stroke, pulmonary embolism, and transient ischemic attacks were found in 31.7%, 21.9%, 13.1%, 9.0%, and 7.0% of cases respectively.

APA are associated with obstetric complications in about 15–20% of cases including fetal loss after 9 weeks' gestation, abruptio placentae, severe preeclampsia, and intrauterine growth restriction (IUGR). Reported ORs for lupus anticoagulant-associated fetal loss range from 3.0 to 4.8, while anticardiolipin antibodies display a wider range of reported ORs of 0.86–20.0.[63] It is unclear whether APA are also associated with recurrent (> 3) early spontaneous abortion in the absence of stillbirth. Fifty percent or more of pregnancy losses in APA patients occur after the 10th week.[69] Patients with APA more often display initial fetal cardiac activity compared with patients with unexplained first trimester spontaneous abortions without APA (86% vs 43%; $P < 0.01$).[70] APA have been commonly found in the general obstetric population, with one survey demonstrating that 2.2% of such patients have either IgM or IgG anticardiolipin antibodies, with most such women having relatively uncomplicated pregnancies.[71] Other factors may play a role in the pathogenesis of APA. Potential mechanism(s) by which APA induce arterial and venous thrombosis as well as adverse pregnancy outcomes include: APA-mediated impairment of endothelial thrombomodulin and APC-mediated anticoagulation; induction of endothelial TF expression; impairment of fibrinolysis and antithrombin activity; augmented platelet activation and/or adhesion; impairment of the anticoagulant effects of the anionic phospholipid binding proteins β2-glycoprotein-1 and annexin V.[72,73] APA induction of complement activation has been suggested to play a role in fetal loss, with heparin preventing such aberrant activation.[74]

Adverse pregnancy outcome and inherited thrombophilias

Inherited thrombophilic conditions have been implicated in a variety of obstetrical complications, including severe preeclampsia and related conditions, late fetal loss (≥ 20 weeks), severe IUGR (< 5th percentile), and abruptio placentae. The frequency, recurrence risks, and impact in subsequent pregnancies for the general population without regard to thrombophilia are listed in Table 47.6.

Severe preeclampsia/syndrome of hemolysis, elevated liver enzymes, and low platelets (HELLP)

Several studies (mostly case–controlled) have evaluated the relationship between heterozygous factor V Leiden and severe preeclampsia. Factor V Leiden was identified in 4.5–26% of patients with severe preeclampsia, eclampsia, or HELLP syndrome (Table 47.7).[75–90] Kupferminc et al.[79] found that a thrombophilic mutation was present in 67% of patients who had previous adverse pregnancy outcome (APO). The system-

Table 47.6 Adverse pregnancy outcomes (APO): prevalence and recurrence.[43]

APO	Prevalence of APO	Recurrence of same APO	Fetal death with APO	Fetal death in next pregnancy
Loss at > 20 weeks	0.5%	8.5%	–	8.5%
SPE	2%	26%	13.5%	5.9%
HELLP	1%	4%	13.5%	4%
Eclampsia	0.5%	3%	13.5%	5.9%
Abruptio placentae	0.8%	5%	26%	2.4%
IUGR < 5%	5.3%	16%	20%	8%
One or more	8%	–	–	6%

HELLP, hemolysis, elevated liver enzymes; SPE, severe preeclampsia.

Table 47.7 Severe preeclampsia and thrombophilic conditions.

Author	Year	No. with SPE	FVL positive (%)	PG mutation positive (%)	PS deficiency (%)	Delivery gestational age, weeks (mean ± SD)	Reference
Dekker	1995	85	–	–	24.7	–	75
Dizon-Townson	1996	158	8.9	–	–	–	76
Nagy	1998	69	18.8	–	–	31.6 ± 3.1	77
Krauss	1999	21	19		4.8	–	78
Kupferminc et al.	1999	34	26.5	5.9	11.8	35.1 ± 3.6	79
van Pampus	1999	284	6.0	–	–	–	80
de Groot	1999	37	5.4	–	–	–	81
Kupferminc et al.	2000	63	23.8	8	8	32.0 ± 4.0	82
Rigo	2000	120	18.3		–	32.8 ± 3.8	83
von Tempelhoff	2000	61	19.7		10	29 (range 22–33)	84
Kupferminc et al.	2000	55		9.1	–	–	85
Kim	2001	187	6.4	–	–	–	86
Livingston	2001	110	4.5	0	–	34.3 ± 5.1	87
Currie	2002	48	8.3	–	–	34.1	88
Benedetto	2002	32	9.3	6.2	–	–	89
Schlembach	2003	36	16.7	0	–	–	90

FVL, factor V Leiden; PG, prothrombin gene; SPE, severe preeclampsia.

atic review by Alfirevic[91] suggested a positive association between factor V Leiden and preeclampsia/eclampsia [OR 1.6, 95% confidence interval (CI) 1.2–2.1)]. Factor V Leiden occurred in 11.4% (95/830) of patients with severe preeclampsia, with an OR of 2.84 (95% CI 1.95–4.14) in the study by Morrison.[92] The prothrombin gene mutation was identified in up to 9.1% of cases, whereas PS deficiency was reported in 5–25% of cases (Table 47.7). Paidas et al.[40] found that there was a significant decrease in PZ levels in patients ($n = 51$) with a variety of APO, including IUGR, preeclampsia, preterm delivery, and bleeding in pregnancy compared with women ($n = 51$) with normal pregnancy outcomes (NPO) (second trimester 1.5 ± 0.4 vs 2.0 ± 0.5 μg/mL, $P < 0.0001$; and third trimester 1.6 ± 0.5 vs 1.9 ± 0.5 μg/mL, $P < 0.0002$). PZ levels at the 20th percentile (1.30 μg/mL) were associated with an increased risk of APO (OR 4.25, 95% CI 1.536–11.759, with a sensitivity of 93%, specificity 32%). In the same group of patients, PS levels were significantly lower in the second and third trimesters among patients with APO compared with patients with NPO (second trimester 34.4 ± 11.8% vs 38.9 ± 10.3%, $P < 0.05$ respectively; and third trimester 27.5 ±8.4 vs 31.2 ± 7.4, $P < 0.025$ respectively). The authors speculate that decreased PZ and PS levels are additional risk factors for APO. These authors also compared first trimester (first trimester) PZ levels in 103 women with subsequent NPO, 106 women with APO, and 20 women known to be thrombophilic, with 6/20 of these women having had APO. The mean first trimester PZ level was significantly lower among patients with APO compared with pregnant control subjects (1.81 ± 0.7 vs 2.21 ± 0.8 μg/mL, respectively, $P < 0.001$). Of patients with known thrombophilia, those with APO had a tendency for lower mean PZ levels compared with those thrombophilic women with NPO (1.5 ± 0.6 vs 2.3 ± 0.9 μg/mL, respectively, $P < 0.0631$). Thus, there is compelling evidence that PZ is another thrombophilic condition associated with pregnancy complications. Further studies are needed to confirm the findings of Paidas et al. who have demonstrated that lower than normal pregnancy-associated PS levels are associated with a variety of adverse pregnancy outcomes.

Abruptio placentae and thrombophilia

The determination of the relationship between thrombophilias and abruptio placentae (decidual hemorrhage) is difficult secondary to the limited number of studies and the confounding variables, including chronic hypertension, and cigarette and cocaine use.[93,94,113,114] de Vries[95] found that 9/31 (29%) patients with abruptio placentae had a PS deficiency, compared with their general population prevalence of 0.2–2%. The prevalence of factor V Leiden, prothrombin gene mutation, and PS deficiency was 22–30%, 18–20%, and 0–29%, respectively (Table 47.8).[79,85,95–97]

IUGR

Infante-Rivard et al.[51] found rates of 4.5% and 2.5% for factor V Leiden and prothrombin gene mutation, respectively, when IUGR was defined as < 10th percentile. In a recent systematic review, factor V Leiden and prothrombin gene mutation were associated with an increased risk of IUGR: OR 2.7 (1.3–5.5), and OR 2.5 (1.3–5.0), respectively, in 10 case–control studies.[98] However, in five cohort studies (three prospective, two retrospective), the relative risk was 0.99 (0.5–1.9). The authors concluded that both factor V Leiden and prothrombin gene

Table 47.8 Abruptio placentae and thrombophilic conditions.

Author	Year	No. of abruptions	FVL positive (%)	PG mutation positive (%)	PS deficiency (%)	Reference
De Vries	1997	31	–	–	29	95
Weiner-Megnangi et al.	1998	27	29.6	–	0	96
Kupferminc et al.	1999	20	25	20	–	79
Kupferminc et al.	2000	27	–	18.5	–	85
Facchinetti	2003	50	22	20	–	97

Table 47.9 Inherited thrombophilia and fetal loss (≥ 20 weeks).

Author	Year	No. of fetal losses	FVL positive (%)	PG mutation positive (%)	PS deficiency (%)	Reference
Preston et al.	1996	141	27	–	29	103
Gris	1999	22	68	28.6	92	100
Dizon–Townson	1997	29	41.4	–	–	104
Kupferminc et al.	1999	12	25	0	–	79
Tal	1999	9	22.2	–	–	105
Lindqvist and Dahlback	2000	269	4.5	–	–	106
Martinelli	2000	11	45.4	–	–	101
Kupferminc et al.	2000	23	–	13.0	–	85
Murphy	2000	16	18.8	–	–	107
Alfirevic	2001	7	–	33.3	42.9	91
Many et al.	2002	6	50	–	–	108
Alonso	2002	110	8	12	–	109
Rey et al.	2003	180	15	–	77.3	99
Hefler et al.	2004	94	10.6	7.4	–	110
Gonen et al.	2005	37	10.8	0	8.1	111

mutation confer an increased risk of giving birth to an IUGR infant, although this may be driven by small, poor-quality studies that demonstrated extreme associations.

Fetal loss

In a meta analysis of 31 studies, Rey et al.[99] found that factor V Leiden was associated with an increased risk of late fetal loss (OR 3.26, 95% CI 1.82–5.83). Gris[100] found a positive correlation between the number of stillbirths and the prevalence of thrombophilias among 232 women with previous late fetal loss (22 weeks) and 464 control subjects. PS deficiency was found in 9 out of 84 (10.7%) with at least two stillbirths, and the presence of factor V Leiden was associated with a high risk of fetal loss at > 22 weeks (OR 7.83, 95% CI 2.83–21.67). Martinelli[101] found that the risk of late fetal death (> 20 weeks) was threefold higher if the patient was a carrier of either factor V Leiden or prothrombin gene mutation. The relative risk of carriers (factor V Leiden, prothrombin gene mutation) for late fetal loss was 3.2 (1.0–10.9) and 3.3 (1.1–10.3) respectively. Martinelli[102] evaluated recurrent late loss and found that factor V Leiden was present in 28.6% of patients with recurrent late loss.

Rey et al.[99] pooled data from nine studies (n = 2087) and found a significant association between fetal loss and the prothrombin gene mutation. Prothrombin gene mutation was associated with recurrent fetal loss before 25 weeks (n = 690 women, OR 2.56, 95% CI 1.04–6.29) and with nonrecurrent fetal loss after 20 weeks (five studies, n = 1299, OR 2.3, 95% CI 1.09–4.87). The prevalence of prothrombin gene mutation ranges from 0 to 33%, and of PS deficiency from 29% to 92% (Table 47.9).[79,85,91,99,100,103–111] On the other hand, Hefler et al.[110] did not find any significant association between factor V Leiden, prothrombin gene mutation, or PS deficiency and fetal death (median gestational age 34 weeks, with range 20–42 weeks). Two other studies that examined recurrent fetal loss and PS deficiency found a significant association (OR 14.7, 95% CI 0.99–218).[100,108] Rey et al.[99] found that PS deficiency was associated with nonrecurrent loss after 22 weeks in three studies (n = 565, OR 7.39, 95% CI 1.28–42.83).

Early pregnancy loss and thrombophilia

The association between early pregnancy loss and thrombophilia has also yielded conflicting results. In three recent systematic reviews, the diversity among the included studies

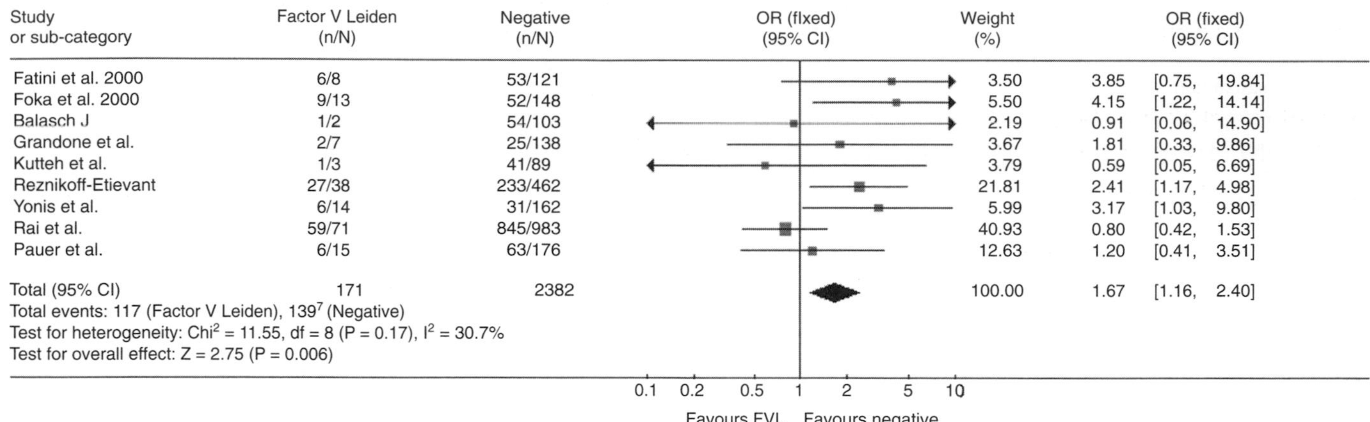

Review: Thrombophilia and early pregnancy loss
Comparison: 01 Factor V Leiden and recurrent fetal loss before 13 weeks
Outcome: 02 Recurrent fetal loss before 13 weeks
Study or sub-category | Factor V Leiden (n/N) | Negative (n/N) | OR (fixed) (95% CI) | Weight (%) | OR (fixed) (95% CI)
Fatini et al. 2000 | 6/8 | 53/121 | 3.50 | 3.85 [0.75, 19.84]
Foka et al. 2000 | 9/13 | 52/148 | 5.50 | 4.15 [1.22, 14.14]
Balasch J | 1/2 | 54/103 | 2.19 | 0.91 [0.06, 14.90]
Grandone et al. | 2/7 | 25/138 | 3.67 | 1.81 [0.33, 9.86]
Kutteh et al. | 1/3 | 41/89 | 3.79 | 0.59 [0.05, 6.69]
Reznikoff-Etievant | 27/38 | 233/462 | 21.81 | 2.41 [1.17, 4.98]
Yonis et al. | 6/14 | 31/162 | 5.99 | 3.17 [1.03, 9.80]
Rai et al. | 59/71 | 845/983 | 40.93 | 0.80 [0.42, 1.53]
Pauer et al. | 6/15 | 63/176 | 12.63 | 1.20 [0.41, 3.51]
Total (95% CI) | 171 | 2382 | 100.00 | 1.67 [1.16, 2.40]
Total events: 117 (Factor V Leiden), 139[7] (Negative)
Test for heterogeneity: Chi² = 11.55, df = 8 (P = 0.17), I² = 30.7%
Test for overall effect: Z = 2.75 (P = 0.006)
0.1 0.2 0.5 1 2 5 10
Favours FVL Favours negative

Figure 47.3 Recurrent first trimester loss and factor V Leiden (from ref. 114). A recent meta-analysis suggests that the factor V Leiden is associated with an increased risk of recurrent first trimester loss (odds ratio 1.67, 95% CI 1.16–2.40).

Review: Thrombophilia and early pregnancy loss
Comparison: 02 Prothrombin mutation and recurrent fetal oss before 13 weeks
Outcome: 01 Recurrent fetal loss before 13 weeks

Study or sub-category	Prothrombin mutation (n/N)	Negative (n/N)	OR (fixed) (95% CI)	Weight (%)	OR (fixed) (95% CI)
Fatini et al. 2000	1/2	58/127		6.48	1.19 [0.07, 19.44]
Foka et al. 2000	4/7	87/150		23.96	0.97 [0.21, 4.47]
Reznikoff-Etievant	20/27	240/463		49.42	2.65 [1.10, 6.40]
Pickering et al.	5/6	70/197		4.97	9.07 [1.04, 79.19]
Pauer et al.	2/5	67/186		15.17	1.18 [0.19, 7.26]
Total (95% CI)	47	1123		100.00	2.25 [1.20, 4.21]

Total events: 32 (Prothrombin mutation), 522 (Negative)
Test for heterogeneity: Chi² = 3.58, df = 4 (P = 0.47), I² = 0%
Test for overall effect: Z = 2.54 (P = 0.01)

0.1 0.2 0.5 1 2 5 10
Favours PTm Favours negative

Figure 47.4 Recurrent first trimester loss and prothrombin gene mutation G20210A (from ref. 114). A recent meta-analysis suggests that the prothrombin gene mutation G2021A is associated with an increased risk of recurrent first trimester loss (odds ratio 2.25, 95% CI 1.20–4.21).

implies that these meta-analyses included heterogeneous studies.[99,112–114] Factors influencing results include inclusion of isolated or recurrent fetal loss, presence or absence of successful live birth in obstetrical history, gestational age cutoff for evaluation, and inclusion of proper control groups. Figures 47.3 and 47.4 demonstrate the latest compilation of data concerning pregnancy loss and factor V Leiden and prothrombin gene mutation respectively.[114] The typical OR for factor V Leiden is 1.67 (1.16–2.40) and, for prothrombin gene mutation, the typical OR is 2.25 (1.20–4.21). There was no increased risk of loss for the MTHFR C677T mutation.[105] Roque et al.[115] reported that the odds of having thrombophilia were actually significantly lower in women with recurrent embryonic losses. In this retrospective cohort study, patients with recurrent early pregnancy loss (two or more) were stratified by gestational age into losses before 9 weeks and 6 days and losses from 10 weeks to 14 weeks and 0 days. Simple correlations between individual factors of thrombophilia and early first trimester loss (below 10 weeks) were mostly nonsignificant and negative for all parameters, when compared with those in late first trimester losses. These authors investigated the association of thrombophilia (anticardiolipin antibodies, lupus anticoagulant, factor V Leiden, prothrombin gene mutation G20210A, homocysteine, deficiencies in PC, PS, or antithrombin, and one measure of thrombophilia or more) and adverse pregnancy outcome in 491 patients with a history of preeclampsia, IUGR < 10th percentile, fetal loss at > 14 weeks, recurrent abortion prior to 14 weeks, abruptio placentae, preterm delivery, and history of thromboembolism. Thrombophilia was associated with an increased risk of fetal loss at > 14 weeks, IUGR, abruptio placentae, and preeclampsia. There was a "dose-dependent" increase in abruptio risk (OR 3.6, 95% CI 1.20–8.6). In those with thrombophilia, preeclampsia was noted in 9%, abruptio in 5.5%, IUGR < 10th percentile in 37%, fetal loss at > 14 weeks in 16.5%, and preterm delivery in 33%. Biological considerations might explain a reduced influence of thrombophilic factors in very early pregnancy losses (< 10 weeks). The blood flow pattern and oxygenation at the placental site change at about 10 weeks of gestation.

Anticoagulation to prevent recurrent adverse pregnancy outcomes in women with thrombophilia

Heparin and aspirin administration is the best strategy for the treatment of recurrent pregnancy loss associated with APS, according to the Cochrane review in 2002.[116] This approach has been associated with a 54% reduction in pregnancy loss and is better than aspirin alone. Steroid administration is associated with an excessive risk of prematurity, and therefore is not recommended as a first-line prevention strategy.

Given that uteroplacental thrombosis is a feature of pregnancies complicated by IUGR, severe preeclampsia and abruptio placentae, and fetal loss in women with thrombophilia, prophylaxis with heparin has been offered to prevent recurrent pregnancy complications in the setting of inherited thrombophilias. The rationale for this approach is that maternal heparin administration will decrease vascular injury and thrombin generation, thereby reducing thrombosis in the uteroplacental circulation.

There are few published studies describing the use of low-molecular-weight heparin (LMWH) with previous adverse pregnancy outcomes (Table 47.10).[117–124] Kupferminc et al.[120] treated 33 women with a history of severe preeclampsia, abruptio placenta, IUGR, or fetal demise and a known thrombophilia with LMWH and low-dose aspirin (LDA). Treated patients had a higher infant birthweight and a higher gestational age at delivery than in the previous pregnancy. Treated pregnancies were not associated with fetal losses or severe preeclampsia. Riyazi et al.[117] found that treatment with LMWH and LDA in patients with previous early-onset preeclampsia and/or severe IUGR and a thrombophilic disorder resulted in a higher infant birthweight than in patients with a comparable history but not receiving this intervention.

Paidas et al.[122] evaluated a cohort of patients carrying either factor V Leiden or prothrombin gene mutation who experi-

Table 47.10 Heparin administration to prevent adverse pregnancy outcome.

Author (reference)	Year	No. of patients	Drug	Patients studied	Outcome
Riyazi et al.[117]	1998	26	Nadroparin + ASA 80 mg	Thrombophilia plus prior preeclampsia or IUGR	Treatment associated with lower rates of preeclampsia/IUGR compared with historical controls
Brenner[118]	2000	50	Enoxaparin	Thrombophilia plus recurrent fetal loss	Treatment associated with higher live birth rates (75% vs 20%) compared with historical controls
Ogueh[119]	2001	24	Unfractionated heparin	Thrombophilia plus IUGR or abruptio placentae	No improvement compared with historical control
Kupferminc et al.[120]	2001	33	Enoxaparin + ASA 100 mg	Thrombophilia plus preeclampsia or IUGR	Higher birthweight and gestational age at delivery
Grandone[121]	2002	25	Unfractionated heparin or enoxaparin	Thrombophilia + APO	Treatment was associated with lower rates of APO in treated (10%) vs untreated (93%)
Paidas et al.[122]	2004	41	Unfractionated or low-molecular-weight heparin	FVL or PGM plus history of fetal loss	Treatment was associated with an 80% reduction in fetal loss (OR 0.21, 95% CI 0.11–0.39)
Gris et al.[123]	2004	160	Enoxaparin or 100 mg aspirin; folic acid 5 mg	Thrombophilia plus fetal loss	Enoxaparin was superior to aspirin. 29% patients treated with LDA and 86% treated with enoxaparin had healthy live birth (OR 15.55, 95% CI 7–34)
Brenner et al.[124]	2004	183	Enoxaparin (40 mg/day or 40 mg b.i.d.)	Thrombophilia + ≥ three losses in the first trimester, or ≥ two losses in the second trimester, or ≥ one loss in the third trimester	Enoxaparin increased the rate of live births (81.4% vs 28.2%, $P < 0.01$ for 40 mg, 76.5% vs 28.3%, $P < 0.01$ for 80 mg), decreased the rate of preeclampsia (3.4% vs 7.1%, $P < 0.01$ for 40 mg; 4.5% vs 15.7%, $P < 0.01$ for 80 mg), and decreased the rate of abruptio placentae (4.4% vs 14.1%, $P < 0.01$ for 40 mg; 3.4% vs 9.6%, $P < 0.1$ for 80 mg)

enced at least one prior APO. A total of 41 patients (28 with factor V Leiden, 13 with prothrombin gene mutation) had 158 pregnancies. They compared the 41 heparin-treated pregnancy outcomes with the remaining 117 untreated pregnancies. Antenatal heparin administration consisted of enoxaparin, dalteparin, or unfractionated heparin. Antenatal heparin administration was associated with an 80% reduction in APO overall (OR 0.21, 95% CI 0.11–0.39, $P < 0.05$). This relationship persisted if first trimester losses were excluded ($n = 111$ total pregnancies, OR 0.46, 95% CI 0.23–0.94, $P < 0.05$).

Brenner et al.[124] reported on the LIVE-ENOX study, a multicenter prospective randomized trial to evaluate the efficacy and safety of two doses of enoxaparin (40 mg/day or 40 mg b.i.d.) in 183 women with recurrent pregnancy loss and thrombophilia. Inclusion criteria were ≥ three losses in the first trimester, ≥ two losses in the second trimester or ≥ one loss in the third trimester. Compared with the patient's historical rates of live birth and pregnancy complications, enoxaparin increased the rate of live birth (81.4% vs 28.2%, $P < 0.01$ for 40 mg, 76.5% vs 28.3%, $P < 0.01$ for 80 mg), decreased the rate of preeclampsia (3.4% vs 7.1%, $P < 0.01$ for 40 mg; 4.5% vs 15.7%, $P < 0.01$ for 80 mg), and decreased the rate of abruptio placentae (4.4% vs 14.1%, $P < 0.01$ for 40 mg; 3.4% vs 9.6%, $P < 0.1$ for 80 mg). The lack of a placebo arm, use of historical control subjects, and the small number of patients are limitations of this study.

Gris et al.[123] compared the administration of LDA 100 mg daily with enoxaparin 40 mg daily from the 8th week of gestation in a cohort of patients with a prior loss after 10 weeks and the presence of heterozygous factor V Leiden, prothrombin gene mutation G20210A, or PS deficiency. The authors found that 23/80 patients treated with aspirin and 69/80 patients treated with enoxaparin had a successful pregnancy (OR 15.5, 95% CI 7–34, $P < 0.0001$). Birthweights were higher, and there were fewer small for gestational age infants in the enoxaparin group.

The small size and inadequate study designs of the published studies do not permit any firm recommendation regarding the antenatal administration of heparin for the sole indication of the prevention of adverse pregnancy outcome.[125] These authors strongly recommended a randomized trial to address the use of anticoagulation for prevention. According to a recent Cochrane review, based upon an extensive literature search from 1966 to 2004 of women with a history of ≥ two spontaneous losses or one fetal demise without apparent cause other than inherited thrombophilia, only two trials were available for review.[126] The other study besides the Gris trial was the trial reported by Tulppala et al.,[127] which involved 82 patients and compared aspirin 50 mg versus placebo in women with three or more unexplained consecutive losses. No differences were noted between the aspirin compared with the placebo group (relative risk 1.00 (0.78–1.29).

Thrombophilia screening: testing and candidates

The selection of suitable patients for thrombophilia screening and the thrombophilia workup continue to evolve. At this time, suitable candidates for thrombophilia screening include those with a history of unexplained fetal loss at > 10 weeks; a history of severe preeclampsia/HELLP at < 36 weeks; a history of abruptio placentae; a history of IUGR ≤ 5th percentile; a personal history of thrombosis; and a family history of thrombosis. Initial thrombophilia evaluation should include: protein C (functional level); PS (functional/free antigen level); antithrombin III (functional level); factor V Leiden [by polymerase chain reaction (PCR)]; prothrombin gene mutation 20210A (PCR); lupus anticoagulant; anticardiolipin antibody IgG, M, A; and platelet count. Other commonly ordered screens include MTHFR C677T mutation, fasting homocysteine level, and β2-glycoprotein-1 IgG, M, A. Depending on the clinical scenario, thrombophilia evaluation can be extended to include other tests, such as PZ, other antiphospholipid antibodies, and the more uncommon factor V mutations, the angiotensin I-converting enzyme (ACE) gene polymorphism, components of the PC system, and PAI-I mutation. Large prospective studies are needed to address the role of the interaction of thrombophilic conditions in the causation of VTE and APO.

Pharmacology of anticoagulation in pregnancy

Thromboembolism and APO management continue to present clinical challenges. The available anticoagulant drugs for the prevention and treatment of VTE include warfarin, unfractionated heparin, LMWH, factor Xa inhibitors, and direct thrombin inhibitors. However, heparins are the mainstay of therapy in pregnancy. Unfractionated heparin enhances antithrombin activity, increases factor Xa inhibitor activity, and inhibits platelet aggregation.[128] LMWH is generated by chemical or enzymatic manipulation of unfractionated heparin from a molecular weight of 15 000 Da to 4000–6500 Da. The smaller size impedes its antithrombin but not antifactor Xa effects. Both LMWH and unfractionated heparin cross the placenta, are considered safe for pregnancy, and are compatible with breastfeeding. Complications associated with heparins include hemorrhage, osteoporosis, and thrombocytopenia. Heparin-induced thrombocytopenia (HIT) occurs in two forms. Type I HIT typically occurs within days of heparin exposure, is self-limited, and is not associated with significant risk of hemorrhage or thrombosis. Type II HIT is an immunoglobulin-mediated syndrome that occurs in the setting of venous or arterial thrombosis, usually 5–14 days following the initiation of heparin therapy. Fortunately, it is quite rare in pregnancy. Type II HIT can be confirmed by serotonin release assays, heparin-induced platelet aggregation assays, flow cytometry, or solid phase immunoassay.[129]

Unfractionated heparin has a short half-life and is administered subcutaneously or via continuous infusion. Usually, patients receiving unfractionated heparin require frequent laboratory monitoring and dosage adjustment. LMWH is administered subcutaneously either once or twice daily. It has advantages over unfractionated heparin including better bioavailability, longer plasma half-life, and more predictable pharmacokinetics and pharmacodynamics. LMWH is much more expensive than unfractionated heparin. A recent review has found that LMWH has a reassuring risk profile, including antenatal bleeding, 0.43 (0.22–0.75); postpartum hemorrhage more than 500 mL, 0.94 (0.61–1.37); wound hematoma, 0.61 (0.36–0.98); thrombocytopenia, 0.11 (0.02–0.32); HIT, 0.00 (0.00–0.11); and osteoporosis, 0.04 (< 0.01–0.20).[130]

Coumarins are vitamin K antagonists that block the generation of vitamin KH2. The latter serves as a cofactor for the post-translational carboxylation of glutamate residues to τ-carboxyglutamates on the N-terminal regions of prothrombin and factors VII, IX, and X as well as the anticlotting agents, PC and PS. The peak effect of warfarin, the most commonly used vitamin K antagonist, occurs 36–72 h after initiating therapy, and it has a half-life of 36–42 h. Aspirin and other nonsteroidal anti-inflammatory drugs, as well as high doses of penicillins and moxolactam, increase the risk of warfarin-associated bleeding by inhibiting platelet function. As PC has a relatively shorter half-life compared with most of the vitamin K-dependent clotting factors, warfarin may initially create a relatively prothrombotic state. Indeed, it may take 6 days to achieve full antithrombotic effects, especially in pregnancy, given the elevated levels of factor VIII and often occurring APC resistance. In pregnancy, it is critical to maintain these women on therapeutic doses of unfractionated heparin or LMWH for 5 days and until the international normalized ratio (INR) reaches the therapeutic range between 2.0 and 3.0 for two successive days.

Several other anticoagulants are now available that may have a role in limited circumstances in pregnancy.[131] Danaparoid is another low-molecular-weight heparinoid that is especially useful in cases of HIT and in cases of heparin allergy. Fondaparinux is a synthetic heparin pentasaccharide that complexes with the antithrombin binding site for heparin to permit the selective inactivation of factor Xa but not thrombin. Given as a once-daily subcutaneous injection, fondaparinux is excreted in the kidney, has a half-life of 15 h, and does not appear to induce HIT. Direct thrombin inhibitors represent another class of anticoagulants.

Hirudin is a 65-amino-acid protein derived the medicinal leech (*Hirudo medicinalis*). It can be used in patients with type II HIT and is readily available in a recombinant form, lepirudin. There is limited use of lepirudin in pregnancy. Argatroban is a synthetic direct thrombin inhibitor that competitively binds to thrombin's active site, has a short half-life (45 min), and is cleared by the liver, making it the direct thrombin inhibitor of choice for patients with renal failure. Bivalirudin is a 20-amino-acid synthetic polypeptide analog of hirudin.

Management of venous thromboembolism in pregnancy: diagnosis of venous thromboembolism

Pregnant patients requiring therapeutic anticoagulation require meticulous care and a thorough understanding of the physiologic changes in pregnancy, underlying pathophysiology, and drug treatment effects. In pregnancy, the diagnosis of VTE is based on history, physical examination, and diagnostic studies. The typically cited signs and symptoms of DVT include erythema, warmth, pain, edema, tenderness, and a positive Homan's sign. However, among patients with these signs and symptoms, the diagnosis of DVT is confirmed in only one-third when reliable objective tests are performed.[132] Venous ultrasound with or without color Doppler has become the primary diagnostic modality for evaluating patients at risk of DVT (Fig. 47.5). The most accurate ultrasonic criterion for diagnosing venous thrombosis is noncompressibility of the venous lumen in a transverse plane under gentle probe pressure using duplex and color flow Doppler.[132] The sensitivity and specificity of venous ultrasound is generally reported to be 90–100% for proximal-vein thromboses, but is thought to be lower with calf-vein thrombosis.[133]

Two other imaging modalities include magnetic resonance imaging (MRI) and impedance plethysmography. The published literature suggests that the range of sensitivity and specificity for MRI in the diagnosis of DVT is 80–100% and 90–100%, respectively, with median published rates of 100% for both.[134] Impedance plethysmography utilizes two sets of electrodes placed around the patient's calf and an oversized blood pressure cuff around the thigh. Published sensitivities and specificities for diagnosing proximal DVT range from 65% to 98% and 83% to 97% respectively.[133] It is expensive, and the test is insensitive (< 20%) for detecting calf-vein and small nonobstructing proximal-vein thromboses. Venography remains the "gold standard" for the diagnosis of DVT with a sensitivity and specificity of 100%, by definition. However, its radiation exposure is a significant disadvantage, and it is not typically used in pregnancy.

Acute pulmonary embolus (APE)

Tachypnea (> 20 breaths/min) and tachycardia (> 100 beats per minute; b.p.m.) are present in 90% of patients with APE, but are nonspecific indices of risk.[135] Symptoms such as dyspnea and pleuritic chest pain are present in up to 90% of

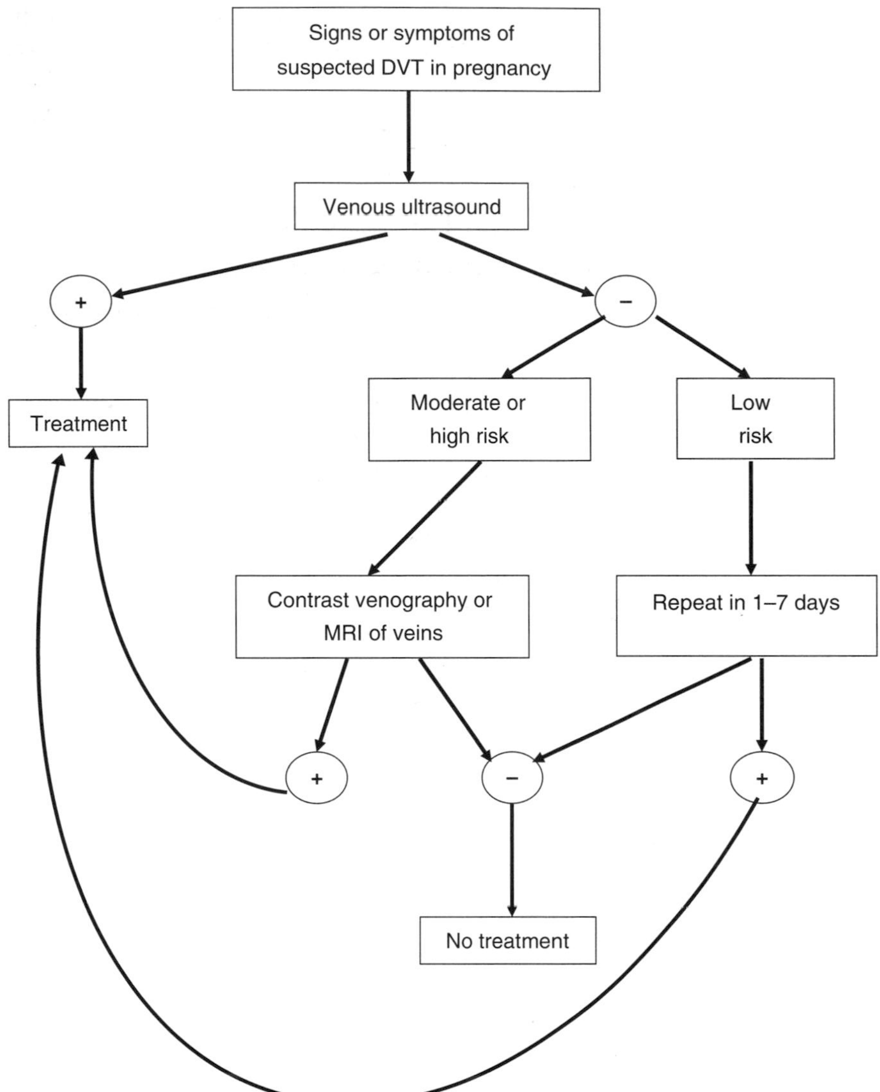

Figure 47.5 Management of suspected DVT in pregnancy. Once a DVT is suspected, a venous ultrasound should be performed to establish the diagnosis of DVT. If positive, anticoagulation should be instituted. If negative, additional testing or repeat venous ultrasound may be indicated, depending upon the level of suspicion for the presence of DVT.

patients with APE, while presyncope and syncope are rarer and indicative of massive emboli.[136]

Electrocardiographic changes may be present in 87% of patients with proven APE who are without underlying cardiopulmonary disease; however, these findings are nonspecific. The Urokinase Pulmonary Embolism Trial found that 26–32% of those with massive APE had electrocardiogram (ECG) manifestations of acute cor pulmonale (S1 Q3 T3 pattern, right-bundle branch block, P-wave pulmonale, or right-axis deviation).[137] Assessments of arterial blood gases and oxygen saturation are also of limited value in APE; pO_2 values of > 80 mmHg are found in 29% of APE patients less than 40 years of age.[138] The alveolar–arterial oxygen tension difference appears to be a more useful indicator of disease with alveolar–arterial differences of > 20 mmHg present in 86% of patients with APE.[135] Chest radiographs may be abnormal in up to 84% of affected patients.[135] Common findings include pleural effusion, pulmonary infiltrates, atelectasis, and elevated hemidiaphragm. A chest radiograph cannot be used to rule out a pulmonary embolism. More than 80% of patients with APE display sonographic imaging or Doppler abnormalities of right-ventricular size or function, including a dilated and hypokinetic right ventricle, tricuspid regurgitation, and absence of pre-existing pulmonary arterial or left-heart pathology.

To confidently diagnose pulmonary embolism, one or more specific diagnostic studies must be performed (Figs 47.6 and 47.7).

Ventilation–perfusion (V/Q) scanning has long been considered a mainstay of the diagnostic evaluation of patients with suspected APE. V/Q scanning is performed by imaging both the pulmonary vascular bed and the airspace. Perfusion scanning is accomplished by injecting isotopically labeled (e.g., technetium-99) human albumin macroaggregates into the bloodstream where they are deposited in the pulmonary capillary bed. Their topographic distribution is then assessed by a photoscanner. Ventilation scanning entails the inhalation of

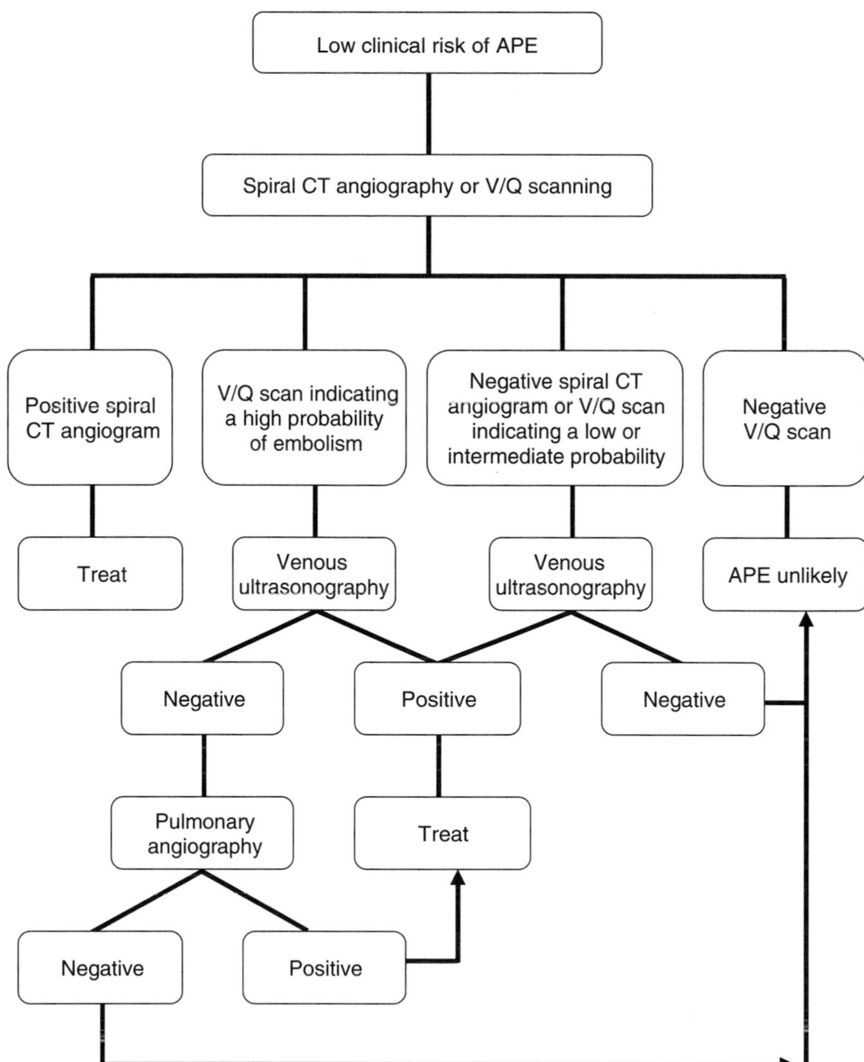

Figure 47.6 Management paradigm for patient at low clinical risk of acute pulmonary embolism. Spiral CT angiography or ventilation/perfusion scanning are indicated as first line imaging modalities. Anticoagulation is indicated in the setting of: a positive spiral CT angiography; a high probability V/Q scan along with a positive venous ultrasound; a positive pulmonary angiogram; negative spiral CT and positive venous ultrasound; low or intermediate V/Q scan and a positive venous ultrasound.

radiolabeled aerosols (e.g., xenon-133), whose distribution in alveolar spaces is assessed by a gamma camera. The combination of perfusion and ventilation scanning allows the discernment of characteristic patterns that can be used to assign diagnostic probabilities. Large mismatched defects (i.e., those associated with abnormal perfusion scans but normal ventilation scans) are associated with APE in 80–96% of high- and moderate-risk patients but in only 50% of low-risk patients.

The Prospective Investigation of Pulmonary Embolism Diagnosis (PIOPED) was a multicenter, collaborative effort designed to determine the sensitivity and specificity of V/Q scanning in patients with signs and symptoms of suspected APE.[139] Patients with high-probability scans had APE in 87.2% of cases, but only 41% of patients with APE had high-probability scans (sensitivity of 41% and specificity of 97%). Patients with intermediate-probability scans had APE in 33.3% of cases, while APE was present in 13.5% of patients with low-probability scans and 3.9% of patients with near-normal or normal scans.

An APE can be present in a substantial percentage of patients with nondiagnostic (low and intermediate probability) V/Q scans if there is a high clinical suspicion of APE. Conversely, 44% of low-risk patients with a high-probability V/Q scan will not ultimately be found to harbor an APE. Spiral (helical) computerized tomographic angiography (spiral CT) is a technique that requires the continuous movement of a patient through a CT scanner as a contrast bolus is administered.[134] It is of limited value with small subsegmental peripheral vessels and horizontally oriented vessels in the right middle lobe. Cross et al.[140] compared spiral CT with V/Q scans for the initial investigation of patients with suspected APE, and observed that a definitive diagnosis was more often possible following spiral CT than with V/Q scanning (90% vs 54%; $P < 0.001$). The principal difference between the two modalities was that spiral CT more often demonstrated nonembolic lesions responsible for the patients' symptoms. However, there was no difference in the prevalence or detection rate of APE in the two groups. The published sensitivi-

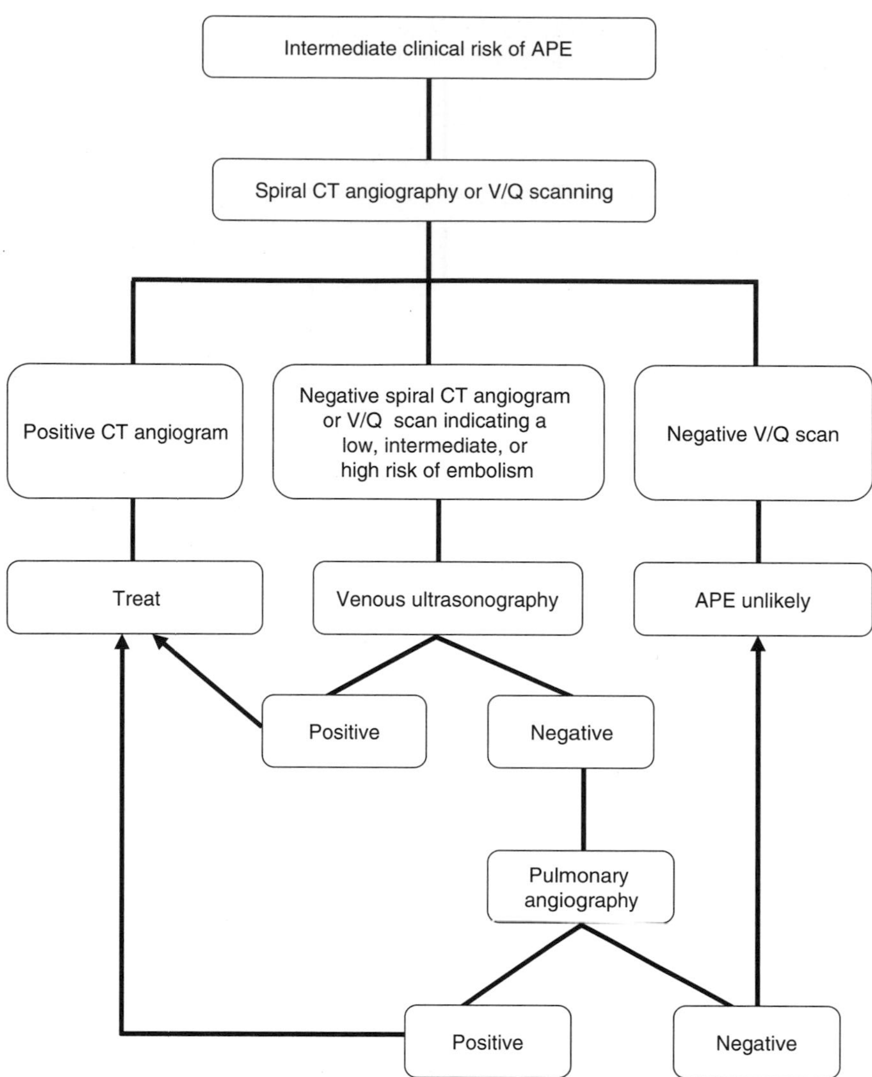

Figure 47.7 Management paradigm for patient at intermediate clinical risk of acute pulmonary embolism. Spiral CT angiography or ventilation/perfusion scanning are indicated as first line imaging modalities. Pulmonary angiography remains the gold standard for the diagnosis of APE. If there is a high clinical risk of acute pulmonary embolism, pulmonary angiography should be performed even if initial tests (spiral CT angiography or V/Q scanning) do not suggest APE.

ties and specificities of spiral CT for the diagnosis of APE range from 53% to 100% (median 87%) and from 78% to 97% (median 95%) respectively.[134]

Conventional pulmonary arteriography

Pulmonary arteriography is considered the gold standard for the diagnosis of APE with sensitivities and specificities of 100% by definition.[134] An APE is diagnosed by the finding of an intraluminal filling defect on two views of a pulmonary artery. The procedure carries with it a 0.5% mortality rate and a complication rate of 3%. The majority (90%) of cases of APE arise from lower extremity DVTs; among patients with APE, 50% will be found to harbor a DVT, including up to 20% of patients without lower extremity signs or symptoms.[136] Finally, the routine use of D-dimer as a screen for thromboembolism is not helpful in pregnancy given the normal hematologic changes in pregnancy (Table 47.1).

Radiation exposure in pregnancy

Concern often arises about the level of radiation exposure to the fetus from the various diagnostic modalities employed in the evaluation of patients at risk for VTE. Limited contrast venography with an abdominal shield generates < 500 μGy (< 0.05 rad). Full venography without a shield exposes the fetus to 3.1 mGy (0.31 rad). Pulmonary arteriography from the brachial vein route generates less than 500 μGy (0.05 rad) but from the femoral vein route, it is 2.2–3.3 mGy (0.22–0.33 rad), making the former the preferable route in pregnancy. V/Q scans expose the fetus to less than 120 μGy (0.012 rad) from the technetium-99 perfusion scan and less than 190 μGy (0.019 rad) from the xenon-133 ventilation scan. Spiral CT angiography exposes the fetus to a maximum of 131 μGy (0.013 rad). Virtually all these exposures are substantially less than 5 rad and thus pose no known risk of spontaneous abortion, teratogenicity, or perinatal morbidity. Doses above 1 rad may create a marginally increased risk of childhood leukemia (from 1 : 3000 baseline to 1 : 2000).[141,142]

Neither mutagenic nor teratogenic effects have been described after the administration of gadolinium or iodinated contrast media.[143] Concerns about fetal goiter following maternal radiographic contrast exposure suggest that fetal heart rates should be assessed to rule out hypothyroidism, and neonatal thyroid function should be checked during the first week of life.[143]

Treatment of venous thromboembolism

Before initiating anticoagulation therapy, a thrombophilia panel should be obtained as noted above. Functional clotting factor testing should be performed well after the cessation of anticoagulant therapy to diagnose a factor deficiency. Women with new-onset VTE during a current pregnancy should receive therapeutic anticoagulation for at least 20 weeks during the pregnancy followed by prophylactic therapy (Table 47.11). After delivery, patients require a minimum of 6 weeks of anticoagulation. During pregnancy, unfractionated heparin and LMWH are the anticoagulants of choice. Postpartum, oral anticoagulation with warfarin may be started and is considered to be safe in breastfeeding mothers. As osteoporosis is more common with doses of heparin greater than 15 000 U/day employed for more than 6 months, all patients treated with heparin should receive 1500 mg of calcium supplementation per day. Postpartum bone densitometry may be appropriate in such patients.

In pregnancy, LMWH from multidose vials containing benzoyl alcohol, which is potentially toxic to the fetus and newborn, should be avoided. The goals of therapy for an acute VTE in pregnancy are to maintain the activated partial thromboplastin time (aPTT) between 1.5 and 2.5 times control when using unfractionated heparin. The dose required may vary greatly between women secondary to interpatient differences in heparin-binding proteins during pregnancy. The aPTT should be evaluated every 4–6 h during the initial phase of therapy and adjustments made in dosage as needed (see Tables 47.9 and 47.10). Intravenous therapeutic unfractionated heparin should be continued for at least 5–10 days or until clinical improvement is noted. Thereafter, therapeutic doses of unfractionated heparin may be administered subcutaneously every 8–12 h in order to maintain the aPTT at 1.5–2 times control levels 6 h after the injection. These should be continued for 20 weeks followed by prophylactic dosages For example, prophylactic doses of unfractionated heparin can range from 5000 to 10 000 U subcutaneously every 12 h titrated to maintain an antifactor Xa level of 0.1–0.2 IU/mL 6 h after the last injection. Patients with highly thrombogenic thrombophilias such as antithrombin deficiency or those homozygous for the factor V Leiden or prothrombin G20210A gene mutations or compound heterozygotes for these mutations require therapeutic anticoagulation throughout pregnancy.

If vaginal or Cesarean delivery occurs more than 4 h after a prophylactic dose of unfractionated heparin, the patient is not at significant risk of hemorrhagic complications. Protamine sulfate may be administered to those patients with an elevated aPTT receiving prophylactic or therapeutic unfractionated heparin who are about to deliver vaginally or by Cesarean section.

Low-molecular-weight heparin

For therapeutic dosing, the antifactor Xa level should be maintained at 0.6–1.0 U/mL 4–6 h after injection (e.g., starting with enoxaparin 1 mg/kg subcutaneously every 12 h). Again, treatment should continue for 20 weeks and then prophylactic dosages should be given (e.g., enoxaparin 40 mg subcutaneously every 12 h, adjusted to maintain antifactor Xa levels at 0.1–0.2 U/mL 4 h after an injection). As noted, patients with highly thrombogenic thrombophilias require therapeutic anticoagulation throughout pregnancy. As regional anesthesia is contraindicated within 18–24 h of LMWH administration, we recommend switching to unfractionated heparin at 36 weeks or earlier if preterm delivery is expected.

If vaginal or Cesarean delivery occurs more than 12 h from prophylactic or 24 h from therapeutic doses of LMWH, the patient should not experience anticoagulation-related problems with delivery. Protamine may partially reverse the anticoagulant effects of LMWH (see previous section).

Postpartum

Either unfractionated heparin or LMWH can be restarted 3–6 h after vaginal delivery or 6–8 h after Cesarean delivery. Warfarin should be started on the first postdelivery day. Therapeutic doses of unfractionated heparin or LMWH are needed for 5 days and until the INR reaches the therapeutic range between 2.0 and 3.0 for 2 successive days.

Surgery and thrombolytic therapy

Pregnancy poses special concerns about such therapy given the risk of abruptio placentae and puerperal hemorrhage. Turrentine et al.,[144] reviewed outcomes among 172 pregnant patients treated with thrombolytic therapy and reported that the maternal mortality rate was 1.2%, the fetal loss rate was 6%, and that maternal complications from hemorrhage occurred in 8%. Recombinant tissue plasminogen activator (rtPA) has been successfully administered to treat a massive pulmonary embolism at a dose of 10 mg intravenous bolus, then 90 mg infusion/2 h, followed by unfractionated heparin for 48 h, then four times/day LMWH (antifactor Xa level 0.5–1.0 U/mL). This approach should be avoided peripartum

Table 47.11 Anticoagulation in pregnancy: indications and dosing.

Indication	Description	Antepartum		Postpartum	
		Therapeutic	Prophylactic	Therapeutic	Prophylactic
VTE current pregnancy		X		*	
High-risk thrombophilia Factor V Leiden homozygous Prothrombin G20210A mutation homozygous Antithrombin III deficiency	History of VTE or APO*	X			X
	No history		X		X
Intermediate-risk thrombophilia Compound heterozygote (FVL/prothrombin G20210A)			X		X
Low-risk thrombophilia Factor V Leiden heterozygous	Prior VTE		X		X
	History of APO† but not VTE		± X‡		X§
Prothrombin G20210A mutation heterozygous Protein C deficiency Protein S deficiency Hyperhomocystein emia (refractory to folate therapy)	No history of VTE or APO†				X§
No thrombophilia	Prior VTE				X
Hyperhomocysteinemia	Prior VTE or		X		X§§

* VTE during current pregnancy should receive therapeutic anticoagulation for 20+ weeks during pregnancy, followed by prophylactic therapy for up to 6 weeks postpartum.

† Adverse pregnancy outcome (APO) includes early-onset severe preeclampsia, unexplained recurrent abruptio placentae, severe IUGR, intrauterine fetal demise (>10 weeks) with placental thrombosis or infarction.

‡ Patients with less thrombogenic thrombophilias and histories of APO should be treated prophylactically in the antepartum period if the clinical scenario suggests a high risk of recurrence or there are other thrombotic risk factors (obesity, immobilization, etc.).

§ If Cesarean delivery or first-degree relative with history of VTE.

§§ Cases of hyperhomocysteinemia unresponsive to folate, vitamin B6, and vitamin B12 therapy.

Notes

Unfractionated heparin (UFH)
- Initial dose of UFH for acute VTE to keep aPTT 1.5–2.5 times control. Thereafter, UFH may be given subcutaneously q 8–12 h to keep aPTT 1.5–2 times control (when tested 6 h after injection) for therapeutic levels.
- Prophylactic doses may range from 5000 to 10 000 units subcutaneously q 12 h and can be titrated to achieve heparin levels (by protamine titration assay) of 0.1–0.2 U/mL.

Low-molecular-weight heparin (LMWH)
- Therapeutic doses of Lovenox (enoxaparin) may start at 1 mg/kg subcutaneously q12 h. Therapeutic doses should be titrated to achieve antifactor Xa levels of 0.6–1.0 U/mL (when tested 4-6 h after injection).
- Prophylactic doses of Lovenox (enoxaparin) may start at 40 mg subcutaneously q12 h. Prophylactic doses should be titrated to achieve antifactor Xa levels of 0.1–0.2 U/mL 4 h after injection.
- Regional anesthesia is contraindicated within 18–24 h of LMWH and thus LMWH should be converted to UFH at 36 weeks or earlier if clinically indicated.

Postpartum
- Heparin anticoagulation (LMWH or UFH) may be restarted 3–6 h after vaginal delivery and 6–8 h after Cesarean.
- Warfarin anticoagulation may be started on postpartum day 1.
- Therapeutic doses of LMWH or UFH must be continued for 5 days and until the INR reaches the therapeutic range (2.0–3.0) for 2 successive days.

Maternal and fetal surveillance
- Fetal growth should be monitored every 4–6 weeks beginning at 20 weeks in all patients on anticoagulation.
- Nonstress tests (NSTs) and biophysical profiles (BPPs) may be appropriate at 36 weeks or earlier as clinically indicated.

because of the hemorrhagic risk from the placental site.[145] However, given the limited evidence of the benefit of such therapy, its use in pregnant patients should be limited.

Anticoagulation in pregnancy: special considerations

Recurrent VTE in women with prior VTE

Antepartum heparin is not necessary in patients without thrombophilia and whose prior VTE is associated with temporary risk factors, based upon the study by Brill-Edwards et al.[146] In a prospective evaluation of 125 women with a single previous episode of VTE, antepartum heparin was withheld. In the 95 patients who did not have a known thrombophilia and whose prior VTE was associated with a temporary risk factor, the recurrence of VTE was 0% (95% CI 0–8.0). In patients with thrombophilia and/or idiopathic prior VTE, the relative risk of recurrent antepartum VTE was 5.9 (1.2–16%). Antepartum prophylaxis is indicated in the latter group of patients. Postpartum anticoagulation is indicated in both groups.

Mechanical heart valves

There is no ideal anticoagulation strategy for this especially high-risk clinical dilemma. Some experts suggest using therapeutic LMWH in this setting, even though failures have occurred with this regimen.[147] One option is enoxaparin 1 mg/kg q 12 h and warfarin discontinued either before or immediately after pregnancy is diagnosed. Trough levels of enoxaparin must be 0.5 IU/mL. Peak antifactor Xa levels should ideally be 0.8–1.0 IU/mL, but levels can safely be obtained with the upper range of the peak antifactor-Xa level being 1.5 IU/mL. Weekly peak and trough antifactor-Xa levels should be obtained.

Antithrombin deficiency

Patients with antithrombin deficiency represent the highest thrombogenic risk. Patients with antithrombin deficiency should receive antithrombin concentrate if they experience an acute arterial or venous thromboembolism. Human antithrombin III (ATIII) is available as Thrombate III® (Bayer Healthcare), a sterile, preservative-free, nonpyrogenic, biologically stable, lyophilized preparation of purified human ATIII. The baseline antithrombin level is expressed as the percentage of the normal level based on the functional ATIII assay. The goal is to increase the antithrombin levels to those found in normal human plasma (around 100%).

Summary

Thromboembolism continues to remain a leading cause of maternal mortality. Prompt diagnosis and initiation of therapy are essential to optimize maternal and perinatal outcome. Doppler ultrasound is a valuable test in the evaluation of patients suspected of having a deep venous thrombosis, while ventilation–perfusion scanning and spiral CT scanning are key diagnostic tests in the evaluation of patients suspected of having a pulmonary embolus. In select cases, pulmonary angiography is a necessary diagnostic test. Suitable candidates for thrombophilia screening include those with a history of unexplained fetal loss at > 10 weeks; a history of severe preeclampsia/HELLP at < 36 weeks; a history of abruptio placentae; a history of IUGR ≤ 5th percentile; a personal history of thrombosis; and a family history of thrombosis. Unfractionated heparin and LMWHs are the mainstay of treatment and prevention strategies to reduce the risk of thrombotic complications. Venous thromboembolism should be treated with therapeutic anticoagulation for a minimum of 20 weeks, with prophylactic dosing extended to a minimum of 6 weeks postpartum. Assessment of risk factors for thromboembolism will optimize treatment and prevention strategies and minimize hemorrhagic complications associated with anticoagulation.

Key points

1. Venous thromboembolism is a leading cause of death in women. It is estimated that VTE complicates 1 in 1000 pregnancies, but the precise frequency of thromboembolism is probably underestimated.
2. Pregnancy is associated with significant elevations in a number of clotting factors. Fibrinogen concentration is doubled, and 20–1000% increases in factors VII, VIII, IX, X, XII, and von Willebrand factor are observed, with maximum levels reached at term. Protein S decreases in pregnancy. Mean protein S free antigen levels have been reported to be 38.9 ± 10.3% and 31.2 ± 7.4% in the second and third trimesters respectively.
3. The high-risk thrombophilias include antithrombin III deficiency, factor V Leiden homozygosity, and prothrombin gene (G20210A) mutation. Heterozygous factor V Leiden is associated with a 0.2% risk of thromboembolism associated with pregnancy, while heterozygous prothrombin gene mutation is associated with a 0.5% risk. Compound heterozygous factor V Leiden and prothrombin gene mutation is associated with a 4.6% risk of thromboembolism.

4 Antiphospholipid antibody syndrome is defined by the combination of VTE, obstetric complications, and antiphospholipid antibodies (APA). Antiphospholipid antibodies must be present on two or more occasions at least 6 weeks apart, and are immunoglobulins directed against proteins bound to negatively charged surfaces, usually anionic phospholipids.

5 Antiphospholipid antibodies have commonly been found in the general obstetric population, with one survey demonstrating that 2.2% of such patients have either IgM or IgG anticardiolipin antibodies, with most such women having relatively uncomplicated pregnancies.

6 There is a 5% risk of VTE during pregnancy and the puerperium among patients with APA despite treatment.

7 Suitable candidates for thrombophilia screening include those with a history of unexplained fetal loss at > 10 weeks; a history of severe preeclampsia/HELLP at < 36 weeks; a history of abruptio placentae; a history of IUGR ≤ 5th percentile; a personal history of thrombosis; and a family history of thrombosis.

8 Initial thrombophilia evaluation should include: protein C (functional level); PS (functional/free antigen level); ATIII (functional level); factor V Leiden (PCR); prothrombin gene mutation 20210A (PCR); lupus anticoagulant; anticardiolipin antibody IgG, M, A; and platelet count. Other commonly ordered screens include MTHFR C677T mutation, fasting homocysteine level, and β2-glycoprotein-I IgG, M, A.

9 Heparin and aspirin administration is the best strategy for the treatment of recurrent pregnancy loss associated with antiphospholipid antibody syndrome.

10 Therapeutic anticoagulation during the antepartum period should be reserved for patients with mechanical heart valves, VTE in the current pregnancy, high-risk thrombophilias [antithrombin III deficiency, factor V Leiden homozygosity, or prothrombin gene (G20210A) mutation] with a history of VTE or adverse pregnancy outcome.

11 Venous thromboembolism should be treated with therapeutic anticoagulation for a minimum of 20 weeks, with prophylactic dosing extended to a minimum of 6 weeks postpartum.

12 Appropriate treatment of the antiphospholipid antibody syndrome includes prophylactic anticoagulation and aspirin in the antepartum period and prophylactic anticoagulation alone in the postpartum period.

13 Dosing of therapeutic anticoagulation should be titrated to keep the PTT between 1.5 and 2.5 times control for unfractionated heparin and antifactor Xa levels between 0.6 and 1.2 U/mL for LMWH.

14 Because of its long half-life and the difficulty in reversing its effects, LMWH should be switched to unfractionated heparin at 36 weeks or earlier (if early delivery is anticipated).

15 Heparin anticoagulation may be restarted 3–6 h after vaginal delivery and 6–8 h after Cesarean delivery. Warfarin may be started postpartum day 1.

16 Therapeutic doses of LMWH or unfractionated heparin must be continued for 5 days and until the INR reaches the therapeutic range (2.0–3.0) for 2 successive days.

17 Heparin anticoagulation has been associated with thrombocytopenia (3%) and osteoporosis and, thus, patients should be managed with periodic platelet counts and calcium supplementation.

18 Fetal surveillance of patients on anticoagulation during pregnancy should include fetal growth evaluation every 4–6 weeks beginning at 20 weeks and fetal testing with nonstress tests and/or biophysical profiles beginning at 36 weeks, or earlier if clinically indicated.

19 Antepartum heparin is not necessary in patients without thrombophilia and prior VTE associated with a temporary risk factor.

20 Two useful agents in pregnancy when heparin cannot be administered are: danaparoid, a low-molecular-weight heparinoid; and fondaparinux, a synthetic heparin pentasaccharide.

References

1 Eldor A. Thrombophilia, thrombosis and pregnancy. *Thromb Haemost* 2001;86:104–111.

2 Gherman RB, Goodwin TM, Leung B, et al. Incidence, clinical characteristics, and timing of objectively diagnosed venous thromboembolism during pregnancy. *Obstet Gynecol* 1999;94:730–734.

3 Andres RL, Miles A. Venous thromboembolism and pregnancy. *Obstet Gynecol Clin North Am* 2001;28:613–630.

4 Nierkegaard A. Incidence and diagnosis of deep venous thrombosis associated with pregnancy. *Acta Obstet Gynecol Scand* 1983;62:239–243.

5 Wessler S. Medical management of venous thrombosis. *Annu Rev Med* 1976;27:313–319.

6 Kakkar V. Prevention of venous thrombosis and pulmonary embolism. *Am J Cardiol* 1990;65:50–54.

7 Villasanta U. Thromboembolic disease in pregnancy. *Am J Obstet Gynecol* 1965;93:142–160.

8 Ruggeri ZM, Dent JA, Saldivar E. Contribution of distinct adhesive interactions to platelet aggregation in flowing blood. *Blood* 1999;94:172–178.

9 Pytela R, Pierschbacher MD, Ginsberg MH, et al. Platelet membrane glycoprotein IIb/IIIa: member of a family of Arg-Gly-Asp-specific adhesion receptors. *Science* 1986;231:1559–1562.

10 Nemerson Y. Tissue factor and hemostasis. *Blood* 1988;71:1–8.

11 Mackman N. Role of tissue factor in hemostasis, thrombosis, and

vascular development. *Arterioscler Thromb Vasc Biol* 2004;24: 1015–1022.

12 Giesen PL, Nemerson Y. Tissue factor on the loose. *Semin Thromb Hemost* 2000;26:379–384.

13 Falati S, Liu Q, Gross P, et al. Accumulation of tissue factor into developing thrombi in vivo is dependent upon microparticle P-selectin glycoprotein ligand 1 and platelet P-selectin. *J Exp Med* 2003;197:1585–1598.

14 Neuenschwander PF, Fiore MM, Morrissey JH. Factor VII autoactivation proceeds via interaction of distinct protease–cofactor and zymogen–cofactor complexes. Implications of a two-dimensional enzyme kinetic mechanism. *J Biol Chem* 1993; 268:21489–21492.

15 Broze GJ, Jr. The rediscovery and isolation of TFPI. *J Thromb Haemost* 2003;1:1671–1675.

16 Dahlback B. Progress in the understanding of the protein C anticoagulant pathway. *Int J Hematol* 2004;79:109–116.

17 Han X, Fiehler R, Broze GJ, Jr. Characterization of the protein Z-dependent protease inhibitor. *Blood* 2000;96:3049–3055.

18 Kemkes-Matthes B, Matthes KJ. Protein Z. *Semin Thromb Hemost* 2001;5:551–556.

19 Broze GJ, Jr. Protein Z-dependent regulation of coagulation. *Thromb Haemost* 2001;86:8–13.

20 Broze GJ, Jr. Protein-Z and thrombosis. *Lancet* 2001;357:933–934.

21 Han X, Huang ZF, Fiehler R, Broze GJ, Jr. The protein Z-dependent protease inhibitor is a serpin. *Biochemistry* 1999;38:11073–11078.

22 Yurdakok M, Gurakan B, Ozbag E, et al. Plasma protein Z levels in healthy newborn infants. *Am J Hematol* 1995;48:206–207.

23 Miletich JP, Broze GJ, Jr. Human plasma protein Z antigen: range in normal subjects and effect of warfarin therapy. *Blood* 1987;69:1580–1586.

24 Kemkes-Matthes B, Nees M, Kuhnel G, et al. Protein Z influences the prothrombotic phenotype in factor V Leiden patients. *Thromb Res* 2002;106;183–185.

25 McColl MD, Deans A, Maclean P, et al. Plasma protein Z deficiency is common in women with antiphospholipid antibodies. *Br J Haematol* 2003;120:913–914.

26 Steffano B, Forastiero R, Martinuzzo M, Kordich L. Low plasma protein Z levels in patients with antiphospholipid antibodies. *Blood Coagul Fibrinolysis* 2001;12:411–412.

27 Gamba G, Bertolino G, Montani N, et al. Bleeding tendency of unknown origin and protein Z levels. *Thromb Res* 1998;90: 291–295.

28 Preissner KT, Zwicker L, Muller-Berhaus G. Formation, characterization and detection of a ternary complex between protein S, thrombin and antithrombin III in serum. *Biochem J* 1987;243: 105–111.

29 Schatz F, Lockwood CJ. Progestin regulation of plasminogen activator inhibitor type-1 in primary cultures of the endometrial stromal and decidual cells. *J Clin Endocrinol Metab* 1993;77: 621–625.

30 Bouma BN, Meijers JC. New insights into factors affecting clot stability: a role for thrombin activatable fibrinolysis inhibitor (TAFI; plasma procarboxypeptidase B, plasma procarboxypeptidase U, procarboxypeptidase R). *Semin Hematol* 2004;41(1 Suppl. 1):13–19.

31 Urano T, Ihara H, Takada Y, et al. The inhibition of human factor Xa by plasminogen activator inhibitor type 1 in the presence of calcium ion, and its enhancement by heparin and vitronectin. *Biochim Biophys Acta* 1996;1298:199–208.

32 Romero A, Alonso C, Rincon M, et al. Risk of venous thromboembolic disease in women: a qualitative systematic review. *Eur J Obstet Gynecol Reprod Biol* 2005;epub ahead of print.

33 Lindqvist P, Dahlback B, Marsal K. Thrombotic risk during pregnancy: a population study. *Obstet Gynecol* 1999;94: 595–599.

34 Danilenko-Dixon DR, Heit JA, Silverstein MD, et al. Risk factors for deep vein thrombosis and pulmonary embolism during pregnancy or post partum: a population-based, case-control study. *Am J Obstet Gynecol* 2001;184:104–110.

35 Anderson FA, Jr, Spencer FA. Risk factors for venous thromboembolism. *Circulation* 2003;107(23 Suppl. 1):I9–16.

36 Lockwood CJ, Krikun G, Schatz F. The decidua regulates hemostasis in the human endometrium. *Semin Reprod Endocrinol* 1999;17:45–51.

37 Erlich J, Parry GC, Fearns C, et al. Tissue factor is required for uterine hemostasis and maintenance of the placental labyrinth during gestation. *Proc Natl Acad Sci USA* 1999;96:8138–8143.

38 Bremme KA. Haemostatic changes in pregnancy. *Best Pract Res Clin Haematol* 2003;16:153–168.

39 Bremme K, Ostlund E, Almqvist I, et al. Enhanced thrombin generation and fibrinolytic activity in normal pregnancy and the puerperium. *Obstet Gynecol* 1992;80:132–137.

40 Paidas MJ, Ku DW, Lee MJ, et al. Protein Z, protein S levels are lower in patients with thrombophilia and subsequent pregnancy complications. *J Thromb Haemost* 2005;3:497–501.

41 Paidas M, Ku DW, Arkel Y, et al. Normal pregnancy is associated with the development of protein S and protein Z antibodies, independent of PS and PZ level. *Am J Obstet Gynecol* 2004;191:S491.

42 Quack Loetscher KC, Stiller R, Roos M, et al. Protein Z in normal pregnancy. *Thromb Haemost* 2005;93:706–709.

43 Paidas MJ, Ku DH, Langhoff-Roos J, Arkel YS. Inherited thrombophilias and adverse pregnancy outcome: screening and management. *Semin Perinatol*, 2005;29:150–163.

44 Dahlback B. Inherited resistance to activated protein C, a major cause of venous thrombosis, is due to a mutation in the factor V gene. *Haemostasis* 1994;24:139–151.

45 Ridker PM, Miletich JP, Hennekens CH, Buring JE. Ethnic distribution of factor V Leiden in 4047 men and women. Implications for venous thromboembolism screening. *JAMA* 1997;277: 1305–1307.

46 Lockwood CJ. Inherited thrombophilias in pregnant patients. *Prenat Neonat Med* 2001;6:3–14.

47 Voorberg J, Roelse J, Koopman R, et al. Association of idiopathic venous thromboembolism with single point-mutation at arg506 of factor V. *Lancet* 1994;343:1535–1536.

48 Poort SR, Rosendaal FR, Reitsma PH, Bertina RM. A common genetic variation in the 3′-untranslated region of the prothrombin gene is associated with elevated plasma prothrombin levels and an increase in venous thrombosis. *Blood* 1996;88: 3698–3703.

49 Gerhardt A, Scharf RE, Beckmann MW, et al. Prothrombin and factor V mutations in women with a history of thrombosis during pregnancy and the puerperium. *N Engl J Med* 2000;342:374–380.

50 Dizon-Townson D. and NICHD MFM U Network. The relationship of the factor V Leiden mutation and pregnancy outcomes for mother and fetus. *Am J Obstet Gynecol* 2002;187:Abstract 363.

51 Infante-Rivard C, Rivard GE, Yotov WV, et al. Absence of association of thrombophilia polymorphisms with intrauterine growth restriction. *N Engl J Med* 2002;347:19–25.

52 Nelen WL, Blom HJ, Steegers EA, et al. Hyperhomocysteinemia and recurrent early pregnancy loss: a meta-analysis. *Fertil Steril* 2000;74:1196–1199.

53 Francis CW. Plasminogen activator inhibitor-1 levels and polymorphisms. *Arch Pathol Lab Med* 2002;126:1401–1404.

54 Juul K, Tybjaerg-Hansen A, Steffensen R, et al. Factor V Leiden: The Copenhagen City Heart Study and 2 meta-analyses. *Blood* 2002;100:3–10.

55 Price DT, Ridker PM. Factor V Leiden mutation and the risks for thromboembolic disease: a clinical perspective. *Ann Intern Med* 1997;127:895–903.

56 Franco RF, Reitsma PH. Genetic risk factors of venous thrombosis. *Hum Genet* 2001;109:369–384.

57 Aznar J, Vaya A, Estelles A, et al. Risk of venous thrombosis in carriers of the prothrombin G20210A variant and factor V Leiden and their interaction with oral contraceptives. *Haematologica* 2000;85:1271–1276.

58 Emmerich J, Rosendaal FR, Cattaneo M, et al. Combined effect of factor V Leiden and prothrombin 20210A on the risk of venous thromboembolism – pooled analysis of 8 case–control studies including 2310 cases and 3204 controls. Study Group for Pooled-Analysis in Venous Thromboembolism. *Thromb Haemost* 2001;86:809–816.

59 Langman LJ, Ray JG, Evrovski J, et al. Hyperhomocyst(e)inemia and the increased risk of venous thromboembolism: more evidence from a case-control study. *Arch Intern Med* 2000;160: 961–964.

60 Vossen CY, Conard J, Fontcuberta J, et al. Familial thrombophilia and lifetime risk of venous thrombosis. *J Thromb Haemost* 2004;2:1526–1532.

61 Goodwin AJ, Rosendaal FR, Kottke-Marchant K, Bovill EG. A review of the technical, diagnostic, and epidemiologic considerations for protein S assays. *Arch Pathol Lab Med* 2002;126:1349–1366.

62 Wilson WA, Gharavi AE, Koike T, et al. International consensus statement on preliminary classification criteria for definite antiphospholipid syndrome. *Arthritis Rheum* 1999;42:1309–1311.

63 Galli M, Barbui T. Antiphospholipid antibodies and thrombosis: strength of association. *Hematol J* 2003;4:180–186.

64 Galli M, Luciani D, Bertolini G, Barbui T. Anti-beta 2-glycoprotein I, antiprothrombin antibodies, and the risk of thrombosis in the antiphospholipid syndrome. *Blood* 2003;102: 2717–2723.

65 Wahl DG, Guillemin F, de Maistre E, et al. Risk for venous thrombosis related to antiphospholipid antibodies in systemic lupus erythematosus – a meta-analysis. *Lupus* 1997;6:467–473.

66 Garcia-Fuster MJ, Fernandez C, Forner MJ, Vaya A. Risk factors and clinical characteristics of thromboembolic venous disease in young patients: a prospective study. *Med Clin (Barc)* 2004;123:217–219.

67 Branch DW, Silver RM, Blackwell JL, et al. Outcome of treated pregnancies in women with antiphospholipid syndrome: an update of the Utah experience. *Obstet Gynecol* 1992;80:614–620.

68 Cervera R, Piette JC, Font JK, et al. Euro-Phospholipid Project Group. Antiphospholipid syndrome: clinical and immunologic manifestations and patterns of disease expression in a cohort of 1,000 patients. *Arthritis Rheum* 2002;46:1019–1027.

69 Branch DW, Silver RM. Criteria for antiphospholipid syndrome: early pregnancy loss, fetal loss or recurrent pregnancy loss? *Lupus* 1996;5:409–413.

70 Rai RS, Clifford K, Cohen H, Regan L. High prospective fetal loss rate in untreated pregnancies of women with recurrent miscarriage and antiphospholipid antibodies. *Hum Reprod* 1995; 10:3301–3304.

71 Lockwood C, Romero R, Feinberg R, et al. The prevalence and biologic significance of lupus anticoagulant and anticardiolipin antibodies in a general obstetric population. *Am J Obstet Gynecol* 1989;161:369–373.

72 Field SL, Brighton TA, McNeil HP, Chesterman CN. Recent insights into antiphospholipid antibody-mediated thrombosis. *Baillieres Best Pract Res Clin Haematol* 1999;12:407–422.

73 Rand JH, Wu XX, Andree HA, et al. Pregnancy loss in the antiphospholipid-antibody syndrome: a possible thrombogenic mechanism. *N Engl J Med* 1997;337:154–160.

74 Girardi G, Redecha P, Salmon JE. Heparin prevents antiphospholipid antibody-induced fetal loss by inhibiting complement activation. *Nature Med* 2004;10:1222–1226.

75 Dekker GA. Underlying disorders associated with severe early-onset preeclampsia. *Am J Obstet Gynecol* 1995;173: 1042–1048.

76 Dizon-Townson D. The factor V Leiden mutation may predispose women to severe preeclampsia. *Am J Obstet Gynecol* 1996;175:902–905.

77 Nagy B. Detection of factor V Leiden mutation in severe preeclamptic Hungarian women. *Clin Genet* 1998;53:478–481.

78 Krauss T. Activated protein C resistance and factor V Leiden in patients with hemolysis, elevated liver enzymes, low platelets syndrome. *Obstet Gynecol* 1998;92:457–460.

79 Kupferminc, MJ, Eldor, A, Steinman, N, et al. Increased frequency of genetic thrombophilia in women with complications of pregnancy. *N Engl J Med* 1999;340:9.

80 VanPampus EC. High prevalence of hemostatic abnormalities in women with a history of severe preeclampsia. *Am J Obstet Gynecol* 1999;180:1146–1150.

81 DeGroot CJ. Preeclampsia and genetic risk factors for thrombosis: a case–control study. *Am J Obstet Gynecol* 1999;181: 975–980.

82 Kupferminc MJ, Fait G, Many A, et al. Severe preeclampsia: high frequency of genetic thrombophilic mutations. *Obstet Gynecol* 2000;96;45–49.

83 Rigo J. Maternal and neonatal outcome of preeclamptic pregnancies: the potential roles of factor V Leiden mutations and 5,10-methylenetrahydrofolate reductase. *Hypertens Pregnancy* 2000;19:163–172.

84 vonTempelhoff GF. Incidence of the factor V Leiden-mutation, coagulation inhibitor deficiency, and elevated antiphospholipid-antibodies in patients with preeclampsia or HELLP-syndrome. Hemolysis, elevated liver-enzymes, low platelets. *Thromb Res* 2000;100:363–365.

85 Kupferminc MJ, Peri H, Zwang E, et al. High prevalence of the prothrombin gene mutation in women with intrauterine growth retardation, abruptio placentae and second trimester loss. *Acta Obstet Gynecol Scand* 2000;79:963–967.

86 Kim YJ. Genetic susceptibility to preeclampsia: roles of cytosineto-thymine substitution at nucleotide 677 of the gene for methylenetetrahydrofolate reductase, 68-base pair insertion at nucleotide 844 of the gene for cystathionine [beta]-synthase, and factor V Leiden mutation. *Am J Obstet Gynecol* 2001;184: 1211–1217.

87 Livingston J. Maternal and fetal inherited thrombophilias are not related to the development of severe preeclampsia. *Am J Obstet Gynecol* 2001;185:153–157.

88 Currie L. Is there an increased maternal–infant prevalence of

Factor V Leiden in association with severe pre-eclampsia? *Br J Obstet Gynaecol* 2002;109:191–196.
89 Benedetto A, Marozio L, Satton L, et al. Factor V Leiden and factor II G20210A in preeclampsia and HELLP syndrome. *Acta Obstet Gynecol* 2002;81:1095–1100.
90 Schlembach D. Association of maternal and/or fetal factor V Leiden and G20210A prothrombin mutation with HELLP syndrome and intrauterine growth restriction. *Clin Sci* 2003;105: 279–285.
91 Alfirevic Z. How strong is the association between maternal thrombophilia and adverse pregnancy outcome? A systematic review. *Eur J Obstet Gynecol Reprod Biol* 2002;101:6–14.
92 Morrison ER. Prothrombotic genotypes are not associated with pre-eclampsia and gestational hypertension: results from a large population-based study and systematic review. *Thromb Haemost* 2002;87:779–785.
93 Ananth CV, Smulian JC, Vintzileos AM. Incidence of placental abruption in relation to cigarette smoking and hypertensive disorders during pregnancy: a meta-analysis of observational studies. *Obstet Gynecol* 1999;93:622–628.
94 Addis A. Fetal effects of cocaine: an updated meta-analysis. *Reprod Toxicol* 2001;15:341–369.
95 deVries JI. Hyperhomocysteinaemia and protein S deficiency in complicated pregnancies. *Br J Obstet Gynaecol* 1997;104: 1248–1254.
96 Wiener-Megnagi Z, et al. Resistance to activated protein C and the leiden mutation: high prevalence in patients with abruptio placentae. *Am J Obstet Gynecol* 1998;179:1565–1567.
97 Faccinetti F. Thrombophilic mutations are a main risk factor for placental abruption. *Haemotologica* 2003;88:785–788.
98 Howley HA. Systematic review: FVL or PGM and IUGR. *Am J Obstet Gynecol* 2005;192:694–708.
99 Rey E, Kahn SR, David M, Shrier I. Thrombophilic disorders and fetal loss: a meta-analysis. *Lancet* 2003;361:901–908.
100 Gris JC. Case–control study of the frequency of thrombophilic disorders in couples with late foetal loss and no thrombotic antecedent – the Nimes Obstetricians and Haematologists Study5 (NOHA5). *Thromb Haemost* 1999;81:891–899.
101 Martinelli I. Mutations in coagulation factors in women with unexplained late fetal loss. *N Engl J Med* 2000;343: 1015–1018.
102 Martinelli I. Recurrent late fetal death in women with and without thrombophilia. *Thromb Haemost* 2002;87:358–359.
103 Preston FE, Rosendaal FR, Walker ID, et al. Increased fetal loss in women with heritable thrombophilia. *Lancet* 1996;348: 913–916.
104 Dizon-Townson D. The incidence of the factor V Leiden mutation in an obstetric population and its relationship to deep vein thrombosis. *Am J Obstet Gynecol* 1997;176:883–886.
105 Tal A. A possible role for activated protein C resistance in patients with first and second trimester pregnancy failure. *Hum Reprod* 1999;14:1624–1627.
106 Lindqvist PG, Dahlback B. Bleeding complications associated with low molecular weight heparin prophylaxis during pregnancy. *Thromb Haemost* 2000;84:140–141.
107 Murphy R. Prospective evaluation of the risk conferred by factor V Leiden and thermolabile methylenetetrahydrofolate reductase polymorphisms in pregnancy. *Arterioscler Thromb Vasc Biol* 2000;20:266–270.
108 Many A, Elad R, Yaron Y, et al. Third trimester unexplained intrauterine fetal death is associated with inherited thrombophilia. *Obstet Gynecol* 2002;99:684–687.
109 Alonso A. Acquired and inherited thrombophilia in women with unexplained fetal losses. *Am J Obstet Gynecol* 2002;187: 1337–1342.
110 Hefler L, Jirecek S, Heim K, et al. Genetic polymorphisms associated with thrombophilia and vascular disease in women with unexplained late intrauterine fetal death: a multicenter study. *J Soc Gynecol Invest* 2004;11:42–44.
111 Gonen R, Lavi N, Attias D, et al. Absence of association of inherited thrombophilia with unexplained third-trimester intrauterine fetal death. *Am J Obstet Gynecol* 2005;192:742–746.
112 Kovalevsky G, Gracia CR, Berlin JA, et al. Evaluation of the association between hereditary thrombophilias and recurrent pregnancy loss. *Arch Intern Med* 2004;164:558–563.
113 Kujovich JL. Thrombophilia and pregnancy complications. *Am J Obstet Gynecol* 2004;191:412–424.
114 Langhoff-Roos J, Paidas MJ, Ku DH, et al. *Immunology of pregnancy*. Mor G, ed. Eurekah.com 2005 and Springer Science + Business Media.
115 Roque H, Paidas MJ, Funai EF, et al. Maternal thrombophilias are not associated with early pregnancy loss. *Thromb Haemost* 2004;91:290–295.
116 Cochrane E. Antiphospholipid antibody and recurrent pregnancy loss. *Obstet Gynecol* 2002;99:135–144.
117 Riyazi N, Leeda M, de Vries JI, Huijgens PC, et al. Low-molecular-weight heparin combined with aspirin in pregnant women with thrombophilia and a history of preeclampsia or fetal growth restriction: a preliminary study. *Eur J Obstet Gynecol Reprod Biol* 1998;80:49–54.
118 Brenner B. Gestational outcome in thrombophilic women with recurrent pregnancy loss treated by enoxaparin. *Thromb Haemost* 2000;83:693–697.
119 Ogueh O. Outcome of pregnancy in women with hereditary thrombophilia. *Int J Gynaecol Obstet* 2001;74:247–253.
120 Kupferminc M, Fait G, Many A, et al. Low molecular weight heparin for the prevention of obstetric complications in women with thrombophilia. *Hypertens Pregnancy* 2001;20:35–44.
121 Grandone E. Preventing adverse obstetric outcomes in women with genetic thrombophilia. *Fertil Steril* 2002;78:371–375.
122 Paidas M, Ku DH, Triche E, et al. Does heparin therapy improve pregnancy outcome in patients with thrombophilias? *J Thromb Haemost* 2004;2:1194–1195.
123 Gris JC, Mercier E, Quere II, et al. Low-molecular-weight heparin versus low-dose aspirin in women with one fetal loss and a constitutional thrombophilic disorder. *Blood* 2004;103: 3695–3699.
124 Brenner B, Hoffman R, Carp H, et al. LIVE-ENOX Investigators. Efficacy and safety of two doses of enoxaparin in women with thrombophilia and recurrent pregnancy loss: the LIVE-ENOX study. *J Thromb Haemost* 2005;3:227–229.
125 Walker MC, Ferguson SE, Allen VM (Cochrane Review). Heparin for pregnant women with acquired or inherited thrombophilias. In: The Cochrane Library, Issue 4, 2003.
126 Nisio M, Peters LW, Middeldorp S. Anticoagulants for the treatment of recurrent pregnancy loss in women without antiphospholipid syndrome (review). *Cochrane Database Syst Rev* 2005;2:CD004734.
127 Tulppala M, Marttunen M, Soderstrom-Anttila V, et al. Low-dose aspirin in prevention of miscarriage in women with unexplained or autoimmune related recurrent miscarriage: effect on prostacyclin and thromboxane A2 production. *Hum Reprod* 1997;12:1567–1572.
128 Hirsh J. Heparin. *N Engl J Med* 1991;324:1565–1574.
129 Walenga JM, Jeske WP, Fasanella AR, et al. Laboratory diagno-

sis of heparin-induced thrombocytopenia. *Clin Appl Thromb Hemost* 1999;5(Suppl. 1):S21–S27.

130 Greer IA, Nelson-Percy C. Safety and efficacy of LMWH: thromboprophylaxis and treatment of venous thromboembolism (64 reports, 2777 pregnancies). *Blood* 2005;106:401–407.

131 Clinical Updates in Women's Health. *Thrombosis, thrombophilia and thromboembolism in women*. American College of Obstetricians and Gynecologists, in press.

132 Hirsh J, Hoak J. Management of deep vein thrombosis and pulmonary embolism : a statement for healthcare professionals from the Council on Thrombosis (in consultation with the Council on Cardiovascular Radiology), American Heart Association. *Circulation* 1996;93:2212–2245.

133 Kassai B, Boissel JP, Cucherat M, et al. A systematic review of the accuracy of ultrasound in the diagnosis of deep venous thrombosis in asymptomatic patients. *Thromb Haemost* 2004; 91:655–666.

134 Tapson VF, Carroll BA, Davidson BL, et al. The diagnostic approach to acute venous thromboembolism. Clinical practice guideline. American Thoracic Society. *Am J Respir Crit Care Med* 1999;160:1043–1066.

135 Stein PD, Terrin ML, Hales CA, et al. Clinical, laboratory, roentgenographic, and electrocardiographic findings in patients with acute pulmonary embolism and no pre-existing cardiac or pulmonary disease. *Chest* 1991;100:598–603.

136 Fedullo PF, Tapson VF. Clinical practice. The evaluation of suspected pulmonary embolism. *N Engl J Med* 2003;349: 1247.

137 The Urokinase Pulmonary Embolism Trial: a national cooperative study. *Circulation* 1973;47(Suppl. II):1–108.

138 Green RM, Meyer TJ, Dunn M, Glassroth J. Pulmonary embolism in younger adults. *Chest* 1992;01:1507–1511.

139 The PIOPED Investigators. Value of the ventilation/perfusion scan in acute pulmonary embolism. Results of the prospective investigation of pulmonary embolism diagnosis (PIOPED). *JAMA* 1990;263:2753–2759.

140 Cross JJ, Kemp PM, Walsh CG, et al. A randomized trial of spiral CT and ventilation perfusion scintigraphy for the diagnosis of pulmonary embolism. *Clin Radiol* 1998;53:177–182.

141 Brent RL. The effect of embryonic and fetal exposure to x-ray, microwaves, and ultrasound: counseling the pregnant and non-pregnant patient about these risks. *Semin Oncol* 1989;16: 347–368.

142 Stewart A, Kneale GW. Radiation dose effects in relation to obstetric x-rays and childhood cancers. *Lancet* 1970;1:1185–1188.

143 Webb JA, Thomsen HS, Morcos SK. Members of Contrast Media Safety Committee of European Society of Urogenital Radiology (ESUR). The use of iodinated and gadolinium contrast media during pregnancy and lactation. *Eur Radiol* 2005;15:1234–1240.

144 Turrentine MA, Braems G, Ramirez MM. Use of thrombolytics for the treatment of thromboembolic disease during pregnancy. *Obstet Gynecol Surv* 1995;50:534–541.

145 Patel RK, Fasan O, Arya R. Thrombolysis in pregnancy. *Thromb Haemost* 2003;90:1216–1217.

146 Brill-Edwards P, Ginsberg JS, Gent M, et al. Safety of withholding heparin in pregnant women with a history of venous thromboembolism. Recurrence of clot in this pregnancy study group. *N Engl J Med* 2000;343:1439–1444.

147 Anticoagulation in Prosthetic Heart Valves and Pregnancy Consensus Report (APPCR). Anticoagulation and enoxaparin use in patients with prosthetic heart valves and/or pregnancy. *Clin Cardiol Consensus Rep* 2002;3:1–20.

48 Coagulation and hematological disorders of pregnancy

Carl P. Weiner and Chien Oh

Red blood cell disorders/anemia

Normal physiological change

Functionally, anemia is defined as an inadequate red blood cell (RBC) mass to deliver the necessary oxygen to peripheral tissues. Clinically, anemia is defined as a hemoglobin (Hgb) or hematocrit below the lower limit of a given range, typically the 10th percentile. Age, gender, race, and pregnancy are all factors influencing the normal range.[1,2] The "normal" hemoglobin value for an adult female is 12–15 g/dL. There is an increase in blood volume during pregnancy with a disproportionate rise in plasma volume, causing a net RBC dilution.[3] The Centers for Disease Control (CDC) defines anemia during pregnancy as a hemoglobin level less than 11 g/dL in the first and third trimesters and less than 10.5 g/dL in the second trimester.[4] This useful definition takes into account the increase in plasma volume, but it does not consider other changes that may increase the hemoglobin, such as smoking or hemoglobin variants.

The effect of anemia on pregnancy is dependent on the severity and the cause of the anemia. It is not cost-effective to test every woman with anemia, given that the vast majority have mild anemia secondary to iron deficiency. A trial of replacement therapy should be initiated if the woman is not already taking prenatal vitamins. At the very least, a follow-up complete blood count should be obtained to insure improvement. In cases of more severe anemia (Hgb < 9.0 g/dL), a careful evaluation may reveal a diagnosis with implications for the mother, fetus, and future children (e.g., a hereditary hemoglobinopathy or a hemolytic anemia).

Laboratory workup of anemia

Anemia may result from decreased RBC production, increased RBC destruction/loss, or dilution. The evaluation of anemia during pregnancy is the same as that in the nonpregnant subject (Fig. 48.1). A complete medical history and physical examination may improve the efficiency of the evaluation. Questions about onset, duration, previous medical history, family history, diet, occupational exposures, and drug history are all potentially important. Physical signs such as fever, bruising, jaundice, hepatomegaly, and splenomegaly will direct the clinician to consider more serious causes of anemia.

The basic laboratory evaluation begins with a reticulocyte count. If the reticulocyte count is low or normal, the assumption is that the anemia is secondary to decreased RBC production. There are three morphological categories: microcytic [mean corpuscular volume (MCV) < 80], normocytic (MCV 80–100), and macrocytic (MCV > 100). Additional laboratory tests are selected based on the grouping. An elevated reticulocyte count suggests an increased RBC loss secondary to either blood loss (acute or chronic) or hemolysis.

The most common cause of microcytic anemia is iron deficiency. Potential iron studies of value may include serum ferritin, total iron-binding capacity (TIBC), and plasma iron levels. Ferritin and plasma iron values are all reduced in iron deficiency anemia, whereas the TIBC may be elevated. Ferritin correlates best with the marrow iron stores. Transferrin levels fluctuate daily and are rarely useful for the evaluation of iron deficiency.[5] In practice, a serum ferritin is all that is necessary. Iron supplementation should be withheld for 24–48 h before testing. A hemoglobin electrophoresis in search of a hemoglobinopathy is the next step should the ferritin suggest adequate iron stores. In general, the MCV is lower in subjects with hemoglobinopathies than in those with iron deficiency anemia. Both the anemia of chronic disease and sideroblastic anemias are also part of the differential.

Macrocytic anemia usually results from nutritional deficiencies of either folate or vitamin B12. Additional causes of macrocytic anemia include specific drugs that interfere with DNA synthesis. The term megaloblastic anemia is not synonymous with macrocytic anemia. Megaloblastic anemia specifically describes the presence of megaloblasts, distinctive large cells with abnormal-appearing nuclear chromatin that reflects aberrant DNA synthesis. Pregnancy increases the demand upon the body's reserve, and a patient with marginal

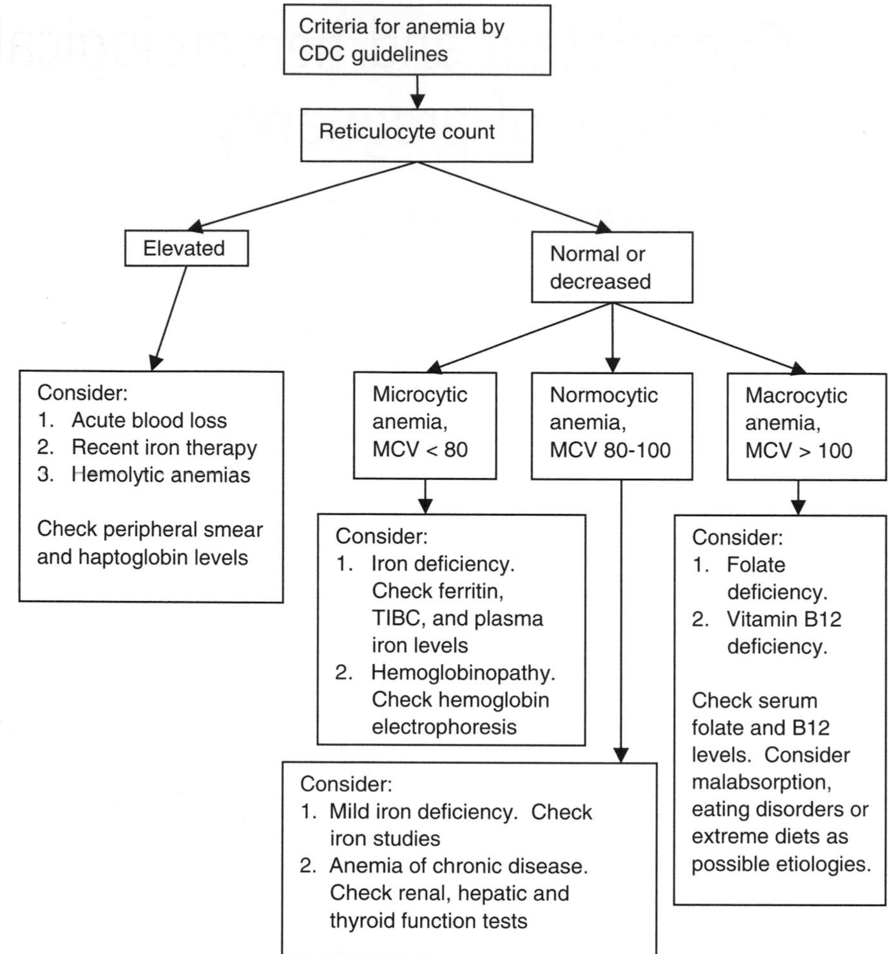

Figure 48.1 Workup algorithm for anemia.

stores may develop megaloblastic anemia. If macrocytic anemia is present, serum levels of B12 and folic acid need to be evaluated.

Normocytic anemia without reticulocytosis is perhaps the most difficult diagnosis because of the long differential. Etiologies include mild iron deficiency and anemia of chronic disease. In the absence of an identifiable, longstanding medical problem, thyroid, renal, and hepatic function tests should be considered.

If the reticulocyte count is elevated, recent blood loss (acute or chronic) or a hemolytic anemia must be considered in the differential diagnosis. Haptoglobin is a glycoprotein that binds free serum hemoglobin. Its level decreases as it binds hemoglobin and is subsequently cleared by the liver. A peripheral smear may also be useful, indicating hemolysis if schizocytes or a hereditary hemolytic anemia (e.g., spherocytosis or sickle cell anemia) are seen. Thus, a low haptoglobin level and an abnormal peripheral smear may indicate hemolysis.

Nutritional anemias

Iron deficiency

The current CDC guidelines recommend 35 mg of elemental iron daily during pregnancy for patients who are not anemic. The effect of iron deficiency on pregnancy outcome is not entirely clear. The iron supplementation in patients who are deficient clearly raises hemoglobin and iron stores, but may not change perinatal outcome.[6] Although several studies suggest an increase in low birthweight and preterm birth when

Table 48.1 Iron dextran protocol.

Indications: treatment of iron deficiency anemia in patients unable to absorb oral iron

Contraindications/precautions:
- Hypersensitivity to iron dextran complex
- Use caution in patients with asthma, hepatic impairment, and rheumatoid arthritis

Dosing recommendations:
- Test dose:
  - Administer 0.5 mL i.v./i.m. prior to starting therapy
  - For the i.v. dose, dilute 25 mg/0.5 mL in 50 mL of NSS and infuse over 15 min
  - Have epinephrine at the bedside. Watch patient for 30 min after test dose for anaphylactic reactions
- Dose (mL):
  - 0.0476 × weight (kg) × (14.8–observed Hgb) + (1 mL/5 kg to maximum of 14 mL for iron stores)
  - Maximum i.v. dose = 3000 mg (60 mL)
  - Dilute total dose in 250–1000 mL of NSS. Usual volume 500 mL
  - Maximum concentration = 50 mg/mL
  - Infuse over 1–6 h (no faster than 50 mg/min). Common infusion time over 2–3 h. Watch patient closely during first 25 mL for allergic reactions
  - Do not add iron dextran to TPN

Adverse effects:

CV	flushing, hypotension, cardiovascular collapse (< 1%)
CNS	dizziness, fever, headache (> 10%), chills (< 1%)
DERM	urticaria, phlebitis (< 1%), staining of skin at i.m. site
GI	nausea, vomiting, metallic taste, discoloration of urine (1–10%)
RESP	diaphoresis (> 10%)

Note: diaphoresis, urticaria, fever, chills, and dizziness may be delayed 24–48 h after i.v. administration and 3–4 days after i.m. administration. Anaphylactic reactions occur generally in the first few minutes after administration

Pregnancy category: C

Monitoring: check blood pressure every 5 min during the test dose. Watch for allergic reactions and side-effects for 3–4 days. Monitor Hgb and reticulocyte count

CV, cardiovascular; CNS, central nervous system; DERM, dermatologic; GI, gastrointestinal; Hgb, hemoglobin; i.m., intramuscularly; i.v., intravenously; NSS, normal saline solution; RESP, respiratory; TPN, total parenteral nutrition.

the mother is iron deficient,[7,8] it is not clear whether there is a cause and effect relationship. Fetal iron stores are not affected in most cases of iron deficiency anemia.[9,10]

Iron deficiency is the most common cause of anemia in women of reproductive age, in part because of menstrual blood loss. The diagnosis is made when the ferritin level is low and the MCV is mildly decreased. Iron can be supplied as either ferrous sulfate (65 mg of elemental iron/325 mg) or ferrous gluconate (38 mg of elemental iron/325 mg) in a dose of 325 mg p.o. q.d. to t.i.d. Gastrointestinal transferrin becomes saturated after 7 days of twice-daily therapy. Supplemental vitamin C may increase iron absorption by enhancing the reduction of the ferrous to the ferric form, which increases intestinal absorption.

While elemental iron is best absorbed on an empty stomach, it may increase maternal nausea and vomiting. Many practitioners recommend taking the iron during or after meals, assuming that any decrease in absorption is offset by the excessive dose given. Constipation is common. There are many over-the-counter formulations that minimize constipation by including stool softeners.

Parenteral iron therapy may be of value when a patient fails to respond adequately to oral therapy. An example of an iron dextran protocol is listed in Table 48.1. A major risk of parenteral iron therapy is anaphylaxis, and anesthesia personnel should be readily available. Because of this risk, a firm diagnosis of severe iron deficiency should be made before administering parenteral iron.

Megaloblastic anemia

Megaloblastic anemia results from impaired DNA synthesis due to a deficiency of a required cofactor, usually either folic acid or vitamin B12. The diagnosis of megaloblastic anemia is suggested when the MCV is greater than 100 and there is hypersegmentation of the polymorphonuclear leukocytes. It is confirmed by serum testing. Folate supplementation with 2–4 mg daily should correct a folate deficiency. A B12 deficiency requires parenteral therapy with 1000 μg weekly for 6 weeks or until the deficiency has corrected. A prolonged vitamin B12 deficiency may lead to neuropathy and pernicious anemia. An isolated deficiency of either folic acid or B12 is

Table 48.2 Hemoglobin nomenclature.

Normal hemoglobins

Hgb A(A/A): normal adult hemoglobin. Composed of two α-chains and two β-chains

Hgb A2 (note: not the same as A/A): a less common, but normal form of adult hemoglobin. Composed of two α-chains and two δ-chains. Will be increased, typically > 3.5% in β-thalassemia

Hgb F: normal fetal hemoglobin. May be elevated in patients with β-thalassemias. Has a different oxygen dissociation curve than Hgb A

Hemoglobinopathies

Hgb SA: sickle cell trait. Defect in the β-chain. Little maternal clinical significance other than an increased risk of urinary tract infections. Obvious genetic implications

Hgb SS: sickle cell anemia. Characterized by painful crises. Both maternal and fetal implications for poor outcome. Genetic implications

Hgb CA: hemoglobin C trait. Defect in the β-chain on one chromosome. No maternal clinical significance, mild microcytic anemia. Genetic implications for fetus if parent has child with partner with SA or SS or β-thalassemia

Hgb CC: hemoglobin C disease. Homozygous for Hgb C. No maternal clinical significance. More microcytic anemia compared with Hgb CA. Genetic implications for fetus if parent has child with partner with SA or SS or β-thalassemia

Hgb SC: hemoglobin SC disease. Milder form of sickle cell anemia, less crises when nonpregnant. Debatable whether maternal and fetal outcomes are worse, the same, or better than Hgb SS. Spleen is more functional, and hemolytic crises may be made worse because of acute splenic sequestration

Hgb EA: hemoglobin E trait. Defect in the β-globulin chain. Like Hgb C, no maternal clinical significance, mild microcytic anemia. Genetic implications for fetus if parent has child with partner with SA or SS or β-thalassemia. Found primarily in South-east Asians

Hgb EE: hemoglobin E disease. No maternal clinical significance. More microcytic anemia compared with Hgb EA. Genetic implications for fetus if parent has child with partner with SA or SS or β-thalassemia

Thalassemia disorders

α-Thalassemia minor. Deletion of one or two α-globulin genes. No maternal clinical significance, mild microcytic anemia. Genetic implications for fetus if parent has child with partner also with α-thalassemia minor

Hgb H: hemoglobin H. Composed of four β-globulin chains because of little α-chain. Hgb H disease patients have a three-gene deletion, and will have a mixture of Hgb H, Hgb A, and Hgb Bart. Severe hemolytic anemia, compatible with extrauterine life. Note that Hgb H disease is separate from Hgb H

Hgb Bart: hemoglobin Bart. Composed of four γ-globulin chains. Hgb Bart disease patients have no α-chain production at all because of a four-gene deletion. Not compatible with extrauterine life. No α-chain production at all

β-Thalassemia: decreased production of β-globulin usually because of a defect in the promoter region of the β-globulin gene. β^0 means that no β-chain is produced. β^+ means that little chain is produced. There are hundreds of mutations, and there is a spectrum of clinical findings and severity

β-Thalassemia major or Cooley's anemia: No fetal significance because Hgb F produced; however, after birth, neonate will fail to thrive and become anemic. Little maternal significance because females do not get pregnant often because of severity of disease

β-Thalassemia minor: heterozygote for β-thalassemia gene. Diagnosed because of elevated Hgb A2 levels (> 3.5%). Hgb A2 has no β-chains

β-Thalassemia intermedia: applied to patients in between minor and major thalassemia in terms of clinical significance and severity

Combined abnormalities

Because the defects in hemoglobinopathies can combine with thalassemias, especially with β-thalassemias, a combined abnormality will be found on occasion, which may cause a hemolytic anemia (such as Hgb C/β-thalassemia or Hgb E/β-thalassemia). If β-thalassemia combines with Hgb S, a sickling hemoglobinopathy will result

rare: an extreme diet or malabsorption should be considered as potential etiologies.

Hemoglobinopathies

Normal adult hemoglobin consists of two α-chains and two β-chains (Hgb A), while the normal fetal hemoglobin consists of two α-chains and two γ-chains (Hgb F). Mutations, whether they result in decreased synthesis of hemoglobin (e.g., the thalassemias) or altered hemoglobin structure (structural hemoglobinopathies), can cause a wide range of problems. Hundreds of hemoglobin variants have been identified. These hemoglobinopathies are genetic; there are implications for future childbearing. Hemoglobinopathy nomenclature can be confusing and is summarized in Table 48.2.

Thalassemias

The thalassemias are classified by the abnormal chain. The α-chain is encoded by four gene copies with two copies on each chromosome 16 (αα/αα). The severity of α-thalassemia depends on the number of gene copies that are deleted or defective. There is no clinical impact if one gene is missing. A mild microcytic anemia results if two genes are lost (α-thalassemia minor). A three gene deletion (hemoglobin H disease)

Blacks

(P) α–, α–

		α-	α-
(M) α–, α–	α-	α– , α–	α–, α–
	α-	α–, α–	α–, α–

All four possibilities of two black a-thallasemia minor parents result in a a-thallassemia minor genotype.

Asians

(P) αα, --

		αα	--
(M) αα, --	αα	αα, αα	αα, —
	--	αα, —	—, —

The four possibilities of two Asian α-thalassemia minor parents result in one normal child, two α-thalassemia minor genotypes, and one Hemoglobin Bart disease.

Figure 48.2 α-Thalassemia. Effects of inheritance in different races.

results in a β-globulin tetramer called hemoglobin H (Hgb H). This disease is compatible with life, but is associated with profound hemolytic anemia. Hemoglobin Bart disease results if all four genes are missing; it is incompatible with life. Affected untreated fetuses die of hydrops, and their mothers often develop severe, early-onset preeclampsia. Survival is possible with repeated fetal transfusions followed by neonatal bone marrow transplantation.

In black people, α-thalassemia minor usually results from the loss of one gene from each chromosome (α–/α–). In Asians, two gene deletions are more likely to occur on one chromosome (αα/– –). As a result, Asians have a higher risk of having a child with hemoglobin Bart or hemoglobin H disease (Fig. 48.2). A specific diagnosis should be made using DNA probes prior to further genetic counseling.

The β-thalassemias reflect mainly an underproduction of the β-globulin chains. Although less common, abnormalities of the β-globulin chain are transmitted in an autosomal dominant fashion.[11] β-Thalassemias occur in many parts of the world including the Mediterranean, Africa, southern China, the Malay Peninsula, and Indonesia. Over 150 mutations have been identified that affect the promoter region of the β-globulin gene.[11]

The severity of the β-thalassemias is subclassified by the quantity of β-globulin produced. β^+ indicates that some β-chains are being produced, whereas β^0 means that no chains are being produced. Homozygote patients for a defective β-thalassemia gene (thalassemia major or Cooley's anemia) have a markedly ineffective erythropoiesis and severe hemolysis. The disease is manifest postnatally, as the fetus produces hemoglobin F, which does not use the β-globulin chain. After birth, the hemoglobin type switches from hemoglobin F to the adult type and β-thalassemia appears. Heterozygotes for β-thalassemia require prenatal counseling, and antenatal diagnosis should be offered. Screening programs are effective in areas where β-thalassemia is prevalent. The combination during pregnancy of β-thalassemia with another abnormal hemoglobin variant can cause hemolytic and sickling anemias that confer higher rates of maternal and fetal morbidities and mortalities.

Sickle cell anemia, disease, and crisis

Sickle cell disease (SCD) is caused by an abnormal β-globulin resulting from a point mutation replacement of glutamic acid with valine at the sixth position (hemoglobin S). In times of stress (e.g., hypoxemia or infection), the abnormal β-globulin chain undergoes a conformational change causing sickling of the RBC. The sickled RBC have reduced deformability, causing microvascular occlusion, hemolysis, and increased susceptibility to infection.

A patient homozygous for hemoglobin S (hemoglobin SS) has sickle cell anemia. Heterozygote individuals (hemoglobin SA) have sickle cell trait. Other sickling hemoglobinopathies of importance during pregnancy include hemoglobin SC disease and hemoglobin S/β-thalassemia. Patients with hemoglobin SC disease are double heterozygotes for both hemoglobin S and hemoglobin C. Hemoglobin C is a β-globulin chain that does not confer as much protection from sickling during pregnancy as does hemoglobin A. Hemoglobin S/β-thalassemia is a "mild" form of sickle cell anemia that is managed similarly to hemoglobin SC disease. Sickle cell crises may occur especially in the third trimester with hemoglobin SC disease. Splenic infarction and vaso-occlusive disease do not occur outside pregnancy; as their spleens function normally, these patients can experience a more rapid and severe anemia than is expected with hemoglobin SS because of acute splenic sequestration. The management is similar to the patient with sickle cell anemia. Sickle cell trait individuals are not at risk of sequestration crises, nor are they at risk of excess obstetric complications with the exception of urinary tract infections.[12]

Pregnancy in a woman with one of these three sickling disorders exposes the mother and fetus to increased complication rates associated with vaso-occlusive disease, such as intrauterine growth restriction (IUGR), preterm labor, preeclampsia, and perinatal mortality.[13–16] Complications of SCD are often exacerbated by pregnancy. The hallmark of disease is the sickle cell crisis in which the main complaint is severe pain in the back, chest, abdomen, and long bones. The treatment of sickle cell crisis has not changed significantly over the past decade, and consists of hydration, oxygenation, and pain relief. Pulmonary and urinary infections are common crisis triggers and must be ruled out. If present, infections must be treated aggressively. Alternative causes of pain should be considered. Symptomatic patients may benefit from transfusion therapy. General indications for transfusion are hemoglobin < 5g/dL, a hemoglobin drop of 30% or more, acute chest syndrome, and hypoxemia. The goal is to keep the hemoglobin S concentration at no more than 30–40% of the total hemoglobin. Regular antepartum fetal testing for fetal well-being and growth is strongly recommended.

Transfusion treatment for acute disease must be differentiated from prophylaxis, which is controversial. The goal of routine prophylactic transfusion therapy is to maintain the hematocrit above 25% and the hemoglobin S concentration below 60%. Two randomized trials compared routine transfusion versus transfusion only for an acute crisis.[17,18] Patients transfused prophylactically had fewer crises and spent less time in hospital. However, perinatal outcome was not improved, and multiple transfusions were associated with a 25% rate of alloimmunization and a 20% prevalence of delayed transfusion reaction. The risks and benefits of routine prophylactic transfusion should be discussed with the patient. The use of prophylactic transfusion seems especially attractive in women with recurrent crises during pregnancy.

There are two particular complications of SCD that may be misdiagnosed during pregnancy. First, patients with SCD have a higher likelihood of a seizure disorder. Neurologic events secondary to SCD must be separated from pregnancy-associated events such as eclampsia. SCD neurologic events may result from thrombosis, hemorrhage, hypoxia, or meperidine use. Imaging studies and other clinical findings may help to differentiate neurologic events from complications of SCD and pregnancy.

The second SCD complication that may be misdiagnosed during pregnancy is acute chest syndrome (ACS). ACS is the leading cause of death in SCD patients and the second most common cause of hospitalization.[19] The presentation is similar to pneumonia and consists of fever, cough, chest pain, pulmonary infiltrates, hypoxemia, and leukocytosis. Differentiation between the two diseases may be impossible. Pneumonia is implicated as a potential cause of ACS, being diagnosed concomitantly in 20% of ACS patients. The exact role of infection, thrombosis, or embolism in the development of ACS remains unclear. Exchange transfusion and antibiotic therapy is recommended if an SCD patient presents with severe respiratory symptoms; consultation with a pulmonologist and/or a hematologist would also be wise.

Routine screening for sickle cell trait is offered to at-risk women. If a woman is found to have sickle cell trait, her partner should be offered testing to determine whether the fetus is at risk of SCD. Women with an 'at-risk' pregnancy should be offered counseling and testing. Prenatal diagnosis can be accomplished by amniocentesis or by chorionic villus sampling (CVS). Many locales of high prevalence have effective postnatal screening programs in place.

Hemoglobin C and hemoglobin E

Hemoglobin C and hemoglobin E are both variants that cause microcytic anemia. Hemoglobin C is common in Africans, while hemoglobin E is more prevalent in South-east Asia. Patients may either have a trait form (hemoglobin CA, hemoglobin EA) or "disease" (hemoglobin CC, hemoglobin EE). The microcytic anemia is mild even in homozygous states and of little clinical significance. No additional maternal treatment or fetal testing is required. However, pregnant women are at higher risk for morbidity if they are a compound heterozygote. Hemoglobin E/β-thalassemia and hemoglobin SE are each reported to cause a hemolytic anemia.[20]

Hemolytic anemias

Structural, immunologic, and enzymopathic hemolytic anemias may each be exacerbated by pregnancy.

Structural hemolytic anemias include hereditary spherocytosis (HS), hereditary elliptocytosis (HE), hereditary pyropoikilocytosis (HPP), South-east Asian ovalocytosis (SAO), hereditary and acquired acanthocytosis, and hereditary and acquired stomatocytosis. These diseases are distinguished by the morphology of the erythrocyte and result from defective erythrocyte membrane skeleton proteins that cause the deformed erythrocytes to be selectively sequestered and destroyed in the spleen.

Over 50 mutations affecting various membrane proteins such as spectrin or ankyrin are recognized. The symptomatology is varied and, in milder cases, the abnormality may not be identified until pregnancy. The diagnosis should be considered when unexplained splenomegaly, anemia, hemolysis, and unconjugated bilirubinemia present during pregnancy. The diagnosis is made using the osmotic fragility test. A peripheral blood smear may be falsely negative during a hemolytic episode when most of the abnormal erythrocytes have been destroyed in the spleen. Splenectomy is the treatment for the more severe forms of structural hemolytic anemia. However, splenectomy may be difficult during pregnancy and, if not feasible, supportive transfusion treatment and folate supplementation are recommended.

Autoimmune hemolytic anemia (AIHA) is caused by the production of antierythrocyte autoantibodies. Three forms of AIHA are described: IgM-mediated (cold-reactive) AIHA; IgG-mediated (warm-reactive) AIHA; and IgG Donath–Landsteiner antibody-mediated (paroxysmal cold-reactive). AIHA may occur as the primary disease, a secondary disease (often associated with hematological malignancy), or after the administration of various drugs. Penicillin, cephalosporins, and methyldopa are all implicated as causes of hemolytic episodes.[21–25] Infection is another known trigger, but often no trigger is identifiable. The rate of autoantibody production increases during pregnancy over age-matched, nonpregnant subjects. Perhaps as a result, hemolytic episodes may be worse during pregnancy and improve after delivery. The diagnosis of AIHA is made after documentation of a hemolytic anemia associated with a positive direct Coombs' test. The treatment is similar to that for immune thrombocytopenic purpura (ITP), and focuses on corticosteroid and intravenous immunoglobulin (IVIG) administration. A RBC transfusion should be performed if indicated, although crossmatching can be difficult because of the autoantibodies.

Glucose 6-phosphate dehydrogenase (G6PD) aids the synthesis of reduced glutathione (GSH), which protects the erythrocyte from oxidative damage. G6PD deficiency causes hemolytic anemia when the erythrocyte is exposed to oxidative stress, and is often associated with certain drugs such as nitrofurantoin and trimethoprim-sulfa, two drugs commonly used in obstetrics. The inheritance is X-linked. Up to 20% of African–American women are heterozygous and 1% homozygous.[26] The G6PD activity of heterozygote individuals ranges between deficient males and normal subjects, although some have little activity because of lyonization. Although rare, hemolytic episodes have been reported through "vertical" transmission.[27] Thus, while there is little chance that exposure to these drugs will cause a hemolytic episode in heterozygous carriers, pregnant and nursing women should avoid them where possible in case their fetus/neonate is either an affected male or a homozygous female. The primary treatment during a hemolytic episode is to discontinue the offending drugs and transfuse if necessary.

Paroxysmal nocturnal hemoglobinuria (PNH) is a hematopoietic stem cell disorder in which the abnormal erythrocytes undergo intravascular complement-mediated hemolysis. The abnormal stem cells also produce abnormal leukocytes and platelets. The degree of hemolysis reflects the size of the abnormal clone, the degree of erythrocyte abnormality, and the amount of complement fixation. These patients are at increased risk for thrombotic events and for bone marrow failure. Prophylactic heparin should be considered beginning in the first trimester. One report described a 6% mortality rate in patients with PNH, primarily due to Budd–Chiari syndrome (thrombosis of the mesenteric vessels). The diagnosis is made after a positive Ham test demonstrates RBC vulnerability to complement. Referral to a hematologist is appropriate.

Coagulation disorders in pregnancy

Pregnancy changes in coagulation factors

Coagulation is a complex process that requires a delicate balance between prothrombotic factors and thrombolytic factors. Pregnancy tips the balance between thrombotic and thrombolytic factors toward a hypercoagulable state. Concentrations of both thrombotic and thrombolytic factors change during pregnancy, and most are estrogen dependent (Table 48.3). Fibrinopeptide A, the first peptide cleaved from

Table 48.3 Relative changes in coagulation factors in pregnancy.

Increased
Fibrinogen
vWF antigen, factor VIII function, and ristocetin cofactor activity
Factors III, XII, X
Fibrinopeptide A
Plasminogen activators: tissue type, urokinase type
Plasminogen activator inhibitor-I and -II
α2-macroglobulin
D-Dimers (not a useful test for diagnosing thromboembolism in pregnancy)
Decreased
Platelets
Protein S
Factors XI, XIII
Unchanged
Factors II, V, IX
Protein C
Antithrombin (some reports indicate that this may be decreased in the third trimester)
Plasminogen
Prekallikrein

vWF, von Willebrand's factor.

fibrinogen during thrombin-mediated fibrin generation, increases before the end of the first trimester.[28] The production of prostacyclin and nitric oxide, two potent inhibitors of platelet adhesion and aggregation, is increased by the endothelium during pregnancy.[29] Having a higher level of clotting activity predisposes the woman to disseminated intravascular coagulation (DIC) in pathologic states. Many of these same changes are observed in women taking oral estrogen-containing contraceptives. During pregnancy, a woman is four times more likely to suffer a thromboembolic event than a woman not taking oral contraceptives.[30] Each point of Virchow's triad is affected by pregnancy. Not only is there a relative hypercoagulable state, but there is also increased venous stasis in dependent limbs and vascular damage during delivery.

Laboratory workup of coagulation

A coagulation panel may include a complete blood count (CBC), prothrombin time (PT), partial thromboplastin time (PTT), fibrinogen, fibrin split products and, occasionally, a bleeding time. The bleeding time is a test of platelet function, and useful only in testing populations at risk of selected disorders. It should not be used as a test of overall coagulation function.[31] The test itself is a poor predictor of surgical bleeding and a poor tool for following the response to therapy.[32] Factors that influence the bleeding time include antiplatelet drugs, skin thickness, technologist skill and experience, and platelet count.

Thrombocytopenia

Thrombocytopenia may have major clinical consequences for the management of the pregnant woman. Although the diagnosis of thrombocytopenia is usually made on a routine CBC, a platelet disorder may be suspected should the patient present with spontaneous bleeding from mucous membranes, petechiae, easy bruising, and epistaxis. Concerns for maternal and fetal bleeding must be considered in determining a need for platelet transfusions, mode of delivery, and anesthesia.

The diagnosis of thrombocytopenia is made when the platelet count is below the lower laboratory reference limit. This value ranges among laboratories from 120 000 to 150 000/μL. However, management is not altered until the count drops below 100 000/μL. The "minimum" platelet count necessary for safely performing invasive procedures is listed in Table 48.4 as per the British Haematological Society.[33] Both they and the Red Cross agree that platelet transfusions are rarely indicated during Cesarean section when the count is above 50 000/μL and then only when there is evidence of abnormal function. Unnecessary platelet transfusion can lead to alloimmunization and may worsen immune-mediated thrombocytopenia.

The differential diagnosis for thrombocytopenia is listed in Table 48.5. The general causes of thrombocytopenia (like anemia) can reflect either increased platelet destruction/consumption or decreased production. Increased destruction/consumption accounts for most thrombocytopenia. The evaluation of thrombocytopenia begins with a careful history attempting to exclude a drug-induced thrombocytopenia, a CBC to rule out a pancytopenia, and a review of the peripheral smear to rule out pseudothrombocytopenia and microangiopathy. In a pregnant woman with no other medical or pregnancy problems, the most common causes of maternal thrombocytopenia are gestational thrombocytopenia (GT) and immune thrombocytopenic purpura (ITP).

Table 48.4 "Minimum" amount of platelets necessary for pregnancy-related procedures.

Procedure	Platelet count (/μL)
Minor surgery	> 50 000
Major surgery	> 80 000
Vaginal delivery	> 50 000
Cesarean section	> 80 000
Regional anesthesia	> 80 000

From the British Committee for Standards in Haematology General Haematology Task Force.[33] Note that these guidelines indicate 80 K as a cutoff. Discuss the use of regional anesthesia with the anesthesiologist who may have a different level of comfort if the platelet count is < 100 000.

Table 48.5 Differential diagnosis for thrombocytopenia.

Gestational thrombocytopenia
Immune thrombocytopenia purpura
Pregnancy-induced hypertension, HELLP syndrome
Drug-related thrombocytopenia (heparin, sulfonamides, see drug inserts)
Antiphospholipid syndrome, systemic lupus erythematosus
HIV infection
DIC, TTP, HUS
Pseudothrombocytopenia (laboratory artifact)

DIC, disseminate intravascular coagulation; HELLP, hemolysis, elevated liver enzymes, and low platelets; HIV, human immunodeficiency virus; HUS, hemolytic uremic syndrome; TTP, thrombotic thrombocytopenic purpura.

Gestational thrombocytopenia

GT affects approximately 8% of all pregnancies.[34] The precise cause is unknown, although some authors attribute it to complement-mediated destruction of platelets as opposed to the antibody-mediated destruction that occurs in ITP.[35] It has no affect on pregnancy outcome. Neuraxial anesthesia is safe for the laboring patient with an unexplained thrombocytopenia with a platelet count from 100 000 to 120 000/μL.[36] Neuraxial anesthesia has also been administered when the platelet count was between 50 000/μL and 100 000/μL without complication,[36] although the anesthesiologist may decline to place an epidural catheter.

Immune thrombocytopenia purpura

ITP is the result of antibody-mediated destruction of platelets. The bone marrow responds to the shortened platelet lifespan by increasing production. The result is megakaryocyte hyperplasia in bone marrow smears and characteristically large (i.e., young) circulating platelets. The definitive cause of ITP was demonstrated by Harrington et al.[37] who observed that plasma from patients with ITP caused a severe thrombocytopenia when transfused into normal subjects. These autoantibodies bind to the platelet membrane glycoprotein, causing the platelets to be destroyed rapidly. The site of clearance is most likely in the spleen, as splenectomy induces a remission in about 60% of patients with chronic ITP, although there is some evidence for intravascular destruction.[38] Splenectomy is not generally recommended during pregnancy, but can be performed in the second trimester. Splenectomy does not remove the perinatal risk, and may actually increase it.

The goal of management during pregnancy is a platelet count of at least 50 000/μL by delivery. A platelet count of less than 20 000/μL is associated with spontaneous bleeding, and some form of treatment is necessary. Treatment of asymptomatic women with platelet counts between 20 000/μL and 50 000/μL who will not be delivering in the near future is unnecessary in most instances.

The first-line treatment is systemic corticosteroid administration. About two-thirds of patients with ITP will respond at least partially to corticosteroids.[39] The mechanism of action is unclear. Corticosteroids both increase the production and reduce the rate of platelet destruction.[40,41] Prednisone is initially given at a dosage of 0.5–1.0 mg/kg/day in divided doses; it may take 3–10 days before a response is noted. If the platelet count rises to acceptable levels, the dose is tapered over a 2- to 4-week interval to the minimal effective dose.

In patients refractory or intolerant to corticosteroids, IVIG will often stimulate a transient increase within 48 s. Some centers use a regimen of IVIG of 1 g/kg/day for 1–2 days (Table 48.6). However, the dose most often described in the obstetric literature is 0.4 g/kg/day for 5 days. A single, randomized trial in nonpregnant subjects observed no difference between the two regimens. Approximately 80% of patients will respond to IVIG, and the duration of the response is 2–3 weeks.[42] Pregnant women who fail corticosteroids and IVIG and who are in need of immediate treatment should be evaluated by a hematologist. Remaining therapeutic options include high-dose intravenous methylprednisolone with or without IVIG or azathioprine or splenectomy.

Many of the antibodies associated with ITP are IgG and can thus cross the placenta. The prevalence of fetal platelet counts at birth of less than 50 000/μL is 10–15%. It is less than 20 000/μL in 5%.[43,44] Unlike alloimmune thrombocytopenia, the fetus of a woman with ITP is at no or minimal risk of a hemorrhagic complication *in utero* and during delivery.[45] ITP is an indication for neither a fetal blood sample nor a Cesarean delivery. However, prudence dictates the avoidance of either vacuum or forceps delivery. The morbidity of ITP occurs in the newborn period. Platelet counts may continue to decline during the first week of life.

Table 48.6 IVIG protocol.

Indications:
- Treatment of ITP refractory to corticosteroid use
- Treatment of neonatal alloimmune thrombocytopenia purpura

Dosing recommendations:
- Usual dosage is 1 g/kg. IVIG solution often comes as 3% solution
- 30 mL/h × 15 min, then
- 60 mL/h × 30 min, then
- 120 mL/h × 30 min, then
- 240 mL/h until completion of infusion.

Monitoring:
- Monitor maternal heart rate, respirations, blood pressure, and fetal heart rate
- Preinfusion baseline, then
- Every 15 min for first hour, then
- 2 × per h, then
- Every 2 h until infusion is complete
- Anaphylaxis precautions: diphenhydramine, epinephrine, and hydrocortisone readily available for each dose

Adverse reactions:
- Chills, nausea, flushing, headache, myalgia, fatigue
- Anaphylaxis: generalized flush, urticaria, apprehension, dizziness, palpitations, respiratory distress, hypotension, arrhythmia

Differentiating between GT and ITP

No test differentiates between GT and ITP. A prior history may suggest ITP, but the diagnosis remains problematic. Testing for antiplatelet antibodies to make the diagnosis of ITP is unreliable and is not recommended by the American College of Obstetricians and Gynecologists (ACOG). Many authors and ACOG take a pragmatic approach and suggest using the platelet count to differentiate between the two.[45] The diagnosis of GT is made when no other maternal disease can be identified and the platelet count is greater than 70 000/μL; the diagnosis of ITP is made when the platelet count is less than 100 000/μL. Although these ranges overlap, it has no clinical relevance. A platelet count of 70 000/μL unassociated with bleeding requires no treatment. The patient may receive routine prenatal care with platelet counts every month or two. A platelet count below 50 000/μL with no other identifiable cause can be attributed to ITP. The diagnosis of ITP is strengthened when the maternal platelet count remains below 100 000/μL for 3 months after delivery, and/or the neonate has thrombocytopenia without a difficult delivery.

Alloimmune thrombocytopenic purpura (AITP)

AITP is the platelet form of rhesus (Rh) disease. However, the behavior of the disease differs from RBC alloimmunization in two key ways. First, approximately half of affected fetuses occur in the first pregnancy. Second, there is no reliable screening method for AITP. The initial diagnosis is often made when a thrombocytopenic neonate is born to a woman with a normal platelet count. On occasion, the presentation is fetal intracranial hemorrhage. It remains unclear as to why the risk of hemorrhage is essentially nonexistent in the fetus affected by ITP and relatively high in the fetus with AITP despite equal platelet counts. The workup for AITP includes maternal and paternal platelet typing for human platelet antigen phenotype. At least 10 platelet antigens have been implicated in AITP, with human platelet antigen 1a accounting for most cases.

Because of the risk of intracranial hemorrhage, aggressive therapy is used to prevent severe fetal thrombocytopenia. Treatment options used in the past include corticosteroids, IVIG administration to both the fetus and the mother, and fetal platelet transfusion. No treatment strategy is perfect, although maternal treatment with high doses of IVIG weekly has consistently eliminated the risk of fetal hemorrhagic events.[46] These patients should be referred to a fetal medicine specialist for management.

The only reliable way to check the fetal platelet count is by cordocentesis. One management approach is to withhold IVIG until a fetal blood sample at 22–24 weeks confirms thrombocytopenia. The fetal platelet type should be determined if the count is normal. An alternative approach is to initiate IVIG around 12 weeks' gestation, and then to check the fetal platelet count around 26 weeks. This allows time for additional therapy if the fetus is found to have thrombocytopenia despite the IVIG. A final fetal platelet count is obtained around the time at which pulmonary maturity is likely and before the onset of labor to determine whether labor is contraindicated (generally considered to be when the count is < 50 000/μL).[47] Should the fetus be thrombocytopenic, a platelet transfusion can be performed and labor induced the following day.

Other causes of thrombocytopenia

Preeclampsia is another common cause of thrombocytopenia during pregnancy. The mechanism here is accelerated platelet destruction, although many potential etiologies have been suggested. The thrombocytopenia associated with hemolysis and elevated hepatic transaminases appears to respond to corticosteroid treatment.[48] Twelve milligrams of either dexamethasone or betamethasone given every 12 h for two doses improves platelet counts.[49] Additional doses of dexamethasone (6 mg intravenously q 12 h for two doses after the initial doses) have also been used. This strategy may help to increase the time available for fetal pulmonary maturity and reduce the risk of delivery. The platelet counts rise within a week of delivery when the explanation is preeclampsia. Preeclampsia is not a cause of fetal thrombocytopenia.

Thrombotic thrombocytopenic purpura (TTP) is characterized by a fever, microangiopathic hemolytic anemia, thrombocytopenia, central nervous system (CNS) symptoms, and renal impairment. Not all elements of the classic pentad must be present simultaneously. Hemolytic uremic syndrome (HUS) is clinically similar to TTP, only having a milder thrombocytopenia, no CNS changes, and worse renal dysfunction. Clearly, the outcomes and response to therapy are different, suggesting that they share only elements of the same pathophysiologic pathway. The diagnosis is often difficult in the third trimester when the default diagnosis is preeclampsia. The principal treatment for both TTP and HUS is plasmapheresis, which has increased survival by up to 90%.[50,51] Plasma exchange should be initiated without delay once the diagnosis is made, exchanging one plasma volume in the first 24 h. If there is no or an inadequate response, corticosteroids (1–2 mg/kg/day of prednisone or equivalent) are added.

Other platelet disorders

Thrombocytosis

Thrombocytosis is defined as a platelet count greater than 450 000/μL. Most thrombocythemias are secondary to another process (Table 48.7). The diagnosis of essential thrombocytosis (ET) is suspected when all other underlying disorders appear to have been ruled out but the thrombocytosis persists. ET is a myeloproliferative disorder, and the diagnosis is made from a bone marrow aspiration. Thrombocytosis has a theoretical adverse effect on pregnancy because of a higher risk of thrombosis, and most reports suggest the use of aspirin (81 mg) to improve pregnancy outcome.[52]

Table 48.7 Differential diagnosis for thrombocytosis.

Primary causes
Myeloproliferative syndromes
Essential thrombocytosis
Polycythemia vera
Chronic myelogenous leukemia
Myelofibrosis
Secondary causes
Infectious diseases
Inflammatory diseases
Rebound after recovery from thrombocytopenia
Asplenia
Iron deficiency
Parturition
Exercise

Platelet qualitative disorders

Poor platelet function can also result from inherited disorders such as Bernard–Soulier syndrome or Glanzmann thrombasthenia. These result from an abnormal platelet surface glycoprotein that interferes with platelet adherence and/or aggregation. These rare diseases are treated by platelet transfusions in case of hemorrhage. Both are identifiable prenatally by DNA studies.

A more common cause of qualitative platelet dysfunction is drug related, notably aspirin ingestion. Aspirin inhibits the platelet release reaction and prevents platelet aggregation by the irreversible acetylation of platelet cyclo-oxygenase (average platelet lifespan is 10 days). Impairment may occur after doses as small as 40 mg.[53] Larger, "clinical" doses of 60 mg/day are used extensively during pregnancy and are not associated with increased rates of maternal or neonatal bleeding complications.[54] This dose is also safe for neuraxial anesthesia. Other commonly used drugs in obstetrics that may affect platelet function include penicillin, cephalosporins, nitrofurantoin, nonsteroidal anti-inflammatory drugs (NSAIDs), calcium channel blockers, and ketanserin.[55]

Inherited bleeding disorders

Inherited disorders of some soluble clotting factors will cause a hemorrhagic coagulopathy of varying degrees. The most commonly encountered inherited coagulopathy during pregnancy is von Willebrand's disease (vWD). Other deficiencies of the coagulation cascade described during pregnancy include deficiencies in factor X, factor XI, and factor XIII. These deficiencies are rare and can be treated with blood products if complicated by clinically significant bleeding (Table 48.8).

von Willebrand's disease

vWD is the most common inherited coagulopathy of clinical significance in the pregnant woman, affecting approximately 0.5–1% of the general population.[56] Von Willebrand's factor (vWF) binds platelets to the damaged endothelium, and is a necessary cofactor for stabilizing factor VIII. vWD is divided into three types. The quantitative deficiency of normal vWF is called type 1. Abnormal structure and function but a normal concentration of vWF is called type 2. It can be further subdivided into type 2A and 2B and differentiated by how effectively the vWF binds to platelets. In type 2B, the vWF binds platelets very effectively, but does not bind endothelium. Type 3 vWD is a complete deficiency of vWF. It is important to differentiate among the three types to facilitate the prevention or treatment of bleeding, especially in labor or postpartum. Bleeding during pregnancy is uncommon. The greatest risk is postpartum as the pregnancy-stimulated rise in factor VIII component factors declines.

Medical management of vWD includes either vasopressin or blood products (cryoprecipitate or fresh frozen plasma). Vasopressin was developed to treat diabetes insipidus, but its extrarenal actions stimulate endothelial cells to release vWF and factor VIII. Type 1 vWD is the most common form of vWD and is responsive to vasopressin. Vasopressin can be administered either parenterally (0.3 μg/kg intravenously over 30 min) or intranasally (150 μg; one spray in each nostril or, if the patient is < 50 kg, one spray in one nostril). It is given at the onset of active labor to women with low vWF levels, and repeated every 12 h. Vasopressin is not as effective in patients with type 2A vWD, and it is contraindicated in patients with type 2B vWD. The administration of vasopressin to these patients will cause thrombocytopenia without improving clot function. Vasopressin has no effect on type 3

Table 48.8 Administration of blood products for coagulation deficiencies with major bleeding.

Disorder	Therapeutic material	Loading dose	Maintenance dose
Hemophilia A (factor VIII deficiency)	Cryoprecipitate	3.5 bags/10 kg	1.75/10 kg every 8 h for 1–2 days, then every 12 h
Hemophilia B (factor IX deficiency)	Purified factor IX	60–70 U/kg	20–40 U/kg every 24 h
vWD	Cryoprecipitate	Not usually required	1 bag/10 kg daily
Fibrinogen deficiency	Cryoprecipitate	1–2 bags/10 kg	1 bag/10 kg every other day
Prothrombin deficiency	FFP	15 mL/kg	5-10 ml/kg daily
Dysprothrombinemia	Purified prothrombin complex	20 U/kg	10 U/kg daily
Factor V deficiency	FFP	20 mL/kg	10 mL/kg q12–24 h
Factor VII deficiency	FFP	20 mL/kg	5 mL/kg q6–24 h
Factor X deficiency	FFP	20 mL/kg	5–10 mL/kg daily
Factor XI deficiency	FFP	20 mL/kg	5 mL/kg q6–24 h
Factor XIII deficiency	FFP	5 mL/kg q1–2 weeks	Not usually required

FFP, fresh frozen plasma.

vWD. The administration of blood products will be necessary for patients in whom vasopressin is ineffective or contraindicated.

Hemophilia

Factor VIII deficiency (hemophilia A) and factor IX deficiency (hemophilia B) are both sex-linked recessive traits and rarely cause significant maternal bleeding. Carriers of hemophilia A and B, however, should have a coagulation profile and factor VIII activity level tested. An activated PTT does not become abnormal until the factor VIII level is < 25%. As a result, some women at risk may be missed. The severity of hemophilia is classified by the activity levels of factors VIII and IX. Individuals with mild hemophilia have activity levels of 6–40%, those with moderate hemophilia 1–5%, and with severe hemophilia < 1%. If a carrier has clinically low factor VIII or IX level, they can be treated with either fresh frozen plasma or cryoprecipitate.

Male infants born to carriers have a 50% chance of having hemophilia. Prenatal detection is possible using DNA-based techniques. Carrier detection is based on family history, coagulation-based assays, and DNA testing. The gene mutation can be determined either by testing a known affected family member or after sequencing the maternal factor VIII or IX. Once the specific gene mutation is known and the mother is determined to be a carrier, amniocentesis or CVS can be performed to determine whether the fetus is affected. Without knowing the specific gene mutation, a hemophilia genetic test is less than ideal because of cost and a delay in results, although 98–99% of the hemophilias can be detected in this way. Known affected fetuses can safely deliver vaginally, but scalp monitoring and operative vaginal delivery should be avoided.

Disseminated intravascular coagulation (DIC)

DIC remains a serious obstetric complication. DIC may be compensated, hypercompensated, or decompensated. Hypercompensated DIC is associated with thrombosis. In decompensated DIC, excess thrombin generation results in the circulation of free thrombin, stimulating widespread microvascular thrombosis. Decompensated DIC can cause tissue ischemia and organ damage. Clinical laboratory findings include prolongation of the PT and activated PTT, decreased fibrinogen, elevated fibrin split products, an abnormal platelet count, and schistocytosis on a peripheral blood smear. A compensated DIC such as that which occurs in women with preeclampsia can become decompensated because of either worsening disease or another complication. Other causes of decompensated DIC include abruptio placentae, amniotic fluid embolus, saline abortion, dead fetus syndrome, and septic shock. Hemorrhage can also trigger a decompensated DIC secondary to hypovolemia/hypoxemia. Management of DIC consists of two general steps. First, identify and remove the underlying pathological process and, second, prevent hypovolemia and hypoxemia. Occasionally, it is necessary to replace coagulation factors.

Abruptio placentae is the most common obstetric cause of decompensated DIC. The direct cause of clotting cascade activation is unclear, but may be related to the process of placental separation itself or the release of tissue thromboplastin. The diagnosis of a placental abruption associated with clinical laboratory abnormalities is an indication for rapid delivery. If the fetus is not in distress and the laboratory abnormalities are mild, a vaginal delivery may be considered, especially if the labor has occurred spontaneously. In cases of more severe laboratory abnormalities, a controlled Cesarean section should be considered with adequate blood replacement products available.

Intrauterine fetal demise (IUFD) routinely causes a compensated DIC that on rare occasions becomes decompensated. Clinical laboratory parameters do not change for at least 3–4 weeks after the demise, and some 80% of women with an IUFD will labor spontaneously within 2–3 weeks.[57] However, most patients do not wish to wait until spontaneous labor, and delay can compromise the search for a cause of the fetal death. Thus, even medically stable patients are typically delivered soon after the diagnosis.

One challenge is the singleton death in a preterm multiple gestation. There is no *a priori* indication for delivery regardless of whether the placentation is monochorionic or dichorionic. Delivery places the surviving fetus at risk from complications of prematurity. Close monitoring of the pregnancy with coagulation panels is recommended as well as other antenatal surveillance techniques. Concerns of neurologic and other organ damage to the surviving fetus from embolizing "thromboplastic" material from the dead fetus have been refuted. Should the placentation be monochorionic, perimortal blood pressure fluctuations cause shunt reversals and hypovolemia/hypotension in the survivor, making the risk of morbidity high.

Amniotic fluid embolism (AFE) is a relatively rare event, complicating approximately 1 in 250 000 pregnancies.[58] Unfortunately, the associated mortality rate ranges from 50% to 80% and has been attributed to 13–30% of all maternal mortality in industrialized countries. The pathophysiology of AFE is not well understood, in great part because of its rarity and unpredictability. The current theory is that the clinical picture of AFE reflects an anaphylactic response to materials present in the amniotic fluid. The term anaphylactoid syndrome of pregnancy is sometimes used synonymously and may represent a more accurate description of the pathophysiology underlying AFE. AFE occurs classically in the late stages of a rapid labor and presents with acute and profound hypotension and hypoxia (phase 1), followed in 0.5–2 h by a coagulopathy (phase 2). Only 50% of patients survive phase 1. A standardized management protocol has not been established, but therapy focuses on cardiovascular and ventilatory support. Basic and then advanced life support protocols should be initiated immediately in phase 1. A pulmonary artery catheter is essential, especially when pressors are needed to maintain the blood pressure and cardiac output. A perimortem Cesarean section or, if possible, an operative vaginal delivery should be considered immediately in phase 1 to preserve the neurologic status of the fetus. If a patient survives phase 1, she is at risk of developing severe coagulopathy and uterine atony. The administration of blood and blood products may be necessary to correct the coagulopathy if the bleeding cannot be controlled.

Septic abortion is another pregnancy-related diagnosis associated with decompensated DIC. Bacterial endotoxin is most likely the initiating mediator of DIC.[59,60] Aggressive antibiotic treatment and evacuation of the uterus are the primary treatments. Removal of the source of infection leads to rapid resolution of the coagulopathy.

Heparin is useful for the treatment of DIC in specific scenarios. It requires a high enough antithrombin III level for function. Heparin is useful with an IUFD and possibly to prevent septic shock after a septic abortion has been evacuated. It is not appropriate in the setting of placental abruption and/or preeclampsia. It is unknown whether the use of heparin will prevent the coagulopathy associated with AFE.[61] The dose of heparin described for the treatment of DIC with IUFD is 5000–10 000 U subcutaneously b.i.d. Therapeutic doses of heparin where the activated PTT is 1.5 time normal may be considered after the treatment of the underlying disorder is completed or if there is evidence of thrombosis causing endorgan damage.[62] Fortunately, this scenario is uncommon, and consultation with a hematologist should be considered first. Other forms of therapy such as antithrombin, gabexate mesilate, and activated protein C are currently being studied as possible options for the treatment of obstetric DIC instead of heparin.[63]

Thrombophilias in pregnancy

The possible effects of thrombophilias on pregnancy outcome have attracted interest and controversy. Unresolved questions include who should be tested, how the results are interpreted, and what therapeutic options are effective and indicated. Thrombophilias have variously been purported to increase the risks of IUGR, placental abruption, severe preeclampsia, fetal death, maternal deep venous thrombosis (DVT), and pulmonary embolus.[64–67] Thrombophilias may be inherited or acquired, and major or minor in their impact.

Acquired thrombophilias

Perhaps the most common acquired thrombophilias are the group of antiphospholipid antibodies that includes the lupus anticoagulant (LAC) and anticardiolipin antibodies (ACA). First identified obstetrically by Nilsson et al. in 1975,[68] these antibodies can be associated with both venous and arterial thrombosis in nonpregnant individuals. The diagnosis is suspected when paradoxically there is an elevated activated PTT that does not correct after a 1:1 mix with normal plasma, or when there is a false-positive rapid plasma reagin (RPR). The definitive diagnosis is made by repeated positive titers of antiphospholipid antibodies. A positive titer does not mandate treatment as there is a subset of women who have no obstetric complications despite a positive test. The diagnosis of obstetric antiphospholipid syndrome (APS) is made only when these antibodies are associated with recurrent pregnancy loss or a history of thrombosis (Table 48.9). The mechanisms responsible for the poor neonatal outcome remain to be determined, although thrombosis (either acute or chronic) at the maternal–fetal interface is believed to be involved.

Women with obstetric APS benefit from treatment. Several regimens have been compared in randomized trials. Lassere and Empson[69] summarized 13 randomized and quasirandomized trials. The studies were hampered by small sample sizes, absence of blinding to treatment, a lack of placebo control subjects, and highly variable disease definitions. The current recommendation based on these trials is to initiate in the early second trimester a combination of heparin (5000 U to 10 000 U subcutaneously b.i.d.) plus low-dose aspirin (81 mg q.d.). Prednisone does not improve outcome and may actually be associated with a higher rate of preeclampsia.

Inherited thrombophilias

The inherited thrombophilias are listed in Table 48.10. They can be subgrouped into major or minor groups depending upon their impact on pregnancy. Inherited thrombophilias include factor V Leiden (activated protein C resistance), deficiencies in protein C, protein S, and antithrombin (III) activity, prothrombin gene mutation (G20210A), and hyperhomocysteinemia. Other inherited thrombophilias exist, such as plasminogen activator inhibitor mutation, elevated factor VIII levels, "sticky platelet" syndrome, and others, but their impact on pregnancy is not well described.

Factor V Leiden is the most studied. This mutation is common in northern Europeans (5–9%) and may well account for the increased risk of thrombosis in women taking third-generation oral contraceptives. This mutation prevents activated factor V from being neutralized by the activated protein C/protein S complex. Other mutations cause activated protein C resistance, and some authors suggest testing for activated protein C resistance, the functional assay, before checking for the factor V Leiden mutation. This suggestion may not be applicable to pregnancy, however, as pregnancy may increase activated protein C resistance, and factor V Leiden accounts for most of the activated protein C resistance mutations.[70,71] The significance of factor V Leiden in pregnancy has been extensively debated. It is generally agreed that heterozygosity increases the likelihood of maternal thrombosis. However,

Table 48.9 Diagnostic criteria for antiphospholipid syndrome (APS).

Definite APS is considered to be present if at least one of the clinical criteria and one of the laboratory criteria are met.

Clinical criteria:

Vascular thrombosis: one or more clinical episodes of arterial, venous, or small-vessel thrombosis in any tissue or organ confirmed by imaging or Doppler studies or histopathology, with the exception of superficial venous thrombosis. For histopathologic confirmation, thrombosis should be present without inflammation in the vessel wall.

Pregnancy morbidity: (1) one or more unexplained deaths of a morphologically normal fetus beyond the 10th week of gestation with normal fetal morphology documented by sonography or by direct examination, or (2) one or more premature births of a morphologically normal neonate at or before the 34th week of gestation because of severe preeclampsia or eclampsia, or severe placental insufficiency, or (3) three or more unexplained consecutive spontaneous abortions before the 10th week of gestation with maternal anatomic or hormonal abnormalities and paternal and maternal chromosomal abnormalities excluded.

Laboratory criteria:

Anticardiolipin antibody of IgG and/or IgM isotype in blood, present in medium or high titer, on two or more occasions, at least 6 weeks apart, measured by a standardized enzyme-linked immunosorbent assay (ELISA) for β2-glycoprotein-I-dependent anticardiolipin antibodies.

Lupus anticoagulant present in plasma on two or more occasions at least 6 weeks apart, detected according to the International Society of Thrombosis and Hemostasis guideline/steps: (1) prolonged phospholipid-dependent coagulation demonstrated on a screening test (activated PTT, kaolin clotting time, dilute Russell's viper venom time, dilute PT, textarin time), (2) failure to correct the prolonged coagulation time on the screening test by mixing with normal platelet poor plasma, (3) shortening or correction of the prolonged coagulation time on the screening test by addition of excess phospholipids, (4) exclusion of other coagulopathies, e.g., factor VIII inhibitor or heparin as appropriate.

Table 48.10 Inherited thrombophilias.

"Greater" thrombophilias: consider therapeutic anticoagulation
- Compound heterozygosity with factor V Leiden and prothrombin G20210A gene mutation
- Homozygosity of factor V Leiden and prothrombin gene mutations
- Antithrombin deficiency (activity levels < 70%)

"Lesser" thrombophilias: consider prophylactic anticoagulation
- Protein C deficiency
- Protein S deficiency
- Factor V Leiden
- Prothrombin G20210A gene mutation
- Antiphospholipid antibodies

Other thrombophilias:
- Hyperhomocysteinemia
- Plasminogen activator inhibitor mutation

there is ongoing debate as to whether heterozygosity is associated with recurrent pregnancy loss, placental abruption, and IUFD.[72] Heterozygosity for factor V Leiden does not diminish life expectancy and, in the absence of thrombosis, nonpregnant individuals do not require lifelong anticoagulation.[73]

Deficiencies in protein C, protein S, and antithrombin decrease the body's ability to impede the coagulation process. Protein C and protein S deficiencies are autosomal-dominant traits that cause either quantitatively or qualitatively decreased activity. They are produced in the liver, and the activity levels are lowered by warfarin or acute thrombosis. Testing protein C and S activities should occur at least 10 days after cessation of warfarin and not in the setting of acute thrombosis. If warfarin is started in a patient who has protein C or S without heparinization, this may cause enough of a decrease in activity to cause thrombosis. For protein C, activity levels of less than 55% off warfarin are suspicious of a genetic abnormality; ranges of 55–65% are borderline.[74] Protein C activity levels are unchanged by pregnancy. However, protein S activity and antigen are decreased by pregnancy; antigen levels < 60% are suspicious of a genetic abnormality in the nonpregnant subject not taking warfarin.[75] The analogous figure during pregnancy is < 20–25%.[76,77]

The antithrombin molecule binds to serine protease clotting factors. After a conformational change, antithrombin becomes a potent anticoagulant, inhibiting factors IXa, Xa, XIa, and XII, and accelerates the dissociation of the tissue factor–factor VIIa complex. The antithrombin deficiency is divided into two types. In type I, there is a quantitative decrease in antithrombin. In type II, there is a mutation affecting the qualitative activity of antithrombin. The activity levels, in general, do not change significantly during pregnancy, although some decrease in activity has been reported in the third trimester. This inherited thrombophilia is considered by many as the most thrombogenic of the inherited thrombophilias. Antithrombin activity levels of heterozygotes range from 40% to 70%. Homozygotes are rare. Acute thrombosis, heparin, and systemic disease may decrease antithrombin activity during pregnancy, whereas warfarin may increase antithrombin activity. Experts disagree about the level of anticoagulation necessary for asymptomatic patients diagnosed because of a positive family history, but most agree that heparin prophylaxis is indicated to prevent maternal thrombosis.

The prothrombin gene mutation increases the gene translation rate, causing elevated prothrombin levels. It may well be the second most common thrombophilia mutation, increasing the risk of thrombosis threefold in the nonpregnant state. This mutation is found in approximately 5–15% of patients being tested for thrombophilia.

Hyperhomocysteinemia (HHC) causes thrombosis by damaging the endothelium. The risk of stillbirth correlates with the homocysteine level. A twofold increase in the rate of stillbirth was reported in women with levels between 10 and 15 μmol/L; it was sevenfold in women with levels greater than 15 μmol/L.[78] There are two general causes of HHC: enzyme deficiencies or nutritional deficiencies. The enzyme deficiency most associated with hyperhomocysteinemia is an enzyme defect in methylenetetrahydrofolate (MTHFR), which clears homocysteine from the blood. Once an elevated hyperhomocysteinemia is documented, one may either check for the MHTFR mutation or simply administer additional folate.

A personal history of thrombosis in a woman of reproductive age requires a thrombophilia workup. However, there is a large group of women between the symptomatic group and those that are completely asymptomatic with no family history of thrombosis. A study evaluating the cost-effectiveness of spending US$1000 or more on the evaluation of every woman who experiences severe preeclampsia, placental abruption, IUGR, or unexplained IUFD needs to be done. No guidelines exist as to who might benefit from an inherited thrombophilia workup.

Existing recommendations are based on small studies and on theoretical grounds. Because of a lack of evidence, a discussion with the patient should take place once a thrombophilia has been diagnosed as to whether anticoagulation is of potential value. Some experts suggest stratifying risk for thrombosis into a "greater" risk and a "lesser" risk category.[79] Patients with a "greater" risk of thrombophilia are those with homozygous gene mutations for prothrombin and factor V Leiden, combined heterozygous mutations for prothrombin and factor V Leiden, and antithrombin deficiency. These patients will likely benefit from therapeutic anticoagulation as if the patient has already had a thrombosis. Those with "lesser" risk of thrombophilias may, in the presence of other risk factors (e.g., Cesarean delivery, preeclampsia), benefit from prophylactic anticoagulation. Treatment with heparin has its own inherent risks such as bleeding and osteoporosis, and these have to be considered and discussed with the patient prior to starting therapy.

Key points

Anemia

1 Pregnancy is subject to a disproportionate rise in plasma volume. The CDC defines anemia as hemoglobin levels less than 11 g/dL in the first and third trimesters and less than 10.5 g/dL in the second.

2 A basic workup depends on the reticulocyte count and MCV of the CBC.

3 The effect of anemia on pregnancy is dependent on the type and severity of anemia diagnosed.

4 Hemoglobinopathies in the mother are important to diagnose even if they have no effect on the pregnancy because of genetic implications.

5 Sickling hemoglobinopathies confer a high risk of maternal and fetal morbidity and mortality, and antepartum surveillance is recommended.

6 Neurologic and pulmonary symptoms of the sickling hemoglobinopathies need to be diagnosed very carefully, and prompt action taken. Acute chest syndrome is the major cause of morbidity in a patient with a sickling hemoglobinopathy.

Coagulation disorders

7 Pregnancy causes a heightened activation of the coagulation system of both the procoagulant and the anticoagulant systems with a tendency toward thrombosis.

8 A coagulation panel may include a CBC, PT, activated PTT, fibrinogen, fibrin split products, and possibly a bleeding time.

Thrombocytopenia/platelet disorders

9 The most common cause of thrombocytopenia during pregnancy is gestational thrombocytopenia (GT), which rarely decreases platelet counts to less than 70 000/μl. GT has little clinical significance.

10 Immune thrombocytopenic purpura (ITP) is another potential cause of thrombocytopenia and may be difficult to distinguish from GT. Treatment includes corticosteroids and IVIG.

11 Alloimmune thrombocytopenia purpura can be a devastating disease for the fetus/neonate. Management should be performed in conjunction with a fetal medicine specialist.

12 Drugs, especially aspirin, can cause platelet dysfunction. Doses higher than 81 mg/day should be used with caution and discussed with an anesthesiologist before regional anesthesia is given.

Inherited bleeding disorders

13 Von Willebrand's disease (vWD) is the most common inherited coagulopathy of clinical significance in the pregnant woman. Knowing the type of vWD has important management implications. Vasopressin should not be given in type 2B and type 3 vWD, and blood products should be given instead.

14 Hemophilia has X-linked inheritance with implications for the male fetus. Genetic counseling and testing are important for proper management.

DIC

15 Abruptio placentae is the most common cause of DIC, and prompt delivery, especially with laboratory abnormalities, should reverse changes. Heparin should not be given before delivery.

16 Intrauterine fetal demise and septic abortion cause DIC, and delivery of the fetus or evacuation of the uterus should be prompt.

17 Amniotic fluid embolus is a devastating complication that is treated with supportive measures.

Thrombophilias in pregnancy

18 There are many issues regarding thrombophilias in pregnancy that still need to be resolved, including impact, screening, and management issues.

19 Thrombophilias can be divided into acquired and inherited. Acquired thrombophilias are diagnosed by certain laboratory and clinical criteria. Inherited thrombophilias are diagnosed by laboratory criteria.

20 Management usually involves placing patients on heparin and aspirin. The amount of heparin (prophylactic versus therapeutic) depends on the thrombophilia and the past medical history.

References

1 Freedman ML, Marcus DL. Anemia and the elderly: is it physiology or pathology? *Am J Med Sci* 1980;280:81.

2 Dallman PR, Yip R, Johnson C. Prevalence and causes of anemia in the United States, 1976 to 1980. *Am J Clin Nutr* 1984;39:437.

3 Caton W, Roby CC, Reid DE, Gibson JG. Plasma volume and extravascular fluid volume during pregnancy and the puerperium. *Am J Obstet Gynecol* 1949;57:471.

4 Centers for Disease Control. Anemia during pregnancy in low-income women – United States, 1987. *Morbid Mortal Weekly Rep* 1990;39:73.

5 Cartwright GE. The anemia of chronic disorders. *Semin Hematol* 1966;3:351.

6 Mahomed K. Iron supplementation in pregnancy. *Cochrane Database Syst Rev* 2000;CD 000117.

7 Turgeon O'Brien H, Sanure M, Maziade J. The association of low and high ferritin levels and anemia with pregnancy outcome. *Can J Diet Pract Res* 2000;61:121.

8 Scholl TO, Hediger ML, Fischer RL, Shearer JW. Anemia vs iron deficiency: increased risk of preterm delivery in a prospective study. *Am J Clin Nutr* 1992;55:985.

9 Lanzkowsky P. The influence of maternal iron-deficiency anemia on the hemoglobin of the infant. *Arch Dis Child* 1961;36:205

10 Murray MJ, Murray AB, Murray NJ, Murray MB. The effect of iron status of Nigerian mothers on that of their infants at birth and six months, and on the concentration of iron in breast milk. *Br J Nutr* 1978;39:627.

11 Olivieri NF. The B-thalassemias. *N Engl J Med* 1999;341:99.

12 Whalley PJ. Bacteriuria of pregnancy. *Am J Obstet Gynecol* 1967;97:723.

13 Milner PF, Jones BR, Dobler J. Outcome of pregnancy in sickle-cell anemia and sickle cell-hemoglobin C disease. *Am J Obstet Gynecol* 1980;138:239.

14 Smith JA, Espeland M, Bellevue R, et al. Pregnancy in sickle cell disease: experience of the cooperative study of sickle cell disease. *Obstet Gynecol* 1996;87:199.

15 Cunningham FG, Pritchard JA, Mason R. Pregnancy and sickle cell hemoglobinopathies: results with and without prophylactic transfusions. *Obstet Gynecol* 1983;62:419.

16 Tuck S. Pregnancy in sickle cell disease in the United Kingdom. *Br J Obstet Gynecol* 1983;90:112.

17 Koshy M, Burd L, Wallace D, et al. Prophylactic red cell transfusion in pregnant patients with sickle cell disease. A randomized cooperative study. *N Engl J Med* 1988;319:1447.

18 Tuck SM, Jones CE, Brewster EM, et al. Prophylactic blood transfusion in maternal sickle cell syndromes. *Br J Obstet Gynaecol* 1987;94:121.

19 Vichinsky EP, Neumayr LD, Earles AN, et al. Causes and outcomes of the acute chest syndrome in sickle cell disease: National Acute Chest Syndrome Study Group. *N Engl J Med* 2000;342:1855.

20 Eichhorn RF, Buurke EJ, Blok P, et al. Sickle cell-like crisis and bone marrow necrosis associated with parvovirus B19 and heterozygosity for Haemoglobins S and E. *J Intern Med* 1999;245:103.

21 Petz LD, Fudenberg HH. Coombs-positive hemolytic anemia caused by penicillin administration. *N Engl J Med* 1966;274:178.

22 Swanson MA, Channongan D, Schwartz RS. Immunohemolytic anemia due to anti-penicillin antibodies. *N Engl J Med* 1966;274:178.

23 Branch DR, Berkowitz LR, Becker RL, et al. Extravascular hemolysis following the administration of cefamandole. *Am J Hematol* 1985;18:213.

24 Worlledge SM, Carstairs KC, Dacie JV. Autoimmune haemolytic anaemias associated with alpha-methyldopa therapy. *Lancet* 1966;2:135.

25 Carstairs KC, Breckenridge A, Dollery CT, et al. Incidence of a positive direct Coombs' test in patients on a-methyldopa. *Lancet* 1966;2:133.

26 Petrakis NL, Wiesenfeld SL, Sams BJ, et al. Prevalence of sickle-cell trait and glucose 6-phosphate dehydrogenase deficiency. *N Engl J Med* 1970;282:767.

27 Brown AK. Hyperbilirubinemia in black infants: role of glucose-6-phosphate dehydrogenase deficiency. *Clin Pediatr (Phila)* 1992; 31:712.

28 Weiner CP, Kwaan H, Hauck WW, et al. Fibrin generation in normal pregnancy. *Obstet Gynecol* 1984;64:46.

29 Moncada S, Vane JR. The role of prostacyclin in vascular tissue. *Fed Proc* 1979;38:66.

30 National Institutes of Health Consensus Development Conference. Prevention of venous thrombosis and pulmonary embolism. *JAMA* 1986;256:744.

31 Lind SE. Prolonged bleeding time. *Am J Med* 1984;77:305.

32 Lind SE. The bleeding time does not predict surgical bleeding. *Blood* 1991;77:2547.

33 British Committee for Standards in Haematology General Haematology Task Force. Guidelines for the investigation and management of idiopathic thrombocytopenic purpura in adults, children and in pregnancy. *Br J Haematol* 2003;120:574.

34 Burrows RF, Kelton JG. Thrombocytopenia at delivery: a prospective survey of 6715 deliveries. *Am J Obstet Gynecol* 1990;163: 731.

35 Freedman J, Musclow E, Garvey B, Abbott D. Unexplained perparturient thrombocytopenia. *Am J Hematol* 1986;21:397.

36 Rolbin SH, Abbott D, Musclow E, et al. Epidural anesthesia in pregnant patients with low platelet counts. *Obstet Gynecol* 1988;71:918.

37 Harrington WJ, Minnich V, Hollingworth JW, Moore CV. Demonstration of a thrombocytopenic factor in the blood of patients with thrombocytopenic purpura. *J Lab Clin Med* 1951;38:1.

38 Stasi R, Stipa E, Masi M, et al. Long-term observation of 208 adults with chronic idiopathic thrombocytopenic purpura. *Am J Med* 1995;98:436.

39 George JN, Woolf SH, Raskob GE, et al. Idiopathic thrombocytopenic purpura: a practice guideline developed by explicit methods for the American Society of Hematology. *Blood* 1996;88:3.

40 Gernsheimer T, Stratton J, Ballem PJ, Slichter SJ. Mechanism of response to treatment in autoimmune thrombocytopenic purpura. *N Engl J Med* 1989;320:974.

41 Fujisawa K, Tani P, Piro L, McMillan R. The effect of therapy on platelet-associated autoantibody in chronic immune thrombocytopenic purpura. *Blood* 1993;81:2872.

42 Bussel JB, Pham LC. Intravenous treatment with gammaglobulin in adults with immune thrombocytopenic purpura: review of the literature. *Vox Sang* 1987;52:206.

43 Iyori H, Fujisawa K, Abatsuka J. Thrombocytopenia in neonates born to women with autoimmune thrombocytopenic purpura. *Pediatr Hematol Oncol* 1997;14:367.

44 Christiaens GC, Nieuwenhuis HK, Bussel JB. Comparison of platelet counts in first and second newborns of mothers with immune thrombocytopenic purpura. *Obstet Gynecol* 1997; 90:516.

45 ACOG Technical Bulletin no. 6, September 1999.

46 Bussel JB, Berkowitz RL, Lynch L, et al. Antenatal management of alloimmune thrombocytopenia with intravenous gamma-globulin: a randomized trial of the addition of low-dose steroid to intravenous gamma-globulin. *Am J Obstet Gynecol* 1996;174: 1414.

47 Kaplan C, Daffos F, Forestier F, et al. Management of alloimmune thrombocytopenia: antenatal diagnosis and in utero transfusion of maternal platelets. *Blood* 1988;72:340.

48 O'Brien JM, Milligan DA, Barton JR. Impact of high-dose corticosteroid therapy for patients with HELLP (hemolysis, elevated liver enzymes, and low platelet count) syndrome. *Am J Obstet Gynecol* 2000;183:921.

49 Tompkins MJ, Thiagarajah S. HELLP (hemolysis, elevated liver enzymes, and low platelet count) syndrome: the benefit of corticosteroids. *Am J Obstet Gynecol* 1999;187:304.

50 Ambrose A, Welham RT, Cefalo RC. TTP in early pregnancy. *Obstet Gynecol* 1985;66:267.

51 Vandeherchove F. TTP mimicking toxemia. *Am J Obstet Gynecol* 1984;150:320.

52 Pagliaro P, Arrigoni L, Muggiasca ML, et al. Primary thrombocythemia and pregnancy: treatment and outcome in fifteen cases. *Am J Hematol* 1998;57:181.

53 Roth GJ, Calvarly DC. Aspirin, platelets, and thrombosis: theory and practice. *Blood* 1994 83:885.

54 Sibai BM, Caritis SN, Thorm E et al. Low dose aspirin in nulliparous women: safety of continuous epidural block and correlation between bleeding time and maternal–neonatal bleeding complications. *Am J Obstet Gynecol* 1995;172:1553.

55 Hoffman R, ed. *Hoffman's hematology: basic principles and practice*, 3rd edn. New York: Churchill Livingstone, 2000.

56 Punnonen R, Nyman D, Gronroos M, Wallen O. Von Willebrand's disease in pregnancy. *Acta Obstet Gynecol Scand* 1981;60: 507.

57 Pritchard JA. Fetal death in utero. *Obstet Gynecol* 1959;14:573.

58 Tuffnell DJ. Amniotic fluid embolism. *Curr Opin Obstet Gynecol* 2003;15:119.

59 McKay KG, Jewett JF, Reid DE. Endotoxin shock and the generalized Schwartzman reaction in pregnancy. *Am J Obstet Gynecol* 1959;78:546.

60 Beller FK, Schoendorf T. Augmentation of endotoxin-induced fibrin deposits by pregnancy and estrogen-progesterone treatment. *Gynecol Obstet Invest* 1972;3:176.

61 Strickland MA, Bates GW, Whitworth NS, Martin JN. Amniotic fluid embolism: prophylaxis with heparin and aspirin. *South Med J* 1985;78:377.

62 Stratta P, Canavese C, Goia F, et al. Clinical and therapeutic correlations in consumption coagulopathy of obstetric acute renal failure. *Clin Exp Obstet Gynecol* 1986;13:43.

63 Kobayashi T, Terao T, Maki M, Ikenoue T. Diagnosis and management of acute obstetrical DIC. *Semin Thromb Hemost* 2001;27:161.

64 Tranquilli AL, Giannubilo SR, Dell'uomo B, Grandone E. Adverse pregnancy outcomes are associated with multiple maternal thrombophilic factors. *Eur J Obstet Gynecol Reprod Biol* 2004; 117:114.

65 Kujovich JL. Thrombophilia and pregnancy complications. *Am J Obstet Gynecol* 2004:19:412.

66 Preston FE, Rosendaal FR, Walker ID, et al. Increased fetal loss in women with heritable thrombophilia. *Lancet* 1996;348: 913.

67 Rey E, Kahn SR, David M, Shrier I. Thrombophilic disorders and fetal loss: a meta-analysis. *Lancet* 2003;361:901.

68 Nilsson IM, Astedt B, Hedner U, Berezin D. Intrauterine death and circulating anticoagulant ("antithromboplastin"). *Acta Med Scand* 1975;197:153.

69 Lassere M, Empson M. Treatment of antiphospholipid syndrome in pregnancy – a systematic review of randomized therapeutic trials. *Thromb Res* 2004;114:419.

70 Faioni EM, Franchi F, Asti D, Mannucci PM. Acquired resistance to activated protein C develops during pregnancy (abstract). *Thromb Haemost* 1995;73:1375.

71 Thomas R. Hypercoagulability syndromes. *Ann Intern Med* 2001;161:2433.

72 Kujovich JL. Thrombophilia and pregnancy complications. *Am J Obstet Gynecol* 2004;191:412.

73 Hille ET, Westenderp RG, Vandenbroucke JP, et al. Mortality and causes of death in families with the factor V Leiden mutation (resistance to activated protein C). *Blood* 1997;89:1963.
74 Bauer K. Hypercoagulable states. In: Hoffman R, Furie B, Cohen H, et al., eds. *Hematology: basic principles and practice*, 2nd edn. London: Churchill Livingstone; 1995:1781.
75 Bick RL, Kaplan H. Syndromes of thrombosis and hypercoagulability. *Med Clin North Am* 1998;82:409.
76 Comp PC, Thurnau GR, Welsh J, Esmon CT. Functional and immunologic protein S levels are decreased during pregnancy. *Blood* 1986;68:881.
77 Malm J, Laurell M, Dahlback B. Changes in the plasma levels of vitamin K-dependent proteins C and S and of C4b-binding protein during pregnancy and oral contraception. *Br J Haematol* 1988;68:437.
78 Gris JC, Perneger TV, Quere I, et al. Antiphospholipid/antiprotein antibodies, hemostasis-related autoantibodies, and plasma homocysteine as risk factors for a first early pregnancy loss: a matched case–control study. *Blood* 2003;102:3504.
79 Lockwood CJ. Inherited thrombophilias in pregnant patients: detection and treatment paradigm. *Obstet Gynecol* 2002;99: 333.

49 Maternal alloimmunization and fetal hemolytic disease

Carl P. Weiner and Anita C. Manogura

Fetal hemolytic disease was first described in 1609 when a hydropic twin died shortly after birth and its co-twin succumbed of kernicterus a few days later. The cause and relationship between hydrops and kernicterus was unrecognized until 1932 when Diamond et al. noted that erythroblastosis fetalis was associated with fetal edema, neonatal anemia, and hyperbilirubinemia. They demonstrated that these were manifestations of a disease characterized by hepatosplenomegaly, extramedullary erythropoiesis, and erythroblastosis. Levine and Stetson in 1939 were the first to suggest that the hemolysis was due to the maternal development of a blood group antibody directed against a fetal blood group antigen. They observed atypical agglutinins in the serum of a woman who had just delivered a hydropic stillborn. These agglutinins were active against her husband's erythrocytes (same ABO blood group). Subsequently, Levine and Stetson postulated that an immunizing agent in the fetus, inherited from the father, entered the maternal circulation and caused her to develop the agglutinin. The discovery of blood group antigens by Landsteiner and Wiener in 1940 laid the foundation for the role of alloimmunization in the pathogenesis of fetal hemolytic disease.

Rhesus (Rh) blood group system

The Rh blood group system is the most common system causing serious alloimmunization. However, other blood group systems (so-called "minor antigens" of the erythrocyte membrane) are of growing importance as the prevalence of Rh alloimmunization declines secondary to prevention programs.

Nomenclature

The Fisher–Race system (first proposed in the 1940s) presumes the presence of three genetic loci, each with two major alleles – Dd, Cc, Ee.[1] An Rh gene complex is described by three letters – Cde, cde, cDE, cDe, Cde, cdE, CDE, CdE (the first three being the most common and the last one yet to be demonstrated).

The antigens produced by these alleles (located on chromosome 1p34–36) were originally identified by specific antisera.[2] No antiserum for the d antigen has been identified, and it is felt that the d antigen reflects in truth the absence of an allelic product. The presence or absence of the D antigen determines the Rh status. Approximately 45% of D-positive individuals are homozygous for D. If the Rh-positive husband of a Rh-negative woman is homozygous, all his children will be D positive; if he is heterozygous, there is an equal chance that the fetus will be D negative or D positive in each pregnancy.

There are alternative classification systems. The Wiener system is based on the theory that a single locus is occupied by a pair of complex agglutinogens.[3] The eight genotypes are designated (in decreasing order of frequency in the white population) R^1, r, R^2, R^0, r′, r″, R^z, and r^y. This system may be the most accurate. The Rosenfield system is based on the belief that neither of the two discussed systems explains the quantitative differences in the expression of Rh antigens.[4] They also note that genetic concepts such as the operon model of gene function with nonlinked regulator genes are poorly accommodated by the mendelian model of Fisher–Race. Rosenfield proposed an updated system of nomenclature that numbered the Rh antigens as Rh1–Rh48.

Diversity and ethnicity

The Rh blood group system is complex; 42 antigens other than the five mentioned have been described.[5] C^w, an allele for C, is relatively common. D^u, an allele for D, is more common in black populations than in other racial groups.

In most white populations, the incidence of Rh negativity is 15–16%. In Finland, it is 10–12%. It is 30–35% in the Basque population, but less than 1% in the Chinese and Japanese populations. Approximately 1–2% of North American Indians and Inuit are Rh negative, as are approximately 2% of Indo-Eurasians. In the black population, the incidence ranges from 4% to 8%, being higher in North American than in African black people.

Immunology

The Rh antigens are embedded in the lipid phase of the erythrocyte membrane, and are expressed on fetal erythrocytes by day 38. Ten different antigenic epitopes have been identified to date. One theory suggests that the different epitopes are variably expressed within the erythrocyte membrane, and that this immunologic variation accounts for the spectrum of fetal hemolytic disease.

Rh functionality

The function of the Rh antigen is unclear, although it may have a role in maintaining erythrocyte integrity, plus contributing to electrolyte and volume flux across the erythrocyte membrane. For example, the red blood cells (RBCs) of individuals with Rh_{null} (lacking all Rh antigens) suffer multiple membrane defects, osmotic fragility, and abnormal shapes.

Pathogenesis of maternal alloimmunization

Blood transfusion was a common cause of Rh alloimmunization before the discovery of the Rh blood group system. It is still a common cause of non-D blood group alloimmunization. Although many non-D blood group antibodies have no clinical significance, some may cause severe erythroblastosis.

For Rh alloimmunization to occur:

1 The woman must be Rh negative and the fetus Rh positive.
2 Fetal erythrocytes must enter the maternal circulation in sufficient quantity.
3 The mother must be immune competent.

Transplacental hemorrhage

The prevalence of Rh alloimmunization declined only slightly after the discovery of the Rh blood group system and the introduction of transfusion of Rh D-compatible blood. In 1954, Chown proved Weiner's hypothesis that fetal-to-maternal transplacental hemorrhage (TPH) caused Rh immunization.[6,7]

The Kleihauer acid elution test is an accurate and sensitive method of detecting TPH.[8] Seventy-five percent of women have a fetal TPH some time during pregnancy or at delivery.[9] The volume of the hemorrhage is usually small, but exceeds 5 mL in 1% and 30 mL in 0.25% of pregnancies. Antepartum hemorrhage, toxemia of pregnancy, Cesarean section, manual removal of the placenta, and external cephalic version each increase the risk and volume of TPH. The prevalence and volume of TPH rises with advancing gestation, from 3% (0.03 mL) in the first trimester to 12% (usually < 0.1 mL) in the second trimester, and to 45% (occasionally up to 25 mL) in the third trimester.[9] Spontaneous abortion has a low risk of TPH (typically < 0.1 mL). However, the risk may be as high as 25% after therapeutic abortion, with volumes exceeding 0.2 mL in 4% of pregnancies.

Maternal response

At least two characteristics affect whether alloimmunization occurs. First, 30% of Rh-negative individuals act as immunologic nonresponders and do not become sensitized regardless of the Rh-antigen load. Second, ABO incompatibility has a protective effect. One explanation for this phenomenon is that the maternal anti-A or anti-B antibodies damage or alter the fetal Rh antigen so that it is no longer immunogenic. Another hypothesis holds that ABO-incompatible fetal cells are more rapidly cleared from the maternal circulation, so that maternal sensitization does not occur. Regardless of the mechanism, ABO incompatibility decreases the risk of alloimmunization to 1.5–2% after the delivery of a Rh-positive neonate.

Rh immune response

The primary Rh immune response develops slowly, typically over 6–12 weeks but sometimes up to 6 months. It is usually weak and predominantly IgM, which does not cross the placenta (molecular weight 900 000 kDa). Most immunized women convert quickly to IgG anti-D (molecular weight 160 000 kDa) production, which can readily cross the placenta. The IgG anti-D coats Rh-positive fetal erythrocytes and triggers hemolysis.

A second TPH, which may be very small, produces a very different secondary immune response. The response is rapid (days) and is usually IgG. Additional episodes of TPH may further increase the antibody titer. Long periods between Rh-positive erythrocyte exposures are associated with marked increases in Rh antibody titer along with increased binding avidity for the D antigen.[10] The greater the avidity, the more severe the disease.

Antibody detection and measurement methods

Methods used to measure and detect antibodies include:

1 Saline – Rh-positive erythrocytes suspended in isotonic saline are agglutinated only by IgM anti-D. IgG anti-D cannot bridge the gap between erythrocytes suspended in saline. This method is no longer in use.
2 Colloid – Rh-positive red cells suspended in albumin are agglutinated by IgG anti-D.[11] Because IgM anti-D also agglutinates colloid-suspended Rh-positive erythrocytes, the albumin titer may not be an accurate measurement of IgG anti-D. Mixing the serum with dithiothreitol disrupts IgM sulfhydryl bonds, destroying IgM but leaving IgG intact. Subsequent titration allows a true measurement of the IgG anti-D level. This method is rarely used.
3 Indirect antiglobulin test (IAT)[12] – antihuman globulin (AHG) antibody (Coombs' serum) is produced by the injection of human serum (or specific human IgG) into an animal.

IgG anti-D, if present, adheres to Rh-positive erythrocytes after incubation with the serum being screened for Rh antibody. The erythrocytes are then washed with isotonic saline and suspended in the AHG antibody serum. The erythrocytes agglutinate if coated with antibody (a positive IAT or indirect Coombs' test). The reciprocal of the highest dilution causing agglutination is the indirect antiglobulin titer. IAT screening is more sensitive than albumin screening. IAT titers are usually one to three dilutions higher than albumin titers. A critical titer is defined as the titer associated with a significant risk of fetal hydrops. This varies with the institution and methodology. Most centers have a critical titer between 8 and 32.

4 Enzyme – the incubation of erythrocytes with various enzymes (papain, trypsin, or bromelin) reduces the negative electrical potential of the cells. As a result, they are closer together in saline and are agglutinated by IgG anti-D. Enzyme techniques are the most sensitive available manual methods for detecting Rh immunization.[13]

5 AutoAnalyzer (AA) (Technicon Instruments Corp., Tarrytown, NY, USA) – AA methods (bromelin[14] and low ionic[15]) are most sensitive for the detection of Rh antibody. They are so sensitive that, if manual methods fail to confirm the presence of Rh antibody, the mother may not be Rh immunized. Erythrocytes are mixed with agents to enhance agglutination by the anti-D antibodies. Agglutinated cells are separated from nonagglutinated cells and lysed. The amount of released hemoglobin is then compared with an international standard. A modification of the bromelin method is used to measure accurately (μg/mL) the amount of serum anti-D.[16]

Prevalence of Rh immunization

Rather small amounts of Rh-positive blood (as little as 0.3 mL) can produce Rh immunization in Rh-negative volunteers.[17] The risk of Rh immunization is antigen-dose dependent: 15% after 1 mL, 33% after 10 mL, and 65% after 50–250 mL of Rh-positive erythrocytes.[18] A secondary immune response may follow a small repeat challenge (0.05 mL of Rh-positive erythrocytes). The incidence of Rh immunization 6 months after delivery is 3% of Rh-negative women who, on serial Kleihauer tests, never had evidence of a TPH above 0.1 mL. If the volume is greater than 0.1 mL, the incidence is 14%;[16] it is 22% if the volume is greater than 0.4 mL.[19]

The incidence of Rh immunization 6 months after delivery of the first Rh-positive ABO-compatible neonate is 8–9%. An equal number of women are immunized during their first pregnancy, but have an undetectable antibody level until challenged again, typically in their next pregnancy ("sensibilization").[20] Therefore, the overall risk of Rh immunization following the first Rh-positive ABO-compatible pregnancy is 16%. An unimmunized Rh-negative woman faces approximately the same risk during a second such pregnancy. As parity increases and the ratio of good responders to poor immune responders decreases, the risk becomes less. There is a 50% likelihood that she will be Rh immunized after five Rh-positive ABO-compatible pregnancies. In one study, five of 3533 Rh-negative women with Rh-positive fetuses (0.14%) were Rh immunized before 28 weeks' gestation, and 1.66% were immunized 3 days postpartum (total 1.8%).[21] Because the total incidence of Rh immunization approximates 13% (16% in the 80% carrying ABO-compatible babies, 1.5–2% in the 20% carrying ABO-incompatible babies), 13–14% of all instances of Rh immunization [1.8 × (100/13)] occur during pregnancy or within 3 days after delivery.

ABO incompatibility

ABO incompatibility between the Rh-positive fetus and the Rh-negative mother reduces the risk of immunization to 1.5–2%.[18] The partial protection reflects, at least in part, rapid intravascular hemolysis of the fetal ABO-incompatible cells and their sequestration in the liver, where there are fewer antibody-forming lymphocytes than in the spleen. ABO incompatibility confers no protection once Rh immunization has developed.[22]

Rh immunization caused by abortion

The woman who becomes Rh immunized after an abortion is a "good responder," and frequently has very severely affected babies. The risk is approximately 2% after spontaneous abortion and 4–5% after therapeutic abortion.

Pathogenesis of fetal hemolytic disease

Fetal blood is produced in the yolk sac as early as the third week. The Rh antigen is detectable on the red cell membrane by the sixth week. Erythropoiesis begins in the yolk sac but moves to the liver and, finally, to the bone marrow by 16 weeks' gestation.

Maternal IgG anti-D crosses the placenta and coats the D-positive fetal red cells. The fetal red cells are destroyed extravascularly, primarily in the spleen, as anti-D does not fix complement. The resulting anemia stimulates fetal erythropoietin synthesis and release. A reticulocytosis occurs when the fetal hemoglobin deficit exceeds 2 g/dL compared with gestational age-appropriate norms. Should marrow red cell production fail to compensate, extramedullary erythropoiesis recurs, initially in the liver and spleen. Hepatomegaly may become extreme. Cardiac output increases, and 2,3-diphosphoglycerate levels are enhanced. Although the blood $P\text{O}_2$ is unaltered, tissue hypoxia results from the decreased carrying capacity. Umbilical arterial lactate begins to rise only after the fetal hemoglobin falls below 8 g/dL, while the umbilical venous lactate begins to rise after the hemoglobin falls below 4 g/dL.[23] Nucleated red cell precursors from normoblasts to primitive erythroblasts are released into the circulation (hence the term erythroblastosis fetalis coined by Diamond).

Degrees of Rh hemolytic disease

The severity of hemolytic disease reflects the amount of maternal IgG anti-D (the titer), its affinity or avidity for the fetal red cell membrane D antigen, and the ability of the fetus to tolerate hypoxemia before developing hydrops secondary to myocardial pump failure. When the globin chain is split from hemoglobin during hemolysis, the remaining heme pigment is converted by heme oxygenase to biliverdin, and then by biliverdin reductase to neurotoxic indirect bilirubin. The fetal and newborn liver is deficient in glucuronyl transferase and Y transport protein. Thus, the increased indirect bilirubin is deposited in the perinate's extravascular fluid compartments.

Indirect bilirubin is water insoluble and can remain in the plasma only when bound to albumin. When the albumin-binding capacity of the perinate's plasma is exceeded, "free" indirect bilirubin appears and diffuses into fatty tissues. The neuron membrane has a high lipid content, and the free indirect bilirubin penetrates the neuron where it interferes with cellular metabolism. Mitochondria swell, then balloon, and the neuron dies. The dead neurons with accumulated bilirubin appear yellow at autopsy (kernicterus).

Mild disease

Approximately 50% of affected fetuses do not require treatment postnatally. Their umbilical cord blood hemoglobin is above 12 g/dL, and their umbilical cord serum bilirubin is less than 68 μmol/L (< 4 mg/100 mL). In the nursery, their hemoglobin does not drop below 11 g/dL, and their serum indirect bilirubin remains below 340 μmol/L (20 mg/dL) or 260–300 μmol/L (15–17.5 mg/dL) if preterm. Postdischarge hemoglobin remains above 7.5 g/dL.

Intermediate disease

Some 25–30% of affected fetuses have intermediate disease. They are born at or near term in good condition, with an umbilical cord blood hemoglobin between 9 g/dL and 12 g/dL. Extramedullary erythropoiesis is modest and liver function normal.

Some of these infants develop severe hyperbilirubinemia; those with kernicterus are deeply jaundiced. They become lethargic by day 3–5 and then hypertonic. They assume an opisthotonic position with their necks hyperextended, backs arched, and knees, wrists, and elbows flexed. Their vegetative reflexes disappear and apneic spells develop. The mortality rate is up to 90%. In the remaining 10%, the jaundice fades and spasticity lessens. However, they show severe central nervous system dysfunction over time with profound neurosensory deafness and choreoathetoid spastic cerebral palsy. Intellectual retardation may be relatively mild, but learning and functioning are hindered by deafness and spastic choreoathetosis.

Severe disease

The 20–25% of most severely affected fetuses, despite maximal RBC production, become progressively more anemic. Ascites with anasarca (generalized edema) occurs. Half these fetuses become hydropic between 18 and 34 weeks' gestation; the other half between 34 weeks and term.

The exact mechanism underlying hydrops has become clear over time. There is always a large hemoglobin deficit.[24] Hemoglobin concentration clearly rises with advancing gestational age. Hydrops, consequently, occurs at higher absolute hemoglobin levels during late compared with early gestation, and is extremely rare before 20 weeks' gestation. Cardiac dysfunction secondary to severe fetal anemia and the resultant inadequate oxygen-carrying capacity is evident in at least 90% of hydropic fetuses. Fetal cardiac dysfunction is characterized by an increase in the biventricular cardiac diameter, systolic atrial–ventricular valve regurgitation, and an elevated umbilical pressure for gestational age.[25] This cardiac dysfunction is detectable prior to the development of hydrops and, within 48 h of a RBC transfusion (and before the hydrops resolves), the umbilical venous pressure decreases into the normal range for gestation.[26,27] Although hepatomegaly was once thought to cause portal hypertension and decrease cardiac return, it is clear that this is not the typical mechanism. Additionally, while hypoalbuminemia (secondary to fetal liver failure) was once thought to be a contributing factor, fetal studies reveal that the albumin concentration is normal for all but premoribund, hydropic fetuses.[28,29]

Monitoring the mother and fetus at risk

A blood sample is obtained from every woman during her first prenatal visit for blood type and antibody screening. Ideally, all women should have two blood type determinations on record that are in agreement. Mistyping of a Rh-negative woman may have occurred in a prior pregnancy, and a Rh-positive woman, particularly if she has been transfused, may have developed a dangerous atypical blood group antibody.

The Rh-positive woman without blood group antibodies at her first prenatal visit is not likely to develop dangerous atypical blood group antibodies later in her pregnancy. Frequent retesting is not cost-effective.[30]

The Rh-negative woman without Rh antibodies should be ABO grouped, and the Rh status of her husband should be determined. If he is Rh negative, her fetus will be Rh negative if paternity is correct. Rh status should, however, be confirmed at birth. If the father is Rh positive, his ABO group and Rh phenotype should be determined. Depending on his Rh phenotype, the likelihood of his Rh zygosity can be determined. If he is heterozygous, there is a 50% chance that the fetus is Rh negative. If the husband is ABO incompatible with his wife, there is roughly a 60% chance that the baby is ABO incompatible. If the fetus is ABO incompatible, the risk of Rh immunization is reduced from 16% to 1.5–2%.

The Rh-negative pregnant woman whose husband is Rh positive should undergo additional testing to exclude isoimmunization during the pregnancy. Cesarean section and manual removal of the placenta increase the frequency and size of fetal–maternal TPH, increasing the risk of immunization if the fetus is Rh positive. Amniocentesis for genetic purposes or for the determination of pulmonary maturity carries a 2% risk of immunization if performed under constant ultrasound guidance.[31] At delivery, umbilical cord and maternal blood are tested: umbilical cord blood for ABO, Rh type and the direct Coombs' status, and maternal blood for the presence of Rh antibody and fetal red cells. Although most instances of Rh immunization occur after small or undetectable fetal TPH [maternal Rh prophylaxis being readily provided by one dose of Rh immune globulin (120–300 μg)], approximately one woman in 400 has a fetal TPH of more than 30 mL of whole blood and will not be protected by a single prophylactic dose.

Predicting the severity of Rh hemolytic disease

History

Hemolytic disease may remain similar from pregnancy to pregnancy (mild, moderate, or severe), but it is more likely to progress with each Rh-positive pregnancy. The risk of hydrops is 8–10% in a first sensitized pregnancy. If a woman has had a hydropic fetus, there is a 90% chance that the next affected fetus will also develop hydrops without intervention, typically at the same or an earlier time in gestation.

Rh antibody titers

If Rh antibody titers are measured in the same laboratory by the same experienced personnel using the same methods, the results are reproducible and of some value in predicting the risk of severe hemolytic disease. Because the binding constant of the Rh antibody varies, as may the density of Rh antigen on the RBC membrane and the ability of the fetus to compensate for RBC hemolysis, the titer indicates only which fetus is at risk. The maternal antibody titer that puts the fetus at risk must be determined for each laboratory. Generally speaking, an albumin titer of 16 or an indirect antiglobulin titer of 32–64 carries a 10% risk that the fetus will become hydropic without intervention. Titers of at-risk women should be repeated monthly after the first prenatal visit.

Maternal history and antibody titer alone are inadequate for the proper management of the Rh-immunized pregnancy. In one study of 426 Rh-immunized women managed at one hospital between 1954 and 1961 using amniocentesis and maternal titers, the severity of disease was predicted accurately in only 62% of the 121 affected fetuses.[32] If prediction of severity of hemolytic disease had been completely accurate, 50% of the 67 deaths would have been prevented by the interventions available at the time.

Amniotic fluid analysis

Amniotic fluid of severely affected fetuses is stained yellow with bilirubin that absorbs visual light at 450 nm. The bilirubin reaches the amniotic fluid primarily by excretion into fetal pulmonary and tracheal secretions and diffusion across the fetal membranes and umbilical cord. Bevis was the first to report that spectrophotometric determinations of amniotic fluid bilirubin correlated with the severity of fetal hemolysis.

Liley reported a method in 1961 that allowed comparisons between one laboratory and another.[33] Although this technique remains important in some locales, it has been largely displaced by noninvasive techniques discussed later.

Optical density readings of centrifuged amniotic fluid (protected from light which can destroy the bilirubin) are made over the visual wavelength spectrum from 700 to 350 nm. The readings are plotted on semilogarithmic graph paper (with wavelength as the horizontal linear coordinate and optical density as the vertical logarithmic coordinate). The deviation from linearity at 450 nm (the ΔOD 450 reading) correlates directly with disease severity. An increase at 405 nm, if present, is due to heme. The heme peak may be another indication of severe disease if the fluid has not been contaminated with blood.

Liley divided a plot of single amniotic fluid sample ΔOD 450 readings from 101 pregnancies after 28 weeks' gestation into three zones and related them to neonatal outcome. Readings in zone 1 indicated mild or no disease, but did not exclude the possibility that treatment would be required after birth. Readings in zone 2 were felt to indicate intermediate disease, increasing in severity as the zone 3 boundary was approached. There was no control group, i.e., women with a Rh-negative fetus. The zone boundaries slope downward because of the diminishing amount of bilirubin normally produced after 25 weeks' gestation. Before 25 weeks, the zone boundaries are almost certainly parabolic rather than linear, probably reaching their highest levels at 24 weeks (Fig. 49.1). Extrapolating the Liley curves to pregnancies before 27 weeks has proved erroneous. Nicolaides et al.,[34] in 1986, correlated fetal hematologic values in 59 Rh D-sensitized pregnancies between 18 and 25 weeks' gestation with ΔOD 450 values on a Liley curve extrapolated to 18 weeks' gestation. If intervention were reserved for fetuses with ΔOD 450 values in zone 3, 70% of anemic fetuses would not have been detected.

A modified ΔOD 450 curve for such situations was proposed by Queenan et al.[35] in 1993 and, in 1998, Scott and Chan[36] conducted a prospective evaluation of this curve. The Queenan curve was predictive of severely affected fetuses (more than 7 g/dL deficit in hemoglobin) with a sensitivity of 100% and a specificity of 79%. The sensitivity for detecting moderate anemia (hemoglobin deficit of 3–7 g/dL) was 83% with a specificity of 94%. With further study, it became clear

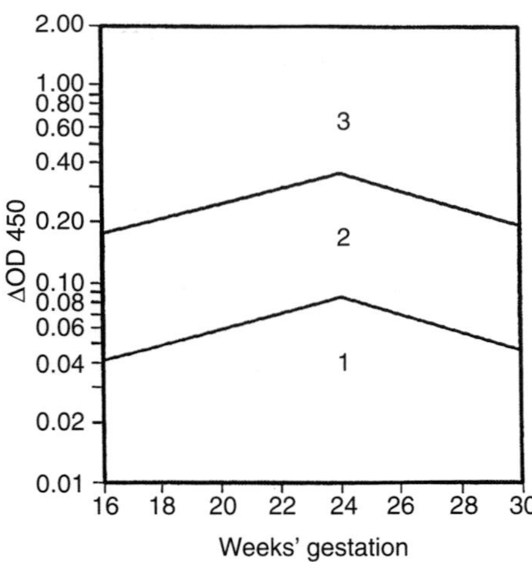

Figure 49.1 Modification of Liley's ΔOD 450 reading zone boundaries before 24 weeks' gestation (From ref. 78).

that a single measurement of ΔOD 450 was poorly predictive of the fetal status unless it was extremely high or extremely low. Liley emphasized the need for repeating the amniotic fluid analyses to establish the ΔOD 450 trend. Thus, a decision to rely on amniotic fluid ΔOD 450 measurements is a decision to do at least two invasive procedures.

Serial ΔOD 450 readings increase the accuracy of the identification of severity. From examination of 3177 amniotic fluids obtained from 1027 immunized women, the following observations can be made:

1 A ΔOD 450 reading of 0.400 or higher at any period of gestation is associated with hydrops fetalis in 65% of instances.

2 Hydrops may be present with readings of 0.200–0.250 at 28 weeks' gestation.

3 Once serial readings reach 80–85% of zone 2, hydrops may be present by the time the reading reaches zone 3 without therapy.

4 Disease may be fulminant. For example, readings of 0.160 at 23 weeks and 0.240 at 27 weeks can be followed 2 weeks later by readings of 0.385 and 0.370 with hydrops present at the time of the second amniocentesis.

5 Conversely, readings of 0.200–0.250 at 20–22 weeks may occur in the presence of a negative, unaffected fetus.

Other spectrophotometric measurements of amniotic fluid have been developed. Bartsch concluded that none is better than the Liley method, and some are worse.[37] The experience and judgment of the individual assessing the amniotic fluid findings are more important than the method of measurement used. Clearly, amniocentesis is a less than desirable tool for the management of Rh disease.

Hazards of amniocentesis

The risks of amniocentesis include placental trauma causing TPH, rising titers, and increasing severity of fetal hemolytic disease, amnionitis, and premature rupture of membranes. Any invasive procedure should be performed under continuous ultrasound visualization.

Sources of error

Maternal or fetal blood produces sharp 580-, 540-, and 415-nm oxyhemoglobin peaks that obscure the ΔOD 450 readings (Fig. 49.2). Small amounts of blood do not mask the ΔOD 450, but small amounts of plasma, particularly fetal plasma, can increase the ΔOD 450 reading, giving a falsely high reading. Heme produces a 405-nm peak, which may obscure the 450-nm peak, but can itself be indicative of severe hemolytic disease. Meconium in amniotic fluid distorts and increases the 450-nm peak. Exposure of the sample to light (particularly fluorescent light) decolorizes bilirubin, reducing the ΔOD 450 peak. Maternal urine produces no ΔOD 450-nm peak. Ascitic fluid is clear, bright yellow, and more viscous than amniotic fluid because of a higher protein level. It has a much higher ΔOD 450 level.

Congenital anomalies, such as anencephaly, open meningomyelocele, and upper gastrointestinal obstruction, produce hydramnios and markedly elevated ΔOD 450 readings, which may be misleading if the mother is immunized.

Fetal blood sampling

Cordocentesis is available in many tertiary perinatal centers.[38] This procedure, which usually precedes fetal intravascular transfusion (IVT), allows the measurement of all blood parameters that can be measured after birth (i.e., hemoglobin, hematocrit, serum bilirubin, direct and indirect platelet count, leukocyte count, serum proteins, and blood gases). Fetal blood sampling is by far the most accurate means of determining the degree of severity of hemolytic disease, in the absence of hydrops fetalis.

Fetal blood sampling has an associated mortality rate of less than 1%[27] (0.2% in the authors' hands for Rh disease using a needle guide). Other morbidity occurs in approximately 5% of patients sampled using a freehand technique: prolonged bradycardia, umbilical cord hematoma, amnionitis with maternal adult respiratory distress syndrome, and placental abruption are each described. Cordocentesis is recommended when a screening tool such as measurement of the middle cerebral artery (MCA) peak velocity is abnormal. Cordocentesis can be performed as early as 16–18 weeks; it is usually feasible by 20–21 weeks.

Ultrasound

Ultrasound has a central role in the management of the alloimmunized pregnancy. First, it is used early to accurately establish gestational age. Second, many investigators have searched for alternative ultrasound parameters that could predict mild to moderate anemia. Such studies include:

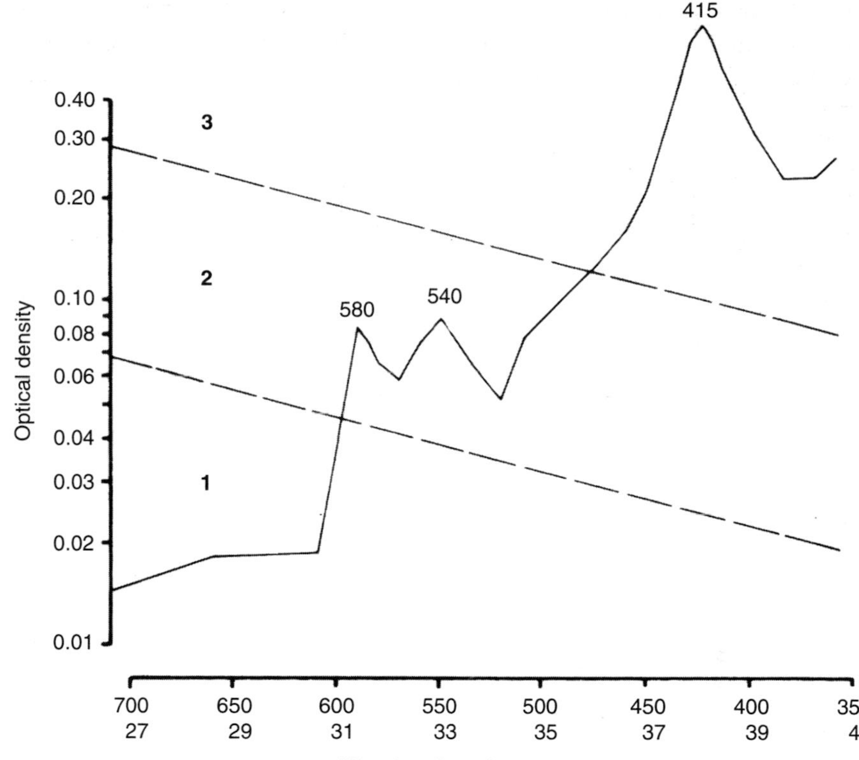

Figure 49.2 Spectrophotometric curve (Liley method) of amniotic fluid grossly contaminated with blood. Note sharp peaks at 580, 540, and 415 nm that obscure the 450-nm rise (Bowman JM. Hemolytic disease of the newborn. In: Conn HF, Conn RB, eds. *Current diagnosis 5*. Philadelphia: W.B. Saunders; 1977:1107).

1 Nicolaides et al.[39] in 1988 investigated the fetal abdominal circumference, head-to-abdomen circumference ratio, intraperitoneal volume, intrahepatic and extrahepatic umbilical vein diameter, and placental thickness to predict a fetal hemoglobin less than 5 g/dL. Placental thickness and intraperitoneal volume detected only 25% of cases; the other parameters detected < 10% of severe cases.

2 Vintzileos et al.[40] in 1986 and Roberts et al.[41] in 2001 used ultrasound to assess the fetal liver, reasoning that it is the principal site of extramedullary hematopoiesis. The length of the right lobe of the liver reportedly detected 93% of anemic fetuses.

3 Oepkes et al.[42] in 1993 and Bahado-Singh et al.[43] in 1998, measured splenic perimeter (length + width × 1.57), reasoning that the spleen is another site of extramedullary hematopoiesis. In two series, a splenic perimeter greater than two standard deviations was predictive of severe fetal anemia (94% and 100% respectively).

Despite this experience, hepatic length and splenic perimeter have not been widely used in alloimmunization management.

Lastly, hydrops fetalis can easily be detected with ultrasound.

Doppler ultrasonography

A number of investigators have reasoned that decreasing fetal hemoglobin levels would be associated with a lower blood viscosity and increased cardiac output, producing higher blood velocities. Sites studied include the descending aorta, the umbilical vein, the splenic artery, the common carotid artery, and the MCA.

Vyas et al.[44] in 1990 was the first to apply MCA Doppler velocity for the detection of fetal anemia. They found the best correlation with fetal hemoglobin levels using the intensity-weighted time-averaged mean velocity of the MCA; unfortunately, only 50% of the anemic fetuses were identified.

The peak systolic velocity in the fetal MCA has proved more accurate. Mari[45] established normative data for gestational age. Using a threshold value of 1.5 multiples of the mean to predict moderate to severe anemia, more than 70% of invasive tests were avoided. Since 2000, multiple reports have confirmed the high sensitivity of the peak MCA velocity in detecting moderate to severe fetal anemia.

The fetal MCA closest to the maternal skin should be evaluated using a minimal angle of insonation. The Doppler gate is placed over the vessel just as it bifurcates from the carotid artery; placement on the more distal aspects of the MCA can falsely depress the real peak systolic velocity.

Detti et al.[46] in 2002 examined the time trend of MCA velocities as a tool to identify fetal anemia. The slope of a regression line based on three consecutive Doppler measurements greater than 1.95 was predictive of the subsequent development of moderate to severe fetal anemia. They proposed the following scheme:

1 Doppler assessment weekly.
2 If the MCA peak velocity remains < 1.5 MoM, calculate the slope of the increase between the three measurements.
3 If the slope is less than 1.95, repeat studies at 10- to 14-day intervals.
4 If the peak MCA velocity is at least 1.5 MoM and there are other ultrasound findings consistent with fetal anemia, proceed with cordocentesis. If there are no sonographic signs of anemia, repeat the peak MCA Doppler measurement within 24 h to confirm elevation; if persistent, proceed with cordocentesis.
5 Do not use the MCA after 35 weeks' gestation.

Cell-mediated maternal antibody functional assays

Because of the relatively poor correlation between blood group antibody and severity of hemolytic disease, various functional assays were developed to reflect the antibody-binding avidity for the RBC membrane antigen. These assays include the monocyte monolayer assay (MMA),[47] antibody-dependent cellular cytotoxicity (ADCC) using lymphocytes,[48] ADCC using monocytes,[49] and monocyte chemiluminescence.[50] Each assay has its proponents. A survey of nine European laboratories revealed that they correctly predicted disease outcome in about half of the cases. The assays are perhaps more helpful in predicting mild disease than very severe disease. In a recent study, there was no correlation between the hematocrit at cordocentesis and the MMA in 41 pregnant women with potentially dangerous blood group antibodies who delivered affected babies.[51] All tests are incapable of differentiating the unaffected antigen-negative fetus from the affected antigen-positive fetus. In summary, these tests appear to have modest clinical value as currently formulated.

Determination of fetal D antigen status by polymerase chain reaction

The cloning of the CcEe and D complementary DNA allows for the determination of the fetal Rh D genotype from DNA obtained by chorionic villus biopsy or amniocentesis.[52] Although highly uncommon, point mutations can result in the occasional incorrect diagnosis. Thus, it is possible to determine the D status of a fetus whose mother is Rh d and whose father appears to be heterozygous for D and, if negative, no further testing will be required. Probes are also available for Kell.

It is also possible to determine D antigen fetal status from maternal blood using the polymerase chain reaction (PCR). The fetal nucleated hematopoietic stem cells present in the maternal circulation are subjected to PCR.[53] Finning et al.[54] in 2002 followed a series of 137 sensitized pregnancies. Fetal typing using DNA from maternal serum was 100% accurate in determining the Rh D type in 94 Rh D-positive and 43 Rh D-negative cases.

Management of the Rh-immunized woman and her fetus

Clinical management is dependent on the available diagnostic tools, the patient and her history of fetal/neonatal manifestations of hemolytic disease, and on the clinical condition of the fetus. As a rule, the patient's first Rh D-sensitized pregnancy results in minimal fetal/neonatal disease; subsequent pregnancies are associated with a worsening outcome.

Nonsensitized women

Management of the newly sensitized woman begins upon identification. The practitioner cannot predict fetal risk accurately relying on the obstetric history and serology. The caregiver must be familiar with their laboratory's maternal indirect Coombs' antibody titers (assuming the results are reproducible) and threshold. Antibody titers have their greatest utility during the first sensitized pregnancy; in later pregnancies, they are of limited value.

When the maternal indirect Coombs' antibody titers are below the threshold (below which severe fetal hemolytic disease does not occur), they should be repeated monthly. Once the critical titer is exceeded, the fetus is followed with serial measurements of the peak MCA velocity. It is important to remember that a determination of the fetal PCR Rh genotype should be standard in any at-risk women undergoing chorionic villus sampling (CVS) or second-trimester amniocentesis because a negative result eliminates the need for further testing.

The timing of invasive fetal testing is now determined by ultrasound evidence of fetal anemia as several investigators have found an association between fetal anemia and increased MCA velocities.[44,45,55]

Invasive fetal evaluation following a positive Doppler finding consists of cordocentesis. With the declining incidence of maternal isoimmunization, these patients should be referred to maternal–fetal medicine specialists with experience in the field.

The principal concern with cordocentesis is safety – vascular accidents and maternal sensitization are known to occur. As described earlier, this technique accounts for at least 30% of fetal losses and, by using a needle guide, the loss rate is decreased to approximately 0.3%.[56] The first cordocentesis should be performed when the peak MCA velocity becomes elevated or (if applicable) a few weeks before the last sensitized fetus required a transfusion. Laboratory tests performed on the first fetal specimen include type and Rh status, direct Coombs' test, complete blood count (CBC), manual reticulocyte count, and total bilirubin. Laboratory tests sent on subsequent fetal specimens include CBC, manual reticulocyte count, and total bilirubin. If the fetus is not anemic when first sampled, a strongly positive direct Coombs' test or a manual reticulocyte count outside the 95% confidence interval are strong risk factors for the development of anemia *in utero*. Approximately 50% of isoimmunized women will require only one cordocentesis and, with the use of Doppler ultrasound, delivery may be safely deferred until term.

Rh-immunized woman with a previously affected fetus or infant

Patients should be referred to a tertiary care center if they have documented isoimmunization. Maternal titers are not predictive of the degree of fetal anemia. If the paternal phenotype is heterozygous, an amniocentesis is performed at 15 weeks to determine fetal Rh D status. If the fetus is antigen positive, initiate serial MCA Doppler measurements by 18 weeks to monitor these pregnancies. Testing should be repeated every 1–2 weeks as long as they are normal. If a rising value for peak MCA Doppler velocity greater than 1.5 MoM is found, a cordocentesis is performed and the fetus transfused if the hematocrit is < 30%.

Intrauterine fetal transfusion

Preterm delivery is associated with increased perinatal morbidity and mortality. This can be avoided for the most part using modern techniques for fetal transfusion. Fetal intraperitoneal transfusion is rarely necessary, and the techniques will only be mentioned briefly. Fetal transfusion therapy should never be undertaken in the absence of hydrops without first confirming that the fetus has significant anemia (fetal hematocrit < 30%, a value less than the 2.5 percentile at all gestational ages above 20 weeks). These procedures should only be performed by individuals with considerable experience.

Intraperitoneal fetal transfusions

This is the original, but least preferred, method of fetal transfusion. Red cells placed in the peritoneal cavity of any animal with a diaphragm are absorbed intact into the circulation via the subdiaphragmatic lymphatics and the right thoracic duct. Diaphragmatic contractions are necessary for the absorption.[57] In the absence of hydrops, 10–12% of transfused red cells are absorbed each day after transfusion. Absorption is greatly diminished and unpredictable in the presence of hydrops.[58]

The volume of blood injected is limited by the capacity of the peritoneal space. If the volume transfused is such that intraperitoneal pressure exceeds umbilical venous pressure, blood flow from the placenta to the fetus stops and the fetus dies.[59] The intraperitoneal transfusion (IPT) volume can be calculated by the following formula: IPT volume = (weeks' gestation–20) × 10 mL (i.e., 50 mL at 25 weeks, 90 mL at 29 weeks). Calculation of residual donor hemoglobin concentration is necessary to space IPTS optimally so that the fetus undergoes the minimal number of procedures. After IPT, 80% of the infused red cells are in the fetoplacental circulation (based on a fetoplacental blood volume of 125 mL/kg fetal body weight). The residual donor hemoglobin concentration is calculated according to the following formula: residual hemoglobin concentration (g/L) = [(0.80 × a)/(125 × b)] × [(120–c)/(120)] where "a" is the amount of donor red cell hemoglobin transfused in grams, "b" is the estimated fetal weight according to gestation (i.e., 1 kg at 27 weeks' gestation, 1.5 kg at 30 weeks' gestation), "c" is the interval in days after the IPT, and 120 days is the lifespan of the donor red cell. For example, 10 days after IPT of 55 mL of blood with a hemoglobin concentration of 280 g into a fetus of 27 weeks' gestation (weight 1 kg), there would be a residual donor hemoglobin concentration of [(0.80 × 55 × 280)/(125 × 1)] × [(120–10)/(120)] = 90.3 g/L. A second IPT is performed as soon as the first is absorbed, and every 4 weeks thereafter.

IPT has several disadvantages. There is slow correction of the fetal anemia and a higher risk of trauma. There is the added risk of obstructing cardiac return if the intra-abdominal pressure becomes too high.

Direct intravascular fetal transfusion

In 1981, Rodeck et al. introduced direct fetal blood sampling and intravascular transfusion (IVT) through a needle introduced down a fetoscope.[60] The presence of blood (common after a first IVT), meconium, or turbidity (common in later gestation) in amniotic fluid creates major problems with visualization of fetal vessels through the fetoscope. Fetal blood sampling and direct IVT are now carried out in most, if not all, tertiary level centers under ultrasound. Transfusion therapy is initiated when the fetal hematocrit is < 30%, a value less than the 2.5 percentile at all gestational ages above 20 weeks.

The blood should be from a fresh donor, group O, and negative for the antigen (or antigens) to which the mother is sensitized (D negative if the mother is Rh negative with anti-D). It should also be negative for hepatitis B surface antigen (HBsAg), anti-human immunodeficiency virus (HIV), anti-hepatitis C virus (HCV), and anti-cytomegalovirus (CMV). Alloimmunized Rh negative women are functional hyperresponders. They frequently develop other blood group antibodies, such as M, S, s, Jk^a, Fy^a, and so on. A second antibody may become manifest after one or two intrauterine transfusions (IUTs), jeopardizing the lifespan of the donor red cells transfused next if not corrected. The blood unit is centrifuged, and the supernatant plasma with its buffy coat is discarded. Gamma irradiation of the donor red cells is recommended. Sterile isotonic saline is added to the packed red cells immediately before the IUT raising the hematocrit to between 70% and 75%. Transfused blood with a higher hematocrit mixes much more slowly.

Technique of intravascular transfusion

The mother is made comfortable with pillows placed under her knees (to take pressure off the lower spine) and a pillow positioned on the left to displace the uterus to avoid supine hypotension. Diazepam 5–10 mg intravenously is used to foster relaxation during the procedure. The maternal abdomen is surgically prepared. Prophylactic antibiotic administration is neither effective nor cost-efficient. The unit of blood at room temperature is attached to a blood filter and then a three-way valve. A length of extension tubing is attached to the stopcock end and filled with donor red cells, taking great care to insure that no air bubbles are in the tubing, stopcock, or syringe.

Once prepared, the operator selects the easiest approach to the umbilical vein and, under real-time ultrasound guidance (the transducer being enclosed in a sterile drape), directs a 10-cm, 22-gauge spinal puncture needle into the umbilical vein. The selected skin site is infiltrated with 1% lidocaine. If the artery is inadvertently punctured, the needle should be removed and redirected to the vein unless there is no other option. When the needle appears within the vessel, the stylet is withdrawn and, upon free return of blood, the fetus is paralyzed with pancuronium, 0.3 mg/kg estimated fetal weight (EFW) intravenously, to insure fetal quiet, as any fetal movement may cause catastrophic events such as vessel laceration or cord hematoma. Pancuronium is also advantageous for transfusion specifically because its sympathomimetic effect helps to maintain cardiac output as the fetus is volume loaded. After fetal paralysis, the umbilical venous pressure is measured. It provides definitive identification of the vessel punctured and allows for the monitoring of the fetal response to volume loading. The author also administers furosemide (3 mg/kg EFW); however, research has failed to show a clear benefit.[61] The donor blood is injected in 20-mL aliquots over 2–3 min. The transfusion is monitored continuously by ultrasound (streaming turbulence is seen as the donor red cells pass down the vein). Meanwhile, the assistant must be ready to halt the infusion if there is any abrupt change in the resistance to flow. Because only 2–3 mm of needle is in the fetal vessel, there is a significant risk of dislodgement, either into the amniotic cavity (easily recognized and not hazardous) or into the cord substance producing a cord hematoma with risk of umbilical venous compression and vasospasm-induced bradycardia. Excluding the first transfusion of a hydropic fetus, the target for the post-transfusion fetal hematocrit is 48–55%. Consequently, the volume infused depends on the gestational age and the initial hematocrit.

A variety of options exist to monitor the fetus during the transfusion. First, many physicians will image the fetal heart to rule out bradycardias, but this is of limited value. A second option is to periodically measure the umbilical venous pressure. If the fetus does not tolerate the transfusion, the umbilical venous pressure will increase (fetal bradycardias also increase the umbilical venous pressure); an increase of > 10 mmHg is associated with increased perinatal mortality, and the transfusion should be stopped and, if needed, blood volume should be removed to reduce the fetal preload. Another option is Doppler ultrasound to evaluate fetal well-being during the transfusion.

The fetal hematocrit declines slowly over time after transfusion therapy is begun. It is more rapid and variable between the first and the second transfusion compared with subsequent transfusions. Except for the hydropic fetus, the second transfusion is generally performed 2 weeks after the first transfusion. The decline in fetal hematocrit thereafter is more predictable and generally, by 34–35 weeks, delivery may be delayed 4–5 weeks without another transfusion.[62]

Transfusion therapy suppresses fetal erythropoiesis, and the average reticulocyte count is usually < 1% by the third transfusion. The complications of hyperbilirubinemia are less if at least two transfusions are performed 3 weeks apart. The last transfusion is done between 34 and 35 weeks' gestation, and delivery is planned at 38–39 weeks. Transfusion therapy is not an indication for Cesarean delivery.

Intrauterine transfusion in the presence of hydrops fetalis

Most hydropic fetuses have myocardial dysfunction. As a result, they frequently fail to tolerate the typical volume load.[28] Thus, their target hematocrit after the first transfusion should be no more than 25%. A day later, the hematocrit can safely be brought up to the target 48–55% with a second transfusion.

Umbilical vein pH (UVpH) maintenance is especially important in the hydropic fetus. During a transfusion, the UVpH normally declines because the pH of the transfused blood is 6.98–7.01. The RBC is the principal buffer in the human fetus. In the authors' experience, all losses of hydropic fetuses after the era of umbilical venous pressure measurement began were associated with profound acidemia and occurred hours after the transfusion. Consequently, the author now infuses bicarbonate in 1-mEq increments to maintain UVpH above 7.30. The overall survival rate for hydrops (since beginning IVT) now exceeds 94%.

The blood volume transfused is dependent on gestational age and the starting hematocrit. Several formulae exist to calculate the volume needed; however, none is reliable enough to terminate the procedure without first checking the hematocrit. Donor blood with a hematocrit < 75% equilibrates rapidly (likely because of the rapid fluid exchange across the placenta) whereas donor blood with a hematocrit > 80% does not equilibrate as rapidly (likely because of increased viscosity).

Survival after fetal transfusion

Survival after IUT varies with center experience and with the presence or absence of hydrops. Overall survival in one review was 84%. However, fewer hydropic fetuses survived after IUT (70%) compared with fetuses who were not hydropic (92%). One treatment center looking at 213 fetuses receiving 599 IUTs had similar results. Survival with any degree of hydrops was 78% compared with 93% for nonhydropic fetuses. These investigators further classified hydrops into mild (mild ascites) and severe (significant ascites with scalp edema, pericardial effusion, or pleural effusion). Mild hydrops reversed in 88% of cases, whereas severe hydrops only reversed in 39%, a finding clearly linked to overall perinatal survival: 98% of fetuses survived after reversal of hydrops. With persistent hydrops, only 39% of fetuses survived; if the hydrops was severe and persisted, only a quarter survived.

Delivery of the fetus after intrauterine transfusion

Generally, the last transfusion is administered around 34–35 weeks' gestation. If the fetal hematocrit at the end of the last transfusion was approximately 50%, then it will still be above 35% at delivery 4 weeks later. Consequently, there is no justification for preterm induction of labor if a transfusion can be performed.

Infants who have received *in utero* transfusion therapy do well after birth. Generally, the neonatal capillary hematocrit increases about 15% within the first few hours of life (likely secondary to fluid shifts) and then decreases slowly to a level at or below the umbilical cord hematocrit level at delivery over the next few days to weeks. As these infants are now delivered at term, they have a higher tolerance to bilirubin levels and can usually be managed with phototherapy alone. The infant may develop anemia by 5 weeks after delivery; this is expected as the transfused blood is nearing the end of its lifespan. This neonatal anemia is also likely indicated by a low reticulocyte count. These neonates should have their hematocrit and reticulocyte count monitored weekly. The therapeutic goal is to maintain them with a modest anemia; small transfusions will keep the infant asymptomatic but leave the erythropoietic stimulus unblunted. Once reticulocytosis is observed, the neonate will no longer need further transfusion therapy.

Suppression of Rh immunization

Plasma exchange

Large amounts of maternal antibody-containing plasma (3 L/day, 5 days/week) are removed and replaced with saline, 5% albumin, and intravenous gammaglobulin to reduce the circulating maternal blood group antibody levels by 75–80%. Such reductions are transient and at best delay the need for IUT by 2–3 weeks. The procedure is costly in both professional time and resources. With the advent of fetal blood sampling and IVT as early as 18–20 weeks' gestation, intensive plasmapheresis is only rarely indicated.

Intravenous immune serum globulin

Intravenous immunoglobulin (IVIG) has been reported to reduce the severity of hemolytic disease.[63] The dose used is 1 g/kg maternal body weight administered weekly. IVIG may exert a beneficial effect by negative feedback, reducing maternal antibody levels by 50%, or by saturating the trophoblastic Fc receptor sites to impede placental transfer of antibody to the fetus, or by saturating fetal splenic Fc receptor sites, preventing the destruction of antibody-coated fetal RBCs.

Prevention of Rh immunization

The development of Rh immunization prophylaxis was a major advance in the management of the Rh-negative pregnant woman. In 1900, Von Dungern showed that administration to rabbits of antibody from ox red cells along with ox red cells prevented the development of rabbit anti-ox red cell antibodies.[64] He proved that the presence of antibodies to an antigen, in sufficient amount, suppresses active immunization to the antigen. This information was used 60 years later in New York,[65] Liverpool,[66] and Winnipeg.[16] In the initial experiments, Rh-negative male volunteers were given Rh-positive red cells and Rh antibody in the form of Rh immune globulin (RhIG, anti-D IgG); the anti-D IgG prevented Rh immunization.

Clinical trials were performed in which Rh-negative unimmunized women were given RhIG after the delivery of a Rh-positive infant. All such trials were successful. As a result of these trials, RhIG was licensed in 1968 for use in North America. The standard dose in the United States is 300 μg given intramuscularly (i.m.). Smaller doses of 100–125 μg i.m. are used in Canada, Europe, and Australia. All these doses appear to be effective.

RhIG prevents Rh immunization with two provisos: it must be given in an adequate amount, and it must be given before Rh immunization has begun. RhIG administration does not suppress Rh immunization once it has begun, no matter how weak the immunization.[67]

RhIG mechanism of action

The precise mechanism of action of RhIG is unknown. There are three theories: antigen deviation, antigen blocking–competitive inhibition, and central inhibition. The first theory, antigen deviation, was proposed by Race and Sanger. Rh-positive cells bound by RhIG succumb to intravascular hemolysis that destroys or alters the Rh antigen so as to prevent anti-D antibody production. It is now known, however, that IgG anti-D does not cause intravascular hemolysis of Rh-positive cells. Instead, the antibody-coated fetal cells are removed from the circulation in the spleen and lymph nodes (the site of antibody production). Consequently, antigen deviation is likely not the mechanism of action of RhIG.

The second theory, antigen blocking–competitive inhi-bition, is also likely not the mechanism of RhIG action. Antibody preparations that lack the Fc portion also avidly bind the antigen, but do not suppress the immune response. Consequently, this also is not the mechanism of action.

The most likely mechanism of action for RhIG is that of central inhibition, proposed by Gorman and elaborated by Pollack. Fetal erythrocytes are coated with anti-D IgG and are filtered out by the spleen and lymph nodes. The increase in local concentrations of anti-D IgG bound to the D antigen appears to suppress the primary immune response by interrupting the commitment of B cells to IgG-producing plasma cell clones. The binding of anti-D–D antigen complexes releases cytokines that inhibit the proliferation of B cells specific for the antigen. This process is dependent on the presence of the IgG Fc receptor.

Because the half-life of RhIG is approximately 16 days, 15–20% of patients receiving it at 28 weeks have a very low anti-D titer at term delivery. It is recommended in the United States that 300 μg of RhIG be administered within 72 h of delivery of a Rh-positive infant. This dose will protect against sensitization from a fetal–maternal hemorrhage (FMH) of 30 mL of fetal whole blood. Approximately 1 in 1000 deliveries will exceed this volume, and risk factors identify only 50%. Therefore, routine screening at delivery for excessive FMH is indicated. The rosette test, a qualitative yet sensitive test for FMH, is performed first. A negative test result implies that the patient should receive only the standard dose of RhIG. A Kleihauer–Betke stain is performed if the rosette test is positive. The percentage of fetal blood cells is multiplied by 50 to estimate the FMH volume, and additional vials of RhIG are administered to prevent maternal sensitization. No more than five units of RhIG should be administered intramuscularly in a 24-h period. Should a large dose of RhIG be required, the entire calculated dose may be given using an intravenous preparation.

Standard Rh prophylaxis recommendations

One prophylactic dose unit of RhIG is administered to a Rh-negative nonimmune woman as soon as her infant is determined to be Rh positive, and no later than 72 h postpartum. If the Rh status of the baby remains unknown at 72 h, the woman should be given RhIG regardless. It is better to treat unnecessarily than to fail to treat an at-risk woman. ABO status is not part of the decision paradigm as ABO incompatibility is only partially protective. If there is a failure to administer RhIG within 72 h, Rh prophylaxis may still be beneficial up to 28 days postpartum, although the experimental evidence suggests that RhIG will provide some protection only up to 13 days after exposure to Rh-positive red cells.[68]

Rh prophylaxis problems

Postpartum Rh prophylaxis programs have greatly reduced, but not entirely eliminated, Rh immunization. Residual problems still exist[69,70] and include the following:

1 Failure of compliance after delivery.
2 Failure to give prophylaxis after abortion.
3 Failure to give prophylaxis after amniocentesis.
4 Failure to protect after massive fetal TPH.
5 Failure to protect against Rh immunization during pregnancy.
6 The question of augmentation of the risk of Rh immunization.
7 The question of Rh immunization during infancy.
8 The question of the D^u mother.
9 The question of suppression of weak Rh immunization.
10 Reactions to i.m. RhIG–ion exchange and RhIG–monoclonal RhIG.

Failure of protection after massive fetal transplacental hemorrhage

The protection provided by RhIG is dose dependent. Experimentally, 300 μg of RhIG given i.m. prevents Rh immunization after an exposure of up to 30 mL of Rh-positive blood (12–15 mL of red cells).[17] The protection is only partial if the volume of blood is greater. Rh immunization occurred in 30% of Rh-negative male volunteers given up to 450 mL of blood with 300 μg of RhIG i.m.[71] Because only about 1 woman in 400 is exposed to more than 30 mL, Rh immunization failure due to undiagnosed massive fetal TPH occurs rarely (1 in 1400 Rh-negative women carrying Rh-positive babies). Nevertheless, screening the Rh-negative woman for massive fetal TPH after delivery is recommended.

If massive TPH is diagnosed after delivery of a Rh-positive baby, 600 μg (two vials) should be administered if the TPH is greater than 25 mL but less than 50 mL, 900 μg (three vials) if the TPH is greater than 50 mL but less than 75 mL, and so on. Up to 1200 μg (four vials) i.m. can be given every 12 h until the total dose has been administered.

Not only is there a risk of Rh immunization, but there is also a risk of fetal exsanguination if a massive TPH occurs antenatally and exceeds 100 mL (nearly always in the third trimester).[72] There is a risk of fetal red cell hemolysis from the large amounts of RhIG that must be given before delivery. If the TPH does not exceed 50 mL of blood, the dose required (600 μg) does not cause significant fetal red cell hemolysis.

It is prudent to consider delivery after the TPH exceeds 50 mL if the fetus is 33 weeks or greater and there is evidence of pulmonary maturity. If the baby is Rh positive, the mother should be given an appropriate amount of RhIG. The baby should be examined immediately and, if pale and shocky or with significant anemia, transfused immediately.

If a fetal TPH greater than 50 mL is diagnosed early in pregnancy before evidence of fetal lung maturity, cordocentesis should be performed, and a transfusion carried out if a significant anemia is discovered. RhIG (600 μg) should be given to the mother if the fetus is Rh positive. Thereafter, the fetus should be followed by serial ultrasound examinations. If gestation and lung maturity are such that delivery is not prudent within 14 days of the transfusion, a second fetal blood sampling procedure should be performed to insure stability of the fetal hematocrit.

Rh immunization during pregnancy

Rh immunization during pregnancy accounts for approximately 13% of all Rh immunization if no prophylaxis is given. In Manitoba, 1.8%[57] of 3533 mothers carrying Rh-positive fetuses who had no evidence of Rh immunization at the beginning of their pregnancies were Rh immunized during pregnancy or within 3 days after delivery.[20] Similar prevalence figures were reported from Hamilton, Ontario,[73] and Sweden.[74] Rh immunization during pregnancy has also been reported in the United States.[75]

A clinical trial of antenatal Rh prophylaxis with 300 µg of RhIG given i.m. at 28 and again at 34 weeks' gestation reduced the incidence of Rh immunization from 1.8% to 0.1%.[20] As a result, antenatal Rh prophylaxis is accepted practice in many locales, although most give a single injection of 300 µg of RhIG at or as close to 28 weeks' gestation as possible. The single dose at 28 weeks' gestation has been highly successful.[76] Universal antenatal prophylaxis combined with universal postpartum, postabortion, and postamniocentesis prophylaxis will reduce the prevalence of Rh immunization by 97% from the preprophylaxis incidence of approximately 13 to 0.27%.[77]

The administration of RhIG during pregnancy does not harm the fetus. When 300 µg is given at 28 and 34 weeks' gestation, one-third of neonates have red cells that are weakly direct antiglobulin positive, but none shows any evidence of anemia or hyperbilirubinemia. Only very rare babies have direct antiglobulin-positive red cells after their mothers have received 300 µg just once, at 28 weeks' gestation.

Reactions to intramuscular RhIG – newer forms of RhIG

Ion-exchange RhIG

RhIG is most often prepared by the Cohn cold ethanol precipitation process. Although it is effective and carries a low risk of adverse reactions, it does contain small amounts of IgA, IgM, and other plasma proteins. Because it is anticomplementary, it can be given i.m. only. The efficacy of yield of anti-D IgG from the starting plasma is quite low (35–45%). Severe anaphylaxis has been reported.[78]

Hoppe et al. prepared RhIG by ion-exchange chromatography.[79] This method produces a very pure product with low total protein, no demonstrable IgM, and an IgA content only 0.3% of that in the Cohn prepared RhIG. It also has very low anticomplementarity and can be given safely intravenously (i.v.). It is twice as effective when given i.v.; thus only half the dose is needed after delivery (120 µg). However, the antenatal prophylaxis dose must be the same (300 µg) because its half-life is the same.

Clinical trials and service programs in which hundreds of thousands of doses of ion-exchange RhIG have been given (either i.v. or i.m.) demonstrate it is at least as successful in preventing Rh immunization as the Cohn prepared RhIG.

The advantages of ion-exchange prepared RhIG are greater purity, less likelihood of an adverse reaction, greater efficiency of yield (and, therefore, lower cost), lower dose, and less discomfort when given i.v.

Monoclonal RhIG

At present, RhIG is manufactured from the plasma of hyperimmunized Rh-negative donors, either from the plasma of sterile women initially immunized by pregnancy or from the plasma of Rh-negative deliberately immunized male donors. The former population, the best source of Rh immune plasma, is decreasing in number because of Rh prophylaxis. Deliberate Rh immunization of male volunteers has been questioned on moral and ethical grounds as the majority of those exposed to Rh-positive red cells do not produce acceptable Rh antibody levels. Within the next few years, RhIG will be produced in tissue culture. Monoclonal anti-D has been produced by Epstein–Barr virus transformation of lymphoblastoid cell lines taken from Rh-immunized donors[80,81] and by the fusion of similarly transformed cell lines with mouse–human heteromyelomas (hybridomas).[82,83] Once sufficient stable monoclonal anti-D is produced, tissue-culture RhIG will replace plasma-prepared RhIG.

Current recommendations for Rh prophylaxis

1 Every Rh-negative unimmunized woman who delivers a Rh-positive baby must be given one prophylactic dose of RhIG as soon as possible after delivery.

2 Every Rh-negative unimmunized woman who aborts or threatens to abort must be given RhIG, unless her husband (or father of the baby) is known to be Rh negative.

3 Every Rh-negative unimmunized woman who undergoes amniocentesis or CVS, unless her husband (or father of the baby) is known to be Rh negative, must be given 300 µg of RhIG at the time of the procedure, with subsequent doses at 12-week intervals until delivery.

4 Every Rh-negative unimmunized woman whose husband (or father of the baby) is either Rh positive or Rh unknown should be given 300 µg of RhIG at 28 weeks' gestation. A second dose should be given 12.5 weeks later if delivery has not taken place, but then need not be repeated postpartum if delivery occurs within 3 weeks.

5 If massive TPH is diagnosed, 300 µg of RhIG should be given i.m. for every 25 mL of fetal blood or fraction thereof in the maternal circulation. The dose may be reduced by one-third if RhIG is given i.v..

6 One prophylactic dose of RhIG should be given antepar-tum to the mother who has an Rh antibody detectable only by AA

methods and again after delivery, if she delivers a Rh-positive baby. If the antibody is detectable by a manual enzyme method, administration of RhIG will not prevent progressive immunization. However, it should be given if there is any question about the specificity of the enzyme reactions.

NonRh D blood group immunization

ABO hemolytic disease

Although ABO-incompatible hemolytic transfusion reactions are intravascular and much more serious than extravascular Rh-incompatible hemolytic transfusion reactions, ABO hemolytic disease is much milder than Rh hemolytic disease. Kernicterus due to ABO hemolytic disease is reported, but hydrops caused by ABO hemolytic disease is extremely rare.[84] In another case, neonatal death due to hydrops fetalis occurred in an ABO-incompatible newborn who had direct antiglobulin-positive red cells but whose umbilical cord blood hematocrit was 43%, rendering it most unlikely that this was alloimmune hydrops fetalis.[85]

ABO hemolytic disease is mild because A and B antigens are not well developed on the fetal red cell membrane, because most anti-A and anti-B is IgM and does not cross the placenta, and because most of the small amounts of IgG anti-A and anti-B that do cross become attached to numerous other tissue and fluid A or B antigens. Thus, only a small amount of A or B antibody traversing the placenta binds to red cell antigenic sites. This explains why the umbilical cord blood direct antiglobulin test is only weakly positive and may even be negative unless a sensitive test is used. Even with the most sensitive test, red cells taken from a 1- or 2-day old baby with ABO hemolytic disease may be direct antiglobulin negative.

ABO hemolytic disease is by far the most common hemolytic disease. From 1954 to 1965, of 45 000 deliveries at the Winnipeg General Hospital, 9000 ABO-incompatible babies were born. Of the 9000, 2500 had weakly direct antiglobulin-positive cord blood red cells and therefore had serologic ABO erythroblastosis. Of those 2500, only 41 (less than 2%) required exchange transfusion.[86] The management of ABO erythroblastosis is entirely a pediatric concern. Amniocentesis and other fetal investigative measures are not required in the ABO-incompatible pregnancy.

Hemolytic disease caused by atypical blood group antibodies

Anti-D in the Rh blood group system remains the most common antibody causing severe hemolytic disease. Rh immunization preventive measures have produced a marked reduction in Rh immunization, however.

In Manitoba (population 1 million), the mean annual occurrence of D alloimmunization in pregnant women dropped from 194 in the 5-year period ending October 31, 1967 to 22 in the 5-year period ending October 31, 1995. In the same two periods, the mean annual occurrence of detected nonD alloimmunization in pregnant women, excluding ABO alloimmunization, increased from 14 to 116. This increase is partly because of the increased screening of pregnant D-positive women. It may also be because of a real increase in the occurrence of nonD alloimmunization because of the increased frequency of blood transfusion (transfused blood being only ABO and D compatible).

NonD alloantibodies, therefore, have assumed greater significance in the etiology of hemolytic disease. The alloantibodies causing hemolytic disease of the newborn outlined by Mollison et al. are numerous.[87] However, the only antibodies implicated in moderate to severe disease are all those in the Rh blood group system plus anti-K, -Jk^a, -Js^a, -Js^b, -Ku, -Fy^a, -M, -N, -s, -U, -PP_1p^k, -Di^b, -Lan, -LW, -Far, -Good, -Wr^a, and-Zd. Although this list seems overwhelming, it must be considered in conjunction with the frequency with which such antibodies occur and the frequency with which they cause significant hemolytic disease of the newborn (Table 49.1).

Of the nonD alloantibodies observed in one hospital during the 34-year period ending September 30, 1996, anti-E and anti-K were the most common, although only 20 of the 171 affected infants due to anti-E and 8 of the 17 affected infants due to anti-K required exchange transfusion or phototherapy. Two, due to anti-Kell, were very severely affected. Anti-C, when present, is more likely to cause hemolytic disease (54% versus 24% and 3.3% for anti-E and anti-K respectively) and, in those affected, is more likely to cause disease requiring treatment than anti-E (29% versus 12%), but not so for anti-Kell, where 47% who were affected required treatment.[88] Anti-C, anti-Kell, and anti-Fy^a were the only nonD alloantibodies in the 34-year period that caused disease so severe that it resulted in either severe

Table 49.1 Association of hemolytic disease with maternal blood group antibodies.

Common	c(cE) – incidence high, disease common, may be severe
	Kell – incidence high, disease uncommon but, if present, may be severe
	E – incidence high, disease uncommon, usually mild, rarely severe
	C(Ce, C^w) – incidence moderate, disease common, usually mild
Uncommon	K – rarely present but, when present, may be very severe
	$Kp^a(Kp^b)$ – rare, disease may require treatment, very rarely severe
	Jk^a – uncommon, may require treatment, rarely severe
	Fy^a – uncommon, usually mild, may require treatment, rarely severe
	S – uncommon, usually mild, may require treatment, rarely severe
Rare	s, U, M, Fy^b, N, Do^a, Di^a, Di^b, Lu^a, Yt^a, Jk^b – rarely cause hemolytic disease
Never	Le^a, Le^b, P – never cause hemolytic disease

anemia requiring IUT or neonates born with hemoglobin levels less than 60 g/dL.

Pregnant women with atypical antibodies [i.e., c(cE), Kell, E, C(Ce, C^w), k, $Kp^a(Kp^b)$, Jk^a, Fy^a, S] should be managed in exactly the same manner as if they were Rh negative and Rh D immunized. Although some of these antibodies are common and only occasionally (or rarely) cause dangerous hemolytic disease (i.e., anti-E), and although others are very rare but, if present, may cause severe disease (i.e., anti-K), the potential remains for severe disease. Antibodies that never cause hemolytic disease (i.e., Le^a, Le^b, P) may be disregarded, as for the most part may those that rarely, if ever, cause hemolytic disease (i.e., s, U, M, Fy^b, N, Do^a, Di^a, Di^b, Lu^a, Yt^a, Jk^b). However, if in the latter group, the antibody appears very potent and of high titer, ultrasound evaluation and possibly amniocentesis or fetal blood sampling is warranted.

Anti-Kell alloimmunization is a special case. There are several reports of severe Kell alloimmune disease with low, misleading ΔOD 450 values.[89,90] Anti-Kell has been postulated to cause destruction of poorly hemoglobinized marrow erythroid precursors,[91] which may explain the reports of more severe Kell hemolytic disease of the newborn than was predicted from the ΔOD 450 readings.[83,84] The management of Kell isoimmunization is the same as for Rh disease, and based on serial MCA peak velocity measurements and cordocentesis when abnormal.

Key points

1 For Rh alloimmunization to occur:
   (a) The woman must be Rh negative and the fetus Rh positive.
   (b) Fetal erythrocytes must enter the maternal circulation in sufficient quantity.
   (c) The mother must be immune competent.

2 The primary maternal Rh immune response is slow (typically over 6–12 weeks) – it is usually weak and predominantly IgM (which does not cross the placenta). The second TPH in an immunized woman produces a rapid (within days) secondary immune response – IgG anti-D, which can readily cross the placenta, coat fetal erythrocytes, and trigger hemolysis.

3 ABO incompatibility between a Rh-positive fetus and a Rh-negative mother reduces the risk of immunization to 1.5–2%. This protection is in part because of rapid intravascular hemolysis of the fetal ABO-incompatible cells and their sequestration in the liver. Remember ABO incompatibility confers no protection once Rh immunization has developed.

4 Fetal blood is produced as early as the third week in the yolk sac, but moves to the liver and, finally, to the bone marrow by 16 weeks' gestation. The Rh antigen is detectable on the red cell membrane by the sixth week.

5 Pathogenesis – maternal IgG anti-D crosses the placenta (TPH) and coats the D-positive fetal red cells. These fetal red cells are destroyed extravascularly, resulting in anemia, which stimulates the synthesis of fetal erythropoietin. Reticulocytosis occurs when fetal hemoglobin deficit exceeds 2 g/dL (compared with gestational age-appropriate norms). Nucleated red cell precursors from normoblasts to primitive erythroblasts are released into the circulation (erythroblastosis fetalis).

6 During hemolysis, the globin chain is split from hemoglobin. The remaining heme pigment is converted by heme oxygenase to biliverdin, and then by biliverdin reductase to neurotoxic indirect bilirubin. The fetal and newborn liver is deficient in glucuronyl transferase and Y transport protein; therefore, the increased indirect bilirubin is deposited in the extravascular fluid. Indirect bilirubin is water insoluble and, when the albumin-binding capacity is exceeded, the excess indirect bilirubin diffuses into fatty tissues (i.e., the neuron), where it interferes with cellular metabolism causing the mitochondria to swell, balloon, and then the neuron dies.

7 Bilirubin reaches the amniotic fluid primarily by excretion into fetal pulmonary and tracheal secretions and diffusion across the fetal membranes and umbilical cord. Spectrophotometric determinations of amniotic fluid bilirubin correlate with the severity of fetal hemolysis. The deviation from linearity at 450 nm (the ΔOD 450 reading) correlates directly with disease severity. (An increase at 405 nm, if present, is due to heme.)

8 The Liley curve emphasizes the need for repeating the amniotic fluid analyses to establish the ΔOD 450 trend. Readings in zone 1 indicate mild or no disease, but did not exclude the possibility that treatment would be required after birth. Readings in zone 2 are felt to indicate intermediate disease, increasing in severity as the zone 3 boundary is approached.

9 Cordocentesis is the most accurate means of determining degree of severity of hemolytic disease, in the absence of hydrops fetalis – it allows the measurement of all blood parameters that can be measured after birth (hemoglobin, hematocrit, serum bilirubin, direct and indirect platelet count, leukocyte count, serum proteins, and blood gases). Cordocentesis has an associated mortality rate of 1% and approximately 5% morbidity (prolonged bradycardia, umbilical cord hematoma, amnionitis with maternal adult respiratory distress syndrome, and placental abruption). Consequently, cordocentesis is recommended when a screening tool such as the measurement of the MCA peak velocity is abnormal.

10 Ultrasound is invaluable in the management of alloimmunization. First, it establishes accurate dating criteria for gestational age. Second, many ultrasound parameters exist that help to predict fetal anemia. Lastly, hydrops fetalis can be detected with ultrasound.

11 Doppler ultrasound – the peak systolic velocity in the fetal MCA has proved very accurate, and normative data have been established for gestational age. Using a threshold value of 1.5 MoM to predict moderate to severe anemia, more than 70% of invasive tests were avoided. The fetal MCA closest to the maternal skin should be evaluated using a minimal angle of insonation. The Doppler gate should be placed over the vessel just as it bifurcates from the carotid artery.

12 Management of the newly sensitized woman begins with identification. If titers are below the threshold (below which severe fetal hemolytic disease does not occur), they should be repeated monthly. Once the critical titer is exceeded, the fetus is followed with serial measurements of the peak MCA velocity. The timing of invasive fetal testing (cordocentesis) is determined by ultrasound evidence of fetal anemia (when the peak MCA velocity becomes elevated).

13 Management of the woman with a previously sensitized fetus again begins with identification. If the fetus is deemed to be at risk, initiate serial MCA Doppler measurements by 18 weeks to monitor these pregnancies. Testing should be repeated every 1–2 weeks as long as they are normal. If a rising value for peak MCA Doppler velocity of more than 1.5 MoM is found, a cordocentesis should be performed and the fetus transfused if the hematocrit is < 30%.

14 Transfusion therapy is initiated when the fetal hematocrit is < 30%, a value less than the 2.5th per centile at all gestational ages above 20 weeks.

15 The blood used for fetal transfusion should be from a fresh donor, group O, and negative for the antigen (or antigens) to which the mother is sensitized. It should also be negative for HBsAg, anti-HIV, anti-HCV, and anti-CMV.

16 Intraperitoneal fetal transfusion is the original, but now least preferred, method of fetal transfusion. It has several disadvantages: there is slow correction of the fetal anemia and a higher risk of trauma. There is the added risk of obstructing cardiac return if the intra-abdominal pressure becomes too high.

17 Transfusion therapy suppresses fetal erythropoiesis, and the average reticulocyte count is usually < 1% by the third transfusion. The complications of hyperbilirubinemia are less if at least two transfusions are performed 3 weeks apart. The last transfusion can be done between 34 and 35 weeks' gestation and delivery planned at 38–39 weeks. (Transfusion therapy is not an indication for Cesarean delivery.)

18 Neonates affected by alloimmunization should have their hematocrit and reticulocyte count monitored weekly. The therapeutic goal is to maintain them with a modest anemia; small transfusions will keep the infant asymptomatic but leave the erythropoietic stimulus unblunted. Once reticulocytosis is observed, the neonate will no longer need further transfusion therapy.

19 RhIG prevents Rh immunization with two provisos: it must be given in adequate amounts, and it must be given before Rh immunization has begun. RhIG administration does not suppress Rh immunization once it has begun, no matter how weak the immunization.

20 In the United States, it is recommended that 300 μg of RhIG be administered within 72 h of delivery of a Rh-positive infant. This dose will protect against sensitization from TPH of 30 mL of fetal whole blood. Approximately 1 in 1000 deliveries will exceed this volume. Therefore, routine screening at delivery for excessive TPH is indicated. The rosette test is performed first; if negative, the patient need only receive the standard dose of RhIG and, if positive, a Kleihauer–Betke stain is performed to determine the number of additional vials of RhIG that are needed to prevent maternal sensitization.

References

1 Race RR. The Rh genotype and Fisher's theory. *Blood* 1948;3:27.

2 Le Van Kim C, Mouro I, Cherif-Zahar B, et al. Molecular cloning and primary structure of the human blood group RhD polypeptide. *Proc Natl Acad Sci USA* 1992;89:10925.

3 Wiener AS, Wexler IB. *Heredity of the blood groups*. New York: Grune & Stratton, 1958.

4 Rosenfield RE, Allan FH, Jr, Swisher SN, Kochwa A. A review of Rh serology and presentation of a new terminology. *Transfusion* 1962;2:287.

5 Issitt PD. The Rh blood group system, 1988: eight new antigens in nine years and some observation on the biochemistry and genetics of the system. *Transfus Med Rev* 1989;3:1.

6 Wiener AS. Diagnosis and treatment of anemia of the newborn caused by occult placental hemorrhage. *Am J Obstet Gynecol* 1948;56:707.

7 Chown B. Anemia from bleeding of the fetus into the mother's circulation. *Lancet* 1954;1:1213.

8 Kleihauer E, Braun H, Betke K. Demonstration von fetalem haemoglobin in den erythrozyten eines blutausstriches. *Klin Wochenschr* 1957;35:637.

9 Bowman JM, Pollock JM, Penston LE. Fetomaternal transplacental hemorrhage during pregnancy and after delivery. *Vox Sang* 1986;51:117.

10 Bowman JM. Maternal alloimmunization and fetal hemolytic disease. In: Reece EA, Hobbins JC, Mahoney MJ, Petrie RH, eds. *Medicine of the fetus and mother*, 2nd edn. Philadelphia: J.B. Lippincott; 1992:1152.

11 Wiener AS. Conglutination test for Rh sensitization. *J Lab Clin Med* 1945;30:662.
12 Coombs RRA, Mourant AE, Race RR. A new test for the detection of weak and "incomplete" Rh agglutinins. *Fr J Exp Pathol* 1945;26;255.
13 Lewis M, Kaita H, Chown B. Kell typing in the capillary tube. *J Lab Clin Med* 1958;52:163.
14 Rosenfield RE, Haber GV. Detection and measurement of homologous human hemagglutinins. Automation in Analytical Chemistry–Technicon Symposia 1965:503.
15 Lalezari P. A polybrene method for the detection of red cell antibodies. *Fed Proc* 1967;26:756.
16 Moore BPL. Automation in the blood transfusion laboratory. I. Antibody detection and quantitation in the Technicon Auto Analyzer. *Can Med Assoc J* 1969;100:381.
17 Zipursky A, Israels LG. The pathogenesis and prevention of Rh immunization. *Can Med Assoc J* 1967;97:1245.
18 Pollack W, Ascari WQ, Kochesky RJ, et al. Studies on Rh prophylaxis. I. Relationship between doses of anti-Rh and size of antigenic stimulus. *Transfusion* 1971;11:333.
19 Woodrow JC. *Rh immunization and its prevention.* Series hematologia. Vol. III. Copenhagen: Munksgaard, 1970.
20 Nevanlinna HR. Factors affecting maternal Rh immunization. *Ann Med Exp Biol* 1953;31(Fenn Suppl. 2):1.
21 Bowman JM, Chown B, Lewis M, Pollock JM. Rh-immunization during pregnancy: antenatal prophylaxis. *Can Med Assoc J* 1978;118:623.
22 Bowman JM. Fetomaternal ABO incompatibility and erythroblastosis fetalis. *Vox Sang* 1986;50:104.
23 Soothill PW, Nicolaides KH, Rodeck CH, et al. Relationship of fetal hemoglobin and oxygen content to lactate concentration in sensitized pregnancies. *Obstet Gynecol* 1987;69:268.
24 Nicolaides KH, Warenski JC, Rodeck CH. The relationship of fetal protein concentration and haemoglobin level to the development of hydrops in rhesus isoimmunization. *Am J Obstet Gynecol* 1985;152:341.
25 Wiener CP, Heilskov J, Pelzer G, et al. Normal values for human umbilical venous and amniotic fluid pressures and their alteration by fetal disease. *Am J Obstet Gynecol* 1989;161:714.
26 Weiner CP, Williamson RA, Wenstrom KD, et al. Management of fetal hemolytic disease by cordocentesis: II. Outcome of treatment. *Am J Obstet Gynecol* 1991;165:1302.
27 Weiner CP, Pelzer GD, Heilskov J, et al. The effect of intravascular transfusion on umbilical venous pressure in anemic fetuses with and without hydrops. *Am J Obstet Gynecol* 1989;161: 149E.
28 Weiner CP, Williamson RA, Wenstrom KD, et al. Management of fetal hemolytic disease by cordocentesis: I. Prediction of fetal anemia. *Am J Obstet Gynecol* 1991;165:546.
29 Weiner CP. Human fetal bilirubin and fetal hemolytic disease. *Am J Obstet Gynecol* 1992,116:1449.
30 Barss VA, Frigoletto FD, Konugres A. The cost of irregular antibody screening. *Am J Obstet Gynecol* 1988;159:428.
31 Bowman JM, Pollock JM. Transplacental fetal hemorrhage after amniocentesis. *Obstet Gynecol* 1985;66:749.
32 Bowman JM, Pollock JM. Amniotic fluid spectrophotometry and early delivery in the management of erythroblastosis fetalis. *Pediatrics* 1965;35:815.
33 Liley AW. Liquor amnii analysis in management of pregnancy complicated by Rhesus immunization. *Am J Obstet Gynecol* 1961;82:1359.
34 Nicolaides KH, Rodeck CH, Mibashan RS, Kemp JR. Have Liley charts outlived their usefulness? *Am J Obstet Gynecol* 1986;155: 90.
35 Queenan JT, Tomai TP, Ural SH, King JC. Deviation in amniotic fluid optical density at a wavelength of 450 nm in Rh-immunized pregnancies from 14 to 40 weeks' gestation: a proposal for clinical management. *Am J Obstet Gynecol* 1993;168:1370.
36 Scott F, Chan FY. Assessment of the clinical usefulness of the 'Queenan' chart versus the 'Liley' chart in predicting severity of rhesus iso-immunization. *Prenat Diagn* 1998;18:1143.
37 Bartsch FK. Bilirubin in the amniotic fluid: a review. In: Robertson JG, Dambrosio F, eds. International symposium on the management of the Rh problem. *Annali Obstet Ginec Milano* 1970; special no. 73.
38 Daffos F, Capella-Pavlovsky M, Forestier F. Fetal blood sampling during pregnancy with use of a needle guided by ultrasound: a study of 606 consecutive cases. *Am J Obstet Gynecol* 1985;153:655.
39 Nicolaides KH, Fontanarosa M, Gabbe SG, Rodeck CH. Failure of ultrasonographic parameters to predict the severity of fetal anemia in rhesus isoimmunization. *Am J Obstet Gynecol* 1988;158:920.
40 Vintzileos AM, Campbell WA, Storlazzi E, et al. Fetal liver ultrasound measurements in isoimmunized pregnancies. *Obstet Gynecol* 1986;68:162.
41 Roberts AB, Mitchell JM, Lake Y, Pattison NS. Ultrasonographic surveillance in red blood cell alloimmunization. *Am J Obstet Gynecol* 2001;184:1251.
42 Oepkes D, Meerman RH, Vandenbussche FP, et al. Ultrasonographic fetal spleen measurements in red blood cell-alloimmunized pregnancies. *Am J Obstet Gynecol* 1993;169:121.
43 Bahado-Singh R, Oz U, Mari G, et al. Fetal splenic size in anemia due to Rh-alloimmunization. *J Ultrasound Med* 2005; 24: 697.
44 Vyas S, Nicolaides KH, Campbell S. Doppler examination of the middle cerebral artery in anemic fetuses. *Am J Obstet Gynecol* 1990;162:1066.
45 Mari G, Adrignolo A, Abuhamad AZ, et al. Diagnosis of feta anemia with Doppler ultrasound in pregnancy complicated by maternal blood group immunization. *Ultrasound Obstet Gynecol* 1995;5:400.
46 Detti L, Mari G, Akiyama M, et al. Longitudinal assessment of the middle cerebral artery peak systolic velocity in healthy fetuses and in fetuses at risk for anemia. *Am J Obstet Gynecol* 2002;187:937.
47 Zupanska B, Brojer E, Richards Y, et al. Serological and immunological characteristics of maternal anti-Rh(D) antibodies in predicting the severity of haemolytic disease of the newborn. *Vox Sang* 1989;56:247.
48 Urbaniak SI, Greiss MA, Crawford RJ, et al. Prediction of the outcome of Rhesus haemolytic disease of the newborn: additional information using an ADCC assay. *Vox Sang* 1984;46:323.
49 Engelfriet CP, Brouwers HAA, Huiskes E, et al. Prognostic value of the ADCC with monocytes and maternal antibodies for haemolytic disease of the newborn. Abstracts of the XXIst Congress ISH and XIXth Congress ISBT, Sydney 1986: 162(abst).
50 Hadley AB, Kumpel BM, Leader KA, et al. Correlation of serological, quantitative and cell-mediated functional assays of maternal alloantibodies with the severity of haemolytic disease of the newborn. *Br J Haematol* 1991;77:221.
51 Brown SJ, Perkins JT, Sosler SD, et al. The monocyte-monolayer

assay does not predict severity of hemolytic disease of the newborn. *Transfusion* 1991;31(Suppl)SI93:53S.

52 Bennett PR, Le Van Kim C, Collin Y, et al. Prenatal determination of fetal RhD type by DNA amplification. *N Engl J Med* 1993;329:607.

53 Lo Y-MD, Bowel PJ, Selinger M, et al. Prenatal determination of fetal RhD status by analysis of peripheral blood of Rhesus negative mothers (letter). *Lancet* 1993;341:1147.

54 Finning KM, Martin PG, Soothill PW, Avent ND. Prediction of fetal D status from maternal plasma: introduction of a new noninvasive fetal RHD genotyping service. *Transfusion* 2002;42:1079.

55 Steiner H, Schaffer J, Spitzer D, et al. The relationship between peak velocity in the fetal descending aorta and hematocrit in rhesus isoimmunization. *Obstet Gynecol* 1995;85:659.

56 Weiner CP, Wenstrom KD, Sipes SL, Williamson RA. Risk factors for cordocentesis and fetal intravascular transfusions. *Am J Obstet Gynecol* 1991;165:1020.

57 Menticoglou SM, Harman CR, Manning FA, Bowman JM. Intraperitoneal fetal transfusion: paralysis inhibits red cell absorption. *Fetal Ther* 1987;2:154.

58 Lewis M, Bowman JM, Pollock JM, Lown B. Absorption of red cells from the peritoneal cavity of a hydropic twin. *Transfusion* 1973;13:37.

59 Crosby WM, Brobmann GF, Chang ACK. Intrauterine transfusion and fetal death; relationship of intraperitoneal pressure to umbilical vein flow. *Am J Obstet Gynecol* 1970;108:135.

60 Rodeck CH, Holman CA, Karnicki J, et al. Direct intravascular fetal blood transfusion by fetoscopy in severe Rhesus isoimmunization. *Lancet* 1981;1:652.

61 Chestnut DH, Pollack KL, Weiner CP, et al. Does furosemide alter the hemodynamic response to rapid intravascular transfusion of the anemic fetal lamb. *Am J Obstet Gynecol* 1989;161:1571.

62 Egberts J, van Kamp IL, Kanhai HH, et al. The disappearance of fetal and donor red blood cells in alloimmunized pregnancies: a reappraisal. *Br J Obstet Gynecol* 1997;104:818.

63 Margulies M, Voto LS, Mathet E, Marguilies M. High-dose intravenous IgG for the treatment of severe Rhesus alloimmunization. *Vox Sang* 1991;61:181.

64 Von Dungern F. Beitrage zur immunitatslehr. *Munch Med Wochenschr* 1900;47:677.

65 Freda VJ, Gorman JG, Pollack W. Successful prevention of experimental Rh sensitization in man with an anti-Rh gamma-2 globulin antibody preparation: a preliminary report. *Transfusion* 1964;4:26.

66 Clarke CA, Donohoe WTA, McConnell RB, et al. Further experimental studies in the prevention of Rh-haemolytic disease. *Br Med J* 1963;1:979.

67 Bowman JM, Pollock JM. Reversal of Rh alloimmunization. Fact or fancy? *Vox Sang* 1984;47:209.

68 Samson D, Mollison PL. Effect on primary Rh-immunization of delayed administration of anti-Rh. *Immunology* 1975;28:349.

69 Bowman JM. Controversies in Rh prophylaxis: who needs Rh immune globulin and when should it be given? *Am J Obstet Gynecol* 1985;151:289.

70 Bowman JM. The prevention of Rh immunization. *Transfus Med Rev* 1988;2:129.

71 Pollack W, Ascari WQ, Crispin JF, et al. Studies on Rh prophylaxis. II. Rh immune prophylaxis after transfusions with Rh-positive blood. *Transfusion* 1971;11:340.

72 De Almeida V, Bowman JM. Massive fetomaternal hemorrhage: Manitoba experience. *Obstet Gynecol* 1994;83:323.

73 Zipursky A, Blajchman M. The Hamilton Rh prevention studies. Presented at McMaster Conference on Prevention of Rh Immunization, 28–30 September, 1977. *Vox Sang* 1979;36:50.

74 Bartsch F, Sandberg L. Incidence of anti-D at delivery in previously non-immunized Rh-negative mothers with Rh-positive babies. Presented at McMaster Conference on Prevention of Rh Immunization, 28–30 September, 1977. *Vox Sang* 1979;36:50.

75 Scott JR. Beer AE, Guy LR, et al. Pathogenesis of Rh immunization in primigravidas. Fetomaternal versus maternofetal bleeding. *Obstet Gynecol* 1977;49:9.

76 Bowman JM, Pollock JM. Antenatal Rh prophylaxis: 28-week gestation service program. *Can Med Assoc J* 1978;118:627.

77 Bowman JM, Pollock JM. Failures of intravenous Rh immune globulin prophylaxis: an analysis of the reasons for such failures. *Transfus Med Rev* 1987;1:101.

78 Rivat L, Rivat C, Parent M, Ropartz C. [Adverse effects of an injection of anti-Rh gamma-globulin due to the presence of anti-gamma A antibodies.] *Presse Med* 1970;78:2072.

79 Hoppe HH, Mester T, Hennig W, Krebs HJ. Prevention of Rh-immunization: modified production of IgG anti Rh for intravenous application by ion exchange chromatography (IEC). *Vox Sang* 1973;25:308.

80 Crawford DH, Barlow MJ, Harrison JF, et al. Production of human monoclonal antibody to Rhesus D antigen. *Lancet* 1983;1:386.

81 Crawford DH, McDougall DCJ, Mulholland N, et al. Further characteristics of a human monoclonal antibody to the Rhesus D antigen produced in vitro. *Boehring Inst Mitt* 1984;74:55.

82 Bron D, Feinberg MB, Teng NNH, Kaplan HS. Production of human monoclonal IgG antibodies against Rhesus (D) antigen. *Proc Natl Acad Sci USA* 1984;81:3214.

83 MacDonald G, Primrose S, Biggins K, et al. Production and characterization of human–human and human–mouse to hybridomas secreting Rh (D)-specific monoclonal antibodies. *Scand J Immunol* 1987;25:477.

84 Miller DF, Petrie SJ. Fatal erythroblastosis fetalis secondary to ABO incompatibility: report of a case. *Obstet Gynecol* 1963;22:773.

85 Gilja BK, Shah VP. Hydrops fetalis due to ABO incompatibility. *Clin Pediatr* 1988;27:210.

86 Bowman JM. Neonatal management. In: Queenan JT, eds. *Modern management of the Rh problem*, 2nd edn. New York: Harper & Row; 1977:209.

87 Mollison PL, Engelfriet CP, Contreras M. Hemolytic disease of the newborn. In: Mollison PL, ed. *Blood transfusion in clinical medicine*, 8th edn. Oxford: Blackwell Scientific Publications; 1987:639.

88 Bowman JM, Pollock JM, Manning FA, et al. Maternal Kell blood group alloimmunization. *Obstet Gynecol* 1992;79:239.

89 Caine ME, Mueller-Heubach E. Kell sensitization in pregnancy. *Am J Obstet Gynecol* 1986;154:85.

80 Hadi HA, Robertson A. Kell sensitization, hydrops, and low delta OD_{450}. *J Matern Fetal Med* 1992;1:293.

91 Vaughan JI, Warwick R, Letsky E, et al. Erythropoietic suppression in fetal anemia because of Kell alloimmunization. *Am J Obstet Gynecol* 1994;171:247.

50 Maternal infections, human immunodeficiency virus infection, and sexually transmitted diseases in pregnancy

Richard L. Sweet and Howard Minkoff

Maternal infections during pregnancy

The altered immune state of pregnancy increases the risk of infection for the adult host. This is a paradox. The blunting of the immunologic response in a pregnancy is beneficial because it permits the maintenance of a foreign protein graft, the placenta and the fetus. At the same time, it can be detrimental to the pregnant women when she is exposed to such foreign antigens as viruses and bacteria. Both the frequency and the severity of infection can be increased.

There are conflicting laboratory data about a reduced immunologic response during pregnancy. For the purposes of this discussion, evaluation of immunity is divided into two categories: humoral and cellular. Most of the studies of humoral immune response in pregnancy show reactions similar to those found in nonpregnant women.[1] In contrast, the cellular immune response has generally been diminished. Although the mechanism remains in question, pregnancy has generally been associated with a depressed cell-mediated immunity.

The most important test of the hypothesis of diminished cell-mediated immunity in pregnancy is clinical observation. If infection in pregnant women is more frequent or severe, this should settle the issue. There have been many studies with a multitude of varied pathogens that document a diminished host response in pregnant women. For example, Finland and Dublin's[2] detailed study, published in 1939, of a large number of Boston women who had a pneumococcal pneumonia documented a death rate that was higher in pregnant than in nonpregnant women, particularly when the disease was contracted in the third trimester. The increased severity of infection in pregnant women is not limited to bacterial infections. Viruses are also a problem. In the influenza pandemic of 1957, death was much more common among pregnant women.[3] Protozoal disease and systemic fungal disease can also be serious. For example, pregnant women have an increase in both the incidence and the complications of malaria and, in endemic regions, coccidioidomycosis is a leading cause of maternal death.[4] All these different disease entities, caused by bacteria, viruses, protozoa, and fungi, share two similar traits: they are normally held in check by cell-mediated immune mechanisms, and all are more serious in pregnancy.

The control of maternal infection during pregnancy requires two strategies. The traditional approach is the treatment of an established infection, and this takes up the bulk of the presentation in this chapter. Of equal or greater importance is prevention. Up to now, this has been a neglected subject for obstetricians. Comprehensive prevention of infection implies two target patient populations: those women before pregnancy (preconception) and those women during pregnancy.

Obstetricians must take a more active role in the immunization of adult women.[5] When young women become sexually active, they switch their primary care from the pediatrician to the obstetrician–gynecologist. In the future, we will need to become more attuned to preventive medicine strategies in women.

The preconception period is a window of opportunity for the prevention of infections in women. This should be a familiar theme for obstetricians because it applies to other problems. For infectious disease control, the strategies fit into three major groupings: treatment, immunization, and prevention strategies.

Treatment is included here as a preventive measure, because of the clinically silent nature of most *Chlamydia trachomatis* infections in women. Screening for *C. trachomatis* should be applied to sexually active women, particularly those younger than age 25 years who are at most risk of acquiring this infection. As discussed in the section on sexually transmitted diseases (STDs), chlamydial infection is associated with adverse prognosis complications. In addition, undetected *C. trachomatis* infection can have myriad untoward long-term effects on the future health of women including infertility,[6] ectopic pregnancy,[7] and abortion.[8] Diagnosis and treatment of chlamydial infections are discussed in the section on STDs.

Immunization of adult women

Immunization programs are a major part of our infectious disease prevention strategy. Of critical importance is the recognition that adult immunization programs are an integral part of this strategy.[9,10] It has been estimated that over 60000 adults die annually in the United States from vaccine-preventable diseases with influenza and pneumococcal disease the most common.[11] Gonik et al.[10] have recently emphasized the important role that obstetrician–gynecologists play in adult immunization.

Tetanus–diphtheria

Tetanus is a rare problem in the United States, with only 50–65 cases per year, but it is a serious disease that can cause death.[9] The Centers for Disease Control (CDC) recommends that adults, including pregnant women with uncertain history of a complete primary vaccination series, should receive a primary series of tetanus and diphtheria (Td).[9] This includes a series of three doses with the first two doses given at least 4 weeks apart and the third dose 6–12 months after the second. For those women who have received the primary series, one booster dose should be administered every 10 years.[9] The most important fact in the physician's care decision is that tetanus can be prevented by immunization. New nonpregnant patients in the childbearing age group should be asked about their tetanus immunization status. If they have not had a booster dose in the last 10 years, they should be given tetanus toxoid. This should be a lifetime concern of obstetrician–gynecologists because 60% of tetanus cases and 75% of deaths occur in the elderly, especially women.[12]

Measles, mumps, and rubella

The next three preventable diseases, measles, mumps, and rubella, are discussed together because a vaccine that protects against them is commercially available. Antibody testing should be done to confirm susceptibility. If the patient has no antibodies, she should be offered immunization. Because this is an attenuated live virus, the patient should be counseled to avoid getting pregnant for 3 months after the immunization. These women should be advised before the injection that adult women have a much higher incidence of migratory arthritis than men.[13] Fortunately, this is a transient, not a permanent, problem. Unfortunately, the symptoms can last up to 9 months.

Hepatitis B

Hepatitis B is an important disease for American women. It occurs with a greater frequency in the United States than other vaccine-preventable communicable diseases.[18] More importantly, it causes short-term illness and, for those chronic carriers of the virus, there is the possibility of serious long-term morbidity with cirrhosis or a hepatic carcinoma. The Advisory Committee on Immunization Practices (ACIP) has developed recommendations for the prevention of hepatitis B virus (HBV) transmission in the United States.[14] Pre-exposure vaccination to prevent HBV infection addresses three groups of patients: (1) routine vaccination of all newborns/infants; (2) catch-up vaccination of susceptible children and adolescents; and (3) vaccination of high-risk adults (Table 50.1).[9,14] Despite the frequency of hepatitis B compared with rubella,[18] American obstetricians are predisposed to immunize against rubella, a very rare disease, but not hepatitis B, which is much more common and a greater threat to the long-term health of women. This is a problem of education and awareness for physicians and patients. This is a three-shot immunization regimen. The first two are given 1 month apart, with the third administered 6 months later.[9] These women should be reassured. This vaccine is a recombinant DNA vaccine derived from yeast and is safe in pregnancy.

Hepatitis B vaccine is recommended for all newborns/infants; those born to mothers who are hepatitis surface antigen-positive should receive the first dose of vaccine within 12 h of birth and a concomitant injection of hepatitis B immune globulin (HBIG).

Varicella

Varicella is a potentially serious illness for adults, resulting in pneumonia in some cases, and progressing to death in a few, especially in pregnant women. In addition, acquisition during pregnancy can be damaging to the fetus. As some women are unclear about a prior history of varicella, susceptibility should be determined by antibody testing. If susceptible, immunization should be offered. It is a live attenuated virus vaccine that is usually well tolerated by adults. For adults, the best response is achieved by two injections, 4–8 weeks apart.

Varicella vaccine is a live attenuated virus vaccine and thus, because of a theoretical risk, should not be given to pregnant women or those planning on becoming pregnant in the next

Table 50.1 Groups at high risk of hepatitis B infection.

Sexually active heterosexual persons with recent STD, identified as prostitutes, having more than one sexual partner in the past 6 months, or seen in STD clinic
Homosexual or bisexual men
Household contacts and sexual partners of HbsAg-positive persons
Intravenous drug abusers
Persons at occupational risk through exposure to blood or infected body fluids (i.e., healthcare workers, public safety workers)
Clients and staff of institutions for the developmentally disabled
Patients on hemodialysis
Patients receiving clotting factor concentrate
Adoptees from countries where HBV infection is endemic
International travelers to areas where HBV is endemic who will have close contact with the local population
Inmates of long-term correctional facilities

STD, sexually transmitted disease; HBsAg, hepatitis B surface antigen; HBV, hepatitis B virus.

1 (ACIP) to 3 (Merck) months.[9,15] However, to date, no evidence of the congenital varicella syndrome has been reported among offspring of mothers inadvertently vaccinated in the first trimester. Breastfeeding is not a contraindication to varicella vaccine.

Influenza

Influenza vaccines are inactivated viral vaccines and, as a result, are safe to use during any trimester of pregnancy.[16] Pregnant women suffered excess deaths due to influenza during the pandemics of 1918–1919 and 1957–1958.[17] Thus, the benefits of influenza vaccination in pregnant women clearly outweigh the potential risks. Women who will be pregnant during the influenza season should be inoculated with the influenza vaccine prior to the influenza season, regardless of the stage of pregnancy.

Pneumococcal pneumonia

Pneumococcal infections caused by *Streptococcus pneumoniae* are a major source of morbidity and mortality.[18] *S. pneumoniae* is the leading cause of community-acquired pneumonia in the United States requiring hospitalization,[18] and is associated with an overall mortality rate of 5–10% and mortality rates as high as 30% in patients ≥ 65 years of age.[19] The ACIP recommends pneumococcal vaccine for all persons ≥ 65 years of age and for those individuals between 2 and 65 years of age who are at increased risk of serious pneumococcal infection.[9] Those at increased risk include: (1) persons with functional or anatomic asplenia; (2) persons with chronic cardiovascular or pulmonary disease; (3) those with diabetes mellitus; (4) alcoholics and those with chronic liver disease; (5) persons with cerebrospinal fluid leaks; and (6) persons living in special environments (e.g., nursing homes, chronic-care facilities, homeless shelters) or social settings (Native Alaskan, Native American).[20] While the safety of pneumococcal vaccine use in pregnancy has not been determined, there is no reason to suspect that the vaccine would have an adverse effect on the fetus or mother, and thus pneumococcal vaccine is not contraindicated during any stage of pregnancy.

Hepatitis A

Hepatitis A vaccine is recommended for those ≥ 2 years of age who are at increased risk of hepatitis A virus (HAV) infection.[9] Those at high risk include: (1) international travelers to countries where hepatitis A is endemic; (2) military personnel; (3) high-risk ethnic or geographic populations (e.g., Native Americans, Native Alaskans); (4) men who have sex with men; (5) intravenous drug abusers; (6) regular recipients of blood or plasma-derived products; (7) persons engaged in high-risk employment (primate handlers, employees of institutions for the developmentally challenged, day-care staff); and (8) persons chronically infected with hepatitis C.

Hepatitis A vaccine is an inactivated virus, and thus is not specifically contraindicated during pregnancy and is safe when breastfeeding. However, it is recommended by the CDC that hepatitis A vaccine should be given in pregnancy only if clearly indicated (e.g., exposure to infected contact or travel to endemic region).[9]

Preventive care for pregnant women

The antepartum time-frame is critical for the obstetrician who practices preventive medicine. Many strategies of prevention are in harmony with preconception care. There are many patients who will first see their healthcare provider when they are pregnant. In these instances, the whole process of education should be part of their care. Finally, preventive strategies that work will be beneficial to the mother and the fetus. For pregnancy, strategy follows three lines: treatment, prevention, and immunization.

Treatment should be directed at silent infections that could adversely affect the pregnant woman. There are eight disease entities that require attention. Two are discussed in this section; six others are presented elsewhere. Asymptomatic bacteriuria and patients with positive skin test results for tuberculosis are discussed under specific organ systems, the urinary and respiratory tract. Human immunodeficiency virus (HIV), *Neisseria gonorrhoeae*, *C. trachomatis*, syphilis, and trichomoniasis and bacterial vaginosis are discussed in other sections.

Although we think of them as symptomatic diseases, both bacterial vaginosis (BV) and *Trichomonas* vaginitis can be asymptomatic in many women. Their discovery is important, because these vaginal infections have been associated with an increased rate of premature labor and delivery.[22,23] There are currently no recommended techniques for screening asymptomatic women for the presence of these diseases. At the time of the initial pelvic examination, a vaginal pH and a whiff test with potassium hydroxide should be done. If both these test results are positive, a microscopic examination of a saline preparation should be done for the presence of clue cells. The positive whiff test and the presence of more than 20% clue cells in the vaginal preparation is the most sensitive screening test for BV.[24] Although the Vaginal Infection in Pregnancy study emphasizes the use of the Gram stain of a vaginal smear and one more recent study supports its sensitivity,[25] it is probably unlikely that this will be a popular screening test for clinicians.

While epidemiologic studies have demonstrated an association between BV and preterm birth, published randomized control studies have been inconsistent. Detection and treatment of asymptomatic BV in pregnant women with a previous preterm birth has significantly reduced the rate of preterm births.[26–28] In contradistinction, treatment of asymptomatic BV in low-risk women (i.e., no previous history of preterm birth) did not reduce the preterm birth rate.[28,29] Currently, the CDC does not recommend screening and treatment of asymptomatic pregnant women for BV.[30] For symptomatic pregnant or high-risk pregnant women, metronidazole 250 mg orally t.i.d. for 7 days or clindamycin 300 mg orally b.i.d. for 7 days is recommended.[30] Intravaginal topical preparations are not recommended for the treatment of BV during pregnancy.

Even less is known about a pregnancy strategy for *Trichomonas*. The hanging drop microscopic examination is not a sensitive test.[31] In contrast, a higher yield of positive test results was obtained in an urban population when the screening was done with the polymerase chain reaction (PCR) technique.[32] Although the presence of *Trichomonas* is associated with an increased rate of preterm delivery, there is no consensus on screening and treatment. Paradoxically, a large prospective, randomized, placebo-controlled treatment trial of asymptomatic *T. vaginalis* infection in pregnancy, by the National Institutes of Health (NIH)-supported Maternal–Fetal Medicine network, reported an increased risk of preterm delivery (< 37 weeks' gestation) in the metronidazole-treated patients.[33]

Screening for asymptomatic bacteriuria and tuberculosis is discussed in the sections on urinary tract and respiratory tract infections.

Toxoplasmosis is not a common disease in pregnancy, but it is important because the first maternal infection during pregnancy can result in fetal infection and morbidity. Any preventive strategy requires knowledge of the patient's susceptibility. For those antibody-negative women, printed recommendations should be provided (Table 50.2).[34] These measures are not difficult to understand or to follow. A similar set of recommendations given in patient education sessions significantly lowered the incidence of toxoplasmosis acquisition in Belgium.[35]

Cytomegalovirus (CMV) requires a very different emphasis by obstetricians because of its frequency. It is the most common cause of congenital viral infections, with an estimated 30 000–40 000 infected newborns born each year in the United States, 9000 of whom have permanent serious sequelae.[36] The starting point of preventive care is to determine the antibody status of the patient. If the patient is susceptible, there is a wide range of behavioral modifications that will decrease the risk of acquisition of this virus during pregnancy (Table 50.3).[34] The first applies to patients who remain in nonmonogamous sexual relationships after they are pregnant. They should have their male sexual partners use condoms. The second measure, handwashing, is especially applicable to the CMV-susceptible working mother who has young children in a childcare center, nursery school, or kindergarten. These procedures should be easily followed. The third reminder is for physicians to remember to counsel patients.

The rest of this chapter addresses problems of maternal infection during pregnancy, with an emphasis on organ systems.

Vulvovaginal infections

A frequent problem for pregnant women is the development of an increased vaginal discharge. Often, this is accompanied by other uncomfortable symptoms, such as itching or vulvar burning.

Changes in physician attitudes are needed to care properly for these women. Altered strategies are needed because of new information now available to physicians. In the past, the defining obstetric dogma was that pregnant women had an increased incidence of yeast vaginitis that was related in theory to a range of events from pregnancy hormonal changes to the glycosuria so commonly seen in pregnant women. The accepted therapeutic pattern among obstetricians was to prescribe a local antifungal agent or to have the patient medicate herself with over-the-counter antifungal preparations. Neither of these strategies mandated a vaginal examination, and it was frequently not done. Instead, the vaginal secretions were evaluated in patients who remained symptomatic despite treatment. This approach is no longer acceptable for a number of reasons. Practitioners have observed and it has been reported that patient self-diagnosis of a yeast vaginitis is often incorrect.[37] Physicians and patients should not assume that a symptomatic vaginal discharge in pregnancy is due to yeast. This is

Table 50.2 Toxoplasmosis, uncommon disease.

Patients should be tested for the presence of *Toxoplasma* antibodies. If the antibody is negative:

Patients should be advised not to eat raw or undercooked meat, particularly pork, lamb, or venison. Specifically, meat should be cooked to an internal temperature of 150°F; meat cooked until no longer pink inside generally has an internal temperature of 165°F.

Patients should be advised to wash their hands after contact with raw meat and after gardening or contact with soil; in addition, they should wash fruit and vegetables well before eating them raw.

If the patient owns a cat, someone else should change the litter box daily; alternatively, the patient should wash her hands thoroughly after changing the litter box. Patients should be encouraged to keep their cats inside and not to adopt or handle stray cats.

Table 50.3 Cytomegalovirus (CMV), common disease.

Patients should be tested for the presence of CMV antibodies. If the antibody is negative:

Patients should be advised that CMV is shed in semen, cervical secretions, and saliva. Latex condoms should be used during sexual contact if the patient is not in a monogamous relationship.

Providers of childcare or parents of children in childcare centers should be informed that they are at increased risk of acquiring a CMV infection. The risk of CMV infection can be diminished by avoiding mouth-to-mouth kissing and by handwashing, particularly after changing diapers.

If a blood transfusion is needed, these patients should receive only CMV antibody-negative blood or leukocyte-reduced cellular blood products in nonemergency situations.

important, because the Vaginal Infection in Pregnancy study noted two outcomes of other vaginal infections that are important to obstetricians. Patients with BV[22] and *Trichomonas* vaginitis[23] have a higher than expected incidence of preterm labor and delivery. These new correlates change the diagnostic demands on physicians caring for pregnant women. A physical examination and necessary laboratory testing need to be done to confirm the etiology of the vaginal discharge.

This physical and laboratory examination of the pregnant patient with a troublesome vaginal discharge does not require any new expensive office equipment or specialized clinical expertise. The approach to these women is simple and straightforward. The physician has to examine the vulva and vagina and do some immediate testing in the office environment. Cotton swabs, pH paper, solutions of saline, potassium hydroxide, and dilute acetic acid, as well as slides, coverslips, and a usable microscope, should be on hand. Physicians have to evaluate the pH paper reading, assay the scent emanating when vaginal secretions are added to the dilute potassium hydroxide solution, and be able to identify fungal forms, trichomonads, white blood cells, vaginal epithelial cells, and survey the bacterial background of the wet mount smears at the time of the immediate microscopic examination. This is the required office workup of every pregnant patient with vulvovaginal symptoms. Unfortunately, as reported by Wiesenfeld and Macio,[38] many obstetrician–gynecologists do not perform these simple office-based tests for determining the etiology of vaginitis symptoms and signs.

A frequent diagnosis of the pregnant patient with a troublesome vaginal discharge is a *Candida* vaginitis. The evaluation of these patients is straightforward. The vaginal pH is tested and is usually acidic. Vaginal secretions are added to a drop of saline on one slide and a drop of dilute potassium hydroxide on another. The physician should determine if an odor is present. A portion of the secretions is put in a sterile microbiological culture kit, which may or may not be sent to the laboratory. The diagnosis is usually made by microscopic examination of the saline and the potassium hydroxide preparation. If this is the first vaginal infection and *Candida* forms can be identified, a culture is not needed. If the diagnosis of *Candida* vaginitis cannot be confirmed on microscopic examination or the patient has recurrent vaginal yeast infections, the culture should be sent to the laboratory,[39] and on the specimen slip, a request made that, if yeast is present, it should be speciated.[40]

Candida albicans vaginitis is usually easy to treat, because it is not resistant to the available, local antifungal agents, nystatin and the azoles, all of which can be prescribed or obtained over the counter. These local agents should be the drugs of choice for pregnant women for three reasons. The systemic absorption of the topical azoles is minimal,[41] their use in the first trimester has been documented with no detectable evidence of teratogenicity,[41] and congenital anomalies (craniofacial, skeletal, and cardiac) have been reported in women who received fluconazole in the first trimester.[42] The reported ossification defects resemble those seen in pregnant animals given fluconazole.[42] There is no evidence that patients with a recurrent *C. albicans* vaginal infection have an improved clinical cure rate if their male sexual partners are treated.[43] Other strains of yeast are a more serious problem, and this is one reason for obtaining cultures in women with recurrent or persistent problems.

Torulopsis glabrata may be resistant to local azole antifungals. Treatment with a local boric acid preparation is often effective in nonpregnant women,[40] but its safety in pregnancy has not been studied. Routine antepartum glucose screening of all obstetric patients will reveal any with a problem of glucose metabolism. Another reason for culture in women with persistent vaginal symptoms is the awareness that some of these symptomatic women do not have a chronic vaginal yeast infection. Many patients become sensitive to the propylene glycol present in most vaginal creams and suppositories[44] and are helped if these local treatments are discontinued.

Another common cause of troublesome vaginal discharge for a pregnant woman is BV. In addition to a persistent copious discharge, many of these women report an unacceptable odor, particularly after intercourse. This is an important entity to recognize because it has been associated with a higher than expected incidence of preterm labor and delivery.[22] The diagnosis is simple and is immediately apparent to the physician at the time of the patient's office visit. The first test to perform is the vaginal pH, which is usually alkaline, that is > 4.5 in women with BV. These women invariably have a positive whiff test result when vaginal secretions are added to the dilute potassium hydroxide solution, and more than 20% of the vaginal squamous cells are clue cells when the saline preparation is examined immediately under the microscope. The two most sensitive tests for an immediate accurate diagnosis are a positive whiff test result and the presence of clue cells on the microscopic examination of the saline preparation.[24]

For symptomatic BV in pregnancy, the CDC recommends metronidazole 250 mg t.i.d. for 7 days or clindamycin 300 mg orally b.i.d. for 7 days.[30]

Some women complain of a troublesome vaginal discharge that is due to the organism *Trichomonas vaginalis*. Although textbooks have in the past described the typical clinical presentation of a patient with this infection, which includes a frothy vaginal discharge and "strawberry" spots on the vaginal surface, the problem for the physician is that these signs are not sensitive indicators of a *Trichomonas* vaginitis.[31] As with previously described vaginal syndromes, the diagnosis is straightforward. The pH of the vagina is usually alkaline, there is often a positive whiff test result and, on microscopic examination of the saline preparation, there is an abundance of white cells, and motile trichomonads are often seen. If trichomonads are not seen, these patients should have either a culture or a PCR test for *T. vaginalis* performed.[32] Unlike BV, the diagnosis may not be obvious at the time of the initial physician evaluation. This is an important diagnosis to confirm because these vaginal infections are associated with a higher than expected incidence of premature delivery.[23] In those women in whom the diagnosis is established, there are two available treatment regimens with metronidazole. The woman can be prescribed either 2.0g orally in a single dose or 500mg b.i.d. for 7 days.[3] Obviously, the male sexual partner should be treated concomitantly with the same dose.

If office pH, microscopy, and selective microbiological studies do not delineate the infection as BV, *Candida* vaginitis, or *Trichomonas* vaginitis, there are a variety of other problems that should be suspected, including vulvar vestibulitis, allergic vaginitis, desquamative vaginitis, and cervicitis.[44] There are signs associated with these alternative diagnoses that are apparent to the physician at the time of seeing the patient. The patient with vulvar vestibulitis has point tenderness with a cotton-tipped applicator applied at the vaginal entry sites of 3:30 and 8:30, if the vaginal entrance is oriented as the face of a clock; the patient with cervicitis has mucous present. None of these patients is helped with local antifungal preparations and, if these women have an allergic vaginitis, their symptoms can be magnified by the use of local preparations containing propylene glycol. Desquamative vaginitis is effectively treated with clindamycin vaginal cream. A patient with cervicitis should have microbiological tests for the presence of *N. gonorrhoeae* or *C. trachomatis*. They should be treated for both gonorrhea and chlamydia if they are a member of a patient population with a high prevalence of infection, treated for chlamydia if the prevalence of gonorrhea is low and the likelihood of chlamydia is substantial, or await test results if the likelihood of either is low.[3] The treatment for both gonorrhea and chlamydia has been noted in the preventive section of this chapter.

Urinary tract infections

Increased stasis of urine during pregnancy and the fact that urine is an excellent growth medium for bacteria makes the urinary tract the most common site of infection. Urinary stasis is caused by the convergence of a number of normal pregnancy changes. The capacity of the urinary tract is usually increased. In spite of the fact that few radiologic observations have been made of the urinary tract in normal pregnant women, the available data indicate that dilation is mild in the first half of pregnancy, but this is not a uniform phenomenon. After midpregnancy, the right side is dilated in three-quarters of cases, and the left side is dilated in a third.[45] There is also expansion of the renal pelves and calices as well as an increase in bladder capacity. While this anatomic expansion occurs, more urine is delivered to this excretion system as renal blood flow and glomerular filtration rate increase. Increased progesterone production also affects urinary tract function. Ureteral peristalsis slows, and the transit time from kidneys to bladder is prolonged. The bladder is hypotonic and has an increase in the residual volume of urine. The sum of these changes results in stagnant urine, an environment that encourages overgrowth of bacteria and subsequent clinical infection. The bacterial nidus for infection is present in the 2–10% of pregnant women with asymptomatic bacteriuria.[46] It is small wonder that urinary tract infections are seen so frequently in pregnant women.

Prevention is the appropriate starting place for any discussion of the therapy of urinary tract infections in pregnancy. Successful prevention eliminates the morbidity of symptomatic infections. This can be achieved in most instances and is described below.

Prevention of pyelonephritis

An estimated 25–30% of women with asymptomatic bacteriuria at the time of their first antepartum visit who are not treated will subsequently develop pyelonephritis in pregnancy.[47] These women are the focus of programs of detection and therapeutic intervention. Eighty percent of all cases of pyelonephritis in pregnancy could be eliminated if this population was identified and treated.[48] Harris[49] reported that, when an effort was made to identify and treat pregnant women with asymptomatic bacteriuria (ASB), there was a fivefold decrease in the annual incidence of acute antepartum pyelonephritis from 4.0% to 0.8%. In addition, ASB has been associated with an increased risk of preterm delivery and low birthweight.[47] Romero et al.[50] performed a meta-analysis that demonstrated a strong association of untreated ASB with preterm delivery or low birthweight.

These results buttress the idea of a uniform approach to all pregnant women seen for the first time. They should have a voided urine culture obtained to screen for significant bacteriuria. The health team caring for these women should advise them on how to produce a clean voided urine sample, and the specimens should be either processed immediately or refrigerated until they can be transported to the laboratory (this prevents bacterial overgrowth and false-positive urine cultures).

Although other screening tests are available, they lack sensitivity, and the standard remains the screening culture. When voided urine culture tests are employed, a significant test result has more than 100000 colonies/mL of one bacterial species. If multiple bacterial isolates are obtained, the specimen was contaminated at the time of collection, and another clean voided urine sample should be obtained and cultured. The treatment of women who are culture positive is based on the recognition that, as in nonpregnant women, *Escherichia coli* is the predominant pathogen isolated (80–90% of cases).[47] Other important pathogens include *Staphylococcus saprophytieus* and group B streptococci. Those women who are positive on urine culture for the group B streptococci early in pregnancy have been identified as a high-risk population for newborn group B streptococcal infection and should be treated with penicillin or ampicillin during labor.[51]

When the presence of ASB is identified, empiric treatment is instituted based on the above described causative microorganisms. Treatment is instituted with a 3-day course of trimethoprim-sulfamethoxazole (TMP-SMX, one double-strength tablet b.i.d.) or nitrofurantoin 100 mg b.i.d. In geographic areas where *E. coli* remains sensitive to ampicillin, amoxicillin 500 mg t.i.d. is an alternative. Continuous monitoring of patients for recurrent or persistent ASB is critical. If infection recurs, treatment should be based on antimicrobial susceptibility studies, and the patient should be maintained on suppressive antimicrobials (nitrofurantoin 100 mg h.s.) for the remainder of the pregnancy.[47]

Cystitis and pyelonephritis

Despite universal screening and treatment of women with ASB, unlike the prevention of pyelonephritis, the incidence of cystitis remains the same.[52] Fortunately, acute cystitis in pregnancy has not been associated with preterm birth, low birthweight, or acute pyelonephritis.[52]

The diagnosis of cystitis should be suspected in any pregnant woman with frequency and dysuria. *E. coli* is the most commonly isolated organism in the urine of patients with acute cystitis, followed by other Gram-negative bacteria such as *Klebsiella* and *Proteus*.[47] Gram-positive organisms, including group B streptococcus and *S. saprophytieus*, are less common.[47] Whereas in nonpregnant women with acute cystitis, empiric treatment without a culture is appropriate, in pregnancy, a culture should be obtained before commencing empiric therapy, and antibiotic therapy adjusted as indicated.[47] While ≥ 100 000 colonies/mL is the gold standard, Stamm et al.[53] demonstrated that, in acutely dysuric women, a quantitative count of 100 organisms/mL was sufficient for diagnosing acute cystitis.

For acute cystitis, the duration of therapy is 3 days. The antimicrobial agents suggested for the treatment of acute cystitis are the same as those utilized for the treatment of ASB including TMP-SMX 160/800 mg b.i.d. for 3 days and nitrofurantoin 100 mg b.i.d. for 3 days.

Acute pyelonephritis is one of the most frequent medical complications of pregnancy, occurring in 1–2.5% of obstetric patients.[47] The treatment of patients with pyelonephritis during pregnancy is much more intense. These patients are sicker and usually benefit from intensive therapy, so that problems of fever, hydration, and electrolyte imbalance, as well as the infection, can be treated. In addition, premature labor can occur in these women. This increase in uterine activity can be due to actions of the bacterial products causing the pyelonephritis, fever, or decreased intravascular volume. Therapy can modify these changes, and the uterus can be monitored to see whether a contraction pattern is becoming established. If necessary, tocolytic therapy may be indicated in addition to the antibiotics. Occasionally, some of these women become critically ill. In a series with a large number of pregnant women with pyelonephritis, 3 out of 99 (3%) had evidence of septic shock.[54] In addition, adult respiratory distress syndrome has been reported in pregnant women with pyelonephritis.[55–57] These women require close medical supervision.

All these potential problems require a broad therapeutic approach to the pregnant patient with pyelonephritis. Clinically, the diagnosis is usually obvious. These patients look ill, are febrile, and usually have flank pain. The uterus should be assessed immediately to be sure there is not a pattern of uterine contractions, and there should be immediate fetal heart rate monitoring to ascertain the health of the fetus. A vaginal examination should be done to insure there is no cervical dilation and cultures obtained to rule out maternal colonization with group B streptococcus, *C. trachomatis*, and *N. gonorrhoeae*. As soon as a voided urine sample can be obtained from the patient, a portion should be examined microscopically for the presence of bacteria. Uncentrifuged urine samples have been used, but a survey of laboratory studies in patients with bacteriuria recommended oil immersion microscopy of a Gram-stained centrifuged urine sample.[58] A portion of the urine should be sent for culture. If the clinical diagnosis has been made, treatment should begin. Fluid replacement should be an important part of therapy because some of these women are dehydrated, which is further aggravated because they are febrile with an increased insensible fluid loss. This is probably the reason why some investigators have noted diminished renal function in the first 24 h of treatment of pregnant women with pyelonephritis.[59] They need sufficient intravenous fluid replacement with a balanced electrolyte solution to insure a urine output of at least 50 mL/h. Because septic shock and respiratory distress have been reported in these women, they should be observed frequently, with regular monitoring of vital signs. In addition, these patients must be monitored for premature labor. If it occurs, tocolytic agents can be employed. Because respiratory distress can occur when these agents are used, an electrocardiogram should be obtained before treatment begins. If the patient has unrelenting flank pain, an ultrasound evaluation for the presence of urinary tract calculi should be done. If electrolyte abnormalities are noted in the initial screening blood chemistries, these can be corrected and repeat electrolyte determinations done until they are normal. Intravenous fluid electrolytes can be modified and repeat electrolyte determinations done until they are normal.

Initially, treatment for acute pyelonephritis is empiric with antimicrobial therapy dictated by knowledge of the most common etiologic organisms and the need for bactericidal drugs. The organisms most commonly recovered from pregnant women with acute pyelonephritis include *E. coli* (80–85%) and, less commonly, the *Klebsiella–Enterobacter* group.[47] Gram-positive bacteria, such as group B streptococcus and enterococci, have increasingly been recognized as pathogens in acute pyelonephritis in pregnant women.[47] Because of increasing resistance to *E. coli*, ampicillin and first-generation cephalosporins, which had been favored regimens for acute pyelonephritis in pregnancy, are generally no longer recommended for empiric therapy.[47,60] The authors recommend that empiric therapy for acute pyelonephritis during pregnancy be instituted with ceftriaxone 1–2 g intravenously as a single daily dose; it provides coverage against most major uropathogens other than *Enterococcus* and, because of once-daily administration, facilitates home parenteral therapy after initial in-hospital treatment and stabilization. TMP-SMX 160/800 mg intravenously b.i.d. is also appropriate in geographic areas where *E. coli* resistance to this agent has not occurred. A combination of either ampicillin (1–2 g intravenous q6h) or cefazolin (1–2 g intravenous q8h) in combination with gentamicin (1 mg/kg q8 h) is an alternative approach. All patients should have a repeat culture done at 48 h after the initiation of treatment. If bacteria are still recovered, consideration should be given to switching antibiotics to an agent more effective against the organism to avoid later recurrence of infection. When patients have been afebrile for 24–48 h, they can be switched to an oral agent or home parenteral therapy to complete 10 days of therapy. All these women should have a post-treatment culture obtained and, if it is positive, they should be treated with a different agent that is effective against the isolates. In those women who remain culture positive after a full course of treatment, an ultrasound examination should check for the presence of urinary tract calculi.

Economic pressures have altered this inpatient treatment emphasis, and there is evidence suggesting that selected patients might be treated as outpatients. Brooks and Garite[61] examined 34 patients as outpatients with uncomplicated initial episodes of pyelonephritis. Low-risk patients were identified by the absence of any sepsis, an oral temperature of greater than 39°C, severe nausea and vomiting, presence of diabetes or HIV infection, concomitant preterm labor, multiple gestation, severe penicillin allergy, history of renal disease or urinary tract anomalies, or the presence of an indwelling bladder catheter. After 2 h of observation, the patients had an initial dose of 2 g of ceftriaxone given intravenously, followed by 2 g of daily outpatient intramuscular ceftriaxone, until resolution of fever and flank pain, followed by a 10-day course of oral antibiotics. These carefully selected low-risk patients did well. Of the 34 in the outpatient treatment group, only four (12%) required subsequent hospital admission and one developed an upper urinary tract recurrence. None had premature delivery or any other serious complications.

Angel et al.[62] suggested that treatment with oral antimicrobial agents only for acute pyelonephritis during pregnancy is appropriate and safe. They reported equal efficacy in a randomized trial of oral cephalexin versus intravenous cephalothin (91% versus 93% respectively). However, 13 (14.4%) of their patients had bacteremia and were excluded from the study. With inclusion of the bacteremic patients, oral therapy was less effective than parenteral therapy (71% versus 87%).[62] Millar et al.[60] undertook a randomized controlled trial comparing inpatient and outpatient management of acute pyelonephritis in pregnancy prior to 24 weeks of gestation. All patients were observed in the emergency department to insure that they were stable and able to tolerate oral intake. The ambulatory group received ceftriaxone 1 g intramuscularly (i.m.) in the emergency department and 1 g i.m. within 18–36 h after discharge, followed by oral cephalexin (500 mg q.i.d.) to complete a 10-day course. In addition, home-health nurses monitored the ambulatory patients for 48–72 h. Patients with severe pyelonephritis were excluded. The rates of persistent or recurrent bacteriuria and recurrent pyelonephritis were similar. However, the study was biased in favor of the outpatient arm because 10% of inpatients required the addition of gentamicin for failure to respond to cefazolin monotherapy; 12% of *E. coli* isolates were resistant to cefazolin.[60] Wing et al.[63] studied pregnant women with pyelonephritis at more than 24 weeks' gestation. After all patients received two 1-g doses of ceftriaxone i.m. during a 24-h observation period, women were discharged (if stable) on oral cephalexin (500 mg q.i.d.) to complete a 10-day course. Inpatients received oral cephalexin until they were afebrile for 48 h and then were discharged to complete a 10-day course of cephalexin. There were no significant differences in clinical response or pregnancy outcomes between the groups.[63] However, 30% of outpatients could not complete their course of therapy, and the majority of women with acute pyelonephritis were excluded because of suspected sepsis, signs of acute respiratory distress syndrome (ARDS), serious underlying medical disorders, renal or urologic abnormalities, or inability to tolerate oral intake.

As a result of the concerns described above with these studies advocating oral ambulatory treatment of acute pyelonephritis in pregnancy, the authors recommend that all pregnant women, at any gestational age, should be hospitalized for initiation of antimicrobial therapy, rehydration, close monitoring for complications, and monitoring for preterm labor. Once stabilized and afebrile for 24–48 h, they may be discharged to complete a 10-day course of oral antibiotics.

If the follow-up culture result is negative, there is controversy about the subsequent care of these women for the rest of the pregnancy. Both antibiotic suppression of these women for the remainder of the pregnancy (i.e., nitrofurantoin, 50–100 mg/day) and urine culture at frequent intervals with short courses of treatment in women who are culture positive have been suggested.[47] Either of these approaches for the prevention of recurrent pyelonephritis is acceptable. The authors utilize the suppression approach for the duration of pregnancy.

Respiratory tract infections

Upper respiratory tract

Upper respiratory infections occur frequently in the winter. Many are viral in origin, and antibiotic treatment will not be beneficial. Women complaining of a sore throat should be examined and, if the throat is inflamed or if tonsillitis is present, a culture for group A streptococcus should be obtained. If the physician suspects a group A infection, penicillin should be prescribed instead of waiting for culture results. If the patient is allergic to penicillin, erythromycin can be given. If the clinician suspects a viral cause for a sore throat, it is appropriate to wait for a culture report before starting therapy.

Lower respiratory tract

The incidence of lower respiratory tract infection varies from service to service, many different risk factors have been determined, current methods of precisely defining the microbiological etiology of this disease are not specific, and there are a multitude of suggested treatment regimens. Clearly, a scientific consensus for a uniform approach to this disease has not been reached. Everyone does agree that this is a serious disease that has associated morbidity and mortality for both the mother and the fetus.[64,65]

The frequency of pneumonia has varied widely over the years but, in general, the incidence has decreased since the introduction of antibiotics into clinical practice. However, there has been an increase in numbers since HIV was identified in women in the mid-1980s. HIV positivity in women is a major risk factor in the high frequency of pneumonia.[66]

Although it is not a common disease in pregnant women, the physician should be alert to risk factors for pneumonia. Several risk subgroups have been identified.[64–68] Poor urban women are at highest risk. In addition to HIV infections, maternal smoking, excessive alcoholic intake, and cocaine crack use are also risk factors. Pneumonia is usually seen in the winter months.

Prevention is the starting point in the respiratory tract care of pregnant women. High-risk patients should be immunized against organisms that can cause serious respiratory infections. All pregnant women should receive the influenza vaccine as discussed previously. For HIV-positive pregnant patients, preventive respiratory tract care is important because lower respiratory infections can be fatal. One strategy is the influenza vaccine. This seems logical except for troubling reports that the viral load of HIV is increased after immunization with an antigen.[69] These women are also candidates for a single dose of 23 valent polysaccharide pneumococcal vaccine.[70] All patients should be skin tested for tuberculosis and, if positive, they should have chest radiography performed with appropriate shielding of the pregnant abdomen. If the chest radiography result is normal, these HIV-positive women should receive 12 months of chemoprophylaxis with isoniazid.[34] For the immunocompetent patient, the treatment interval is 6 months. TMP-SMX administered daily can be effective as an agent for *Pneumocystis carinii* pneumonia prophylaxis in HIV-positive women. All these preventive strategies should reduce their risk of developing pneumonia.

In those patients who develop pneumonia, the prognosis has markedly improved since the introduction of antibiotics. In the preantibiotic era, maternal death from pneumococcal pneumonia occurred in approximately one-third of cases.[2] In another series, the death rate in pregnant women with all types of pneumonia was 20%.[70] Since antibiotics have become available, the death rate is much lower, ranging from 0% to 8.6%.[64–68,71,72] Part of this improvement was due to early diagnosis and less severe disease. Additional therapeutic advantages include better ventilatory aids and more precise techniques to monitor vital signs and fluid balance. Because of the increasing numbers of HIV-positive women in the childbearing age groups, more seriously ill patients with pneumonias will be seen by obstetricians in the future.

There is no consensus about the care of patients with a community-acquired pneumonia.[70] There is concern that increasing numbers of *S. pneumoniae* strains in the United States are resistant to penicillin.[73] This fact, combined with a diverse variety of encountered pneumonia pathogens, has resulted in conflicting opinions about the care of pregnant patients with community-acquired pneumonia.

The key to the care of women with pneumonia in pregnancy is an early and accurate diagnosis. Patients with respiratory symptoms need a meticulous evaluation to determine if they have a lower respiratory tract infection. The evaluation begins with careful percussion and auscultation. A carefully obtained sputum sample for microscopic examination and culture before treatment is advised. A microscopic examination of a Gram-stained specimen showing polymorphonuclear leukocytes and the absence of squamous epithelial cells indicates that the specimen is expectorate and not saliva. A chest radiograph should be obtained with appropriate shielding of the abdomen. This serves as a guide to both the diagnosis and the severity of the disease. Blood studies should include a complete blood count and an arterial P_{O_2}. Patients sick enough to require hospitalization should have a blood chemistry panel performed and blood cultures before antibiotics are begun.

In general, the most frequent organism causing a community-acquired pneumonia is *S. pneumoniae*. This pathogen should be suspected at the time of admission in the febrile patient with lobar consolidation on chest radiography and white cells with Gram-positive diplococci present on microscopic examination of a smear of sputum.

In immunocompetent nonpregnant patients with community-acquired pneumonia, the decision whether to treat on an ambulatory or a hospitalized basis remains a key clinical decision that determines both the selection and the route of administration of antimicrobial agents.[74] However, pregnant women with this diagnosis should be admitted because of the potential for premature labor. In one study of 22 women with pneumonia, preterm labor was seen in five, and three had a preterm delivery.[72] They will need intravenous hydration and close monitoring of uterine activity.

Currently, the Infectious Disease Society of America's recommendation for hospitalized patients with community-acquired pneumonia, with no recent antibiotic therapy, includes an advanced macrolide (e.g., azithromycin or clarithromycin) plus a beta-lactam antibiotic such as cefotaxime, ceftriaxone, or ampicillin-sulbactam.[74] For those with a history of recent antibiotic use, similar type antibiotics are recommended with selection dependent on the nature of recent antibiotic use.[74] While respiratory fluroquinolones are an alternative recommended therapy in nonpregnant patients, these agents are best not used in pregnancy.

A variety of other organisms can be implicated in the patient with pneumonia in pregnancy who is febrile. Three other pathogens are isolated with some frequency and should be considered by the physician: *Haemophilus influenzae*, the coagulase-positive staphylococcus, and Gram-negative bacilli.[73,75] *H. influenzae* and Gram-negative bacilli should be suspected if Gram-negative rods are seen on the Gram stain of the expectorate. *H. influenzae* is a fastidious organism and will not be isolated if the culture specimen is obtained after antibiotic therapy has begun. Because 30% of the strains of *H. influenzae* are resistant to ampicillin, the cephalosporins are a good choice for treatment if this organism is suspected.[73] Pneumonia due to the coagulase-positive staphylococcus can be serious. It should be considered as a potential pathogen as a complication of influenza.[75] This organism should be suspected when clumps of Gram-positive cocci are seen on the Gram stain. In this situation, the drug of choice is a cephalosporin. Pneumonia due to the group A beta-hemolytic streptococcus is quite rare, but it should be suspected if chains of Gram-positive cocci are seen on the Gram stain of the expectorate and if a pleural effusion is seen on chest radiography, which when aspirated is found to be an empyema.[76]

Another category of patients, which constitutes a segment of pregnant women with pneumonia, is made up of those with an atypical clinical presentation. These are the patients with roentgenographic evidence of pneumonia who may not be febrile. The most important diagnostic clue to these atypical pneumonias is the microscopic examination of the expectorate. If few or no bacteria are found, *Legionella pneumophila*,[77] *Mycoplasma*,[78] and *Chlamydia pneumoniae*[70] are prime concerns. Despite physician awareness, these are difficult diagnoses to make. The positive culture result confirms the diagnosis of *Legionella*, but it requires invasive procedures to get appropriate culture material.[77] For *Mycoplasma* and *C. pneumoniae*, culture and PCR testing are available. Other testing is available to help confirm the diagnosis. Blood can be drawn for serologic testing for *Legionella*, *Mycoplasma*, and *C. pneumoniae*. Repeat titers should be drawn in 4 weeks. The antibiotics of choice for these organisms are erythromycin, clarithromycin, and azithromycin. All these are safe for use during pregnancy.

There are other rare pneumonias that will tax the diagnostic and therapeutic skills of the obstetrician. Varicella is a serious disease for susceptible pregnant women. Antepartum antibody screening and a history to determine whether they have received the varicella vaccine will identify susceptible women. Although a varicella pneumonia can be life-threatening, acyclovir is a potent antiviral agent for treatment during pregnancy. Oral acyclovir can be given to pregnant women when they first develop cutaneous manifestations of varicella to lessen the frequency and severity of a subsequent pneumonia.[79] In women with respiratory symptoms, the diagnosis of pneumonia can be confirmed by roentgenographic examination.[47] These seriously ill women should be admitted and given intravenous acyclovir and assisted ventilation if indicated. The fetus will receive passive immunity from the transplacental passage of IgG from the mother, so long as the delivery occurs at an interval long enough from the maternal viral exposure for maternal antibody formation to occur.

There are other pneumonias that are not as immediate a threat to the mother but have serious implications. The first is tuberculosis. This disease is a threat to pregnant women even though a recent study showed no evidence that pregnancy increased the risk that a woman of childbearing age infected with *Mycobacterium tuberculosis* will develop active tuberculosis.[80] In the United States, the incidence of tuberculosis has increased over the past 20 years, particularly among poor urban women. In this population, a tuberculin skin test will be performed and, in those women who have positive skin test results, a chest roentgenographic examination should be performed. In HIV-positive patients, a screening chest roentgenographic examination should be performed in patients who have negative skin test results if chest roentgenography has not been done in the past year. If there are apical changes, sputum should be sent for *M. tuberculosis* culture. The organisms isolated need to be evaluated for antibiotic susceptibilities. This will determine the combination of antibiotics to be prescribed. The most popular combination treatment now in use is isoniazid and ethambutol, but antibiotic susceptibility studies may alter the choice.[81,82] Multidrug-resistant tuberculosis (MDR-TB) has become a major public health problem.[82,83] Unfortunately, little information is available about the safety of the drugs used to treat MDR-TB during pregnancy. In a small study, Shin et al.[83] reported that, in seven cases of MDR-TB during pregnancy, excellent treatment outcomes were obtained for all seven women and their children. As a result, these authors stressed that MDR-TB can be successfully treated during pregnancy. The reader is referred to references 84 and 85 for more details on the treatment of MDR-TB. *P. carinii* pneumonia is seen with some frequency in urban obstetric services with a high incidence of HIV-positive pregnant patients. These patients usually have high fever, a lowered Po_2, and can have no changes initially on chest radiography, but are subsequently found to have diffuse bilateral alveolar disease. A definitive diagnosis is made by isolation of the organism from material from the lung. The usual treatment is TMP-SMX, but trimethoprim–dapsone, clindamycin–primaquine, and atovaquone can be used. In endemic areas, pulmonary infection due to a yeast can occur. The most common pathogens in these patients are *Coccidioides immitis* and *Histoplasma capsulatum*. The diagnosis can be confirmed by specific culture techniques. In the case of *Coccidioides*, systemic treatment with antifungal agents such as amphotericin B can be life-saving.[4]

Central nervous system infections

Central nervous system infections during pregnancy are uncommon but can be life-threatening when they occur. Because they are infrequent, the obstetrician has to be alert for early signs and symptoms. Treatment is most successful when initiated early. A physician's suspicion of a central nervous system infection should be high in any patient who has had general malaise for a period of time, followed by headache, nausea, vomiting, and hyperthermia. A serious sign is convulsions in a woman with normal blood pressure and no history of epilepsy.

Recent medical advances have increased our ability to make an accurate diagnosis of central nervous system pathology. Imaging techniques, such as the computed tomographic study (CT scan) or magnetic resonance imaging (MRI) give detailed views of the brain, in which brain abscesses can be diagnosed and evidence of ventricular enlargement can be documented. In the febrile patient without any gross imaging abnormalities who has nuchal rigidity, a diagnostic spinal tap should be performed. The fluid should be examined immediately under the microscope after Gram staining, and a portion of the sample sent for culture and biochemical studies. If the Gram stain reveals Gram-negative diplococci, the presumptive diagnosis is *Neisseria meningitides* meningitis, and a broad-spectrum cephalosporin should be prescribed.[84] If Gram-positive diplococci are seen, the presumptive diagnosis is *Streptococcus pneumoniae* meningitis, and vancomycin and a cephalosporin should be begun.[84] *H. influenzae* meningitis, common in children, is rarely seen in adults.

There are some cases in which the spinal fluid examination is not diagnostic. In these women, bacteria are not present in the fluid, and the glucose level is not reduced. There are a number of possible pathogens. One differential diagnosis is a viral meningitis such as coxsackievirus B_2. Viral cultures should be done on the cerebrospinal fluid and antibiotics discontinued if the study results of the fluid are positive for a virus.

If a brain abscess is found on imaging studies of a woman with central nervous system symptoms, the HIV antibody status of the patient should be investigated if it is not known, and *Toxoplasma gondii* should be suspected.[85] The treatment is spiramycin and TMP-SMX or clindamycin.

In endemic areas, cryptococcal meningitis should be considered. The diagnosis should be suspected if encapsulated organisms are present on an India ink preparation and confirmed by culture. The treatment of choice is amphotericin given intravenously.[86]

Bacterial endocarditis

Bacterial endocarditis is another rare, but serious infection for a pregnant woman. In 1983, Pastorek et al.[87] reported three cases and estimated an incidence of 1 in 4000 deliveries. In 1988, Cox et al.[88] reported seven cases, of whom four were from their clinic population, with an incidence of 1 in 16 500 deliveries. Both these reports stress the increasing frequency of this disease in urban pregnant women with an increasing number of intravenous drug abusers.

The starting point in the care of these patients is prevention. There are no prospective clinical studies to demonstrate the effectiveness of antibiotic prophylaxis.[89] Observations indicate that endocarditis follows bacteremia, and the bacteria that cause endocarditis are usually susceptible to antibiotics. Making a decision about prophylaxis usually involves two considerations. The first is the risk of infective endocarditis associated with pre-existing cardiac disorders. For the obstetrician, the largest single category of patients for consideration is those with mitral valve prolapse without regurgitation, a low-risk population, but the risk is not zero. The second consideration is the procedure. While bacteremia can occur in 1–5% of women during uncomplicated delivery, most medical authorities recommend prophylaxis only for vaginal delivery complicated by infection.[90,91]

The American Heart Association (AHA) issued revised guidelines for antibiotic prophylaxis of bacterial endocarditis in 1997.[92] These guidelines stratify cardiac conditions into high-, moderate-, and negligible-risk categories according to the potential outcome if endocarditis occurs. Endocarditis prophylaxis is recommended for the high- and moderate-risk groups. In the high-risk group are those with: (1) prosthetic cardiac valves (bioprosthetic and homograft); (2) previous bacterial endocarditis; (3) complex cyanotic congenital heart disease (e.g., transposition of the great vessels, tetralogy of Fallot); and (4) surgically constructed systemic pulmonary shunts or conduits. The moderate-risk category includes: (1) most other congenital cardiac malformations; (2) acquired valvar dysfunction (e.g., rheumatic heart disease); (3) hypertrophic cardiomyopathy; and (4) mitral valve prolapse with valvar regurgitation or thickened leaflets. Endocarditis prophylaxis is not recommended for the negligible-risk group which includes: (1) isolated secundum atrial septal defect; (2) surgical repair of atrial septal defect, ventricular septal defect or patent ductus arteriosus; (3) previous coronary bypass surgery; (4) mitral valve prolapse without valvar regurgitation; (5) physiologic, functional, or innocent heart murmurs; (6) previous Kawasaki disease without valvar dysfunction; (7) previous rheumatic fever without valvar dysfunction; and (8) cardiac pacemakers (intravascular and epicardial) and implanted defibrillators.

Mitral valve prolapse is the most common cardiac abnormality seen in obstetric and gynecologic patients. The AHA guidelines provide for a clinical approach to determining the need for bacterial endocarditis prophylaxis.[92] If there is a murmur of mitral regurgitation, prophylaxis is recommended. In instances in which the presence or absence of mitral regurgitation is not determined or unknown, and if confirmation is not available, prophylaxis is indicated when an immediate need for the procedure exists. In nonemergency situations, referral to a cardiologist for echocardiography and/or Doppler flow studies should be done for evaluation and determination of the need for prophylaxis.

For obstetric or gynecologic procedures, the AHA recommends that women undergoing cystoscopy or urethral dilation receive endocarditis prophylaxis.[92] Prophylaxis is not recommended for vaginal delivery, Cesarean section, vaginal hysterectomy, or procedures involving uninfected tissues including: (1) urethral catheterization; (2) dilation and curettage (D&C); (3) therapeutic abortions; (4) sterilization procedures; and (5) insertion or removal of intrauterine devices (IUDs).[92] However, the AHA notes that, for high-risk women undergoing vaginal delivery or Cesarean section, prophylaxis is optional. Obviously, for patients with infected intrauterine tissue undergoing D&C or for removal of an IUD in the presence of pelvic inflammatory disease (PID), prophylaxis is indicated.

Endocarditis prophylaxis for obstetric and gynecologic procedures is primarily directed against enterococci (e.g., *Streptococcus faecalis*). While Gram-negative bacteria are commonly the cause of bacteremia in obstetric and gynecologic patients, they rarely cause endocarditis. According to the AHA recommendations, high-risk patients should receive ampicillin plus gentamicin as follows: ampicillin 2 g i.m. or i.v. plus gentamicin 1.5 mg/kg within 30 min of starting the procedure; 6 h later, ampicillin 1 g i.m. or i.v. or amoxicillin 1 g orally. High-risk patients allergic to ampicillin should receive vancomycin plus gentamicin with vancomycin given 1.0 g i.v. over 1–2 h within 30 min of the procedure. Moderate-risk patients should be prophylaxed with amoxicillin or ampicillin with amoxicillin 2.0 g orally 1 h prior to the procedure or ampicillin 50 mg/kg i.m. or i.v. within 30 min of the procedure. For those allergic to ampicillin, vancomycin 1.0 g i.v. over 1–2 h with infusion complete within 30 min of the procedure is recommended.

The population of pregnant women who develop bacterial endocarditis is different than it was in the past. Formerly, we focused on women with rheumatic or congenital heart disease. Now, our concerns have to include women with mitral valve prolapse and those patients who are intravenous drug users. Although rarely seen, bacterial endocarditis is life-threatening; maternal death has been reported in pregnant women with this infection.[87] This is a difficult diagnosis for the obstetrician. It is an uncommon disease, and the clinical and laboratory findings are subtle. It should be suspected in a febrile patient who is lethargic with no localizing signs of infection. There are clues that bacterial endocarditis could be the problem. The patient should be questioned and examined for evidence of intravenous drug abuse. Cutaneous manifestations can be seen, particularly splinter hemorrhages under the fingernails or nontender purpuric spots on the heels or palms. A diagnostic sign of significance is a new or changing heart murmur. A number of tests should be employed to confirm the diagnosis. At least three blood cultures should be drawn, 30–60 min apart. An electrocardiogram and an echocardiogram should be done to determine if there is any vegetation on any of the heart valves.

The treatment of these women is much more intense than the usual antibacterial regimens in pregnancy. These are difficult infections to treat successfully. Cure requires eradication of all the organisms. The usual strategy involves the use of penicillins, cephalosporins, or vancomycin intravenously for 2–6 weeks. The length of time of treatment depends on the susceptibility of the bacteria. The addition of aminoglycosides produces synergistic killing of streptococci, particularly the enterococci. Women with bacterial endocarditis are at risk of preterm labor and the delivery of a premature infant.[90] In addition to the focus on the mother, careful monitoring of uterine activity and fetal well-being is important in this population.

Antepartum mastitis

In contrast to postpartum mastitis, antepartum mastitis is a rare event. Reports of this entity appear as case reports.[93] Because it is so rare, it is difficult to identify predisposing factors, although many of these women have skin disorders in which the skin surface is not intact. When mastitis occurs, cultures should be obtained. The initial choice of antibiotics is empirical, but a cephalosporin is a good starting point. Susceptibility studies can dictate changes. The formation of an abscess requires operative drainage.

Gastrointestinal infections

Gastrointestinal infections in a pregnant woman present in many forms. Physicians can be asked to evaluate chronic cases, for example a persistent diarrhea, or, at the other end of the spectrum, a woman with an acute life-threatening emergency, such as a ruptured appendix.

Appendicitis

Acute appendicitis is an illustration of how pregnancy can modify the clinical manifestations of intra-abdominal disease. The large uterus, hormonal changes, and immunologic suppression change patient symptomatology. For example, a pregnant patient with appendicitis usually presents with no fever, no leukocytosis, and right midquadrant pain, instead of right lower quadrant pain.[94] New imaging techniques such as a CT scan are not applicable to the pregnant patient. Based on clinical acumen and imaging findings, an operative exploration should be carried out if appendicitis is suspected. It is far better to explore a few patients with inconclusive signs and subsequently discover a ruptured appendix. If intraperitoneal rupture does occur, these women are at high risk of premature labor and delivery.

Cholecystitis

Acute cholecystitis is another gastrointestinal problem sometimes seen in pregnant women. It should be suspected in the patient with nausea, vomiting, and right upper quadrant pain. New imaging techniques (e.g., ultrasound) without radiation can be used to detect the presence of stones in the gallbladder or the collecting ducts.

Infections of the liver

Hepatitis is an infection caused by a broad range of microbiological agents that can cause morbidity for both the mother and the fetus. Except for hepatitis E, viral hepatitis does not occur with more frequency or severity during pregnancy.[95,96] Physicians associate hepatitis with the various hepatitis viruses, but this condition has been seen with other viruses and bacteria. The underlying health of the pregnant woman influences maternal morbidity.

Hepatitis A is a significant infectious disease that occurs worldwide. Transmission of the virus is usually by the fecal–oral route. It is unique among the hepatitis viruses because the infection resolves without a carrier state. The impact of this disease on pregnant women varies. In the United States, no increase in maternal mortality with hepatitis A has been noted,[95] whereas in the Third World countries, an increase in maternal death rate has been documented. Prevention is now possible with the development of an inactivated virus vaccine. The selection of pregnant patients for the administration of the vaccine is limited to high-risk groups as previously described.

Hepatitis B is a serious medical problem for pregnant women. It is still a common disease in the United States. It can cause serious maternal morbidity, although maternal mortality is rarely seen. Approximately 5% of women become chronic carriers of the virus and, in turn, have the capability of infecting their newborn with this virus. This risk applies to women infected with the virus before they become pregnant. As mentioned earlier in this chapter, prevention is the starting point of care. The hepatitis B vaccine is available and should be made available to pregnant women. Because this is not a live virus vaccine, it can be administered during pregnancy.

Obstetricians have become cognizant of hepatitis C. In 1989, the genome of the hepatitis C virus[97] was cloned, and tests were developed for antibodies against this agent. Subsequent studies have demonstrated that 88–90% of posttransfusion nonA, nonB hepatitis is due to hepatitis C.[98] The acute hepatitis C infection poses few problems for the obstetrician, for it is usually a subclinical infection. In prospective studies, only 20–30% of the patients have symptoms, and only half of this symptomatic group develop jaundice.[99] There are exceptions. Fulminant hepatitis secondary to hepatitis C virus infection can occur in pregnancy.[100] In these seriously ill women, hepatitis A, B, and C antibody testing should be done to determine the etiology. Supportive medical care should be offered until the symptoms of hepatitis resolve. The main problem with hepatitis C virus is that chronic infection results in a majority of cases, with progressive chronic liver disease leading to hepatocellular carcinoma.[100] Clearly, prevention is the preferred approach to this problem. Blood is the most important source of spread. Although transfusion-associated hepatitis C still occurs, its incidence has been dramatically reduced through the screening of blood for hepatitis C virus antibody.[101] Intravenous drug abusers remain at risk. Although the risk of sexual transmission of hepatitis C virus is small, there is evidence that it occurs,[102] as does mother-to-child vertical transmission,[103] particularly among women co-infected with HIV. Each of these modes of transmission is less than with hepatitis B. For prevention, condoms can be suggested.

Hepatitis D infection is sometimes a concern among patients who are positive for hepatitis B antigen. When this occurs, the acute infection resembles uncomplicated hepatitis B. In fewer than 15% of these cases, the disease may be severe, and fatalities have been reported.[104] Treatment is supportive.

Other hepatitis viruses have been identified, and more will be known to us in the future. Outside of hepatitis A, B, C, and D, hepatitis due to hepatitis E virus is more dangerous in pregnant women, with a reported mortality rate of 15–20%. To date, this disease has been reported in India, Africa, and the Middle East.[105,106]

Hepatitis can be caused by other viruses, notably herpes simplex virus (HSV), CMV, Epstein–Barr virus, and coxsackie B virus. HSV hepatitis is uncommon, with fewer than 20 cases reported in the literature,[107,108] but it is a serious disease with a maternal mortality rate of close to 50%.[107] This is a difficult disease to diagnose, because of its rarity, but it should be included in the differential diagnosis of a patient with hepatic dysfunction in the third trimester.[108] The physician's suspicions should be aroused by the patient presenting with onset of disease in the third trimester, a prodromal illness, vulvar or pharyngeal vesicular lesions, and an anicteric presentation. It is important to confirm the diagnosis by liver biopsy[108] and begin treatment with acyclovir. This significantly reduces maternal mortality.[107] Hepatitis due to CMV, Epstein–Barr virus, and coxsackievirus can be suspected when other causes of hepatitis cannot be confirmed. Liver biopsy and culture help to confirm the diagnosis.

Occasionally, a pregnant woman will be seen with a liver abscess secondary to *Entamoeba histolytica* (amebiasis). They usually present with a sudden onset with right upper quadrant pain and a fever. Ultrasound confirms the diagnosis. These abscesses respond to medical treatment with metronidazole. This avoids intraperitoneal rupture and usually results in a cure.

Peritonitis

Primary bacterial peritonitis is a rare but life-threatening condition in pregnant women. In nonpregnant women, such problems are usually secondary to bacteremia with Gram-positive aerobic cocci, such as group A β-hemolytic streptococci or pneumococci. In pregnant women, it has been associated with underlying disease or acute salpingitis.[109,110] The diagnosis should be considered in any pregnant woman with fever and abdominal tenderness. If more common entities such as chorioamnionitis and appendicitis have been ruled out and if the patient has evidence of liver disease, primary peritonitis should be considered as a diagnosis. Paracentesis and microscopic examination of peritoneal fluid should confirm this diagnosis, and the treatment should be with systemic antibiotics. Some of these women are critically ill and should be monitored closely for evidence of premature labor.

Diarrhea

Diarrhea is seen with some frequency in any large obstetric practice. Fortunately, it is usually self-limited and without complications. When it is explosive in nature or persists beyond 24 h, the associated dehydration can be accompanied by premature labor. Close communication must be kept with these patients.

The diagnostic and therapeutic care of these patients requires a knowledge of the etiologies and pathophysiology of diarrheal disease. Table 50.4 provides an outline of the physician considerations when viewing these patients.[111]

The obstetrician can adapt a wait and see approach to pregnant patients who have diarrhea. The patients should be advised to take adequate oral fluids, solid food as tolerated, and to limit the use of medications in the first 24 h to nonabsorbed local medications such as loperamide (Kaopectate), which do not alter intestinal motility. Because most cases have a mild self-limited course, neither a stool culture nor treatment is necessary. Antimicrobial therapy should be based on antibiotic susceptibility studies. Antimotility drugs, such as loperamide, can be used to control moderate to severe diarrhea. In patients beyond the 12th week of pregnancy, without a contraindication to the use of salicylates, bismuth subsalicylate can be used. It is helpful for it has antimicrobial properties because of the bismuth and antisecretory properties of the salicylate moiety. Nearly all these women will be managed as outpatients because it is rare in the United States to have a case so severe that admission is needed.

Table 50.4 Classification of diarrhea.

Toxigenic diarrhea	Caused by *Vibrio cholerae* and toxigenic *Escherichia coli*
Invasive bacterial diarrhea	Caused by *Shigella* species, nontyphoidal *Salmonella* species, enterohemorrhagic *E. coli*, enteroinvasive *E. coli*, *Campylobacter jejuni*, *Vibrio parahaemolyticus*, *Yersinia enterocolitica*, noncholera vibrios
Viral diarrhea	Caused by rotavirus, caliciviruses, including the Norwalk virus, astrovirus, and enteric adenovirus
Parasitic diarrhea	Caused by *Giardia lamblia*, *Entamoeba histolytica*, *Cryptosporidium parvum*, *Cyclospora cayetanensis*, *Isospora belli*, and *Balantidium coli*

Women with chronic diarrhea need to be evaluated for ova and parasites, particularly *Giardia lamblia* and *E. histolytica*. These symptomatic women should be treated with quinacrine and metronidazole, respectively, after the 12th week of pregnancy.[112,113] The influx of refugees from South-east Asia, the Caribbean, and Central America, plus immigrants from South America, has increased the pool of pregnant patients in the United States with intestinal parasites.[112,113] In one evaluation of 97 South-east Asian refugees in Philadelphia, 65% were colonized with gastrointestinal parasites. The most common isolates in the study were hookworm, *Trichuris trichiura*, *Clonorchis sinesis*, *Ascarisa lumbricoides*, *Strongyloides stercoralis*, *E. histolytica*, *G. lamblia*, *Endolimax nana*, *Taenia*, and *Plasmodium vivax*.[112] Despite the high infection rate, this population had uncomplicated pregnancy outcomes with the usual pregnancy care and treatment of symptomatic patients. Lee[114] counsels therapeutic conservatism if obstetricians discover intestinal parasites in their pregnant patients. He suggests two major indications for therapy: gastrointestinal problems that persist and interfere with maternal health; and parasite-related extraintestinal abnormalities. A detailed description of treatment for parasitic diseases in pregnancy is reviewed in reference 112.

Malaria

Malaria is a serious infection in pregnant women. In endemic areas, peripartum infection increases the risk of perinatal death and low birthweight.[112,115] Chloroquine prophylaxis protected against maternal and fetal malaria, low birthweight, and perinatal death, even in areas where chloroquine-resistant *Plasmodium falciparum* is endemic.[115] Fortunately, this is a rare disease in the United States. In these days, when more people are involved in international travel, more cases will be seen by American physicians.

Lyme disease

Lyme disease is a new infection for obstetricians. It was first described in 1977 and given its name because of a clustering of children with suspected juvenile rheumatoid arthritis in Lyme, CT, USA.[116] It is caused by a tick-borne spirochete, *Borrelia burgdorferi*, and is spread by the bite of infected ticks, including *Ixodes dammini*, or related ixodid ticks.[117] It is a multisystem disorder that usually begins in the summer with a spreading skin eruption to be followed weeks to months later by cardiac, neurologic, or arthritic abnormalities. Unfortunately for the obstetrician, this is a transplacental infection that can result in intrauterine fetal death or impairment of cerebral function because of *in utero*-acquired central nervous system infection.[118,119] Fortunately, this pathogen is susceptible to antibiotics so that cure can be achieved, particularly when an early diagnosis is made.

The diagnosis of Lyme disease depends on the obstetrician's clinical awareness, backed up by appropriate laboratory testing. In the United States, most of the cases to date have been clustered in three areas: the north-east, from Massachusetts to Maryland; the Midwest in Wisconsin and Minnesota; and the west in California and Oregon. Clinically, the disease begins as a red macule or papule at the site of the tick bite, and this lesion spreads. Concomitant with this, the patient complains of malaise, fatigue, headache, chills, and fever. This is not the flu to be dismissed by physician admonitions "to take fluids and acetaminophen, get to bed, and let nature take its course." These women need to be examined meticulously for skin lesions. Blood should be drawn for IgM antibodies. One study indicated that immunoblotting was superior to indirect enzyme-linked immunosorbent assay (ELISA) tests for diagnosing early Lyme disease.[120] Patients with Lyme disease do not have a positive regain test result for syphilis (e.g., a Venereal Disease Research Laboratory test), but they can crossreact with other treponemal tests and have a positive fluorescent treponemal antibody absorption test result.[121] In nonpregnant women, the treatment of choice would seem to be tetracycline, which gives superior results to erythromycin, particularly in the prevention of the major late complications, myocarditis, meningitis, and arthritis.[122] In pregnancy, phenoxymethyl penicillin would seem to be the drug of choice for early disease. For patients who are first diagnosed with late-onset arthritis, ceftriaxone seems to be the drug of choice because of its long half-life.[123]

Other tick-borne diseases

There are a number of other tick-borne diseases seen in the United States. These are identified in Table 50.5.[124] Prevention is the approach of choice. Pregnant women should be advised to wear long-sleeved shirts, long pants, and closed-toe shoes in areas where tick exposure is likely. Walking on cleared trails away from bush vegetation is also helpful. If a tick bite occurs, an embedded tick should be removed by tweezers, with a slow steady pressure, perpendicular to the skin. If symptoms occur, the obstetrician should be consulted. Table 50.5 provides some general treatment guidelines. Tetracycline, frequently the drug of first choice, is not used in pregnant women.

HIV in pregnancy

A quarter of a century after first coming to national attention, the HIV epidemic has entered a phase that can be described in a paraphrase of the famous opening line of Dickens' *Tale of Two Cities*, "it is the best of times, it is the worst of times." This is particularly true of maternal–child issues. In the developed world, where access to the full array of antiviral therapies can be assured, the prognosis for infected individuals has improved dramatically, and the birth of an HIV-infected child has become a relative rarity. Unfortunately, the same cannot be said for those areas of the world where 95% of HIV-infected individuals reside. In those settings, where the epidemic continues to expand, most HIV-infected individuals are condemned to substandard care and a concomitant poor prognosis. However, great efforts are being expended to alter that trend, and there are success stories even in the developing world. Obstetricians in the United States, by dint of their ability to utilize the most effective therapies, have an obligation to keep abreast of this rapidly changing field in order to guarantee their patients the best prognosis and the greatest likelihood of giving birth to an uninfected child. In this section, we will briefly review the epidemiology and pathophysiology of HIV, but will focus on the clinical aspects of the disease in order to enable clinicians to provide state of the art care to their patients.

Epidemiology

According to United Nation statistics, close to 30 million people were alive with HIV infection in 2003. During that year, nearly five million new infections were recorded, and almost three million people died. Women now comprise about half of all HIV-infected individuals, and there are approximately 2000 new infections of children under the age of 15 years (the vast majority secondary to mother-to-child transmission) every day. These infections are not evenly dispersed across the globe. Over 95% of infections occur in sub-Saharan Africa. However, if recent projections prove correct, the bulk of new infections will be occurring in other parts of the world by the end of this decade. It is now predicted that India,

Table 50.5 Other tick-borne diseases in the USA.

Disease	Causative agent	Classification	Region	Treatment
Rocky Mountain spotted fever	*Rickettsia rickettsii*	Bacteria	South-east, West, south central	Chloramphenicol
Ehrlichiosis	*Ehrlichia chafeenis*	Bacteria	south central, south Atlantic	Chloramphenicol
Relapsing fever	*Borrelia* sp.	Bacteria	West	Erythromycin
Tularemia	*Francisella tularensis*	Bacteria	Arkansas, Missouri, Oklahoma	Gentamicin
Colorado tick fever	*Coltivirus* sp.	Virus	West	Supportive care
Babesiosis	*Babesia* sp.	Protozoa	North-east	Oral quinine plus clindamycin
Tick paralysis	Toxin	Neurotoxin	North-west, south	Removal of tick

Nigeria, China, Ethiopia, and Russia (in decreasing order of new infections) will have as many as 70 million infected individuals within 5 years.

Perhaps as important as these numbers are the opportunities that exist to alter the course of the epidemic. It has been projected that, if several preventive steps are taken, as many as 29 million infections (63% of all new infections) can be avoided by the year 2010.[125] These interventions include voluntary HIV counseling and testing in order to raise awareness of the need for risk reduction and to help to bring the disease into the open, behavioral interventions to build motivation and risk-reduction skills, treatment of sexually transmitted diseases to reduce the likelihood that unprotected sex will result in HIV transmission, antenatal antiretroviral regimens to decrease mother-to-child transmission (MTCT), and drug treatment and programs to distribute sterile needles and syringes to help prevent the spread of HIV among injecting drug users. It is estimated that preventive services currently reach only a small minority of people at risk in developing countries. Achieving the aforementioned preventive goals will require at least a fourfold increase in global spending to US$4.8 billion in developing countries by 2005, and US$5.85 billion by 2007. In contrast, total spending from all sources in 2002 on HIV prevention efforts in those countries was approximately US$1.2 billion.

In the United States, the CDC estimates that 40 000 new HIV infections occur every year.[126] From the beginning of the epidemic in 1981 to 2000, an estimated 1.3–1.4 million Americans have been infected with HIV, and approximately one-third (450 000) of those have died. Despite declines in the number of new infections since the 1990s, the number of individuals alive with HIV infection is greater than ever before. It is further estimated that, as of 2000, between 850 000 and 950 000 people are alive with HIV. While the number of HIV-infected children born in the United States has dropped dramatically in the wake of new antiretroviral therapies and modifications in obstetrical practices (*vide infra*), challenges remain. As many as one in eight HIV-infected women do not receive prenatal care, and one in nine is not tested for HIV before giving birth.

Virology and pathophysiology

HIV-1 and HIV-2 are members of the lentivirus subfamily of Retroviridae and are single-stranded ribonucleic acid (RNA) enveloped viruses that have the ability to become incorporated into cellular deoxyribonucleic acid (DNA).[127] HIV preferentially infects cells with the CD4 antigen, particularly helper lymphocytes, but also macrophages, cells of the central nervous system and, according to some evidence, cells of the placenta.[128] At least two other cell-surface molecules help HIV to enter the cells. These coreceptors for HIV, called CXCR4 and CCR5, are receptors for chemokines.[129] It has also been reported that individuals who are homozygous for a 32-basepair deletion at the CCR5 gene are less likely to acquire HIV, while those who are heterozygous for the deletion progress less rapidly if infected. Once the virus is internalized, its RNA is released from the nucleocapsid, and is reverse transcribed into proviral DNA. The provirus is inserted into the genome and then transcribed into RNA; the RNA is translated, and virions assemble and are extruded from the cell membrane by budding. The virus is composed of core (p18, p24, and p27) and surface (gp120 and gp41) proteins, genomic RNA, and the reverse transcriptase enzyme surrounded by a lipid bilayer envelope.

Untreated, HIV infection leads to progressive debilitation of the immune system, rendering infected individuals susceptible to opportunistic infections (e.g., *Pneumocystis carinii* pneumonia and central nervous system toxoplasmosis) and neoplasias (e.g., Kaposi's sarcoma) that rarely afflict patients with intact immune systems. For an HIV-infected patient with one of several specific opportunistic infections, neoplasia, dementia encephalopathy, or wasting syndrome, the diagnosis of acquired immunodeficiency syndrome (AIDS) is assigned. In 1993, the CDC changed the case definition to include all individuals with HIV infection whose CD4 counts drop below 200 CD4 lymphocytes/μL as well as HIV-infected individuals with advanced cervical cancer, pulmonary tuberculosis, and recurrent pneumonia.[130]

At the time of initial infection, there is an immediate viremia of substantive proportions (up to a billion viral particles turned over per day) and an equally impressive immune response with similar levels of T-cell turnover.[131] After the initial viremia, the level of virus returns to a "set point." The level of virus in the plasma at that time can provide an estimate of the probability that an individual, if left untreated, will develop AIDS within 5 years. Antibodies are usually detectable 1 month after infection and are almost always detectable within 3 months. Evidence of immune dysfunction may be followed by clinical conditions ranging from fever, weight loss, malaise, lymphadenopathy, and central nervous system dysfunction to infections such as herpes simplex virus or oral candidiasis. Studies of infected individuals have noted that, 5 years after infection was confirmed, up to 35% had progressed to AIDS.[132,133] It should be noted that these statistics antedate the use of highly active antiretroviral therapy (HAART), which has been shown to have a significant effect on the course of HIV disease.

Management of the HIV-infected pregnant women

Appropriate management of HIV-infected pregnant women requires an understanding of testing, monitoring, and medical therapy. The last issue is the most complex and the most rapidly changing. In order to stay abreast of those changes, the International AIDS Society[134] and the Public Health Service[135] provide continuing updates, the latter on a website, to which the reader should refer as new drugs and protocols emerge. The Public Health Service ("AIDSinfo") website also provides guidelines specifically for the care of pregnant women.

Testing

A great deal can now be offered to HIV-infected individuals. As will be detailed below, therapy is now available that can reliably reduce both disease progression and MTCT. All the available treatments work best when they are initiated before clinical disease or advanced immune compromise occurs. It is a bit disheartening to realize that many people still do not learn their serostatus until they have reached an advanced stage of illness. Similarly, while some MTCT can be prevented even when HIV infection is not diagnosed until labor, success rates are much higher if longer term therapy is employed. Thus, it is essential that obstetricians ascertain the serostatus of all their patients as early in pregnancy as possible. "Opt-in" testing is the most common testing strategy employed in the United States. It requires counseling and written consent. However, it is neither the most successful nor the currently recommended strategy for testing. In the antepartum setting, identification of infected women is best accomplished using a "routine" right-of-refusal approach and employing standard ELISA and Western blot technologies. The use of standard testing technologies provides among the most sensitive and specific testing algorithms available for any infection. The right-of-refusal ("opt-out") approach respects pregnant women's autonomy, but does not explicitly or implicitly either stigmatize women who are offered the test or dissuade women from being tested. The opt-out approach is associated with greater testing rates than the opt-in approach. Medical record surveys, laboratory data, and population-based surveys (1998–2001) report 85–98% HIV testing rates in surveyed areas using the opt-out approach, compared with testing rates ranging from 25% to 83% in surveyed areas using the opt-in approach.[136]

Despite the implementation of routine testing protocols in prenatal settings, there will still be circumstances in which rapid testing will play an important role. It is estimated that 40–85% of infants infected with HIV are born to women whose HIV infection is unknown prior to delivery.[137] A number of studies have been published that demonstrate the ability of antiretroviral therapy, even when first introduced in the intrapartum or immediate neonatal period, to prevent some cases of pediatric HIV infection.[138] In the intrapartum period, the testing technology involves rapid testing. A rapid test is an HIV screening test with results available within hours. When selecting a rapid HIV test for use during labor and delivery, it is important to consider the accuracy of the test and the site (i.e., hospital laboratory versus point of care testing in labor and delivery) at which testing will be performed. Tests that require serum or plasma (e.g., Reveal) are more suitable for use in the laboratory, whereas tests that can be performed with whole blood (e.g., OraQuick, Uni-Gold) without specimen processing can be performed more easily in the labor and delivery unit.[139] Performance evaluations on three United States Food and Drug Administration (FDA)-approved rapid HIV tests (OraQuick, Reveal, and Uni-Gold) indicate a sensitivity of 100%, 99.8%, and 100% [95% confidence interval (CI)], respectively, and a specificity of 99.9%, 99.1% (serum), and 99.7% (95% CI) respectively.[140] Despite the fact that rapid tests may be associated with more false-positive results than standard tests (particularly in low-prevalence communities), there are several steps that should be taken whenever a positive result is received. The patient should be informed that the preliminary screen suggests that she might be positive and her neonate might therefore be exposed so that a follow-up is being performed. Consent should be obtained to initiate therapy immediately for her and her neonate, and advice should be offered not to breastfeed. Finally, her pediatrician should be informed of her status.

Monitoring

The advent of HAART has made HIV, in many ways, a chronic illness similar to diabetes. Just as no clinician would think about managing a diabetic woman without ongoing assessments of their disease state and the impact of their therapy (e.g., monitoring of blood glucose levels), so no HIV specialist would be able to manage his/her patient without tracking their immune status, viral status, and viral resistance as appropriate. The first two measures let the provider know how far advanced the disease is and how rapidly it is progressing. The last test, used in circumstances in which there is evidence that treatment is not being met with complete success, can help the clinician to choose the best regimen to use in a variety of clinical circumstances.

During pregnancy, viral load status should be determined every month until the virus is no longer detectable. Viral load should drop by approximately 1–2 logs per month if effective therapy is being used. Once the virus is no longer detectable, testing can be performed every 3 months. The higher the viral load, the longer it will take to become undetectable. However, in all circumstances, the viral load should become undetectable within 6 months of starting therapy. The CD4 count can be used to decide when it is necessary to institute prophylaxis for opportunistic infections. No such medications are required if the CD4 count is higher than 200/μL. If such therapy is begun at a lower count, but the CD4 count rises back above 200/μL consequent to HAART, the prophylaxis can be discontinued once the count has remained over that threshold for 6 months.

Failure to achieve the "undetectable" benchmark often reflects the development of a resistant organism. The life cycle of HIV predisposes to mutations and, hence, resistance because of the combination of the rapid turnover of HIV (10^7–10^8 rounds of replication/day) and the high error rate of reverse transcriptase when replicating the nearly 10 000 nucleotides present in the HIV genome. When incompletely suppressive drug regimens are used, they provide the evolutionary pressure that selects those mutations that cause resistance to antiretroviral agents. The number of mutations required to cause a clinically relevant effect varies with the agent in question. Thus, the rate at which resistance develops will depend on the number of mutations necessary to create a significant change in susceptibility.

While obstetricians have often used culture and sensitivity testing in order to choose appropriate antimicrobials, antiviral resistance testing can be a bit more complicated. However, as randomized trials have demonstrated that individuals assigned to study arms with access to resistance test results have a greater reduction in viral load after the initiation of salvage therapy, obstetricians should familiarize themselves with these tools.[141] Currently, two types of testing are available, genotypic and phenotypic, each with distinct advantages and disadvantages.[142]

Phenotypic testing is a measure of the activity of the virus under a particular set of conditions, whereas genotyping provides a molecular biologic snapshot of the viral structure. Phenotypic tests compare the ability of the virus to replicate in various concentrations of an antiretroviral drug with its ability to replicate in the absence of the drug.[143] Resistance is related to the ability of the virus to overcome treatments aimed at viral activities needed for replication, i.e., reverse transcription and at the protease gene. Genotypic testing seeks to detect mutations in the genes that encode reverse transcriptase and protease formation by the virus. These tests establish the nucleotide sequence (ergo the amino acid sequence) of the portion of the viral genome coding for reverse transcriptase and protease. Point mutations in the virus result in the substitution of amino acids in the proteins produced, i.e., reverse transcriptase or protease. The significance of these point mutations is determined by correlating specific mutations with phenotypic resistance, as measured by viral susceptibility assays and correlation with clinical response to therapy. Obstetricians should interpret and act upon the results from both types of tests in consultation with an expert in the field.

Certain limitations are present for both genotypic and phenotypic assays. As most HIV-infected individuals have several circulating viral quasispecies, the assays may not detect resistant species that constitute 20% or less of the population. This issue may be especially important for evaluating resistance to drugs that a person took in the past but is no longer receiving, as wild-type virus, being fitter, may have overgrown the mutant strain in the interim. It also means that resistance testing is more useful for ruling out, than for ruling in, therapies to be utilized in a given patient. That is because the absence of resistance may merely reflect the re-emergence of the wild-type strain. In that circumstance, the assays will not detect the minority mutant strain. However, if the patient is re-exposed to the offending agent, the resistant strain may again attain dominance. Drug resistance testing is not advised for persons with viral load of < 1000 copies/mL, as amplification of the virus is unreliable.

There are several defined circumstances in which clinicians should utilize these tests. The most common indication for testing is treatment failure. Treatment failure is defined as the failure to attain an undetectable level of virus or the persistent presence of virus after it had become undetectable. If it has been determined that failure has occurred, resistance testing should be performed *before* the failing regimen is discontinued. This is to prevent the overgrowth of wild-type strains that might occur after the regimen is discontinued, such that resistant strains would not be detected even though they might be "lying in wait" for the reinstitution of some components of the regimen. Resistance testing can also be helpful in the setting of an individual who has recently seroconverted. It has been reported that a substantial percentage of new infections are with organisms that are resistant.[144] If testing can be performed before a wild-type virus overgrows the infecting strain, the clinician will have an opportunity to choose an initial regimen that will have a high probability of success against the infecting virus.

Medical therapy: when to start

Once a diagnosis of HIV infection has been made and the individual's clinical, virologic, and immune status has been assessed, the clinician must determine whether antiretroviral therapy is appropriate. Given the cost, toxicities, and inconveniences of therapy, a clear advantage in prognosis should be shown before the commitment to lifetime treatment is made.

If the patient has severe immune compromise or a clinical diagnosis of AIDS, then the decision is clear. Randomized clinical trials have demonstrated a survival benefit with the use of antiretroviral therapy in those circumstances.[145] For less severely compromised individuals (i.e., asymptomatic individuals with CD4 cell counts ≥ 200/μL), the data are not as clear cut; there are no definitive data from prospective, randomized, controlled studies. Instead, inferences must be drawn from observational studies, as well as what is known about the consequences of moderate degrees of immune deficiency, and the long-term safety of antiretroviral drugs. The largest study, which analyzed data from more than 10 000 patients, concluded that prognosis could be best predicted by CD4 cell count and HIV RNA response after 6 months of treatment, independent of pretreatment values.[146,147] Another study analyzed data from 1464 patients from several clinics in the United States and found that, after 4 years of follow-up, patients with baseline CD4 cell counts between 200/μL and 350/μL who started antiretroviral therapy had lower mortality rates than those who waited until their CD4 cell count was below 200/μL.[148] These data agreed with the results of another study that reported the outcomes of 1173 patients who had received therapy for at least 90 days.[149] Again, those who initiated therapy with a CD4 cell count below 200/μL had a higher risk of disease progression even if a durable virologic suppression was achieved. A Canadian cohort found a similar association between lower CD4 cell count and prognosis, but also noted that a baseline HIV RNA level higher than 100 000 copies/mL was independently associated with death.[150]

Thus, delay in the initiation of therapy carries with it some risk of poorer prognosis. However, there are countervailing considerations. These include concerns over the long-term safety of therapy, toxic effects, potential cardiovascular consequences, and the negative impact of fat maldistribution on quality of life. These outcomes may be present at different frequencies dependent upon the drug regimen employed.[151,152] Additionally, some treatment complications (e.g., lipoatrophy) may be more frequent and severe when therapy is initiated at lower CD4 cell counts.[153]

In sum, these data from observational cohorts strongly suggest that antiretroviral therapy may decrease the incidence of potentially life-threatening conditions. That finding in conjunction with long-term safety data on some regimens, and the availability of newer drugs that are safer and easier to take, would support the initiation of therapy before HIV-related disease becomes clinically manifest.

In reviewing all the aforementioned data, the International AIDS Society drew several conclusions.[134] They felt that therapy should be recommended for all patients with symptomatic HIV disease, although in rare circumstances initiation can be delayed. For example, treatment of potentially life-threatening opportunistic diseases, or conditions that require drugs that are difficult to co-administer with antiretroviral drugs (e.g., tuberculosis or hepatitis C virus co-infection), or can lead to an immune reconstitution syndrome following the initial CD4 cell count increase, may take precedence over immediate initiation of antiretroviral therapy. They also recommend antiretroviral treatment initiation before CD4 cell counts reach 200/μL. However, initiation of therapy in patients with CD4 cell counts below 350/μL but above 200/μL should be individualized. They cite as an example of an individual in whom it would be reasonable to defer therapy, someone with a low HIV RNA level, stable CD4 cell count (or one that is declining slowly, e.g., a loss of fewer than 50/μL per year), and someone who is reluctant to start therapy. Conversely, they would be more aggressive with an individual with plasma HIV RNA levels above 100 000 copies/mL or a CD4 cell count loss of more than 100 μL/year. Finally initiation of therapy is generally not recommended for patients with CD4 cell counts between 350/μL and 500/μL, but it may be considered in cases with high plasma viral load or a rapid decline in CD4 cell count.

More recently, the Panel on Clinical Practices for Treatment of HIV Infection convened by the Department of Health and Human Services[135] modified their recommendations for when to initiate therapy for asymptomatic treatment-naïve patients with CD4 cell counts > 350 cells/μL. The viral load recommendation at which to defer or to consider therapy was increased from 55 000 to 100 000 copies/mL. They based this change on the belief that, even at those CD4 and viral load levels, the chance of disease progression is relatively low.

Medical therapy: what to start (see Table 50.6)

Over the last several years, arrays of antiretroviral therapies have come on the market. They vary in price, efficacy, and toxicity. Some are inappropriate for use in pregnancy. The obstetrician should be comfortable with a few regimens that are most appropriate for use in pregnancy and be liberal in consulting with experts in HIV infection in those circumstances (e.g., resistance) in which their usual choices are no longer appropriate.

While the choice of initial regimen is influenced by several factors that may be unique to a given patient, including comorbid conditions and concomitant medications, in general, certain initial regimens are preferable to others, at least as evidenced by data from controlled clinical trials. Additionally, some of the newer formulations of medications should improve adherence.

A HAART regimen using a non-nucleoside reverse transcriptase inhibitor (NNRTI) is often the initial regimen of choice because of convenience, superior virological suppression, lower rates of toxic effects, and fewer interactions between drugs than seen with regimens that utilize a boosted

Table 50.6 Currently used antiretroviral drugs.

Drug	Dosage	Side effects	Pregnancy category
Zidovudine	100 mg 6 times per day	Anemia, gastrointestinal upset, headache, myopathy	C
Didanosine	> 60 kg: 200 mg b.i.d.; < 60 kg: 125 mg b.i.d.	Pancreatitis, diarrhea, peripheral neuropathy	B
Zalcitabine	0.75 mg t.i.d.	Peripheral neuropathy, pancreatitis, stomatitis	C
Lamivudine	150 or 300 mg b.i.d.	Minimal toxicity	C
Stavudine	> 60 kg: 40 mg b.i.d.; < 60 kg: 30 mg b.i.d.	Peripheral neuropathy, pancreatitis	C
Indinavir sulfate	800 mg q8h	Nephrolithiasis, drug interactions, hyperbilirubinemia	C
Saquinavir mesylate	600 mg t.i.d.	Gastrointestinal disturbances	B
Ritonavir	600 mg b.i.d.	Gastrointestinal disturbances, paresthesias, drug interactions	B

Reprinted from ref. 21, with permission.

protease inhibitor. However, during pregnancy, that approach may require modification because the preferred NNRTI, efavirenz, is contraindicated in women who are or wish to become pregnant because of potential teratogenicity. Nevirapine (NVP), which is a reasonable option under other circumstances, has the disadvantage of potential toxic effects that are particularly common among pregnant women with relatively high CD4 counts (> 250/μL). Delavirdine, another NNRTI, is not generally recommended for initial regimens because of insufficient data.

The alternative to an NNRTI backbone in a HAART regimen is a protease inhibitor backbone. Some of these regimens involve two PIs with one drug acting to "boost" the availability of the other. Regimens that are ritonavir boosted are often recommended because of the improvement in PI pharmacokinetics and potency. That combination has good rates of sustained response and low rates of viral resistance. The boosted regimen with the most supporting literature is lopinavir/ritonavir,[154] although there is no compelling evidence that this combination is dramatically superior to other boosted regimens such as atazanavir and low-dose ritonavir, and the latter regimen may have less metabolic toxicities (plasma lipid abnormalities). Other choices such as nelfinavir, unboosted atazanavir, and the combination of fosamprenavir and low-dose ritonavir have lower potencies and, consequently, less utility as first-line therapy.

A large number of nucleoside reverse transcriptase inhibitor (NRTI) combinations are available for use as the backbone of HAART regimens in nonpregnant women. These include zidovudine (ZDV) plus lamivudine or emtricitabine, tenofovir plus lamivudine or emtricitabine, or emtricitabine plus didanosine. In pregnancy, the first choice is ZDV plus lamivudine. There are a few combinations that should be avoided. Combining stavudine and ZDV is contraindicated; combinations of stavudine and didanosine or combinations with zalcitabine are not recommended because of increased toxic effects.

Prevention of transmission

Drugs

Since the results of ACTG 076 were first reported in 1994 (monotherapy with ZDV reduced MTCT from 25.5% to 8.3%), it has been apparent that antiretroviral therapy can substantially reduce the rate of MTCT. Those initial reports demonstrated that single drug therapy that is administered over a long period of time (it was administered from 14 weeks' gestation until term) could prevent two-thirds of transmissions. Since that time, research has advanced in two directions. In the developing world, there have been a large number of studies designed to see whether cheaper, shorter regimens could have benefits similar to those seen with more expensive, cumbersome approaches. In the developed world, the focus has been on improved efficacy, as opposed to reduced cost. Both avenues of research have borne fruit.

Abbreviated regimens of ZDV alone, as well as ZDV in conjunction with 3TC (lamivudine), have been shown to prevent some cases of MTCT.[155] The most dramatic result, from the perspective of simplicity and cost, came from the HIVNET 012 trial, which documented the efficacy of oral NVP when given just twice, once in the intrapartum period and once to the neonate.[156] Subsequent studies have highlighted the public health risks attendant on this approach. Fairly high frequencies of resistant virus in the postpartum period have been reported among mothers who have used NVP in the intrapartum period and, more alarmingly, there is some evidence that women who took NVP to prevent MTCT were more likely to fail NVP-based HAART when they became eligible for treatment later in life.[157]

In the United States, data accumulated fairly quickly demonstrating that the results obtained with monotherapy could be exceeded with more aggressive antiretroviral therapy. As HAART became the standard of care for HIV infection, several authors noted that those pregnant women who were on HAART for their own care had remarkably low rates of MTCT, independent of the mode of delivery (*vide infra*). These data were all the more dramatic because those women on HAART were, by definition, women with more advanced disease and thus those who would otherwise be expected to have relatively high rates of MTCT. In fact, there are now preliminary data, summarized in the next section, indicating that HAART therapy *per se* may be as efficacious as Cesarean section in preventing MTCT.

In determining which regimen should be used for the prevention of MTCT, the first question to be asked is what regimen does the mother need for her own health, and is there any need to modify that regimen in order to minimize rates of MTCT? If the patient meets the criteria for antiretroviral therapy (as detailed above), then she should be on a HAART regimen. There is no place for monotherapy for women who have advanced immune compromise, high viral load, or clinical illness. The obstetrician should review the regimen that the patient is taking. If it is effective (viral load is undetectable), then it should only be changed if some component of the regimen is contraindicated in pregnancy (e.g., efavirnez). If it is failing, then it should be changed, taking into consideration both the results of resistance testing and the safety of individual agents for use during pregnancy.

Mode of delivery

When considering the optimal mode of therapy for HIV-infected women, the obstetrician must be cognizant of both maternal interests and fetal interests. Therefore, the clinician must consider minimizing the risks of both perinatal transmission of HIV-1 and the potential for maternal and neonatal complications. Evidence of the potential benefit of Cesarean section for reducing MTCT antedates the use of antiretroviral therapy. Studies from that era showed substantive reductions in transmission (55–80%) when surgery was performed before labor or rupture of membranes occurred.

The most compelling data from that time were observational data from a meta-analysis and from an international randomized study. The former included observations from 15 prospective cohort studies, including more than 7800 mother–child pairs, and found that the rate of perinatal HIV-1 transmission among women undergoing elective Cesarean delivery was significantly lower than that among similar women having either nonelective Cesarean or vaginal delivery, regardless of whether they received ZDV, the only antiretroviral in use at the time.[158] In the latter, transmission was 1.8% among women randomized to elective Cesarean delivery, many of whom received ZDV.[159] Because the trial was underpowered (it began prior to ZDV treatment, and a background rate of transmission of 25% was anticipated), significant differences in the subgroup analysis (mode of delivery stratified by receipt of ZDV) could not be obtained. However, in all analyses, the differences between rates of transmission by mode of delivery were dramatic and consistent. Finally, in both the meta-analysis and the trial, nonelective Cesarean delivery (performed after the onset of labor or rupture of membranes) was not associated with a significant decrease in transmission compared with vaginal delivery. The American College of Obstetricians and Gynecologists' (ACOG) Committee on Obstetric Practice, after reviewing these data, issued a Committee Opinion concerning route of delivery recommending consideration of scheduled Cesarean delivery for HIV-1-infected pregnant women. However, as data were also available demonstrating low rates of transmission, independent of mode of delivery, when the viral load was < 1000 copies/mL, the committee limited their recommendation to those women with HIV-1 RNA levels > 1000 copies/mL near the time of delivery.[160]

Transmission, viral load, and combination antiretroviral therapy

As noted, the studies mentioned above were performed on the cusp of the era of HAART. Give the dramatic reductions in MTCT that have followed in the wake of these therapies, it is becoming increasingly difficult to document an effect of operative delivery above and beyond that which can be obtained with medical therapy alone. For example, independent of the specific regimen used, when a woman has a viral load under 1000 copies/mL and is on some therapy, her transmission rate apparently drops into the low single digits. In a study of women with HIV RNA levels below 1000 copies/mL at or near delivery, maternal antiretroviral therapy, primarily ZDV, was the most significant predictor of transmission risk [adjusted odds ratio (AOR) 0.12, $P < 0.001$], but any Cesarean delivery, scheduled or urgent, was also associated with a reduced risk of transmission (AOR 0.09, $P = 0.028$).[161] The association between Cesarean section and lower transmission did not control for the receipt of ZDV, and it is not counterintuitive to think that those providers who used Cesarean section may also have been more likely to employ antiretroviral therapy. However, current standard for medical therapy is no longer ZDV alone, and it is far from certain that HAART cannot replicate the benefits of operative delivery.

That is not to say that there are not some data that continue to suggest a benefit for Cesarean section even in the HAART era. In an Italian study evaluating risk factors for transmission, the risk of transmission was reduced with elective Cesarean delivery (AOR 0.54, 95% CI 0.29–1.02) compared with other modes of delivery even after adjustment for type of antiretroviral therapy and other risk factors, but not including HIV RNA levels. Among women receiving any antiretroviral therapy, transmission occurred among 13 (2.4%) of 553 women undergoing elective Cesarean delivery and 10 (4.4%) of 229 with other modes of delivery ($P = 0.13$).[162] In the European Collaborative Study, elective Cesarean delivery was associated with a reduced risk of transmission (AOR 0.42, 95% CI 0.27–0.67) even after adjustment for antiretroviral therapy and maternal CD4+ lymphocyte count. HIV RNA levels were not included in the model. Of note, the transmission rate among women on combination antiretroviral therapy regardless of mode of delivery was 1.7% (2/118).[163] Taken together, these studies suggest a benefit from elective Cesarean delivery among women on antiretroviral therapy, but the majority of the women in all these studies were receiving ZDV monotherapy rather than current combination regimens. Where specified, the risk of transmission among women on HAART was under 2%, making it difficult to detect potential differences in transmission by mode of delivery in this subset.

Even the most recent data fail to clarify the proper role for Cesarean section in the era of HAART, with some suggesting a role for Cesarean section even in the presence of HART, and others seeming to demonstrate that HAART alone will have maximal benefits. Thus, data from PACTG 367,[164] including 2756 women, do not demonstrate any benefit from elective Cesarean delivery among either women with HIV RNA levels below 1000 copies/mL or those on multiagent antiretroviral therapy. Specifically, women with HIV RNA levels under 1000 copies/mL on multiagent therapy had transmission rates of 0.8% with elective Cesarean delivery and 0.5% with all other delivery modes (OR 1.4, 95% CI 0.2–6.4), and those on single-agent therapy, usually ZDV, had a transmission rate of 4.3% after elective Cesarean delivery and 1.8% with all other delivery modes (OR 2.5, 95% CI 0.04–50.0). Women on multiagent therapy with HIV RNA levels over 1000 copies/mL near delivery had a transmission rate of 3.6% with elective Cesarean and 2.3% with other delivery modes (OR 1.6, 95% CI 0.6–4.3). The transmission rate among all women on multiagent antiretroviral therapy was 1.3% (34/2539). Data from the 4377 women who participated in the European Collaborative Study[165] yielded strikingly divergent results, suggesting a reduction in perinatal transmission of HIV with scheduled Cesarean delivery even among women on HAART or with undetectable HIV RNA levels. While the overall transmission rate among women on HAART was a reassuringly low 10 out of 678 (1.5%), a logistic regression, adjusting for antenatal antiretroviral therapy, CD4+ lymphocyte count, gender, and time period, revealed that scheduled Cesarean delivery was still associated with a reduced risk of transmission (AOR 0.51, 95% CI 0.31–0.82). Even among the 481 women with undetectable HIV RNA levels at delivery, 51% of whom were on HAART, scheduled Cesarean delivery was associated with an OR of transmission of 0.11 (95% CI 0.03–0.37). Thus, despite accumulating experience with Cesarean section in the HAART era, it is still unclear whether there are uniform benefits of elective Cesarean delivery. Hence, consideration must be given to the increased risk to the mother of Cesarean compared with vaginal delivery.

Maternal risks by mode of delivery

Obstetricians are fully familiar with a rich literature that details the excess morbidity, specifically infectious and hemorrhagic, attendant on Cesarean birth relative to vaginal delivery among HIV-uninfected women. In general, postpartum infections are approximately five to seven times more common after Cesarean delivery performed after labor or membrane rupture compared with vaginal delivery.[166,167] The risks associated with elective surgery, while still greater than for vaginal deliveries, are much less dramatic, to the point that more and more women are electing that mode even for uncomplicated births.[168]

In recent years, the types of studies that demonstrated the relative risk of morbidity associated with Cesarean section have been repeated among HIV-infected women. Not surprisingly, Cesarean section was still associated with greater rates of infectious morbidity, although the severity of the morbidity was not remarkable. For example, in the European trial in which HIV-1-infected women were randomized to Cesarean section or vaginal delivery, no major complications occurred in either the Cesarean or the vaginal delivery group, although postpartum fever occurred in fewer women who delivered vaginally (1.1%) than in women who delivered by Cesarean delivery (6.7%; $P = 0.002$).[159] Similarly, an analysis of nearly 1200 women enrolled in an American cohort of HIV-infected pregnant women (WITS) demonstrated an increased rate of postpartum fever among women undergoing elective Cesarean delivery compared with spontaneous vaginal delivery, but hemorrhage, severe anemia, endometritis, or urinary tract infections were not increased.[169] In PACTG 185, only endometritis, wound infection, and pneumonia were increased among women delivered by scheduled or urgent Cesarean delivery, compared with vaginal delivery.[170] In these studies, elective Cesarean sections were performed for obstetrical indications (e.g., previous Cesarean delivery or severe preeclampsia), not for prevention of HIV-1 transmission. That factor may have contributed to higher complication rates than might be seen when scheduled Cesarean delivery is performed solely to reduce perinatal transmission. However, even in cohorts weighted toward women who underwent elective surgery expressly to reduce rates of MTCT, fever was still increased after Cesarean compared with vaginal delivery.[171] In a multivariate analysis adjusted for maternal CD4+ count and antepartum hemorrhage, the relative risk of any postpartum complication was 1.85 (95% CI 1.00–3.39) after elective Cesarean delivery and 4.17 (95% CI 2.32–7.49) after emergency Cesarean delivery, compared with that for women delivering vaginally. Febrile morbidity was increased among women with low CD4+ counts.

Some researchers have now included comparisons of HIV-infected and -uninfected women in their assessments of operative risk. A European study performing such an analysis found that, among HIV-infected subjects, minor complications (anemia, fever, wound infection, curettage, endometritis, urinary tract infection) occurred in 16.8% of women delivering vaginally and 48.7% of those with Cesarean delivery, while major complications occurred in none of the women with vaginal delivery and 3.2% (5/158) of those with elective Cesarean delivery.[172] These frequencies were increased compared with matched HIV-uninfected women, but the relative difference between vaginal and Cesarean deliveries was similar in HIV-infected and HIV-uninfected women.

Several other studies have compared postoperative complications between HIV-infected women and similar HIV-uninfected women.[172–179] While two studies found similar outcomes among HIV-infected women compared with control subjects,[180,181] many more detected an increased risk of one or more complications, albeit predominantly minor complications, among the HIV-infected women. Cases of pneumonia were seen among HIV-infected women in four of the studies, while no cases occurred in the HIV-negative women. In those studies that included an assessment of immune status, an increased risk of complications was seen among women with a lower CD4+ lymphocyte count or percentage.

Timing of scheduled Cesarean delivery

Once a decision has been made to perform an elective Cesarean delivery for the purpose of preventing HIV-1 transmission, it should be scheduled at 38 weeks, as per current ACOG guidelines. This recommendation stands in contrast to that organization's recommendations for HIV-1-uninfected women, in which case ACOG recommends that scheduled Cesarean delivery without confirmation of fetal lung maturity should be scheduled at 39 completed weeks or the onset of labor in order to minimize the chance of complications in the neonate.[182] Delivery at 38 weeks, as is currently recommended for HIV-infected women, rather than at 39 weeks, entails a small absolute increase in risk of development of infant respiratory distress requiring mechanical ventilation.[183,184] This increased risk must be balanced against the potential risk of labor or membrane rupture, and attendant increased rates of MTCT, if delivery is delayed until 39 weeks of gestation. Theoretically, the risks associated with births a week earlier than standard could be mitigated by maturity studies. However, amniocentesis in not recommended in these circumstances for fear of contamination of the amniotic sac by maternal HIV, which could pose a risk of consequent fetal infection. Thus,

ACOG also recommends that the timing of delivery be based on the best clinical estimate of dating.[160] Women should be informed of the potential risks and benefits to themselves and their infants in choosing the timing and mode of delivery.

Intrapartum management

If a decision has been made to effect delivery via scheduled Cesarean delivery, then antiretroviral therapy should be part of the preoperative protocol. Intravenous ZDV should begin 3 h before surgery, according to standard dosing recommendations, and the infant should receive ZDV for 6 weeks after birth.[185] Other maternal drugs should be continued on schedule as much as possible to provide maximal effect and minimize the chance of development of viral resistance. Oral medications may be continued preoperatively with sips of water. Medications requiring food ingestion for absorption could be taken with liquid dietary supplements, but consultation with the attending anesthesiologist should be obtained before administering in the preoperative period. If maternal antiretroviral therapy must be interrupted temporarily in the peripartum period, all drugs (except for intrapartum intravenous ZDV) should be stopped and reinstituted simultaneously to minimize the chance of resistance developing.

As noted above, infectious morbidity is an important consideration, and consideration should be given to the initiation of prophylactic antibiotics. If vaginal delivery is planned, and if labor is progressing and membranes are intact, artificial rupture of membranes or invasive monitoring should be avoided. These procedures should be considered only when obstetrically indicated, and the length of time for ruptured membranes or monitoring is anticipated to be short.

The most problematic clinical dilemmas involve circumstances in which the fetus may be exposed to prolonged periods of membrane rupture. If a vaginal delivery had been planned, i.e., the viral load is low, then continuing antiviral therapy and aggressively moving toward vaginal delivery seems the most appropriate management plan. However, if a Cesarean section was planned, it is unclear how long after membranes rupture that Cesarean section will continue to offer a benefit with regard to a lowered MTCT rate. Much of the data linking duration of rupture to increased risk of transmission antedate the use of antiretroviral therapy, and their utility for predicting events in the HAART era is therefore limited.[186,187] The data from more recent studies are less uniform in conclusion. Among women receiving ZDV, some studies have shown an increased risk of transmission with ruptured membranes for four or more hours before delivery,[188] but others have not.[189] If a Cesarean section had been indicated and the patient appears shortly after ruptured membranes, it would seem reasonable to proceed expeditiously toward operative delivery, making sure that intravenous ZDV is started as quickly as possible. If the patient ruptures membranes when she is preterm, then the clinician must balance the potential gain in reduced prematurity-related morbidity from an anticipated latent phase versus the risk of MTCT that would be encountered by waiting. The further forward from the time of periviability the rupture occurs, the more Cesarean delivery shortly after rupture would be favored.

Postpartum management

The first management decision that the obstetrician and parturient confront in the immediate postpartum period is whether to continue the medications the woman had been on during pregnancy. If the woman had been on HAART prior to pregnancy and her viral load had continued to be suppressed throughout gestation, then she should be maintained on the same regimen at least until she re-establishes contact with her primary HIV care provider. Alternatively, if the patient had not met criteria for HAART during the prepregnancy period, but had been started merely as part of a strategy to reduce the risk of MTCT, the discontinuation of therapy would be appropriate. In that circumstance, all medications should be discontinued simultaneously to avoid prolonged exposure to monotherapy and the consequent risk of development of resistant virus. It should be noted that certain agents have much longer half-lives than others so that, even if all drugs are stopped concurrently, the possibility of a period of *de facto* monotherapy cannot be completely dismissed.

After the patient has been discharged, with suitable instructions about antiviral medication, the obstetrician must assure appropriate follow-up both by an HIV specialist and by a provider who can provide family planning advice.

Summary recommendations

- All pregnant women should be given the opportunity to ascertain their HIV serostatus as early in pregnancy as possible. The preferred testing algorithm involves the "opt-out" approach, in which women are routinely informed that they will be tested unless they specifically request to opt out.
- The physician's primary responsibility is to maximize the health of his/her pregnant patient. Women's viral load and CD4 counts should be monitored and HAART administered per standard recommendations. If her viral load and CD4 results do not, unto themselves, justify HAART therapy, consideration should still be given to aggressive therapy in order to minimize the likelihood of MTCT.
- While HAART is probably the most effective regimen for MTCT prevention, there are circumstances (e.g., viral load less than 1000 copies/mL) in which alternatives might be acceptable. As a minimum for the reduction of perinatal HIV-1 transmission, ZDV prophylaxis according to the PACTG 076 regimen is recommended unless the woman is intolerant of ZDV.
- Plasma HIV-1 RNA levels should be monitored during pregnancy according to the guidelines for management of HIV-1-infected adults. The most recently determined viral load value should be used when counseling a woman regarding mode of delivery.
- Perinatal HIV-1 transmission is reduced by scheduled

Cesarean delivery among women with unknown or high HIV-1 RNA levels who are not receiving antiretroviral therapy or are receiving only ZDV for prophylaxis of perinatal transmission. The benefit among women on HAART is unproven. Given the low rate of transmission among this group, it is unlikely that scheduled Cesarean delivery would confer additional benefit in the reduction of transmission.

• Management of women originally scheduled for Cesarean delivery who present with ruptured membranes or in labor must be individualized based on duration of rupture, progress of labor, plasma HIV-1 RNA level, current antiretroviral therapy, and other clinical factors. The woman's autonomy to make an informed decision regarding route of delivery should be respected and honored.

Sexually transmitted diseases in pregnancy

Although STDs have been recognized for more than three millennia and have played major roles in the history of civilization, the last three decades have brought the greatest progress in our understanding of this rapidly expanding field. Advances in microbiology and immunology have made our comprehension of their pathogenesis and amplified treatment options more sophisticated.

Despite these breakthroughs, the epidemic of STDs remains unabated in America.[190–192] In 1993, the Institute of Medicine (IOM) in their report, *The Hidden Epidemic: Confronting Sexually Transmitted Diseases*, estimated that 12 million new cases of STDs occurred annually in the United States at an estimated annual cost of US$17 billion.[190] Subsequently, in 1998, the American Social Health Association (ASHA) suggested that 15 million new cases of STDs were occurring each year in the United States.[191] Recently, Weinstock et al.[192] increased the estimate of new STD cases to nearly 19 million annually. In particular, this trend has had far-reaching implications on the reproductive health of women.

Not only is there a resurgence of traditional STDs, but new ones have been added to the list (Table 50.7). Unfortunately, many of these new STDs are either incurable or associated with serious sequelae in women. *Chlamydia trachomatis* has been associated with infertility,[193] ectopic pregnancy,[191,194–196] and a host of adverse perinatal outcomes;[197] human papillomavirus (HPV) is associated with genital squamous cell carcinomas;[198] HSV becomes a chronic infection; and HIV is ultimately fatal and had become one of the five leading causes of death in women of reproductive age by 1991.[199] Many of these infections have been associated with abortion, preterm delivery, premature ruptured membranes, and amnionitis. Finally, many of these agents, including HIV, HSV, *N. gonorrhoeae*, *Chlamydia*, and *Treponema pallidum*, can be transmitted to the fetus or newborn.

As might be expected, all the STDs regularly occur in pregnancy, with varying effects on mother, fetus, and neonate. This section focuses on issues related to gonorrhea, syphilis, *Chlamydia,* HPV, HSV, and *Trichomonas* in pregnant women and their fetuses.

Table 50.7 Sexually transmitted pathogens.

Bacterial agents
Neisseria gonorrhoeae
Chlamydia trachomatis
Gardnerella vaginalis
Haemophilus ducreyi
Shigella sp.
Group B streptococci
Treponema pallidum
Mycoplasma agents
Mycoplasma hominis
Ureaplasma urealyticum
Ectoparasites
Phthirius pubis
Sarcoptes scabiei
Viral agents
Human papillomavirus
Herpes simplex virus
Hepatitis B virus
Cytomegalovirus
Molluscum contagiosum virus
Human immunodeficiency virus
Protozoan agents
Trichomonas vaginalis
Entamoeba histolytica
Giardia lamblia
Fungal agents
Candida albicans

Gonorrhea

Gonorrhea is perhaps the oldest known STD, with references to its symptoms dating back to numerous ancient civilizations. It was not until relatively recent times that the disease's effects in women were first described.

Gonorrhea, caused by the Gram-negative diplococcus, *Neisseria gonorrhoeae*, is the second most commonly reported communicable disease in the United States with over 335 000 cases reported in 2003.[200] As a result of under-reporting, it is estimated that approximately 750 000 cases actually occur annually in the United States. In 2003, for the first time, the reported gonorrhea rate among women (118.8 per 100 000) was greater than that reported for men (113 per 100 000).[200]

N. gonorrhoeae infects both columnar and transitional epithelium, including the endocervix, urethra, anal canal, pharynx, and conjunctivae. Local spread in women results in endometritis, salpingitis, and bartholinitis; systemic manifestations include arthritis, dermatitis, endocarditis, meningitis, myocarditis, and hepatitis. Humans are the only natural host for this organism, and the only known forms of transmission are sexual and vertical.

Epidemiology

A number of risk markers for gonorrhea have been identified. These include young age (younger than 25 years), nonwhite race, early onset of sexual activity, low socioeconomic status, unmarried status, urban dwelling, illicit drug use, and prostitution. According to the CDC, 60% of reported cases of gonorrhea occur in the 15- to 24-year age group with the gonorrhea rate among women (125/100 000) similar to that of men (124/100 000).[200] From 1975 through 1997, a dramatic (74%) decrease in gonorrhea was reported. However, in 1998, an 8.9% increase occurred and, since that time, rates have plateaued until 2003 when they began to increase again.

Increasingly resistant strains of *N. gonorrhoeae* have occurred.[201] These resistant strains include penicillinase-producing *N. gonorrhoeae* (PPNG), high-level chromosomal resistance to penicillin, plasmid-mediated tetracycline resistance (TRNG), chromosomally mediated resistance to cephalosporins, tetracycline, spectinomycin, and aminoglycosides and, most recently, *N. gonorrhoeae* resistant to fluoroquinolones.

Pathogenesis

Similarly to other infections, the initial step in the pathogenesis of gonococcal infection is adherence of *N. gonorrhoeae* to mucosal cells lining the genitourinary tract. Pili and other surface proteins, including porin protein (Por), opacity-associated proteins (Opa), and reduction modifiable protein (RmP), mediate this attachment.[202–204] Additional gonococcal virulence factors include lipopolysaccharides,[204] immunoglobulin A,[202] and iron-repressible proteins involved in iron uptake.[204] After the organism attaches to mucosal cells, it enters the cell by endocytosis. It releases endotoxins, causing widespread cell damage.

Clinical manifestations

The clinical presentation depends on the site of inoculation, duration of infection, and whether the infection has remained local or has spread systemically. The percentage of women with asymptomatic infection ranges between 25% and 80%.[205,206] Gonococcal infections in pregnant patients are commonly asymptomatic.

Anogenital gonorrhea

Acute symptomatic anogenital infections in women are characterized by dysuria, increased urinary frequency, increased vaginal discharge secondary to an exudative endocervicitis, abnormal menstrual bleeding, or anorectal discomfort. Most women who become symptomatic do so within 3–5 days of inoculation or during menstruation. Inflammation of the Skene's or Bartholin's glands is usually unilateral and acute in nature. Only 15% of all women with gonorrhea have extension of infection to the upper genital tract, although this is rarely seen during pregnancy.

Localized extragenital gonorrhea

The majority of patients with pharyngeal infections are asymptomatic. The most common signal is a mild sore throat, and erythema, lesions, and a tonsillar or pharyngeal exudate may be present. Pharyngeal infection is more common during gestation.[207]

Gonococcal conjunctivitis, as the result of direct sexual contact or indirect autoinoculation, is rare and heralded by the acute onset of severe inflammation and purulent exudate.

Disseminated gonococcal infection

Disseminated gonococcal infection (DGI) occurs in 1–3% of adult infections, and 80% of these cases are in women.[208,209] Most women with DGI develop symptoms either during pregnancy or while menstruating. The majority of *N. gonorrhoeae* isolates recovered from patients with DGI are sensitive to antibiotics but resistant to complement-mediated bactericidal activity in normal serum.

There are two distinct clinical syndromes found in DGI: an early bacteremic and a later arthritic stage. Patients with disseminated infection rarely complain of genital symptoms. Bacteremic patients complain of fever, chills, malaise, and skin lesions. The initial dermatologic manifestation most frequently involves the distal extremities, including the palms and soles, with up to 20 lesions. Lesions are characterized as small vesicles that become first pustular, then necrotic, and finally heal spontaneously. Endocarditis, meningitis, and toxic hepatitis are infrequent complications of this phase. The arthritic phase is typically symptomatic and involves the knees, ankles, and wrists, with purulent tenosynovitis. The pain is thought to be secondary to deposition of immune complexes. Without treatment, symptoms usually resolve in approximately a week; the infection may either become chronic or progress to septic arthritis and joint destruction.

Maternal and fetal risks

The association between maternal gonorrheal infection and ophthalmia neonatorum has been appreciated for over a century. Before routine administration of silver nitrate, this disease occurred in 10% of newborns. The institution of routine neonatal prophylaxis reduced this rate dramatically. Gonococcal infection is transmitted to 30–35% of babies who pass through an infected cervix.[210] After an incubation period of between 4 and 21 days, bilateral purulent conjunctivitis is the usual manifestation, with rapid progression to corneal ulceration, scarring, and blindness in the absence of treatment.

Subsequently, gonococcal infection during gestation has been linked to a wide variety of perinatal complications. Postabortal and postpartum endometritis occur more frequently in women with untreated gonococcal cervicitis at the time of delivery. Intra-amniotic infection has also been described and is characterized by inflammation of the fetal membranes, placenta, and umbilical cord; it results in maternal fever, leukocytosis, and fetal infection.[211–214] A chronic, low-grade infection may ensue, with resultant intrauterine growth retardation (IUGR).[214] Whether infection predisposes to or is the result of premature rupture of the membranes (PROM) remains controversial. Preterm delivery is the customary outcome, and both mother and infant are at risk of continued infection and sepsis. The incidence of preterm delivery in women with untreated cervical gonorrhea has been recorded to be as high as 67%.[211]

Laboratory diagnosis

Although the Gram stain of urethral discharge is both sensitive and specific in men, it has two major disadvantages in women: asymptomatic patients are not tested, and the test has poor sensitivity in women. Thus, the diagnosis of gonococcal infection in women requires the identification of *N. gonorrhoeae* at infected sites. Available methods include culture, immunochemical detection, or molecular diagnostic techniques.

Selective plates, such as Thayer–Martin, provide optimal conditions for isolation of the organism. *N. gonorrhoeae* forms oxidase-positive colonies that can be differentiated from other *Neisseria* species by their ability to dissimulate glucose but not maltose, sucrose, or lactose.

The traditional method of gonorrhea detection in women was culture of the cervix and any other symptomatic site. During pregnancy, cultures should be obtained from all patients at the first antenatal visit and again in the third trimester in those at high risk of infection. Factors identifying those at high risk include sex with a symptomatic partner, multiple sex partners, other STDs, bleeding induced by cervical swab, Medicaid as a method of payment, age at first intercourse less than 16 years of age, and low abdominal or pelvic pain.[215]

With the introduction of nonculture assays for the detection of *N. gonorrhoeae*, these newer methodologies have replaced culture.[204] Nonamplified DNA probe tests (e.g., Gen-Probe Pace 2) were the first widely accepted alternative to culture and became the most common nonculture method for the detection of *N. gonorrhoeae* in the United States.[204] Nonamplified DNA probes have a sensitivity of 89–97% and a specificity of 99%. Nucleic acid amplification tests have become available more recently and include PCR, ligase chain reaction (LCR), and transcription-mediated amplification (TMA). These amplification methods have excellent sensitivity and specificity.

Treatment

Anogenital and pharyngeal infection

The factors to consider in the treatment of uncomplicated anogenital gonococcal infection are: (1) the incidence in many urban areas of resistant strains of *N. gonorrhoeae*; (2) the availability of effective single-dose agents against *N. gonorrhoeae*; (3) the coexistence of chlamydial infection in up to 30% of patients; and (4) the absence of a rapid, reliable, inexpensive means of making the diagnosis of *C. trachomatis*.[216] Patients with gonococcal infections should be treated with regimens effective against both pathogens. The CDC recommendations are listed in Table 50.8.[201] For pregnant women, the recommended regimens include ceftriaxone or cefixime plus erythromycin.

Alternative cephalosporins for the pregnant patient include cefotaxime, ceftizoxime, cefotetan, and cefoxitin. For patients who cannot tolerate cephalosporins, spectinomycin is the preferred alternative. It covers resistant strains of *N. gonorrhoeae*; unfortunately, it is ineffective against pharyngeal infection. Both doxycycline and the quinolones are contraindicated during pregnancy because of their effects on the fetus.

The incidence of treatment failure among those treated with ceftriaxone or cefixime is extremely rare, obviating the need for test-of-cure for *N. gonorrhoeae*. These women should be screened for reinfection after 2–3 months. Women undergoing other treatment regimens should have follow-up cultures performed 7–14 days after completion of therapy. These cultures should be obtained from the rectum as well as the cervix, because 25% of female treatment failures harbor organisms only in the rectum. Any gonococcal isolate recovered after treatment failure should be tested for antibiotic sensitivity, because the incidence of resistance is high. These patients should be treated with a single dose of ceftriaxone.

All women diagnosed with gonorrhea should undergo serologic testing for syphilis and screening for *C. trachomatis*, and be offered confidential counseling and testing for HIV infection.

Extragenital disseminated infection

Inpatient treatment is advisable for patients with DGI, particularly those with endocarditis, meningitis, synovial effusions,

Table 50.8 Centers for Disease Control 2002 recommended treatment guidelines for uncomplicated anogenital gonorrhea during pregnancy.

Regimens
Recommended regimens
Ceftriaxone, 125 mg i.m. once
or
Cefixime, 400 mg p.o. in a single dose
plus
Erythromycin, 500 mg p.o. q.i.d. for 7 days
or
Amoxicillin 500 mg p.o. q.i.d. for 7 days
Alternative regimens
Spectinomycin, 2 g i.m. in a single dose
Cefotaxime, 500 mg i.m. once
Ceftizoxime, 500 mg i.m. once
Cefotetan, 1 g i.m. once
Cefoxitin, 2 g i.m. once

Table 50.9 Centers for Disease Control 2002 recommended treatment guidelines for disseminated gonococcal infection during pregnancy.

Recommended inpatient regimen
Ceftriaxone, 1 g i.m. or i.v. q.d.
Alternative inpatient regimen
Ceftizoxime, 1 g i.v. q8 h
or
Cefotaxime, 1 g i.v. q8 h
or
Spectinomycin, 2 g i.m. q12 h
Recommended ambulatory follow-up regimen
Cefixime, 400 mg p.o. b.i.d.

or compliance problems. CDC recommendations for treatment include ceftriaxone, ceftizoxime, cefotaxime, or spectinomycin (Table 50.9).[201] All regimens should be continued for 24–48 h after improvement begins. Therapy can then be switched to oral cefixime to complete a 7-day course. Although the value of continued inpatient observation of pregnant patients to reduce the risk of adverse perinatal outcomes has not been demonstrated, it may be advisable. The treatment of meningitis and endocarditis infections due to *N. gonorrhoeae* involves high-dose intravenous treatment with ceftriaxone (1–2 g every 12 h) for 2 and 4 weeks respectively.

Syphilis

Syphilis is a chronic, debilitating systemic infection caused by the spirochete *Treponema pallidum* and characterized by infrequent but severe and varied exacerbations.

When untreated, the natural history of this infection may encompass several decades. Two major stages are designated, early and late, and each of these is further separated. The phases of early syphilis are incubating, primary, secondary, and early latent. Late syphilis progresses from late latent to tertiary.

Epidemiology

Globally, there has been a steady decline in the incidence of syphilis since 1960. Both the United States and Europe experienced syphilis epidemics during World War II. Starting in 1982, there was an overall reduction in its incidence, due primarily to the fear of HIV and the use of safer sexual practices in men having sex with men.[217] Alarmingly, the incidence among inner city heterosexuals, particularly in New York City, Florida, Texas, and California, began rising in 1987 and peaked in 1990.[217] A disproportionate number of these cases were women, which led to a dramatic rise in the prevalence of congenital syphilis.[218–220] Since the peak in 1990, the reported primary and secondary syphilis rates declined by 90% from 20.34 cases per 100 000 population to 2.12 per 100 000.[200] The 2000 rate was the lowest since reporting of syphilis began in 1941. Unfortunately, since 2000, the rate of primary and secondary syphilis has increased for three consecutive years, and the 2003 rate (2.5 per 100 000) was 19% higher than that reported for 2000.[200] The good news is that, despite a 62% increase among men, there has been a 43% decrease among women.[221] In 2003, there were 34 270 total reported cases of syphilis in the United States.[200]

Gestational and congenital syphilis tend to occur in young, nonwhite, unmarried, poor, inner city dwellers with insufficient antenatal care.

As with primary and secondary syphilis, the rate of congenital syphilis declined sharply from the peak of 107.3 per 100 000 population in 1991.[221] During 2003, a total of 413 cases of congenital syphilis were reported in the United States compared with 412 cases in 2002.[200]

Pathogenesis

Syphilis is efficiently transmitted during sexual contact, with 60% of partners acquiring the infection after a single sexual encounter. Spirochetes require a break in the integument in order to gain access to the host. Microscopic tears in genital mucosa occur almost universally during sexual intercourse. There follows a mean incubation period of 21 days, with a range of 10–90 days. The organism sets up a local infection and eventually disseminates widely via lymphatic drainage. Wherever it lodges, it stimulates an immune response.

Clinical manifestations

The manifestations of syphilis are wide ranging, involving nearly every organ system. The degree of clinical expression clearly reflects the immune status of the host. With an intact immune system, 60% of patients remain in the latent phase.

Primary

The first sign of primary infection is the development of a single, nontender lesion (chancre) at the site of entry. The most customary sites of infection in women include the vulva, introitus, or cervix. Extragenital sites include the lips, tongue, tonsils, breasts, and fingers. The syphilitic chancre is a painless, dull red macule, which becomes a papule and then ulcerates. Ulcers are rounded, with a well-defined margin and a rubbery, indurated, weeping base. The ulcer persists for 3–6 weeks without treatment and then heals spontaneously. Painless unilateral or bilateral inguinal lymphadenopathy often develops a week after the appearance of the lesion. Nodes are small, rubbery, and nonsuppurative.

Secondary

The symptoms of secondary syphilis typically emerge 3–6 weeks later. By this time, the infection is widely disseminated, and most symptoms are due to immune complex deposition. Nonspecific complaints include fever, malaise, sore throat, headache, musculoskeletal pains, and weight loss.

A classic faint macular rash develops over the trunk and flexor surfaces in the vast majority of infected individuals. Its lesions are pink, rounded, and ordinarily less than 1 cm in diameter. The rash spreads over the whole body, including the palms and soles, and becomes first dull red and papular, then squamous. Superficial ulcerations called mucous patches appear in the mucous membranes in 30% of patients. Also, generalized lymphadenopathy is present in the majority.

Latent

By definition, this stage lacks clinical manifestations. The early latent phase (less than 1 year) has been associated with recurrence of secondary mucocutaneous lesions, and these lesions are infectious. Although late latent syphilis (more than 1 year) cannot be transmitted sexually, vertical transmission to the fetus persists.

Tertiary

One-third of untreated patients develop tertiary syphilis. This is characterized by involvement of the cardiovascular, central nervous, or musculoskeletal systems. The presence of gummas in various tissues designates late benign tertiary syphilis. Aortic aneurysms and aortic insufficiency are characteristic cardiovascular lesions, whereas generalized paresis, tabes dorsalis, and optic atrophy with the Argyll Robertson pupil that accommodates, but does not react to, light are all features of neurosyphilis.

Laboratory diagnosis

The gold standard for diagnosis of early syphilis is the detection of treponemes on darkfield examination of ulcer scrapings or tissue samples. The test is inexpensive and easy, and provides immediate results. The reliability of this test is proportional to the skill of the person performing it. The lesion should be cleansed thoroughly with saline and scraped firmly to collect serum. If no spirochetes are apparent, the test should be repeated twice to increase sensitivity. Although a positive test result is diagnostic, a negative one does not preclude the possibility of infection.

Indirect diagnosis of syphilis can be made with the use of two types of serologic tests. Nontreponemal tests such as the Venereal Disease Research Laboratory (VDRL) test and rapid plasma regain (RPR) show reactive results approximately 2 weeks after development of the initial lesion. Both measure anticardiolipin antibody. In secondary syphilis, the VDRL titer is usually greater than or equal to 1 to 16. After successful treatment, the VDRL should decrease fourfold in 3 months and eightfold in 6 months. It should be nonreactive 1 year after therapy for primary infection, and 2 years for secondary disease.

Treponemal-specific tests include the fluorescent treponemal antibody absorbed (FTA-ABS) assay and microhemagglutination assay for antibody to *T. pallidum* (MHATP). More sensitive (70–90%) than nontreponemal tests, these tests become reactive at approximately the same time as the primary lesion develops and are used to confirm the serologic diagnosis of syphilis. Unfortunately, these test results remain positive for life.

The diagnosis of latent syphilis is made on the basis of two elevated nontreponemal serologic test results taken at least 1 year apart. A further diagnostic workup includes evaluation of the cerebrospinal fluid (CSF).

The CDC recommends that all pregnant women should be screened for syphilis at their first prenatal visit.[201] Where prenatal care is problematic, the RPR card test screening (a rapid screen for syphilis) is recommended when pregnancy is diagnosed and treatment given if positive.[201] For women at high risk of syphilis and in populations with a high prevalence of syphilis, additional serologic testing at 28 weeks' gestation and at delivery is recommended.[201]

Patients with neurologic or ophthalmic signs of symptoms, evidence of tertiary syphilis, treatment failure, or HIV infection with late latent syphilis of unknown duration should have CSF obtained to test for neurosyphilis.

The diagnosis of neurosyphilis is challenging, because no one test is reliable. The CSF should be tested for cell count, protein, and with the VDRL test. An elevated count of greater than 5 white blood cells/μL is a relatively sensitive indicator of active infection. A positive CSF VDRL result is diagnostic for neurosyphilis.

Treatment

In 1943, penicillin was found to be effective in treating syphilis. To date, no resistance has developed. The goal in therapy is to provide continuous, low-level concentrations of penicillin in infected tissues. It is still the preferred drug in gestational and congenital syphilis, as well as neurosyphilis. Women with history of penicillin allergy should undergo skin testing to validate the sensitivity and proceed with desensitization and penicillin therapy for optimal results.[222,223]

Treatment regimens in pregnancy are listed in Table 50.10. Alternative regimens in nonpregnant patients include tetracy-

Table 50.10 Centers for Disease Control 2002 recommended treatment guidelines for syphilis in pregnancy.

Early syphilis recommended regimen (primary, secondary, and early latent syphilis)
Benzathine penicillin G, 2.4 million units (U) i.m. once (1.2 million U in each buttock)
Late latent and tertiary syphilis recommended regimen
Benzathine penicillin G, 7.2 million U total administered as three doses of 2.4 million U i.m. given 1 week apart for three consecutive weeks
Neurosyphilis recommended regimen
Aqueous crystalline penicillin G, 12–24 million U administered 2–4 million U i.v. q4h for 10–14 days
Neurosyphilis alternative regimen
Procaine penicillin, 2.4 million U i.m. daily with
Probenecid, 500 mg p.o. q.i.d., both for 10–14 days

cline and doxycycline, both contraindicated during pregnancy. Pregnant patients who are allergic to penicillin should be treated with penicillin after desensitization.[222,223]

The Jarisch–Herxheimer reaction is an acute reaction, apparently provoked by the release of prostaglandins during the initiation of treatment for primary or secondary infection.[224] The reaction must be differentiated from penicillin allergy. It occurs within 24h of receiving the first dose of antibiotic and is characterized by fever, malaise, headache, musculoskeletal pain, nausea, tachycardia, and exacerbation of skin lesions. Although the reaction is more common in primary disease, its symptoms are more severe with secondary disease. Fluids and antipyretics are recommended for symptomatic relief. Pregnant women are at risk of preterm labor and intrauterine fetal demise.

Maternal and fetal risks

Pregnancy does not appear to alter the course of syphilis; however, *T. pallidum* adversely affects pregnancy. It crosses the placenta and has been associated with preterm delivery, stillbirth, congenital infection, and neonatal death, depending on the timing of infection. The majority of infants with congenital syphilis are born to mothers with early syphilis or secondary infection. Fetal infection during the first and second trimesters carries significant morbidity, whereas third-trimester exposure results in asymptomatic infection.[225,226] Paley[225] initially reported that approximately 50% of the pregnancies in which the untreated syphilitic infection was of less than 2 years' duration resulted in living nonsyphilitic infants. On the other hand, Fiumara et al.[227] reported that, with untreated primary or secondary syphilis, 50% of the infants were premature, stillborn, or died as neonates, and the remaining 50% developed congenital syphilis. With early latent syphilis, 20–60% of infants were normal, 20% premature, and 16% stillborn; 40% had congenital syphilis. For late untreated syphilis, the congenital syphilis rate was 10%, stillbirth rate was 10%, premature rate was 9%, and healthy infants made up 70%. More recently, studies have confirmed the significant adverse effect of untreated syphilis on pregnancy outcome.[228,229] Rici et al.,[228] in Miami, reported a 34% incidence of stillbirth, 85% prematurity, and 21% IUGR. Overall, 68% of liveborn infants in this series had significant clinical disease. MacFarlin et al.,[229] in Detroit, noted a 28% incidence of preterm birth. In this report, eight (75%) out of 12 women who received no antibiotic treatment for syphilis were delivered of stillborn infants; overall, stillbirth complicated 10 out of 72 (13.9%) women in the congenital syphilis group. These authors also documented an alarmingly high rate of failure of current therapy to prevent the development of congenital syphilis.

Infants with early congenital syphilis are usually asymptomatic at birth, but develop symptoms at 10–14 days of life. A maculopapular rash arises and often desquamates or becomes vesicular. Many develop a flu-like syndrome with a copious nasal discharge, commonly referred to as "snuffles." Other symptoms include oropharyngeal mucous patches, lymphadenopathy, hepatosplenomegaly, jaundice, osteochondritis, iritis, and chorioretinitis.[226,227] Untreated early congenital syphilis progresses to the late phase, marked by Hutchinson teeth, mulberry molars, deafness, saddle nose, saber shins, mental retardation, hydrocephalus, general paresis, and optic nerve atrophy.

Pregnant women undergoing treatment for syphilis are at minimal risk of intrauterine fetal demise. Those who develop Jarisch–Herxheimer reactions are at increased risk of preterm labor.

Prevention

As noted previously, the accessibility of early and complete antenatal care with routine screening and adequate treatment for this infection is critical for prevention. Careful post-treatment follow-up is essential for controlling the spread of syphilis. Treatment failure is difficult to distinguish from reinfection. Patients should be examined and tested serologically at 3 and 6 months. If signs and symptoms persist or if nontreponemal antibody test results have not decreased appropriately after therapy, patients should undergo evaluation of their CSF and be retreated as warranted.

Partner tracing is particularly important in syphilis, given its prolonged course and multiple asymptomatic phases. In women with primary syphilis, all partners in the last 3 months should be evaluated; this time period should extend to 12 months for those diagnosed with secondary syphilis.

All patients with syphilis should be screened for other STDs, including confidential counseling and testing for HIV. Patients with coexistent HIV infection should be evaluated more frequently and treated for neurosyphilis in the event of any signs of persistent infection.

Chlamydial infections

Chlamydia trachomatis is the most frequently diagnosed bacterial STD in the United States, with an estimated prevalence of more than 4 million cases and an annual cost of more than US$1 billion.[200,230,231] In addition, chlamydia is the most commonly reported infectious disease in the United States with 877478 cases of genital chlamydial infection reported in 2003.[200] Lower genital tract infection predisposes nonpregnant women to pelvic inflammatory disease (PID), and pregnant women to a variety of maternal and neonatal infections.

Epidemiology

C. trachomatis is the causative agent of trachoma, the leading preventable cause of blindness in the developing world. In the United States, it is most frequently manifested as genital tract infections in the adult and inclusion conjunctivitis and pneumonia in the neonate.

It has been estimated that between 20% and 40% of sexually active women in the United States have been exposed to *C. trachomatis*. Cervical infection rates range from 5.5–22.5%

of asymptomatic women attending family planning clinics to 34–63% of women with mucopurulent cervicitis.[232] The prevalence among pregnant women depends on the population sampled, varying from 2% to 37%.[232]

Chlamydial infections tend to occur in women at high risk of other STDs, with infection rates proportional to the number of sexual partners and inversely proportional to age. Risk markers in pregnant women include age less than 20 years, unmarried status, low socioeconomic status, residence in inner cities, late presentation for prenatal care, the presence of other STDs, and the findings of mucopurulent endocervicitis or nonbacteriuric pyuria.[233–236] Up to two-thirds of women with cervical chlamydial infection are asymptomatic, creating a large reservoir for both horizontal and vertical transmission.[232]

Pathogenesis

There are 15 recognized *C. trachomatis* serotypes, eight of which appear to cause oculogenital infection.[233] The organism is classified as an obligate intracellular bacterium, requiring viable columnar or pseudostratified columnar epithelial cells for survival and multiplication. The bacterium has an interesting life cycle lasting 48–72 h. The elementary body is the form of the organism capable of infecting cells, whereas the reticulate body is the metabolically active, multiplying form responsible for producing the characteristic inclusions. The long growth cycle of *C. trachomatis* requires long-term therapy.

Clinical manifestations

The incubation period for genital chlamydial infections ranges from 6 to 14 days. A variety of clinical manifestations, from bartholinitis to PID with peritonitis and perihepatitis, have been described. The most common perinatal syndromes are described briefly here.

Endocervicitis

The most commonly infected site in the female genital tract is the endocervix. As mentioned previously, the majority of infected women are asymptomatic. Findings on physical examination extend from normal to cervical erosion and mucopurulent cervicitis. Requisite components of the diagnosis of mucopurulent cervicitis include endocervical friability, erythema or edema, the presence of yellow or green endocervical mucopus, and more than 10 polymorphonuclear leukocytes (PMNs) per high-power field of a cervical Gram stain.

Acute urethral syndrome

Chlamydial infection has also been implicated in the etiology of 25% of patients with acute urethral syndrome. Such women present with dysuria and increased urinary frequency in the face of sterile urine. Also, many report oral contraceptive use, recent contact with a new sexual partner, and a prolonged symptom duration of up to 14 days.[237] Although *C. trachomatis* can sometimes be cultured from the urethra, it is more frequently recovered from the endocervix of these patients.

Endometritis

It has been well established that the incidence of postabortion endometritis is higher among women with chlamydial cervicitis.[238–242] Because up to 35% of women with chlamydial cervical infection who undergo elective termination develop endometritis, antibiotic prophylaxis is recommended for high-risk women.

The association between chlamydial infection and postpartum endometritis is more controversial. Although some authors have found such an association,[243–246] others have not.[247–249]

Acute pelvic inflammatory disease

The association between maternal lower genital tract *C. trachomatis* infection, neonatal inclusion conjunctivitis, and the subsequent development of postpartum PID has been recognized for 70 years.[250] Chlamydial PID can also occur during pregnancy, although its incidence appears to be extremely rare.[251–254] Pregnancy confounds the diagnosis, given the frequency of adverse gastrointestinal complaints and a physiologic leukocytosis among normal pregnant women, and the low prevalence of gestational PID. Because the rate of fetal wastage approximates 50% in pregnancies complicated by PID, prompt administration of appropriate broad-spectrum antibiotic coverage should be initiated once the diagnosis has been entertained.[254]

Maternal and fetal risks

Vertical transmission rates secondary to passage through an infected cervix are as high as 60–70%.[232] Inclusion conjunctivitis develops during the first 2 weeks of life in 25–50% of these neonates, whereas another 10–20% develop chlamydial pneumonia within 4 months of birth. Although the use of erythromycin eye prophylaxis has markedly decreased the incidence of conjunctivitis, this topical preparation gives no protection against pneumonia.

The role of endocervical *C. trachomatis* infection in the development of spontaneous abortion, fetal death, PROM, preterm delivery, and IUGR is debated. An association with spontaneous abortion, preterm delivery, and perinatal mortality was initially noted by Martin et al.[255] These contentions have remained unsubstantiated in subsequent larger studies.[247,248,256] Interestingly, however, both Harrison et al.[248] and Sweet et al.[257] have identified a subgroup of pregnant women with chlamydial infection, those with IgM seropositivity, who may be at increased risk of PROM and preterm delivery. One recent retrospective study compared the pregnancy outcomes of women with chlamydial infection who underwent successful treatment with both untreated infected and uninfected women and found a higher incidence of PROM and preterm delivery in the untreated infected group.[258] Ryan et al.[259] reported that pregnant women with chlamydial infection treated with erythromycin had significantly lower incidences of PROM, low birthweight and perinatal death compared with untreated infected women or uninfected control subjects.

Laboratory diagnosis

The diagnosis of chlamydia has seen phenomenal evolution. In the past, culture was considered the optimal means of making the diagnosis of chlamydial infection. However, isolation of *C. trachomatis* was challenging, because the organism requires a susceptible tissue culture cell line, using a technically arduous procedure whereby these cells are inoculated with specimen and then examined 24–72 h later for the development of inclusions.

The first major advancement in making *Chlamydia* testing more available was the introduction of chlamydial antigen detection products in the late 1980s. One is fluorescent monoclonal antibody staining of chlamydial elementary bodies (MicrotracSyva Co., Palo Alto, CA, USA), and the other is an ELISA (Chlamydiazyme, Abbott Laboratories, Chicago, IL, USA). The sensitivities and specificities of both products are comparable, at more than 90%.[232] Their most appropriate use is in populations with a high prevalence of chlamydial infection because their positive predictive value decreases markedly in low-prevalence populations.

These antigen detection tests were largely replaced in the 1990s by methods using DNA probe hybridization (PACE 2 test; Gen. Probe, San Diego, CA, USA). An important advantage of the DNA probe is that it can be used in conjunction with a probe for the detection of *N. gonorrhoeae* in a single swab. As a result, it became the most widely used diagnostic test for *C. trachomatis* in the United States.[260]

Most recently, DNA amplification methodology has been introduced into clinical practice. Both PCR and LCR tests for *C. trachomatis* have excellent sensitivity, specificity, and positive predictive value.[261–263] In comparative studies, PCR and LCR have performed better than culture, antigen detection, or DNA probe techniques for the detection of *Chlamydia*. A major advantage of these amplification techniques is that they identify patients with a low inoculum of *C. trachomatis*.

Treatment

The CDC recommendations for the treatment of chlamydial genital tract infection during pregnancy are provided in Table 50.11.[201] As doxycycline and fluoroquinolones are contraindicated for pregnant women, erythromycin base and amoxicillin are the CDC-recommended regimens for the treatment of chlamydial infection during pregnancy. Crombleholme et al.[264] were the first group to demonstrate the efficacy of amoxicillin in preventing vertical transmission of *C. trachomatis*. In addition, amoxicillin was well tolerated. Subsequent, randomized, prospective trials comparing amoxicillin and erythromycin for the treatment of chlamydial infection in pregnancy demonstrated treatment success in 85–99% of amoxicillin-treated patients compared with 72–88% of erythromycin-treated cases (Table 50.12). At the time when the current CDC guidelines for the treatment of chlamydial infection were published, the safety and efficacy of azithromycin in pregnant and lactating women had not been established.[201] Thus, azithromycin was suggested as an alternative regimen for pregnant women. Other alternatives include erythromycin ethylsuccinate or the option of reducing by half the dose of erythromycin base or ethylsuccinate but doubling the length of therapy for patients not able to tolerate the larger dose of erythromycin.[201] Erythromycin estolate is contraindicated in pregnancy because it is associated with drug-induced hepatotoxicity.[201]

Table 50.11 Centers for Disease Control 2002 recommended treatment guidelines for chlamydial infections in pregnancy.

Recommended regimen
Erythromycin base, 500 mg p.o. q.i.d. for 7 days
or
Amoxicillin 500 mg p.o. t.i.d. for 7 days
Alternative regimens
Erythromycin base, 250 mg p.o. q.i.d. for 14 days
or
Erythromycin ethylsuccinate, 800 mg p.o. q.i.d. for 7 days
or
Azithromycin 1 g p.o. as a single dose

Prevention

The risks of vertical transmission to newborns, horizontal transmission to sexual partners, and possible adverse perinatal outcomes underscore the need for large-scale screening programs to detect and eradicate cervical chlamydial infections. The CDC recommends diagnostic testing for *C. trachomatis* at the first prenatal visit and, for those at high risk of contracting this infection, again during the third trimester. Finally, as with other STDs, it is important to emphasize the importance of partner screening and treatment, as well as education about safe sexual practices to avert reinfection.

Human papillomavirus

HPV is a member of the papovavirus family and is composed of double-stranded DNA. More than 100 types have been identified, of which 35 primarily infect the genital tract. Genital HPV types are generally divided into two major groups based upon their oncogenic potential.[265,266] The high-risk or oncogenic group includes HPV types 16, 18, 31, 33, 35, and 39. The low-risk group includes HPV types 6, 11, 42, 43, and 44. These low-risk HPV types are associated with genital warts (condyloma acuminata), cervical condyloma, and some cases of low-grade squamous intraepithelial lesions (LGSIL).

Table 50.12 Amoxicillin versus erythromycin for the treatment of antenatal *Chlamydia* infection.

Authors	Percentage with treatment success		
	Amoxicillin	Erythromycin	*P*-value
Crombleholme et al. 1990[264]	63/64 (98%)	55/58 (95%)	NS
Magat et al. 1993[327]	55/65 (85%)	47/65 (72%)	NS
Alray et al. 1994[328]	99/100 (99%)	87/99 (88%)	< 0.01
Silverman et al. 1994[329]	33/39 (85%)	32/38 (84%)	NS
Turrentine et al. 1995[330]	50/55 (91%)	45/53 (85%)	NS
Total	300/323 (93%)	266/313 (85%)	–

NS, not significant.

Among women in the United States today, genital warts caused by HPV is the most common viral STD.[190] Difficulties in deciphering the molecular biology of HPV slowed our progress in understanding this infection. Since the 1970s, however, the association of HPV with genital intraepithelial neoplasias and squamous cell carcinomas has been widely publicized, resulting in an increased public awareness of the problem.

Epidemiology

Sexual transmission of HPV is the primary route of transmission and results in urogenital and anorectal lesions. The highest risk groups are sexually active teenagers and young adults. Transmission rates are high, with 65% of sexual contacts becoming infected.[267] Although sexual transmission predominates, vertical transmission can occur, particularly with HPV types 6 and 11.

According to the CDC, an estimated 24 million Americans are infected with HPV and between 500 000 and one million new cases of HPV-induced genital warts occur each year in the United States.[268] Use of PCR technology has shown that the prevalence of subclinical HPV is higher, and recent studies have suggested that at least 50% of sexually active women have been infected with one or more HPV types.[265,269] Host immunity plays an important role in the development of this infection. Immunosuppressed patients, such as renal transplant recipients and pregnant women, have a higher incidence of genital warts, and their symptoms are more severe.[270]

Clinical manifestations

The majority of HPV lesions are subclinical, identified only with colposcopy, cytology, tissue examination, or *in situ* hybridization techniques. They can be found on the vulva, vagina, cervix, and anorectal region. More recently, PCR technology has been utilized for the detection of HPV. Exophytic warts, also called condyloma acuminata, are typically caused by HPV types 6 and 11. They appear as friable, pink, fleshy skin appendages that vary greatly in size and are either broad based or pedunculated. Many lesions, however, are not visible to the naked eye. These flat endophytic condylomata are found with the use of colposcopy on the cervix, vagina, and vulva.

Colposcopy uses a lighted, magnification system to view genital epithelium. A 3–5% solution of acetic acid is applied to the area to be examined and allowed to absorb. Common colposcopic findings in HPV infection are irregularly defined patches that appear shiny and white and are not confined to the transformation zone. Any suspicious lesion should be biopsied.

Laboratory diagnosis

The diagnosis of condyloma acuminata is usually made on clinical grounds. Given the high prevalence of subclinical disease, cytology, tissue biopsy, and *in situ* hybridization techniques are often necessary to make the diagnosis.

In the least sensitive of laboratory methods available, cytologic evidence in the form of koilocytosis has been found in approximately 2% of women receiving Pap smears.[271] Cervical biopsies tested for both koilocytosis and HPV antigen found that 20% were positive by both methods.[272] The most sensitive detection method for HPV has been DNA *in situ* hybridization. One study tested routine Pap smears using this technique and found that 16% had evidence of HPV types 6, 11, 16, or 18.[273]

Treatment

Treatment for HPV infection of the genital tract depends upon the anatomic location of disease (external genitalia/perianal, cervical, vaginal, or urethral), the clinical presentation of disease (clinical versus subclinical), and the extent of disease. The primary goal of treatment of external genital warts (condyloma accuminata) is to eliminate warts that cause physical or psychological symptoms or distress.[273] However, elimination of genital warts may or may not decrease infectivity because internal sites (vagina or cervix) and clinically normal skin may act as reservoirs for infection.[274]

In most patients, treatment will include wart-free periods of varying lengths. The CDC notes that there is no evidence indicating that currently available treatment modalities eradicate

Table 50.13 Centers for Disease Control 2002 recommendations for treatment of external genital warts.

Recommended treatments
Patient applied
Podofilox 0.5% solution or gel. Apply podofilox solution with a cotton swab, or podofilox gel with a finger, to visible genital warts twice a day for 3 days, followed by 4 days of no therapy. Cycle may be repeated as necessary for a total of four cycles
or
Imiquimod 5% cream. Apply with finger at bedtime, three times a week for up to 16 weeks

Provider administered
Cryotherapy with liquid nitrogen or cryoprobe. Repeat every 1–2 weeks
or
Podophyllin resin 10–25% in compound tincture of benzoin. Repeat weekly if necessary
or
TCA or BCA 80–90%. Repeat weekly if necessary
or
Surgical removal by tangential scissors excision, tangential shave excision, curettage, or electrosurgery

Alternative treatments
Intralesional interferon
or
Laser surgery

or affect the natural history of HPV infection.[201] Visible genital warts that are not treated may resolve spontaneously, remain unchanged, or increase in size or number.

For external genital/perianal warts (condyloma acuminata), the recommended therapeutic measures are listed in Table 50.13. According to the CDC, none of the currently available treatments is superior to other treatments, and no single treatment is ideal for all patients or all warts.[201] Available treatments for visible genital warts are divided into two categories: (1) patient-applied therapies (i.e., podofilox and imiquimod); and (2) provider-administered treatments (i.e., cryotherapy, podophyllin resin, trichloroacetic acid (TCA), bichloroacetic acid (BCA), interferon, and surgery). Factors influencing choice of treatment include wart size, wart number, anatomic site, wart morphology, patient preference, cost of treatment, convenience, side-effects, and provider experience.[201] Many patients require a course of therapy rather than a single treatment and, thus, it is important that providers have a treatment plan or protocol for the management of genital warts. The CDC suggests that the treatment modality should be changed if the patient has not improved substantially after three provider-administered treatments or if warts have not completely cleared following six treatments.[201]

The use of podophyllin, podofilox, and imiquimod are contraindicated in pregnancy. During pregnancy, the best approach to treatment is removal of lesions by excision, electrocautery, or cryosurgery. TCA application has been used in pregnancy without adverse effects.[275] Laser therapy is another alternative among pregnant women with extensive disease.

For the treatment of vaginal exophytic warts, the recommendations include: (1) cryotherapy with liquid nitrogen; (2) TCA or BCA 80–90%; or (3) podophyllin 10–25% in compound tincture of benzoin.[201] Because of concern about potential systemic absorptions, it is best not to use podophyllin in the vagina. Podophyllin is contraindicated in pregnancy. Podofilox is not approved for vaginal use as the patient cannot visualize the lesions for application. For urethral meatus warts, either cryotherapy with liquid nitrogen or podophyllin is recommended.[201]

Maternal and fetal risks

Warty lesions have a tendency to grow and become more vascularized during pregnancy. The only contraindications to a vaginal delivery are extensive lesions that might result in dystocia and lesions that might bleed heavily with birth trauma. Although some suggest removal of large warts during pregnancy, this practice is of uncertain benefit. Vertical transmission of HPV is rare, but can result in respiratory papillomatosis in the exposed infant. The exact mode of spread is unknown. Thus, Cesarean section is not recommended in the presence of genital warts in order to prevent vertical transmission of HPV.

Prevention

Given the fact that transmission rates are low, and adverse perinatal outcome unknown, it is not recommended that pregnant patients be routinely screened for HPV. Sexual partners of infected women should be examined for the presence of warts, and those infected should be schooled in safe sexual practices to avoid transmission to uninfected partners.

Herpes simplex virus

HSV is a double-stranded DNA virus that is a member of the Herpesviridae family. Two major serotypes are recognized: HSV-1 and HSV-2. Genital herpes is an infection caused by sexual transmission of HSV-1 and HSV-2. Following primary infection, HSV ascends to the dorsal root ganglion where it persists in a latent form throughout the host's lifetime. Subsequently, active viral replication and recurrent infection may or may not occur.

Epidemiology

There are an estimated one million new cases of genital HSV in the United States each year.[191] While approximately 5 million American adults have a history of genital herpes, serologic surveys utilizing type-specific HSV-2 antibodies to glycoprotein G have demonstrated a seroprevalence for HSV-2 in 30% of adults; thus, an estimated 45 million Americans have been infected with HSV-2.[191,276–278]

Three types of genital herpes infections are recognized on the basis of clinical history, serologic testing, and HSV typing. Primary infection is an initial infection with either HSV-1 or HSV-2 in an individual without serologic evidence of prior exposure to either HSV-1 or HSV-2. Nonprimary first clinical episode is an initial episode (clinical or subclinical) with HSV-1 or HSV-2 in an individual with serologic evidence of prior exposure to the other serotype. Recurrent genital herpes is reactivation of latent virus.

The prevalence of genital herpes based on culture of HSV in the obstetric population has been estimated at 0.1–4.0%.[279–282] However, as noted above, use of specific HSV-2 antibody has demonstrated that 30% of adults in the United States have had genital herpes infection. Thus, these older studies underestimate the prevalence in pregnant women. A concomitant increase in the incidence of neonatal herpes infections paralleled the sharp rise in genital herpes infection among adults in the United States.[283] Risk markers for herpes describe a population much different from the ones at risk for other STDs; this infection tends to occur in older, well-educated, married, white individuals.

Pathogenesis

The majority of genital herpetic infections are caused by HSV-2, although up to 15% may be due to HSV-1.[284,285] HSV infects susceptible mucosal surfaces. It has an incubation period of 2–10 days, which is followed by a primary infection characterized by focal vesicle formation and a pronounced cellular immune response. The infection enters a latent phase, with the virus ascending peripheral sensory nerves and coming to rest in nerve root ganglia. Recurrent exacerbations occur intermittently, stimulated by poorly understood mechanisms.

Clinical manifestations

As noted above, there are three types of herpetic episodes. Primary infections occur in previously unexposed hosts and are characterized by multiple, painful, vesicular lesions that ulcerate, with inguinal lymphadenopathy and flu-like symptoms, including fever, malaise, nausea, headaches, and myalgias. Symptoms usually persist for approximately 2 weeks, with viral shedding for approximately 12 days. Nearly 4% progress to viral meningitis.[286]

First-episode nonprimary genital herpes occurs in an individual with previous nongenital exposure to HSV-1 or HSV-2. Its presentation is generally much milder than primary infections.

Recurrent HSV is more frequent after HSV-2 infection. Approximately one-half of infected individuals experience a recurrence within 6 months.[286] Most of these episodes are prefaced by a 1- or 2-day prodrome consisting of localized pruritus, pain, and paresthesias. Systemic manifestations are absent. The episode usually lasts approximately half as long as the primary outbreak, with only 4–5 days of viral shedding.

Laboratory diagnosis

Until recently, viral culture was the gold standard for diagnosis of HSV infection. HSV grows rapidly, and results are generally available within 48–72 h. Cultures are more likely to be positive among patients with first episodes of HSV infection and those with vesicles or pustules rather than ulcerative or crusted lesions. Detection of HSV in culture has been facilitated by the use of monoclonal antibodies in immunofluorescence or immunoassay tests.[287]

The introduction of nucleic acid amplification tests such as PCR has revolutionized the laboratory diagnosis of HSV. Compared with culture, PCR has excellent sensitivity and specificity for the detection of HSV. The clinical implications of PCR detection of low viral load, especially among pregnant women at term, remain to be determined.

Diagnosis of HSV infection has been further enhanced by the introduction of type-specific serology.[286,288] Identifiable proteins for each HSV type are present in a characteristic protein coat; glycoprotein G-1 is associated with HSV-1 and glycoprotein G-2 with HSV-2. Detection of HSV-2 antibodies using glycoprotein G technology is virtually diagnostic of genital herpes infection. Type-specific serologic assays are now commercially available. United States FDA-approved type-specific assays include HerpeSelect-1 ELISA IgG and HerpeSelect-2 ELISA IgG and HerpeSelect 1 and 2 Immunoblot IgG (Focus Technologies, Cypress, CA, USA).

While serologic screening for HSV-1 and HSV-2 infection in the general population is not recommended,[201] screening may be useful in counseling couples in which one partner has a history of genital herpes and the other does not, especially preconception or in pregnant couples.

Maternal and fetal risks

Neither the frequency nor the severity of recurrent genital herpes is increased during pregnancy.[289] Primary episodes of genital herpes may be more severe during pregnancy.[289] Initial reports demonstrated a threefold increase in spontaneous abortion with primary maternal HSV infection in early pregnancy.[290] This association has been questioned more recently.[291] In 1997, Brown et al.[291] reported no overall differences in mean birthweight, gestational age at birth, incidence of IUGR, stillbirth, or neonatal death with acquisition of HSV infection during pregnancy. However, these investigators did demonstrate that acquisition of primary genital herpes in the third trimester of pregnancy was associated with preterm birth, IUGR, and substantial risk of neonatal herpes infection.[291]

The major adverse impact of genital herpes in pregnancy is the development of neonatal herpes infection. An estimated 700–1000 cases of neonatal herpes infection occur each year in the United States, resulting in an incidence ranging from 1 in 3500 to 1 in 5000 births.[289] Infection may be transmitted vertically either transplacentally or perinatally. Fortunately, transplacental transmission is rare. Neonatal symptoms typically arise during the first 7 days of life. Death occurs in approximately one-third of infants, and neurologic sequelae are noted in most survivors.[293] Perinatal acquisition occurs either with passage through an infected birth canal or from contact with orolabial lesions in the parents or hospital workers.[289] The vast majority (> 85%) of neonatal herpes infection is acquired from an infected maternal genital tract during the process of labor and delivery.[292]

During the past two decades, risk factors associated with transmission of HSV from mother to neonate have been elucidated.[289,292] These include: (1) HSV type (HSV-2 > HSV-1); (2) maternal clinical stage of infection (primary > recurrent); (3) anatomic site of viral shedding (cervix > labia); (4) use of fetal scalp electrode; and (5) presence and specificity of transplacental passively transferred HSV antibodies from mother to infant. With recently acquired first-episode genital HSV infection, neonates have a 10-fold greater risk of acquiring HSV infection than infants born to mothers with recurrent infection. First-episode genital herpes infection, whether primary or nonprimary, is associated with neonatal infection rates of 40% and 31% respectively. Prober et al.[294] demonstrated that passive transplacental passage of maternal antibodies to HSV-2 (but not HSV-1) are protective in a study reporting that, following exposure to HSV during labor and delivery, none of 34 infants with antibody present developed neonatal herpes infection (95% CI 0–8).

Primary HSV infection during pregnancy ranges from asymptomatic to severe, and may result in transplacental or intrapartum neonatal infection. It results in a 40% or higher risk of neonatal HSV infection, depending upon the presence or absence of maternal antibody to heterologous HSV type.[289] With nonprimary first-episode genital herpes, maternal symptoms also range from asymptomatic to severe. However, mainly intrapartum acquisition occurs, and the risk of neonatal HSV infection is up to 40%.[289] While with recurrent genital herpes symptoms also range from asymptomatic to severe, only neonatal infection secondary to intrapartum or postpartum acquisition occurs, and the estimated risk of neonatal infection is < 1–4%.[289] The estimated risk of neonatal herpes occurring from an asymptomatic mother with a history of recurrent genital HSV is less than 1 in 1000.[289]

Until the mid-1980s, the approach for prevention of neonatal herpes focused on the use of weekly cultures for HSV starting at 34–36 weeks' gestation in women with a history of recurrent genital herpes.

Because weekly maternal vaginal cultures in the third trimester do not predict viral shedding at the time of delivery, this approach was abandoned. The Infectious Disease Society for Obstetrics and Gynecology developed a position paper on the peripartum management of women with a history of HSV.[295] They made the following suggestions:

- Weekly antenatal cultures should be abandoned.
- In the absence of genital lesions, Cesarean sections should be performed for obstetric considerations only.
- A culture should be obtained from mother or neonate at delivery in order to identify exposed infants.
- Women with genital lesions should undergo Cesarean section, preferably within 6 h of membrane rupture, to prevent HSV exposure in the neonate.
- The mother should not be isolated from her infant.

Shortly thereafter (November, 1988), the ACOG issued a Technical Bulletin, which basically concurred with these recommendations.[296] ACOG stated: (1) cultures should be done when a woman has active HSV lesions during pregnancy to confirm the diagnosis; (2) if there are no visible lesions at the onset of labor, vaginal delivery is acceptable; (3) weekly surveillance cultures of pregnant women with a history of HSV infection, but no visible lesions, are not necessary and vaginal delivery is acceptable; and (4) amniocentesis, in an attempt to rule out intrauterine infection, is not recommended for mothers with HSV infection at any stage of gestation. Until recently, limited experience with active herpetic lesions in the face of preterm premature rupture of membranes (PPROM) suggested that expectant management may be successful.[297,298] More recently, Major[299] reported a series of 29 patients with PPROM complicated by active recurrent genital HSV infection. The mean gestational age of the women was 28.7 weeks (range 24.6–31 weeks), and the mean latency from development of herpes lesions to delivery was 13.2 days (range 1–35 days). There were no cases of neonatal herpes infection among the delivered newborns, and all neonatal cultures for HSV were negative (95% CI 0–10.4).

Treatment

Because there is no known cure for this virus, HSV becomes a chronic and usually recurrent infection. Fortunately, there are antiviral medications now available that reduce the duration and frequency of HSV outbreaks, reduce symptomatic HSV shedding, and reduce the transmission of HSV.[300–304] Acyclovir (Zovirax) is an antiviral agent that inhibits viral DNA synthesis by interfering selectively with viral thymidine kinase. Because of its selectivity for HSV-infected cells, acyclovir has a high margin of safety. It has been shown to ameliorate the symptoms of primary infections and, when given prophylactically, may reduce the frequency and intensity of recurrences. The drug is available in three forms: topical, oral, and intravenous. The oral preparation is considerably more effective than its topical counterpart. Oral acyclovir is recommended by the CDC for the treatment of genital herpes.[300] Intravenous treatment should be reserved for severe infection or immunocompromised hosts. More recently, two additional antiviral agents, valacyclovir and famciclovir, have been approved for the treatment and suppression of HSV infection.[300]

The current CDC-recommended treatment guidelines for herpes simplex virus infections are listed in Table 50.14. If lesions of first-episode herpes infection are not fully healed, treatment with antiviral agents can be extended beyond 10 days. Intravenous acyclovir should be reserved for severe primary outbreaks or disseminated herpes infections. In these instances, the recommended treatment is acyclovir i.v.

Table 50.14 Centers for Disease Control and Prevention 2002 recommended treatment guidelines for genital herpes.

Recommended regimens: first clinical episode
Acyclovir 400 mg orally, three times a day for 7–10 days
Acyclovir 200 mg orally, five times a day for 7–10 days
Famciclovir 250 mg orally, three times a day for 7–10 days
Valacyclovir 1 g orally, twice a day for 7–10 days
Recommended regimens: episodic recurrent regimens
Acyclovir 400 mg orally, three times a day for 5 days
Acyclovir 200 mg orally, five times a day for 5 days
Acyclovir 800 mg orally, twice a day for 5 days
Famciclovir 125 mg orally, twice a day for 5 days
Valacyclovir 500 mg orally, twice a day for 3–5 days
Valacyclovir 1 g orally, once a day for 5 days
Recommended regimens: suppression of recurrent episodes
Acyclovir 400 mg orally, twice a day
Famciclovir 250 mg orally, twice a day
Valacyclovir 500 mg orally, once a day*
Valacyclovir 1 g orally, once a day

*Valacyclovir 500 mg once a day might be less effective than other dosing regimens in patients who have frequent (≥ 10 episodes per year) recurrences.

5–10 mg/kg every 8 h for 2–7 days or until clinical improvement followed by oral antiviral therapy to complete at least 10 days of therapy.[300]

Following the first clinical episode of genital herpes, two alternative approaches are available: episodic therapy with signs of recurrent outbreak or continuous suppressive therapy. Episodic treatment has been shown to decrease the proportion of patients with outbreaks, reduce the duration of symptoms, and shorten the duration of viral shedding.[288] Suppressive therapy reduces the frequency of genital herpes recurrences by 70–80% among patients with frequent recurrences and, in many patients, no symptomatic outbreaks occur.[288]

Interest has focused on the use of acyclovir prophylaxis during late pregnancy to prevent recurrent herpes simplex virus infection at delivery.[305] Acyclovir is well tolerated in pregnancy with minimal fetal drug accumulation.[306] The Acyclovir in Pregnancy Registry assessed data from over 1200 pregnant women exposed to acyclovir with no increases in drug-related fetal abnormalities attributed to acyclovir use.[305] However, long-term developmental outcomes were not evaluated. While the CDC suggested that insufficient data exist to recommend prophylaxis in pregnancy,[300] the ACOG suggest that use of acyclovir to suppress recurrent HSV infection in late pregnancy is acceptable.[307] ACOG notes that, for women at or beyond 36 weeks of gestation who are at risk of recurrent HSV infection, antiviral therapy may be considered. However, they caution that such therapy may not reduce the likelihood of Cesarean delivery. Recently, Sheffield and colleagues[305] performed a meta-analysis of acyclovir prophylaxis to prevent HSV recurrence at delivery. They demonstrated that acyclovir prophylaxis commencing at 36 weeks' gestation was effective in reducing clinical HSV recurrences at the time of delivery [odds ratio (OR) 0.25, 95% CI 0.15–0.40], Cesarean deliveries for clinical recurrence of genital herpes (OR 0.30; 95% CI. 0.13–0.67), total HSV detection at delivery (OR 0.11; 95% CI 0.04–0.31), and asymptomatic HSV shedding at delivery (OR 0.09; 95% CI 0.02–0.39).

Prevention

The following recommendations have been suggested for the management of genital herpes infection in pregnancy.[289]

- Women with primary HSV infection during pregnancy should be treated with antiviral therapy.
- Cesarean delivery should be performed on women with first-episode HSV infection who have active lesions at the time of delivery.
- For women ≥ 36 weeks' gestation with a first episode of HSV infection during the current pregnancy, antiviral therapy should be considered.
- Cesarean delivery should be performed on women with recurrent herpes who have active lesions or prodrome at labor and delivery.
- Expectant management of patients with preterm labor or PPROM and active HSV lesion(s) may be warranted.
- For women ≥ 36 weeks' gestation who are at risk of recurrent HSV infection, antiviral therapy may also be considered.
- In women with no active lesions or prodrome during labor, Cesarean delivery should not be performed on the basis of a history of recurrent herpes.

Trichomonas vaginalis

Trichomoniasis is a localized genitourinary infection caused by the protozoon *Trichomonas vaginalis*.[308] It was first described in 1836 by Donne[308] as a nonpathogenic resident of the genital tract. Its pathogenicity was recognized during the twentieth century in a novel set of experiments in which healthy male and female volunteers were inoculated with organisms and followed to describe the natural history of the infection.[309,310] One of the most prevalent parasites in humans, it has been found in nearly 10% of healthy women and in up to 50% of patients screened at STD clinics. It has been estimated that 2–3 million women in the United States contract the infection annually.[311] More recently, Cates[191] estimated that 5 million new cases of trichomoniasis occur each year in the United States.

Epidemiology

Sexual contact is the primary mode of transmission for *T. vaginalis*, although the infection can be passed from mother to female infants during vaginal delivery. Because trichomoniasis is not a reportable infection, its epidemiology is difficult to ascertain. As noted above, as many as 5 million new cases of trichomoniasis occur annually in the United States.[191] Screening studies comparing various populations have discerned that prevalence parallels the degree of sexual activity ranging from 2–3% in middle-class women to over 50% in women attending STD clinics.[312,313] Prior to the introduction of metronidazole, *T. vaginalis* was responsible for approximately 25% of clinically evident cases of vulvovaginitis.[314] As a result of effective therapy, approximately 5–10% of vulvovaginitis is currently attributed to *T. vaginalis*.[313] As might be expected, barrier contraception has a protective effect, as do oral contraceptives.

It appears that asymptomatic infected men may serve as reservoirs for their female partners. Although only 30–40% of male partners of infected women carried *T. vaginalis*, it was recovered in 85% of female partners of infected men.[315] Finally, carriage of this STD is a risk marker for other STDs, especially gonorrhea, which is 1.4–3.0 times more frequent among women with trichomoniasis.[315,316]

Pathogenesis

T. vaginalis is an oval-shaped, moderately anaerobic protozoon. The presence of four flagella and an undulating membrane render it motile. Multiple serotypes, which may correlate with virulence, have been identified. The parasite attaches to mucous membranes, but neither enters nor kills the cells. Instead, it induces a moderate cellular immune response.

Clinical manifestations

It appears that this pathogen confines itself to the genitourinary system. Although most men are asymptomatic, anywhere from 50% to 90% of infected women become symptomatic at some time. Host factors, such as vaginal pH, circulating hormonal levels, the integrity of the normal vaginal flora, and the presence of menstrual blood, appear to play important roles in the development of symptoms.

An abnormal vaginal discharge is noted by 50–75% of symptomatic women. In only 10% of these women is the exudate malodorous. Pruritus, dysuria, and dyspareunia are experienced in up to half of them. Low abdominal pain and lymphadenitis are relatively uncommon complaints.[313,315]

Physical examination findings are normal in 15% of infected patients. Vaginal erythema and an excessive vaginal discharge are present in up to 75%, whereas vulvar inflammation is much less common. The so-called classic findings of a yellowish-green frothy discharge and strawberry cervix are relatively uncommon, seen in 25% and 2% respectively.[313,315]

Laboratory diagnosis

Because clinical manifestations are so nonspecific, the clinician must rely on laboratory parameters to make the diagnosis. Most commonly, the diagnosis is made by light microscopic examination of a saline wet mount. The vaginal pH is ≥ 4.5 in the majority of patients. Performance of a Pap smear makes the diagnosis nearly 70% of the time.[313,315,316]

Collection of a sample of vaginal discharge for wet mount or culture is the diagnostic procedure of choice. Because the organism attaches only to squamous cells, evaluation of the endocervical columnar epithelium is positive in only 13% of women. A cotton swab should be used to wipe both anterior and posterior fornices. In the preparation of a wet mount, the swab should then be rubbed across a slide containing a drop of sodium chloride and immediately overlaid with a coverslip. Low to medium (100–400 ×) magnification with a light- or darkfield microscope should be used to examine the material. More recently, *T. vaginalis* has been identified as a risk factor facilitating the transmission and acquisition of HIV.[317] Large numbers of PMNs are generally present. *T. vaginalis* can be seen as motile ovoids that appear slightly larger than PMNs.[318] The sensitivity of the wet mount ranges between 40% and 80%, matching that of the Pap smear.[313,319,320] Culture is the optimum method currently available for detecting the presence of *T. vaginalis*.[313] While easily performed, culture for *T. vaginalis* requires the use of special medium such as Diamond or Kupferberg. Culture, using a number of selective media, promotes growth in 2–7 days, and is 95% sensitive.[313] PCR technology has also been demonstrated to be an effective method for the diagnosis of trichomoniasis. However, no FDA-approved PCR test for *T. vaginalis* is currently available. An FDA-approved DNA probe-based test for *T. vaginalis* (Affirm VP III; Becton Dickinson, Sparks, MD, USA) is also available.[321]

Treatment

Until 40 years ago, trichomoniasis was a chronic, relapsing urogenital infection. In the 1960s, the 5-nitroimidazoles, including metronidazole, were developed and found to be effective in the treatment of this infection.[322] Recent years have seen the development of isolated clusters of resistant organisms.[323]

Given the colonization of both genital and urinary tracts, a systemic agent is needed. The original regimen for metronidazole therapy lasted 7 days. This has been shortened to a single oral dose in order to improve compliance, decrease the total dose, and deal with the problems of alcohol use during treatment (Table 50.15). Cure with this regimen is achieved in 82–88% of cases, and this increases to 95% when partners are treated empirically.

Relative resistance of *T. vaginalis* to metronidazole is documented.[324] For treatment failures, the CDC recommends

Table 50.15 Centers for Disease Control 2002 recommended treatment guidelines for trichomoniasis in pregnancy.

Recommended regimen
Metronidazole,* 2 g orally in a single dose
Alternative regimen
Metronidazole,* 500 mg twice daily for 7 days

*Metronidazole cannot be recommended for use in the first trimester.

retreatment with metronidazole 500 mg twice daily for 7 days.[201] If failure occurs again, a single 2-g dose once daily for 3–5 days is recommended. For patients still having persistent trichomoniasis, the CDC suggests excluding reinfection, evaluating the *in vitro* susceptibility of the isolate, and managing in consultation with an expert.[201] In May 2004, tinidazole (Tindamax) was approved by the FDA for the treatment of trichomoniasis with a suggested treatment regimen of a single 2-g oral dose.

Metronidazole freely crosses the placenta. Studies of limited numbers of pregnant women have shown no increased risk of spontaneous abortion or adverse perinatal outcomes.[313] Thus, the use of metronidazole in pregnancy appears to be safe. However, some experts prefer to wait until the second trimester to use metronidazole.[201]

Maternal and fetal risks

Studies with conflicting results have been published on the potential association of *T. vaginalis* with adverse pregnancy outcomes. In an adolescent, inner-city population with a *T. vaginalis* prevalence of 34%, Hardy et al.[312] noted that *T. vaginalis* was associated with low birthweight and preterm birth. In contradistinction, Mason and Brown,[325] in a similar high-prevalence population, found no association with adverse pregnancy outcome. In a similar vein, Minkoff et al.[326] failed to find a significant association between *T. vaginalis* and preterm labor. Conversely, the Vaginal Infection and Prematurity Study demonstrated that *T. vaginalis* in midpregnancy was significantly associated with preterm low birthweight (OR 1.6, 95% CI 1.3–1.9).[313] However, a recent prospective randomized trial of metronidazole versus placebo sponsored by the NIH demonstrated that metronidazole treatment of asymptomatic pregnant women with trichomoniasis (identified by culture) during the midtrimester resulted in an increased risk of preterm birth.[33]

Prevention

Because this infection is sexually transmitted, its diagnosis should serve as a reminder to test carefully for the coexistence of other, more dangerous STDs.

Key points

1. Determine the HIV serostatus of all women as early in pregnancy as possible. The preferred testing algorithm involves the "opt-out" approach, in which women are routinely informed that they will be tested unless they specifically request to opt out.
2. Women's viral load and CD4 counts should be monitored and HAART administered per standard recommendations. If the woman's viral load and CD4 results do not, unto themselves, justify HAART therapy, consideration should still be given to aggressive therapy in order to minimize the likelihood of MTCT.
3. While HAART is probably the most effective regimen for MTCT prevention, there are circumstances (e.g., viral load less than 1000) when alternatives might be acceptable. At a minimum, for the reduction of perinatal HIV-1 transmission, ZDV prophylaxis according to the PACTG 076 regimen is recommended unless the woman is intolerant of ZDV.
4. Plasma HIV-1 RNA levels should be monitored during pregnancy according to the guidelines for the management of HIV-1-infected adults. The most recently determined viral load value should be used when counseling a woman regarding mode of delivery.
5. If HAART is successful, then viral load will drop by more than 1 log per month, not rebound, and be undetectable within 6 months.
6. If HAART fails, resistance testing should be performed before discontinuing the initial regimen and choosing a new one.
7. Perinatal HIV-1 transmission is reduced by scheduled Cesarean delivery among women with unknown or high HIV-1 RNA levels who are not receiving antiretroviral therapy or are receiving only ZDV for prophylaxis of perinatal transmission. The benefit among women on HAART is unproven. Given the low rate of transmission among this group, particularly among those with a low viral load, it is unlikely that scheduled Cesarean delivery would confer additional benefit in reduction of transmission.
8. Management of women originally scheduled for Cesarean delivery who present with ruptured membranes or in labor must be individualized based on duration of rupture, progress of labor, plasma HIV-1 RNA level, current antiretroviral therapy, and other clinical factors. The woman's autonomy to make an informed decision regarding route of delivery should be respected and honored.
9. Women who present in labor with unknown HIV status should be offered rapid HIV testing.
10. If a woman was placed on antiretroviral therapy solely to prevent MTCT (i.e., she did not meet the criteria for therapy based on her own clinical, immunologic, or virologic status), then all medications should be discontinued once she has given birth.

References

1 Brabin BJ. Epidemiology of infection in pregnancy. *Rev Infect Dis* 1985;7:579.
2 Finland M, Dublin TD. Pneumococcal pneumonias complicating pregnancy and the puerperium. *JAMA* 1939;122:1027.
3 Greenberg M, Jacobziner H, Pakter J, et al. Maternal mortality in the epidemic of Asian influenza, New York City, 1957. *Am J Obstet Gynecol* 1 958;76:897.
4 Smale LE, Waechter KG. Dissemination of coccidioidomycosis in pregnancy. *Am J Obstet Gynecol* 1970;107:356.
5 American College of Obstetricians and Gynecologists. Immunization during pregnancy. ACOG Committee Opinion No. 282. *Obstet Gynecol* 2003;101:207.
6 Brunham RC, Maclean IW, Binns B, et al. *Chlamydia trachomatis*: its role in tubal infertility. *J Infect Dis* 1985;152:1275.
7 Brunham RC, Binns B, McDowell J, et al. *Chlamydia trachomatis* infection in women with ectopic pregnancy. *Obstet Gynecol* 1986;67:722.
8 Licciardi F, Grifo JA, Rosenwaks Z, et al. Relation between antibodies to *Chlamydia trachomatis* and spontaneous abortion following in vitro fertilization. *J Assist Reprod Genet* 1992;9: 207.
9 Centers for Disease Control and Prevention. Recommended Adult Immunization Schedule – Untied States, October 2004–September 2004. *Morbid Mortal Wkly Rep* 2004;53: Q1–4.
10 Gonik B, Fasahn N, Foster S. The obstetrician-gynecologist's role in adult immunization. *Am J Obstet Gynecol* 2002;1887: 984.
11 Gardner P, Schaffner W. Immunization of adults. *N Engl J Med* 1993;328:1252.
12 Bentley DW. Immunizations in older adults. *Infect Dis Clin Pract* 1996;5:490.
13 Mitchell LA, Zhang T, Tingle AJ. Differential antibody responses to Rubella virus infections in males and females. *J Infect Dis* 1992;166:1258.
14 Centers for Disease Control and Prevention. Hepatitis B virus: a comprehensive strategy for eliminating transmission in the United States through universal childhood vaccination. Recommendations of the Advisory Committee on Immunization Practices (ACIP). *Morbid Mortal Wkly Rep* 1991;40.
15 Gershon AA, Takahashi M, White CJ. Varicella vaccine. In: Plotkin SA, Orenstein WA, eds. *Vaccines*. Philadelphia, PA: W.B. Saunders; 1999:475.
16 Centers for Disease Control and Prevention. Prevention and control of influenza: recommendations of the Advisory Committee on Immunization Practices (ACIP). *Morbid Mortal Wkly Rep* 2000;49:1.
17 Sweet RL, Gibbs RS. Immunization. In: Sweet RL, Gibbs RS, eds. *Infectious diseases of the female genital tract*. Philadelphia, PA: Lippincott Williams and Wilkins; 2002:673.
18 Musher DM. Streptococcus pneumoniae. In: Maudel GI, Bennett JE, Dolin R, eds. *Principles and practice of infectious diseases*. New York: Churchill Livingstone; 2000:2128.
19 Markowitz JS, Pashko S, Gutterman EM, et al. Death rates among patients hospitalized with community-acquired pneumonia: an examination with data from three states. *Am J Public Health* 1996;86:1152.
20 Centers for Disease Control and Prevention. Prevention of pneumococcal disease: recommendations of the Advisory Committee on Immunization Practices (ACIP). *Morbid Mortal Wkly Rep* 1997;46:1.
21 Fedson DS, Musher DM, Eskola J. Pneumococcal vaccine. In: Plotkin SA, Orenstein WA, eds. *Vaccines*. Philadelphia, PA: W.B. Saunders; 1999:553.
22 Hillier SL, Nugent RP, Eschenback DA, et al. Association between bacterial vaginosis and preterm delivery of a low birth weight infant. *N Engl J Med* 1995;333:1737.
23 Pastorek JG, Cotch MF, Martin DH, et al. Clinical and microbiological correlates of vaginal trichomoniasis during pregnancy. *Clin Infect Dis* 1996;23:1075.
24 Thomason JL, Gelbart SM, Anderson RJ, et al. Statistical evaluation of diagnostic criteria for bacterial vaginosis. *Am J Obstet Gynecol* 1990;162:155.
25 Schwebke JR, Hillier SL, Sobel JD, et al. Validity of the vaginal Gram stain for the diagnosis of bacterial vaginosis. *Obstet Gynecol* 1996;88:573.
26 Morales WJ, Schorr J, Albretton J. Effect of metronidazole in patients with preterm birth on preceding pregnancy and bacterial vaginosis: a placebo-controlled double blind study. *Am J Obstet Gynecol* 1994;171:345.
27 Hauth JC, Goldenberg RL, Andrews WW, et al. Reduced incidence of preterm delivery with metronidazole and erythromycin in women with bacterial vaginosis. *N Engl J Med* 1995;333: 1732.
28 McDonald HM, O'Loughlin JA, Vigneswaran R, et al. Impact of metronidazole therapy on preterm birth in women with bacterial vaginosis flora: a randomized, placebo-controlled trial. *Br J Obstet Gynecol* 1997;104:1391.
29 Carey JC, Klebanoff MA, Hauth JC, et al. Metronidazole to prevent preterm delivery in pregnant women with asymptomatic bacterial vaginosis. *N Engl J Med* 2000;342:534.
30 Centers for Disease Control and Prevention. 2002 Sexually Transmitted Diseases Treatment Guidelines. *Morbid Mortal Wkly Rep* 2002;51:1.
31 Fouts AC, Kraus SJ. *Trichomonas vaginalis*: reevaluation of its clinical presentation and laboratory diagnosis. *J Infect Dis* 1980;141:137.
32 Jeremias J, Draper D, Ziegert M, et al. Detection of *Trichomonas vaginalis* using the polymerase chain reaction in pregnant and non-pregnant women. *Infect Dis Obstet Gynecol* 1994;2:16.
33 Klebanoff MA, Carey JC, Hauth JC, et al. Failure of metronidazole to prevent preterm delivery among pregnant women with asymptomatic *Trichomonas vaginalis* infection. *N Engl J Med* 2001;345:487.
34 Centers for Disease Control. US PHS/IDSA guidelines for the prevention of opportunistic infections in persons infected with human immunodeficiency virus: a summary. *Morbid Mortal Wkly Rep* 1995;44:1.
35 Foulon W, Naessens A, Derde MP. Evaluation of the possibilities for preventing congenital toxoplasmosis. *Am J Perinatol* 1994;11:57.
36 Demmler GJ. Summary of a workshop on surveillance for congenital cytomegalovirus disease. *Rev Infect Dis* 1991;13:315.
37 Hillier S. Self-diagnosis and over-the-counter treatment. *Clinician* 1994;12:12.
38 Wiesenfeld H, Macio I. The infrequent use of office-based diagnostic tests for vaginitis. *Am J Obstet Gynecol* 1999;181:39.
39 McCormack WM, Starko KM, Zinner SH. Symptoms associated with vaginal colonization with yeast. *Am J Obstet Gynecol* 1988;158:31.
40 Nyirjesy P, Seeney SM, Grody MHT, et al. Chronic fungal vaginitis: the value of cultures. *Am J Obstet Gynecol* 1995;173:820.

41 Reef SE, Levine WC, McNeil MM, et al. Treatment options for vulvovaginal candidosis, 1993. *Clin Infect Dis* 1995;20:80.
42 Pursley TJ, Blomquist IK, Abraham J, et al. Fluconazole-induced congenital anomalies in three infants. *Clin Infect Dis* 1996;22:336.
43 Sobel JD. Pathogenesis and treatment of recurrent vulvovaginal candidosis. *Clin Infect Dis* 1992;14:148.
44 Ledger WJ. Chronic vulvovaginitis. *Infect Dis Clin Pract* 1993;2:60.
45 Schulman A, Herlinger H. Urinary tract dilatation in pregnancy. *Br J Radiol* 1975;48:638.
46 Nicolle LE, Friesen D, Harding GKM, et al. Hospitalization for acute pyelonephritis in Manitoba, Canada, during the period from 1989 to 1992: impact of diabetes, pregnancy, and aboriginal origin. *Clin Infect Dis* 1996;22:1051.
47 Sweet RL, Gibbs RS. Urinary tract infection. In: Sweet RL, Gibbs RS, eds. *Infectious diseases of the female genital tract*. Philadelphia, PA: Lippincott Williams and Wilkins; 2002;413.
48 Whalley PJ. Bacteriuria of pregnancy. *Am J Obstet Gynecol* 1967;97:723.
49 Harris RE. The significance of eradication of bacteriuria during pregnancy. *Obstet Gynecol* 1979;53:71.
50 Romero R, Oyarzun E, Mazor M, et al. Meta-analysis of the relationship between asymptomatic bacteriuria and preterm delivery/low birth weight. *Obstet Gynecol* 1989;73:576.
51 Centers for Disease Control and Prevention. Prevention of perinatal group B streptococcal disease: a public health prospective. *Morbid Mortal Wkly Rep* 1996;45:1.
52 Millar LK, Cox SM. Urinary tract infections complicating pregnancy. *Infect Dis Clin North Am* 1997;11:13.
53 Stamm WE, Counts CW, Running KR, et al. Diagnosis of coliform infection in acutely dysuric women. *N Engl J Med* 1982;307:463.
54 Cunningham FG, Morris GB, Mickal A. Acute pyelonephritis of pregnancy: a clinical review. *Obstet Gynecol* 1973;42:112.
55 Cunningham FG, Leveno KJ, Hankins GOV, et al. Respiratory insufficiency associated with pyelonephritis during pregnancy. *Obstet Gynecol* 1984;63:121.
56 Purett K, Faro S. Pyelonephritis associated with respiratory distress. *Obstet Gynecol* 1987;69:444.
57 Elkington KW, Greb LC. Adult respiratory distress syndrome as a complication of acute pyelonephritis during pregnancy; case report and discussion. *Obstet Gynecol* 1986;67:185.
58 Jenkins RD, Fenn JP, Matson JM. Review of urine microscopy for bacteriuria. *JAMA* 1986;255:3397.
59 Whalley PJ, Cunningham FG, Martin F. Transient renal dysfunction associated with acute pyelonephritis of pregnancy. *Obstet Gynecol* 1975;46:174.
60 Millar LK, Wing DA, Paul RH, et al. Outpatient treatment of acute pyelonephritis in pregnancy: a randomized controlled trial. *Obstet Gynecol* 1995;86:560.
61 Brooks AM, Garite TJ. Clinical trial of the outpatient management of pyelonephritis in pregnancy. *Infect Dis Obstet Gynecol* 1955;3:50.
62 Angel JL, O'Brien WF, Finan MA, et al. Acute pyelonephritis: a prospective study of oral versus intravenous antibiotic therapy. *Obstet Gynecol* 1990;76:28.
63 Wing DA, Hendershott CM, Debuque L, et al. Outpatient management of acute pyelonephritis in pregnancy after 24 weeks. *Obstet Gynecol* 1999;94:683.
64 Benedetti TJ, Valle R, Ledger WJ. Antepartum pneumonia in pregnancy. *Am J Obstet Gynecol* 1982;144:413.
65 Madinger NE, Greenspoon JS, Ellrodt AG. Pneumonia during pregnancy: has modern technology improved maternal and fetal outcome? *Am J Obstet Gynecol* 1989;161:657.
66 Berkowitz K, La Sala A. Risk factors associated with the increasing prevalence of pneumonia during pregnancy. *Am J Obstet Gynecol* 1990;163:981.
67 Hopwood HG. Pneumonia in pregnancy. *Obstet Gynecol* 1965;28:875.
68 Richey SD, Roberts SW, Ramin KD, et al. Pneumonia complicating pregnancy. *Obstet Gynecol* 1994;84:525.
69 Stanley SK, Ostrowski MA, Justement JS, et al. Effect of immunization with a common recall antigen on viral expression in patients infected with human immunodeficiency virus types. *N Engl J Med* 1996;334:1222.
70 Bartlett JG, Mundy LM. Community acquired pneumonia. *N Engl J Med* 1995;333:1618.
71 Oxorn H. The changing aspects of pneumonia complicating pregnancy. *Am J Obstet Gynecol* 1955;70:1057.
72 Maccato ML, Pinell P, Martens MG, et al. Preterm labor and maternal hypoxia in patients with community-acquired pneumonia. *Infect Dis Obstet Gynecol* 1996;4:221.
73 Butler JC, Hofmann J, Cetron MS, et al. The continued emergence of drug-resistant *Streptococcus pneumoniae* in the United States: an update from the Centers for Disease Control and Prevention's pneumococcal sentinel surveillance system. *J Infect Dis* 1996;174:986.
74 Mandell LA, Bartlett JG, Dowell SF, et al. Update of practice guidelines for the management of community-acquired pneumonia in immunocompetent adults. *Clin Infect Dis* 2003;37: 1405.
75 Robertson L, Caley JP, Moore J. Importance of *Staphylococcus aureus* in pneumonia in the 1957 epidemic of influenza A. *Lancet* 1958;2:233.
76 Henschke C, Liberman L. Streptococcal empyema: the role of cross-sectional diagnostic imaging. *Infect Surg* 1989;8:11.
77 Soper DE, Melone PJ, Conover WB. Legionnaire disease complicating pregnancy. *Obstet Gynecol* 1986;67:10S.
78 Couch RB. Mycoplasma pneumonia (primary atypical pneumonia). In: Mandell GL, Douglas RG, Jr, Bennett JE, eds. *Principles and practices of infectious diseases*, 2nd edn. New York: Wiley, 1985.
79 Landsberger EJ, Hager WD, Grossman JH. Successful management of varicella pneumonia complicating pregnancy. A report of three cases. *J Reprod Med* 1986;31:311.
80 Espinal MA, Reingold AL, Lavander M. Effect of pregnancy on the risk of developing active tuberculosis. *J Infect Dis* 1996;173:488.
81 Telzak EE, Sepkowitz K, Alpert P, et al. Multidrug-resistant tuberculosis in patients without HIV infection. *N Engl J Med* 1995;333:907.
82 Centers for Disease Control and Prevention. Treatment of tuberculosis. *Morbid Mortal Wkly Rep* 2003;52:1.
83 Shin S, Guerra D, Rich M, et al. Treatment of multidrug-resistant tuberculosis during pregnancy: a report of 7 cases. *Clin Infect Dis* 2003;36:996.
84 Quagliarello VJ, Scheld WM. Drug therapy: treatment of bacterial meningitis. *N Engl J Med* 1997;336:708.
85 Luft BJ, Remington JS. Toxoplasmic encephalitis in AIDS. *Clin Infect Dis* 1992;5:211.
86 Stafford CR, Fisher JF, Fadel HE, et al. Cryptococcal meningitis in pregnancy. *Obstet Gynecol* 1983;62:355.
87 Pastorek JG, Plauche WC, Faro S. Acute bacterial endocarditis

in pregnancy. A report of three cases. *J Reprod Med* 1983;28:611.
88 Cox SM, Hankins GDV, Leveno KJ, et al. Bacterial endocarditis. *J Reprod Med* 1988;33:671.
89 Durack DT. Prevention of infective endocarditis. *N Engl J Med* 1995;332:38.
90 Boggess KA, Watts DH, Hillier SL, et al. Bacteremia shortly after placental separation during Cesarean delivery. *Obstet Gynecol* 1996;87:779.
91. Sweet RL, Gibbs RS. Antibiotic prophylaxis in obstetrics and gynecology. In: Sweet RL, Gibbs RS, eds. *Infectious diseases of the female genital tract*. Philadelphia, PA: Lippincott Williams and Wilkins; 2002:661.
92 Dajani AS, Taubert KA, Wilson W, et al. Prevention of bacterial endocarditis. Recommendations by the American Heart Association. *JAMA* 1997;277:1795.
93 Smith-Levitin M, Skupski DW. Antepartum mastitis: a case report. *Infect Dis Obstet Gynecol* 1995;3:34.
94 Reed C, Killackey M. The acute surgical abdomen in pregnancy. *Infect Surg* 1982;1:126.
95 Sweet RL, Gibbs RS. Hepatitis infection. In: Sweet RL, Gibbs RS, eds. *Infectious diseases of the female genital tract*. Philadelphia, PA: Lippincott Williams and Wilkins; 2002:207.
96 Snydman D. Hepatitis in pregnancy. *N Engl J Med* 1985;313: 1398.
97 Kuo, G, Choo HJ, Alter GL, et al. An essay for circulatory antibodies to a major etiologic virus of human non-A non-B hepatitis. *Science* 1989;244:362.
98 Esteban JI, Gonzalez A, Hernandes JM, et al. Evaluation of antibodies to hepatitis C virus in a study of transfusion associated hepatitis. *N Engl J Med* 1990;323:1107.
99 Iworson S, Norkrans G, Wejstäl R. Hepatitis C: natural history of a unique infection. *Clin Infect Dis* 1995;20:1361.
100 Joffe GM. Hepatitis C virus in pregnancy: case reports and literature review. *Infect Dis Obstet Gynecol* 1995;3:248.
101 Donahue JG, Munoz A, Ness PM, et al. The declining risk of post-transfusion hepatitis C virus infection. *N Engl J Med* 1992;327:369.
102 Kao J-H, Chen P-J, Yang P-M, et al. Intrafamilial transmission of hepatitis C virus: the important role of infection between spouses. *J Infect Dis* 1992;166:900.
103 Novati R, Thiers V, Monforte Ad'A, et al. Mother-to-child transmission of hepatitis C virus detected by nested polymerase chain reaction. *J Infect Dis* 1992;165:720.
104 Caredda F, Rossi E, Monforte A, et al. Hepatitis B virus-associated coinfection and superinfection with della agent: indistinguishable disease with different outcome. *J Infect Dis* 1985;151: 925.
105 Centers for Disease Control. Hepatitis E among US travelers, 1989–1992. *Morbid Mortal Wkly Rep* 1993;42:1.
106 Krawczynski K. Hepatitis E. *Hepatology* 1993;17:932.
107 Klein NA, Mabie WC, Shaver DC, et al. Herpes simplex virus hepatitis. *Gastroenterology* 1991;100:239.
108 Chatelain S, Neumann DE, Alexander SM. Fatal herpetic hepatitis in pregnancy. *Infect Dis Obstet Gynecol* 1994;1:246.
109 Stauffer RA, Wygal J, Lavery JP. Spontaneous bacterial peritonitis in pregnancy. *Am J Obstet Gynecol* 1982;144:104.
110 Browne MK, Cassie R. Spontaneous bacterial peritonitis during pregnancy. *Br J Obstet Gynaecol* 1981;88:1150.
111 Hamer DH. IDCP guidelines: infectious diarrhea: part 1. *Infect Dis Clin Pract* 1997;6:68.
112 Sweet RL, Gibbs RS. Parasitic diseases in pregnancy. In: Sweet RL, Gibbs RS, eds. *Infectious diseases of the female genital tract*. Philadelphia, PA: Lippincott Williams and Wilkins; 2002: 570.
113 Roberts NS, Copel JA, Bhutani V, et al. Intestinal parasites and other infections during pregnancy in Southeast Asian refugees. *J Reprod Med* 1985;30:720.
114 Lee RV. G.I. parasites: how hazardous in pregnancy? *Contemp Gynecol Obstet* 1987;29:137.
115 Nyirjesy P, Kauasya T, Axelrod P, et al. Malaria during pregnancy: neonatal morbidity and mortality and the efficacy of chloroquine chemoprophylaxis. *Clin Infect Dis* 1993;16:127.
116 Steere AC, Malawista SE, Snydman DR, et al. Lyme arthritis: an epidemic of oligoarticular arthritis in children and adults in three Connecticut communities. *Arthritis Rheum* 1977;20:7.
117 Burgdorfer W, Barbour AG, Hayes SF, et al. Lyme disease – a tick borne spirochetosia? *Science* 1982;216:1317.
118 Schlesinger PA, Duray PH, Burke BA, et al. Maternal–fetal transmission of the Lyme disease spirochete: *Borrelia burgdorferi*. *Ann Intern Med* 1985;103:67.
119 Markowitz LE, Steere AC, Benach JL. Lyme disease during pregnancy. *JAMA* 1986;255:3394.
120 Grodzicki RL, Steere AC. Comparison of immunoblotting and indirect enzyme linked immunoabsorbent assay using different antigen preparations for diagnosing early Lyme disease. *J Infect Dis* 1988;157:790.
121 Magnarelli LA, Anderson JF, Johnson RC. Cross reactivity in serological tests for Lyme disease and other spirochetal infections. *J Infect Dis* 1987;156:183.
122 Steere AC, Hutchinson GW, Rahn DW, et al. Treatment of the early manifestation of Lyme disease. *Ann Intern Med* 1983;99:22.
123 Dattwyler RJ, Halperin JJ, Puss H, et al. Ceftriaxone as effective therapy in refractory Lyme disease. *J Infect Dis* 1987;155:1322.
124 Spack DH, Liles WC, Campbell GL, et al. Tick borne diseases in the United States. *N Engl J Med* 1993;329:936.
125 Gayle HD. Curbing the global AIDS epidemic. *N Engl J Med* 2003;348:1802.
126 *HIV/AIDS update: a glance at the HIV epidemic*. Atlanta, GA: Centers for Disease Control and Prevention. Available at http//www.cdc.gov/nchstp/od/news/At-a-Glance.pdf. Retrieved November 22, 2004.
127 Fauci AS, Lane HC. Human immunodeficiency virus (HIV) disease: AIDS and related disorders. In: Brunwald E, Fauci AS, Isselbecher KJ, et al., eds. *Harrison's textbook of medicine*. New York. McGraw-Hill, Chapter 309.
128 Maury W, Potts BJ, Rabson AB. HIV-1 infection of the first-trimester and term human placental tissue: a possible mode of maternal-fetal transmission. *J Infect Dis* 1989;160:583.
129 Levy JA. Infection by human immunodeficiency virus: CD4 is not enough. *N Engl J Med* 1996;335:1528.
130 Centers for Disease Control. 1993 Revised classification system for HIV infection and expanded surveillance case definition for AIDS among adolescents and adults. *Morbid Mortal Wkly Rep* 1992;41:1.
131 Ho DD, Neumann AU, Perelson AS, et al. Rapid turnover of plasma virions and CD4 lymphocytes in HIV-1 infection. *Nature* 1995;373:123.
132 Lifson AR, Rutherford GW, Jaffe HW. The natural history of human immunodeficiency virus infection. *J Infect Dis* 1988;158:1360.
133 Goedert JJ, Kessler CM, Aledort LM, et al. A prospective study of human immunodeficiency virus type 1 infection and the

development of AIDS in subjects with hemophilia. *N Engl J Med* 1989;321:1141.

134 Yenni PG, Hammer SM, Hirsch MS, et al. Treatment for adult HIV infection. 2004 recommendations of the International AIDS Society–USA Panel. *JAMA* 2004;292:251.

135 AIDSinfo.nih.gov.

136 HIV testing among pregnant women – United States and Canada, 1998–2001. *Morbid Mortal Wkly Rep* 2002;51:1013.

137 American College of Obstetricians and Gynecologists. Prenatal and perinatal human immunodeficiency virus testing: expanded recommendations. ACOG Committee Opinion No. 304. *Obstet Gynecol* 2004;104:1119.

138 Wade NA, Birkhead GS, Warren BL, et al. Abbreviated regimens of zidovudine prophylaxis and perinatal transmission of the human immunodeficiency virus. *N Engl J Med* 1998;339: 1409.

139 *Rapid HIV antibody testing during labor and delivery for women of unknown HIV status: a practical guide and model protocol.* Centers for Disease Control and Prevention. Atlanta, GA: CDC; 2004. Available at http://www.cdc.gov/hiv/rapid/testing/materials/.

140 Bulterys M, Jamieson DJ, O'Sullivan MJ, et al. Rapid HIV-1 testing during labor: a multicenter study. Mother–Infant Rapid Intervention at Delivery (MIRIAD) Study Group. *JAMA* 2004; 292:219.

141 Durant J, Clevenbergh P, Halfon P, et al. Drug-resistance in HIV-1 therapy: the VIRADAPT randomized control trial. *Lancet* 1999;353:2195.

142 Minkoff H. HIV Infections in pregnancy. *Obstet Gynecol* 2003;101:797.

143 Watts H, Minkoff H. Managing pregnant patients. In: Dolin R, Masur H, Saag M, eds. *AIDS therapy*, 2nd edn. New York: Churchill Livingstone, 2002.

144 Hirsch MS, Brun-Vezinet F, D'Auila RT, et al. Antiretroviral drug resistance testing in adult HIV-1 infection: recommendations of an International AIDS Society–USA Panel. *JAMA* 2000,283: 2417.

145 Yeni PG, Hammer SM, Carpenter CCJ, et al. Antiretroviral treatment for adult HIV-1 infection in 2002: updated recommendations of the International AIDS Society–USA panel. *JAMA* 2002;288:222.

146 Chene G, Sterne JA, May M, et al. Prognostic importance of initial response in HIV-1 infected patients starting potent antiretroviral therapy: analysis of prospective studies. *Lancet* 2003;362:679.

147 Egger M, May M, Chene G, et al. Prognosis of HIV-1 infected drug naive patients starting potent antiretroviral therapy: a collaborative analysis of prospective studies. *Lancet* 2002;360: 119.

148 Palella FJ, Deloria-Knoll M, Chmiel JS, et al. Survival benefit of initiating antiretroviral therapy in HIV-infected persons in different CD4+ cell strata. *Ann Intern Med* 2003;138:620.

149 Sterling TR, Chaisson RE, Keruly J, Moore RD. Improved outcomes with earlier initiation of highly active antiretroviral therapy among human immunodeficiency virus-infected patients who achieve durable virologic suppression: longer follow-up of an observational cohort study. *J Infect Dis* 2003;188: 1659.

150 Wood E, Hogg RS, Yip B, et al. Higher baseline levels of plasma human immunodeficiency virus type 1 RNA are associated with increased mortality after initiation of triple-drug antiretroviral therapy. *J Infect Dis* 2003;188:1421.

151 Robbins GK, De Gruttola V, Shafer RW, et al. Comparison of sequential three-drug regimens as initial therapy for HIV-1 infection. *N Engl J Med* 2003;349:2293.

152 Shafer RW, Smeaton LM, Robbins GK, et al. Comparison of four-drug regimens and pairs of sequential three-drug regimens as initial therapy for HIV-1 infection. *N Engl J Med* 2003;349:2304.

153 Lichtenstein KA, Delaney KM, Armon C, et al. Incidence of and risk factors for lipoatrophy (abnormal fat loss) in ambulatory HIV-1-infected patients. *J Acquir Immune Defic Syndr* 2003;32:48.

154 Carr A, Samaras K, Burton S, et al. A syndrome of peripheral lipodystrophy, hyperlipidaemia and insulin resistance in patients receiving HIV protease inhibitors. *AIDS* 1998;12:51.

155 Study Team. Efficacy of three short-course regimens of zidovudine and lamivudine in preventing early and late transmission of HIV-1 from mother to child in Tanzania, South Africa, and Uganda (Petra study): a randomized, double-blind, placebo-controlled trial. *Lancet* 2002;359:1178.

156 Guay LA, Musoke P, Fleming T, et al. Intrapartum and neonatal single-dose nevirapine compared with zidovudine for prevention of mother-to-child transmission of HIV-1 in Kampala, Uganda: HIVNET 012 randomized trial. *Lancet* 1999;354: 795.

157 Jourdaine G, Ngo-Giang-Huong N, Le Couer S, et al. Intrapartum exposure to nevirpaine and subsequent maternal responses to nevirapine based antiretroviral therapy. *N Engl J Med* 2004;351:229.

158 The International Perinatal HIV Group. The mode of delivery and the risk of vertical transmission of human immunodeficiency virus type 1 – a meta-analysis of 15 prospective cohort studies. *N Engl J Med* 1999;340:977.

159 The European Mode of Delivery Collaboration. Elective Cesarean section versus vaginal delivery in prevention of vertical HIV-1 transmission: a randomized clinical trial. *Lancet* 199;353:1035.

160 ACOG Committee on Obstetric Practice. Scheduled Cesarean delivery and the prevention of vertical transmission of HIV infection. ACOG Committee Opinion 1999;219.

161 Ioannidis JPA, Abrams EJ, Ammann A, et al. Perinatal transmission of human immunodeficiency virus type 1 by pregnant women with RNA virus loads <1000 copies/ml. *J Infect Dis* 2001;183:539.

162 The Italian Register for Human Immunodeficiency Virus Infection in Children. Determinants of mother-to-infant human immunodeficiency virus 1 transmission before and after the introduction of zidovudine prophylaxis. *Arch Pediatr Adolesc Med* 2002;156:915.

163 European Collaborative Study. HIV-infected pregnant women and vertical transmission in Europe since 1986. *AIDS* 2001;15:761.

164 Shapiro D, Tuomala R, Pollack H, et al. Mother-to child HIV transmission risk according to antiretroviral therapy, mode of delivery, and viral load in 2895 US women (PACTG 367). Oral presentation at the 11th Conference on Retroviruses and Opportunistic Infections, San Francisco, CA, February, 2004. Abstract 99.

165 Thorne C, Newell ML, for the European Collaborative Study. The continuing conundrum of mode of delivery in HIV-infected women in the HAART era. Oral presentation at the XV International AIDS Conference, Bangkok, Thailand, July, 2004. Abstract ThOrC1419.

166 Nielsen TF, Hokegard KH. Postoperative Cesarean section morbidity: a prospective study. *Am J Obstet Gynecol* 1983;146: 911.

167 Hebert PR, Reed G, Entman SS, et al. Serious maternal morbidity after childbirth: prolonged hospital stays and readmissions. *Obstet Gynecol* 1999;99:942.

168 Minkoff H, Chervenak F. Elective primary Cesarean delivery. *N Engl J Med* 2003;348:946.

169 Read JS, Tuomala R, Kpamegan E, et al. Mode of delivery and postpartum morbidity among HIV-infected women: the Women and Infants Transmission Study. *J Acquir Immune Defic Syndr* 2001;26:236.

170 Watts DH, Lambert JS, Stiehm ER, et al. Complications according to mode of delivery among human immunodeficiency virus infected women with CD4 lymphocyte counts of < or = 500/microL. *Am J Obstet Gynecol* 2000; 183:100.

171 Marcollet A, Goffinet F, Firtion G, et al. Differences in postpartum morbidity in women who are infected with the human immunodeficiency virus after elective Cesarean delivery, emergency Cesarean delivery, or vaginal delivery. *Am J Obstet Gynecol* 2002;186:784.

172 European HIV in Obstetrics Group. Higher rates of post-partum complications in HIV-infected than in uninfected women irrespective of mode of delivery. *AIDS* 2004;18:933.

173 Semprini AE, Castagna C, Ravizza M, et al. The incidence of complications after caesarean section in 156 HIV-positive women. *AIDS* 1995;9:913.

174 Grubert TA, Reindell D, Kastner R, et al. Complications after caesarean section in HIV-1-infected women not taking antiretroviral treatment. *Lancet* 1999;354:1612.

175 Maiques-Montesinos V, Cervera-Sanchez J, Bellver-Pradas J, et al. Post-Cesarean section morbidity in HIV-positive women. *Acta Obstet Gynecol Scand* 1999;78:789.

176 Vimercati A, Greco P, Loverro G, et al. Maternal complications after caesarean section in HIV infected women. *Eur J Obstet Gynecol Reprod Biol* 2000;90:73.

177 Rodriguez EJ, Spann C, Jamieson D, et al. Postoperative morbidity associated with Cesarean delivery among human immunodeficiency virus-seropositive women. *Am J Obstet Gynecol* 2001;184:1108.

178 Urbani G, de Vries MMJ, Cronje HS, et al. Complications associated with Cesarean section in HIV-infected patients. *Int J Gynecol Obstet* 2001;74:9.

179 Avidan MS, Ferrero S, Bentivoglio G. Post-operative complications after caesarean section in HIV-infected women. *Arch Gynecol Obstet* 2003;268:268.

180 Avidan MS, Panburana P, Groves P, et al. Low complication rate associated with Cesarean section under spinal anesthesia for HIV-1-infected women on antiretroviral therapy. *Anesthesiology* 2002;97:320.

181 Panburana P, Phaupradit W, Tantisirin O, et al. Maternal complications after caesarean section in HIV-infected pregnant women. *Aust NZ J Obstet Gynaecol* 2003;43:160.

182 ACOG Educational Bulletin. Assessment of fetal lung maturity. No. 230, November, 1996. Committee on Educational Bulletins of the American College of Obstetricians and Gynecologists. *Int J Gynaecol Obstet* 1997;56:191.

183 Parilla BV, Dooley SL, Jansen RD, Socol ML. Iatrogenic respiratory distress syndrome following elective repeat Cesarean delivery. *Obstet Gynecol* 1993;81:392.

184 Madar J, Richmond S, Hey E. Surfactant-deficient respiratory distress after elective delivery at "term". *Acta Pediatr* 1999;88:1244.

185 Centers for Disease Control. Recommendations of the Public Health Service Task Force on use of zidovudine to reduce perinatal transmission of human immunodeficiency virus. *Morbid Mortal Wkly Rep* 1994;43:1.

186 Minkoff H, Burns DN, Landesman S, et al. The relationship of the duration of ruptured membranes to vertical transmission of human immunodeficiency virus. *Am J Obstet Gynecol* 1995;173:585.

187 Landesman SH, Kalish LA, Burns DN, et al. Obstetrical factors and the transmission of human immunodeficiency virus type 1 from mother to child. *N Engl J Med* 1996;34: 1617.

188 Garcia PM, Kalish LA, Pitt J, et al. Maternal levels of plasma human immunodeficiency virus type 1 RNA and the risk of perinatal transmission. *N Engl J Med* 1999;341:394.

189 Mofenson LM, Lambert JS, Stiehm ER, et al. Risk factors for perinatal transmission of human immunodeficiency virus type 1 in women treated with zidovudine. Pediatric AIDS Clinical Trials Group Study 185 Team. *N Engl J Med* 1999;341: 385.

190 Eng TR, Butler WT, eds. *The hidden epidemic: confronting sexually transmitted diseases.* Committee on Prevention and Control of Sexually Transmitted Diseases. Washington, DC: Institute of Medicine National Academy Press, 1997.

191 Cates W and The American Social Health Panel. Estimates of the incidence and prevalence of sexually transmitted diseases in the United States. *Sex Transm Dis* 1999;26(Suppl.):S2.

192 Weinstock H, Berman S, Cates W, Jr. Sexually transmitted diseases among American youth: incidence and prevalence estimates, 2000. *Perspect Sexual Reprod Health* 2004;36:1. http://www.guttmacher-org/pubs/.

193 Westrom L. Incidence, prevalence and trends of acute pelvic inflammatory disease and its consequences in industrialized countries. *Am J Obstet Gynecol* 1980;38:880.

194 Chow JM. Yonekura ML, Richwald GA, et al. The association between *Chlamydia trachomatis* and ectopic pregnancy: a matched-pair, case-control study. *JAMA* 1990;26:3164.

195 Svensson L, Mardh P-A, Ahlgren M, et al. Ectopic pregnancy and antibodies to *Chlamydia trachomatis*. *Fertil Steril* 1984;44: 313.

196 Brunham RC, Binns B, McDowell J, et al. *Chlamydia trachomatis* infection in women with ectopic pregnancy. *Obstet Gynecol* 1986;67:722.

197 Martin DH, Koutsky L, Eschenbach DA, et al. Prematurity and perinatal mortality in pregnancies complicated by maternal *Chlamydia trachomatis* infections. *JAMA* 1982;247:1585.

198 zur Hansen H, Schneider A. The role of papillomaviruses in human anogenital cancer. In: Salzmann NP, Howley PM, eds. *The papovaviridae, the papillomaviruses*, Vol. 2. New York: Plenum; 1987:245.

199 Chu SY, Buehler JW, Berkelman RL. Impact of the human immunodeficiency virus epidemic on mortality in women of reproductive age. United States. *JAMA* 1990;26:4225.

200 Centers for Disease Control Summary of Notifiable Diseases – United States, 2003. *Morbid Mortal Wkly Rep* 2005;52:1.

201 Centers for Disease Control and Prevention. 2002 sexually transmitted diseases treatment guidelines. *Morbid Mortal Wkly Rep* 2002;51:1.

202 Meyer TF. Pathogenic Neisseriae: complexity of pathogen–host cell interplay. *Clin Infect Dis* 1999;28:433.

203 Kellogg DS, Jr, Peacock WL, Jr, Deacon WE, et al: Neisseria gonorrhoeae. I. Virulence genetically linked to clonal variation. *J Bacteriol* 1963;85:1274.
204 Hook EW, Handsfield HH. Gonococcal infections in adults. In: Holmes KK, Sparling PF, Mardh P-A, et al, eds. *Sexually transmitted diseases*. New York: McGraw-Hill; 1999:451.
205 Pedersen AHB, Bonin P. Screening females for asymptomatic gonorrhea infection. *Northwest Med* 1971;70:255.
206 McCormack WM, Stumacher RJ, Johnson K, Donner A. Clinical spectrum of gonococcal infection in women. *Lancet* 1977;2:1182.
207 Corman LC, Levison ME, Knight R, et al. The high frequency of pharyngeal gonococcal infection in a prenatal clinic population. *JAMA* 1974;230:568.
208 Holmes KK, Counts GW, Beaty HN. Disseminated gonococcal infection. *Ann Intern Med* 1971;74:979.
209 Suleiman SA, Grimes EM, Jones HS. Disseminated gonococcal infections. *Obstet Gynecol* 1983;61;48.
210 Holmes KK. Gonococcal infection. In: Remington JS, Klein JO, eds. *Infectious diseases of the fetus and newborn infant*. Philadelphia, PA: W.B. Saunders; 1983:616.
211 Amstey MS, Steadman KT. Symptomatic gonorrhea and pregnancy. *J Am Vener Dis Assoc* 1976;3:14.
212 Sarrel PM, Pruett KA. Symptomatic gonorrhea during pregnancy. *Obstet Gynecol* 1968;32:670.
213 Handsfield HH, Hodson A, Holmes KK. Neonatal gonococcal infection. 1. Orogastric contamination with *Neisseria gonorrhoeae*. *JAMA* 1973;22:56.
214 Edwards LE, Barrada MI, Hamann AA, Hakanson EY. Gonorrhea in pregnancy. *Am J Obstet Gynecol* 1978;13:26.
215 Phillips RS, Hanff PA, Wertheimer A, Aronson MD. Gonorrhea in women seen for routine gynecologic care: criteria for testing. *Am J Med* 1988;85:177.
216 Sweet RL, Gibbs RS. Sexually transmitted diseases. In: Sweet RL, Gibbs RS, eds. *Infectious diseases of the female genital tract*. Philadelphia, PA: Lippincott-Williams & Wilkins; 2002:118.
217 Nakashim AK, Rolfs RT, Flock MC, et al. Epidemiology of syphilis in the United States 1941–1993. *Sex Transm Dis* 1996;23:16.
218 Centers for Disease Control. Congenital syphilis, United States, 1983–1985. *Morbid Mortal Wkly Rep* 1986;35:625.
219 Centers for Disease Control. Increases in primary and secondary syphilis, United States. *Morbid Mortal Wkly Rep* 1987;36:393.
220 Centers for Disease Control. Summary of notifiable diseases, United States 1995. *Morbid Mortal Wkly Rep* 1995;44.
221 Centers for Disease Control. Sexually transmitted disease surveillance, 2003. Atlanta, GA: US Department of Health and Human Services, CDC, 2004.
222 Ziya PR, Hankins DV, Gilstrap LC, Halsey AB. Intravenous penicillin desensitization and treatment during pregnancy. *JAMA* 1986;256:2561.
223 Wendel GD, Stark BJ, Jamison RB, et al. Penicillin allergy and desensitization in serious maternal/fetal infections. *N Engl J Med* 1985;312:1299.
224 Cox SM, Klein VR, Wendel GD. *The Jarisch–Herxheimer reaction in pregnancy*. San Antonio: Society of Perinatal Obstetricians; 1987:abstract 106.
225 Paley SS. Syphilis in pregnancy. *NY J Med* 1937;37:585.
226 Ingall D, Sanchez PJ, Musher D. Syphilis. In: Remington JS, Klein JO, eds. *Infectious diseases of the fetus and newborn infant*. Philadelphia, PA: W.B. Saunders; 1995:529.
227 Fiumara NJ, Fleming WL, Downing JG, Good FL. The incidence of prenatal syphilis at the Boston City Hospital. *N Engl J Med* 1952;247:48.
228 Ricci JM, Fojaco RM, O'Sullivan MJ. Congenital syphilis: the University of Miami/Jackson Memorial Medical Center Experience 1986–1988. *Obstet Gynecol* 1989;74:687.
229 McFarlin BL, Bottoms SF, Dock BS, Isada NB. Epidemic syphilis: maternal factors associated with congenital infection. *Am J Obstet Gynecol* 1994;170:535.
230 Cates W, Jr, Wasserheit JN. Genital chlamydial infections: epidemiology and reproductive sequelae. *Am J Obstet Gynecol* 1991;164:1771.
231 Washington AE, Johnson RE, Sanders LL. *Chlamydia trachomatis* infections in the United States: what are they costing us? *JAMA* 1987;157:2070.
232 Sweet RL, Gibbs RS. Chlamydial infections. In: Sweet RL, Gibbs RS, eds. *Infectious diseases of the female genital tract*. Philadelphia, PA: Lippincott-Williams & Wilkins; 2002:57.
233 Thompson SE, Washington AE. Epidemiology of sexually transmitted *Chlamydia trachomatis* infections. *Epidemiol Rev* 1983;5:96.
234 Schachter J, Stoner E, Moncoda J. Screening for chlamydial infections in women attending family planning clinics: evaluations of presumptive indicators for therapy. *West J Med* 1983;138:375.
235 Arya OP, Mallinson H, Goddaard AD. Epidemiological and clinical correlates of chlamydial infection of the cervix. *Br J Venereal Dis* 1981;57:118.
236 Chacko MR, Louchik JC. *Chlamydia trachomatis* infection in sexually active adolescents: prevalence and risk factors. *Pediatrics* 1984;73:836.
237 Stamm WE, Wagner KF, Ansel R, et al. Causes of the acute urethral syndrome in women. *N Engl J Med* 1980;303:409.
238 Moller BR, Ahoms S, Laurin J, Mardh P-A. Pelvic infection after elective abortion associated with *Chlamydia trachomatis*. *Obstet Gynecol* 1982;59:210.
239 Westergard L, Philipson T, Scheibel J. Significance of cervical *Chlamydia trachomatis* infection in postabortal pelvic inflammatory disease. *Obstet Gynecol* 1982;60:322.
240 Quigstad E, Skaug K, Jerve F, et al. Pelvic inflammatory disease associated with *Chlamydia trachomatis* infection after therapeutic abortion. *Br J Venereal Dis* 1983;59:189.
241 Osser S, Persson K. Postabortal pelvic infection associated with *Chlamydia trachomatis* and the influence of humoral immunity. *Am J Obstet Gynecol* 1984;150:699.
242 Barbacci MB, Spence MR, Kappus EW, et al. Postabortal endometritis and isolation of trachomatis. *Obstet Gynecol* 1986;68:686.
243 Ismail MA, Chandler AE, Beem MO, Moawad AH. *Chlamydia* colonization of the cervix in pregnant adolescents. *J Reprod Med* 1985;30:549.
244 Wager GP, Martin DH, Koutsky L, et al. Puerperal infectious morbidity: relationship to route of delivery and to antepartum *Chlamydia trachomatis* infection. *Am J Obstet Gynecol* 1980;138:1028.
245 Cytryn A, Sen P, Haingsub R, et al. Severe pelvic infection from *Chlamydia trachomatis* after Cesarean section. *JAMA* 1982;247:1732.
246 Hoyme UB, Kiviat N, Eschenbach DA. Microbiology and treatment of late postpartum endometritis. *Obstet Gynecol* 1986;68:226.
247 Thompson S, Lopez B, Wong KG, et al. A prospective study of chlamydial and mycoplasmal infections during pregnancy. In:

Mardh P-A, Holmes KK, Oriel JD, et al, eds. *Chlamydial infections*, Vol. 2. Fernstrom Foundation Series. Amsterdam: Elsevier; 1982:155.

248 Harrison HR, Alexander ER, Weinstein L, et al. Cervical *Chlamydia trachomatis* and mycoplasmal infections in pregnancy. Epidemiology and outcomes. *JAMA* 1983;250:1721.

249 Sweet RL, Landers DV, Walker C, Schachter J. *Chlamydia trachomatis* infection and pregnancy outcome. *Am J Obstet Gynecol* 1987;156:824.

250 Thygeson P, Mengert WF. The virus of inclusion conjunctivitis: further observations. *Arch Ophthalmol* 1936;15:377.

251 Lennon GG. Acute salpingitis during pregnancy. *J Obstet Gynaecol Br Commonw* 1948;56:1035.

252 McCord M, Simmons CM. Acute purulent salpingitis during pregnancy. *Am J Obstet Gynecol* 1953;65:1136.

253 Acosta AA, Mabray CR, Kaurman RH. Intrauterine pregnancy and coexistent pelvic inflammatory disease. *Obstet Gynecol* 1971;37:282.

254 Blanchard AC, Pastorek JG, II, Weeks T. Pelvic inflammatory disease during pregnancy. *South Med J* 1987;80:1363.

255 Martin DH, Koutsky L, Eschenbach DA, et al. Prematurity and perinatal mortality in pregnancies complicated by maternal *Chlamydia trachomatis* infections. *JAMA* 1982;247:1585.

256 Hardy PH, Hardy JB, Nell EE, et al. Prevalence of six sexually transmitted disease agents among pregnant inner-city adolescents and pregnancy outcome. *Lancet* 1984;2:333.

257 Sweet RL, Landers DV, Walker C, Schachter J. *Chlamydia trachomatis* infection and pregnancy outcome. *Am J Obstet Gynecol* 1987;156:824.

258 Cohen I, Veille JC, Calkins BM. Improved pregnancy outcome following successful treatment of chlamydial infection. *JAMA* 1990;263:3160.

259 Ryan GM, Abdella JN, McNeeley SG, et al. *Chlamydia trachomatis* infection in pregnancy and effect of treatment on outcome. *Am J Obstet Gynecol* 1990;162:34.

260 Black CM. Current methods of laboratory diagnosis of *Chlamydia trachomatis* infections. *Clin Microbiol Rev* 1997;10:160.

261 Sweet RL, Wiesenfeld HC, Uhrin M, Dixon B. Comparison of EIA, culture, and polymerase chain reaction for *Chlamydia trachomatis* in a sexually transmitted disease clinic. *J Infect Dis* 1994;170:500.

262 Loeffelholz MS, Lewinski CA, Silver SR, et al. Detection of *Chlamydia trachomatis* in endocervical specimens by polymerase chain reaction. *J Clin Microbiol* 1992;30:2847.

263 Schachter J. Noninvasive tests for diagnosis of *Chlamydia trachomatis* infection: application of ligase chain reaction to first-catch urine specimens in women. *J Infect Dis* 1995;172: 1411.

264 Crombleholme WR, Schacter J, Grossman M, et al. Amoxicillin therapy for *Chlamydia trachomatis* in pregnancy. *Obstet Gynecol* 1990;75:752.

265 Koutsky LA, Kiviat NB. Genital human papillomavirus. In: Holmes KK, Sparling PF, Mardh P-A, et al., eds. *Sexually transmitted diseases*. New York: McGraw-Hill; 1999:347.

266 Institute of Medicine Committee on Prevention and Control of Sexually Transmitted Diseases. *The hidden epidemic: confronting sexually transmitted diseases*. Washington, DC: National Academy Press, 1997.

267 Oriel JD. Natural history of genital warts. *Br J Venereal Dis* 1971;47:1.

268 US Centers for Disease Control, Division of STD Prevention. *Sexually transmitted disease surveillance, 1995*. Atlanta: Centers for Disease Control and Prevention. US Department of Health Service, Public Health Service, 1996.

269 Winer RL, Lee S-K, Hughes JP, et al: Genital human papillomavirus infection: incidence and risk factors in a cohort of female university students. *Am J Epidemiol* 2003;157:218.

270 Halpert R, Fruchter RG, Sedlis A, et al. Human papillomavirus and lower genital neoplasia in renal transplant patients. *Obstet Gynecol* 1986;68:251.

271 Byrne P, Woodman C, Meanwell C, et al. Koilocytes and cervical human papillomavirus infection. *Lancet* 1986;1:205.

272 Singer A, Wilter J, Walker P, et al. Comparison of prevalence of human papillomavirus antigen in biopsies from women with cervical intraepithelial neoplasia. *J Clin Pathol* 1985;38:855.

273 Lorinez AT, Temple GF, Patterson JA, et al. Correlation of cellular atypia and human papillomavirus DNA in exfoliated cells of the uterine cervix. *Obstet Gynecol* 1986;68:508.

274 Beutner KR, Wiley DJ, Douglas JM, et al: Genital warts and their treatment. *Clin Infect Dis* 1999;28(Suppl.):S37.

275 Chamberlain MJ, Reynolds AL, Yeomen WB. Toxic effects of podophyllin application in pregnancy. *Br Med J* 1972;3:391.

276 Centers for Disease Control. National Disease and Therapeutic Index (IMS American Ltd.) CDC website.

277 Fleming DT, McQuillian GM, Johnson RE, et al. Herpes simplex virus type 2 in the United States, 1976 to 1994. *N Engl J Med* 1997;337:1105.

278 Langenberg AGM, Corey L, Ashley RL, et al. for the Chiron HSV Vaccine Study Group. A prospective study of new infections with herpes simplex virus type 1 and 2. *N Engl J Med* 1999;341: 1432.

279 Bolognese RJ, Cosen SL, Fuccillo DA, et al. Herpes virus hominis type II infections in asymptomatic pregnant women. *Obstet Gynecol* 1976;48:507.

280 Tejani N, Klein SW, Kaplan M. Subclinical herpes simplex genitalis infections in the perinatal period. *Am J Obstet Gynecol* 1979;135:547.

281 Scher J, Bottone E, Desmond E, Simons W. The incidence and outcome of asymptomatic herpes simplex genitalis in an obstetric population. *Am J Obstet Gynecol* 1982;144:906.

282 Nahmias AJ, Roczman B. Infection with herpes simplex virus I and II. *N Engl J Med* 1973;289:781.

283 Sullivan-Bolyai J, Hull HF, Wilson C, Corey L. Neonatal herpes simplex infection in King County, Washington. Increasing incidence and epidemiological correlates. *JAMA* 1983;250:3059.

284 Whitley RJ, Nahmias AJ, Visintine AM, et al. the natural history of herpes simplex virus infection of mother and newborn. *Pediatrics* 1980;66:489.

285 Rooney JF, Felser JM, Ostrove JM, et al. Medical intelligence: acquisition of genital herpes from an asymptomatic sexual partner. *N Engl J Med* 1986;314:1561.

286 Corey L, Wald A. Genital herpes. In: Holmes KK, Sparling PF, Mardh P-A, et al., eds. *Sexually transmitted diseases*. New York: McGraw-Hill; 1999;285.

287 Baker DA. Herpes simplex virus infections. *Curr Opin Obstet Gynecol* 1992;4:676.

288 Hollier LM, Workowski K. Treatment of sexually transmitted diseases in women. *Obstet Gynecol Clin North Am* 2003;30:751.

289 Sweet RL, Gibbs RS. Herpes simplex virus infection. In: Sweet RL, Gibbs RS, eds. *Infectious diseases of the female genital tract*. Philadelphia, PA: Lippincott Williams & Wilkins, 2002.

290 Nahmias AJ, Josey WE, Naib ZM, et al. Perinatal risk associated with maternal genital herpes simplex virus infection. *Am J Obstet Gynecol* 1971;110–185.

291 Brown ZA, Selke S, Zeh J, et al. The acquisition of herpes simplex virus during pregnancy. *N Engl J Med* 1997;337:509.

292 Arvin AM, Whitley RJ. Herpes simplex virus infection. In: Remington JS, Klein JV, eds. *Infectious diseases of the fetus and newborn infant*. Philadelphia, PA: W.B. Saunders; 2001:425.

293 Hutto C, Arvin A, Jacobs R, et al. Intrauterine herpes simplex virus infections. *J Pediatr* 1987;110:97.

294 Prober CG, Sullender WM, Yasukawa LL, et al. Low risk of herpes simplex virus infections in neonates exposed to the virus at the same time of vaginal delivery to mothers with recurrent genital herpes simplex virus infections. *N Engl J Med* 1987;316:240.

295 Gibbs RS, Amstey MS, Sweet RL, et al. Management of genital herpes infection in pregnancy. *Obstet Gynecol* 1988;71:779.

296 American College of Obstetricians and Gynecologists. Perinatal herpes simplex virus infections. ACOG Technical Bulletin 122. Washington, DC: American College of Obstetricians and Gynecologists, November, 1988.

297 Ray DA, Evans AT, Elliott JP, et al. Maternal herpes infection complicated by prolonged premature rupture of membranes. *Am J Perinatol* 1985;2:96.

298 Utley K, Bromberger P, Wagner L, et al. Management of primary herpes in pregnancy complicated by ruptured membranes and extreme prematurity: case report. *Obstet Gynecol* 1987;69: 471.

299 Major C, Towers CV, Lewis DF, Garite TJ. Expectant management of preterm premature rupture of membranes complicated by active recurrent genital herpes. *Am J Obstet Gynecol* 2003;188:1551.

300 Centers for Disease Control and Prevention. 2002 Sexually transmitted diseases treatment guidelines. *Morbid Mortal Wkly Rep* 2002;51:1.

301 Bryson YJ, Dillon M, Lovett M, et al. Treatment of first episodes of genital herpes simplex virus infection with oral acyclovir. *N Engl J Med* 1983;308:916.

302 Reichman RC, Badger GJ, Mertz GJ, et al. Treatment of recurrent genital herpes simplex infections with oral acyclovir. *JAMA* 1984;251:2103.

303 Kaplowitz LG, Baker D, Gelb L, et al. Prolonged continuous acyclovir treatment of normal adults with frequently recurring genital herpes simplex infection. *JAMA* 1991;265:747.

304 Corey L. Wald A, Patel R, et al. Once-daily valacyclovir to reduce the risk of transmission of genital herpes. *N Engl J Med* 2004;350:11.

305 Sheffield JS, Hollier LM, Hill JB, et al. Acyclovir prophylaxis to prevent herpes simplex virus recurrence at delivery: a systemic review. *Obstet Gynecol* 2003;102:1396.

306 Haddad J, Langer B, Astruc D, et al. Oral acyclovir and recurrent genital herpes during pregnancy. *Obstet Gynecol* 1993;82: 102.

307 American College of Obstetricians and Gynecologists. *Management of herpes in pregnancy*. ACOG Practice Bulletin 8. Washington, DC: ACOG, October 1999.

308 Kampmeier RH. Description *of Trichomonas vaginalis* by M.A. Donne. *Sex Transm Dis* 1978;5:119.

309 Hesseltine HC, et al. Experimental human vaginal trichomoniasis. *J Infect Dis* 1942;71:127.

310 Lancely F, MacEntegart MC. *Trichomonas vaginalis* in the male: the experimental infection of a few volunteers. *Lancet* 1953;4: 668.

311 Rein MF, Chapel TA. Trichomoniasis candidiasis, and the minor venereal disease. *Clin Obstet Gynecol* 1975;18:73.

312 Hardy PH, Nell EE, Spence MR, et al. Prevalence of six sexually transmitted disease agents among pregnant inner city adolescents and pregnancy outcome. *Lancet* 1984;8:333.

313 Sweet RL, Gibbs RS. Infectious vulvovaginitis. In: Sweet RL, Gibbs RS, eds. *Infectious diseases of the female genital tract*. Philadelphia, PA: Lippincott, Williams and Wilkins; 2002: 337.

314 Gardner H, Dukes CD. *Haemophilus vaginalis* vaginitis: a newly defined specific infection previously classified "nonspecific" vaginitis. *Am J Obstet Gynecol* 1955;69:962.

315 Wolner-Hanssen P, Krieger JN, Stevens CE, et al. Clinical manifestations of vaginal Trichomoniasis. *JAMA* 1989;26:45.

316 Honigberg B. Trichomonads of importance in human medicine. In: Kreier JP, ed. *Parasitic protozoa*, Vol. 2. New York: Academic Press; 1978:275.

317 Laga M, Manoka A, Kivuvu M, et al. Nonulcerative sexually transmitted diseases as risk factors for HIV-1 transmission in women: results from a cohort study. *AIDS* 1993;7:95.

318 Rein MF. Clinical manifestations of urogenital trichomoniasis in women. In: Honigberg BM, ed. *Trichomonads parasitic in humans*. New York: Springer; 1989:227.

319 Fouts AC, Kraus SJ. *Trichomonas vaginalis*: reevaluation of its clinical presentation and laboratory diagnosis. *J Infect Dis* 1980;141:137.

320 Krieger JM. Diagnosis of trichomoniasis. Comparison of conventional wet mount preparation with cytologic studies, cultures, and monoclonal antibody staining of direct specimens. *JAMA* 1988;259:1233.

321 Spence MR, Hollander DH, Smith J, McCaig L, et al. The clinical and laboratory diagnosis of *Trichomonas vaginalis* infection. *Sex Transm Dis* 1980;7:168.

322 Lossick JG. Treatment of *Trichomonas vaginalis* infections. *Rev Infect Dis* 1982;4:801.

323 Lossick JG, Muller M, Gorrell TE. In vitro drug susceptibility and doses of metronidazole required for cure in cases of refractory vaginal Trichomoniasis. *J Infect Dis* 1986;153: 948.

324 Muller M, Lossick JG, Gorrell TE, et al. In vitro susceptibility of *Trichomonas vaginalis* to metronidazole and treatment outcome in vaginal Trichomoniasis. *Sex Trans Dis* 1988; 15:17.

325 Mason PR, Brown I. Trichomonas in pregnancy (letter). *Lancet* 1980;11:1025.

326 Minkoff H, Grunebaum AN, Schwarz RH, et al. Risk factors for prematurity and premature rupture of membranes: a prospective study of the vaginal flora in pregnancy. *Am J Obstet Gynecol* 1984;150:965.

327 Magat AH, Alger LS, Nagey DA, et al. Double-blinded randomized study comparing amoxicillin and erythromycin for the treatment of *Chlamydia trachomatis* infection in pregnancy. *Obstet Gynecol* 1993;81:745.

328 Alray M, Jolly JR, Moutguin J-M, et al. Randomized comparison of amoxicillin and erythromycin treatment of genital chlamydial infection in pregnancy. *Lancet* 1993;344:1461.

329 Silverman NS, Sullivan M, Hochman M, et al. A randomized prospective trial comparing amoxicillin and erythromycin for the treatment of *Chlamydia trachomatis* in pregnancy. *Am J Obstet Gynecol* 1994;170:829.

330 Turrentine MA, Newton ER. Amoxicillin or erythromycin for the treatment of antenatal chlamydia infection: a meta-analysis. *Obstet Gynecol* 1995;86:1021.

51 Rheumatologic and connective tissue disorders in pregnancy

Gustavo F. Leguizamón and E. Albert Reece

Rheumatologic and connective tissue disorders are multisystem conditions that occur most commonly in women of reproductive age. Therefore, it is not unusual for the obstetrician to be challenged by patients with autoimmune disorders seeking preconception counseling or antenatal care. This chapter addresses the effect of systemic lupus erythematosus, scleroderma, rheumatoid arthritis, and ankylosing spondylitis on perinatal outcomes as well as the impact of pregnancy on the natural course of these conditions. Furthermore, drugs commonly used to treat these disorders during pregnancy and lactation are reviewed.

Systemic lupus erythematosus

Systemic lupus erythematosus (SLE) is a chronic autoimmune disorder of unknown etiology. It has an overall incidence in the United States of approximately 7 per 100 000.[1] A strong predilection for women is observed with a female to male ratio of 7:1. Furthermore, African–Americans and Hispanics have an excess risk of two- to fourfold over the background population.[2]

The onset of SLE is often subtle and can compromise one or multiple organ systems. Frequently, the disease is characterized by periods of disease activity alternating with quiescence. Systemic signs and symptoms are common and usually involve fatigue, fever, malaise, and weight loss. The frequency of involvement of major systems is depicted in Table 51.1.

Recently, the American College of Rheumatology (ACR) has reviewed and modified the 1982 revised criteria for the diagnosis of SLE (Table 51.2). Positive LE cell preparation was removed from the classification, and "positive finding of antiphospholipid antibodies" was included among the immunologic criteria.[3,4] If at least four of the 11 ACR criteria are met (either simultaneously or serially), the diagnosis of SLE is achieved.

Laboratory evaluation

Antinuclear antibodies (ANA) are the most sensitive screening laboratory tool for evaluating patients with the clinical suspicion of SLE. Approximately 90% of patients with SLE will present a positive test for ANA. False positives have been reported in normal subjects and those with chronic inflammatory disorders, other autoimmune diseases, certain drugs, and viral infections. A negative ANA result makes the diagnosis of lupus very unlikely, whereas a positive result (> 1/80) favors the diagnosis. Antibodies directed against double-stranded DNA (ds DNA) and Sm have better specificity; however, they are present in a minority of the patients. Antibodies against ds DNA are present in approximately 60% of patients suffering from lupus and have been associated with disease activity and nephritis.[5,6] Anti-Sm antibodies are present in Caucasian and black populations with SLE in approximately 10% and 30% of the population respectively. It has also been suggested that these antibodies are associated with disease activity as well as renal and neurological involvement.[7] Although the ability of antibody testing to predict disease activity is controversial, in general, rising titers of anti-ds DNA antibodies suggest a two- to threefold increased risk of flare in the following 3–4 months.[6] In some patients, however, decreasing plasma complement together with other laboratory abnormalities such as microscopic hematuria, decreased leukocyte count, and increasing proteinuria are better predictors of lupus exacerbation.[7]

The presence of anti-Ro (SS-A) and anti-LA (SS-B) antibodies is of recognized clinical significance as they were consistently associated with neonatal lupus. These antibodies are present in 20–60% of patients with SLE depending on the techniques used for their detection. Table 51.3 depicts relevant clinical information for different ANA.

Effects of pregnancy on systemic lupus erythematosus

The impact of pregnancy on SLE is not fully elucidated. The fact that this disorder has a clear predilection for female subjects raises the notion that estrogen levels are involved in the pathophysiology of SLE. Therefore, high estrogen level conditions, such as pregnancy, generate significant concern.[8] Overall, the incidence of lupus flares during pregnancy ranges from 15% to 63%.[9] Early uncontrolled studies suggested exacerbations during pregnancy or the puerperium. More

Table 51.1 Frequency of organ system involvement in SLE.

System involved	Frequency (%)
Systemic	95
Musculoskeletal	95
Cutaneous	80
Hematologic	85
Neurologic	60
Cardiopulmonary	60
Renal	50
Gastrointestinal	45
Vascular	15

recent reports have shown contradictory results. While some authors report no differences in lupus flares during pregnancy,[10–13] others observed disease exacerbation.[14–17]

Lockshin et al.[13] compared different clinical markers of disease activity in 33 pregnancies of women with SLE with nonpregnant women with SLE matched for age, race, organ involvement, and disease severity. Both groups were followed for periods of up to 1 year after delivery. No differences between pregnant and nonpregnant patients were observed; however, new-onset proteinuria occurred in four pregnant patients compared with one nonpregnant patient, and SLE-related thrombocytopenia occurred more frequently in pregnant patients. The authors concluded that, although

Table 51.2 The 1982 revised criteria for the classification of systemic lupus erythematosus.

Criterion	Definition
1. Malar rash	Fixed erythema, flat or raised, over the malar eminences, tending to spare the nasolabial folds
2. Discoid rash	Erythematous raised patches with adherent keratotic scaling and follicular plugging; atrophic scarring may occur in older lesions
3. Photosensitivity	Skin rash as a result of unusual reaction to sunlight, by patient history or physician observation
4. Oral ulcers	Oral or nasopharyngeal ulceration, usually painless, observed by physician
5. Arthritis	Nonerosive arthritis involving two or more peripheral joints, characterized by tenderness, swelling, or effusion
6. Serositis	a) Pleuritis – convincing history of pleuritic pain or rubbing heard by a physician or evidence of pleural effusion or b) Pericarditis – documented by ECG or rub or evidence of pericardial effusion
7. Renal disorder	a) Persistent proteinuria >0.5 g/day or > 3+ if quantitation not performed or b) Cellular casts – may be red cell, hemoglobin, granular, tubular, or mixed
8. Neurologic disorder	a) Seizures – in the absence of offending drugs or known metabolic derangements, e.g., uremia, ketoacidosis, or electrolyte imbalance or b) Psychosis – in the absence of offending drugs or known metabolic derangements, e.g., uremia, ketoacidosis, or electrolyte imbalance
9. Hematologic disorder	a) Hemolytic anemia – with reticulocytosis or b) Leukopenia – < 4000/mm^3 total on two or more occasions or c) Lymphopenia – < 1500/mm^3 on two or more occasions or d) Thrombocytopenia – less than 100 000/mm^3 in the absence of offending drugs
10. Immunologic disorder	a) Anti-DNA: antibody to native DNA in abnormal titer or b) Anti-Sm: presence of antibody to Sm nuclear antigen or c) Positive finding of antiphospholipid antibodies based on: an abnormal serum level of IgG or IgM anticardiolipin antibodies or a positive test result for lupus anticoagulant using a standard method or a false-positive serologic test for syphilis known to be positive for at least 6 months and confirmed by *Treponema pallidum* immobilization or fluorescent treponemal antibody absorption test
11. Antinuclear antibody	An abnormal titer of antinuclear antibody by immunofluorescence or an equivalent assay at any point in time and in the absence of drugs known to be associated with "drug-induced lupus" syndrome

From ref 3.
ECG, electrocardiogram.

pregnancy complications are frequent, the assertion that pregnancy causes exacerbation of SLE remains unproven. In a subsequent publication concerning 80 women whose pregnancies were complicated by SLE, these authors observed that, if only SLE-specific abnormalities were counted, disease exacerbation occurred in less than 13%.

Other investigators concluded that pregnancy increases the frequency of flare. Ruiz-Irastorza et al.[16] compared the incidence of flare during pregnancy and puerperium in 78 SLE-complicated pregnancies and 50 consecutive, nonpregnant, age-matched SLE patients. Additionally, 43 of the pregnant patients continued attending the lupus clinic for the year after puerperium, and their course was compared with their course during pregnancy. The incidence of flare was 65% during pregnancy and/or the puerperium and 42% in the control group. The 43 patients controlled after the puerperium flared more frequently during pregnancy than thereafter. Kidney and central nervous system involvement was not different between the pregnancy and control groups. The authors concluded that SLE tends to flare during pregnancy, especially during the second and third trimesters and the puerperium. Finally, when flares occurred, they were not more severe than in non-pregnant patients. Similarly, Petri et al.[15] and Wong et al.[14] observed a significant increase in flare incidence associated with pregnancy. Numerous reasons can explain this lack of consistency: inadequate control, differences in patient characteristics, proportion of patients with antiphospholipid syndrome (APS), inconsistencies in flare definition, and methods of assessment of disease activity. Furthermore, physiologic changes of pregnancy such as palmar erythema, increased urinary protein excretion secondary to increased renal blood plasma flow, and changes in facial skin pigmentation can often lead to overdiagnoses of lupus flare in pregnancy.[18] Table 51.4 summarizes current studies evaluating the impact of pregnancy on the occurrence of lupus flare.

Patients with lupus nephritis have a small but crucial risk of permanent renal function deterioration following pregnancy. Burkett[19] reviewed six retrospective studies including over 200 pregnancies with lupus nephritis. The authors observed that 7% of the patients had permanent renal failure, 26% had transient renal function deterioration, and 60% had no significant change in renal function parameters. Conditions associated with improved outcomes include prepregnancy remission of at least 6 months, serum creatinine less than 1.5 mg/dL, creatinine clearance of 60 mL/min or more, or proteinuria of 3 g/24 h or less. In a case–control study, Urowitz et al.[12] concluded that inactive disease at conception was protective against the occurrence of flare during pregnancy.

Table 51.5 summarizes relevant information about pregnancy influencing the natural course of SLE.

Table 51.3 Antibodies of clinical significance in SLE.

Antibody	Frequency (%)	Feature
Anti-ds DNA	60–90	Specific for SLE Associated with activity and nephritis
Anti-Sm	10–30	Specific for SLE Lupus nephritis?
Anti-La	20–40	Neonatal lupus
Anti-Ro	20–40	Neonatal lupus
Anti-RNP	10	Mixed connective tissue disorder

Effects of systemic lupus erythematosus on pregnancy

SLE can affect pregnancy in different ways. It increases the risk of early and late pregnancy losses owing to hypertension, renal dysfunction, placental insufficiency, and its association with antiphospholipid syndrome APS. Furthermore, it is an important cause of fetal and neonatal heart block. Finally, it also increases the risk of spontaneous as well as medically indicated preterm labor. In the following sections, the relevant aspects of such complications are discussed.

Preeclampsia

Women with SLE have an increased risk of developing preeclampsia with an incidence of 15–32%.[11,12,20] Several risk factors have been identified, such as lupus nephritis, APAS,

Table 51.4 Impact of pregnancy on lupus flare.

Authors	Publication year	Patients (n)	Design	Flare incidence
Lockshin et al.	1984	28	Matched	Equal
Mintz et al.	1986	75	Unmatched	Equal
Urowitz et al.	1993	46	Matched	Equal
Wong et al.	1991	22	Unmatched	Increased
Petri et al.	1991	37	Unmatched	Increased
Ruiz-Irastorza et al.	1996	68	Matched	Increased

Table 51.5 Effects of pregnancy on the natural course of SLE.

Increased incidence of flare during pregnancy and puerperium is controversial
Flare is frequent and can occur throughout pregnancy and puerperium
Women with quiescent disease at conception could have better outcome
Although onset of definitive renal failure can occur in pregnancy, patients with lupus nephritis and normal renal function usually have no long-term effects

and chronic hypertension. However, making the differential diagnosis between the onset of preeclampsia and the occurrence of lupus flare could be a difficult challenge for the obstetrician. Making the differential diagnosis is of utmost importance because the therapeutic approach differs substantially; while the lupus flare is treated with high doses of steroids, preeclampsia is most likely treated with seizure prophylaxis, control of hypertension and, eventually, delivery. Both conditions can coexist in a patient with SLE and, even when they present as a single complication, both can cause hypertension, deteriorating renal function, proteinuria, and edema. Laboratory evaluation can be helpful in making the differential diagnosis. Mainly, decreased complement levels (C3-C4-CH50), increased anti-ds DNA, leukopenia, hematuria, and the presence of casts in urine raise the suspicion for SLE flare, while the presence of microangiopathic hemolytic anemia, abnormal liver function tests, and hyperuricemia most likely indicate preeclampsia.

Fetal outcome

Most investigations are consistent with the notion that women with SLE present an excess risk of pregnancy loss. Early retrospective studies[21–24] as well as more recent prospective investigations are consistent with this finding. Petri et al.[25] conducted a case–control study to compare the incidence of pregnancy loss (including spontaneous abortion, miscarriage, or stillbirth) between women whose pregnancies were complicated with SLE and two control groups. The authors found a significantly increased risk of 21% versus 14% and 8% in the control groups. Prospective studies addressing this issue are in agreement with a median incidence of pregnancy loss of approximately 20%.[11,14,26–31] The incidence of preterm labor in this population has been reported to be from 20% to 50%.[32] In a case–control study, Johnson et al.[32] evaluated the causes of increased preterm delivery in this population. The authors found that premature rupture of membranes was the most frequent associated finding, and was present in 39% of gestations between 24 and 36 weeks' gestation. The incidence of intrauterine growth restriction (IUGR) is also increased, and has been reported in 12–32% of pregnancies complicated by SLE.[14,28,33]

SLE complicating pregnancy constitutes a rather heterogeneous population, and several risk factors for poor fetal outcome have been described. Cortes-Hernandez et al.[34] recently evaluated clinical and laboratory markers of fetal outcomes in 60 patients with SLE and 103 pregnancies. In a multiple regression model, the authors observed that increased levels of anti-β2 glycoprotein I, hypertension at conception, and hypocomplementemia were significantly associated with pregnancy loss (spontaneous abortions and stillbirth), occurring in 74%, 22%, and 44% of the cases respectively. Furthermore, the presence of anticardiolipin antibodies and hypertension during pregnancy as well as lupus nephritis was associated with IUGR and prematurity. Rahman et al.[35] also concluded that hypertension and maternal renal disease are predictors of poor fetal outcomes. In summary, although most pregnancies in women with SLE do well, those presenting with risk factors need to be monitored aggressively throughout pregnancy.

Selected patients with immune diseases have an excess risk of perinatal morbidity and mortality. The most significant factors influencing outcome are most likely activity of disease at conception, renal involvement, and the presence of APAS.

Antiphospholipid syndrome: definition, classification, and epidemiology

APS is an autoimmune disorder frequently associated with other immunologic-related diseases with significant impact on perinatal and maternal outcomes. Primary APS occurs in patients without other immune disorders, whereas the so-called secondary APS occurs in conjunction with autoimmune disease, mainly SLE.

Its diagnosis has been a matter of controversy and is still an ongoing process. Recently, an international consensus has been generated to orient research efforts and aid in clinical diagnosis (Table 51.6).[36] At least one clinical and one laboratory criterion must be met to achieve the diagnosis of APS. Clinical criteria consist of either vascular thrombosis or pregnancy complications, such as one or more unexplained deaths of a morphologically normal fetus at or beyond the 10th week of gestation, one or more premature births before 34 weeks of a morphologically normal neonate, or three or more unexplained consecutive spontaneous abortions before 10 weeks of gestation.

Although many antiphospholipid antibodies have been described, only lupus anticoagulant (LAC) and moderate to high levels of IgG and IgM anticardiolipins detected on two occasions separated by no less than 6 weeks are recognized criteria from the 1999 consensus conference. Laboratory detection of LAC must follow the guidelines of the International Society of Thrombosis and Hemostasis[37] including: (1) prolongation of at least one phospholipid-dependent coagulation test (e.g., activated partial thromboplastin time, dilute Rusell's viper venom time, kaolin clotting time); (2) failure to correct the initial phospholipid-dependent clotting test when mixed with normal plasma; and (3) correction of the abnormal coagulation assay when excess phospholipid is added.

Table 51.6 International consensus statement on preliminary criteria for the classification of the antiphospholipid syndrome.

Clinical criteria
Vascular thrombosis: one or more episodes of arterial, venous, or small vessel thrombosis
Complication of pregnancy:
One or more unexplained deaths of a morphologically normal fetus at or beyond the 10th week of gestation or
One or more premature births before 34 weeks of a morphologically normal neonate or
Three or more unexplained consecutive spontaneous abortions before 10 weeks of gestation
Laboratory criteria
Anticardiolipin antibodies IgG or IgM present in blood at moderate or high levels on two or more occasions at least 6 weeks apart
Lupus anticoagulant antibodies detected in blood on two or more occasions at least 6 weeks apart, according to the guidelines of the International Society of Thrombosis and Hemostasis

From ref. 36.

Among patients with antiphospholipid antibodies, excess vascular and obstetric morbidity is observed when these antibodies react against the phospholipid-binding protein β2 glycoprotein I. In contrast, antibodies reacting directly against negatively charged phospholipids are commonly transient and associated with intravenous drug exposure.[38] Therefore, laboratory detection of the anticardiolipin antibodies must be performed by standardized enzyme-linked immunosorbent assay (ELISA) methods measuring β2 glycoprotein I-dependent anticardiolipin antibodies.[39]

To test the Sapporo classification criteria, Lockshin et al.[40] studied a total of 243 consecutive patients with the clinical diagnoses of primary APS, secondary APS, SLE without clinical APS, and lupus-like disease without clinical APS. The authors reported a sensitivity and specificity of 71% and 98% respectively. Overall, studies show that concordance of antibodies is not always found. In fact, among patients with the syndrome, between 50% and 70% have both LAC and APS.[39,41] Anticardiolipin antibodies (ACLA) tend to be more sensitive, whereas LAC is more specific. Specificity of ACLA increases with increasing titers and when IgG is present.[39] Five percent of healthy individuals present with ACLA;[42] however, patients with SLE present with these autoantibodies more frequently than the general population, with an incidence of approximately 12–30%.[43,44] Furthermore, among this group, the occurrence of thrombosis or pregnancy complications has been reported to be between 50% and 70% at long-term follow-up.[42,45]

Fetal loss in the antiphospholipid syndrome

The association of pregnancy loss and APS has been reported consistently among patients with both primary and secondary APS.[9,46] Rai et al.[46] studied the incidence of miscarriages (median 4) among 20 women with APAS and history of recurrent pregnancy loss who declined treatment in the next pregnancy and compared them with 100 consecutive women with recurrent miscarriage (median 4) of unknown etiology. The authors found a pregnancy loss rate of 90% among untreated women with APS versus 34% in the control group. In a cross-sectional study, Ginsberg et al.[47] evaluated the association between pregnancy loss and secondary APS among 42 women. Patients were considered to be positive for LAC and/or ACLA only when at least two tests were positive on separate occasions. Significant associations were found between previous pregnancy loss and both presence of LAC [odds ratio (OR) 4.8] and ACLA (OR 20). Importantly, when patients showed only transient LAC and/or ACLA, this association was lost.[47] Finally, when fetal loss occurs in association with APS, a high proportion of late (second and third trimester) fetal losses are observed.[48]

Complications secondary to placental insufficiency such as IUGR, stillbirth, preeclampsia, and preterm labor are also commonly observed in this population.[9,39,49] IUGR has been reported in 15–30% of pregnancies affected by APS.[50,51] Abnormalities in tests of fetal well-being have been observed in as many as 50% of pregnancies with APS,[52–54] leading to a preterm delivery rate of approximately 32–65%.[52,53,55–57] Lockshin et al.[58] prospectively studied the relationship between ACLA and the presence of midpregnancy fetal distress among women with SLE. The authors found that all women with lupus presenting with abnormal antenatal fetal testing had abnormal ACLA values, while patients with normal antenatal test results had low antibody levels.[58] Loizou et al.[59] studied the impact of ACLA on fetal outcome among 84 women with SLE. The authors observed that, when antibodies were present, fetal loss tended to occur at a later gestational age (17.4 ± 7.1 weeks) and that 30% of the pregnancy losses occurred in the third trimester.[59]

Finally, preeclampsia complicates pregnancies in women with APS with a frequency of 32–50%.[52,53,55–57,60] Although some authors have observed elevated antiphospholipid antibodies among women who develop preeclampsia, especially at early gestational age,[50] others have not.[61]

Neonatal lupus syndrome (NLS)

This syndrome occurs rarely in neonates born to mothers with SLE. It has been described in 1 in 20000 live births in the general population.[62] One or more of the following findings are characteristic: congenital heart block (CHB), cardiomyopathy, cutaneous lesions, thrombocytopenia, and hepatobiliary disease. The most frequent and severe finding in NLS is CHB. The occurrence of this complication is correlated with the presence of anti-SS-A/Ro and anti-SS-B/La antibodies. Among mothers with SLE, Ramsey-Goldman et al.[63] estimated a risk for CHB of 1 in 60; however, when anti-SS-A antibodies were present, the risk increased to 1 in 20. Furthermore, 85% of the mothers whose fetuses had CHB and structurally normal hearts presented with anti-SS-A/Ro and anti-SS-B/La antibodies.[64,65] In a large series of data obtained from the

National Neonatal Lupus Registry, Buyon et al.[66] exposed relevant information to both support clinical management and counsel parents. Among 87 pregnancies with CHB and positive anti-SS-A/Ro and anti-SS-B/La antibodies, no major structural abnormalities were observed. The majority of abnormalities (82%) were diagnosed by ultrasound before 30 weeks of gestation. A significant mortality was found (19%), most likely occurring in the first 3 months of life. Although the cumulative 3-year survival was 79%, significant morbidity was present as 63% required pacemaker placement. Finally, for women with a previous child with CHB, the recurrence rate was 16%.[66]

The frequency and characteristics of hepatobiliary disease were reviewed by Lee et al.[67] Among 219 cases, 19 (9%) had a diagnosis of hepatic disease. Most of them (16) were combined with either cardiac or cutaneous manifestations, and only three were isolated. Three clinical forms were observed: (1) severe liver failure present during gestation or in the neonatal period; (2) conjugated hyperbilirubinemia with mild or no elevations of aminotransferases, occurring in the first few weeks of life; and (3) mild elevations of aminotransferases occurring at approximately 2–3 months of life.

Neiman et al.[68] reviewed the feature of cutaneous manifestations in 57 infants born to 47 women who were positive for anti-SS-A/Ro, anti-SS-B/La, and/or anti-U1-ribonucleoprotein antibodies. Skin lesions usually emerged after ultraviolet (UV) exposure around 6 weeks of age and lasted an average of 17 weeks. Most frequently, it was manifested as a periorbital rash with secondary extension to the scalp, trunk, and extremities. Most (65%) resolved without sequelae, but 25% had chronic manifestations such as telangiectasia and skin dyspigmentation. Importantly, mothers who delivered a child with a cutaneous lupus manifestation had an increased risk of having a newborn with CHB in future pregnancies.[68]

Clinical management of systemic lupus erythematosus in pregnancy

Preconception period

Frequently, patients seeking preconception counseling have been exposed to cyclophosphamide. This cytotoxic drug has been associated with decreased fertility as well as teratogenicity. Overall, the rate of permanent amenorrhea is approximately 25%,[69] and certain risk factors have been recognized as being associated with a higher risk. Ioannidis et al.[70] found that age (≥ 32 years) was a strong predictor of ovarian failure secondary to cyclophosphamide use. Furthermore, the cumulative dose was associated with the successive fertility rate.[71] For those patients under treatment, an adequate method of contraception is mandatory as this drug has been associated with spontaneous abortion and teratogenicity when used during the first trimester.[72]

Evaluation of renal function is of significant relevance during the preconception period. A 24-h urine collection for proteinuria and creatinine clearance should be obtained. Furthermore, blood samples for complete blood count (CBC), platelet count, serum creatinine, and liver function tests are recommended. Disease activity should be determined on clinical grounds as well as with laboratory values such as the previously mentioned renal function, ANA, C3, C4, and anti-ds DNA. A remission period of no less than 6 months is recommended. A significant impact on pregnancy management is determined by the presence of APAS; therefore, anticardiolipins and lupus anticoagulant need to be evaluated. Finally, anti-SS-A/SS-B antibodies need to be measured as fetal cardiac conduction anomalies will increase the risk of perinatal death, especially if they are not recognized.

Prenatal care

Although there are no prospective randomized trials assessing the best strategy to enhance fetal and maternal well-being, some general conclusions can be made from the available information. During the first two trimesters of pregnancy, women should be evaluated every 2 weeks and weekly during the last trimester. At each visit, a urinalysis, blood pressure measurements, maternal weight, and evaluation for signs of flare should be obtained. A 24-h urine collection for proteinuria and creatinine clearance as well as serum creatinine and uric acid should be obtained every 1–3 months. Although there is no consistent evidence of the clinical value of serial ANA and complement determinations, some authorities recommend this approach. Normally, complement levels increase during pregnancy and with preeclampsia; therefore, this measurement could help in the early diagnosis of a flare, especially when the differential diagnosis is preeclampsia.[73,74] An early ultrasound to establish heart activity and accurately date gestational age as well as an anomaly screen between 18 and 22 weeks is recommended. After 22–24 weeks of gestation, fetal growth should be followed with ultrasound every 4–6 weeks. Initiation of nonstress testing is advisable from 28 to 32 weeks according to individual risk factors. Patients who are at increased risk of fetal heart block need to undergo echocardiogram starting during the second trimester. Some authorities recommend performing a serial evaluation every 2 weeks between 16 and 24 weeks of gestation.[66] In general, the mode of delivery is determined by obstetric indications, and vaginal delivery should be attempted. An exception could be the delivery of the fetus with bradycardia secondary to CHB. In this case, fetal pulse oximetry should be considered for fetal monitoring during labor.[75] Figure 51.1 describes different levels of intervention in patients with SLE.

Drug therapy

The drugs most commonly used in the treatment of SLE are aspirin and other nonsteroidal anti-inflammatory drugs (NSAIDs), antimalarials such as hydroxychloroquine, corticosteroids, and cytotoxic agents. Many of these drugs present fetal side-effects and, therefore, the benefits should outweigh the risks for them to be administered during pregnancy.

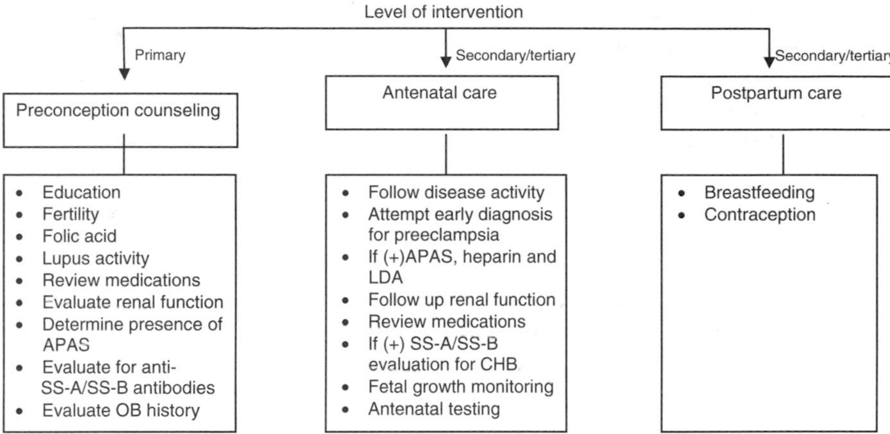

Figure 51.1 Levels of intervention in SLE.

Aspirin is commonly used as an analgesic for patients with rheumatic conditions, and the effects on pregnancy have been studied extensively. When used during the first trimester, no teratogenic effect has been identified;[76–78] however, aspirin has been associated with increased incidence of miscarriages. Acetaminophen, on the other hand, appears to be safe during the first trimester.[79]

In a population-based cohort study of 1055 pregnant patients recruited immediately after a positive pregnancy test, Li et al.[79] evaluated the effects of aspirin, NSAIDs, and acetaminophen on pregnancy loss. The authors found an 80% increased risk of miscarriage among women taking NSAIDs and aspirin. The association was stronger if the initial NSAID use was around the time of conception or if NSAID use lasted more than a week. Prenatal use of acetaminophen was not associated with an increased risk of miscarriage regardless of timing and duration of use.[79] During late gestation, NSAIDs and aspirin have been associated with a reduction in amniotic fluid levels and constriction of the fetal ductus arteriosus.[80] Therefore, acetaminophen appears to be safe at any trimester during pregnancy, and NSAIDs as well as aspirin are better avoided during the first trimester and after 32 weeks of gestation.

Corticosteroids are the other agents frequently used during pregnancy for patients with SLE. Maternal side-effects secondary to corticosteroids are gastrointestinal discomfort, fluid retention and hypertension secondary to the mineralocorticoid activity, bone demineralization, avascular necrosis, acne, and gestation diabetes. No teratogenic effect in humans has been described with these drugs.[18] In fact, prednisone, prednisolone, and methylprednisone only minimally (~ 10%) cross the placenta, as an enzyme with 11-β-ol hydroxylase activity inactivates these drugs. Fluorinated steriods (β-methasone and dexamethasone) should be avoided when steroids are administered for maternal indications as they readily cross the placenta. Although theoretical risks exist for suppression of the hypothalamic–pituitary axis, no such effect has been consistently described in the literature. Finally, when a pregnant patient receives steroids for at least a month in the year previous to the delivery, she should receive a stress dose (100 mg of hydrocortisone intravenously) of steroids every 6 h to prevent acute adrenal failure.

Hydroxychloroquine (HCQ) is an antimalarial that has been used in pregnancy and lactation. This drug interferes with phagocytic function, leading to interference in antigen processing. Early reports raised concern regarding potential fetal ear and ocular side-effects;[81] however, recent studies have shown a lack of teratogenicity or other significant fetal effects.[82–85] Furthermore, recent reports suggest that discontinuing HCQ in high-risk patients may be associated with a poorer prognosis. Levy et al.[86] randomized 20 pregnant women with SLE to receive either HCQ or placebo. The authors found improvement in clinical disease scores as well as fewer flares and lower prednisone doses in the HCQ group. Gestational age at delivery and Apgar scores were higher in the HCQ-treated group. Finally, no congenital anomalies as well as normal neuro-ophthalmologic and auditory evaluations were observed at 1.5–3 years of age. Based on these data, it would appear prudent to continue HCQ therapy in pregnant patients with SLE.[86]

In general, cytotoxic drugs are contraindicated during pregnancy. Azathioprine, however, has been widely used throughout gestation in patients with renal transplants and is the only cytotoxic agent that can be considered safe during pregnancy. For patients with SLE, azathioprine could be indicated when nephritis is present or in women without renal involvement requiring maintenance therapy of 15 mg or more of prednisone as well as those who have experienced recurrent flares. It is also effective for patients with skin lesions, pneumonitis, thrombocytopenia, or hemolytic anemia.[87] Early animal[88] as well as clinical studies[89,90] suggested an increased incidence of IUGR; however, most recent series have demonstrated that azathioprine is well tolerated during pregnancy[91] with no significant increase in congenital malformations or growth restrictions.[71] Although hematological abnormalities in the offspring such as neonatal lymphopenia have been described, they are transient and disappear as the infant ages.[92] Cyclosporine A has also been used in pregnant women with renal transplants and continued during pregnancy in patients with rheumatic disease when other agents failed. Although some degree of fetal growth restriction was reported, no teratogenic effect was observed.[72] Table 51.7 depicts the maternal and fetal toxicities of frequently used drugs.

Scleroderma

Systemic sclerosis is a connective tissue disorder that affects women four times more frequently than men with the mean age of onset in the early forties. This multisystem disorder is characterized by fibrosis of the skin, blood vessels, gastrointestinal tract, lungs, kidneys, and heart. Different degrees of organ involvement are associated with a wide range of clinical scenarios. Generally, two subsets can be described. In the diffuse cutaneous scleroderma form, symmetric skin thickening of extremities, face, and trunk is observed, frequently accompanied by kidney and other visceral involvement. On the other hand, in limited cutaneous scleroderma, fibrosis is usually confined to the skin of the proximal extremities and face, presenting a symmetrical distribution, and frequently has features of the CREST syndrome (calcinosis, Raynaud's phenomenon, esophageal dysmotility, sclerodactyly, and telangiectasia). In general, the prognosis of the limited form is more positive.

Early data, mainly from case reports, suggested that scleroderma complicating pregnancy carried an ominous prognosis.[93] More recent and larger studies suggest that, with careful planning and intensive monitoring, maternal and fetal prognosis are in general favorable.[94] Generally, scleroderma symptoms remain unchanged or even improve during pregnancy.[95] Gastroesophageal reflux commonly worsens and, if present, Raynaud's phenomenon tends to improve.[95] Although some authors suggested that skin thickening could increase postpartum,[72] others found no evidence to support this belief.[95] Among pregnant patients with scleroderma, renal crisis is probably the most problematic complication, and its diagnosis represents a difficult challenge. It usually occurs during the first years following the diagnosis of diffuse scleroderma and presents with acute onset of severe hypertension, rapidly progressing renal impairment, daily increases in serum creatinine, and thrombocytopenia. The differential diagnosis includes preeclampsia–hemolysis, elevated liver function, and low platelets (HELLP) syndrome and is based on normal liver function tests, the rapid progression of renal deterioration with daily increases in serum creatinine, lack of proteinuria, as well as a history of diffuse scleroderma diagnosed within 5 years.[72,95] Although the use of angiotensin-converting enzyme (ACE) inhibitors during the second and third trimesters has been associated with severe fetal toxicity,[96,97] these drugs dramatically improve short- and long-term outcomes after a renal crisis in patients with scleroderma. Specifically, they increase survival and decrease the need for long-term dialysis after a renal crisis.[98] Furthermore, if treatment is delayed, irreversible kidney damage or death can still occur.[99] Steen and Medsger[99] suggested that, if renal crisis is suspected, treatment should be started with a serum creatinine of less than 3 mg/dL. Finally, there is no evidence suggesting that abortion will reverse renal crisis.[70] Based on these findings, most authorities suggest that, if renal crisis is diagnosed in pregnancy, the parents should be counseled and ACE inhibitors offered as these therapies could be life-saving.

It is currently not possible to determine the impact of pregnancy on the development of renal crisis in patients with systemic sclerosis.[95]

Overall, perinatal outcomes are good for women who demonstrate stable disease before conception, especially for patients with localized forms. Preterm labor is the most frequent complication, and recent studies show an incidence of approximately 30%.[95] Although some series have shown an increased incidence of growth restriction,[100] others have not confirmed this finding.[95] The rate of miscarriages was reported to be increased in older studies. Silman and Black[101] in a retrospective study, described a twofold increase in the rate of spontaneous abortion. Recently, Steen and Medsger[102] compared perinatal outcomes in 214 women with systemic sclerosis, in 167 women with rheumatoid arthritis (RA) and 105 healthy control subjects, and found no significant differences in the rate of first-trimester spontaneous abortion.

Rheumatoid arthritis

RA affects approximately 1% of the adult population and is three times more common in women, predominantly of reproductive age, complicating 1 in every 1000–2000 pregnancies.[103] It is a systemic, autoimmune, and inflammatory disorder that primarily affects synovial tissues. Its etiology is unknown, and it is characterized by symmetric involvement of peripheral joints such as metacarpophalangeal, proximal interphalangeal, wrist, and metatarsophalangeal, with characteristic cartilage destruction and eventual joint distortion. The affected joints characteristically present with swelling, and are warm and tender with limitation of movement and morning stiffness (Fig. 51.2A and B). Extra-articular involvement can occur including rheumatoid nodules, vasculitis, uveitis, interstitial lung disease, serositis, and Felty's syndrome. Usually, it has an insidious onset associated with fatigue, weakness, and anorexia. The disease has a chronic fluctuating course with variable degrees of compromise, with some patients having only a few joints affected and others presenting with significant disability. The diagnosis is not made by a single finding, but rather by the combination of clinical and laboratory findings together with the clinical course. The ACR published the revised criteria depicted in Table 51.8. These guidelines have a sensitivity and a specificity of 91–94% and 84%, respectively,[104] and are based on the presence of the following characteristics: morning stiffness, arthritis of three or more joint areas, arthritis of hand joints, symmetric arthritis, rheumatoid

Table 51.7 Side-effects of drugs commonly used in rheumatologic and connective tissue disorders.

Drug	FDA codes for use in pregnancy	Major maternal toxicities	Fetal toxicities	Lactation
Aspirin	C; D in third trimester	Anemia, peripartum hemorrhage, prolonged labor	Premature closure of ductus hypertension	Use cautiously; excreted at low concentration; doses >1 tablet (325 mg) result in high concentrations in infant plasma
NSAIDs	B; D in third trimester	As for aspirin	As for aspirin	Compatible according to AAP
Corticosteroids				
Prednisone	B	Exacerbation of diabetes and hypertension, PROM	IUGR	5–20% of maternal dose excreted in breast milk; compatible, but wait 4 h if dose >20 mg
Dexamethasone	C			
Hydroxychloroquine	C	Few	Few	Contraindicated (slow elimination rate, potential for accumulation)
Gold	C	No data	One report of cleft palate and severe CNS abnormalities	Excreted into breast milk (20% of maternal dose); rash, hepatitis, and hematologic abnormalities reported, but AAP considers it compatible
D-Penicillamine	D	No data	Cutis laxa connective tissue abnormalities	No data
Sulfasalazine	B; D if near term	No data	No increase in congenital malformations, kernicterus if administered near term	Excreted into breast milk (40–60% maternal dose); bloody diarrhea in one infant; AAP recommends caution
Azathioprine	D	No data	IUGR (rate up to 40%) and prematurity, transient immunosuppression in neonate, possible effect on germlines of offspring	No data; hypothetical risk of immunosuppression outweighs benefit
Chlorambucil	D	No data	Renal angiogenesis	Contraindicated
Methotrexate	X	Spontaneous abortion	Fetal abnormalities (including cleft palate and hydrocephalus)	Contraindicated; small amounts excreted with potential to accumulate in fetal tissues
Cyclophosphamide	D	No data	Severe abnormalities; case report: male twin developed thyroid papillary cancer at 11 years and neuroblastoma at 14 years	Contraindicated; has caused bone marrow depression
Cyclosporine A	C	No data	IUGR and prematurity; one case report: hypoplasia of right leg; not an animal teratogen and unlikely to be a human one	Contraindicated because of potential for immunosuppression

ICH, intracranial hemorrhage; AAP, American Academy of Pediatrics; PROM, premature rupture of membranes; IUGR, intrauterine growth retardation; CNS, central nervous system; IUD, intrauterine device.

Food and Drug Administration (FDA) codes used in pregnancy ratings are as follows: A, controlled studies show no risk. Adequate, well-controlled studies in pregnant women have failed to demonstrate risk to the fetus; B, no evidence of risk in humans. Either animal findings show risk but human findings do not or, if no adequate human studies have been performed, animal findings are negative; C, risk cannot be ruled out. Human studies are lacking, and results from animal studies are either positive for fetal risk or lacking as well. However, potential benefits may justify the potential risk; D, positive evidence of risk. Investigational or postmarketing data show risk to the fetus. Nevertheless, potential benefits may outweigh the potential risk; X, contraindicated in pregnancy. Studies in animals or humans, or investigational or postmarketing reports, have shown fetal risk that clearly outweighs any possible benefit to the patient.

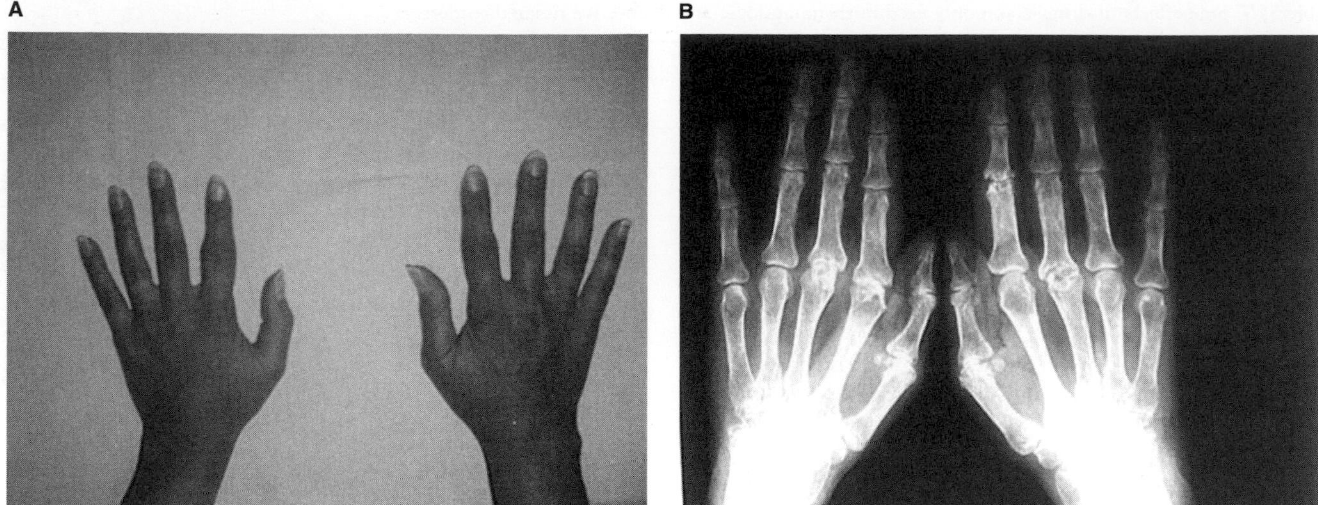

Figures 51.2 Clinical (A) and radiological (B) evidence of RA lesions. Courtesy of Dr Carlos Perandones, Rheumatology Division, CEMIC, Buenos Aires, Argentina.

Table 51.8 1987 criteria for the classification of acute arthritis of rheumatoid arthritis.

Criterion	Definition
1. Morning stiffness	Morning stiffness in and around the joints, lasting at least 1 h before maximal improvement
2. Arthritis of three or more joint areas	At least three joint areas simultaneously have had soft-tissue swelling or fluid (not bony overgrowth alone) observed by a physician. The 14 possible areas are right or left PIP, MCP, wrist, elbow, knee, ankle, and MTP joints
3. Arthritis of hand joints	At least one area swollen (as defined above) in a wrist, MCP, or PIP joint
4. Symmetric arthritis	Simultaneous involvement of the same joint areas (as defined in 2) on both sides of the body (bilateral involvement of PIPs, MCPs, or MTPs is acceptable without absolute symmetry)
5. Rheumatoid nodules	Subcutaneous nodules, over bony prominences, or extensor surfaces, or in juxta-articular regions, observed by a physician
6. Serum rheumatoid factor	Demonstration of abnormal amounts of serum rheumatoid factor by any method for which the result has been positive in < 5% of normal control subjects
7. Radiographic changes	Radiographic changes typical of rheumatoid arthritis on posteroanterior hand and wrist radiographs, which must include erosions or unequivocal bony decalcification localized in or most marked adjacent to the involved joints (osteoarthritis changes alone do not qualify)

From Arnett FC, Edworthy SM, Bloch DA, et al. The American Rheumatism Association 1987 revised criteria for the classification of rheumatoid arthritis. Arthritis Rheum 1988;31:315–324.
MCP, metacarpophalangeal; MTP, metatarsophalangeal; PIP, proximal interphalangeal. For classification purposes, a patient shall be said to have rheumatoid arthritis if he/she has satisfied at least four or these seven criteria. Criteria 1 through 4 must have been present for at least 6 weeks. Patients with two clinical diagnoses are not excluded. Designation as classic, definite, or probable rheumatoid arthritis is *not* to be made.

nodules, serum rheumatoid factor, and radiographic changes. Early radiologic changes are less specific and mainly demonstrate joint effusion and evidence of soft-tissue swelling. Later on in the course of the disease, more characteristic findings are observed, such as symmetric involvement, juxta-articular osteopenia, and loss of cartilages with narrowing of joint spaces. Serum rheumatoid factor is present in approximately 80% of affected patients,[103] but it is not specific. In fact, it is present in 5% of healthy individuals as well as in patients with SLE, Sjogren syndrome, and syphilis among others. Other frequent laboratory findings during periods of disease activity are normocytic normochronic anemia, increased erythrocyte sedimentation rate, C-reactive protein, as well as other acute-phase reactants.

The beneficial effect of pregnancy on the course of RA has been known for many years.[105] It has been reported that pregnancy induces improvement in RA symptoms in approximately 75% of women.[106] Recently, Barrett et al.[107] examined the influence of pregnancy on disease activity. The authors prospectively analyzed 140 women, of whom two-thirds reported decreased joint swelling and pain, while 16% experienced total remission during pregnancy. However, the authors considered that the influence of pregnancy on disease activity showed widespread variability. The mechanism for these improvements is complex and still under investigation. One of the leading hypotheses is related to the immunologic changes observed in pregnancy with increased T-helper type 2 responses, which could potentially counterbalance the exacerbated T-helper type 1 response observed in RA.[105] During the puerperium, however, the relapse rate is approximately 90%.[108] Silman et al.[109] conducted a case–control study to determine the relationship between the onset of RA and parturition in 88 women with recent-onset RA and 144 age-matched control subjects. There was an increase during th first 3 months postpartum [OR 5.6, 95% confidence interval (CI) 1.8–17.6], which was greater when RA onset occurred after the first pregnancy. Other investigators have linked this increased risk specifically with breastfeeding.[110,111] Barrett et al.[111] prospectively followed and compared disease activity during pregnancy and 6 months postpartum among 49 nonbreastfeeders, 38 first-time breastfeeders, and 50 repeat breastfeeders. The authors found that women breastfeeding for the first time had increased disease activity at 6 months postpartum.[111] The considerable increase in prolactin secretion during breastfeeding together with its immunoregulatory activity are thought to be involved in the increase in disease activity or onset among susceptible women.[112] Finally, the risk of adverse perinatal outcome does not seem to be increased in women with RA.[113] The fertility rate as well as the miscarriage rate is similar to that in the general population,[113] and perinatal outcome is not different from that of healthy women.[114] If general anesthesia is needed in patients with upper spinal involvement, caution must be exerted as atlanto-occipital joint luxation is an infrequent but severe complication. As perinatal outcome is not affected and RA activity tends to ameliorate during pregnancy, most concerns during the preconception and antenatal period focus on the safety of the medications.

Treatment

Treatment of RA is usually delivered by a healthcare team involving a primary-care physician, rheumatologist, and a physical therapist. The goal of the treatment is initially to attain remission of symptoms and maintenance of such remission over time together with adequate joint function.[115] Nonpharmacologic treatment consists of education regarding the disease and psychological support to help patients to cope with the chronicity of this condition. Physical therapy is necessary to maintain adequate joint range of motion and includes supervised physical activity to improve muscle strength and improvement in emotional adjustment.[104]

In nonpregnant individuals, three groups of agents are available for the treatment of RA: NSAIDs, corticosteroids, and the so-called DMARDs (disease-modifying antirheumatic drugs), most commonly hydroxychloroquine, sulfasalazine, methotrexate, leflunomide, etanercept, and infliximab. Optimal treatment of RA in nonpregnant individuals consists of starting DMARD therapy within the first 3 months following diagnosis as these agents can arrest or delay the progression of the disease.[116] NSAIDs are useful in decreasing symptoms especially during the first weeks until a definitive diagnosis is achieved and DMARDs start acting. However, these drugs do not decelerate the rate of disease progression.[115] Low-dose oral glucocorticoids (< 10 mg/day) are effective in relieving symptoms[116] as well as in slowing joint damage.[117,118] However, their dose-dependent side-effects limit their long-term effectiveness. During pregnancy and the preconception period, patient education and guidance regarding drug side-effects are of utmost importance in achieving a good perinatal outcome. Frequently, the decreased disease activity during gestation allows patients to treat mild symptoms with analgesics such as acetaminophen, which have been shown to be safe for the fetus.[79] If NSAIDs are needed, they can be used with caution after the first trimester and up to 32 weeks. As the potential risk of decreased amniotic fluid is well proven, it is recommended that follow-up should include the assessment of amniotic fluid volume with ultrasonography during treatment. When steroids are required to control the symptoms of arthritis, they are generally considered to be safe for use in pregnancy and during lactation. Most DMARDs are contraindicated during pregnancy, lactation, and the preconception period.[104] Methotrexate and leflunomide have significant teratogenicity[114,119] and therefore should be avoided during pregnancy. If pregnancy is detected in a woman already taking these agents, the agents should be discontinued immediately. When preconception planning is possible, either leflunomide should be stopped 2 years before conception or cholestyramine washout should be attempted in those women who desire to conceive sooner.[120] Methotrexate should be discontinued 3 months before conception.[120] Hydroxychloroquine and sulfasalazine can be used cautiously during pregnancy and lactation.[121]

Ankylosing spondylitis

Ankylosing spondylitis is an inflammatory condition with unknown etiology, strong genetic predisposition, and a remarkable association with human leukocyte antigen (HLA)-B27. It most frequently affects the axial skeleton; however, 30% of patients can develop peripheral arthritis.[122] Its onset usually occurs during the reproductive years from adolescence to early adulthood. Characteristically, symptoms arise with insidious lumbar pain and morning stiffness. Later in the disease course, decreased spinal mobility can be observed. Laboratory evaluation has poor specificity and is not diagnostic. If isolated, rheumatoid factor and ANA are negative. Usually, patients are positive for HLA-B27[123] and for

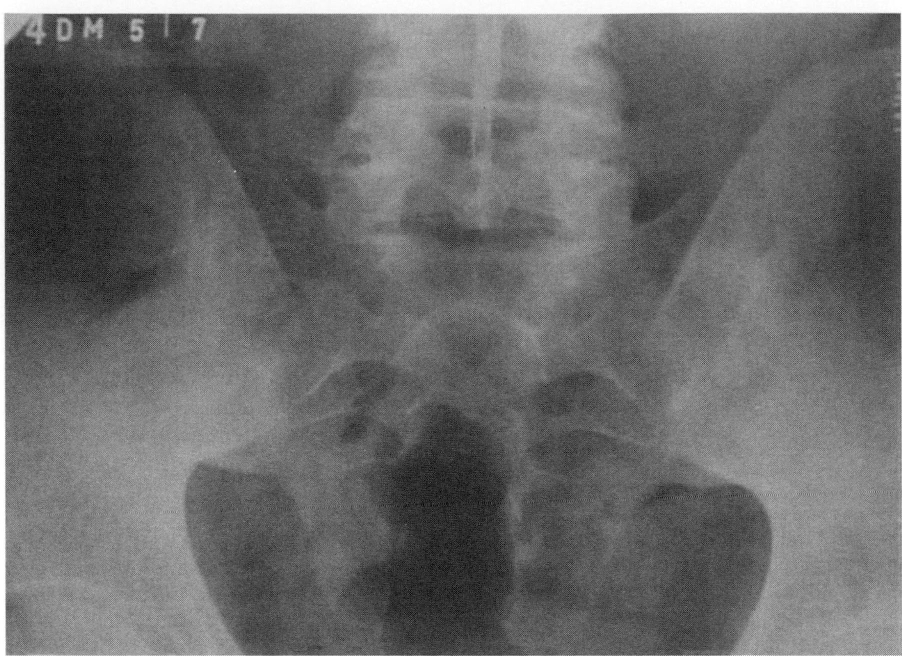

Figure 51.3 Radiological evidence of sacroiliitis in a patient with ankylosing spondylitis. Courtesy of Dr Carlos Perandones, Rheumatology Division, CEMIC, Buenos Aires, Argentina.

active-phase reactants such as C-reactive protein. Chest radiographs are characteristic, when the disease is well established, demonstrating evidence of symmetric erosions and sclerosis of sacroiliac joints (Fig. 51.3). Furthermore, loss of the normal spine lordosis and squaring of vertebral bodies with calcification of the outer fibers of the annulus fibrosus giving the "bamboo spine" appearance can be seen. Diagnosis of ankylosing spondylitis is based on the modified New York criteria of 1984 including: (1) history of inflammatory back pain; (2) limitation of motion of the lumbar spine in the sagittal and frontal planes; (3) limited chest expansion; and (4) evidence of radiographic sacroiliitis. The presence of the first with any of the other criteria is sufficient for diagnosis.[124]

Unlike rheumatoid arthritis, ankylosing spondilitis does not usually undergo remission during pregnancy. Ostensen and Ostensen[125] studied pregnancy performance in 930 patients with ankylosing spondylitis. The authors found that the mean age of onset was 23 years, and 21% had onset during pregnancy. Disease activity was unchanged in 33%, improved in 31%, and worsened in 33%. Interestingly, the group of patients with symptomatic improvement had a previous history of peripheral arthritis and gave birth to a female fetus. Among patients with active disease at conception, 60% presented with postpartum flares within 6 months of delivery.[125] Women with ankylosing spondylitis can be reassured that the perinatal outcome is not significantly affected by the disease.[125,126] Ostensen and Ostensen[125] observed a rate of miscarriage of 15%, with 93% of the deliveries being at term with a mean birthweight of 3340 g. Cesarean section was performed in 58% of cases. Finally, the authors found no evidence of an increased rate of infertility among women with ankylosing spondylitis.[125] Among offspring of women with ankylosing spondylitis, 12% had the disease by the age of 18 years. Therefore, children of women with ankylosing spondylitis seem to have an increased incidence of the disease over the general population.[127]

Treatment during pregnancy is oriented to maintaining functional capacity as well as to ameliorating pain. NSAIDs can be used with caution, but must be avoided during the first trimester and during the last 8 weeks of pregnancy.

Key points

1 SLE is diagnosed when at least four of the 11 ACR criteria are met. Approximately 90% of the patients will be positive for ANA.

2 Either anti-Ro (SS-A) and/or anti-LA (SS-B) antibodies are present in 20–40% patients with the diagnosis of lupus, and they are associated with the occurrence of congenital heart block.

3 Whether pregnancy causes exacerbation of SLE is still under debate. However, flares occur frequently during pregnancy and the puerperium, and are not more severe than in nonpregnant patients.

4 Although most women with lupus nephritis have no permanent renal deterioration secondary to pregnancy (60%), some will develop permanent renal failure

(7%). Inactive disease as well as mild renal dysfunction at conception are associated with improved outcome.

5 SLE is associated with an increased risk of poor perinatal outcome, such as early and late pregnancy loss, IUGR, preeclampsia, preterm labor, and neonatal complications secondary to complete heart block.

6 The most significant factors influencing outcome are probably activity of disease at conception, renal involvement, and the presence of antiphospholipid syndrome (APS).

7 Primary APS occurs in patients without other immune disorders, and secondary APS occurs in conjunction with autoimmune disease.

8 At least one clinical and one laboratory criteria must be met to achieve the diagnosis of APS. Lupus anticoagulant (LAC) and moderate to high levels of IgG and IgM anticardiolipins detected on two occasions separated by no less than 6 weeks must be present to consider diagnosis.

9 APS complicating SLE increases fetal risks of spontaneous abortion, stillbirth, IUGR, preeclampsia, abnormalities in tests of fetal well-being, and preterm delivery.

10 During prenatal care, efforts should be directed to early detection of maternal complications, such as preeclampsia, lupus flare, renal function deterioration, and to fetal well-being including adequate growth, placental function, and normal heart rate.

11 Women exposed to cyclophosphamide have a rate of permanent amenorrhea of approximately 25% and an increased incidence of infertility. Patient's age at exposure is an important risk factor. Adequate contraception is mandatory while undergoing treatment as this drug is teratogenic.

12 NSAIDs can be used with caution during the second trimester and up to 32 weeks of gestation to relieve symptoms.

13 Corticosteroids have no teratogenic effects. When required, prednisone or prednisolone can be utilized as only 10% of these drugs cross the placenta.

14 When necessary, hydroxychloroquine can be used during pregnancy. It has been shown to have no teratogenic effect or significant neonatal morbidity.

15 Azathioprine can be considered in pregnancy when a cytotoxic drug is necessary. Recent studies demonstrated that it is fairly well tolerated in pregnancy.

16 In general, with careful planning and intensive monitoring, maternal and fetal outcomes are good in women with scleroderma.

17 Among patients with scleroderma, renal crisis is the most severe complication. Although ACE inhibitors have significant fetal toxicity, these drugs could be life-saving and should be offered to pregnant women with scleroderma and renal crisis.

18 The diagnosis of rheumatoid arthritis is based on the modified criteria of the ACR that evaluate the presence of the following characteristics: morning stiffness, arthritis of three or more joint areas, arthritis of hand joints, symmetric arthritis, rheumatoid nodules, serum rheumatoid factor, and radiographic changes.

19 The course of rheumatoid arthritis shows significant improvements throughout pregnancy in the majority of women. However, most (90%) relapse in the puerperium and during breastfeeding.

20 The fertility rate as well as the incidence of miscarriage is not increased in women with rheumatoid arthritis. Furthermore, perinatal outcome is similar to that in the general population.

21 When preconception planning is possible, either leflunomide should be stopped 2 years before conception or cholestyramine washout should be attempted in those women who desire to conceive sooner. Methotrexate should be discontinued 3 months before conception. Hydroxychloroquine and sulfasalazine can be used cautiously during pregnancy and lactation.

22 Diagnosis of ankylosing spondylitis is based on the modified New York criteria of 1984 including: (1) history of inflammatory back pain; (2) limitation of motion of the lumbar spine in sagittal and frontal planes; (3) limited chest expansion; and (4) evidence of radiographic sacroiliitis. The presence of the first with any of the other criteria is sufficient for the diagnosis.

23 Ankylosing spondylitis does not generally undergo remission during pregnancy, and the few exceptions are observed in patients with involvement of the peripheral joints. Fertility and perinatal outcome are not significantly altered by the disease.

References

1 Jacobson DL, Gange SJ, Rose NR, et al. Epidemiology and estimated population burden of selected autoimmune diseases in the United States. *Clin Immunol Immunopathol* 1997;84:223–243.

2 Kotzin BL. Systemic lupus erythematosus. *Cell* 1996;85: 303–306.

3 Tan EM, Cohen AS, Fries JF, et al. The 1982 revised criteria for the classification of systemic lupus erythematosus. *Arthritis Rheum* 1982;25:1271–1277.

4 Hochberg MC. Updating the American College of Rheumatology revised criteria for the classification of systemic lupus erythematosus. *Arthritis Rheum* 1997;40:1725.

5 Smeenk RJT, van den Brink HG, Brinkman K, et al. Anti-dsDNA: choice of assay in relation to clinical value. *Rheumatol Int* 1991;11:101–107.

6 Ter Borg EJ, Horst G, Hummel EJ, et al. Measurement of increases in anti-double-stranded DNA antibody levels as a predictor of disease exacerbation in systemic lupus erythematosus:

a long-term, prospective study. *Arthritis Rheum* 1990;33:634–643.
7 Hahn BH. Mechanism of disease: antibodies to DNA. *N Engl J Med* 1998;338:1359–1368.
8 Ahlenius I, Floberg J, Thomassen P. Sixty-six cases of intrauterine fetal death. A prospective study with an extensive test protocol. *Acta Obstet Gynecol Scand* 1995;74:109–117.
9 Warren JB, Silver RM. Autoimmune disease in pregnancy: systemic lupus erythematosus and antiphospholipid syndrome. *Obstet Gynecol Clin North Am* 2004;31:345–372.
10 Mintz G, Niz J, Gutierrez G, et al. Prospective study of pregnancy in systemic lupus erythematosus. Results of a multidisciplinary approach. *J Rheumatol* 1986;13:732–739.
11 Lockshin MD. Pregnancy does not cause systemic lupus erythematosus to worsen. *Arthritis Rheum* 1989;32:665–670.
12 Urowitz MB, Gladman DD, Farewell VT, et al. Lupus and pregnancy studies. *Arthritis Rheum* 1993;36:1392–1397.
13 Lockshin MD, Reinitz E, Druzin ML, et al. Lupus pregnancy. Case–control prospective study demonstrating absence of lupus exacerbation during or after pregnancy. *Am J Med* 1984;77:893–898.
14 Wong KL, Chan FY, Lee CP. Outcome of pregnancy in patients with systemic lupus erythematosus. A prospective study. *Arch Intern Med* 1991;151:269–273.
15 Petri M, Howard D, Repke J. Frequency of lupus flare in pregnancy. The Hopkins Lupus Pregnancy Center experience. *Arthritis Rheum* 1991;34:1538–1545.
16 Ruiz-Irastorza G, Lima F, Alves J, et al. Increased rate of lupus flare during pregnancy and the puerperium: a prospective study of 78 pregnancies. *Br J Rheumatol* 1996;35:133–138.
17 Garsenstein M, Pollak VE, Kark RM. Systemic lupus erythematosus and pregnancy. *N Engl J Med* 1962;267:165–169.
18 Mock CC, Wong RWS. Pregnancy in systemic lupus erythematosus. *Postgrad Med J* 2001;77:157–165.
19 Burkett G. Lupus nephropathy and pregnancy. *Clin Obstet Gynecol* 1985;28:310–323.
20 Yasmeen S, Wilkins EE, Field NT, et al. Pregnancy outcomes in women with systemic lupus erythematosus. *J Matern Fetal Med* 2001;10:91–96.
21 Hayslett JP, Lynn RI. Effect of pregnancy in patients with lupus nephropathy. *Kidney Int* 1980;18:207–220.
22 Gimovsky ML, Montoro M, Paul RH. Pregnancy outcome in women with systemic lupus erythematosus. *Obstet Gynecol* 1984;63:686–692.
23 Meehan RT, Dorsey JK. Pregnancy among patients with systemic lupus erythematosus receiving immunosuppressive therapy. *J Rheumatol* 1987;14:252–258.
24 McHugh NJ, Reilly PA, McHugh LA. Pregnancy outcome and autoantibodies in connective tissue disease. *J Rheumatol* 1989;16:42–46.
25 Petri M, Allbritton J. Fetal outcome of lupus pregnancy: a retrospective case-control study of the Hopkins Lupus Cohort. *J Rheumatol* 1993;20:650–656.
26 Devoe LD, Taylor RL. Systemic lupus erythematosus in pregnancy. *Am J Obstet Gynecol* 1979;135:473–479.
27 Deng JS, Bair LW, Jr, Shen-Schwarz S, et al. Localization of Ro (SS-A) antigen in the cardiac conduction system. *Arthritis Rheum* 1987;30:1232–1238.
28 Nossent HC, Swaak TJ. Systemic lupus erythematosus. VI. Analysis of the interrelationship with pregnancy. *J Rheumatol* 1990;17:771–776.
29 Derksen RH, Bruinse HW, de Groot PG, Kater L. Pregnancy in systemic lupus erythematosus: a prospective study. *Lupus* 1994;3:149–155.
30 Huong DLT, Weschsler B, Piette JC. Pregnancy and its outcome in systemic lupus erythematosus. *Q J Med* 1994;87:721–729.
31 Lima F, Buchanan NM, Khamashta MA, et al. Obstetric outcome in systemic lupus erythematosus. *Semin Arthritis Rheum* 1995;25:184–192.
32 Johnson MJ, Petri M, Witter FR, Repke JT. Evaluation of preterm delivery in a systemic lupus erythematosus pregnancy clinic. *Obstet Gynecol* 1995;86:396–399.
33 Englert HJ, Derue GM, Loizou S, et al. Pregnancy and lupus: prognostic indicators and response to treatment. *Q J Med* 1988;66:125–136.
34 Cortes-Hernandez J, Ordi-Ros J, Paredes F, et al. Clinical predictors of fetal and maternal outcome in systemic lupus erythematosus: a prospective study of 103 pregnancies. *Rheumatology (Oxford)* 2002;41:643–650.
35 Rahman P, Gladman DD, Urowitz MB. Clinical predictors of fetal outcomes in systemic lupus erythematosus. *J Rheumatol* 1998;25:1526–1530.
36 Wilson WA, Gharavi AE, Koike T, et al. International consensus statement on preliminary classification criteria for definite antiphospholipid syndrome: report of an international workshop. *Arthritis Rheum* 1999;42:1309–1311.
37 Brandt JT, Barna LK, Triplett DA. Laboratory identification of lupus anticoagulants: results of the Second International Workshop for Identification of Lupus Anticoagulants. On behalf of the Subcommittee on Lupus Anticoagulants/Antiphospholipid Antibodies of the ISTH. *Thromb Haemost* 1995;74:1597–1603.
38 Hanly JG. Antiphospholipid syndrome: an overview. *Can Med Assoc J* 2003;168:1675–1682.
39 Branch DW, Khamashta MA. Antiphospholipid syndrome: obstetric diagnosis, management, and controversies *Obstet Gynecol* 2003;101:1333–1344.
40 Lockshin MD, Sammartino LR, Schwatzman S. Validation of the Sapporo criteria for antiphospholipid syndrome. *Arthritis Rheum* 2000;43:440–443.
41 Ninomiya C, Taniguchi O, Kato T, et al. Distribution and clinical significance of lupus anticoagulant and anticardiolipin antibody in 349 patients with systemic lupus erythematosus. *Intern Med* 1992;31:194–199.
42 Petri M. Epidemiology of the antiphospholipid antibody syndrome. *J Autoimmun* 2000;15:145–151.
43 Merkel PA, Chang Y, Pierangeli SS, et al. The prevalence and clinical associations of anticardiolipin antibodies in a large inception cohort of patients with connective tissue diseases. *Am J Med* 1996;101:576–583.
44 Cervera R, Khamashta MA, Font J, et al. Systemic lupus erythematosus: clinical and immunologic patterns of disease expression in a cohort of 1,000 patients. The European Working Party on Systemic Lupus Erythematosus. *Medicine (Baltimore)* 1993;72:113–124.
45 Alarcon-Segovia D, Perez-Vazquez ME, Villa AR, et al. Preliminary classification criteria for the antiphospholipid syndrome within systemic lupus erythematosus. *Semin Arthritis Rheum* 1992;21:275–286.
46 Rai RS, Clifford K, Cohen H, Regan L. High prospective fetal loss rate in untreated pregnancies of women with recurrent miscarriage and antiphospholipid antibodies. *Hum Reprod* 1995;10:3301–3304.
47 Ginsberg JS, Brill-Edwards P, Johnston M, et al. Relationship of

antiphospholipid antibodies to pregnancy loss in patients with systemic lupus erythematosus: a cross-sectional study. *Blood* 1992;80:975–980.

48 Oshiro BT, Silver RM, Scott JR, et al. Antiphospholipid antibodies and fetal death. *Obstet Gynecol* 1996;87:489–493.

49 Ruiz-Irastorza G, Khamashta MA, Castellino G. Systemic lupus erythematosus. *Lancet* 2001;357:1027–1032.

50 Branch DW, Andres R, Digre KB, et al. The association of antiphospholipid antibodies with severe preeclampsia. *Obstet Gynecol* 1989;73:541–545.

51 Milliez J, Lelong F, Bayani N, et al. The prevalence of autoantibodies during third-trimester pregnancy complicated by hypertension or idiopathic fetal growth retardation. *Am J Obstet Gynecol* 1991;165:51–56.

52 Caruso A, De Carolis S, Ferrazzani S, et al. Pregnancy outcome in relation to uterine artery flow velocity waveforms and clinical characteristics in women with antiphospholipid syndrome. *Obstet Gynecol* 1993;82:970–977.

53 Branch DW, Silver RM, Blackwell JL, et al. Outcome of treated pregnancies in women with antiphospholipid syndrome: an update of the Utah experience. *Obstet Gynecol* 1992;80:614–620.

54 Branch DW, Scott JR, Kochenour NK, Hershgold E. Obstetric complications associated with the lupus anticoagulant. *N Engl J Med* 1985;313:1322–1326.

55 Lima F, Khamashta MA, Buchanan NM, et al. A study of sixty pregnancies in patients with the antiphospholipid syndrome. *Clin Exp Rheumatol* 1996;14:131–136.

56 Lockshin MD, Druzin ML, Qamar T. Prednisone does not prevent recurrent fetal death in women with antiphospholipid antibody. *Am J Obstet Gynecol.* 1989;160:439–443.

57 Huong DL, Wechsler B, Bletry O, et al. A study of 75 pregnancies in patients with antiphospholipid syndrome. *J Rheumatol* 2001;28:2025–2030.

58 Lockshin MD, Druzin ML, Goei S, et al. Antibody to cardiolipin as a predictor of fetal distress or death in pregnant patients with systemic lupus erythematosus. *N Engl J Med* 1985;313: 152–156.

59 Loizou S, Byron MA, Englert HJ, et al. Association of quantitative anticardiolipin antibody levels with fetal loss and time of loss in systemic lupus erythematosus. *Q J Med* 1998;68: 525–531.

60 Pauzner R, Dulitzki M, Langevitz P, et al. Low molecular weight heparin and warfarin in the treatment of patients with antiphospholipid syndrome during pregnancy. *Thromb Haemost* 2001;86:1379–1384.

61 Lee RM, Brown MA, Branch DW, et al. Anticardiolipin and anti-beta2-glycoprotein-I antibodies in preeclampsia. *Obstet Gynecol* 2003;102:294–300.

62 Lee LA. Neonatal lupus erythematosus. *J Invest Dermatol* 1993;100:9S–13S.

63 Ramsey-Goldman R, Hom D, Deng JS, Ziegler GC, et al. Anti-SS-A antibodies and fetal outcome in maternal systemic lupus erythematosus. *Arthritis Rheum* 1986;29:1269–1273.

64 Brucato A, Doria A, Frassi M, et al. Pregnancy outcome in 100 women with autoimmune diseases and anti-Ro/SSA antibodies: a prospective controlled study. *Lupus* 2002,11:716–721.

65 Brucato A, Frassi M, Franceschini F, et al. Risk of congenital complete heart block in newborns of mothers with anti-Ro/SSA antibodies detected by counterimmunoelectrophoresis: a prospective study of 100 women. *Arthritis Rheum* 2001,44: 1832–1835.

66 Buyon JP, Hiebert R, Copel J. Autoimmune-associated congenital heart block: demographics, mortality, morbidity and recurrence rates obtained from a national neonatal lupus registry. *J Am Coll Cardiol* 1998;31:1658–1666.

67 Lee LA, Sokol RJ, Buyon JP. Hepatobiliary disease in neonatal lupus: prevalence and clinical characteristics in cases enrolled in a national registry. *Pediatrics* 2002;109:E11.

68 Neiman AR, Lee LA, Weston WL, Buyon JP. Cutaneous manifestations of neonatal lupus without heart block: characteristics of mothers and children enrolled in a national registry. *J Pediatr* 2000;137:674–680.

69 Boumpas DT, Austin HA, 3rd, Vaughan EM, Yarboro CH. Risk for sustained amenorrhea in patients with systemic lupus erythematosus receiving intermittent pulse cyclophosphamide therapy. *Ann Intern Med* 1993;119:366–369.

70 Ioannidis JP, Katsifis GE, Tzioufas AG. Predictors of sustained amenorrhea from pulsed intravenous cyclophosphamide in premenopausal women with systemic lupus erythematosus. *J Rheumatol* 2002;29:2129–2135.

71 Wang CL, Wang F, Bosco JJ. Ovarian failure in oral cyclophosphamide treatment for systemic lupus erythematosus. *Lupus* 1995;4:11–14.

72 Gordon C. Pregnancy and autoimmune diseases. *Best Pract Res Clin Rheumatol* 2004;18:359–379.

73 Massobrio M, Benedetto C, Bertini E. Immune complexes in preeclampsia and normal pregnancy. *Am J Obstet Gynecol* 1985;152:578–583.

74 de Messias-Reason IJ, Aleixo V, de Freitas H. Complement activation in Brazilian patients with preeclampsia. *J Invest Allergol Clin Immunol* 2000;10:209–214.

75 Begg L, East C, Chan FY. Intrapartum fetal oxygen saturation monitoring in congenital fetal heart block. *Aust NZ J Obstet Gynaecol* 1998;38:271–274.

76 Buckfield P. Major congenital faults in newborn infants: a pilot study in New Zealand. *NZ Med J* 1973;778:195.

77 Slone D, Siskind V, Heinonen OP, et al. Aspirin and congenital malformations. *Lancet* 1976;11:1373.

78 Turner G, Collins E. Fetal effects of regular salicylate ingestion in pregnancy. *Lancet* 1975;2:238.

79 Li DK, Liu L, Odouli R. Exposure to non-steroidal anti-inflammatory drugs during pregnancy and risk of miscarriage: population based cohort study. *Br Med J* 2003;327:368.

80 Stika CS, Gross GA, Leguizamon G, et al. A prospective randomized safety trial of celecoxib for treatment of preterm labor. *Am J Obstet Gynecol* 2002;187:653–660.

81 Carr RE, Henkind P, Rothfield N, Siegel IM. Ocular toxicity of antimalarial drugs. Long-term follow-up. *Am J Ophthalmol* 1968;66:738–744.

82 Parke AL, Rothfield NF. Antimalarial drugs in pregnancy – the North American experience. *Lupus* 1996;5(Suppl.1):S67–69.

83 Khamashta MA, Buchanan NM, Hughes GR. The use of hydroxychloroquine in lupus pregnancy: the British experience. *Lupus* 1996;5(Suppl. 1):S65–66.

84 Motta M, Tincani A, Faden D, et al. Follow-up of infants exposed to hydroxychloroquine given to mothers during pregnancy and lactation. *J Perinatol* 2005;25:86–89.

85 Costedoat-Chlumeau N, Amoura Z, Duhaut P, et al. Safety of hydroxychloroquine in pregnant patients with connective tissue diseases: a study of one hundred thirty-three cases compared with a control group. *Arthritis Rheum* 2003;48:3207–3211.

86 Levy RA, Vilela VS, Cataldo MJ, et al. Hydroxychloroquine

(HCQ) in lupus pregnancy: double-blind and placebo-controlled study. *Lupus* 2001;10:401–404.
87 Abu-Shakra M, Shoenfeld Y. Azathioprine therapy for patients with systemic lupus erythematosus. *Lupus* 2001;10:152–153.
88 Scott JR. Fetal growth retardation associated with maternal administration of immunosuppressive drugs *Am J Obstet Gynecol* 1977;128:668–667.
89 Armenti VT, Ahlswede KM, Ahlswede BA, et al. National Transplantation Pregnancy Registry: analysis of outcome/risks of 394 pregnancies in kidney transplant recipients. *Transplant Proc* 1994;26:2535.
90 Pirson Y, Van Lierde M, Ghysen J, et al. Retardation of fetal growth in patients receiving immunosuppressive therapy. *N Engl J Med* 1985;313:328.
91 Ramsey-Goldman R, Mientus JM, Kutzer JE, et al. Pregnancy outcome in women with systemic lupus erythematosus treated with immunosuppressive drugs. *J Rheumatol* 1993;20:1152–1157.
92 Cote CJ, Meuwissen HJ, Pickering RJ. Effects on the neonate of prednisone and azathioprine administered to the mother during pregnancy. *J Pediatr* 1974;85:324–328.
93 Black CM, Stevens WM. Scleroderma. *Rheum Dis Clin North Am* 1989;15:193–212.
94 Steen VD. Scleroderma and pregnancy. *Rheum Dis Clin North Am* 1997;23:133–147.
95 Steen VD. Pregnancy in women with systemic sclerosis. *Obstet Gynecol* 1999;94:15–20.
96 Tabacova S, Little R, Tsong Y, et al Adverse pregnancy outcomes associated with maternal enalapril antihypertensive treatment. *Pharmacoepidemiol Drug Safety* 2003;12:633–646.
97 Piper JM, Ray WA, Rosa FW. Pregnancy outcome following exposure to angiotensin converting enzyme inhibitors. *Obstet Gynecol* 1992;80:429–432.
98 Steen VD, Costantino JP, Shapiro AP. Outcome of renal crisis in systemic sclerosis: relation to availability of angiotensin converting enzyme (ACE) inhibitors *Ann Intern Med* 1990;113:352–357.
99 Steen VD, Medsger TA, Jr. Long-term outcomes of scleroderma renal crisis. *Ann Intern Med* 2000;133:600–603.
100 Steen VD, Conte C, Day N, et al. Pregnancy in women with systemic sclerosis. *Arthritis Rheum* 1989;32:151–157.
101 Silman AJ, Black C. Increased incidence of spontaneous abortion and infertility in women with scleroderma before disease onset: a controlled study. *Ann Rheum Dis* 1988;47:441–444.
102 Steen VD, Medsger TA, Jr. Fertility and pregnancy outcome in women with systemic sclerosis. *Arthritis Rheum* 1999;42:763–768.
103 Shehata HA, Nelson-Piercy C. Connective tissue and skin disorders in pregnancy. *Curr Obstet Gynecol* 2001;II:329–335.
104 American College of Rheumatology Subcommittee on Rheumatoid Arthritis Guidelines. Guidelines for the management of rheumatoid arthritis: 2002 Update. *Arthritis Rheum* 2002;46:328–346.
105 Hench PS. The ameliorating effect of pregnancy on chronic atrophic (infectious rheumatoid) arthritis, fibrositis, and intermittent hydrarthosis. *Mayo Clin Proc* 1938;13:161–167.
106 Ostensen M, Villieger PM. Immunology of pregnancy-pregnancy as a remission inducing agent in rheumatoid arthritis. *Transpl Immunol* 2002;9:155–160.
107 Barrett JH, Brennan P, Fiddler M, Silman AJ. Does rheumatoid arthritis remit during pregnancy and relapse postpartum? Results from a nationwide study in the United Kingdom performed prospectively from late pregnancy. *Arthritis Rheum* 1999;42:1219–1227.
108 Ostensen M. Sex hormones and pregnancy in rheumatoid arthritis and systemic lupus erythematosus. *Ann NY Acad Sci* 1999;876:131–144.
109 Silman A, Kay A, Brennan P. Timing of pregnancy in relation to the onset of rheumatoid arthritis. *Arthritis Rheum* 1992;35:152–155.
110 Brennan P, Silman A. Breast-feeding and the onset of rheumatoid arthritis. *Arthritis Rheum* 1994;6:808–813.
111 Barrett JH, Brennan P, Fiddler M, Silman A. Breast-feeding and postpartum relapse in women with rheumatoid arthritis and inflammatory arthritis. *Arthritis Rheum* 2000;43:1010–1015.
112 Hampl JS, Papa DJ. Breastfeeding-related onset, flare, and relapse of rheumatoid arthritis. *Nutr Rev* 2001;59:264–268.
113 Nelson JL, Ostensen M. Pregnancy and rheumatoid arthritis. *Rheum Dis Clin North Am* 1997;23:195–212.
114 Klipple GL, Cecere FA. Rheumatoid arthritis and pregnancy. *Rheum Dis Clin North Am* 1989;15:213–239.
115 O'Dell JR. Therapeutic strategies for rheumatoid arthritis. *N Engl J Med* 2004;350:2591–2602.
116 Felson DT, Anderson JJ, Meenan RF. The comparative efficacy and toxicity of second-line drugs in rheumatoid arthritis: results of two metaanalyses. *Arthritis Rheum* 1990;33:1449–1461.
117 No authors listed. A comparison of prednisolone with aspirin or other analgesics in the treatment of rheumatoid arthritis. *Ann Rheum Dis* 1959; 18:173–188.
118 No authors listed. A comparison of prednisolone with aspirin or other analgesics in the treatment of rheumatoid arthritis: a second report by the joint committee of the Medical Research Council and Nuffield Foundation on clinical trials of cortisone, ACTH, and other therapeutic measures in chronic rheumatic diseases. *Ann Rheum Dis* 1960;19:331–337.
119 Janssen NM, Genta MS. The effects of immunosuppressive and anti-inflammatory medications on fertility, pregnancy, and lactation. *Arch Intern Med* 2000;160:610–619.
120 Bresnihan B. Treating early rheumatoid arthritis in the younger patient. *J Rheumatol* 2001;62(Suppl.):4–9.
121 Janssen NM, Genta MS. The effects of immunosuppressive and anti-inflammatory medications on fertility, pregnancy, and lactation. *Arch Intern Med* 2000;160:610–619.
122 Calin A. Seronegative spondyloarthritides. *Med Clin North Am* 1986;70:323–336.
123 Calin A, Fries JF. Striking prevalence of ankylosing spondylitis in "healthy" w27 positive males and females. *N Engl J Med* 1975;293:835–839.
124 van der Linden S, Valkenburg HA, Cats A. Evaluation of diagnostic criteria for ankylosing spondylitis. A proposal for modification of the New York criteria. *Arthritis Rheum* 1984;27:361–368.
125 Ostensen M, Ostensen H. Ankylosing spondylitis – the female aspect *J Rheumatol* 1998;25:120–124.
126 Ostensen M. The effect of pregnancy on ankylosing spondylitis, psoriatic arthritis, and juvenile rheumatoid arthritis. *Am J Reprod Immunol* 1992;28:235–237.
127 Ostensen M, Romberg O, Husby G. Ankylosing spondylitis and motherhood. *Arthritis Rheum* 1982;25:140–143.

52 Dermatologic disorders during pregnancy

Thomas D. Horn and Jerri Hoskyn

Pigmentary alterations

The most common change in the skin during pregnancy is hyperpigmentation, which is most noticeable in more darkly complexioned individuals.[1] While darkening may affect the normal skin, it is more pronounced in scars, melanocytic nevi, and ephelides, and particularly in skin and mucosal surfaces that contain more melanin – genital and axillary skin, areolae, and the perineum. The linea alba may darken, becoming the linea nigra.

Melasma or chloasma, the latter term confined to pregnant women, occurs commonly in pregnancy or in patients taking oral contraceptive medications. Well-defined hyperpigmented macules arise on the face in a symmetric distribution, particularly on the cheeks and forehead. Wood's lamp examination highlights the affected skin, but is rarely necessary to establish the diagnosis. Ultraviolet light exposure enhances the hyperpigmentation; thus, treatment is directed toward bleaching the epidermal melanin and protecting the skin with sunscreens. Combinations of 4% hydroquinone (pregnancy category C) and sunscreens exist in various formulations. Topical retinoids (pregnancy category C) and azelaic acid (pregnancy category B) are reported to possess bleaching effects beneficial in the treatment of melasma. Delay of treatment until well after delivery is reasonable, as melasma resolves spontaneously in the majority of patients.

Melanocytic nevi, including Spitz nevi, are reported to increase in size during pregnancy. One prospectively performed study of photographic documentation of melanocytic nevi during pregnancy disputes this generally accepted notion by showing that only a small number of nevi change in size, with some nevi decreasing in surface area.[2] Thus, any melanocytic nevus undergoing significant change should be sampled to explore the possibility of melanoma. The exact incidence of melanoma arising in pregnancy is uncertain, but the event is rare. Prognosis appears to be the same, based upon the characteristics of the tumor, as in nonpregnant women (Tables 52.1 and 52.2).[3] Melanoma is the most common cause of placental metastasis. The risk of fetal metastasis is estimated to be 22%. This level of disease portends a poor prognosis for mother and fetus.[4,5]

Vascular alterations

Spider angioma, capillary hemangioma, pyogenic granuloma, palmar erythema, varicosities and hemorrhoids, livedo reticularis, gingival hyperemia and hyperplasia, and dependent edema may arise in pregnancy. Spider angiomas are characterized by a central dilated arteriole with a fine meshwork of radiating capillary-sized vessels forming a blanching macule several millimeters in width. Firm pressure on the lesion followed by quick release reveals refilling of the lesion from the central arteriole with rapid spread outward. Persistent lesions may be destroyed using electric current or vascular laser. Pyogenic granuloma is a misnomer for a vascular tumor arising after minor trauma. The lesion is a lobular capillary hemangioma that is exophytic, beefy, and friable. These lesions may arise on mucosal and skin surfaces. Treatment is indicated to stop the nearly constant erosion and bleeding, and is best accomplished by removing the bulk of the tumor surgically followed by destruction of the feeder vessel. Left alone, pyogenic granulomas decrease in size and may involute. Livedo reticularis is asymptomatic, and is recognized by a lacy network of red–purple macules with intervening normal skin. The erythema blanches with pressure. Cold temperatures exacerbate the appearance of livedo reticularis.

Connective tissue alterations

Striae (striae distensae) arise from stretching of the skin from various causes and are common in pregnancy. Initially, they appear as symmetric reddish/purple linear macules with evolution to depressed skin-colored patches. Striae may itch. In

Table 52.1 Melanoma TNM classification.

T classification	*Thickness*	*Ulceration status*
T1	≤1.0 mm	a: Without ulceration and level II/III b: With ulceration or level IV/V
T2	1.01–2.0 mm	a: Without ulceration b: With ulceration
T3	2.01–4.0 mm	a: Without ulceration b: With ulceration
T4	>4.0 mm	a: Without ulceration b: With ulceration
N classification	*No. of metastatic nodes*	*Nodal metastatic mass*
N1	1 node	a: Micrometastasis* b: Macrometastasis†
N2	2–3 nodes	a: Micrometastasis* b: Macrometastasis† c: In transit met(s)/satellite(s) without metastatic node(s)
N3	4 or more metastatic nodes, or matted nodes, or in transit met(s)/satellite(s) with metastatic node(s)	
M classification	*Site*	*Serum lactate dehydrogenase*
M1a	Distant skin, subcutaneous, or nodal metastases	Normal
M1b	Lung metastases	Normal
M1c	All other visceral metastases	Normal
	Any distant metastasis	Elevated

Reprinted with permission from Bolognia JL, Jorizzo JL, Rapini RP, et al. *Dermatology*. London: Mosby, 2003.

*Micrometastases are diagnosed after sentinel or elective lymphadenectomy.

†Macrometastases are defined as clinically detectable nodal metastases confirmed by therapeutic lymphadenectomy or when nodal metastasis exhibits gross extracapsular extension.

association with pregnancy, the lesions arise most commonly on the abdomen, but they may develop on other sites, including breasts, thighs, hips, and buttocks. Striae arise most commonly in the third trimester and have been associated with vaginal lacerations during delivery.[6] While striae may fade over time, topical therapy with tretinoin cream 0.1% and application of pulsed-dye laser at 585 nm may improve their appearance.[7,8] Unrelated to the appearance of striae, skin tags, or acrochordons, may proliferate during pregnancy. Skin of the neck, axillae, and groin are typical sites.

Hair and nail alterations

Hirsutism is defined as the development of a male pattern of hair growth (terminal and/or vellus) in a woman, while hypertrichosis is defined as an increased amount of hair. Both conditions may arise during pregnancy, but neither condition warrants concern or treatment. For persistent hair abnormalities after delivery, topical application of eflornithine or the use of hair removal lasers may provide benefit.

Telogen effluvium is a shedding of hair that begins roughly 2–4 months after delivery, lasts for 2–4 months, and resolves over many months without intervention. A minority of patients progress to chronic telogen effluvium. In this disorder, anagen hairs, which normally account for 90–95% of all hairs, cycle into telogen. Telogen hair shafts are wispy, small, and nonpigmented and, thus, the appearance of hair loss ensues.

Changes in the appearance of the nail plate of fingers and toes are common. The nail plate may become brittle, and some patients report an increased rate of nail growth. The most common nail plate abnormality of significance is the development of Beau's lines in one or, more typically, several nails. Beau's lines are transverse depressions in the surface of the nail plate that arise from physiologic changes in the nail matrix. The Beau's lines will grow distally with continued nail growth, resulting in a normal nail plate after many months.

Table 52.2 Proposed stage groupings for cutaneous melanoma.

	Survival (%)*	Clinical staging†			Pathologic staging‡		
		T	N	M	T	N	M
0		Tis	N0	M0	Tis	N0	M0
IA	95	T1a	N0	M0	T1a	N0	M0
IB	90	T1b	N0	M0	T1b	N0	M0
		T2a			T2a		
IIA	78	T2b	N0	M0	T2b	N0	M0
		T3a			T3a		
IIB	65	T3b	N0	M0	T3b	N0	M0
		T4a			T4a		
IIC	45	T4b	N0	M0	T4b	N0	M0
III§		Any T	N1	M0			M0
			N2				
			N3				
IIIA	66				T1	N1a	M0
					T1	N2a	
IIIB	52				T1-4b	N1a	M0
					T1-4b	N2a	
					T1-4a	N1b	
					T1-4a	N2b	
					T1-4a/b	N2c	
IIIC	26				T1-4b	N1b	M0
					T1-4b	N2b	
					Any T	N3	
IV	7.5–11	Any T	Any N	Any M1	Any T	Any N	Any M1

Reprinted with permission from Bolognia JL, Jorizzo JL, Rapini RP, et al. *Dermatology*. London: Mosby, 2003.

*Approximate 5-year survival as a percentage.

†Clinical staging includes microstaging of the primary melanoma and clinical/radiologic evaluation for metastases. By convention, it should be used after complete excision of the primary melanoma with clinical assessment for regional and distant metastases.

‡Pathologic staging includes microstaging of the primary melanoma and pathologic information about the regional lymph nodes after partial or complete lymphadenectomy. Pathologic stage 0 or stage IA patients are the exception.

§There are no stage III subgroups for clinical staging.

Dermatoses of pregnancy

The dermatoses of pregnancy are a group of skin conditions unique to pregnancy or directly related to the products of conception (Table 52.3).

Polymorphic eruption of pregnancy

Polymorphic eruption of pregnancy (PEP), also known as pruritic urticarial papules and plaques of pregnancy, is the most common of the pregnancy dermatoses.

Clinical presentation

Pruritic urticarial papules appear first on the abdomen, often in the striae gravidarum, then progress to involve the thighs, buttocks, arms, and trunk (Fig. 52.1).[9] Periumbilical skin is characteristically spared, as are the face, palms, soles, and mucous membranes. Papules may coalesce into plaques, sometimes surrounded by a pale halo[10] and occasionally surmounted by pinpoint vesicles that do not progress to bullae.[11] In some cases, there are annular or target-like lesions. Excoriations are unusual despite the often marked pruritus. PEP presents in the third trimester, most commonly around the 35th week.[9,10] Occasionally, the presentation is postpartum, usually within 10 days,[12] although in one case, PEP appeared 4 weeks after delivery.[13] Primigravidas comprise about three-quarters of PEP cases.[9,11,14] In multiple pregnancies, PEP appears to be more common, and may occur earlier and be more severe.[10,15–17]

Table 52.3 Key features of the dermatoses of pregnancy.

	Incidence	Key signs/ symptoms	Presentation	Diagnosis	Course	Risks to mother or fetus	Recurrence	Treatment
PEP	1:150–160	Abdominal urticarial papules favoring striae, periumbilical sparing	36–39 weeks, rarely postpartum	Clinical Negative DIF	Self-limited, with resolution in 6 weeks	No	No	Symptomatic Systemic steroids in severe cases
CP	1:100–200	Pruritus ± jaundice	>30 weeks in 80%	Clinical Elevated serum bile salts	Resolution with delivery. Pruritus remits before laboratory values normalize	Yes, fetal distress	Yes	Symptomatic UDCA Delivery
PG	1:40 000–60 000	Periumbilical urticarial papules, vesicles, bullae	Second and third trimesters	Clinical Skin biopsy Positive DIF	Remission in third trimester with postpartum flare. Resolution in 2–6 months	Yes, low birthweight, small for dates, prematurity	Yes Flare with OCP or menses	Systemic steroids
IH	Rare (case reports)	Grouped sterile pustules, favor flexural areas, constitutional symptoms	Second and third trimesters	Clinical Skin biopsy Negative DIF	Resolution with delivery	Yes, placental insufficiency	Yes Flare with OCP or menses	Systemic steroids Delivery or termination
PP	1:300	Red papules, most excoriated, on trunk and extremities	Third trimester	Clinical	Resolution by 3 months postpartum	No	Rare	Symptomatic
PFP	Case reports	Small follicular papules and pustules on the trunk	Third trimester	Clinical	Resolution with delivery	No	Unknown	Symptomatic

PEP, polymorphic eruption of pregnancy; CP, cholestasis of pregnancy; PG, pemphigoid gestationis; IH, impetigo herpetiformis; PP, prurigo of pregnancy; PFP, pruritic folliculitis of pregnancy; DIF, direct immunofluorescence; OCP, oral contraceptive pills; UDCA, ursodeoxycholic acid.

Course

PEP is self-limited, with most cases clearing prior to or within 1 week of delivery. In a typical course, the eruption evolves over 1–2 weeks and fades over the following 2–4 weeks. PEP rarely lasts beyond 6 weeks postpartum.[12] Resolution is not clearly tied to delivery,[18] although in one severe case, early delivery led to prompt resolution of symptoms.[19] PEP rarely, if ever, recurs in subsequent pregnancies.

Epidemiologic features

With an estimated incidence ranging from 1:150 to 1:240 pregnancies,[11,20] PEP is the most common of the pregnancy-specific dermatoses. PEP is not thought to be familial, although there is one case report of its occurrence in two sets of sisters.[21] There has been no association with particular human leukocyte antigen (HLA) subtypes.[10]

Pathogenesis

The pathogenesis of PEP is unknown. Given its association with abdominal striae and presentation late in pregnancy, maternal and/or fetal weight gain have been theorized to play a role, but the evidence for this has been contradictory.[14,22,23]

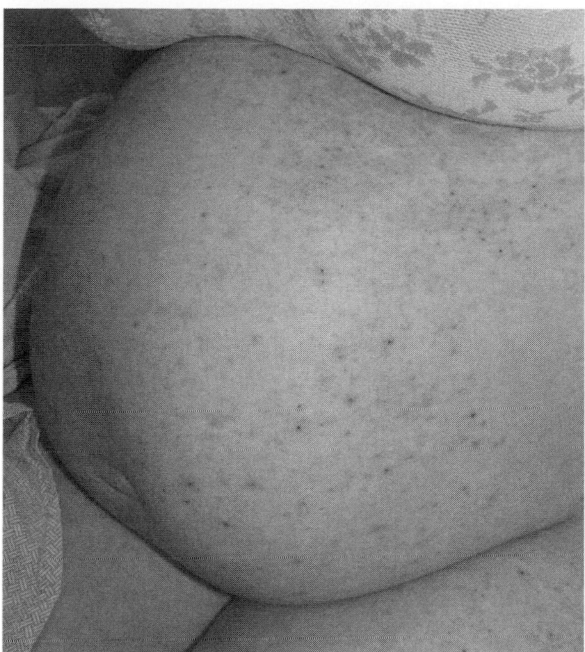

Figure 52.1 Polymorphic eruption of pregnancy. Erythematous papules on the abdomen, sparing the umbilicus. Excoriations are present here, but are not typical. Image courtesy of Susan Mallory, MD.

Fetal DNA has been identified in the skin lesions of PEP, suggesting that a maternal immune reaction to fetal DNA may play a role in PEP, but this has not been proven.[24] Interestingly, fetal microchimerism has been detected in the blood of nonpregnant women as much as 27 years postpartum,[25] and there is one report of PEP-like lesions 28 years postpartum in a woman with a prior history of PEP.[26]

Diagnosis and differential diagnosis

The diagnosis of PEP is a clinical one, as there is no confirmatory diagnostic test. No consistent laboratory or hormonal abnormalities have been associated with PEP,[27] and the histopathology is nonspecific, with negative direct immunofluorescence (DIF). The most important differential diagnosis is pemphigoid gestationis (PG), as the urticarial lesions of PG can be clinically and histopathologically indistinguishable from PEP. Only DIF can reliably distinguish these entities when the clinical picture is unclear. Other differential diagnoses include contact dermatitis, drug eruptions, erythema multiforme, and viral exanthems.

Prognosis

The prognosis for mother and baby is excellent. Aside from pruritus, there appear to be no risks to the mother. Likewise, there have been no reports of adverse outcomes for the babies of mothers with PEP. To date, there has been a single case report of a transient PEP-like eruption in a newborn whose mother was diagnosed clinically with PEP; however, because DIF was not done on either the mother or the baby, PG could not be definitively ruled out.[28]

Management

As PEP is self-limited, treatment is aimed at controlling symptoms. Moderate- to high-potency topical steroids are helpful in the majority of cases. Antihistamines have been variably helpful. In severe cases, systemic steroids may be required. One severe case of PEP was delivered early via Cesarean section, with resolution of symptoms within hours.[19]

Pemphigoid gestationis

PG, also known as herpes gestationis and gestational pemphigoid, is an autoimmune blistering disorder similar to bullous pemphigoid, but is unique to pregnancy.

Clinical presentation

In classic PG, pruritic urticarial papules and plaques appear on the periumbilical skin and evolve into vesicles and tense bullae within days to weeks (Figs 52.2–52.5). Eventual palmoplantar involvement is common, but the face and mucous membranes are usually spared. Acute onset has been reported infrequently.[29] In some cases, pruritus may precede the rash, or the rash may consist only of urticarial lesions, never developing typical vesiculobullous lesions.[29] Barring secondary infection, the lesions typically heal without scarring.[30]

PG typically presents in the second or third trimester, with an average onset at 21 weeks.[11] Up to 20% of cases may begin in the postpartum period, usually within 3–5 days after delivery. Although there are case reports of PG presenting up to 35 days postpartum, the diagnosis of PG is suspect if presentation is delayed for more than a few days.[30–32]

Course

In the third trimester, there may be relative remission or even clearance of the rash, but the vast majority will flare after delivery.[11,29,30] Most cases will clear within 2–6 months, although postpartum duration of disease varies.[31,32] In exceptional cases, disease activity has been reported to last one to several years after delivery.[11,33–35] PG may appear in any pregnancy, but generally recurs thereafter, skipping fewer than 10% of subsequent pregnancies.[29–31] Thirty percent of PG cases occur in primigravidas.[11] Recurrent episodes tend to occur earlier and to be more severe and prolonged.[30] Recurrent eruptions may or may not share the same morphology. In

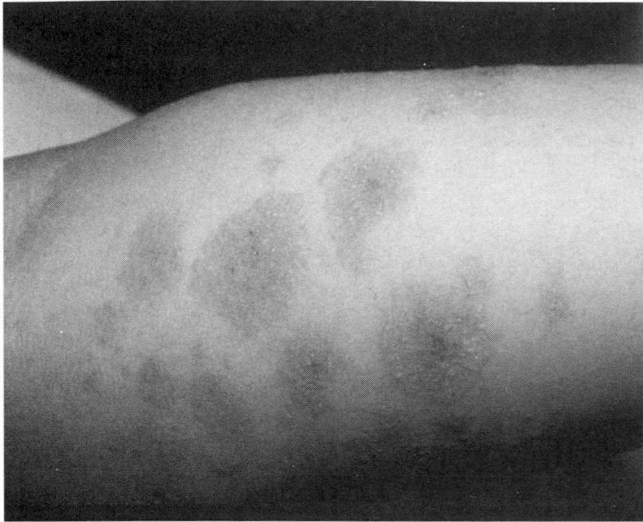

Figure 52.2 Pemphigoid gestationis. Urticarial plaques with small vesicles. Image courtesy of Susan Mallory, MD.

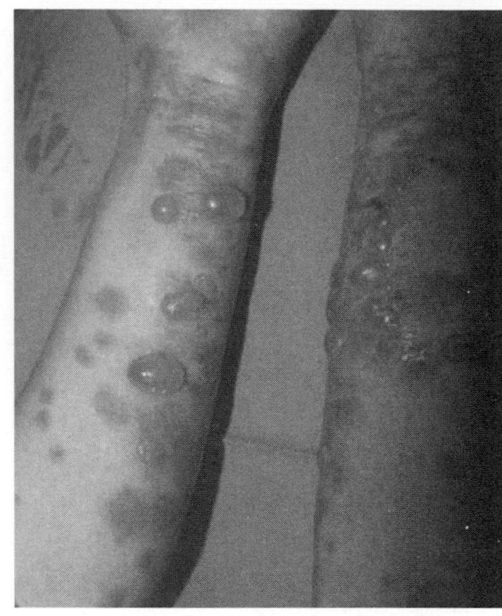

Figure 52.4 Pemphigoid gestationis. Urticarial plaques surmounted by tense bullae. Image courtesy of Jeffrey Callen, MD.

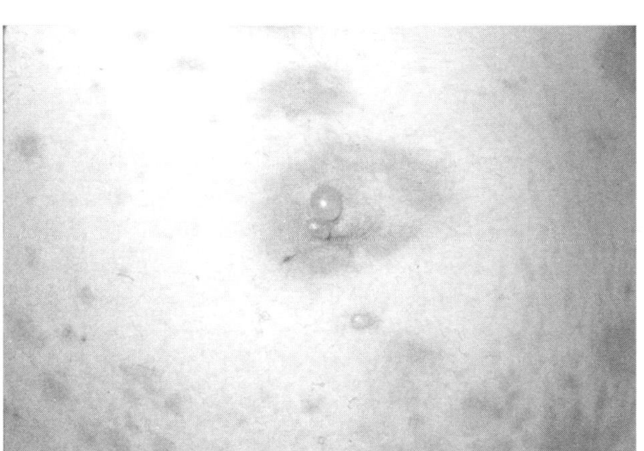

Figure 52.3 Pemphigoid gestationis. Typical periumbilical involvement. Image courtesy of Jeffrey Callen, MD.

other words, a typical eruption may be followed by one with urticarial lesions only, and vice versa.[30] Flares may occur with oral contraceptive pills and menses.[36]

Epidemiologic features

PG is a relatively rare disorder, and estimations of its incidence have varied widely from 1:1700[20] to 1:50 000–60 000 pregnancies,[29,30] the latter being the more recent estimates. The incidence has been estimated at 1 : 4500 in Mexicans,[37] and PG is reported to be distinctly uncommon in African–Americans.[30] The incidence in different populations appears partly to reflect the prevalence of the HLA haplotypes that have been associated with PG, most prominently the DR3 and DR4 alleles.[38] Some authors have reported an increase in other autoimmune diseases in PG patients, particularly Graves' disease.[39] PG has also been reported in association with hydatidiform mole and choriocarcinoma,[40,41] suggesting that placental tissue is a prerequisite for the development of PG.[30]

Pathogenesis

PG is caused by an autoantibody to a component of the basement membrane zone. Most patients with PG have an antibody to collagen XVII, a hemidesmosomal protein also known as bullous pemphigoid antigen 2. It is unclear what leads to the development of these autoantibodies in pregnancy, but the finding of anti-HLA antibodies in women with PG suggests that a maternal response to the placenta may play a role.[42,43] Some theorize that abnormal expression of major histocompatibility complex (MHC) class II molecules on the placenta may lead to a maternal immune response against the

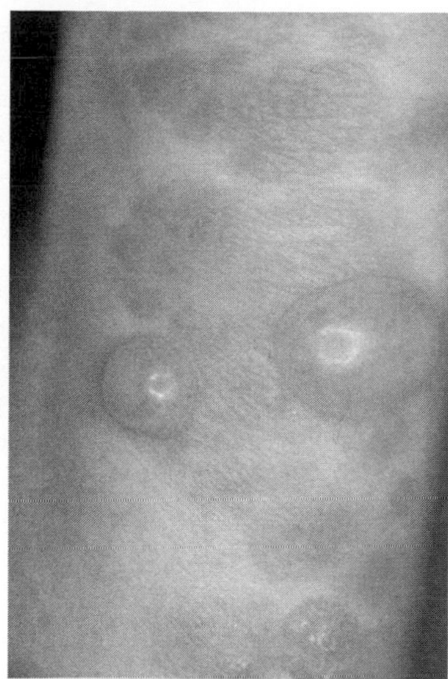

Figure 52.5 Pemphigoid gestationis. The characteristic tense bullae seen in PG. Image courtesy of Jeffrey Callen, MD.

placental basement membrane zone, which then leads to cross-reaction in the skin.[44]

Diagnosis and differential diagnosis

Clinically, the diagnosis of PG can suggest itself readily in a case with classic features; however, not all cases are straightforward, and routine laboratory and histopathology data can be unrevealing. The main source of confusion can be in distinguishing the urticarial lesions of PG from those of PEP. Laboratory values tend to be normal in PG, although there may be peripheral eosinophilia.[30] Routine histopathology may reveal typical subepidermal bullae with eosinophils, but the urticarial lesions of PG are only reliably distinguished from PEP on the basis of DIF.[45] DIF reveals C3 deposited in a linear fashion along the basement membrane zone in 100% of patients, and immunoglobulin (Ig)G can be seen in up to 25%.[46] The main differential diagnosis is PEP, but urticaria, contact dermatitis, erythema multiforme, bullous drug eruption, and other autoimmune blistering disorders such as bullous pemphigoid or dermatitis herpetiformis may also be considered depending on the clinical setting.

Prognosis

Maternal risks include the postpartum flare, sometimes severe, and a high likelihood of recurrence with subsequent pregnancies. But, most importantly, PG has been associated with an increased incidence of fetal risks, including prematurity, low birthweight, and small size for gestational age.[36,46,47] Early onset or severity of maternal disease does not appear to predict fetal outcome.[47] In addition, up to 10% of newborns may get a transient, nonscarring bullous eruption[11] that usually resolves within 2 weeks.[29,31,47,48] The eruption in the newborn is thought to be due to passive transfer of the maternal anti-basement membrane zone antibodies, which are eventually cleared from the baby's circulation.

Management

Systemic steroids are usually required to control symptoms during pregnancy and the postpartum flare, and may be required for up to 6–10 weeks postpartum.[29] In milder cases or in newborns, topical steroids alone may be sufficient. A variety of therapies have been reported to be helpful in severe or refractory cases, including plasmapheresis,[49,50] immunoapheresis (a variant of plasmapheresis),[51] high-dose intravenous immunoglobulin (IVIG),[52] IVIG in combination with cyclosporine,[53] goserelin,[54] cyclophosphamide,[55] ritodrine,[56] and minocycline[57] or doxycycline[58] with nicotinamide.

Impetigo herpetiformis

Impetigo herpetiformis (IH) is an extremely rare noninfectious pustular dermatosis that occurs exclusively in pregnancy. There has been considerable debate regarding its status as a disease *sui generis* or variant of pustular psoriasis.[59]

Clinical features

Erythematous patches with groups of pinpoint pustules at the margins appear first in the groin, axillae, and neck, and later generalize. The face, hands, and feet are usually spared, but mucous membranes may be involved. Subungual pustules may lead to nail plate separation and fragmentation.[60] Pruritus is not prominent. The patient with IH is systemically ill, and may have fever, malaise, diarrhea, and vomiting. IH typically presents early in the third trimester, although presentation in the first trimester[61] and 1 day postpartum[62] has been reported. Patients with IH rarely provide a personal or family history of psoriasis.

Course

IH typically resolves with delivery, but postpartum exacerbation was reported in one case.[63] Lesions dry, then desquamate, and heal without scarring, but postinflammatory hyperpigmentation is typical. Recurrences are common in subsequent pregnancies and generally occur earlier and are more severe than the initial episode.[60,64] Oral contraceptives may also precipitate a recurrence.[65]

Epidemiologic features

IH is extremely rare, with less than 200 cases reported in the world literature. Although IH has not generally been considered to be a genetic disorder, there have been a handful of familial cases.[66–68]

Pathogenesis

The etiology of IH is unknown. Although hypocalcemic states, including hypoparathyroidism,[64,69] have been associated with both IH and pustular psoriasis, it is unclear what role hypocalcemia plays in the disease.

Diagnosis and differential diagnosis

The diagnosis can be confirmed by biopsy, which shows features identical to that of pustular psoriasis. DIF is negative. Elevated leukocyte counts and erythrocyte sedimentation rates are common, with hypocalcemia and hypoalbuminemia less frequently noted. Cultures from intact pustules are negative, although secondary infection can occur. Differential diagnoses may include herpes gestationis, pustular psoriasis, drug eruption, subcorneal pustular dermatosis, dermatitis herpetiformis, and infections. Interestingly, acrodermatitis enteropathica was eventually diagnosed in one patient who was initially thought to have IH.[70]

Prognosis

Patients with IH can be quite ill and must be monitored for secondary infection. When present, hypocalcemia can lead to tetany, seizures, and delirium. With subsequent pregnancies, patients risk earlier and more severe recurrences. In some cases, patients with IH have gone on to develop more typical pustular psoriasis.[59,71] Risks to the fetus are considerable and are those associated with placental insufficiency, namely stillbirth, neonatal death, and fetal abnormalities.[60]

Management

Systemic steroids are the treatment of choice, along with appropriate supportive care and treatment of secondary infection. Severe or refractory cases may necessitate early delivery or termination.[72,73] Other treatments reported to be effective have included cyclosporine,[74] etretinate,[75] photochemotherapy,[76] isotretinoin with photochemotherapy,[59,63,73] methotrexate,[62] and a mestranol–ethynodiol combination.[61] One patient with hypocalcemia was treated with systemic steroids but improved only after calcium and vitamin D were administered.[64]

Cholestasis of pregnancy

Cholestasis of pregnancy (CP), also known as intrahepatic cholestasis of pregnancy, gestational cholestasis, and prurigo gravidarum, is a condition characterized by pruritus and intrahepatic cholestasis, with or without jaundice, occurring late in pregnancy.

Clinical presentation

Unlike the other dermatoses of pregnancy, CP has no primary skin lesions, but may present with excoriations in more severe cases. CP typically presents with pruritus on the palms and soles that later spreads to include the trunk, extremities, and face. Pruritus can be mild or severe and is often worse at night. There may or may not be associated biochemical abnormalities. In a minority of patients, jaundice can follow the pruritus by 2–4 weeks.[77] CP presents in the third trimester, with over 80% of cases presenting after 30 weeks,[77,78] and may follow a previous pregnancy without CP. A personal or family history of gallbladder disease is sometimes noted.[78]

Course

CP usually remits within 1–2 weeks of delivery, with the pruritus resolving before the biochemical abnormalities, which can take 4–6 weeks to normalize. Up to 70% of subsequent pregnancies may be affected by CP.[77]

Epidemiologic features

CP is present in populations worldwide, but with significant geographic variation in frequency. In most European and North American countries, the incidence has ranged from 0.5% to 1%.[20,79,80] Higher rates have historically been reported in Sweden and Chile,[77] but this is now thought to reflect nutritional factors.[81,82]

Diagnosis and differential diagnosis

The diagnosis of CP is largely clinical, with laboratory tests used to support the diagnosis and rule out other diseases. Elevated serum bile acids are the most sensitive and most commonly seen laboratory finding,[83] but elevations in transaminases, alkaline phosphatase, and conjugated bilirubin may also be present. Because pruritus can precede laboratory abnormalities by several weeks, repeat testing may be warranted.[78,84] Skin biopsy is not useful, as there are no primary lesions. A few patients with CP have had liver biopsies, which have showed only mild cholestasis without significant inflammation or necrosis.[81] The differential diagnosis is broad and, depending on the clinical presentation, may include entities such as scabies, eczema, hepatitis, urticaria, other liver or biliary disease, early PEP, or early PG. When jaundice is present, it is essential to rule out viral hepatitis, which is the most common cause of jaundice in pregnancy.[85]

Pathogenesis

The pathogenesis of CP is unclear, but likely to be multifactorial. A genetic component is suggested by the observation of familial clusters of cases[77] and the finding that sisters and mothers of patients with CP are 12 times more likely to develop CP than control subjects.[86] In addition, recent work has pointed to an association with the multidrug resistance protein 3 (MDR3) gene.[87] Hormonal factors are also likely to be important in CP, as estrogens can reduce hepatocyte bile acid secretion, and progesterone metabolites can intensify the estrogen effect by reducing hepatic clearance of estrogens.[88] Finally, dietary factors have been implicated in studies in Chile, where the seasonal and yearly incidence of CP has correlated with selenium levels.[82]

Prognosis

The risks to the mother are generally minimal and limited to severe pruritus. However, postpartum hemorrhage has been reported, likely due to vitamin K deficiency as a result of malabsorption in the setting of prolonged cholestasis.[89] The risk of fetal complications is substantial and may include fetal distress, meconium staining, and preterm labor (up to 44%).[89,90]

Perinatal mortality has ranged from 3% to 11% of cases.[89,90] A recent report describes possible "bile acid pneumonia" causing respiratory distress in three newborns born to mothers with severe CP, and suggests that bile acid accumulation may impair the function of surfactant in the lungs.[91] The severity of maternal disease does not predict fetal outcome,[89] but earlier onset of pruritus has been associated with spontaneous prematurity.[92]

Management

The goal of treatment is to control the pruritus and minimize fetal complications. In mild cases, symptomatic treatment with emollients, anti-itch lotions, and antihistamines may suffice. In more severe cases, systemic therapy may be required, and those aimed at reducing serum bile acids have had the most success in treating the pruritus and normalizing the laboratory abnormalities. Several recent studies have documented the efficacy of ursodeoxycholic acid (UDCA) in this regard.[93–97] It remains to be seen whether treatment with UDCA will affect fetal outcome. Other treatments have been variably effective in reducing pruritus and/or bile acid levels, including *S*-adenosyl-L-methionine,[93] ultraviolet light (UVB),[88] activated charcoal,[98] dexamethasone,[99] cholestyramine,[100,101] phenobarbital,[100,101] ondansetron,[102] and guar gum.[103,104] Prophylactic vitamin K may decrease the rate of postpartum hemorrhage.[78] Some authors advocate elective early delivery, as most singleton intrauterine deaths have occurred after 37 weeks of gestation.[92]

Miscellaneous eruptions in pregnancy

These entities are less well characterized, and it is unclear whether they represent truly separate diseases or are part of a poorly understood spectrum of overlapping disorders.

Pruritic folliculitis of pregnancy

Pruritic folliculitis (PF) of pregnancy was first described in 1981 in six patients with sterile follicular pustules appearing on the trunk in the latter half of pregnancy.[105] No maternal or fetal morbidity has been reported, and the rash has cleared spontaneously after delivery in all cases. The etiology is unknown. Serum androgen levels were elevated in one case,[106] but a more recent study reported normal androgen levels in 12 PF patients.[107] Treatment is symptomatic.

Prurigo of pregnancy

Prurigo of pregnancy (PP) is usually a diagnosis of exclusion. PP presents in the second or third trimester with excoriated papules predominantly on the trunk and extensor aspects of the extremities. Resolution may come quickly after delivery or occur more slowly over weeks to months. The etiology is unknown, but some cases may represent other undiagnosed pregnancy- and nonpregnancy-related dermatoses. Treatment is symptomatic.

Approach to the patient

Pruritus is common in pregnancy,[108] and the differential diagnosis is broad, encompassing not only the specific dermatoses of pregnancy, but many conditions that cause pruritus with or without rash in the nonpregnant population (Tables 52.4 and 52.5). It is especially important to exclude the dermatoses of pregnancy that are associated with fetal complications, chiefly PG and CP (see Fig. 52.6). Given the fetal risks associated with PG and CP, some have recommended a laboratory evaluation in all patients with itching during pregnancy, and a skin biopsy with DIF when there is an associated rash.[20]

Table 52.4 Common skin disorders that may cause pruritus in pregnancy.

Category	Skin disorder	Clinical features
Allergic/atopic	Urticaria (hives)	Transient wheals
	Atopic dermatitis	Scaly plaques with lichenification. Often coexists with allergic rhinitis and asthma
	Contact dermatitis	Pattern of rash often suggestive
	Drug reactions	History of drug ingestion or change in medication. Morphology varies
Infection/infestation	Scabies	Excoriated papules favor fingerwebs, areola. Burrow is diagnostic
	Infectious folliculitis	Follicle-based pustules. May follow hot-tub exposure
	Tinea (ringworm)	Annular or round scaly plaques. May have affected child or pet
	Other arthropod bites	Scattered excoriated or urticarial papules. Flea bites usually on legs. Chigger bites favor areas where clothing fits tightly. Head or pubic lice in characteristic location
Others	Psoriasis	Scaly red plaques on extensor limbs, scalp. May be generalized
	Pityriasis rosea	Oval plaques with fine scale on trunk. May be preceded by a larger "herald patch"
	Miliaria (prickly heat)	Tiny vesicles appear in hot weather
	Polymorphous light eruption	Pink papules, papulovesicles on sun-exposed areas of arms, chest. Appears in spring or after sunny vacation in winter. Improves over summer
	Xerosis	Dry skin

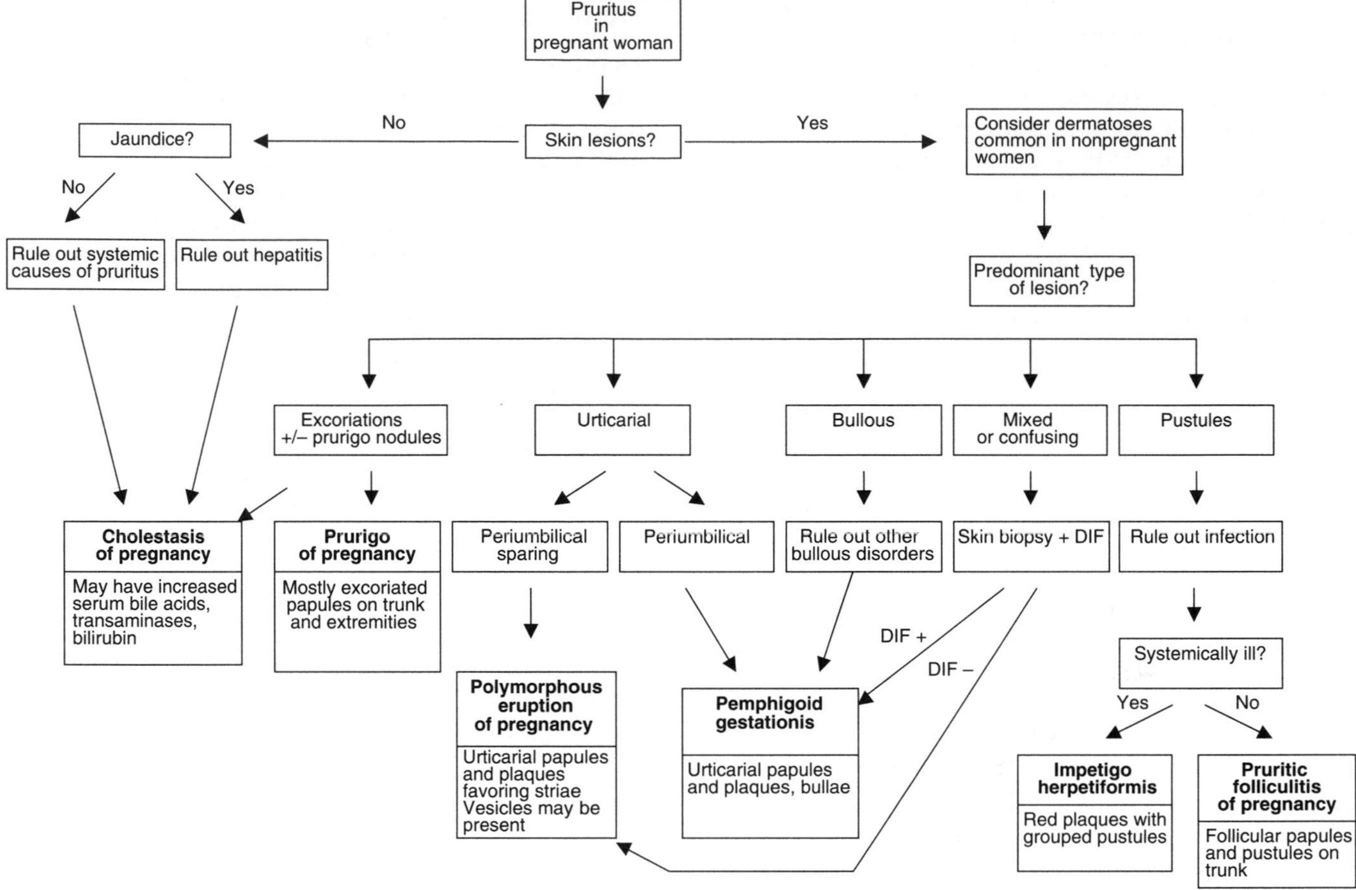

Figure 52.6 Approach to the pregnant patient with pruritus.

Table 52.5 Some causes of pruritus without rash.

Medications (e.g., opiates)
Drug reactions
Hepatitis
Cholestatic or obstructive biliary disease
Chronic renal failure
Malignancy (especially lymphoma)
Hyperthyroidism
Iron deficiency
Acquired immunodeficiency syndrome

58 Amato L, Coronella G, Berti S, et al. Successful treatment with doxycycline and nicotinamide of two cases of persistent pemphigoid gestationis. *J Dermatol Treat* 2002;13(3):143–146.

59 Chang SE, Kim HH, Choi JH, et al. Impetigo herpetiformis followed by generalized pustular psoriasis: more evidence of same disease entity. *Int J Dermatol* 2003;42(9):754–755.

60 Beveridge GW, Harkness RA, Livingstone JR. Impetigo herpetiformis in two successive pregnancies. *Br J Dermatol* 1966; 78(2):106–112.

61 Gligora M, Kolacio Z. Hormonal treatment of impetigo herpetiformis. *Br J Dermatol* 1982;107(2):253.

62 Katsambas A, Stavropoulos PG, Katsiboulas V, et al. Impetigo herpetiformis during the puerperium. *Dermatology* 1999;198(4): 400–402.

63 Breier-Maly J, Ortel B, Breier F, et al. Generalized pustular psoriasis of pregnancy (impetigo herpetiformis). *Dermatology* 1999;198(1):61–64.

64 Bajaj AK, Swarup V, Gupta OP, Gupta SC. Impetigo herpetiformis. *Dermatologica* 1977;155(5):292–295.

65 Oumeish OY, Farraj SE, Batainch AS. Some aspects of impetigo herpetiformis. *Arch Dermatol* 1982;118(2):103–105.

66 Erbagci Z, Erkilic S. A case of recurrent impetigo herpetiformis with a positive family history. *Int J Clin Pract* 2000;54(9): 619–620.

67 Alli N, Lenk N. Twins with impetigo herpetiformis. *Int J Dermatol* 1996;35(2):149–150.

68 Tada J, Fukushiro S, Fujiwara Y, et al. Two sisters with impetigo herpetiformis. *Clin Exp Dermatol* 1989;14(1):82–84.

69 Moynihan GD, Ruppe JP, Jr. Impetigo herpetiformis and hypoparathyroidism. *Arch Dermatol* 1985;121(10):1330–1331.

70 Bronson DM, Barsky R, Barsky S. Acrodermatitis enteropathica. *J Am Acad Dermatol* 1983;9(1):140–144.

71 Sahin HG, Sahin HA, Metin A, et al. Recurrent impetigo herpetiformis in a pregnant adolescent: case report. *Eur J Obstet Gynecol Reprod Biol* 2002;101(2):201–203.

72 Arslanpence I, Dede FS, Gokcu M, Gelisen O. Impetigo herpetiformis unresponsive to therapy in a pregnant adolescent. *J Pediatr Adolesc Gynecol* 2003;16(3):129–132.

73 Chang SE, Cho SY, Bae JY, et al. A case of impetigo herpetiformis with unusual clinical features. *J Dermatol* 2001;28(6):335–337.

74 Imai N, Watanabe R, Fujiwara H, et al. Successful treatment of impetigo herpetiformis with oral cyclosporine during pregnancy. *Arch Dermatol* 2002;138(1):128–129.

75 Bukhari IA. Impetigo herpetiformis in a primigravida: successful treatment with etretinate. *J Drugs Dermatol* 2004;3(4):449–451.

76 El-Din Selim MM, Rehak A, Abdel-Hafez K, Al-Saleh K. Impetigo herpetiformis. Report of a case treated with photochemotherapy (PUVA). *Dermatol Monatsschr* 1982;168(1): 44–48.

77 Reyes H. The spectrum of liver and gastrointestinal disease seen in cholestasis of pregnancy. *Gastroenterol Clin North Am* 1992;21(4):905–921.

78 Kenyon AP, Piercy CN, Girling J, et al. Obstetric cholestasis, outcome with active management: a series of 70 cases. *Br J Obstet Gynaecol* 2002;109(3):282–288.

79 Mela M, Mancuso A, Burroughs AK. Review article: pruritus in cholestatic and other liver diseases. *Aliment Pharmacol Ther* 2003;17(7):857–870.

80 Paternoster DM, Fabris F, Palu G, et al. Intra-hepatic cholestasis of pregnancy in hepatitis C virus infection. *Acta Obstet Gynecol Scand* 2002;81(2):99–103.

81 Reyes H. Review: intrahepatic cholestasis. A puzzling disorder of pregnancy. *J Gastroenterol Hepatol* 1997;12(3):211–216.

82 Reyes H, Baez ME, Gonzalez MC, et al. Selenium, zinc and copper plasma levels in intrahepatic cholestasis of pregnancy, in normal pregnancies and in healthy individuals, in Chile. *J Hepatol* 2000;32(4):542–549.

83 Kroumpouzos G, Cohen LM. Dermatoses of pregnancy. *J Am Acad Dermatol* 2001;45(1):1–19.

84 Kenyon AP, Piercy CN, Girling J, et al. Pruritus may precede abnormal liver function tests in pregnant women with obstetric cholestasis: a longitudinal analysis. *Br J Obstet Gynaecol* 2001;108(11):1190–1192.

85 Rustgi VK. Liver disease in pregnancy. *Med Clin North Am* 1989;73(4):1041–1046.

86 Eloranta ML, Heinonen S, Mononen T, Saarikoski S. Risk of obstetric cholestasis in sisters of index patients. *Clin Genet* 2001; 60(1):42–45.

87 Pauli-Magnus C, Lang T, Meier Y, et al. Sequence analysis of bile salt export pump (ABCB11) and multidrug resistance p-glycoprotein 3 (ABCB4, MDR3) in patients with intrahepatic cholestasis of pregnancy. *Pharmacogenetics* 2004;14(2):91–102.

88 Kroumpouzos G. Intrahepatic cholestasis of pregnancy: what's new. *J Eur Acad Dermatol Venereol* 2002;16(4):316–318.

89 Reid R, Ivey KJ, Rencoret RH, Storey B. Fetal complications of obstetric cholestasis. *Br Med J* 1976;1(6014):870–872.

90 Fisk NM, Storey GN. Fetal outcome in obstetric cholestasis. *Br J Obstet Gynaecol* 1988;95(11):1137–1143.

91 Zecca E, Costa S, Lauriola V, et al. Bile acid pneumonia: a "new" form of neonatal respiratory distress syndrome? *Pediatrics* 2004;114(1):269–272.

92 Williamson C, Hems LM, Goulis DG, et al. Clinical outcome in a series of cases of obstetric cholestasis identified via a patient support group. *Br J Obstet Gynaecol* 2004;111(7):676–681.

93 Roncaglia N, Locatelli A, Arreghini A, et al. A randomised controlled trial of ursodeoxycholic acid and S-adenosyl-l-methionine in the treatment of gestational cholestasis. *Br J Obstet Gynaecol* 2004;111(1):17–21.

94 Nicastri PL, Diaferia A, Tartagni M, et al. A randomised placebo-controlled trial of ursodeoxycholic acid and S-adenosylmethionine in the treatment of intrahepatic cholestasis of pregnancy. *Br J Obstet Gynaecol* 1998;105(11):1205–1207.

95 Diaferia A, Nicastri PL, Tartagni M, et al. Ursodeoxycholic acid therapy in pregnant women with cholestasis. *Int J Gynaecol Obstet* 1996;52(2):133–140.

96 Floreani A, Paternoster D, Melis A, Grella PV. S-adenosylmethionine versus ursodeoxycholic acid in the treatment of intrahepatic cholestasis of pregnancy: preliminary results of a controlled trial. *Eur J Obstet Gynecol Reprod Biol* 1996;67(2):109–113.

97 Palma J, Reyes H, Ribalta J, et al. Ursodeoxycholic acid in the treatment of cholestasis of pregnancy: a randomized, double-blind study controlled with placebo. *J Hepatol* 1997; 27(6):1022–1028.

98 Kaaja RJ, Kontula KK, Raiha A, Laatikainen T. Treatment of cholestasis of pregnancy with peroral activated charcoal. A preliminary study. *Scand J Gastroenterol* 1994;29(2):178–181.

99 Hirvioja ML, Tuimala R, Vuori J. The treatment of intrahepatic cholestasis of pregnancy by dexamethasone. *Br J Obstet Gynaecol* 1992;99(2):109–111.

100 Laatikainen T. Effect of cholestyramine and phenobarbital on pruritus and serum bile acid levels in cholestasis of pregnancy. *Am J Obstet Gynecol* 1978;132(5):501–506.

101 Heikkinen J, Maentausta O, Ylostalo P, Janne O. Serum bile acid levels in intrahepatic cholestasis of pregnancy during treatment with phenobarbital or cholestyramine. *Eur J Obstet Gynecol Reprod Biol* 1982;14(3):153–162.
102 Schumann R, Hudcova J. Cholestasis of pregnancy, pruritus and 5-hydroxytryptamine 3 receptor antagonists. *Acta Obstet Gynecol Scand* 2004;83(9):861–862.
103 Gylling H, Riikonen S, Nikkila K, et al. Oral guar gum treatment of intrahepatic cholestasis and pruritus in pregnant women: effects on serum cholestanol and other non-cholesterol sterols. *Eur J Clin Invest* 1998;28(5):359–363.
104 Riikonen S, Savonius H, Gylling H, et al. Oral guar gum, a gel-forming dietary fiber relieves pruritus in intrahepatic cholestasis of pregnancy. *Acta Obstet Gynecol Scand* 2000;79(4):260–264.
105 Zoberman E, Farmer ER. Pruritic folliculitis of pregnancy. *Arch Dermatol* 1981;117:20–22.
106 Wilkinson SM, Buckler H, Wilkinson N, et al. Androgen levels in pruritic folliculitis of pregnancy. *Clin Exp Dermatol* 1995;20:234–236.
107 Vaughan Jones SA, Hern S, Black MM. Neutrophil folliculitis and serum androgen levels. *Clin Exp Dermatol* 1999;24: 392–395.
108 Dacus JV. Pruritus in pregnancy. *Clin Obstet Gynecol* 1990; 33(4):738–745.

53 Cancer and other neoplasms in pregnancy

Peter E. Schwartz and Masoud Azodi

In the USA, benign gynecologic masses account for more than 1 million hospital admissions per year.[1] Benign masses may occur in pregnancy, and their management is complicated by the risk to the fetus. Knowledge of the natural history of these masses during pregnancy is essential to their proper management. Cancer during pregnancy is unusual. As a result of physiologic changes that normally occur in pregnancy, cancer during pregnancy may be more advanced because the diagnosis is not recognized as early as it might otherwise have been. However, stage-for-stage, cancer during pregnancy is no more virulent than cancer occurring in the nonpregnant state. The routine interruption of pregnancy to influence cancer progression has not been established.

Benign masses in pregnancy

Uterine myomas

Myomas are very common in the general population, especially in nonwhite women.[1] They are a frequent cause of infertility, and are less prevalent among pregnant women than among the same age group of nonpregnant women. Myomas that cause hospitalization are mostly seen in women aged 40–45 years. Complications occur in about 10% of pregnancies with uterine myomas.[2]

Estrogen receptors are amplified in myomas compared with normal myometrium.[3] Several other hormone receptors also appear to be amplified in myomas. Estrogen has been thought to stimulate the growth of uterine myomas, but the precise mechanism is not well understood. Traditionally, it was believed that uterine myomas will grow during pregnancy, but this has been challenged by several prospective studies.[4–6] Nongrowing myomas can cause symptoms during pregnancy as a result of the enlarging uterus displacing them out of the pelvis. Symptoms may develop as asymptomatic myomas compress abdominal organs.

Uterine myomas can undergo central necrosis and degeneration, causing localized pain at the site of known myoma. Degenerating myomas can provide a culture medium for pathogenic organisms with occasional leukocytosis and superimposed infection. Myomas are thought to increase the frequency of preterm labor and premature rupture of membranes. They have been implicated in first-trimester spontaneous abortions,[7,8] and large cervical and lower uterine segment myomas can cause obstructed labor.[6,9]

Placental abruption, postpartum hemorrhage, and retained placenta are thought to be complications of uterine myomas during pregnancy. However, several studies failed to show statistically different rates of these complications compared with the general population.[6,9] One study showed that women with leiomyomata are at increased risk of second-trimester spontaneous abortion.[10]

Management of myomas in pregnancy

Myomas can cause pain through degenerative changes or by direct compression of adjacent organs. Most of the symptoms can be managed medically in pregnant women. Symptomatic treatment with acetaminophen or opioid analgesics usually provides relief. Several studies have shown that nonsteroidal anti-inflammatory drugs can be used successfully in pregnancy for management of the symptoms.[2,11] However, these drugs have known fetal risks and should be used with caution during pregnancy.[12] Hydration and antibiotics can be used if infection is suspected. Medical management is the primary means of treatment in pregnancy. Surgical management is usually avoided during pregnancy. There are very few studies and no randomized trials available on the safety of myomectomy in pregnancy.[13–15] Myomectomy during pregnancy is best avoided in all but the most extreme circumstances, such as torsion of a pedunculated myoma or when a malignancy is suspected.

Adnexal masses in pregnancy

Benign adnexal tumors are sometimes associated with normal pregnancies. Clinical features suspicious for malignancy, particularly ovarian cancer, include the presence of a fixed mass, lymphadenopathy, ascites, and constitutional symptoms such as pain, abdominal distention, dyspareunia, frequency, or constipation.[16,17] Sonographic features of adnexal masses suspicious for malignancy include size greater than 6 cm, thick septations, papillary projections, complex echogenicity, and the presence of ascites.[18,19] The negative predictive value of sonography as a method of excluding malignancy appears to improve in pregnancy.[20] Magnetic resonance imaging (MRI) and computed tomography (CT) have been used to distinguish benign from malignant ovarian masses in pregnancy. These modalities may prove particularly useful in the evaluation of adenopathy and tumor invasion. To date, there is little evidence to link exposure to diagnostic MRI with adverse fetal effects.[21,22]

The most common benign pelvic masses in pregnancy are persistent corpus luteum cysts, benign cystic teratomas, paratubal cysts, cystadenomas, and pedunculated myomas. Although the vast majority of benign pelvic neoplasms discovered during pregnancy are present before the beginning of the pregnancy, the hormonal changes of pregnancy, particularly the production of human chorionic gonadotropin (hCG), are associated with luteomas, theca-lutein cysts, hyperreactio luteinalis, and large solitary luteinized follicular cyst of pregnancy.

Corpus luteum of pregnancy

The corpus luteum is the most common hormone-producing tumor of pregnancy. The corpus luteum of pregnancy is a physiologic cyst in which granulosa-lutein cells in the postovulatory ovarian follicle are stimulated by placental chorionic gonadotropin production to produce progesterone. The corpus luteum maintains progesterone production until approximately 9 weeks' gestation, when placental progesterone production is sufficient to maintain the pregnancy. They are unilateral, sonolucent structures contiguous with the ovary. Corpus luteum cysts can complicate pregnancy if they undergo torsion or spontaneous rupture. Asymptomatic corpus luteum cysts typically regress during the second trimester and are completely absent by the third trimester. If a corpus luteum is removed before 9 weeks' gestation, exogenous progesterone is administered.

Luteoma

Luteomas of pregnancy are solid tumors that are characterized by hypertrophy of ovarian stroma. This hypertrophy may be secondary to stimulation by hCG. They are frequently bilateral and multinodular. Elevated levels of testosterone accompany luteomas in at least 25% of cases, although other hormones may be responsible for maternal virilization.[23–25] When maternal virilization is present, female fetuses are at risk of virilization. The female fetus is usually not at significant risk of labioscrotal fusion because placental aromatization of maternal androgens is not usually overwhelmed by androgen production until fusion is complete.[26,27] There does not appear to be any association between luteomas and multiple gestation or gestational trophoblastic disease. Expectant management is recommended.[28] Luteomas can occasionally recur; therefore, preconception counseling is necessary for women with a history of luteoma.[29]

Hyperreactio luteinalis

Hyperreactio luteinalis is a benign, non-neoplastic enlargement of theca-lutein cysts, most likely due to stimulation by hCG.[30] Hyperreactio luteinalis is strongly associated with conditions that produce abnormally elevated hCG, such as multiple gestation, gestational trophoblastic disease, and ovarian hyperstimulation syndrome.[31] Hyperreactio luteinalis is usually bilateral and multicystic with stromal edema. Ovarian enlargement can be massive. Although maternal androgen excess is occasionally present, virilization of female fetuses rarely occurs.[32,33] Life-threatening ascites, electrolyte abnormalities, thromboembolism, intravascular depletion, hemoconcentration, renal failure, and pleural effusion with respiratory difficulties may be present when hyperreactio luteinalis complicates ovarian hyperstimulation syndrome or gestational trophoblastic disease. In addition to supportive measures, uterine evacuation may be necessary to reverse hCG-induced ovarian stimulation in such cases. In milder cases, expectant management is appropriate because hyperreactio luteinalis and theca-lutein cysts usually resolve shortly after delivery.

Cancers in pregnancy

Incidence

Data reflecting the incidence of cancers during pregnancy are scant because of a lack of information accrued by population-based tumor registries. Estimates of cancer during pregnancy vary considerably (Table 53.1). The uterine cervix remains the most common site for neoplasia to develop in pregnancy.[34] The breast is the second most common site for malignancy that occurs during pregnancy.[35] The frequency distribution of other cancers during pregnancy such as leukemia, lymphoma, and cancers of the ovary, vulva, vagina, skin (melanoma), brain, and gastrointestinal tract reflects that of cancer occurring in all women in their reproductive years.[36]

The study by Haas[37] reporting the incidence of cancer during pregnancy compared with that in control nonpregnant women suggested that there may be a significantly reduced incidence of cancer in pregnancy. These data were from a population-based epidemiologic study in the German Democratic Republic. As women grew older, the 5-year age group observed-to-expected ratios of pregnancy-associated cancers increased from 0.22 for women aged 15–19 years (1.9 cancers per 100000 live births) to 1.40 (232.4 cancers per 100000

Table 53.1 Estimate of cancers occurring in pregnancy.

Site	Estimated incidence	Authors
Skin, melanoma	2.8/1000	Smith and Randal[237]
Cervix		
Carcinoma *in situ*	1/767	Sokol and Lessmann[34]
Invasive	1/2205	Sokol and Lessmann[34]
Breast	1/3000	Benedet et al.[35]
	10–39/100 000	Wallack et al.[47]
Vulva	1/8000	Nugent and O'Connell[229]
Ovary	1/9000	Nugent and O'Connell[229]
	1/25 000	Ribeiro and Palmer[230]
Leukemia	Less than 1/75 000	Applewhite et al.[231]
	1/100 000	Haas[37]
Hodgkin's disease	1/1000	Riva et al.[234]
	1/6000	Morgan et al.;[235] Stewart and Monto[236]
Colorectal	1/100 000	Fisher et al.;[232] Clark et al.[233]

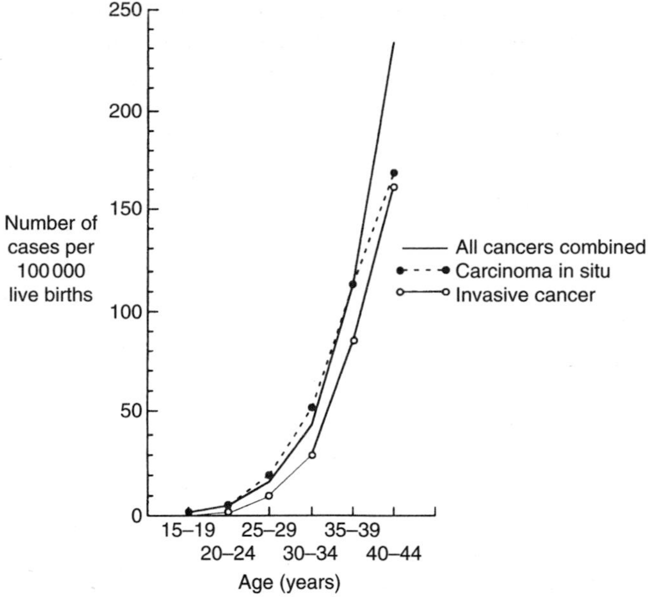

Figure 53.1 Overall incidence of cancer occurring in pregnancy by age and incidence of carinoma *in situ* and invasive cervical cancer (modified from ref. 37).

live births) for those aged 40–44 years (Fig. 53.1). The frequency of occurrence, in descending order, was cervical cancer, breast cancer, ovarian cancer, lymphoma, melanoma, brain cancer, and leukemia.

A fear expressed by pregnant patients is that the cancer might spread to the fetus. Information collected during the past two decades suggests that transplacental metastasis is extremely unusual, and metastases to the fetus are so rare as to preclude this as an indication for termination of a pregnancy. The most common malignancy to be associated with fetal metastases is malignant melanoma. The reported number of cases in the literature of such an event is fewer than 30.[38]

Surgery in pregnancy

Patients may undergo successful surgical procedures when they are pregnant without jeopardizing the fetus. In general, surgery should be delayed until the second trimester, which seems to be the safest time in terms of avoiding patients going into labor. Spontaneous abortion frequently occurs when surgery is performed in the first trimester, and premature labor has been associated with surgery in the third trimester. Corpus luteum function is replaced by the placenta after the 12th week of gestation. Pathologic ovaries may be removed safely once the patient has entered into the second trimester.

In preparing the patient for a surgical procedure, simple technical considerations may have an important impact on the success of the operation. For example, placing the patient in a lateral position to avoid vena cava and aortic compression is an important factor in considering the anesthetic consequences of surgery.[39,40] Anesthesiologists must always act as if a pregnant woman has a full stomach, as progesterone relaxes the gastroesophageal sphincter, and pyloric displacement by the gravid uterus impedes gastric emptying.[41]

Radiation in pregnancy

Radiation is commonly employed in the routine management of cancers that may occur in pregnancy. Deleterious effects that the fetus may experience from being exposed to radiation therapy have been recognized for many years.[42–44] Production of genetic mutations by radiation in the laboratory was documented as early as 1927, but data directly applicable to humans are scant.[45] Three phases of pregnancy must be considered with regard to radiation damage.[46] The preimplantation phase lasts for approximately 7–10 days and represents the time from fertilization to the implantation of the blastocyst into the uterine wall. Spontaneous abortion is the most likely consequence of an embryo being exposed to radiation in the preimplantation phase. For many patients, the pregnancy may not be clinically recognized.[47] Organogenesis, the period from the first to the 10th week of gestation, represents the most sensitive time for the fetus with regard to radiation injury.[46] This is the time of major organ formation and the time when the fetus is most susceptible to teratogenic agents.

However, the central nervous system, the eyes, and the hematopoietic system remain highly sensitive to the effects of radiation throughout the entire pregnancy. Radiation has been associated with microcephaly, the most common malformation observed in humans exposed to high-dose radiation during pregnancy, and mental retardation.[48] In general, such effects are seen in fetuses exposed to amounts greater than 50 rad of low-energy-transfer (LET) radiation. Embryonic exposure to 5 rad or less is rarely associated with anomalies.[48] The actual radiation dose rates are extremely important in assessing the risks to the fetus for developing growth retardation, malformations, or death.

Pregnant women exposed to radiation therapy of 250 rad or greater during the first 2–3 weeks of gestation have an increased risk of spontaneous abortion but not a dramatic risk of severe congenital anomalies.[49] However, once patients are exposed to such radiation during the third to 10th weeks of gestation, multiple congenital anomalies including low birthweight, microcephaly, mental retardation, retinal degeneration, cataracts, and genital and skeletal malformations have been reported.[49] Radiation exposure between the 11th and 20th weeks has been associated with a significant decline in anomalies. Exposure after the 20th week of gestation is usually limited to anemia, skin pigmentation changes, and dermal erythema. The risks of growth retardation and abnormalities of the eye and central nervous system (CNS) increase throughout the latter period of fetal radiation exposure. It has been suggested that fetuses exposed to radiation doses higher than 10 rad should be considered for therapeutic abortion.[46]

Pelvic irradiation for the management of malignancies, particularly cervical lesions in pregnancy, will result in fetal demise and will usually lead to spontaneous abortion. The fetus may receive only minor exposure when supradiaphragmatic irradiation is given, particularly if such radiation is tapered so that the internal scatter is minimal during the first trimester of pregnancy. Proper shielding equipment can significantly reduce the radiation dose to the fetus.[50] However, as the fetus grows, its exposure to supradiaphragmatic radiation increases. Such radiation may not be appropriate in the more advanced stages of pregnancy.

Chemotherapy and pregnancy

Prior experience supported the concept that cytotoxic chemotherapy should not be administered to patients, especially during the first trimester of pregnancy. This was because of the high incidence of spontaneous abortion following exposure to chemotherapy and the teratogenic effects of these agents on the developing fetus.[51,52] However, as anecdotal and small series reports have accumulated, it appears that, although certain drugs must be avoided during early pregnancy, others might be life-saving and might not cause congenital anomalies in the fetus[53–56] (Table 53.2). Prematurity and low birthweight are frequent complications of chemotherapy exposure in any trimester of pregnancy. However, the fear of exposure in the second and third trimesters of pregnancy resulting in congenital anomalies no longer appears to be a major concern, provided that the selection of drugs is appropriate.[51,52] The long-term neurologic consequences of intrauterine exposure to chemotherapeutic agents has yet to be established. Children who have been born after *in utero* exposure to chemotherapeutic agents during the second and third trimesters have not been noted to have significant congenital abnormalities. One study of 17 children exposed *in utero* to chemotherapy for the management of maternal acute leukemia revealed no fetal malformations. The children's growth and development, school performance, intelligence tests, neurologic examinations, and hematologic evaluations (with a follow-up period ranging from 4 to 22 years) were normal.[56] Another study of 16 pregnant women treated for non-Hodgkin's lymphoma reported similar results.[54]

Physiologic effects of pregnancy may have an impact on the efficacy and toxicity of chemotherapeutic agents. For example, renal blood flow, glomerular filtration rate, and creatinine clearance increases may lead to increased clearance of drugs from the body.[57] It has been suggested that amniotic fluid may act as a pharmacologic third space for such drugs as methotrexate, analogous to ascites or pleural effusions which may then increase methotrexate toxicity.[58] Gastrointestinal absorption of drugs may be decreased owing to delayed gastric motility. The distribution and kinetics of antineoplastic agents may be substantially affected by the physiologic increase in body water in a pregnant woman in association with a 15% increase in plasma volume and changes in plasma protein concentrations.[59] Drugs that cross the placenta have low molecular weight, high lipid solubility, are nonionized, and are loosely bound to plasma proteins.[58,60,61]

In assessing the teratogenic effects of chemotherapeutic agents administered in pregnancy, it must be kept in mind that up to 3% of children have associated major congenital anomalies and 9% have minor anomalies in pregnancies not complicated by cancer treatments or exposure to a chemotherapeutic agent.[62]

Congenital anomalies have been noted in patients treated with alkylating agents in the first trimester of pregnancy but not in the second and third trimesters.[51] Cisplatin has become the most important drug in the management of gynecologic malignancies.[63]

Antimetabolites are cell cycle specific and interfere with DNA, RNA, and some coenzymes. Aminopterin and methotrexate act as abortifacients for patients when administered during the first trimester.[34,51] Only one congenital anomaly was observed in 56 patients exposed to other antimetabolites during pregnancy.[52] Second- and third-trimester exposure to a variety of antimetabolites resulted in no congenital anomalies in 37 fetuses. Thus, antimetabolites other than amethopterin and aminopterin may be relatively

Table 53.2 Chemotherapeutic agents and reported associated anomalies by trimester.

Chemotherapeutic agents	Mechanism of action	Reported significant anomalies by trimester*		
		1st	2nd	3rd
Alkylating agents				
Melphalan, chlorambucil, cyclophosphamide, triethylene thiophosphoramide, cisplatin, carboplatin, carmustine (BCNU), chloroethylcyclohexyl nitrosourea, methyl-CCNU, busulfan	Cell-cycle nonspecific; forms cross linkages with DNA	Yes†	No	No
Antimetabolites				
Amethopterin (methotrexate),‡ aminopterin, 5-fluorouracil,‡ cytosine arabinoside, 6-thioguanine, 5-azacytidine, hydroxyurea, hexamethylmelamine, L-asparaginase	Cell-cycle specific; structural analogue of precursor purine and pyrimidine bases; lead to nonfunctional DNA and cell death	Yes$	No	No
Antibiotics				
Actinomycin D, doxorubicin, daunorubicin, bleomycin, mitomycin C, mithramycin	Cell-cycle nonspecific; interferes with DNA-dependent RNA synthesis; cell death from lack of RNA and an inability to produce cell proteins	No	No	No
Vinca alkaloids				
Vincristine, vinblastine, etoposide (VP-16), teniposide (VM-26)	Cell phase specific	Yes	No	No
Glucocorticoids				
Cortisone, prednisolone, prednisone, methylprednisolone, dexamethasone	Inhibition of DNA, RNA, and protein synthesis	Yes¶	No	No

*Reports of anomalies are limited and should be viewed with caution.

†Chlorambucil syndrome: renal aplasia, cleft palate, skeletal abnormalities.

‡Abortifacients in first trimester.

$Aminopterin syndrome: cranial dysostosis, hypertelorism, anomalies of the external ears, micrognathia, cleft palate.

¶Cleft lip, cleft palate.

safely used in the management of cancer during pregnancy.

Antibiotics such as actinomycin D, doxorubicin, daunorubicin, bleomycin, mitomycin C, and mithramycin have been used relatively safely in the second and third trimesters of pregnancy. Recent data suggest that doxorubicin and daunorubicin may be relatively safe when used in the first trimester of pregnancy, but the follow-up information on children exposed *in utero* remains extremely limited.[64,65]

Vinca alkaloids are cell phase-specific agents that cause mitotic arrest. These agents include vincristine, vinblastine, VP-16, and VM-26. A limited experience with exposure to vinca alkaloids suggests that only one of 15 pregnancies exposed during the first trimester was associated with a congenital anomaly. No anomalies were seen in 11 patients treated later in pregnancy.[51,52]

The reported rate of fetal malformations when exposed to combination chemotherapy in the first trimester (16%) is similar to that of single-agent therapy.[51,66–68] Theoretically, the incidence could be reduced to 6% by removing folate antagonists in common with radiation therapy.[53] Doll and colleagues[53] summarized the findings of 71 patients treated with single-agent therapy in the last two trimesters and of 79 patients treated with combination therapy; they identified one child in each treatment group with a congenital anomaly. Thus, second- and third-trimester chemotherapy appears to be safe with regard to teratogenicity in the fetus.[53] Nevertheless, a 40% incidence of low birthweight was reported by Nicholson[51] when fetuses were exposed to chemotherapy *in utero*. Other complications may occur in the fetus exposed to cytotoxic chemotherapy in addition to teratogenicity, death, and stunted growth.[69] Anemia, leukopenia, and thrombocytopenia may occur in the fetus as a result of bone marrow suppression and leukopenia, or immune suppression may lead to secondary infection.[55] Timing of chemotherapy in relation to the anticipated delivery must be carefully assessed. Deliveries should occur when the mother is not bone marrow suppressed. Breastfeeding is discouraged in patients who are receiving cytotoxic chemotherapy, although the data supporting this are weak.[69] To date, there have been no reports of children developing leukemia after *in utero* exposure to chemotherapeutic agents.

Assessing fetal maturity

The early delivery of a child has been incorporated into the management strategy in treating pregnant cancer patients. This strategy requires that sophisticated newborn special care units be available for maintaining premature infants. The survival rate for infants treated in the Newborn Special Care Unit at Yale–New Haven Children's Hospital for the years 1994 through 2003 is presented in Fig. 53.2. The data presented are typical of those reported from newborn intensive care units in the United States.

Antenatal corticosteroid therapy has been shown to decrease complications related to organ immaturity such as respiratory distress syndrome, intraventricular hemorrhage, and necrotizing enterocolitis. They are most effective if delivery occurs from 1 to 7 days after the initiation of therapy. Tests of fetal lung maturity, such as the lecithin/sphingomyelin (L/S) ratio, are important in determining the timing of delivery.[70]

Cervical cancer

Invasive cervical cancer is on the decline in the United States. Effective Pap smear screening techniques in combination with colposcopy for directed biopsies have allowed physicians to recognize the presence of malignancy early and to treat patients with simple office procedures. Although the decline in invasive cancer is evident in the United States, an increase in cervical intraepithelial neoplasia (CIN) has occurred as a result of widescale cytologic screening.[71,72] The cervix remains the most common site for precancerous and cancerous changes in pregnancy (see Table 53.1 and Fig. 53.1). Epidemiologic studies suggest that women who develop CIN and invasive cancer in pregnancy tend to be married at an earlier age, have an earlier age of diagnosis of CIN and invasive cancer, and have a higher parity than a control population.[73–75] The most common histologic types of cancer occurring in the cervix are squamous cell. Four case reports of a small cell neuroendocrine carcinoma arising in the uterine cervix in pregnancy have been reported.[76]

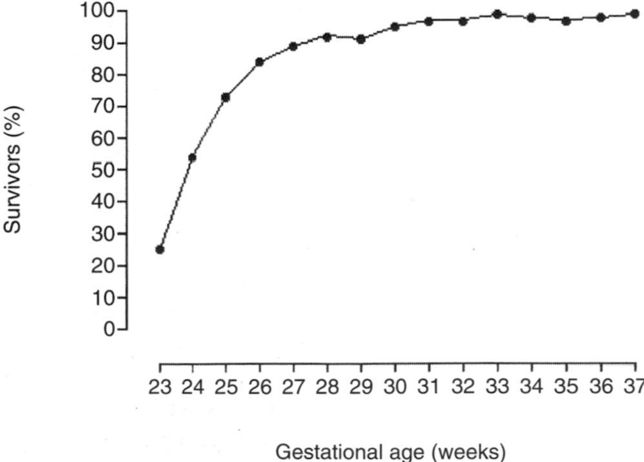

Figure 53.2 Newborn special care unit survival statistics, Yale–New Haven Hospital.

Cervical intraepithelial neoplasia

The presence of CIN in pregnancy is usually identified by Pap smear and confirmed by colposcopically directed biopsies. It is the policy at Yale–New Haven Hospital to use colposcopy to evaluate patients with abnormal Pap smears in pregnancy and to limit the biopsy to the site that has the worst colposcopic appearance. In general, colposcopy will show the entire transformation zone, as the squamocolumnar junction tends to be present well out on the exocervix during pregnancy. Cone biopsies of the cervix are avoided, as they are associated with hemorrhage, abortion, and premature labor.[77] It has been a successful policy at Yale–New Haven Hospital to biopsy the worst colposcopically identified site and, if the cervical biopsy and Pap smear are consistent, to follow the patient throughout the pregnancy with Pap smears every 3 months. Patients are reevaluated at approximately 36 weeks' gestation with repeat colposcopy and Pap smears to be as certain as possible that the lesion has not progressed. Cotton-tip applicator sticks are used to obtain endocervical cytologic specimens in pregnancy. The preference for the cotton-tip applicator stick is to avoid disrupting the fetal membranes with the wire-like tip of the cytobrush. Adenocarcinomas arising in association with carcinoma *in situ* of the exocervix are easily visualized in pregnancy and may be readily biopsied.[77] In the 30 years that this policy has been practiced, only one case of a stage IB cancer of the cervix has occurred in a patient initially assessed to have a precancerous lesion. That patient was recognized at delivery to have an invasive lesion and was subsequently successfully managed with a type III radical hysterectomy and bilateral deep pelvic lymphadenectomy.

If the assessment at 36 weeks remains consistent with CIN, the patient and her physician are advised that the patient may deliver vaginally. No attempt is made routinely to perform Cesarean hysterectomies in the management of CIN if further pregnancies are desired. Assessment of precancerous changes can be readily carried out 8–12 weeks following delivery.

Microinvasive cancer of the cervix

Microinvasive cancer of the cervix is defined as a lesion that has only microscopically penetrated through the basement membrane. The current International Federation of Gynecology and Obstetrics (FIGO) staging system is seen in Table 53.3. Confirmation of the presence of stage IA1 or stage IA2 microinvasive cancer is important in distinguishing it from

Table 53.3 International Federation of Gynecology and Obstetrics (FIGO) cervical cancer staging classification.

0	Carcinoma *in situ*, intraepithelial carcinoma; cases of stage 0 should not be included in any therapeutic statistics for invasive carcinoma
I	Carcinoma is strictly confined to the cervix (extension to the corpus should be disregarded)
Ia	Preclinical carcinoma of the cervix, i.e., those diagnosed only by microscopy
Ia1	Minimal microscopically evident stromal invasion
Ia2	Lesions detected microscopically that can be measured; the upper limit of the measurement should not show a depth of invasion of more than 5 mm taken from the base of the epithelium, either surface or glandular, from which it originates; a second dimension, the horizontal spread, must not exceed 7 mm; larger should be staged as Ib
Ib	Lesions of greater dimension than stage Ia2, whether seen clinically or not; preformed space involvement should not alter the staging but should be specifically recorded so as to determine whether it should affect treatment decisions in the future
II	Carcinoma extends beyond the cervix but has not extended onto the pelvic wall; the carcinoma involves the vagina, but not as far as the lower third
IIa	No obvious parametrial involvement
IIb	Obvious parametrial involvement
III	Carcinoma has extended onto the pelvic wall; on rectal examination there is no cancer-free space between the tumor and the pelvic wall; the tumor involves the lower third of the vagina; all cases with a hydronephrosis or nonfunctioning kidney should be included, unless they are known to be due to another cause
IIIa	No extension onto the pelvic wall, but involvement of the lower third of the vagina
IIIb	Extension onto the pelvic wall or hydronephrosis or nonfunctioning kidney
IV	Carcinoma has extended beyond the true pelvis or has clinically involved the mucosa of the bladder or rectum
IVa	Spread of the growth to adjacent organs
IVb	Spread to distant organs

Reprinted from Staging Announcement: FIGO Cancer Committee. *Gynecol Oncol* 1986;25:383, with permission.

frankly invasive cancer. In general, patients with microinvasive cancer identified by abnormal Pap smears should undergo routine colposcopic assessment. The confirmation of the extent of disease is extremely important in pregnancy and may require a more extensive biopsy in the form of a hemicone biopsy or a cone biopsy of the cervix. If surgical margins are histologically free of disease on the cervical biopsy, patients may safely continue with the pregnancy as long as they are willing to be assessed with frequent Pap smears and colposcopy. Stage IA2 patients have more extensive microinvasive cancer. Once again, the issue is related to the margins of the biopsy used to establish the diagnosis and the patient's desire to preserve the pregnancy and her fertility. Those patients with stage IA1 microinvasive cancer who wish to undergo prompt therapy are usually successfully managed with a simple hysterectomy and leaving the ovaries in place. Those with stage IA2 cervical cancer are recommended to undergo a type II modified radical hysterectomy. Patients who wish to have definitive surgery performed following completion of pregnancy may be delivered vaginally with a subsequent hysterectomy (stage IA1) or may be delivered by Cesarean section followed by modified radical hysterectomy (stage IA2).

Invasive cancer

The identification of invasive cancer of the cervix requires prompt treatment, except for patients in the late second or third trimester, when one may briefly delay therapy until fetal viability is established. Sood et al.[78] reported on 11 women with cervical cancer diagnosed in pregnancy who underwent surgical treatment in the third trimester with a mean planned delay in therapy of 16 weeks. None of these patients experienced a recurrence. Patients with stage IB and stage IIA cervical cancer recognized in the first trimester of pregnancy are routinely recommended to be treated with a type III radical hysterectomy and bilateral deep pelvic lymphadenectomies. This approach affords the patient the opportunity to preserve ovarian function and have a more pliable vagina compared with patients treated with radiation therapy.

Patients with more advanced cervical cancer are routinely recommended to be treated with radiation therapy concurrent with weekly cisplatin.[79–81] External beam radiation therapy has generally been employed first and will induce spontaneous abortion. Intracavitary radiation follows completion of the external beam radiation regimen. Radiation therapy is a known abortifacient when treating pelvic malignancies. Abortion following initiation of radiation exposure occurs more rapidly in the first trimester than in the second.[82] In general, the plan of management at Yale–New Haven Hospital for cervical cancer is to use external beam radiation first and not to attempt to deliver the fetus prior to initiation of therapy. There are no data to suggest that delivering the fetus through an irradiated cervix affects the course of the disease. However, 13 pregnant women with squamous cell carcinoma who delivered vaginally were subsequently diagnosed to have the same type of malignancy in episiotomy sites.[83,84]

Advanced stage cervical cancer has a particularly poor response to standard radiation therapy. A major effort in the past few years has resulted in the development of neoadjuvant chemotherapy protocols for the management of such disease.[85] It may be appropriate to consider a role for neoadjuvant chemotherapy in the management of locally advanced cervical cancer, particularly in situations where definitive treatment will be excessively delayed in order for the fetus to reach viability. In reviewing the 5-year survival for pregnant women with stage I and II cancers treated in pregnancy compared with those patients not pregnant at diagnosis, the survivals were 74.5% and 47.8%, respectively, compared with 76.5% and 55% for overall 5-year survival in the FIGO annual report.[86] Stage III and IV disease did worse in pregnancy, with 16.2% compared with 27.9% survival in the FIGO annual report.[86] The treatment for cervical cancer remains unsatisfactory in the advanced stages, particularly in pregnancy, and bold new initiatives will be necessary for managing this common cancer in pregnant women.

Breast cancer

Breast cancer may be difficult to diagnose during pregnancy and lactation due to the anatomic changes in the breast parenchyma associated with the preparation for lactation. Only 3% of breast cancers occur during pregnancy, but it is the second most common site for invasive cancer in a pregnant woman.[87]

Pregnancy-associated cancers are defined as those diagnosed simultaneously or within 1 year after pregnancy. A number of studies have demonstrated that breast cancer presents at a more advanced stage because of the delay in diagnosis.[81,88–90] The median duration of symptoms before treatment is 15 months in the pregnant patient compared with 9 months in nonpregnant premenopausal women.[91]

The breasts should be examined at the first prenatal visit and thereafter if there have been any concerns noted either by the patient or by the physician during the initial examination. With rare exceptions, any mass discovered during pregnancy should be evaluated.

An ultrasound evaluation may be helpful. If the mass is obvious, a fine needle aspiration (FNA) can be performed.[92] For most patients, an open biopsy on a day surgery basis under local anesthesia is appropriate. Sedation is not necessary and, therefore, there is no risk to the developing fetus. Because of the increased engorgement and vascularity during pregnancy, absolute hemostasis must be achieved, and a pressure dressing should be applied and left in place for 48 h. Open biopsy can also be performed during lactation. The breasts are emptied early in the morning of the day of surgery, and the procedure is again performed under local anesthesia. A pressure dressing is left in place for a few hours. Temporary leakage may occur during breastfeeding, but this soon disappears.

Biopsy material should be sent to the pathologist in a fresh state, and the tissue should be submitted for estrogen and progestin receptor analysis as well as DNA studies. Steroid hormone receptors may not be detected during pregnancy. Pregnancy, in fact, may depress levels of detectable estrogen and progestin receptors, resulting in a false-negative study because high circulating levels of estrogen and progesterone hormones associated with pregnancy result in many more occupied receptor sites.[93]

Earlier studies of breast cancer diagnosed during pregnancy uniformly suggested a poor prognosis. Data now show a similar prognosis for breast cancer patients who are pregnant compared with their nonpregnant counterparts when controlled for stage.[94–98] Other studies have noted that younger women with shorter intervals from pregnancy to cancer diagnosis appear to have a poorer prognosis.[88] Guinee et al.[99] evaluated 407 women younger than 30 years of age and found that those cancer patients who were diagnosed during pregnancy had a significantly greater risk of dying from breast cancer than those who had never been pregnant. When adjusted for tumor size and axillary node status, the risk was reduced only slightly.[97] The authors concluded that concurrent or recent previous pregnancy adversely affects survival of breast cancer in young women. Chung et al.[100] evaluated 6571 breast cancer patients in Rhode Island and divided them into age groups of 10-year intervals. These researchers concluded that women 40 years of age and younger had a worse 5-year cancer-specific survival rate compared with their older counterparts, except in stage I breast cancers (Table 53.4). Anderson et al.[101] conducted a retrospective analysis of young women (younger than 30 years of age) and observed them throughout 20-year intervals. Improved survival rates were found in patients treated during the "modern era," probably as a result of less extensive surgical procedures and the introduction of cytotoxic chemotherapy.[101]

Once the diagnosis of carcinoma has been confirmed, prompt treatment is essential. During the first trimester, modified radical mastectomy is the treatment of choice. Breast conservation treatment poses several problems including potential fetal injury from the effects of radiation.[102] If the patient insists on breast conservation, wide local excision and axillary dissection may be performed and radiation postponed until after delivery. The alternative is termination of the pregnancy and immediate institution of radiation therapy.

During the third trimester, it may be more reasonable to complete local treatment, i.e., wide local excision and axillary dissection, and to delay radiation therapy until after delivery. If the patient chooses modified radical mastectomy, this can be delayed until after delivery if the cancer was diagnosed during the third trimester. Appropriate tests should be obtained to insure maturity of the fetus before delivery. The role of sentinel node evaluation during pregnancy needs to be defined.

If axillary dissection reveals lymph node involvement, adjuvant therapy must be considered. This is standard treatment

Table 53.4 International Union Against Cancer and the American Joint Commission on Cancer Staging and End Results Reporting breast cancer staging classification.

T	Primary tumors		
T1	Tumor 2 cm or less in its greatest dimension a. No fixation to underlying pectoral fascia or muscle b. Fixation to underlying pectoral fascia or muscle		
T2	Tumor more than 2 cm but not more than 5 cm in its greatest dimension		
T3	Tumor more than 5 cm in its greatest dimension a. No fixation to underlying pectoral fascia or muscle b. Fixation to underlying pectoral fascia or muscle		
T4	Tumor of any size with direct extension to chest wall or skin Note: chest wall includes ribs, intercostal muscles, and serratus anterior muscle, but not the pectoral muscle a. Fixation to chest wall b. Edema (including peau d'orange), ulceration of the skin of the breast, or satellite skin nodules confined to the same breast c. Both of the above (a and b) d. Inflammatory carcinoma		
Dimpling of the skin, nipple retraction, or any other skin changes except those in T4b may occur in T1, T2, or T3 without affecting the classification			
N	Regional lymph nodes		
N0	No palpable homolateral axillary nodes		
N1	Movable homolateral axillary nodes a. Nodes not considered to contain growth b. Nodes considered to contain growth		
N2	Homolateral axillary nodes containing growth and fixed to one another or to other structures		
N3	Homolateral supraclavicular or infraclavicular nodes containing growth or edema of the arm		
M	Distant metastasis		
M0	No evidence of distant metastasis		
M1	Distant metastasis present, including skin involvement beyond the breast area		
Clinical stage grouping			
Stage I	T1a or T1b	N0 or N1a	M0
Stage II	T0	N1b	M0
	T1a or T1b	N1b	M0
	T2a or T2b	N0, N1a, or N1b	M0
Stage III	T1a or T1b	N2	M0
	T2a or T2b	N2	M0
T3a or T3b	N0, N1, or N2	M0	
Stage IV	T4	Any N	Any M
	Any T	N3	Any M
	Any T	Any N	M1

Reprinted from DeVita VT Jr, Hellman S, Rosenberg SA, eds. *Cancer: principles and practice of oncology*, 3rd edn. Philadelphia, PA: Lippincott–Raven, with permission.

for node-positive premenopausal patients and may be considered in selected node-negative patients. Biologic response modifiers have been administered in pregnancy without adverse effects.[103–106]

The final decision whether to use adjuvant chemotherapy rests with the patient after she has received appropriate counseling. In cases of locally advanced cancer, the decisions are even more difficult because chemotherapy and radiotherapy may be required for palliation. In this situation, pregnancy termination would be recommended. This is a difficult decision, and there are no absolutely correct answers. In most of these patients, life expectancy is severely limited, and a frank discussion of the issues involved is imperative.

With prompt diagnosis and appropriate treatment, many patients survive the disease and desire further pregnancies. Most recurrences of breast cancer appear within the first 2 years, and pregnancy should be avoided during this period. Some studies have shown no adverse effect of a subsequent pregnancy even in patients with positive nodes or patients in whom pregnancy occurred earlier than 2 years after completion of treatment.[107–111] Abortion has not improved survival.[108]

Ovarian cancer

Most ovarian cancers complicating pregnancy are either borderline malignant potential epithelial cancers or germ cell malignancies. Invasive epithelial cancers are rare in pregnancy, and sex cord–stromal tumors occur extremely infrequently. It can be expected that the incidence of ovarian neoplasms recognized in pregnancy will increase with the routine use of diagnostic ultrasound in pregnancy. As a result, more patients are now being seen in our institution with ovarian masses. A recent series of adnexal masses reported from the Yale–New Haven Hospital suggests that ultrasound evaluation is a very successful way of assessing the nature of an ovarian tumor.[112] MRI is useful in further delineating the nature of the ovarian neoplasm.[112,113] Our experience suggests, however, that for most patients an ultrasound assessment of an adnexal mass is likely to establish the benign nature of the lesion, with MRI being used in those patients in whom the ultrasound findings are equivocal or the lesion cannot be distinguished from a uterine neoplasm, in particular a uterine leiomyoma.[112] Figure 53.3 demonstrates an MRI confirming a uterine fibroid that was ultrasonographically indistinguishable from an ovarian tumor associated with a 15-week pregnancy. Figure 53.4 demonstrates a benign cystic teratoma diagnosed in pregnancy by MRI techniques.

Ovarian malignancies occurring in pregnancy are estimated to complicate 1 in 9000 to 1 in 25 000 pregnancies.[114] Ovarian neoplasms are usually observed in the first trimester and are operated upon in the second trimester. These lesions tend to be asymptomatic when recognized. However, torsion is a relatively frequent presentation for a germ cell malignancy of the ovary and requires prompt surgical intervention. Simple cysts of the ovary may be followed with serial ultrasound examinations until the cysts resolve. Lesions greater than 6 cm in diameter, complex cysts (i.e., cysts containing both solid and cystic elements), and solid tumors are the usual indications for operative intervention in pregnancy. Figure 53.5 demonstrates a complex ovarian cyst that proved to be a mucinous carcinoma of the ovary. Germ cell ovarian malignancies occur relatively infrequently in younger women, but must be considered in the differential diagnosis of solid or solid and cystic pelvic masses occurring in pregnancy.[115] The more rapidly growing tumors (i.e., the endodermal sinus tumors and embryonal carcinoma) may be associated with hemorrhage and necrosis, giving a rather inhomogeneous appearance to the mass on ultrasound or MRI scans. Elevated levels of circulating tumor markers may help to distinguish germ cell tumors from other ovarian neoplasms. However, elevated α-fetoprotein (AFP) and β-hCG titers are routine in pregnancy, and such assays may be more confusing than informative in the preoperative evaluation of patients with pelvic masses. Similarly, serum lactic dehydrogenase (SLDH) and other liver enzyme levels may be elevated in nonpregnant women with solid adnexal tumors that prove to be dysgerminoma.[116] However, SLDH and other liver enzymes may be elevated in the pregnant state unrelated to the presence of a dysgerminoma. CA 125, an antigenic determinant made by approximately 80% of ovarian cancers, may be elevated in early pregnancy for reasons unrelated to the presence of a malignancy.[117–119]

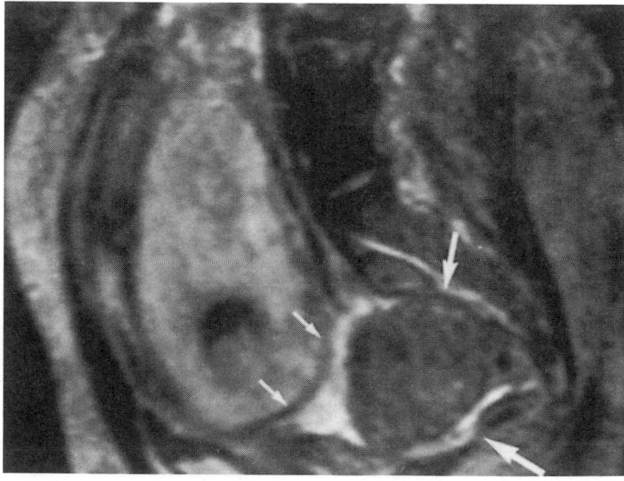

Figure 53.3 Uterine leiomyoma, T2-weighted sagittal magnetic resonance image. The low signal intensity of this well-circumscribed mass (*large arrows*) and origin from the posterior wall of the gravid uterus (*small arrows*) permit a confident diagnosis of a uterine leiomyoma. (Courtesy of Dr. R. Kier.)

In general, surgical management of ovarian neoplasms occurring in pregnancy is delayed until the second trimester, provided the patient is asymptomatic and the tumor is not suspicious for malignancy by diagnostic imaging techniques. Symptomatic patients and patients with tumors suspicious for malignancy should promptly undergo surgery to diagnose and initiate the treatment of the cancer.

Surgical staging

Surgical staging for ovarian cancer in pregnancy should be the same as that recommended for surgical staging in the nonpregnant state. However, the pregnant uterus makes assessment of the retroperitoneum much more difficult. A vertical incision should be used. On entering the abdomen, any free fluid should be aspirated and sent for cytology. If no free fluid is present, washings of the paracolic spaces, the pelvis, and subdiaphragmatic spaces should be obtained. The ovarian lesion should then be removed and sent for frozen section histologic analysis. Every effort should be made to remove the tumor intact. The remaining ovary should be carefully inspected and biopsied. Any peritoneal abnormalities should

A

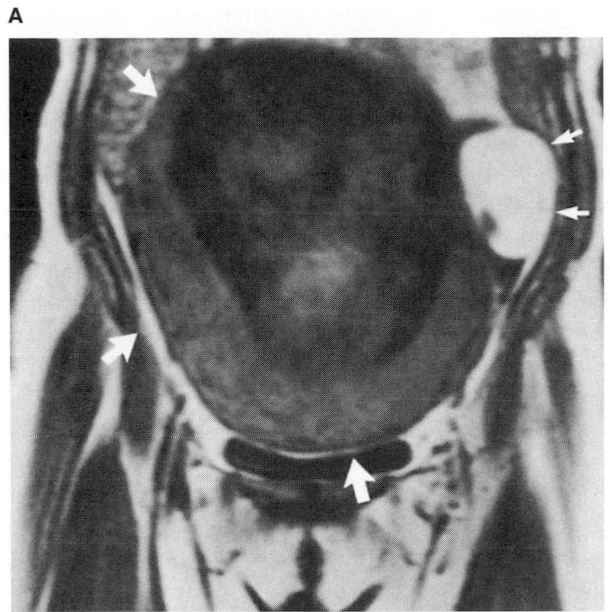

B

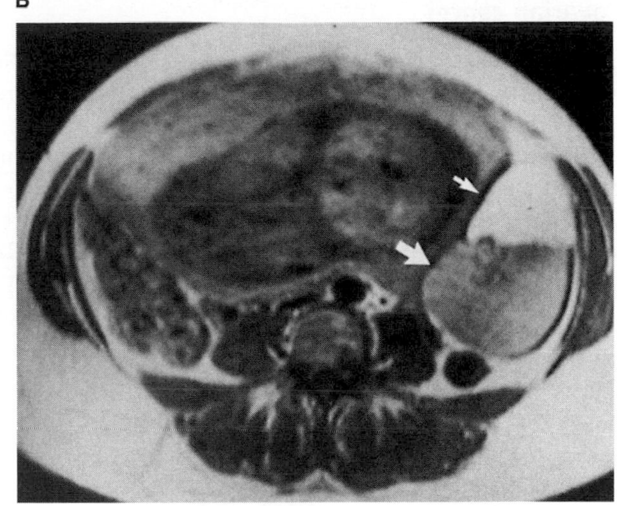

C

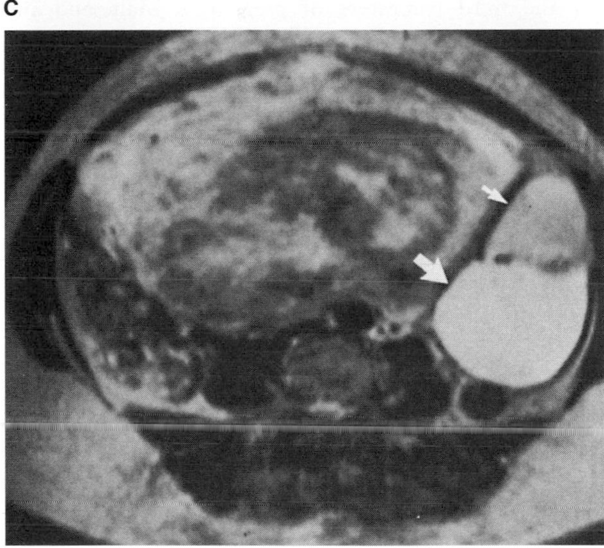

Figure 53.4 Mature cystic teratoma of the left ovary. (**A**) Coronal T1-weighted magnetic resonance image demonstrates a left ovarian mass (*small arrows*) next to the gravid uterus (*large arrows*). High signal intensity on T1-weighted images is consistent with the presence of fat within the tumor. (**B**) T2-weighted axial image again demonstrates the fatty component of the tumor (*small arrow*) floating above fluid (*large arrow*). On T2-weighted images, the fat becomes of intermediate signal intensity, whereas the serum becomes high signal intensity. (**C**) Axial T1-weighted image demonstrates the left ovarian mass next to the gravid uterus. Fat floats in the nondependent portion of the mass (*small arrow*), whereas fluid within the mass (*large arrow*) is dependent within the mass. (Courtesy of Dr. R. Kier.)

be sampled. Any retroperitoneal nodularities should also be sampled. Sampling of periaortic lymph nodes should be attempted. This can be the most difficult part of the procedure in pregnancy because of the bulk of the gravid uterus. It is inappropriate to remove both ovaries when a germ cell ovarian malignancy is diagnosed by frozen section techniques. The most common neoplasm in the contralateral ovary of a woman with a germ cell malignancy is a benign cystic teratoma. However, if both ovaries are involved with malignant growths and the patient is in the second trimester of pregnancy, each ovary should be removed, as the pregnancy will sustain itself in the second and third trimesters without ovaries being present.[77] Germ cell ovarian malignancies are almost invariably unilateral. Removing the contralateral ovary does not affect prognosis for the patient. Recent evidence suggests that occult dysgerminomas may be present in a grossly normal contralateral ovary.[120] In such a circumstance, it is not necessary to remove the entire ovary. Nonpregnant women with microscopic dysgerminoma in the contralateral ovary have subsequently been treated with chemotherapy and have gone on to conceive normal healthy children. The current FIGO staging system for ovarian cancer is presented in Table 53.5.

Epithelial ovarian cancer

Borderline malignant potential tumors are the most common epithelial ovarian cancers in pregnancy.[121] Patients with stage IA and IB borderline malignant potential tumors are adequately treated with surgery alone. More advanced stage ovarian borderline malignant potential tumors are also treated surgically, chemotherapy being reserved only for the unusual group of patients with invasive metastases in association with borderline malignant potential tumors of the ovary.[122]

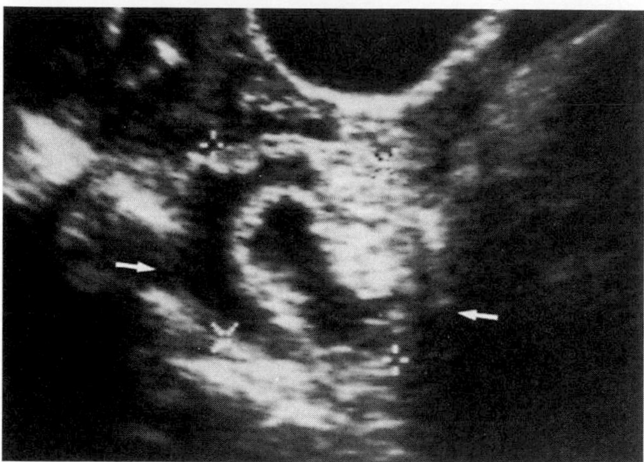

Figure 53.5 Mucinous carcinoma of the ovary. Sagittal ultrasonogram demonstrates a complex ovarian mass (*arrows*) posterior to the lower uterine segment of the gravid uterus. (Courtesy of Dr. M. G. Tompkins.)

Patients found to have stage I invasive cancers of the ovary are generally managed conservatively, and the pregnancy is allowed to go to term. Recent data suggest that, in a non-pregnant state, patients with stages IA and IB, grades 1 and 2, epithelial cancers of the ovary are adequately treated with surgery alone.[123] Additional adjuvant chemotherapy appears to play no significant role in improving a very high disease-free survival. Once the cancer is more advanced than stage IB, aggressive cytoreductive surgery is necessary. In general, a total abdominal hysterectomy and bilateral salpingo-oophorectomy, omentectomy, and para-aortic and pelvic lymph node sampling, and resection of all gross tumor is recommended in early-stage ovarian cancer. The patient is subsequently treated with platinum-based combination chemotherapy.

Recent studies with germ cell ovarian malignancies suggest that platinum-based chemotherapy may be given successfully in the second and third trimester prior to the fetus reaching viability.[124] Such a strategy may be employed for common epithelial cancers as well, first recognized to be present in the second and third trimesters of pregnancy. Malfetano and Goldkrand[125] treated one patient successfully with cisplatin-based chemotherapy after conservative surgery at 16 weeks' gestation confirmed the presence of an advanced-stage epithelial ovarian cancer. That patient went on to a vaginal delivery and a postpartum laparotomy that revealed no evidence of persistent cancer. In turn, Buckley et al.[126] reported on a pregnant woman with an advanced ovarian cancer in a pregnancy complicated by human immunodeficiency virus (HIV) infection who failed to respond to cytoreductive surgery and

Table 53.5 International Federation of Gynecology and Obstetrics (FIGO) ovarian cancer staging classification.

I	Growth limited to the ovaries
Ia	Growth limited to one ovary; no ascites; no tumor on the external surface; capsule intact
Ib	Growth limited to both ovaries; no ascites; no tumor on the external surfaces; capsule intact
Ic	Tumor either stage Ia or Ib, but with tumor on the surface of one or both ovaries; or with the capsule ruptured; or with ascites containing malignant cells; or with positive peritoneal washings
II	Growth involving one or both ovaries with pelvic extension
IIa	Extension, metastases, or both to the uterus, tubes, or both
IIb	Extension to other pelvic tissue
IIc	Tumor either stage IIa or IIb but with tumor on the surface of one or both ovaries; or with the capsule ruptured; or with ascites present containing malignant cells; or with positive peritoneal washings
III	Tumor involving one or both ovaries with peritoneal implants outside the pelvis and/or positive retroperitoneal or inguinal nodes; superficial liver metastases equals stage III; tumor is limited to the true pelvis but with histologically proven malignant extension to the small bowel or omentum
IIIa	Tumor grossly limited to the true pelvis with negative nodes but with histologically confirmed microscopic seeding of abdominal peritoneal surfaces
IIIb	Tumor involving one or both ovaries with histologically confirmed implants of abdominal peritoneal surfaces, none exceeding 2 cm in diameter; nodes are negative
IIIc	Abdominal implants greater than 2 cm in diameter and/or positive retroperitoneal or inguinal nodes
IV	Growth involving one or both ovaries with distant metastases. If pleural effusion is present, there must be positive cytology to allot a case to stage IV; parenchymal liver metastasis equals stage IV

Reprinted from Staging Announcement: FIGO Cancer Committee. *Gynecol Oncol* 1986;25:383, with permission.

cytotoxic chemotherapy and who died within 13 months of her cancer diagnosis.

Germ cell ovarian malignancies

Germ cell ovarian malignancies are infrequently occurring tumors that present in women in their second and third decades of life. The dysgerminoma is the most common malignancy in pregnancy.[127] Management of dysgerminoma requires removal of the primary tumor and careful surgical staging, as described earlier. Dysgerminomas are the only germ cell malignancies of the ovary to frequently (5–15%) involve both ovaries. Thus, biopsying the contralateral ovary is appropriate even if it appears to be grossly normal. Dysgerminomas also have a tendency to spread to the para-aortic nodes. Every effort should be made to sample the para-aortic lymph nodes surgically at the time of the extirpation for the dysgerminoma.

Dysgerminomas are exquisitely sensitive to radiation therapy and chemotherapy.[115] Vincristine, actinomycin D, and cyclophosphamide (VAC) and bleomycin, etoposide, and platinum (BEP) are extremely effective regimens for the management of dysgerminomas.[128] Stage IA dysgerminoma may be treated very effectively with surgery alone.[115] Advanced-stage dysgerminoma should be treated with postoperative chemotherapy.[115] Pregnant women should be given the chance to maintain the pregnancy if a dysgerminoma is present. Chemotherapy may be given in the second or third trimesters. BEP and VAC chemotherapy regimens require only short-term administration and are given every 3–4 weeks. A Cesarean section is used to deliver the fetus at the time of fetal viability. A second-look procedure may also be performed at that surgery. The endodermal sinus tumor is the most virulent of all the germ cell ovarian malignancies. It was associated with a 2-year survival of 12–19% in the prechemotherapy era. Our current recommendation for this disease is the BEP regimen.

Other germ cell malignancies include the embryonal carcinoma, the immature teratoma, choriocarcinoma, and mixed germ cell tumors. Their management is based on both the stage of disease and the presence or absence of circulating oncofetal proteins that can be used as markers for response to therapy. In general, these malignancies require aggressive therapy in the form of resection of all viable tumor followed by intense combination chemotherapy.[115] Pregnant women found to have these tumors in the second and third trimesters of pregnancy should be offered the opportunity of receiving chemotherapy during pregnancy as a way of being treated and not terminating the pregnancy. Christman and colleagues[129] have reported a patient with a stage IC, grade 3, immature teratoma who was successfully treated with a unilateral salpingo-oophorectomy at 15 weeks' gestation and one course of cisplatin, vinblastine, and bleomycin in her 19th week of gestation.[129] The patient delivered a normal term infant, received four more cycles of therapy postpartum, and is alive and well 61 months from diagnosis. The child has developed normally.

Sex cord–stromal tumors

Sex cord–stromal tumors are rare tumors that may complicate pregnancy. The granulosa theca cell tumor is the most common member of this category and is associated with estrogen production.[130] The Sertoli–Leydig cell tumor is rare and is associated with androgen production. Young and colleagues[131] reported on 36 sex cord–stromal tumors diagnosed in pregnancy. Treatment was limited to removing the tumor. Only one of these patients has subsequently recurred. Advanced-stage sex cord–stromal tumors require more aggressive chemotherapy. Our current recommendation in the nonpregnant state is a carboplatin and paclitaxel combination.

Hodgkin's disease

Hodgkin's disease generally occurs during the reproductive years, the peak incidence being between the ages of 18 and 30 years.[132] It is estimated that one-third of women with Hodgkin's disease are pregnant or have delivered within 1 year of the diagnosis.[133,134] As with almost all malignancies associated with pregnancy, Hodgkin's disease has not been reported to be affected by the pregnancy.[135–137] It is a disease that is extremely sensitive to therapy. The cure rate for localized disease treated with radiation therapy is 80%, and patients with advanced disease treated with chemotherapy can anticipate a long-term disease-free survival of 65%.[138,139] Peripheral lymphadenopathy is the most common presenting symptom for patients with Hodgkin's disease. Between 60% and 80% of Hodgkin's disease patients have enlarged cervical lymph nodes. In addition, patients may be asymptomatic or may have a history of fever, night sweats, weight loss, malaise, and pruritus.[140]

Selection of local radiation or systemic chemotherapy is based on the staging system (Table 53.6). Staging studies recommended for a patient with Hodgkin's disease are done in an attempt to identify extranodal disease. Pregnant women may undergo ultrasound or MRI studies of the liver, spleen, and retroperitoneal lymph nodes to avoid the hazard of diagnostic imaging radiation exposure to the fetus. Strategies for treating patients with stage I and stage II Hodgkin's disease are usually radiotherapeutic, with reported 5-year survivals of 89% and 67% respectively.[140] Radiation is the only modality necessary for patients with stage IIIA lymphocyte-predominant or nodular-sclerosing Hodgkin's disease. Stage IIIA disease with other histologic types is treated with radiation and combination chemotherapy. More advanced disease is treated with combination chemotherapy.[141]

The standard mantle field for midline mediastinal radiation to doses of 4000 rad results in fetal exposure to a degree that is greater than acceptable.[142] It has been recommended that, in the first trimester of pregnancy, the fetus should not be exposed to more than 10 rad (0.1 cGy). Internal radiation

Table 53.6 Ann Arbor staging classification for Hodgkin's disease.

I	Involvement of a single lymph node region (I) or a single extralymphatic organ or site (I_E)
II	Involvement of two or more lymph node regions on the same side of the diaphragm (II) or localized involvement of an extralymphatic organ or site (II_E)
III	Involvement of lymph node regions on both sides of the diaphragm (III) or localized involvement of an extralymphatic organ or site (III_E), spleen (III_S), or both (III_{SE})
IV	Diffuse or disseminated involvement of one or more extralymphatic organs with or without associated lymph node involvement. The organ(s) involved should be identified by a symbol
	A = Asymptomatic
	B = Fever, sweats, weight loss >10% of body weight

Reprinted from DeVita VT Jr, Hellman S, Rosenberg SA, eds. *Cancer: principles and practice of oncology*, 3rd edn. Philadelphia, PA: Lippincott–Raven, 1989; with permission.

scatter from standard mantle fields cannot be shielded and would result in a greater exposure rate to the fetus than the dose recommended for continuation of the pregnancy.[141] Patients with pelvic disease or disease localized to the inguinal or abdominal region should undergo therapeutic abortion prior to radiation therapy. Similar disease first recognized in the third trimester would be treated with localized radiation therapy once fetal maturity was achieved and the infant delivered. Patients found to have rapidly progressing disease routinely receive chemotherapy, with the decision for initiating treatment based on the trimester of pregnancy and the patient's desires.

Advanced (stage III and stage IV) Hodgkin's disease has been successfully treated with the MOPP regimen – Mustargen (nitrogen mustard), Oncovin (vincristine), procarbazine, and prednisone.[140] Eighty-one percent of patients in the National Cancer Institute series with previously untreated stage III and stage IV disease were successfully managed with only 6 months of treatment.[139] The role for chemotherapy in the management of Hodgkin's disease in the first trimester of pregnancy is only beginning to become defined.[137] Therapeutic abortion should be offered to those patients in the first half of pregnancy who are unwilling to accept an increase in risk of adverse fetal outcome potentially attributable to treatment.

Non-Hodgkin's lymphoma

Fewer than 50 cases of non-Hodgkin's lymphomas during pregnancy have been published.[54,140,143] The mean age of patients with non-Hodgkin's lymphoma is 42 years, suggesting that most patients are past their childbearing years or are in a subfertile period of their reproductive life. The most important prognostic features for non-Hodgkin's lymphoma are the histologic type and the stage of disease.[141] Non-Hodgkin's lymphomas tend to be widely disseminated at the time of diagnosis and therefore require less elaborate staging than Hodgkin's disease. Breast and ovarian involvement is frequent, and breast metastases have a particularly bad prognosis.[144,145]

Localized non-Hodgkin's lymphoma is treated with radiation and has a 50% cure rate. Chemotherapy may also be curative in this disease.[146] Disseminated nodular lymphoma and chronic lymphocytic leukemia fall into a favorable group of disseminated non-Hodgkin's lymphomas. They tend to be relatively indolent.[141] Palliative treatment results in survivals of about 5 years. The unfavorable types of non-Hodgkin's lymphoma have a much shorter life expectancy, although occasional complete remissions and prolonged survival with chemotherapy have been reported.[147] Because of the aggressive nature of diffuse non-Hodgkin's lymphoma, aggressive therapy should not be delayed until fetal maturity. Aviles and colleagues published the largest experience treating non-Hodgkin's lymphoma in pregnancy.[54]

Acute leukemia

Acute leukemia rarely complicates pregnancy, the incidence being less than one case in 75 000 pregnancies.[57,148] The disease is usually first recognized in the second or third trimester.[149] A recent review of 72 women with leukemia in pregnancy from 1975 to 1988 revealed that 64 (89%) had acute leukemia. Of these 72 women, 44 had acute myelogenous leukemia, 20 had acute lymphocytic leukemia, five had chronic myelogenous leukemia, one had a hairy cell leukemia, and two had unspecified leukemias.[150] Sixteen (22%) were detected in the first trimester, 26 (36%) were detected in the second trimester, and 30 (42%) were detected in the third trimester of pregnancy. Presenting symptoms are becoming easily fatigued, bleeding diathesis, or recurrent infections that reflect bone marrow failure. Specific physical findings associated with acute leukemia include sternal tenderness, skin pallor, petechiae, ecchymoses, and hepatosplenomegaly. Patients with acute lymphocytic, myelocytic, or monocytic leukemia usually have normocytic anemia, normochromic anemia, mild to marked thrombocytopenia, and leukocytosis.[140]

Pregnancy does not influence the natural history of acute leukemia.[55,150] Substantial improvement in the survival of women with acute leukemia in pregnancy has occurred with the use of chemotherapy, radiation therapy, and supportive care, including blood products, antibiotics, and autologous bone marrow transplantation.[151] Virtually all women treated with chemotherapy in pregnancy will survive to delivery, and 87% of the fetuses will also survive.[140] Intense combination chemotherapy leads to multiple complications, including severe infections secondary to bone marrow suppression and the risk of central nervous system leukemia. The latter is treated with whole brain radiation, intrathecal methotrexate, or cytosine arabinoside. Hyperuricemia is usually treated with allopurinol.[152]

Chronic myelocytic leukemia

Chronic myelocytic leukemia makes up 90% of the chronic leukemias complicating pregnancy.[153,154] Pregnancy does not adversely affect the natural history of chronic myelocytic leukemia. Treatment is palliative. Median survival is 45 months. All patients eventually die, most from an acute blastic crisis resembling myeloblastic leukemia.[141] The median survival is less than 1 year following the development of an acute blastic crisis.[140] Eighty-five percent of chronic myelocytic leukemia patients have a Philadelphia chromosome, a 9:22 translocation.[140] Approximately 96% of pregnant women with chronic myelocytic leukemia survive to delivery. Fetal survival throughout the gestation is 84%.[140]

Melanoma

Pigment-producing melanocytes are found in the base layer of the epidermis, the mucosa of the gastrointestinal tract, the vagina, and the pigmented portion of the retina. Malignant melanoma derives from such cells and, in 90% of cases, originates in the skin in pre-existing pigmented nevi.[155] Malignant melanoma localized to superficial layers of the skin is associated with a 50–80% cure rate. Lesions that have infiltrated into the lowest third of the dermis or that have metastasized to regional lymph nodes have a 20% cure rate.[140]

Pregnancy frequently induces a darkening in the appearance of pigmented nevi, but a bluish or slightly gray appearance to a nevus requires immediate excisional biopsy. Indeed, pigmented nevi that have become darker or irregular in outline and elevated should always be promptly excised in pregnancy under local anesthesia. Pregnancy does not change the natural history of melanoma.[156,157] McNammy and colleagues[156] reported on 23 patients pregnant at the time of the diagnosis of melanoma and were unable to show that pregnancy had any significant influence on the survival of those patients. They did recommend that subsequent pregnancies be avoided for the first 3 years following excision of a malignant melanoma. Wong and colleagues reviewed 66 patients with stage I melanoma diagnosed during pregnancy and were unable to identify any significant difference between the pregnant population and a control population with regard to the location of the primary tumor, the age of diagnosis, Clark's level, mean depth of invasion, and histologic type.[157] The 5-year survival for women with melanoma during pregnancy and for the entire population was 86% and 87% respectively. Thus, the pregnancy did not influence the survival of the patients.[157] Terminating a pregnancy will not initiate a remission.[158] The clinical significance of estrogen receptor protein found in malignant melanoma has yet to be established. Clinical trials with an estrogen agonist–antagonist have yet to demonstrate any benefit in the treatment of malignant melanoma.[140,159,160]

Most patients with malignant melanoma present with stage I disease, disease limited to a primary cutaneous lesion. Stage I disease is pathologically staged according to Clark's level of deepest anatomic invasion or the Breslow system.[161,162] Stage I lesions are usually treated with wide local excisions. Adjuvant immunotherapy for completely resected stage I and stage II disease has not shown definite benefit.[155] Surgery should be performed promptly in patients with stage I and stage II disease, whereas patients with stage III disease can only be palliated. Early delivery of the fetus in the third trimester once fetal lung maturation has been achieved should be considered routinely for stage III patients.

Placental or fetal metastases have been reported only 16 times, with four fetal deaths due to transplacental metastases of malignant melanoma.[158] Although malignant melanoma is the most common malignancy to metastasize to the placenta and fetus, this is such a rare event as to preclude the recommendation of pregnancy termination for the management of the disease to avoid transplacental carcinogenesis or to induce a remission.

Gastrointestinal cancer

Colorectal cancers

Cancers of the gastrointestinal tract rarely complicate pregnancy.[163] There is no evidence that pregnancy changes the natural history of colorectal cancer, the most common of these neoplasms.[164–168] Most pregnant patients with gastrointestinal cancers have rectal carcinomas. Approximately 20% of patients have carcinoma presenting in the sigmoid colon.[169] Unfortunately, diagnosis is frequently difficult in pregnancy, and there is a considerable delay in diagnosis. Typical presenting symptoms include severe constipation, abdominal distention, and rectal bleeding. As most diagnoses can be made by rectal examination, these symptoms should be promptly evaluated. Delay in diagnosis can be associated with intussusception, obstruction, or perforation.[168] Carcinoembryonic antigen (CEA) is routinely elevated in pregnancy and is of little use in diagnosing colorectal cancers in the gravid state.[170]

Early-stage colorectal cancers diagnosed in the first and second trimester should be treated with prompt surgery, and the pregnancy should be allowed to go to term.[168,171] Patients with large colorectal lesions with metastases suspected or present have been allowed to carry the pregnancy until fetal maturity and have then undergone a Cesarean section and bowel resection, provided they remained relatively asymptomatic.[169] Most colorectal cancer patients are delivered by Cesarean section, as labor may result in dystocia or hemorrhage. Lesions initially identified in the third trimester are not usually treated until fetal maturity is achieved.[171] Standard therapy for curable lesions is definitive surgery, including standard bowel resections, low anterior resections, or abdominal perineal resections.[172]

Pancreatic tumors

Pancreatic carcinoma rarely complicates pregnancy and is difficult to diagnose in the presence of pancreatitis.[173,174] Three cases of pancreatic carcinoma have been diagnosed in pregnancy, with the mothers dying soon after delivery.[173,174]

Stomach tumors

Gastric cancers rarely complicate pregnancy, and their symptoms are similar to those normally experienced in pregnancy, including gastrointestinal discomfort, nausea, and vomiting.[175–178] Diagnosis may be made by gastroscopy, which avoids diagnostic radiation exposure. Maeta[179] reported 14 cases of gastric cancer occurring in pregnancy.

Liver tumors

Hepatocellular carcinomas are rare in women and usually present in postmenopausal women. A literature review revealed only 28 cases of hepatocellular carcinoma reported through 1995.[179] Hepatocellular carcinoma predominantly occurs in males, tends to present at a later age in women, and decreased fertility is associated with advanced cirrhosis (a predisposing factor for hepatocellular carcinoma).[180] One case report of a hepatocellular carcinoma resulted in a maternal death in pregnancy.[181] A single case of an extrahepatic biliary tract carcinoma complicating pregnancy has been reported.[182]

Gynecologic malignancies

Uterine carcinoma

Adenocarcinoma of the endometrium is an extremely unusual disease in pregnant women, as only 8% of endometrial cancers have been reported to occur in women under age 40 years.[183] Infertility has been a factor associated with women who develop adenocarcinoma of the endometrium. Eleven cases of adenocarcinoma of the endometrium associated with pregnancy have been reported.[184–188] The cases were generally associated with vaginal bleeding and were found to be well-differentiated adenocarcinomas. Only one of the patients has died to date. Standard therapy for patients with adenocarcinoma of the endometrium is a total abdominal hysterectomy and bilateral salpingo-oophorectomy. One patient with a mixed mesodermal tumor of the uterus has also been reported from Yale–New Haven Hospital.[189]

Vulvar cancer

Vulvar carcinoma *in situ* has been increasing, according to data from the Connecticut Tumor Registry.[190] Forty percent of patients with vulvar carcinoma *in situ* are under age 40 years. Thus, it can be anticipated that more women will be diagnosed in pregnancy to have vulvar carcinoma *in situ*. The management of a vulvar lesion in pregnancy is a wide local excision. Vulvar carcinoma *in situ* does not progress rapidly to invasive cancer unless associated with an immune deficiency. Definitive therapy in terms of a wide local excision or vulvectomy can be delayed in most cases until after completion of the pregnancy.

Lutz and colleagues[191] reported that 5% of women with carcinoma of the vulva seen at the Medical University of South Carolina were diagnosed in pregnancy or within 2–6 months postpartum. Invasive cancer is usually treated with a radical vulvectomy. Recently, less extensive surgery has been quite effective if the tumor is only superficially invasive.[192] Extensive vulvectomies may be performed in pregnancy, but the current trend in the nonpregnant state is to manage microinvasive cancer with wide local excision.[192,193]

Vaginal cancer

Carcinoma of the vagina occurs infrequently and is usually a squamous carcinoma presenting in a peri- or postmenopausal woman. Its management is similar to that of cervical cancer. Senekjian and colleagues[194] reported on 20 patients who developed clear cell adenocarcinomas of the vagina in pregnancy. These women had been exposed *in utero* to diethylstilbestrol. It was noted that the pregnancy did not have an adverse effect on clear cell carcinomas of the vagina or cervix. Perhaps this is due to the fact that, in a previous report, clear cell carcinomas did not have estrogen and progestin receptors.[195]

Soft tissue sarcoma

Soft tissue sarcomas rarely complicate pregnancy. The overall prognosis is poor. No evidence suggests that, if they were successfully managed, subsequent pregnancies would be deleterious to the patient's health.[196,197] Osteogenic sarcoma is the most frequent sarcoma reported in pregnancy. No survival differences were noted in 18 cases of osteogenic sarcoma managed in pregnancy when they were matched with nonpregnant women for skeletal tumor location, histologic appearance, and age.[198] Therapeutic abortion has been recommended in the first trimester for patients exposed to intense cytotoxic chemotherapy.[199] However, it is usually recommended that patients diagnosed in the third trimester undergo early delivery once fetal maturity has been established.[199] A case of a Ewing's sarcoma involving the iliac wing diagnosed at 25 weeks' gestation appears to have been successfully treated with multiagent chemotherapy in pregnancy followed by a Cesarean section at 34 weeks' gestation.[200]

Endocrine tumors

Thyroid cancer

Disorders of the thyroid gland are common in pregnancy, and thyroid nodules are frequently diagnosed in pregnancy.[201] However, the thyroid is an infrequent site for cancer to develop in pregnancy. Tan et al.[201] found three thyroid cancers among 40 nodules assessed in pregnancy. As the population delays childbearing, it is possible that more papillary adenocarcinomas of the thyroid will be diagnosed in the future, as the peak distribution for papillary adenocarcinomas occurs in women aged 30–34 years.[202] Patients at high risk of thyroid cancer include women exposed to radiation therapy to the head, neck, or chest during childhood.[203,204] Most cancers of the thyroid present as solitary nodules. Most thyroid nodules appear in the first and third trimester of pregnancy and are benign.[205]

The most common type of thyroid cancer to be diagnosed in pregnancy is the papillary carcinoma or mixed papillary follicular carcinoma. Prognosis is not affected by subclinical metastases to regional lymph nodes, which are present in 50–70% of patients. Women under age 49 years are expected to have a 15-year survival rate of 90–95%.[203,204] Anaplastic carcinomas have fulminant courses and rarely complicate pregnancy, as they occur most commonly in women over 50 years of age. Medullary carcinomas can occur in association with the multiple endocrine neoplasia type II syndrome (medullary thyroid carcinoma, pheochromocytoma, and parathyroid adenoma), are bilateral, and have only once been reported in pregnancy.[206]

Fine needle aspiration biopsies are used to diagnose thyroid cancer in pregnancy.[201,207] Radionuclide scans are contraindicated in pregnancy because of the theoretical risk of destroying the fetal thyroid. Fine needle aspiration biopsy is associated with a false-negative rate of only 6%.[201,208]

As the overwhelming number of thyroid cancers presenting in pregnancy are histologically well differentiated, there is no reason to terminate pregnancy or avoid future pregnancies.[209,210] Pregnancy does not appear to influence the course of well-differentiated thyroid cancer.[210,211] Thyroid suppression therapy may be administered until delivery, regardless of the trimester in which the cancer was diagnosed.[202] Patients should undergo prompt surgery if metastases develop in regional lymph nodes during suppression therapy or the tumor is fixed to surrounding tissue and enlarges during suppression therapy. A subtotal thyroidectomy is usually performed, and ^{131}I should be administered postpartum to avoid the surgical complication of permanent hypoparathyroidism.[212] Extensive surgery should be avoided during pregnancy, as there is a chance of miscarriage occurring as a result.[213]

Patients diagnosed in the first two trimesters of pregnancy as having a medullary carcinoma should undergo prompt total thyroidectomy and prophylactic neck dissection, whereas those diagnosed in the third trimester can await fetal maturity before definitive surgery. Patients undergoing thyroidectomy in pregnancy are recommended to receive levothyroxine postoperatively in a dose sufficient to keep serum thyroid-stimulating hormone (TSH) low.[214]

Adrenal tumors

Pheochromocytoma is the most common tumor arising in the adrenal gland in pregnancy. In the past, it has been associated with a high maternal mortality (58%) and fetal mortality (55%).[168] However, Harper and colleagues[215] reviewed the literature from 1980 to 1987 and presented 47 cases with pheochromocytoma diagnosed in pregnancy. The overall mortality was 17% and fetal loss was 26%. MRI may be used to confirm the presence, laterality, and location of the pheochromocytoma.[216] Figure 53.6 shows a pheochromocytoma diagnosed by MRI in a 25-week-pregnant patient. Provocative tests should not be performed, because these might lead to maternal fatality.[217]

The management of pheochromocytoma has been surgical in the first two trimesters and delivery by Cesarean section followed by tumor resection in the third trimester.[168] Medical management of the disease includes preoperative adrenergic blockade with oral phenoxybenzamine, to lower the blood pressure, and propranolol to reduce the heart rate and prevent arrhythmias through the adrenergic receptor blockade.[218,219] Stenstrom and Swolin[220] have recommended using alpha receptor-blocking agents for the treatment of patients diagnosed as having pheochromocytomas in the second and third trimester and delaying surgery until fetal viability is accomplished. Armaroli and colleagues[221] also reported on the successful management of a mother in this fashion. Lyons and Colmorgen[222] managed a patient throughout her entire pregnancy with adrenergic blockade.

Parathyroid carcinoma

One case of a parathyroid carcinoma complicating pregnancy has been reported.[223] That patient presented with acute pancreatitis at 31 weeks' gestation, underwent a left parathyroidectomy, subsequently delivered a viable infant, and then had an additional pregnancy.[223]

Urinary tract malignancies

Kidney tumors

Renal cell carcinoma is the most common malignancy arising in the urinary tract in pregnancy. Tydings and colleagues[224] reviewed 37 cases of renal tumors, 22 of which were renal cell

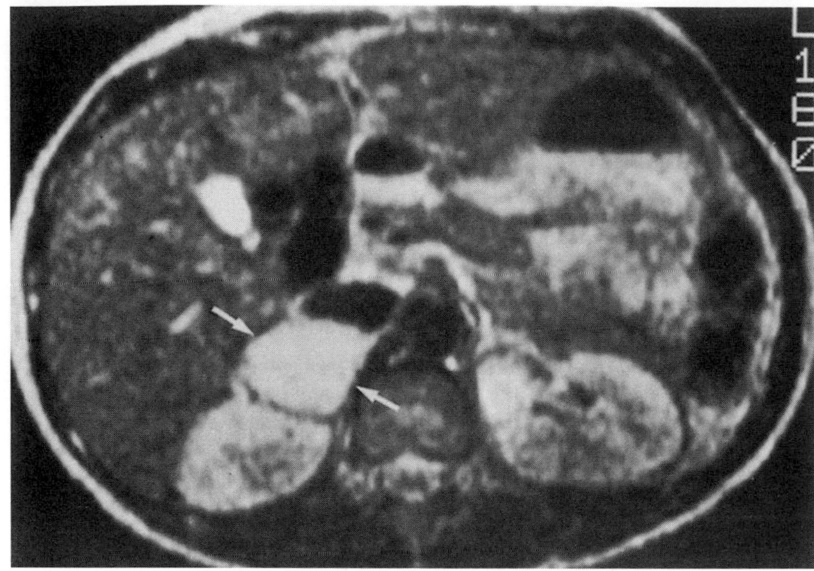

Figure 53.6 Pheochromocytoma in a pregnant patient. The right adrenal mass (*arrows*) is very high signal intensity on this T2-weighted image, consistent with a diagnosis of pheochromocytoma. (Courtesy of Dr. R. Kier.)

carcinoma. Hematuria is the most common presenting symptom. Nephrectomy with or without radiation therapy is standard treatment.

Bladder cancers

Bladder cancers have infrequently been reported in pregnancy.[225–227] The histologic distribution is similar to that in the nonpregnant state, with an overwhelming majority being transitional cell carcinoma followed by squamous cell and adenocarcinomas.

Central nervous system tumors

Central nervous system tumors rarely complicate pregnancy.[228] Patients present with headaches and visual disturbances. MRI allows for rapid evaluation without radiation exposure. The overall maternal mortality for patients with central nervous system tumors is 60%. Therapeutic abortions have been recommended for patients diagnosed in the first trimester as having malignant brain tumors because of the rapid course of such tumors.

Key points

1 Medical management is the primary means of treatment of myoma in pregnancy.

2 The hormonal changes of pregnancy, particularly the production of human chorionic gonadotropin (hCG), are associated with luteomas, theca-lutein cyst, hyperreactio luteinalis, and large solitary luteinized follicular cyst of pregnancy.

3 Radiation and chemotherapy are commonly employed in the routine management of cancers that may occur in pregnancy, such as cervical cancer, breast cancer, ovarian cancer, uterine cancer, vaginal carcinoma, vulvar cancer, and urinary tract malignancies.

4 Surgical staging for ovarian cancer in pregnancy should be the same as that recommended in the nonpregnant state.

5 Dysgerminoma is a germ cell ovarian cancer, and is the most common ovarian malignancy in pregnancy.

6 Sex cord–stromal tumors, such as Sertoli–Leydig cell tumors, are rare during pregnancy.

7 It is estimated that one-third of women with Hodgkin's disease are pregnant or have delivered within 1 year of diagnosis.

8 Non-Hodgkin's lymphoma, acute leukemia, gastrointestinal cancers, and thyroid cancers are rare during pregnancy.

References

1 Velebil P, Wingo PA, Xia Z, et al. Rate of hospitalization for gynecologic disorders among reproductive-age women in the United States. *Obstet Gynecol* 1995;86:764.

2 Katz VL, Dotters DJ, Drogemuller W. Complication of uterine leiomyomas in pregnancy. *Obstet Gynecol* 1989;73:593

3 Brandon DD, Erickson TE, Keenan EJ, et al. Estrogen receptor gene expression in human uterine leiomyomata. *J Clin Endocrinol Metab* 1995;80:1876

4 Strobelt N, Ghidini A, Cavallone M, et al. Natural history of uterine leiomyomas in pregnancy. *J Ultrasound Med* 1994;13:399.

5 Aharoni A, Reiter A, Golan D, et al. Patterns of growth of uterine leiomyomas during pregnancy: a prospective longitudinal study. *Br J Obstet Gynaecol* 1988;95:510.

6 Lev-Toaff AS, Coleman BG, Arger PH, et al. Leiomyomas in pregnancy: sonographic study. *Radiology* 1987:164:375.

7 Droegmuller W, Herbest AL, Mishell DR, Stenchever MA. *Comprehensive gynecology*. St Louis: Mosby; 1987:1059.

8 Jabiry-Zieniewicz Z, Gajewska M. The pregnancy and delivery course with pregnant women with uterine myomas. *Ginekol Pol* 2002;73(4):271.

9 Vergani P, Ghidini A, Strobelt N, et al. Do uterine leiomyomas influence pregnancy outcome? *Am J Perinatol* 1994;11:356.

10 Salvador E, Bienstock J, Blackemore KJ, Pressman E. Leiomyoma uteri, genetic amniocentesis, and the risk of second-trimester spontaneous abortion. *Am J Obstet Gynecol* 2002;186(5):913.

11 Dildy GA, Moise KJ, Smith LG, et al. Indomethacin for the treatment of symptomatic uterine leiomyoma during pregnancy. *Am J Perinatol* 1992;9:185.

12 Norton ME, Merrill J, Cooper BAB, et al. Neonatal complications after the administration of indomethacin for preterm labor. *N Engl J Med* 1993;329:1602.

13 Exacoustos C, Rosati P. Ultrasound diagnosis of uterine myomas and complications in pregnancy. *Obstet Gynecol* 1993;82:97.

14 Lolis DE, Kalantoridou SN, Makrydimas G, et al. Successful myomectomy during pregnancy. *Hum Reprod* 2003 Aug; 18(8):1699.

15 Burton CA, Grimes DA, March CM. Surgical management of leiomyomata during pregnancy. *Obstet Gynecol* 1989;5:707.

16 Berek JS, Haker NF. *Practical gynecologic oncology*. Baltimore: Williams & Wilkins; 1994:331.

17 Webb PM, Purdie DM, Grover S, et al. Symptoms and diagnosis of borderline, early and advanced epithelial ovarian cancer. *Gynecol Oncol* 2004;92(1):232.

18 Goldstein S, Timor-Tritsch IE. *Ultrasound in gynecology*. New York: Churchill Livingstone, 1995.

19 Rulin MC, Preston AL. Adnexal masses in postmenopausal women. *Obstet Gynecol* 1987;70:678.

20 Bromley B, Benacerraf BR. Maternal adnexal masses in pregnancy: accuracy of diagnosis and perinatal outcome. *J Ultrasound Med* 1996;16:S25.

21 Kanal E, Gillen J, Evans JA, et al. Survey of reproductive health among female MR workers. *Radiology* 1993;187:395.

22 De Wilde JP, Rivers AW, Price DL. A review of the current use of magnetic resonance imaging in pregnancy and safety implications for the fetus. *Prog Biophys Mol Biol* 2005;87(2–3):335.

23 Kurman RJ. *Blaustein's pathology of the female genital tract*. New York: Springer-Verlag; 1987;495.

24 Norris HJ, Taylor HB. Virilization associated with cystic granulose tumors. *Obstet Gynecol* 1989;34:629.

25 Choi JR, Levine D, Finberg H. Luteoma of pregnancy: sonographic findings in two cases. *J Ultrasound Med* 2000;19(12):877.

26 Van Slooten AJ, Rechner SF, Dodds WG. Recurrent maternal virilization during pregnancy caused by benign androgen-producing ovarian lesions. *Am J Obstet Gynecol* 1992;167: 1342.

27 Joshi R, Dunaif A. Ovarian disorders of pregnancy. *Endocrinol Metab Clin North Am* 1995;24:153.

28 Baxi L, Holub D, Hembree W. Bilateral luteomas of pregnancy in a patient with diabetes. *Am J Obstet Gynecol* 1988;159:454.

29 Shortle BE, Warren MP, Tsin D. Recurrent androgenicity in pregnancy. *Obstet Gynecol* 1987;70:462.

30 Schnorr JA, Miller H, Davis JR, et al. Hyperreactio luteinalis associated with pregnancy: a case report and review of the literature. *Am J Perinatol* 1996;13:95.

31 Berkowitz RS, Goldstein DP. Chorionic tumors (review). *N Engl J Med* 1996;335:1740.

32 Suzuki S. Comparison between spontaneous ovarian hyperstimulation syndrome and hyperreactio luteinalis. *Arch Gynecol Obstet* 2004;269(3):227.

33 Bradshaw KD, Santos-Ramos R, Rawlins SC, et al. Endocrine studies in a pregnancy complicated by ovarian theca lutein cysts and hyperreactio luteinalis. *Obstet Gynecol* 1986;67:66S.

34 Sokal JE, Lessmann EM. Effect of cancer chemotherapeutic agents on the human fetus. *JAMA* 1960;172:151.

35 Benedet JL, Boyes DA, Nichols TM, et al. Colposcopic evaluation of pregnancy patients with abnormal cervical smears. *Br J Obstet Gynaecol* 1976;84:517.

36 Jemal A, Tiwari RC, Murray T, et al. Cancer statistics, 2004. *Cancer* 2004;54:8.

37 Haas JF. Pregnancy in association with a newly diagnosed cancer: a population based epidemiologic assessment. *Int J Cancer* 1984;34:229.

38 Potter JF, Schoeneman M. Metastasis of maternal cancer to the placenta and fetus. *Cancer* 1970;25:380.

39 Goodlin RC. Importance of the lateral position during labor. *Obstet Gynecol* 1971;37:698.

40 Eckstein K, Marx GF. Aortocaval compression and uterine displacement. *Anesthesiology* 1974;40:92.

41 Roberts RB, Shirley MA. Reducing the risk of acid aspiration during cesarean section. *Anesth Analg* 1979;53:859.

42 Streffer C, Shore R, Konermann G, Meadows A, et al. Biological effects after prenatal irradiation (embryo and fetus). A report of International Commission on Radiological Protection. *Ann ICRP* 2003;33(1–2):5.

43 Bailey H, Bragg HJ. Effects of irradiation on fetal development. *Am J Obstet Gynecol* 1923;5:461.

44 Brill AB, Forgotson EH. Radiation and congenital malformations. *Am J Obstet Gynecol* 1964;90:1149.

45 Muller HJ. Artificial transmutation of the gene. *Science* 1927;66:84.

46 Orr JW Jr, Shingleton HM. Cancer in pregnancy. *Curr Prob Cancer* 1983;8:1.

47 Wallack MK, Wolf JA Jr, Bedwinek J, et al. Gestational carcinoma of the female breast. *Curr Prob Cancer* 1983;7:1.

48 Brent RC. The effect of embryonic and fetal exposure to x-ray, microwaves, and ultrasound: counseling the pregnant and nonpregnant patient about these risks. *Semin Oncol* 1989;16:347.

49 Dekaban A. Abnormalities in children exposed to x-irradiation during various stages of gestation: tentative timetable of radiation injury to the human fetus. Part I. *J Nucl Med* 1968;9:471.
50 Stovall M, Blackwell CR, Cundiff J, et al. Fetal dose from radiotherapy with photon beams: report of AAPM Radiation Therapy Committee Task Force Group No. 36. *Med Phys* 1995; 22:63.
51 Nicholson HD. Cytotoxic drugs in pregnancy. *J Obstet Gynecol Br Commonw* 1968;75:307.
52 Sweet DL, Kinzie J. Consequences of radiotherapy and antineoplastic therapy for the fetus. *J Reprod Med* 1976;17:241.
53 Doll DC, Ringenberg S, Yarbro JW. Antineoplastic agents and cancer. *Semin Oncol* 1989;16:337.
54 Aviles A, Diaz-Maqueo JC, Torra V, et al. Non-Hodgkin's lymphomas and pregnancy: presentation of 16 cases. *Gynecol Oncol* 1990;37:335.
55 Reynoso EE, Shepherd FA, Messner HA, et al. Acute leukemia during pregnancy: the Toronto leukemia study group experience with long-term follow-up of children exposed *in utero* to chemotherapeutic agents. *J Clin Oncol* 1987;5:1098.
56 Aviles A, Niz J. Long-term follow-up of children born to mothers with acute leukemia during pregnancy. *Med Pediatr Oncol* 1988;16:3.
57 Redmond GP. Physiologic changes during pregnancy and their implications for pharmacologic treatment. *Clin Invest Med* 1985;8:317.
58 Wan SH, Huffman DH, Azarnoff DL, et al. Effect of route of administration and effusions on methotrexate pharmacokinetics. *Cancer Res* 1974;34:3487.
59 Pirani BBK, Campbell DM, MacGillivray I. Plasma volume in normal first pregnancy. *J Obstet Gynecol Br Commonw* 1973;80:884.
60 Muckcow JC. The fate of drugs in pregnancy. *Clin Obstet Gynecol* 1986;13:161.
61 Powis G. Anticancer drug pharmacodynamics. *Cancer Chemother Pharmacol* 1985;14:177.
62 Krepart GV, Lotocki RJ. Chemotherapy during pregnancy. In: Allen HH, Nisker JA, eds. *Cancer in pregnancy*. Mt Kisco, NY: Futura Publishing; 1986:69.
63 Zemlickis D, Klein J, Moselhy G, et al. Cisplatin protein binding in pregnancy and the neonatal period. *Med Pediatr Oncol* 1994; 23:476.
64 Willemse PHB, vd Sijde R, Sleijfer DT. Combination chemotherapy and radiation for stage IV breast cancer during pregnancy. *Gynecol Oncol* 1990;36:281.
65 Garber JE. Long-term follow-up of children exposed *in utero* to antineoplastic agents. *Semin Oncol* 1989:16:437.
66 Mulvihill JJ, McKeen EA, Rosner F, et al. Pregnancy outcome in cancer patients. *Cancer* 1987;60:1143.
67 Jones RT, Weinterman BH. MOPP (nitrogen mustard, vincristine, procarbazine and prednisone) given during pregnancy. *Obstet Gynecol* 1979;54:477.
68 Lowenthal RM, Funnell CF, Hope DM, et al. Normal infant after combination chemotherapy including teniposide for Burkitt's lymphoma in pregnancy. *Med Pediatr Oncol* 1982;10:165.
69 Barber HRK. Fetal and neonatal effects of cytotoxic agents. *Obstet Gynecol* 1981;58(Suppl):41.
70 Collaborative Group of Antenatal Steroid Therapy. Effect of antenatal dexamethasone administration on prevention of respiratory distress syndrome. *Am J Obstet Gynecol* 1981;141: 276.
71 Stone ML, Weingold AB, Sall S. Cervical carcinoma in pregnancy. *Am J Obstet Gynecol* 1965;93:479.
72 Kaplan KJ, Dainty LA, Dolinsky B, et al. Prognosis and recurrence risk for patients with cervical squamous intraepithelial lesions diagnosed during pregnancy. *Cancer* 2004;102(4): 228.
73 Kinch RA. Factors affecting the prognosis of cancer of the cervix in pregnancy. *Am J Obstet Gynecol* 1961;82:43.
74 Creasman WT, Rutledge FN, Fletcher GH. Carcinoma of the cervix associated with pregnancy. *Obstet Gynecol* 1970;36:495.
75 Seltzer V, Sall S, Castadot M, et al. Glassy cell cervical carcinoma. *Gynecol Oncol* 1979;8:141.
76 Turner WA, Gallup DG, Talledo OE, et al. Neuroendocrine carcinoma of the uterine cervix complicated by pregnancy. Case report and review of the literature. *Obstet Gynecol* 1986; 67(Suppl):80.
77 Schwartz PE. Cancer in pregnancy. In: Gusberg SB, Shingleton HM, Deppe G, eds. *Female genital cancer*. New York: Churchill Livingstone; 1988;725.
78 Sood AK, Sorosky JI, Krogman S, et al. Surgical management of cervical cancer complicating pregnancy: a case–control study. *Gynecol Oncol* 1996; 63:294.
79 Rose PG. Combined-modality therapy of locally advanced cervical cancer. *J Clin Oncol* 2003;21(10 Suppl):211.
80 ACOG Practice Bulletin. Diagnosis and treatment of cervical carcinoma. No. 35, May 2002. *Int J Gynecol Obstet* 2002 l;78(1): 79.
81 Rose PG, Lappas PT. Pharmacoeconomics of cisplatin-based chemoradiation in cervical cancer: a review. *Expert Opin Pharmacother* 2002;3(9):1245.
82 Prem KA, Makowski EL, McKelvey JL. Carcinoma of the cervix associated with pregnancy. *Am J Obstet Gynecol* 1966;95: 99.
83 Gordon AN, Jensen R, Jones HW III. Squamous carcinoma of the cervix complicating pregnancy: recurrence in episiotomy after vaginal delivery. *Obstet Gynecol* 1989;73:850.
84 Cliby WA, Dodson MF, Podratz KC. Cervical cancer complicated by pregnancy: episiotomy site recurrences following vaginal delivery. *Obstet Gynecol* 1994; 84:179.
85 Sardi JE, Guillermo R, DiPaola MD, et al. A possible new trend in the management of the carcinoma of the cervix uteri. *Gynecol Oncol* 1986;25:139.
86 Hacker NF, Berek JS, LaGasse LD, et al. Carcinoma of the cervix associated with pregnancy. *Obstet Gynecol* 1982;59:735.
87 Wingo PA, Tong T, Bolden S. Cancer statistics, 1995. *Cancer J Clin* 1995;45:8–30.
88 Petrek JA, Dukoff R Rogatko A. Prognosis of pregnancy-associated breast cancer. *Cancer* 1991;67:869.
89 Zemlickis D, Lishner M. Degendorfer P, et al. Maternal and fetal outcome after breast cancer in pregnancy. *Am J Obstet Gynecol* 1992;166:781.
90 Jackisch C, Schwenkhagen A, Louwen F, et al. Breast cancer in pregnancy. *Proc Ann Meet Am Soc Clin Oncol* 1995;14:228.
91 Peters MV. The effect of pregnancy in breast cancer. In: Forrest APM, Kunkler PB, eds. *Prognostic factors in breast cancer*. Baltimore: Williams & Wilkins; 1968:65.
92 Bottles K, Taylor RN. Diagnosis of breast masses in pregnancy and lactating women by aspiration cytology. *Obstet Gynecol* 1985;66:76S.
93 Read LD, Greene GL, Katzenellenbogen BS. Regulation of estrogen receptor messenger ribonucleic acid and protein levels in human breast cancer cell lines by sex steroid hormones, their antagonists and growth factors. *Mol Endocrinol* 1989;3: L295.

94 Higgins S, Haffty BG. Pregnancy and lactation after breast-conserving surgery for early stage breast cancer. *Cancer* 1994;78:2175–2180.
95 Marchant DJ. Breast cancer in pregnancy. *Clin Obstet Gynecol* 1994;37:993.
96 Petrek JA. Breast cancer during pregnancy. *Monogr Natl Cancer Inst* 1994;16:113.
97 Petrek JA. Breast cancer during pregnancy. *Cancer* 1994;74:518.
98 Tretli S, Kvalheim G, Thorensen S, et al. Survival of breast cancer patents diagnosed during pregnancy or lactation. *Br J Cancer* 1988;58:382.
99 Guinee VF, Olsson H, Moller T, et al. Effects of pregnancy on prognosis for young women with breast cancer. *Lancet* 1984;343:157.
100 Chung M, Chang HR, Bland KI, et al. Younger women with breast carcinoma have a poorer prognosis than older women. *Cancer* 1996;77:97.
101 Anderson BO, Petrek JA, Byrd DR, et al. Pregnancy influences breast cancer stage at diagnosis in women 30 and younger. *Ann Surg Oncol* 1996;3:204.
102 Stovall M, Blackwell CR, Condiff J, et al. Fetal dose from radiotherapy with photon beams: Report AAPM Radiation Therapy Committee Task Group 36. *Med Phys* 1995;22:63.
103 Doll DC, Ringenberg S, Yarbro JW. Management of cancer during pregnancy. *Arch Intern Med* 1988;148:2058.
104 Shapiro CL, Mayer RJ. Breast cancer during pregnancy. *Adv Oncol* 1992;8:25.
105 Arango HA, Kalter CS, DeCesare SL, et al. Management of chemotherapy in a pregnancy complicated by a large neuroblastoma. *Obstet Gynecol* 1994;84:665.
106 Garber JE. Long term follow-up of children exposed *in utero* to antineoplastic agents. *Semin Oncol* 1989;16:437.
107 Clark RM, Chua AT. Breast cancer and pregnancy: the ultimate challenge. *Clin Oncol* 1989;1:11.
108 Danforth DN. How subsequent pregnancy affects outcome in women with prior breast cancer. *Oncology* 1991;5:2823.
109 Dow KH. Having children after breast cancer. *Cancer Pract* 1994;2:407.
110 Sankila R, Heinaavra S, Hakulinen T. Survival of breast cancer patients after a subsequent term pregnancy: "Health mother effect." *Am J Obstet Gynecol* 1994;170:813.
111 Antonella S, Petrek JA. Childbearing issues in breast cancer survivors. *Cancer* 1997;79:1271.
112 Kier R, McCarthy SM, Scoutt LM, et al. Pelvic masses in pregnancy: MR imaging. *Radiology* 1990;176:709.
113 Chang SD, Cooperberg PL, Wong AD, et al. Limited-sequence magnetic resonance imaging in the evaluation of the ultrasonographically indeterminate pelvic mass. *Can Assoc Radiol J* 2004;55(2):87.
114 Chung A, Birnbaum SJ. Ovarian cancer associated with pregnancy. *Obstet Gynecol* 1973;41:211.
115 Schwartz PE. Combination chemotherapy in the management of ovarian germ cell malignancies. *Obstet Gynecol* 1984;64:564.
116 Schwartz PE, Morris JMcl. Serum lactic dehydrogenase, a tumor marker for dysgerminoma. *Obstet Gynecol* 1988;72:511.
117 Bast RC Jr, Klug TL, St John E, et al. A radioimmuno-assay using a monoclonal antibody to monitor the course of epithelial ovarian cancer. *N Engl J Med* 1983;309:883.
118 Schwartz PE, Chambers SK, Chambers JT, et al. Circulating tumor markers in the monitoring of gynecologic malignancies. *Cancer* 1987;60:353.
119 Niloff JM, Knapp RC, Schaetzl E, et al. CA 125 antigen levels in obstetrics and gynecologic patients. *Obstet Gynecol* 1985;64:703.
120 Bianchi UA, Sartori E, Favall G, et al. New trends in treatment of ovarian dysgerminoma. *Gynecol Oncol* 1986;23:246.
121 Dgani R, Shoham Z, Atar E, et al. Ovarian carcinoma during pregnancy: a study of 23 cases in Israel between the years 1960 and 1984. *Gynecol Oncol* 1989;33:326.
122 Chambers JT, Merino MJ, Kohorn EI, Schwartz PE. Borderline ovarian tumors. *Am J Obstet Gynecol* 1988;159:1088.
123 Young RC, Walton LA, Ellenburgss, et al. Adjuvant therapy in stage I and stage III epithelial ovarian cancer: results of two prospective randomized trials. *N Engl J Med* 1990;322:1021.
124 Malone JM, Gershenson DM, Creasy RK, et al. Endodermal sinus tumor of the ovary associated with pregnancy. *Obstet Gynecol* 1986;68(Suppl):86.
125 Malfetano JH, Goldkrand JW. Cis-platinum combination chemotherapy during pregnancy for advanced epithelial ovarian cancer. *Obstet Gynecol* 1990;75:545.
126 Buckley SL, Molphus K, Carr MB, et al. Advanced ovarian carcinoma diagnosed during pregnancy in a patient with human immunodeficiency virus infection. *Gynecol Oncol* 1993;50:352.
127 Karlen JR, Akbari A, Cook WA. Dysgerminoma associated with pregnancy. *Obstet Gynecol* 1979;53:330.
128 Gershensen DM, Morris M, Cangir A, et al. Treatment of malignant germ cell tumors of the ovary with bleomycin, etoposide, and cisplatin. *J Clin Oncol* 1990;8:715.
129 Christman JE, Teng NNH, Lebovic GS, Sikic BI. Delivery of a normal infant following cisplatin, vinblastine, and bleomycin (PVB) chemotherapy for malignant teratoma of the ovary during pregnancy. *Gynecol Oncol* 1990;37:292.
130 Schwartz PE. Sex cord–stromal tumors of the ovary. In: Piver S, ed. *Ovarian cancer*. London: Churchill Livingstone; 1986:251.
131 Young RH, Dudley AG, Scully RF. Granulosa cell, Sertoli–Leydig cell and unclassified sex cord–stromal tumors associated with pregnancy. A clinicopathological analysis of thirty-six cases. *Gynecol Oncol* 1984;18:181.
132 Desforges JF, Rutherford CJ, Piro A. Hodgkin's disease. *N Engl J Med* 1979;301:1212.
133 Chapman RM, Sutcliffe SV, Malpas JS. Cytotoxic-induced ovarian failure in women with Hodgkin's disease. I. Hormone function. *JAMA* 1979;242:1877.
134 Smith RBW, Sheehy TW, Rothberg H. Hodgkin's disease and pregnancy. *Arch Intern Med* 1958;102:777.
135 Sweet DL Jr. Malignant lymphoma: implications during the reproductive years and pregnancy. *J Reprod Med* 1976;17:198.
136 Tawil E, Mercier JP, Dondavino A. Hodgkin's disease complicating pregnancy. *J Can Assoc Radiol* 1985;36:133.
137 Ward FT, Weiss RB. Lymphoma and pregnancy. *Semin Oncol* 1989;16:397.
138 Sutcliffe SB, Wrigley PFM, Peto J, et al. MVPP chemotherapy regimen for advanced Hodgkin's disease. *Br Med J* 1978;1:679.
139 Devita VT, Simon RM, Hubbard SM, et al. Curability of advanced Hodgkin disease with chemotherapy. *Ann Intern Med* 1980;92:587.
140 Mitchell MS, Capizzi RL. Neoplastic disease. In: Burrow GN, Ferris TF, eds. *Medical complications during pregnancy*. Philadelphia: W.B. Saunders; 1982:510.
141 Sutcliffe SB, Chapman RM. Lymphomas and leukemias. In: Allen HH, Nisker JA, eds. *Cancer in pregnancy*. Mt Kisco, NY: Futura Publishing; 1986:135.
142 Meruk ML, Green JP, Nussbaum H, et al. Phantom dosimetry

study of shaped colbalt-60 fields in treatment of Hodgkin's disease. *Radiology* 1968;91:554.
143 Steiner-Salz D, Yahalon J, Samuelov A, et al. Non-Hodgkin's lymphoma associated with pregnancy. A report of 6 cases with a review of the literature. *Cancer* 1985;56:2087.
144 Armitages JD, Feagler JR, Skoog DP. Burkitt's lymphoma during pregnancy with bilateral breast involvement. *JAMA* 1977; 237:151.
145 Armon PJ. Burkitt's lymphoma of the ovary in association with pregnancy: two case reports. *Br J Obstet Gynaecol* 1976;83:169.
146 Miller TP, Jones SE. Chemotherapy of localized histiocytic lymphoma. *Lancet* 1979;1:358.
147 Devita VT Jr, Chabner B, Hubbard SP, et al. Advanced diffuse histiocytic lymphoma, a potentially curable disease. *Lancet* 1975;1:248.
148 Yahia C, Hyman GA, Phillips LL. Acute leukemia and pregnancy. *Obstet Gynecol Surv* 1958;13:1.
149 Hoover BA, Schumacher HR. Acute leukemia in pregnancy. *Am J Obstet Gynecol* 1966;96:316.
150 Caligiuri MA, Mayer RJ. Pregnancy and leukemia. *Semin Oncol* 1989;16;388.
151 Roy V, Gutteridge CN, Hysenbaum A, Newliand AC. Combination chemotherapy with conservative obstetric management in the treatment of pregnant patients with acute myeloblastic leukemia. *Clin Lab Haematol* 1989;11:171.
152 Henderson EJ. Acute leukemia: general considerations. In: Williams WJ, Beutler E, Erslev AJ, Rundles RW, eds. *Hematology*, 2nd edn. New York: McGraw-Hill; 1977:108.
153 McLain CR Jr. Leukemia in pregnancy. *Clin Obstet Gynecol* 1974;17:185.
154 Moloney WC. Management of leukemia in pregnancy. *Ann NY Acad Sci* 1964;114:857.
155 McCulloch PB, Dent PB. Melanoma. In: Allen AA, Nisker JA, eds. *Cancer in pregnancy*. Mt Kisco, NY: Futura Publishing; 1986:205.
156 McNamny DS, Moss AL, Pocock PV, Briggs JC. Melanoma and pregnancy: a long-term follow-up. *Br J Obstet Gynaecol* 1989;96:1419.
157 Wong JH, Sterns EE, Kopald KH, et al. Prognostic significance of pregnancy in stage I melanoma. *Arch Surg* 1989;124:1227.
158 Colbourn DS, Nathanson L, Belilos E. Pregnancy and malignant melanoma. *Semin Oncol* 1989;16:377.
159 Toma S, Ugolini D, Palumbo R. Tamoxifen in the treatment of metastatic malignant melanoma: still a controversy? (review). *Int J Oncol* 1999;15(2):321.
160 Dobos J, Timor J, Bossi J, et al. In vitro and in vivo anti-tumor effect of 2-methoxyestradiol on human melanoma. *Int J Cancer* 2004;112(5):771.
161 Clark WH, From L, Bernardino EA, et al. The histogenesis and biologic behavior of primary malignant melanomas of skin. *Cancer Res* 1969;29:705.
162 Broslow AL. Tumor thickness, level of invasion and node dissection in stage I cutaneous melanoma. *Ann Surg* 1975;182:572.
163 Byers T, Graham S, Swanson M. Parity and colorectal cancer risk in women. *J Natl Cancer Inst* 1982;69:1059.
164 Barber HRK, Brunschwig A. Carcinoma of the bowel. *Am J Obstet Gynecol* 1968;100:926.
165 Zaridze DG. Environmental etiology of large bowel cancer. *J Natl Cancer Inst* 1983;70:389.
166 Girard RM, Lamarche J, Baillot R. Carcinoma of the colon associated with pregnancy. Report of a case. *Dis Colon Rectum* 1981;24:473.
167 Bernstein MA, Madoff RD, Caushaj PF. Colon and rectal cancer in pregnancy. *Dis Colon Rectum* 1993;36:172.
168 Cappell MS. Colon cancer during pregnancy. *Gastroenterol Clin North Am* 2003;32(1):34.
169 Allen HH, Nisker JA. Colorectal cancer in pregnancy. In: Allen HH, Nisker JA, eds. *Cancer in pregnancy*. Mt Kisco, NY: Futura Publishing; 1986:281.
170 Lamerz R, Ruider H. Significance of CEA determinations in patients with cancer of the colon–rectum and the mammary glands in comparison to physiological states in connection with pregnancy. *Bull Cancer* 1976;63:575.
171 Parry BR, Tan BK, Chan WB, et al. Rectal carcinoma during pregnancy. *Aust NZ Surg* 1994;64:618.
172 O'Leary JA, Pratt JH, Symmonds RE. Rectal carcinoma in pregnancy. A review of 17 cases. *Obstet Gynecol* 1967;30:862.
173 Gamberdella FR. Pancreatic cancer in pregnancy. A case report. *Am J Obstet Gynecol* 1984;149:15.
174 Boyle JM, McLeod ME. Pancreatic cancer presenting as pancreatitis in pregnancy. Case report. *Am J Gastroenterol* 1979; 70:371.
175 Skokos CK, Lipshitz J. Adenocarcinoma of the stomach associated with pregnancy. *J Tenn Med Assoc* 1982;75:103.
176 Sims EH, Schlater TL, Sims M, et al. Obstructing gastric carcinoma complicating pregnancy. *J Natl Med Assoc* 1980;72;21.
177 Bowers RH, Walters W. Carcinoma of the stomach complicated by pregnancy. Report of an unusual case. *Minn Med* 1958;41:30.
178 Dai D, Chen J, Wang S. Stomach cancer in pregnancy and breast feeding: report of 17 cases. *Chinese J Surg* 1995;33:768.
179 Maeta M, Yamashiro H, Oka A, et al. Gastric cancer in the young, with special reference to 14 pregnancy-associated cases: analysis based on 2,325 consecutive cases of gastric cancer. *J Surg Oncol* 1995;58:191.
180 Au WY, Leung WT, Ho S, et al. Hepatocellular carcinoma during pregnancy and its comparison with other pregnancy-associated malignancies. *Cancer* 1995;75:2669.
181 Goncalves CS, Pereira FE, deVargas PR, et al. Hepatocellular carcinoma positive in pregnancy. *Arq Gastroenterol* 1984;21:75.
182 Devoe LD, Moosa AR, Levin B. Pregnancy complicated by an extrahepatic biliary tract carcinoma. *J Reprod Med* 1983;28:153.
183 Kempson RL, Pokorny GE. Adenocarcinoma of the endometrium in women aged forty and younger. *Cancer* 1968;21:650.
184 Sandstrom RE, Welch WR, Green TH Jr. Adenocarcinoma of the endometrium in pregnancy. *Obstet Gynecol* 1979;53(Suppl):73.
185 Zirkin HJ, Krugliak L, Katz M. Endometrial adenocarcinoma coincident with intrauterine pregnancy. A case report. *J Reprod Med* 1983;28:624.
186 Suzuki A, Konishi I, Okamura H, et al. Adenocarcinoma of the endometrium associated with intrauterine pregnancy. *Gynecol Oncol* 1984;18:261.
187 Hoffman MS, Cavanagh D, Walter TS, et al. Adenocarcinoma of the endometrium and endometrioid carcinoma of the ovary association with pregnancy. *Gynecol Oncol* 1989;32:82.
188 Kovacs AG, Csernig G. Endometrial adenocarcinoma in early pregnancy. *Gynecol Obstet Invest* 1996;41:70.
189 Scoscia A, Merino MJ, Haas M, et al. Malignant mixed mullerian tumor of the uterus arising in associated with a viable gestation. *Obstet Gynecol* 1988;71:1047.
190 Schwartz PE, Naftolin F. Type 2 herpes simplex virus and vulvar carcinoma in situ. *N Engl J Med* 1981;305:517.
191 Lutz M, Underwood PB Jr, Rozier JC, et al. Genital malignancy in pregnancy. *Am J Obstet Gynecol* 1977;129:536.

192 Schwartz PE. Gynecologic cancer. In: Spittell JA Jr, ed. *Clinical medicine*. Philadelphia: Harper & Row; 1985:1.
193 Gitsch G, Van Eijkeren M, Hacker NF. Surgical therapy of vulvar cancer in pregnancy. *Gynecol Oncol* 1995;56:312.
194 Senekjian EK, Hubby M, Herbst AL. Clear cell adenocarcinoma (CCA) of the cervix and vagina associated with pregnancy. *Gynecol Oncol* 1985;20:250.
195 Eisenfeld AJ, Schwartz PE, Morris JMcl. Estrogen and progesterone receptors in vaginal and uterine adenocarcinomas following estrogen use. *Gynecol Oncol* 1980;10:63.
196 Cantin J, McNeer GP. The effect of pregnancy on the clinical course of sarcoma of the soft somatic tissues. *Surg Gynecol Obstet* 1967;125:28.
197 Lysyj A, Berquist JR. Pregnancy complicated by sarcoma. Report of two cases. *Obstet Gynecol* 1963;21:506.
198 Huvos AG, Butler A, Bretsky SS. Osteogenic sarcoma in pregnant women. Prognosis, therapeutic implications, and literature review. *Cancer* 1985;56:2326.
199 Simon MA, Phillips WA, Bonfiglio M. Pregnancy and aggressive or malignant bone tumors. *Cancer* 1984;53:2564.
200 Haerr RW, Pratt AT. Multiagent chemotherapy for sarcoma diagnosed during pregnancy. *Cancer* 1985;56:1028.
201 Tan GH, Gharib H, Gohllner JR, et al. Management of thyroid nodules in pregnancy. *Arch Intern Med* 1996;156:2317.
202 Stuart GCE, Temple WJ. Thyroid cancer in pregnancy. In: Allen NH, Nisker JA, eds. *Cancer in pregnancy*. Mt Kisco, NY: Futura Publishing; 1986;191.
203 Cady B, Sedwick CE, Meissner WA. Changing clinical, pathologic, therapeutic and survival patterns in differentiated thyroid carcinoma. *Ann Surg* 1976;184:541.
204 Cady B, Sedwick CE, Meissner WA. Risk factor analysis in differentiated thyroid cancer. *Cancer* 1979;43:810.
205 Rosen IB, Walfish PG. Pregnancy as a predisposing factor in thyroid neoplasia. *Arch Surg* 1986;121:1287.
206 Chodander CM, Abhyankar SC, Deodhar KP. Sipple's syndrome (multiple endocrine neoplasia) in pregnancy (case report). *Aust NZ J Obstet Gynecol* 1982;22:243.
207 Goldman MH, Tisch B, Chattock AG. Fine needle biopsy of a solitary nodule arising during pregnancy. *J Med Soc NJ* 1983;80:525.
208 Schwartz AE, Nieburgs HE, Davis TF. The place of fine needle biopsy in the diagnosis of nodules of the thyroid. *Surg Gynecol Obstet* 1982;155:54.
209 Rosvoll RV, Winship T. Thyroid carcinoma and pregnancy. *Surg Gynecol Obstet* 1965;121:1039.
210 Herzon FS, Morris DM, Segal MN, et al. Coexistent thyroid cancer and pregnancy. *Arch Otolaryngol Head Neck Surg* 1994; 120:1191.
211 Hill CS, Clark RL, Wolf M. The effect of subsequent pregnancy in patients with thyroid carcinoma. *Surg Gynecol Obstet* 1966;122:1219.
212 Farrar WB, Cooperman M, James AG. Surgical management of papillary and follicular carcinoma of the thyroid. *Am Surg* 1980;192:701.
213 Cunningham MP, Slaughter DP. Surgical treatment of diseases of the thyroid gland in pregnancy. *Surg Gynecol Obstet* 1970; 131:486.
214 Choe W, McDougall IR. Thyroid cancer in pregnancy women: diagnostic and therapeutic management. *Thyroid* 1994; 4:433.
215 Harper MA, Murnaghan GA, Kennedy L, et al. Pheochromocytoma in pregnancy. Five cases and a review of the literature. *Br J Obstet Gynaecol* 1989;96:594.
216 Greenberg M, Moawad AH, Wieties BM, et al. Extraadrenal pheochromocytoma: detection during pregnancy using MR imaging. *Radiology* 1986;161:475.
217 Ellison GT, Mansberger JA, Mansberger AR Jr. Malignant recurrent pheochromocytoma during pregnancy. Case report and review of the literature. *Surgery* 1988;103:484.
218 Fusge TL, McKinnon WMP, Geary WL. Current surgical management of pheochromocytoma during pregnancy. *Arch Surg* 1980;115:1224.
219 Leak D, Carroll JJ, Robinson DC, et al. Management of pheochromocytoma during pregnancy. *Obstet Gynecol Surv* 1977;32:583.
220 Stenstrom G, Swolin K. Pheochromocytoma in pregnancy. Experience of treatment with phenoxybenzamine in three patients. *Acta Obstet Gynecol Scand* 1985;64:357.
221 Armaroli R, Simoni S, Artuso S, Mattioli G. Pheochromocytoma during pregnancy. *Ital J Surg Sci* 1989;19:75.
222 Lyons CW, Colmorgan GH. Medical management of pheochromocytoma in pregnancy. *Obstet Gynecol* 1988;72:450.
223 Hess HM, Dickson J, Fox HE. Hyperfunctioning parathyroid carcinoma presenting as acute pancreatitis in pregnancy. *J Reprod Med* 1980;25:83.
224 Tydings A, Weiss RR, Lin JH, et al. Renal cell carcinoma and mesangiocapillary glomerulonephritis. *NY State J Med* 1978; 78:1950.
225 Stanhope CR. Management of the obstetric patient with malignancy. In: Sciarra JJ, ed. *Gynecology and obstetrics*, Vol. 2. New York: Harper & Row; 1984:1.
226 Keegan GT, Forkowitz MJ. Transitional cell carcinoma of the bladder during pregnancy. A case report. *Texas Med* 1982;78:44.
227 Cruikshank SH, McNellis TM. Carcinoma of the bladder in pregnancy. *Am J Obstet Gynecol* 1983;145:768.
228 Carmel PN. Neurologic surgery in pregnancy. In: Barber HRK, ed. *Surgical disease in pregnancy*. Philadelphia: W.B. Saunders; 1974:207.
229 Nugent P, O'Connell TX. Breast cancer and pregnancy. *Arch Surg* 1985;120:1221.
230 Ribeiro GG, Palmer MK. Breast cancer associated with pregnancy: a clinician's dilemma. *Br Med J* 1977;2:1524.
231 Applewhite RR, Smith IR, DiVincenti F. Carcinoma of the breast associated with pregnancy and lactation. *Am Surg* 1973;39:101.
232 Fisher RI, Neifeld JP, Lippman ME. Estrogen receptors in human malignant melanoma. *Lancet* 1976;2:237.
233 Clark WH, From L, Bernardino EA, et al. The histogenesis and biologic behavior of primary malignant melanomas of skin. *Cancer Res* 1969;29:705.
234 Riva HL, Anderson PS, Grady JW. Pregnancy and Hodgkin's disease: a report of 8 cases. *Am J Obstet Gynecol* 1953;66:866.
235 Morgan DS, Hall SE, Gibbs WN. Hodgkin's disease in pregnancy: a report of three cases. *West Indian Med J* 1976;25:121.
236 Stewart HL, Monto RW. Hodgkin's disease and pregnancy. *Am J Obstet Gynecol* 1952;63:570.
237 Smith RS, Randal P. Melanoma during pregnancy. *Obstet Gynecol* 1969;34:825.

Part XI

Medicosocial Considerations in Pregnancy

54 Pregnancy before age 20 years and after age 35 years

Helen H. Kay

The problem with pregnancies in younger and older women

The optimal age for childbearing is debatable. Younger and older maternal age are considered to be suboptimal for childbearing, but it is uncertain whether that adversity is due to age itself, to biologic factors, or to socioeconomic factors. It has been taught that older women have more complications because of an increase in medical complications and risks from aneuploidy. Younger parous teens have difficulties because of socioeconomic pressures and, possibly, immature pelvises. In Fig. 54.1, the relative risks of maternal mortality by age in the United States from 1979 to 1986 is demonstrated by a J-shaped distribution with slightly increased risk mortality for those less than 20 years of age and for those beyond 24 years of age, rising exponentially.[1,2] In actual numbers, pregnancy complications kill 70 000 teenagers a year worldwide.[3] At ages greater than 40 years, risk of mortality is 8.6 times that for women between the ages of 20 and 24 years. Additionally, low birthweight is more closely linked with age less than 15 years and age 40 years and older in New Jersey.[4] Maternal age, either low or high, was included among the list of high-risk factors that Creasy and colleagues suggested using in a screening protocol to identify pregnant women at risk of preterm delivery.[5] Therefore, pregnancy for women at the extremes of reproductive potential may be more hazardous. Physicians should be aware when counseling patients regarding the optimal timing of pregnancy. A realistic understanding of the true risks and reassurances by healthcare providers would be valuable to women in those reproductive years.

At the same time, it is important to determine whether adverse outcomes are related to physiology, genetics, or psychosocial behaviors. Many epidemiologic studies have not been able to control for a multitude of variables such as smoking, education, socioeconomic status, and race. Consequently, only associations have been identified without direct cause and effect relationships. Even a focused analysis of outcomes in Nigeria suggests that poor obstetric outcomes are a reflection of poor utilization of prenatal care rather than a biologic factor from maternal age.[6]

The literature also contains studies from a variety of countries with a multitude of unique problems. Therefore, is the problem of obstructed labor due to a patient's young age or to the inability to perform a Cesarean section, which is a problem unique to an environment? Reported complications in the literature worldwide may not be pertinent to the US-based population in our current healthcare system. In this chapter, we will discuss the primary issues pertinent to pregnancies complicated by teenage mothers and women over the age of 35 years, drawing data and experience primarily from Westernized countries' experiences.

Adolescent pregnancies are a cost to society. Public aid programs through Aid to Families with Dependent Children, Medicaid, Food Stamps, WIC programs, home visiting nurses, and others increase costs; these costs add up to billions of dollars per annum.[7] Older women having pregnancies are also a cost to society, although these mothers tend to be more financially secure. Costs accrued to them include those related to infertility, prenatal diagnosis, and care resulting from medical complications such as diabetes, chronic hypertension, and other medical illnesses. The amount is also likely to be in the billions of dollars annually.

We as physicians should understand the scope of these problems because we will be asked for consultation. During our routine practices, we will have opportunities to identify those at risk of pregnancy at either an early age or a mature age. We should also be aware of those who are deciding whether to proceed or not to proceed with a conception. We should be prepared to provide proper consultation and guidance through wise counsel. Ultimately, whether our advice is heeded or not, it is our responsibility to provide appropriate prenatal care tailored to the age group in order to ensure the best neonatal outcomes.

Adolescent pregnancies

Many resources have been spent on preventing and reducing the incidence of teenage births. The primary reason for doing so is the high-risk nature of these pregnancies, resulting in physical and psychosocial ill-effects to the young mothers. In addition, there are long-term socioeconomic burdens to society from the offspring of these often unplanned pregnancies. One other outcome, not well known, is the ill-effect among the offspring of adolescent mothers. In Sweden, risks of attempted and completed suicide attempts were higher among those offspring of teenage mothers (hazard ratio of 2.09 compared with those age 20 years or older, $P < 0.0001$).[8] These risks deserve further study.

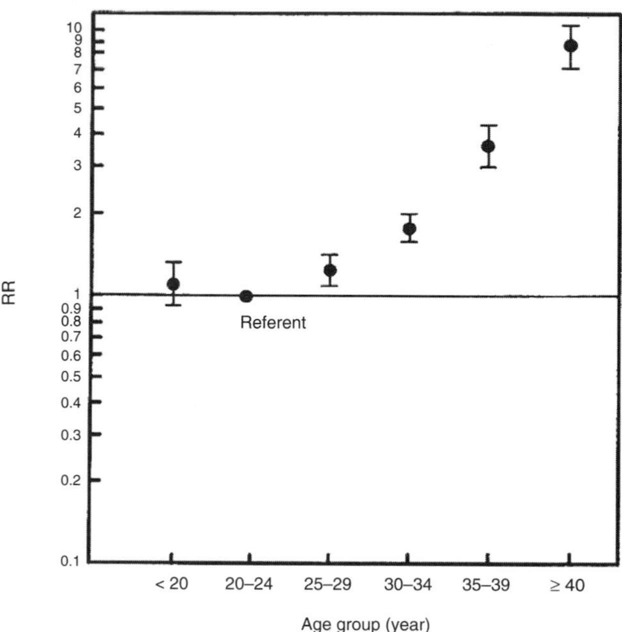

Figure 54.1 Relative risk (RR) of maternal death by age group in the United States, 1979–1986 (from ref. 1 with permission).

Incidence

Teenage pregnancy, often termed adolescent pregnancy, is, by definition, pregnancy in a patient who is between the ages of 13 and 20 years. In the USA, teenage births peaked in the 1950s and have declined since then[9] (Table 54.1). However, over one million teenagers still become pregnant in the US each year.[10] This is a very high rate for an advanced society and underscores the inadequate educational efforts that have been put forth[11] (Fig. 54.2). The incidence of unplanned and unwanted pregnancies among the black teenage population is 51.2%.[13] Approximately half are aborted[14] (Table 54.2). In 2002, Hispanic teenagers had the highest pregnancy rate (82.9 per 1000) compared with other ethnic groups, surpassing black women for the first time[17] (Fig. 54.3). The proportion of births to unmarried Hispanic women increased to 43.4% from 2001 to 2002. In California, Hispanics accounted for the largest percentage of early and late teenage pregnancies (65% and 60% respectively). This phenomenon should be recognized and appreciated in order to better understand its socioeconomic impact.[18]

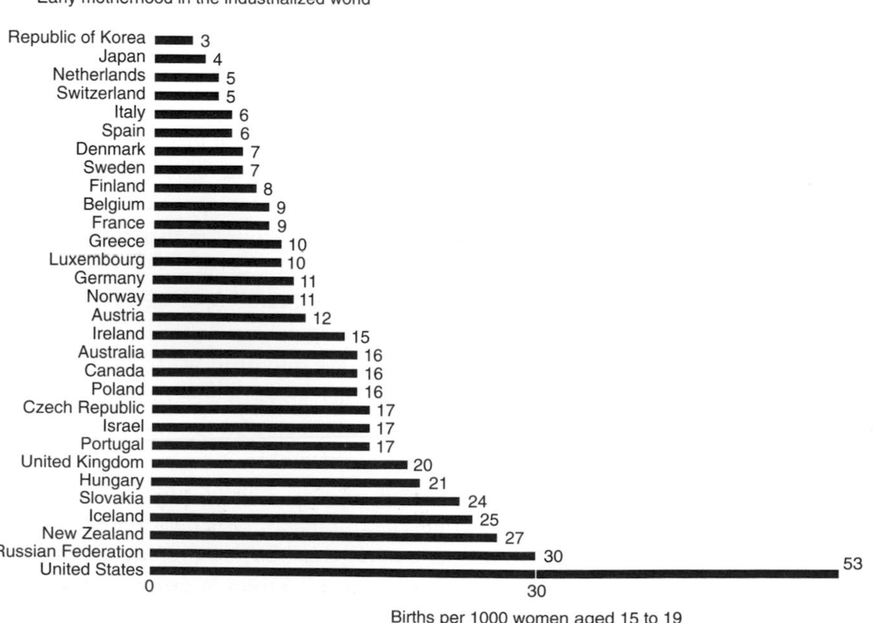

Figure 54.2 UNICEF data. Births per 1000 women aged 15–19 years per country in the industrialized world (from ref. 12).

Table 54.1 Teenage birth rates in the USA.

Year and age of woman	Birth rate	Abortion rate	Pregnancy rate
Women under age 20 years*			
1920	51.4	u.	u.
1930	60.1	u.	u.
1940	47.9	u.	u.
1950	72.3	u.	u.
1960	71.8	u.	u.
1972	62.9	u.	u.
1973	60.5	23.9	98.9
1974	58.7	28.3	101.6
1975	56.8	32.7	104.2
1976	53.9	35.8	104.1
1977	53.9	39.0	107.6
1978	52.5	41.1	108.2
1979	53.4	43.9	112.3
1980	54.2	44.3	113.8
1981	53.2	44.4	112.7
1982	53.4	44.2	112.6
1983	52.4	44.9	112.4
1984	51.6	44.8	111.2
1985	52.1	45.4	112.4
1986	51.3	44.0	109.9
1987	51.7	43.3	109.7
1988	54.2	45.0	114.5
1989	58.6	43.4	118.1
1990	61.6	42.0	120.2
1991	63.2	38.8	118.6
1992	61.7	36.7	114.5
1993	60.5	35.3	111.4
1994	59.7	33.0	107.9
1995	57.4	30.7	102.5
1996	54.7	29.7	98.3
1997	52.3	28.1	93.8
1998	51.3	26.8	91.0
1999	49.7	25.6	87.8
2000	48.6	24.8	85.6
2001	46.1	u.	u.

*Statistically significant; u., unavailable data. National Center for Health Statistics (NCHS) of the US Department of Health and Human Services.

Some more recent reports on teenage pregnancies are positive. The teenage birth rate for women aged 15–19 years was 61.8/1000 women in 1991, but declined to 43.0/1000 women in 2002. This is a 30% decrease. In 2002, the teenage birth rate decreased by 50% among the highest risk ages of 15–17 years; rates for black teenagers decreased by 40%. According to recent statistics from national surveys in 2001, sexual activity decreased by 16% from 1991 (54.1%) to 2001 (45.6%); the prevalence of multiple partners decreased by 24%; condom use increased; and sexually transmitted diseases (STD) decreased.[15]

Risk behaviors and social factors leading to teenage pregnancies

Health risk behaviors

In contrast to older mothers, who often obtain prepregnancy consultation, teenagers rarely seek advice prior to getting pregnant. Therefore, abusive habits such as alcohol, cigarette, and drug abuse are not addressed and resolved prior to conception. Although younger teenagers less than 15 years of age

Table 54.2 Facts about teenage pregnancies.[7,9,15,16]

Pessimistic facts about teenage pregnancies
Approximately one million teenage pregnancies occur each year in the United States
75–95% are unplanned or unwanted
Approximately 50% give birth
13% of all US births are to teenagers
Teenage birthrate in 2002 was 28.5/1000 aged 15–19 years among whites, 68.3/1000 aged 15–19 years among blacks, and 83.4/1000 aged 15–19 years among Hispanics
Approximately 1 in 16 teenage girls has a baby each year
Birth rate is rising the fastest among girls aged 15–17 years
Approximately one-third to one-half are aborted
18% of teenage girls are sexually active before age 15 years
66% of teenage girls are sexually active by age 19 years
35% do not use contraception at first intercourse
Adolescent girls tend to delay using contraception until 1 year after initiation of sexual intercourse
The illegitimacy rate is 29.7 per 1000 teenagers

Optimistic facts about teenage pregnancies
Teenage birth rate has declined by 30% over past decade
Black teenage births are down by 40% over past decade
The younger 15- to 17-year-old black teenage births are down by 50% in 2002
Between 1990 and 1999, there was a 22% drop in the abortion rate
Sexual activity among teenage girls decreased by 16% from 1990 to 2001
Prevalence of multiple partners decreased by 24%

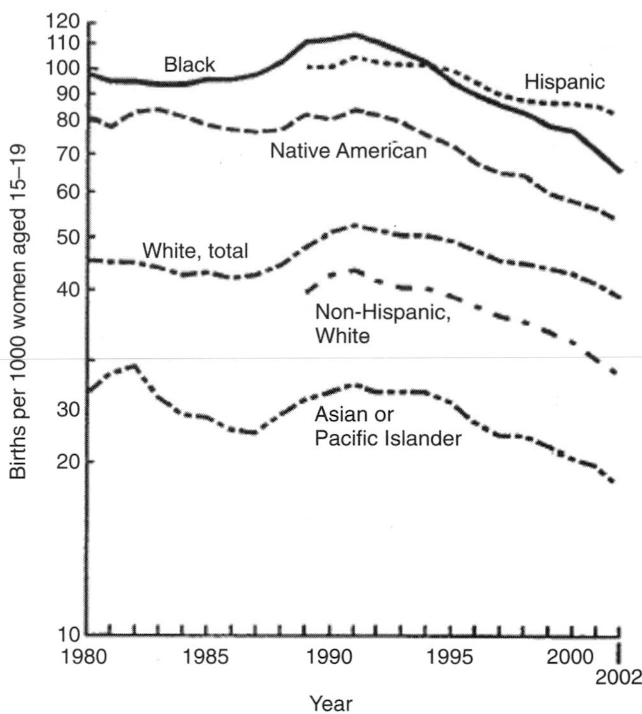

Figure 54.3 Birth rate for teenagers aged 15–19 years by race and Hispanic origin, United States, 1980–2002. Note: data for 2001 are preliminary. Rates are plotted on a log scale.

have inadequate prenatal care, it is the older teenagers, between the ages of 15 and 17 years, who have a higher incidence of drug and cigarette use as well as a higher incidence of sexually transmitted disease.[19,20] Twenty-five percent of teenagers report cigarette smoking of more than half a pack per day,[21] and there was a higher correlation between cigarette smoking and sexual activity. Youths who began using alcohol and drugs were also more likely to initiate sexual activity within a year.[22]

As illegal drug use is prevalent among adolescents and may account for some adverse outcomes, this relationship was evaluated in an Australian study of 456 teenage antenatal patients. Comparisons were made between a control group, a marijuana-only group, and a multidrug group. After controlling for significant covariates, and in the setting of good antenatal care, the only difference in outcome was a significant linear trend toward an increased incidence of threatened preterm labor ($P = 0.02$) in those using illegal drugs.[23] There was no increase in preterm deliveries, preterm rupture of membranes, or poor neonatal outcomes. It is reassuring that, although illegal drug use and associated behaviors may increase the likelihood of teenage pregnancies, once pregnant, those individuals appear not to have significant adverse outcomes when provided with good antenatal care.

Low socioeconomic status

There is no doubt that low socioeconomic status promotes adolescent pregnancies because it is a vicious cycle. Poverty leads to a loss of opportunities, which promotes a lack of upward social mobility, leading to higher crime and adverse behaviors such as drug and alcohol abuse. Poverty also promotes poor self-esteem. All this leads to a lack of incentive to avoid parenthood. Adolescents surrounded by other pregnant adolescents will consider pregnancy to be the norm, further promoting adolescent childbearing.[7]

Poor support from parents or the father of the baby

Many teenagers do not obtain psychological support at home. The needs of teenagers are often not addressed at school and are inadequately addressed at home. With a national divorce rate of 50%, it is no surprise that teenagers are not getting the support they need. Others have shown that those teenagers with significant support from families through adult role models, family communication, religion, community involvement, good health practices, some aspirations for the future, and an ability to make responsible choices had an overall lower incidence of sexual intercourse or delayed first intercourse, and had used birth control measures at last sexual intercourse. Clearly, a strong and meaningful social structure could have an impact on the timing of teenage behaviors that lead to pregnancy. Teenagers with strong parental and community support are less likely to become teenage parents, whereas those whose parents do not openly discuss contraception and sexual behavior with their children tend not to use contraception and are more likely to be teenage parents.[24]

Poor self-esteem/low achievement in school

It is difficult to determine why some teenagers have low self-esteem but, when present, it fosters psychosocial behaviors resulting in teenage pregnancies. Women with low self-esteem also tend to be poor achievers or underachievers at school. They also tend to have a higher rate of drug, alcohol, and tobacco use.[25,26] Such individuals are more likely to be influenced by their surroundings and engage in destructive behaviors. In today's society, there are many forces influencing young, moldable individuals. Most of it comes through the commercial mass media, movies, TV shows, and magazines. The perceived accepted norm of sexual freedom is rampant. It is not surprising that many teenagers believe that premarital sexual intercourse is the social norm. This type of peer pressure pervades, and it is difficult for unguided teenagers to sort out what is important for them as an individual. By the age of 19 years, 80% of young women and 87% of young men have had sexual intercourse.[27] Women with low self-esteem are also less likely to use contraception.

Many girls with poor self-esteem have had a prior history of sexual or physical abuse, as high as 33%.[28–31] This history, combined with depression, probably increases their willingness to engage in childbearing, perhaps as a means to overcome their past history and negative feelings. Healthcare providers should routinely inquire about a history of abuse when taking care of pregnant adolescents.

Racial factors

Half of all teenage births are to non-Hispanic whites, but blacks and Hispanic teenagers have almost twice the pregnancy rates of whites.[32] Blacks have a higher proportion of preterm and low birthweight births than whites or Hispanics. At the same time, however, blacks also have a higher mortality rate among term, post-term, normal birthweight, and macrosomic infants.[33] Hispanics have the lowest risks of neonatal mortality at term (Table 54.3). Efforts to address the teenage pregnancy rate, however, should recognize that there are major differences between racial groups within the United States, and there needs to be some understanding of the cultural differences that contribute to perinatal and neonatal adverse outcomes.

In the final analysis, there are several basic facts as to why teenagers become pregnant: (1) poverty; (2) lack of education, both higher education and sex education; (3) lack of stable home environments and caring parents who discuss contraception and sexual behavior with teenagers; (4) health risk behaviors; (5) poor self-esteem; and (6) race.

Table 54.3 Odds ratios (ORs) and 99% confidence intervals (CIs) for pregnancy outcomes of non-Hispanic white, Hispanic, African–American (AA), and Asian women compared with white women aged 20–29 years.[18]

Pregnancy outcome	ORs (CIs)	ORs (CIs)	ORs (CIs)	ORs (CIs)	ORs (CIs)	ORs (CIs)
	White 11–15	*White 16–19*	*White 20–29*	*Hispanic 11–15*	*Hispanic 16–19*	*Hispanic 20–29*
Infant death	3.1 (2.1, 4.7)	1.9 (1.6, 2.2)	Reference	2.0 (1.5, 2.6)	1.3 (1.2, 1.5)	1.1 (0.98, 1.3)
Neonatal death	2.7 (1.6, 4.7)	1.8 (1.4, 2.2)	Reference	2.1 (1.5, 2.9)	1.4 (1.2, 1.7)	1.3 (1.1, 1.5)
Preterm delivery	1.9 (1.7, 2.1)	1.33 (1.3, 1.4)	Reference	2.3 (2.1, 2.4)	1.55 (1.5, 1.6)	1.24 (1.2, 1.3)
Low birthweight (< 2500 g)	1.8 (1.6, 2.1)	1.3 (1.27, 1.4)	Reference	1.8 (1.7, 1.9)	1.4 (1.3, 1.42)	1.2 (1.19, 1.3)
Preeclampsia	1.5 (0.8, 2.8)	1.0 (0.9, 1.1)	Reference	0.5 (0.3, 0.8)	0.7 (0.6, 0.8)	0.7 (0.6, 0.9)
Severe preeclampsia	0.5 (0.03, 6.3)	0.9 (0.5, 1.6)	Reference	0.4 (0.1, 1.6)	0.6 (0.4, 0.9)	0.7 (0.5, 1.0)
Eclampsia	2.8 (0.2, 39.5)	1.7 (2.3, 2,7)	Reference	1.3 (0.2, 9.0)	0.7 (0.2, 1.9)	0.5 (0.2, 1.4)
Pyelonephritis	2.8 (2.1, 3.6)	2.5 (2.3, 2.7)	Reference	2.6 (2.2, 3.0)	2.3 (2.2, 2.5)	1.6 (1.5, 1.7)
Infectious complications	3.6 (0.3, 51.9)	2.9 (1.0, 8.3)	Reference	2.5 (0.5,13.0)	2.4 (1.0, 5.8)	1.6 (0.7, 3.6)
	AA 11–15	*AA 16–19*	*AA 20–29*	*Asian 11–15*	*Asian 16–19*	*Asian 20–29*
Infant death	3.4 (2.3, 5.1)	2.5 (2.0,3.1)	2.6 (2.1, 3.1)	1.9 (0.7, 5.2)	1.3 (0.7, 2.2)	1.0 (0.8, 1.2)
Neonatal death	3.2 (1.9, 5.5)	2.3 (1.8, 3.1)	3.2 (2.6, 4.0)	2.8 (0.97, 8.1)	1.5 (0.8, 2.8)	0.9 (0.7, 1.2)
Preterm delivery	3.1 (2.8, 3.5)	2.0 (1.9, 2.1)	1.7 (1.6, 1.8)	3.0 (2.5, 3.6)	2.2 (2.0, 2.4)	1.05 (1.0, 1.1)
Low birthweight (< 2500 g)	2.8 (2.4, 3.1)	2.5 (2.3, 2.6)	2.3 (2.2, 2.5)	3.1 (2.5, 3.9)	2.2 (2.0, 2.5)	1.3 (1.2, 1.4)
Preeclampsia	1.3 (0.6, 2.6)	0.9 (0.6, 1.3)	1.2 (0.9, 1.5)	0.7 (0.1, 4.4)	0.1 (0.05, 0.9)	0.3 (0.2, 0.5)
Severe preeclampsia	0.5 (0.04, 6.9)	0.8 (0.3, 1.9)	1.1 (0.6, 2.1)	NA	NA	0.2 (0.1, 0.7)
Eclampsia	NA	0.9 (0.1, 6.4)	1.0 (0.2, 5.1)	NA	NA	0.5 (0.1, 3.4)
Pyelonephritis	2.1 (1.6, 2.9)	2.5 (2.3, 2.9)	1.9 (1.7, 2.1)	1.1 (0.5, 2.4)	1.3 (0.9, 1.7)	0.6 (0.5, 1.7)
Infectious complications	NA	12.1 (4.9, 29.7)	11.0 (4.6, 25.9)	NA	NA	0.3 (0.02, 4.7)

Adverse outcomes of teenage pregnancies

In the medical literature, the incidence and types of adverse outcomes resulting from teenage pregnancies vary and remain inconsistent (Table 54.4). Older literature may not apply to current practice. The primary reason is that the populations studied tended to be heterogeneous and, unless there is proper control of factors such as race, socioeconomic status, and type of healthcare system, the findings and conditions will likely be variable. Unlike older patients, adverse outcomes in teenage pregnancies are not the result of maternal medical illness, as the majority are young and healthy. Instead, the current literature supports the understanding that adverse outcomes in teenagers result from poor psychosocial environments rather than biologic risks inherent to the adolescent. In other words, adverse outcomes are more a reflection of a social problem than a medical problem.

Teenage mortality

Mortality to a teenager secondary to pregnancy is extremely low. In the past, one of the major causes of maternal mortality was eclampsia. However, with better recognition of hypertension and early intervention, these cases of maternal mortality are drastically reduced. The mortality ratio (pregnancy-related deaths per 100 000 live births) for preeclampsia and eclampsia for all women <20 years of age from 1979 to 1992 was 1.6 compared with 1.5 for all age groups, 3.3 for women aged 35–39 years, and 6.0 for women aged 40–49 years.[34]

Table 54.4 Adverse pregnancy outcomes for adolescents.

Event	Risk	Reference
Preterm delivery	OR 1.41 (1.203–1.90)*	38
	RR 1.12 (1.04–1.21)*	40
	OR 1.5 (1.2–1.9)*	41
	OR 1.02 (0.66–1.58)*	20
	OR 1.5 (1.0–2.2)	42
Gestational hypertension	OR 2.57 (2.14–3.07)*	46
Gestational diabetes	OR 0.19 (0.07–0.50)*	38
Preeclampsia	RR 1.33 (1.15–1.54)*	40
	RR 1.30 (0.94–1.82)	38
Eclampsia	RR 2.23 (1.37–3.66)*	40
Emergency Cesarean section	OR 0.45 (0.38–0.58)*	38
Operative vaginal delivery	OR 0.46 (0.41–0.56)*	38
Induction of labor	OR 0.83 (0.75–0.92)*	38
Postpartum hemorrhage	OR 0.83 (0.72–0.95)*	38
Abruption	OR 0.71 (0.36–1.24)	38
Placenta previa	OR 0.48 (0.15–1.52)	38

OR, odds ratio; RR, relative risk; *significant difference.

Perinatal mortality

In California, USA, teenagers had a higher rate of infant and neonatal deaths than an older control group of white women irrespective of race, except that Asians had a similar rate to the control group.[18] However, in another study, the perinatal mortality rate was not increased in adolescents compared with older women and, in some reports, the data were inconsistent.[20,35,36] In a large retrospective review of 21 610 873 single births between 1995 and 2000, the overall fetal death rate after 24 weeks' gestation was 2.7 per 1000 total births and was not increased in younger aged women.[37]

Preterm labor

The incidence of preterm labor in a teenage population is variable. There was no difference between young or older adolescents compared with women over 20 years of age[36] in one controlled study from Texas, whereas others reported a higher incidence.[38,39]

Preterm birth

In a large inner city hospital on the east coast of the USA, younger adolescents and older adolescents were also found to have a high risk of preterm delivery compared with older control subjects.[40] A slightly lower rate of preterm birth (14.5% vs. 17.4%) was seen when black adolescents were compared with black women in general.[19] In a Californian study that controlled for parity, race, and healthcare systems, adolescents also demonstrated greater risks for preterm delivery at less than 37 weeks' gestation than an older control group.[18] Younger adolescents had a higher rate of preterm delivery than older adolescents.[41,42] In contrast, in a military population in which there was equal access to a tertiary care center, young maternal age was not an independent risk factor for prematurity.[43] This was also the case in an ultraorthodox Jewish population with social support and medical care.[44] In another controlled study, there was no difference in preterm labor in those aged 16–17 years compared with those aged 20–22 years.[36] Thus, it appears that the data for preterm delivery risk are mixed, although there is a trend toward an increased risk, most likely reflecting a lack of control in some studies for factors that influence the access to, or quality of, medical care.

Preterm rupture of membranes

Despite being high-risk pregnancies, teenage pregnancies do not appear to have an increased incidence of preterm premature rupture of membranes.[36,45]

Low birthweight

Most studies, but not all, reported a higher risk of low birthweight and very low birthweight infants from teenage

Table 54.5 Adverse neonatal outcomes for adolescents.

Event	Risk	Reference
Low birthweight	OR 0.93 (0.55–1.57)	20
	RR 1.47 (1.31–1.64)*	40
	OR 1.25 (1.00–1.56)*	46
	OR 2.0 (1.2–3.1)*	42
Very low birthweight	RR 1.25 (1.01–1.56)*	40
Perinatal mortality	OR 1.83 (0.73–4.60)	20

OR, odds ratio; RR, relative risk; *significant difference.

women.[18,40,42,46] There is a U-shaped distribution of small babies, with the highest percentages for teenagers and women over 40 years.[47] Other studies, however, do not show an increased rate of low birthweight infants in populations in which there was a commitment to prenatal care.[19,36,43,44] There was only a modest difference between blacks and whites (16% vs. 9% respectively)[47] (Table 54.5).

Preeclampsia/eclampsia

Gestational hypertension has not been definitively shown to be increased among adolescents when variables such as access to healthcare are controlled.[36,45] However, one serious concern is the high incidence of preeclampsia. When eclampsia is also involved, the mortality rate is significantly increased to 1.5 per 100 000 live births. Rates of preeclampsia (6.3%) were higher in teenagers than in adult black (2.5%) and white women (2.2%) in an inner city, black population on the east coast.[19] This was also true for an Atlanta inner city population.[40] It was not true, however, on the west coast, primarily in California, where there was more standardized healthcare and a higher standard of living than in inner city Baltimore or Atlanta.[18] Clearly, the environment is an important issue, but it appears that adolescents, if given proper care, may not be at increased risk of hypertensive disorders of pregnancy compared with older women of similar race.[38] Until the etiology of preeclampsia is identified, we may not be able to assess risks unique to the age of a population because of many confounding variables.

Cesarean section

It would appear that the Cesarean section rate in teenagers should be higher because of their immature pelvises. However, this has not been proven. Although it has been reported by Moerman[48] that the pelvises of girls at menarche had room to grow, it is not certain that this leads to an obstructed pelvis. In Moerman's study, measurements were taken in an anteroposterior (AP) direction and only three planes at the sacrum, inlet, and interspinous diameter. These measurements could not accurately determine differences in the AP diameter or the curvature of the iliac wings, thus negating their conclusion.[48] In another study, bone age was determined by radiographs of the hand and wrist in adolescents during the puerperium, and found not to correlate with adverse perinatal or neonatal outcomes. Therefore, there are no anatomic risks associated with adolescent childbearing.[49]

When girls of < 15 years of age were compared with those between 20 and 22 years, the incidence of Cesarean delivery was not higher; in fact, it was lower.[18,36] The lower rates in this population would suggest that dystocia or cephalopelvic disproportion that could result from these less mature pelvises does not happen often and that these pelvises are not "abnormal" with regard to the ability to deliver a fetus vaginally. Cesarean delivery, if performed, appears to result from other causes but not an immature pelvis.

In Nigeria, where there is a very high incidence of adolescent pregnancies, the incidence of symphysiotomies for an immature, dystotic pelvis is not high. Out of a total of 1013 symphysiotomy procedures performed in Nigeria (3.7%), the rate was not higher among adolescents, but was actually higher among older women. In 87.7%, the primary reason for performing a symphysiotomy was for cephalopelvic disproportion. This suggests that symphysiotomy was not indicated in a higher percentage of adolescents because of an immature pelvis.[50] Therefore, the concern for an increased risk of dystocia or cephalopelvic disproportion among adolescents may need to be revisited, perhaps with imaging studies.

Risk factors contributing to adverse pregnancy outcomes among teenagers

Anemia

Social pressures have influenced outcomes related to weight gain and nutrition. Anemia among adolescents is rampant, most likely secondary to poor nutrition. Many studies have demonstrated a significant incidence of anemia among African–American adolescents.[51] However, adverse pregnancy outcomes have been inconsistently demonstrated. One study did find fewer adverse outcomes among those with mild to moderate anemia, but much more among those with severe anemia.[36,52] There is an equal amount of negative impact from either low hemoglobin or high hemoglobin levels, i.e., there is a U-shaped distribution correlating low birthweight neonates with low and high degrees of anemia compared with those with normal blood count levels.[51] In these cases, the lack of normal plasma volume expansion, which leads to the higher hemoglobin levels, causes poor uteroplacental perfusion, resulting in the low birthweights.[52]

Poor nutrition

Nutritional intake is clearly a significant problem among teenagers. Across the nation, there is a serious problem with eating disorders. The incidence of anorexia among females is

15 per 100 000 person-years compared with 1.5 per 100 000 among males. It tends to be higher among younger females.[53] It is more common among white adolescents than blacks or Hispanics. This may explain why there is a higher risk of excessive weight gain among non-Hispanic white adolescents,[54] and that there are more girls below ideal body weight at the start of pregnancy. Because this disorder is often associated with the individual's poor body image and low self-esteem, provision of psychological care is also important in antenatal clinics. Excess weight gain may induce further hazards to the fetus if macrosomia is present and there is an increased risk of long-term health problems and obesity for the mothers.

In contrast, obesity is an extremely prevalent health issue in the United States that may be seen with poor weight gain. It is extremely important for our healthcare system to recognize the need for skilled providers who can recognize disorders in the pregnant teenager, provide the appropriate immediate intervention, and initiate a lifelong educational process.

Late prenatal care

As many as 55% of pregnant adolescents in the United States do not receive early prenatal care. Factors influencing late entry to care include unemployment (1.9; 95% CI 1.1–3.5) lower educational level (1.2; 95% CI 1.04–1.4), and race, blacks compared with whites or Hispanics (1.9; 95% CI 1.2–3.2).[55] There is a clear racial difference, with white women usually reporting more prenatal visits than black women.[56] Unplanned pregnancy is also a risk factor for late prenatal care.[57] Finally, in a study from South Carolina, prenatal care sought by adolescents correlated with the school term, with a diminished seeking of care when school was not in session.[58] Understanding and accepting these risk factors will enable the medical and social community to better design clinics that would successfully encourage adolescents to seek prenatal care.

Drug use

Cigarettes, alcohol, and illegal drug use among teenagers contribute to adverse pregnancy outcomes for a variety of reasons, including bleeding in pregnancy, fetal alcohol syndrome, and the socioeconomic issues related to the drug scene. Although use has declined since the 1970s,[59] a large number of teenagers still admit to partaking, 17% by questionnaire self-report and 11% by urine screen[60] (Fig. 54.4). Binge drinking and heavy drinking are particularly high among white teenagers. Black teenagers do not have a significantly higher rate of drug abuse than white teenagers.[61] Healthcare providers need to question pregnant teenagers regarding drug abuse and be able to provide treatment and psychosocial support if needed.

Infection

Infectious complications are higher in teenage pregnancies for all ethnic groups except for Asians.[18] One of the more common complications is pyelonephritis, highlighting the need for increased surveillance for subclinical urinary tract bacterial colonization. No difference in chorioamnionitis was observed between adolescents and older patients.[36]

Teenagers have a high rate of sexually transmitted diseases. At the first prenatal visit, as many as 23.5% tested positive for *Neisseria gonorrhoeae* (1.2%), *Chlamydia trachomatis* (13%), *Trichomonas vaginalis* (8.9%), or *Treponema pallidum* (1.2%).[62] Other investigators found a comparably high incidence of gonorrhea and chlamydia.[63–66] Risk-taking behaviors such as inconsistent condom use, concomitant alcohol abuse, multiple sexual partners, sex with older partners, nationality, and foreigner status place them at high risk, particularly for human immunodeficiency virus (HIV) infection.[62,67] Healthcare providers for pregnant teenagers should routinely screen for sexually transmitted disease, screen care-

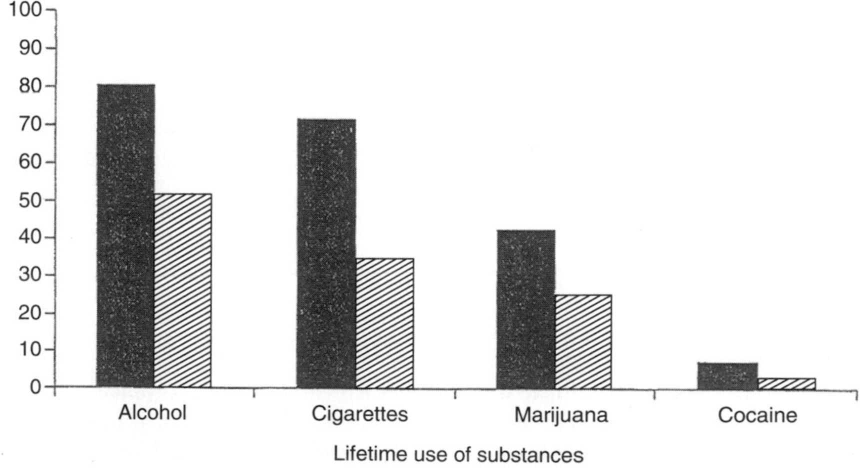

Figure 54.4 Percentage of students reporting lifetime use of substances (solid bars) and use during the past 30 days (hatched bars) (from ref. 32 with permission).

fully for high-risk behavior, be able to provide counseling, and encourage condom use. Commitment to condom use among these adolescents would clearly be increased if they had a good understanding that lack of use could lead to adverse effects on their own health.[68] Subsequent evaluation of teenagers with abnormal Pap smears showing human papillomavirus infection is important because of the possibility of developing cervical dysplasia.

One very sobering reason to work toward educating adolescents against unplanned childbearing is the very real issue that HIV-positive adolescents are becoming pregnant. This will be an increasing concern as the number of parentless adolescents continues to increase (estimated that there will be 20 million orphans in Africa by the year 2010) and as they reach childbearing age. Currently, 33.5 million people globally are HIV infected. If pregnancies are planned and wanted, women will continue their HIV treatments and decrease the risks of transmission. One recent study of Puerto Rican adolescents reported that all five liveborns from HIV-infected mothers were HIV negative because the mothers had been on antiviral agents.[69] It is uncertain how successful worldwide attempts will be to curb this spread.

What can be done about reducing the incidence of teenage pregnancies?

Sex education

Although unpopular among certain groups in the USA, school sex education is one of the best means of preventing teenage pregnancies and their recurrence. Sex education is usually required in schools. However, to be fully effective, sex education in schools should include coverage of the topics of reproductive biology, sexual development, birth control, and other means of prevention such as abortion.[70] Perhaps one of the reasons for failure is the timing of this education. Marsiglio and Mott[71] reported that 52% of 15-year-old girls have already initiated coitus before taking sex education classes.

Educational interventions during pregnancy and postpartum may be effective in reducing future teenage pregnancies for this population. In general, efforts to prevent repeat pregnancies have been disappointing, because educational programs have not targeted these high-risk populations well.[72] A study evaluating five structured postnatal home visits by nurse-midwives in Australia found a reduced incidence in adverse neonatal outcomes and a significant increase in contraception knowledge.[73] As an educational approach is assumed to be longlasting, it may perhaps be more effective in the long term in preventing repeat teenage pregnancy. Although it may be difficult to implement in a large and diverse society, such programs may be more successful because we know that, without any intervention, the subsequent pregnancy would likely occur within 2 years in approximately half of those studied.[72]

School-based clinics

The school environment is one of the best locations in which to establish classes to educate teenagers about responsibilities related to sexual freedom.[74] It is an environment that reaches those in the neediest age groups, students will be learning among their peers, both female and male students can be reached, and it resides within an atmosphere of learning and training. Finally, within that environment, interventions may be undertaken in the form of additional education, counseling, or introduction to prevention programs. Even more successful are those programs in which the community is actively engaged and contributes.[27] Although such programs have been criticized as a means of encouraging teenagers to take advantage of the welfare system, recent legislation in many areas of the USA, such as the mandated 2-year return to work program in Wisconsin, is curtailing and discouraging such behavior. In time, this will become an ineffective criticism.

Another tested concept is providing care in a specialized teenage pregnancy clinic where nutritional and social issues are more carefully addressed, where infection is more often screened for, and where patients are seen with their peers. One study reported a decreased incidence of preterm labor, preterm delivery, and preterm premature rupture of the membranes among those provided with prenatal care at a teenage pregnancy clinic. In addition, there was a higher incidence of breastfeeding and a higher rate of discharge on effective contraception. Although not a randomized trial, this effort again highlights the positive success through close, direct educational efforts with adolescents.[75] A teenage mother is also less likely to finish her secondary school education and, without that education, teenagers are likely to continue the vicious cycle of poverty, social isolation, and repeat teenage pregnancies. Therefore, school-based prenatal care, which has been shown to reduce the absenteeism and dropout rates (adjusted OR 0.39; 95% CI 0.15–0.99, $P = 0.048$), is also a positive thing.[76] It is only through education that teenage pregnancies can be reduced. Knowledge imparted from school-based clinics should be fully supported to further decrease the current teenage pregnancy rate.

Emergency contraception

Although it is debated whether access to emergency contraception promotes unprotected intercourse, it has been shown that this is not the case as there is no decrease in the age at first intercourse, nor is there an increase in the incidence of sexually transmitted diseases. The provision of emergency contraception may actually encourage young teenagers to seek pelvic examinations and Pap smear screening.[77]

Emergency contraception may be taken in the form of combination pills, in two doses 12 hours apart, or progestin-only pills, in one dose or in two doses 12 hours apart. They are most effective when taken within 72 hours of unprotected

Table 54.6 Emergency contraception.

Pill brand	Manufacturer	First dose	Second dose (12 h later)
Combination hormone pills			
Alesse®	Wyeth-Ayerst	5 pink pills	5 pink pills
Aviane®	Duramed	5 orange pills	5 orange pills
Cryselle®	Barr	4 white pills	4 white pills
Enpresse®	Barr	4 orange pills	4 orange pills
Lessina®	Barr	5 pink pills	5 pink pills
Levlen®	Berlex	4 light orange pills	4 light orange pills
Levlite®	Berlex	5 pink pills	5 pink pills
Levora®	Watson	4 white pills	4 white pills
Lo/Ovral®	Wyeth-Ayerst	4 white pills	4 white pills
LowOgestrel®	Watson	4 white pills	4 white pills
Nordette®	Wyeth-Ayerst	4 light orange pills	4 light orange pills
Ogestrel®	Watson	2 white pills	2 white pills
Ovral®	Wyeth-Ayerst	2 white pills	2 white pills
Portia®	Barr	4 pink pills	4 pink pills
Preven®	Gynetics	2 blue pills	2 blue pills
Seasonale®	Barr	4 pink pills	4 pink pills
Tri-Levlen®	Berlex	4 yellow pills	4 yellow pills
Triphasil®	Wyeth-Ayerst	4 yellow pills	4 yellow pills
Trivora®	Watson	4 pink pills	4 pink pills
Progestin-only pills			
Ovrette®	Wyeth-Ayerst	20 yellow pills or 40 yellow pills in one dose	20 yellow pills
Plan B®	Barr	1 white pill or 2 white pills in one dose	1 white pill

sexual intercourse but may be taken up to 120 hours after intercourse. They reduce the risk of pregnancy by 75–89%. Another form of emergency contraception includes intrauterine device (IUD) insertion, usually with a Copper T 380A IUD (Paragard), which is left in place until the patient is certain she is not pregnant (Table 54.6).

Abortion

Abortion has been practiced as a very effective means of contraception for teenagers. Abortion rates increased dramatically from the mid-1970s to the mid-1980s, from 29% to 42%.[7] The proportion of black and white adolescents who obtain abortions is similar but, because there is a higher pregnancy rate among blacks, the rate of abortion is higher among blacks than among whites. Adolescents who obtain abortions tend to be better students from higher socioeconomic backgrounds with a lower dropout rate and higher education goals.[7]

Factors that influence abortions include perceptions that there is a lack of continued involvement from the father of the baby, a lack of a satisfying relationship with the father of the baby, a lack of parental involvement, and an existing child.[13] Recognizing those teenagers who perceive their pregnancies as unplanned and unwanted may enable programs to provide better support for them. Adoption remains a viable option for teenagers, and information should be given (Table 54.7).

Table 54.7 Useful resources for pregnant teenagers.

Planned Parenthood 1-800-230-PLAN, www.plannedparenthood.org
American's Pregnancy Helpline 1-888-4-OPTIONS
Emergency Contraception Information Project 1-888-NOT-2-LATE
National Abortion Federation 1-800-772-9100
National Adoption Center 1-800-862-3678
Rosie Adoptions 1-800-841-0804
For adoption options and information, www.adoption.com

Contraception

In order to achieve postpartum and continued health for these teenage mothers, one important issue to address is the contraceptive needs of these patients. These teenagers should be educated regarding their reproductive options and childbearing options. Older studies support the fact that adolescents are capable of using contraception effectively provided there is a supportive environment from their mothers and the babies' fathers. In those cases, subsequent pregnancies were planned because there was a closer relationship with their boyfriends, who provided sufficient support.[78]

Taking care of pregnant adolescents

When an adolescent is first seen for a pregnancy, it is important to screen for sexually transmitted diseases, a history of any physical or sexual abuse, and a history of substance abuse. The social environment should be investigated when possible to determine appropriateness for the future newborn. A good dietary history is also important and should be an opportunity to address nutritional issues, particularly common ones such as iron and vitamin deficiency. They should be encouraged to gain the higher acceptable amount of weight gain if they are starting at below ideal body weight. Although medically less complex than an older patient, teenagers are still at risk for pregnancy complications, primarily preterm labor and intrauterine growth restriction. These should be monitored closely and carefully. In the postpartum period, close attention should be provided to insure that the new adolescent mother has proper support for herself and her fetus, in terms of both financial and nutritional support as well as psychosocial support. Effective contraception should be encouraged and education provided to help those with histories of drug abuse to stay clean for as long as possible. Proper referrals to support groups will be particularly important for these teenagers.

Pregnancy in older women aged > 35 years

Advanced maternal age is defined as greater than age 35 years based on higher perinatal morbidity and mortality after that age. That consensus derives from older studies from the 1980s. Within the past decade, there has been a rise in the number of births to women over 35 years, and it is now not uncommon to see women over the age of 40 years having pregnancies. There is even an increasing number of pregnant women over the age of 50 years (Fig. 54.5). Perhaps advanced maternal age should be redefined as greater than 40 years based on maternal morbidity and mortality, both of which continue to drop. Many studies have focused on such an age group, but few studies, if any, have compared the differences between women over 35 years and those over 40 years. For women interested in future childbearing, they should be informed that their pregnancy risks and fertility do start to decline after the age of 35 years and, hence, it would be prudent to keep the definition of advanced maternal age as age greater than 35 years in order to initiate awareness for this older population without an undue false sense of security.

In a study using a database of 94 346 deliveries in Montreal, the average maternal age at delivery increased from

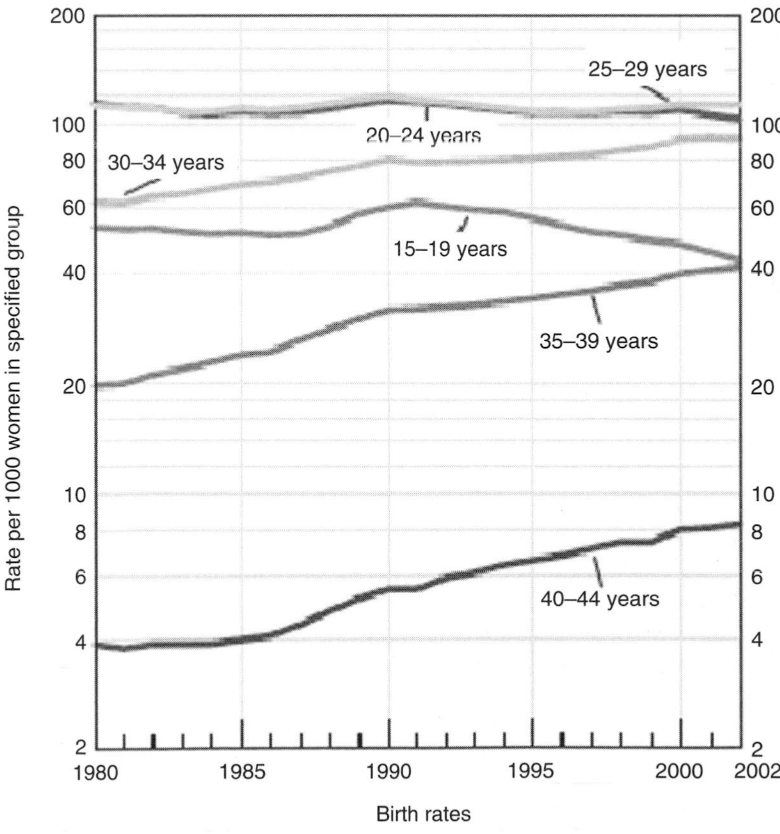

Figure 54.5 Birth rates by age of mother: United States, 1980–2002. Note: rates are plotted on a log scale. Denominations for population-based ratios for 1991–2002 are inter- and postcensal estimates that incorporate the 2000 results. Rates for 1991–2001 have been revised and may differ from those previously published.

27 years in the 1960s to 30 years from 1990 through 1993. The proportion of pregnant women 40 years of age or older was 2.5% in the 1960s and doubled from the 1970s to the 1990s.[79] Women are either delaying their childbearing or extending their childbearing in order to account for the increasing numbers of elderly gravid women. The primary reasons are social changes that have taken place over the past four decades, including the acceptance of oral contraceptive technologies, the legalization of abortions, the availability of prenatal diagnosis, and the improvements in medical care overall such that women with diabetes or hypertension are now well controlled and able to consider pregnancy options.

Risks to older women having pregnancies

There are some unique risks to pregnancy at an older age, issues that a woman should know before embarking on a pregnancy and physicians should discuss with them in anticipation. Physicians should recognize that these older women will enter pregnancy with more medical complications than the younger patient.[80] Women greater than 35 years of age have a higher incidence of hypertension (2.7%), pre-existing diabetes (0.7%), and obesity (6.9%) at the beginning of pregnancy.[81] Gestational diabetes was also identified in 6.9% of older women.

Although some older literature suggests that women of advanced age have more complications, the more recent literature refutes this. In a study in which women had access to good medical care within an urban setting and where there was a higher educational level, adverse pregnancy outcomes including small for gestational age, perinatal death, and preterm delivery were not increased compared with younger women.[82]

Declining fertility

One of the most important facts that older women should know, particularly the older nulliparous women, is that fertility is expected to decline (Fig. 54.6) dramatically after the age of 35 years.[84] Oocyte numbers in a woman's ovary decline from several million before birth to only 200 000–300 000 at birth, but this decline and its link to infertility are not well understood. Today, the options for a woman desiring fertility have increased through assisted reproductive technologies and include *in vitro* fertilization (IVF), intracytoplasmic sperm injection (ICSI), gamete intrafallopian transfer (GIFT), zygote intrafallopian transfer (ZIFT), oocyte donation, embryo donation, and surrogacy, each with a varied but optimistic success rate.

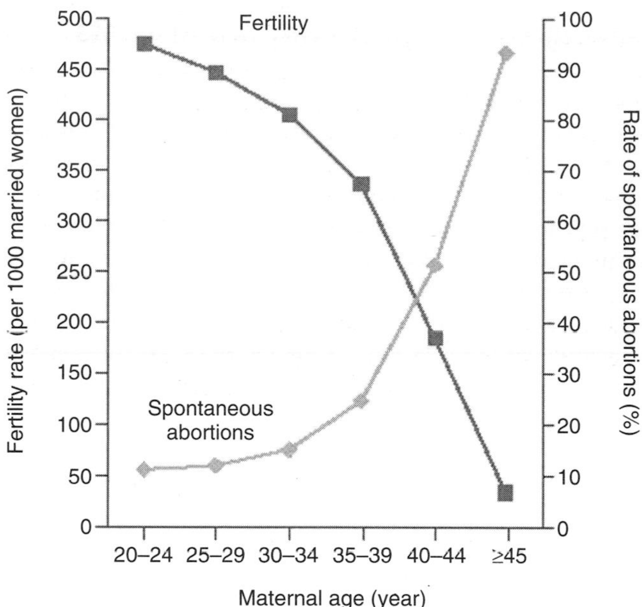

Figure 54.6 Fertility and miscarriage rates as a function of maternal age (from ref. 83 with permission).

Risks for aneuploidy

It is well known that, with advancing age, a woman's risk of nondysjunction within the chromatids in her oocytes increases, leading to trisomies. Other forms of aneuploidy such as deletions and translocations also increase. In part, this explains the higher incidence of spontaneous abortions to women over the age of 35 years.[84,85] Several options for prenatal diagnosis are available, and proper counseling, from either subspecialists or genetic counselors, is mandatory (Tables 54.8 and 54.9).

Multiple gestation

Dizygotic multiples are increased among gestations from older women (Fig. 54.7). This is influenced by a higher incidence undergoing assisted reproductive technologies. Among women aged 50–54 years, the rates of low and very low birthweight, preterm and very preterm delivery, small for gestational age, and mortality were higher, but the risks were lower than for single pregnancies, perhaps because of the higher levels of healthcare and socioeconomic status in these older women.[87]

Mortality

Maternal mortality for women over 40 years was 50 per 100 000 in 1954, 10 per 100 000 in 1985,[88] and 8.9 per 100 000 live births in the year 2002.[89] Recent medical advances in the past few decades have decreased maternal mortality significantly. The most common causes of mortality now are hypertensive disorders, hemorrhage, and infection. Pulmonary embolism is also a major cause. The fact that older women have higher mortality is not surprising because, as they age, women will have a higher incidence and a prolonged duration of hypertensive diseases and diabetes and, hence, a higher likelihood of complications such as hemorrhage and infection. Some of the mortality risks may also be influenced by women who have complications after corrected congenital heart disease, a problem not encountered previously in past decades.

Maternal mortality clearly rises with increasing maternal age: 1.4/100 000 deliveries for age 20–29 years; 22.1/100 000 deliveries for age group 40–44 years, OR 16.2 (95% CI 6.38–41.2); and 166/100 000 deliveries for age group ≥ 45 years, OR 121 (95% CI 27–542).[90] Mortality is also influenced by race. Black women over 40 years of age have the highest pregnancy-related mortality risk ratio, 5.6, compared with white 40+-year-old women, 2.4 (Table 54.1).[91] For older black women, the most common cause of death was hypertensive disorders of pregnancy followed by hemorrhage and embolism.[2,34]

Table 54.8 Risk of Down syndrome in relation to maternal age (live births).[86]

Maternal age at delivery (years)	Risk	Maternal age at delivery (years)	Risk
15	1:1580	33	1:575
16	1:1570	34	1:475
17	1:1565	35	1:385
18	1:1560	36	1:305
19	1:1540	37	1:240
20	1:1530	38	1:190
21	1:1510	39	1:145
22	1:1480	40	1:110
23	1:1450	41	1:85
24	1:1400	42	1:65
25	1:1350	43	1:49
26	1:1290	44	1:37
27	1:1210	45	1:28
28	1:1120	46	1:21
29	1:1020	47	1:15
30	1:901	48	1:11
31	1:795	49	1:8
32	1:680	50	1:6

Maternal obstetric complications due to advanced age

Cesarean sections

Cesarean sections are increased among women over 40 years;[82,92–94] in one study, by a factor of 2, 24.3% vs. 11.7%.[95] In another study addressing older women aged 40 years and beyond in 24 032 cases, the Cesarean section rate was also higher among these women than among the control population aged 20–29 years (47% vs. 30%). The reasons for the increased rate of Cesarean sections are not fully understood. There are other increased findings in study groups such as birth asphyxia, fetal growth restriction, malpresentation, and gestational diabetes that may explain the higher rates for surgical delivery.[96] Mean gestational age were also

Table 54.9 Options for prenatal diagnosis.

Nuchal translucency
First trimester screening
Chorionic villus sampling
Preimplantation genetic diagnosis
Second trimester serum biochemical marker screening
Ultrasound to evaluate for markers of aneuploidy
Amniocentesis
Percutaneous fetal blood sampling

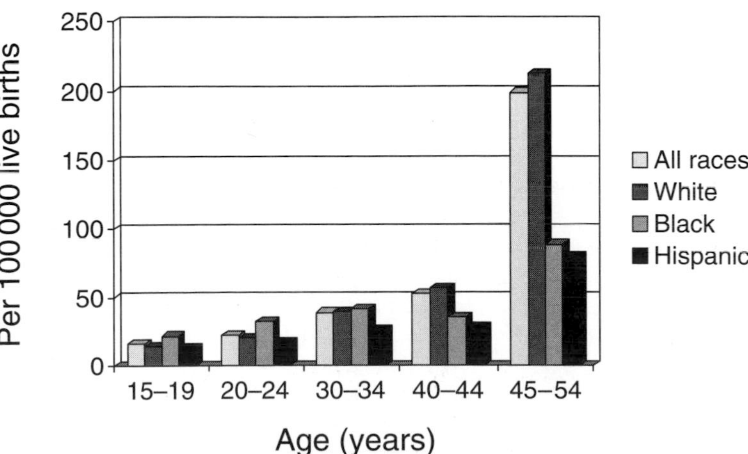

Figure 54.7 Twin births by age and race (adapted from ref. 16).

significantly lower. Other reasons could include higher rates of hypertensive diseases, fetal growth restriction leading to a higher incidence of fetal distress, or more dysfunctional labor due to higher parity. Indeed, a retrospective study reported that risks for emergency Cesarean sections and a need for oxytocin utilization were higher in nulliparous women age 35 years or older than in a younger group of women aged between 25 and 29 years, suggesting that there was more fetal distress and dysfunctional labor.[81,97] In addition, there may be a higher incidence of infertility and perhaps a higher incidence of Cesarean deliveries because of these assumed "premium" pregnancies and a higher unwillingness to take riskier approaches such as forceps deliveries. It is less likely to be related to differences in the maternal pelvis, but other factors such as dysfunctional labor from multiparity and more macrosomic babies could contribute. The rate of Cesarean sections will need to be monitored as more older women become pregnant, and counseling regarding this higher rate should be provided to women in advance of pregnancy (Table 54.10).

Increased operative vaginal deliveries

Operative vaginal deliveries are higher in older women of > 35 years of age than in younger women.[94,97] In older women, the need for oxytocin utilization is also higher.[81] The causes of these findings are uncertain, but may be due to a higher rate of dysfunctional labor, as with the higher Cesarean section rates, or they may be related to a higher chance of maternal exhaustion, but that variable is difficult to quantify.

Table 54.10 Adverse pregnancy outcomes for women aged > 35 years.

Event	Risk	Reference
Preterm delivery	OR 1.41 (1.24–1.61)*	97
	OR 2.0 (1.5–2.8)*	80
	OR 1.9 (1.2–2.9)*	101
	OR 1.1 (0.5–2.6)	82
Chronic hypertension	OR 3.4 (1.6–7.2)*	80
Preeclampsia	OR 1.19 (1.01–1.40)*	97
Diabetes	OR 2.2 (0.2–20.7)	80
	OR 2.63 (2.40–2.89)*	97
Emergency Cesarean section	OR 1.59 (1.52–1.67)*	97
Cesarean section	OR 7.3 (2.2–16.7)*	94
Operative vaginal delivery	OR 1.5 (1.43–1.57)*	97
	OR 7.5 (2.2–25.0)*	94
Induction of labor	OR 1.04 (1.00–1.08)*	97
	RR 1.3 (1.0–1.6)*	100
	OR 2.4 (1.6–3.7)*	80
Postpartum hemorrhage	OR 1.14 (1.09–1.19)*	97
Placenta previa	OR 1.93 (1.58–2.35)*	97
	OR 1.37 (1.25–1.50)*	100
Abruptions	OR 2.3 (1.3–3.9)*	102

OR, odds ratio; RR, relative risk; *significant difference.

Preeclampsia/eclampsia

Older women tend to have a higher incidence of preeclampsia and eclampsia. In a Swedish study, women aged 40 years and older had higher risks of severe preeclampsia.[90] Other retrospective studies also found a higher incidence in women aged over 40 years.[81,97,98] In 1997, the National Center for Health Statistics started recording vital data on pregnant women aged 50–54 years. Their results indicate that women over 50 years, compared with women aged 20–29 years, 30–39 years, and 40–49 years, have a higher incidence of chronic hypertension and eclampsia.[87] Clearly, hypertensive diseases, which are more prevalent among older women, contribute to the incidence of preeclampsia and eclampsia, most likely from the underlying vasculopathy associated with chronic hypertension.

Postpartum hemorrhage

In a study from London, with a database containing more than 80% of all deliveries in a region with > 3.5 million population, increasing maternal age grouped from 18–34 years, 35–40 years, and > 40 years was studied, and odds ratios for postpartum hemorrhage were higher for women aged 35 years and older.[97]

Dysfunctional labor

An association between advanced maternal age and dysfunctional labor is not well established. In a retrospective cohort study of women over the age of 40 years, maternal morbidities included a higher incidence of abnormal labor patterns.[98] However, others reported no increased risk for prolonged labor or arrest in the second stage secondary to advanced maternal age.[82,99]

Induction of labor

The odds for induction of labor are higher for older women than for younger women.[80,97,100] In a study from Ireland, induction of labor was 28% for women over the age of 40 years, double the rate for the younger women (12.5%).[95] In a retrospective cohort study of women over the age of 40 years, maternal morbidities included a higher incidence of labor induction. There were also more abnormal labor patterns, suggesting that older women had more pregnancy complications near term and labor was more dysfunctional, requiring more oxytocin.[98] The causes of this higher incidence could not be defined within their clinical setting, as it is not clear that dysfunctional labor is increased in this age group.

It may be influenced by the physicians' desire to deliver older women by their due date because of concerns over the higher rates of adverse outcomes in older women.

Preterm labor/preterm delivery

Adverse perinatal outcomes for older women were studied and reported from a Swedish Medical Birth Register in a population-based cohort study. Although taken from a Scandinavian country where 95% or more of pregnant women receive antenatal care, confounding factors related to medical and socioeconomic factors were controlled. Preterm delivery was found to be increased among older women.[101] In another Swedish study, women aged 40 years and older had higher risks of preterm labor and preterm birth.[90] In retrospective cohort studies of women over the ages of 35 or 40 years, preterm premature rupture of membranes and preterm labor were identified more frequently compared with younger women.[80,81,96,97] Some of this may be attributable to assisted reproductive technologies, which are more commonly utilized among older women, as well as the higher rates of multiple gestations resulting from this utilization. However, one study of well-educated women with higher socioeconomic status did not identify an increased risk of delivery prior to 33 weeks' gestation.[82]

Placenta previa

The incidence of placenta previa is increased for women over the age of 40 years, 3% vs. 0.92%.[95] This accounts for a higher incidence of antepartum hemorrhage. In another Swedish study, women aged 40 years and older had a higher risk of placenta previa.[90] In a study from London, higher odds ratios were noted for placenta previa and postpartum hemorrhage in older women.[97] Data from the National Center for Health Statistics on pregnant women aged 50–54 years also reported a higher incidence of placenta previa.[87] These findings reflect a higher incidence of multiparity,[98] uterine myomas, or uterine scarring from prior surgeries, which could explain the higher incidence of placenta previa.[99,101]

Antepartum bleeding

Antepartum bleeding is more frequent for women over 40 years (8.23% vs. 2.8%).[95] This was also reported in other retrospective cohort studies.[81,98,102] Because abruptions are more frequent among women aged over 40 years than among younger patients, 2.03% vs. 0.13%,[95] and placenta previa is more common, they could contribute to this higher rate of bleeding. Older women also have higher risks for vasculopathy, and recognized bleeding from abruptions and placenta previa may occur more frequently.[100]

Adverse perinatal outcomes due to advanced maternal age

Early and late fetal loss

Early pregnancy loss is more common among older women because of the increased risk of aneuploidy (Fig. 54.6). As many as 50% of first-trimester spontaneous abortions are the result of chromosomal abnormalities.[103] Although first-trimester loss is approximately 15% after recognized pregnancy in younger women, it may be as high as 25% in women aged over 40 years.[104]

Although the fetal death rate decreased from the 1960s to the 1990s, the fetal death rate increased with increasing maternal age. Women aged 40 years or older had twice the fetal death rate compared with women younger than 30 years, even after controlling for recognized coexisting conditions that contribute to fetal death.[79] This death rate included congenital malformations. Factors contributing to fetal death are influenced by maternal age because those factors include multiple gestation, hypertension, diabetes mellitus, placenta previa, placenta abruption, previous abortion, and previous fetal death. The cause of these fetal deaths is uncertain, but it is very possibly related to increasing maternal vascular disease with increasing age.

Low birthweight

Low birthweight is another adverse perinatal outcome for older women studied and reported from the Swedish Medical Birth Register in a population-based cohort study. As stated earlier, although taken from a Scandinavian country where 95% or more of pregnant women receive antenatal care, confounding factors related to medical and socioeconomic factors were controlled. Adverse outcomes included very low birthweight and very preterm delivery.[97,101] Others have reported a rate of 10.15% for low birthweight infants in older women versus 5.92% for those less than 40 years of age.[95] Women over 50 years, compared with women aged 20–29 years, 30–39 years, and 40–49 years, had an increasing incidence of low birthweight infants. The rates of very preterm and small for gestational age neonates as well as fetal mortality were significantly higher for women aged over 50 years, possibly related to assisted reproductive technologies.[87] In another retrospective study of nulliparous women aged 35 years or older and a younger group of women between the ages of 25 and 29 years, the older aged women had higher incidences of neonatal complications, including lower birthweight and neonatal intensive care unit (NICU) admissions.[81] This is not surprising because older women tend to have a higher incidence of medical complications. Whether this is enhanced by age itself is still somewhat controversial, although there are several studies suggesting that age, in and of itself, is a predisposing factor, perhaps resulting from suboptimal uteroplacental blood flow from underlying maternal vascular disease.[101] In most of these studies, smoking was a controlled variable. One other complication is placenta previa, which may be increased in multiparous women related to increased parity, uterine myomas, and uterine scarring from prior surgeries, and may be responsible for low birthweight infants (Fig. 54.8, Table 54.11).

Fetal death

Perinatal mortality rate (500 g and over in the first week of life) was 28.6 per 1000 live births for older women compared with 10.8/1000 for younger women. This persisted even when corrected for congenital malformations (18.7 vs. 7.5%).[95] Others have confirmed higher adjusted odds ratios for perinatal mortality, perinatal death, and intrauterine fetal death with increasing maternal age.[37,90,97] Suboptimal uteroplacental blood flow from underlying maternal vascular disease may be responsible for the increase in perinatal mortality[101] as well as the increase in chromosomally abnormal fetuses.

Table 54.11 Adverse neonatal outcomes for women aged > 35 years.

Event	Risk	Reference
Fetal death at > 24 weeks		
Age 35–39 years	RR 1.23 (1.17–1.30)*	37
Age 40–44 years	RR 1.62 (1.48–1.76)*	37
Age 45–49 years	RR 2.40 (1.77–3.27)*	37
Fetal death	OR 1.41 (1.17–1.70)*	97
Low birthweight	OR 1.28 (1.20–1.36)*	97

OR, odds ratio; RR, relative risk; *significant difference.

Other adverse outcomes

Other more common adverse outcomes include admission to the intensive care unit in 16.2% of neonates from women over 40 years compared with 12.5% of neonates born to women aged less than 40 years.[81,98] Low Apgar scores and meconium were also found among these neonates from older women.[98] Intrapartum late decelerations or scalp pH of less than 7.2 are more frequent among women aged over 40 years (16.1% vs. 8.6%).[95]

Taking care of older patients

The elderly gravida deserves special attention. First of all, genetic counseling should be provided to all gravidas over 35 years of age at delivery. Options for prenatal diagnosis should be discussed in detail and offered in a timely manner. A detailed history and physical examination should be performed to determine the presence of other medical disorders and family history that may place the patient at increased risk of complications, i.e., cardiovascular disease, autoimmune disease. Any medical illness or chronic disease should be evaluated and followed closely, e.g., elevated blood pressure. Appropriate consultation with medical specialists should be

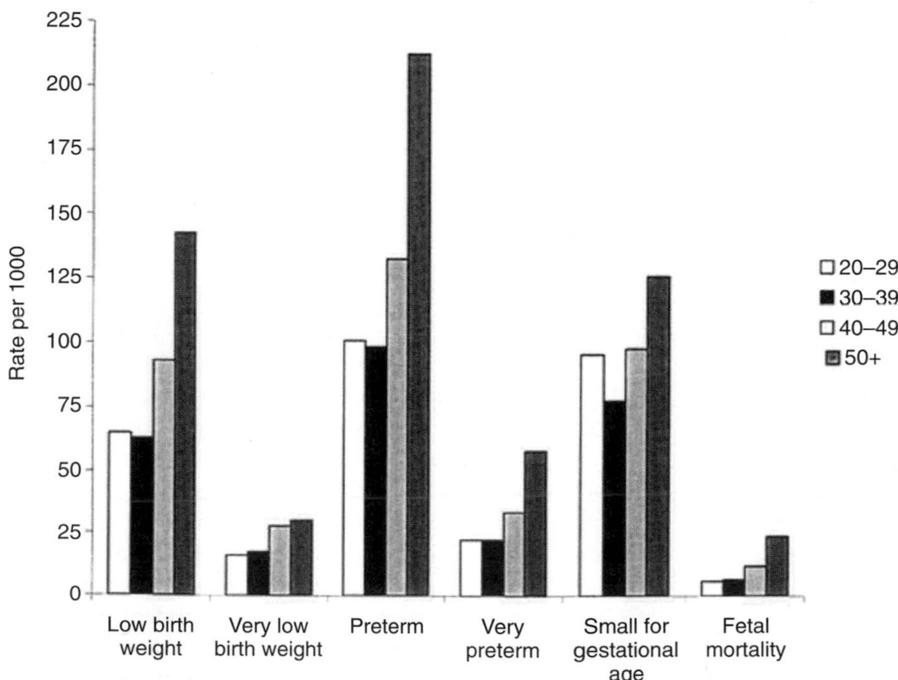

Figure 54.8 Crude rates for fetal morbidity and mortality among singletons by maternal age in the United States, 1997–1999 (from ref. 87 with permission).

obtained when necessary and in conjunction with a maternal–fetal medicine subspecialist. There should be a low threshold to screen for disorders such as diabetes and thyroid disease. Carers should be knowledgeable about their patients' medications and impact on the fetus and pregnancy. Fortunately, most older patients have more normal balanced diets, and the more educated patient will be easily convinced to abandon bad habits such as cigarette smoking. It should not be forgotten that psychosocial support is as important for the older gravida as it is for the adolescent patient. Perhaps it is even more important as there is a tendency to believe that older women have planned pregnancies and therefore do not require additional psychosocial support. However, fear of an abnormal fetus, concerns about raising a child at an older age, and anxiety over the integration of a child into an established career path may be encountered more often in today's times. Finally, preparation for the birth and subsequent childrearing issues should not be forgotten when taking care of the elderly gravida.

Key points

1 Pregnancy at the extremes of reproductive age is more hazardous than that not at extreme ages.

2 Adverse outcomes from pregnancies at the extremes of maternal age are influenced by a multitude of variables that must be controlled in order to determine the real risks from younger or older maternal age.

3 Over one million teenagers become pregnant in the USA each year.

4 The teenage pregnancy rate in the USA far exceeds that in most developed countries.

5 The teenage birth rate decreased to 43/1000 women in 2002.

6 The highest rise in teenage pregnancies is among Hispanics.

7 Adverse pregnancy outcomes among adolescents are not due to biologic risks secondary to their age, but to poor psychosocial environments.

8 Risk factors that contribute to teenage pregnancies include black and Hispanic race, substance abuse, low socioeconomic status, lack of support from parents or the father of the baby, poor self-esteem, and poor school performance.

9 The major risk to adolescents from pregnancy is preeclampsia.

10 Adverse outcomes not clearly shown to be increased in adolescents include maternal mortality, perinatal mortality, preterm labor, preterm birth, preterm rupture of membranes, low birthweight, and Cesarean section.

11 Risk factors contributing to adverse pregnancy outcomes in teenagers include anemia, poor nutrition, late prenatal care, drug use, and infection.

12 Teenage pregnancies may be reduced through sex education, school-based clinics, emergency contraception, regular contraception, and abortion.

13 Delayed childbearing is more acceptable today because women have better access to contraception, abortion is a realistic option, prenatal diagnosis minimizes the risks of having an abnormal child, and improvements in medical care enable older women to consider pregnancy.

14 Risks to older gravidas result primarily from underlying medical illnesses such as hypertension and diabetes.

15 Access to good healthcare will minimize an older woman's pregnancy risks.

16 Older women have a clear and well-documented decline in fertility, whereas their risk of aneuploidy rises.

17 Older gravidas need to be counseled that they have an increased risk of multiple gestation, mortality, Cesarean section delivery, operative vaginal delivery, preeclampsia, eclampsia, postpartum hemorrhage, dysfunctional labor, induction of labor, preterm delivery, placenta previa, and antepartum bleeding.

18 The increased risk to older women of Cesarean section delivery is not clear, but could be related to higher rates of fetal growth restriction, maternal medical illness complications, failed inductions, and possibly a lower threshold for operative delivery from a perceived concern for the older pregnant woman.

19 Older gravidas need to be informed that they have increased neonatal risks, including early fetal loss, low birthweight, fetal death, admission to the intensive care nursery, low Apgar scores, meconium, and fetal distress in labor.

20 Older pregnant women would benefit from care from a team of physicians, including maternal–fetal subspecialists, internal medicine subspecialists, and social workers.

References

1 Grimes DA. The morbidity and mortality of pregnancy: still risky business. *Am J Obstet Gynecol* 1994;170(5):1489–1494.
2 Chang J, Elam-Evans LD, Berg CJ, et al. Pregnancy-related mortality surveillance – United States, 1991–1999. *MMWR Surveill Summ* 2003;52(2):1–8.
3 Ahmad K. Pregnancy complications kill 70 000 teenagers a year. *Lancet* 2004;363(9421):1616.
4 Reichman NE, Pagnini DL. Maternal age and birth outcomes: data from New Jersey. *Fam Plann Perspect* 1997;29(6):268–272.
5 Creasy RK, Gummer BA, Liggins GC. A system for predicting spontaneous preterm birth. *Obstet Gynecol* 1980;55:692.
6 Loto OM, Ezechi OC, Kalu BK, et al. Poor obstetric performance of teenagers: is it age- or quality of care-related? *J Obstet Gynecol* 2004;24(4):395–398.
7 Alexander CS, Guyer B. Adolescent pregnancy: occurrence and consequences. *Pediatr Ann* 1993;22(2):85–88.
8 Mittendorfer-Rutz E, Rasmussen F, Wasserman D. Restricted fetal growth and adverse maternal psychosocial and socioeconomic conditions as risk factors for suicidal behaviour of offspring: a cohort study. *Lancet* 2004;364(9440):1135–1140.
9 Hollingsworth DR, Felice M. Teenage pregnancy: a multiracial sociologic problem. *Am J Obstet Gynecol* 1986;155(4):741–746.
10 Morgan C, Chapar GN, Fisher M. Psychosocial variables associated with teenage pregnancy. *Adolescence* 1995;30(118): 277–289.
11 Singh S, Darroch JE. Adolescent pregnancy and childbearing: levels and trends in developed countries. *Fam Plann Perspect* 2000;32(1):14–23.
12 UNICEF. *A league table of teenage births in rich nations*. Innocenti Report Card No. 3. Florence: UNICEF Innocenti Research Centre, 2001.
13 Crosby RA, DiClemente RJ, Wingood GM, et al. Correlates of unplanned and unwanted pregnancy among African–American female teens. *Am J Prev Med* 2003;25(3):255–258.
14 Trad PV. Abortion and pregnant adolescents. *Fam Soc* 1993;74(7):397–409.
15 Centers for Disease Control and Prevention. Trends in sexual risk behaviors among high school students – United States, 1991–2001. *Morb Mortal Wkly Rep* 2002;51:856–859.
16 Martin JA, Hamilton BE, Sutton PD, et al. *Births: final data for 2002*. National Vital Statistics Reports, Vol. 52, No. 10, December 17, 2003.
17 Arias E, MacDorman MF, Strobino DM, Guyer B. Annual summary of vital statistics – 2002. *Pediatrics* 112(8): 1215–1230.
18 Gilbert W, Jandial D, Field N, et al. Birth outcomes in teenage pregnancies. *J Matern Fetal Neonatal Med* 2004; 16(5):265–270.
19 Chang SC, O'Brien KO, Nathanson MS, et al. Characteristics and risk factors for adverse birth outcomes in pregnant black adolescents. *J Pediatr* 2003;143(2):250–257.
20 Hemminki E, Gissler M. Births by younger and older mothers in a population with late and regulated childbearing: Finland 1991. *Acta Obstet Gynecol Scand* 1996:75(1):19–27.
21 Zabin LS, Hardy JB, Smith EA. Substance use and its relation to sexual activity among inner-city adolescents. *J Adolesc Health Care* 1986;7:320–331.
22 Mott FL, Haurin RJ. Linkages between sexual activity and alcohol and drug use among American adolescents. *Fam Plann Perspect* 1988;20:128–136.
23 Quinlivan JA, Evans SF. The impact of continuing illegal drug use on teenage pregnancy outcomes – a prospective cohort study. *Br J Obstet Gynaecol* 2002;109(10):1148–1153.
24 Oman RF, Vesely SK, Aspy CB, et al. The association between multiple youth assets and sexual behavior. *Am J Health Promot* 2004;19(1):12–18.
25 Durant R, Knight J, Goodman E. Factors associated with aggressive and delinquent behaviors among patients attending an adolescent medicine clinic. *J Adolesc Health* 1997;21(5):303–308.
26 Paulson MJ, Coombs RH, Richardson MA. School performance, academic aspirations, and drug use among children and adolescents. *J Drug Educ* 1990;20:289–303.
27 Kaufman J. Teenage parents and their offspring. *Ann NY Acad Sci* 1996; 789:17–30.
28 Rainey DY, Steven-Simon C, Kaplan DW. Are adolescents who report prior sexual abuse are at high risk for pregnancy. *Child Abuse Negl* 1995;19:1283–1288.
29 Stevens-Simon C, McAnarney E. Childhood victimization relationship to adolescent pregnancy outcome. *Child Abuse Negl* 1994;18:569–575.
30 Stevens-Simon C, Reichert S. Sexual abuse adolescent pregnancy and child abuse. *Arch Pediatr Adolesc Med* 1994;148:23–27.
31 Roberts R, O'Connor T, Dunn J, Golding J. The effects of child sexual abuse in later family life; mental heath, parenting and adjustment of offspring. *Child Abuse Negl* 2004:28(5):525–545.
32 Flanagan P, Kokotailo P. Adolescent pregnancy and substance use. *Clin Perinatol* 1999; 26(1):185–200.
33 Alexander GR, Kogan M, Bader D, et al. US birth weight/gestational age-specific neonatal mortality: 1995–1997 rates for whites, Hispanics and blacks. *Pediatrics* 2003;111:61–66.
34 Mackay AP, Berg CJ, Atrash HK. Pregnancy-related mortality from preeclampsia and eclampsia. *Obstet Gynecol* 2001; 97:533–538.
35 Cunnington AJ. What's so bad about teenage pregnancy? *J Fam Plann Reprod Health Care* 2001;27(1):36–41.
36 Berenson AB, Wiemann CM, McCombs SL. Adverse perinatal outcomes in young adolescents. *J Reprod Med* 1997;42(9): 559–564.
37 Canterino JC, Ananth CV, Smulian J, et al. Maternal age and risk of fetal death in singleton gestations: United States, 1995–2000. *J Matern Fetal Neonatal Med* 2004; 15:193–197.
38 Jolly MC, Sebire N, Harris J, et al. Obstetric risks of pregnancy in women less than 18 years old. *Obstet Gynecol* 2000; 96:962–966.
39 Hediger ML, Scholl TO, Schall JI, Krueger PM. Young maternal age and preterm labor. *Ann Epidemiol* 1997;7(6):400–406.
40 Eure CR, Lindsay MK, Graves WL. Risk of adverse pregnancy outcomes in young adolescent parturients in an inner-city hospital. *Am J Obstet Gynecol* 2002; 186(5):918–920.
41 Olausson PM, Cnattingius S, Goldenberg RL. Determinants of poor pregnancy outcomes among teenagers in Sweden. *Obstet Gynecol* 1997;89(3):451–457.
42 Fraser AM, Brockert JE, Ward RH. Association of young maternal age with adverse reproductive outcomes. *N Engl J Med* 1995;332 (17):113–117.
43 Yoder BA, Young MK. Neonatal outcomes of teenage pregnancy in a military population. *Obstet Gynecol* 1997;90:500–506.
44 Gale R, Seidman DS, Dollberg S, et al. Is teenage pregnancy a neonatal risk factor? *J Adolesc Health Care* 1989;10:404–408.
45 Perry RL, Mannino B, Hediger ML, Scholl TO. Pregnancy in early adolescence: are there obstetric risks? *J Matern Fetal Med* 1996;5(6):333–339.

46 Gortzak-Uzan L, Hallak M, Press F, et al. Teenage pregnancy: risk factors for adverse perinatal outcome. *J Matern Fetal Med* 2001;10(6):393–397.
47 Ananth CV, Balasubramanian B, Demissie K, Kinzler WL. Small-for-gestational-age births in the United States: an age-period-cohort analysis. *Epidemiology* 2004;15(1):28–35.
48 Moerman ML. Growth of the birth canal in adolescent girls. *Am J Obstet Gynecol* 1982;143(5):528–532.
49 Stevens-Simon C, McAnarney ER. Skeletal maturity and growth of adolescent mothers: relationship to pregnancy outcome. *J Adolesc Health* 1993;14(6):428–432.
50 Sunday-Adeoye IM, Okonta P, Twomey D. Symphysiotomy at the Mater Misericordiae Hospital Afikpo, Ebonyi State of Nigeria (1982–1999): a review of 1013 cases. *J Obstet Gynaecol* 2004;24(5):525–529.
51 Chang SC, O'Brien KO, Nathanson MS, et al. Hemoglobin concentrations influence birth outcomes in pregnant African–American adolescents. *J Nutr* 2003;133(7):2348–2355.
52 Steer PJ. Maternal hemoglobin concentration and birth weight. *Am J Clin Nutr* 2000;71(Suppl):1285S–1287S.
53 Lucas AR, Crowson CS, O'Fallon WM, Melton LJ 3rd. The ups and downs of anorexia nervosa. *Int J Eat Disord* 1999;26(4): 397–405.
54 Howie LD, Parker JD, Schoendord KC. Excessive maternal weight gain patterns in adolescents. *J Am Diet Assoc* 2003; 103(2):1653–1657.
55 Wiemann CM, Berenson AB, Pino LG, McCombs SL. Factors associated with adolescents' risk for late entry into prenatal care. *Fam Plann Perspect* 1997;29(6):273 276.
56 Kogan MD, Kotelchuck M, Johnson S. Racial differences in late prenatal care visits. *J Perinatol* 1993;13(1):14–21.
57 Kost K, Landry DJ, Darroch JE. Predicting maternal behaviors during pregnancy: does intention status matter? *Fam Plann Perspect* 1998;30(2):79–88.
58 Petersen DJ, Alexander GR. Seasonal variation in adolescent conceptions, induced abortions, and late initiation of prenatal care. *Public Health Rep* 1992;107(6):701–706.
59 Johnston LD, O'Malley PM, Bachman JG. *Drug use among American high school seniors, college students and young adults, 1975–1990.* Vol. 1, High school seniors. US Department of Health and Human Services Publication (ADM) 91-1813. Rockville, MD: National Institute on Drug Abuse, 1991.
60 Kokotailo PK, Adger H Jr, Duggan AK, et al. Cigarette, alcohol, and other drug use by school-age pregnant adolescents: prevalence, detection, and associated risk factors. *Pediatrics* 1992;90: 328–334.
61 Cornelius MD, Richarson GA, Day NL, et al. A comparison of prenatal drinking in two recent samples of adolescents and adults. *J Stud Alcohol* 1994;55:412.
62 Diclemente RJ, Wingood GM, Sionean C, et al. Association of adolescents' history of sexually transmitted disease (STD) and their current high-risk behavior and STD status: a case for intensifying clinic-based prevention efforts. *Sex Transm Dis* 2002;29(9):503–509.
63 Matson SC, Pomeranz AJ, Kamps KA. Early detection and treatment of sexually transmitted disease in pregnant adolescents of low socioeconomic status. *Clin Pediatr* 1993;32(10):609–612.
64 Niccolai LM, Ethier KA, Kershaw TS, et al. Pregnant adolescents at risk: sexual behaviors and sexually transmitted disease prevalence. *Am J Obstet Gynecol* 2003;188(1):63–70.
65 Chokephaibulkit K, Patamasucon P, List M, et al. Genital *Chlamydia trachomatis* infection in pregnant adolescents in east Tennessee: a 7-year case–control study. *J Pediatr Adolesc Gynecol* 1997;10(2):95–100.
66 Diclemente RJ, Wingood GM, Crosby RA, et al. A descriptive analysis of STD prevalence among urban pregnant African-American teens: data from a pilot study. *J Adolesc Health* 2004;34(5):376–583.
67 Berger DK, Rivera M, Perez G, Fierman A. Risk assessment for human immunodeficiency virus among pregnant Hispanic adolescents. *Adolescence* 1993;28(111):597–607.
68 Shrier LA, Goodman E, Emans SJ. Partner condom use among adolescent girls with sexually transmitted diseases. *J Adolesc Health* 1999;24(5):357–361.
69 Zorrilla C, Febo I, Ortiz I, et al. Pregnancy in perinatally HIV infected adolescents and young adults, Puerto Rico, 2002. *Morbid Mortal Wkly Rep* 2003;52(08):149–151.
70 Fielding JE, Williams CA. Adolescent pregnancy in the United States: a review and recommendations for clinicians and research needs. *Am J Prev Med* 1991;7(1):47–52.
71 Marsiglio W, Mott FL. The impact of sex education on sexual activity, contraceptive use and premarital pregnancy among American teenagers. *Fam Plann Perspect* 1986;18(4):151–162.
72 Polit DF, Kahn JR. Early subsequent pregnancy among economically disadvantaged teenage mothers. *Am J Public Health* 1986;76:167–171.
73 Quinlivan JA, Evans SF. Teenage antenatal clinics may reduce the rate of preterm birth: prospective study. *Br J Obstet Gynaecol* 2004;111:571–578.
74 Davis S. Pregnancy in adolescents. *Pediatr Clin North Am* 1989;36(3):665–680.
75 Quinlivan JA, Box H, Evans SF. Postnatal home visits in teenage mothers: a randomised controlled trial. *Lancet* 2003;361(9361): 893–900.
76 Barnet B, Arroyo C, Devoe M, Duggan AK. Reduced school dropout rates among adolescent mothers receiving school-based prenatal care. *Arch Pediatr Adolesc Med* 2004;158(3):262–268.
77 Stewart HE, Gold MA, Parker AM. The impact of using emergency contraception on reproductive health outcomes: a retrospective review in an urban adolescent clinic. *J Pediatr Adolesc Gynecol* 2003;16(5):313–318.
78 Freeman EW, Rickels K, Sondheimer SJ. The impact of medical and social factors in teenage pregnancy. *Am J Gynecol Health* 1988;2(1):5–14.
79 Fretts RC, Schmittdiel J, McLean FH, et al. Increased maternal age and the risk of fetal death. *N Engl J Med* 1995;333(15): 953–957.
80 Roberts CL, Algert CS, March LM. Delayed childbearing – are there any risks? *Med J Aust* 1994;160(9):539–544.
81 Prysak M, Lorenz RP, Kisly A. Pregnancy outcome in nulliparous women 35 years and older. *Obstet Gynecol* 1995;85(1):65–70.
82 Berkowitz GS, Skovron ML, Lapinski RH, Berkowitz RL. Delayed childbearing and the outcome of pregnancy. *N Engl J Med* 1990;322(10):659–664.
83 Heffner LJ. Advanced maternal age – how old is too old? *N Engl J Med* 2004;351(19):1927–1929.
84 Stein ZA. A woman's age: childbearing and child rearing. *Am J* Epidemiol 1985;121(3):327–342.
85 Hassold T, Chiu D. Maternal age-specific rates of numerical chromosome abnormalities with special reference to trisomy. *Hum Genet* 1985;70:11–17.
86 Cuckle HS, Wald NJ, Thompson SG. Estimating a woman's risk of having a pregnancy associated with Down's syndrome using

her age and serum alpha-fetoprotein level. *Br J Obstet Gynaecol* 1987;94(5):387–402.

87 Salihu HM, Shumpert MN, Slay M, et al. Childbearing beyond maternal age 50 and fetal outcomes in the United States. *Obstet Gynecol* 2003;102(5):1006–1014.

88 O'Reilly-Green C, Cohen WR. Pregnancy in women aged 40 and older. *Obstet Gynecol Clin North Am* 1993;20(2):313–331.

89 Kochanek KD, Murphy SL, Anderson RN, Scott C. Deaths: final data for 2002. *Natl Vital Stat Rep* 2004;53(5):1–115.

90 Jacobsson B, Ladfors L, Milsom I. Advanced maternal age and adverse perinatal outcome. *Obstet Gynecol* 2004;104(4): 727–733.

91 Callaghan WM, Berg CJ. Pregnancy-related mortality among women aged 35 years and older, United States, 1991–1997. *Obstet Gynecol* 2003;102:1015–1021.

92 Heffner LJ, Elkin E. Fretts RC. Impact of labor induction, gestational age, and maternal age on cesarean delivery rates. *Obstet Gynecol* 2003;102(2):287–293.

93 Ecker JL, Chen KT, Cohen AP, et al. Increased risk of cesarean delivery with advancing maternal age indications and associated factors in nulliparous women. *Am J Obstet Gynecol* 2001; 185(4):883–887.

94 Dulitzki M, Soriano D, Schiff E, et al. Effect of very advanced maternal age on pregnancy outcome and rate of cesarean delivery. *Obstet Gynecol* 1998;92(6):935–939.

95 Milner M, Barry-Kinsella C, Unwin A, Harrison RF. The impact of maternal age on pregnancy and its outcome. *Int J Gynaecol Obstet* 1992;38(4):281–286.

96 Gilbert WM, Nesbitt TS, Danielsen B. Childbearing beyond age 40: pregnancy outcome in 24,032 cases. *Obstet Gynecol* 1999;93:9–14.

97 Jolly M, Sebire N, Harris J, et al. The risks associated with pregnancy in women aged 35 years or older. *Hum Reprod* 2000;15(11):2433–2437.

98 Bianco A, Stone J, Lynch L, et al. Pregnancy outcome at age 40 and older. *Obstet Gynecol* 1996;87(6):917–922.

99 Friedman EA, Sachtleben MR. Relation of maternal age to the course of labor. *Am J Obstet Gynecol* 1965;91:915–924.

100 Ananth CV, Wilcox AJ, Savitz DA, et al. Effect of maternal age and parity on the risk of uteroplacental bleeding disorders in pregnancy. *Obstet Gynecol* 1996;88:511–516.

101 Cnattingius S, Forman MR, Berendes HW, Isotalo L. Delayed childbearing and risk of adverse perinatal outcome. *JAMA* 1992;268:886–890.

102 Williams MA, Lieberman E, Mittendord R, et al. Risk factors for abruptio placentae. *Am J Epidemiol* 1991;134(9):965–972.

103 Kajii T, Ferrier A, Niikawa N, et al. Anatomic and chromosomal abnormalities in 639 spontaneous abortuses. *Hum Genet* 1980;55:87.

104 Newcomb WW, Rodriguez M, Johnson JW. Reproduction in the older gravida. A literature review. *J Reprod Med* 1991; 36(12):839–845.

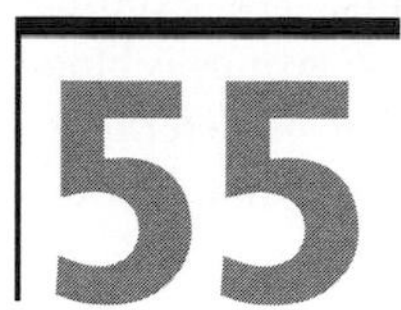

Essentials in biostatistics and perinatal epidemiology

Paula K. Roberson and Benjamin P. Sachs

The ability to evaluate the medical literature and to incorporate findings into clinical practice has become a cornerstone of medical education. Increasingly, practice guidelines are based on reliable evidence of clinical efficacy and cost-effectiveness. Evidence-based medicine is the process of systematically finding, appraising, and using contemporaneous research findings as the basis for clinical practice.[1] The purpose of this chapter is to review the epidemiologic and statistical tools needed to evaluate medical literature. Clinicians can then recommend practice patterns based on the strength of the evidence.

Epidemiology

Understanding the strengths and weaknesses of study design and the quality of evidence provided is critical in evaluating a research article. Epidemiology is concerned with the assessment of exposure and outcome. Exposure may be to a drug, treatment, therapy, surgical procedure, or genetic factor and the related outcome may be disease, morbidity, mortality, or side-effects. The basic design strategies used in epidemiologic research can be broadly characterized according to whether the investigation focuses on describing the distributions of disease (descriptive epidemiology) or on elucidating the determinants of disease (analytic epidemiology).

Descriptive epidemiology describes the general characteristics of exposure and outcome, particularly in relation to person, place, and time. Indices of person include basic demographic factors such as age, race, sex, marital status, or occupation as well as lifestyle factors such as diet or use of medication. Characteristics of place refer to the geographic distribution of an outcome such as variations among or within countries or between urban and rural areas. Descriptive studies may examine seasonal patterns or compare outcomes from different time periods. Data for descriptive studies come from diverse sources such as census records, vital statistics records, and hospital charts and office records (clinical data). Because information about many of the characteristics of person, place, and time is readily available, descriptive studies can be performed relatively quickly and inexpensively. There are three main types of descriptive study: correlational studies, case reports (or case series), and cross-sectional studies.

Correlational studies use data from entire populations to compare exposures and outcomes among different groups during the same period of time or in the same population at different times. An example is the evaluation of folic acid intake and incidence of neural tube defects. Although correlational studies are useful for the formulation of hypotheses, they cannot be used to test hypotheses because of a number of limitations inherent in their design. Correlational studies refer to whole populations rather than individuals, so it is impossible to link an exposure to an outcome in an individual person. To test a hypothesis, it is necessary to carry out analytic studies of individuals.

A *case study* is the most basic type of descriptive study of an individual, consisting of a careful, detailed report of an intervention and outcome in a single patient. The simple case report can be expanded into a case series, describing the characteristics of a number of patients with a given exposure and outcome. Although case studies and series may suggest a correlation between exposure and outcome, it is impossible to distinguish among alternative explanations without studying an adequate sample of individuals using an appropriate comparison group.

Cross-sectional surveys simultaneously assess the status of individuals with respect to the presence or absence of exposure and outcome. Because exposure and outcome are assessed simultaneously, cross-sectional surveys cannot always identify the time sequence of exposure and outcome. As with the other types of descriptive studies, cross-sectional surveys are useful for raising the possibility of an association rather than for testing a hypothesis.

Analytic epidemiology explicitly compares exposure and outcome. The investigator assembles a group of individuals for the express purpose of systematically determining whether the outcome is different in individuals who are exposed or not exposed to a factor of interest. The use of an appropriate comparison group allows the testing of epidemiologic hypotheses in analytic study designs. Analytic epidemiology can be further divided into two strategies: observational and interventional. The major difference lies in the investigator's role. In *observational studies*, the investigator merely observes the natural course of events, recording the exposure and outcome status of each individual. In *interventional studies*, the investigator allocates the exposure and then follows the subjects for the development of the outcome. Observational studies can be further divided into case–control and cohort studies.

In a case–control study, the levels of exposure of a case group or series of patients who have a particular outcome of interest are compared with those of a control group who do not have the outcome. Cohort studies classify subjects based on their exposure to a particular factor, and then study each group for the development of a particular outcome. An example of a cohort study is the examination of a potential relationship between diabetic control in the first trimester of pregnancy and the incidence of congenital anomalies. The risk factor is an abnormal glucose level in the first trimester, and the disease outcome is the presence or absence of a congenital anomaly. A relationship between blood sugar control in the first trimester and birth defects can also be examined using the case–control method. The cases are women with diabetes who had babies with congenital anomalies; control subjects are diabetic women who deliver normal infants. The exposure (outcome measure) to be compared in the two groups is blood sugar control in the first trimester, which can be determined by measuring hemoglobin A_{1c} levels, for example. In this example, although the hemoglobin A_{1c} levels are collected prospectively, the study is still analyzed as a case–control (retrospective) study.

Table 55.1 gives the basic design details of cohort and case–control studies, and Table 55.2 summarizes their relative strengths and weaknesses. Although often maligned, the case–control method has many advantages. There is a potential for bias in a case–control study but, if it is well constructed and executed, it has a great potential for economically yielding valid conclusions.

Interventional studies, often referred to as clinical trials, are studies in which the investigator assigns exposure and then follows the subjects for outcome. A comparison group is used, which may involve subjects under another treatment, test, or placebo.

Randomized controlled clinical trials, considered to be most reliable in terms of the evidence they provide, involve an investigator assigning subjects at random into an experimental group and a control (placebo or standard therapy) group. If an alternative experimental treatment is given to the comparison group, the study is called a *(randomized) comparative clinical trial*. Randomization minimizes any potential con-

Table 55.1 Study design.

	Cohort study				Case–control study	
	Disease	No disease	Total		Disease	No disease
Risk factors	A	B	A + B	Risk factors	a	b
No risk factors	C	D	C + D	No risk factors	c	d
	Total				a + c	b + d
Cohort studies compare	A/(A + B) vs. C/(C + D)			Case–control studies compare	a/(a + c) vs. b/(b + d)	

By convention, A, B, C, and D represent the total population; a, b, c, and d represent samples of the population.

Table 55.2 Relative strengths and weaknesses of observational study design.

	Cohort studies	Case–control studies
Strengths	Enable direct estimation of disease rates Less subject to recall bias	More economical Can be completed in shorter time-frame
Weaknesses	More likely to be biased in determining disease frequency Require large sample size, particularly if disease is rare More expensive May require very long time if induction time for disease development is long May pose ethical dilemmas if exposure could be removed Subject to losing subjects in follow-up	Greater risk of recall bias Identification of appropriate control group may be more difficult

founding factors and ensures that participants are as similar as possible with respect to all variables except for the intervention of interest.

Evaluation of epidemiological studies

Precision, validity, and bias

Both precision and validity are important concepts in a critical literature review of study design. *Validity* refers to the extent that the outcome variable actually measures the effect of interest. High validity implies a lack of systematic error or *bias*. *Precision* refers to the consistency or closeness of repeated measurements of outcome to each other. Note that it is possible to have high precision and poor validity or vice versa. Kleinbaum and colleagues[2] helped to clarify the concepts of precision and validity with a target-shooting analogy: "Validity is concerned with whether or not one is aiming at the correct bull's-eye; precision is concerned with individual variation from shot to shot, given the actual bull's-eye that is being considered."

Assessments of validity often refer to indicators of internal and external validity. *Internal validity* generally refers to validity within the study group itself and the larger group from which it is drawn. It is influenced by aspects of study design that include the subject selection, quality and appropriateness of exposure and outcome measures, and the presence of confounding factors. Limitations in internal validity most often result from selection, information, or confounding biases. *External validity* refers to the extent to which findings can be generalized to a wider population. External validity is most influenced by the comparability of the pool of potential study participants with the population for whom the generalization is intended. For example, the findings of a study conducted in an academic medical center may not apply to other clinical settings. Some investigators view external validity as nonexistent, believing that little justification exists for generalizing study results beyond the study population.

There are a seemingly infinite number of potential sources of bias that can arise in epidemiological studies. Much of an epidemiologist's effort is spent in attempting to identify and overcome sources of bias. Sackett[3] discusses a number of the most frequently encountered causes of bias.

Confounding

A *confounding factor* (or *confounder*) can be defined as a risk factor for disease, other than the exposure under study, that is unequally distributed between the cases and the comparison or control groups. Confounding is a form of bias that can occur in both case–control and cohort studies and can lead the unwary investigator to inaccurate conclusions. Table 55.3 gives four characteristics of a potential confounding variable, as described by Rothman.[4] Many factors, including age, race, and socioeconomic status, are risk factors for prematurity.

Table 55.3 Rothman's four characteristics of a potential confounding variable.[4]

A risk factor for disease but not necessarily an actual cause of the disease
Linked to the exposure under study
Cannot be an intermediate step in the chain of events between the exposure and the disease outcome
Must be associated with both the disease and the exposure under study

Table 55.4 Techniques to reduce confounding effects.

Restriction limits the admission criteria into the study with respect to known potential confounding factors
Matching involves comparison (control) groups that are identical to cases with respect to the matched variables (this approach may be very costly and requires a specialized matched analysis)
Randomization involves assigning subjects to different study groups on a random basis, in an effort to distribute known and unknown confounding factors equally among groups

When these risk factors are linked with the exposure of interest they may be confounding factors. For example, in a study of the efficacy of home uterine contraction monitoring in preventing prematurity, women who have insurance may be more likely to use such a device and, therefore, without careful development of eligibility criteria, the control group might include more women of a lower socioeconomic status. Because socioeconomic status is an index of risk for prematurity and, in this study, is linked with the exposure of interest (home monitoring), such a study would be confounded by the distribution of socioeconomic status. Table 55.4 lists techniques that can be used in the design or analysis stages of a study to reduce the effects of confounding.

Screening tests

Screening tests are the basic tools of the clinician. The fundamental concepts of screening tests are the same regardless of the test, e.g., an analysis of a hematocrit or the identification of patients at risk for premature labor. In any population, some people have a certain disease and others do not; the challenge is to identify the diseased individuals at the earliest opportunity.

Sensitivity is the probability of correctly identifying a sick individual. *Specificity* is the probability of correctly identifying a healthy individual. For example, if a normal hematocrit is defined as being above 40%, the specificity of the test is poor because many healthy people would be missed. Conversely, if an abnormal hematocrit is defined as being less than

Table 55.5 Relationship of sensitivity, specificity, and predictive values.

Risk factors	Disease	No disease
Yes	a	b
No	c	d

Predictive value negative = d/(c + d); predictive value positive = a/(a + b); sensitivity = a/(a + c); specificity = d/(d + b).

30%, the sensitivity is poor because many anemic people would be excluded. Defining the normal cutoff value affects both the sensitivity and specificity of a screening test but in opposite directions.

The *positive predictive value* is defined as the proportion of individuals with a specific risk factor who have the disease. The *negative predicative value* is the converse, i.e., the proportion of those without the risk factor who are disease free. The relationship between sensitivity, specificity, and predictive values is shown in Table 55.5. The predictive value of a screening test depends on the sensitivity and specificity of the test as well as the prevalence of the disease in question. Thus, the predictive value is not a measure of the test's accuracy. The positive predictive value may be low because the test results do not adequately reflect the true disease status *or* because the disease prevalence is low. The same statistical measures are used to evaluate diagnostic tests, although the numeric values for a given test will differ in the two settings because the applicable population will be different. For a full discussion of the statistical principles of screening and diagnostic tests, including the design of studies to evaluate them, see Pepe.[5]

Null hypothesis: type I and type II errors

The null hypothesis is the focus of statistical testing in biomedical research. In two-group comparisons, this hypothesis generally stipulates that there is no difference between the two groups with respect to the mean of a variable of interest. Thus, rejection of the null hypothesis implies an identifiable difference in the group means beyond what might be reasonably attributed to chance.

The common decision-making tool for evaluating the null hypothesis is the *P*-value, i.e., the probability that a difference at least as great as that observed would occur by chance if the null hypothesis were true. Although other criteria may be used, the most frequently applied convention is that a *P*-value of less than 0.05 leads to rejection of the null hypothesis. If the *P*-value is greater than 0.05, and therefore not significant, the null hypothesis is not rejected. The maximum *P*-value that will be declared significant is called the *alpha level* of the hypothesis test. Table 55.6 defines the possible errors in decision-making that can occur. Type I and type II errors have a clear relationship. The level of either error depends on the cutoff value chosen to define significance. Thus, the type II error is larger if the type I error is reduced and vice versa.

Table 55.6 Possible types of error associated with hypothesis testing.

Statistical testing decision	Truth (null hypothesis true)	Truth (null hypothesis false)
Do not reject null hypothesis	No error	Type II error (β)
Reject null hypothesis	Type I error (α)	No error ($1 - \beta =$ power)

Table 55.7 Factors relating to power and required sample size of a specific statistical test.

Alpha level (type I error)
Power (1 – type II error)
Difference to detect at specified power
Standard deviation
Sample size

Power and sample size

The *power* of a test is its ability to detect a difference between the groups being tested at a given level of statistical significance. In other words, it is the probability of rejecting the null hypothesis given that the alternative is true. For a given statistical probability distribution, the five factors listed in Table 55.7 are related such that, given four of the five, one can solve for the fifth. This implies that the power is not an absolute value but, for fixed alpha, standard deviation and detectable difference is a (non-linear) function of sample size (and vice versa).

The major factor under the control of the cohort study investigator is generally the sample size. As the sample size is increased, it is possible to detect smaller differences with a given power. In a case–control study, both increasing the sample size and improving the ratio of control subjects to case subjects enhance study power.[6–8] In some settings, the measurement procedures can be modified in ways that reduce the variance.

The failure to consider statistical power is one of the most frequent errors in study design.[9,10] Freiman and colleagues[11] reported an analysis of 71 "negative" randomized controlled clinical trials published in peer review journals and found that 50 (70%) of the trials used had insufficient power to detect a 50% improvement in outcome with the treatment. Similarly, DerSimonian and colleagues[12] reported the results of a survey of methods in 67 clinical trials published in four prestigious journals; the statistical power of the trial for detecting treatment effect was discussed in only 12% of the articles. For practical purposes, sample size and power calculations are most often derived from commercial computer software programs or existing references.[7,8,13–16] These calculations should always be based on the same statistical methods that the investigator plans to use for data analysis at the conclusion of the study.

Comparative measures of effect

In epidemiology, common comparative measures of effect include the absolute risk difference, the risk ratio (relative risk), the odds ratio, and the attributable proportion. These might be used, for example, to assess the effect of maternal smoking (exposure) on the risk of premature birth.

The *risk difference* is the proportion of diseased individuals among the exposed subjects minus the proportion of diseased individuals among the unexposed subjects.

The *risk ratio* is the proportion of diseased individuals among the exposed subjects divided by the proportion of diseased individuals among the unexposed subjects.

The *odds ratio* (OR), or relative odds, is the ratio of the odds of disease in exposed individuals relative to the unexposed, or, equivalently, the ratio of the odds of exposure among diseased individuals relative to healthy individuals. The OR is often used as an approximation of the risk ratio for case–control studies, in which the risk ratio cannot be measured directly. This approximation is a good one when the prevalence of the disease is low (the "rare disease assumption"). For further details, see Cornfield's landmark publication[17] or most epidemiologic texts.

The *attributable proportion* (or *etiologic fraction*) is an expression of the proportion of the cases of disease resulting from exposure. It combines risk factor prevalence with the risk ratio to better assess the public health impact of the association. A full discussion may be found in Benichou.[18]

The null value for the risk difference and attributable risk is 0, whereas the null value for the risk ratio and OR is 1. When a confidence interval crosses these values, the null hypothesis is not rejected at the given level of significance. For example, a relative risk of 3.2 (95% confidence limits from 0.8 to 4.0) is not statistically significant at a *P*-value of less than 0.05.

Statistical testing and confidence intervals

A number of factors must be taken into account in selecting the best statistical test or group of tests. All statistical test procedures are founded in probability theory, and the validity of each test is intimately linked to assumptions about how the data relate to the probability underlying the test. Features of the study design and data are also important in statistical testing, including the nature of the exposure and outcome variables, the distribution of values of the variables under study, whether matching was included in the study design, whether measures are independent or repeated for a particular individual, and the potential confounding factors for each association tested.

For the purposes of critical literature review, Table 55.8 outlines categories of statistical tests that are used in examining various combinations of exposure (explanatory) and outcome (response) data or variables. A categorical or discrete variable is able to assume only a finite or countable number of outcomes. One example is marital status, where the outcome can be single, married, divorced, or widowed. A continuous variable such as weight, height, or gestational age can take on any value within a specified interval or continuum. Although Table 55.8 helps to narrow the choice of statistical tests to the appropriate group, the process of selecting the best test requires a

Table 55.8 Alternative univariate and multivariate statistical methods used in hypothesis testing of continuous and/or categorical data.

Exposure (explanatory) variables	Outcome (response) variables	
	Categorical	Continuous
Single		
Categorical	Contingency table (chi-squared or Fisher's exact text) or normal approximation (Z-statistic)	Z-statistic, Student's *t*-test, ANOVA, or nonparametric analogs
Continuous	Z-statistic, Student's *t*-test, ANOVA, or nonparametric	Linear regression, correlation coefficient
Multiple*		
Categorical	Stratification or loglinear analysis or logistic regression	ANOVA
Continuous	Logistic regression	Multiple regression
Mixed	Logistic regression	ANCOVA

ANCOVA, analysis of covariance; ANOVA, analysis of variance.
*Adapted from ref. 29.

broader knowledge of the principles of study design and biostatistical testing.

To choose the optimal statistical test, the investigator must consider the question being asked, the study design, the nature of the variables, and the assumptions of the different statistical test procedures. Because the appropriate use of statistical tests is not a trivial task, we recommend that statistical testing be performed by an individual with expertise in biostatistics and that investigators actively cultivate a collaboration with such an individual. A number of excellent general texts cogently discuss the principles of biostatistics that are relevant to clinical research.[19–24] The take-home message concerning epidemiologic analyses was stated well by Schoolman et al:[25] "Good answers come from good questions, not from esoteric analyses."

Some authors argue that confidence intervals should be reported to the exclusion of hypothesis testing and *P*-values. However, there is a one-to-one relationship between confidence intervals and hypothesis testing, and the choice of which to report should be tailored to the context of the study. Measures of effect and 95% confidence intervals (consistent with $P = 0.05$) offer the advantage of being more informative than *P*-values alone but, given the point estimate and standard error, it is possible to calculate confidence intervals of whatever confidence limit is desired. A more extensive discussion is provided by van Belle et al.[24]

Multiple comparisons

Some investigators appear to approach each epidemiologic study as a series of statistical tests in the quest for a *P*-value less than 0.05. These "fishing expeditions" are often characterized by indiscriminate statistical comparisons that are frequently unfounded in prior hypotheses or biological plausibility. The criticism of this approach is based on the increasing probability that a "statistically significant" *P*-value is likely to be obtained by chance alone (i.e., in the absence of biological significance) if repetitive statistical tests are performed. This phenomenon is called an alpha (type I) error. If the significance level is set at 5% ($P < 0.05$), the expected frequency of this event is 1 in 20 tests performed. Incomplete reporting of statistical methods further complicates the interpretation of "significant" *P*-values; there is an apparent publication bias favoring positive results and leading to a reluctance to report the multiple "insignificant" comparisons that may accompany a single statistically significant association.

The multiple comparison criticism is best avoided by limiting statistical testing to factors about which a hypothesis has been formulated a priori and for which a biologically plausible explanation exists. Investigators are also encouraged: (1) to include detailed descriptions of the statistical methods and negative results as part of manuscripts that might otherwise focus only on a positive association,[26] and/or (2) to make more stringent requirements for significance or adjustments to the *P*-value obtained through multiple comparisons.[23]

Some epidemiologists view these comparisons as instrumental in the generation of new hypotheses. Feinstein and Horwitz[27] state: "Although agreement has not been reached on when and how to adjust the statistical levels of significance in a study in which multiple agents have been investigated without preceding hypotheses about them, the results of such studies should be viewed not as conclusions but as tentative hypotheses to be confirmed by further research."

Suggestions by Pocock and colleagues[28] for hypothesis testing in the clinical trial may be useful in avoiding the issue of multiple comparisons and other statistical considerations. All the preceding recommendations imply that investigators must define a priori a coordinated policy for the statistical aspects of a clinical trial; this should reflect a consistency of intent throughout the trial (beginning with trial design) on issues such as the primary study question and endpoint definitions, and throughout its conduct, analysis, interpretation, and reporting.

Multivariate analysis

Stratification is one of the major approaches used in controlling confounding factors in categorical data analysis. This approach offers the dual advantages of straightforward calculable results and ease of visual inspection of the data. Stratified data may be analyzed by standardization (standardized mortality–morbidity ratios) or summary (Mantel–Haenszel test) methods. Limitations of stratified analyses include their dependence on categorical delineation of the confounders and (given a finite number of subjects) their difficulty in accommodating more than a few factors simultaneously without the data becoming too sparse. For example, if one wished to stratify an analysis of birthweight by the mother's socioeconomic status (SES), insurance type, and a dichotomous indicator of whether or not she received regular prenatal care, the stratum representing low SES, no health insurance, and regular prenatal care might have very few infants whose data would then unduly influence the results of the analysis.

Multivariate analyses, most appropriately used as complements to stratified analysis, offer a number of potential benefits. They can control for a greater number of variables simultaneously, facilitate the exploration of interrelationships between covariates, and provide a model that enables the calculation of the odds of disease for a particular individual.

Advances in computing technology in the past three decades have led to advances in the statistical methodology and accessibility of multivariate procedures. Among the methods encountered frequently in the clinical and epidemiologic literature are multiple linear regression, logistic regression, loglinear analysis, mixed-effects models and generalized estimating equations (GEE) for longitudinal data, and the (Cox) proportional hazards model for censored time-to-event data. General information about the appropriate application and interpretation of each of these procedures is discussed in van Belle and

Table 55.9 Hill's causal criteria.[31]

Strength of association
Consistency
Temporality
Biologic gradient
Plausibility
Coherence
Experimental evidence
Analogy

colleagues.[24] Care is needed when assessing the adequacy of data to meet the assumptions underlying the various methods, as well as when evaluating model fit and interpreting the results. It is strongly recommended that investigators requiring analysis using these methods engage the collaboration of a statistician who is well versed in the procedures.

Causal inference

A widely accepted principle of epidemiology is that "the most one can hope to show, even with several studies, is that an apparent association cannot be explained either by design bias or by confounding effects of other known risk factors."[30] Investigators are often cautioned with the maxim: "association does not imply causation." Nevertheless, criteria for assessing the likelihood that a given association is causal are often helpful.

Most students of medicine first become familiar with the concept of assessing causality when they are exposed to Koch's postulates. Hill proposed the epidemiologic criteria for causality shown in Table 55.9,[31] partially in response to a discussion of Koch's work. The merits of these criteria have been subject to considerable academic debate, but Hill's guidelines provide a reasonable starting point when considering causal inference.

Breslow and Day's text[30] discusses the derivation of Hill's criteria that are thought to be most relevant to clinical studies, i.e., dose–response, specificity of risk to disease subgroups, specificity of risk to exposure subcategories, strength of association, temporal relation of risk to exposure, lack of alternative explanations, and considerations external to the study.

A brief introduction to the causal criteria relevant to clinical studies cannot begin to address the many thought-provoking historic and contemporary discussions on the subject of causality and causal inference. Some theorists have proposed alternative criteria, whereas others believe that no role exists for causal criteria. Rothman[32] has provided a stimulating debate on causality by contemporary thinkers who refer to Popperian (deductivist), Bayesian (subjective probabilist), and frequentist (statistical) viewpoints. Additional discussion is presented in a recent paper by Rothman and Greenland.[33]

Key points

1 Understanding a study's strengths and weaknesses of design and the quality of evidence that it provides is critical in evaluating a research article.

2 The basic design strategies used in epidemiologic research can be broadly divided into descriptive epidemiology or analytic epidemiology.

3 *Descriptive epidemiology* describes the general characteristics of exposure and outcome, particularly in relation to person, place, and time.

4 *Analytic epidemiology* explicitly compares exposure and outcome.

5 Analytic epidemiology can be further divided into two strategies: observational and interventional.

6 Observational studies can be further divided into case–control and cohort studies.

7 *Interventional studies*, often referred to as clinical trials, are studies in which the investigator assigns exposure and then follows the subjects for outcome.

8 Randomization minimizes potential confounding factors and ensures that participants are as similar as possible with respect to all variables except for the intervention of interest.

9 *Validity* refers to the extent that the outcome variable actually measures the effect of interest.

10 *Precision* refers to the consistency or closeness of repeated measurements of outcome to each other.

11 A *confounding factor* (or *confounder*) can be defined as a risk factor for disease, other than the exposure under study, that is unequally distributed between the cases and the comparison or control groups. The effects of confounding can sometimes be reduced by careful study design and analytic methods.

12 The predictive value of a screening test (or diagnostic test) depends on the sensitivity and specificity of the test as well as the prevalence of the disease in question.

13 The *P*-value associated with a test of hypothesis is the probability that a result at least as great as that observed would occur by chance if the null hypothesis were true.

14 The *power* of a test is its ability to detect a difference between the groups being compared at a given level of

statistical significance. In other words, it is the probability of rejecting the null hypothesis given that the alternative is true. The failure to consider statistical power is one of the most frequent errors in study design.

15 The odds ratio is often used as an approximation of the risk ratio for case–control studies, in which the risk ratio cannot be measured directly. This approximation is a good one when the prevalence of the disease is low (the "rare disease assumption").

16 The process of selecting the best statistical test requires a broader knowledge of the principles of study design and biostatistical testing. Because the appropriate use of statistical tests is not a trivial task, it is recommended that statistical testing be performed by an individual with expertise in biostatistics and that investigators actively cultivate a collaboration with such an individual.

17 There is a one-to-one relationship between confidence intervals and hypothesis tests; the context should provide a guide as to which is appropriate to report in a given situation. The former emphasizes the estimation of effect size, whereas the latter is a decision-making tool.

18 Investigators should define a coordinated policy for the statistical aspects of a clinical trial that reflects a consistency of intent from the design of a trial through its conduct, analysis, interpretation, and reporting.

19 Multivariate modeling is complex. Care is needed when assessing the adequacy of data to meet the assumptions underlying the various methods, as well as when evaluating model fit and interpreting the results. It is strongly recommended that investigators requiring analysis using these methods engage the collaboration of a statistician well versed in the procedures.

20 Although investigators are cautioned to always keep in mind the maxim "association does not imply causation," criteria exist for evaluating the likelihood that a relationship between a risk factor and a disease is causal.

References

1 Rosenberg W, Donald A. Evidence based medicine: an approach to clinical problem-solving. *Br Med J* 1995;310:1122.
2 Kleinbaum D, Kupper L, Morgenstern H. *Epidemiology research: principles and quantitative methods*. Belmont, CA: Lifetime Learning Publications, 1981.
3 Sackett DL. Bias in analytic research. *J Chronic Dis* 1978;32: 51.
4 Rothman K. A pictorial representation of confounding in epidemiological studies. *J Chronic Dis* 1975;32:101.
5 Pepe MS. *The statistical evaluation of medical tests for classification and prediction*. New York: Oxford University Press, 2003.
6 Lubin J. Some efficiency comments on group size in study design. *Am J Epidemiol* 1980;111:453.
7 Schlessman J. Sample size requirements in cohort and case–control studies of disease. *Am J Epidemiol* 1974;99:381.
8 Ury H. Efficiency of case–control studies with multiple controls per case: continuous or dichotomous data. *Biometrics* 1975;31: 643.
9 Hennekens C, Buring J. Need for large sample sizes in randomized trials. *Pediatrics* 1987;79:569.
10 Rennie D. Vive la difference. *N Engl J Med* 1978;299:828.
11 Freiman J, Chalmers T, Smith H, et al. The importance of beta, the type II error and sample size in the design and interpretation of the randomized control trial. *N Engl J Med* 1978;299:690.
12 DerSimonian R, Charette L, McPeek B, et al. Reporting on methods in clinical trials. *N Engl J Med* 1982;306:1332.
13 Van Marter LJ, Bowich DM, Torday J, et al. Interpretation of indices of fetal pulmonary maturity by gestational age. *N Engl J Med* 1988;2:360.
14 Cohen J. *Statistical power analysis for the behavioral sciences*. New York: Academic Press, 1977.
15 Pasternack B, Shore R. Sample size for group sequential cohort and case–control study designs. *Am J Epidemiol* 1981;113: 182.
16 Walter S. Determination of significant relative risks and optimal sampling procedure in prospective and retrospective comparative studies of various sizes. *Am J Epidemiol* 1977;105:387.
17 Cornfield J. A method of estimating comparative rates from clinical data: applications to cancer of the lung, breast, and cervix. *J Natl Cancer Inst* 1951;11:1269.
18 Benichou J. Attributal risk. In: Gail MH, Benichou J, eds. *Encyclopedia of epidemiologic methods*. Chichester: John Wiley & Sons Ltd; 2000:50.
19 Godfrey K. Comparing the means of several groups. *N Engl J Med* 1985;313:1450.
20 Smith E. Analysis of repeated measure designs. *J Pediatr* 1987;111:723.
21 Glantz S. Primer of biostatistics. New York: McGraw-Hill, 1981.
22 Ingelfinger J, Mosteller F, Thibodeau L, et al. *Biostatistics in clinical medicine*. New York: Macmillan, 1983.
23 Koopmans L. *An introduction to contemporary statistics*. Boston, MA: PWS Publishers, 1981.
24 van Belle G, Fisher LD, Heagerty PJ, et al. *Biostatistics: a methodology for the health sciences*, 2nd edn. Hoboken, NJ: John Wiley & Sons, 2004.
25 Schoolman H, Becktel J, Best W, et al. Clinical and experimental statistics in medical research: principles versus practices. *J Lab Clin Med* 1968;71:357.
26 Rothman K. *Modern epidemiology*. Boston, MA: Little, Brown, 1986.
27 Feinstein A, Horwitz R. Double standards, scientific methods, and epidemiological research. *N Engl J Med* 1982;307:1611.
28 Pocock S, Hughes M, Lee R. Statistical problems in the reporting of clinical trials. A survey of three medical journals. *N Engl J Med* 1987;317:426.
29 Louis T, Fineberg H, Mosteller F. Findings for public health from meta-analyses. *Annu Rev Public Health* 1985;6:1.

30 Breslow N, Day N. *Statistical methods in cancer research. I: the analysis of case–control studies*. Lyon, France: IARC Scientific Publications, 1987.
31 Hill A. The environment and disease: association or causations. *Proc R Soc Med* 1965;58:295.
32 Rothman K, ed. Casual inference. *Epidemiology resources*. Boston, MA: Little, Brown, 1988.
33 Rothman K, Greenland S. Causation and causal inference in epidemiology. *Am J Public Health* 2005;95:S144.

56 Sexuality in pregnancy and the postpartum period

Kirsten von Sydow

Sexual relations of expectant and new parents are of great medical and psychological significance. Sexual activity during pregnancy might harm the fetus, and pregnancy, birth, and breastfeeding might impair maternal sexual health. Sexuality can be a problem for (expectant) parents, but becoming a mother or a father can also improve sexual health and relationships.

This chapter presents information from several recent reviews[1–7] and new publications.

Sexual development during pregnancy and the first year postpartum

Genital physiology and sexual responsiveness

In the first trimester of pregnancy, breasts are very sensitive and may hurt easily. In the first and second trimesters, genital vasocongestion increases during sexual excitement and leakage of urine with orgasm is not unusual. In the third trimester, vasocongestion is generally increased and influenced little by sexual excitement. Lubrication and orgasm are intensified in pregnancy, but climax may sometimes be accompanied by cramps. In the third trimester, vaginal contractions are weaker and sometimes tonic muscle spasms occur. Postorgasmic contractions usually stop after about 15 min.[1,4]

In the first 6–8 weeks postpartum and during breastfeeding, the sexual arousability of mothers is physiologically reduced, the walls of the vagina are thinner, and orgasm is less intense. Breastfeeding women may ejaculate milk during climax. After about 3 months, or on cessation of breastfeeding, these changes regress; some women then experience orgasm more intensely than before. On resumption of intercourse, women mostly perceive their vaginal tension to be unchanged or tighter; at 3–4 months postpartum, vaginal tension is mostly unchanged but is reduced in about 20% of women. About 6–12 months after birth, sexual responsiveness is reduced in 40–50% of mothers and in about 20% of fathers.[1,6]

Sexual interest and initiative

Generally, female sexual interest remains unchanged or decreases slightly in the first trimester of pregnancy, and decreases sharply at the end of the third trimester; however, it is remarkably variable, especially in the second trimester.[5] Male sexual interest mostly remains unchanged until the end of the second trimester, when it decreases sharply. Female interest in tenderness remains unchanged or increases in pregnancy. The preferred erotic and sexual activities tend to remain unchanged during pregnancy and after birth, but vaginal stimulation becomes less important in the second and third trimesters.[1] At 3–4 months postpartum, female sexual interest is reduced in most cases compared with the time before pregnancy, but is subsequently very variable. Men appear to be sexually uninterested postpartum more often than women.[1]

With most couples, men show more sexual initiative before, during, and after pregnancy than women.[1] Female coital activity during pregnancy and postpartum is sometimes motivated by a concern about the partner's sexual satisfaction and faithfulness.[1]

Sexual activity

Coital activity in pregnancy declines slightly in the first trimester, is variable in the second trimester, and declines sharply in the third trimester. Most couples practice intercourse up to the seventh month, with coital activity occurring in about one-half to three-quarters in the eighth month, and around one-third in the ninth month. On average, the last coitus occurs 1 month before delivery. About 10% of women abstain from coitus once pregnancy is confirmed. The use of the male superior position declines during pregnancy, and other positions are practiced more often (side-by-side; rear entry; female superior, but only in the second trimester). In the second trimester of pregnancy, sexual intercourse occurs about 4–5 times per month.[1,8,9]

On average, intercourse is resumed 6–8 weeks after the birth in Europe and the USA (16.5 weeks in Nigeria). In the third month postpartum, 88–95% of couples practice intercourse, and, by the 13th month, coital activity occurs in 97% of couples. Coital activity postpartum is highly variable. Compared with the prepregnancy period, coital frequency is reduced during the first year after the birth. About 84–90% of couples use contraceptives postpartum, mostly the oral contraceptive pill or condoms.[1,8–10]

Nongenital physical tenderness is first unchanged and then decreases continuously from the sixth month of pregnancy until 3 years postpartum. On average, noncoital sexual contact is resumed 3 weeks after the birth, usually before intercourse is resumed. Anal intercourse is practiced by only a minority during pregnancy. The course of most heterosexual activity (e.g., coital activity, French kissing, manual genital stimulation) and female masturbation mostly follows a "standard pattern" characterized by a decrease during pregnancy (especially during the third trimester) and no or very low activity in the first 3 months postpartum; this is then followed by a slight increase. During late pregnancy and the first weeks postpartum, fellatio is practiced more often than cunnilingus. Male masturbation activity is stable throughout pregnancy and the postpartum period.[1,8,9]

Sexual enjoyment and orgasm

Before pregnancy, 76–79% of women enjoy intercourse (7–21% do not enjoy intercourse at all). In the first trimester of pregnancy, this decreases to 59%; in the second trimester, it increases to 75–84%; and in the last trimester, it decreases again to 40–41%. More than one-half of women enjoy sexual intimacy with their partner in the first year after giving birth, with 18–20% partially enjoying it and 24–30% not enjoying it at all. Father reports the same data.[1]

Before pregnancy, or in women aged under 30 years, the cumulative incidence of orgasm varies from 51% to 87%, with 10–26% of all women remaining nonorgasmic during their entire lives. Results describing female orgasm in pregnancy are contradictory. In the third trimester, 54% of sexually active women report having an orgasm with the last coitus.[1] On average, the first orgasm postpartum occurs after 7 weeks. Only 20% of women have a climax during the first coitus postpartum, rising to 75% (about the same as before pregnancy) 3–6 months after the birth. The preferred methods for reaching orgasm mostly remain unchanged. Both genders prefer manual stimulation, oral stimulation, intercourse, and masturbation.[1,11]

Erotic aspects of the parent–infant relationship

Touching is necessary for the baby and, for both baby and mother, mostly pleasurable (data regarding fathers are not available). The physical contact with the baby can be accompanied by erotic feelings, especially during breastfeeding. One-third to one-half of breastfeeding mothers describe it as an erotic experience. One-quarter have guilt feelings resulting from their sexual excitement, and some even stop nursing because they are afraid of the sexual stimulation.[1]

Risks and benefits of sexual activity during pregnancy

Large representative studies have observed no overall association between birth complications (perinatal mortality, preterm birth, premature rupture of the membranes, low birthweight) and either coital activity or orgasmic frequency. However, intercourse using the male superior position and intercourse in women with certain genital infections are associated with an elevated risk of preterm delivery.[1,4,12–18] In healthy women, there is no significant relationship between the frequency of intercourse and genital infections. Pregnant women whose partners have a sexually transmitted disease (STD), have extramarital relationships, or inject drugs should use condoms; unfortunately, however, they usually do not.[4] Few studies[4,6,19,20] associate cunnilingus during pregnancy with the very rare complication of venous air embolism, which can occur if air is blown into the vagina.

The benefits of sexual activity during pregnancy have only occasionally been researched, but at least one study[1] has found that sexual activity and enjoyment in pregnancy is associated with higher subsequent evaluations of relationship stability, tenderness, and communication at 4 months and 3 years postpartum.

Sexual problems and dysfunctions

Epidemiology

During pregnancy, one-third to one-half of all expectant parents fear harming their baby. Men also fear harming their partner, and women worry about the sexual satisfaction of their partner or about orgasmic uterine contractions (only during the third trimester). Less frequently, expectant mothers suffer from dyspareunia (painful intercourse) or men report difficulty in ejaculating during intercourse.[1,6,21,22]

Only 12–14% of both partners report having no sexual problems postpartum. Many mothers and fathers are afraid to resume intercourse. More than 50% of all women experience pain during their first intercourse after birth, with 41% still suffering from dyspareunia at 3 months postpartum. This is reduced to 22% at 6 months postpartum, and remains at this level until 13 months postpartum. About 57% of women are worried about the sexual satisfaction of their partners, and around one-fifth of couples have problems with contraception or milk leakage from breastfeeding mothers. Long term, the sexual relationship of at least one-third of all couples

Table 56.1 Factors associated with decreased sexual interest, activity, and enjoyment and increased sexual problems during pregnancy.

Biomedical factors
Tiredness
Worry that the fetus could be hurt during intercourse
Dyspareunia
Backache
Woman's low physical attractiveness (self and partner evaluation)
Psychosocial factors
Mental symptoms (depressed mood, emotional lability)
Prepregnancy sexual history and sexual symptoms (e.g., dyspareunia)
Negative or ambivalent feelings about the pregnancy
Couple/relationship factors
Low relationship satisfaction

Table 56.2 Factors associated with decreased sexual interest, activity, and enjoyment and increased sexual problems during the postpartum period.

Biomedical factors
Degree of perineal birth trauma (tears, episiotomy)
Assisted vaginal delivery
Tiredness
Kegel exercises not performed
No reliable method of contraception
Psychosocial factors
Mental symptoms (depressed mood, emotional lability)
Prepregnancy sexual history and sexual symptoms (e.g., dyspareunia)
Poor childhood relationship with father (e.g., good relationship only with mother)
Couple/relationship factors
Low relationship satisfaction (in women and men)
Attributes of the baby and the mother–child relationship
Male babies: mothers of boys are perceived by their partners as being less tender during the postpartum months than mothers of girls
Mothers with a rigid and overprotective relationship to their baby
Breastfeeding

worsens, although it improves for one-quarter of new mothers.[23]

About 4–28% of fathers have extramarital relationships during pregnancy and in the first months postpartum, whereas women do so only rarely. In West Africa, postnatal marital coital abstinence is associated with an increased risk of male extramarital affairs and unprotected extramarital sex.[1,23–25]

Etiology of sexual problems and dysfunctions

It would appear that female sexual problems and decreases in sexual activity, interest, and enjoyment during pregnancy and the postpartum period are related to the physical processes of pregnancy, delivery, and breastfeeding. However, only some of the observable changes can be attributed to physiological processes. Sexual behavior and problems during the transition to parenthood are influenced by a complex interplay of biomedical, psychological, and social–marital factors, similar to the situation in other phases of the life cycle (Tables 56.1 and 56.2[1,7,10,23,25–28]).

The degree of perineal trauma is strongly related to postnatal dyspareunia in a dose-dependent manner (no perineal damage, 11% coital pain; unstitched tears, 15% pain; stitched tears, 21% pain; episiotomy, 40% pain) and is also associated with sexual behavior postpartum. The risk of postbirth dyspareunia is highest for women who undergo assisted vaginal deliveries (vacuum extractor, forceps), intermediate for women with spontaneous vaginal deliveries, and lowest following Cesarean sections. Women who undergo a Cesarean section resume intercourse somewhat earlier than women who deliver vaginally.[1,2,8,10,23,29–32]

Breastfeeding (at months 1–4 postpartum) is accompanied by reduced coital activity, sexual desire, and sexual satisfaction in women and their male partners. Mothers who breastfeed long term resume intercourse at a later time, are slightly less sexually interested, suffer from coital pain more often, and enjoy intercourse to a lesser degree. The cessation of breastfeeding has a positive effect on sexual activity, but no effect on sexual responsiveness or orgasm. The negative impact of breastfeeding on maternal (and paternal) sexuality results from changes in the hormonal status of the mother, which influences desire and lubrication, and from the changed "meaning" of the breasts (nutritional versus sexual) for both partners.[1,8,10,23,33]

It should be borne in mind that sexual activity, tenderness, and sexual satisfaction generally decline with increasing relationship duration, in childless couples as well as in parents.[1]

Diagnosis of sexual problems and dysfunctions, their prevention and treatment

Gynecological and obstetrical intervention and advice

The use of an episiotomy is strongly related to postbirth dyspareunia, even more so than spontaneous perineal tears, and its use should be reduced and restricted as far as possible to specified indications.[1,31]

Although the majority of gynecologists believe that they spontaneously discuss sexuality with their pregnant patients, two-thirds of all women questioned in various industrialized countries do not remember discussing sexuality in pregnancy with their gynecologist. About 76% of expectant mothers feel that sexuality should be discussed, with 45% finding that the information given by medical staff about sex during pregnancy was insufficient. Approximately 49% of women who talked to their doctor about sexuality in pregnancy raised the issue first, with 34% feeling uncomfortable in bringing up the topic themselves. Women who do not ask their gynecologists sexual questions during pregnancy more often experience an intensification of their sexual feelings than women who do ask because doctors often give restrictive advice. Alternative coital positions or alternatives to intercourse (e.g., mutual hand stimulation) are only very rarely mentioned by doctors. No doctor mentioned that sex could improve during pregnancy, and only 8–10% of women abstained from intercourse because of medical advice.[1,4,11,21]

Intercourse and/or orgasm should be avoided by expectant mothers who have certain pregnancy complications (Table 56.3). If a woman's partner may be infected with an STD, including HIV, a condom should always be used. STD infection in the mother can lead to miscarriage or stillbirth, or can be harmful to the embryo/fetus. However, for the majority of healthy pregnant women and their partners, there is no reason to "forbid" sex, even in the last weeks before birth.[1,4,6]

Many gynecologists are uncertain about what sexual advice to give when problems occur in pregnancy. Nearly all agree that intercourse should be avoided during and after bleeding, but there is no agreement as to how long the period of abstinence should be and when the ban on intercourse can be reversed, e.g., after vaginal bleeding has stopped. Similarly, recommendations vary with regard to the sexual consequences of premature contractions, and some doctors fail to give restrictive advice when it is necessary, e.g., in cases of incompetent cervix or vaginal infection. There is a lack of medical knowledge concerning sexuality and the management of pregnancy complications, and medical textbooks rarely contain information on this subject.[4,21] Uncertainty and a lack of training in couple/sexual counseling might be reasons why doctors neglect this topic. Discussions about sexual problems are not included in routine antenatal care and, if they do occur, the male partner is usually not included.[1,4]

Post birth, maternal and child health services in Europe and the USA focus more on the child than on the mother. Health professionals do not always have the awareness, knowledge, and skills to deal with postnatal sexual problems.[29] Postbirth medical advice about sexuality usually focuses only on contraception, which is discussed at 76% of 6-week postnatal visits; topics such as intercourse, perineal problems, pain, and sexual interest are not mentioned and these problems are not recognized in the great majority of women.[29] About 22% of new mothers desire medical advice because of perineal or coital problems; three-quarters who need help actively seek it, whereas 8% feel that they have not received adequate help.[10] Many couples wish to receive more information about bodily changes and sexuality postpartum, and 30% say that sexual counseling might have been helpful.[1]

Practical recommendations for giving medical advice about sexuality during pregnancy and postpartum are summarized in Table 56.4.[1,4]

Healthcare policy and prevention

At the final 6- to 8-week postnatal visit, only about one-half of all new mothers have resumed sexual intercourse. Women's sexual health problems extend well into the first postnatal year

Table 56.3 Indications for coital and orgasmic abstinence during pregnancy.

Vaginal bleeding
Abdominal pains
Rupture of the membranes
Premature dilation of the cervix
History of premature delivery, heightened risk of premature labor
Placenta previa
Placental insufficiency
Incompetent cervix
Multiple pregnancy

Table 56.4 Recommendations for taking a sexual history and giving the patient sexual information.

If possible, include the partner

Put open questions and listen to the answers

Pregnancy: the current emotional, marital, and sexual situation, and the information needs of the woman and her partner

Postpartum: sexual interest, behavior, coital pain, or incontinence

Give information about normal changes during the transition to parenthood

Pregnancy: some women (and men) have no sexual interest, whereas, in others, sexual interest is intensified

Postpartum: some mothers experience erotic feelings during breastfeeding and some fathers are jealous about breastfeeding. Vaginal dryness may be associated with breastfeeding

Acknowledge patients' and partners' fears and uncertainties and respect their inner limitations

The aim is a sexual life that both partners and, from the medical and parental point of view, the baby are contented with. This also includes the option of sexual abstinence

Give technical advice about the range of sexual options

Tenderness, noncoital sexual activities (e.g., manual and oral stimulation, masturbation) and, during pregnancy, alternative coital positions (female superior, rear entry/"spoon," use of pillows)

Instruct the patient in self-help

Post birth: self-inspection of the vulva with a hand mirror and insertion of a finger to test for healing; vaginal muscle-toning (Kegel) exercises

Be sensitive for sexual and nonsexual domestic violence

and sometimes even longer.[1,29,30] Consequently, a 6-month postbirth checkup that includes questions about sexuality, for example "Have you already resumed intercourse?," "How did it feel?," "Do you have any perineal problems?," and other taboo topics such as incontinence would be more helpful in identifying the full range of problems women may experience after childbirth.

A new prenatal program designed to decrease the potentially negative effects of parenthood on the quality of marital relationships had positive effects on postpartum satisfaction and the sexual aspects of marriage compared with a traditional prenatal education program.[34]

Counseling, psychotherapy, and intervention

Perineal pain may be decreased by the resolution of inflammatory processes using therapeutic ultrasound.[35] If sexual problems persist after gynecological treatment has been successfully completed (e.g., coital pain from episiotomy scars) and the woman has terminated breastfeeding, a closer look at the psychological situation and the relationship of both partners is necessary. It is also helpful if the doctor or midwife is able to assess the psychosocial and sexual situation of patients and, if necessary, refer them to mental health professionals for marital counseling or psychotherapy. This is in the interests not only of the parents but also of the newborn baby, whose life may be affected if his/her parents live in an unhappy relationship or get divorced.

Research implications can be found in two extensive reviews.[1,7]

Conclusion

In summary, sex is of little relevance for most new breastfeeding mothers during the first 3 months postpartum because adaptation to motherhood requires all of their energy, involves profound psychosocial and hormonal changes, and results in a lack of sleep. Male sexual activity is also reduced during this phase of life but to a lesser degree. There is remarkable variation in female and male sexual behavior during pregnancy and the later postpartum stages (months 4–12). On average, all heterosexual activities tend to decline during pregnancy; they reach a point near zero in the immediate postpartum period and then slowly start to increase again.

Key points

1 During the last weeks of pregnancy and the first 2 or 3 months postpartum, female sexual activity is universally very low or nonexistent.

2 In every other phase of the transition to parenthood, female sexual activity is very variable depending on the physical and mental health of the (expectant) mother, her sexual and nonsexual biography, the relationship of the couple, and her life circumstances.

3 Healthy women and their partners can stay sexually active during the entire pregnancy; however, sexual activity in pregnancy should be discouraged if certain problems occur (e.g., vaginal bleeding).

4 Intercourse is resumed on average about 6–8 weeks post birth, but it can be many months later.

5 Sexual problems (e.g., dyspareunia) are very common during the first year postpartum but are often not recognized by doctors, nurses, and midwives.

6 Postbirth sexual problems are often related to perineal trauma (assisted deliveries, episiotomy, tears), breastfeeding, marital problems, and prebirth sexual problems of the couple.

7 Patients feel that doctors rarely discuss sexual issues during pregnancy and the postpartum period, although most gynecologists believe that they have done so.

References

1 von Sydow K. Sexuality during pregnancy and after childbirth: a meta-content-analysis of 59 studies. *J Psychosom Res* 1999;47: 27–49.

2 Barrett G, Victor C. Incidence of postnatal dyspareunia. *Br J Sex Med* 1996;23:6–8.

3 Hobbs K, Bramwell R, May K. Sexuality, sexual behavior and pregnancy. *Sex Marital Ther* 1999;14:371–383.

4 Leeners B, Brandenburg U, Rath W. Sexualität in der Schwangerschaft: risiko oder Schutzfaktor? (Sexual activity during pregnancy: risk factor or protection?). *Geburtshilfe Frauenheilkd* 2000;60:536–543.

5 Regan PC, Lyle JL, Otto AL, et al. Pregnancy and changes in female sexual desire: a review. *Soc Behav Pers* 2003;31:603–611.

6 Sarrel, PM, Sellgren UM. Sexuality in pregnancy and the puerperium. In: EA Reece, JC Hobbins (eds) *Medicine of the fetus and mother*, 2nd edn. Philadelphia, PA: Lippincott-Raven: 1999;1451–1459.

7 von Sydow K. Female sexual dysfunction: pregnancy, childbirth and postpartum period. In: Goldstein I, Meston CM, Davis S, et al. (eds) *Women's sexual function and dysfunction*. London: Taylor & Francis, 2006.

8 Hyde JS, DeLamater JD, Plant EA, et al. Sexuality during pregnancy and the year postpartum. *J Sex Res* 1996;33:143–151.

9 von Sydow K, Ullmeyer M, Happ N. Sexual activity during pregnancy and after childbirth: results from the Sexual Preferences Questionnaire. *J Psychosom Obstet Gynecol* 2001;22:29–40.

10 Glazener CMA. Sexual function after childbirth: women's experiences, persistent morbidity and lack of professional recognition. *Br J Obstet Gynaecol* 1997;104:330–335.

11 von Sydow K. Sexual enjoyment and orgasm postpartum: sex differences and perceptual accuracy concerning partners' sexual experience. *J Psychosom Obstet Gynecol* 2002;23:147–155.
12 Naeye RL. Coitus and associated amniotic-fluid infections. *N Engl J Med* 1979;301:1198–1200.
13 Mills JL, Harlap S, Harley EE. Should coitus late in pregnancy be discouraged? *Lancet* 1981;2:136–138.
14 Klebanoff MA, Nugent RP, Rhoads GG. Coitus during pregnancy: is it safe? *Lancet* 1984;2:914–917.
15 Read JS, Klebanoff MA, the VIP Study Group. Sexual intercourse during pregnancy and preterm delivery: effects of cervicovaginal microflora. *Paediatr Perinat Epidemiol* 1996;7:A1-A2.
16 Read JS, Klebanoff MA. Sexual intercourse during pregnancy and preterm delivery: effects of vaginal microorganisms. *Am J Obstet Gynecol* 1993;168:514–519.
17 Berghella V, Klebanoff M, McPherson C, et al. Sexual intercourse association with asymptomatic bacterial vaginosis and *Trichomonas vaginalis* treatment in relationship to preterm birth. *Am J Obstet Gynecol* 2002;187:1277–1282.
18 Ekwo EE, Gosselink CA, Woolson R, et al. Coitus late in pregnancy: risk of preterm rupture of amniotic sac membranes. *Am J Obstet Gynecol* 1993;168:22–31.
19 Bray P, Myers R, Cowley RA. Orogenital sex as a cause of nonfatal air embolism in pregnancy. *Obstet Gynecol* 1983;61:653–657.
20 Hill BF, Jones JS. Venous air embolism following orogenital sex during pregnancy. *Am J Emerg Med* 1993;11:155–157.
21 Bartellas E, Crane JM, Daley M, et al. Sexuality and sexual activity in pregnancy. *Br J Obstet Gynaecol* 2000;107:964–968.
22 Oruc S, Esen A, Lacin S, et al. Sexual behavior during pregnancy. *Aust NZ J Obstet Gynaecol* 1999;39:48–50.
23 Signorello LB, Harlow BL, Chekos AK, et al. Postpartum sexual functioning and its relationship to perineal trauma: a retrospective cohort study of primiparous women. *Am J Obstet Gynecol* 2001;184:881–890.
24 Ali MM, Cleland JG. The link between postnatal abstinence and extramarital sex in Cote d'Ivoire. *Stud Fam Plann* 2001;32:214–219.
25 Onah HE, Ilobachie GC, Obi SN, et al. Nigerian male sexual activity during pregnancy. *Int J Obstet Gynecol* 2002;76:219–223.
26 De Judicibus MA, McCabe MP. Psychological factors and the sexuality of pregnant and postpartum women. *J Sex Res* 2002;39:94–103.
27 Morof D, Barrett G, Peacock J, et al. Postnatal depression and sexual health after childbirth. *Obstet Gynecol* 2003;102:1318–1325.
28 Bogren LY. Changes in sexuality in women and men during pregnancy. *Arch Sex Behav* 1991;20:35–45.
29 Barrett G, Victor C. Postnatal sexual health (Letters). *Br Med J* 1994;309:1584–1585.
30 Barrett G, Victor C. Postnatal sexual health. *Br J Gen Pract* 1996;46:47–48.
31 Klein MC, Gauthier RJ, Robbins JM, et al. Relationship of episiotomy to perineal trauma and morbidity, sexual dysfunction, and pelvic floor relaxation. *Am J Obstet Gynecol* 1994;171:591–598.
32 Wenderlein JM, Merkle F. Beschwerden infolge Episiotomie: Studie an 413 Frauen mit komplikationsloser Spontangeburt (Complaints caused by episiotomy: study of 413 women with spontaneous complication-free labor). *Geburtshilfe Frauenheilkd* 1983;43:625–628.
33 Avery MD, Duckett L, Frantzich CR. The experience of sexuality during breastfeeding. *J Midwifery Wom Health* 2000;45:227–237.
34 Kermeen P. Improving postpartum marital relationships. *Psychol Rep* 1995;76:831–834.
35 Hay-Smith EJ. Therapeutic ultrasound for postpartum perineal pain and dyspareunia. *Cochrane Database Syst Rev* 2000;2. CD000495.

57 Psychiatric problems during pregnancy and the puerperium

Linda L.M. Worley and Jennifer L. Melville

Psychiatric disorders are common in pregnant and postpartum women yet they often go undiagnosed and untreated. Approximately one-quarter of pregnant and postpartum women may have a psychiatric disorder, but the majority of these patients do not receive adequate treatment as part of their obstetric care. In addition to the distress associated with mental illness, pregnant women with psychiatric disorders report more somatic symptoms and are at an increased risk for poor obstetrical and neonatal outcomes. Women suffering from a severe depressive illness or psychosis are also at risk for suicide, the leading cause of maternal death through the first postpartum year.

All women should be asked early in pregnancy about any history of psychiatric disorders and use of psychiatric medications, and screened for current psychiatric disorders. If present, management plans should be initiated to decrease both complications from the illness and the high risk of recurrence following delivery. Management of psychiatric disorders is complicated by pregnancy and the potential risk to the fetus, but collaboration between obstetric providers and psychiatrists can provide effective treatments.

This chapter will provide obstetricians and perinatologists with a clinically relevant overview of psychiatric issues that may be confronted in caring for pregnant and postpartum women. It covers depressive disorders, anxiety disorders, psychiatric emergencies, and special treatment challenges including bipolar disorder, somatization, denial of pregnancy, capacity to parent, and pregnancy after loss.

Depressive disorders

Epidemiology

Depressive disorders are common in pregnancy, affecting 9–23% of antepartum women[1–6] and 12–16% of postpartum women.[7,8] Of these, an estimated 3–11% suffer from the most serious form of depression, major depressive disorder.[5,6] Although these prevalence rates are similar to those seen in nonpregnant women of childbearing age, pregnant women are more likely to be seen by a physician, increasing the opportunity for diagnosis and treatment. Table 57.1 lists the depressive disorders that an obstetrician is likely to encounter.

There are common risk factors for the development of antenatal and postpartum depression (see Table 57.2), with additional risks for postpartum depression based on prior depressive episodes. Women with a history of depression have a 25% risk of developing postpartum depression,[5] whereas those with a history of postpartum depression have a 50% chance of it recurring and should be monitored closely throughout pregnancy and the postpartum period.

Untreated antenatal and postpartum depression have been shown to have a detrimental effect on both maternal and fetal outcomes (Table 57.3). Direct and indirect mechanisms of association have been hypothesized. Maternal psychosocial factors have been shown to affect neuroendocrine activity[9,10] and uterine blood flow,[11] both of which may play a direct role in adverse outcomes such as low birthweight, prematurity, and preeclampsia. Both maternal depression and anxiety have been linked to adverse health behaviors (e.g., poor nutrition and smoking),[12] which in turn contribute to adverse pregnancy outcomes. In one study,[13] depressed pregnant women were 4.1 times more likely to be smokers than nondepressed pregnant women. Attempts to quit smoking during pregnancy may be thwarted in the presence of comorbid depression,[13,14] and cessation attempts may increase the risk for relapse of depression in individuals with a previous history.[15]

Clinical presentation

Table 57.1 lists the typical course and features of the disorders outlined below.

Antenatal depression

Antenatal depression is characterized by classic depressive symptoms (Fig. 57.1, DSM-IV[16]); however, it may be overlooked because many of the symptoms of depression (e.g., sleep and appetite disturbance and low energy) are also normal symptoms of pregnancy. Clinical features that are not symptoms of normal pregnancy and which support the

Table 57.1 Depressive disorders.

Syndrome	Onset/course	Possible features	Management
Antenatal depression: 9–23% of pregnant women	Before conception or during pregnancy May progress to postpartum depression	Must have depressed mood or anhedonia lasting at least 2 weeks Loss of interest and pleasure, sleep disturbance, appetite change, guilt, decreased concentration, suicidal ideation	For mild to moderate depression with minimal role impairment, refer for counseling or bright light therapy For depression with significant role impairment, add treatment with an antidepressant
Postpartum blues: 50–70% of postpartum women	Peaks 3–5 days after delivery Resolves <2 weeks	Crying spells, emotional lability, irritability, anxiety,[141] hypochrondriasis[141]	Reassure and educate Monitor for resolution[141] Encourage family to offer emotional and social support
Postpartum depression: 12–16% of postpartum women[7,8]	Within 6 months of delivery Insidious onset	Classic depression symptoms lasting at least 2 weeks (same as antenatal depression above) May also include intrusive thoughts or fears of harming infant	For mild to moderate depression with minimal role impairment, refer for counseling or bright light therapy For depression with significant role impairment, add treatment with an antidepressant Hospitalization when warranted
Postpartum psychosis:* 0.5% of postpartum women	Within 3 weeks of childbirth Abrupt onset Women with bipolar disorder are at high risk	Delusions, confusion, hallucinations, agitation, insomnia, disorganized thinking	Emergency referral to psychiatrist Medical workup to rule out underlying etiology

*See section on psychiatric emergencies.

Table 57.2 Risk factors for developing antenatal and postpartum depression.[10]

Family or personal history of depression, anxiety disorder, or bipolar disorder
Limited social support
History of physical, emotional, or sexual abuse
Cigarette smoking or alcohol or substance use
Current financial, occupational, health, or relationship stressors
Abrupt discontinuation of an antidepressant before completing a full course of treatment

diagnosis of depression include depressed mood, anhedonia, guilt, hopelessness, and suicidal thoughts.

Postpartum depression

Postpartum depression is also characterized by classic depressive symptoms (Fig. 57.1, DSM-IV) and often has an insidious onset in the 6 months following delivery. Patients may be ashamed to reveal how badly they are feeling to their doctor as the postpartum period is expected to be a joyful time for the new mother. Postpartum depression is a serious form of

Table 57.3 Risks of untreated depression

Antepartum risks
Increased physical pain and discomfort[115]
Increased use of cigarettes, alcohol, and other drugs[124,125]
Inadequate self-care and poor compliance with prenatal care[28]
Peripartum risks
Low birthweight (< 2500 g)[126,127] and SGA infants[127]
Preeclampsia[128]
Preterm delivery (< 37 weeks)[127]
Operative delivery[129]
Postpartum risks
Difficulty breastfeeding[130]
Poor growth and failure to thrive[131,132]
Decreased IQ in infants and children[42]
Missed pediatric outpatient appointments and increased emergency room visits[133]
Marital and relationship difficulties[134]
Depression in children[43]

SGA, small for gestational age.

A *Five (or more)* of the following symptoms have been present during the *same 2-week period* and represent a *change* from previous functioning. At least one of the symptoms is either (1) *depressed mood* or (2) *loss of interest or pleasure (anhedonia)*

Note: do not include symptoms that are clearly due to a general medical condition (*or pregnancy*)

(1) *Depressed mood nearly every day for most of the day*, as indicated by either subjective report (e.g., feels sad or empty) or observation made by others (e.g., appears tearful). Note: in children and adolescents, can present as irritable mood
(2) *Markedly diminished interest or pleasure in all, or almost all, activities nearly every day for most of the day* (as indicated by either subjective account or observation made by others)
(3) Significant weight loss when not dieting or weight gain (e.g., a change of more than 5% of body weight in a month), or decrease or increase in appetite nearly every day. Note: in children (and pregnancy), consider failure to make expected weight gain
(4) Insomnia or hypersomnia nearly every day
(5) Psychomotor agitation or retardation nearly every day (observable by others, not merely subjective feelings of restlessness or being slowed down)
(6) Fatigue or loss of energy nearly every day
(7) Feelings of worthlessness or excessive or inappropriate guilt (which may be delusional) nearly every day (not merely self-reproach or guilt about being sick)
(8) Diminished ability to think or concentrate, or indecisiveness nearly every day (either by subjective account or as observed by others)
(9) Recurrent thoughts of death (not just fear of dying), recurrent suicidal ideation without a specific plan, or attempted suicide or a specific plan for committing suicide

In addition:

B The symptoms do not meet criteria for a mixed episode (of bipolar disorder with simultaneous mania and depression)
C The symptoms cause clinically significant distress or impairment in social, occupational, or other important areas of functioning
D The symptoms do not result from the direct physiological effects of a substance (e.g., a drug of abuse, medication) or a general medical condition (hypothyroidism)
E The symptoms are not better accounted for by bereavement, i.e., after the loss of a loved one, the symptoms persist for longer than 2 months or are characterized by marked functional impairment, morbid preoccupation with worthlessness, suicidal ideation, psychotic symptoms, or psychomotor retardation

Figure 57.1 DSM-IVR diagnostic criteria for a major depressive episode.[16]

depressive illness that requires management and should not be confused with the "baby blues."

Postpartum blues

Postpartum blues, or "baby blues," are a common phenomenon, affecting 50–70% of postpartum women. Characteristic symptoms include crying spells, emotional lability, and irritability, peaking 3–5 days post delivery. These symptoms are usually mild and self-limited, usually resolving within 2 weeks.

Management

The high prevalence of depressive disorders warrants screening of all pregnant and postpartum women. Self-report screening instruments, such as the PRIME-MD Patient Health Questionnaire 9-item (PHQ-9; Fig. 57.2A), can easily be incorporated into obstetric care to facilitate diagnosis and treatment or referral. When establishing a diagnosis, potential underlying etiologies such as hypothyroidism, nicotine withdrawal, substance use, and current abuse must be considered.

Management of depression during pregnancy depends on both the severity of symptoms and degree of impairment (Fig. 57.2A and B). The optimal treatment for antenatal and postpartum depression minimizes the risk to the fetus and neonate while limiting morbidity from untreated psychiatric illness in the mother.[17] Support groups and interpersonal psychotherapy [with a counselor such as a licensed clinical social worker (LCSW) or a PhD psychologist] have been found to be effective in cases of mild depression with minimal impairment.[8,18–20] Additionally, a trial of light therapy (e.g., sitting in front of a broad-spectrum light each morning for approximately 15–60 min) may be warranted.[21–23] The duration of exposure should be decreased if side-effects of hypomania or nausea emerge. Social support for the patient is also very important, with the involvement of family and friends if possible.

Antidepressant treatment may be necessary in cases of major depression with impaired role functioning. Carefully conducted observational studies of human fetal and neonatal exposure to therapeutic doses of many psychotropic medications in pregnancy and lactation have been largely reassuring,[24–28] although no randomized trials of antidepressants in pregnancy have been conducted. For many antidepressants that have been studied[29,30] there has been no reported increase in the frequency of major malformations over the baseline rate of 2–4% found in the general population. However, first-trimester exposure to the most anticholinergic selective serotonin reuptake inhibitor (SSRI), paroxetine (Paxil), may be associated with a mildly increased risk for major congenital malformations, particularly cardiovascular malformations.[31] SSRIs are widely used in pregnancy; prescribing information for commonly used SSRIs for which antenatal exposure data are available are listed in Table 57.4. Tricyclic antidepressants (TCAs) have also been widely used in pregnancy. Certain TCAs have been labeled as pregnancy category D by the Food and Drug Administration (FDA), but pooled available data suggest that these drugs are likely to be safe for use during pregnancy.[25,26] Among the TCAs, desipramine and nortriptyline are preferred because they are less anticholinergic and the least likely to exacerbate the orthostatic hypotension that may occur during pregnancy. Avoid using TCAS in patients prone to taking impulsive overdoses or in patients with cardiac conduction delays. Prospective data on the use of mirtazapine,

(A)

Over the *last 2 weeks*, how often have you been bothered by any of the following problems?
Please check the box that corresponds to your response:

	Not at all <0>	*Several days* <1>	*More than half the days* <2>	*Nearly every day* <3>
a. Little interest or pleasure in doing things	☐	☐	☐	☐
b. Feeling down, depressed, or hopeless	☐	☐	☐	☐
c. Trouble falling or staying asleep, or sleeping too much	☐	☐	☐	☐
d. Feeling tired or having little energy	☐	☐	☐	☐
e. Poor appetite or overeating	☐	☐	☐	☐
f. Feeling bad about yourself – or that you are a failure or have let yourself or your family down	☐	☐	☐	☐
g. Trouble concentrating on things, such as reading the newspaper or watching television	☐	☐	☐	☐
h. Moving or speaking so slowly that other people could have noticed? Or the opposite – being so fidgety or restless that you have been moving around a lot more than usual	☐	☐	☐	☐
i. Thoughts that you would be better off dead or of hurting yourself in some way	☐	☐	☐	☐

Scoring instructions:
If at least one of 3a and 3b in dark gray area is checked <☐YES> ***and*** *at least five total of 3a through 3i in total shaded area are checked <☐YES> 'you' may benefit from treatment for depression.*

(B)

If you checked off any problems on questions above, how difficult have these problems made it for you to do your work, take care of things at home, or get along with other people?

Not difficult at all	*Somewhat difficult*	*Very difficult*	*Extremely difficult*
☐	☐	☐	☐

Figure 57.2 (A) PHQ-9: depression screen; (B) role impairment screen.

nefazodone, and trazodone are not currently available.[28] Monoamine oxidase inhibitors (MAOIs) are generally avoided during pregnancy because of their potential to precipitate a hypertensive crisis in the event that tocolytic medications are necessary.[28] Severely depressed patients with acute suicidality or psychosis, or women who wish to avoid extended exposure to psychotropic medications during pregnancy, may also be effectively treated with electroconvulsive therapy (ECT).[32,33]

A transient neonatal discontinuation syndrome has been reported in babies born to women taking antidepressants at term.[34] Although this syndrome is rare, it is recommended that newborns with recent *in utero* antidepressant exposure be monitored for symptoms of tachypnea, respiratory distress, desaturation upon feeding, hypoglycemia, poor tone, and weak or absent cry for at least 48 h after birth,[31,35] and that supportive care be appropriately administered. If the risk of maternal illness does not outweigh the risk of neonatal withdrawal, a tapering of the maternal antidepressant dose in the days or weeks before birth may help minimize the risk of symptoms from neonatal discontinuation syndrome. If this is done, the normal antidepressant dose should be resumed immediately following delivery. Neonates of smokers are at an additional risk for withdrawal from nicotine.[36,37]

The decision whether to breastfeed while taking antidepressants should be discussed with the patient before delivery. The American Academy of Pediatrics endorses breast milk as the ideal form of nutrition for the newborn, citing both physical and emotional benefits.[38] Significant data exist documenting the low excretion of SSRI and TCA[39] antidepressants in breast milk (see Table 57.4).[40] Minimal concentrations of sertraline, paroxetine, and nortriptyline in breast milk make them the preferred antidepressants in breastfeeding.[40] If women take an antidepressant in pregnancy, it is recommended that the same antidepressant be continued during lactation to limit the infant's exposure to a single medication.[41]

Antidepressant medication may be initiated and monitored by the obstetrical provider or the consulting psychiatrist (see antidepressant treatment tips, Table 57.5). Treatment choices must balance the risks associated with untreated depression[42,43] against the potential risks from treatment with antidepressants. It is the treating physician's responsibility to give accurate and up-to-date information on the reproductive safety of pharmacological treatment and to help the patient make an informed decision regarding treatment.[28] A resource list at the end of this chapter includes registries that maintain up-to-date information on antidepressant use in pregnancy. If medication is initiated, depressive symptoms should be reassessed at each appointment (with the PHQ-9) and the dose adjusted accordingly (see Table 57.4). Once the depression is in remission (a score < 5 on the PHQ-9), treatment should be continued for a full 6–9 months.[44,45] After a full course of treatment, medication should be gradually tapered and discontinued over 2–4 weeks with careful observation for reemergence of symptoms. A patient who has experienced more than two major depressive episodes may require maintenance antidepressant treatment to remain depression free.[46,47]

Table 57.4 Administration schedule for selected SSRI antidepressants.

Antidepressants	Dose range (mg/day)	Initial suggested dose	Characteristics and administration schedule
Fluoxetine (Prozac): pregnancy class C	10–40	10–20 mg every morning with food (10 mg if ↑ anxiety)	Activating: not first choice in patients with ↑ anxiety, but can be beneficial for patients with fatigue Increase in 10-mg increments at intervals of 7 days Maintain 20 mg for 4–6 weeks before dose increase Monitor maternal and neonatal weight gain; decrease dose in week before delivery to aid in neonatal clearance
Sertraline (Zoloft): pregnancy class C	50–150	25–50 mg q.d. with food (25 mg if ↑ anxiety)	Increase in 25–50 mg increments at intervals of 7 days as tolerated Maintain 100 mg for 4–6 weeks before dose increase Extensively studied for use in breastfeeding; minimal amounts transfer into breast milk, and milk can be discarded 8–9 h after dose to further minimize exposure[142]
Paroxetine (Paxil): pregnancy class D*	10–50	10–20 mg q.d. with food (10 mg if ↑ anxiety, every morning)	The most anticholinergic of the SSRIs Avoid first-trimester exposure when possible* Sedating: good choice for patients with ↑ anxiety Increase in 10-mg increments at intervals of 7 days up to a maximum of 40 mg/day Maintain 20 mg for 4–6 weeks before dose increase Monitor the newborn for transient neonatal discontinuation syndrome[143,144] Of the SSRIs, this passes least into breast milk and is virtually undetectable[145]
Citalopram (Celexa): pregnancy class C	10–40	10–20 mg every morning with food (10 mg if ↑anxiety)	Increase in 10-mg increments every 7 days as tolerated Maintain 20 mg for 4–6 weeks before dose increase This medication has been widely prescribed in Europe during pregnancy and lactation

*Preliminary results of two recent studies indicate that paroxetine increases the risk of congenital malformations, particularly cardiovascular malformations. Patients taking paroxetine who become pregnant or who are currently in the first trimester of pregnancy should be alerted to the potential risk to the fetus. Discontinuing paroxetine therapy or switching to another antidepressant should be considered for these patients. For individual patients, however, the benefits of continuing paroxetine may outweigh the potential risk to the fetus. Paroxetine should generally not be initiated in women who are in the first trimester of pregnancy or in women who plan to become pregnant.[31]

Table 57.5 Antidepressant treatment tips.

Rule out bipolar disorder (e.g., episodes of high energy, little need for sleep, excessive spending); if present, refer to psychiatry for management
For *anxious* patients, begin with lowest possible dose and increase *very* slowly
Resume a medication that worked previously (*if safe in pregnancy*)
Use a *single* antidepressant medication[41]
Use the same medication in pregnancy and lactation[24]

Table 57.6 Risks of untreated antepartum anxiety.

Low birthweight[136]
Preeclampsia[128]
Premature rupture of membranes[137]
Preterm delivery[138]
Operative delivery[137,139]
Increased risk for behavioral/emotional problems in children[140]

Anxiety disorders

The most common psychiatric disorder in women is anxiety disorder; approximately one in three women suffer from an anxiety disorder at some time in their life.[48] Anxiety disorders include generalized anxiety disorder, panic disorder, obsessive–compulsive disorder, social and other phobias, and posttraumatic stress disorder. Although the evidence shows that untreated anxiety disorders are associated with poor obstetrical outcomes[49] (see Table 57.6), limited data exist that examine the impact of pregnancy and the postpartum period on the course of many of these disorders. It does appear that the postpartum period is a time of elevated risk for an exacerbation of anxiety-related symptoms.[50] Obstetricians need to recognize these disorders and understand their management.[49] The anxiety disorders for which data exist are discussed below.

Panic disorder in pregnancy

Epidemiology

The prevalence of panic disorder in women is approximately 1–3% in community samples and 3–8% in primary care samples.[51] Pregnancy does not appear to be protective; panic symptoms often continue throughout pregnancy and worsen postpartum without treatment.[49,52–54] Approximately 50% of patients with panic disorder have comorbid major depression. In some cases, the first symptoms of panic disorder begin following birth.[55] In a prospective study[56] of pregnant women with pre-existing panic disorder, 7 out of 10 continued to have symptoms throughout pregnancy. In this study, treatment with an SSRI during the third trimester and postpartum was effective in preventing postpartum exacerbation of the disorder.[57]

Clinical presentation

A panic attack is characterized by "out of the blue" episodes of terror and may be indistinguishable from symptoms of a heart attack with a pounding heart, chest pain, shortness of breath, sweating, and nausea.[16] Classically, panic attacks occur without warning and often wake an individual from sleep. The location where an attack occurs may become associated with precipitating the episode, and phobias and avoidance may ensue in an effort to avert further attacks.

Management

The obstetrician generally refers a patient with panic disorder for treatment. Treatment with medication during pregnancy generally consists of an SSRI, beginning with a very low dose. When initiating SSRI treatment, some psychiatrists will also provide benzodiazepines for breakthrough panic attacks. In addition, cognitive behavioral therapy has been shown to be as effective as medication (SSRIs, high-potency benzodiazepines, and tricyclic antidepressants) and more effective than placebo in multiple randomized controlled trials.

Obsessive–compulsive disorder

Epidemiology

Obsessive–compulsive disorder (OCD) has a lifetime prevalence of approximately 2.5% for both women and men,[58] but prospective studies identifying the prevalence in pregnant and postpartum women are lacking.[59] A connection between pregnancy, childbirth, and obsessional states has long been recognized,[60,61] and women are more vulnerable to the onset of OCD during pregnancy and following childbirth.[62–65] In addition, women with pre-existing OCD who miscarry are at a significant risk for an exacerbation of symptoms.[66]

Clinical presentation

OCD is characterized by the presence of obsessions (e.g., excessive concern with dirt or germs)[59] and compulsions (e.g., checking locks and windows, repetitive handwashing, or other ritualistic behaviors).[16] In the postpartum state, the obsessions can include unwanted aggressive thoughts toward the infant. To relieve the distress caused by the obsessions, the patient feels compelled to perform ritual behaviors to prevent bad things from happening.

Management

Patients with OCD should be referred for psychiatric treatment. Treatment will usually include higher doses of SSRIs and behavioral therapy to help the patient decrease her compulsions.[67]

Post-traumatic stress disorder

Epidemiology

Lifetime rates of post-traumatic stress disorder (PTSD) in women range from 10.4% to 13.8%.[49,51,68] The exact rates in pregnancy are unknown, but one study[69] found a 7.7% prevalence of PTSD in economically disadvantaged pregnant women. PTSD in pregnancy has been associated with an increased incidence of miscarriage, hyperemesis, and preterm labor.[70] PTSD often occurs alongside generalized anxiety disorder,[69] depression, and substance abuse.[49] PTSD in women is most often a sequela of sexual assault,[51,68] and women with a history of sexual assault may attempt to avoid reminders of the trauma such as intrusive procedures in prenatal care.[69]

Clinical presentation

Women with PTSD suffer from intrusive recollections of an experienced or witnessed life-threatening traumatic event. Recollections can present as flashbacks, nightmares, sympathetic nervous system arousal, emotional numbing, or global hyperarousal, and patients will make great efforts to avoid stimuli that trigger reminders of the trauma.[16] In pregnancy, labor pains may induce flashbacks and dissociative exacerbations.[71]

Management

Evidence-based treatment for PTSD includes SSRIs, which have been shown to be more effective than placebo. Cognitive behavioral therapy (CBT) and eye movement desensitization have also been shown in randomized controlled trials to be effective. The obstetrician should avoid precipitating trauma by intrusive medical procedures whenever possible,[69] and should provide the patient with verbal information before the initiation of any procedure or touch.

Psychiatric emergencies

Psychiatric emergencies are most likely to occur in the first month postpartum,[72,73] but may arise at any point in the course of obstetric care. Four major conditions should be regarded as emergencies requiring immediate psychiatric consultation: psychosis, delirium, suicidal ideation, and homicidal ideation.

Psychosis and psychotic disorders

The term psychosis refers to a gross impairment in reality testing characterized by the presence of auditory or visual hallucinations or a false fixed belief system.[16] Psychosis may occur as a result of an organic precipitant or a major mental illness (e.g., schizophrenia, schizoaffective disorder, bipolar disorder, major depression, and delusional disorders). The evaluation for a primary episode of psychosis must rule out any underlying medical illness (e.g., metastatic brain tumor, endocrine or metabolic disorder, electrolyte disturbance, medication- or substance-induced effect).

Epidemiology

Psychotic psychiatric disorders occur in less than 2% of women aged from 18 to 44,[74] and the prevalence is similar in pregnant and nonpregnant women of childbearing age.[75] The annual incidence in pregnancy is 7.1 cases per 100 000 pregnancies.[76] Because newer antipsychotic medications induce less hyperprolactinemia, more women taking antipsychotics are now becoming pregnant. Schizophrenia has been associated with preterm delivery, low birthweight, and small for gestational age (SGA) infants.[77–79] In addition, there is an increased risk of stillbirth[80] and neonatal death.[78,79,81] Offspring of women with schizophrenia have an 8- to 10-fold higher risk of developing the disorder than the general population.[82]

Postpartum psychosis affects 2 out of 1000 new mothers[72] and most often has an abrupt onset within the first 2 weeks after birth. Women with bipolar affective disorder have a 100-fold greater risk of developing a postpartum psychosis than women with no previous psychiatric history.[83–86] In addition, women with bipolar disorder are at a higher risk for postpartum depression than women with a history of unipolar depression. Postpartum psychotic exacerbations occur in 25% of women with a prior history of schizophrenia,[87] and for women with a prior episode of postpartum psychosis the estimates of recurrence in subsequent pregnancies range from 20% to 90%.[88,89]

Clinical presentation

The essential features of a psychosis are hallucinations or delusions. Psychotic individuals may behave bizarrely and have disorganized thoughts and speech but generally remain cognitively oriented to person, place, time, and situation. The majority of postpartum psychoses are affective (i.e., manic or depressive psychoses) and may present with perplexity, confusion, and prominent delusions and hallucinations.[90–94] Family members may report waxing and waning episodes (generally more characteristic of delirium), with the patient appearing well one moment and psychotic the next.[88] The patient may also experience somatic psychotic symptoms (e.g., tactile, olfactory, and visual hallucinations) that are generally more characteristic of a psychosis precipitated by a brain tumor or withdrawal from a substance.[93] Mothers with postpartum psychosis rarely express hostility toward the newborn but may harbor potentially dangerous delusional thoughts (e.g., believing that the infant is "evil" or "would be better off dead").

Management

Regardless of the underlying etiology, the presence of psychosis constitutes a psychiatric emergency. Judgment is so seriously impaired in the presence of delusions or hallucinations that the obstetrician should be concerned about the risk for suicide or homicide. Command auditory hallucinations, in which a patient hears a voice directing her actions, are particularly worrying. In addition to requesting an immediate psychiatric evaluation to assess the current risk for suicide or homicide, the obstetrician should contact a concerned family member who can assist with a history and disposition. The patient must not be left unsupervised while awaiting psychiatric evaluation and appropriate disposition. A thorough medical workup including vital signs, electrolytes, urine drug screen, and physical and neurological examinations is necessary. Obtaining an accurate past psychiatric and substance use history is also critical in guiding the appropriate intervention and treatment. Tables 57.7 and 57.8 list the pharmacological treatment considerations in psychosis.

Ideally, a woman with a past history of psychotic disorder will obtain a preconception consultation with both an obstetrician and a psychiatrist to evaluate whether she should remain on antipsychotic medication throughout the pregnancy or discontinue it during gestational periods of highest risk.[95] Typical antipsychotics, including chlorpromazine and thioridazine, have the longest history of use in pregnancy; there are fewer safety data available for the newer atypical antipsychotics, including olanzapine and clozapine, and these drugs have been associated with an increased risk of glucose intol-

Table 57.7 Treatment considerations in psychosis.[94]

Infants born to psychotic women (on no medication) have twice the normal rate of malformations[25]
No treatment regimen is completely safe[146]
The risks of harm associated with exposure to antipsychotics *in utero* or through breastfeeding are unknown[146,147]
Discontinuing antipsychotic treatment during pregnancy is associated with a 65% relapse rate[148]
The risk of avoiding medication may outweigh any treatment-associated danger
Avoid neuroleptics during the first trimester when possible[149,150]
Avoid low-potency antipsychotics (chlorpromazine) with orthostatic hypotension and sedation[146]
Use high-potency traditional antipsychotics (haloperidol or flupenazine) at the lowest effective dose
Use a single antipsychotic medication
Monitor newborn for perinatal syndrome; motor restlessness, tremor, hypertonicity, abnormal movements, and difficulty with feeding[151]

Table 57.8 Specific pharmacological treatment considerations in psychosis.[94]

	Exposure data
Conventional (typical) antipsychotics[152]	
Phenothiazines	
Thorazine (clorpromazine)	Long history of use in pregnancy for hyperemesis gravidarum Use between weeks 4 and 10 increases risk of anomalies to 4 in 1000[153,154]
Thioridazine (Mellaril)	Not associated with a higher rate of malformations[154]
Fluphenazine (Prolixin)	Not associated with a higher rate of malformations[154]
Trifluoperazine (Stelazine)	Not associated with a higher rate of malformations[154]
Perphenazine (Trilafon)	Not associated with a higher rate of malformations[154]
Buterophenone	*Exposure data*
Haloperidol (Haldol)	Low dose used in hyperemesis not associated with malformations[155,156] Elevates prolactin
New (atypical) antipsychotics: limited data available	
Clozapine (Clozaril),[157] used in treatment of refractory schizophrenia	Does not appear to increase teratogenic risk[94] Risks for agranulocytosis in fetus are unknown Contraindicated in breastfeeding; may cause sedation, decreased suckling, restlessness or irritability, seizures, and cardiovascular instability[157,158] Monitor for hyperglycemia and excessive weight gain Accumulates in fetal serum and breast milk more than maternal serum[159]
Olanzapine (Zyprexa)	Does not appear to increase teratogenic risk[94] Lower prolactin levels than with other antipsychotics; increases fertility Monitor for hyperglycemia and excessive weight gain
Risperidone (Risperdal)	Elevates prolactin Limited data available
Quetiapine (Seroquel)	Limited data available
Aripiprazole (Abilify)	Limited data available
Ziprasidone (Geodon)	Limited data available

erance and weight gain during gestation. All antipsychotics have been placed in pregnancy category C by the FDA. At present, the newer atypical agents do not demonstrate any evident safety advantages in pregnancy and lactation compared with older, more typical neuroleptic agents.[94]

If an acutely psychotic patient conceives, her mental state may deteriorate resulting from the stress of pregnancy. She is at risk for incorporating her bodily changes into her delusional thinking such as believing that fetal movement is caused by "snakes growing in her belly." In circumstances of acute psychosis, the risk of deterioration and noncompliance with prenatal care must be weighed against the risk of exposure of the fetus to medication. Generally, symptoms are rapidly controlled with antipsychotic medication, keeping the patient and fetus safe. Once stable, the medication dose can be gradually reduced.[96] For patients with treatment-resistant psychosis during pregnancy or those who do not wish to expose the fetus to medication, ECT has been used and appears safe if both the mother and fetus are carefully monitored.[97] Women with postpartum psychosis who are at risk of harm to themselves or others require immediate psychiatric hospitalization. Ideally, they should be admitted with their infants whenever possible.

Delirium

Delirium refers to a state of acute cerebral insufficiency resulting from an underlying medical emergency and is associated with high morbidity and mortality. Delirium is rare in obstetrics but may be seen in cases of sepsis, severe anemia, hypoxia, and electrolyte disturbance. Alcohol and benzodiazepine withdrawal may also precipitate a potentially life-threatening delirium with elevated vital signs. The classic symptoms of delirium are a waxing and waning course of disorientation, bizarre perceptual disturbances, and psychomotor agitation or retardation. Patients with delirium will often be unable to draw the hands on the face of a clock.

Suicidal ideation

Suicide is the leading cause of maternal death in the first postpartum year.[98,99] Patients with delirium, psychosis, bipolar disorder, and severe depressive illness are at a heightened risk for suicide.[98] Delirium and psychosis pose a serious risk of suicide as the patient may act swiftly with little or no warning. In one study, nearly one-half of mothers who committed suicide had been admitted to a psychiatric hospital following a previous childbirth, but healthcare providers caring for them in subsequent pregnancies were frequently unaware of their histories. Suicidal ideation may be expressed passively ("I'd be better off dead") or actively ("I would like to drive my car off the bridge"). It is important to inquire as to whether the patient has envisioned a method by which to take her own life, whether she has the means to do so, what has prevented her from acting on her feelings, and whether she feels safe not to act on them now. The obstetrician should request an emergency psychiatric consultation to evaluate the need for medication and/or hospitalization.

Homicidal ideation

As with suicide, homicide is a serious risk in delirium and other psychotic states because the patient may act suddenly and without warning, often in response to command hallucinations. In general, the expression of homicidal thoughts should be taken at face value as a plea for immediate help. The obstetrician should request an emergency psychiatric consultation as to the need for hospitalization and the application of the mandatory duty to warn potential adult victims and protect potential child victims.[100]

Miscellaneous treatment challenges

Bipolar disorder (manic depressive disorder)

Epidemiology

Bipolar disorder is a serious, recurrent psychiatric illness with a lifetime prevalence of above 1% for women and men.[48] Studies examining the specific prevalence of this disorder in pregnancy do not exist. The postpartum period represents the time of highest risk for symptom exacerbation and 40% of women with bipolar disorder experience postpartum mania or depression.[85,101] A history of postpartum exacerbation increases the risk of postpartum episodes in subsequent pregnancies. Recent studies have shown that puerperal prophylaxis with a mood stabilizer reduces the rate of recurrence to 10%.[102–104] Given the risks associated with a postpartum bipolar episode for both mother and newborn, the use of prophylactic mood stabilizers is advised.[85] Suicide is also a grave concern, with actual suicide carried out by 10–15% of individuals with the most severe form of bipolar disorder.[99]

Clinical presentation

Bipolar disorder is characterized by alternating episodes of depression and mania. Symptoms of mania may include an elated or irritable mood, having high energy and requiring little sleep, grandiose ideas of self-importance, rapid and pressured speech, spending excessive amounts of money, a high libido, and poor impulse control.[16]

Management

The management of bipolar disorder during pregnancy and postpartum is challenging and should be undertaken by a psychiatrist with expertise in women's mental health, in close collaboration with the patient's obstetrician. Mood stabilizers such as valproic acid (Depakote) and carbamazepine (Tegretol), which are routinely prescribed to manage bipolar disorder, are neurotoxic (see Table 57.9) and associated with significant rates of malformation (e.g., neural tube defects, craniofacial anomalies, growth retardation, microcephaly, and heart defects).[105,106] Lithium, although less teratogenic than once thought, is associated with a 0.1–0.2% risk for Ebstein's anomaly when taken during the first trimester. To date, lamotrigine (Lamictal) appears to be the safest mood stabilizer in pregnancy but data are limited. Antipsychotics are safer than most other mood stabilizers. Mood stabilizers are frequently discontinued during conception and early pregnancy in an attempt to avoid the windows of greatest risk to the developing fetus (see Table 57.10); the mother should be closely monitored during this time. For women who wish to breastfeed, proactive planning should be undertaken by the patient, psychiatrist, and pediatrician, who will review the latest evidence regarding the potential risks and benefits. The cautious approach[85] for a bipolar woman who wishes to breastfeed (on a mood stabilizer during the final weeks of pregnancy) is to pump and discard her breast milk for the first 2 days following delivery. This allows a "washout" period for the infant's immature system before initiating breastfeeding. After these first 2 days, lactation consultants and supportive pediatricians are instrumental in assisting the newborn to take the breast rather than a bottle. The breastfeeding mother must be knowledgeable about the signs and management of potential toxicity in her newborn.

Eating disorders

Anorexia nervosa and bulimia complicate approximately 1% of pregnancies;[107] they affect 4.5 million American women overall[108] and are a risk factor for hyperemesis gravidarim. Most women attempt to hide their eating disorder and may not spontaneously reveal their behavior to the obstetrician. Detection is important, however, as eating disorders are associated with miscarriage, low birthweight, intrauterine growth retardation (IUGR), preterm delivery, Cesarean birth, low Apgar scores,[108] and a higher frequency of postpartum depression.[109] Anorexia is also associated with a high mortality rate, which is frequently attributed to cardiac failure and severe electrolyte abnormalities.[108] All women with hyperemesis gravidarim should be screened for comorbid eating disorders.

Clinical presentation

The prevalence of anorexia nervosa in women between the ages of 15 and 29 is approximately 0.1%[110] and appears to be increasing. It is characterized by a 15% reduction in weight below the normal range, an intense fear of gaining weight, and

Table 57.9 Pharmacological treatment considerations in bipolar disorder.

Medication	Organ dysgenesis	Clinical management	Breastfeeding[85]
Lithium: considered first-line treatment option in pregnancy[101,160]	Ebstein's anomaly occurs in 1 in 20 000 of the general population, and 1 or 2 in 1000 offspring of lithium users, although the absolute risk remains small[161,162]	High-resolution ultrasound with fetal echocardiography at 16–18 weeks to aid in decision-making[163] Increase dose in second trimester Decrease dose in labor Maintain adequate hydration Observe the neonate for signs of toxicity,[163] and "floppy baby" syndrome, and manage supportively	Expert opinion ranges from strong statements against breastfeeding while taking lithium to supporting a mother's informed choice[122] Many have breast fed without complication with careful monitoring of infant's and mother's blood levels, complete blood count (CBC) and thyroid status, and a rapid reduction in dose exposure when infant has fever, dehydration, or diarrhea[164]
Valproate: avoid in pregnancy if possible	First-trimester exposure associated with neural tube defect (5–9%) Effect occurs 17–30 days post conception Risk is dose related	4 mg of folic acid per day before and during pregnancy[105] Measure B12 level before folate supplementation[101] Observe neonate for heart rate decelerations;[165] withdrawal symptoms of irritability, jitteriness, feeding difficulties, abnormal tone;[166] liver toxicity,[167] hypoglycemia,[168] and low fibrinogen levels[169]	Usually compatible with breastfeeding[164,170] Infant serum levels range from undetectable to 40% of maternal serum levels Half-life in neonates is 47 h; in infants from 10 days to 2 months, half-life is 9–22 h[171]
Carbamazepine: avoid in pregnancy if possible	Neural tube defect (0.5–1%),[172,173] craniofacial defects (11%), fingernail hypoplasia (26%), and developmental delay (20%)[172] Risk worse when co-administered with valproate[173]	20 mg of oral vitamin K per day in the last month of pregnancy[174] Can cause fetal vitamin K deficiency; administer 1 mg i.m. of vitamin K to exposed neonates[101]	Usually compatible with breastfeeding[164,170] Infant serum levels range from 6% to 65% of maternal serum concentrations[85] Monitor for hepatic dysfunction[164,175,176]
Lamotrigine: approved as a maintenance therapy for bipolar disorder	Risk for major malformation appears to be similar to the general population rate (about 2%)	Increase dose in second trimester Decrease dose in labor[177] Observe neonate for hepatotoxicity and skin rash	Infant serum levels range from 23% to 33% of maternal serum concentrations
Gabapentin	More research is needed before safety in pregnancy and breastfeeding can be clarified[178]		
Oxcarbazepine	More research is needed before safety in pregnancy and breastfeeding can be clarified[178]		

Table 57.10 Associated risks in bipolar disorder.[101]

Potential risks of pharmacotherapy in pregnancy
Neural tube defects (window of risk: 17–30 days after conception)
Heart defects (window of risk: 21–56 days after conception)
Lip/palate defects (window of risk: 8–11 weeks after conception)
Craniofacial defects (window of risk: 8–20 weeks after conception)
Neurobehavioral teratogenicity from exposure after the first trimester

Pregnancy and recurrence risks
Abrupt discontinuation of a mood stabilizer (1–14 days) led to a 100% relapse of illness
Slow taper over more than 2 weeks (15–30 days) led to a 62% risk for relapse

a distorted body image. In nonpregnant women, one criterion for diagnosis is the lack of menses for 3 months.[16] Binging, purging, and laxative use are often present and increase the risk for cardiac irregularities. Women may attempt to conceal their weight loss from healthcare providers and may try to wear shoes or have heavy items in their clothing when being weighed.

The prevalence of bulimia in women ranges from 1% to 3.8%[111,112] and consists of recurrent episodes (at least two times per week for 3 months) of uncontrollable binge eating with inappropriate compensatory behavior to prevent weight gain. These compensatory behaviors include self-induced vomiting; misuse of laxatives, diuretics, enemas, or other medications; and excessive exercise.[16] Women with bulimia may be of normal weight, underweight, or slightly overweight.

An atypical eating disorder occurs in women with diabetes who withhold their insulin to lose weight. Clinical signs include disparate hemoglobin A_{1c} levels and dramatic weight fluctuations over time. Recognition of this maladaptive pattern of weight control is of critical importance as it is associated with extremely high rates of diabetic complications.[108]

Management

Obstetricians should routinely calculate prepregnancy body mass index (BMI)[113] and ask patients about any current or past history of eating disorders. Women with a BMI below 18 kg/m^2 before pregnancy will need to gain extra weight in the early part of pregnancy to prevent fetal growth restriction.[114] For pregnant women with an eating disorder, it is important to screen for comorbid depression.[109] It is also helpful to query the patient about her preferences for weight measurements (e.g., allowing the patient to face away from the scale or not informing her of the result unless it is significantly low).[113] The patient should be comanaged with a team of eating disorder specialists in dietetics and mental health.

Somatization

Patients with multiple physical complaints who lack organic findings are challenging to the physician. Pregnant women with current depressive and anxiety disorders have significantly more somatic symptoms such as nausea, headaches, shortness of breath, and discomfort with intercourse than pregnant women without these disorders.[115] In addition, depression and anxiety are associated with a general amplification of the normal physical symptoms of pregnancy (both pregnancy-related and other physical symptoms).[115]

When a patient complains of multiple unexplained physical symptoms and she does not have depression or an anxiety disorder, she may have somatization disorder. The DSM-IV criteria for somatization disorder include a history of many physical complaints beginning before the age of 30 and occurring over a period of several years, resulting in the seeking of treatment or significant impairment in social, occupational, or other important areas of functioning. The symptoms must include: (1) pain in at least four different parts of the body; (2) at least two gastrointestinal symptoms; (3) at least one sexual symptom; and (4) one neurological symptom. The physical symptoms cannot be fully explained by a known medical condition or substance, or are in excess of what would be expected.[16] Management should include avoiding unnecessary medical tests, offering reassurance, and scheduling additional time for patient visits to allow time to address her physical complaints through physical examination. Healthcare providers should avoid prescribing analgesic and anxiolytic substances. In addition, the healthcare provider may offer nonjudgmental education that the patient's body may be exquisitely sensitive and "oversignaling" the normal physical changes associated with pregnancy. Some patients benefit from CBT where they relearn how to interpret bodily cues.

Denial of pregnancy

Denial of pregnancy[116] is a heterogeneous condition called an "adjustment disorder with a maladaptive denial of a physical condition."[117] It can be associated with continued menstruation-like bleeding (use of oral contraceptives may contribute) throughout the pregnancy, causing the woman to believe she cannot be pregnant. Denial, an unconscious defense mechanism, can appear when a woman is confronted with an unwanted or unintended pregnancy. This defense mechanism is common in children and immature adults during times of severe external stress and internal conflict.

When a woman beyond 20 weeks' gestation is informed of a pregnancy for which she has been completely unaware, she may feel embarrassment and guilt.[118] The patient may feel that she has put her fetus at risk by not seeking prenatal care and by failing to alter her lifestyle appropriately. Immediately following the diagnosis, the care team should address the psychosocial stressors associated with the denial. Psychiatric assessment and counseling are indicated to evaluate the patient's parenting skills and support network, and whether she is prepared and capable of caring for her child.

Capacity to parent

When it is feared that a newborn will be at risk if a parent is allowed to take the child home and/or a previous history of child abuse or neglect exists, a maternal competency evaluation in the immediate postpartum period may be warranted. Risk factors involve both maternal and newborn features (see Tables 57.11–57.13). A comprehensive assessment including evaluations by psychiatry,[119] nursing, neonatology, and social work departments will provide a better understanding of the mother's capacity to parent and will guide appropriate interventions for the future.[120]

Pregnancy after loss

Carrying a pregnancy following a previous pregnancy or neonatal loss is associated with significant distress and anxiety for the woman and her partner.[55,66,121] Table 57.14 lists recommendations for managing a pregnancy following a previous loss.

Resources

The following websites can be accessed to obtain further information:

1 AED (Antiepileptic Drug) Pregnancy Registry, Genetics & Teratology Unit.[85] Registry for pregnant women who are using antiepileptic drugs. World Wide Web URL: http://www.aedpregnancyregistry.org.

2 The Motherisk Program.[122,123] A counseling service for pregnant and lactating mothers on the safety and risk of drugs,

chemicals, radiation, and infections to the fetus and neonate. World Wide Web URL: http://www.motherisk.org.

3 Emory Women's Program.[41] A website with links to many support groups, reproductive safety registries, or other women's health websites. World Wide Web URL: http://www.emorywomensprogram.org.

Table 57.11 Risk factors for maternal incompetence.[120]

Psychiatric problems
Major mental illness with lack of insight
Munchausen syndrome by proxy
Drug or alcohol dependence
Severe personality disorder
Cognitive problems
Mental retardation
Medical and neurological problems
Major medical illness (e.g., heart failure or AIDS)
Motor deficit (e.g., stroke, spinal cord injury)
Sensory impairment (e.g., blindness or deafness without adequate compensation)
Problems with maternal–infant relationship
History of child abuse or removal of child from custody
Unwanted or unplanned pregnancy
Lack of interest in infant and verbal threats
Lack of support
Homelessness
Social isolation
No heat or utilities
Past problems in social/family relationships
Maternal childhood history of abuse
History of violence
Previous infanticide

Table 57.12 Risk factors for maltreatment of infants.[120]

Major medical problems requiring constant medical attention
Cardiorespiratory monitoring
Tube feeding or poor feeders
Oxygen needed at home
Difficult temperament
Physical or intellectual defects
Prematurity

Table 57.13 Predictors of good parenting.[120]

A positive attitude toward the pregnancy
Prepared for infant
Supportive partner
Good parental role models
Realistic expectations of an infant
Appropriate response to infant's cues

Table 57.14 Management of pregnancy following previous loss.

Acknowledge the distress[55]
Address fears about the current pregnancy
Frequent prenatal visits[121]
Additional support through telephone contact[121]
Reassuring check of fetal heart tones
Reassuring ultrasound

Key points

1. Women suffering from a severe depressive illness or psychosis are at risk for suicide, the leading cause of maternal death through the first postpartum year.[98]
2. About 9–23% of antepartum women suffer from depression characterized by feelings of anhedonia, guilt, hopelessness, and possible suicidal thoughts.
3. Antepartum depression is associated with increased physical pain and discomfort,[115] smoking, alcohol and other drug use,[124,125] and poor participation in prenatal care.[28]
4. Antepartum depression is associated with low birthweight,[126,127] SGA infants,[127] preeclampsia,[128] preterm delivery,[127] and operative delivery.[129]
5. During the postpartum period, 50–70% of women experience transient postpartum blues.
6. During the postpartum period, 12–16% of women suffer from postpartum depression.
7. Women with a previous history of depression have a 25% risk for developing postpartum depression.
8. The abrupt discontinuation of an antidepressant before a full course of treatment is associated with a significant risk for the relapse of depression.
9. Women with a history of postpartum depression have a 50% chance of it recurring and should be monitored closely throughout pregnancy.
10. Postpartum depression is associated with difficulty in breastfeeding,[130] poor growth of the infant as well as failure to thrive,[131,132] decreased IQ in infants and children,[42] missed pediatric outpatient appointments and increased emergency room visits,[133] marital and relationship difficulties,[134] depression,[43] and violence in children.[135]
11. Minimal concentrations of sertraline, paroxetine, and nortriptyline in breastmilk make them preferred antidepressants in breastfeeding.[40]

12 Anxiety disorders are common in women and are associated with low birthweight,[136] preeclampsia,[128] premature rupture of membranes,[137] preterm delivery,[138] operative delivery,[137,139] and increased risk for behavioral/emotional problems in children.[140]

13 Women with bipolar disorder have a significant risk for postpartum psychosis, depression, and mania.

14 Puerperal prophylaxis with a mood stabilizer decreases the rates of postpartum bipolar exacerbations to 10%.

15 Prescribing an antidepressant medication to a woman with bipolar disorder who is not on an antimanic agent can precipitate mania.

16 Eating disorders are associated with miscarriage, low birthweight, IUGR, preterm delivery, Cesarean birth, low Apgar scores, and postpartum depression.

17 An atypical eating disorder in diabetics who withhold their insulin for weight control is associated with widely fluctuating weight and hemoglobin A_{1c} levels, and significant morbidity and mortality.

18 The onset of OCD often occurs in the postpartum period.

19 Women with post-traumatic stress disorder may experience flashbacks and dissociative episodes during obstetrical procedures and labor.

20 Schizophrenia is associated with preterm delivery, low birthweight, SGA infants, stillbirth, and neonatal death.

References

1 Holcomb WL, Jr, et al. Screening for depression in pregnancy: characteristics of the Beck Depression Inventory. *Obstet Gynecol* 1996;88:1021–1025.

2 Johanson R, et al. The North Staffordshire Maternity Hospital prospective study of pregnancy-associated depression. *J Psychosom Obstet Gynecol* 2000;21:93–97.

3 Spitzer RL, et al. Validity and utility of the PRIME-MD patient health questionnaire in assessment of 3000 obstetric-gynecologic patients: the PRIME-MD Patient Health Questionnaire Obstetrics–Gynecology Study. *Am J Obstet Gynecol* 2000;183:759–769.

4 Kelly R, et al. The detection and treatment of psychiatric disorders and substance use among pregnant women cared for in obstetrics. *Am J Psychiatry* 2001;158:213–219.

5 Smith M, et al. Screening for and detection of depression, panic disorder, and PTSD in public-sector obstetric clinics. *Psychiatr Serv* 2004;55:407–414.

6 Andersson L, et al. Neonatal outcome following maternal antenatal depression and anxiety: a population-based study. *Am J Epidemiol* 2004;159:872–881.

7 O'Hara MW, et al. Rates and risk of postpartum depression: a meta-analysis. *Int Rev Psychiatry* 1996;8:37–54.

8 Wisner KL, et al. Clinical practice. Postpartum depression (see Comment). *N Engl J Med* 2002;347:194–199.

9 Wadhwa PD, et al. Prenatal psychosocial factors and the neuroendocrine axis in human pregnancy. *Psychosom Med* 1996; 58:432–446.

10 Hobel CJ, et al. Maternal plasma corticotropin-releasing hormone associated with stress at 20 weeks' gestation in pregnancies ending in preterm delivery. *Am J Obstet Gynecol* 1999;180:S257–S263.

11 Teixeira JM, et al. Association between maternal anxiety in pregnancy and increased uterine artery resistance index: cohort based study (see Comment). *Br Med J* 1999;318:153–157.

12 Martin JA, et al. Births: final data for 2002. *Natl Vital Stat Rep* 2003;52:1–113.

13 Zhu SH, et al. Depression and smoking during pregnancy. *Addict Behav* 2002;27:649–658.

14 Anda RF, et al. Depression and the dynamics of smoking. A national perspective (see Comment). *JAMA* 1990;264:1541–1545.

15 Dierker LC, et al. Smoking and depression: an examination of mechanisms of comorbidity. *Am J Psychiatry* 2002;159:947–953.

16 American Psychiatric Association. *Diagnostic and statistical manual of mental disorders*, 4th edn revised. Washington, DC: American Psychiatric Press, 2000.

17 Newport DJ, et al. Maternal depression: a child's first adverse life event. *Semin Clin Neuropsychiatry* 2002;7:113–119.

18 Altschuler LL, et al. Treatment of depression in women: a summary of the expert consensus guidelines. *J Psychiatric Pract* 2001:185–208.

19 Stuart S, et al. The prevention and psychotherapeutic treatment of postpartum depression. *Arch Wom Ment Health* 2003; 6(Suppl.2):57–69.

20 Spinelli MG. Interpersonal psychotherapy for depressed antepartum women: a pilot study. *Am J Psychiatry* 1997;154:1028–1030.

21 Oren DA, et al. An open trial of morning light therapy for treatment of antepartum depression. *Am J Psychiatry* 2002;159: 666–669.

22 Epperson CN, et al. Randomized clinical trial of bright light therapy for antepartum depression: preliminary findings. *J Clin Psychiatry* 2004;65:421–425.

23 Freeman MP, et al. Selected integrative medicine treatments for depression: considerations for women. *J Am Med Wom Assoc* 2004;59:216–224.

24 Stowe Z. *Ob/gyn grand rounds: depression and anxiety disorders in women across the reproductive life: identification and treatment*. Little Rock, AR:2004.

25 Altshuler LL, et al. Pharmacologic management of psychiatric illness during pregnancy: dilemmas and guidelines. *Am J Psychiatry* 1996;153:592–606.

26 Cohen L, et al. Pharmacologic management of psychiatric illness during pregnancy and the postpartum period. In: Rosenbaum J, ed. *Psychiatric clinics of North America: annual of drug therapy*. Philadelphia, PA: WB Saunders; 1997:21–60.

27 Wisner KL, et al. Pharmacologic treatment of depression during pregnancy. *JAMA* 1999;282:1264–1269.

28 Nonacs R, et al. Assessment and treatment of depression during pregnancy: an update. *Psychiatr Clin North Am* 2003;26: 547–562.

29 Koren G, et al. Drugs in pregnancy. *N Engl J Psychiatry* 1996;338:1128–1137.

30 Ostrer H. Etiology of birth defects. *Up To Date*, 2004;13.2.

31 FDA, FDA Alert. *Increase in the risk of birth defects. Paroxetine hydrochloride (marketed as Paxil) information*. US Food and Drug Administration. Center for Drug Evaluation and Research, 2005.

32 Ferrill MJ, et al. ECT during pregnancy: physiologic and pharmacologic considerations. *Convulsive Ther* 1992;8:186–200.

33 Miller LJ. Use of electroconvulsive therapy during pregnancy. *Hosp Community Psychiatry* 1994;45:444–450.

34 Chambers D, et al. Birth outcomes in pregnant women taking fluoxetine. *N Engl J Med* 1996;335:1010–1015.

35 Koren G. Discontinuation syndrome following late pregnancy exposure to antidepressants. *Arch Pediatr Adolesc Med* 2004;158:307–308.

36 Godding V, et al. Does in utero exposure to heavy maternal smoking induce nicotine withdrawal symptoms in neonates? *Pediatr Res* 2004;55:645–651.

37 Law KL, et al. Smoking during pregnancy and newborn neurobehavior (see Comment). *Pediatrics* 2003;111:1318–1323.

38 American Academy of Pediatrics. The promotion of breastfeeding. Policy statement based on task force report. *Pediatrics* 1982;69:654–661.

39 Yoshida K, et al. Investigation of pharmacokinetics and of possible adverse effects in infants exposed to tricyclic antidepressants in breast-milk. *J Affective Disord* 1997;43:225–237.

40 Weissman AM, et al. Pooled analysis of antidepressant levels in lactating mothers, breast milk, and nursing infants. *Am J Psychiatry* 2004;161:1066–1078.

41 Levey L, et al. Psychiatric disorders in pregnancy. *Neurol Clin* 2004;22:863–893.

42 Hay DF, et al. Intellectual problems shown by 11-year-old children whose mothers had postnatal depression. *J Child Psychol Psychiatry Allied Disciplines* 2001;42:871–889.

43 Halligan SL, et al. Exposure to postnatal depression predicts elevated cortisol in adolescent offspring. *Biol Psychiatry* 2004;55:376–381.

44 Schulberg HC, et al. Treating major depression in primary care practice. Eight-month clinical outcomes. *Arch Gen Psychiatry* 1996;53:913–919.

45 Kocsis JH, et al. Stability of remission during tricyclic antidepressant continuation therapy for dysthymia. *Psychopharmacol Bull* 1995;31:213–216.

46 Keller MB, et al. Maintenance phase efficacy of sertraline for chronic depression: a randomized controlled trial (see Comment). *JAMA* 1998;280:1665–1672.

47 Kocsis JH, et al. Maintenance therapy for chronic depression: a controlled clinical trial of desipramine. *Arch Gen Psychiatry* 1996;53:769–774.

48 Kessler RC, et al. Lifetime and 12-month prevalence of DSM-III-R psychiatric disorders in the United States. Results from the National Comorbidity Survey. *Arch Gen Psychiatry* 1994;51: 8–19.

49 Levine RE, et al. Anxiety disorders during pregnancy and postpartum. *Am J Perinatol* 2003;20:239–248.

50 Wenzel A, et al. Prevalence of generalized anxiety at eight weeks postpartum. *Arch Wom Ment Health* 2003;6:43–49.

51 Kessler RC, et al. Posttraumatic stress disorder in the National Comorbidity Survey. *Arch Gen Psychiatry* 1995;52:1048–1060.

52 George DT, et al. Effect of pregnancy on panic attacks. *Am J Psychiatry* 1987;144:1078–1079.

53 Villeponteaux VA, et al. The effects of pregnancy on preexisting panic disorder. *J Clin Psychiatry* 1992;53:201–203.

54 Northcott CJ, et al. Panic disorder in pregnancy. *J Clin Psychiatry* 1994;55:539–542.

55 Geller PA, et al. Anxiety following miscarriage and the subsequent pregnancy: a review of the literature and future directions. *J Psychosom Res* 2004;56:35–45.

56 Cohen LS, et al. Course of panic disorder during pregnancy and the puerperium: a preliminary study. *Biol Psychiatry* 1996;39: 950–954.

57 Cohen LS, et al. Postpartum course in women with preexisting panic disorder. *J Clin Psychiatry* 1994;55:289–292.

58 Karno M, et al. The epidemiology of obsessive-compulsive disorder in five US communities. *Arch Gen Psychiatry* 1988;45: 1094–1099.

59 Abramowitz JS, et al. Obsessive-compulsive symptoms in pregnancy and the puerperium: a review of the literature. *J Anxiety Disord* 2003;17:461–478.

60 Pollitt J. Natural history of obsessional states; a study of 150 cases. *Br Med J* 1957;32:194–198.

61 Ingram IM. Obsessional illness in mental hospital patients. *J Ment Sci* 1961;107:382–402.

62 Brandt KR,et al. Obsessive-compulsive disorder exacerbated during pregnancy: a case report. *Int J Psychiatry Med* 1987; 17:361–366.

63 Neziroglu F, et al. Onset of obsessive-compulsive disorder in pregnancy. *Am J Psychiatry* 1992;149:947–950.

64 Williams KE, et al. Obsessive-compulsive disorder in pregnancy, the puerperium, and the premenstruum. *J Clin Psychiatry* 1997;58:330–334.

65 Neziroglu F, et al. Onset of obsessive-compulsive disorder in pregnancy (see Comment). *Am J Psychiatry* 1992;149:947–950.

66 Geller PA, et al. Anxiety disorders following miscarriage. *J Clin Psychiatry* 2001;62:432–438.

67 Diaz SF, et al. Obsessive-compulsive disorder in pregnancy and the puerperium. In: Dickstein LJ, et al. (eds) *American Psychiatric Press review of psychiatry*, vol 16. Washington, DC: American Psychiatric Press; 1997:97-112.

68 Resnick HS, et al. Prevalence of civilian trauma and posttraumatic stress disorder in a representative national sample of women. *J Consult Clin Psychol* 1993;61:984–991.

69 Loveland Cook CA, et al. Posttraumatic stress disorder in pregnancy: prevalence, risk factors, and treatment. *Obstet Gynecol* 2004;103:710–717.

70 Yehuda R. Post-traumatic stress disorder (see Comment). *N Engl J Med* 2002;346:108–114.

71 Rhodes N, et al. Labor experiences of childhood sexual abuse survivors. *Birth* 1994;21:213–220.

72 Paffenbarger RS. Epidemiological aspects of mental illness associated with childbearing. In: Brockington IF, Kumar R, eds. *Motherhood and mental illness*. London, UK: Academic Press; 1982:21–36.

73 Kendell RE, et al. Epidemiology of puerperal psychoses [erratum appears in *Br J Psychiatry* 1987;151:135]. *Br J Psychiatry* 1987;150:662–673.

74 Robins LN, et al. Lifetime prevalence of specific psychiatric disorders in three sites. *Arch Gen Psychiatry* 1984;41:949–958.

75 McNeil TF, et al. Women with nonorganic psychosis: pregnancy's effect on mental health during pregnancy. *Acta Psychiatr Scand* 1984;70:140–148.

76 Nurnberg HG. An overview of somatic treatment of psychosis during pregnancy and postpartum. *Gen Hosp Psychiatry* 1989;11:328–338.

77 Sacker A, et al. Obstetrics complications in children born to parents with schizophrenia: a meta-analysis of case-control studies. *Psychol Med* 1996;26:279–287.
78 Bennedsen BE, et al. Obstetric complications in women with schizophrenia. *Schizophr Res* 2001;47:167–175.
79 Bennedsen BE, et al. Preterm birth and intra-uterine growth retardation among children of women with schizophrenia. *Br J Psychiatry* 1999;175:239–245.
80 Nilsson, E, et al. Women with schizophrenia: pregnancy outcome and infant death among their offspring. *Schizophr Res* 2002; 58:221–229.
81 Howard LM, et al. Medical outcome of pregnancy in women with psychotic disorders and their infants in the first year after birth. *Br J Psychiatry* 2003;182:63–67.
82 Gottesman II, et al. Clinical genetics as clues to the "real" genetics of schizophrenia: a decade of modest gains while playing for time. *Schizophr Bull* 1987;13:23–47.
83 Pariser, SF. Women and mood disorders. Menarche to menopause. *Ann Clin Psychiatry* 1993;5:249–254.
84 Jefferson J, et al. *Lithium encyclopedia for clinical practice*. American Psychiatric Press: Washington, DC; 1987:504–525.
85 Chaudron LH, et al. Mood stabilizers during breastfeeding: a review. *J Clin Psychiatry* 2000;61:79–90.
86 Chaudron LH, et al. The relationship between postpartum psychosis and bipolar disorder: a review. *J Clin Psychiatry* 2003;64:1284–1292.
87 Bosanac P, et al. Motherhood and schizophrenic illnesses: a review of the literature. *Aust NZ J Psychiatry* 2003;37:24–30.
88 Spinelli MG. Maternal infanticide associated with mental illness: prevention and the promise of saved lives. *Am J Psychiatry* 2004;161:1548–1557.
89 Viguera AC, et al. Managing bipolar disorder during pregnancy: weighing the risks and benefits. *Can J Psychiatry* [*Revue Canadienne de Psychiatrie*] 2002;47:426–436.
90 Rhode A, et al. Postpartum psychoses: onset and long-term course. *Psychopathol* 1993;26:203–209.
91 Videbech P, et al. First admission with puerperal psychosis: 7–14 years of follow-up. *Acta Psychiatr Scand* 1995;91:167–173.
92 Wisner KL, et al. Symptomatology of affective and psychotic illnesses related to childbearing. *J Affective Disord* 1994;30: 77–87.
93 Wisner K, et al. Postpartum disorders: phenomenology, treatment approaches, and relationship to infanticide. In: Spinelli M, ed. *Infanticide: psychosocial and legal perspectives on mothers who kill*. Washington, DC: American Psychiatric Publishing; 2002: 36–60.
94 Gentile S. Clinical utilization of atypical antipsychotics in pregnancy and lactation. *Ann Pharmacother* 2004;38:1265–1271.
95 Altshuler LL, et al. Course of psychiatric disorders in pregnancy. Dilemmas in pharmacologic management. *Neurol Clin* 1994;12:613–635.
96 Oates M. The treatment of psychiatric disorders in pregnancy and the puerperium. *Clin Obstet Gynecol* 1986;13:385–395.
97 Wise MG, et al. Case report of ECT during high-risk pregnancy. *Am J Psychiatry* 1984;141:99–101.
98 Oates M. Perinatal psychiatric disorders: a leading cause of maternal morbidity and mortality. *Br Med Bull* 2003;67: 219–229.
99 Dell DL, et al. Suicide in pregnancy. *Obstet Gynecol* 2003;102: 1306–1309.
100 Simon R. *Clinical psychiatry and the law*. Washington, DC: American Psychiatric Press, 1986.
101 Yonkers KA, et al. Management of bipolar disorder during pregnancy and the postpartum period. *Am J Psychiatry* 2004;161: 608–620.
102 Cohen LS, et al. Postpartum prophylaxis for women with bipolar disorder (see Comment). *Am J Psychiatry*, 1995;152: 641–645.
103 Stewart DE, et al. Prophylactic lithium in puerperal psychosis. The experience of three centres. *Br J Psychiatry* 1991;158: 393–397.
104 Austin MP. Puerperal affective psychosis: is there a case for lithium prophylaxis? (see Comment). *Br J Psychiatry* 1992;161: 692–694.
105 Crawford P, et al. Best practice guidelines for the managment of women with epilepsy. *Seizure* 1999;8:201–217.
106 Baldessarini RJ, et al. Is lithium still worth using? An update of selected recent research. *Harvard Rev Psychiatry* 2002;10:59–75.
107 Morgan JF, et al. Impact of pregnancy on bulimia nervosa [erratum appears in *Br J Psychiatry* 1999;174:278]. *Br J Psychiatry* 1999;174:135–140.
108 James DC. Eating disorders, fertility, and pregnancy: relationships and complications. *J Perinat Neonat Nurs* 2001;15:36–48.
109 Franko DL, et al. Pregnancy complications and neonatal outcomes in women with eating disorders (see Comment). *Am J Psychiatry* 2001;158:1461–1466.
110 Rooney B, et al. The incidence and prevalence of anorexia nervosa in three suburban health districts in south west London, U.K. *Int J Eating Disord* 1995;18:299–307.
111 Hart KJ, et al. Prevalence of bulimia in working and university women. *Am J Psychiatry* 1985;142:851–854.
112 Schotte DE, et al. Bulimia vs bulimic behaviors on a college campus. *JAMA* 1987;258:1213–1215.
113 Abraham S. Obstetricians and maternal body weight and eating disorders during pregnancy. *J Psychosom Obstet Gynecol* 2001;22:159–163.
114 Conti J, et al. Eating behavior and pregnancy outcome. *J Psychosom Res* 1998;44:465–477.
115 Kelly RH, et al. Somatic complaints among pregnant women cared for in obstetrics: normal pregnancy or depressive and anxiety symptom amplification revisited? *Gen Hosp Psychiatry* 2001;23:107–113.
116 Wessel J, et al. Elevated risk for neonatal outcome following denial of pregnancy: results of a one-year prospective study compared with control groups. *J Perinat Med* 2003;31:29–35.
117 Kaplan R, et al. Denied pregnancy. *Aust NZ J Psychiatry* 1996;30:861–863.
118 Spielvogel A, et al. Denial of pregnancy: a review and case reports. *Birth* 1995;22:220.
119 Schindler BA. Maternal "competency." In: *Academy of Psychosomatic Medicine*. Marco Island, Florida: 2004.
120 Nair S, et al. The evaluation of maternal competency. *Psychosom* 2000;41:523–530.
121 Cote-Arsenault D. The influence of perinatal loss on anxiety in multigravidas. *J Obstet Gynecol Neonat Nurs* 2003;32: 623–629.
122 Moretti ME, et al. Monitoring lithium in breast milk: an individualized approach for breast-feeding mothers. *Ther Drug Monitoring* 2003;25:364–366.
123 Einarson A, et al. How physicians perceive and utilize information from a teratogen information service: the Motherisk Program. *BMC Med Educ* 2004;4:5.
124 Zuckerman B, et al. Depressive symptoms during pregnancy: relationship to poor health behaviors. *Am J Obstet Gynecol* 1989;160:1107–1111.

125 Ludman EJ, et al. Stress, depressive symptoms, and smoking cessation among pregnant women. *Health Psychol* 2000;19:21–27.

126 Paarlberg KM, et al. Psychosocial predictors of low birthweight: a prospective study. *Br J Obstet Gynaecol* 1999;106:834–841.

127 Steer RA, et al. Self-reported depression and negative pregnancy outcomes. *J Clin Epidemiol* 1992;45:1093–1099.

128 Kurki T, et al. Depression and anxiety in early pregnancy and risk for preeclampsia. *Obstet Gynecol* 2000;95:487–490.

129 Chun TK, et al. Antepartum depressive symptomatology is associated with adverse obstetric and neonatal outcomes. *Psychosom Med* 2001;63:830–834.

130 Henderson JJ, et al. Impact of postnatal depression on breastfeeding duration [erratum appears in *Birth* 2004;31:76]. *Birth* 2003;30:175–180.

131 Rahman A, et al. Impact of maternal depression on infant nutritional status and illness: a cohort study. *Arch Gen Psychiatry* 2004;61:946–952.

132 O'Brien LM, et al. Postnatal depression and faltering growth: a community study. *Pediatrics* 2004;113:1242–1247.

133 Flynn HA, et al. Rates of maternal depression in pediatric emergency department and relationship to child service utilization. *Gen Hosp Psychiatry* 2004;26:316–322.

134 Burke L. The impact of maternal depression on familial relationships. *Int Rev Psychiatry* 2003;15:243–255.

135 Hay DF, et al. Pathways to violence in the children of mothers who were depressed postpartum. *Dev Psychol* 2003;39:1083–1094.

136 Wadhwa PD, et al. The association between prenatal stress and infant birth weight and gestational age at birth: a prospective investigation. *Am J Obstet Gynecol* 1993;169:858–865.

137 Rizzardo R, et al. Variations in anxiety levels during pregnancy and psychosocial factors in relation to obstetric complications. *Psychother Psychosom* 1988;49:10–16.

138 Mancuso RA, et al. Maternal prenatal anxiety and corticotropin-releasing hormone associated with timing of delivery. *Psychosom Med* 2004;66:762–769.

139 Ryding EL, et al. Fear of childbirth during pregnancy may increase the risk of emergency cesarean section. *Acta Obstet Gynecol Scand* 1998;77:542–547.

140 O'Connor TG, et al. Maternal antenatal anxiety and behavioural/emotional problems in children: a test of a programming hypothesis. *J Child Psychol Psychiatry* 2003;44:1025–1036.

141 O'Hara MW, et al. Prospective study of postpartum blues. Biologic and psychosocial factors. *Arch Gen Psychiatry* 1991;48:801–806.

142 Stowe ZN, et al. The pharmacokinetics of sertraline excretion into human breast milk: determinants of infant serum concentrations. *J Clin Psychiatry* 2003;64:73–80.

143 Nordeng H, et al. Neonatal withdrawal syndrome after in utero exposure to selective serotonin reuptake inhibitors. *Acta Paediatr* 2001;90:288–291.

144 Dahl ML, et al. Paroxetine withdrawal syndrome in a neonate. *Br J Psychiatry* 1997;171:391–392.

145 Stowe ZN, et al. Paroxetine in human breast milk and nursing infants (see Comment). *Am J Psychiatry* 2000;157:185–189.

146 Pinkofsky HB. Effects of antipsychotics on the unborn child: what is known and how should this influence prescribing? *Paediatr Drugs* 2000;2:83–90.

147 Webb RT, et al. Antipsychotic drugs for non-affective psychosis during pregnancy and postpartum. *Cochrane Database Syst Rev* 2004;2:CD004411.

148 Casiano M, et al. Major mental illness and child bearing: a role for the consultation-liaison psychiatrist in obstetrics. *Psychiatr Clin North Am* 1987;10:35–51.

149 Mortola J. The use of psychotropic agents in pregnancy and lactation. *Psychiatr Clin North Am* 1989;12:69–87.

150 Green T, et al. Determinants of drug disposition and effects in fetus. *Annu Rev Pharmacol Toxicol* 1979;19:285–322.

151 Auerbach J, et al. Maternal psychotropic medication and neonatal behavior. *Neurotoxicol Teratol* 1992;14:399–405.

152 Maguire GA. Prolactin elevation with antipsychotic medications: mechanisms of action and clinical consequences. *J Clin Psychiatry* 2002;63(Suppl.4):56–62.

153 Edlund M, et al. Antipsychotic drug use and birth defects: an epidemiologic reassessment. *Compr Psychiatry* 1984;25:32–38.

154 Rumeau-Rouquette C, et al. Possible teratogenic effects of phenothiazines in human beings. *Teratology* 1977;15:57–64.

155 Hanson J, et al. Haloperidol and limb deformity (Letter). *JAMA* 1975;231:26.

156 van Waes A, et al. Safety evaluation of haloperidol in the treatment of hyperemesis gravidum. *J Clin Pharmacol* 1969;9:224–237.

157 Iqbal MM, et al. Clozapine: a clinical review of adverse effects and management. *Ann Clin Psychiatry* 2003;15:33–48.

158 USP *Drug information for the health care professional.* Rockville, MD: United States Pharmacopeial Convention, 1998.

159 Barnas C, et al. Clozapine concentrations in maternal and fetal plasma, amniotic fluid, and breast milk. *Am J Psychiatry* 1994;151:945.

160 Cohen L. Bipolar disorder in pregnancy. *Clin Psychiatry News* 2002;30:20.

161 Jacobson SJ, et al. Prospective multicentre study of pregnancy outcome after lithium exposure during first trimester (see Comment). *Lancet* 1992;339:530–533.

162 Cohen LS, et al. A reevaluation of risk of in utero exposure to lithium (see Comment) [erratum appears in *JAMA* 1994;271:1485]. *JAMA* 1994;271:146–50.

163 Pinelli JM, et al. Case report and review of the perinatal implications of maternal lithium use. *Am J Obstet Gynecol* 2002;187:245–249.

164 AAP, American Academy of Pediatrics Committee on Drugs. Transfer of drugs and other chemicals into human milk (see Comment). *Pediatrics* 2001;108:776–789.

165 Jager-Roman, E. Fetal growth, major malformations and minor anomalies in infants born to women receiving valproic acid. *J Pediatr* 1986;108:997–1004.

166 Kennedy D, et al. Valproic acid use in psychiatry: issues in treating women of reproductive age. *J Psychiatry Neurosci* 1998;23:223–228.

167 Felding I, et al. Congenital liver damage after treatment of mother with valproic acid and phenytoin. *Acta Paediatr Scand* 1984;73:565–568.

168 Thisted E, et al. Malformations, withdrawal manifestations, and hypoglycaemia after exposure to valproate in utero. *Arch Dis Child* 1993;69:288–291.

169 Majer R, et al. Neonatal afibrinogenaemia due to sodium valproate. *Lancet* 1987;2:740–741.

170 AAP, American Academy of Pediatrics Committee on Drugs. The transfer of drugs and other chemical into human milk. *Pediatrics* 1994;93:137–150.

171 Nau H, et al. Anticonvulsants during pregnancy and lactation. Transplacental, maternal and neonatal pharmacokinetics. *Clin Pharmacokinet* 1982;7:508–543.

172 Jones K, et al. Pattern of malformations in the children of women treated with carbamazepine during pregnancy. *N Engl J Med* 1989;320:1661–1666.
173 Rosa F. Spina bifida in infants of women treated with carbamazepine during pregnancy. *N Engl J Med* 1991;324:674–677.
174 Karceski S, et al. The expert consensus guideline series: treatment of epilepsy. *Epilepsy Behav* 2001;2:A1–A50.
175 Merlob P, et al. Transient hepatic dysfunction in an infant of an epileptic mother treated with carbamazepine during pregnancy and breastfeeding. *Ann Pharmacother* 1563;26:1563–1565.
176 Frey B, et al. Transient cholestatic hepatitis in a neonate associated with carbamazepine exposure during pregnancy and breastfeeding. *Eur J Pediatr* 1990;150:136–138.
177 Tran T, et al. Lamotrigine clearance during pregnancy. *Neurology* 2002;59:251–255.
178 Dodd S, et al. The pharmacology of bipolar disorder during pregnancy and breastfeeding. *Expert Opinion Drug Safety* 2004;3: 221–229.

58 Ethical and legal dimensions of medicine of the pregnant woman and fetus

Judith L. Chervenak, Frank A. Chervenak, and Laurence B. McCullough

Ethics is an essential dimension of maternal–fetal medicine.[1–3] In this chapter, we develop a framework for physicians' clinical judgment and decision-making regarding the ethical dimensions of the medical care of pregnant women and fetuses. We explain the ethical concept of the fetus as a patient and identify its implications for maternal–fetal medicine in a preventive ethics approach. This approach appreciates the potential for ethical conflict and adopts ethically justified strategies to prevent those conflicts from occurring. Because the professional liability crisis has become the dominant legal concern for obstetrician–gynecologists, our discussion of legal issues focuses on medical malpractice.

Medical ethics and law

Ethics is the disciplined study of morality. Medical ethics is the disciplined study of morality in medicine and concerns the ethical obligations of physicians and healthcare organizations to patients as well as the obligations of patients themselves.[4] The approach to medical ethics has been secular since the eighteenth-century European and American Enlightenments;[5] it makes no reference to God or revealed tradition, but focuses on what rational discourse requires and produces. Therefore, medical ethical principles (Figs 58.1–58.3) should be understood to apply to all physicians, regardless of their personal religious and spiritual beliefs.[6] Medical ethics and law have been closely related since Thomas Percival's *Medical Ethics* appeared in 1803.[7] Percival's early version of this text was entitled *Medical Jurisprudence*.[8] Criminal law sets the boundaries of acceptable behavior, whereas civil law plays a large role in regulating drugs and devices, licensing physicians and healthcare organizations, regulating insurance companies and employer-provided health plans, and regulating medical practice.

The informed consent process

The close relationship of ethics and law is illustrated by informed consent. This process involves three sequential autonomy-based behaviors on the part of the patient: (1) absorbing and retaining information about her condition and the alternative diagnostic and therapeutic responses to it; (2) understanding the information (i.e., evaluating and rank-ordering those responses, and appreciating that there could be benefits and risks of treatment); and (3) expressing a value-based preference. The physician has a role to play in each of these three behaviors. They are respectively: (1) to recognize the capacity of each patient to deal with medical information (and not underestimate that capacity), provide information (disclose and explain all medically reasonable alternatives, i.e., supported in beneficence based clinical judgment), and recognize the validity of the values and beliefs of the patient; (2) to not interfere with but, when necessary, assist the patient in her evaluation and ranking of diagnostic and therapeutic alternatives for managing her condition; and (3) to elicit and implement the patient's value-based preference.[4]

The legal obligations of the physician regarding informed consent were established in a series of cases during the twentieth century. In 1914, *Schloendorff* v. *The Society of The New York Hospital* established the concept of simple consent, i.e., whether the patient says "yes" or "no" to medical intervention.[9,10] This decision is still quoted today in the medical and bioethics literature: "Every human being of adult years and sound mind has the right to determine what shall be done with his body, and a surgeon who performs an operation without his patient's consent commits an assault for which he is liable in damages."[9] The legal requirement of consent further evolved to include disclosure of sufficient information to enable patients to make informed decisions about whether to say "yes" or "no" to medical intervention.[9,10]

There are two legal standards for such disclosure. The professional community standard defines adequate disclosure in the context of what the relevantly trained and experienced physician tells patients. The reasonable person standard, which has been adopted by most states, goes further and requires the physician to disclose "material" information, i.e., what any patient with that particular condition needs to know and what the lay person of average sophistication should not be expected to know.[10] The reasonable person standard has

The principle of beneficence

The principle of beneficence requires one to act in a way that is expected reliably to produce the greater balance of benefits over harms in the lives of others. To put this principle into clinical practice requires a reliable account of the benefits and harms relevant to the care of the patient and of how those goods and harms should be reasonably balanced against each other when not all of them can be achieved in a particular clinical situation, such as a request for an elective Cesarean delivery. In medicine, the principle of beneficence requires the physician to act in a way that is reliably expected to produce the greater balance of clinical benefits over harms for the patient.

Figure 58.1 The principle of beneficence.

Nonmaleficence

Nonmaleficence means that the physician should prevent causing harm and is best understood as expressing the limits of beneficence. This is also known as "*primum non nocere*" or "first do no harm." This commonly invoked dogma is really a latinized misinterpretation of the Hippocratic texts that emphasized beneficence while avoiding harm when approaching the limits of medicine.

Figure 58.2 Nonmaleficence.

The principle of respect for autonomy

The principle of respect for autonomy requires one always to acknowledge and carry out the value-based preferences of the competent adult patient, unless there is compelling ethical justification for not doing so, e.g., prescribing antibiotics for viral respiratory infections. The female or pregnant patient increasingly brings to her medical care her own perspective on what is in her interest. The principle of respect for autonomy translates this fact into autonomy-based clinical judgment. Because each patient's perspective on her interests is a function of her values and beliefs, it is impossible to specify the benefits and harms of autonomy-based clinical judgment in advance. Indeed, it would be inappropriate for the physician to do so, because the definition of her benefits and harms, and their balancing, are the prerogative of the patient. Not surprisingly, autonomy-based clinical judgment is strongly antipaternalistic in nature.

Figure 58.3 The principle of respect for autonomy.

emerged as the ethical standard, and specialists in maternal–fetal medicine are urged to adopt it.[4] Using this standard, the physician should disclose to the patient: (1) her diagnosis or that of the fetus (including differential diagnosis when only that is known); (2) the medically reasonable alternatives to diagnose and manage the condition; and (3) the short-term and long-term benefits and risks of each alternative.

As a rule, the result of the informed consent process should be implemented. When the patient refuses to accept any of the alternatives supported in beneficence-based clinical judgment, the physician is ethically and legally obligated to engage in what is known as "informed refusal." This legal and ethical obligation arose from the 1980 case of *Truman* v. *Thomas* in California.[10,11] Dr. Thomas had delivered several of Mrs Truman's babies and, on the delivery of her last child, recommended that she have a Pap smear. She refused to have this test until she could pay for it and did not accept Dr. Thomas's offer to perform it without charge. Mrs Truman subsequently presented to Dr. Thomas with advanced cervical cancer from which she died. In the malpractice action brought by her survivors, Dr. Thomas stated that he did not tell Mrs Truman about detectable presymptomatic changes in her cervix indicative of cervical cancer or that he was concerned that she could die from such disease. The California Supreme Court ruled that, because the risks were of clinical salience to Dr. Thomas (they were the motivation for his offering the Pap smear), he should have informed Mrs Truman about these risks so that her refusal would be informed. This case changed practice and introduced the concept of informed refusal into medical law and ethics.

The ethical and legal obligation of the physician in the matter of informed refusal is very clear and not difficult to fulfill. The law requires that the patient be informed about the medical risks he or she is taking by the refusal of treatment. The risks that should be disclosed are those that are salient in clinical judgment: if they are important to the physician, i.e., they motivate the physician to offer or recommend a diagnostic test or therapy, they are salient. Any discussion, especially regarding the risks of refusal, should be thoroughly documented in the patient's chart. Preventive ethics requires that disclosure of risks be followed by a strong recommendation that the patient reconsider his or her refusal. This preventive ethics approach avoids the need to abandon the patient, keeps lines of communication open, and sends a powerful signal of concern to the patient from the physician about the medical folly of refusal.

The fetus as a patient

The ethical principles of beneficence and respect for autonomy play a complex role in maternal fetal medicine. There are obviously beneficence- and autonomy-based obligations to the pregnant patient: the physician's perspective on the pregnant woman's health-related interests provides the basis for the physician's beneficence-based obligations to her, whereas her own perspective on those interests provides the basis for the physician's autonomy-based obligations to her. The fetus cannot meaningfully be said to possess values and beliefs because of an insufficiently developed central nervous system. Thus, there is no basis for saying that a fetus has a perspective on its interests and there can be no autonomy-based obligations to the fetus. Hence, the language of fetal rights has no meaning and therefore no application to the fetus in obstetric clinical judgment and practice despite its popularity in public and political discourse in the USA and other countries.[4] Obviously, the physician has a perspective on the fetus's health-related interests and can have beneficence-based obligations to the fetus, *but only when the fetus is a patient.*

One prominent approach for establishing if the fetus is a patient has involved attempts to show whether the fetus has independent moral status; this is the first sense of the concept of the fetus as a patient. For the fetus to have independent moral status, one or more characteristics that the fetus possesses, in and of itself and therefore independently of the pregnant woman or any other factor, must generate and therefore ground obligations to the fetus on the part of the pregnant woman and the physician. Many fetal characteristics have been nominated for this role, including the moment of conception, implantation, central nervous system development, quickening, and birth. There is considerable variation among ethical arguments about when the fetus acquires independent moral status. Some take the view that the fetus has independent moral status from the moment of conception or implantation.[12] Others believe that independent moral status is acquired in degrees, resulting in "graded" moral status,[13] or that the fetus never has independent moral status while it is *in utero*.[14]

Despite the ever-expanding theological and philosophical literature on this subject, there is no single authoritative account of the independent moral status of the fetus. This is not surprising because there is no single method that would be authoritative for all of the markedly diverse theological and philosophical schools of thought involved in this endless debate; debates about such a final authority within and between theological and philosophical traditions would have to be resolved in a way satisfactory to all, an inconceivable intellectual and cultural event. Therefore, there is no stable or clinically applicable meaning of the fetus as a patient in terms of its independent moral status. As a result, we abandon these futile attempts to understand the fetus as a patient in terms of its independent moral status and turn to an alternative approach that makes it possible to identify ethically distinct senses of the fetus as a patient and their clinical implications for directive and nondirective counseling.

Analysis of this second sense of the concept of the fetus as a patient begins with the recognition that it is not necessary to possess independent moral status to be a patient. Rather, being a patient means that one can benefit from the applications of the clinical skills of the physician. Put more precisely, a human being without independent moral status is properly regarded as a patient when two conditions are met: (1) that human being is presented to the physician, and (2) clinical interventions exist that are reliably expected to be efficacious, i.e., they are expected to result in a greater balance of clinical benefits over harm for the human being in question.[15] This second sense of the concept of the fetus as a patient is called the dependent moral status of the fetus.

The authors have argued elsewhere[4] that beneficence-based obligations to the fetus exist when the fetus is reliably expected to later achieve independent moral status as a child and person. In other words, the fetus is a patient when the fetus is presented for medical interventions, whether diagnostic or therapeutic, that can be reasonably expected to result in a greater balance of good over harm for the child and person the fetus can become during early childhood. The ethical significance of the concept of the fetus as a patient, therefore, depends on links that can be established between the fetus and it later achieving independent moral status.

The viable fetal patient

Viability is one such link between the fetus and it later achieving independent moral status. However, it must be understood in terms of both biological and technological factors; it is only by virtue of both factors that a viable fetus can exist *ex utero* and thus achieve independent moral status. The fetus is a patient when it is viable, i.e., when it is of sufficient maturity that it can survive into the neonatal period and achieve independent moral status with the requisite technological support and when it is presented to the physician.

Viability exists as a function of biomedical and technological capacities, which are different in different parts of the world. Consequently, there is no worldwide uniform gestational age to define viability at the present time. In the USA, we believe viability presently occurs at approximately 24 weeks' gestation.[16]

When the fetus is a patient, directive counseling for fetal benefit is ethically justified. In clinical practice, this involves one or more of the following: recommending against the termination of pregnancy; recommending against nonaggressive management; or recommending aggressive management. Aggressive obstetric management includes interventions such as fetal surveillance, tocolysis, Cesarean delivery, or delivery in a tertiary care center when indicated. Nonaggressive obstetric management excludes such interventions. Directive counseling for fetal benefit, however, must also take into account the presence and severity of fetal anomalies, extreme prematurity, and obligations to the pregnant woman.

It is crucial to appreciate that, in obstetric clinical judgment and practice, the strength of directive counseling for fetal benefit varies according to the presence and severity of anomalies. As a rule, the more severe the fetal anomaly, the less directive counseling should be for fetal benefit. In particular, when lethal anomalies such as anencephaly can be diagnosed with certainty, there are no beneficence-based obligations to provide aggressive management. Such fetuses are dying patients; counseling should be nondirective in recommending between nonaggressive management and termination of pregnancy, but directive in recommending against aggressive management for the sake of maternal benefit.[17] By contrast, third-trimester abortion for Down syndrome or achondroplasia is not ethically justifiable because there is a high probability that the future child will have the capacity to grow and develop as a human being.[18,19]

Any directive counseling for fetal benefit must occur in the context of balancing beneficence-based obligations to the fetus against beneficence- and autonomy-based obligations to the pregnant woman. Any such balancing must recognize that a pregnant woman is obligated only to take reasonable risks of medical interventions that are reliably expected to benefit the viable fetus or later child. A unique feature of obstetric ethics is that the pregnant woman's autonomy influences whether, in a particular case, the viable fetus ought to be regarded as being presented to the physician.

Obviously, any strategy for directive counseling for fetal benefit that takes into account obligations to the pregnant woman must be open to the possibility of conflict between the physician's recommendation and a pregnant woman's autonomous decision to the contrary. Such conflict is best managed preventively through the informed consent process as an ongoing dialogue throughout a woman's pregnancy, augmented as necessary by negotiation and respectful persuasion.[4,20]

The previable fetal patient

As technological factors cannot result in the previable fetus becoming a child, the only possible link between the previable fetus and the child it can become is the pregnant woman's autonomy. The previable fetus has no claim to the status of being a patient independently of the pregnant woman's autonomy; the link between the previable fetus and the child it can become can only be established by the pregnant woman's decision to confer the status of being a patient on her previable fetus. The pregnant woman is free to withhold, confer, or, having once conferred, withdraw the status of being a patient on or from her previable fetus according to her own values and beliefs. The previable fetus is presented to the physician as a function of the pregnant woman's autonomy.[4]

If a pregnant woman refuses to confer the status of being a patient on her previable fetus, counseling regarding the management of her pregnancy should be nondirective in terms of continuing the pregnancy or having an abortion. If she does confer such status in a settled way, beneficence-based obligations to her fetus come into existence and directive counseling for fetal benefit becomes appropriate. Just as for viable fetuses, counseling must take into account the presence and severity of fetal anomalies, extreme prematurity, and obligations owed to the pregnant woman.

For pregnancies in which the woman is uncertain about whether to confer such status, the authors propose that the fetus be provisionally regarded as a patient. This justifies directive counseling against behavior that can harm a fetus in significant and irreversible ways, for example substance abuse, especially of alcohol, until the woman decides whether to confer the status of being a patient on the fetus.

In particular, nondirective counseling is appropriate in cases of what we term near-viable fetuses, i.e., those that are 22–23 weeks of gestational age, for which there are anecdotal reports of survival. In our view, aggressive obstetric and neonatal management should be regarded as clinical investigation (i.e., a form of medical experimentation) and not a standard of care. There is no obligation on the part of a pregnant woman to confer the status of being a patient on a near-viable fetus because the efficacy of aggressive obstetric and neonatal management has yet to be proven.

Legal considerations

Black's Law Dictionary defines malpractice as "an instance of negligence on the part of a professional."[21] Negligence is a tort or civil wrong whose elements are: (1) a duty recognized by the law; (2) a failure on the part of the person to conform to the standard required; (3) a reasonably close connection between the conduct and the resulting injury, known as the "proximate or legal cause;" and (4) actual loss or damage to the interests of another.[22] The court provides a remedy for this civil wrong in the form of equity or money damages.

The duty to the patient arises from the physician–patient relationship and is generally considered to be a contractual duty implied from the actions of the parties rather than one expressed in written form.[22] This relationship ends with the consent of both parties, dismissal of the physician, or when the services of the physician are no longer needed.[22]

Good Samaritan legislation has been enacted in 49 US states and the District of Columbia to encourage physicians to render aid in emergency situations.[23] In general, these statutes were designed to safeguard the physician by "protecting them from liability for any injury they cause or enhance." These statutes generally do not apply to doctors who provide emergency services in the ordinary course of their activities or to doctors who have a pre-existing duty to the injured party. Often, these laws also do not protect an obstetrician who attends the emergency delivery of a woman with whom the physician has no physician–patient relationship if that delivery occurs in a hospital setting.[24]

Standard of care

In a medical malpractice action, the standard of conduct for the physician is usually expressed as "the minimum knowledge, skill and care ordinarily possessed and employed by members of the profession in good standing."[22] For those who are specialists, the standard is modified accordingly.[22] Therefore, a physician who has met the applicable legal standard will not be liable for an honest mistake in judgment even if the clinical outcome is poor.

The standard of care in a medical malpractice action is usually established by expert testimony of other physicians who are limited by the state of medical knowledge at the time of the incident.[25] In contrast, after-acquired knowledge is admissible when assessing causation of the injury.[26] In the early 1960s, courts recognized that, because of the wide dissemination of medical information by journals and at specialty conferences, the practice of medicine was similar throughout the country.[26]

Most medical malpractice cases require the testimony of an expert to establish the standard of care. Expert testimony is very different from that given by a lay witness; lay witnesses are allowed to testify only to that which they actually perceived through their own senses. This allows jurors to use their own life experiences to better assess whether witnesses' testimonies are credible. Experts, however, are allowed to testify about events that they have not witnessed and about matters that are outside the general knowledge of most jurors.[27] Therefore, courts have sought to prevent abuses by establishing criteria for the reliability of medical testimony.

The Supreme Court's decision in the case of *Daubert* v. *Merrill Dow* established what have become known as the *Daubert* factors for the admissibility of medical testimony in federal courts.[28] These are: (1) whether the expert's technique or theory can be or has been tested; (2) whether the technique or theory has been subject to peer review and publication; (3) the known or potential rate of error of the technique or theory when applied; (4) the existence and maintenance of standards and controls; and (5) whether the technique or theory has been generally accepted in the scientific community.[28] Before *Daubert*, which was based on the federal rules of evidence, courts used what was known as the Frye standard, under which expert testimony was admissible only if it was based upon techniques or procedures that were "generally accepted in the medical community."[29] In the case of *Daubert*, the plaintiffs offered the testimony of eight expert witnesses regarding the teratogenicity of Bendectin (an antinausea drug), whereas the medical literature was overwhelmingly adverse to the plaintiff's position.[28] The Supreme Court opined that courts should act as gatekeepers to exclude expert testimony that is unreliable. *Daubert* challenges can take two forms.[28] The first is a challenge made to the expert in a motion for summary judgment (a motion to dismiss the case because there are no triable issues of fact). In this motion, the defense asks the court to dismiss the case by arguing that the plaintiff's case has no merit because it is based on an expert's opinion or theory that is not scientifically reliable. The second form is a pretrial motion (motion *in limine*) to preclude the expert from testifying.[28] In either case, the court can decide to hold a separate hearing either before or even during a trial before deciding whether to allow the expert to testify before the jury.[28]

In cases in which the jury is considered capable of determining whether negligence occurred without the benefit of an expert opinion, the doctrine of *res ipsa loquitur* applies.[30] In such cases, the harm to the patient could not ordinarily have occurred without the negligent conduct of the defendant, and the thing or things that caused the harm must have been in the exclusive control of the defendant. The burden in such cases then shifts to the defendant to prove that he or she did not commit the negligent act.[30] An example of this type of case would be an instrument left in an abdomen during a surgical procedure.

Causation

There must also be a causal link between the conduct and the harm that results. The proximate or legal cause in a medical malpractice action is usually expressed as a "reasonable medical probability" that the conduct was a "substantial factor" in bringing about the harm.[31] Most jurisdictions require that there is more than a 50% probability that the alleged conduct caused the harm,[31] e.g., in a typical cerebral palsy case, plaintiffs will allege that, despite other potential causes, the damage to the infant was most likely the result of hypoxia at birth. The requirement is often not met when the plaintiff has a pre-existing condition and alleges a lost opportunity for cure, such as an obstetrician's failure to recognize premature labor or failure to treat a woman who suffered from an amniotic fluid embolism. In *Falcon* v. *Memorial Hospital*, a Michigan court held that a woman who suffered an amniotic fluid embolism could recover for negligent treatment even though there was testimony that, had she been given the proper treatment, she would have had only a 33% chance of survival.[32]

Other birth-based causes of action are wrongful pregnancy, wrongful birth, and wrongful life. In a wrongful pregnancy action, one or both parents of a child born following a negligently performed sterilization procedure can bring suit on their own behalf for the costs of having an unplanned child. Most US jurisdictions recognize this cause of action.[33] In a wrongful birth action, the parents of an unhealthy child born following negligent genetic counseling or negligent failure to diagnose a fetal defect or disease bring suit for the costs of having to raise and care for an impaired child, arguing that they were wrongfully deprived of the ability to avoid or terminate a pregnancy to prevent the birth of a child with the defect or disease.[34] Most states allow recovery for the "extraordinary expenses of raising a child with a birth defect."[34] In a wrongful life action, an unhealthy child born following either a negligently performed sterilization of one of his or her parents, or negligent genetic counseling or testing, argues that he or she has been damaged by being born at all.[34] To date, most courts have rejected this cause of action.

New York has recently recognized a separate cause of action for emotional distress on behalf of the mother in the absence of an independent injury to her. In *Broadnax*,[35] the Court of Appeals (the highest New York state court) held that medical malpractice resulting in miscarriage or stillbirth entitled the mother to damages for emotional harm. In *Sheppard-Mobley* v. *King*, the Supreme Court, Second Department, Appellate Division, held that malpractice resulting in the birth of a severely impaired child was a violation of the duty of care to the mother and also entitled her to damages for emotional harm.[36] The Court of Appeals later rejected this cause of action.[37]

Damages

The monetary damages awarded in an obstetrical malpractice suit involving a child with cerebral palsy can be enormous. In New York, recent jury verdicts of $90 million and $112 million in brain-damaged baby cases have made headlines and are frequently cited as evidence of a crisis.[38] It should be recognized that many, if not all, of these large verdicts are reduced on appeal.[38] Many trial lawyers also enter into what is known as a "high–low" agreement whereby the parties agree on a high settlement value in the event of a plaintiff's verdict and a low value for a defendant's verdict.[38] Such agreements protect plaintiffs from a lengthy appeals process and are typically set close to the limits of the insurance policy available for that case. In the case of the $112 million jury verdict noted above, the plaintiffs actually received $6 million because such an agreement was made just prior to jury deliberations.[38]

Impact of obstetrical malpractice on physicians

In 2003, a professional liability survey by the American College of Obstetricians and Gynecologists (ACOG) found that 76.3% of obstetricians had a least one claim filed against them during their career. The average number of claims against all respondents was 2.64, and 29.6% had at least one claim filed during their residency.[39] In the same survey, 14% of respondents said that they no longer practice obstetrics, and 12.3% had decreased the level of high-risk obstetrical cases that they take because of liability concerns.[39]

Tort reform

Tort reform in the medical malpractice context has primarily focused on enacting legislation designed to discourage lawsuits by placing a cap on pain and suffering or by making it more difficult to file a claim, as well as by replacing litigation with another system of compensation for injured parties such as a no-fault system.[40] In California, the use of a $250 000 cap has resulted in insurance premium increases that are less than one-third of those in states not using caps.[41] In Florida, a no-fault system for compensation reduced the number of tort claims for premature labor and delivery, injury, and death by 16–32%, but the total claims frequency rose by 11–38% when no-fault claims were added to tort claims.[42] It should be noted that because of the narrow statutory definition for "birth-related neurological injury," many children, including many premature infants, did not qualify for coverage.

As most medical malpractice lawsuits are brought in state rather than federal courts because of jurisdictional issues, procedural reforms enacted in the different states and influenced heavily by political support from various interest groups will undoubtedly influence obstetrical malpractice insurance premiums in the future.

Conclusion

In this chapter we have provided a general ethical and legal framework for maternal–fetal medicine. Implementing this framework on a daily basis is essential for creating and sustaining the physician–patient relationship in obstetrics and gynecology. This framework emphasizes preventive ethics, i.e., an appreciation that the potential for ethical conflict is built into clinical practice, and the use of such clinical tools as informed consent and negotiation to prevent such conflict from occurring.

Key points

1. Medical ethics and law have been closely related since at least the early nineteenth century.
2. The informed consent process implements the ethical principle of respect for autonomy in the decision-making process between physicians and patients.
3. Simple consent concerns whether the patient accepts or refuses treatment.
4. Informed consent concerns whether the patient's decision about treatment is adequately informed and is voluntary.
5. The professional community standard requires the physician to provide information to the patient that any adequately trained and experienced physician would provide.
6. The reasonable person standard requires the physician to provide information that any patient with that particular diagnosis needs in order to make an informed decision.
7. The previable fetus is a patient solely as a function of the pregnant woman's autonomy and has no independent claim to this moral status.
8. The viable fetus is a patient when it is able to exist *ex utero*, with full technological support, and when it is presented to the physician.
9. When the fetus is a not a patient, counseling about the management of pregnancy should be nondirective.
10. When the fetus is a patient, counseling about the management of pregnancy should be directive with the weight of recommendations a function of both the fetal patient's and the pregnant woman's interests.
11. Malpractice is an instance of negligence on the part of a professional. The elements of malpractice are duty, breach, causation, and damages.
12. The duty to the patient arises from the physician–patient relationship and is generally considered to be a contractual duty implied from the actions of the parties rather than one expressed in written form.
13. Good Samaritan legislation may not protect an obstetrician who attends the emergency delivery of a woman in a hospital setting.
14. In a medical malpractice action, the standard of conduct for the physician is usually expressed as "the minimum knowledge, skill and care ordinarily possessed and employed by members of the profession in good standing."
15. For those who are specialists, the standard is modified accordingly.
16. Most medical malpractice cases require the testimony of an expert to establish the standard of care.
17. In the case of *Daubert* v. *Merrill Dow*, the Supreme Court established what have become known as the *Daubert* factors for the admissibility of medical testimony in federal courts.
18. *Daubert* challenges can take two forms: (1) a motion for summary judgment, or (2) a pretrial motion to prevent the expert from testifying.
19. The proximate or legal cause in a medical malpractice action is usually expressed as a "reasonable medical probability" that the conduct was a "substantial factor" in bringing about the harm.
20. Wrongful pregnancy is an action brought on behalf of one or both parents for the costs of raising an unplanned child and is often brought after a negligent sterilization procedure.
21. Wrongful birth actions are brought on behalf of the parents of a child who is unhealthy and who claim that they were wrongfully denied the chance to terminate the pregnancy. Most states allow recovery for the extraordinary expenses associated with raising such a child.
22. Most states have rejected wrongful life actions where an unhealthy child argues that he or she has been damaged by being born at all.

References

1 American College of Obstetricians and Gynecologists. *Ethics in obstetrics and gynecology*. Washington, DC: ACOG, 2002.
2 Association of Professors of Gynecology and Obstetrics. *Exploring medical-legal issues in obstetrics and gynecology*. Washington, DC: APGO Medical Education Foundation, 1994.
3 FIGO Committee for the Study of Ethical Aspects of Human Reproduction. *Recommendations of ethical issues in obstetrics and gynecology*. London: International Federation of Gynecology and Obstetrics, 1997.
4 McCullough LB, Chervenak FA. *Ethics in obstetrics and gynecology*. New York: Oxford University Press, 1994.
5 Engelhardt HT, Jr. *The foundations of bioethics*, 2nd edn. New York: Oxford University Press, 1995.
6 Beauchamp TL, Childress JF. *Principles of biomedical ethics*, 5th edn. New York: Oxford University Press, 2001.
7 Percival T. *Medical ethics, or a code of institutes and precepts, adapted to the professional conduct of physicians and surgeons*. London: Johnson and Bickerstaff, 1803.
8 Percival, T. *Medical jurisprudence; or a code of ethics and institutes, adapted to the professions of physic and surgery*. Manchester, UK: Johnson and Bickerstaff, 1794.
9 *Schloendorff* v. *The Society of The New York Hospital*, 211 N.Y. 125, 126, 105 N.E. 92, 93 (1914).
10 Faden RR, Beauchamp TL. *A history and theory of informed consent*. New York: Oxford University Press, 1986.
11 *Truman* v. *Thomas* 611 P.2d 902 (Cal. 1980).
12 Callahan S, Callahan D, eds. *Abortion: understanding differences*. New York: Plenum Press, 1984.
13 Strong C. *Ethics in reproductive medicine: a new framework*. New Haven, CT: Yale University Press, 1997.
14 Annas GJ. Protecting the liberty of pregnant patient. *N Engl J Med* 1988;316:1213–1214.
15 Chervenak FA, McCullough LB. Ethics in obstetrics and gynecology: an overview. *Eur J Obstet Gynecol Reprod Med* 1997;75: 91–94.
16 Chervenak FA, McCullough LB. The limits of viability. *J Perinat Med* 1997;25:418–420.
17 Chervenak FA, McCullough LB. An ethically justified, clinically comprehensive management strategy for third-trimester pregnancies complicated by fetal anomalies. *Obstet Gynecol* 1990;75: 311–316.
18 Chervenak FA, McCullough LB, Campbell S. Is third trimester abortion justified? *Br J Obstet Gynaecol* 1995;102:434–435.
19 Chervenak FA, McCullough LB, Campbell S. Third trimester abortion: is compassion enough? *Br J Obstet Gynaecol* 1999;106:293–296.
20 Chervenak FA, McCullough LB. Clinical guides to preventing ethical conflicts between pregnant women and their physicians. *Am J Obstet Gynecol* 1990;162:303–307.
21 Garner BA, ed. *Black's law dictionary*, 8th edn. St Paul, MN: West Publishing Group; 2004:1061.
22 Prosser W, Keeton WP, Dobbs DB, et al. *Prosser and Keeton on the law of torts*, 5th edn. St Paul, MN: West Publishing Group; 1984.
23 Furrow BR, Greaney TL, Johnson SH, et al. *Health law; cases, materials and problems*, 4th edn. St Paul, MN: West Publishing Group; 2001:231.
24 American College of Obstetricians and Gynecologists. 2005 Legislative Program: district II website. info@nyacog.org.
25 Moore T, Gaier M. Medical malpractice. *New York Law Journal* December 7 2004:1.
26 Furrow BR, Greaney TL, Johnson SH, et al. *Health law; cases, materials and problems*, 4th edn. St Paul, MN: West Publishing Group; 2001:171–173.
27 Gebauer ME. The "what" and "how" of Daubert challenges to expert testimony under the new federal rule of evidence 702. *Pennsylvania Bar Quarterly* 2002;73:76–85.
28 *Daubert* v. *Merrill Dow*, 509 U.S. 579(1993).
29 *Frye* v. *US* 293 F. 1013(1923).
30 Furrow BR, Greaney TL, Johnson SH, et al. *Health law; cases, materials and problems*, 4th edn. St Paul, MN: West Publishing Group; 2001:189–192.
31 Prosser W, Keeton WP, Dobbs DB, et al. *Prosser and Keeton on the law of torts*, 5th edn. St Paul, MN: West Publishing Group, 1984.
32 *Falcon* v. *Memorial Hospital*, 462 N.W. 2d 44 (Mich. 1990).
33 Furrow BR, Greaney TL, Johnson SH, et al. *Health law; cases, materials and problems*, 4th edn. St Paul, MN: West Publishing Group; 2001:1170–1171.
34 Abrams FR, Barclay ML, Cain JM, et al. eds. *APGO task force on medical ethics. Exploring medical-legal issues in obstetrics and gynecology*. Washington, DC: Association of Professors of Gynecology and Obstetrics, 1994;53–55.
35 *Broadnax* v. *Gonzalez,* 809 N.E. 2d 645; 2 N.Y. 3d 148 (2004).
36 *Sheppard-Mobley et al.* v. *King*, 778 N.Y.S. 2d 98; 2004 N.Y. App. Div. LEXIS 7819.
37 *Sheppard-Mobley et al.* v. *King*, 4 N.Y. 3d 627 (2005).
38 Hallinan JT. Malpractice trials, juries rarely have the last word. *Wall Street Journal*, November 30 2004:A1, A6.
39 Strunk AL, Esser L. Editorial: overview of the 2003 ACOG Professional Liability Survey. *ACOG Clin Rev* 2004;9:1, 13.
40 Burke TF. *Lawyers, lawsuits and legal rights*. California: University of California Press; 2004:27.
41 Lockwood CA, Auerbach R, Scott J, et al. Roundtable: The ob/gyn and legal liability: condition critical, part 2. *Contemporary Ob/Gyn* 2005;50:57–72.
42 Sloan FA, Whetten-Goldstein K, Stout SS, et al. No-fault system of compensation for obstetric injury: winners and losers. *Obstet Gynecol* 1998;91:437–443.

Part XII

Obstetric and Peripartal Events

59 Bleeding in the third trimester

Lawrence W. Oppenheimer and the late Carl A. Nimrod

Bleeding in the third trimester is common. The most important cause is placental abruption (also called *abruptio placentae*), which has an incidence of approximately 0.6% in the USA and an associated risk of stillbirth of 12%. Placenta previa, which can also cause bleeding in the third trimester, occurs with a frequency of 0.3%. There is a significant association of Cesarean section with placenta previa and placenta accreta. Vasa previa is a rare but important cause of vaginal bleeding and occurs in 1 in 3000 to 5000 pregnancies. However, in approximately 50% of cases of vaginal bleeding, the etiology is either unexplained or assumed to result from local lesions.

Placenta previa

Introduction

Placenta previa is defined as a placenta implanted in the lower segment of the uterus presenting ahead of the leading pole of the fetus. It occurs in 2.8 to 4.0 out of 1000 singleton pregnancies[1,2] and 3.9 out of 1000 twin pregnancies[1] and represents a significant clinical problem in terms of the need for hospitalization, potential need for blood transfusion, and risk of premature delivery. The incidence of hysterectomy in women who have undergone a Cesarean section because of placenta previa is 5.3%, which represents a relative risk of 33 compared with women undergoing Cesarean section without placenta previa.[3] Perinatal mortality rates are 3–4 times higher than in normal pregnancies.[4] This is principally because of the association of placenta previa with preterm birth;[5] however, even after 37 weeks' gestation, the risk of neonatal mortality from placenta previa is still double that of babies born without previa.[6] The risk factors for placenta previa[2,7,8] are listed in Table 59.1. Placenta previa does not appear to be associated with significant fetal growth restriction[4,8] and has a negative association with pregnancy-induced hypertension.[8]

Diagnosis

Placenta previa classically presents with painless vaginal bleeding. The traditional classification of placenta previa describes the degree to which the placenta encroaches upon the cervix. This categorization into low-lying, marginal, partial, or complete placenta previa[9] was originally based on digital palpitation through the cervix. In modern practice, the diagnosis of placenta previa is usually made in asymptomatic women found to have a low-lying placenta on routine ultrasonography, and digital vaginal examination may be completely avoided.[9] The superior accuracy of transvaginal sonography (TVS), which can measure the actual distance between the placental edge and the internal cervical os, has rendered the traditional classification obsolete,[10] and the "sonic" finger obviates the need for the "double-setup" examination except in very rare circumstances.[11] Transvaginal sonography enables reclassification of placental position in up to 60% of cases compared with transabdominal sonography (TAS).[12–15] The inherent inaccuracies of TAS include poor visualization of the posterior placenta,[16] interference of the fetal head with visualization of the lower segment,[17] obesity,[18] and under- or overfilling of the bladder.[19,20] For these reasons, the diagnosis of placenta previa by TAS is associated with a false-positive rate of up to 25%[21] (Figs 59.1 and 59.2). Accuracy rates for TVS are high (sensitivity 87.5%, specificity 98.8%, positive predictive value 93.3%, negative predictive value 97.6%), establishing it as the "gold standard" for the diagnosis of placenta previa.[22] A small randomized trial[23] has confirmed the benefit of TVS compared with TAS. TVS has also been shown to be safe in the presence of placenta previa,[22,24] even when there is established vaginal bleeding. It is also possible to accurately image the placenta using magnetic resonance imaging (MRI), a superior technique to TAS,[25] but MRI may not provide any benefit over TVS.

Prediction of placenta previa at delivery

The occurrence of placenta previa is common in the first half of pregnancy (Fig. 59.3) and its persistence to term will depend

Table 59.1 Selected risk factors for placenta previa.

Risk factor	Typical odds ratio (OR)
Maternal age ≥ 40 (vs. < 20)	9.1
Illicit drugs	2.8
≥ 1 previous Cesarean section	2.7
Parity ≥ 5 (vs. para 0)	2.3
Parity 2–4 (vs. para 0)	1.9
Prior abortion	1.9
Smoking	1.6
Congenital anomalies	1.7
Male fetus (vs. female)	1.1
Pregnancy-induced hypertension	0.4

on the gestational age at diagnosis and the definition employed for the exact relationship of the internal cervical os to the placental edge on TVS.[20,26–31] The results of these studies are summarized in Table 59.2. The data suggest that a placental edge that overlaps the internal os by less than 10 mm on TVS at any time before 24 weeks is highly unlikely to be associated with a placenta previa at term. The process of placental "migration," or relative upward shift of the placenta as a result of differential growth of the lower segment, is continuous into the late third trimester.[20,23,32] (Fig 59.4). For this reason, it is reasonable to carry out repeated imaging every 4 weeks until delivery. Vaginal delivery is possible when, at any gestational age, the distance from the placental edge to the internal os is greater than 20 mm.[10,32] Transperineal or

Table 59.2 Persistence of placenta previa at delivery based on various gestational ages at TVS and overlap distances of the placental edge.

Reference no.	Number of patients	Gestational age (weeks)	Overlap (mm)	Incidence [n (%)]	Previa at delivery (%)
27	1252	9–13	≥ 16	20 (1.6)	25
29	2158	10–16	≥ 14	34 (1.6)	18
28	6428	12–16	≥ 15	156 (2.4)	5.1
26	351	11–14	≥ 23	–	8
20	2910	15–24	≥ 10	–	38
30	3696	18–23	≥ 15	57 (1.5)	19
		18–23	≥ 25	10 (0.3)	40
31	8650	20–23	> 0–10	99 (1.14)	50
			11–24	–	63
			≥ 25	–	100

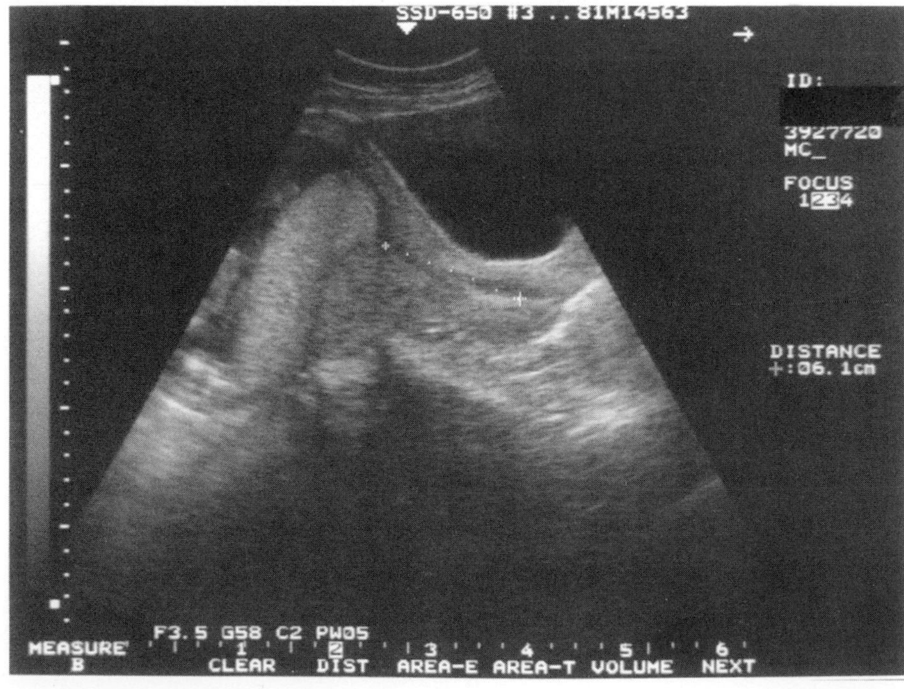

Figure 59.1 Transabdominal scan of placenta covering cervical os at 28 weeks' gestation. Note the full bladder at top right.

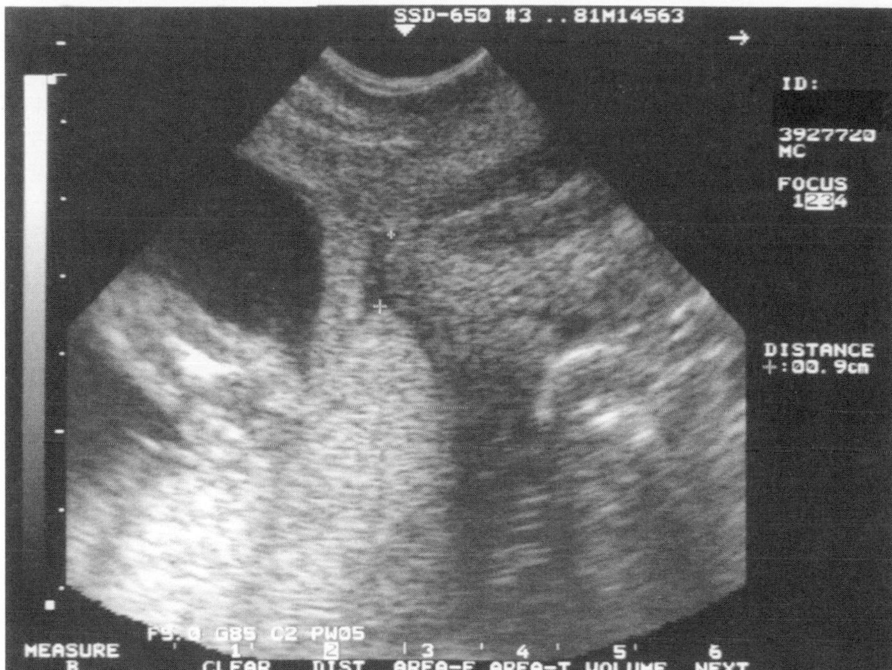

Figure 59.2 Transvaginal scan of the above case with an empty bladder. The placental edge no longer covers the os. At follow-up, the placental edge moved further away and resulted in vaginal delivery.

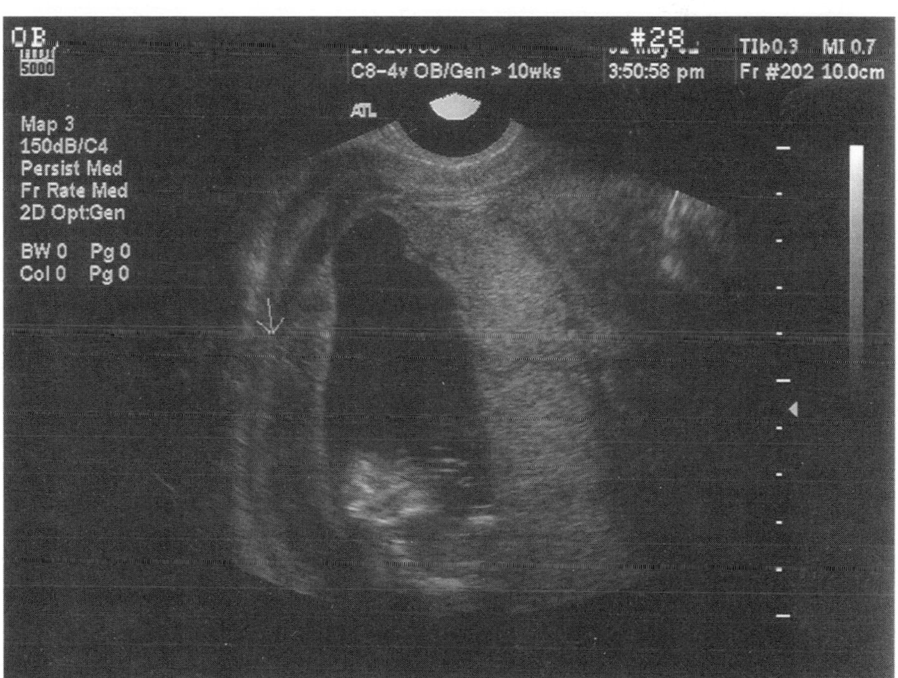

Figure 59.3 Transvaginal scan at 16 weeks showing a 20-mm overlap of the placental edge. By 25 weeks, the placenta was no longer low lying.

translabial ultrasound can provide a higher diagnostic accuracy than TAS and may be a useful alternative when TVS is not available.[33]

The need for Cesarean section at term is predicated by the distance from the os to the placental edge, and by clinical features (e.g., presence of unstable lie and/or bleeding). Four studies have examined the likelihood of Cesarean section in cases of placenta previa based on the distance from the os to the placental edge on the last ultrasound before delivery.[10,33–35] The last scan was performed at a mean of 35–36 weeks' gestation, and a distance of > 20 mm was associated with a high likelihood of vaginal delivery (range 63–100%). It has been suggested that below this cutoff distance of 20 mm, the placenta should be defined as "low-lying" rather than as a previa;

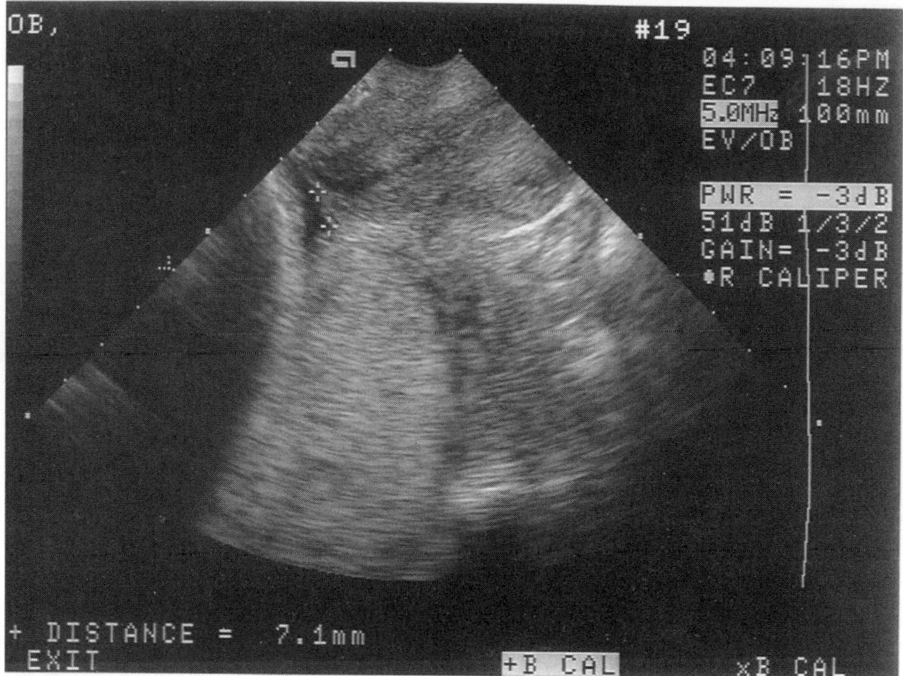

Figure 59.4 Transvaginal scan of placental edge 7 mm from the internal os posteriorly at 30 weeks' gestation in a woman presenting with vaginal bleeding. The fetal head is on the left. Migration continued and vaginal delivery occurred at 39 weeks.

this is to avoid the bias of physicians performing an elective Cesarean section based on the report of a previa,[34] and to enable these cases to be managed in the high expectation of a vaginal delivery.

A distance of between 20 and 0 mm from the os to the placental edge on the last scan results in a higher likelihood of Cesarean section. This distance may be further subdivided: from 10 to 0 mm, a Cesarean section is required in most cases but vaginal delivery is possible depending on clinical features; and from 20 to 11 mm, the likelihood of significant hemorrhage is reduced, and delivery by Cesarean section varies and may be driven by the physician's prior knowledge of the ultrasound finding.[34,35] In this latter group, trial of labor may be appropriate in the absence of an unstable lie or bleeding,[34] although more data in the form of prospective studies are required. In all cases where the placenta overlaps the os by any amount (greater than 0 mm) on the last scan before delivery, delivery by Cesarean section is necessary.[32–35] This group may be defined as "complete placenta previa." A classification of placenta previa is given in Table 59.3, describing the likelihood of Cesarean section according to the distance from the placental edge to the internal os near term.

Table 59.3 Likelihood of Cesarean section based on placental-edge to internal-os distance on last scan prior to delivery performed at an average of 35 weeks' gestation.

Distance	Cesarean section
Overlapping	100%
< 10 mm	84%
> 10 mm and < 20 mm	40%
> 20 mm	16%

Management

A policy of expectant management, pioneered by MacAfee,[36] continues to be the standard with the focus on bedrest and avoiding preterm birth. This approach has reduced preterm birth and perinatal mortality;[37] however, preterm delivery remains a problem with 46% of women diagnosed with placenta previa delivering preterm.[4] The requirement for prolonged bedrest in hospital associated with this conservative approach is very stressful for women[38] and is increasingly being questioned. The difficulty lies in predicting the likelihood of bleeding in the individual patient.[39] Almost three-quarters of all women with placenta previa experience at least one episode of bleeding, at a median gestational age of 29 weeks, but the majority remain stable for a prolonged period and will not deliver until a median of 36 weeks.[40] However, the clinical outcomes of placenta previa are highly variable and cannot be predicted confidently from antenatal events.[41] A number of retrospective studies[40] have provided evidence for the safety and cost-effectiveness of outpatient management of placenta previa[41,42,43] culminating in a randomized controlled trial of inpatient versus outpatient management of placenta previa.[44] The evidence suggests that outpatient management is an acceptable alternative for selected patients.

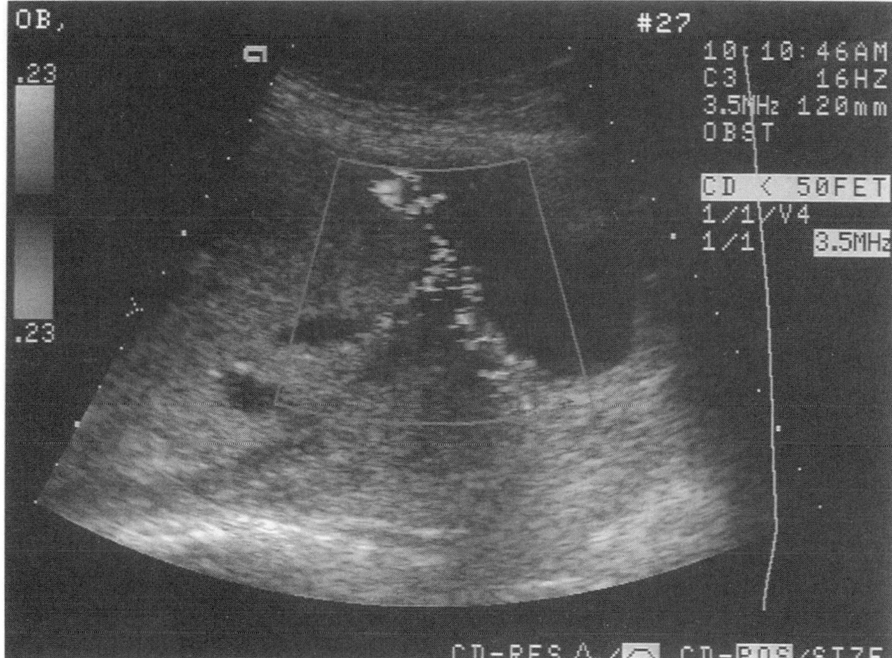

Figure 59.5 Transabdominal scan of placenta accreta. There is loss of the hypolucent zone between the placenta and myometrium, multiple lacunae (Swiss cheese appearance), and abnormal vasculature extending into the bladder wall. The case was managed by classical Cesarean section; the placenta was left *in situ* and resorbed spontaneously.

Tocolytic therapy has been shown to prolong pregnancy in symptomatic women.[45,46] However, in a small study using home uterine monitoring, uterine contractions did not appear to be a major factor in the onset of bleeding, and tocolytic therapy did not alter the clinical course.[47] Further studies into the potential benefits of prolonging pregnancy using cervical cerclage are required.[48–50]

When carrying out a Cesarean section, a low transverse uterine incision is usually possible. If available immediately prior to incision, an examination by ultrasound will allow the operator to avoid cutting through the placenta, which can then be peeled aside and the nearest window of membranes located and entered. The frequency of blood transfusion, either antenatally or peripartum, is fairly low, and autologous blood donation is not feasible for most patients.[51] Two retrospective studies have concluded that regional anesthesia is safe for Cesarean section,[52,53] and one small randomized trial has suggested that epidural anesthesia is superior to general anesthesia with regard to maternal hemodynamics.[54]

Placenta previa/accreta

The association between a previous Cesarean section and placenta previa and placenta accreta/percreta (pathological adherence of the placenta) is well recognized. The incidence of placenta previa increases with the number of previous deliveries by Cesarean section,[55,56] and there is a suggestion that the incidence of previa is rising because of the increasing Cesarean section rate.[57] The mechanism of causation of previa by a previous scar is poorly understood but may be the result of reduced differential growth of the lower segment, resulting in less upward shift in placental position as pregnancy advances.[58] Certainly, the increasing Cesarean section rate has resulted in an increased incidence of placenta accreta which, in a 1997 study,[57] occurred in 1 in 2500 deliveries. The relative risk of placenta accreta in the presence of placenta previa is 2065-fold higher than in women who have a normally situated placenta.[57] The risk of placenta accreta in the presence of placenta previa increases dramatically with the number of previous Cesarean sections, with a 25% risk for one prior Cesarean section and more than a 40% risk for two prior Cesarean sections.[56] Placenta accreta is a significant condition with a high potential risk for hysterectomy and a maternal death rate reported at 7%. Prenatal diagnosis may be beneficial in preparing for delivery.[59–61] A number of imaging techniques including ultrasonography[61–63] and color Doppler[64–67] (Fig. 59.5) are helpful in making a prenatal diagnosis of placenta accreta. Dynamic contrast MRI can differentiate chorionic villi and decidua basalis, and can provide excellent contrast between the placenta and myometrium anywhere within the uterus[68–70] (Fig. 59.6).

The key diagnostic imaging features described in placenta accreta are summarized in Table 59.4. Conservative treatment, leaving the placenta *in situ*, may be a useful management option[71] (Table 59.5).

Vasa previa

In vasa previa, the fetal vessels cross within the membranes between the internal os and the presenting part, usually the

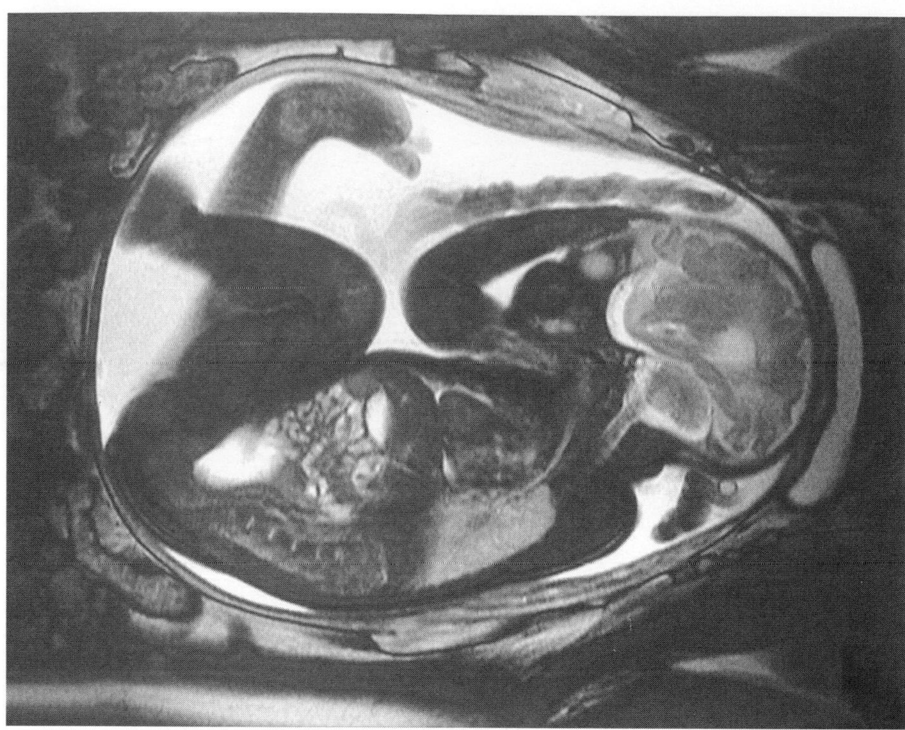

Figure 59.6 MRI of anterior placenta with loss of the retroplacental space and invasion of the placenta into the myometrium superior to the bladder.

Table 59.4 Ultrasound features of placenta accreta.

Hypoechoic zone between myometrium and placenta less than 2 mm
Disruption of the hyperechoic uterine serosa–bladder interface
Lacunar spaces (Swiss cheese) in placental parenchyma
Prominent vessels extending from placental base to uterine wall
Dilated blood vessels and turbulent blood flow in lacunae
Abnormal blood vessels linking the placenta and bladder with diastolic flow
Focal extension of placental tissue beyond the uterine serosa

Table 59.5 Management options in placenta accreta/percreta.

Hysterectomy
Avoid incision of placenta or attempted removal
Use of cell saver
Deliberate cystotomy to assist bladder mobilization
Placement of ureteral stents
Hypogastric artery ligation or embolization/balloon occlusion
Uterine conservation
Classical Cesarean section avoiding placenta
Leave placenta *in situ* if no hemorrhage
Prophylactic radiological hypogastric artery embolization/balloon occlusion
Attempt placental removal if bleeding occurs
Control bleeding by: circumferential sutures over placental site, prostoglandin F2-alpha myometrial injection, ligating uterine pedicles and/or ovarian vessels, uterine packing

fetal head. It is an uncommon form of placental anatomy, occurring in 1 out of 3000–5000 pregnancies.[72] It primarily occurs in two settings: a velamentous cord insertion or a succenturiate lobe on the opposite side of the internal os from the main placental structure. Because fetal vessels within the membranes are unprotected by Wharton's jelly, they are prone to compression during labor and may tear when the membranes rupture, resulting in severe fetal heart rate abnormalities accompanied by slight or moderate vaginal bleeding leading to fetal exsanguination.

Vasa previa is strongly associated with a low-lying placenta,[73] even when a second-trimester placental location subsequently converts to normal.[74] Ultrasound imaging including Doppler, color Doppler, and power Doppler technology with TVS, now offers the possibility of predicting vasa previa well before the onset of labor although, at present, screening for vasa previa would not be considered to be part of routine care. In two large case series, the specificity and sensitivity of a prenatal diagnosis was excellent.[72,75] The survival rates of infants with a prenatal diagnosis was 97% compared with 44% in those not diagnosed before delivery.[76] The protocol for ultrasound identification and management of vasa previa is shown in Table 59.6.

Placental abruption

Placental abruption is defined as a complete or partial separation of the placenta prior to delivery and is accompanied by hemorrhage into the decidua basalis. The incidence of placental abruption is approximately 0.6% in singleton preg-

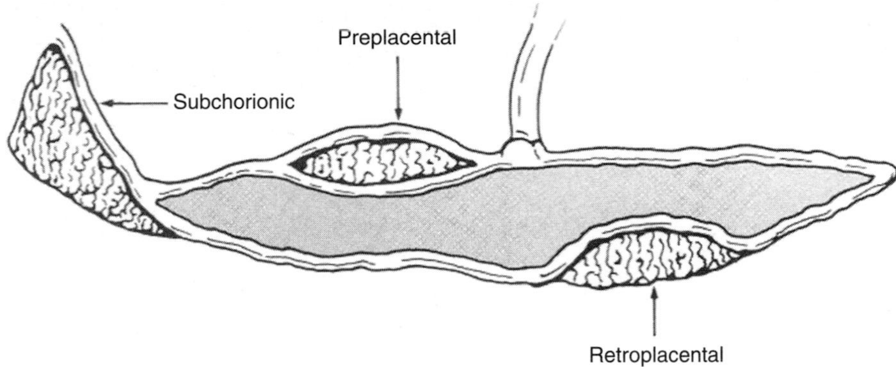

Figure 59.7 Sites of periplacental hemorrhage that have been described sonographically. Subchorionic hemorrhage may be remote from the placenta but is thought to arise from marginal abruptions. The term *preplacental hemorrhage* has been chosen to describe both subamniotic hematoma and massive subchorial thrombosis. Intraplacental hemorrhages (intervillous thrombi) may also be identified but are difficult to distinguish from placental lakes or other intraplacental sonolucencies.

Table 59.6 Protocol for diagnosis of vasa previa.[52]

Attempt to visualize cord insertion in all cases
High index of suspicion with low-lying placenta or succenturiate lobe
Sweep across the lower uterine segment to look for velamentous vessels
Color or power Doppler with TVS to further investigate suspicious cases
Ascertain whether pulse rate maternal or fetal on Doppler
Follow-up sonograms if vessels identified over or near the cervix
Cesarean delivery if vasa previa confirmed in later pregnancy

nancies and 1% in twin pregnancies,[77] although quoted rates vary widely from 0.1% to 2.7%.[78] The wide range of reported incidences may be explained by the different criteria used for diagnosing placental abruption as well as the increased recognition of milder forms, for example complete, partial, or marginal placental detachment (Fig. 59.7). Perinatal mortality occurs in 11.9% of cases of abruption compared with 0.8% of all other births.[79] Older case series report a perinatal mortality rate of up to 21%.[80] Abruption is associated with a nearly ninefold increase in the risk of stillbirth;[81] the case fatality rate, expressed as the number of abruptio-stillbirth cases per 100 total placental abruption cases, is reported to be 5.3%[80] to 7%.[87] Abruption accounts for more than 8% of all cases of perinatal mortality.[79] The high mortality rate results, in part, from its strong association with preterm delivery; in a large population study, 55% of the excess perinatal deaths with abruption resulted from early delivery.[79] Placental abruption appears to be occurring more frequently probably because of increased ascertainment and reporting.[82–84] The risk of preterm birth in women with abruption ranges from 39.6%[80] to 50%[79] compared with 9.1% for women without abruption. Abruption is also significantly associated with fetal growth restriction, which occurs in 14.3% of cases of placental abruption and 8.1% of cases without abruption;[80] this association is stronger for term than for preterm babies. At each gestational age, the relative risk of abruption is highest among babies in the lowest weight percentile and progressively

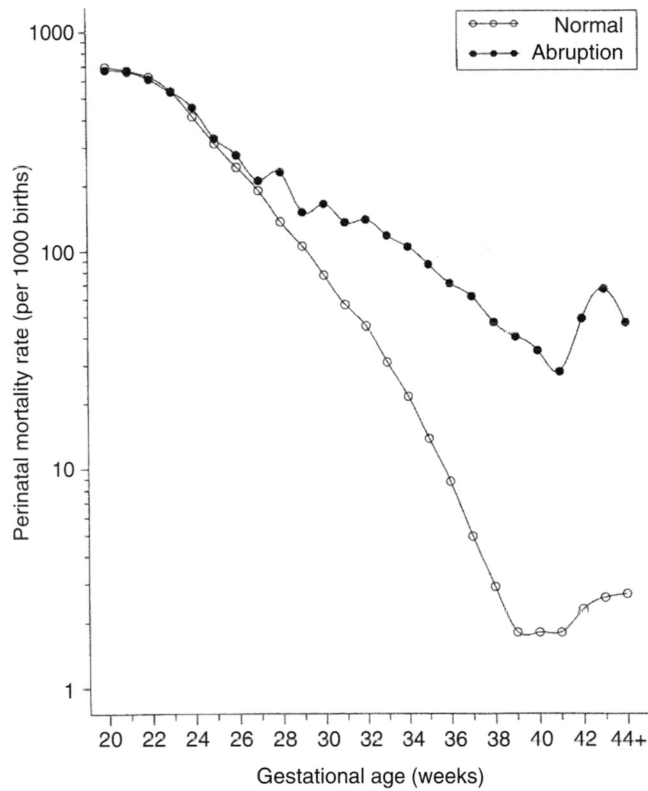

Figure 59.8 Gestational age-specific perinatal mortality rate (plotted on a logarithmic scale) in pregnancies with and without abruption, in the USA, in 1995 and 1996 (reproduced from ref. 79, with permission).

declines with increasing weight. This effect is slightly greater for term babies than for preterm babies, thus, at about 36 weeks' gestation, a baby weighing less than those within the first percentile for weight had a relative risk of abruption of 9.8 compared with a baby weighing more than those in the 90th percentile.[79] The excess in perinatal mortality rate in cases of abruption increases toward term both in relation to gestational age[79] (Fig. 59.8) and to birthweight[79] (Fig 59.9) compared with pregnancies without abruption. Even in babies weighing around 4000 g, who have the best chance of

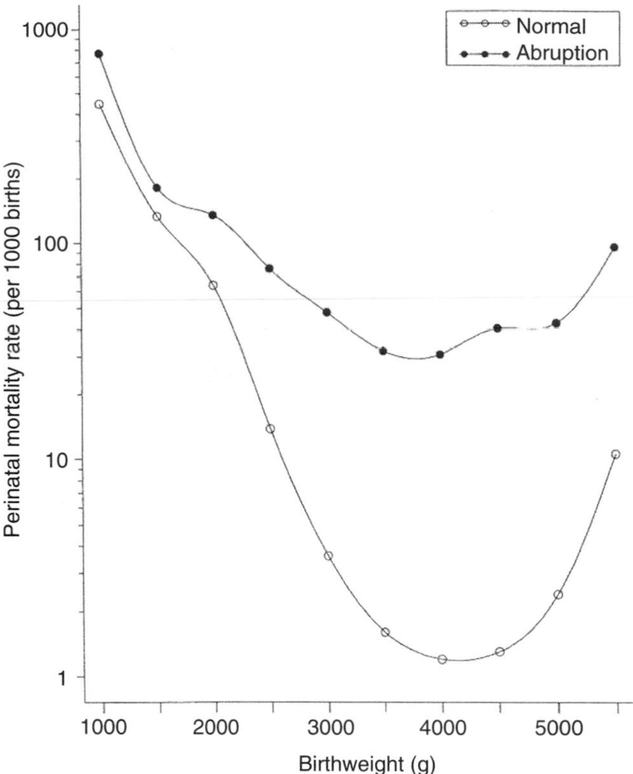

Figure 59.9 Birthweight-specific perinatal mortality rates (plotted on a logarithmic scale) in term pregnancies (≥ 37 weeks) with and without placental abruption, in the USA, in 1995 and 1996 (reproduced from ref. 79, with permission).

survival, the excess perinatal mortality rate due to abruption is increased 25-fold.

Risk factors

Table 59.7 shows the etiological fractions for a number of factors that are significantly associated with the occurrence of abruption.[85] The factor in this study with the highest etiological fraction is the presence of a male fetus, which has an associated risk of 16.3%. The next most important determinant is severe growth restriction. The association between placental abruption and advanced maternal age is inconsistent and may be more a factor of parity.[86] Smoking is an important preventable cause of abruption;[77,87–89] a meta-analysis of a large number of studies on smoking in pregnancy[90] showed that there was a strong concordance in the finding of a twofold increased risk of abruption in women who smoke. The results suggest that between 15% and 25% of placental abruption episodes could be prevented if women stopped smoking cigarettes during pregnancy. The analysis included five studies where dose–response relationships showed a two- to threefold increase in the incidence of abruption in women who smoked more than 20 cigarettes per day (Table 59.8).

Table 59.7 Etiological fractions for significant determinants of abruption.

Determinant	Etiological fraction
Male fetus	0.163
Severely small for gestational age	0.064
Unmarried	0.054
Age > 35 years	0.053
Smoking > 10 cigarettes per day	0.042
Preeclampsia	0.038
Rupture of membranes > 24 h	0.032
Chorioamnionitis	0.026
Prepregnancy hypertension	0.015
Pregnancy-induced hypertension without albuminuria	0.010

From ref. 85, with permission.

Table 59.8 Meta-analysis of the joint effects of cigarette smoking and hypertensive disorders on the risk of placental abruption.

Hypertensive disorder	Nonsmokers	Smokers
None	1.0 (referent)	1.4 (1.2, 1.5)
Chronic hypertension	2.8 (2.5, 3.2)	5.2 (2.7, 10.0)
Mild preeclampsia	0.9 (0.6, 1.2)	2.3 (1.6, 3.3)
Severe preeclampsia	4.1 (2.8, 6.0)	5.9 (3.4, 10.3)
Chronic hypertension with preeclampsia	2.0 (0.7, 5.4)	7.8 (2.4, 25.9)

From ref. 90, with permission.

Data are given as odds ratio (95% confidence interval).

Maternal hypertension is a major risk factor for placental abruption,[77,78,85,91,92] and women with preeclampsia are twice as likely to develop placental abruption as normotensive women.[78] At least two studies[91,92] did not find an increased risk of abruption in chronically hypertensive women, although they did confirm the important effect of severe preeclampsia and superimposed preeclampsia. An interaction between smoking and hypertensive disorders is also well known. Overall, the incidence of placental abruption in women with hypertensive disorders in pregnancy is 10%.[93] In severe preeclampsia or eclampsia, quantitative proteinuria and degree of blood pressure elevation are not predictive of placental abruption.[94] A paradoxical effect of smoking is also well known in that the risk of mild and severe preeclampsia is reduced by one-half in smokers.[95] However, women who smoked and were hypertensive had an almost eightfold increased risk of abruption compared to women who had neither condition.[90,91,95] Cocaine is a potent cause of placental abruption and may have a high prevalence in some areas.[96] Up to 10% of women using cocaine may experience abruption,[97]

Table 59.9 Factors significantly associated with placental abruption.

Factor	Typical odds ratios
Severely small for gestational age	3.99
Cocaine use	3.92
Chorioamnionitis	2.61
Premature rupture of membranes	2.44
Alcohol	2.29
Chronic hypertension	2.21
Oligohydramnios	2.09
Twins	2.06
Smoking	2.00
Preeclampsia	1.9
Parity > 3	1.6
Maternal age > 35	1.37
Unmarried	1.27

and its effect appears to be related to vasoconstriction in the placental bed.[98] Rupture of the membranes,[77,99] and associated chorioamnionitis, and birthweight discordance in twins also have a significant impact on the likelihood of abruption.[100] The typical odds ratios (ORs) for factors associated with abruption are given in Table 59.9. Overall, however, an etiological factor is present in less than one-half of cases[85] and the majority of placental abruption occurs in women with no established risk factors. Placental abruption remains, therefore, difficult to predict and is largely unpreventable. A combination of risk factors may allow the identification of a group of women at high risk of abruption in whom increased surveillance may be appropriate.[101]

Pathogenesis

The association of abruption with poor fetal growth suggests that the origins of abruption may extend back to the earliest stages of pregnancy. The chronic process underlying abruption may also contribute to the risk of preterm delivery.[3] Pathological studies suggest that abruption is associated with abnormal placental vasculature, thrombosis, and reduced placental perfusion.[102] A high incidence of inherited thrombophilias is noted in patients with abruption, and in particular there is an increased prevalence of mutations in the genes coding for Factor V Leiden, homocysteine, activated protein C resistance, and antiphospholipid antibodies.[103,104] Postpartum women who have experienced placental abruption should be considered for screening for the presence of these factors.[105]

For women who have experienced placental abruption, the risk of recurrence in subsequent pregnancies is observed to be 10–15% (i.e., 30-fold increased risk),[78] although in one study the risk was found to be increased 100-fold.[106] In cases with two previous abruptions, the OR of a third abruption was 36.5.[107]

Table 59.10 Clinical presentation in 59 cases of moderate to severe abruption.

Vaginal bleeding	78%
Fetal distress	50%
Uterine tenderness/back pain	66%
High-frequency contractions	17%
Uterine hypertonus	17%
Unexplained preterm labor	22%
Dead fetus at admission	15%
Perinatal death of fetus alive at admission	18% (9 out of 50)

Adapted from ref. 108.

Management of moderate to severe abruption

Approximately 30% of women presenting with bleeding in the third trimester are diagnosed with definitive placental abruption.[108] Hurd and co-workers[108] reported the outcome of 59 cases of abruption prospectively managed in a selective manner; the clinical features are described in Table 59.10. The mean diagnosis to delivery time in patients with a clinical presentation consistent with abruption was 2 h and 54 min, and the Cesarean section rate was 52%.[109] Clinical management decisions in cases of moderate to severe placental abruption must be individualized and aggressive plans for delivery made if there is evidence of fetal distress or maternal hemodynamic instability or coagulation disorders. Minimizing the interval between presentation and delivery may be important.[110] Knab[111] found that almost 70% of all cases of perinatal mortality occurred in infants who were delivered more than 2 h from the time of diagnosis. In one series of 33 women with clinically overt placental abruption associated with fetal bradycardia, death or cerebral palsy occurred in 33% of the cases; a diagnosis to delivery interval of 20 min or less was associated with substantially reduced neonatal morbidity and mortality compared with delivery at 30 min (OR of 0.44).[108] There is some evidence that women diagnosed with concealed abruption, with an absence of vaginal bleeding, have a higher stillbirth rate, perhaps because of a delay in diagnosis.[111] In most cases, blood eventually escapes from behind the membranes or past an impacted fetal head and bleeding occurs. Fetal heart rate abnormalities are common in abruption, occurring in 58% of cases.[112] Cesarean section rates in this study were 71%, and undergoing a Cesarean section significantly reduced the odds of perinatal death to 0.1. Abruption may also present as backache associated with a nontender uterus.[113] Although being a very subjective clinical measure, the estimation of degree of placental separation can be used to assess the risk of stillbirth and preterm delivery[80] (Fig. 59.10). Women with severe hemorrhage are more likely to be classified as having over 50% placental separation. The presence of severe hemorrhage may serve as a reliable marker for the severity of placental abruption.[80] Management principles for severe abruption are given in Table 59.11.

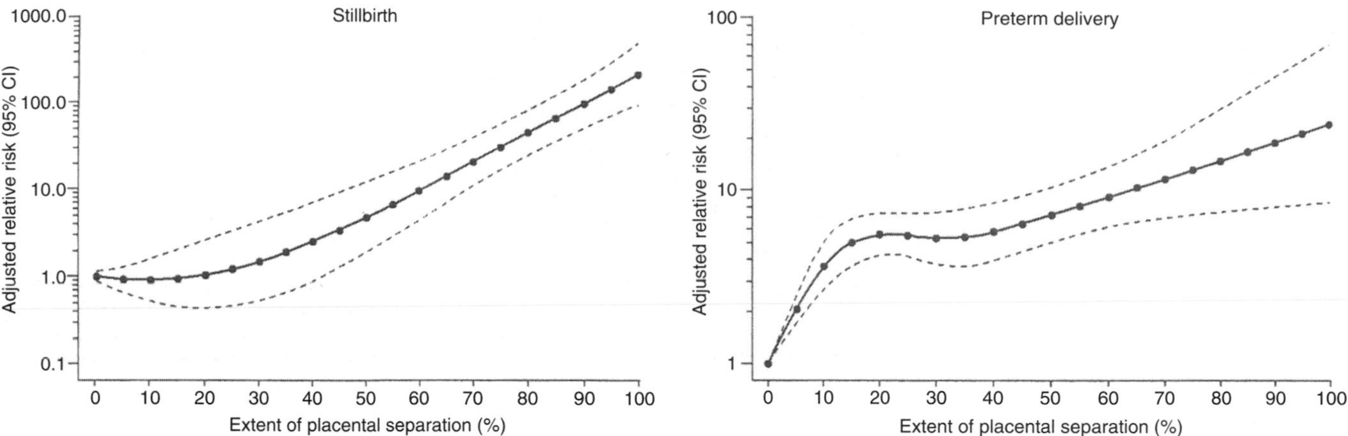

Figure 59.10 Adjusted relative risks with 95% confidence intervals of the association between extent of placental separation and stillbirth and preterm delivery, Mount Sinai Hospital, NY, 1989–1996 (reproduced from ref. 80, with permission).

Table 59.11 Management principles for severe abruption.

Fetal assessment for viability, welfare, and size (growth restriction is common)
Estimate severity of abruption (uterine tone, hardness, pain, amount of vaginal bleeding)
Maternal assessment for hypovolemia and coagulation status
Early aggressive treatment of suspected disseminated intravascular coagulation[114]
Kleihauer–Betke test and Rhesus status should be checked as fetal–maternal hemorrhage is present in up to 30% of cases, particularly in traumatic abruption[115]
Expedite delivery of a live fetus with a low threshold for Cesarean section

Mild abruption

A rapid Cesarean section appears to be beneficial for acute cases of placental abruption; however, less severe cases, particularly those presenting well before term, may be managed more conservatively.[109,116] In women presenting preterm, either with vaginal bleeding in the absence of uterine tenderness, or fetal distress, or in whom there was a retrospective diagnosis of abruption, 26% delivered on the day of admission, 50% delivered within 3 days and, of the remainder, about one-half delivered 15 or more days after admission. Some were treated with tocolytics although this practice is controversial and no benefit was seen in an uncontrolled study of 95 preterm women.[117] Bond and co-workers[118] expectantly managed 43 cases of abruption at less than 35 weeks' gestation and achieved a mean prolongation of pregnancy of 12 days, but the Cesarean section rate was still high at 75%.

Where vaginal delivery is pursued, amniotomy may be beneficial in hastening delivery. Oxytocin may likewise be helpful and there is no evidence that the latter increases complications.[118,119] Many cases of unexplained vaginal bleeding, which occur in up to 6% of the obstetric population, may result from marginal placental separation.[88] Vaginal and cervical lesions should also be excluded. The prognosis is generally good although patients should be followed in case of recurrence. Unlike abruption, the lack of association with smoking suggests the possibility of a distinct pathological process in these cases.[88]

Ultrasound diagnosis

Negative findings on ultrasound do not exclude the possibility of significant placental abruption. Scholl[116] reported ultrasound visualization of a clot in only 25% of placental abruption cases and found that ultrasound was unhelpful in management. In a series of 110 women who underwent ultrasonic examination for suspected abruption after 22 weeks' gestation, umbilical artery resistance indices on Doppler were in the normal range in 79% of cases and direct visualization of abruption was only possible in 20%.[120]

Glantz and Purnell[121] found a sonographic detection rate of only 11% for abruption but, in general, abnormal ultrasound findings were predictive of a more adverse outcome. Abruption may appear as a sonolucent area of blood (Fig. 59.11) or as a more echogenic picture of an organized blood clot (Figs 59.12 and 59.13). Fetal mortality may be as high as 75% when a retroplacental hemorrhage of greater than 60 mL is present.[122]

Trauma

Fetal death occurring as a result of injury during pregnancy is often preceded by placental abruption.[123] Abruption was diagnosed in 6.8% of injured pregnant women and fetal death occurred in 3.4% of trauma victims.[124] However, the injury

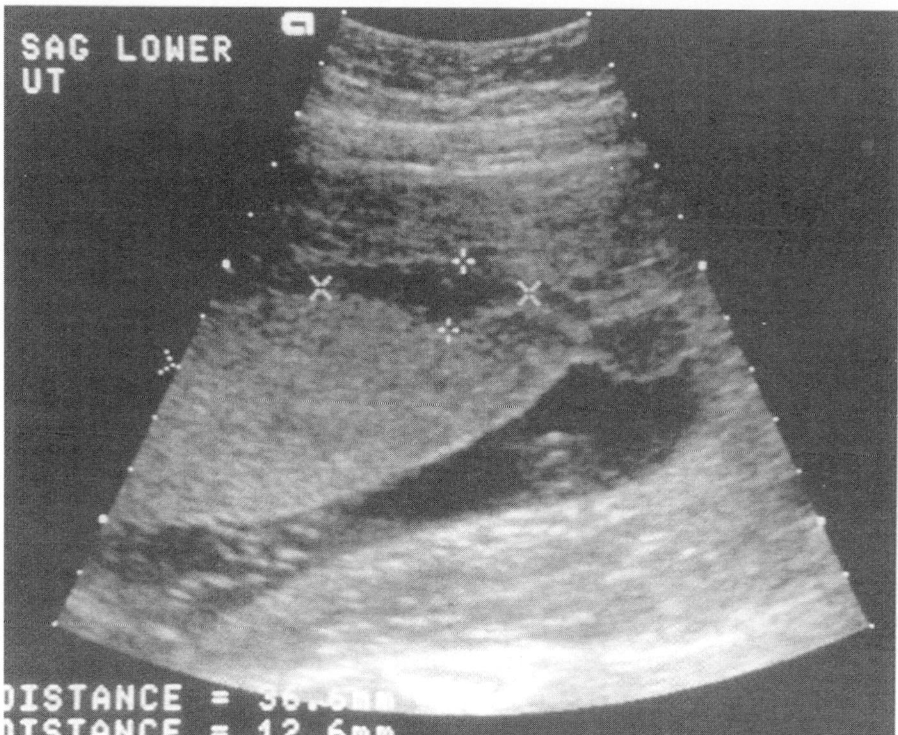

Figure 59.11 Sonolucent, retroplacental portion of the placenta identified by the markers '+' and '×', indicative of an area of abruption at least 2 weeks after the occurrence.

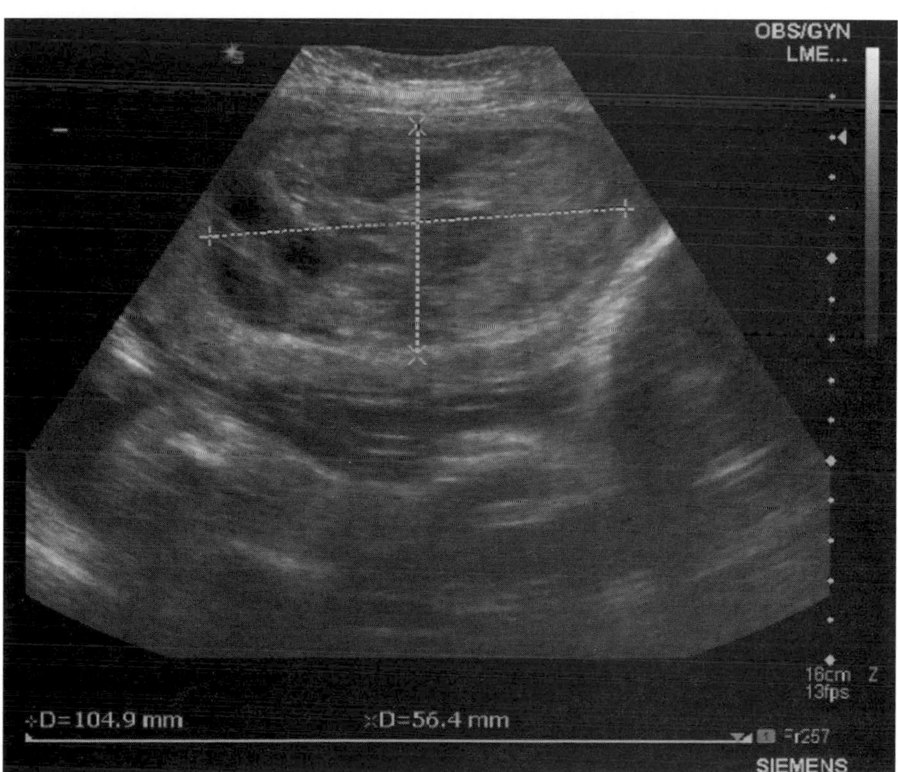

Figure 59.12 A large organizing hematoma in the placenta anteriorly at 29 weeks' gestation. The fetal head is in the lower right of the picture. Emergency Cesarean section was performed shortly after this picture was taken because of spontaneous fetal heart rate decelerations and a healthy fetus was delivered.

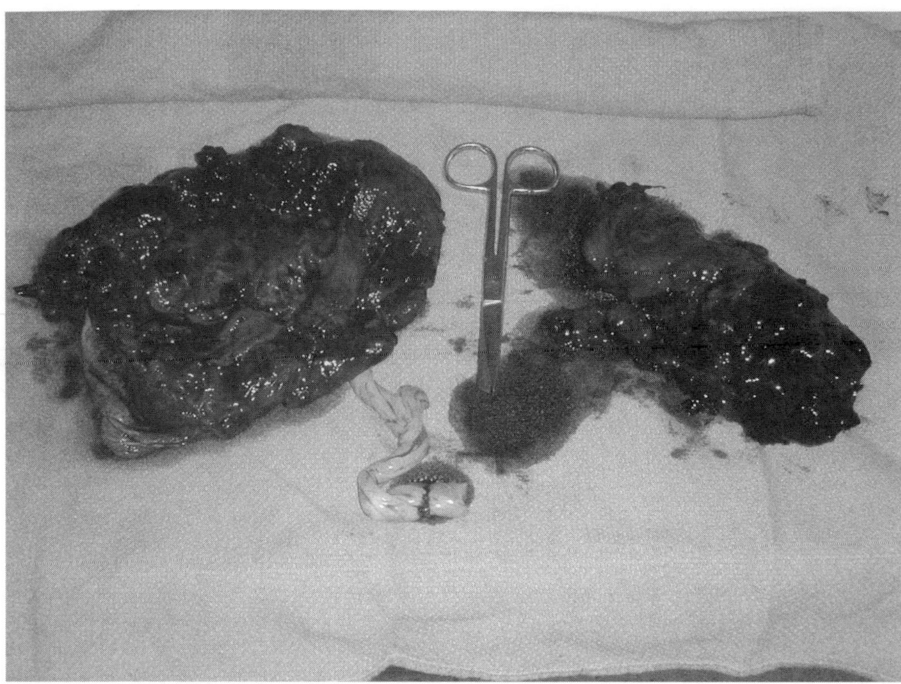

Figure 59.13 Placenta and 225 mL of retroplacental blood clot from the same case as in Fig. 59.11.

severity score in pregnant trauma victims is poorly predictive of placental abruption and fetal death. Even relatively minor injuries were associated with adverse pregnancy outcomes.[124] Traumatic abruption was more likely in car accidents occurring at speeds above 30 miles per hour.[125] The importance of correct seatbelt restraints for pregnant women should be emphasized.[126,127] Placental abruption following trauma may be asymptomatic and a high index of suspicion should be maintained;[128] it is recommended to carry out fetal monitoring for a minimum of 4 h.[115]

Key points

1 The most important cause of bleeding in the third trimester is placental abruption (with an incidence of approximately 0.6%), followed by placenta previa (with an incidence of 0.3%).

2 Major risk factors for placenta previa include: maternal age with an odds ratio (OR) of 9.1, prior Cesarean section (OR 2.7), multiparity (OR 2.3), and smoking (OR 1.6).

3 Transvaginal sonography (TVS) obviates the need for the "double-setup" examination and has become the "gold standard" for the diagnosis of placenta previa.

4 Vaginal delivery is possible when the distance from the placental edge to internal os is greater than 20 mm on TVS at any gestational age.

5 A Cesarean section is necessary when the placenta overlaps the internal os by any amount after approximately 35 weeks' gestation.

6 A placental edge lying within 20 mm of the os but not overlapping requires individualized management but vaginal delivery is possible.

7 The risk of placenta previa in any pregnancy increases with the number of previous deliveries by Cesarean section.

8 In any pregnancy, the risk of placenta accreta in the presence of placenta previa increases dramatically with the number of previous deliveries by Cesarean section with a 25% risk for one Cesarean section and more than a 40% risk for two.

9 Prenatal diagnosis of placenta accreta by ultrasound or magnetic resonance imaging (MRI) may be beneficial in preparing for delivery.

10 Vasa previa is strongly associated with a low-lying placenta, and color Doppler with TVS now offers the possibility of prediction of vasa previa well before the onset of delivery.

11 Placental abruption is associated with a nearly ninefold increase in the risk of stillbirth compared with pregnancies without abruption.

12 Major risk factors for placental abruption include: cocaine use (OR 3.9), chorioamnionitis (OR 2.6),

chronic hypertension (OR 2.8), severe preeclampsia (OR 4.1), twins (OR 2.1), and smoking (OR 2).

13 Between 15% and 25% of placental abruption episodes could be prevented if women stopped smoking cigarettes during pregnancy.

14 The majority of placental abruption occurs in women with no established risk factors.

15 A high incidence of inherited thrombophilias, in particular Factor V Leiden, homocysteine, activated protein C resistance, and antiphospholipid antibodies are found in patients with abruption.

16 In subsequent pregnancies, the risk of recurrence of placental abruption is observed to be 10–15% (i.e., 30-fold increase in risk).

17 70% of all perinatal mortality occurred in infants who delivered more than 2 h from the time of diagnosis of abruption.

18 Negative findings on ultrasound do not exclude the possibility of significant placental abruption.

19 The injury severity score in pregnant trauma victims is poorly predictive of placental abruption and fetal death.

20 Kleihauer–Betke test and Rhesus status should be checked as fetal–maternal hemorrhage is present in up to 30% of cases, particularly in traumatic abruption.

References

1 Ananth CV, Demissie K, Smulian JC, et al. Placenta previa in singleton and twin births in the United States, 1989 through 1998: a comparison of risk factor profiles and associated conditions. *Am J Obstet Gynecol* 2003;188:275–281.

2 Faiz AS, Ananth CV. Etiology and risk factors for placenta previa: an overview and meta-analysis of observational studies. *J Maternal–Fetal Neo Med* 2003;13:175–190.

3 Crane JM, Van den Hof MC, Dodds L, et al. Maternal complications with placenta previa. *Am J Perinatol* 2000;17:101–105.

4 Crane JM, Van den Hof MC, Dodds L, et al. Neonatal outcomes with placenta previa. *Obstet Gynecol* 1997;177:210–214.

5 Salihu HM, Li Q, Rouse DJ, et al. Placenta previa: neonatal death after live births in the United States. *Am J Obstet Gynecol* 2003;188:1305–1309.

6 Ananth CV, Smulian JC, Vintzileos AM. The effect of placenta previa on neonatal mortality: a population-based study in the United States, 1989 through 1997. *Am J Obstet Gynecol* 2003;188:1299–1304.

7 Rasmussen S, Albrechtsen S, Dalaker K. Obstetric history and the risk of placenta previa. *Acta Obstet Gynecol Scand* 2000;79:502–507.

8 Ananth CV, Demissie K, Smulian JC, et al. Relationship among placenta previa, fetal growth restriction, and preterm delivery: a population based study. *Obstet Gynecol* 2001;98:299–306.

9 Obstetrical hemorrhage. In: Cunningham FG, Gant NF, Leveno KJ, et al., eds. *Williams obstetrics*, 21st edn. Norwalk, CT: Appleton & Lange; 2001:619–669.

10 Oppenheimer L, Farine D, Ritchie K, et al. What is a low-lying placenta? *Am J Obstet Gynecol* 1991;165:1036–1038.

11 Oppenheimer LW, Farine D, Ritchie JWK. The classification of placenta praevia: time for a change? *Fetal Maternal Med Rev* 1992;4:73–78.

12 Farine D, Fox HE, Timor-Tritsch I. Vaginal ultrasound for ruling out placenta previa. *Br J Obstet Gynaecol* 1989;96:117–119.

13 Smith RS, Lauria MR, Comstock CH, et al. Transvaginal ultrasonography for all placentas that appear to be low-lying or over the internal cervical os. *Ultrasound Obstet Gynecol* 1997;9:22–24.

14 Farine D, Fox HE, Jakobson S, et al. Vaginal ultrasound for diagnosis of placenta previa. *Am J Obstet Gynecol* 1988;159:566–569.

15 Oyelese KO, Holden D, Awadh A, et al. Placenta previa: the case for transvaginal sonography. *Cont Rev Obstet Gynaecol* 1999;11:257–261.

16 Edlestone DI. Placental localization by ultrasound. *Clin Obstet Gynecol* 1977;20:285–287.

17 King DL. Placental ultrasonography. *J Clin Ultrasound* 1973;1:21–26.

18 Timor-Tritsch IE, Rottem S. *Transvaginal sonography*. New York: Elsevier; 1987:1–13.

19 Townsend RR, Laing FC, Nyberg DA, et al. Technical factors responsible for placental migration: sonographic assessment. *Radiology* 1986;160:105–108.

20 Lauria MR, Smith RS, Treadwell MC, et al. The use of second-trimester transvaginal sonography to predict placenta previa. *Ultrasound Obstet Gynecol* 1996;8:337–340.

21 McClure N, Dorman JC. Early identification of placenta praevia. *Br J Obstet Gynaecol* 1990;97:959–961.

22 Leerentveld RA, Gilberts ECAM, Arnold KJCW, et al. Accuracy and safety of transvaginal sonographic placental localization. *Obstet Gynecol* 1990;76:759–762.

23 Sherman SJ, Carlson DE, Platt LD, et al. Transvaginal ultrasound: does it help in the diagnosis of placenta praevia? *Ultrasound Obstet Gynecol* 1992;2:256–260.

24 Timor-Tritsch IE, Yunis RA. Confirming the safety of transvaginal sonography in patients suspected of placenta previa. *Obstet Gynecol* 1993;81:742–744.

25 Powell MC, Buckley J, Price H, et al. Magnetic resonance imaging and placenta praevia. *Am J Obstet Gynecol* 1986;154:656–659.

26 Mustafa SA, Brizot ML, Carvalho MHB, et al. Transvaginal ultrasonography in predicting placenta previa at delivery: a longitudinal study. *Ultrasound Obstet Gynecol* 2002;20:356–359.

27 Hill LM, Di Nofrio DM, Chenevey P. Transvaginal sonographic elvauation of first-trimester placenta previa. *Ultrasound Obstet Gynecol* 1995;5:301–303.

28 Taipale P, Hiilesmaa V, Ylostalo P. Diagnosis of placenta previa by transvaginal sonographic screening at 12–16 weeks in a non-selected population. *Obstet Gynecol* 1997;89:364–367.

29 Rosati P, Guariglia L. Clinical significance of placenta previa detected at early routine transvaginal scan. *Ultrasound Med* 2000;19:581–585.

30 Taipale P, Hiilesmaa V, Ylostalo P. Transvaginal ultrasonography at 18–23 weeks in predicting placenta previa at delivery. *Ultrasound Obstet Gynecol* 1998;12:422–425.

31 Becker RH, Vonk R, Mende BC, et al. The relevance of placental location at 20–23 gestational weeks for prediction of placenta previa at delivery: evaluation of 8650 cases. *Ultrasound Obstet Gynecol* 2001;17:496–501.
32 Oppenheimer L, Holmes P, Simpson N, et al. Diagnosis of low-lying placenta: can migration in the third trimester predict outcome. *Ultrasound Obstet Gynecol* 2001;8:100–102.
33 Dawson WB, Dumas MD, Romano WM, et al. Translabial ultrasonography and placenta previa: does measurement of the os-placental distance predict outcome? *J Ultrasound Med* 1996;15: 441–446.
34 Sallout B, Oppenheimer LW. The classification of placenta previa based on os-placental edge distance at transvaginal sonography. *Am J Obstet Gynecol* 2002;187:S94.
35 Bhide A, Prefumo F, Moore J, et al. Placental edge to internal os distance in the late third trimester and mode of delivery in placenta previa. *Br J Obstet Gynaecol* 2003;110:860–864.
36 MacAfee CHG. Placenta previa: a study of 174 cases. *J Obstet Gynaecol Br Commonwealth* 1945;52:313–317.
37 Cotton DB, Read JA, Paul RH, et al. The conservative aggressive management of placenta previa. *Am J Obstet Gynecol* 1980;137:687–695.
38 Katz A. Waiting for something to happen: hospitalization with placenta previa. *Birth* 2001;28:186–191.
39 Dola CP, Garite TJ, Dowling DD, et al. Placenta previa: does its type affect pregnancy outcome? *Am J Perinatol* 2003;20:353–360.
40 Love CDB, Wallace EM. Pregnancies complicated by placenta previa: what is appropriate management? *Br J Obstet Gynaecol* 1996;103:864–867.
41 Rosen DMB, Peek MJ. Do women with placenta praevia without antepartum haemorrhage require hospitalization? *Aust NZ J Obstet Gynaecol* 1994;34:130–134.
42 Mouer JR. Placenta previa: antepartum conservative management, inpatient versus outpatient. *Am J Obstet Gynecol* 1994; 170:1683–1686.
43 Droste S, Keil K. Expectant management of placenta previa: cost benefit analysis of outpatient treatment. *Am J Obstet Gynecol* 1994;170:1254–1257.
44 Wing DA, Paul RH, Millar LK. Management of the symptomatic placenta praevia: a randomised, controlled trial of inpatient versus outpatient expectant management. *Am J Obstet Gynecol* 1996;175:806–811.
45 Besinger RE, Monial CW, Paskiewicz LS, et al. The effect of tocolytic use in the management of symptomatic placenta previa. *Am J Obstet Gynecol* 1995;172:1770–1778.
46 Sharma A, Suri V, Gupta I. Tocolytic therapy in conservative management of symptomatic placenta previa. *Int J Gynaecol Obstet* 2004;84:109–113.
47 Magnam EF, Johnson CA, Gookin KS, et al. Placenta previa: does uterine activity cause bleeding? *Aust NZ J Obstet Gynaecol* 1993;33:22–24.
48 Nelson JP. Interventions for suspected placenta praevia. *Cochrane Database Syst Rev* 2003;2. Oxford: Update Software.
49 Arias F. Cervical cerclage for the temporary treatment of patients with placenta praevia. *Obstet Gynecol* 1988;71:545–548.
50 Cobo E, Conde-Agudelo A, Delgado J, et al. Cervical cerclage: an alternative for the management of placenta praevia. *Am J Obstet Gynecol* 1998;179:122–125.
51 Toedt ME. Feasibility of autologous blood donation in patients with placenta previa. *J Fam Pract* 1999;48:219–221.
52 Parekh N, Husaini SW, Russel IF. Caesarean section for placenta praevia: a retrospective study of anaesthetic management. *Br J Anaesth* 2000;84:725–730.
53 Frederiksen MC, Glasenberg R, Stika CS. Placenta previa: a 22-year analysis. *Am J Obstet Gynecol* 1999;180:1432–1437.
54 Hong JY, Jee YS, Yoon HJ, et al. Comparison of epidural and general anesthesia in cesarean section for placenta previa. *Int J Obstet Anesth* 2003;12:12–16.
55 Gilliam M, Rosenberg D, Davis F. The likelihood of placenta previa with greater number of cesarean deliveries and higher parity. *Obstet Gynecol* 2002;99:976–980.
56 Clark SL, Koonings PP, Phelan JP. Placenta praevia/accreta and prior caesarean section. *Obstet Gynecol* 1985;66:89–92.
57 Miller DA, Chollet JA, Goodwin TM. Clinical risk factors for placenta praevia/placenta accreta. *Am J Obstet Gynecol* 1997; 177:210–214.
58 Dashe JS, McIntire DD, Ramus RM, et al. Persistence of placenta previa according to gestational age at ultrasound detection. *Obstet Gynecol* 2002;99:692–697.
59 O'Brien JM, Barton JR, Donaldson ES. The management of placenta percreta: conservative and operative strategies. *Am J Obstet Gynecol* 1996;75:1632–1638.
60 Hudon L, Belfort MA, Broome DR. Diagnosis and management of placenta percreta: a review. *Obstet Gynecol Surv* 1998; 8:509–517.
61 Jurcevic P, Grover S, Henderson J. A reassessment of options for the management of placenta previa percreta. *Aust NZ J Obstet Gynaecol* 2002;42:91–94.
62 Finberg H, Williams J. Placenta accreta: prospective sonographic diagnosis in patients with placenta previa and prior cesarean section. *J Ultrasound Med* 1992;11:333–343.
63 Guy GP, Peisner DB, Timor-Tritsch IE. Ultrasonographic evaluation of uteroplacental blood flow patterns of abnormally located and adherent placenta. *Am J Obstet Gynecol* 1990;164:723–727.
64 Chou MM, Ho ESC. Prenatal diagnosis of placenta praevia accreta with power amplitude ultrasonic angiography. *Am J Obstet Gynecol* 1997;177:1523–1525.
65 Hoffman-Tretin F, Koenigsberg M, Rabin A. Placenta accreta; additional sonographic observations. *J Ultrasound Med* 1992; 11:29–34.
66 Levine D, Hulka CA, Ludmir J, et al. Placenta accreta: evaluation with color Doppler US, power Doppler US, and MR imaging. *Radiology* 1997;205:773–776.
67 Chou MM, Ho ESC, Lee YH. Prenatal diagnosis of placenta previa accreta by transabdominal color Doppler ultrasound. *Ultrasound Obstet Gynecol* 2000;15:28–35.
68 Maldjian C, Adem R, Pelosi M, et al. MRI appearance of placenta percreta and placenta accreta. *Magn Reson Imaging* 1999;17:965–971.
69 Lam G, Kuller J, McMahon M. Use of magnetic resonance imaging and ultrasound in the antenatal diagnosis of placenta accreta. *J Soc Gynecol Invest* 2002;9:37–40.
70 Tanaka YO, Sohda S, Shigemitsu S, et al. High temporal resolution contrast MRI in high risk group for placenta accreta. *Magn Reson Imaging* 2001;19:635–642.
71 Ouellette A, Sallout B, Oppenheimer L. Outcomes of conservative versus surgical management of placenta accreta-percreta: a systematic review. *Am J Obstet Gynecol* 2003;89:S130.
72 Catanzarite V, Maida C, Thomas W, et al. Prenatal sonographic diagnosis of vasa previa: ultrasound findings and obstetric outcome in ten cases. *Ultrasound Obstet Gynecol* 2001; 18:109–115.
73 Lee W, Lee V, Kirk JS, et al. Vasa previa. Prenatal diagnosis, natural evolution, and clinical outcome. *Obstet Gynecol* 2000; 95:572–576.

74 Francois K, Mayer S, Harris C, et al. Association of vasa previa at delivery with a history of second-trimester placenta previa. *J Reprod Med* 2003;48:771–774.

75 Fung TY, Lau TK. Poor prenatal outcome associated with vasa previa: is it preventable? Report of three cases and review of the literature. *Ultrasound Obstet Gynecol* 1998;12:430–433.

76 Oyelese Y, Catanzarite V, Prefumo F, et al. Vasa previa: the impact of prenatal diagnosis on outcomes *Obstet Gynecol* 2004;103:937–942.

77 Ananth CV, Smulian JC, Demissie K, et al. Placental abruption among singleton and twin births in the United States: risk factor profiles. *Am J Epidemiol* 2001;153:771–778.

78 Ananth CV, Savitz DA, Williams MA. Placental abruption and its association with hypertension and prolonged rupture of membranes: a methodologic review and meta-analysis. *Obstet Gynecol* 1996;88:309–318.

79 Ananth CV, Wilcox AJ. Placental abruption and perinatal mortality in the United States. *Am J Epidemiol* 2001;153:332–337.

80 Ananth CV, Berkowitz GS, Savitz DA, et al. Placental abruption and adverse perinatal outcomes. *JAMA* 1999;282:1646–1651.

81 Krohn M, Voigt L, McKnight B, et al. Correlates of placental abruption. *Br J Obstet Gynaecol* 1987;94:333–340.

82 Broers, T, King WD, Arbuckle TE, et al. The occurrence of abruptio placentae in Canada: 1990 to 1997. *Chronic Dis Can* 2004;25:16–20.

83 Rassmussen S, Irgens LM, Bergsjo P, et al. The occurrence of placental abruption in Norway 1967–1991. *Acta Obstet Gynecol Scand* 1996;75:222–228.

84 Saftlas AF, Olson DR, Atrash HK, et al. National trends in the incidence of abruptio placentae, 1979–1987. *Obstet Gynecol* 1991;78:1081–1086.

85 Kramer MS, Usher RH, Pollack R, et al. Etiologic determinants of abruptio placentae. *Obstet Gynecol* 1997;89:221–226.

86 Ananth CV, Wilcox AJ, Savitz DA, et al. Effect of maternal age and parity on the risk of uteroplacental bleeding disorders in pregnancy. *Obstet Gynecol* 1996;88:511–516.

87 Andres RL. The association of cigarette smoking with placenta previa and abruptio placentae. *Semin Perinatol* 1996;20: 154–159.

88 Ananth CV, Savitz DA, Luther ER. Maternal cigarette smoking as a risk factor for placental abruption, placenta previa, and uterine bleeding in pregnancy. *Am J Epidemiol* 1996;144: 881–889.

89 Mortensen JT, Thulstrup AM, Larsen H, et al. Smoking, sex of the offspring, and risk of placental abruption, placenta previa, and preeclampsia: a population-based cohort study. *Acta Obstet Gynecol Scand* 2001;80:894–898.

90 Ananth CV, Smulian JC, Vintzileos AM. Incidence of placental abruption in relation to cigarette smoking and hypertensive disorders during pregnancy: a meta-analysis of observational studies. *Obstet Gynecol* 1999;93:622–628.

91 Ananth CV, Savitz DA, Bowes WA, Jr, et al. Influence of hypertensive disorders and cigarette smoking on placental abruption and uterine bleeding during pregnancy. *Br J Obstet Gynaecol* 1997;104:572–578.

92 Sibai BM, Lindheimer M, Hauth J, et al. Risk factors for preeclampsia, abruptio placentae, and adverse neonatal outcomes among women with chronic hypertension. *N Engl J Med* 1998;339:667–671.

93 Sibai BM. Diagnosis and management of chronic hypertension in pregnancy. *Obstet Gynecol* 1991;78:451–461.

94 Witlin AG, Saade GR, Mattar F, et al. Risk factors for abruptio placentae and eclampsia: analysis of 445 consecutively managed women with severe preeclampsia and eclampsia. *Am J Obstet Gynecol* 1999;180:1322–1329.

95 Cnattingius S, Mills JL, Yuen J, et al. The paradoxical effect of smoking in preeclamptic pregnancies: smoking reduces the incidence but increases the rates of perinatal mortality, abruptio placentae, and intrauterine growth restriction. *Am J Obstet Gynecol* 1997;177:156–161.

96 Hulse GK, Milne E, English DR, et al. Assessing the relationship between maternal cocaine use and abruptio placentae. *Addiction* 1997;92:1547–1551.

97 Hoskins IA, Friedman DA, Frieden FJ, et al. Relationship between antepartum cocaine abuse, abnormal umbilical artery Doppler velosymetry and placental abruption. *Obstet Gynecol* 1991;78:279–283.

98 Addis A, Moretti ME, Ahmed SF, et al. Fetal effects of cocaine: an updated metro anyalsis. *Reprod Toxicol* 2001;15:341–348.

99 Ananth CV, Oyelese Y, Srinivas N, et al. Preterm premature rupture of membranes, intrauterine infection, and oligohydramnios: risk factors for placental abruption. *Obstet Gynecol* 2004;104:71–77.

100 Ananth CV, Demissie K, Hanley ML. Birth weight discordancy and adverse perinatal outcomes among twin gestations in the United States: the effect of placental abruption. *Am J Obstet Gynecol* 2003;188:954–960.

101 Baumann P, Blackwell SC, Schild C, et al. Mathematic modeling to predict abruptio placentae. *Am J Obstet Gynecol* 2000;183: 815–822.

102 Alfirevic Z, Roberts D, Martlew V. How strong is the association between maternal thrombophilia and adverse pregnancy outcome? A systematic review. *Eur J Obstet Gynecol Reprod Biol* 2002;101:6–14.

103 Alfirevic Z, Mousa HA, Martlew V, et al. Postnatal screening for thrombophilia in women with severe pregnancy complications. *Obstet Gynecol* 2001;97:753–759.

104 Kupferminc MJ, Eldor A, Steinman N, et al. Increased frequency of genetic thrombophilia in women with complications of pregnancy. *N Engl J Med* 1999;340:9–13.

105 Prochazka M, Happach C, Marsal K, et al. Factor V leiden in pregnancies complicated by placental abruption. *Br J Obstet Gynaecol* 2003;110:462–466.

106 Pritchard JA, Cunningham G, Pritchard SA. On reducing the frequency of severe abruptio placentae. *Am J Obstet Gynecol* 1991;165:1345–1351.

107 Rasmussen S, Irgens LM, Dalaker K. The effect on the likelihood of further pregnancy of placental abruption and the rate of its recurrence. *Br J Obstet Gynaecol* 1997;104:1292–1295.

108 Hurd WW, Miodovnik M, Hertzberg V, et al. Selective management of abruptio placentae: a prospective study. *Obstet Gynecol* 1983;61:467–473.

109 Kayani SI, Walkinshaw SA, Preston C. Pregnancy outcome in severe placental abruption. *Br J Obstet Gynaecol* 2003; 110:679–683.

110 Chang YL, Chang SD, Cheng PJ. Perinatal outcome in patients with placental abruption with and without antepartum hemorrhage. *Int J Gynaecol Obstet* 2001;75:193–194.

111 Knab DR. Abruptio placentae. An assessment of the time and method of delivery. *Obstet Gynecol* 1978;52:625–629.

112 Witlin AG, Sibai BM. Perinatal and maternal outcome following abruptio placentae. *Hypertens Pregnancy* 2001;20: 195–203.

113 Notelovitz M, Bottoms SF, Dase DF, et al. Painless abruptio placentae. *Obstet Gynecol* 1979;53:270–272.

114 Kobayashi T, Toshihiko T, Maki M, et al. Diagnosis and management of acute obstetrical DIC. *Semin Thromb Hemost* 2001;27:161–167.
115 Pearlman MD, Tintanilli JE, Lorenz RP. A prospective controlled study of outcome after trauma in pregnancy. *Am J Obstet Gynecol* 1990;162:1502–1510.
116 Scholl JS. Abruptio placentae: clinical management in nonacute cases. *Am J Obstet Gynecol* 1987;156:40–51.
117 Towers CV, Pircon RA, Heppard M. Is tocolysis safe in the management of third-trimester bleeding? *Am J Obstet Gynecol* 1999;180:1572–1578.
118 Bond AL, Edersheim TG, Curry L, et al. Expectant management of abruptio placentae before 35 weeks gestation. *Am J Perinatol* 1989;6:121–126.
119 Clark SL, Hankins GDV, Dudley DA, et al. Amniotic fluid embolism: analysis of the national registry. *Am J Obstet Gynecol* 1995;172:1159–1173.
120 Toivonen S, Heinonen S, Anttila M, et al. Reproductive risk factors, Doppler findings, and outcome of affected births in placental abruption: a population-based analysis. *Am J Perinatol* 2002;19:451–460.
121 Glantz C, Purnell L. Clinical utility of sonography in the diagnosis and treatment of placental abruption. *J Ultrasound Med* 2002;21:837–840.
122 Nyberg DA, Mack LA, Benedetti TJ, et al. Placental abruption and placental hemorrhage: correlation of sonographic findings with fetal outcome. *Radiology* 1987;164:357–361.
123 Corsi PR, Rasslan S, Du Oliveira LB, et al. Trauma and pregnant women: analysis of maternal and fetal mortality. *Injury* 1999;30:239–243.
124 Schiff MA, Holt VL. The injury severity score in pregnant trauma patients: predicting placental abruption and fetal death. *J Trauma-Inj Infect Crit Care* 2002;53:946–949.
125 Reis PM, Sander CM, Pearlman MD. Abruptio placentae after auto accidents. A case-control study. *J Reprod Med* 2000;45:6–10.
126 Pearlman MD, Philips ME. Safety belt use during pregnancy. *Obstet Gynecol* 1996;88:1026–1029.
127 McGwin G, Jr, Russell SR, Rux RL, et al. Knowledge, beliefs, and practices concerning seat belt use during pregnancy. *J Trauma* 2004;57:682–683.
128 Kettle LM, Branch VW, Scott JR. Occult placental abruption after maternal trauma. *Obstet Gynecol* 1988;71:449–452.

60 Normal and abnormal labor

Wayne R. Cohen

All approaches to the systematic assessment of labor are grounded in the concept that it is possible to evaluate the progress of labor by analyzing the relationships among cervical dilation, fetal descent, and elapsed hours in labor.[1–7] This kind of graphic analysis forms the basis for clinical decision-making in dysfunctional labor but it must be used in conjunction with other obstetric data. Thus, information about pelvic architecture, uterine contractility, fetal size, position, and attitude, and the state of fetal oxygenation must be integrated with labor curve data if the obstetrician is to make the most informed and appropriate clinical judgments.

To a large extent, intrapartum decision-making is a process of estimating *seriatim* the probability of a safe vaginal delivery as updated information is obtained during the course of labor. All of the clinical data used in reaching decisions about obstetric interventions (especially the use of oxytocin, conduction anesthesia, Cesarean section, and instrumental delivery) should be viewed from this perspective.

Normal cervical dilation

The relationship between cervical dilation and the time elapsed in labor is described by a sigmoid shaped curve (Fig. 60.1).[1–3] Dilation is traditionally divided into a latent phase and an active phase. The latent phase extends from the onset of labor until the upward inflection in the curve and is associated with little incremental change in dilation. Enhancement in the rate of dilation begins at the onset of the active phase, during which most cervical dilation occurs. A gradual increase in dilation (the acceleration phase) initiates the active phase and leads, usually in about an hour, to a period of more rapid and linear dilation (the phase of maximum slope). During the terminal part of the active phase, the deceleration phase, dilation appears to slow. In fact, the cervix continues to open at a constant rate but, as it retracts around the head (which has begun to descend) to achieve complete dilation, its movement is directed cephalolaterally. This change cannot be appreciated readily by examination with the fingers, because only radial changes in distance can be determined.

By convention, full cervical dilation is considered to be 10 cm. This is a clinically useful approximation; however, because the cervix does not generally dilate to more than the largest diameter of the object passing through it, full dilation for most term babies is somewhat less, whereas for exceptionally large babies it may be more. This issue is of particular importance when interpreting the labor curves of very premature fetuses whose head diameter may be considerably less than 10 cm; in these cases, the curve of dilation is necessarily foreshortened.

In general, the labors of multiparas are shorter than those of nulliparas, with a shorter latent phase and more rapid rates of dilation and descent in the active phase and second stage.[3] Criteria for all multiparas are the same, irrespective of how many babies they have had.[1–3] Multiparas who have had all previous babies by Cesarean section should be judged by nulliparous criteria during labor.[8]

Latent phase

During the latent phase, the cervix is prepared for the more rapid dilation that will occur later.[3,9,10] Physical changes take place that can be appreciated clinically; these constitute what has been referred to as ripening or maturation of the cervix and, in some patients (particularly nulliparas), occur largely or completely before the onset of labor. The duration of the latent phase is inversely proportional to the degree of prelabor cervical maturation. The palpable softening, effacement, and anterior rotation of the cervix in the pelvic axis that occur during the latent phase are prerequisites for entering active phase dilation.

Measurement of the duration of the latent phase requires knowledge of the time of onset of labor, which cannot always be determined with certainty. It is reasonable to use the time at which the patient began to perceive regular uterine contractions as an approximation. The latent phase tends to be shorter in multiparas than in nulliparas, a consequence, at

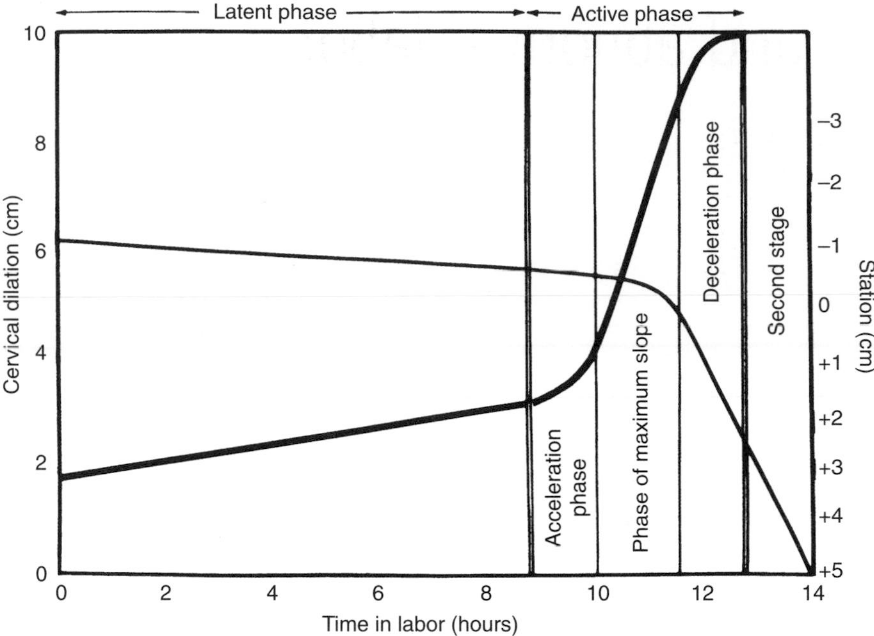

Figure 60.1 Composite of normal cervical dilation and fetal descent curves showing their interrelations and components. From Cohen WR, Friedman EA, eds. *Management of labor*. Rockville, MD: Aspen Publishers, 1983.

least in part, of the fact that multiparas tend to begin labor with more cervical dilation. For the same reason, the latent phase is often shorter in multiple gestations, hydramnios, or after removal of a cervical cerclage.

During the latent phase, the cervix dilates slowly (maximally 0.5 cm/h) or not at all. The shift to active phase often occurs at approximately 5 cm of cervical dilation,[11] but it can be misleading to identify this transition by the absolute degree of dilation. For example, the conversion from latent to active phase may occur at 3 cm of dilation, especially for patients who began labor with the cervix closed. The transition to active phase may not occur until about 6 or 7 cm of dilation in multiparas who began labor with the cervix dilated 4 or 5 cm.

Active phase

Except for the usually brief acceleration and deceleration periods, cervical dilation during the active phase is linear and much more rapid than in the latent phase. To determine normality, clinical assessment of labor requires measuring the speed at which the cervix dilates during the active phase. When two observations of cervical dilation have been made during this period of linear change, the slope of the dilation line can be calculated. Once established, this rate tends to be constant for each individual (i.e., if the labor is normal, dilation continues at the same rate until the deceleration phase is reached). Abnormalities of active phase are defined by deviations from this projected rate of dilation. These deviations can be readily identified if serial observations of cervical dilation and fetal station are plotted on square-ruled graph paper. Observation and calculation of slopes are relatively simple.[1] Paradigms exist in order to use the graphic system without the need for calculations;[4–6] some electronic medical records automate these calculations.

Full cervical dilation occurs when the cervix retracts to the widest diameter of the presenting part. Usually the cervix retracts symmetrically but sometimes a segment lingers, particularly anteriorly, in the presence of deflexed attitudes of the head. Full dilation should not be diagnosed until the entire cervix has retracted spontaneously to or beyond the widest diameter of the leading part of the fetus.

As indicated previously, during the phase of maximum slope of dilation, descent of the fetus normally begins; during the terminal period of dilation, descent of the fetus tends to accelerate as the widely dilated cervix retracts around the presenting part.

Normal fetal descent

As the cervix dilates in late active phase, resistance to fetal descent decreases and the force of uterine contractions, coupled after complete dilation with active maternal bearing-down efforts, begins the expulsion of the fetus. By the time of complete cervical dilation, descent has usually become linear and, during the second stage, normally proceeds in this way until the presenting part encounters the pelvic floor. The efficiency and normality of the descent mechanism can be judged from the rate of descent. If the relationship between fetal descent and elapsed time in labor is plotted graphically, it is apparent that descent also has a latent phase during which little in the way of descent occurs under most circumstances (Fig. 60.1). The degree of descent that has occurred before the onset of labor has prognostic importance for the probability of vaginal delivery. In fact, an unengaged head at the onset of labor is associated with a considerably increased risk for Cesarean delivery.[12]

Considerable descent may sometimes occur during the latent phase. Multiparas often commence labor with the presenting part at a relatively high station, and appreciable descent takes place in the latent phase. Of utmost importance in this regard is that lack of fetal descent before active phase labor is not evidence of a labor aberration or of fetopelvic disproportion.

Uterine activity in labor

Initially, contractions are often mild and somewhat irregular; they become progressively more intense, frequent, and regular as the latent phase progresses. However, this is not always the case and a broad range of contraction patterns may be observed in the normal latent phase, including very intense and frequent contractions. It is usually impossible to identify the transition from latent phase to active phase labor solely on the basis of uterine activity.

During the active phase, contractions are generally more frequent and of greater amplitude and duration than in the latent phase. However, a large spectrum of contractile patterns exists during normal labor[13] and there is no reliable or predictive means to identify dysfunctional dilation or descent by observing uterine activity. Consequently, the clinical identification of dysfunctional labor should be based primarily on aberrations in the graphic patterns of labor. This approach allows a continuous assessment of and provides an unequivocal language for communicating labor progress.[14]

Abnormal labor

Latent phase dysfunction

A prolonged latent phase (Figs 60.2 and 60.3; Table 60.1) is diagnosed when the latent phase exceeds 20 h in nulliparas or 14 h in multiparas.[3,10,15] It is most likely to occur when labor begins with the cervix minimally effaced and dilated. The latent phase is particularly susceptible to the inhibitory effects of narcotics and anesthetics, which may predispose to prolongation of this period of labor.

The diagnosis of a prolonged latent phase may lack precision because of the difficulty in ascertaining the exact time of labor onset. It is important to recognize that the latent phase may normally be quite long. A prolonged latent phase is not a predictor of active phase disorders, nor does it have a strong association with cephalopelvic disproportion. It may sometimes occur as a result of a contractile abnormality that could become apparent later. Ignorance about the normal course of the latent phase may lead to unnecessary Cesarean section under the erroneous assumption that continuous progress should be expected in all phases of labor or that very long labors are always abnormal.

Treatment of prolonged latent phase consists of maternal sedation or active efforts to stimulate uterine contractility (Fig. 60.3). Stimulation with oxytocin effectively converts a prolonged latent phase to an active phase in 85% of cases and this response generally occurs within 3 h. A similar proportion of patients respond favorably to narcotic sedation ("therapeutic rest"). After a dose of morphine sulfate, the patient

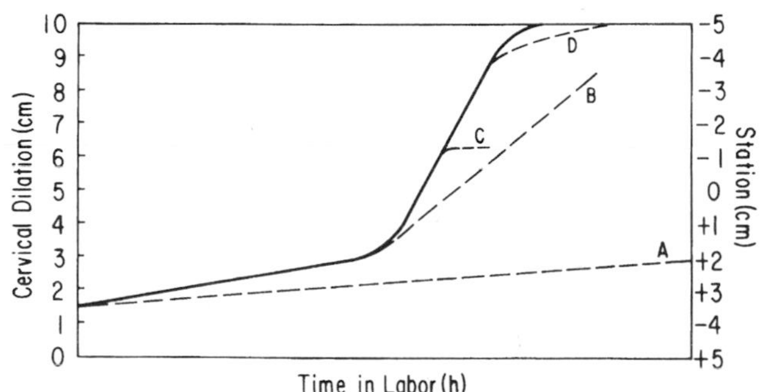

Figure 60.2 Schematic showing various disorders of dilation (broken lines) compared to a normal pattern of dilation (solid line). (A) prolonged latent phase; (B) protracted active phase; (C) arrest of dilation; (D) prolonged deceleration phase.

Table 60.1 Dysfunctional labor patterns.

Dysfunction	Nulliparas	Multiparas
Disorders of dilation		
Prolonged latent phase	> 20 h duration	> 14 h duration
Protracted active phase	Dilation at < 1.2 cm/h	Dilation at < 1.5 cm/h
Arrest of dilation	2 h without progress in active phase	2 h without progress in active phase
Prolonged deceleration phase	> 3 h duration	> 1 h duration
Disorders of descent		
Protracted descent	Descent at < 1 cm/h	Descent at < 2 cm/h
Arrest of descent	1 h without progress after active descent has begun	1 h without progress after active descent has begun
Failure of descent	No descent by deceleration phase or second stage onset	No descent by deceleration phase or second stage onset

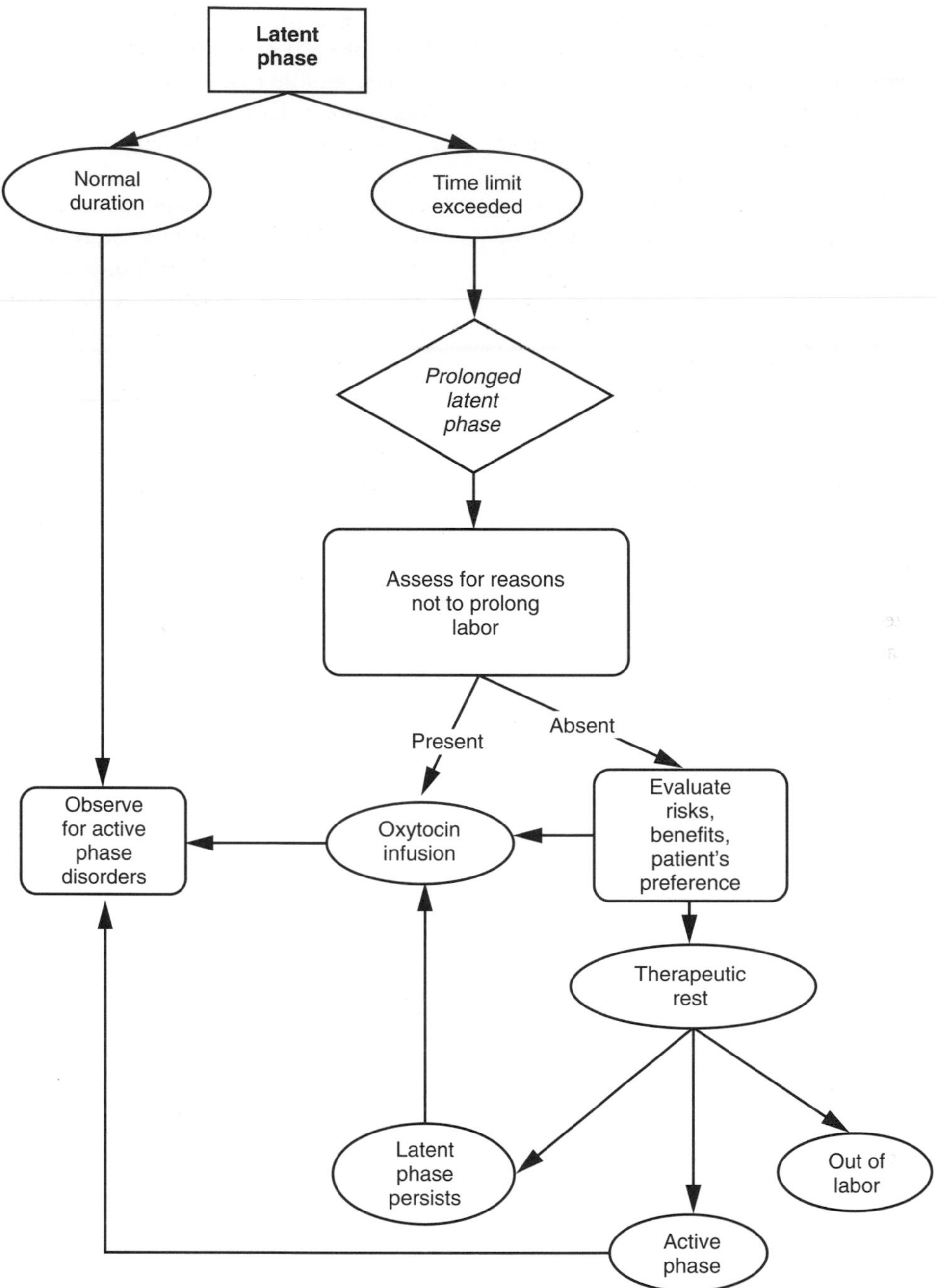

Figure 60.3 Paradigm for management of prolonged latent phase, diagnosed when the latent phase exceeds 20 h in a nullipara and 14 h in a multipara. Oxytocin stimulation and narcotic sedation are equally effective. Choice depends on the patient's preference and the presence of risks that would accrue if the labor were prolonged.

often sleeps for several hours and awakens in active phase labor. Having had a respite from many hours of painful contractions, she may be more eager and better prepared to cope with the physical and emotional demands of the active phase. Approximately 10% of women persist in a desultory latent phase after the effects of the narcotic have abated; in these cases oxytocin stimulation is still necessary. Another advantage of therapeutic rest is that it allows the identification of the approximately 5% of women diagnosed with prolonged latent phase who are in false labor;[3,15] their contractions abate completely after narcotic treatment.

The choice between uterine stimulation and therapeutic rest depends on the clinical situation. There are concerns that fetal deoxygenation may occur after treatment with some narcotic drugs;[16,17] however, no adverse outcomes have been reported after treatment of prolonged latent phase with narcotics, and the approach does not seem to be associated with an increased rate of neonatal depression. Active intervention with oxytocin should be used whenever a fetal or maternal condition exists that could be jeopardized by prolonging the labor, unless there is a clear contraindication to its administration. Similarly, when there is a reason to minimize the duration of labor, it is reasonable to intervene during the latent phase, even before the normal endpoint. The presence of prolonged rupture of membranes, preeclampsia, early intrauterine infection, or certain acute maternal illnesses favors an approach of active stimulation of labor. Finally, the mother's wishes should be taken into consideration; some women prefer oxytocin stimulation, whereas others prefer the interposition of some rest into the arduous and stressful experience of birth.

Active phase dysfunction

Two abnormalities of active phase dilation have been identified (Figs 60.2, 60.4, and 60.5; Table 60.1). A protracted active phase is diagnosed when cervical dilation progresses linearly after commencement of the active phase but at a rate below the established limits of normal.[18] Arrest of dilation occurs when cervical dilation ceases for 2 h during the active phase[19] (although this is the standard definition, there is evidence that even an hour of well documented arrest may be of clinical importance and should prompt evaluation[20]). The term prolonged deceleration phase may be used to describe protracted or arrested labor during the terminal period of cervical dilation.[3] The time limits for the duration of the deceleration phase are 3 h in nulliparas and 1 h in multiparas. The obstetric conditions associated with protraction and arrest disorders are similar, but the therapeutic approaches differ (Figs 60.3 and 60.4). All active phase disorders commonly occur in association with cephalopelvic disproportion, malpositions (especially persistent occiput posterior or transverse), excessive sedation or anesthesia, chorioamnionitis, or deciduitis. Myometrial dysfunction, which may be primary or a consequence of the preceding factors, also contributes.

In the evaluation of any active phase dysfunction, a thorough examination of the patient is necessary to identify any associated or predisposing conditions. Clinical cephalopelvimetry is useful in ascertaining the likelihood of disproportion. An experienced clinician can accurately evaluate the dynamic as well as the static aspects of fetopelvic fit. In addition to determining the architectural characteristics of the pelvis, this examination should confirm the fetal position and attitude, along with the degree of cranial bone molding and caput succedaneum formation. Use of the Müller–Hillis maneuver (vaginal examination during the peak of a contraction, in advanced cervical dilation, with gentle fundal pressure applied) provides a useful assessment of the degree of descent, rotational tendencies, and attitudinal changes that are likely to occur with subsequent contractions.[21] If disproportion seems unlikely and fetal head position is normal, it is necessary to carry out an assessment of uterine contractility and search for infection and possible pharmacological inhibition of labor. The risk of dysfunctional active phase labor may be increased in older mothers[22] but diagnosis and therapy should not be influenced by maternal age.

Available evidence suggests that when protraction disorders arise *de novo*, they are not amenable to correction by stimulating uterine contractions.[3] If, however, the protraction disorder has resulted from some inhibitory influence, oxytocin may prove beneficial. For example, if the protraction disorder was provoked by conduction anesthesia or by other drugs that have the potential to inhibit contractility, oxytocin infusion may override these inhibitory influences and restore normal dilation. By contrast, a protraction disorder that has arisen in the absence of these inhibitory factors probably would not benefit from uterine stimulation, irrespective of the degree of contractility present.

Protraction disorders are sensitive to many inhibitory factors and may be exacerbated or even converted to arrest disorders under some circumstances, for example after an excessively large dose of analgesia or conduction anesthesia. Deliberate rupture of the fetal membranes (amniotomy) as a treatment for protraction disorders has not been proven to be beneficial, and it may sometimes worsen the situation by precipitating an arrest of dilation.[3,23]

Arrest of dilation may evolve during a protracted or a previously normal active phase. This dysfunction requires the same kind of evaluation as for protraction disorders, with the understanding that an arrest of labor is more commonly associated (at least 40%) with cephalopelvic disproportion.[3,19] Therapy also differs because arrest disorders may respond to oxytocin augmentation of uterine activity. In the presence of an arrest, cephalopelvic relationships must be evaluated carefully and a judgment made about the probability of disproportion. If the evidence for fetopelvic disproportion is considerable, especially if uterine activity is normal, it may be appropriate to deliver by Cesarean section. If the pelvis is deemed probably adequate, stimulation of uterine activity with close maternal and fetal surveillance is reasonable.

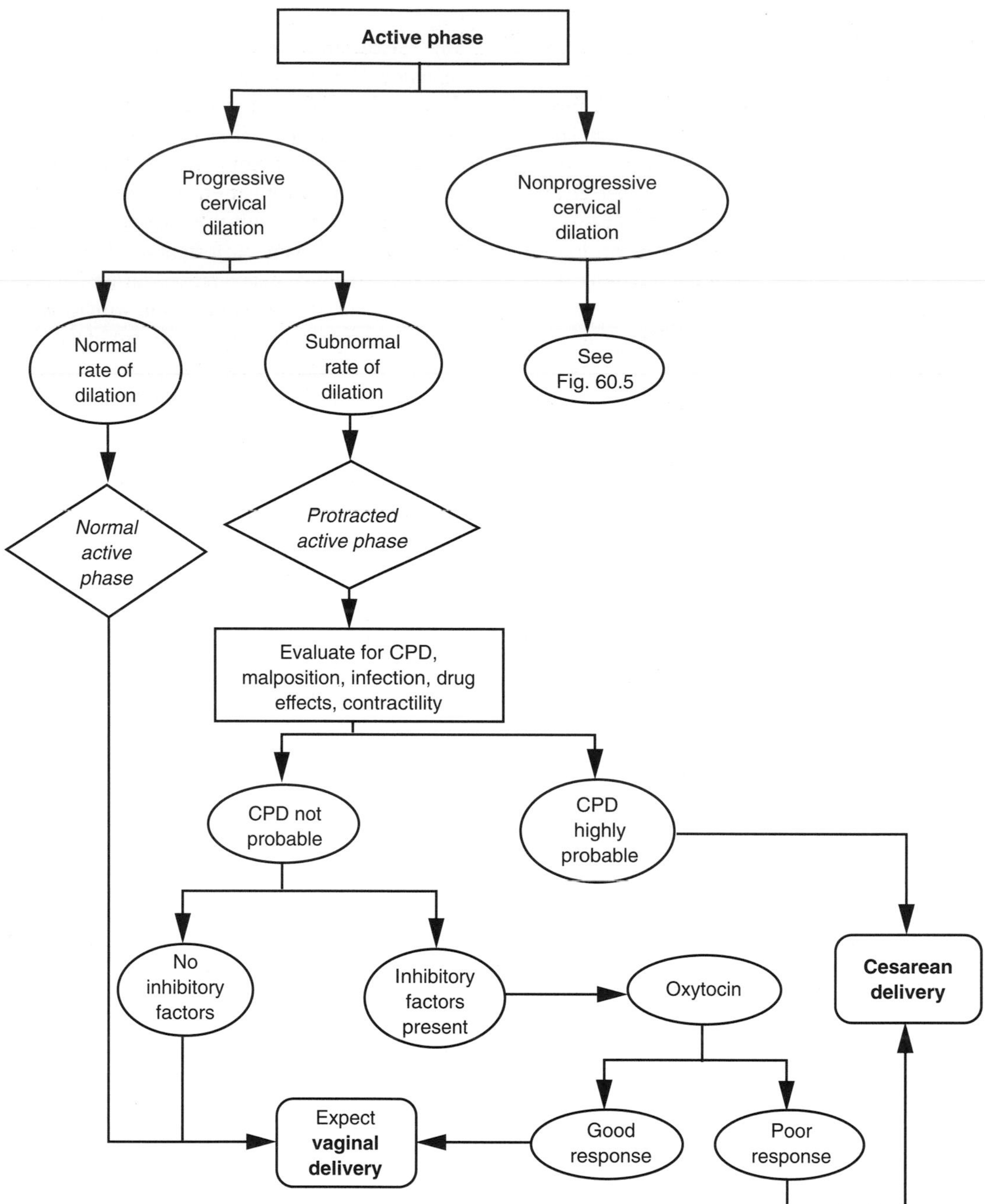

Figure 60.4 Paradigm for management of protracted active phase, diagnosed when dilation is progressive but occurs at < 1.2 cm/h in nulliparas and < 1.5 cm/h in multiparas. A good response to oxytocin is defined as one in which dilation is maintained at the same or improved rate. Oxytocin is useful in this disorder when the slow progress is related to the presence of factors that may inhibit contractility (e.g., infection, drug effects). CPD, cephalopelvic disproportion.

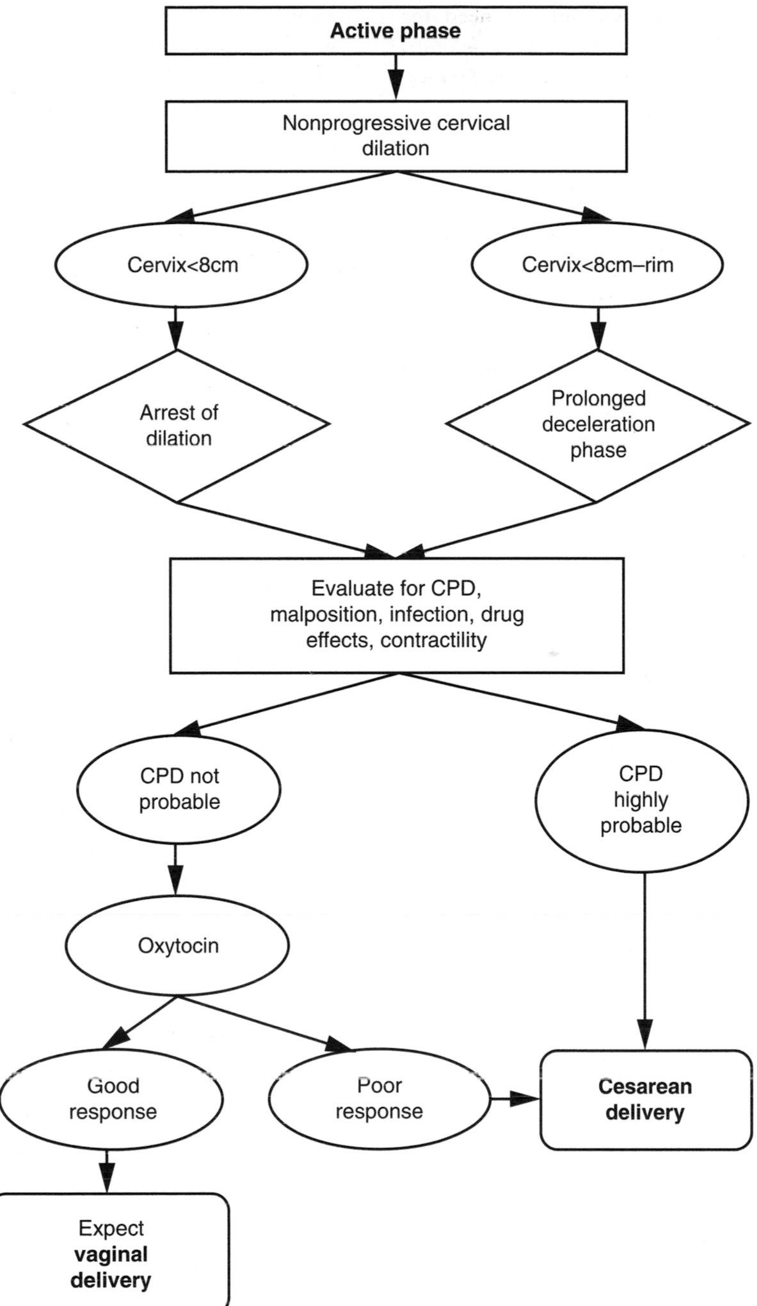

Figure 60.5 Paradigm for management of arrest of dilation, defined as an absence of progress in dilation for 2 h once the active phase has begun. When progress is abnormally slow or ceases at the end of the active phase, prolonged deceleration phase is diagnosed (> 3 h in nulliparas; > 1 h in multiparas). There is a strong association with cephalopelvic disproportion (CPD). A good response to oxytocin is defined as a postarrest slope that is equal to or greater than the prearrest slope. A poor response usually requires Cesarean delivery.

Sometimes arrest disorders resolve without the need for oxytocin or operative intervention. This may occur spontaneously or as the result of an abatement of inhibitory factors. The use of maternal ambulation, warm baths, anxiolytic drugs, or psychoprophylactic techniques has advocates, but the efficacy of these techniques has not been proven.

There are three possible outcomes of oxytocin infusion for an arrest disorder: absence of any further change in dilation or descent, progress that is as good as or better than that before the arrest, or progress at a rate that is lower than the prearrest rate. About 85% of the patients who respond to oxytocin do so within 3 h of treatment.[3,24] If there has been no return to the prearrest slope after this interval, delivery by Cesarean section is usually necessary.

If oxytocin results in cervical dilation that is at least as rapid as before the arrest, the likelihood of eventual vaginal delivery is high. If dilation resumes at a rate slower than before the arrest, it is likely that disproportion or an insurmountable problem with uterine contractility is present. The use of an intrauterine pressure catheter is often desirable to document the change in uterine activity in response to oxytocin and to warn when excessive stimulation is occurring. The goal of any treatment must be individualized but, in general, firm contractions (approximately 50 mmHg at peak intensity) that occur every 2–3 min indicate sufficient contractility. Quantitative measures of contractility, such as Montevideo units, are thought by some to be helpful in guiding oxytocin therapy, but the relationship between these assessments of contractility and the likelihood of a change in cervical dilation or fetal descent is not reliably predictable. Whatever approach to the assessment of contractility is used, it is important to remember that the use of oxytocin may increase the likelihood of fetal hypoxemia. Therefore, continuous fetal heart rate monitoring and close observation of uterine contractility are required when uterotonic drugs are used. It also appears that dysfunctional labor may precipitate abnormal fetal heart rate patterns.[25]

The potential benefit of artificial rupture of membranes in labor is controversial. Although rupture of membranes can induce labor in many individuals, its influence on labor that is already established is less certain. Some studies have shown a modest shortening of active phase labor in response to rupture of membranes.[23,26] Although amniotomy may increase uterine work,[27] a beneficial effect on dysfunctional labor has not been proven. Many clinicians believe that rupture of the membranes is effective in terminating arrest disorders but objective data have failed to verify this.[28] It is, nevertheless, reasonable to rupture membranes when an arrest disorder has been identified. The few patients who respond do so promptly; it is therefore generally inappropriate to wait longer than approximately 60 min to determine whether rupture of membranes has been successful in altering the pattern of labor progress.

When conduction anesthesia is employed, it should generally begin during the active phase of dilation. To have a minimal effect on labor progress and provide pain relief when most required, an epidural anesthetic should be given during the acceleration phase of labor. When it is properly administered, it has little or no inhibitory effect on the progress of normal cervical dilation or fetal descent. Anesthesia is more likely to slow labor progress if administered during the latent phase or in the presence of a protraction or arrest disorder. This does not mean that conduction anesthesia is contraindicated in such circumstances; it may be beneficial for pain relief but it should also be recognized that it might prolong the latent phase or create an active phase abnormality requiring the administration of oxytocin.

Although there is evidence that the use of epidural analgesia is associated with an enhanced likelihood of Cesarean section, this has not been a universal finding.[29,30] Epidural anesthetics do have the potential to prolong labor or even to induce abnormalities in dilation or descent but these effects depend to a large extent on the anesthetic technique. The type of drug used, the dose given, and the time and method of administration all determine the influence on labor. Furthermore, the outcome is determined largely by the clinical attitude of the obstetrician. For example, if the physician believes that the second stage of labor must always be terminated after 2 h, operative delivery would be more common in patients whose second stage is prolonged by epidural analgesia. However, a physician who understands that such prolongations are usually innocuous would not feel compelled to intervene. Therefore, epidural analgesia administered with a proper regard for the clinical situation will generally have no significant adverse impact on labor progress or mode of delivery.

The second stage of labor

The first stage of labor, which extends from the onset of labor to complete cervical dilation, serves to ready the parturient for expulsion of the fetus from the uterus. Having been prepared by the physical and biochemical changes that result in cervical ripening, uterine contractions produce rapid cervical dilation. The cervix retracts around the presenting part in order to dilate maximally and descent begins. Thus, during the second stage of labor (from complete dilation to delivery), the focus of interest changes from cervical dilation to descent of the fetus. The process of fetal expulsion is evaluated from the characteristics of the descent curve. The rate at which active descent occurs is influenced by several factors including: uterine contractile force; voluntary maternal expulsive efforts; fetal size, position, and attitude; deformability of the fetal head; pelvic architecture; and the characteristics of the pelvic floor.

Three descent disorders have been identified: protracted descent, arrest of descent, and failure of descent[3,7,31,32] (Fig. 60.7; Table 60.1). All are associated with similar obstetric conditions and are, in many respects, analogous to the protraction and arrest disorders of dilation. Ascertainment of the

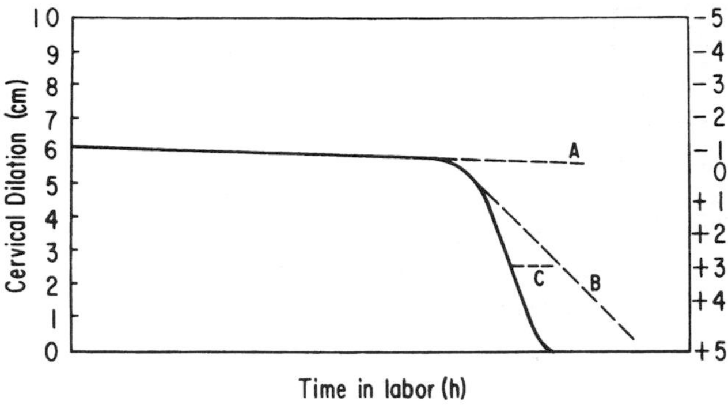

Figure 60.6 Schematic showing possible disorders of descent. (A) failure of descent; (B) protracted descent; (C) arrest of descent.

significance of descent abnormalities requires considerable clinical insight and experience because assessment must include determination of fetal position and attitude, molding, and the evolving mechanism of labor in relation to the patient's pelvic form. Identification of the station of the presenting part may be difficult if considerable scalp edema or molding of the head is present. Suprapubic palpation of the head, as well as vaginal examination, may be necessary to determine whether true descent of the head has occurred as opposed to molding with advancement to the leading edge but no descent of the biparietal diameter.

Thorough cephalopelvimetry and an evaluation for other associated obstetric problems are both necessary when descent disorders are diagnosed. Analogous to disorders of active phase dilation, the best evidence suggests that oxytocin stimulation of uterine activity is generally not beneficial in the presence of protracted descent, but an arrest or failure of descent may respond.

Cephalopelvimetry

Clinically astute obstetricians and midwives take pride in their knowledge of pelvic architecture and its influence on labor. Although radiographic pelvimetry is now used infrequently, accurate clinical pelvimetry is still required to make proper judgments about labor.

The knowledge of pelvic architecture and its relationship to labor should be used as a complementary technique to the analysis of labor curves. This approach makes it possible to explain the observed mechanism of labor, to judge the effects of labor on the fetal skull, and helps to make a reasonable and informed judgment concerning the advisability of uterine stimulation or operative intervention.

The value of an interpretation of cephalopelvic relationships and an evaluation of the labor curves cannot be overestimated as a means of providing a safe outcome of dysfunctional labor. For an optimal assessment of labor, both cephalopelvic relationships and labor curves must be considered together rather than individually. For example, a narrowed midpelvis with a molded head impinging on the inlet in the presence of a failure of descent makes the probability of safe vaginal delivery remote. Similarly, an arrest of descent with a posterior position in a midpelvis with prominent ischial spines (making internal rotation difficult) and a forward lower sacrum (resisting further descent without rotation) also suggests an insurmountable problem. The use of oxytocin would not be recommended in either case. If these disorders of labor occurred in the presence of a more favorable pelvic structure, spontaneous delivery would be more likely and uterine stimulation safer.

Duration

The question of whether the length of the second stage should be a consideration in the timing of delivery has been a persistent theme in obstetrics. Although some data appear to show a direct relationship between duration and morbidity, several lines of evidence suggest that it is not appropriate to terminate labor merely because an arbitrary period of time has passed in the second stage, as long as the labor progress and fetal heart rate patterns are normal.[33–35] This does not imply that long second stages are always innocuous; they are more commonly associated with dysfunctional descent patterns that often require prompt evaluation and treatment. Decisions about management in the second stage must be based on a careful evaluation of the maternal and fetal condition and of the progress of descent.

The possible influence of epidural analgesia on the progress of descent during the second stage is of particular importance. Epidural anesthetics can potentially delay descent in three ways: by inhibiting perineal sensation and the mother's reflexive urge to bear down; by reducing uterine contractility; or by compromising motor function and reducing the effectiveness of the mother's voluntary pushing efforts. Any potential delay of descent will depend on several factors including the dose and nature of the anesthetic agent and the mode of administration. When the minimum effective dose of epidural anesthetic is used (with an appropriate consideration of the clinical situation), few significant inhibitory effects on labor should be anticipated except for a modest lengthening of the second stage in some cases. As long as fetal oxygenation remains adequate, there is no danger in allowing such prolongation.

Concerns about the long-term health of the pelvic floor have also led some obstetricians to minimize second stage duration. There is conflicting evidence as to whether there is a relationship between the length of the second stage and the likelihood of pelvic floor problems later in life.[36,37] Alternatives to a long second stage instrumental vaginal delivery (or Cesarean section) confer other risks to the mother and fetus, and the optimal approach to prevent the development of pelvic floor problems later in life is yet unclear.

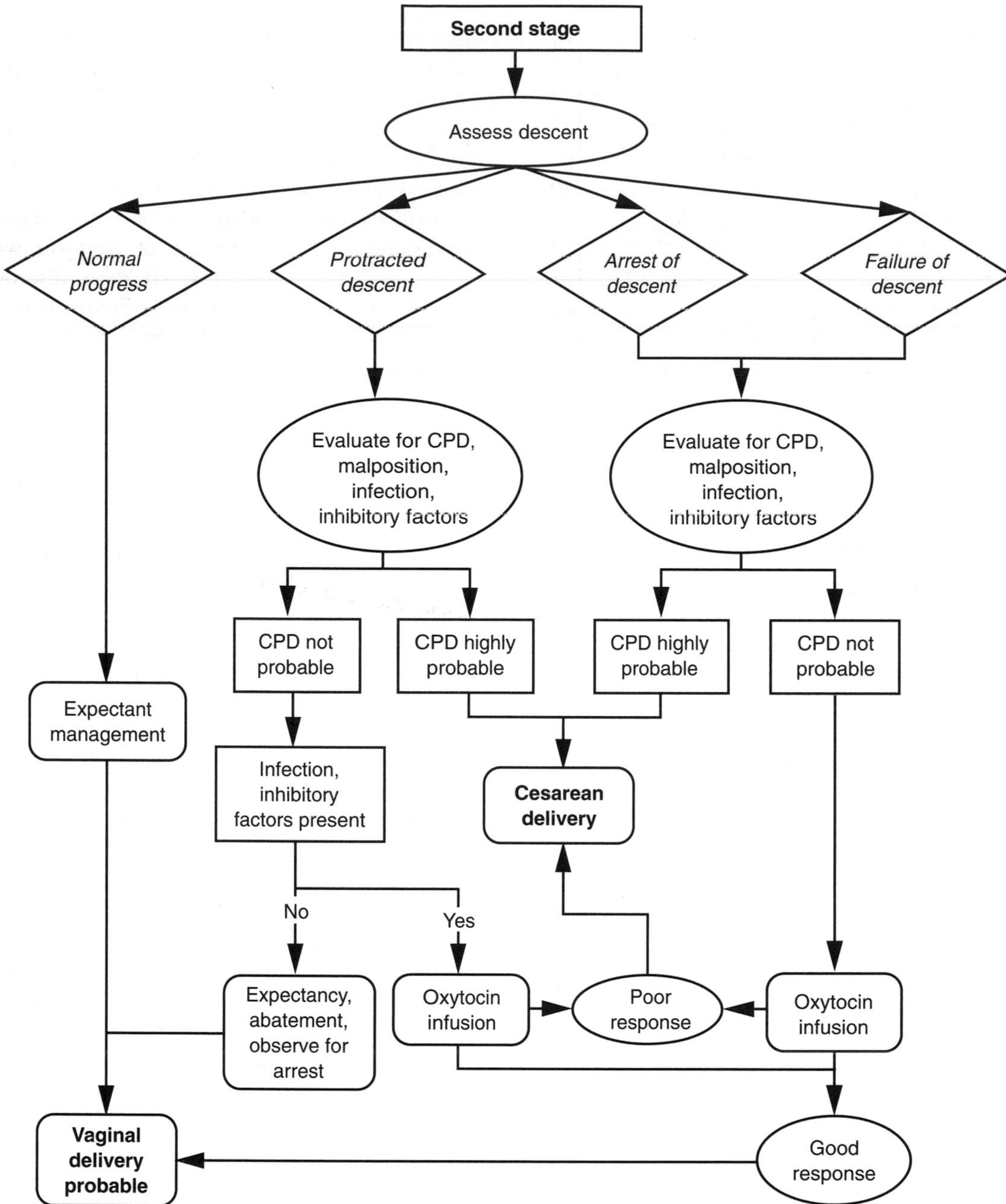

Figure 60.7 Paradigm for management of the second stage. Progress is assessed by the rate of descent rather than elapsed time. Fetal position, station, attitude, and molding should be determined at each examination. A good response to oxytocin given for arrest of descent is defined as a postarrest slope equal to or greater than the prearrest slope. CPD, cephalopelvic disproportion.

Conclusions

The disciplined approach to the management of labor advocated in this chapter emphasizes the need to use objective clinical information to optimize decision-making.[38] It is evident, nevertheless, that the process of assisting women with childbirth requires the practitioner to integrate such objective data with the spectrum of psychosocial features unique to each individual's labor. A woman's attitudes and expectations concerning pregnancy are conditioned by her social and cultural background and by her experiences during gestation. Consequently, no universal formula exists for the provision of emotional support; rather, the practitioner must respond to the patient's needs, encouraging her to express her questions, fears, or concerns and discussing them in an honest and reassuring way.

The obstetrician cannot guarantee a good outcome for every childbirth but, through the application of the principles expressed in this chapter, can promise to seek the best outcome possible for the mother and fetus in the safest possible way. This should occur in the context of a birth experience that is emotionally enriching for the parturient and her family and that treats the laboring mother with the requisite gentleness, dignity, and compassion demanded by the process of giving birth.

Key points

1 A graphic analysis of dilation and descent is required to determine whether or not labor progress is normal.

2 Intrapartum decision-making is a process of continuously reassessing the probability of safe vaginal delivery.

3 Factors involved in estimating the feasibility of safe delivery include: the pattern of dilation and descent; uterine contractility; fetal size, position, and attitude; and the state of fetal oxygenation.

4 The first stage of labor includes the latent phase and the active phase.

5 The latent phase extends from labor onset to the beginning of the active phase, which is marked by an increase in the rate of cervical dilation.

6 The active phase ends with complete cervical dilation. This signals the start of the second stage of labor, which ends with delivery of the fetus.

7 In a normal labor, dilation will be linear through most of the active phase.

8 A prolonged latent phase is one that is longer than 20 h in a nullipara or 14 h in a multipara.

9 A prolonged latent phase is treated by stimulation with oxytocin or by maternal sedation.

10 A protracted active phase is one in which dilation is progressive and linear, but at a rate below normal.

11 A protracted descent is one in which active descent is progressive and linear, but at a rate below normal.

12 Protraction disorders do not respond to oxytocin except when they have been caused by some inhibitory factor such as anesthesia or infection.

13 A prolonged deceleration phase is one that is longer than 3 h in nulliparas and 1 h in multiparas.

14 Cephalopelvic disproportion, second stage disorders, and shoulder dystocia should be considered in cases of prolonged deceleration.

15 A failure of descent occurs when no descent is observed from early labor to the onset of the deceleration phase or the second stage. It is the labor disorder that has the strongest association with cephalopelvic disproportion.

16 The normality of dilation and descent cannot be ascertained from the pattern of uterine contractility.

17 All protraction and arrest disorders may be associated with cephalopelvic disproportion, malposition, intrauterine infection, excess analgesia or anesthesia, or deficient uterine contractility.

18 Most patients with arrest disorders who respond to oxytocin will do so within 3 h of treatment.

19 Artificial rupture of membranes can induce labor; however, it is not certain whether it can reliably enhance an established labor dysfunction.

20 Properly administered epidural anesthesia should have little effect on the course of labor except for some lengthening of the second stage.

21 It is not appropriate to terminate labor simply because an arbitrary period of time has elapsed in the second stage.

22 Upright or squatting postures may enhance descent in some labors.

References

1 Friedman EA. Graphic analysis of labor. *Am J Obstet Gynecol* 1954;68:1568.
2 Friedman EA. Evolution of graphic analysis of labor. *Am J Obstet Gynecol* 1978;132:824.
3 Friedman EA. *Labor: clinical evaluation and management*, 2nd edn. New York: Appleton-Century-Crofts, 1978.
4 Philpott RH, Castle WM. Cervicographs in the management of labour in primigravidae. II. The action line and treatment of abnormal labour. *J Obstet Gynaecol Br Commonw* 1972;79:599.
5 Drouin P, Nasah BT, Nkounawa F. The value of the partogramme in the management of labor *Obstet Gynecol* 1979;53:741.
6 Kwast BE, Lennox CE, Farley TMM. World Health Organization partograph in management of labour. *Lancet* 1994;343:1399.
7 Cohen WR, Acker DB, Friedman EA. *Management of labor*, 2nd edn. Rockville, MD: Aspen Publishers, 1989.
8 Chazotte C, Madden R, Cohen WR. Labor patterns in women with previous cesareans. *Obstet Gynecol* 1990;75:350.
9 Friedman EA. The functional divisions of labor. *Am J Obstet Gynecol* 1971;109:274.
10 Peisner DB, Rosen MG. Latent phase of labor in normal patients: a reassessment. *Obstet Gynecol* 1985;66:644.
11 Peisner DB, Rosen MG. Transition from latent to active phase labor. *Obstet Gynecol* 1985;68:448.
12 Murphy K, Shah L, Cohen WR. Labor and delivery in nulliparas who present with an unengaged fetal head. *J Perinatol* 1998; 18:122.
13 Shulman H, Romney S. Variability of uterine contractions in normal human parturition. *Obstet Gynecol* 1970;36:215.
14 Schifrin BS, Cohen WR. Labor's dysfunctional lexicon. *Obstet Gynecol* 1989;74:123.
15 Friedman EA, Sachtleben MR. Dysfunctional labor: I. Prolonged latent phase in the nullipara. *Obstet Gynecol* 1961;17:135.
16 Baxi L, Petrie RH, James LS. Human fetal oxygenation (tcPO2), heart rate variability, and uterine activity following maternal administration of meperidine. *J Perinat Med* 1988;16:23.
17 Kopecky EA, Ryan ML, Barrett JFR, et al. Fetal response to maternally administered morphine. *Am J Obstet Gynecol* 2000;183: 424.
18 Friedman EA, Sachtleben MR. Dysfunctional labor: II. Protracted active phase dilatation in the nullipara. *Obstet Gynecol* 1961; 17:566.
19 Friedman EA, Sachtleben MR. Dysfunctional labor: III. Secondary arrest of dilatation in the nullipara. *Obstet Gynecol* 1962;19:576.
20 Bottoms SF, Sokol RJ, Rosen MG. Short arrest of cervical dilatation: a risk for maternal/fetal/infant morbidity. *Am J Obstet Gynecol* 1981;140:108.
21 Hillis DS. Diagnosis of contracted pelvis. *Illinois Med J* 1938; 74:131.
22 Cohen WR, Newman L, Friedman EA. Frequency of labor disorders with advancing maternal age. *Obstet Gynecol* 1980;55: 414.
23 Laros RK, Work BA, Witting WC. Amniotomy during the active phase of labor. *Obstet Gynecol* 1972;39:702.
24 Rouse DJ, Owen J, Hauth JC. Active-phase labor arrest: oxytocin augmentation for at least 4 hours. *Obstet Gynecol* 1999;93:323.
25 Porreco RP, Boehm FH, Dildy GA, et al. Dystocia in nulliparous patients monitored with fetal pulse oximetry. *Am J Obstet Gynecol* 2004;190:113.
26 Stuart P, Kennedy JH, Calder AA. Spontaneous labour: when should the membranes be ruptured? *Br J Obstet Gynaecol* 1982:89:39.
27 Van Praagh I, Hendricks CH. The effect of amniotomy during labor in multiparas. *Obstet Gynecol* 1964;24:258.
28 Friedman EA, Sachtleben MR. Amniotomy and the course of labor. *Obstet Gynecol* 1963;22:755.
29 Impey L, MacQuillan K, Robson M. Epidural analgesia need not increase operative delivery rates. *Am J Obstet Gynecol* 2000; 182:358.
30 Halpern SH, Leighton BL, Ohlsson A, et al. Effect of epidural vs parenteral opoid analgesia on the progress of labor. *JAMA* 1998;280:2105.
31 Friedman EA, Sachtleben MR. Station of the fetal presenting part: V. Protracted descent patterns. *Obstet Gynecol* 1970;36: 558.
32 Friedman EA, Sachtleben MR. Station of the fetal presenting part: VI. Arrest of descent in nulliparas. *Obstet Gynecol* 1976;47: 129.
33 Cohen WR. Influence of the duration of second stage labor on perinatal outcome and puerperal morbidity. *Obstet Gynecol* 1977;49:266.
34 Cohen WR, Mahon T, Chazotte C. *The very long second stage of labor*. Proceedings of the Third World Congress on labor and delivery. New York: Parthenon Publishing; 1998:348.
35 Menticoglou SM, Manning F, Harman C, et al. Perinatal outcome in relation to second-stage duration. *Am J Obstet Gynecol* 1995;173:906.
36 Van Kessel K, Reed S, Newton K, et al. The second stage of labor and stress urinary incontinence. *Am J Obstet Gynecol* 2001; 184:1571.
37 Cohen WR, Romero R. Childbirth and the pelvic floor. In: Kurjak A, Chervenak F, eds. *Textbook of perinatal medicine*, 2nd edn. London, UK: Taylor & Francis, 2006.
38 Garrett K, Butler A, Cohen WR. Cesarean delivery in the second stage: characteristics and diagnostic accuracy. *J Maternal–Fetal Neonat Med* 2005;17:49.

61 Operative vaginal delivery

Edward R. Yeomans

Operative vaginal delivery (OVD) is an endangered species. In the animal kingdom, the label of "endangered species" implies that, unless special measures are adopted, extinction may result. Metaphorically, OVD may become extinct if current statistical trends continue unabated. Proper training in OVD techniques during residency is necessary but not sufficient. Those techniques, once learned, must be practiced to maintain this vitally important skill. The purpose of this chapter is to present the current status of both forceps delivery and vacuum extraction as options intermediate between spontaneous vaginal and Cesarean delivery. Recommendations regarding how to interdict the progression toward extinction of OVD will be made at the close of the chapter, but a return to the "halcyon days" (of even a decade ago) is unlikely.

History

It is instructive, in view of the above-stated purpose of examining the current status of OVD, to briefly review the past. The use of forceps dates back some 400+ years, whereas the use of the vacuum extractor (VE) began only in the 1950s (although James Young Simpson, after whom Simpson forceps are named, experimented with a VE device in the mid-1800s). A glance at the crude design (Fig. 61.1) of the original Chamberlen forceps can give the modern practitioner some perspective on the improvements introduced over four centuries. During the 1700s, Levret and Smellie contributed the pelvic curve, and Tarnier elucidated the principle of axis traction in the 1800s. Kielland, Barton, and Piper designed and "field tested" their special instruments in the 1900s. More subtle design changes such as the pseudofenestrated blades developed by Luikart[1] and the divergent forceps proposed and used by Laufe also occurred in the last century. In the mid-1950s, Malmstrom invented a practical VE device, which included rigid steel cups of various sizes. In 1973, Kobayashi introduced a soft-cup product made of silicone rubber. Subtle refinements in cup design and construction as well as vacuum-generating equipment took place over the next three decades. Importantly, the commercialization and marketing of VE devices vastly exceeded anything that ever characterized the development of a new forceps. It is interesting to consider whether business interests affected the reversal of the ratio of forceps to vacuum operations between 1980 and 2000, or whether this was based solely on scientific or clinical grounds. In 1980, the rates of forceps to VE procedures in the United States was 18 to 1.[2] By 1990, it was 3 to 2 and, in 2000, it was 1 to 2, and will likely swing further to the VE side. In 1952, more than half of all the babies in the United States were delivered by forceps. By 2002, that proportion had fallen to 2.3%! In fact, even combining forceps and VE accounted for only 5.9% of all deliveries in 2002,[3] and it is this datum that prompted the "endangered species" analogy. The steady, even precipitous, decline in OVD paralleled an unprecedented increase in Cesarean deliveries worldwide, but especially in the United States. However, it is naïve to attribute the former to the latter without examining the problem more closely.

In the first half of the twentieth century, Cesarean delivery was dangerous for mothers. Refinements in blood banking, anesthesia, antibiotic availability, and hospital-based childbirth all made possible a 1950 report[4] of 1000 consecutive Cesarean deliveries without a maternal death. By 1980,[5] that number had grown to 10 000 consecutive Cesareans with no maternal mortality. The focus of care shifted from maternal outcome to perinatal outcome, and difficult instrumental vaginal deliveries came under scrutiny. Even by 1950, Cesarean delivery was an option that only minimally increased maternal risk, but reduced the neonatal risk associated with difficult vaginal delivery. In the 1970s and 1980s, the Cesarean rate escalated by far more than could be accounted for by the small number of difficult vaginal deliveries. The threat of litigation began to influence capable, well-trained practitioners to consider their own risk in addition to those of mother and baby in choosing a route of delivery when it appeared that spontaneous delivery was not an option. Studies conducted in the last 10–15 years called attention to pelvic floor damage with OVD,[6] to risk associated with vaginal breech delivery[7] and vaginal birth after Cesarean section (VBAC),[8] and to infant birth trauma associated with OVD.[9] The contribution of other factors, such as regional anesthesia and the presence

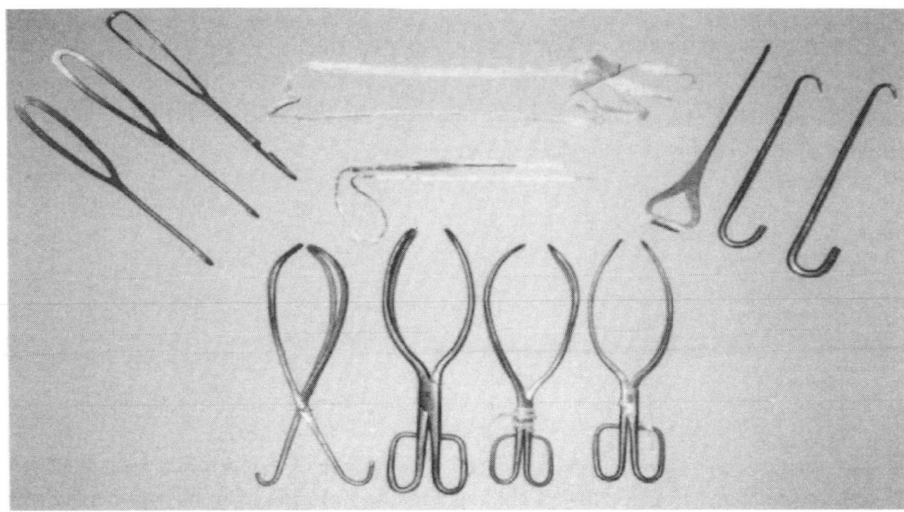

Figure 61.1 Chamberlen forceps.

of family members in the delivery room, to the declining frequency of OVD is difficult to evaluate. Pediatricians and neonatologists focus on only one of the two patients whose interests must be considered in selecting the route of delivery, so they may favor Cesarean delivery to improve the outcome for the neonate. More recently, women themselves have requested elective repeat and even elective primary Cesarean delivery. All of these factors, and more that have not been cited, account for the shrinking percentage of OVD performed in 2005. Are these few procedures sufficient to train residents, and later to maintain proficiency?

Training

The written word (this chapter, for example) can impact on an operator's skill to only a limited degree. In the foreword to his renowned textbook on forceps,[10] Dr Edward Dennen advised that the trainee be given a series of "painstaking lectures" on the subject of forceps delivery, then "drilled extensively" on the manikin. Then the intern is allowed to do an easy case under direct supervision. After that, the volume of work would increase according to the individual's ability and interest. In Dennen's practice lifetime, the "volume of work" was enormous. He reported on over 13 000 forceps deliveries. The problem now is obvious: there is no volume of work. Residents in training perform few procedures. Then, when they graduate, most perform even fewer. The median number of OVD procedures in 1 year reported by candidates preparing to take their oral board examination was five![11]

Some opinion leaders in the field of obstetrics and gynecology[12] have written that elective forceps is no longer considered to be an indication. Others defend the practice, some when conditions for outlet forceps are met, others who sanction elective low forceps as well. This author strongly supports the performance of elective outlet forceps both in residency training and after graduation, to acquire and maintain proficiency, respectively. Support for this procedure is predicated on adherence to the definitions outlined in Table 61.1.

Table 61.1 1988 American College of Obstetricians and Gynecologists' classification of forceps and vacuum.

Outlet forceps
Scalp is visible at introitus without separating labia
Fetal skull has reached pelvic floor
Sagittal suture is in anteroposterior diameter or right or left occiput anterior or posterior position
Fetal head is at or on perineum
Rotation does not exceed 45°
Low forceps
Leading point of fetal skull is at station ≥ +2 cm* and not on the pelvic floor
Rotation of ≤ 45° (left or right occiput anterior to occiput anterior, or left or right occiput posterior to occiput posterior)
Rotation of > 45°
Midforceps
Station above + 2 cm but head engaged
High forceps
Not included in classification

*Station is measured in cm from the ischial spines to the perineum (0 to +5 cm).

It has been said that "experience is not a substitute for training; it serves only to increase confidence, not skill."[13] This is a thought-provoking criticism of an accreditation system that places undue emphasis on numbers of procedures of whatever type rather than the quality of training in that procedure. Admittedly, the latter is harder to evaluate.

A regimental approach to training is advocated by the author, following the recommendation of the senior Dr Dennen: lectures (e.g., those outlined in Table 61.2), manikin practice, followed by graduated degree of difficulty progressing from easy outlet forceps, then to low forceps without rota-

Table 61.2 Sample lecture schedule for operative vaginal delivery (repeat every 2 years).

1 Clinical pelvimetry
2 Basic forceps
3 Advanced forceps
4 Forceps you almost never see
5 Principles of vacuum extraction
6 Maternal and perinatal complications

Table 61.3 Indications for forceps or vacuum delivery.

Fetal indications
Nonreassuring fetal heart rate pattern
Premature separation of placenta
Prolapsed cord

Maternal indications
Protracted second stage
Maternal exhaustion
Certain maternal conditions

tion; from there, to low forceps with 45–90° rotation and, finally, to low forceps with 90–180° rotation and carefully selected midforceps procedures. Augmenting this training approach is instruction in the use of forceps at Cesarean delivery for fetuses in cephalic or breech presentation and the routine use of Piper forceps to the aftercoming head at vaginal breech delivery. Some clinicians believe that experience with both forceps and VE should be provided to residents and, if clinical volume is adequate, such an approach has merit. At the University of Texas-Houston LBJ Hospital residency program, experience with forceps is disproportionately emphasized. This stems from the author's firm belief that a graduate proficient in the use of forceps can readily master the technique of VE with only a few cases, whereas the reverse is not achievable.

Case selection and choice of instrument

These two areas are closely related, and they require a working knowledge of both the art and the science of OVD. Indications and prerequisites are readily tabulated (Tables 61.3 and 61.4), but the art demands more than running through a "pilot's checklist." [14] The course of labor, maternal and fetal status, adequacy of anesthesia, exact diagnosis of the position of the fetal head (including attitude, caput, molding, asynclitism, and station of the presenting part) and, of great importance, the maternal pelvic architecture must all be assessed and integrated to arrive at a decision to attempt OVD. It is highly recommended to document this assessment, especially the clinical pelvimetry, in the maternal medical record prior to embarking on the procedure, if time permits.[15] As part of the

Table 61.4 Prerequisites for forceps application.

Experienced operator in attendance
Engagement of the fetal head
Knowledge of the position of the fetal head
Completely dilated cervix
Clinically adequate pelvis
Adequate anesthesia

OVD training at the author's institution, the position of the fetal head is ascertained at every vaginal examination from 6 cm right up to the time of application of an instrument or, more commonly, just prior to spontaneous delivery of the head. Moreover, clinical pelvimetry is recorded for the majority of laboring women, but especially for those diagnosed with a labor abnormality or candidates for OVD. Dr Dennen referred to this as "constant alertness;" without it, inaccurate assessments are made and the risk of injury to either patient increases.

The art of clinical pelvimetry is vanishing from modern training programs. In all but a small percentage of cases, the inability to deliver spontaneously is followed by immediate resort to Cesarean delivery without considering an attempt at OVD. Pursuing such a course perforce renders clinical pelvimetry meaningless. In his article[16] entitled "Midforceps delivery: a vanishing art" (parenthetically, if it was vanishing in 1963, it is of historical interest only in many programs today), Danforth meticulously describes the characteristics of the four pelvic types of Caldwell and Moloy, not only at the inlet but at all levels traversed by the presenting part. This article is strongly recommended for required reading in a modern OVD training program.

From the foregoing discussion, case selection can be a daunting task, literally requiring years of practice. It would be naïve to think, given the complexity of the case selection process, that a single instrument could be chosen for all clinical problems. In the randomized clinical trials comparing forceps with VE, the student of OVD is led to believe that there are only two choices. However, there are 5–10 commonly used forceps from which to select. Vacuum proponents can select from a number of different cup designs, tailored in some cases to the position of the fetal head. The choice of an instrument for OVD is different for the trainee than for the experienced operator. If the trainee is exposed to one or only a few instruments during residency, he or she is likely to rely on that instrument even when better choices are available. Trainees should be encouraged to make the instrument fit the clinical situation, not vice versa. Table 61.5 contains some elementary guidance with respect to choosing an instrument. Only after residency is it reasonable to allow experience or "comfort" to be a major factor in instrument selection. In addition to Table 61.5, the following clinical case scenario is included to illustrate the combined tasks of case selection and choice of instrument.

Table 61.5 Selection of instrument.

Outlet or low, parous woman, no molding – Tucker–McLane
Outlet or low, nullipara, molding – Simpson, Simpson–Luikart
Low or mid with asynclitism – Luikart
Low with rotation – Kielland, Barton
Aftercoming head – Piper, Laufe, Kielland
Face – Simpson, Kielland

A primigravid woman at 41 weeks' gestation is admitted to labor and delivery with a diagnosis of premature rupture of membranes at term. Oxytocin induction is begun. The active phase of labor is protracted and, after 2 h of the second stage, the fetal head is at +2 station, 60° LOA, with moderate asynclitism. Caput is present over the anterior parietal bone, but molding is insignificant. Clinical pelvimetry confirms a gynecoid pelvis with blunt ischial spines and a hollow sacrum. The estimated fetal weight is 3600 g and fetal heart tones are reassuring. After counseling, the woman states that she would like to avoid a Cesarean delivery if possible (yes, women still do say this). Her pain relief is satisfactory with an effective epidural anesthetic. She is fatigued from 2 h of voluntary expulsive effort that began immediately after complete dilation was diagnosed. Is this case appropriate for OVD? The woman is unlikely to achieve spontaneous delivery secondary to fatigue. She would like to avoid Cesarean section. Factors such as asynclitism and epidural are amenable to operative correction. A VE would be likely to fail because of the difficulty of obtaining proper cup placement and a resulting tendency to pop off. Luikart forceps represent an ideal choice. The pseudofenestrated blades are unlikely to leave forceps marks on the fetal face. The sliding lock permits correction of asynclitism. The overlapping shanks do not distend the perineum the way that parallel shanks would. The bar built into the handle of the left branch prevents undue compression of the fetal head. All these advantages were cited by Luikart in his 1940 article.[17] Interestingly, several major birthing centers in the city of Houston do not even have Luikart forceps in their armamentarium!

It should be obvious that case selection and choice of instrument require sound clinical judgment and broad experience. Even under favorable circumstances, all these intricacies only set the stage for the most critical step: proper execution of the delivery.

Technique – forceps

This section can only serve as a springboard to provide both the resident and the young practitioner with the impetus to read more and practice more in an effort to develop and refine their clinical skills. Procedure-specific textbooks are available to enrich the knowledge of proper technique but, analogous to hitting a golf ball or playing the piano, there is no substitute for practice. A few pointers are suggested to guide the beginner through narrow straits (pun intended) that have been encountered by all who claim to be experienced in OVD. To intrigue the reader with more than a modicum of experience, some of these points are not available in other sources.

As noted in a now superseded ACOG Technical Bulletin on OVD,[18] the ART of forceps is an acronym that stands for application, rotation, and traction. Of these, application is the most important, for inability to apply the forceps effectively sabotages the whole procedure. A decidedly worse circumstance is to place the forceps inaccurately and fail to recognize the error prior to either rotation or traction. Three of the previously referenced "pointers" pertain to application:

1 For a head that is at 60° LOA, as in the example, the posterior, in this case left, blade should be applied first. The fingers of the protecting (right) hand should extend beyond the toe of the blade and should assist in maintaining the cephalic curve of the blade in contact with the contour of the fetal skull. Once the blade has been inserted to the appropriate depth, pressure with the index and middle fingers of the right hand on top of the blade should direct it to a position slightly inferior to the posterior (left) lambdoid suture. This is the easy blade to place! The anterior (right) blade should be held obliquely, not vertically, with the handle in the right hand extending toward the left groin of the woman. The handle should then be lowered in contact with the woman's left thigh as the thumb of the left hand advances the heel of the blade into the pelvis. Almost immediately, the right cephalic prominence of the fetal head will be encountered and this structure (not really a structure but a feature of the fetal frontal bone) will cause difficulty in rotating the blade into the anterior, right upper quadrant of the pelvis where it needs to be. The secret is to press the handle laterally and inferiorly with the right hand, thereby bringing the blade away from the forehead of the baby. Simultaneously, the index and middle fingers of the left hand positioned under the right blade should lift it into its final position just below the anterior (right) lambdoid suture. Prior to checking the application, asynclitism (if present) should be corrected using a sliding lock, a key feature of Luikart and Kielland forceps.

2 The three standard checks proposed by Dennen presuppose the use of a fenestrated blade in order to check depth of application. No more than one fingerbreadth should be able to be inserted into the posterior aspect of the fenestra (window) of the blade. This check cannot be performed with either a solid blade or a pseudofenestrated blade. Therefore, gauging depth of insertion requires assessment of the distance between the upper border of the heel of the blade and the bony head. This distance should be < 2 cm. The other two checks should be made as recommended by Dennen: the sagittal suture should bisect the plane of the shanks, and the posterior fontanelle should be one fingerbreadth above (anterior to) the plane of the shanks.

3 Not mentioned by Dennen, but readily accessible to the operator, is the relationship of the upper aspect of each blade to the lambdoid sutures. The lambdoid suture on each side should be palpable above the upper aspect of the blade for occiput ante-

rior positions. Furthermore, the distance from the upper aspect of the blade to the lambdoid sutures should be equal and symmetric. When either lambdoid suture cannot be palpated separately from the top of the blade, the possibility of an undesirable, brow–mastoid application should be considered. Traction should not be initiated until the application is corrected.

Once a proper application has been achieved, checked, and determined to be correct, rotation to the anterior (OA) can be undertaken. For conventional forceps with a pelvic curve, the handles should transcribe a wide arc, while the toes of the blades (out of view of the operator) transcribe a narrow arc. Two pointers are relevant:

1 The handles should not occupy the midsagittal plane prior to attempting rotation. Instead they should point to the maternal leg on the same side as the fetal occiput.

2 Rotation of the handles in a wide arc can be accomplished with one hand. The fingers of the other hand should be placed in the lambdoid suture adjacent to the posterior aspect of the anterior lambdoid suture to assist with and monitor the rotation.

Last but not least is traction. Modern forceps have no strain gauge attached to them, and the size and strength of modern operators vary substantially. Force can be wasted against the posterior aspect of the pubic bone, or force may be directed too far posteriorly for too long, thus putting the external anal sphincter at risk of tearing. Two very important pointers apply to traction on the forceps:

1 Every operator, regardless of experience, should use a Bill's axis traction handle on at least a few occasions to gain an appreciation of how descent of the fetal head affects the direction of traction. This principle is illustrated diagrammatically in the 1994 ACOG Technical Bulletin.[18]

2 The control of the delivery once the occiput is under the symphysis is the responsibility of the operator. Raising the handles too high risks vaginal sulcus as well as periurethral lacerations. Failure to raise the handles enough puts the anal sphincter at risk. Forceps add 8% to the volume of the fetal head passing through the introitus. Once the fingers of the dominant hand have secured the chin of the fetus through the maternal soft tissue, the forceps should be removed, ideally in the opposite order to the way they were placed, before completing the delivery of the head. An episiotomy of appropriate size and type can aid in decreasing traction force and protecting maternal anatomy. Maternal morbidity such as deep perineal lacerations (third- and fourth-degree extensions) can be significantly diminished by the skill of the operator. Some reports attribute morbidity to the instrument and neglect the fact that the instrument may not have been used properly to effect delivery.

Technique – vacuum extraction

Just as with forceps, proper technique with the VE can minimize maternal and neonatal morbidity. Proper cup placement over the vertex of the fetal skull, symmetrically covering the skull both side-to-side and anteriorly to posteriorly, is a critical aspect of VE. Asymmetric cup placement may inappropriately extend the head and present a larger diameter to the maternal pelvis, thereby leading to detachment of the cup and possibly failure of the procedure. Most series in the literature report a higher failure rate for VE than for forceps delivery. Imparting torque to the cup, even the soft cup, should be avoided. Excluding maternal soft tissue from the suction cup is essential. Traction perpendicular to the plane of the biparietal diameter (BPD) of the fetal head requires practice. Total duration of the extraction as well as number of pop-offs should be monitored carefully. Traction should be intermittent, as with forceps, and coordinated with the woman's voluntary expulsive effort. Most importantly, traction should be associated with visible progress in descent of the fetal head. Despite its increasing popularity, there is the potential for serious neonatal morbidity with the use of the VE. Some of this serious morbidity is related to poor technique, and other morbidity is related to reluctance on the part of the operator to abandon the procedure when problems are encountered. The very serious subaponeurotic hemorrhage will be considered later in the chapter.

Maternal and perinatal outcome for OVD

At present, both forceps and vacuum extractors are acceptable and safe instruments for OVD.[19] Better quality evidence than currently exists is needed to determine the proper place for OVD in the future. For example, there are no randomized controlled trials (RCTs) of OVD with Cesarean delivery, the logical comparison group. In contrast, there are RCTs for vacuum versus forceps, but these trials are hampered by small sample size, by the incorrect assumption that there are only two instruments being compared (vacuum and forceps, but not which vacuum or which forceps), and by the unprovable notion that operators have equal skill and experience with both instruments. There are also some studies classified as level II evidence that will be reviewed. Regrettably, much of the literature on OVD is consigned to level III evidence, and much of that is limited by small sample size. Analyses of large databases also suffer from potentially serious limitations: the reliability of the data collection, the omission in the database of an important datum such as indication for OVD, and the span of time covered by the database, which could obscure important changes in practice.

There are several additional considerations in examining outcomes of OVD:

1 What are the important outcomes?

2 What is the appropriate comparison group?

3 When was the study done? Does it reflect current practice?

4 Where was the study conducted? In a country with a comparable threat of litigations? In an institution where most OVDs are performed by residents?

Table 61.6 Maternal and neonatal morbidity from OVD.

Maternal	Neonatal	
Short term	*Short term*	
Deep perineal lacerations (third and fourth degree)	Low Apgar score	Skull fracture
Vaginal lacerations	Acidosis	Ocular injury
Cervical lacerations	Facial nerve palsy	Scalp trauma
Urinary retention	Brachial plexus palsy	Jaundice
Vulvovaginal hematomas	Intracranial hemorrhage	Cephalohematoma
Symphyseal separation	Subgaleal hemorrhage	Cervical spine injury
Lumbosacral plexopathies		
Long term	*Long term*	
Damage to pelvic floor resulting in:	Intellectual handicap	
Urinary incontinence	Cerebral palsy	
Fecal incontinence	Other permanent neurologic handicap	
Pelvic prolapse		
Cystocele		
Rectocele		
Enterocele		
Uterine prolapse		

Note: Cesarean delivery is also associated with significant maternal and neonatal morbidity.

Clearly, there are more questions than answers, but it is still necessary to examine and critique what evidence exists. One significant restriction is imposed on this literature review: only studies reported after the 1988 ACOG classification of forceps deliveries was adopted will be considered.

Table 61.6 contains the maternal and neonatal outcomes most commonly cited as morbidity in reports on OVD. The frequency of the complications listed in the table is highly variable among reported studies, and also variable according to the method of delivery, forceps versus vacuum. Moreover, the morbidity is not only attributable to the instrument but also to the skill of the operator, maternal and fetal characteristics, and indication for delivery. Some generalizations reported in the literature regarding the morbidity of forceps and VE procedures fail to account for skill, degree of difficulty, and severity of the injury. Selected examples from recent publications serve to illustrate these points.

Maternal morbidity

A systematic review of 10 randomized trials of forceps versus vacuum concluded that VE is associated with less maternal trauma than forceps.[20] The largest single trial[21] in that review confirmed that maternal injuries were more common with forceps. However, in that study, all deliveries were performed by residents supervised by maternal–fetal medicine fellows. Nineteen cases assigned to the forceps group were abandoned because of poor forceps application. Whether injuries that occurred should be attributed to the instrument or to operator skill is unclear.

In a retrospective study,[22] Damron and Capeless reported that third- and fourth-degree lacerations occurred more often with forceps (54%) than with VE (27%). In contrast, de Parades et al.[23] noted anal sphincter injury in less than 13% of forceps deliveries, but did not compare their results with VE procedures. In the latter report, all deliveries were performed by trained obstetricians. Operator skill likely contributes more to the outcome than the instrument used.

A small RCT by Fitzpatrick and colleagues[24] found that "altered fecal continence" was more common in the forceps group at a follow-up visit 3 months postpartum. Conversely, at 5-year follow-up, Johanson et al.[25] found no significant differences in either bowel or urinary dysfunction between women delivered by forceps or those delivered by VE. Thus, length of follow-up also affects the frequency of maternal morbidity. If maternal morbidity was consistently worse for forceps, which some of the above-mentioned reports refute, one would still have to weigh the neonatal morbidity prior to recommending "the instrument of first choice."

Neonatal morbidity

A large database analysis by Towner and colleagues[9] confirmed that the frequency of neonatal intracranial hemorrhage is nearly the same for VE as for forceps. However, most cases of subgaleal hemorrhage reported have been associated with VE. As opposed to maternal perineal trauma, subgaleal bleeding is a potentially life-threatening complication in the infant. Cephalohematomas do not cross suture lines because they are limited by the periosteum of individual cranial bones. Subgaleal bleeds involve the subaponeurotic layer of the scalp, can expand in all directions, and can even extend downward into the neck. This space can accommodate almost the entire circulating blood volume of the infant. Most concerning is the fact that subgaleal hemorrhage can complicate VE deliveries that are described as easy with no pop-offs and involving no prolonged traction.

Shoulder dystocia is associated with brachial plexus injury. Several studies show that shoulder dystocia occurs more frequently after VE than after forceps deliveries. Once again, the explanation for this observation may not lie with the instrument itself, but rather with such variables as indication for use, starting station, or inability to successfully apply forceps.

Clearly, the selection of an instrument for OVD is more complex than balancing maternal and neonatal morbidity. The clinical situation and the training and experience of the operator should be the primary determinants of choice of instrument. Nevertheless, studies that compare the results of forceps with VE deliveries are valuable, and further investigation is needed.

OVD versus Cesarean delivery

In the author's opinion, a more important question is the comparison of OVD with Cesarean delivery. As noted previously, there has never been an RCT conducted to resolve this dilemma. The most frequent indication for OVD in the past was elective or prophylactic vaginal delivery. Now, with OVD numbers dwindling substantially, most are indicated, not elective. Drife[26] raised the concern that indicated OVDs are not all difficult and, further, that many easy deliveries were enrolled in clinical trials.

Only two investigations have attempted to compare difficult vaginal delivery with Cesarean delivery. The first, by Bashore et al.,[27] compared 358 forceps deliveries with 486 Cesarean deliveries for similar indications. Maternal febrile morbidity occurred in 25% of the Cesarean group, compared with 4% in the forceps group, and women undergoing Cesarean were transfused more frequently. All infants in the forceps group were occiput transverse or occiput posterior at the start of the procedure and, except for two, were at +2 to +3 station (on a 5-cm scale). Thus, most were low forceps according to the ACOG classification, and easy outlet forceps were completely excluded. A more recent attempt to define "difficult" forceps is the study by Murphy and colleagues[28] from the UK. All women in both the vaginal and the Cesarean delivery groups were completely dilated. The study design was retrospective. Only those women whose deliveries took place "in theater" (in the operating room) were included. Thus, difficulty was not defined specifically by either station or rotation. Women in the Cesarean group (n = 209) experienced major hemorrhage more often than those in the OVD group (n = 184); within the OVD group were 58 forceps, 67 VE, and 59 combined forceps and VE deliveries. Overall neonatal morbidity was low.

Conclusions

In the introduction to this chapter, it was stated that recommendations would be made to preserve the performance of indicated OVD and prevent what clearly appears to be a pathway toward extinction. Elective instrumental delivery should continue to be offered to women who meet the requirements. This experience should be supplemented in training programs by instruction from the podium and on manikins. The graduate obstetrician should insure that hard-earned skills do not diminish over time; therefore, he or she should continue to perform both indicated and elective procedures and monitor the results. Only through training and practice can we confidently offer our patients an option intermittent between spontaneous vaginal delivery and Cesarean section.

Key points

1. The frequency of operative vaginal delivery has declined steadily over the last 40 years.
2. The use of elective outlet forceps is still justifiable today.
3. It is advisable to write a preoperative note that includes pelvic examination findings before performing operative vaginal delivery.
4. Luikart forceps are an appropriate choice to correct asynclitism.
5. One important prerequisite for forceps application is an exact knowledge of the fetal position.
6. The most important check to confirm proper forceps application is to ascertain that the sagittal suture bisects the plane of the shanks.
7. Use of a Bill's axis traction device is recommended for the new operator to appreciate the direction of traction.
8. Forceps should be removed prior to delivery of the fetal head.
9. The critical principle in vacuum extraction is proper cup placement.

10 The frequency of neonatal intracranial hemorrhage is approximately the same for both vacuum and forceps.

11 At 5-year follow-up, there were no significant differences in either fecal or urinary incontinence for women delivered by forceps compared with those delivered by vacuum.

12 Randomized trials of forceps versus vacuum did not demonstrate conclusively which should be the "instrument of first choice."

13 The most important variables in classifying forceps or vacuum deliveries are station and rotation.

14 The primary function of Kielland forceps is rotation.

15 Vacuum extraction is associated with a much greater risk of subgaleal bleeding than forceps.

16 Twice as many vacuum procedures are performed in the United States compared with forceps deliveries.

17 One of the hazards of OVD is damage to the pelvic floor.

18 Selective use of episiotomy rather than routine use is advocated for operative vaginal delivery.

19 Candidates for the oral board examination report minimal (< five procedures/year) experience with operative vaginal delivery.

20 The most important requirement for operative vaginal delivery is proper training during residency.

References

1 Luikart R. A modification of the Kielland, Simpson, and Tucker–McLane forceps to simplify their use and improve function and safety. *Am J Obstet Gynecol* 1937;686–687.

2 Kozak LJ, Weeks JD. US trends in obstetric procedures, 1990–2000. *Birth* 2002;29:157–161.

3 Martin JA, Hamilton BE, Sutton PD, et al. Births: final data for 2002. *Natl Vital Stat Rep* 2003;52:1–113.

4 D'Esopo DA. A review of cesarean section at Sloane Hospital for Women 1942–1947. *Am J Obstet Gynecol* 1950;59:77–95.

5 Frigoletto FD, Jr, Ryan KJ, Phillippe M. Maternal mortality rate associated with cesarean section: an appraisal. *Am J Obstet Gynecol* 1980;136:969–970.

6 Sultan AH, Kamm MA, Hudson CN, et al. Anal-sphincter disruption during vaginal delivery. *N Engl J Med* 1993;329: 1905–1911.

7 Hannah ME, Hannah WJ, Hewson SA, et al. Planned caesarean section versus planned vaginal birth for breech presentation at term: a randomized multicentre trial. Term Breech Trial Collaborative Group. *Lancet* 2000;356:1375–1383.

8 Landon MB, Hauth JC, Leveno KJ, et al. Maternal and perinatal outcomes associated with a trial of labor after prior cesarean delivery. *N Engl J Med* 2004;351:2581–2589.

9 Towner D, Castro MA, Eby-Wilkens E, Gilbert WM. Effect of mode of delivery in nulliparous women on neonatal intracranial injury. *N Engl J Med* 1999;341:1709–1714.

10 Dennen EH. *Forceps deliveries*. Philadelphia, PA: F.A. Davis Company, 1955.

11 Chez RA, Droegemueller W, Grant NF, Jr, O'Sullivan MJ. Clinical experience reported by candidates for the American Board of Obstetrics and Gynecology 1995 and 1997 oral examinations. *Am J Obstet Gynecol* 2001;185:1429–1432.

12 Dennen PC. *Dennen's forceps deliveries*. Washington, DC: The American College of Obstetricians and Gynecologists, 2001.

13 Ennis M. Training and supervision of obstetric senior house officers. *Br Med J* 1991;303:1442–1443.

14 Belfort MA. Shoulder dystocia and flying airplanes! *Obstet Gynecol* 2004;104:658–660.

15 Leung WC, Lam HS, Lam KW, et al. Unexpected reduction in the incidence of birth trauma and birth asphyxia related to instrumental deliveries during the study period: was this the Hawthorne effect? *Br J Obstet Gynaecol* 2003;110:319–322.

16 Danforth DN, Ellis AH. Midforceps delivery – a vanishing art? *Am J Obstet Gynecol* 1963;86:29–37.

17 Luikart R. A new forceps possessing a sliding lock, modified fenestra, with improved handle and axis traction attachment. *Am J Obstet Gynecol* 1940;1058–1060.

18 ACOG Technical Bulletin. *An educational aid to obstetrician–gynecologists. Operative vaginal delivery*. No. 196, August 1994.

19 ACOG Practice Bulletin. *Clinical management guidelines for obstetrician–gynecologists. Operative vaginal delivery*. No. 17, June 2000.

20 Johanson RB, Menon VJ. Vacuum extraction versus forceps for assisted vaginal delivery. *Cochrane Database Syst Rev* 2000;2: CD000224.

21 Bofill JA, Fust OA, Schorr SJ, et al. A randomized prospective trial of the obstetric forceps versus the M-cup vacuum extractor. *Am J Obstet Gynecol* 1996;175:1325–1330.

22 Damron DP, Capeless EL. Operative vaginal delivery: A comparison of forceps and vacuum for success rate and risk of rectal sphincter injury. *Am J Obstet Gynecol* 2004;191:907–910.

23 de Parades V, Etienney I, Thabut D, et al. Anal sphincter injury after forceps delivery: myth or reality? *Dis Colon Rectum* 2004;47:24–34.

24 Fitzpatrick M, Behan M, O'Connell R, O'Herlihy C. Randomised clinical trial to assess anal sphincter function following forceps or vacuum-assisted vaginal delivery. *Br J Obstet Gynaecol* 2003; 110:424–429.

25 Johanson RB, Heycock E, Carter J, et al. Maternal and child health after assisted vaginal delivery: five-year follow up of a randomized controlled study comparing forceps and ventouse. *Br J Obstet Gynaecol* 1999;106:544–549.

26 Drife JO. Choice and instrumental delivery. *Br J Obstet Gynaecol* 1996;103:608–611.

27 Bashore RA, Phillips WH, Jr, Brinkman CR. A comparison of the morbidity of midforceps and cesarean delivery. *Am J Obstet Gynecol* 1990;162:1428–1435.

28 Murphy DJ, Leibling RE, Patel R, et al. Cohort study of operative delivery in the second stage of labour and standard of obstetric care. *Br J Obstet Gynaecol* 2003;110:610–615.

62 Preterm labor

Erol Amon and Thomas D. Myles

Epidemiology and demography

Definitions

Traditionally, pediatricians have defined prematurity as having a birthweight of 2500g or less. Today, this is more commonly known as *low birthweight* (*LBW*) in a liveborn infant.[1] According to the World Health Organization, a preterm birth is any birth, regardless of birthweight, which occurs up to 37 menstrual weeks' gestation.[2] *Williams Obstetrics* defines preterm birth as a birth occurring before 38 menstrual weeks' gestation.[3] In this chapter, preterm is used to describe a fetus or pregnancy up to 37 weeks' gestation, based on the best obstetric criteria.

The lower gestational age limit for a preterm birth, whether the baby is born alive or dead, is 20 weeks. This lower limit is based on traditional medical definitions[3] and some statutory legal definitions of stillbirth,[4] rather than on clinical utility (i.e., the neonate's ability to survive).[5,6]

Importance of subject

Preterm birth is one of the most important issues in reproductive medicine; in 2002, the preterm delivery rate was 12%.[7] It is directly responsible for 75–90% of all neonatal deaths that are caused by lethal congenital malformations.[8,9] Preterm birth also accounts for the vast majority of perinatal mortality and both short- and long-term neonatal morbidity. The major diseases of the preterm infant result from organ immaturity, and the incidence and severity of disease are inversely related to gestational age.[10] These conditions include respiratory distress syndrome (RDS), patent ductus arteriosus, necrotizing enterocolitis (NEC), hyperbilirubinemia, intraventricular hemorrhage (IVH), retinopathy of prematurity, and neonatal sepsis. Previously, if preterm infants survived, they faced a high risk of significant long-term handicap (blindness, deafness, cerebral palsy, or mental retardation). Today, only 7.5% of very LBW (VLBW) infants (less than 1500g) have a condition that results in a major handicap. Neonatal survival has been reported as early as 22–23 weeks' gestation. In the last 20 years, the break-even or 50% survival rate dropped from 25–26 weeks' gestation or a birthweight of 750g,[11] to 24 weeks or 600g;[12,13] the mortality rate in infants weighing from 501 to 600g was 71%, whereas it was 89% for infants weighing from 401 to 500g[13] (Fig. 62.1). Although the overall handicap rate of these infants was high, the severe handicap rate in survivors was about 30%.[13]

Epidemiology

LBW is a surrogate measure for the health of any community or nation. LBW is one of the strongest determinants of infant mortality and morbidity; thus, it continues to be closely monitored. The classification of LBW births is summarized in Table 62.1.[11] Many mildly preterm infants have birthweights of 2500g or more (35–36 weeks); conversely, many moderately LBW infants (1500–2499g) are actually full term. In some series, nearly one-half of LBW infants were considered term.[14] The concepts of preterm birth and LBW differ in their pathogenesis but share many predisposing factors (Table 62.2)[15] and, as such, these phenomena are often considered together. It is noteworthy that impaired fetal growth does not exert the same force on neonatal and infant mortality as early gestational age.

The national distributions of LBW and prematurity are markedly skewed.[16] More than 60% of all LBW infants weigh 2000g or more at birth, a time when survival is extremely high and neonatal morbidity is very low. Moreover, nearly 85% of preterm births occur at 32 weeks or more,[17] a time when uncorrected gestational age-specific mortality is 4% or less. Neonatal mortality and severe morbidity tend to be most prevalent in the late second trimester and early third trimester, a period that accounts for fewer than one in six preterm births.

Despite decades of advances in reproductive medicine and large reductions in the rates of neonatal and infant mortality, the incidence of LBW and VLBW births has not decreased (Fig. 62.2).[7] The rate of LBW births declined during the 1970s and early 1980s. From a low of 6.7% in 1984, it increased to a rate of 8% in 2002, its highest level since 1975.[16] The incidence of VLBW births also increased from 1.2% to 1.5%,

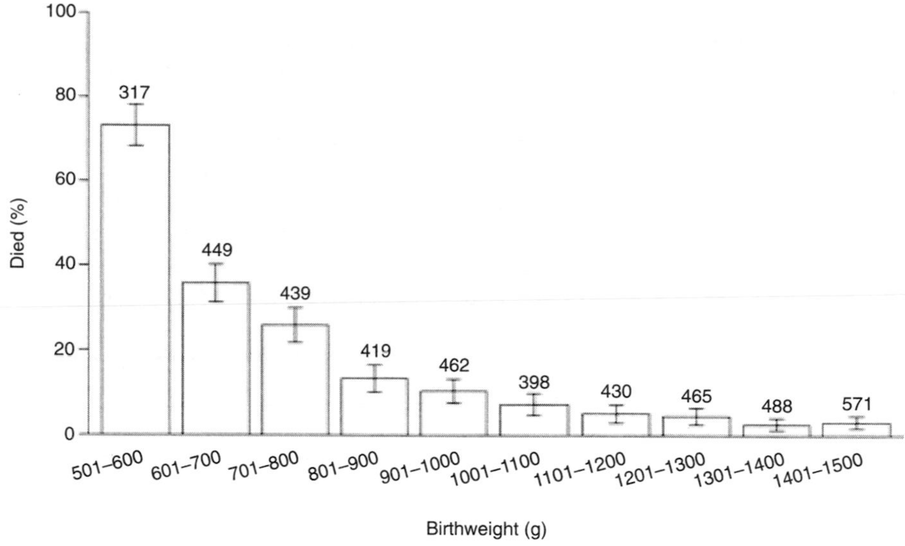

Figure 62.1 Mortality before discharge by birthweight among infants born in NICHD Neonatal Research Network Centers between 1 January 1995 and 31 December 1996. Data expressed as percentage died and 95% confidence intervals for each 100-g birth weight interval. From ref. 13, with permission.

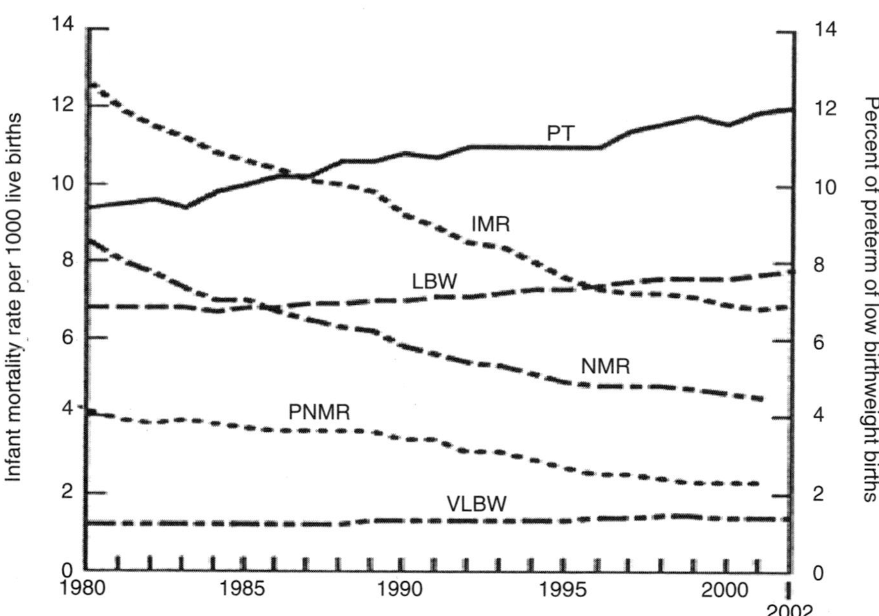

Figure 62.2 Infant, neonatal, and postneonatal mortality; LBW and VLBW; and preterm delivery, United States, 1980 to 2002. From ref. 7 with permission.

Table 62.1 Birthweight categories.

Category	Weight (g)
Low birthweight	< 2500
Very low birthweight	< 1500
Extremely low birthweight or very, very low birthweight	≤ 1000
Incredibly low birthweight	≤ 750

From ref. 11, with permission.

whereas the national preterm birth rate increased steadily from 10.2% to 12%.[7]

Racial disparity between black people and white people

The incidence of LBW and VLBW infants differs substantially between black people and white people.[17] The incidence of preterm birth is 17.4% in black people and 11.0% in white people,[17] and this racial disparity increases as gestational age at delivery decreases (Fig. 62.3).[17]

The reasons for these demographic differences are complex and relate to socioeconomic and biological differences between races. It had been assumed that socioeconomic disadvantages

Table 62.2 Categories of maternal risk for low birthweight.

Economic
Poverty
Unemployment
Maternal father's poor socioeconomic status
Uninsured, underinsured
Poor access to prenatal care
Poor access to food
Cultural–behavioral
Low educational status
Poor healthcare attitudes
No or inadequate prenatal care
Cigarette, alcohol, drug abuse
Age of < 16 years or > 35 years
Unmarried
Short interpregnancy interval
Lack of support group (husband, family, church)
Stress (physical, psychological)
Poor weight gain during pregnancy
Black race*
Biological–genetic–medical
Previous low birthweight infant
Mother low weight at birth
Black race*
Low weight for height
Short stature
Poor nutrition
Chronic medical illness
Inbreeding (autosomal recessive?)
Intergenerational effects
Reproductive
Multiple gestation
Premature rupture of membranes
Infections (systemic, amniotic, extra-amniotic, cervical)
Preeclampsia or eclampsia
Uterine bleeding (placental abruption, placenta previa)
Parity (0 or > 5)
Uterocervical anomalies
Fetal disease
Anemia or high hemoglobin
Idiopathic premature labor
Iatrogenic prematurity

From ref. 15 with permission.

* Black race is a risk factor for both growth retardation and premature birth. The risk is twice that for white people and remains present when confounding social and economic variables are controlled. Classification of risk for black people as cultural and biological is due to the uncertainty of the role of these variables.

were primarily responsible for the substantial difference in rates but, after controlling for some confounding socioeconomic variables, investigators found that the twofold increase in the relative risk for LBW infants remained.[15] In fact, the rate of VLBW births in low-risk black women was 1.7 times higher than that of high-risk white women. According to Papiernik and colleagues,[18] these differences can be explained, in part, by biological differences in gestational length.

According to Naeye,[19] urogenital infections represent the largest single category of black–white disparity in perinatal mortality. Black women have higher rates of lower urogenital tract infection than other ethnic groups. These infections include sexually transmitted infections such as syphilis, gonorrhea, chlamydia, and trichomoniasis.[20] Black women also have a higher incidence of nonsexually transmitted urogenital tract colonization and infections, including bacteriuria, bacterial vaginosis, group B streptococcal infections, and genital mycoplasmas;[21] the rate of bacterial vaginosis in black women ranges from 20% to 50% compared with 7% to 30% in white women. Although these infections may account for up to 35% of the difference in perinatal mortality between black people and white people, racial differences in reported sexual behavior do not account for the difference in rates of infections.

Epidemiology and etiology

Many epidemiological risk factors are not etiological *per se*, but are simply markers identifying patients at increased risk for preterm birth. Table 62.3 lists the identifiable causes most proximate to preterm birth. Most spontaneous preterm births do not belong to the idiopathic category; only after known or suspected causes are eliminated should patients be diagnosed with idiopathic preterm labor. More recent studies have shown that clinically evident membrane rupture, medical or obstetric maternal complications, or fetal complications account for approximately 70% of preterm births.[9,22,23]

A study by Amon and colleagues[9] showed that most infants at highest risk (less than or equal to 1000 g) are born prematurely as a result of etiological factors that are currently not preventable. Although placental pathology was not systematically studied, 82% had a major identifiable associated finding, thus classifying only 18% as idiopathic preterm birth.[9]

Subclinical intra-amniotic infection or accelerated fetal pulmonary maturation remain undiagnosed unless an assessment is carried out by amniocentesis;[24–26] the incidence of idiopathic preterm labor would be lower than the 30–50% that is often quoted if amniocentesis were performed more often. When a comprehensive evaluation, including placental pathology, immunopathology, and intrauterine infection, is combined with clinical factors, up to 96% of patients have a potentially identifiable etiology and more than 50% of patients have two or more proximate causes.[27] The remainder of this chapter focuses on spontaneous preterm labor with intact membranes, a small portion of which is idiopathic.

Pathophysiology

The pathophysiology of preterm labor is unknown. This is not surprising because the normal mechanisms that initiate parturition spontaneously at term are also unknown. However,

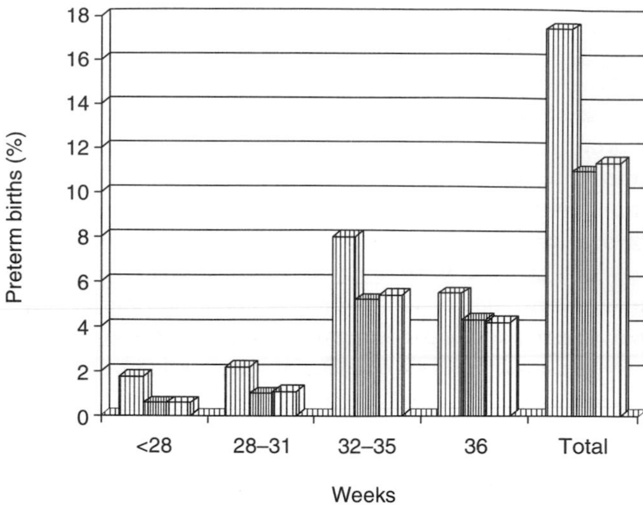

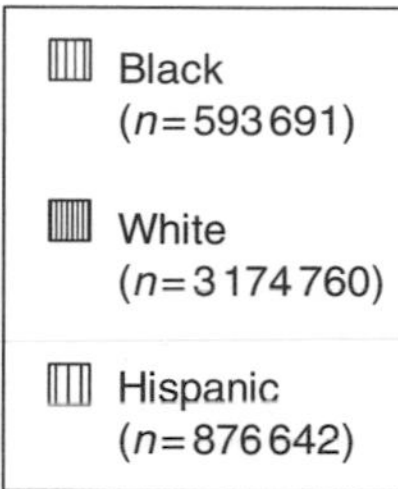

Figure 62.3 Percentage of live preterm births by race. Created from data from ref. 17.

Table 62.3 Proximate factors and causes associated with preterm birth.

Iatrogenic preterm delivery
Physician error
Maternal causes
Significant systemic medical illness
Significant nonobstetric abdominal pathology
Illicit drug abuse
Severe preeclampsia or eclampsia
Trauma
Uterine causes
Malformation
Acute overdistention
Large myomata, degenerating myomata
Deciduitis, decidual thrombosis and hemorrhage
Idiopathic uterine activity
Placental causes
Placental abruption
Placenta previa
Marginal placental bleeding
Large chorioangioma
Amniotic fluid causes
Oligohydramnios with intact membranes
Preterm rupture of chorioamniotic membranes
Polyhydramnios
Subclinical intra-amniotic infection
Clinical chorioamnionitis
Fetal causes
Fetal malformation
Multifetal gestation
Fetal hydrops
Fetal growth retardation
Fetal distress
Fetal demise
Cervical causes
Cervical incompetence
Cervical foreshortening
Acute cervicitis or vaginitis

there is extensive literature available on the biomolecular processes closely involved with the phenomenon of labor. Factors produced locally within the placenta, chorioamniotic membranes, and decidua, together with biochemical messages from the fetus, act in some complex manner to initiate normal spontaneous labor.

In all mammalian species tested, prostaglandin production increases during and perhaps even before labor. In many species, the three most temporally related uterine events antecedent to the onset of spontaneous labor are cervical ripening, formation of gap junctions, and an increase in oxytocin receptors. Fundamentally, these mechanisms must bring about myometrial contraction by regulating the free intracellular cytosolic calcium concentration in myometrial cells. Myometrial cells contract when the concentration of calcium increases, and relax when the concentration decreases.[28]

Another key regulator of myometrial contractility is the phosphorylation (causing contraction) and dephosphorylation (causing relaxation) of myosin light chains. Cellular tocolytic mechanisms include the regulation of myosin phosphorylation, cyclic adenosine monophosphate (cAMP) regulation of myosin light-chain kinase, regulation of intracellular free calcium levels, and regulation of adenylate-cyclase activity.[29]

Organ communication

Up to 30% of preterm labor may be caused by infection. The generation of cytokines is considered to be the normal response to a variety of infectious mediators. One of the host tissues generating such responses is maternal decidua. Inflammatory cytokines are elevated in the amniotic fluid and plasma of women in preterm labor. Notably, anti-inflammatory cytokines such as interleukin 10 (IL-10) do not appear to be present in substantial quantities. Animal models have verified that bacteria, bacterial cell-wall products, and inflammatory cytokines such as IL-1 and tumor necrosis factor can stimulate preterm labor. IL-6 is subsequently released and can mediate a systemic response. Healing of the inflammatory process may occur through the actions of IL-10, IL-4, and transforming growth factors. Dysregulation of the normal host defense inflammatory response could result in preterm labor and delivery.[30] Placental histology indicates that inflammation only accounts for 30–40% of cases of preterm labor. The most common noninflammatory lesion of the placenta is decidual thrombosis and acute atherosis, which may lead to uteroplacental ischemia and subsequent initiation of preterm labor.[31] This may explain the subset of patients who have complications of fetal growth restriction and placental abnormalities.

Other factors such as fetal stress and decidual hemorrhage are also important in preterm labor. Initiators such as peptide hormones (e.g., corticotropin-releasing hormone) and inflammatory mediators may promote the production of uterotonic factors (e.g., prostanoids and endothelin) that result in contractions and the release of proteases (e.g., collagenases and elastases), which in turn initiate membrane rupture and cervical change. Accordingly, extracellular matrix proteins [e.g., fetal fibronectin (fFN), also known as oncofetal fibronectin, and prolactin] in cervicovaginal secretions are elevated. Such release may lead to further cervical change and disruption of the tightly regulated maternal–fetal interface, ultimately resulting in preterm delivery.[32]

Biochemistry of cervical change

The structure and function of the cervix has been well described.[33] The underlying stroma is predominantly an extracellular connective tissue matrix, mainly made up of type I and type III collagen. Other important constituents of the matrix are water, glycosaminoglycans, proteoglycans, dermatan sulfate, hyaluronic acid, and heparin sulfate. Elastin, the functional protein of elastic fibers, runs longitudinally between bundles of collagen fibers. The ratio of elastin to collagen is highest at the internal os. Smooth muscle cells make up 10–15% of cervical tissue, with the greatest number of cells located just below the internal os, and fewer found toward the external os.

Controversy exists over whether cervical ripening is primarily a biochemical rearrangement of the extracellular matrix related to biomechanical factors such as increased intrauterine pressure at the lower segment from the presenting fetal part or uterine activity, or whether it is due to an inflammatory reaction in which macrophages and polymorphonuclear cells release enzymes to degrade collagen, which then leads to proteolytic rearrangement.[34] It may be that both theories of initiation are correct, but one may predominate over the other, especially in view of the different biomolecular mechanisms for labor. Apoptosis is a genetically timed event; it may also be an intrinsic cause of preterm labor, explaining the many cases of preterm labor in certain families.[35]

Therapeutic implications of pathophysiological subsets

Recognizing the etiological heterogeneity, complexity, and interactive nature of the underlying biomolecular processes of preterm labor, Keelan and colleagues[36] have elegantly proposed that future therapeutic trials be tailored to the specific etiological mechanism determined by a battery of preterm labor tests (Table 62.4). Preterm labor *per se* is not a disease in itself but an aberration of timing with diverse underlying heterogeneity. Consequently, in the future, a careful strategy of specific biomolecular diagnosis and treatment for preterm labor will be necessary.

Clinical antecedents to preterm labor and delivery

Many risk factors antedate the diagnosis of preterm labor, but unfortunately these factors are not very specific. This lack of specificity is further compounded by the inability to accurately diagnose preterm labor. True preterm labor, if left untreated, implies cervical progression and prompt preterm delivery. Unfortunately, the overlap with false, nonprogressive, and episodic preterm labor is considerable.

Traditional risk factor scoring and prevention programs

In general, risk scoring quantitatively screens a population for factors associated with a given outcome or disease. One of the fundamental principles underlying a screening program of any type is that there be safe and effective management plans for identified patients. If individuals can be identified before the onset of their condition or early in the course of their disease, preventive measures may be employed to eliminate, lessen, or even stabilize a condition. Unfortunately, preterm labor and delivery have been resistant to most prevention and management efforts. Methods used to prevent preterm birth are quite inconsistent and of limited clinical value.[37] There are limitations to screening, regionalization, eleventh-hour care, prophylactic and therapeutic antibiotics, bedrest, social and psychological support, and educational programs.[38] Furthermore, there are inconsistencies and a lack of effectiveness, even among well-staffed, well-funded, and well-organized comprehensive prematurity prevention programs.[39]

Nonetheless, risk scoring can clearly identify a group of pregnant individuals who are at an increased risk for spontaneous preterm labor and birth, and these individual high-risk patients can then receive high-risk care. Various clinically based risk scoring systems have been developed to identify women who have an above-average risk for preterm birth. However, although spontaneous preterm labor with intact membranes is treatable with tocolytic agents, it is important to note that there are still many other proximate causes of

Table 62.4 Potential applications of newer therapeautic options for the treatment of preterm labor.

Cause of preterm labor	Diagnostic indicators	Treatment options
Clinical chorioamnionitis	↑ fFN, IL-6, and ECM proteases Normal free CRH Positive clinical indicators	Deliver if maternal or fetal condition compromised Antibiotics, glucocorticoids
Subclinical chorioamnionitis	↑ fFN, IL-6, and ECM proteases Bacterial vaginosis Normal free CRH	Antibiotics, PGHS inhibitors/β-mimetics Glucocorticoids Deliver if maternal or fetal condition compromised
Lower genital tract infection	↑ Vaginal fFN, IL-6, and ECM proteases Bacterial vaginosis Normal free CRH	Antibiotics with regular review
Idiopathic endocrinopathies	↑ Free CRH, ?↑ fFN ?↑ Salivary E_3 Normal cytokines	Prophylactic progesterone/glucocorticoids Oxytocin antagonists if presenting with PTL ?No donor therapy
High risk for PTL (i.e., previous PTL)	History/social factors ↑ Free CRH at 26 wks ?↑ fFn/salivary E_3	Prophylactic progesterone Prophylactic glucocorticoids If presenting with PTL: OT antagonist/NO/β-mimetics
Decidual hemorrhage	Clinical indicators Normal free CRH/salivary E_3 ↑ ECM proteases	Glucocorticoids If in PTL: glucocorticoids, tocolysis (β-mimetics/PGHS inhibitors) unless otherwise contraindicated
Fetal hypoxia/stress	↑ Free CRH ↑ Salivary E_3	Glucocorticoids OT antagonist/(β-mimetics/PGHS inhibitors)
Cervical incompetence	↓ fFN, IL-6, and ECM proteases Normal free CRH	Cervical cerclage

From ref. 36, with permission.

↓, Decreased; ↑ increased; ?, query/possible; CRH, corticotropin-releasing hormone; E_3, estrone; ECM, extracellular matrix; fFN, fetal fibronectin; IL-6, interleukin 6; NO, nitric oxide; OT, oxytocin; PGHS, prostaglandin H synthase; PTL, preterm labor.

preterm birth for which short- and long-term tocolysis is contraindicated (e.g., antepartum stillbirth, significant maternal hemorrhage, chorioamnionitis, lethal congenital abnormalities, and eclampsia).

In the USA, Creasy and colleagues[40] first popularized a scoring system of risk factors to predict spontaneous preterm birth. More than 30 items are divided into four categories: socioeconomic, prior medical history, daily habits, and current pregnancy problems. Screening is performed at the initial prenatal visit and repeated near the end of the second trimester. Patients with a score of 10 points or more are considered to be at high risk.

This system (modified from that of Papiernik[41]) identified 9% of the study population as high risk at the initial screening and 13% at the second screening. The prevalence of preterm birth in this population was 6.1%. The sensitivity of the high-risk score was 64%, with a positive predictive value of 30%. This system relies heavily on past obstetric history; consequently, it is more effective in the multiparous than the nulliparous patient. The Creasy score was later used in a hospital obstetric population in San Francisco as one part of a comprehensive preterm birth prevention program with impressive results although they acknowledged the limitations of historical controls and the potential for major population differences.[42]

Holbrook and colleagues[43] reduced the number of items in their simplified risk scoring system for the prediction of preterm labor (not preterm birth) from 37 to 18 without any significant statistical loss of identification, prevalence, sensitivity, or positive predictive value (Table 62.5). Some 14% of patients were identified as high risk; the sensitivity was 41% and the positive predictive value 25%. The modified system does not require the calculation of a risk score. Twelve factors are defined as major (any one indicating high risk) and six as minor (two or more indicating high risk).

Main and colleagues[23] performed a similar combined risk scoring and intervention study. In their prospective study, 132 of 380 patients (35%) were classified as high risk. In the study population the prevalence of preterm birth was 16.3%. In the low-risk control subjects the preterm delivery rate was 12.9%, of whom 78% had preterm labor or premature rupture of membranes. The sensitivity of the high-risk score was 48%; the positive predictive value of the high-risk score was 27%. Of note, of preterm deliveries due to preterm labor in women

Table 62.5 Major and minor risk factors of the modified scoring system for spontaneous preterm labor.

*Major factors**
Multiple gestation
Previous preterm delivery
Previous preterm labor, term delivery
Abdominal surgery during pregnancy
Diethylstilbestrol exposure
Hydramnios
Uterine anomaly
History of cone biopsy
Uterine irritability (admission to rule out preterm labor)
More than one second-trimester abortion
Cervical dilation (> 1 cm) at 32 weeks
Cervical effacement (< 1 cm) at 32 weeks
Minor factors†
Febrile illness during pregnancy
Bleeding after 12 weeks
History of pyelonephritis
Cigarette smoking (>10 per day)
One second-trimester abortion
More than two first-trimester abortions

From ref. 43, with permission.

*Presence of one or more indicates high risk.

†Presence of two or more indicates high risk.

with candidacy for tocolysis, more than 50% were classified as low risk.

In the same report, high-risk patients were randomly assigned to a comprehensive preterm birth prevention program or standard high-risk care.[23] Unfortunately, the extensive intervention program *failed* to lower the incidence of preterm birth. Preterm delivery occurred in 25% of the patients in the preterm birth prevention program, compared with 21% of the high-risk control patients. The authors attributed these unfavorable results to the high incidence (70%) of proximate causes of preterm birth not amenable to tocolytic therapy.

After evaluating 31 studies describing preterm birth prevention programs, Hueston and colleagues[44] found that only six studies had controlled for scientific bias. A meta-analysis on these studies did not find any benefit for preterm birth education programs in preventing neonatal mortality or preterm birth. However, there was an increase in the diagnosis of preterm labor.

In a more complex screening process that also includes race, low prepregnant body mass index (BMI; underweight), and a poor work environment, the positive predictive value for spontaneous preterm birth for nulliparous patients was 28% and for multiparous patients was 33%.[45]

Despite the limitations for prevention of spontaneous preterm labor and birth, risk scoring is an inexpensive index that can be used readily to identify individual pregnant women at risk in clinical practice. After identification these women deserve a more intense workup and ongoing individualized medical attention. Such women may actually modify their behavior (e.g., stop smoking and illicit drug use) and decrease somewhat their risk status. Moreover, such women are motivated to learn how to effectively access health care as and when their symptoms arise.

Table 62.6 Risk for recurrent preterm labor.

First birth preterm	Second birth preterm	Risk for preterm birth
No	–	4.6
No	No	2.6
No	Yes	11.1
Yes	–	17.2
Yes	No	5.7
Yes	Yes	28.4

Modified from ref. 52.

Recurrence risk for preterm labor and preterm birth

In a middle-class population, a second-trimester abortion was associated with an increased risk of preterm labor (14%) in subsequent pregnancies.[43] In an indigent population, if the second-trimester loss occurred between 19 and 24 weeks, the subsequent preterm delivery rate was approximately 50%.[46] One or two first-trimester abortions are not associated with subsequent preterm labor, but three first-trimester abortions are associated with an increased risk of preterm labor (12%).[43]

The recurrence risk for preterm birth varies from 15% to 40% after one previous premature delivery.[14,47–50] An intervening term pregnancy markedly decreases the risk of a subsequent preterm birth. The recurrence risk significantly increases with two or more previous preterm births (Table 62.6).[51] The more premature the delivery, the less likely the subsequent pregnancy is to deliver at term.[52]

Digital cervical examination

Asymptomatic cervical dilation may represent silent preterm labor, cervical incompetence, or a normal anatomic variation. In the general obstetric population, the frequency of preterm asymptomatic cervical dilation increases as gestation advances. The risk of preterm birth by gestational age at cervical dilation was studied by Papiernik and colleagues (Table 62.7).[53] In two other studies,[54,55] cervical dilation was found to be associated with preterm birth, with a positive predictive value of 27–28%. In a low-risk population, Stubbs and colleagues[56] found an association between preterm birth and cervical dilation at 28–32 weeks' gestation (positive predictive value 12%). The relative risk for preterm birth with asymptomatic cervical dilation was two- to fourfold higher than the risk for preterm birth with an undilated cervix. Conversely, at least three previous reports have emphasized that such dilation is a normal anatomic variant, particularly in the multiparous patient.[57–59] These studies showed no significant increase in the rate of preterm birth with cervical dilation.

A large multicenter randomized controlled trial in seven European countries compared the use of "routine" cervical examination at every prenatal visit with a clinically "indicated" examination in a general obstetric population of more than 5600 patients.[60] There were no significant differences in the rates of preterm birth, LBW, premature rupture of membranes, admission to neonatal intensive care units, or perinatal mortality between the two groups. Although routine cervical examinations and associated interventions appear logical to the clinician, this powerful clinical study does not support routine digital cervical evaluation.

Sonographic cervical evaluation

Digital examination is prone to subjectivity and variation between examiners. If the cervix is closed, funneling at the internal os cannot be evaluated digitally. If the cervix is dilated, placement of the examining finger next to the fetal membranes may increase the risk of infection or membrane rupture. Transvaginal sonography appears to provide a relatively noninvasive, more reproducible, accurate, and quantitative description of cervical anatomy. Cervical sonography is also a better predictor of preterm birth resulting from preterm labor.[61] Transvaginal scanning is preferred to transabdominal or translabial scanning because of cervical proximity, lack of obscurity, and increased accuracy; the technique is well described by Sonek and colleagues.[62] The biological variation in the endocervical length of the cervix resembles a normal bell-shaped curve. A length of approximately 35 mm represents the 50th percentile, whereas lengths of 25 and 45 mm represent the 10th and 90th percentiles respectively. The relative risk of spontaneous preterm delivery before 35 weeks is inversely related to transvaginal sonographic cervical length.[63] A more thorough ultrasound description of the cervix includes the parameters shown in Fig. 62.4.[64]

In a group of expectantly managed patients with funneling diagnosed at less than 25 weeks' gestation, a sonographic funneling percentage of more than 50% had a sensitivity, specificity, and positive and negative predictive values of 80–85% for the development of preterm birth. In patients with 25–50% funneling, only 30% delivered preterm.[65] In this group, clinical interventions did occur and so the natural history of funneling was unknown; however, treatment, when effective, decreases the magnitude of the positive predictive value.

In practice, it is rare to see a clinically significant funnel if the functional (residual) cervical length is 30 mm or more.[66] Thus, measurement of the degree of funneling becomes more important as the sonographically apposed endocervical length shortens. The technique of cervical sonography is comprehensively reviewed by Iams[66] and Doyle and Monga.[67]

Table 62.7 Percentage of general obstetric patients with cervical dilatation of the internal os > 1 cm.

Weeks of gestation	Percent	Total	Preterm birth (%)
19–24	2.4	2124	17.3
25–28	4.4	2415	23.4
29–31	10.6	1750	21.6
32–34	12.4	2967	17.4
35–36	22.5	1921	11.1
37–38	32.8	2693	–

Modified from ref. 53.

Home uterine activity monitoring

Home uterine activity monitoring (HUAM) allows the patient at risk to be physically monitored at home with external tocodynamometers. The data are transmitted by telephone to a central viewing station, where the pattern of uterine activity is assessed by a nursing service. The nursing service contacts the patient once or twice daily and prepares a detailed history on the patient's current status. Should the service detect abnormalities, the physician is notified immediately.

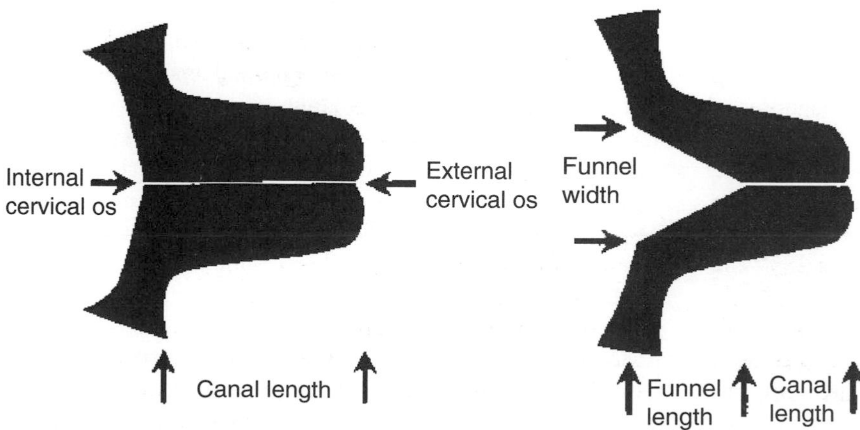

Figure 62.4 Cervical length with and without funneling (from ref. 64 with permission).

The principal variable that is monitored is the frequency of uterine activity. Studies have shown that the mean frequency of uterine contractions per hour rises with increasing time of gestation.[68,69] Some believe that there is a further increase in frequency from 24 h to 48 h before the onset of true labor.[69] However, in a prospective evaluation, Iams and colleagues[70] found that the "window of opportunity" for early tocolysis does not extend beyond 12–24 h before overtly symptomatic preterm labor occurs. The mean contraction frequency for women destined to have preterm labor is higher than for those who deliver at the normal time, but the overlap between these two groups is high, limiting its positive predictive value.[69]

Some monitoring devices are extremely sensitive, and mothers cannot always perceive the measured uterine activity. In one study,[71] only 10% of women correctly perceived their contractions more than half of the time, whereas in another study[72] that used a different monitor, 54% of high-risk patients perceived more than 75% of their contractions.

Initially, a few randomized and nonrandomized trials indicated that preterm birth might be prevented by twice-daily monitoring of high-risk women together with daily nursing support and high-quality obstetric care.[69,73–75] These studies demonstrated that the use of HUAM decreased the preterm birth rate over traditional outpatient care. However, Iams and colleagues[76] and Porto and colleagues[77] found that provider-initiated nursing education and clinical support was the primary beneficial component of the HUAM program.

The results of some more recent randomized controlled studies[78,79] have shown a benefit of HUAM, whereas others have shown no benefit.[76,80–82] A critical review of the literature[83,84] suggests multiple study design problems including: the accuracy and reliability of the HUAM device; management of the control group; the use of intermediate endpoints rather than preterm delivery or neonatal morbidity or mortality; double counting of twins; and limiting analysis to subgroups who developed preterm labor. Accordingly, Corwin and colleagues[85] reanalyzed all of the patients who were enrolled in their earlier trial and addressed some of the study design problems. They found that HUAM resulted in improved pregnancy outcome, decreased preterm birth and a decreased need for neonatal intensive care.[85]

A powerful and meaningful study by Dyson and colleagues[86] of a large number of high-risk pregnant women (n = 2422) investigated whether: (1) adding the HUAM device to daily nursing contact could reduce the rate of spontaneous preterm delivery at less than 35 weeks' gestation; and (2) daily nursing contact, irrespective of monitor use, would be more effective than weekly nursing contact. The authors found that adding the HUAM device to daily contact with the nurse did not improve either the early detection of preterm labor or the pregnancy outcome. Moreover, daily nursing contact did not improve any measure of outcome compared with weekly nursing contact. The authors concluded that the similarity in outcome among the three groups was a result of three factors: (1) the patients received thorough training and a checklist was used for consistency; (2) women were asked to palpate their uteri twice daily and to keep a daily log of the number of contractions and symptoms of labor; and (3) each woman was scheduled for weekly contact with a designated nurse who reviewed her daily logs and encouraged her to seek assistance as and when needed.

In conclusion, the bulk of the scientific evidence available does not suggest that HUAM be considered as the standard of care, and the American College of Obstetricians and Gynecologists do not recommend this system.[87] However, controversy exists as to whether HUAM has an important role to play in outpatient management.[88] Incorporating the time of day and diurnal pattern of uterine activity into a HUAM program may provide more accurate and predictive information in addition to an assessment of contraction frequency.[89] There may be patient subsets that could benefit from HUAM programs, such as those with advanced dilation and those in rural settings, who may not have quick access to a perinatal center.

Fetal fibronectin

Fibronectins are a group of proteins found in plasma, extracellular tissue, and amniotic fluid. Plasma fibronectin helps regulate oncotic pressure, coagulation, and bacterial opsonization. fFN is a unique fibronectin found in the basement membrane near the choriodecidual interface. It is produced by fetal membranes and is likely to function as an adhesive binding the placenta and membranes to the decidua. Fibronectin found in the cervical stroma is distinct from fFN.

fFN is commonly found in cervicovaginal secretions before 20 weeks' gestation and at term. Its clinical detection at 22–34 weeks at concentrations greater than 50 mg/mL is considered abnormal and indicates choriodecidual disruption. Because fFN is also found in amniotic fluid, its presence in the vagina may indicate the presence of amniotic fluid in cervicovaginal secretions. fFN may leak into the vagina by at least three other possible mechanisms. First, during the early process of uteroplacental membrane development, fFN is found in the vagina before completion of the choriodecidual interface. Second, cervical ripening during preterm and term labor, as a result of biomechanical stress caused by uterine contractions, promotes the loss of fFN from the interface. Third, inflammation at the interface may occur during preterm and term labor resulting in fFN expression in the cervicovaginal fluid.

There is a relationship between the presence of fFN in cervicovaginal secretions and spontaneous preterm birth. Three categories of patients have been evaluated: symptomatic patients hospitalized for evaluation of preterm labor, high-risk asymptomatic patients, and asymptomatic patients taken from the general obstetric population.[90–93]

In a large study of patients (n = 763) presenting with symptoms of preterm labor, almost 20% tested positive for fFN.[94] In these circumstances, the most pressing concern for the physician is the likelihood of imminent preterm birth;

therefore, delivery within 1 week is an appropriate measure of preterm birth in symptomatic patients. Rapid testing has increased the usefulness of fFN measurements, with similar positive and negative predictive values.[93] The clinical implications of this test are summarized in Fig. 62.5. It is important to note the differences between the pretest positive and negative predictive values and the post-test positive and negative predictive values. From a clinical viewpoint, it remains unclear as to how clinical management should be affected. With a negative result or with no test at all, the odds of delivering within a week are extremely low. Correspondingly, 1% of the fFN-negative group (6 out of 613) delivered a VLBW infant, which is similar to the expected incidence (1.5%) of VLBW births from all causes in the total US obstetric population.

Testing for fFN produces numerous false-positive results. Lukes and colleagues[94] found that cervical dilation or manipulation can explain some of the false-positive results, specifically: cervical dilation, recent sexual intercourse, vaginal bleeding, recent cervical examination, and uterine contractions. To improve the accuracy of positive results, specimens should be obtained before any cervical manipulation and before advanced dilation or increased uterine activity has occurred. Faron and colleagues[95] noted that test results were more frequently positive among multiparous than nulliparous women. The collection technique is illustrated in Fig. 62.6.

The overall rate of fFN positivity in low-risk populations was found to be 3–4%.[96] More than one-half of spontaneous preterm births before 28 weeks were associated with a positive fFN test result at 24 weeks.[96] This isolated finding appeared to be promising for the prevention of extremely LBW births. However, there was also an extremely high false-positive rate in that 83% of fFN-positive subjects delivered after 28 weeks, and 75% of fFN-positive patients delivered after 34 weeks.[96] The association of a positive fFN test result at the 24-week visit with spontaneous preterm birth before 34 weeks was as follows: sensitivity, 23%; specificity, 97%; positive predictive value, 25%; and negative predictive value 96%.[96]

fFN has also been proposed as a marker for upper genital tract infections. In women who delivered very preterm infants, a positive fFN test result was highly associated with clinical chorioamnionitis, histological chorioamnionitis, and neonatal sepsis, all of which were increased further in the presence of bacterial vaginosis.[97] Subsequently, a randomized multicenter trial with antibiotics was carried out. Unfortunately, of the asymptomatic women with a positive cervical or vaginal fFN test between 21 and 25 weeks' gestation, treatment with metronidazole plus erythromycin did not decrease the risk of spontaneous delivery or result in improved neonatal outcomes.[98]

	fFN+	fFN−	
Delivery ≤ 7 days	19	3	22
Delivery > 7 days	131	610	741
	150	613	763

Test	Predictive value +	Predictive value −
Without test	2.9%	97.1%
fFN negative	0.5%	99.5%
fFN positive	12.7%	88.3%

Figure 62.5 The predictive value within 1 week of fFN. The primary endpoint delivery is less than or equal to 7 days. (Modified from data in ref. 91.)

Urogenital tract infections

There is increasing evidence that urogenital tract infection, inflammation, or both are associated with and causative of many cases of preterm labor.[99] The association between asymptomatic bacteriuria and preterm birth is clear;[100] untreated asymptomatic bacteriuria may lead to pyelonephritis during pregnancy. In one study,[101] treatment of group B

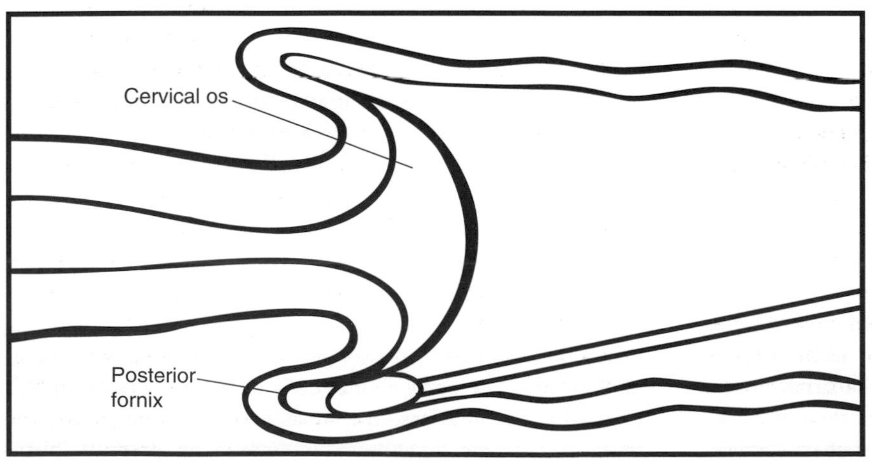

Figure 62.6 Specimen collection for fFN testing. Lightly rotate swab across either the posterior fornix of the vagina or the ectocervical region of the external cervical os for 10 seconds. This must be done prior to digital examination; alternatively, wait another 24 h.

streptococcal bacteria, which indicate heavy colonization of the lower urogenital tract, resulted in a decreased incidence of preterm birth. However, in a separate study,[102] prenatal treatment of group B streptococci with erythromycin was ineffective in preventing preterm birth.

Histological chorioamnionitis is more often seen in cases of preterm birth. Intra-amniotic positive culture results are also associated with preterm labor and birth and, in many cases, the same organism is also cultured from the vagina. Therefore, ascending cervicovaginal bacteria seem to cause deciduitis and upper genital tract infections.[99]

The association between bacterial vaginosis and preterm birth has been clearly demonstrated.[103] The relative risk of preterm delivery is 1.5–3 times higher in patients with bacterial vaginosis than in patients without. Studies have demonstrated that bacterial vaginosis may be a marker for a treatable and preventable cause of spontaneous preterm labor. Hauth and colleagues[104] evaluated 624 women at high risk for spontaneous preterm labor as defined by one of two clinical characteristics: a previous spontaneous preterm birth and a weight of less than 50 kg before pregnancy. Out of these high-risk women, more than 40% had bacterial vaginosis. In this double-blind placebo-controlled randomized trial, patients were treated with a 7-day course of oral metronidazole (500 mg, twice daily) and enteric coated erythromycin (300 mg, twice daily). Bacterial vaginosis was associated with a significantly higher rate of preterm delivery at less than 37, 34, or 32 weeks' gestation, regardless of treatment assignment. Antibiotic therapy was only associated with a lower rate of spontaneous preterm birth at less than 37 weeks and only in women with bacterial vaginosis. Thus, there appears to be no benefit in treating women without bacterial vaginosis and who have a very preterm birth (i.e., < 32 weeks).

These findings were similar to those of Morales and colleagues[105] who studied women with both bacterial vaginosis and a previous preterm birth, treated with either oral metronidazole or placebo. In these two randomized studies, the beneficial effects were demonstrated in asymptomatic women. Symptomatic patients were not treated within these protocols.

However, contrary to these conclusions and other meta-analyses, a recent systematic review of *all* of the literature found no evidence to support the use of antibiotic treatment for bacterial vaginosis or *Trichomonas vaginalis* in reducing the risk of preterm birth or its associated morbidities in low- or high-risk women. In fact, for women with *T. vaginalis*, the use of metronidazole reduced the risk of persistent infection but increased the incidence of preterm birth.[106]

Major symptoms of preterm labor

A host of complaints may herald preterm labor (Table 62.8) but many of these symptoms are common in normal pregnancy and are often dismissed by prenatal care providers; however, a study comparing the symptoms of women in preterm labor with the normal symptoms of pregnant women indicated that there was significant overlap.[107] Contractions or menstrual-like cramps are often the most conspicuous complaint, with only 13% of preterm labor patients giving a negative response to all questions about these symptoms. Approximately 10% of normal pregnant women complained of painful contractions.

Table 62.8 Chief symptoms of preterm labor.

Abdominal pain
Back pain
Pelvic pain
"Gas pain"
Menstrual-like cramps
Vaginal bleeding
Pinkish staining
Increased vaginal discharge
Pelvic pressure
Urinary frequency
Diarrhea

A common set of complaints relates to painless uterine activity, described as "balling up" and tightening of the uterus. Some complaints are misinterpreted and consequently misreported by the patient, thus misleading both physician and patient. These include "gas pains," intestinal cramps, constipation, and an increase in fetal movements, any of which may represent undiagnosed actual preterm labor.

In a study of outpatients at increased risk for preterm labor being monitored by a HUAM program ($n = 51$), Iams and colleagues[108] found that only 67% of those who developed preterm labor were symptomatic. Uterine activity recordings *per se* without patient symptoms prompted diagnosis in 24%. A further subgroup (9%) were asymptomatic and were discovered only when silent cervical dilation was found during routine cervical examination. However, the numbers in this study were small and further research is needed.

Vague constitutional symptoms relating to the abdomen and pelvis may also indicate preterm labor, and it is generally a good idea to inform patients, especially those at increased risk, about these vague signs. In addition, a bloody vaginal discharge (bright red, pink, brown, or other discoloration) may well be the signal of a cervical change. Patients experiencing any of these preceding symptoms should be encouraged to contact the physician as soon as possible.

Diagnosis

An accurate diagnosis of preterm labor is difficult until labor has obviously advanced beyond the point of successful tocolysis. With this caveat in mind, preterm labor can be classified as threatened or actual. The basis for such a classification is the difference in prognosis. Approximately 85% of patients with threatened preterm labor deliver at term, whereas

40–50% of all patients in actual preterm labor deliver at term.

The hallmark of threatened preterm labor is uterine activity. Threatened preterm labor is diagnosed when the patient has uterine activity but no evidence of cervical changes. Previously, many of these patients may have been diagnosed as having painful Braxton Hicks contractions. The change in terminology is clinically important because it raises an index of suspicion. The recurrence rate of threatened preterm labor in a pregnancy is approximately 30%; of these women, approximately one-half deliver preterm.[109]

Usually, patients with threatened preterm labor respond to simple conservative measures (bedrest, hydration, sedation, or limited doses of subcutaneous terbutaline or nifedipine). Less commonly, continuous infusion of a tocolytic agent may be required for unrelenting, significant uterine activity. The prognosis of a term delivery appears to be improved if preterm labor begins in the third trimester rather than in the second trimester.

During actual preterm labor (as diagnosed by Ingemarsson's criteria[110] – Table 62.9), approximately 20% (3 out of 15) of placebo-treated patients delivered at term, compared with 80% (12 out of 15) of terbutaline-treated patients.[110] Patients with bleeding, uterine malformations, fever, multiple gestation, and other known causes of preterm labor were excluded. All patients were given 10 mg of diazepam intramuscularly; if this had no obvious effect on contractions, treatment was continued with either terbutaline or placebo.

Creasy[111] has modified the Ingemarsson criteria (Table 62.10); these diagnostic criteria are well accepted for nulliparous women; however, although there is general agreement that the same diagnostic criteria can be used for multiparous women, their prognostic value may be less.

Documenting cervical change requires serial documentation of cervical status, ideally by the same examiner and under similar circumstances (e.g., during a contraction). One method of determining cervical change is by noting changes in the Bishop score.[112] Dilation of the internal cervical os or effacement of cervical length are most significant; other measures of change, such as consistency and position, seem to be clinically inadequate for an accurate diagnosis.

Table 62.9 Ingemarsson's criteria for diagnosing preterm labor.

Gestation of 28–36 weeks
Painful, regular, uterine contractions occurring at intervals of less than 10 min, for at least 30 min, by external tocography
Intact membranes
Cervix effaced or almost effaced and dilated between 1 and 4 cm

Adapted from information in ref 110.

Table 62.10 Creasy criteria for diagnosing preterm labor.

Gestation of 20–37 weeks
Documented uterine contractions (4 in 20 min or 8 in 60 min)
Documented cervical change or cervical effacement of 80% or cervical dilation of 2 cm (or more)
Intact membranes

Adapted from information in ref. 111.

Although not part of the diagnostic criteria for actual preterm labor, fetal station has a prognostic value: the lower the station, the greater the risk of spontaneous preterm delivery. A patient who has a lower frequency of documented uterine contractions with a higher degree of cervical compliance based on the Bishop scoring criteria or transvaginal cervical sonography is at an increased risk for premature delivery.

To be most successful, many practitioners believe that tocolytic therapy should be started before serial cervical change is documented. However, a report by Utter and colleagues[113] disputes this idea of early tocolysis. The authors compared the preterm delivery rates before tocolysis in 98 patients without serial cervical changes in dilation or effacement (group 1) and 75 patients with serial cervical changes (group 2). In both groups, the mean dilation before ritodrine therapy, as well as other risk factors, were the same. The outcomes of each group were not statistically different, with 50% of group 2 patients and 40% of group 1 patients delivering at term. The authors concluded that, even with significant cervical dilation (up to 3 cm), observation was a reasonable alternative until subsequent uterine activity and cervical change could be determined to indicate ritodrine therapy.

The use of cervical sonography and fFN measurements may further define who could benefit from tocolysis as the combination of both a positive fFN and a short cervix was strongly associated with preterm delivery (Fig. 62.7).[114]

Managing preterm labor

After a diagnosis of preterm labor is made, appropriate evaluations and initial management plans are instituted. The evaluation phase has two major parts: first, the need for tocolytic therapy is assessed, focusing on the specific nature of the agents to be used and, second, an etiological diagnostic workup is carried out.

During evaluation, the physician seeks contraindications to substantially prolonging the pregnancy (Table 62.11). Temporary efforts to inhibit uterine activity (so that antenatal corticosteroids can be given, the mother can be transported to a tertiary care center, and conditions for maternal and fetal well-being can be optimized) must be weighed against the relative urgency and necessity of delivery.

Ideally, tocolysis should not be given to patients with threatened preterm labor who resolve their uterine activity with conservative therapy. In these patients, testing for fFN and evaluating the cervix for anatomical changes by digital and sonographic examination may help prevent patients from undergoing prolonged surveillance and tocolysis. The fundamental issue involved in withholding tocolytic agents because

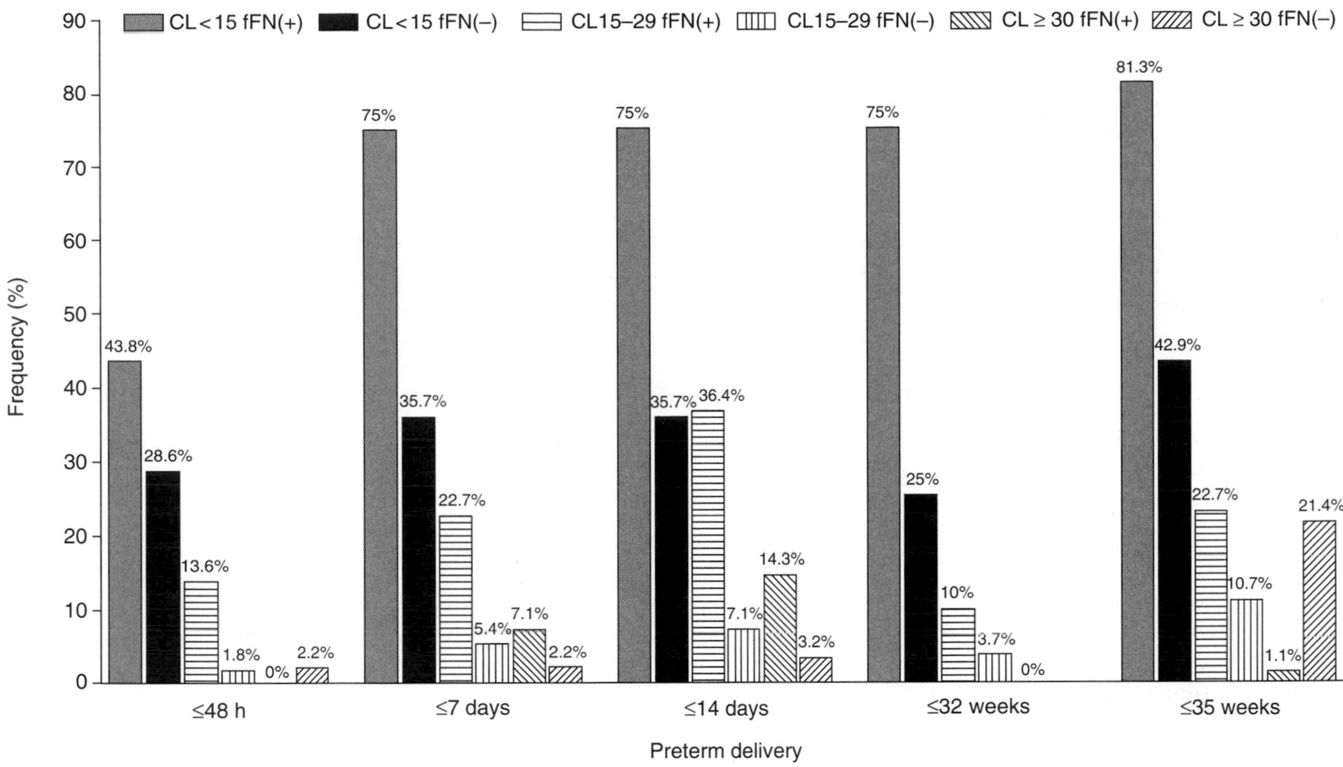

Figure 62.7 Frequency of spontaneous preterm delivery according to cervical length (CL), categorized as < 15 mm, 15–29 mm, and ≥ 30 mm, and vaginal fFN measurement. (From ref. 113.)

Table 62.11 Contraindications to tocolysis.

Absolute contraindications	Relative contraindications
Fetal demise	Fetal heart rate abnormalities
Lethal fetal anomaly	Fetal growth restriction
Severe preeclampsia or eclampsia requiring immediate delivery	Preeclampsia not requiring immediate delivery
Chorioamnionitis	Stable late second or third trimester vaginal bleeding
Severe hemorrhage	Significant maternal disease
	Cervical dilation ≥ 5.0 cm
	Progressive structural but nonlethal fetal anomalies

of contraindications to therapy is whether the odds of delivery and its attendant maternal and perinatal risks outweigh the odds of prolonging the pregnancy with medical interventions and its attendant maternal and perinatal risks.

The lower limit for initiating tocolysis in a favorable candidate is approximately 17–20 weeks' gestation. Different opinions exist as to what are the upper limits of fetal age and weight for appropriate tocolytic therapy. In "uncomplicated" patients, some physicians initiate tocolytic therapy at 36 weeks' gestation.[115] Based on changes in the vascular intracranial anatomy and nursery performance of cardiovascular, pulmonary, and gastrointestinal systems, few data support an overly aggressive tocolytic approach at tertiary care centers beyond the beginning of the 35th week, or an estimated fetal weight of 2000 g, particularly if fetal lung maturity is present. Once the appropriateness of therapy has been determined, the physician must take a number of factors into account before deciding which tocolytic agent to give (Table 62.12).

During the initial evaluation period, some authors recommend performing microbiological cultures (including amniotic fluid), urine toxicology, and baseline maternal cardiac, hematological, and electrolyte evaluations. While these test results are pending and the mother and fetus are deemed stable, a thorough ultrasound examination is done to complete the etiological and prognostic evaluation. Table 62.13 lists the factors to be assessed by ultrasonography; many of these factors have a tremendous influence on clinical management.

Fetal age, weight, and growth status

Gestational age is one of the most important determinations that must be made. Of course, gestational age is not one number but rather a range of numbers based on the best obstetric estimate. At best, sonographic fetal age, based on biometry, is an estimate determined by the mean for a population of normally grown and uncomplicated fetuses.

Routine fetal biometric measurements should be performed including the biparietal diameter (BPD), head circumference,

Table 62.12 Agent-specific contraindications.

Beta-agonist
New York Heart Classification 2 or higher
Cardiac arrhythmias or maternal tachycardia
Severe hypertension
Thyrotoxicosis
Asymmetric septal hypertrophy
Uncontrolled diabetes mellitus
Adrenal tumors
Neurological thromboembolic phenomena
Magnesium sulfate
Myasthenia gravis
Heart block
Certain cardiac rhythm disturbances
Myocardial damage
Severe renal disease (may be used with specific precautions)
Prostaglandin synthesis inhibitors
Maternal:
Hepatic insufficiency
Coagulation disorder
Peptic ulcer disease
Uncontrolled hypertension
Renal disease
Aspirin sensitivity
Fetal:
Oligohydramnios
Gestational age > 32–34 weeks
Monozygotic twins
Discordant twins
Ductal dependent cardiac defect

Table 62.13 Fetal and maternal assessment via ultrasonography.

Fetal evaluation
Age, weight, and growth status
Life and fetal number
Lie, presentation, and position
Well-being
Behavior
Anatomy and sex
Blood and sampling (funicentesis) for rapid karyotype, blood gases, disease-specific hematologic profiles
Amniotic fluid evaluation
Polyhydramnios
Oligohydramnios
Amniocentesis for infection, fetal pulmonary maturation, fetal hemolysis
Placental and funic evaluation
Previa
Abruption
Marginal bleed with membrane separation
Location, internal anatomy, contour, thickness, and grade
Umbilical cord insertion sites
Funic presentation
Umbilical artery Doppler
Uterine and cervical evaluation
Defective uterine scar
Uterine septum
Weak lower uterine segment
Cervical length
Cervical dilation
Myomatous uterus

occipitofrontal diameter (OFD), cephalic index, abdominal circumference (AC), and femur length (FL). After the gestational age has been assigned, the estimated fetal weight (EFW) should be calculated; it is recommended to use the formulae of Shepard and colleagues[116] or Hadlock and colleagues[117] to calculate the EFW. In cases of dolichocephaly, fetal age and weight are underestimated and this finding should be included in any decision-making.

The determination of EFW also becomes important at the lower limits of viability. As with gestational age, estimating fetal weight by sonography carries an inherent error. At the lower limits of viability, a 10% error in predicted birthweight usually corresponds to less than 75 g. Assuming a fetal weight gain of 15 g per day at 24–25 weeks' gestation, this is equivalent to ±5 days of average fetal growth. Although some patients have marked fetal growth restriction, birthweight is still the cornerstone of immediate neonatal prognosis, particularly for infants who weigh less than 1000 g.[5] Accordingly, a determination of fetal weight is useful for predelivery counseling regarding prognosis and is superior, at times, to standard determinations of gestational age at predicting survival.[118] In the same study,[118] BPD was even more reliable than EFW in determining neonatal prognosis, and performed as well as actual birthweight.

After age and weight have been assigned, intrauterine growth status should be assessed. Several investigators have suggested that fetal growth restriction is more common than expected in the setting of preterm labor.[119,120] Westgren and colleagues[121] studied the relationship of idiopathic preterm labor to fetal growth retardation by assessing the ratio of femur length to abdominal circumference (FL/AC). Previously, two groups had found that, between 21 and 42 weeks' gestation, the FL/AC was constant (22 ± 2%) and independent of gestational age.[122,123] Westgren and colleagues[121] found that 41% of infants who were delivered prematurely after failed tocolysis had an FL/AC above 23.5 (indicating asymmetric fetal growth restriction) compared with 5% of patients in preterm labor who responded well to tocolytic therapy.

A finding of fetal growth restriction is of great clinical relevance and importance in management at the lower limits of fetal viability (i.e., 22–25 weeks). In these situations, sonographic measurements may underestimate fetal age secondary to suboptimal growth, and the infant may be erroneously declared previable. In cases of fetal growth restriction at the other end of the prematurity spectrum (32 to 36 weeks), it is not uncommon to find fetal pulmonary maturity when performing transabdominal amniocentesis.

Fetal number

Preterm labor is at least 12 times more common in multiple pregnancies than in singleton pregnancies.[8] In the USA, there is a 50% chance that a multiple gestation will be delivered before 37 weeks.[7] More than 50% of all twins and 90% of all triplets are delivered with LBWs compared with 6% of all singletons.[7]

Assisted reproductive technology has led to an increase in the numbers of twins and higher order multiple gestations. Twins resulting from selective reduction of higher order multifetal gestations are born earlier and weigh less than twins who began their pregnancy as twins. It is not clear why this occurs but reduced pregnancies have a higher incidence of placental abruption and spontaneous preterm labor.[124,125]

Multiple gestations also have a higher incidence of many other maternal and fetal complications that strongly influence the management of preterm labor and delivery. These include complications such as preeclampsia (incidence of 20–33%), severe polyhydramnios, fetal growth restriction, fetal malformation, nonimmune hydrops, and twin–twin transfusion syndrome. Therefore, a complete sonographic evaluation is required for appropriate decision-making and choice of drug therapy in multiple gestations that are complicated by preterm labor. When using tocolysis combined with fluid therapy, the risk of pulmonary edema is higher in multiple gestation than in singleton pregnancies. To prevent pulmonary edema, total fluid intake should be restricted to 3000 mL of salt-free or salt-poor solutions per 24 h.

Malpresentation

Fetal malpresentation is common in patients with preterm labor and delivery; the incidence of malpresentation is inversely related to gestational age. Using sonography, it is possible to detect an associated uterine malformation, placental abnormality, polyhydramnios, oligohydramnios, or fetal abnormality. Suspicion of a fetal malformation or genetic syndrome is warranted in cases of malpresentation as there is a higher incidence of fetal malformation in the preterm breech infant; Nisell and colleagues[126] reported an incidence of fetal malformation of 13.6% in all breech infants born after 28 weeks' gestation and weighing less than 2500 g at birth. Additionally, Braun and colleagues[127] reported a higher incidence of breech-presenting fetuses in a variety of cases of fetal malformation or neuromuscular dysfunction. These included hydrocephalus, neural tube defects, trisomy syndromes 18, 13, and 21, myotonic dystrophy, and other uncommon syndromes.

When faced with preterm delivery (from 25 to 34 weeks) of a breech-presenting fetus in the absence of other clinically pertinent maternal or fetal complications, most specialists in maternal–fetal medicine usually perform a Cesarean section, despite the fact that there is little scientific proof to justify this approach.[128,129] It is appropriate to consider performing a Cesarean section for singleton breech-presenting fetuses estimated to weigh between 600 and 1500 g with a gestational age of 24–32 weeks. At less than 600 g or less than 24 weeks' gestation, inherent fetal biology is thought to be a better predictor of survival or intraventricular hemorrhage (IVH) than delivery mode.

Individualization of care is necessary regarding the delivery mode of extremely LBW preterm breech infants. Head entrapment, which has a reported incidence of 5–10%, may occur in both vaginal and Cesarean deliveries.[130] However, management of this complication is thought to be easier at Cesarean section than at vaginal delivery.

Fetal well-being

Fetal well-being during the course of preterm labor is most commonly assessed using the nonstress test. A classically reactive test is most widely defined as at least two accelerations of fetal heart rate of 15 beats per minute (b.p.m.) for 15 s during a 20-min monitoring period. If the criteria for reactivity are not met, the test is considered nonreactive; this is usually as a result of fetal sleep cycles, medication, or prematurity, especially at less than 32 weeks' gestation. Once sleep cycles or drugs are eliminated then a further assessment of well-being is indicated.

Because the contraction stress test is strongly contraindicated in the presence of preterm labor, the test of choice for further fetal evaluation is the biophysical profile. Fetal tone, fetal movement, amniotic fluid volume, and fetal breathing movements (FBMs) are all usually manifested weeks before classic fetal heart reactivity.[131] According to the criteria of Manning and colleagues,[132] fetal oxygenation is sufficient if these four parameters are present, regardless of reactivity.

In the setting of preterm labor, modifications of classical criteria for a reactive nonstress test have been described by Castillo and colleagues.[133] By defining reactivity as three accelerations of 10 b.p.m., all fetuses tested at 26 weeks were reactive at the end of the 60-min monitoring period, and approximately 90% of the 24-week fetuses were reactive.

Umbilical artery reverse diastolic flow can be ominous and indicates little time for conservative management. Other noninvasive data are prone to high false-positive rates. Accordingly, if noninvasive data are contradictory with regard to oxygenation status, particularly in fetuses at high risk for acidosis yet remote from term, funicentesis (percutaneous umbilical cord sampling) can be helpful in the optimal management of preterm labor. This technique has been well described by Amon and colleagues.[134] If the results of fetal acid–base status are within the normal range, a few days of expectant management may be helpful to enable antenatal glucocorticoid administration.[135]

Fetal breathing movements

There seems to be a significant decrease in FBMs during true labor. Several investigators have observed that the presence or absence of FBMs may identify the patients in preterm labor destined to deliver within 2–7 days of diagnosis.[136–138] This prediction is most accurate in uncomplicated preterm labor without membrane rupture, antepartum hemorrhage, or multiple gestation, and before the initiation of tocolytic therapy.

In a comparison with fFN testing, measurements of FBMs were a less reliable indicator of preterm labor than a negative fFN result or a Bishop score of less than 2.[139] The use of indomethacin for tocolysis is clearly associated with an increase in FBMs,[140] whereas magnesium sulfate may be associated with a decrease in FBMs.

In patients who delivered at less than 32 weeks and within 24 h of a FBM test, Sherer and colleagues[141] found that severe umbilical vasculitis was less frequent in cases in which FBMs were present compared with cases in which FBMs were absent [8 out of 55 (15%) versus 18 out of 56 (32%)]. They concluded that histological evidence of fetal inflammation is associated with an absence of fetal breathing but not chorioamnionitis, even in cases with intact membranes.

Fetal malformation

There is an increased incidence of fetal malformations in patients with preterm labor.[142] Often, these patients have advanced preterm labor, spontaneous rupture of membranes, or vaginal bleeding. In a study of more than 30 000 women who had experienced three singleton births,[49] fetal malformation was most common in infants born prematurely. It was not uncommon to find multiple congenital anomalies, and the rate of central nervous system malformations was as high as 8 per 1000 pregnancies. Overall, the relative risk that an infant with a congenital malformation would be born preterm was 2.0.

Therefore, it is important to perform a complete fetal malformation screen during preterm labor. If sonographic evidence suggests aneuploidy, a rapid fetal karyotype may be useful for optimal medical and obstetric management of labor, mode of delivery, place of delivery, and neonatal resuscitation.[143] If a lethal karyotype is found, tocolysis should be discontinued.

Polyhydramnios

Polyhydramnios is an uncommon but important cause of preterm labor. It occurs as a result of uterine overdistention and has been defined as an amniotic fluid volume of more than 2000 mL. It is usually diagnosed when uterine enlargement is greater than expected for gestational age and there is an inability to palpate fetal parts. Massive uterine overdistention may result in maternal respiratory compromise and postrenal obstruction. As many as 40% of patients with polyhydramnios experience preterm labor and delivery.[144] Sonography is used to confirm the diagnosis, to help determine the proximate cause, and to guide therapeutic mechanical relief via reduction amniocentesis.

Polyhydramnios may be caused by maternal, fetal, or placental factors, or by a combination of factors. In one study,[145] approximately 60% of cases were idiopathic. Maternal causes include diabetes mellitus and red cell alloimmunization (anti-D, anti-Kell, etc.); these conditions can be readily excluded using laboratory tests. Fetal etiologies include a complicated multiple gestation, nonimmune hydrops, and structural congenital malformations. Fetal malformations were found in 75% of cases with severe polyhydramnios compared with 29% of mild cases.[145] Central nervous system defects account for approximately 45–50% of all fetal malformations, upper gastrointestinal defects represent approximately 30%, and circulatory abnormalities account for approximately 7%. A placental cause of polyhydramnios is a large chorioangioma, a benign vascular malformation that acts like an arteriovenous shunt. Tumors that are large enough to produce polyhydramnios and cause preterm labor are rare and associated with fetal hydrops.

The rate of preterm labor and delivery is related to the underlying cause rather than to the degree of polyhydramnios: fetuses with congenital abnormalities [16 out of 41 (39%)] and those of diabetic mothers [10 out of 45 (22%)] had a significantly higher incidence of preterm birth than those with idiopathic polyhydramnios. In contrast, for mild cases of polyhydramnios, preterm delivery occurred in 37 of 199 (19%), in moderate cases, 12 out of 55 (22%), and in severe cases, 3 of 21 (14%)], thus indicating no significant differences in prematurity for varying degrees of polyhydramnios.[146]

Oligohydramnios

Oligohydramnios is caused by a significant reduction in amniotic fluid volume and is easily diagnosed with ultrasound. In the setting of preterm labor, it may occur as a result of premature rupture of the membranes, maternal intake of nonsteroidal anti-inflammatory agents, severe intrauterine growth retardation, or a genitourinary malformation in which fetal urination into the amniotic cavity is absent. Serial sonography and invasive procedures can differentiate between these causes.

The diagnosis of lethal renal diseases is important because many of these cases may present with fetal distress or malpresentation during preterm labor; these are the two most common fetal indications for Cesarean section. Approximately 60% of patients with Potter's syndrome develop preterm labor, and 40–60% are in breech presentation.[147] In these situations, Cesarean section is performed solely for maternal indications. Tocolysis is not indicated except for possible diagnostic evaluation and maternal transfer.

Fetal gender

A curiosity of preterm birth is an excess of male fetuses, which has been demonstrated in multiple studies. A more recent analysis[148] found a 7.2% excess of male fetuses among singleton preterm births of white women with an increased effect in married women. Male excess was also found in twins born prematurely to white women but to a lesser degree than singletons. Out of 14948 low-risk singleton pregnancies included in the RADIUS study, male fetuses accounted for a 13.6% population–attributable risk for spontaneous preterm labor, an even stronger effect than a positive urine culture.[149] These data suggest the existence of a mechanism of preterm birth that is influenced by fetal gender.

Fetal gender has important prognostic significance; female infants weighing less than 1000g have a significant survival advantage.[5] By regression analysis, Fleisher and colleagues[150] found that the lecithin–sphingomyelin (L/S) ratio in female fetuses reached 2:1 at 33.7 weeks, 1.4 weeks earlier than in male fetuses. Phosphatidylglycerol first appeared at 34 weeks in female and at 35 weeks in male fetuses.

Amniocentesis and neonatal outcome

In experienced hands, amniocentesis carries a minimal risk in the late second trimester or third trimester, and there is no scientific evidence that it stimulates labor. Leigh and Garite[26] used amniocentesis during preterm labor to detect subclinical infection and fetal pulmonary maturity and found that 12% had positive culture results. These patients presented at earlier gestational ages and were more likely to have ruptured membranes and to deliver within 48 h of admission than those with negative culture results. One-third of the patients at 31–32 weeks' and 50% of those at 33 weeks' gestation or more had mature L/S ratios.

The amniotic cavity is normally sterile; thus, isolation of any organism indicates microbial invasion. Microorganisms can gain access to the cavity by ascending from the lower genital tract, maternal hematogenous spread, retrograde fallopian tube spread, and iatrogenic introduction during invasive prenatal diagnostic and therapeutic procedures. The most common organisms found in the amniotic fluid are *Ureaplasma urealyticum*, *Mycoplasma hominis*, and *Fusobacterium* species.

In a review of 11 studies of transabdominal amniocentesis in patients with preterm labor and intact membranes, Romero and Mazor[25] found a positive culture rate of 16%. In the patients with positive culture results, 58% had clinical chorioamnionitis, 65% were refractory to tocolysis, and 40% had membrane rupture. The respective rates of these complications in patients with negative culture results were 7%, 16%, and 4%. Although a large percentage of the microbes recovered were anaerobic, neonates rarely developed significant anaerobic infections. A review of preterm labor patients with intact membranes found that amniotic fluid infection occurred at a rate of approximately 13%.[149] Approximately 10–15% of neonates in the positive culture group developed sepsis compared with approximately 2% in the negative culture group.[151]

Rapid amniotic fluid tests for infection have been studied. The most common tests in order of descending sensitivity are measurements of IL-6 levels, a glucose concentration of less than or equal to 15 mg/dL, a white blood cell count greater than or equal to 50 cells/μL, and Gram's stain.[152] Leukocyte esterase and catalase tests have also been performed.[153] The false-positive rates for glucose concentration and white blood cell counts are high.

The appropriate management of patients with positive intra-amniotic culture results remains controversial. Some regimens include antibiotics and immediate delivery but, in others, the fetus is delivered only when there is clear clinical evidence of infection, particularly in fetuses of 25–26 weeks or less. For fetuses of 34 weeks' gestation or more, delivery in the setting of a positive amniotic fluid culture result appears reasonable.

In 1990, we analyzed neonatal morbidity in preterm infants born with mature amniotic fluid tests (Table 62.14).[154] The mothers presented with spontaneous preterm labor and were potential candidates for tocolytic therapy. We found that despite pulmonary maturity, RDS and other morbidities still occurred as an inverse function of gestational age. Hence, prolongation of pregnancy should still be attempted even in the presence of mature amniotic fluid indices for selected patients at less than 34 weeks' gestation. It should be noted that none of the infants had significant RDS at 34 weeks or more. In 1993, Wigton and colleagues[155] confirmed our findings regarding the high false maturity rate of pulmonary maturity tests in the preterm infant with resultant neonatal morbidity.

Konte and colleagues[156] found a similar inverse relationship between neonatal morbidity and gestational age (Table 62.15). In a more indigent population, Lewis and colleagues[157] found a lower rate of RDS of approximately 15% at 34 weeks, with a negligible incidence at 35 weeks or beyond. They recommended that delivery be delayed through the 34th week. At 34–36 weeks, Myers and colleagues[158] found that fetal lung maturity testing was a cost-effective procedure. Testing of fetal lung maturity is biochemically similar between twin and singleton pregnancies and has the same neonatal prognostic value for a given gestational age.[159]

Uterine malformations

A review of pregnancy outcome in 182 women with uterine anomalies found that preterm labor occurred in approximately 25% of 265 pregnancies.[160] Patients with complete bicornuate uteri had the highest incidence of preterm labor (66%), but the number of such patients studied was small (n = 6). Didelphia and all varieties of bicornuate uteri were associated with a greater than 20% incidence of preterm labor, whereas preterm labor occurred in up to 37.5% of patients

Table 62.14 Neonatal morbidity in infants born with mature amniotic fluid tests.

Complication	Gestational age (weeks)			
	< 33 (*n* = 15)	33 (*n* = 13)	34 (*n* = 19)	35–36 (*n* = 35)
RDS	7 (47)	2 (15)	0	0
Air leak	2 (13)	1 (8)	0	0
NEC	1 (7)	3 (23)	0	0
IVH	4 (27)	1 (8)	2 (11)	0
Sepsis	7 (47)	2 (15)	0	0
Blood transfusion	8 (53)	4 (31)	2 (11)	1 (3)
TPN	8 (53)	5 (39)	1 (5)	1 (3)
BWT (mean ± SD)	1563 ± 489	1925 ± 283	2177 ± 259	2442 ± 333

From ref. 154, with permission.

Percentages (in parentheses) are rounded to nearest percent.

BWT, birthweight (g); IVH, intraventricular hemorrhage; NEC, necrotizing enterocolitis; RDS, respiratory distress syndrome; SD, standard deviation; TPN, total parenteral nutrition.

Table 62.15 Neonatal morbidity rates by gestational age at birth.

Complication	Gestational age (weeks)					
	26–27 (*n* = 16)	28–29 (*n* = 32)	30–31 (*n* = 33)	32–33 (*n* = 44)	34 (*n* = 40)	35 (*n* = 36)
Intensive care nursery	16 (100)	32 (100)	31 (94)	40 (91)	29 (73)	8 (22)
RDS	13 (81)	19 (59)	10 (30)	13 (30)	9 (23)	1 (3)
Patent ductus arteriosus	8 (50)	16 (50)	7 (21)	6 (14)	5 (13)	–
Sepsis	5 (31)	8 (25)	5 (15)	3 (7)	2 (5)	2 (6)
IVH	5 (31)	4 (13)	1 (3)	–	–	–
NEC	4 (29)	2 (6)	2 (6)	1 (2)	–	–

From ref. 156, with permission.

Percentages (in parentheses) are rounded to nearest percent.

with unicornuate uteri.[161] The best fetal survival rate was found in women with complete septate uteri (86%), whereas the worst rates were found in women with complete bicornuate (50%) and unicornuate uteri (40%). Uterine anomalies may be associated with cervical incompetence, malpresentation, and maternal genitourinary malformations.

Management decisions at the lower end of viability

Managing preterm delivery at the lower limits of viability (currently 22–24 weeks' gestation) is a vexing problem. The biological and clinical variables associated with obstetric and neonatal management that favorably influence neonatal outcome have been reviewed.[5,11,12,118,162–164] It is optimal for delivery in such cases to occur in immediate proximity to a neonatal intensive care center.[165] When conditions permit, decisions regarding delivery of a severely preterm fetus (i.e., 22–26 weeks' gestation by best obstetric estimate) are ideally made after the mother has been transported to a tertiary care center. Highly coordinated predelivery family counseling by obstetricians and neonatal physicians is recommended to discuss the prognosis and plan management, thereby minimizing anxiety, confusion, and fear.

Survival rates increase as a function of gestational age and birthweight. Gestational age-specific survival rates and management recommendations have been reviewed.[166,167] The survival rate is 50% at 24 weeks' gestation, between 60% and 70% at 25 weeks, and between 70% and 80% at 26 weeks.[13,167–169] Improvements in birthweight-specific survival from 1983 to 1996 are shown in Table 62.16. Literature reviews have found that subsequent severe handicap rates in extremely preterm survivors are about 30%.[167,170,171] Of all extremely LBW nonsurvivors, 70–80% die in the first week of postnatal life, most in the first few days.[11,172]

Consideration of Cesarean section for fetal distress should begin at an estimated gestational age of 24 weeks, an estimated weight of 600 g, or both. In infants weighing less than 1000 g, survival based on birthweight has tighter confidence

Table 62.16 Improvements in neonatal survival with increasing birthweight in extremely low birthweight infants.

Birthweight (g)	Neonatal survival (%)					
	University of Tennessee at Memphis (1983–1985)*	St. Louis University (1986–1991)†	NIH Neonatal Network (1988–1989)‡	NIH Neonatal Network (1989–1990)‡	NIHCD Centers (1995–1996)§	St. Louis University (1992–1996)¶
400–499	–	–	–	–	11	–
500–599	9	25	18	20	27	48
600–699	23	52	30	41	63	62
700–799	43	59	56	65	74	71
800–899	66	–	65	76	–	85
900–999	64	–	–	–	–	89

*From ref. 11: $n = 263$, 500–1000 g.

†From ref. 12: $n = 156$, 500–750 g.

‡From ref. 167: $n = 752$, 500–1000 g.

§From ref. 166: $n = 4438$, 401–800 g.

¶Data from Barbara Cohlan MD, Director of Nurseries, St. Mary's Health Center, and William Keenan MD, Director of Neonatology: $n = 398$, 500–1000 g.

intervals than that based on gestational age.[168] Accordingly, intervention based on EFW is a reasonable approach at the borderline of viability. Outcome based on BPD assessment is even more superior to EFW and is in line with birthweight.[118]

An obstetric willingness to perform Cesarean delivery for fetal indications is associated with an increased rate of survival and a virtual absence of intrapartum stillbirth.[173] This willingness was an even better predictor of survival than either the obstetrician's opinion of viability or actual Cesarean section;[174,175] it results in both a greater likelihood of intact survival and survival with serious morbidity.

Because of inherent inaccuracies in estimating fetal age and weight, survival considerations on behalf of the fetus should begin at between 22 and 23 weeks' gestation and 450–500 g. The likelihood for survival in these instances is very low (i.e., less than 10–20%); therefore, Cesarean section for fetal indications is best avoided. Survival, if it occurs, generally occurs regardless of the delivery mode. To protect the mother from an undue risk of Cesarean section, which has little potential benefit for the newborn, the mother should be offered all other available options including transfer to a tertiary care center, family counseling, standard hydration, fetal monitoring, maternal positioning, maternal oxygenation, controlled sterile delivery, and the presence of one or two neonatologists at delivery. Additional measures include transcervical amnioinfusion and acute tocolysis for uterine relaxation.[176,177]

Tocolytic agents

In the last five decades, a host of drugs have been used in the attempt to inhibit preterm labor. These include relaxin, beta-sympathomimetic agents, ethanol, prostaglandin synthetase inhibitors, organic calcium-channel blockers, magnesium sulfate, diazoxide, aminophylline, progestogens, and, more recently, oxytocin analogs that block oxytocin receptors and nitric oxide donors. Many of the older agents had high success rates initially, but subsequent reports have shown a reduced and somewhat limited efficacy.

Beta-sympathomimetic agents

Beta adrenergic receptors have been described by Lands and colleagues.[178] Beta-1 receptors are predominately found in the heart, small intestine, and adipose tissue, whereas beta-2 receptors are predominately found in the uterus, blood vessels, bronchioles, and liver. Some agents (e.g., ritodrine) have been promoted as having selective beta-2 activity.[179] Beta-2 selective sympathomimetic amines are structurally related to catecholamines and stimulate all beta receptors throughout the entire body.[180] Tachyphylaxis is seen with continued use;[181,182] however, a short course of intermittent therapy may provide a sustained myometrial response.

The side-effects of these agents represent an exaggeration of their physiological effects. The following complications of the cardiovascular system are found: peripheral vasodilation with a decrease in diastolic blood pressure, a positive chronotropic effect with decreased ventricular filling time, a positive inotropic effect, and a tendency toward arrhythmogenesis.[183] Supraventricular tachycardia, nonspecific T-wave changes, and transient ST-segment depression all resolve with discontinuation of drug therapy. It is not uncommon to find chest pain with parenteral administration. These drugs increase oxygen demand and decrease coronary artery perfusion. They may cause myocardial ischemia; however, levels of cardiac isoenzymes are not increased. These clinical and electrocardiographic findings may relate directly to drug therapy or indirectly to electrolyte disturbance *per se*, rather than to ischemia.[184] Maternal cardiac death has also been reported.[185–187]

Pulmonary edema may occur in a small percentage of patients treated with parenteral beta-sympathomimetic agents.[183] This life-threatening complication has several predisposing factors: multiple gestation, a positive fluid balance, blood transfusion, anemia, infection, associated hypertension, polyhydramnios, and underlying cardiac disease. Ritodrine causes the retention of salt and water at the level of the kidney;[180] plasma volume expands and the hematocrit level drops by 10–15%.[188] These findings highlight the importance of refraining from using isotonic fluids throughout ritodrine therapy, restricting total fluids to less than 3000 mL/day, and maintaining a meticulous fluid intake and output record. Because betamethasone and dexamethasone are almost devoid of mineralocorticoid activity, they may be used safely with beta-mimetics.[189]

Metabolic complications, such as hypokalemia resulting from increases in glucose and insulin, hyperglycemia resulting from glucagon stimulation and glycogenolysis, and an increase in free fatty acids as a result of lipolysis, are common with intravenous therapy.[190,191] Less common is lactic acidosis and ketosis,[192] and occasionally there have been cases of diabetic ketoacidosis.[193] Ritodrine has less effect on glucose intolerance than does oral terbutaline.[194–196]

The effects on uteroplacental perfusion are controversial; some studies have shown an increase, whereas others have shown a decrease.[197,198] Placental transfer does occur and it is not uncommon for the fetus to develop a mild tachycardia. Common effects on the neonate have been limited primarily to hypoglycemia, occasional ileus, hypocalcemia, and hyperbilirubinemia.[199] Apgar scores are not significantly affected,[200] and long-term follow-up studies have revealed no significant problems in child development.[201–205]

Controversy exists as to whether there is an association between beta-agonist tocolysis and neonatal IVH.[206–208] However, a large and very well-designed prospective randomized placebo-controlled Canadian study of ritodrine tocolysis could not demonstrate any increased risk of IVH in the group given ritodrine.[209] Sinclair[210] noted no difference in the treatment arms of this study with regard to corticosteroid usage, supporting the view that beta-agonist tocolysis with and without corticosteroid therapy does not increase the risk of IVH.

Ritodrine

Favorable reports in 1980 by Barden and colleagues[185] and Merkatz and colleagues[211] promulgated the clinical use of ritodrine in the USA. Ritodrine became the first drug approved by the Food and Drug Administration (FDA) for the inhibition of preterm labor. It was reported to have a similar efficacy but fewer side-effects than previously used tocolytic agents and, generally, the side-effects were thought to be acceptable. There was evidence that it prolonged pregnancy and, when compared with control subjects, there was a significant reduction in the incidence of neonatal death and RDS.[211]

A subsequent meta-analysis of ritodrine efficacy was performed on 890 women who participated in 16 scientifically acceptable controlled trials.[212] There were significantly fewer deliveries in the beta-mimetic group during the first 24 and 48 h of therapy, and there was a slight reduction in the percentage of preterm deliveries in the group receiving beta-mimetic therapy. However, there was no significant reduction in the incidence of LBW infants, respiratory distress morbidity, or perinatal mortality. The Canadian trial found a statistically significant 48-h delay in labor in women receiving ritodrine as opposed to placebo, and there was a trend toward improved neonatal survival in women receiving ritodrine who were randomized at between 24 and 27 weeks.[209]

Ritodrine infusions should be given according to the guidelines in the manufacturer's package insert[185] or according to the method of Caritis and colleagues.[213] Attention should be paid to contraindications as shown in Table 62.12. Intramuscular ritodrine administration has been described[214] and consists of three injections of 5–10 mg of ritodrine at 2-h intervals. This method appears to be a safe and effective alternate route to intravenous therapy.[215]

To date, beta-agonists have not been shown to be effective when given as a prophylactic agent. In fact, one meta-analysis has indicated the lack of tocolytic efficacy of standard oral beta-agonist maintenance therapy.[216]

A European report of a randomized, double-blind, placebo-controlled trial of a sustained release ritodrine capsule resulting in three daily doses of 80 mg of ritodrine found significant benefits compared with the control group.[217] Recurrent preterm labor occurred much less often in the treatment group [1 out of 50 (2%) compared with 11 out of 45 (25%) patients]; and spontaneous preterm delivery occurred less often (0 out of 50 compared with 4 out of 45 patients).

Terbutaline

Terbutaline is commonly used in the initial management of preterm labor. Initially, its efficacy was thought to be quite significant but subsequent studies have found that it is limited.[110,218,219] Terbutaline has significant, potentially life-threatening side-effects, similar to those of ritodrine, especially when given intravenously.[183,220]

Terbutaline can also be given subcutaneously; the effect is rapid and there are fewer side-effects.[221–223] The ease of administration and the avoidance of intravenous hydration makes the subcutaneous route a reasonable alternative. In a commonly used regimen, 0.25 mg is given subcutaneously every 20–60 min until contractions have subsided. Close attention is paid to the maternal heart rate and other symptoms, in order to prevent serious complications. Oral administration of terbutaline results in widely varying serum concentrations.[224] The usual daily dose ranges from 10 to 30 mg, with a maximum daily dose of approximately 40 mg. Cardiovascular collapse and peripartum heart failure have been rarely associated with oral terbutaline therapy.[225,226]

A more recent development in terbutaline administration is the use of a continuous subcutaneous infusion pump, although controversy exists regarding the efficacy of this therapy.[227–230] It should be noted that the numbers involved in most of these studies were small and the results inconclusive. This type of outpatient therapy is very expensive and invasive; nonetheless, it has unique features and does ensure round-the-clock compliance.

Prostaglandin synthetase inhibitors

Prostaglandin synthetase inhibitors are among the most effective drugs known for inhibiting preterm labor.[231] They are easily administered and well tolerated by the mother. However, they have only a limited window of human application because of fetal safety.

Out of all the traditional tocolytic agents available, indomethacin is likely to have the greatest efficacy. Zuckerman and colleagues[232] first reported its clinical use as a tocolytic agent in the treatment of preterm labor in 1974. Around 80% of patients responded to 100 mg of indomethacin administered rectally followed by 25 mg given orally every 6 h. Other studies showed similar results.[233,234] When randomized placebo-controlled studies as well as comparison studies were performed, indomethacin (daily dose range from 100 to 200 mg) was found to be significantly more effective than placebo[235,236] or beta-agonists.[237–239] More recent trials indicate that beta-agonists[240–242] and magnesium sulfate[243] have similar efficacy.

Maternal side-effects are minimal and primarily consist of a gastrointestinal upset, which may require the use of calcium carbonate (Maalox). Indomethacin is contraindicated in patients with hematological dysfunction, peptic ulcer disease, and known allergies; it appears to increase the bleeding time. It is relatively contraindicated in maternal renal disease. Indomethacin does not significantly affect uteroplacental perfusion[244] or Apgar scores.[236]

The most significant potential complications in the fetus relate to the premature closure of the ductus arteriosus, right-sided heart failure, and fetal death.[245] The prostaglandin E series allows the ductus arteriosus to remain patent, whereas indomethacin tends to transiently constrict the ductus;[246,247] it is much more likely to reversibly constrict the ductus after 31 weeks.[248] Irreversible closure of the ductus is more likely at a much later gestational age, closer to the time of physiological closure; however, there are case reports of fetal deaths resulting from complete ductal closure.[249] Sonographic evaluation of structural fetal anatomy to rule out a ductal-dependent lesion is thus important before and during therapy of preterm labor with indomethacin. Use for more than 72 h should prompt a further evaluation of the ductus and an investigation to rule out fetal heart failure. Nonetheless, fetal echocardiography reports have suggested the relative cardiovascular safety of indomethacin.[250]

In the neonate, the most feared complication is persistent pulmonary hypertension.[251] Fetal and neonatal oliguria is not uncommon;[252–254] in fact, idiopathic polyhydramnios may be treated effectively with indomethacin.[255,256] Sonographic surveillance for oligohydramnios is indicated when indomethacin is used for more than 72 h. There are case reports of neonatal bowel perforation,[257] and hyperbilirubinemia may occur because indomethacin can displace bilirubin from the binding sites of albumin.[258] Indomethacin use may also predispose to NEC and IVH.[254,259] However, others[260–262] have found no increase in neonatal complications in prenatally exposed infants delivered at less than 32 weeks' gestation. Because of the variance in fetal safety, one could consider these agents as second-line therapy, using proper precautions to minimize fetal and neonatal effects.

The 1980s database suggested that the selective use of indomethacin before 34 weeks' gestation caused no substantial and permanent side-effects to the fetus or neonate.[263,264] However, since that time, there have been reports that suggest both short- and long-term side-effects.[265,266] More recent findings suggest that sulindac has a more favorable safety profile than indomethacin, although both have similar degrees of efficacy.[267–269]

More data are being accumulated using cyclo-oxygenase-2-selective inhibitors (COXIBs), and there may also be a role for the newly developed prostaglandin F2 alpha-receptor antagonists.[270]

Magnesium sulfate

In 1985, magnesium sulfate was the second most commonly prescribed parenteral agent for tocolytic therapy in the USA after beta-sympathomimetic agents.[271] More recent evidence and clinical experience favor magnesium over beta-sympathomimetics with regard to safety and tocolytic efficacy.[272] Magnesium sulfate has become the first-line agent of choice for continuous intravenous tocolytic therapy.

Properly used, magnesium sulfate is safe for both tocolysis and seizure prophylaxis. Most clinicians monitor reflexes, respiration, urine output, and intermittent serum magnesium levels to prevent the serious complication of hypermagnesemia. A diminished glomerular filtration rate diminishes the excretion of magnesium, and continued administration of parenteral magnesium sulfate may result in toxicity as serum levels rise. Fortunately, a fast-acting and safe antidote is readily available; intravenous injection of calcium gluconate or chloride rapidly antagonizes the actions of excessive magnesium.

Pharmacology

Only 30% of the normal daily intake of oral magnesium is absorbed; this absorption occurs in the upper small bowel by an active process. The National Research Council's recommended dietary allowance of magnesium for pregnant women is 450 mg daily. Dietary sources of magnesium are meat, milk, dark-green vegetables, seafood, and chocolate. The kidney is the major regulator of the serum magnesium concentration because magnesium is principally excreted in the urine.[273]

The mechanism by which hypermagnesemia exerts its relaxant effects on smooth muscle differs from that of skeletal muscle. Smooth muscle undergoes pharmacomechanical coupling mediated by various agonists rather than the electromechanical coupling characteristic of skeletal muscle. Excess magnesium depresses the peripheral neuromuscular system by inhibiting acetylcholine release and reducing the sensitivity of the motor end plate potential. Acetylcholine is unnecessary for spontaneous contractility of smooth muscle.

The exact mechanism by which magnesium diminishes or abolishes uterine activity remains unclear. Experimental data support the view that the extracellular magnesium ion concentration affects the uptake, binding, and distribution of intracellular calcium in vascular smooth muscle.[274] Similar mechanisms may operate in gravid uterine smooth muscle. Calcium uptake into postpartum myometrial cells appears to be inhibited by high extracellular magnesium concentrations.[275] The extracellular excess of magnesium results in an increase of 50% in intracellular magnesium concentrations. The inhibition of calcium channel currents appears to be related to magnesium-induced tocolysis.[276]

In general, maternal magnesium sulfate-induced hypermagnesemia is associated with increased urinary excretion of both magnesium and calcium. In the study of Hoff and colleagues,[277] three-fourths of the elemental magnesium infused was excreted during the infusion and 90% was excreted within 24 h of the end of the infusion. The urinary excretion of calcium was three times that observed in control subjects; the mean total maternal serum calcium decreased by 12% and the mean serum ionized calcium by 25%. Acutely, phosphate and calcitonin levels did not change significantly, but the mean parathyroid hormone level increased by approximately 25% from baseline to the end of the infusion.

Maternal side-effects

Tables 62.17 summarizes the major clinical side-effects of maternal hypermagnesemia, and Table 62.18 gives the critical serum levels of magnesium needed for some of these effects to occur. Clinically, respiratory depression from hypermagnesemia does not occur before the disappearance of the deep tendon reflexes. The absence of the reflex arc should therefore serve as a warning sign of impending magnesium toxicity. For patients who inadvertently receive high doses of magnesium intravenously over a short period, the initial clinical presentation may be respiratory or cardiac arrest.[278–280]

One of the most important side-effects encountered during standard tocolytic therapy with magnesium sulfate is chest pain, possibly due to myocardial ischemia. This uncommonly occurs as a result of magnesium sulfate therapy alone, but more often there are additional factors. A higher incidence of cardiorespiratory side-effects occurs in patients undergoing supplemental drug therapy after failed single-agent therapy.[281,282]

A potentially lethal side-effect encountered during magnesium sulfate tocolytic therapy is pulmonary edema. It occurs with an incidence of approximately 1%, compared with 5% in patients receiving beta-sympathomimetics.[283,284] Generally, these cases are complicated by other factors associated with pulmonary edema including multiple gestation, polyhydramnios, preeclampsia, anemia, blood transfusion, chorioam-

Table 62.17 Potential maternal effects of hypermagnesemia.

Common side-effects
Loss of deep tendon reflexes
Warmth during infusion
Mild central hypothermic effects
Increase in skin temperature
Cutaneous vasodilation
Nausea, possible emesis
Not uncommon side-effects seen with moderately elevated serum levels
Somnolence, lethargy, lightheadedness
Visual blurring, diplopia
Dysarthria
Nystagmus
Constipation and dyspepsia
Uncommon side-effects
Potentiation of other neuromuscular blockers
Lengthening of the P-R and QRS interval
Controversial effect on the T wave
Chest pain
Pulmonary edema
Effects seen at very high serum concentrations
Respiratory depression
Cardiac arrest
Profound muscular paralysis
Amnesia
Decreased rate of impulse formation of the sinoatrial node
Rare side-effects
Profound hypotension
Maternal tetany
Hypersensitivity: urticarial reaction
Paralytic ileus

Table 62.18 Critical serum levels for magnesium sulfate.

Therapeutic range	6–8 mg/dL
Loss of deep tendon reflexes	8–12 mg/dL
Respiratory paralysis	12–15 mg/dL
Cardiac arrest	> 20 mg/dL

Based in part on information obtained from ref. 277.

Table 62.19 Potential fetal and neonatal effects of hypermagnesemia.

Controversial effects on fetal heart rate variability
Lack of significant effect on fetal umbilical Doppler studies
Fetal breathing movements decrease
Mean baseline fetal heart rate decreases
Flaccidity, hyporeflexia
Need for assisted ventilation
Weak or absent cry
Transient decreased active tone of neck extensors
Possible transient radiographic bony changes

Modified from ref. 289.

nionitis, positive fluid balance, operative delivery, dual-agent therapy, and prolonged therapy.[285–287] With proper patient selection, judicious therapy, and close monitoring, the risk of pulmonary edema can be minimized.[209]

Perinatal side-effects

Neonatal and fetal side-effects of magnesium sulfate therapy are summarized in Table 62.19.[287] None of the neonatal effects appears to be due to magnesium alone; they may be related to confounding variables such as maternal illness, fetal growth retardation, and prematurity. A decreased bone density is seen in magnesium-treated patients compared with control subjects.[288,289]

Reports of the effect of magnesium sulfate on fetal behavior are inconsistent.[287] Gray and colleagues[290] found no significant decrease in FBMs after intravenous magnesium sulfate therapy. Indeed, they found no significant changes in any characteristic of the fetal biophysical profile when magnesium was used for tocolysis over a 12-h period. However, Sherer[291] demonstrated a blunted fetal response to vibroacoustic stimulation in a study of five pregnant women treated with magnesium sulfate for tocolysis.

Because of both maternal heat loss from peripheral vasodilation and a blunted shivering ability, a maternal central hypothermic effect can occur, with the temperature dropping as low as 94°F (34.4°C). The baseline fetal heart rate changes accordingly as it is very sensitive to maternal temperature, and a temporary benign fetal bradycardia occurs. Concomitant accelerations are reassuring and delivery is not indicated.

Efficacy and relative safety

In 1966, Rusu and colleagues[292] performed the first therapeutic trials of magnesium as a tocolytic agent. In 1977, Steer and Petrie[293] were the first investigators to publish the results of a clinical trial evaluating such therapy in English. They studied 71 patients in preterm labor with intact membranes who had a painful, identifiable contraction pattern with a frequency of 5 min or less. Out of these patients, 31 received ethanol and 31 received intravenous magnesium sulfate; the remaining nine received an infusion of 5% dextrose in water. The magnesium group were given a 4-g loading dose of a 10% solution intravenously, followed by 2 g/h. Successful treatment was defined as the absence of contractions for a 24-h interval. The success rate was higher in the magnesium group (77%) than in both the alcohol group (45%) and the control group (44%). In patients with cervical dilation of 1 cm or less, the respective success rates were 96%, 72%, and 60%. The respective frequencies of patients remaining undelivered for at least 1 week were 74%, 42%, and 33%. The authors concluded that magnesium sulfate may become an alternate method of controlling preterm labor.

In 1982, three studies were published. In a randomized trial of tocolytic therapy with magnesium sulfate versus intravenous terbutaline, Miller and colleagues[294] found that magnesium was equally as effective as terbutaline but resulted in fewer side-effects. Spisso and colleagues[295] reported on a large case series that used magnesium sulfate as the primary tocolytic agent and concluded that it is effective and has minimal adverse effects in patients at risk for preterm delivery. Valenzuela and Cline[296] reported on five patients who, after failing to respond to beta-mimetic agents, were treated successfully with intravenous magnesium sulfate.

In 1983, Elliott[297] reported on 355 patients with and without intact membranes who were treated with magnesium sulfate as the primary tocolytic agent. The author found that magnesium sulfate had a similar efficacy to ritodrine. Failure to respond to magnesium was often as a result of chorioamnionitis, advanced cervical dilation, and placental abruption. Around 7% of patients experienced side-effects but, of these, only 2% required discontinuation of medication.

In 1984, Tchilinguirian and colleagues[298] performed a randomized trial of magnesium sulfate versus intravenous ritodrine and found a similar efficacy. Beall and colleagues[299] performed a randomized trial of ritodrine versus terbutaline versus magnesium sulfate, using each as a primary agent. A crossover arm was used when single-agent primary therapy was unsuccessful. They concluded that, in a busy service, magnesium sulfate was the primary tocolytic agent of choice.

In 1987, Hollander and colleagues[271] carried out an excellent prospective randomized study analyzing the efficacy and safety of magnesium sulfate versus ritodrine. All patients were in preterm labor with intact membranes and associated cervical changes. Successful tocolysis was defined as cessation of uterine activity and delay in delivery for 72 h or more from the onset of treatment. The success rates of ritodrine and magnesium sulfate as primary agents were 83% and 91% respectively. When administered as either a primary or secondary agent, the success rate of ritodrine was 79% and magnesium sulfate was 88%. A delay in delivery of 1 week or more occurred in 72% of patients given ritodrine and 75% of those given magnesium sulfate. The mean serum level of magnesium required to achieve tocolysis was 6.6 mg per 100 mL. The authors concluded that magnesium sulfate was easy to administer and clinically efficacious, and that the side-effects were less alarming than those of ritodrine. They recommended that magnesium sulfate be used as the primary agent for tocolytic therapy, with ritodrine as a back-up.

In 1990, Cox and colleagues[300] published a randomized trial comparing magnesium sulfate therapy with no tocolytic therapy in 156 women thought to be in preterm labor. They found no significant prolongation of pregnancy in the group receiving magnesium. Cox and other authors of tocolytic efficacy studies concluded that magnesium sulfate was ineffective in preventing preterm birth. However, this was not a blind study. In the control group, only 28% delivered within 24 h. Almost two-thirds of the control patients had a delay in delivery of at least 1 week, with most remaining undelivered for more than 28 days. Because the majority of the control group did not readily deliver soon after admission, most patients in this study were not in true actual preterm labor. This finding renders the conclusions of ineffectiveness of magnesium sulfate therapy as speculative at best.

In 1992, Chau and colleagues[301] compared intravenous and oral magnesium therapy versus subcutaneous and oral terbutaline therapy. For short-term tocolysis, no significant differences were found between the groups. However, magnesium was associated with a higher rate of term delivery.

In 1995, Hales and colleagues[302] evaluated the efficacy and safety of magnesium sulfate therapy in twins compared with singletons. The same dosing regimen was used in both groups, and no differences were found between them in terms of efficacy. Areflexia was less common in the twin group, but other side-effects were similar. They concluded that higher dosing was not required in twin gestations. However, tocolysis in higher order multifetal gestations does appear to require higher doses.[303]

When moving the inpatient that responded to intravenous magnesium therapy to an outpatient situation, many practitioners slowly discontinue drug therapy. In fact, a randomized trial found that a weaning period was not necessary; retocolysis within 24 h was actually more common in the group undergoing slow weaning.[304]

Dual-agent therapy

In 1984, Ferguson and colleagues[283] performed the first trial comparing dual-agent primary therapy of magnesium sulfate and intravenous ritodrine with intravenous ritodrine and noted serious side-effects. The study was randomized and the administration of magnesium versus intravenous fluids was blinded. The authors concluded that the adjunctive use of magnesium sulfate with ritodrine was associated with an unacceptable increase in serious side-effects and probably no increase in efficacy.

In 1984, Hatjis and colleagues[305] performed a slightly different evaluation comparing primary ritodrine therapy with dual-agent ritodrine plus magnesium sulfate in those who failed primary ritodrine therapy. Treatment-related maternal–fetal complications after dual-agent secondary therapy did not differ among the groups. The authors concluded that adding magnesium in pharmacological doses to conventional ritodrine therapy improved pregnancy outcome in those not responding to primary ritodrine therapy.

In a 1987 study, Hatjis and colleagues[306] randomly assigned patients in preterm labor to one of two treatment groups. One group of 32 women initially received ritodrine alone, while another group of 32 received ritodrine and magnesium sulfate concurrently. The authors concluded that concurrent administration of ritodrine and magnesium sulfate was more efficacious than ritodrine alone and caused no apparent increase in adverse side-effects. However, the efficacy conclusion is debatable because the ultimate success rates of tocolysis in both groups were similar.

Diamond and colleagues[286] reported on 11 patients who received additional magnesium therapy for preterm labor after unsuccessful therapy with ritodrine alone. One patient developed cardiovascular complications, and pulmonary edema developed in a patient with a twin pregnancy.

Ogburn and colleagues[285] studied the effect on preterm labor of a combination of magnesium sulfate and ritodrine or terbutaline in 23 high-risk patients. Pregnancy was prolonged for at least 1 week in six of the patients (26%). Five (22%) developed pulmonary edema and, of these, three had twin gestations with intact membranes, and two had premature rupture of membranes. The authors concluded that combination therapy may be effective in prolonging some pregnancies with preterm labor, but only with an increase in maternal risk. Wilkins and colleagues[281] also found significant risks with dual-agent intravenous therapy.

Careful titration of dual-agent therapy appears to be safe in some hands.[307,308] In one of these studies,[307] the increased safety may have resulted from the low initial drug infusion rates of intravenous terbutaline and the elimination of the magnesium bolus.

Other empirical drug combinations containing magnesium sulfate have been used quite successfully and safely in our hands (e.g., magnesium sulfate and intermittent oral or subcutaneous terbutaline or oral nifedipine). We and others have found that the combination of magnesium sulfate and indomethacin was relatively safe and advocated its use for patients with advanced cervical dilation.[309,310]

Long-term therapy

In 1986, Wilkins and colleagues[281] reported a normal outcome in two patients in preterm labor who had been treated continuously for 6 and 13 weeks with intravenous magnesium sulfate for tocolysis. In each case, conventional therapy with intravenous and oral ritodrine failed to abate uterine contractions and attempts to wean the patients off magnesium sulfate were unsuccessful. In 1989, Dudley and colleagues[311] added 51 patients to the database, successfully supporting long-term magnesium sulfate therapy. They concluded that there need be no time limit for treatment and that magnesium sulfate tocolysis may be continued as clinically indicated. However, some reports have implicated long-term continuous infusion of magnesium sulfate for tocolysis in the genesis of transient neonatal radiographic bony lesions.[288,312]

Oral magnesium as prophylaxis for preterm delivery

Serum magnesium levels are usually lower in pregnancy than in the nonpregnant state, and during preterm labor levels appear to drop still further.[313,314] Some authors have suggested an etiological relationship between low magnesium concentrations and preterm delivery.[315–317] Oral tocolysis with magnesium oxide and gluconate has been used.[318] The mean serum concentration of magnesium may increase from 1.44 ± 0.22 mg per 100 mL before oral therapy to 2.16 ± 0.32 mg per 100 mL after therapy.[319]

In 1987, Martin and colleagues[319] reported on 50 patients in preterm labor who had undergone successful tocolysis. One-half received magnesium sulfate followed by oral magnesium gluconate, and the other one-half received intravenous ritodrine followed by oral ritodrine. The number of patients who progressed to 37 weeks' gestation was similar in both groups, but more of the ritodrine patients suffered side-effects (40% versus 16% of the non-ritodrine group). The authors concluded that both oral agents were equally as effective in prolonging pregnancy to term.

A randomized trial comparing oral terbutaline with magnesium oxide for the maintenance of tocolysis revealed no significant difference in efficacy.[320] The authors did find fewer side-effects and a significant cost advantage was apparent with the magnesium therapy. Another study compared tocolysis with oral ritodrine, oral magnesium, and no oral maintenance;[321] the investigators were unable to demonstrate any pregnancy prolongation as a result of oral therapy.

Sibai and colleagues[322] performed a double-blind randomized controlled study of 400 young primigravid normotensive patients in whom oral daily administration of 365 mg of magnesium aspartate hydrochloride was compared with an aspartic acid placebo. There were no significant differences between the two groups regarding the incidences of preterm labor, preterm delivery, placental abruption, fetal growth retardation, preeclampsia, or admissions to the neonatal intensive care unit. They concluded that magnesium supplements had no demonstrable benefit in the population tested; even with a sample size 10 times larger, no decrease in preterm labor would have been detected in the magnesium group.

Recommended clinical protocol

Most published studies have used a loading dose of 4 g of intravenous magnesium sulfate followed by doses of 2 g/h, but others[323–326] have advocated a 6-g loading dose. The clinical protocol in Table 62.20, modified from Petrie, allows for fine-tuning of infusion rates with decreased potential for fluid overload and is well tolerated by most patients. Paying careful attention to contraindications (Table 62.12), and to fluid intake and output, diminishes the risk of pulmonary edema and magnesium toxicity.

Magnesium sulfate, cerebral palsy, and infant mortality

Can cerebral palsy be prevented by the use of magnesium sulfate? In a retrospective epidemiological study, antenatal exposure to magnesium sulfate in VLBW infants was found to reduce the incidence of cerebral palsy at 3 years of age or more.[327] However, other investigators have not been able to find an association between magnesium and a reduced risk of cerebral palsy.[328] Some clinical investigators have found that the cerebroprotective effect is a result of the underlying indication for treatment rather than magnesium *per se*. They reported fewer neurological impairments in infants born to magnesium-treated women with preeclampsia than infants born to magnesium-treated women with spontaneous preterm labor.[329] Infection, a common underlying mechanism in patients with preterm labor, may be the real predisposing factor.[330,331] Animal models indicate that magnesium deficiency is related to higher levels of IL-1, IL-6, tumor necrosis factor-alpha, endothelin, and inflammatory neuropeptides.[332]

A report from Mittendorf and colleagues[333] found an alarming increase in total pediatric mortality in infants born to women in spontaneous preterm labor who were randomized to receive prenatal exposure to magnesium sulfate. After a preliminary analysis, nine out of 10 pediatric deaths were found to have occurred in the magnesium-exposed group. The causes of the nine deaths could be categorized as follows: post neonatal (4); severe twin transfusion syndrome in a 26-week pregnancy (2); multiple congenital anomalies (1); subepicardial hemorrhage in an 885-g infant who underwent cardiopulmonary resuscitation in labor and delivery (1); and neonatal apnea treated after discharge home (1).

The study by Mittendorf and colleagues had tremendous implications for the use of magnesium sulfate therapy for tocolysis. Importantly, the authors should have provided a clear description of all other potentially confounding variables to make sure the process of randomization actually functioned as it should in theory; however, they presented very few data regarding other potential confounders or risk factors. A barrage of criticism was unleashed from centers around the world,[334–337] and there was general disfavor by guest editorial writers. Methodological problems of the Mittendorf study included: scientific bias because the study was not blind, the presence of deaths not easily related to magnesium, double counting as a result of an excess number of twins in the magnesium group, the inclusion of randomized patients who did not actually receive magnesium, and incomplete data on the control group. Data from other studies have shown no positive association between magnesium sulfate and neonatal mortality.[338,339] In fact, the authors found a strong negative association and stated that magnesium actually conferred a degree of protection against neonatal death. The Australian study[339] concluded that the pediatric outcome for very low birthweight infants was improved in women given magnesium sulfate for preterm labor.

Table 62.20 A clinical recipe to administer magnesium sulfate.

1. 100 mL of a 50% solution of magnesium sulfate is easily obtained from readily available products. This volume contains 50 g of magnesium sulfate.
2. 100 mL is sterilely removed from a 500-mL bag of 5% dextrose in water. Fifty grams of magnesium sulfate is injected into the remaining 400 mL of fluid for intravenous infusion. It should be noted that 10 mL of this final solution equals 1 g of magnesium sulfate.
3. A loading dose of 6 g is infused over 30 min. Perspiration and flushing are observed and occur with a feeling of warmth due to vasodilatation. These findings are usually noted early during the intravenous infusion and continue to a greater or lesser degree throughout the infusion. The face, neck, and hands are particularly affected. Nausea and emesis may occur.
4. The initial continuous maintenance rate is 2–3 g/h for 60 min. One or two doses of subcutaneous terbutaline 0.25 mg per dose, may be used during this interval if there are no contraindications and rapid diminution in uterine activity is desired.
5. Complete and rapid uterine quiescence is unnecessary.
6. The infusion rate is increased in increments of 0.5 g/h every 30 min until uterine activity begins to decrease or signs and symptoms of hypermagnesemia occur. These findings include lethargy, somnolence, diplopia, dysarthria, blurred vision, dry mouth, dizziness, and nystagmus. These effects generally occur at a dose of greater than 2 g/h (2.5–4.0 g/h). Downward adjustments in the rate by half-gram increments are generally all that is needed; discontinuation of therapy for side-effects is rarely needed. If necessary, intravenous injection of 1 g of calcium gluconate can be used in the symptomatic patient; this will be followed by rapid symptomatic relief.
7. The infusion is continued at the lowest effective rate of 2 g/h, whichever is greater, for at least 12 h of relative uterine quiescence.
8. Oral beta-sympathomimetic therapy is administered and the magnesium infusion is discontinued. Should uterine activity begin to increase during this interval, magnesium sulfate infusion should be increased to the effective rate.
9. If the patient cannot be successfully weaned from intravenous magnesium therapy, continuous short-term therapy (24–72 h) may be safely administered, usually at rates of 2–3 g/h. During this interval, another attempt at weaning may be attempted.
10. If uterine activity recurs coincident with the conversion from intravenous magnesium therapy to oral beta-sympathomimetic, attempts to use other tocolytic agents may be instituted.
11. Should discontinuation of magnesium infusion and conversion to an oral tocolytic agent fail to abate increasing uterine activity, continuous intermediate-term to long-term therapy with magnesium sulfate may be given. In general, cervical dilation will not change significantly during these therapeutic maneuvers. During long-term magnesium sulfate infusion therapy, the patient can be managed safely in a step-down unit. The healthcare team should be ready to provide emotional and moral support for patients requiring long-term hospitalization.
12. Most true failures of magnesium sulfate therapy and progressive preterm labor are due to cervical dilatation of >4 cm, placental abruption, or chorioamnionitis.
13. The occasional patient continues to have increased uterine activity, yet has no associated cervical changes while on magnesium sulfate therapy. Other tocolytic agents may be tried in these cases in an attempt to quiet the uterus.
14. Patients who are refractory to treatment for preterm labor are likely to have an identifiable pathophysiologic process, most notably amniotic infection or abruptio placentae. An amniocentesis for studies of infection and pulmonary maturity are indicated.
15. Dual-agent combination therapy with intravenous magnesium sulfate and intravenous beta-sympathomimetic agents is not recommended due to a significantly increased risk of side-effects. However, dual therapy magnesium with oral or subcutaneous tocolytic agents is reasonable. Combined use of magnesium with nifedipine, indomethacin, or oxytocin analogs may be used but needs further study.
16. In the severely preterm gestation with inevitable delivery due to advanced cervical dilation (4–8 cm), aggressive magnesium tocolysis alone or in combination with other tocolytic agents may be extremely useful in delaying delivery for 24–48 h to improve the neonatal survival advantage by giving antenatal betamethasone.

Modified from ref. 289.

Nifedipine

A better term for calcium-channel blockers is *calcium antagonists* because they do not completely block calcium influx into the cell; such an action would be incompatible with life. Rather, calcium antagonists are used to normalize excessive pathological muscle contractility and pacemaker activity at the cardiac, vascular, and uterine tissue and organ levels.[340]

Nifedipine inhibits uterine activity and has less of an effect on the cardiac conduction system than verapamil, another calcium channel antagonist. The mechanism of action of nifedipine appears to be limited to the inhibition of the slow voltage-dependent channels regulating calcium influx. Adverse pharmacological effects include vasodilation, negative inotropism, and sinoatrial or atrioventricular node conduction disturbances. Because it is a potent vasodilator, nifedipine may cause dizziness, lightheadedness, flushing, headaches, and peripheral edema.[341] Although the overall incidence of side-effects is 17%, severe effects necessitating discontinuation of therapy occur in 2–5% of patients.[342] The negative inotropic and dromotropic (affecting cardiac nodal conduction) effects of nifedipine are minimal. This is largely because of the heart's baroreflex response to peripheral vasodilation. Idiosyncratic reactions to nifedipine are rare.

Nifedipine is rapidly and almost completely absorbed from the gastrointestinal tract. Absorption after sublingual administration is rapid but less complete, with levels being measurable in the plasma within 5 min.[343] The rate of absorption of oral and sublingual capsules varies widely among patients. Ferguson and colleagues[344] have shown that the mean elimination half-life of nifedipine is 81 ± 26 min (range 24–156 min) in patients with preterm labor treated with sublingual nifedipine (bitten and held between molars). Prevost and colleagues[345] found that the elimination half-life of nifedipine is 78 ± 30 min (range 24–156 min) when it is given as oral capsules in preeclamptic patients. Within 360 min of receiving a 10-mg oral dose, plasma nifedipine concentrations were undetectable in 12 out of 15 preeclamptic patients. The lower limit of detection for nifedipine in their assay was 10 ng/mL. The mean ratio of fetal cord to maternal serum nifedipine was 0.93 ± .20, whereas the mean amniotic fluid concentration was 53% ± 15% in simultaneously obtained maternal vein samples.

Clinical experience

In 1978, Andersson and Ulmsten[346] observed that nifedipine produced significant pain relief and a decrease in uterine activity in patients with severe primary dysmenorrhea. A significant reduction in uterine activity during menses in normal women was also observed. In 1980, Ulmsten and colleagues[347] first reported on the clinical use of nifedipine for tocolysis, with favorable results, while in 1985, Kaul and colleagues[348] reported on the combined use of nifedipine and oral terbutaline for tocolysis. In 1986, Read and Wellby[349] performed a small randomized trial of oral nifedipine versus intravenous ritodrine versus no treatment, with favorable results in the nifedipine group.

More recent prospective randomized studies have supported nifedipine as having a similar efficacy to more commonly used tocolytic agents. When compared with intravenous ritodrine, several authors[350–353] found that nifedipine was equally as effective and had diminished adverse effects, namely, nausea, chest pain, tachycardia, and palpitations. In normotensive patients, nifedipine caused a statistical decrement in blood pressure, but one of unlikely clinical significance; this decrease was much less than that associated with ritodrine. However, nifedipine was associated with more flushing.

In a study comparing nifedipine with magnesium sulfate as a first-line agent, Glock and Morales[354] found that both treatment regimens were equally as effective and associated with the same frequency of side-effects. However, patients in the magnesium group experienced chest pain more often and needed to discontinue drug therapy. More patients in the nifedipine group experienced episodes of transient hypotension, although none was clinically significant. The authors stressed the need for adequate hydration before the use of nifedipine tocolysis. Initially, a 10-mg capsule of nifedipine was given sublingually; if uterine activity persisted, this dose was repeated every 20 min, up to a maximum of 40 mg during the first hour. If tocolysis was successful, oral therapy was initiated for 48 h with a 20-mg dose every 4 h. Patients were then maintained on oral nifedipine, with a 10-mg dose every 8 h. Comparing nifedipine with intravenous ritodrine, Papatsonis and collegues[355] demonstrated the safety and efficacy of nifedipine. These authors used higher dosages of nifedipine than all previous studies; short-acting nifedipine was used initially with up to 40 mg in the first hour, followed by a slow release formulation in dosages of up to 160 mg daily.

In the triage treatment of premature uterine irritability and contractions, a one-time, 30-mg dose of oral nifedipine compared favorably with a subcutaneous terbutaline injection protocol.[356] A tendency toward fewer side-effects was noted in the nifedipine group.

Nifedipine, as well as terbutaline and ritodrine, has been associated with drug-induced hepatitis.[357] In combination with magnesium, nifedipine has been rarely associated with neuroblockade, an effect that is reversible on administration of calcium and discontinuation of magnesium.[358,359] Rarely, hypocalcemia can also occur;[360] however, combined usage with magnesium is not contraindicated.

Circulatory effects

Based on animal studies, concerns about the potentially untoward effects on uteroplacental blood flow in humans initially limited the clinical application of nifedipine during pregnancy.[361–363] However, the advent of Doppler velocity waveform analysis has enabled uteroplacental and fetal blood circulation to be evaluated. Studies of the effect of nifedipine in 21 pregnant women with preterm labor using continuous wave Doppler revealed no significant changes in the pulsatility index of the fetal middle cerebral artery, umbilical artery, and the uteroplacental vessels.[364,365] Other studies[366,367] found that oral nifedipine reduced blood pressure in preeclamptic patients remote from term, but this was not associated with any adverse effects on fetal or uteroplacental circulation when measured by the Doppler technique.

Clinical implications

Nifedipine has an efficacy profile that is at least as good as that of beta-agonists and magnesium sulfate. More recently, it has been reported that nifedipine has an improved efficacy over ritodrine.[355] Its safety profile renders it quite favorable in comparison with other tocolytic agents.

Progestational agents

Progestational agents have been widely used to prolong pregnancy in women who are judged to be at an increased risk of miscarriage or preterm birth. The most commonly used agent is 17α-hydroxyprogesterone caproate (17P). Keirse[368] reviewed the literature and noted a significant decrease in the preterm labor and birth rate in patients given drug therapy. There was no significant effect on neonatal morbidity or mortality. This drug was primarily given weekly in doses of 250–1000 mg.

Meis and colleagues[369] noted a significant reduction in preterm delivery with a weekly injection of 250 mg of 17P. The data are summarized in Fig. 62.8. Therapy was initiated at 16–20 weeks' gestation in multiparous singleton patients with a history of a spontaneous preterm delivery. Therapy was more useful for prophylaxis than for inhibiting active preterm labor. A similar study by da Fonseca and colleagues[370] noted both decreased uterine activity and preterm birth when a 100-mg progesterone suppository was given daily to high-risk patients.

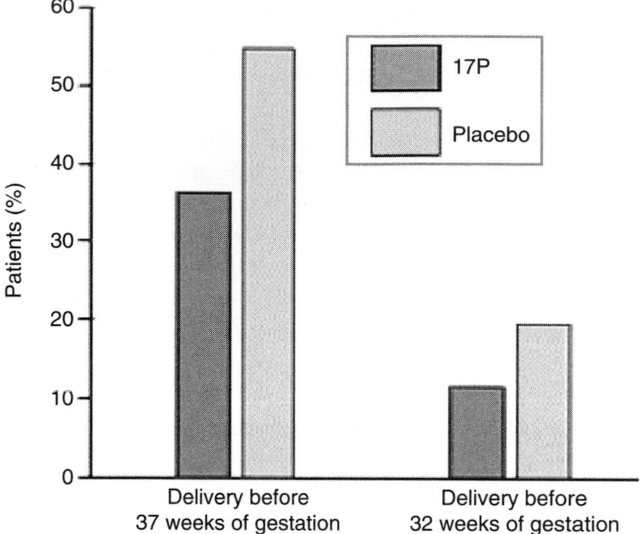

Figure 62.8 Effects of 17P on preterm delivery at 32 and 37 weeks' gestation. Patients had a previous history of spontaneous preterm delivery, and were given weekly injections of 250 mg of 17P. There was a decreased incidence of preterm delivery at < 37 weeks [RR 0.66 (0.54–0.81)] and < 32 weeks [RR 0.58 (0.37–0.91)]. Decreased incidences of both LBW births and IVH (RR 0.25 (0.08–0.82) were observed. (From ref. 369.)

A randomized double-blind trial of 29 women by Erny and colleagues[371] compared the effect of a placebo with four capsules of 100 mg each of an oral progesterone formulation. Oral micronized progesterone decreased uterine activity in 80% of the test group compared with 42% of the placebo group.

A recent meta-analysis noted that one needs to treat a minimum of eight patients with 17P to prevent one preterm birth (Table 62.21).[372]

Oxytocin receptor blockade

The concentration of oxytocin receptors in uterine tissue increases dramatically just before and during labor.[373] Augmented uterine sensitivity to constant serum levels of oxytocin may result in an increase in uterine activity. Oxytocin receptors are also found in the decidua and stimulation at this level produces prostaglandins. Consequently, the potential role of oxytocin antagonists as tocolytic agents has been studied; theoretically, they may offer greater specificity with fewer side-effects than agents in current use.[374–376]

In randomized placebo-controlled trials of women with threatened preterm labor, atosiban, a specific competitive inhibitor of oxytocin-binding oxytocin, reduced and abolished uterine activity more often than a placebo. Side-effects were uncommon and consisted of nausea, vomiting, headache, chest

Table 62.21 Pooled estimates of premature delivery according to treatment assignment.

Study	Treatment group	Comparison/control	Odds ratio (95% CI)
17P			
Papiernik	2/50 (4.0)	9/49 (18.4)	0.18 (0.04–0.91)
Hartikainen-Sorri et al.	15/39 (38.5)	9/38 (23.7)	2.01 (0.75–5.41)
Yemini et al.	5/39 (12.8)	14/40 (35.0)	0.27 (0.09–0.85)
LeVine	2/15 (13.3)	3/15 (20.0)	0.61 (0.09–4.34)
Johnson et al.	2/18 (11.1)	12/25 (48.0)	0.13 (0.03–0.72)
Meis et al.	11/306 (36.3)	84/153 (54.9)	0.47 (0.31–0.69)
Subtotal	137/467 (29.3)	131/320 (40.9)	
Fixed-effects model			0.48 (0.35–0.66)
Random-effects model			0.45 (0.22–0.93)
NNT	8 (5–19)		
Other progestational agents			
da Fonseca et al.	10/72 (13.9)	20/70 (28.6)	0.40 (0.17–0.94)
Goldzieher	0/23	0/31	Excluded
Total	147/562 (26.2)	151/421 (35.9)	
Fixed-effects model			0.47 (0.35–0.63)
Random-effects model			0.45 (0.25–0.80)
NNT	10 (6–24)		

From ref. 372, with permission.

CI, confidence interval; NNT, number needed to treat (95% CI).

Data are presented as *n* (%).

pain, and dysgeusia.[377–379] Additional trials to compare the effects of atosiban with beta-agonists revealed that it has a similar efficacy but produces a lower frequency of maternal side-effects.[380,381] As it is only available in a parenteral form, maintenance therapy using a subcutaneous atosiban pump appears to be the most favorable method of administration.[382]

Nitroglycerin

Nitric oxide is a potent smooth muscle relaxant, and decreased synthesis of nitric oxide in the uterus is associated with initiation of labor in animal models.[383] *In vitro*, cyclic guanosine monophosphate (cGMP) induces myometrial relaxation. Glyceryl trinitrate, also known as nitroglycerin, is a nitric oxide donor.[384] Abouleish and Corn[385] presented data on the role of nitroglycerin in labor and reviewed the literature regarding its obstetric uses. It has been used effectively in external version and breech extraction, in cases of retained placenta, in relieving entrapment of the after-coming head, and in the management of uterine inversion. The drug has a rapid onset and a very short duration of action; it has an extremely short half-life of approximately 2 min. In obstetric situations, intravenous nitroglycerin, in doses of 50–500 μg, promoted uterine relaxation within 45–75 s and without clinically significant side-effects. The drug is available in many forms, including sublingual tablets, sublingual aerosol, transdermal patch, ointment, and the intravenous route. An extended release oral capsule is also marketed. Fetal perfusion does not appear to be effected.[386]

Lees and colleagues[387] reported on 13 consecutive patients who were treated with 10-mg transdermal patches for 24 h after 1 h of preterm labor. If uterine activity continued, an additional patch was applied. Uterine activity generally abated within 24–48 h, with no adverse effect on maternal vital signs and fetal heart rate. Headache was a relatively common side-effect.[388,389] Nitroglycerin appears to have less serious maternal and fetal cardiovascular side-effects than intravenous ritodrine.[390,391] Recent studies have found nitroglycerin to be less effective than either magnesium sulfate or beta-agonists, but better than placebo.[392,393]

Antenatal glucocorticoids

An initial report by Liggins and Howie[394] in 1972 revealed a significant decrease in RDS and neonatal death in patients receiving two doses of 12 mg of betamethasone 24 h apart. Several subsequent trials have found similar results. The optimal glucocorticoid preparation and the ideal dose are unknown, although most studies have used betamethasone or dexamethasone. These two agents are identical except for a 16-methyl group which is in the alpha position in dexamethasone and the beta position in betamethasone. Neither agent has significant mineralocorticoid activity (as opposed to hydrocortisone or methylprednisolone). Both drugs result in elevated plasma glucocorticoid activities for approximately 60–72 h and both readily cross the placenta.

Benefits

Data from 12 controlled trials involving more than 3000 participants demonstrated that corticosteroids reduced the incidence of RDS in each subgroup examined.[395] Reductions in respiratory morbidity were also associated with reductions in IVH, NEC, and neonatal death. Fortunately, these beneficial effects occurred in the absence of strong evidence for adverse effects of corticosteroids. Patients with premature rupture of membranes were included in the analysis.

The meta-analysis was updated in 1995, as part of the National Institutes of Health (NIH) Consensus Conference.[396] Beneficial effects were found with a 50% reduction in RDS in the group receiving antenatal corticosteroids between 29 and 34 weeks. The most dramatic effects (i.e., a 70% reduction) were noted in infants born 24 h after but within 7 days of the last dose of corticosteroids. A lesser effect (i.e., a 30% reduction) was noted in those infants who were delivered within 24 h of the initial treatment. Neonatal mortality was substantially reduced (i.e., a 40% reduction), particularly in patients less than 28 weeks, especially when the case fatality for RDS was high, as seen pre-1980. In this meta-analysis, both male and female infants benefited and maternal race did not seem to adversely influence any beneficial response to corticosteroids; however, in the largest single randomized study carried out (the 1981 US Collaborative study[397]), there were no benefits for male or white infants. In the meta-analysis, reductions were also noted in the rates of periventricular and intraventricular hemorrhage (i.e., a 50% reduction), and NEC (i.e., a 65% reduction).

Nonrandomized trials have also supported the use of corticosteroids in preventing mortality in very preterm gestations and extremely LBW infants.[5,396] Randomized data indicated a decrease in the severity of RDS before 28 weeks, but not a decrease in incidence.[398]

Risks

Data from more than 30 000 patients from five large observational databases in the multicenter network[399] reveal that antenatal corticosteroid exposure was associated with a significant increase (30–50%) in neonatal sepsis and NEC, a finding at odds with the meta-analysis[396] and two early randomized trials, one of which was in patients with membrane rupture.[400,401] Sinclair[210] incisively critiqued Crowley's meta-analysis,[396] indicating that many of the substantive randomized trials excluded some patients from analysis. This important critique found that 135 out of 739 infants (almost 20%) were excluded postrandomization from analysis.[400]

Ohlsson and Fox[402] also constructively critiqued the meta-analysis with regard to IVH; they found missing data, inaccuracies, and outcome ascertainment bias. They recommended

Table 62.22 Absolute risk of RDS (%) based on TDx-FLM (fetal lung maturity) II ratio and gestational age.*

TDx-FLM II ratio (mg/g)	Gestational age (weeks)										
	29	30	31	32	33	34	35	36	37	38	39
10	98	97	96	95	92	89	85	80	73	–	–
20	94	92	89	85	80	73	65	57	47	38	–
30	85	79	73	65	56	47	38	30	23	17	12
40	64	55	46	37	29	22	17	12	8.7	6.2	4.4
50	37	29	22	16	12	8.5	6.1	4.3	3.0	2.1	1.5
60	16	12	8.4	6.0	4.2	3.0	2.1	1.4	1.0	0.70	0.49
70	5.8	4.1	2.9	2.0	1.4	0.98	0.68	0.47	0.33	0.23	0.16
80	2.0	1.4	0.96	0.67	0.46	0.32	0.22	0.16	0.11	0.07	0.05
90	–	0.45	0.31	0.22	0.15	0.11	0.07	0.05	0.04	0.02	0.02
100	–	–	0.10	0.07	0.05	0.03	0.02	0.02	0.01	< 0.01	< 0.01

From ref. 407, with permission.

*These risk estimates reflect the prevalence pattern of RDS across the gestational age range observed in the current study data. The overall prevalence of RDS in a clinical setting depends on both the prevalence of RDS at each gestational age and the distribution of gestational ages encountered.

that a best-evidence synthesis be used as an intelligent alternative to meta-analysis, with a detailed description of each study.[403]

Before the 1994 consensus statement,[404] concern about the harmful effects of corticosteroids limited the widespread application of this therapy.[404] Animal data have suggested that corticosteroids result in alterations in immune response, neurological development, and fetal growth. These harmful effects seem to be limited to studies in which large pharmacological doses of corticosteroids were used in early gestation, and they have not been replicated to any significant degree in the human database. Data from trials with long-term follow-up for up to 12 years have indicated that antenatal corticosteroids do not adversely affect physical growth or psychomotor development.[404]

Short-term effects of transient adrenal suppression, by feedback inhibition of adrenocorticotropic hormone, have been demonstrated in the mother and newborn after prenatal exposure to a single course of corticosteroids.[405] Maternal cortisol levels returned to normal within 48 h of the last dose, and fetal cortisol levels returned to baseline within 6 days of the last dose. Other hormones are also transiently suppressed after a single course of prenatal corticosteroids. Neonatal adrenal suppression occurs for less than a week as measured by reduced levels of dehydroepiandrosterone, hydroxyprogesterone, estrogens, and growth hormone. Nonetheless, the neonate has a normal cortisol response to stress after one course of prenatal corticosteroids. It is not known how hormone levels and the neonatal response to stress are affected after the longer periods of adrenal suppression that occur with multiple corticosteroid courses.

Clinical caveats

The benefit of antenatal corticosteroids *per se* in patients with preeclampsia and multiple gestations is unknown. In higher order multifetal gestations, antenatal corticosteroids are associated with an increase in uterine contractions.[406] In patients with premature rupture of membranes, a benefit of antenatal corticosteroids has been demonstrated, but the benefit–risk ratio was controversial. In general, the benefits from corticosteroids for reducing RDS and mortality were additive to those derived from surfactant. However, it should be noted that an absence of amniocentesis-determined pulmonary maturity was not used in any of these trials as a basis for the administration of corticosteroids; rather, the basis for administration was gestational age. The risk for RDS varied greatly with gestational age even with documentation of fetal lung maturity (Table 62.22).[407]

The NIH consensus statement concluded that all fetuses between 24 and 34 weeks' gestation at risk for preterm delivery are candidates for antenatal corticosteroid therapy.[403] However, to avoid the overuse of corticosteroids in the presence of risk factors for preterm delivery, some important caveats are suggested. As a general rule, neither initial nor repeat corticosteroid injections are indicated for at-risk pregnant women whose pregnancies are stable enough to be managed on an outpatient basis. Initial corticosteroids are indicated for patients who require hospitalization and have an increased risk of delivering prematurely in a relatively emergent setting, but repeat courses are generally not. This has been demonstrated in a large randomized trial.[408] For patients who received their steroids in the remote past, a single rescue dose may be of benefit.[409] For patients who may deliver precipitously, a benefit has been shown if steroids are given as little as 4 h before delivery.[410] Patients with active peptic ulcer disease, active viral infection, active tuberculosis, and either active or suspected chorioamnionitis should probably not receive antenatal corticosteroids.

Thoughtful consideration must be exercised in gestational and pregestational diabetic women. Glucocorticoid therapy is likely to provoke insulin resistance and a deterioration in diabetic control, and the combination of beta-agonists and corticosteroids may well have an even more marked effect. As such, fetal hyperinsulinism resulting from hyperglycemia may actually block surfactant production of type 2 pneumocytes.[396] In addition, a case of glucocorticoid-induced ketoacidosis has been reported in a patient with gestational diabetes in the setting of preterm labor.[411] Glucose values should be closely monitored and insulin should be either added or significantly increased to cover the acute effect of antenatal corticosteroids, which lasts approximately 72 h.

Steroids can also affect fetal biophysical parameters. Changes in the fetal heart rate pattern can occur,[412,413] and fetal movement and breathing can be temporarily affected by betamethasone.[413]

Adjunctive therapy

Adjunctive therapy to optimize the perinatal outcome of impending preterm delivery is fourfold:

1 Administering antenatal corticosteroids together with thyroxin or thyrotropin-releasing hormone (TRH) has been advocated to further decrease the risk of RDS, chronic lung disease, and the number of ventilator days in the neonatal intensive care nursery.[414,415] However, recent studies have demonstrated that a combination of TRH and corticosteroids provides no benefit beyond the use of corticosteroids alone.[416–418]

2 Initial studies have shown that medical therapies, such as the antenatal administration of phenobarbital and vitamin K, are useful in the prevention of IVH; however, further confirmation is required before they can be accepted as clinically valuable adjunctive therapies.[419–423]

3 Administering antenatal antibiotics to patients in preterm labor, to prolong "subclinically" infected pregnancies and to prevent neonatal sepsis, outside the accepted standard antibiotic regimen for intrapartum chemoprophylaxis for group B streptococci, is still controversial and is not established practice.[424,425] In the NIH randomized double-blind placebo-controlled study,[426] treatment with ampicillin and erythromycin during preterm labor with intact membranes was ineffective in prolonging pregnancy or decreasing neonatal morbidity. A meta-analysis[427] found no statistically significant differences in neonatal morbidity or mortality, a finding at variance with the use of antibiotics in patients with premature rupture of membranes.[428] The meta-analysis[427] did find a favorable trend toward the reduction of neonatal pneumonia and NEC, but also a trend toward an increase in neonatal mortality. They concluded that the data do not support the routine use of adjunctive antibiotics in patients with preterm labor. However, most of the studies compared used differing regimens of antibiotics, rendering the meta-analysis itself somewhat questionable. In a more recent randomized blind clinical trial, treatment of patients with threatened preterm labor between 26 and 34 weeks with a combination of ampicillin and metronidazole significantly prolonged gestation and decreased admission to the neonatal intensive care unit.[429] There were no demonstrable effects on maternal and neonatal infectious morbidity. However, several large multicenter studies have failed to demonstrate a benefit of prophylactic antibiotics in the prevention of preterm labor in at-risk patients.[430–432]

4 Operative delivery of the very preterm fetus using procedures such as episiotomy, prophylactic forceps, and prophylactic Cesarean section has been studied as a means to prevent neonatal birth trauma and IVH.[433–437] However, prophylactic operative delivery in the vertex-presenting preterm fetus has not been scientifically proven to decrease mortality or be of any significant benefit to the neurological status of the infant, be it related to intracranial hemorrhage, seizures, or traumatic injury. Major surgical maneuvers strictly on behalf of the fetus are best reserved for established indications such as nonreassuring fetal heart rate patterns and malpresentation. Even although Cesarean section is commonly practiced for the breech preterm fetus, there are no randomized studies that have shown a benefit from operative delivery.[128,129,438,439] As such, selective vaginal breech delivery, with uterine relaxation to prevent or treat head entrapment, is not an unreasonable option in experienced hands.

Preventing preterm birth

Most preterm births result from spontaneous but not idiopathic preterm labor. To be able to prevent preterm birth, it is crucial to be able to predict when it will occur. Predictions based on risk scoring systems, biochemical markers, and cervical examination are still of limited value; prophylaxis with bedrest, cerclage, and tocolytic and progestational agents is also of limited value, and HUAM remains highly controversial, with the bulk of evidence not being very supportive. Programs for the prevention and early detection of preterm labor are still being developed because preterm birth remains the major problem facing modern perinatal medicine.

Advances in risk factor assessment have identified several of the strongest known predictors of spontaneous preterm birth.[440] These are a previous spontaneous preterm birth, black race, low BMI (thinness), a positive fFN test, a foreshortened cervical length on sonographic evaluation, and the presence of bacterial vaginosis in women at high risk for spontaneous preterm birth. A previous spontaneous preterm birth is strongly associated with a short cervix. Bacterial vaginosis may be a causal factor or a marker for a causal factor such as upper genital tract infection. A positive fFN test and a short cervix are not simple independent antepartum markers of

Table 62.23 Preterm prelabor management matrix.

Cervical length	Symptoms of preterm cervical effacement (+1)	Increased uterine activity or funneling (+2)	Increased uterine activity and funneling (+3)
40 mm or more (–1)	0	+1	+2
30–39 mm (0)	+1	+2	+3
20–29 mm (+1)	+2	+3	+4
10–19 mm (+2)	+3	+4	+5

From ref. 445, with permission.

The preterm prelabor profile was derived by adding the number in the row heading category to the number in the appropriate column heading category. For score of 0, no action was required. For score +1, rest was advised. For score of +2, rest and oral tocolysis were prescribed. For score of +3, rest and oral tocolysis were begun, with tocolysis via subcutaneous pump if symptoms and transvaginal ultrasound findings were not stabilized. For score of +4, rest and tocolysis via subcutaneous pump were prescribed. For score of +5, hospital admission for intravenous tocolysis with magnesium sulfate was advised.

distinct causal pathology; in fact, they are intimately involved in the process of labor itself.

Factors that decrease the risk of preterm birth are also important. Measurement of cervical length using transvaginal ultrasound was carried out in 85 twin pregnancies at 24–26 weeks' gestation.[441] A cervical length of more than 35 mm retrospectively identified a group of 34 women with a low-risk twin pregnancy. Only one of these patients was delivered before 34 weeks, indicating a high positive predictive value of 97%. Identification of twin gestations at low risk allows physicians to be more selective in choosing interventions. More research on risk-decreasing factors is merited.

Preterm birth prevention programs

Because there is no single treatable factor that can prevent preterm birth, many investigators have developed comprehensive preterm birth prevention programs. These programs exist at the national, community, and individual physician level. Papiernik and Breart[442] were among the first to institute such a program; its fundamental components include universal preterm birth and preterm labor education of patients, families, staff, and payor sources. Critical to the program's success is 24-h access to care, provider-initiated contact, and a continued commitment to the program. Results are not achieved overnight and, in fact, may take years to develop; the French national program was gradually implemented in 1971. Educational efforts to increase the detection of uterine activity and decrease physical activity were also provided by the mass media. Temporary maternity leave with guaranteed job security supplemented with homecare assistance were integral to the success of the program.

Although most preterm birth prevention programs have been ineffective, particularly in indigent populations, a model community-wide program from West Los Angeles has had promising results.[443] This preterm birth prevention project even targets women with mildly high-risk factors, and is reported to be cost-effective in the prevention of prematurity.[444]

Individualized programs, even in the private practice arena, seem to have potential value. In a nonrandomized intervention study,[445] patients were assigned in rotation to one of five private practice offices for prenatal care and delivery. In four offices, standard obstetric care was provided while, in the remaining office, a prematurity prevention program was used. Features of the program included visit-by-visit screening, patient education, transvaginal cervical ultrasound as indicated, outpatient modification of physical activity, graded outpatient oral and subcutaneous tocolysis, and inpatient tocolysis for failed outpatient therapy. A preterm prelabor management matrix was designed for use in the study office (Table 62.23).[445] Infants in the prematurity prevention group (n = 374) were compared with infants from the other four groups (n = 1391). Significantly fewer VLBW births [0 out of 374 (0%) versus 23 out of 1391 (1.65%), $P < 0.008$] and LBW births [11 out of 374 (2.9%) versus 89 out of 1391 (6.4%), $P < 0.008$] were reported in the study office.

Prevention strategies and policies

Prevention strategies can be viewed from either the obstetricians' or the pediatricians' viewpoint. There are three levels of prevention strategy for the mother. Primary prevention focuses on the entire reproductive-age population and seeks to eliminate known factors associated with preterm birth. Some of these are summarized in Table 62.24. In addition, it is clear that there is a benefit in limiting artificial reproductive technology to single or twin gestations.

The study by Miller and Merritt[446] is a prime example of the potential impact of behavior modification on prematurity. They studied six modifiable behavioral risk factors that are significantly related to LBW: low prepregnant maternal weight for height, low maternal weight gain, lack of prenatal care, age younger than 17 or older than 35 at delivery, cigarette smoking, and the use of drugs and alcohol. Among white women, the risk of a LBW birth was 29% if three of these variables were present; 10% if two variables were

Table 62.24 Primary prevention strategies.

Delay childbearing until age 17 years
Delay interpregnancy interval
Eliminate low maternal weight for height
Smoking prevention and cessation
Prevent and detect sexually transmitted diseases, and treat to cure
Detect bacteriuria and treat to cure
Manage fertility to avoid multifetal gestation
Provide or refer for preconceptional counseling
Detect and treat iron-deficiency anemia
Provide or refer for drug abuse prevention and treatment

Table 62.25 Secondary prevention strategies.

Risk assessment in prenatal care
Improved sufficiency of the content of prenatal care
Repeated education regarding warning signs and symptoms of preterm labor
Early-diagnosis programs
Home uterine activity monitoring, cervical length, oncofetal fibronectin
Early medical intervention
Medications, surgery, early referral
Reduced maternal physical activity
Maternal work leave
Eliminate barriers to care (access, access, access)
Education, education, education

present; 6.7% if one was present; and 1% if none was present.

Secondary prevention identifies pregnant patients who are at increased risk for preterm labor. It then provides education, monitoring of uterine activity and cervical changes, ready access to medical care, and medical interventions as necessary to prolong gestation. These include the use of progesterone prophylaxis. Some of these strategies are identified in Table 62.25.

Tertiary prevention focuses on 11th-hour intensive perinatal care. This includes tocolysis, the use of antibiotics and corticosteroids, maternal transport to a tertiary care center, emergency cerclage, the appropriate mode of delivery, and neonatal intensive care.

Despite scientific advances and the implementation of various prevention and treatment programs, most proximate causes of preterm birth remain unpreventable. Even if all of the appropriately eligible patients (ideally, previous spontaneous preterm birth presenting for prenatal care between 16 and 20 weeks) were treated with 17P, there would only be a very modest reduction in national prematurity.[447] Therefore, large reductions in prematurity are not a reasonable expectation in the foreseeable future.

Prematurity prevention programs have been applied to 20 million pregnant women in France since the early 1970s, with women at low risk gaining the greatest benefits. In the USA, most premature births still occur in low-risk pregnant women because of factors which are, as yet, unidentifiable; therefore, prevention strategies may provide the greatest benefits for these low-risk women.

Key points

1. At 24 weeks' gestation, the neonatal survival rate is more than 50%.
2. The risk of preterm birth and/or delivery of a LBW infant is affected by race.
3. The prediction of a preterm birth is difficult, but risk-scoring cervical ultrasound and fFN testing can help determine which patients are at risk.
4. Preterm labor symptoms are often not specific, and contractions experienced are not always 'textbook' contractions.
5. A history of previous preterm birth is a strong risk factor for recurrent preterm birth.
6. Urogenital tract infections can play a causative role in preterm labor.
7. Tocolysis may provide neonatal benefits by allowing maternal administration of steroids and/or transfer to a tertiary care center.
8. Care should be taken to exclude contraindications to tocolysis early in the management of preterm labor; a complete medical history and physical examination is recommended in order to select the most appropriate agent.
9. The management of multiple gestations requires additional precautions to be taken when using tocolysis.
10. An ultrasound provides important information in the management of preterm labor.
11. Amniocentesis can be of benefit in the analysis of patients presenting with preterm labor.
12. Long-term usage of indomethacin requires close monitoring of the amniotic fluid index (AFI) and frequent Doppler studies of the fetal ductus arteriosus flow.
13. Magnesium sulfate is currently the drug of choice for tocolysis at most institutions.

14 Combination therapy for tocolysis should be used cautiously, but may allow for prolongation of pregnancy.

15 Oral nifedipine has a similar tocolytic efficacy to magnesium sulfate and beta-agonists.

16 17P may decrease the incidence of preterm delivery in patients with a history of spontaneous preterm birth.

17 Steroids decrease the neonatal incidence of RDS, IVH, and possibly NEC, and are best administered at between 24 and 34 weeks' gestation.

18 Steroid administration can negatively affect glucose control in diabetics.

19 A single course of steroids has been shown to be of benefit; repeat dosing is not clinically indicated unless the patient is remote from her last treatment.

20 There is no proven advantage of an elective Cesarean delivery for the vertex preterm infant.

References

1 Schlesinger ER, Allaway NC. The combined effect of birth weight and length of gestation on neonatal mortality among single premature births. *Pediatrics* 1955;15:698.

2 World Health Organization. The incidence of low birth weight: a critical review of available information. *World Health Stat Q* 1980;33:197.

3 Pritchard JA, MacDonald PC, Gant NF, eds. Preterm and post-term pregnancies and fetal growth retardation. In: *Williams' obstetrics,* 17th edn. Connecticut: Appleton-Century-Crofts; 1985:745.

4 Missouri Revised Statutes. RSMO chapter 193:165.

5 Amon E, Sibai BM, Anderson GD, et al. Obstetric variables predicting survival of the immature newborn (<1000 gm.): a five year experience at a single perinatal center. *Am J Obstet Gynecol* 1987;156:1380.

6 Yu VYH, Downe L, Astbury J, et al. Perinatal factors and adverse outcome in extremely low birthweight infants. *Arch Dis Child* 1986;293:1200.

7 Arias E, MacDorman MF, Strobino DM, et al. Annual summary of vital statistics, 2002. *Pediatrics* 2003;112:1215.

8 Rush RW, Keirse MJNC, Howat P, et al. Contribution of preterm delivery to perinatal mortality. *Br Med J* 1976:2:965.

9 Amon E, Anderson GD, Sibai BM, et al. Factors responsible for a preterm delivery of the immature newborn infant (<1000 gm.). *Am J Obstet Gynecol* 1987;156:1143.

10 Robertson PA, Sniderman SH, Laros RK, et al. Neonatal morbidity according to gestational age and birthweight from five tertiary care centers in the United States, 1983–1986. *Am J Obstet Gynecol* 1992;166:1629.

11 Amon E. Limits of fetal viability: obstetric considerations regarding the management and delivery of the extremely premature baby. *Obstet Gynecol Clin North Am* 1988;15:321.

12 Amon E, Steigerwald J, Winn HN. Obstetric factors associated with survival of the borderline viable liveborn infant (500–750 gm) (Abstract). *Am J Obstet Gynecol* 1995;172:418.

13 Lemons JA, Bauer CR, Oh W, et al. Very low birth weight outcomes of the National Institute of Child Health and Human Development Neonatal Research Network, January 1995 through December 1996. NICHD Neonatal Research Network. *Pediatrics* 2001;107(1):E1.

14 Fedrick J, Anderson ABM. Factors associated with spontaneous preterm birth. *Br J Obstet Gynaecol* 1976;83:342.

15 Kliegman RM, Rottman CJ, Behrman RE. Strategies for the prevention of low birth weight infants. *Am J Obstet Gynecol* 1990;162:1073.

16 Mathews TJ, Menacker F, MacDorman MF. Infant mortality statistics from 2002 period linked birth/infant death data set. *National Vital Statistics* November 24, 2004;53:1.

17 Martin JA, Hamilton BE, Sutton PD, et al. Births: final data for 2002. *Natl Vital Stat Department* 2003;52:1.

18 Papiernik E, Alexander GR, Paneth N. Racial differences in pregnancy duration and its implications for prenatal care. *Med Hypothesis* 1990;33:181.

19 Naeye R. Causes of fetal and neonatal mortality by race in a selected US population. *Am J Public Health* 1979;69: 857.

20 Fiscella K. Racial disparities in preterm births. *Public Health Rep* 1996;111:104.

21 Goldenberg RL, Klebanoff MA, Nugent R, et al. Bacterial colonization of the vagina during pregnancy in four ethnic groups. *Am J Obstet Gynecol* 1999;174:1618.

22 Arias F, Tomich P. Etiology and outcome of low birth weight and preterm infants. *Obstet Gynceol* 1982;14:361.

23 Main DM, Gabbe SG, Richardson D. Can preterm deliveries be prevented? *Am J Obstet Gynecol* 1985;151:892.

24 Hameed C, Tejani N, Verma UL, et al. Silent chorioamnionitis as a cause of preterm labor refractory to tocolytic therapy. *Am J Obstet Gynecol* 1984;149:726.

25 Romero R, Mazor M. Infection and preterm labor. *Clin Obstet Gynecol* 1988;31:533.

26 Leigh J, Garite TJ. Amniocentesis and the management of preterm labor. *Obstet Gynecol* 1986;67:500.

27 Lettieri L, Vintzileos AM, Rodis JF, et al. Does "idiopathic" preterm labor resulting in preterm birth exist? *Am J Obstet Gynecol* 1993;168:1480.

28 Carsten ME, Miller JD. Regulation of myometrial contractions. In: MacDonald PC, Porter J, eds. *Initiation of parturition: prevention.* Ohio: Ross Laboratories; 1983:166.

29 Huszar G. Cellular regulation of myometrial contractility and essentials of tocolytic therapy. In: Huszar G, ed. *The physiology and biochemistry of the uterus in pregnancy and labor.* Boca Raton, FL: CRC Press, 1986.

30 Dudly DJ. Preterm labor: an intrauterine inflammatory response syndrome? *J Reprod Immunol* 1997;36:93.

31 Arias F, Rodriguez L, Rayne SC, et al. Maternal placental vasculopathy and infection: two distinct subgroups among patients with preterm labor and preterm ruptured membranes. *Am J Obstet Gynecol* 1993;168:585.

32 Lockwood CJ. The diagnosis of preterm labor and the prediction of preterm delivery. *Clin Obstet Gynecol* 1995;38:675.

33 Leppert PC, Woessner JF, eds. *The extracellular matrix of the uterus, cervix, and fetal membranes.* Ithaca, NY: Perinatology Press, 1991.

34 Leppert PC. Cervical shortening, effacement, and dilation: a complex biochemical cascade. *J Maternal Med* 1992;1:213.
35 Wildschut H, Lumey KH, Lun PW. Is preterm delivery genetically determined? *Paediatr Perinat Epidemiol* 1991;5:363.
36 Keelan JA, Coleman M, Mitchell MD. The molecular mechanisms of term and preterm labor: recent progress and clinical implications. *Clin Obstet Gynecol* 1997;40:460.
37 Creasy RK. Preterm birth prevention; where are we? *Am J Obstet Gynecol* 1993;168:1223.
38 Fuchs AR, Fuchs F, Stubblefield PG, eds. *Preterm birth: causes, prevention, and management*, 2nd edn. New York: McGraw-Hill, 1993.
39 Collaborative Group on preterm birth prevention. Multicenter randomized, controlled trial of a preterm birth prevention program. *Am J Obstet Gynecol* 1993;169:352.
40 Creasy RK, Gummer BA, Liggins GC. System for predicting spontaneous preterm birth. *Obstet Gynecol* 1980;55:692.
41 Papiernik-Berkhauer E. Coefficient de risqué d'accouchement premature. *Presse Med* 1969;77:793.
42 Herron MA, Katz M, Creasy RK. Evaluation of a preterm birth prevention program: preliminary report. *Obstet Gynecol* 1982;59:452.
43 Holbrook RH, Laros RK, Creasy RK. Evaluation of a risk-scoring system for prediction of preterm labor. *Am J Perinatol* 1989;6:62.
44 Hueston WJ, Knox MA, Eilers G, et al. The effectiveness of preterm birth prevention educational programs for high risk women: a meta-analysis. *Obstet Gynecol* 1995;86:705.
45 Mercer BM, Goldenberg RL, Das A, et al. The preterm birth prediction study: a clinical risk assessment system. *Am J Obstet Gynecol* 1996;174:1885.
46 Goldenberg RL, Mayberry SK, Copper RL, et al. Pregnancy outcome following a second trimester loss. *Obstet Gynecol* 1993;81:444.
47 Funderburk S, Guthrie D, Meldrum D. Suboptimal pregnancy outcome among women with prior abortions and premature births. *Am J Obstet Gynecol* 1976;126:55.
48 Carr-Hill RA, Hall MH. The repetition of spontaneous preterm labour. *Br J Obstet Gynaecol* 1985;92:921.
49 Bakketeig LS, Hoffman HJ. The epidemiology of preterm birth: results from a longitudinal study of births in Norway. In: Elder MG, Hendricks CH, eds. *Preterm labor*. London: Butterworth, 1981.
50 Keirse M, Rush R, Anderson A, et al. Risk of preterm delivery in patients with previous preterm delivery and/or abortion. *Br J Obstet Gynaecol* 1978;85:81.
51 Mercer BM, Goldenberg RL, Moawad AH, et al. The Preterm Prediction Study: effect of gestational age and cause of preterm birth on subsequent obstetric outcome. *Am J Obstet Gynecol* 1999;181:1216.
52 Bakketeig LS, Hoffman HJ, Harley EE. The tendency to repeat gestational age and birth weight in successive births. *Am J Obstet Gynecol* 1979;135:1086.
53 Papiernik E, Bouyer J, Collin D, et al. Precocious cervical ripening and preterm labor. *Obstet Gynecol* 1986;67:238.
54 Wood C, Bannerman RHO, Booth RT, et al. The prediction of premature labor by observation of the cervix and external tocography. *Am J Obstet Gynecol* 1965;91:396.
55 Leveno KJ, Cox K, Roark ML. Cervical dilation and prematurity revisited. *Am J Obstet Gynecol* 1986,68:434.
56 Stubbs TM, Van Dorsten P, Miller MC. The preterm cervix and preterm labor: relative risks, predictive values, and change over time. *Am J Obstet Gynecol* 1986;155:829.
57 Parikh MN, Mehta AC. Internal cervical os during the second half of pregnancy. *J Obstet Gynaecol Br Commonw* 1961;68:818.
58 Schafner F, Schanzer SN. Cervical dilation in the early third trimester. *Obstet Gynecol* 1966;27:130.
59 Floyd WS. Cervical dilation in the mid-trimester of pregnancy. *Obstet Gynecol* 1961;18:380.
60 Buekens P, Alexander S, Boutsen M, et al. Randomized controlled trial of routine cervical examinations in pregnancy. *Lancet* 1994;344:841.
61 Gomez R, Galasso M, Romero R, et al. Ultrasonographic examination of the uterine cervix is better than cervical digital examination as a predictor of the likelihood of premature delivery in patients with preterm labor and intact membranes. *Am J Obstet Gynecol* 1994;71:956.
62 Sonek JD, Iams JD, Blumenfeld M, et al. Measurement of cervical length in pregnancy: comparison between vaginal ultrasonography and digital examination. *Obstet Gynecol* 1990;76:172.
63 Iams JD, Golderberg RL, Meis PJ, et al. The length of the cervix and the risk of spontaneous delivery. *N Engl J Med* 1996;334:567.
64 Fuchs IB, Henrich W, Osthues K, et al. Sonographic cervical length in singleton pregnancies with intact membranes presenting with threatened preterm labor. *Ultrasound Obstet Gynecol* 2004;24:554.
65 Bergehella V, Kuhlman K, Weiner S, et al. Cervical funneling: sonographic criteria predictive of preterm delivery. *Ultrasound Obstet Gynecol* 1997;10:161.
66 Iams JD. Opinion: cervical ultrasonography. *Ultrasound Obstet Gynecol* 1997;10:156.
67 Doyle NM, Monga M. Role of ultrasound in screening patients at risk for preterm delivery. *Obstet Gynecol Clin North Am* 2004;31:125.
68 Moore T, Iams JD, Creasy RK, et al. Diurnal and gestational patterns of uterine activity in normal human pregnancy. *Obstet Gynecol* 1994;83:517.
69 Katz M, Newman RB, Gill PJ. Assessment of uterine activity in ambulatory patients at high risk of preterm labor and delivery. *Am J Obstet Gynecol* 1986;154:44.
70 Iams JD, Johnson F, Parker M. A prospective evaluation of the signs and symptoms of preterm labor. *Obstet Gynecol* 1994;84:227.
71 Newman RB, Gill PJ, Wittreich P, et al. Maternal perception of prelabor uterine activity. *Obstet Gynecol* 1986;68:765.
72 Faustin D, Klein S, Spector I, et al. Maternal perception of preterm labor: is it reliable? *J Maternal Fetal Med* 1997;6:1984.
73 Morrison JC, Martin JN, Jr, Martin RW, et al. Prevention of preterm birth by ambulatory assessment of uterine activity: a randomized study. *Am J Obstet Gynecol* 1987;156:536.
74 Hill WC, Fleming AD, Martin RW, et al. Home uterine activity monitoring is associated with a reduction in preterm birth. *Obstet Gynecol* 1990;76:13S.
75 Knuppel RA, Lake MF, Watson DL, et al. Preventing preterm birth in twin gestation: home uterine activity monitoring and perinatal nursing support. *Obstet Gynecol* 1990;76:24S.
76 Iams JD, Johnson FF, O' Shaughnessy RW, et al. A prospective random trial of home uterine activity monitoring in pregnancies at increased risk of preterm labor II. *Am J Obstet Gynecol* 1987;159:595.
77 Porto M, Nageotte MP, Hill O, et al. The role of home uterine monitoring in the prevention of preterm birth (Abstract).

Proceedings of the Society of Perinatal Obstetricians, February 1987, Orlando, FL.
78 Mou SM, Sunderji SG, Gall S, et al. Multicenter randomized clinical trial of home uterine activity monitoring for detection of preterm labor. *Am J Obstet Gynecol* 1991;165:858.
79 Dyson DC, Crites YM, Ray DA, et al. Prevention of preterm birth in high-risk patients: the role of education and provider contact versus home uterine monitoring. *Am J Obstet Gynecol* 199;14:56.
80 Blondel B, Breart G, Berthoux Y, et al. Home uterine activity monitoring in France: a randomized, controlled trial *Am J Obstet Gynecol* 1992;167:424.
81 Nagey DA, Bailey-Jones C, Herman AA. Randomized comparison of home uterine activity monitoring and routine care in patients discharged after treatment for preterm labor. *Obstet Gynecol* 1993;82:319.
82 The Collaborative Home Uterine Monitoring Study Group. A multicenter randomized controlled trial of home uterine monitoring: active versus sham device. *Am J Obstet Gynecol* 1995;173:1120.
83 Grimes DA, Schulz KF. Randomized controlled trials of home uterine activity monitoring: a review and critique. *Obstet Gynecol* 1992;79:137.
84 US Preventive Services Task Force. Home uterine activity monitoring for preterm labor. Review article. *JAMA* 1993;270:371.
85 Corwin MJ, Mou SM, Sunderji SG, et al. Multicenter randomized clinical trial of home uterine activity monitoring: pregnancy outcomes for all women randomized. *Am J Obstet Gynecol* 1996;175:1281.
86 Dyson DC, Danbe KH, Bamber JA, et al. Monitoring women at risk for preterm labor. *N Engl J Med* 1998;338:15.
87 American College of Obstetricians and Gynecologists. ACOG Committee Opinion no. 172. Home uterine activity monitoring. *Int J Gynecol Obstet* 1996;54:71
88 Morrison JC, Chauhan SP. Current status of home uterine activity monitoring. *Clin Perinatol* 2003;30:757.
89 Germain AM, Valenzuela GJ, Ivankovic M. Relationship of circadian rhythms of uterine activity with term and preterm delivery. *Am J Obstet Gynecol* 1993;168:1271.
90 Chien PF, Kahn KS, Ogston S, et al. The diagnostic accuracy of cervico-vaginal fetal fibronectin in predicting preterm delivery: an overview. *Br J Obstet Gynaecol* 1997;104:436.
91 Peaceman AM, Andrews WW, Thorp JM, et al. Fetal fibronectin as a predictor of preterm birth in patients with symptoms: a multicenter trial. *Am J Obstet Gynecol* 1997;177:13.
92 Ascarelli MH, Morrison JC. Use of fetal fibronectin in clinical practice. *Obstet Gynecol Surv* 1997;52:S1.
93 Tekesesin I, Marek S, Hellmeyer L, et al. Assessment of rapid fetal fibronectin in predicting preterm delivery. *Obstet Gynecol* 2005;105:280.
94 Lukes AS, Thorp JM, Eucker BSN, et al. Predictors of positivity for fetal fibronectin in patients with symptoms of preterm labor. *Am J Obstet Gynecol* 1997;176:639.
95 Faron G, Boulvain M, Lescrainier JP, et al. A single fetal fibronectin screening test in a population at low risk for preterm delivery: an improvement on clinical indicators? *Br J Obstet Gynaecol* 1997;104:697.
96 Goldenberg RL, Mercer BM, Meis PJ, et al. The preterm prediction study: fetal fibronectin testing and spontaneous preterm birth. *Obstet Gynecol* 1996;87:643.
97 Goldenberg RL, Thom E, Moawad AH, et al. The preterm prediction study: fetal fibronectin, bacterial vaginosis, and peripartum infection. *Obstet Gynecol* 1996;87:656.
98 Andrews WW, Sibai BM, Thom EA, et al. Randomized clinical trial of metronidazole plus erythromycin to prevent spontaneous preterm delivery in fetal fibronectin-positive women. *Obstet Gynecol* 2003;101:847.
99 Gibbs RS, Romero R, Hillier SL, et al. A review of premature birth and subclinical infection. *Am J Obstet Gynecol* 1992;166: 1515.
100 Romero R, Oyarzun E, Mazor M, et al. Meta-analysis of the relationship between symptomatic bacteriuria and preterm delivery/low birthweight. *Obstet Gynecol* 1989;73:576.
101 Thomsen AC, Morup L, Hansen KB. Antibiotic elimination of group B streptococci in urine in prevention of preterm labor. *Lancet* 1987;1:591.
102 Klebanoff MA, Regan JA, Rao AV, et al. Outcome of the vaginal infections and prematurity study: results of a clinical trial of erythromycin among pregnant women colonized with group B streptococci. *Am J Obstet Gynecol* 1995;172:1540.
103 Hillier SL, Nugent RP, Eschenbach DA, et al. Association between bacterial vaginosis and preterm delivery of a low birth weight infant. *N Engl J Med* 1995;333:1737.
104 Hauth JC, Goldenberg RL, Andrews WW, et al. Reduced incidence of preterm delivery with metronidazole and erythromycin in women with bacterial vaginosis. *N Engl J Med* 1995;333: 1732.
105 Morales WJ, Schoor S, Albritton J. Effect of metronidazole in patients with preterm birth in preceding pregnancy and bacterial vaginosis: a placebo controlled double blind trial. *Am J Obstet Gynecol* 1994;171:345.
106 Okun N, Gronau KA, Hannah ME. Antibiotics for bacterial vaginosis or Trichomonas vaginalis in pregnancy: a systematic review. *Obstet Gynecol* 2005;105:857.
107 Iams JD, Stilson R, Johnson FF, et al. Symptoms that precede preterm labor and preterm premature rupture of the membranes. *Am J Obstet Gynecol* 1990;162:486.
108 Iams JD, Johnson FF, Hamer C. Uterine activity and symptoms as predictors of preterm labor. *Obstet Gynecol* 1990;76:42S.
109 Valenzuela G, Cline S, Hayashi R. Follow-up of hydration and sedation in the pretherapy of premature labor. *Am J Obstet Gynecol* 1983;147:396.
110 Ingemarsson I. Effect of terbutaline on premature labor: a double-blind placebo-controlled study. *Am J Obstet Gynecol* 1976;125:520.
111 Creasy RK. Implications of treatment of preterm labor. In: MacDonald PC, Porter J, eds. *Initiation of parturition: prevention of prematurity*. Ohio: Ross Laboratories; 1983:73.
112 Catalano PM, Ashikaga T, Mann LI. Cervical change and uterine activity as predictors of preterm delivery. *Am J Perinatol* 1989;6:185.
113 Utter GO, Dooley SL, Tamura RK, et al. Awaiting cervical change for the diagnosis of preterm labor does not compromise the efficacy of ritodrine tocolysis. *Am J Obstet Gynecol* 1990;163:882.
114 Gomez R, Romero R, Medina L, et al. Cervical fibronectin improves the prediction of pretem delivery based on sonographic cervical length in patients with uterine contractions and intact membranes. *Am J Obstet* 2005;192:350.
115 Gonik B, Creasy RK. Preterm labor: its diagnosis and management. *Am J Obstet Gynecol* 1986;154:3.
116 Shepard MJ, Richards VA, Berkowitz RL, et al. An evaluation of two equations for predicting fetal weight by ultrasound. *Am J Obstet Gynecol* 1982;142:47.
117 Hadlock FP, Harrist RB, Carpenter RJ. Sonographic estimation of fetal weight. *Radiology* 1984;150:535.

118 Smith RS, Bottoms SF. Ultrasonographic prediction of neonatal survival in extremely low birth weight infants. *Am J Obstet Gynecol* 1939;169:490.
119 Tamura RK, Sabbagha RE, Depp R, et al. Diminished growth in fetuses born preterm after spontaneous labor or rupture of membranes. *Am J Obstet Gynecol* 1984;148:1105.
120 Weiner CP, Sabbagha RE, Visrub N, et al. A hypothetical model suggesting suboptimal intrauterine growth in infants delivered preterm. *Obstet Gynecol* 1985;65:323.
121 Westgren M, Beall M, Divon M, et al. Fetal femur length/abdominal circumference ratio in preterm labor patients with and without successful tocolytic therapy. *J Ultrasound Med* 1986; 5:243.
122 Hadlock FP, Deter RL, Harrist RB, et al. A date-independent predictor of intrauterine growth retardation: femur length/abdominal circumference ratio. *Am J Roentgenol* 1983;141:979.
123 Ott WJ. Fetal femur length, neonatal crown-heel length, and screening for intrauterine growth retardation. *Obstet Gynecol* 1985;65:460.
124 Ricciotti HA, Chen K, Sachs BP. The role of obstetrical medical technology in preventing low birth weight. In: Behrman R, ed. *The future of children: low birth weight.* Los Altos, CA: Center for the Future of Children, 1995;5:78.
125 Silver RK, Helfand BT, Russell TL, et al. Multifetal reduction increases the risk of preterm delivery and fetal growth restriction in twins: a case-control study. *Fertil Steril* 1997;67:30.
126 Nisell H, Bistoletti P, Palme C. Preterm breech delivery: early and late complications. *Acta Obstet Gynecol Scand* 1981;60: 36.
127 Braun FHT, Jones KL, Smith DW. Breech presentation as an indicator of fetal abnormality. *J Pediatr* 1975;86:419.
128 Amon E, Sibai BM, Anderson GD. How perinatologists manage the problem of the presenting breech fetus. *Am J Perinatol* 1988;5:247.
129 Penn ZJ, Steer PJ. How obstetricians manage the problem of preterm delivery with special reference to the preterm breech. *Br J Obstet Gynaecol* 1991;98:531.
130 Robertson PA, Foran CM, Croughan-Minimane MS, et al. Head entrapment and neonatal outcome by mode of delivery in breech deliveries from 24 to 27 weeks of gestation. *Am J Obstet Gynecol* 1995;173:1171.
131 Vintzileos AM, Campbell WA, Nochimson DJ, et al. The use and misuse of the fetal biophysical profile. *Am J Obstet Gynecol* 1987;156:527.
132 Manning FA, Morrison I, Harman CR, et al. Fetal assessment based on fetal biophysical profile scoring: experience in 19,221 referred high risk pregnancies. II. An analysis of false negative results. *Am J Obstet Gynecol* 1987;157:880.
133 Castillo RA, Devoe LD, Arthur M, et al. The preterm nonstress test: effects of gestational age and length of study. *Am J Obstet Gynecol* 1989;160:172.
134 Amon E, Dacus JV, Mabie BC, et al. Ultrasonically guided direct umbilical cord blood sampling, *J Reprod Med* 1987;32: 851.
135 Shalev E, Blondheim O, Peleg D. Use of cordocentesis in the management of preterm or growth-restricted fetuses with abnormal monitoring. *Obstet Gynecol Surv* 1995;50:839.
136 Castle BM, Turnbull AC. The presence or absence of fetal breathing movements predicts the outcome of preterm labour. *Lancet* 1987;2:471.
137 Boylan P, O'Donovan P, Owens OJ. Fetal breathing movements and the diagnosis of labor: a prospective analysis of 100 cases. *Obstet Gynecol* 1985;66:517.
138 Besinger RE, Compton AA, Hayashi RH. The presence or absence of fetal breathing movements as a predictor of outcome in preterm labor. *Am J Obstet Gynecol* 1987;153:753.
139 Senden IP, Owen P. Comparison of cervical assessment, fetal fibronectin, and fetal breathing in the diagnosis of preterm labour. *Clin Exp Obstet Gynaecol* 1996;23:5.
140 Hallak M, Moise KJ, Lira N, et al. The effect of tocolytic agents (indomethacin and terbutaline) on fetal breathing and body movements: a prospective, randomized, double-blind, placebo-controlled clinical trial. *Am J Gynecol* 1992;167:1059.
141 Sherer DM, Spong CY, Salafia AM. Fetal breathing movements within 24 hours of delivery in prematurity are related to histologic and clinical evidence of amnionitis. *Am J Perinatol* 1997; 14:337.
142 Stubblefield PG. Causes and prevention of premature birth: an overview. In: Fuchs AR, Fuchs F, Stubblefield PG, eds. *Preterm birth: causes, prevention, and management.* New York: McGraw-Hill; 1993:3.
143 Donnenfeld AE, Mennuti MT. Sonographic findings in fetuses with common chromosome abnormalities. *Clin Obstet Gynecol* 1988;31:80.
144 Kirbinen P, Jouppila P. Polyhydramnios: a clinical study. *Ann Chir Gynaecol* 1978;67:117.
145 Barkin SZ, Pretorious DH, Beckett MN, et al. Severe polyhydramnios: incidence of anomalies. *Am J Roentgenol* 1987;148: 155.
146 Many A, Hill LM, Lazebnik N. The association between polyhydramnios and preterm delivery. *Obstet Gynecol* 1995;86:389.
147 Ratten GJ, Beischer NA, Fortune DW. Obstetric complications when the fetus has Potter's syndrome. *Am J Obstet Gynecol* 1973;115:890.
148 Cooperstock M, Campbell J. Excess males in preterm birth: interactions with gestational age, race, and multiple birth. *Obstet Gynecol* 1996;88:189.
149 Harlow BL, Frigoletto FD, Cramer DW, et al. Determinants of preterm delivery in low-risk pregnancies. *J Clin Epidemiol* 1996;49:441.
150 Fleisher B, Kulovich MV, Hallman M, et al. Lung profile: sex differences in normal pregnancies. *Obstet Gynecol* 1985;66:327.
151 Romero R, Munoz H, Gomez R, et al. Does infection cause preterm labor and delivery? *Semin Reprod Endocrinol* 1994; 12:227.
152 Romero R, Yoon BH, Mazor M, et al. The diagnostic and prognostic value of amniotic fluid glucose, white blood cell count, interleukin-6, and gram stain in patients with preterm labor and intact membranes. *Am J Obstet Gynecol* 1993;169:805.
153 Font GE, Gauthier DW, Meyer WJ, et al. Catalase activity as a predictor of amniotic fluid culture results in preterm labor or premature rupture of membranes. *Obstet Gynecol* 1995;85: 656.
154 Amon E, Leventhal S, Allen GS, et al. Neonatal outcome following spontaneous preterm labor after demonstrated lung maturity by amniocentesis (Abstract 169). Society for Gynecologic Investigation, 37th Annual Meeting. St. Louis, MO, 1990.
155 Wigton TR, Tamura RK, Wickstrom E, et al. Neonatal morbidity after preterm delivery in the presence of documented lung maturity. *Am J Obstet Gynecol* 1993;169:951.
156 Konte JM, Holbrook RH, Laros RK, et al. Short-term neonatal morbidity. *Am J Perinatol* 1986;3:285.
157 Lewis DF, Futayyeh S, Towers CV, et al. Preterm delivery from 34 to 37 weeks of gestation: is respiratory distress syndrome a problem? *Am J Obstet Gynecol* 1996;147:525.

158 Myers ER, Alvarez JG, Richardson DK. Cost-effectiveness of fetal lung maturity testing in preterm labor. *Obstet Gynecol* 1997;90:824.

159 Winn HN, Romero R, Roberts A, et al. Comparisons of fetal lung maturation in preterm singleton and twin pregnancies. *Am J Perinatol* 1992;9:326.

160 Heinonen PK, Saarikoski S, Pystynen P. Reproductive performance of women with uterine anomalies: an evaluation of 182 cases. *Acta Obstet Gynecol Scand* 1982;61:157.

161 Fedele L, Zamberletti D, Vercellini P, et al. Reproductive performance of women with unicornuate uterus. *Fertil Steril* 1987;47:416.

162 Yu VHY, Downe L, Astbury J, et al. Perinatal factors and adverse outcome in extremely low birthweight infants. *Arch Dis Child* 1986;61:554.

163 Bottoms S, Paul R, Iams J, et al. Obstetrical determinants of neonatal survival in extremely low birth weight infants (Abstract). *Am J Obstet Gynecol* 1994;107:38.

164 Kitchen W, Ford G, Orgill A, et al. Outcome of extremely low birth weight infants in relation to the hospital of birth. *Aust NZ J Obstet Gynaecol* 1984;24:1.

165 Morrison JJ, Rennie JM. Clinical scientific and ethical aspects of fetal and neonatal care at extremely preterm periods of gestation. *Br J Obstet Gynaecol* 1997;104:1341.

166 MacDonald H. American Academy of Pediatrics' Committee on Fetus and Newborn. Perinatal care at the threshold of viability. *Pediatrics* 2002;110:1024.

167 Hack M, Wright LL, Shankaran S, et al. Very low-birthweight outcomes of the National Institute of Child Health and Human Development Neonatal Network, November 1989 to October 1990. *Am J Obstet Gynecol* 1995;172:457.

168 AAP and ACOG combined statement. Perinatal care at the threshold of viability. *Pediatrics* 1995;96:974.

169 Kramer WB, Saade GR, Goodrum L, et al. Neonatal outcome after active perinatal management of the very premature infant between 23 and 27 weeks' gestation. *J Perinatol* 1997;17: 439.

170 Gultom E, Doyle LW, Davis P, et al. Changes over time in attitudes to treatment and survival rates for extremely preterm infants (23–27 weeks' gestational age). *Aust NZ J Obstet Gynaecol* 1997;37:56.

171 Hack M, Friedman H, Fanaroff AA. Outcomes of extremely low birth weight infants. *Pediatrics* 1996;98:931.

172 Hack M, Fanaroff AA. How small is too small? Considerations in evaluating the outcome of the tiny infant. *Clin Perinatol* 1988;15:773.

173 Yu VYH, Wong PY, Bajuk B, et al. Outcome of extremely low birthweight infants. *Br J Obstet Gynaecol* 1986;93:196.

174 Bottoms SF, Paul RH, Iams JD, et al. Obstetric determinants of neonatal survival: influence of willingness to perform cesarean delivery on survival of extremely low-birth weight infants. *Am J Obstet Gynecol* 1997;176:960.

175 Bottoms SF, Paul RH, Iams JD, et al. Obstetrician's attitude and neonatal survival of extremely low-birth weight infants (Abstract). *Am J Obstet Gynecol* 1994;170:296.

176 Miyazaki FS, Taylor NA. Saline amnioinfusion for relief of variable or prolonged decelerations. *Am J Obstet* 1983;146:670.

177 Mendez-Bauer C, Shekarloo A, Cook V, et al. Treatment of acute intrapartum fetal distress by beta2 sympathomimetics. *Am J Obstet* 1987;156:638.

178 Lands AM, Arnold A, McAuliff JP, et al. Differentiation of receptor systems by sympathomimetic amines. *Nature* 1967;214: 597.

179 Lipshitz J, Bailie P. Uterine and cardiovascular effects of beta2-selective sympathomimetic drugs administered as an intravenous infusion. *S Afr Med J* 1976;50:1973.

180 Grospietsch G, Kuhn W. Effects of β-mimetics on maternal physiology. In: Fuchs F, Stubblefield PG, eds. *Preterm birth: causes, prevention, and management.* New York: Macmillan; 1984: 171.

181 Caritis SN, Chiao JP, Moore JJ, et al. Myometrial desensitization after ritodrine infusion. *Am J Physiol* 1987;253:E410.

182 Berg G, Anderson RGG, Ryden G. β-adrenergic receptors in human myometrium during pregnancy. Changes in the numbers of receptors after β-mimetic treatment. *Am J Obstet Gynecol* 1985;151:392.

183 Benedetti TJ. Maternal complications of parenteral beta-sympathomimetic therapy for preterm labor. *Am J Obstet Gynecol* 1983;145:1.

184 Hendricks SK, Keroes J, Katz M. Electrocardiographic changes associated with ritodrine-induced maternal tachycardia and hypokalemia. *Am J Obstet Gynecol* 1986;154:921.

185 Barden TP, Peter JB, Merkatz IR. Ritodrine hydrochloride: a betamimetic agent for use in preterm labor. I. Pharmacology, clinical history, administration, side effects, and safety. *Obstet Gynecol* 1980;56:1.

186 Milliez S, Blot PH, Sureau C. A case report of maternal death associated with betamimetic and betamethasone administration in premature labor. *Eur J Obstet Gynecol Reprod Biol* 1980; 2:95.

187 Hudgens DR, Conradi SE. Sudden death associated with terbutaline sulfate administration. *Am J Obstet Gynecol* 1993;172: 416.

188 Philipsen T, Eriksen PS, Lynggaard F. Pulmonary edema following ritodrine-saline infusion in premature labor. *Obstet Gynecol* 1981;58:304.

189 Haynes RC, Larner J. Adrenocorticotropic hormone; adrenocortical steroids and their synthetic analogs; inhibitors of adrenocortical steroid biosynthesis. In: Goodman LS, Gilman A, eds. *The pharmacological basis of therapeutics*, 5th edn. New York: Macmillan; 1975;1491.

190 Spellacy WN, Cruz AC, Buhi WC, et al. The acute effects of ritodrine infusion on maternal metabolism: measurements of levels of glucose, insulin, glucagons, triglycerides, cholesterol, placental lactogen, and chronic gonadotropin. *Am J Obstet Gynecol* 1978;131:637.

191 Lipschitz J, Vinik AI. The effects of hexoprenaline, a beta2-sympathomimetic drug, on maternal glucose, insulin, glucagons, and free fatty acid levels. *Am J Obstet Gynecol* 1978;130: 761.

192 Lenz S, Kuhl C, Wang P, et al. The effect of ritodrine on carbohydrate and lipid metabolism in normal and diabetic pregnant women. *Acta Endocrinol* 1979;92:669.

193 Wager J, Fredholm B, Lunell N, et al. Metabolic and circulatory effects of intravenous and oral salbutamol in late pregnancy in diabetic and non-diabetic women. *Acta Obstet Gynecol Scand* 1982;108(Suppl.):41.

194 Main DM, Main EK, Strong SE, et al. The effect of oral ritodrine therapy on glucose tolerance in pregnancy. *Am J Obstet Gynecol* 1985;152:1031.

195 Main EK, Maon DM, Gabbe SG. Chronic oral terbutaline tocolytic therapy is associated with maternal glucose intolerance. *Am J Obstet Gynecol* 1987;157:644.

196 Angel JL, O'Brien WF, Knuppel RA, et al. Carbohydrate intolerance in patients receiving oral tocolytics. *Am J Obstet Gynecol* 1988;159:76.

197 Lippert TH, DeGrandi PB, Fridrich R. Actions of the uterine relaxant, fenoterol, on uteroplacental hemodynamics in human subjects. *Am J Obstet Gynecol* 1976;125:1093.

198 Lunell NO, Joelsson I, Lewander R, et al. Uteroplacental blood flow and the effect of beta2-adrenoceptor stimulating drugs. *Acta Obstet Gynecol Scand* 1982;108(Suppl.):25.

199 Huisjes JH, Touwen BC. Neonatal outcome after treatment with ritodrine: a controlled study. *Am J Obstet Gynecol* 1983; 147:250.

200 Hancock PJ, Setzer ES, Beydoun SN. Physiologic and biochemical effects of ritodrine therapy in the mother and perinate. *Am J Perinatol* 1985;2:1.

201 Brazy JE, Eckerman CO, Gross SJ. Clinical and laboratory observations. Follow-up of infants of <1500 gram birth weight with antenatal isoxsuprine exposure. *J Pediatr* 1983;102: 611.

202 Haddengra M, Touwen BCL, Huisjes JH. Longterm follow-up of children prenatally exposed to ritodrine. *Br J Obstet Gynaecol* 1986;1:156.

203 Freysz H, Williard D, Lehr A, et al. A long term evaluation of infants who received a beta-mimetic drug while in utero. *J Perinat Med* 1977;5:94.

204 Svenningsen NW. Follow-up studies on preterm infants after maternal beta-receptor agonist treatment. *Acta Obstet Gynecol Scand* 1982;108(Suppl.):67.

205 Polowczyk D, Tejani N, Lauersen N, et al. Evaluation of seven-to-nine-year old children exposed to ritodrine in utero. *Obstet Gynecol* 1984;64:485.

206 Groome LJ, Golderbert RL, Cliver SP, et al. Neonatal periventricular–intraventricular hemorrhage after maternal beta-sympathetic tocolysis. The March of Dimes Study Group. *Am J Obstet Gynecol* 1991;167:873.

207 Ozcan T, Turan C, Ekici E, et al. Ritodrine tocolysis and neonatal intraventricular-periventricular hemorrhage. *Gynecol Obstet Invest* 1995;39:60.

208 Atkinson MW, Goldenberg RL, Gaudier FL, et al. Maternal corticosteroid and tocolytic treatment and morbidity and mortality in very low birth weight infants, *Am J Obstet Gynecol* 1995;173:302.

209 Canadian preterm labor investigators group. Treatment of preterm labor with the beta-adrenergic agonist ritodrine. *N Engl J Med* 1992;327:308.

210 Sinclair JC. Meta-analysis of randomized controlled trials of antenatal corticosteroid for the prevention of respiratory distress syndrome: discussion. *Am J Obstet Gynecol* 1995;173: 339.

211 Merkatz IR, Peter JB, Barden TP. Ritodrine hydrochloride: a betamimetic agent for use in preterm labor. II. Evidence of efficacy. *Obstet Gynecol* 1980;56:7.

212 King JF, Grand A, Keirse MJN, et al. Betamimetics in preterm labour: an overview of randomized controlled trials. *Br J Obstet Gynaecol* 1988;965:21.

213 Caritis SN, Venkataramanan R, Darby MJ, et al. Pharmacokinetics of ritodrine administered intravenously. Recommendations for changes in the current regimen. *Am J Obstet Gynecol* 1990;162:429.

214 Gonik B, Benedetti TJ, Creasy RK, et al. Intramuscular versus intravenous ritodrine hydrochloride for preterm labor management. *Am J Obstet Gynecol* 1988;159:323.

215 Benedetti TJ, Gonik B, Hayashi RH, et al. A multicenter evaluation of intramuscular ritodrine hydrochloride as initial parenteral therapy for preterm labor management. *J Perinatol* 1994;14:403.

216 Macones GA, Berlin M, Berlin JA. Efficacy of oral beta-agonist maintenance therapy in preterm labor: a meta-analysis. *Obstet Gynecol* 1995;85:313.

217 Holleboom CAG, Merkus JMWM, van Elferen LWM, et al. Double-blind evaluation of ritodrine sustained release for oral maintenance of tocolysis after active preterm labour. *Br J Obstet Gynaecol* 1996;103:702.

218 Howard TE, Killam AP, Penny LL, et al. A double blind randomized study of terbutaline in premature labor. *Milit Med* 1982;147:305.

219 Cotton DB, Strassner HT, Hill LM, et al. Comparison of magnesium sulfate, terbutaline and a placebo for inhibition of preterm labor. A randomized study. *J Reprod Med* 1984;29:92.

220 Caritis SN, Tolg G, Heddinger LA, et al. A double-blind study comparing ritodrine and terbutaline in the treatment of preterm labor. *J Obstet Gynecol* 1984;150:7.

221 Stubblefield PG, Heyl PS. Treatment of premature labor with subcutaneous terbutaline. *Obstet Gynecol* 1982;59:457.

222 Moise KJ, Dorman K, Giebel R, et al. A randomized study of intravenous versus subcutaneous/oral terbutaline in the treatment of preterm labor (Abstract 276). Presented at the Seventh Annual Meeting of the Society of Perinatal Obstetricians, Lake Buena Vista, FL, February 1987.

223 Leferink JG, Lamont H, Wagenmaker-Engles I, et al. Pharmacokinetics of terbutaline after subcutaneous administration. *Int J Clin Pharmacol Biopharmacol* 1979;17:181.

224 Lyrenas S, Grahnen A, Lindberg B, et al. Pharmacokinetics of terbutaline during pregnancy. *Eur J Clin Pharmacol* 1986;29: 619.

225 Carpenter RJ, Jr, Decuir P. Cardiovascular collapse associated with oral terbutaline tocolytic therapy. *Am J Obstet Gynecol* 1984;146:821.

226 Lampert MB, Hibbard J, Weinert L, et al. Peripartum heart failure associated with prolonged tocolytic therapy. *Am J Obstet Gynecol* 1993;168:493.

227 Lam F, Gill P, Smith, et al. Use of the subcutaneous terbutaline pump for long-term tocolysis. *Obstet Gynecol* 1988;72:810.

228 Albert JR, Johnson C, Roberts WE, et al. Tocolysis for recurrent preterm labor using a continuous subcutaneous infusion pump. *J Reprod Med* 1994;39:614.

229 Moise KJ, Jr, Sala DJ, Zurawin RK, et al. Continuous subcutaneous terbutaline pump therapy for premature labor: safety and efficacy. *South Med J* 1992; 85:255.

230 Wenstrom K, Weiner C, Merrill D, et al. A placebo-controlled randomized trial of the terbutaline pump for prevention of preterm delivery. *Am J Perinatol* 1997;14:87.

231 Repke JR, Niebyl JR. Role of prostaglandin synthetase inhibitors in the treatment of preterm labor. *Semin Reprod Endocrinol* 1985;3:29.

232 Zuckerman H, Reiss U, Rubinstein I. Inhibition of human premature labor by indomethacin. *Obstet Gynecol* 1974;44:787.

233 Wigvist N, Lundstrom V, Green K. Premature labor and indomethacin. *Prostaglandins* 1975;10:515.

234 Greila P, Zanor P. Premature labor and indomethacin. *Prostaglandins* 1978;16:1007.

235 Niebyl JR, Blake DA, White RD, et al. The inhibition of premature labor with indomethacin. *Am J Obstet Gynecol* 1980;136: 1014.

236 Zuckerman H, Shaley E, Gilad G, et al. Further study of the inhibition of premature labor by indomethacin. Part II. Double-blind study. *J Perinat Med* 1984;12:25.

237 Spearing G. Alcohol, indomethacin, and salbutamol. *Obstet Gynecol* 1979;53:171.

238 Gamissans O, Canas E, Cararach V, et al. A study of indomethacin combined with ritodrine in threatened preterm labor. *Eur J Obstet Gynecol Reprod Biol* 1978;8:123.
239 Katz Z, Lancet M, Yemini M, et al. Treatment of premature labor contractions with combined ritodrine and indomethacin. *Int J Gynaecol Obstet* 1983;21:337.
240 Morales WJ, Smith SG, Angel JL, et al. Efficacy and safety of indomethacin versus ritodrine in the management of preterm labor: a randomized study. *Obstet Gynecol* 1989;74:567.
241 Kurki T, Eronen M, Lumme R, et al. A randomized double-dummy comparison between indomethacin and nylidrin in threatened preterm labor. *Am J Obstet Gynecol* 1991;164:981.
242 Besinger RE, Niebyl JR, Keyes WG. Randomized comparative trial of indomethacin and ritodrine for the long-term treatment of preterm labor. *Am J Obstet Gynecol* 1991;164:981.
243 Morales WJ, Madhav H. Efficacy and safety of indomethacin compared with magnesium sulfate in the management of preterm labor: a randomized study. *Am J Obstet Gynecol* 1993;169:97.
244 Novy MS. Effects of indomethacin on labor, fetal oxygenation, and fetal development in rhesus monkeys. *Adv Prostaglandin Thromboxane Res* 1978;4:285.
245 Moise KJ, Huhta JC, Sharif DS, et al. Indomethacin in the treatment of preterm labor: effects on the human fetal ductus arteriosus. *N Engl J Med* 1988;319:327.
246 Clyman RI, Mauray F, Roman C, et al. Circulating prostaglandin E2 concentrations and patent ductus arteriosus in fetal and neonatal lambs. *J Pediatr* 1980;97:455.
247 Van den Veyer IB, Moise KJ. Prostaglandin synthetase inhibitor in pregnancy. *Obstet Gynecol Surv* 199;48:493.
248 Vermillion ST, Scardo JA, Lashus AG, et al. The effect of indomethacin tocolysis on fetal ductus arteriosus constriction with advancing gestational age. *Am J Obstet Gynecol* 1997;177:256.
249 Ben-David Y, Hallak M, Rotschild A. Indomethacin and fetal ductus arteriosus: complete closure after cessation of prolonged therapeutic course. *Fetal Diagn Ther* 1996;11:341.
250 Respondek M, Weil SR, Huhta JC. Fetal echocardiography during indomethacin treatment. *Ultrasound Obstet Gynecol* 1995;5:86.
251 Itskovitz J, Abramovich H, Brandes JM. Oligohydramnios, meconium and perinatal death concurrent with indomethacin treatment in human pregnancy. *J Reprod Med* 1980;24:137.
252 Cantor B, Tyler T, Nelson RM, et al. Oligohydramnios and transient neonatal anuria: a possible association with the maternal use of prostaglandin synthetase inhibitors. *J Reprod Med* 1980;24:220.
253 Kirshon B, Moise KJ, Wasserstrum N, et al. Influence of short-term indomethacin therapy on fetal urine output. *Obstet Gynecol* 1988;72:51.
254 Norton ME, Merrill J, Cooper BAB, et al. Neonatal complications after the administration of indomethacin for preterm labor. *N Engl J Med* 1993;329:160.
255 Kirshon B, Mari G, Moise KJ. Indomethacin therapy in the treatment of symptomatic polyhydramnios. *Obstet Gynecol* 1990;75:202.
256 Moise KJ. Indomethacin as treatment of symptomatic polyhydramnios. *Contemp Obstet Gynecol* 1995;40:53.
257 Vanhaesebrouck P, Thiery M, Leroy JG, et al. Oligohydramnios, renal insufficiency, and ileal perforation in preterm infants after uterine exposure to indomethacin. *J Pediatr* 1988;113:737.
258 Rasmussen LF, Wennberger RP. Displacement of bilirubin from albumin binding sites by indomethacin. *Clin Res* 1977;25:2.
259 Major CA, Lewis DF, Harding JA, et al. Tocolysis with indomethacin increases the incidence of necrotizing enterocolitis in the low birth weight neonate. *Am J Obstet Gynecol* 1994;170:102.
260 Gardner MO, Owen J, Skelly S, et al. Preterm delivery after indomethacin: a risk factor for neonatal complications? *J Reprod Med* 1996;41:903.
261 Vermillion ST, Newman RB. Recent indomethacin tocolysis is not associated with neonatal complications in preterm infants. *Am J Obstet Gynecol* 1999;181:1083.
262 Abbasi S, Gerdes JS, Sehdev HM, et al. Neonatal outcome after exposure to indomethacin in utero: a retrospective case cohort study. *Am J Obstet Gynecol* 2003;189:782.
263 Dudly DKL, Hardie NJ. Fetal and neonatal effects of indomethacin used as a tocolytic agent. *Am J Obstet Gynecol* 1985;151:181.
264 Niebyl JR, Witter FR. Neonatal outcome after indomethacin treatment of preterm labor. *Am J Obstet Gynecol* 1986;155:747.
265 Marpeau L, Bouillie J, Barrat J, et al. Obstetrical advantages and perinatal risks of indomethacin: a report of 818 cases. *Fetal Diagn Ther* 1994;9:110.
266 Salokorpi T, Eronen M, von Wendt L. Growth and development until 18 months of children exposed to tocolytics indomethacin or nylidrin. *Neuropediatrics* 1996;27:147.
267 Carlan SJ, O'Brien WF, Jones MH, et al. Outpatient oral sulindac to prevent recurrence of preterm labor. *Obstet Gynecol* 1995;85:769.
268 Carlan SJ, O'Brien WF, O'Leary TD, et al. Randomized comparative trial of indomethacin and sulindac for the treatment of refractory preterm labor. *Obstet Gynecol* 1992;79:223.
269 Sawdy RJ, Lye S, Fisk NM, et al. A double-blind randomized study of fetal side effects during and after the short-term maternal administration of indomethacin, sulindac, and nimesulide for the treatment of preterm labor. *Am J Obstet Gynecol* 2003;188:1046.
270 Cole S, Smith R, Giles W. Tocolysis: current controversies, future directions. *Curr Opin Invest Drugs* 2004;5:424.
271 Hollander DI, Nagy DA, Pupkin MJ. Magnesium sulfate and ritodrine hydrochloride. *Am J Obstet Gynecol* 1987;156:631.
272 Gilman AG, Goodman L, Gilman A, eds. *Goodman and Gilman's the pharmacologic basis of therapeutics*, 6th edn. New York: Macmillan, 1980.
273 Altura BM, Altura BT, Carella A, et al. Mg^{+2}-Ca^{+2} interacts in contractility of smooth muscle: magnesium versus organic calcium channel blockers on myogenic tone and agonist-induced responsiveness of blood vessels. *Can J Physiol Pharmacol* 1987;65:729.
274 Mizuki J, Deiich T, Masumoto N, et al. Magnesium sulfate inhibits oxytocin-induced calcium mobilization in human puerperal myometrial cells; possible involvement of intracellular free magnesium concentration. *Am J Obstet Gynecol* 1993;169:134.
275 Sperelakis N, Inoue Y, Ohya Y. Fast Na^+ channels and slow Ca^+ current in smooth muscle from pregnant rat uterus. *Mol Cell Biochem* 1992; 114:79.
276 Cruikshank DP, Pitkin RM, Donnelly E, et al. Urinary magnesium, calcium, and phosphate excretion during magnesium sulfate infusion. *Obstet Gynecol* 1981:58:430.
277 Hoff HE, Smith PK, Winkler AW. Effects of magnesium on nervous system in relation to its concentration in serum. *Am J Physiol* 1940:130:292.
278 Winkler AW, Smith PK, Hoff HE. Intravenous magnesium sulfate in the treatment of nephritic convulsions in adults. *J Clin Invest* 1942:21:207.

279 Chesley LC. Parenteral magnesium sulfate and the distribution, plasma levels, and excretion of magnesium. *Am J Obstet Gynecol* 1979:133:1.
280 McCubbln JH, Sibai BM, Abdella TN, et al. Cardiopulmonary arrest due to acute maternal hypermagnesaemia. *Lancet* 1981:1:1058.
281 Wilkins IA, Lynch L, Mehalek KE, et al. Efficacy and side effects of magnesium sulfate and ritodrine as tocolytic agents. *Am J Obstet Gynecol* 1988:159:685.
282 Wilkins IA, Goldberg JD, Phillips RN, et al. Long-term use of magnesium sulfate as a tocolytic agent. *Obstet Gynecol* 1986:67:385.
283 Ferguson JE, II, Hensleigh PA, Kredenster D. Adjunctive use of magnesium sulfate with ritodrine for preterm labor tocolysis. *Am J Obstet Gynecol* 1984:148:166.
284 Katz M, Robertson PA, Creasy RK. Cardiovascular complications associated with terbutaline treatment for preterm labor. *Am J Obstet Gynecol* 1981:139:605.
285 Ogburn PL, Hansen CA, Williams PP, et al. Magnesium sulfate and β-mimetic dual-agent tocolysis in preterm labor after single-agent failure. *J Reprod Med* 1985;30:583.
286 Diamond MP, Mulloy MK, Entman SS. Combined use of ritodrine and magnesium sulfate for tocolysis of preterm labor (Letter). *Am J Obstet Gynecol* 1985;148:827.
287 Amon E, Petrie RH. Magnesium sulfate, nifedipine, and other calcium antagonists. In: Fuchs AR, Fuchs F, Stubblefield PG, eds. *Preterm birth: causes, prevention, and management.* New York: McGraw-Hill; 1993:333.
288 Holcomb WL, Schackelford GD, Petrie RH. Magnesium tocolysis and neonatal bone abnormalities. *Obstet Gynecol* 1991; 78:611.
289 Smith LG, Burns PA, Schanler RF. Calcium homeostasis in pregnant women receiving long-term magnesium sulfate therapy for preterm labor. *Am J Obstet Gynecol* 1992;167:45.
290 Gray SE, Rodis JF, Lettieri L, et al. Effect of intravenous magnesium sulfate on the biophysical profile of the healthy preterm fetus. *Am J Obstet Gynecol* 1994;170:1131.
291 Sherer DM. Blunted fetal response to vibroacoustic stimulation associated with maternal intravenous magnesium sulfate therapy. *Am J Perinatol* 1994;11:401.
292 Rusu O, Lupan C, Baltescu V. MagnezivI serie in sarcina normala la termen si nasterea prematura. Rolvl magneziterapiei in combatera nasterii premature. *Obstet Gynecol* 1966;14:215.
293 Steer CM, Petrie RH. A comparison of magnesium sulfate and alcohol for the prevention of premature labor. *Am J Obstet Gynecol* 1977;129:1.
294 Miller JM, Keane MW, Horger EO. A comparison of magnesium sulfate and terbutaline for the arrest of premature labor. *J Reprod Med* 1982;27:348.
295 Spisso KR, Harbert GM, Thiagarajah S. The use of magnesium sulfate as the primary tocolytic agent to prevent premature delivery. *Am J Obstet Gynecol* 1982;112:840.
296 Valenzuela G, Cline S. Use of magnesium sulfate in premature labor that fails to respond to β-mimetic drugs. *Am J Obstet Gynecol* 1982;143:718.
297 Elliott JP. Magnesium sulfate as a tocolytic agent. *Am J Obstet Gynecol* 1983:147:277.
298 Tchilinguirian NG, Najem R, Sullivan GB, et al. The use of ritodrine and magnesium sulfate in the arrest of premature labor. *Int J Gynaecol Obstet* 1984;22:117.
299 Beall MH, Edgar BW, Paul AH, et al. A comparison of ritodrine, terbutaline, and magnesium sulfate for the suppression of preterm labor. *Am J Obstet Gynecol* 1985;153:854.
300 Cox SM, Sherman ML, Leveno KJ. Randomized investigation of magnesium sulfate for prevention of preterm birth. *Am J Obstet Gynecol* 1990;163:767.
301 Chau AC, Gabert HA, Miller JM, Jr. A prospective comparison of terbutaline and magnesium for tocolysis. *Obstet Gynecol* 1991;80:847.
302 Hales KA, Matthews JP, Rayburn WE, et al. Intravenous magnesium sulfate for premature labor: comparison between twin and singleton gestations. *Am J Perinatol* 1995:12:7.
303 Elliott JP, Radin TG. Serum magnesium levels during magnesium sulfate tocolysis in high-order multiple gestations. *J Reprod Med* 1995;40:450.
304 Lewis DF, Bergstedt S, Edwards MS, et al. Successful magnesium sulfate tocolysis: is "weaning" the drug necessary? *Am J Obstet Gynecol* 1997;177:742.
305 Hatjis CG, Nelson LH, Meis PJ, et al. Addition of magnesium sulfate improves effectiveness of ritodrine in preventing premature delivery. *Am J Obstet Gynecol* 1984;150:142.
306 Hatjis CG, Swain M, Nelson LH, et al. Efficacy of combined administration of magnesium sulfate and ritodrine in the treatment of premature labor. *Obstet Gynecol* 1987:69:317.
307 Kosasa TS, Busse R, Wahl N, et al. Long-term tocolysis with combined intravenous terbutaline and magnesium sulfate: a 10-year study of 1000 patients. *Obstet Gynecol* 1994;84:369.
308 Coleman TH. Safety and efficacy of combined ritodrine and magnesium sulfate for preterm labor: a method for reduction of complications. *Am J Perinatol* 1990:7:366.
309 Amon E, Midkiff C, Winn HN, et al. Tocolysis with advanced cervical dilatation. *Obstet Gynecol* 2000;95:358.
310 Lewis DF, Grimshaw A, Brooks G, et al. A comparison of magnesium sulfate and indomethacin to magnesium sulfate to magnesium sulfate only for tocolysis in preterm labor with advanced cervical dilatation. *South Med J* 1995:88:737.
311 Dudley D, Gagnon D, Varner M. Long-term tocolysis with intravenous magnesium sulfate. *Obstet Gynecol* 1989:73:373.
312 Cumming WA, Thomas VJ. Hypermagnesemia. A cause of abnormal metaphyses in the neonate. *Am J Roentgenol* 1989;152:1071.
313 Hall DG. Serum magnesium in pregnancy. *Obstet Gynecol* 1957;9:158.
314 Martin RW, Martin IN, Pryor JA, et al. Comparison of oral ritodrine and magnesium gluconate for ambulatory tocolysis. *Am J Obstet Gynecol* 1988:158:1440.
315 Kiss D, Stoke B. Rolle des Magnesiums bei der verhuttung des frühgeburt. *Zentralb Gynakol* 1975:97:924.
316 Kiss V, Balasz M, Morvav F, et al. Effect of maternal magnesium supply on spontaneous abortion and premature birth and on intrauterine foetal development: experimental epidemiological study. *Mag Bull* 1988:3:73.
317 Spatling L, Spading G. Magnesium supplementation in pregnancy: a double-blind study. *Br J Obstet Gynaecol* 1988:95:120.
318 Woljicicka-Jagodzinska J, Romejko E, Piekarski P, et al. Second trimester calcium–phosphorus–magnesium homeostasis in women with threatened preterm delivery. *Int J Gynaecol Obstet* 1998:61:121.
319 Martin RW, Gaddy DK, Martin JN, et al. Tocolysis with oral magnesium. *Am J Obstet Gynecol* 1987:156:433.
320 Ridgeway LE, Moise K, Wright JW, et al. A prospective randomized comparison of oral terbutaline and magnesium oxide for the maintenance of tocolysis. *Am J Obstet Gynecol* 1990: 163:879.
321 Ricci J, Hariharan S, Helfgott A, et al. Oral tocolysis with magnesium chloride: a randomized controlled prospective clinical trial. *Am J Obstet Gynecol* 1991:165:603.

322 Sibai AM, Villar MA, Bray E. Magnesium supplementation during pregnancy: a double-blind randomized controlled clinical trial. *Am J Obstet Gynecol* 1989:161:115.
323 Sibai BM. The use of magnesium sulfate in preeclampsia-eclampsia. In: Petrie RH, ed. *Perinatal pharmacology*. Oradell, NJ: Medical Economics, 1989.
324 Petrie RH. Tocolysis using magnesium sulfate. *Semin Perinatol* 1981:5:266.
325 Elliott JP. Magnesium sulfate for tocolysis. In: Petrie RH, ed. *Perinatal pharmacology*. Oradell, NJ: Medical Economics, 1989.
326 Amon E, Petrie RH. Magnesium as a tocolytic agent. *Clin Consult Obstet Gynecol* 1991:3:231.
327 Nelson KB, Grether JK. Can magnesium sulfate reduce the risk of cerebral palsy in very low birthweight infants? *Pediatrics* 1995:95:263
328 Paneth N, Jetton J, Pintomartin J, et al. Magnesium sulfate in labor and risk of neonatal brain lesions and cerebral palsy in low birthweight infants. *Pediatrics* 1997:99:E11.
329 Canterino J, Verma U, Jeanty M, et al. Magnesium sulfate is not neuroprotective. Preeclampsia is! (Abstract). *Am J Obstet Gynecol* 1997;176:S31.
330 Verma U, Tejani N, Klein S, et al. Obstetric antecedents of intraventricular hemorrhage and periventricular leukomalacia in the low birth weight neonate. *Am J Obstet Gynecol* 1997:176: 275.
331 Wu YW, Escobar GJ, Grether JK, et al. Chorioamnionitis and cerebral palsy in term and near-term infants. *JAMA* 2003; 290:2677.
332 Weglicki WB, Phillips TM, Freedman AM, et al. Magnesium-deficiency elevates circulating levels of inflammatory cytokines and endothelin. *Mol Cell Biochem* 1992:110:169.
333 Mittendorf R, Covert R, Boman J, et al. Is tocolytic magnesium sulphate associated with increased total pediatric mortality? *Lancet* 1997:350:117.
334 Benichou J, Zupan V, Fernandez H, et al. Tocolytic magnesium sulphate and paediatric mortality (Letter). *Lancet* 1998:351: 290.
335 Crowther CA, Hiller J, Doyle L. Tocolytic magnesium sulphate and paediatric mortality (Letter). *Lancet* 1998:351:291.
336 Leveno KJ. Tocolytic magnesium sulphate and paediatric mortality (Letter). *Lancet* 1998:351:292.
337 Grether JK, Hirtz D, McNellis D. Tocolytic magnesium sulphate and paediatric mortality (Letter). *Lancet* 1998:351:292.
338 Grether JK, Hoogstrate J, Selvin S, et al. Magnesium sulfate tocolysis and risk of neonatal death. *Am J Obstet Gynecol* 1998;178:1.
339 Crowther CA, Hiller JE, Doyle LW, et al. Effect of magnesium sulfate given for neuroprotection before preterm birth: a randomized controlled trial. *JAMA* 2003;26;2669.
340 Fleckenstein A. History of calcium antagonists. *Circ Res* 1983:52(Suppl. 1):3.
341 Lewis JG. Adverse reactions to calcium antagonists. *Drugs* 1983:25:196.
342 Talbert RL, Bussey HI. Update on calcium channel blocking agents. *Clin Pharmacol* 1983:2:403.
343 Raemsch KD, Sommer J. Pharmacokinetics and metabolism of nifedipine. *Hypertension* 1983;5(Suppl. 2):18.
344 Ferguson JE, II, Schutz T, Pershe R, et al. Nifedipine pharmacokinetics during preterm labor tocolysis. *Am J Obstet Gynecol* 1989;161:1485.
345 Prevost RR, Akl SA, Sibai BM, et al. Oral nifedipine pharmacokinetics in pregnancy induced hypertension. *Pharmacotherapy,* 1992;12:174.
346 Andersson KE, Ulmsten U. Effects of nifedipine on myometrial activity and lower abdominal pain in women with primary dysmenorrhoea. *Br J Obstet Gynaecol* 1978:85:142.
347 Ulmsten U, Andersson KE, Wingerup L. Treatment of premature labor with the calcium antagonist nifedipine. *Arch Gynecol* 1980:229:1.
348 Kaul AF, Osathanondh R, Safon LE, et al. The management of preterm labor with the calcium channel blocking agent nifedipine combined with the beta mimetic terbutaline. *Drug Intell Clin Pharm* 1985;5:369.
349 Read MD, Wellby DE. The use of a calcium antagonist (nifedipine) to suppress preterm labor. *Br J Obstet Gynaecol* 1986; 93:933.
350 Meyer WR, Randall HW, Graves WL. Nifedipine versus ritodrine for suppressing preterm labor. *J Reprod Med* 1990:35:649.
351 Ferguson JE, Dyson DC, Schutz T, et al. A comparison of tocolysis with nifedipine or ritodrine: analysis of efficacy and maternal, fetal, and neonatal outcome. *Am J Obstet Gynecol* 1990:163:105.
352 Ferguson JE, II, Dyson DC, Holbrook RH, Jr, et al. Cardiovascular and metabolic effects associated with nifedipine and ritodrine tocolysis. *Am J Obstet Gynecol* 1989;161:788.
353 Kupferminc M, Lessing JB, Yaron Y. Nifedipine vs ritodrine for suppression of preterm labour. *Br J Obstet Gynaecol* 1993; 100:1090.
354 Glock JL, Morales WJ. Efficacy and safety of nifedipine vs magnesium sulfate in the management of preterm labor: a randomized study. *Am J Obstet Gynecol* 1993:169:960.
355 Papatsonis DN, Van Geijn HP, Ader HJ, et al. Nifedipine and ritodrine in the management of preterm labor: a randomized multicenter trial. *Obstet Gynecol* 1997:90:230
356 Smith CS, Woodland MB. Clinical comparison of oral nifedipine and subcutaneous terbutaline for initial tocolysis. *Am J Perinatol* 1993:10:280.
357 Sawaya GE, Robertson PA. Hepatotoxicity with the administration of nifedipine for treatment of preterm labor. *Am J Obstet Gynecol* 1992;167:512.
358 Snyder SW, Cardwell MS. Neuromuscular blockade with magnesium sulfate and nifedipine. *Am J Obstet Gynecol* 1989:161: 35.
359 Ben-ami M, Giladi Y, Shalev E. The combination of magnesium sulfate and nifedipine: a cause of neuromuscular blockade. *Br J Obstet Gynaecol* 1994:101:262.
360 Koontz SL, Friedman SA, Schwartz ML. Symptomatic hypocalcemia after tocolytic therapy with magnesium sulfate and nifedipine. *Am J Obstet Gynecol* 2004;190:1773.
361 Ducsay CA, Thompson JS, Wu AT, et al. Effects of calcium entry blocker (nicardipine) tocolysis in rhesus macaques: fetal plasma concentrations and cardiorespiratory changes. *Am J Obstet Gynecol* 1987:157:1482.
362 Harake B, Gilbert RD, Ashwal S, et al. Nifedipine. Effects on fetal and maternal hemodynamics in pregnant sheep. *Am J Obstet Gynecol* 1987;157:1003.
363 Parisi VM, Salinas J, Stockmar EJ. Fetal vascular responses to maternal nicardipine administration in the hypertensive ewe. *Am J Obstet Gynecol* 1989:161:1035.
364 Mari G, Kirshon B, Moise KJ, Jr, et al. Doppler assessment of the fetal and uteroplacental circulation during nifedipine therapy for preterm labor. *Am J Obstet Gynecol* 198;161:1514.
365 Guclu S, Saygili U, Dogan E, et al. The short-term effect of nifedipine tocolysis on placental, fetal cerebral, and atrioventricular Doppler waveforms. *Obstet Gynecol Surv* 2005;60: 287.

366 Hanretty KR, Whittle MJ, Howie CA, et al. Effect of nifedipine on Doppler flow velocity waveforms in severe preeclampsia. *Br Med J* 1989:299:1205.
367 Moretti M, Fairle FM, Aki S, et al. The effect of nifedipine therapy on fetal and placental Doppler waveforms in preeclampsia remote from term. *Am J Obstet Gynecol* 1990:163:1844.
368 Keirse MJNC. Progestogen administration in pregnancy may prevent preterm delivery. *Br J Obstet Gynaecol* 1990:97: 149.
369 Meis PJ, Klebanoff M, Thom E, et al. Prevention of recurrent preterm delivery by 17 alpha-hydroxyprogesterone caproate. *N Engl J Med* 2003;348:2379.
370 da Fonseca EB, Bittar RE, Carvalho MH, et al. Prophylactic administration of progesterone by vaginal suppository to reduce the incidence of spontaneous preterm birth in women at increased risk: a randomized placebo-controlled double blind study. *Am J Obstet Gynecol* 2003;188:419.
371 Erny R, Pigne A, Prouvost C, et al. The effects of oral administration of progesterone for premature labor. *Am J Obstet Gynecol* 1986:154:525.
372 Sanchez-Ramos L, Kaunitz AM, Delke I. Progestational agents to prevent preterm birth: a meta-analysis of randomized controlled trials. *Obstet Gynecol* 2005;105:273.
373 Fuchs AR, Fuchs F, Husslein P, et al. Oxytocin receptors in the human uterus during pregnancy and parturition. *Am J Obstet Gynecol* 1984:150:734.
374 Akerlund M, Stromberg P, Hauksson A, et al. Inhibition of uterine contractions of premature labour with an oxytocin analogue. Results from a pilot study. *Br J Obstet Gynaecol* 1987:94:1040.
375 Wilson L, Parsons MT, Quano L, et al. A new tocolytic agent: development of an oxytocin antagonist for inhibiting uterine contractions. *Am J Obstet Gynecol* 1990;163:195.
376 Andersen LF, Lyndrup J, Akerlund M, et al. Oxytocin receptor blockade: a new principle in the treatment of preterm labor? *Am J Perinatol* 1989;6:196.
377 Goodwin TM, Paul RH, Silver H, et al. The effect of the oxytocin antagonist atosiban on preterm uterine activity in the human. *Am J Obstet Gynecol* 1994:170:474.
378 Goodwin TM, Valenzuela G, Silver H, et al. Treatment of preterm labor with the oxytocin antagonist atosiban. *Am J Perinatol* 1996:13:143.
379 Romero R, Sibai BM, Sanchez-Ramos L, et al. An oxytocin receptor antagonist (antosiban) in the treatment of preterm labor: a randomized, double-blind, placebo-controlled trial with tocolytic rescue. *Am J Obstet Gynecol* 2000;182:1173.
380 European Atosiban Study Group. The oxytocin antagonist atosiban versus the beta-agonist terbutaline in the treatment of preterm labor. A randomized, double-blind, controlled study. *Acta Obstet Gynecol Scand* 2001;80:413.
381 Moutquin JM, Sherman D, Cohen H, et al. Double-blind, randomized, controlled trial of antosiban and ritodrine in the treatment of preterm labor: a multicenter effectiveness and safety study. *Am J Obstet Gynecol* 2000;182:1191.
382 The Atosiban PTL-098 Study Group. Maintenance treatment of preterm labor with the oxytocin antagonist atosiban. *Am J Obstet Gynecol* 2000;182:1184.
383 Sladek SM, Regenstein AC, Lykins D, et al. Nitric oxide synthetase activity in pregnant rabbit uterus decreases on the last day of pregnancy. *Am J Obstet Gynecol* 1993:169:1285.
384 Izumi H, Yallampalli C, Garfield RE. Gestational changes in l-arginine induced relaxation of pregnant rat and human myometrial smooth muscle. *Am J Obstet Gynecol* 1993:169:1327.
385 Abouleish AE, Corn SB. Intravenous nitroglycerin for intrapartum external version of the second twin. *Anesth Analg* 1994:78:808.
386 Kahler C, Schleussner E, Moller A, et al. Nitric oxide donors: effects on fetoplacental blood flow. *Eur J Obstet Gynecol Reprod Biol* 2004;115:10.
387 Lees C, Campbell S, Janlaux E, et al. Arrest of preterm labour and prolongation of gestation with glyceryl trinitrate, a nitric acid donor. *Lancet* 1994:343:1325.
388 Schleussner E, Moller A, Gross W, et al. Maternal and fetal side effects of tocolysis using transdermal nitroglycerin or intravenous fenoterol combined with magnesium sulfate. *Eur J Obstet Gynecol Reprod Biol* 2003;106:14.
389 de Spirlet M, Treluyer JM, Chevret S, et al. Tocolytic effects of intravenous nitroglycerin. *Fundam Clin Pharmacol* 2004;18: 207.
390 Black RS, Lees C, Thompson C, et al. Maternal and fetal cardiovascular effects of transdermal glyceryl trinitrate and intravenous ritodrine. *Obstet Gynecol* 1999;94:572.
391 Bisits A, Madsen G, Knox M, et al. The Randomized Nitric Oxide Tocolysis Trial (RNOTT) for the treatment of preterm labor. *Am J Obstet Gynecol* 2004;191:683.
392 El-Sayed YY, Riley ET, Holbrook RH, Jr, et al. Randomized comparison of intravenous nitroglycerin and magnesium sulfate for treatment of preterm labor. *Obstet Gynecol* 1999;93:79.
393 Smith GN, Walker MC, McGrath MJ. Randomized, double-blind, placebo controlled pilot study assessing nitroglycerin as a tocolytic. *Br J Obstet Gynaecol* 1999;106:736.
394 Liggins GC, Howie RN. A controlled trial of antepartum glucocorticoid treatment for prevention of the respiratory distress syndrome in premature infants. *Pediatrics* 1972:50:515.
395 Crowley PA, Chalmers L, Keirse MJNC. The effects of corticosteroid administration before preterm delivery: an overview of the evidence from controlled trials. *Br J Obstet Gynaecol* 1990:97:11.
396 Crowley PA. Antenatal corticosteroid therapy: a meta analysis of the randomized trials, 1972–1994. *Am J Obstet Gynecol* 1995:173:322.
397 US Department of Health and Human Services. *Prevention of respiratory distress syndrome. Effect of antenatal dexamethasone administration.* Washington, DC: US Government Printing Office. NIH Publication no. 85–2695, August 1985.
398 Doyle LW, Kitchen WH, Ford GW, et al. Effects of antenatal steroid therapy on mortality and morbidity in very low birth weight infants. *Pediatrics* 1986:108:287.
399 Garite TJ, Rumney PJ, Briggs GG, et al. A randomized placebo controlled trial of betamethasone for the prevention of respiratory distress syndrome at 24 to 28 weeks gestation. *Am J Obstet Gynecol* 1992:166:646.
400 Wright LL, Horbar JD, Gunkel H, et al. Evidence from the multicenter networks on the current use and effectiveness of antenatal corticosteroids in low birth weight infants. *Am J Obstet Gynecol* 1995:173:263.
401 Bauer CR, Morrison JC, Poole K. A decreased incidence of necrotizing enterocolitis after prenatal glucocorticoid therapy. *Pediatrics* 1984:73:682.
402 Ohlsson A, Fox GF. Letter to the editor and response. *Am J Obstet Gynecol* 1996:174:1078.
403 Slavin RE. Best evidence synthesis: an intelligent alternative to meta-analysis. *J Clin Epidemiol* 1995:48:9.
404 NIH Consensus Statement. Effect of corticosteroids for fetal maturation on prenatal outcomes, February 28 to March 2, 1994. *Am J Obstet Gynecol* 1995:173:246.

405 Ballard PL, Ballard RA. Scientific basis and therapeutic regimens for use of antenatal glucocorticoids. *Am J Obstet Gynecol* 1995:173:253.

406 Elliott JP, Radin TG. The effect of corticosteroid administration on uterine activity and preterm labor in high-order multiple gestations. *Obstet Gynecol* 1995:85:250.

407 Parvin CA, Kaplan LA, Chapman JF, et al. Predicting respiratory distress syndrome using gestational age and fetal lung maturity by fluorescent polarization. *Am J Obstet Gynecol* 2005;192:199.

408 Guinn DA, Atkinson MW, Sullivan L, et al. Single vs weekly courses of antenatal corticosteroids for women at risk of preterm delivery: a randomized controlled trial. *JAMA* 2001;286:1581.

409 Vermillion ST, Bland ML, Soper DE. Effectiveness of a rescue dose of antenatal betamethasone after an initial single dose. *Am J Obstet Gynecol* 2001;185:1086.

410 Sen S, Reghu A, Ferguson SD. Efficacy of a single dose of antenatal steroid in surfactant-treated babies under 31 weeks' gestation. *J Maternal Fetal Neonatal Med* 2002;12:298.

411 Bedalov A, Balasubramanyarn A. Glucocorticoid-induced ketoacidosis in gestational diabetes: a sequela of the acute treatment of preterm labor. *Diabetes Care* 1997:20:922.

412 Mushkat Y, Ascher-Landsberg J, Keider R, et al. The effect of betamethasone versus dexamethasone on fetal biophysical parameter. *Eur J Obstet Gynecol Reprod Biol* 2001;97:50.

413 Magee LA, Dawes GS, Moulden M, et al. A randomized controlled comparison of betamethasone with dexamethasone: effects on the antenatal fetal heart rate. *Br J Obstet Gynecol* 1997;104:1233.

414 Maschiach S, Barkai G, Sach J, et al. Enhancement of fetal lung maturity by intra-amniotic administration of thyroid hormone. *Am J Obstet Gynecol* 1978:130:289.

415 Morales WJ, O'Brien WE, Angel JL, et al. Fetal lung maturation: the combined use of corticosteroids and thyrotropin-releasing hormone. *Obstet Gynecol* 1989:73:111.

416 Ballard RA, Ballard PL, Cnaan A, et al. Antenatal thyrotropin-releasing hormone to prevent lung disease in preterm infants. North American Thyrotropin-Releasing Hormone Study Group. *N Engl J Med* 1998;338:493.

417 Collaborative Santiago Surfactant Group. Collaborative trial of prenatal thyrotropin-releasing hormone and corticosteroids for prevention of respiratory distress syndrome. *Am J Obstet Gynecol* 1998;178:33.

418 Crowther CA, Alfirevic Z, Haslam RR. Thyrotropin-releasing hormone added to corticosteroids for women at risk of preterm birth for preventing neonatal respiratory disease. *Cochrane Database Syst Rev* 2004;2:CD000019.

419 Shankaran S, Cepeda EE, Hagarn M, et al. Antenatal phenobarbital for the prevention of neonatal intracerebral hemorrhage. *Am J Obstet Gynecol* 1986:154:53.

420 Morales WJ, Koerten J. Prevention of intraventricular hemorrhage in very low birth weight infants by maternally administered phenobarbital. *Obstet Gynecol* 1986:68:295.

421 Pomerance JJ, Teal JG, Gegolok JF, et al. Maternally administered antenatal vitamin K: effect on neonatal prothrombin activity. Partial thromboplastin time and intraventricular hemorrhage. *Obstet Gynecol* 1987:70:295.

422 Morales WJ, Angel JL, O'Brien WE, et al. The use of antenatal vitamin K in the prevention of early neonatal intraventricular hemorrhage. *Am J Obstet Gynecol* 1988:159:774.

423 Kazzi NH, Hagan NH, Liang KC, et al. Maternal administration of vitamin K does not improve the coagulation profile of preterm infants. *Pediatrics* 1989:84:1045.

424 Morales WL, Angel JF, O'Brien WF, et al. A randomized study of antibiotic therapy in idiopathic preterm labor. *Obstet Gynecol* 1988:72:829.

425 Newton ER, Dinsmoor MJ, Gibbs RS. A randomized blinded placebo-controlled trial of antibiotics in idiopathic preterm labor. *Obstet Gynecol* 1989:74:562.

426 Romero R, Sibai BM, Caritis S, et al. Antibiotic treatment of preterm labor and intact membranes: a multicenter, randomized. double blinded, placebo-controlled trial in the NIH randomized double blinded, placebo-controlled study. *Am J Obstet Gynecol* 1993:169:764.

427 Egarter C, Leitch H, Hussein P, et al. Adjunctive antibiotic treatment in preterm labor and neonatal morbidity: a meta-analysis. *Obstet Gynecol* 1996:88:303.

428 Mercer BM, Arheart KL. Antimicrobial therapy in expectant management of preterm premature rupture of membranes. *Lancet* 1995:346:1271.

429 Svare J, Langanoff-Roos J, Andersen LF, et al. Ampicillin-metronidazole treatment in idiopathic preterm labour: a randomized controlled multicentre trial. *Br J Obstet Gynaecol* 1997:104:892.

430 Vermeulen GM, Bruinse HW. Prophylactic administration of clindamycin 2% vaginal cream to reduce the incidence of spontaneous preterm birth in women with an increased recurrence risk: a randomised placebo-controlled double-blind trial. *Br J Obstet Gynaecol* 1999;106:652.

431 Carey JC, Klebanoff MA, Hauth JC, et al. Metronidazole to prevent preterm delivery in pregnant women with asymptomatic bacterial vaginosis. National Institute of Child Health and Human Development Network of Maternal-Fetal Medicine Units. *N Engl J Med.* 2000;342:534.

432 Huff DL, Thurnau GR, Sheldon R. The outcome of protective forceps deliveries of 26–33 week infants. *Proc Soc Perinatal Obstet* 1987:Abstract 45.

433 Anderson GC, Bada HS, Sibai BM, et al. The relationship between labor and route of delivery in the preterm infant. *Am J Obstet Gynecol* 1988:158:1382.

434 Tejani N, Verma U, Hameed C. Chayen B. Method and route of delivery in the low birth weight vertex presentation correlated with early periventricular/intraventricular hemorrhage. *Obstet Gynecol* 1987:69:1.

435 Schwartz D, Miodovnik M, Lavin J. Neonatal outcome among low birth weight infants delivered spontaneously or by low forceps. *Obstet Gynecol* 1983:62:283.

436 Died J, Arnold H, Mentzel H, et al. Effect of cesarean section on outcome in high- and low-risk very preterm infants. *Arch Gynecol Obstet* 1989:246:91.

437 Grant A, Glazener CM. Elective caesarean section versus expectant management for delivery of the small baby. *Cochrane Database Syst Rev* 2001;2:CD000078.

438 Penn ZJ, Steer PJ, Grant A. A multicentre randomised controlled trial comparing elective and selective caesarean section for the delivery of the preterm breech infant. *Br J Obstet Gynaecol* 1996;103:684.

439 Grant A, Penn ZJ, Steer PJ. Elective or selective caesarean delivery of the small baby? A systematic review of the controlled trials. *Br J Obstet Gynaecol* 1996;103:1197.

440 Goldenberg RL, Iams JD, Mercer BM, et al. The preterm birth prediction study: the value of new vs old risk factors in predicting early and all spontaneous preterm births. *Am J Public Health* 1998:88:233.

441 Imseis HM, Albert TA, Iams JD. Identifying twin gestations at low risk for preterm birth with a transvaginal ultrasonographic

cervical measurement at 24 to 26 weeks gestation. *Am J Obstet Gynecol* 1997:177:1149.

442 Papiernik E, Breart G. Should a prevention program be proposed to high risk patients or all patients? *Am J Obstet Gynecol* 1994:171:1676.

443 Hobel CJ, Ross MG, Bemis RL, et al. The West Los Angeles Preterm Birth Prevention Project II. Program impact on high risk women. *Am J Obstet Gynecol* 1994:170:54.

444 Ross MG, Sanhu M, Bemis R, et al. The West Los Angeles Preterm Birth Prevention Project II. Cost-effectiveness analysis of high risk pregnancy interventions. *Obstet Gynecol* 1994:83: 506.

445 Zalar RW. Transvaginal ultrasound and preterm prelabor: a non-randomized intervention study. *Obstet Gynecol* 1996:88:20.

446 Miller HC, Merritt TA. *Fetal growth in humans.* Chicago: Year Book Medical Publishers, 1977.

447 Petrini KR, Callaghan WM, Klebanoff M, et al. Estimated effect of 17 alpha-hydroxyprogesterone caproate on preterm birth in the United States. *Obstet Gynecol* 2005;105:267.

63 Prelabor rupture of the membranes

Joaquin Santolaya-Forgas, Roberto Romero, Jimmy Espinoza, Offer Erez, Lara A. Friel, Juan Pedro Kusanovic, Ray Bahado-Singh, and Jyh Kae Nien

Definitions

Prelabor rupture of the membranes (PROM) refers to rupture of the chorioamniotic membranes before the onset of labor.[1] The "latency period" is the interval between PROM and the onset of labor. There is no agreement about the length of the interval between rupture of the membranes and the onset of labor required to diagnose PROM. This period of time has been proposed in different reports, to last from 1 to 12 h.[2–9] Some authors have suggested the term "prolonged PROM" to describe a latency period longer than 24 h, but such usage is uncommon.[2,10,11] The consequences of PROM depend on the gestational age. Therefore, this condition has been classified as "preterm PROM" or "term PROM," depending upon whether the episode occurs prior to or after 37 weeks of gestation.[2–12] The term "previable PROM" has been applied to gestations in which this complication occurs before 23 weeks,[12] while "preterm PROM remote from term" refers to the time-frame between viability to about 32 weeks, and "PROM near term" is that which occurs between 32 and 36 weeks.[12]

Frequency, timing, and site of membrane rupture

Frequency

Term PROM occurs in approximately 10% of patients, while the frequency of preterm PROM is 2–3.5%.[5,13–17] Preterm PROM accounts for 30–40% of preterm deliveries and therefore is a leading clinically identifiable cause of preterm birth as well as a major contributor to perinatal morbidity and mortality.[2,5,13,14,16–19] It has been estimated that, in the United States, approximately 150 000 women experience preterm PROM every year.[20]

When do membranes normally rupture?

This question was addressed by a collaborative study in which an effort was made to avoid artificial rupture of the fetal membranes during labor.[21] Figure 63.1 shows the proportion of women with spontaneous rupture of membranes as a function of cervical dilatation. Most patients had spontaneous rupture of membranes at the end of the first stage of labor; hence, the rationale for defining PROM as rupture of membranes before the onset of labor.

Where is the site of membrane rupture?

The site of rupture is generally located in the most dependent part of the uterine cavity in close proximity to the cervix. This has been demonstrated using endoscopy in patients with preterm PROM.[22] After invasive procedures such as fetoscopy, rupture of membranes can occur away from the cervix. However, the frequency with which spontaneous rupture of membranes occurs away from the most dependent part of the uterus ("high leak") is unknown.

Fetal membranes

What are the fetal membranes?

The term "fetal membranes" is applied to an anatomic structure that includes amnion and chorion (which are of fetal origin) and portions of decidua (of maternal origin). Bell and McParland proposed to refer to this structure as the "amniochorial–decidual unit."[23] Figure 63.2 displays the microscopic anatomy of the human amnion and chorion, as described by Bourne in 1960.[24] The amnion is derived from the cytotrophoblast and consists of an epithelium, which faces the amniotic cavity, a compact layer responsible for most of the strength of the amnion, as well as a spongy layer interposed between the amnion and chorion.[25–27] The spongy layer allows the amnion to slide over the fixed chorion. The chorion contains several connective tissue layers, of which the outermost is closely attached to, and often indistinguishable from, the decidua capsularis. The amniochorial–decidual unit is fundamentally an extracellular matrix structure endowed with unique cellular components: amnion, chorion, and decidua. Figure 63.3 displays the distribution of collagen and other extracellular matrix components in the different layers of the amniochorial–decidual unit.

What are the changes in the fetal membranes during spontaneous rupture of membranes?

Examination of the chorioamniotic membranes from patients undergoing elective Cesarean delivery at term with intact membranes has demonstrated that membranes apposed to the cervix have localized morphologic changes which have been referred to as a "zone of altered morphology" (ZAM).[28] ZAM is proposed to encompass an area of about 119 ± 21 cm^2 [29] and is characterized by marked swelling and disruption of the connective tissue, thinning of the trophoblast layer, and thinning or absence of the decidua.[28] Moreover, Bell and McParland[23] demonstrated that the ZAM has increased programmed cell death (apoptosis). A population of mesenchymal cells in the chorion switches their phenotype to activated myofibroblasts.[30] This phenotype has been proposed to emerge when the extracellular matrix is exposed to stress forces caused by stretching of the membranes during uterine growth and uterine contractions. Myofibroblasts are thought to provide a counteractive contractile force to protect the membranes. Changes in extracellular matrix composition in the ZAM include a significant decrease in the density of collagens I, III, and V, and increased expression of tenascin-C[31] and osteonectin.[32] These proteins are expressed during tissue remodeling and wound healing, suggesting that the membranes exhibit a similar response. Increased intrauterine pressure during labor is likely to exert pressure over this weakened area of the membranes (ZAM), resulting in membrane rupture. Preliminary observations by Bell and Malak suggest that the changes in the ZAM are more extensive in preterm PROM.[28,33,34]

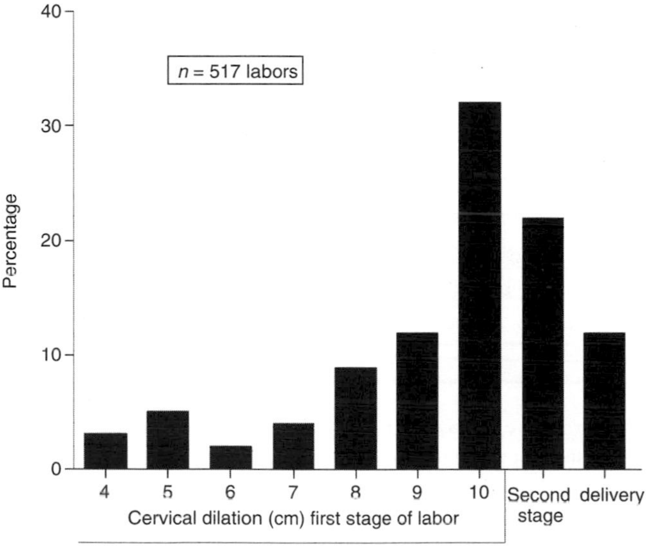

Figure 63.1 Rupture of membranes as a function of cervical dilatation and state of labor. Percentage distribution for 517 normal spontaneous deliveries without medication or maneuvers; vertex presentation. From ref. 21 with permission from the World Health Organization.

Biophysical properties of membranes that rupture prematurely

A critical question is whether the membranes that rupture prematurely are inherently weaker, and whether such weakness is generalized or localized. The earliest experiments designed to investigate this question were probably those performed by Poppel in 1863[35] and Duncan in 1869.[36] Duncan dropped cannonballs onto membranes stretched over a ring to determine their tensile strength. Since that time, most investigators have hypothesized that membranes rupturing prematurely are inherently weaker.

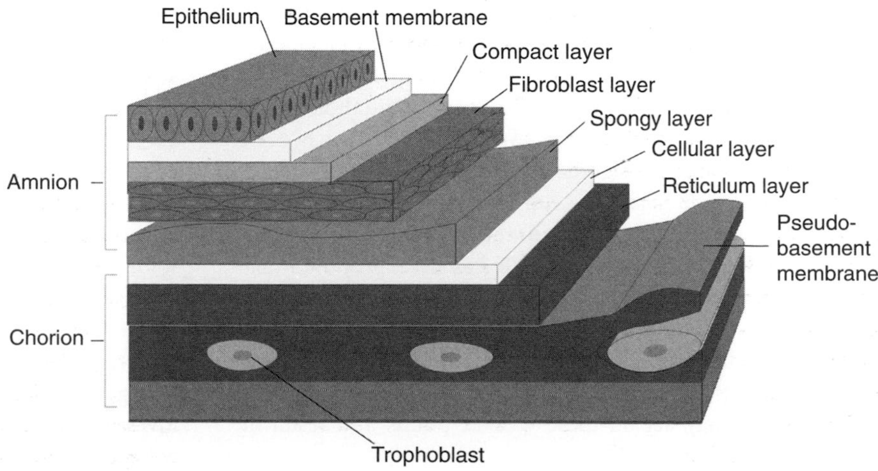

Figure 63.2 Histological layers of the amniochorionic membranes. From ref. 24 with permission from Elsevier.

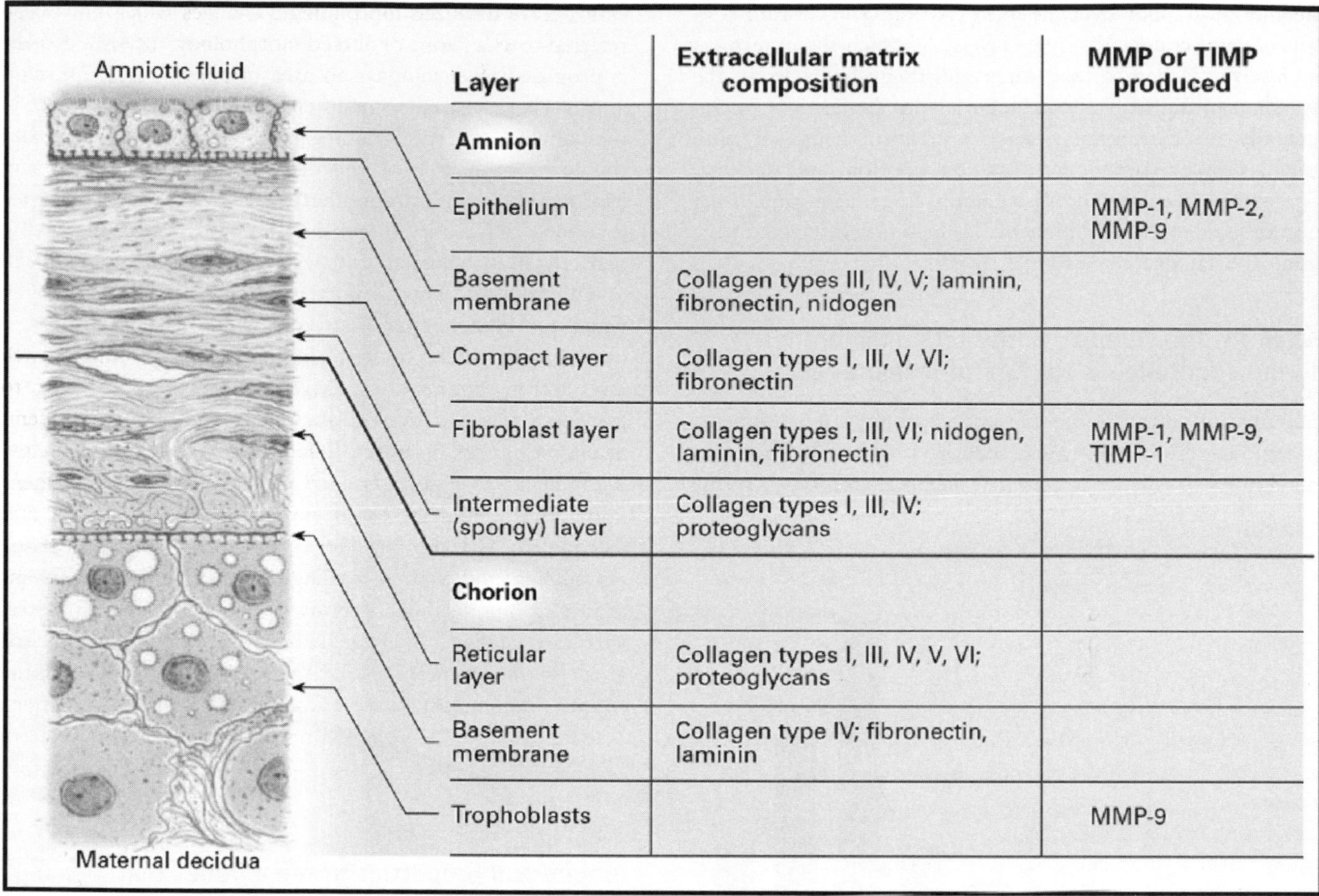

Layer	Extracellular matrix composition	MMP or TIMP produced
Amnion		
Epithelium		MMP-1, MMP-2, MMP-9
Basement membrane	Collagen types III, IV, V; laminin, fibronectin, nidogen	
Compact layer	Collagen types I, III, V, VI; fibronectin	
Fibroblast layer	Collagen types I, III, VI; nidogen, laminin, fibronectin	MMP-1, MMP-9, TIMP-1
Intermediate (spongy) layer	Collagen types I, III, IV; proteoglycans	
Chorion		
Reticular layer	Collagen types I, III, IV, V, VI; proteoglycans	
Basement membrane	Collagen type IV; fibronectin, laminin	
Trophoblasts		MMP-9

Figure 63.3 Schematic representation of the structure of the fetal membranes at term. The extracellular matrix composition of each layer and the production sites of matrix metalloproteinases (MMP) and tissue inhibitors of metalloproteinases (TIMP) are shown. From ref. 38 with permission from the Massachusetts Medical Society.

Indeed, during pregnancy, the chorioamniotic membranes undergo elastic distention or stretch. The intrauterine surface area increases during gestation (as measured by ultrasound *in vivo*); however, the surface area of the membranes, as measured *in vitro*, increases to a lesser extent.[37] During labor, membrane rupture has been attributed to a generalized weakening of the membranes due to repeated stretching.[38] Evidence in support of this view is that the tensile strength of membrane specimens obtained after labor is lower than that of those obtained by Cesarean delivery in the absence of labor.[39]

However, despite testing with various devices, it has been difficult to demonstrate significant differences in the bursting tension between prematurely ruptured and nonprematurely ruptured membranes.[40–48] Membranes that rupture before labor have decreased elasticity.[41,46] It has been proposed that these membranes have focal areas of weakness rather than a generalized weakening.[38,47–50] The use of computer modeling of the biomechanical properties of the chorioamniotic membranes (Lavery's computer model) suggests that acute or chronic stress may act on these weaker points and result in rupture of membranes.[47,48]

Biochemical studies

Collagen concentration of fetal membranes and PROM

The chorioamniotic membranes are essentially connective tissue structures.[34,51,52] As collagen determines the tensile strength of fibrous connective tissue, there has been considerable interest in investigating collagen biochemistry in the setting of PROM. Two studies have shown that total collagen content is reduced in the amnion of women with preterm PROM.[51,52] Skinner and coworkers[51] found that total collagen concentration was lower in the amnion of women with PROM than in that of women with intact membranes.

Subsequently, Kanayama and colleagues[52] reported that total collagen content was lower in the amnion of patients with preterm PROM than in those with preterm delivery with intact membranes. The difference in collagen content in preterm PROM was attributed to a decrease in type III collagen, which provides elastic tensility to tissues. These investigators could not demonstrate a decrease in total collagen content in the amnion of patients with term PROM,

delivery. They found that patients with preterm PROM were more likely to have had sexual intercourse in the missionary position during the previous 4 weeks when compared with matched control subjects (adjusted OR 2.4, 95% CI 1.2–5.0). Other sexual activities were not associated with an increased risk of preterm PROM. Moreover, no connection was found between sexual activity and term PROM. We conclude that, with the possible exception of intercourse in the missionary position late in pregnancy, little evidence implicates coitus *per se* in the etiology of PROM. However, to the extent that sexual intercourse may be the method of transmission for sexually transmitted diseases associated with PROM (i.e., *Neisseria gonorrhoeae*), this behavior may confer some risk.

Vitamin C and trace elements

Vitamin C is involved in the metabolism of collagen and has been proposed to play an important role in the maintenance of the integrity of the chorioamniotic membranes.[169] Evidence in support of this view includes: (1) the rate of PROM is higher among patients with low maternal plasma ascorbic acid concentrations than among those with normal plasma concentrations [14.6% (13/89) in patients with a level of 0.20 mg/dL or less versus 1.4% (1/69) in patients with a level of 0.60 mg/dL or more];[170] (2) decreased concentrations of vitamin C in leukocytes at 20 weeks of gestation have been associated with the subsequent development of PROM;[145] (3) *in vitro* studies demonstrated that increasing concentrations of vitamin C in culture media decreased MMP-1, MMP-2, and MMP-9 enzymatic activity and concentrations;[171] (4) Barrett et al.[146] reported a decreased amniotic fluid concentration of vitamin C in women with PROM; and (5) the total ascorbic acid concentration is significantly lower in the amniotic membranes from patients with preterm PROM than from control subjects (PROM median: 0.0265 mol/g tissue, range 0.008–0.129 versus control median: 0.034 mol/g tissue, range 0.009–0.135; $P = 0.01$).[172]

Casanueva et al.[169] reported a randomized, double-blind controlled study of vitamin C supplementation, in which women with singleton gestations at less than 20 weeks were randomized to vitamin C supplementation (100 mg/day) ($n = 52$) or placebo ($n = 57$).[169] Supplementation with vitamin C was associated with a reduction in the rate of PROM of 74% (RR 0.26, 95% CI 0.078–0.837).

Copper deficiency has been shown to inhibit the maturation of collagen and elastin, although studies of the association of copper levels during pregnancy and PROM have shown conflicting results. Artal et al.[173] reported that, while patients with term PROM had lower copper concentrations in maternal and umbilical cord sera than patients with artificial rupture of membranes during labor, there was no difference in membrane copper content. These findings were not confirmed by a subsequent study by Kiilholma and colleagues,[174] who found no differences in maternal or fetal serum copper concentrations between term patients with and without PROM. On the other hand, umbilical cord (but not maternal) serum copper and ceruloplasmin levels were significantly lower in patients with preterm PROM than in those with preterm delivery without PROM.

Two studies have addressed the relationship between zinc and PROM. Kiilholma and colleagues[174] found no significant difference in maternal and umbilical cord zinc serum concentrations between patients with preterm PROM and those with preterm delivery with intact membranes. A limitation of this study is that serum zinc reflects only a minor proportion of the total body zinc. In another study, a maternal zinc index was calculated (a sum of measurements of zinc in maternal blood, scalp and pubic hair, and colostrum) and was found to be lower in patients with term PROM than in those without this condition.[174,175] On the other hand, magnesium[176] and calcium[177] supplementation in pregnancy has no effect on the incidence of preterm PROM.[176,177]

Elevated maternal serum alpha-fetoprotein concentration (MSAFP)

One study reported that women with an elevated second-trimester MSAFP (more than 2.0 multiples of the median) have a significantly increased risk of subsequent preterm PROM (OR 10.4, 95% CI 3.6–29.4),[178] while two other studies demonstrated no such association.[179,180] The possible association between preterm PROM and elevated MSAFP suggests that leakage of fetal proteins into the maternal circulation may predispose to PROM. This, however, remains speculative.

Previous operations on the genital tract

There are no consistent results on the effect of cervical surgery on the risk of PROM.[181,182] While some studies demonstrated a higher frequency of PROM among patients with a history of cervical conization or dilation and curettage (D&C),[135,136,183] other studies could not demonstrate an association between a history of surgical manipulation and PROM after controlling for confounding variables.[147,181,182]

Pelvic examinations and PROM

Lenihan[184] reported a randomized prospective trial in which women at 37 weeks of gestation were randomized to either weekly pelvic examinations or none at all. PROM was more common in women who underwent repeated pelvic examinations than in the control group [18% (32/174) versus 6% (10/175), $P < 0.001$]. In contrast, McDuffie et al.[185] performed a prospective randomized trial of weekly cervical examinations beginning at the 37th week of gestation versus none at all, and found no differences in the rate of PROM, chorioamnionitis, or neonatal infectious morbidity between the two management policies.

Main et al.[186] reported the results of a preterm delivery prevention program in which women at risk of preterm delivery were randomized to either biweekly pelvic examinations or standard obstetric care. No significant difference in the frequency of PROM was noted between the two groups [50%

(8/16) versus 28.6% (4/14)]. This observation was subsequently confirmed with a larger sample size.[187] Holbrook et al.,[188] in a retrospective review of patients enrolled in a preterm birth prevention program that called for weekly cervical examinations between 20 and 37 weeks, found no increase in rates of preterm PROM, chorioamnionitis, or postpartum endometritis. While most reports do not seem to support an etiologic role for digital examination of the cervix in PROM, the technique of the digital examination is probably important. An examination in which the endocervical canal is probed with the examining finger may dislodge or damage the mucus plug and carry bacteria into close proximity to the membranes. An examination limited to the fornix and external os would not carry a risk of this kind. However, such examination is uninformative for effacement. Sonographic examination can provide information regarding cervical length without the risk of dislodging the mucus plug. We, therefore, do not see the justification for performing repeated cervical examinations during pregnancy if ultrasound is available.

Colonization and infection of the lower genital tract with selective microorganisms

Evidence supports an association between endocervical infection with *Chlamydia trachomatis* and *N. gonorrhoeae* and the development of PROM, but not with colonization with group B *Streptococcus*, genital *Mycoplasmas*, or the presence of bacterial vaginosis in low-risk populations and the development of PROM.[111,189] The relationship between colonization/infection or a change in the bacterial ecosystem and the subsequent development of preterm PROM is reviewed below.

Bacterial vaginosis and vaginal inflammation

An association between bacterial vaginosis (BV) and preterm PROM has been reported in some studies, largely in high-risk patients. However, the results are not consistent. For example, Kurki et al.[115] reported that women with a diagnosis of bacterial vaginosis (BV) between 8 and 17 weeks of gestation had a high risk of preterm PROM (OR 7.3, 95% CI 1.8–29.4). In the Prediction of Prematurity Study, BV was found to be a modest risk factor for preterm PROM before 37 weeks[108] (see Table 63.3). These results contrast with those of a large cohort study of 10 397 women at low risk of preterm delivery, in which no association was found between BV and PROM.[190]

An explanation for the inconsistent results is that only a subset of patients with BV is at risk of preterm birth. Such a subset may represent patients with vaginal inflammation, which can be detected by determining the number of neutrophils in vaginal fluid. The conventional diagnosis of BV relies only on the classification of the microbial flora of the vagina. Using these criteria, approximately 20% of women will have BV, and most will not deliver a preterm neonate or have preterm PROM. There is evidence that patients with vaginal inflammation (with or without BV) may be at risk of subsequent preterm delivery. For example, Simhan et al.[116] reported that patients with vaginal inflammation (defined as vaginal pH > 5 and more than five neutrophils per oil field) in the midtrimester had a higher risk of preterm PROM remote from term in the index pregnancy (for preterm PROM between 24 and 32 weeks: OR 11.7, 95% CI 2.8–49.5). A full discussion of the subject is available for interested readers.[191]

As BV confers a modest risk of spontaneous preterm birth and preterm PROM, it is not surprising that recent trials in low-risk patients have not demonstrated that antibiotic treatment can reduce the rate of spontaneous preterm delivery. For example, a randomized clinical trial conducted by the Network of Maternal Fetal Medicine Units concluded that treatment of asymptomatic BV with metronidazole during pregnancy did not prevent spontaneous preterm deliveries [metronidazole 5.1% (48/953) versus placebo 5.7% (55/966), RR 0.9, 95% CI 0.6–1.3] or spontaneous rupture of the membranes [4.2% (40/953) versus 3.7 (36/966), RR 1.1, 95% CI 0.7–1.8].[192]

In contrast, a recent systematic review conducted by McDonald et al.[193] reported that, among patients with a history of preterm delivery, treatment for BV during pregnancy reduced the risk of preterm PROM (OR 0.14, 95% CI 0.05–0.38). We interpret the conclusions of this systematic review as indicating that a subgroup of patients with BV may benefit from treatment. Such patients may be those who deploy an exaggerated proinflammatory response (hyper-responders) to BV in the vaginal mucosa or the hyporesponders.[116,191]

Group B Streptococcus (GBS)

Colonization with GBS is not a risk factor for spontaneous preterm delivery or preterm PROM. However, once preterm delivery is impending, colonization is a risk factor for adverse neonatal outcome.

Regan and colleagues[194] reported that PROM before the onset of labor or contractions was more common in women with cervical colonization of GBS at the time of delivery than in noncarriers [15.3% (134/877) versus 7% (411/5829), $P < 0.005$]. Matorras et al.[195] reported that patients with positive perineal GBS cultures had a higher rate of PROM than patients with negative cultures [26.4% (32/121) versus 17.8% (158/890), $P < 0.05$]. Among GBS carriers, those who also had a positive cervical culture had a higher rate of PROM than those with a negative cervical culture [41.7% (10/24) versus 19% (8/42), $P < 0.05$].

Patients with PROM had a higher frequency of positive cultures for GBS on admission than those with intact membranes [15.6% (7/45) versus 3.8% (3/80), $P < 0.05$].[196] Women with PROM colonized with GBS had increased incidence of chorioamnionitis, endometritis, and neonatal infections, as opposed to women with PROM and negative GBS cultures.[197] There are inconsistent reports concerning the effect of GBS colonization and the duration of the latency period in patients with PROM.[197,198] Maxwell and Watson[199] reported that antibiotic treatment of patients with preterm PROM

(26–33 weeks) and positive cultures for *N. gonorrhoeae*, GBS, or both resulted in a similar latency period until delivery and frequency of postpartum fever as in patients with negative cultures. However, the incidence of pneumonia was higher in infants born to mothers with positive cervical cultures (OR 6.9, 95% CI 2.1–22.8).[199] In conclusion, GBS colonization is not associated with an increased risk of preterm PROM.[200] Therefore, treatment of colonized patients will not reduce the rate of PROM.

Chlamydia trachomatis

A positive endocervical culture for *C. trachomatis* is an indication for treatment. In pregnant women, the rate of positive cultures has been reported to be 8%.[201] Among patients with positive *C. trachomatis* cultures, PROM was more common in those with positive serum IgM than in those with negative IgM [41.1% (7/17) versus 7.0% (4/53), $P < 0.01$].[201] Similar findings were reported by Sweet et al.[202] A positive *C. trachomatis* culture at the first perinatal visit was associated with a relative risk of 2 for preterm PROM and a population attributed risk of 9%.[202] Moreover, Alger et al.[196] reported that *C. trachomatis* was isolated more frequently from patients with preterm PROM than from women in the control group [44% (23/52) versus 15% (13/84), $P < 0.01$]. Collectively, this evidence suggests that infection with *C. trachomatis* with a humoral immune response (positive IgM) is a risk factor for preterm PROM.

Neisseria gonorrhoeae (NG)

The precise risk for preterm PROM conferred by NG endocervicitis is unknown. This is probably attributable to a long history of screening and treatment of NG during pregnancy. An association between NG and PROM has been recognized clinically based on studies examining the frequency of NG isolation at the time of the diagnosis of PROM. For example, Amstey and Steadman[203] reported an association between PROM and preterm delivery and maternal colonization with NG. Positive cultures for NG were found in 4.4% of patients (222/5065). The prevalence of prolonged PROM (more than 24 h) was significantly higher in women with positive endocervical, endometrial, or placental cultures for NG than in women with negative cultures [75% (9/12) versus 37% (18/49), $P < 0.05$].[204] PROM was more common in women with positive cultures than in those with negative cultures [26% (52/198) versus 19% (799/4246), $P < 0.01$].[203,205] However, the prevalence of PROM in women with positive cervical cultures during pregnancy was not significantly higher than in a matched control group [28.1% (50/178) versus 25.4% (98/386), not significant].[7] Given the standard of practice to screen and treat for NG, calculations of the attributable risk and magnitude of risk for preterm PROM are difficult to make and have limited practical value.

Trichomonas vaginalis (TV)

There is controversy concerning whether colonization with TV and symptomatic vaginitis caused by this organism predispose to preterm PROM. For example, Minkoff et al.[206] reported a study in which 233 patients had cultures performed at the time of their first prenatal visit (mean 13.8 ± 3.6 weeks). The frequency of positive cultures for TV was 14.6% (34/233). Women who subsequently developed PROM (term and preterm) had a higher rate of positive cultures for TV in early pregnancy than women with intact membranes [27.5% (11/40) versus 12.8% (19/148), $P < 0.03$]. Stepwise logistic regression analysis showed that a positive culture for TV was associated with an "estimated probability" of 1.42 for PROM ($P < 0.03$). In the same study, patients with positive vaginal cultures for *Bacteroides* species had an estimated probability of 2.8 ($P < 0.03$) for preterm PROM. *Staphylococcus epidermidis* was associated with an estimated probability of 1.57 ($P < 0.02$) for PROM.[206]

Even though a positive culture for TV may be associated with a modest increase in the risk for spontaneous preterm delivery, perhaps through preterm PROM, randomized clinical trials of antimicrobial agents in women with positive cultures for TV have not reduced the rate of preterm birth. A randomized clinical trial in which women ($n = 617$) were allocated to receive either metronidazole or placebo reported no differences in the rates of preterm delivery (< 37 weeks) with PROM between the two study groups [metronidazole 4.4% (14/315) versus placebo 4.2% (12/289), RR 1.1, 95% CI 0.5–2.3].[207] In contrast, the rates of preterm delivery due to preterm labor and intact membranes were significantly higher in the metronidazole group [metronidazole 10.2% (32/315) versus placebo 3.5% (10/289); RR 3.0, 95% CI 1.5–5.9].[207] Unexpectedly, a recent study reported that treatment of low-risk patients with positive vaginal culture for TV at 23–26 weeks increases the risk of preterm PROM (OR 1.4, 95% CI 1.03–1.8).[208] The authors concluded that treatment of low-risk asymptomatic pregnant women with positive cultures for TV is not recommended.[207] Perhaps there is a difference between asymptomatic women with a positive culture and patients who have clinical manifestations of vaginitis caused by TV.

Genetic factors

Preterm PROM could be considered a "common complex disorder," a term used in modern genetics to refer to a condition resulting from the interaction of genes and the environment. A complex disorder does not follow the pattern of mendelian inheritance. The likelihood of the phenotype (i.e., PROM) may result from gene–gene interaction, gene–environment interaction, and a combination thereof.

Evidence in support of the genetic predisposition for preterm PROM is the association between preterm PROM and Ehler–Danlos syndrome. Barabas[209] reported a retrospective study to determine the birth characteristics of patients with Ehler–Danlos syndrome. Birth histories were available for 18 of these patients. The rate of prematurity was 77% (14/18), and preterm PROM occurred in 92% (13/14) of those neonates delivered preterm. Of note, only one of the 16 unaffected siblings had preterm PROM, and this occurred in a twin gestation in which one of the twins was affected. In a recent study, the pregnancy outcome of 46 women with Ehler–Danlos syndrome was compared with that of 33 unaffected women. There were no significant differences in the frequency of preterm PROM between affected and unaffected women. In contrast, preterm PROM occurred in 34% (31/91) of the affected fetuses, compared with 18% (10/55) of the unaffected fetuses ($P = 0.03$).[143] Several candidate genes have been associated with preterm PROM, and the results of these studies are presented in Table 63.5. Collectively, these data provide additional evidence that the fetal genotype plays an important role in the occurrence of preterm PROM.

Midtrimester fetal heart rate deceleration and subsequent preterm PROM

Decelerations in the second trimester may be associated with the subsequent occurrence of preterm PROM. Indeed, among patients with a singleton gestation who delivered before 32 weeks, those with decelerations between 24 and 27 weeks of gestation had a higher frequency of subsequent PROM than those without decelerations [60.0% (39/65) versus 37.1% (13/35), $P < 0.05$].[210] The authors concluded that periodic or episodic decelerations during the late second trimester were associated with the occurrence of preterm PROM in the index pregnancy.[210] It is unclear why patients destined to have preterm PROM have a higher frequency of second-trimester decelerations.

Consequences of premature rupture of the membranes

The main consequences of preterm PROM are spontaneous onset of labor leading to prematurity,[211–213] infection,[120] abruptio placentae,[214] fetal death,[215] and the oligohydramnios sequence. This section will review, in detail, these conditions. One concept that has been generally overlooked is that PROM carries a risk of maternal death. The prevalence of maternal death associated with PROM was 0.2% in 1959 and decreased to 0.03% (1/3400) in 1982.[18,216]

Preterm parturition

Preterm PROM is associated with impending preterm delivery in most cases.[211–213] Cox and associates[211] managed 298 patients with preterm PROM expectantly (no steroids, tocolytics, and prophylactic antibiotics were administered), and amniocenteses were not performed. Of the 267 patients who gave birth to infants weighing ≥ 750 g, only 7% remained undelivered for more than 48 h after admission.

Wilson and coworkers[212] reported on the outcome of 143 patients with preterm PROM managed expectantly. Eighteen percent of patients remained undelivered after 1 week of admission. Maternal febrile infectious morbidity (antepartum and postpartum) occurred in 10% of patients. The neonatal death rate was 13.1% (18/137).

The most comprehensive study of the natural history of preterm PROM was reported by Nelson et al.,[213] who evaluated the outcome following expectant management of 511 women with a singleton gestation and preterm PROM between 20 and 36 weeks. Fifty-two percent of patients delivered within 48 h, whereas 12.9% remained undelivered after 1 week. The perinatal death rate was 8.4% (43/511). Not surprisingly, most deaths occurred at gestational ages of less than 28 weeks [42.7% (35/82)]. Maternal infection occurred in 21.7%, and the occurrence of fetal death was strongly associated with infection. The perinatal mortality was higher in neonates born to infected mothers with preterm PROM before 28 weeks than after 28 weeks [46.6% (14/30) versus 1.2% (1/81)], as was also true for infection-related morbidity (36% versus 19.8%).

Infection

Rupture of membranes may be associated with maternal or fetal infection. Maternal infection can be expressed as clinical chorioamnionitis. However, most women who have MIAC do not have clinical evidence of infection,[217] such as fever, leukocytosis, etc. This section will review the prevalence, microbiology, fetal attack rate, frequency of fetal inflammation, and short- and long-term consequences of infection/inflammation in preterm PROM.

What is the prevalence of MIAC in PROM?

The prevalence of positive amniotic fluid cultures in women with preterm PROM is 32.4% (473/1462)[120] (see Table 63.6), and is 34.3% (11/32) in term PROM.[218] However, this represents a minimum estimate of the frequency of infection, because: (1) Frequency is dependent upon isolation of microorganisms with standard microbiologic techniques, which underestimate the true rate of infection. The application of molecular microbiologic techniques (cultivation independent) has yielded a higher rate of microbial footprints. Moreover, patients who have a positive polymerase chain reaction (PCR) result for microorganisms, but a negative culture, have comparable outcomes to those who have a positive amniotic fluid culture for microorganisms;[219] (2) Amniocentesis is rarely performed if the patient presents in labor. Yet, there is evidence that patients with preterm PROM and labor have a higher rate of MIAC than patients with preterm PROM without labor;[121] and (3) Amniocentesis is less frequently performed in patients who have reduced volumes of amniotic fluid. Several studies have demonstrated that the lower the volume of amniotic fluid, the higher the rate of positive amniotic fluid cultures.[220–222] Normal amniotic fluid has antimicrobial properties that have been attributed to the presence of natural antimicrobial peptides,[223–226] such as epithelial[227] and neutrophil defensins.[224] Oligohydramnios may be associated with decreased availability of these antimicrobial peptides

Table 63.5 Candidate gene association studies and preterm PROM.

First author	Cases (*n*)	Controls (*n*)	Ethnic group	Mother	Child	Gene	Polymorphism	*P*-value	Odds ratio	95% confidence interval	Comments
Ferrand[549]	246	131	African-American	No	Yes	CARD15	2936insC	0.01	–	–	–
Fujimoto[112]	235	75	African-American	No	Yes	MMP1	G/GG −1607	0.02	2.29	1.09–4.82	–
Ferrand[113]	215	74	African-American	No	Yes	MMP9	CA repeat	<0.0001	3.06	1.77–5.27	–
Ferrand[549]	246	131	African-American	No	Yes	TKR4	A896G	0.75	–	–	–
Roberts[117]	26	110	African-American	Yes	No	TNFA1	G/A −308	0.00	3.18	1.33–7.83	–
Kalish[550]	15	36	United States (New York)	Yes	Yes	IL1RN	IL1RN*2 240-bp tandem repeat	0.005	8.00	1.65–50.34	Multifetal
Wang[114]	168	216	African-American	No	Yes	MMP8	C/T −799 A/G −381 C/G +17	<0.0001	4.63	2.01–11.94	–
Kalish[551]	27	67	United States (New York)	Yes	Yes	TNFα hsp70	G/A −308	Firstborn 0.003	4.85	1.5–16.1	Multifetal
							A/G +1267	<0.05	1.94	1.0–3.9	
								Combo 0.001	7.81	1.9–35.1	
Kalish[552]	33	77	United States (New York)	Yes	Yes	TNFRSF6	A/G −670	Mat GG 0.01	3.046	1.249–7.429	Multifetal
								Mat all G 0.02	2.020	1.120–3.645	
								Firstborn GG 0.04	2.614	1.040–6.573	
Annells[553]	129	185	Australian	Yes	No	IL10	G −1082 C −819 C −592	0.01	1.9	1.1–3.3	Homozygosity
Annells[553]	129	185	Australian	Yes	No	TNF	G +488 G −238 G −308	0.03	0.7	0.5–1.0	–
Fuks[554]	18	18	United States (New York)	No	Yes	TNFRSF6	A/G −670	Fetal AG 0.003	–	–	–
						Fas ligand	A/G −124	NS			

NS, nonsignificant.

Table 63.6 Microbial invasion of the amniotic cavity in women with preterm premature rupture of membranes as determined by amniotic fluid studies obtained by transabdominal amniocentesis.

Author	Number of patients	Positive culture numbers (%)	*Mycoplasma* culture	Success rate (%)	Clinical chorioamnionitis numbers (%)	Neonatal infection numbers (%)
Garite et al.[231]	59	9/30 (30.0)	No	51	6 (66.6)	2 (22.2)
Garite and Freeman[237]	207	20/86 (23.2)	No	42	11 (55.0)	5 (25.0)
Cotton et al.[229]	61	6/41 (14.6)	No	67	6 (100.0)	1 (16.6)
Broekhuizen et al.[233]	79	15/53 (28.3)	No	67	3 (20.0)	8 (53.3)
Vintzileos et al.[220]	54	12/54 (22, 2)	No	–	2 (16.7)	4 (33.3)
Feinstein et al.[235]	73	12/50 (20.0)	No	68	2 (16.7)	5 (41.6)
Romero et al.[121]	230	65/221 (29.4)	Yes	96	–	5 (7.7)
Gauthier et al.[238]	91	49/91 (53.8)	Yes	–	–	–
Coultrip et al.[230]	29	12/29 (41.4)	Yes	–	3 (25.0)	–
Gauthier and Meyer[239]	117	56/117 (47.9)	Yes	–	–	–
Romero et al.[241]	110	42/110 (38.2)	Yes	–	5 (11.9)	20 (47.6)
Font et al.[236]	74	21/37 (56.8)	Yes	–	–	–
Averbuch et al.[228]	90	32/90 (35.5)	Yes	–	–	7 (21.9)
Carroll et al.[111]	97	30/82 (36.6)	Yes	–	–	–
Gomez et al.[250]	52	30/52 (57.7)	Yes	–	–	–
Hussey et al.[555]	26	4/26 (15.4)	Yes	–	–	–
Rizzo et al.[139]	124	21/124 (16.9)	Yes	–	–	–
Yoon et al.[219]	154	37/154 (24.0)	Yes	–	7 (18.9)	10/32 (31.2)
Total	1727	473/1462 (32.4)			49/165 (29.7)	67/277 (24.2)

From ref. 120 with permission of Wiley-Liss, Inc., a subsidiary of John Wiley & Sons, Inc.

and, therefore, impaired innate immunity. Alternatively, fetal infection/inflammation may lead to redistribution of fetal blood flow, reduction in fetal urine production, and oligohydramnios. The net effect is that oligohydramnios is associated with an increased frequency of intra-amniotic infection and inflammation.

What are the microorganisms isolated in MIAC?

In preterm PROM, genital mycoplasmas (*Ureaplasma urealyticum* and *Mycoplasma hominis*) are the most frequent isolates from the amniotic fluid, followed by *Streptococcus agalactiae*, *Fusobacterium* species, and *Gardnerella vaginalis*. Polymicrobial infection is found in 26.7% (43/161) of cases[111,121,228–232] and an inoculum size greater than 10^5 colony-forming units/mL is found in 23% (6/26) of patients for whom quantitative microbiology was performed.[232] The most common microorganisms isolated from women with term PROM are *U. urealyticum*, *Peptostreptococcus*, *Lactobacillus*, *Bacteroides* species, and *Fusobacterium*.[218] Microorganisms isolated from the amniotic fluid in women with term and preterm PROM are qualitatively similar.

What are the consequences of MIAC?

Patients with MIAC are more likely to develop chorioamnionitis, endometritis, and neonatal sepsis than patients with negative amniotic fluid cultures on admission.[65,111,121,220,228–241] Table 63.7 shows the rate of these complications in studies in which antibiotics were not used before delivery. Garite and Freeman[237] reported that the frequency of respiratory distress syndrome (RDS) was twofold higher in neonates born to women with positive amniotic fluid cultures than in those born to women with negative cultures. Two explanations for these findings can be considered. First, patients with a positive amniotic fluid culture are generally at a lower gestational age than those with a negative amniotic fluid culture. Therefore, the higher incidence of RDS may reflect a greater degree of prematurity. Second, some cases of respiratory difficulty may be due to pneumonia rather than RDS.[242–244]

Is MIAC related to the onset of labor in preterm PROM?

The onset of labor in the setting of PROM has traditionally been considered an early sign of intrauterine infection. One study has examined the relationship between MIAC and the onset of preterm labor in women with PROM.[121] Patients in labor on admission had a higher rate of positive amniotic fluid cultures than women admitted with preterm PROM but not in labor [39% (24/61) versus 26% (41/160), $P = 0.049$]. Moreover, 75% of patients who were not in labor on admission, but subsequently went into spontaneous labor, had a positive amniotic fluid culture around the time of onset of labor.

Zlatnik et al.[232] conducted a unique study in which the results of amniotic fluid cultures were not used in patient management. A higher proportion of patients with positive amniotic fluid cultures delivered within 7 days, compared with those with negative cultures [positive cultures 89% (8/9) versus negative cultures: 45% (9/20), $P = 0.04$]. These data support a relationship between MIAC and the onset of preterm labor.

Table 63.7 Rate of infectious complications in premature rupture of membranes.

Main author	Amniotic fluid culture positive				Amniotic fluid culture negative			
	Number	Chorioamnionitis (%)	Endometritis (%)	Documented neonatal sepsis (%)	Number	Chorioamnionitis (%)	Endometritis (%)	Documented neonatal sepsis (%)
Romero[121]	65	–	–	7.7	156	–	–	0.7
Garite[231]	9	66.6	33.3	22.2	21	4.7	4.7	0
Vintzileos[220]	12	16.6	–	33.3	42	9.5	–	0
Broekhuizen[233]	15	20	33	–	38	0	3	–
Cotton[229]	6	100	*	17	35	9	*	3
Feinstein[235]	12	17	–	17	38	5	–	3
Zlatnik[232]	9	66.6	0	11	20	15	10	0

*Inclusive of chorioamnionitis and endometritis.

Are there differences in the inoculum size and type of microorganisms between women in labor and not in labor with preterm PROM?

Zlatnik et al.[232] reported that four of six patients with a colony count greater than 10^4/mL were delivered within 72 h, compared with none of three with counts lower than 10^4/mL. However, this difference did not reach statistical significance. Similarly, Romero et al.[121] reported that patients with preterm PROM in active labor on admission had a higher inoculum size than women not in labor [colony counts higher than 10^5 were found in 55% (10/18) versus 23% (6/26) respectively; $P < 0.05$]. These data suggest a possible relationship between proliferation of microorganisms and the onset of preterm labor. On the other hand, the rate of polymicrobial infection was not different between the two groups. Microbial invasion limited to *Mycoplasma* was found in only 8% of patients in labor versus 20% not in labor.

Can intra-amniotic infection resolve without treatment?

Romero et al.[121] performed a second amniocentesis in 12 women who originally had a negative Gram stain of the amniotic fluid but a positive amniotic fluid culture. One patient had a first amniotic fluid culture positive for *Fusobacterium* species, but the second amniotic fluid culture obtained at the time of the spontaneous initiation of labor showed no growth. It is unclear whether this observation represents a failure of culture or a true resolution of MIAC. The initiation of labor and the observation that this patient had histologic chorioamnionitis makes the second possibility less likely. In 11 patients, the microorganisms recovered from the second amniocentesis were the same as those retrieved from the first, but the colony count was higher in all instances. This indicates that, once MIAC has occurred, it has a progressive course. Whether this is the natural history of intra-amniotic infection in the midtrimester of pregnancy or in patients who have viral colonization of the amniotic fluid is unknown.

Can treatment with antibiotics in patients with intra-amniotic infection alter the natural history?

This question was addressed by Romero et al.,[245] who reported that the latency period was shorter and the neonatal morbidity higher in a cohort of patients with preterm PROM who had a positive culture for *U. urealyticum* (without antibiotic treatment) than in those with sterile amniotic fluid. Gauthier et al.[246] treated patients with preterm PROM and positive amniotic fluid cultures for *U. urealyticum* with a 1-week course of erythromycin. The latency period and the frequency of chorioamnionitis and neonatal sepsis in the treated group were not different from those of patients with sterile amniotic fluid. The observation that patients undergoing midtrimester amniocenteses who had a positive fluid culture or positive antibodies for *U. urealyticum* followed by preterm delivery, low birthweight infants, and fetal death suggests that some infections are chronic in nature.[247]

Does antibiotic administration to patients with preterm PROM prevent subsequent microbial invasion or eradicate existing infection at the time of initiation of treatment?

A recent study investigated the course of MIAC in 46 patients with preterm PROM.[248] All underwent amniocentesis upon admission, with an 18% prevalence of intra-amniotic inflammation (defined as an amniotic fluid white blood cell count $\geq 100/mm^3$) and a 15% prevalence of MIAC. Patients without evidence of intra-amniotic inflammation or MIAC were treated with ampicillin and erythromycin for 7 days. Those with intra-amniotic inflammation or MIAC were treated with ceftriaxone, clindamycin, and erythromycin for 10–14 days. At the time of the second amniocentesis, six of the seven patients with a prior diagnosis of MIAC were again positive for microorganisms. Of 18 patients with intra-amniotic inflammation, only three showed no evidence of inflammation after antibiotic treatment. Of note, among patients with no evidence of intra-amniotic inflammation or MIAC at admission, 32% (9/28) developed inflammation despite therapy. Five of the nine patients in question had positive amniotic fluid cultures. These observations suggest that systemic treatment with these antibiotics may not alter the natural course of MIAC in preterm PROM.

Can the fetus be infected *in utero*? Does this influence the latency period?

Evidence of fetal infection was provided by Carroll et al.,[249] who performed amniocentesis and cordocentesis at the time of presentation with PROM. The frequency of positive fetal blood culture was 10.3% (10/97). The authors found that, for patients with positive amniotic fluid and fetal blood cultures, the median time to delivery was 2 days (range 1–5 days), compared with 41 days (range 1–161 days) for patients with negative cultures in both amniotic fluid and fetal blood. In the case of patients with MIAC and negative fetal blood cultures, the median interval to delivery was 9 days (range 1–37 days).[249]

It is noteworthy that the microorganisms isolated from septic newborns are similar to those found in the amniotic fluid. In a study of 221 patients with preterm PROM, six cases with culture-proven neonatal sepsis were found.[121] In five of these cases, the microorganisms were the same as those found in the amniotic fluid; in the remaining case, the amniotic fluid culture 48 h before delivery had been negative.[121] The practical implication of this observation is that an amniocentesis performed before delivery may provide microbiological information helpful in guiding antibiotic choice in the newborn.

Can the fetus deploy an inflammatory response?

The first evidence that the fetus can mount an inflammatory response was reported some years ago.[250] The authors coined the term "fetal inflammatory response syndrome" (FIRS) to refer to an elevation in the fetal plasma concentration of IL-6 (> 11 pg/mL) that was associated with severe neonatal morbidity[250] and a shorter cordocentesis-to-delivery interval.[251]

Fetal microbial invasion or other insults result in a systemic fetal inflammatory response that can progress toward multiple organ dysfunction, septic shock, and perhaps death in the absence of timely delivery. Evidence of multisystemic involvement in cases of FIRS includes increased concentrations of fetal plasma MMP-9,[100] an enzyme involved in the digestion of type IV collagen and in the pathophysiology of preterm PROM.[252] Moreover, several fetal organs including the hematopoietic system,[253–255] adrenals,[256] heart,[257] brain,[258,259] lungs,[260,261] and skin[262] have been proposed to be target organs during FIRS.

Pathologic examination of the umbilical cord is an easy approach to determine whether fetal inflammation was present before birth. Funisitis and chorionic vasculitis are the histopathologic hallmarks of FIRS.[263] Funisitis is associated with endothelial activation, a key mechanism in the development of organ damage,[264] and neonates with funisitis are at increased risk of neonatal sepsis[265] and long-term handicaps, such as bronchopulmonary dysplasia[259] and cerebral palsy.[261] Indeed, newborns with funisitis are at more than a twofold increased risk of IVH[266] and have an 11-fold risk of development of periventricular echolucencies.[267] In the context of FIRS, the combination of inflammatory changes in the brain and fetal systemic hypotension may increase the likelihood of brain injury.[268] Collectively, these observations suggest that a subset of fetuses presenting with preterm PROM have bacteremia and/or FIRS that may contribute to fetal organ damage.

Microbial invasion: cause or consequence of premature rupture of the membranes?

The traditional view has been that MIAC is the consequence of membrane rupture. However, evidence suggests that PROM may be the result of subclinical infection and inflammation. Naeye and Peters[164] reported in 1980 that patients with preterm PROM 1–4 h before the onset of labor had a higher prevalence of histologic chorioamnionitis than patients who delivered preterm without PROM (Table 63.8). Because it is unlikely that inflammation of the chorioamniotic membranes develops in 4 h, these data suggest that, in these cases, histologic chorioamnionitis precedes rather than follows PROM. Several lines of evidence suggest that the most likely cause of histologic chorioamnionitis is subclinical infection. Bacteria have been recovered from 72% of placentas with histologic chorioamnionitis.[269] Furthermore, we have demonstrated a good correlation between a positive amniotic fluid culture for microorganisms and histologic chorioamnionitis.[270]

MIAC can also be the consequence of PROM. The frequency of positive amniotic fluid cultures increases with time. Indeed, 75% of patients who were quiescent on admission and subsequently went into labor had a positive amniotic fluid culture.[121] However, only 25% of these patients had a positive culture on admission, and the remaining 50% became positive during the latency period.[121] These observations are consistent with those of Naeye and Peters,[164] who showed that the incidence of histologic chorioamnionitis increases with the duration of the latency period.

The authors reported that histologic chorioamnionitis (defined as the presence of 4–15 neutrophils in the chorionic plate) in PROM was two- to threefold more common when rupture of membranes occurred just before the onset of labor

Table 63.8 Gestational age at membrane rupture and frequency of histopathologic chorioamnionitis.[164]

	20–28 weeks (%)	29–32 weeks (%)	33–37 weeks (%)
Rupture of membranes after onset of labor	23	15	11
Premature rupture of membranes 1–4 h before onset of labor	48	29	32

than when it occurred after labor began.[164] This suggests that inflammation (and probably infection) is in many cases not only a consequence of PROM, but it may also be its cause.

Abruptio placentae

Abruptio placentae occurs more frequently in patients with preterm PROM than in those with preterm labor and intact membranes (2.29% versus 0.86% respectively; RR 3.58, 95% CI 1.74–7.39).[214] The same conclusion has been previously reported in a systematic review[271] and a population-based epidemiologic study.[272] The mechanisms responsible for separation of the placenta in preterm PROM have not been determined. Nelson and associates[273] proposed that leakage of fluid after PROM may lead to a disproportion between the placental and uterine surfaces that would favor placental separation. Evidence in support of this concept is the observation that, in the context of preterm PROM, the incidence of abruptio placentae increases with the severity of oligohydramnios (12.3% for patients with a vertical pocket of 1–2 cm versus 3.5% among those with a vertical pocket > 2 cm).[274] However, two groups of investigators using subjective means to estimate amniotic fluid volume could not confirm this observation.[275,276]

An alternative hypothesis to explain the relationship between abruptio placentae and preterm PROM postulates that a disorder of decidual hemostasis leads to separation of the membranes from the decidua, with subsequent compromise of their nutritive support, weakening of the membranes, and eventual rupture. Indeed, patients with abruptio placentae after preterm PROM have a higher incidence of vaginal bleeding before rupture and during the latency period than patients without abruptio placentae. In order to evaluate the mechanism of abruption-related preterm delivery, Mackenzie et al.[130] studied MMP-3 production and expression in primary decidual cell cultures incubated in a medium of steroids plus or minus thrombin. MMP-3, as well as its mRNA, was significantly inhibited by estradiol plus progestin versus estradiol alone. Interestingly, thrombin elicited a dose-dependent reversal of this progesterone inhibition of MMP-3.

Infection/inflammation within the decidua could also facilitate premature placental detachment. Indeed, there is an association between histologic chorioamnionitis and abruptio placentae.[134,277] The relative risk of abruption is 9.03 (95% CI 2.80–29.15) when chorioamnionitis is associated with preterm PROM.[214] One mechanism for this link has been proposed by Lockwood et al.[278] Thrombin, an enzyme released during hemostasis, can enhance IL-8 expression by decidual cells. IL-8 is a chemokine able to recruit neutrophils. The inflammatory process resulting from neutrophil infiltration could induce degradation of extracellular matrix and membrane rupture.

Pulmonary hypoplasia

Pulmonary hypoplasia is characterized by a decrease in the number of lung cells, airways, and alveoli.[279,280] Its frequency is related to gestational age at the time of membrane rupture, and its presence increases the risk of neonatal death and other complications such as pneumothorax and persistent pulmonary hypertension.

Three studies looked specifically at pulmonary hypoplasia in the context of PROM. Vergani et al.[281] conducted a prospective study of patients with PROM before 28 weeks of gestation managed conservatively. Pulmonary hypoplasia was diagnosed at autopsy or in the neonates based on radiographic findings. The frequency of pulmonary hypoplasia was 28% (15/54). Gestational age at the time of PROM and presence of oligohydramnios, but not the latency period, were independent predictors of the subsequent development of pulmonary hypoplasia.[281]

Rotschild et al.[280] studied 88 neonates born to mothers with PROM occurring before 29 weeks and a latency period of at least 1 week (Table 63.9). The prevalence of pulmonary hypoplasia was 16% (14/88). Gestational age at the time of PROM, but not the duration of the latency period or the severity of oligohydramnios, was associated with pulmonary hypoplasia. The risk of pulmonary hypoplasia when PROM occurs at 19 weeks was 50%, whereas it was only 10% when the membranes ruptured at 25 weeks (Fig. 63.5). This has been confirmed by animal experimentation.[282]

Winn et al.[283] prospectively studied 163 patients with preterm PROM from 15 to 28 weeks of gestation. Pulmonary hypoplasia was diagnosed at autopsy or by radiographic findings using the same criteria as Vergani et al.[281] The incidence of pulmonary hypoplasia was 12.9% (21/163). The authors reported that gestational age at rupture of the membranes, latency period, and either the initial or the average amniotic fluid index (AFI) had significant influence on the development of pulmonary hypoplasia.

Table 63.9 Role of pulmonary hypoplasia in neonatal morbidity and mortality.[280]

	Pulmonary hypoplasia % (no.)	No pulmonary hypoplasia % (no.)	Odds ratio (95% confidence interval)	*P*-value (by Fisher's exact test)
Neonatal death	71 (10/14)	11 (8/74)	20.6 (4.5–105)	< 0.001
Pneumothorax	64 (9/14)	15 (11/74)	10.3 (2.5–44.8)	< 0.001
Persistent pulmonary hypertension	43 (6/14)	11 (8/74)	6.2 (1.4–27.2)	< 0.01

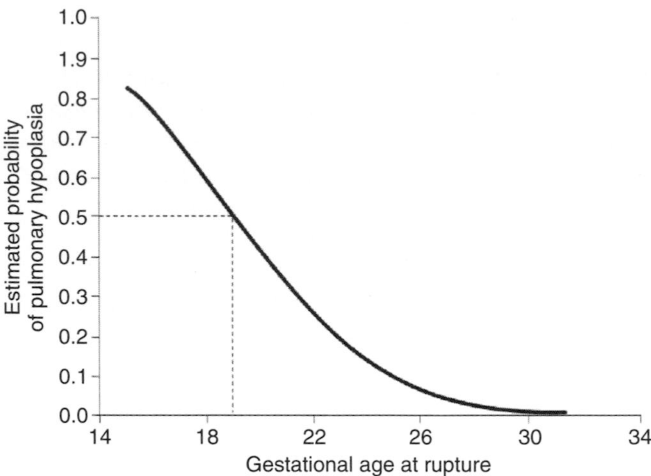

Figure 63.5 Curve relating probability of pulmonary hypoplasia to gestational age at rupture of membranes derived from estimated logistic equation: Probability of pulmonary hypoplasia = $1/(1 + e^{-7.27 + 0.38\ GAR})$. From ref. 280 with permission from Elsevier.

The role of duration of rupture of membranes in the development of pulmonary hypoplasia is not clear. Univariate analysis demonstrated an association between the duration of rupture of membranes and the occurrence of pulmonary hypoplasia.[281,284–286] However, there is an inverse relationship between the duration of the latency period and the gestational age at the time of membrane rupture. Multivariate analysis has not shown a significant effect of the duration of PROM in the development of pulmonary hypoplasia.[281]

Whereas Rotschild et al.[280] reported that the severity of oligohydramnios was not a factor in the development of pulmonary hypoplasia, both Vergani et al.[281] and Winn et al.[283] reported that amniotic fluid volume was an independent predictor of the development of pulmonary hypoplasia. The discrepancy between studies may be explained by the: (1) determination of amniotic fluid volume; (2) exclusion of patients; and (3) definition of pulmonary hypoplasia.

The mechanisms responsible for pulmonary hypoplasia in PROM are poorly understood.[287–296] Experimental evidence suggests that oligohydramnios caused by drainage of the amniotic cavity leads to pulmonary hypoplasia. Traditionally, oligohydramnios has been thought to lead to extrinsic compression of the fetal thorax, impairing lung growth. An alternative view is that oligohydramnios reduces lung fluid volume, and this in turn is responsible for pulmonary hypoplasia. Experimental and clinical evidence supporting the importance of lung fluid in the pathogenesis of pulmonary hypoplasia includes the following: (1) chronic tracheal drainage causes pulmonary hypoplasia in fetal sheep;[289] (2) laryngeal atresia associated with renal agenesis (Fraser syndrome) results in normal pulmonary development despite severe oligohydramnios;[294] and (3) oligohydramnios is often associated with decreased intra-amniotic fluid pressure.[295]

Several biometric and biophysical parameters have been used for the antenatal prediction of pulmonary hypoplasia, including thoracic circumference,[296] thoracic circumference compared with femoral length,[297,298] or abdominal circumference.[299,300] Other methods used include lung length,[301] perinasal fluid flow during fetal breathing movements,[302] breathing-related modulation of ductus arteriosus flow,[303] amniotic fluid volume,[281] pulmonary artery Doppler velocimetry,[304] and various formulas.[300,305,306] No single index has been confirmed independently to have adequate sensitivity and specificity to make it clinically useful.

Serial amnioinfusion has been proposed for the prevention of pulmonary hypoplasia. Fisk et al.[307] performed serial transabdominal amnioinfusion in nine women with midtrimester oligohydramnios (six with preterm PROM and three whose fetuses had lower urinary tract obstructions). Preterm labor occurred in four women between 3 and 12 weeks after the last procedure. One patient developed clinical chorioamnionitis 2 days after her sixth infusion; there was one case of placental abruption. At delivery, three of nine fetuses survived, and five of six neonates who died had normal lung-to-body ratios, suggesting that this management may decrease the risk of pulmonary hypoplasia. Evidence of lung hypoplasia was present in one infant who died and in one who lived. Nakayama et al.[308] have generated experimental evidence that maintenance of amniotic fluid volume by saline infusion in pregnant rabbits could prevent pulmonary hypoplasia. The role of serial amnioinfusion in the clinical management of PROM remains experimental.

Fetal compression syndrome

The fetal compression syndrome was originally described in the context of oligohydramnios and renal agenesis.[309] Classically, it includes limb position deformities and craniofacial defects that are thought to result from physical compression inhibiting fetal growth and movement.[310,311] Nimrod et al.[285] reported an incidence of 12% in women with preterm PROM, most occurring when the latency period was longer than 5 weeks. Blott et al.[287] found that 46% (14/30) of infants born after prolonged membrane rupture (more than 4 weeks) had limb deformities. The median duration of rupture in the group with deformities was 28 days, compared with 9 days in infants without deformities.

Fetal growth restriction

Preterm delivery resulting from patients with preterm labor and intact membranes or preterm PROM has been associated with "fetal growth restriction." Most studies are cross-sectional and have not separated preterm PROM from preterm labor with intact membranes.[312,313] One interesting study determined the fetal growth rate for biometric parameters in a cohort of 69 singleton pregnancies complicated with preterm PROM (24–31 weeks) and who remained undelivered for more than 14 days. The mean growth velocity of the head and abdominal circumference was significantly lower than that of the control group (n = 345 normal pregnancies). Neonates who had intraventricular hemorrhage (IVH), periventricular leukomalacia (PVL), or cerebral palsy had a lower growth velocity than those not affected by these disorders.[314]

Fetal death

The rate of fetal death in preterm PROM is approximately 1% when this complication is diagnosed after 24 weeks and 15% if PROM occurs before.[20] The etiology of fetal death remains unknown. Fetal infection, placental abruption, fetal growth restriction and umbilical cord prolapse or accident (resulting from compression in cases of severe oligohydramnios) have been implicated.

Fetal death, in the context of intrauterine infection, has been attributed to microbial invasion of the fetus, where the unborn child fails to deploy an inflammatory response sufficiently intense to stimulate labor. Indeed, histologic chorioamnionitis (maternal inflammatory response) is nine times more frequent than funisitis (a fetal inflammatory response) in patients with stillbirth.[315] In this case, *in utero* fetal death would represent failure of the host response mechanisms dealing with intrauterine infection. This concept is supported by a genetic association study which demonstrated that fetal carriage of the allele 2 of the gene encoding for the IL-1 receptor antagonist (IL-1ra) is associated with fetal death.[316] An excess of IL-1ra in the fetal compartment may limit the ability of the fetus to deploy a proinflammatory response and limit the effectiveness of the mechanisms available for host defense, including the ability to initiate labor to exit a hostile intrauterine environment.

Diagnosis of prelabor rupture of the membranes

Traditionally, the diagnosis of PROM has been based on clinical findings and bedside tests. The following section will review the accuracy of these tests in the diagnosis of PROM.

Presenting symptoms

The most common presentation of PROM is a watery vaginal discharge or a sudden gush of fluid from the vagina, as reported by the patient. Questioning the patient about the timing of the initial loss of vaginal fluid, color and consistency of the discharge, and any odor may help to differentiate PROM from loss of the mucus plug in early labor, vaginal discharge associated with infection, normal leukorrhea of pregnancy, and urinary incontinence (sometimes present in pregnancy), as well as to determine the presence of blood or meconium in the amniotic fluid.

Vaginal examination

Evaluation of the patient begins with a sterile speculum examination. Visualization of a vaginal pool or obvious leakage of fluid from the cervix into the posterior fornix is considered to be evidence that PROM has occurred. Increasing intra-abdominal pressure may assist in the visualization of this sign. If no fluid is present in the posterior fornix, the patient can be re-examined after resting in the supine position to allow for accumulation of fluid in the posterior fornix. Additionally, a speculum examination allows for collection of vaginal and cervical cultures and amniotic fluid to assess fetal lung maturity, while ruling out cord prolapse.

A sterile swab of fluid should be obtained from the posterior fornix and placed on a clean glass slide and on a piece of nitrazine paper. Amniotic fluid, when put on a slide and allowed to dry, will show arborization ("ferning") under the microscope at low magnification.[317] This method has an overall accuracy of 95%.[318] Rare false-positive ferning results have been described in association with fingerprints on the slide or contamination with semen and cervical mucus.[319,320] False-negative results (5–10%) may be caused by dry swabs or by contamination with blood.[317,321,322] The slide should be evaluated after at least 10 min of drying to decrease the false-negative rate.[323]

Does a digital examination increase the risk of infection?

The traditional view has been that "once an examination has been performed, the clock of infection starts to tick." Several studies have addressed the clinical consequences of digital examination in the setting of PROM.[324–327]

Adoni and coworkers[324] reported a study in which the latency period and incidence of chorioamnionitis were evaluated in patients with preterm PROM (26–34 weeks) who underwent a digital examination or a sterile speculum examination. The latency period was longer in patients undergoing speculum examination than in those examined digitally (9.5 ± 1.5 days versus 3.1 ± 0.5 days, $P < 0.005$). No significant difference in the incidence of chorioamnionitis was found. Lewis and associates[325] prospectively collected data on 271 singleton pregnancies with preterm PROM. The authors reported that patients who underwent digital examination had shorter latency periods than those who had speculum examination (digital examination 2.1 ± 4.0 days versus speculum examination 11.3 ± 13.4 days, $P < 0.0001$) (Fig. 63.6).

Sukcharoen et al.[327] performed a retrospective study in which women with preterm PROM had digital examinations (n = 50) or speculum examinations (n = 65). The authors reported no differences in latency periods or neonatal outcomes in the study groups. However, patients who underwent digital examinations had a higher frequency of chorioamnionitis [digital examination 12% (6/50) versus speculum examination 3.1% (2/65), $P < 0.05$].

Schutte and colleagues[326] retrospectively examined the incidence of neonatal infection in patients with PROM according

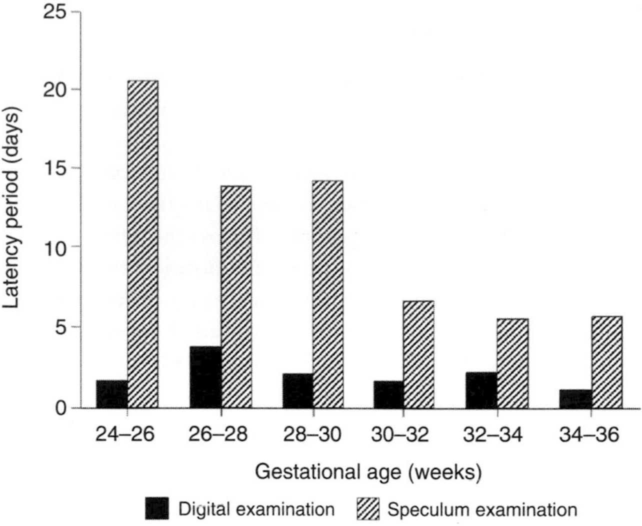

Figure 63.6 Effect of digital examination on latency period ($P < 0.001$ for all groups).[325]

to the interval between initial digital vaginal examination and delivery. The incidence of neonatal infection was higher in patients examined more than 24 h before delivery than in those whose first vaginal examination occurred less than 24 h before delivery [33% (11/33) versus 5% (14/280), $P < 0.0001$]. Although this study has been widely cited in support of the view that digital vaginal examination increases the risk of infection, the design of this study constrains the strength of this conclusion. For example, the policy at the institution in which the study was performed was not to perform digital examinations in patients with PROM unless delivery was anticipated within 24 h. Uterine contractions may have been an early sign of infection, rather than labor, in some patients.

The only justification for performing a digital examination is to determine cervical status. In the preterm gestation, this information rarely alters clinical management but, in the term gestation, the cervical state may be a factor influencing decisions regarding induction. There is a strong relationship between the results of sterile speculum examination and digital examination of the cervix. This was demonstrated in a study in which visual speculum and digital cervical examinations in women in labor were performed by two separate blinded examiners within 5 min of each other. Visual examination underestimated actual cervical dilation by only 0.6 cm (95% CI 0.58–0.62).[328–330] The major objection to a digital examination in the setting of PROM is that it may unnecessarily increase the risk of ascending infection, and the information it provides can be obtained by sterile speculum examination.

Biochemical studies for the detection of amniotic fluid in the vagina

The biochemical properties of the amniotic fluid are the basis in distinguishing it from other fluids that can be observed in the vagina (i.e., cervical secretions, urine, and semen). The normal pH of the vagina during gestation is 4.5–5.5, and that of the amniotic fluid is 7.0–7.5. Nitrazine paper turns from yellow to blue when exposed to any alkaline fluid (i.e., pH of 7.0 or more), and the use of nitrazine paper has been reported to have an accuracy of 93.3%[318] in determining the presence of amniotic fluid in the vagina. False-positive results range from 1% to 17% and can result from alkaline urine, blood, semen, vaginal discharge in cases of bacterial vaginosis, or *Trichomonas* infection.[331] False negatives may occur in up to 10% of cases.

Additional biochemical tests for the diagnosis of PROM include diamine oxidase (DAO) activity,[332] prolactin levels,[333–335] alpha-fetoprotein (AFP; sensitivity 94.5% and specificity 95.4%),[333,336] and insulin-like growth factor-binding protein-1 (IGFBP-1).[337] AFP has been reported to be better than prolactin and more practical than DAO assay with an overall accuracy of 98%.[337,338] IGFBP-1 determinations have a sensitivity of 74.4% and a specificity of 92.6%.[339] Overall, the sensitivity, specificity, positive and negative predictive values of the different diagnostic tests presented today in comparison with the nitrazine test are good (Table 63.10).[340–345] However, the lack of available bedside kits for these tests hampers their clinical use.

The assay for FFN is useful in the identification of patients at risk of preterm and term labor and imminent delivery. However, doubts still exist about its diagnostic value in PROM.[346] Eriksen et al.[347] reported that, for the detection of term PROM, FFN had a sensitivity of 98.2%, but a specificity of only 26.8%. Although the authors proposed that the false positives were the result of the detection of small amounts of amniotic fluid not detected by clinical tests (pool, nitrazine, and ferning), an alternative explanation is that a positive FFN detects degradation of the extracellular matrix in the fetal–maternal interface that precedes the clinical onset of labor rather than PROM. Support for the hypothesis derives from the observation that patients without PROM but with positive cervical FFN are more likely to deliver within 72 h than those with negative cervical FFN.[346,348–355] In conclusion, the detection of cervicovaginal FFN is not specific for PROM.

Transabdominal injection of dye

When the diagnosis of preterm PROM is not clear, a transabdominal injection of dye (indigo carmine, Evans blue, fluorescein) into the amniotic cavity may be used for confirmation.[356–359] Methylene blue should not be used as it may cause fetal methemoglobinemia.[360–362] A tampon in the vagina can document subsequent dye leakage in cases of PROM.

Initial assessment of patients presenting with preterm prelabor rupture of the membranes

The initial evaluation of a patient with preterm PROM includes: (1) accurate assessment of gestational age; (2) exclu-

Table 63.10 Diagnostic indices of detection methods for diagnosis of PROM.

First author	Number of patients	Site of inspection	Method	Timing	Sensitivity (%)	Specificity (%)	Positive predictive value (%)	Negative predictive value (%)
Kishida[344]	46	Vagina	AFP	16–36 weeks	96.9	92.9	96.9	92.9
			Fibronectin		87.5	92.9	96.6	76.5
			Nitrazine test		81.3	100	100	70
		Cervix	AFP		100	85.7	94.1	100
			Nitrazine test		96.9	57.1	83.8	88.9
Anai[343]	204	Vagina	hCG	First trimester	100	64.3	61.5	100
				Second trimester	100	91.8	82.8	100
				Third trimester	100	96.5	88.9	100
Esim[341]	141	Vagina	hCG	Second trimester	86	93	67	97
				Third trimester	60	94	79	86
Erdemoglu[342]	151	Vagina	IGFBP-1	20–42 weeks	97	97	–	–
			Nitrazine test		97	16	–	–
			AFI < 80 mm		94	91	–	–
Buyukbayrak[340]	70	Vagina	Prolactin	First trimester	25	100	100	0.57
				Second trimester	0.66	0.95	0.94	0.74
				Third trimester	0.71	0.97	0.96	0.77

AFP, alpha-fetoprotein; hCG, human chorionic gonadotropin; IGFBP, insulin-like growth factor-binding protein; AFI, amniotic fluid index.

sion of occult cord prolapse; (3) estimation of fetal weight and presentation; (4) evaluation of the risk of infection; (5) determination of lung maturity; and (6) assessment of fetal well-being.

Ultrasound examination in the evaluation of patients with preterm PROM

The initial ultrasound examination aims to: (1) assess fetal viability, biometry, and presentation; (2) quantify amniotic fluid volume; (3) rule out fetal anomalies; and (4) confirm gestational age. The sonographic examination of fetuses with PROM is challenging due to the reduced amniotic fluid volume. For example, sonographic estimates of fetal weight have been shown to underestimate the birthweight.[363–365]

Diagnosis of intrauterine infection in preterm PROM

Amniocentesis is used for the evaluation of the microbiological state of the amniotic cavity and of fetal lung maturity in the patient with preterm PROM.[366] Results of amniotic fluid analysis provide a rational approach to the management of preterm PROM. Patients without evidence of infection/inflammation and lung immaturity could be managed expectantly, whereas those with evidence of infection could be managed using algorithms tailored to the gestational age (see section on Management).

Garite and coworkers[231] were the first to propose the use of amniocentesis in the evaluation of the microbiological state of the amniotic cavity and of fetal lung maturity in the patient with preterm PROM. Subsequently, several investigators reported studies in which amniocentesis had been used in the management of PROM. Relevant issues are the success rate of fluid retrieval, the value of the information obtained, and the risk associated with the procedure.

Table 63.6 gives the success rate of amniotic fluid retrieval by transabdominal amniocentesis in the published reports.[121,229,231,233–235,237,245] Retrieval rates vary from 49% to 96% in published series. The wide disparity in retrieval rates is probably attributable to differences in practice among institutions (e.g., although Garite and associates excluded all patients with anterior placentas and oligohydramnios, subsequent studies have not considered these conditions as contraindications for amniocentesis). Better ultrasound technology, color Doppler, and a skilled maternal–fetal medicine specialist make amniocentesis possible in most cases of PROM.

One randomized clinical trial examined the value of amniocentesis in preterm PROM.[367] Forty-seven patients (26–34 weeks of gestation with an accessible amniotic fluid pocket) were randomized to amniocentesis or no amniocentesis. Indications for induction of labor included positive Gram stain of amniotic fluid or mature fetal lungs, as determined by a lecithin-to-sphingomyelin (L/S) ratio of more than 2.0 or positive phosphatidylglycerol (PG). Neonates born to women who had amniocenteses had a lower incidence of "fetal stress" during labor (diagnosed by fetal heart rate tracing) and a shorter hospital stay than those born to women who were randomized not to have amniocenteses ["fetal distress": 4% (1/24) versus 32% (7/22), $P < 0.05$; hospital stay (median): 8.5 days versus 22 days, $P < 0.01$]. No

Table 63.11 Diagnostic indices and predictive values of different amniotic fluid tests in the detection of positive amniotic fluid culture in patients with premature rupture of the fetal membranes.[241,556]

Amniotic fluid tests	Sensitivity (%)	Specificity (%)	Positive predictive value (%)	Negative predictive value (%)
Gram stain[556]	34.8	96.4	88.9	63.9
IL-6 (≥ 7.9 ng/mL)[241]	80.9	75	66.7	86.4
MMP-8 (> 30 ng/mL)[556]	76.1	61.8	62.5	75.6
WBC count (≥ 30 cells/μL)[556]	55.6	76.4	65.8	67.7
WBC count (≥ 50 cells/μL)[241]	52.4	83.8	66.7	74
Glucose (< 10 mg/dL)[241]	57.1	73.5	57.1	73.5
Glucose (< 14 mg/dL)[241]	71.4	51.5	47.6	74.5
Gram stain + WBC count (≥ 30 cells/μL)[556]	62.2	76.4	68.3	82.5
Gram stain + glucose (< 10 mg/dL)[241]	66.7	73.5	60.9	78.1
Gram stain + IL-6 (≥ 7.9 ng/mL)[241]	80.9	75	66.7	86.4
Gram stain + MMP-8 (> 30 ng/mL)[556]	82.6	61.8	64.4	81
WBC count (≥ 30 cells/μL) + MMP-8 (> 30 ng/mL)[556]	80	60	62.1	78.6
Gram stain + WBC count (≥ 30 cells/μL) + glucose (< 10 mg/dL)[241]	76.2	60.3	54.2	80.4
Gram stain + WBC count (≥ 30 cells/μL) + IL-6 (≥ 7.9 ng/mL)[241]	85.7	61.8	58.1	87.5
Gram stain + WBC count (≥ 30 cells/μL) + MMP-8 (> 30 ng/mL)[556]	84.4	60	63.3	82.5
Gram stain + glucose (< 10 mg/dL) + IL-6 (≥ 7.9 ng/mL)[241]	85.7	52.9	52.9	85.7
Gram stain + WBC count (≥ 30 cells/μL) + glucose (< 10 mg/dL) + IL-6 (≥ 7.9 ng/mL)[241]	92.9	47.1	52	91.4

IL, interleukin; WBC, white blood cell; MMP, matrix metalloproteinase. From ref. 241 with permission from Elsevier.

differences in the rate of neonatal sepsis, maternal chorioamnionitis, or endometritis were noted between the two groups. This study had limited power to detect differences in neonatal morbidity.

The analyses of amniotic fluid used to detect the presence of MIAC or intra-amniotic inflammation include: (1) Gram stain; (2) a quantitative white blood cell (WBC) count; (3) glucose concentration (Table 63.11); and (4) microbial cultures for aerobic and anaerobic bacteria, as well as genital mycoplasmas. Patients with a negative Gram stain (read by experienced personnel) and a high WBC count (more than 30 cells/μL) are at high risk of having microbial invasion with genital mycoplasmas, which are not visible on Gram stain examination. Lower concentrations of glucose in amniotic fluid (< 10 mg/dL) can serve as an additional marker for MIAC. The results of amniotic fluid culture may take days to be available. Therefore, most centers rely on the determination of intra-amniotic inflammation because the outcome of preterm PROM in patients with intra-amniotic inflammation is similar to those with MIAC proven with standard microbiological techniques.[368] Table 63.11 summarizes the diagnostic criteria and predictive values of different amniotic fluid tests in detecting positive amniotic fluid cultures in patients with preterm PROM.[241] Amniotic fluid IL-6 performed best in detecting MIAC, as well as in identifying patients at risk of impending preterm delivery and neonatal complications. We have shown that amniotic fluid IL-6 is a sensitive test for the prospective diagnosis of acute histologic chorioamnionitis [IL-6 of more than 17 ng/mL had a sensitivity of 79% (23/29) and specificity of 100% (21/21)], significant neonatal morbidity (sepsis, RDS, pneumonia, IVH, BPD, and necrotizing enterocolitis), and neonatal mortality [IL-6 of more than 17 ng/mL had a sensitivity of 69% (18/26) and a specificity of 79% (19/24)].[369] Other rapid tests reported for the detection of MIAC include amniotic fluid catalase,[236] alpha$_1$-antitrypsin,[65] limulus amebocyte lysate test,[240] and bacterial PCR.[370]

Recently, a novel diagnostic test, a rapid bedside enzyme-linked immunosorbent assay (ELISA) for the detection of MMP-8 in amniotic fluid, was developed. This kit has been reported to have high accuracy in the identification of patients with MIAC and inflammation among patients with preterm labor and intact membranes.[371] Future studies may determine the utility of this test in the identification of patients with intra-amniotic infection/inflammation among those with preterm PROM.

The risk of amniocentesis, when performed by experienced individuals, appears to be extremely low. Yeast and colleagues[372] specifically addressed this issue in 91 patients with preterm PROM in whom amniocenteses were performed. A retrospective review of neonatal records uncovered no evidence of fetal trauma with any procedure. This study also found that the incidence of spontaneous labor in patients who underwent amniocentesis was no different from that of patients who did not undergo amniocentesis secondary to oligohydramnios or an anterior placenta. The authors concluded that their study failed to show that amniocentesis may induce labor.

Assessment of lung maturity

Lung maturity can be assessed from the amniotic fluid obtained by amniocentesis or from the vaginal pool. The latter has the advantage of being less invasive and more feasible in patients with oligohydramnios. Amniotic fluid from the vaginal pool can be collected in three ways: (1) from the posterior vaginal fornix by sterile speculum examination; (2) in a clean bedpan maintained under the patient; or (3) using obstetric perineal pads left in place for 12–24 h to ensure saturation.[373–376] The success rate in obtaining fluid within 48 h with these noninvasive techniques ranges from 54% to 100%.[375,376] Using a vulval pad to detect PG, Estol et al.[377] found a sensitivity of 88%, specificity of 76%, positive predictive value of 34%, and negative predictive value of 98%. Lewis et al.[378] investigated the value of a rapid antibody agglutination method (Amniostat FLM) to detect PG in vaginal pool samples. Thirty-six of 201 patients between 26 and 36 weeks of gestation had positive PG, and none of the infants born to these mothers developed RDS. PG was detectable only after 30 weeks of gestation.

The reliability of lung maturity tests from amniotic fluid collected vaginally has been challenged.[379,380] This section reviews the correlation between the L/S ratio and PG results in amniotic fluid obtained by amniocentesis and from the vaginal pool. Shaver and associates[373] compared the phospholipid profile of paired amniotic fluid samples in 28 patients with preterm PROM. No significant difference was found in the concentrations of PG, phosphatidylinositol, phosphatidylethanolamine, and phosphatidylserine in amniotic fluid obtained by the two sampling methods. The L/S ratio was higher in fluid collected transvaginally than in fluid collected transabdominally, but this difference did not reach statistical significance (Fig. 63.7). The only phospholipid clearly increased by vaginal contamination was lysolecithin.

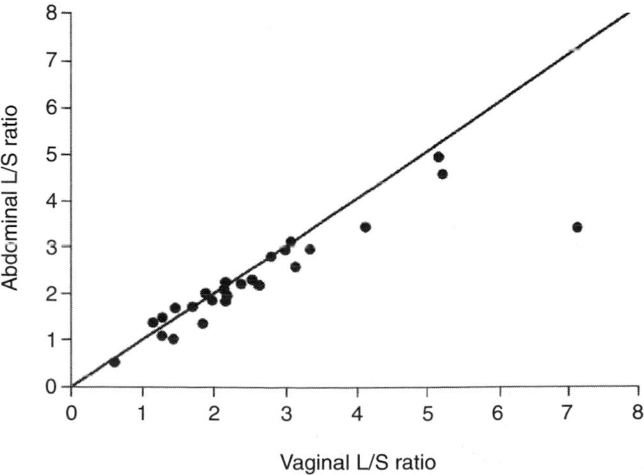

Figure 63.7 Scatterplot showing the relationship between lecithin/sphingomyelin (L/S) ratios of vaginal and amniocentesis fluid. From ref. 373 with permission from Elsevier.

Dombroski et al.[381] reported a study in which amniotic fluid was obtained by amniocentesis in patients at term in labor. Thirty minutes after artificial rupture of membranes, a vaginal sample of amniotic fluid was collected. L/S ratios obtained from amniotic fluid in the vaginal pool samples were significantly lower than those obtained by amniocentesis. However, in 22% (6/27) of cases, L/S ratios were higher in the vaginal pool samples than in amniocentesis.

Several studies have examined the value of PG determinations in amniotic fluid obtained transvaginally. Stedman et al.[374] reported that, of 25 patients with PROM between 26 and 34 weeks, 60% (15/25) had positive PG and none of their neonates developed RDS (within 72 h of the test). Among the newborns of the 10 patients with negative PG, four developed RDS. Similarly, Brame and MacKenna[375] reported no cases of neonatal RDS in 36 patients with PG found in vaginal fluid. Table 63.12 shows the frequency of the presence of PG in fluid obtained from the vaginal pool according to gestational age. Twelve percent of patients with a gestational age of less than 32 weeks had PG present.[378]

The possibility that bacterial contamination from vaginal secretions may lead to false-positive PG results has been raised by Schumacher and associates,[380] who reported that one patient had PG detected in the fluid from the vaginal pool, but not in fluid retrieved by transabdominal amniocentesis. The neonate developed respiratory insufficiency that was attributed to either RDS or pneumonia (the amniotic fluid culture was positive for bacteria). These investigators also demonstrated that bacteria might be a source of PG. Therefore, excessive bacterial contamination may alter the results of PG determinations. It would seem prudent to minimize the interval between sample collection and assay in the hope of preventing bacterial growth in the sample.

Three studies have reported neonatal outcome and L/S ratio results in preterm PROM (Table 63.13).[375,376,382] In two of the studies, a mature L/S ratio was an indication for delivery.[376,382] In the third study, the presence of PG was used as an indication for delivery.[375] The data are consistent: with a mature L/S ratio, the risk of RDS is extraordinarily small. An L/S ratio of more than 2.0 was found in 103 patients, and none of the neonates developed RDS.

Table 63.12 Frequency of positive phosphatidylglycerol in vaginal pool samples.

Gestational age (weeks)	*n* (%)	Gestational age (weeks)	*n* (%)
≤ 28	2/15 (13.3)	26–29	0/16 (0)
29–30	2/19 (10.5)	30	1/14 (7.1)
31–32	4/42 (9.5)	31–32	6/47 (12.8)
33–34	19/97 (19.6)	33–34	16/80 (20)
35–36	20/41 (48.7)	35–36	13/34 (38.2)
Total[375]	47/214 (22)	Total[378]	36/191 (19)

Table 63.13 Vaginal pool lecithin/sphingomyelin (L/S) ratio and neonatal outcome.

First author	L/S ratio	No respiratory distress syndrome	Respiratory distress syndrome
Goldstein[382]	≥ 2, < 2	5, 0	0, 3
Golde[376]	≥ 2, < 2	26, –	0, –
Brame[375]	≥ 2, < 2	72, 36	0, 19

In addition to these clinical studies, data generated from experimental observations provide further support for the lack of effect of vaginal contamination on the L/S ratio results. Sbarra and colleagues[383] demonstrated that cervical and vaginal washings are generally devoid of lecithin and sphingomyelin (in 9/10 cases) and, thus, these secretions are unlikely to alter L/S results. Two studies determined that the introduction of amniotic fluid (obtained by transabdominal amniocentesis) into the vagina results in little change in the L/S ratio.[383,384] In most cases (21/23), amniotic fluid had L/S ratios of more than 2.0 and, therefore, the effect of vaginal contamination in immature L/S ratios was not adequately tested.

The available evidence indicates that fetal lung maturity studies can be performed on amniotic fluid obtained from the vagina, and that a mature L/S ratio or the presence of PG is associated with a very low risk of RDS. Moreover, this noninvasive, low-risk approach allows for serial L/S and PG determinations.

What is the optimal management of patients with a mature phospholipid profile?

A mature phospholipid test has been demonstrated in approximately 50% of patients with preterm PROM at gestational ages of less than 34 weeks.[229,231,367] Garite and associates[231] reported that none of the neonates with an L/S ratio of 1.8 or greater developed RDS. The incidence of this complication in neonates with immature L/S ratios was 33% (5/15).

Two randomized clinical trials have been reported thus far. In the first, 47 patients with preterm PROM (less than 36 weeks) and mature amniotic fluid indices were randomized to either prompt delivery (n = 26) or expectant management (n = 21).[385] A mature test was defined as an L/S ratio above 2.0 or a foam stability index (FSI) of 47 or more (often from vaginal fluid). There was no difference in perinatal mortality between the two groups. There were no cases of RDS in the expectant management group, but two in the prompt delivery group. One newborn died from severe hyaline membrane disease (birthweight 900 g, vaginal FSI = 48), whereas the other neonate survived (birthweight 1700 g, vaginal L/S = 2.0). There were no differences in the rate of neonatal sepsis or other neonatal complications in the two groups. However, the only two cases of intracranial hemorrhage (grade not stated) occurred in the prompt delivery group. Maternal chorioamnionitis was more common in the expectantly managed group than in the delivery group [38% (8/21) versus 8% (2/26), $P < 0.02$]. The predictive value of a mature test based on the FSI was 97% (94/97).

Mercer et al.[386] reported the results of a randomized clinical trial in which 93 women with mature amniotic fluid phospholipid studies (vaginal or transabdominal amniocentesis FSI ≥ 47) were randomized to induction of labor with oxytocin or expectant management (bedrest). Maternal chorioamnionitis was more frequent in the expectant group. However, this difference did not reach significance [27.7% (13/47) versus 10.9% (5/46), $P = 0.06$]. There were no significant differences in the Cesarean delivery rate or in the incidence of confirmed neonatal sepsis between the groups. Suspected sepsis was higher in neonates born to women in the expectant group [59.6% (28/47) versus 28.3% (13/46), $P = 0.003$], as was antibiotic administration and septic workups. However, neonatologists were not blinded to treatment allocation.

Assessment of fetal well-being

The goal of fetal evaluation is to identify fetal infection/inflammation or a pathologic process that increases the risk of antepartum or neonatal death. Methods of fetal surveillance include nonstress test and the components of the biophysical profile. This section will examine the experience with each test in preterm PROM.

Nonstress test (NST)

The differential diagnosis of a nonreactive NST is: (1) prematurity; (2) infection; and (3) hypoxia. The interpretation and significance and management of fetal heart rate decelerations associated with umbilical cord compression due to oligohydramnios are also a challenge.

Are fetuses of mothers with preterm PROM expected to have nonreactive NSTs?

Surprisingly, fetuses with preterm PROM between 24 and 37 weeks have a significantly higher incidence of reactive tracings than gestational age-matched counterparts with intact membranes.[387–389] This has been attributed to "accelerated fetal central nervous system maturation" and umbilical vein compression with resulting fetal heart rate accelerations.[390] Thus, lack of reactivity should not be ascribed to prematurity without further investigation.

A nonreactive NST is frequently observed in fetuses with MIAC. Table 63.14 presents the diagnostic indices of a nonreactive NST in the prediction of total infectious morbidity (i.e., proven or suspected neonatal sepsis, MIAC, and maternal chorioamnionitis). Three studies[391–393] have found the NST to be an insensitive predictor of infection-related outcome. A major issue is the high false-positive rate (approximately 35%) of the NST for the detection of infection. Therefore, a nonreactive NST is not sufficient to diagnose infection. Evaluation of other biophysical parameters and the results of

Table 63.14 Diagnostic indices of a nonreactive nonstress test (NST) in predicting infectious outcomes.

First author	Index of infection	Number of patients	Sensitivity	Specificity	Positive predictive value	Negative predictive value	Prevalence of infection (%)
Vintzileos[403]	Suspected and documented neonatal sepsis	53	0.94	0.7	0.58	0.96	30
Vintzileos[403]	Documented neonatal sepsis	53	1	0.59	0.27	1	13
Romero[557]	Positive amniotic fluid culture	86	0.88	0.75	0.6	0.94	30
Goldstein[558]	Positive amniotic fluid culture	45	0.89	0.75	0.61	0.94	49
Goldstein[558]	Last positive amniotic fluid culture before delivery	45	0.85	0.7	0.75	0.82	49
Carroll[391]	Positive amniotic fluid culture	74	0.39	0.36	0.28	0.5	38
Carroll[391]	Positive fetal blood culture	89	0.5	0.41	0.14	0.18	16
*Asrat[559]	Positive amniotic fluid Gram stain	108	0.71	0.76	0.55	0.87	29
DelValle[392]	Chorioamnionitis, suspected and documented neonatal sepsis	68	0.38	0.84	0.36	0.15	24
Roussis[413]	Chorioamnionitis, suspected and documented neonatal sepsis	99	0.75	0.66	0.3	0.93	16
Gauthier[393]	Positive amniotic fluid culture	111	0.39	0.77	0.7	0.59	49

*Fetal tachycardia >150 b.p.m. and nonreactive NST were used.

Table 63.15 Relationship between amniotic fluid volume and duration of latent period, incidence of chorioamnionitis, and neonatal sepsis.[395]

Amniotic fluid volume	No. of patients	Chorioamnionitis	Neonatal sepsis	Latency of > 48 h	Latency of > 7 days
2 cm or more	54	5/54 (9.2%)*	1/54 (1.8%)*	37/35 (82.2%)*	13/45 (28.8%)*
< 1 cm	19	6/19 (13.5%)	6/19 (13.5%)	5/11 (45.4%)	1/11 (9.0%)

*$P < 0.05$.

amniocentesis are recommended before delivery can be indicated (see below).

Assessment of amniotic fluid volume

Is oligohydramnios always present in PROM?

Contrary to what is generally believed, rupture of membranes is not necessarily associated with oligohydramnios. Jackson et al.[394] noted that the AFI in patients with preterm PROM remains stable after the membranes rupture, with the mean AFI on admission being 5.9 ± 2.5 cm and on the day of delivery 5.4 ± 2.0 cm. Moreover, Vintzileos et al.[395] reported that 65.5% (59/90) of patients with PROM had a vertical pocket of amniotic fluid > 2 cm, while 15.5% (14/90) had a vertical pocket between 1 and 2 cm. Only 19% (17/90) had a vertical pocket of < 1 cm.

Is amniotic fluid volume assessed with ultrasound an index of impending preterm delivery and infection?

Several studies have examined the relationship between oligohydramnios and outcomes in PROM. Patients with a vertical amniotic fluid pocket < 1 cm have a shorter latency period and a higher incidence of chorioamnionitis and neonatal sepsis than those with a vertical pocket > 2 cm (Table 63.15).[395] Similar findings were reported by Gonik et al.[221] Women with a vertical amniotic fluid pocket of < 1 cm had a higher incidence of chorioamnionitis and endometritis than those with an amniotic fluid pocket of > 1 cm. No difference in the duration of the latency period was found between the two groups.[221]

Hadi et al.[396] reported that chorioamnionitis occurred in 26.4% of women with an amniotic fluid pocket < 2 cm. Similarly, Lao and Cheung[397] used a cutoff of 2 cm as the largest pocket of amniotic fluid to define oligohydramnios, and found that the frequency of chorioamnionitis and funisitis was higher in patients with oligohydramnios than in those without reduced amniotic fluid volume (chorioamnionitis: 55.3% versus 29.3%; funisitis: 44.7% versus 16.7%). A reduction in amniotic fluid volume was also associated with MIAC.

The diagnostic indices of oligohydramnios in predicting infection in both the mother and fetus are presented in Table 63.16. Collectively, these data indicate that there is an association between reduced amniotic fluid volume and maternal or neonatal infection-related morbidity and MIAC. The reason

Table 63.16 Diagnostic indices of oligohydramnios in predicting microbial invasion of the amniotic cavity (defined by positive amniotic fluid cultures) and sepsis.

First author	Diagnostic criteria	Sensitivity	Specificity	Positive predictive value	Negative predictive value
Microbial invasion of the amniotic cavity					
Romero[557]	Largest pocket < 1 cm	0.77 (21/27)	0.66 (39/59)	0.51 (21/41)	0.87 (39/45)
Gauthier[393]	Largest pocket < 2 cm	0.43 (23/54)	0.81 (46/57)	0.68 (23/34)	0.6 (46/77)
Romero[560]	Amniotic fluid index < 5	0.71 (12/17)	0.89 (32/36)	0.75 (12/16)	0.87 (32/37)
Carroll[391]	Amniotic fluid index < 5	0.82 (23/28)	0.22 (10/456)	0.39 (23/59)	0.33 (5/15)
Neonatal sepsis					
*Vintzileos[395]	Chorioamnionitis, documented and possible neonatal sepsis	0.54 (13/24)	0.9 (60/66)	0.68 (13/19)	0.84 (60/71)
*Vintzileos[395]	Documented neonatal sepsis	0.75 (6/8)	0.84 (69/82)	0.31 (6/19)	0.68 (13/19)
†Gonik[221]	Clinical chorioamnionitis	0.73 (8/11)	0.68 (19/28)	0.47 (8/17)	0.86 (19/22)
†Gonik[221]	Documented neonatal sepsis	0.5 (3/6)	0.58 (19/33)	0.18 (3/17)	0.86 (19/22)
†Carroll[391]	Positive fetal blood culture	1 (14/14)	0.76 (57/74)	0.78 (14/18)	1 (57/57)

*Largest amniotic fluid pocket < 1 cm.

†Amniotic fluid index < 5 cm.

for the high rate of infection in patients with oligohydramnios is unknown. One possibility is that decreased amniotic fluid volume may deprive patients of the antibacterial properties of normal amniotic fluid[223–226,398] and, therefore, predispose them to infection. Alternatively, intra-amniotic infection may alter amniotic fluid dynamics, leading to a reduction in fluid volume. Yoon et al.[399] proposed that redistribution of blood flow away from the kidneys may take place as part of the host response to microbial products, perhaps leading to oligohydramnios.

Fetal heart rate decelerations and amniotic fluid index

Patients with decelerations have a lower AFI than those without decelerations (4.32 ± 1.67 cm versus 6.47 ± 3.59 cm, $P < 0.01$).[400] This observation suggests that cord compression due to oligohydramnios may be the mechanism behind variable decelerations observed in patients with PROM.

Fetal breathing movements

Preterm PROM is associated with a significant and prolonged reduction in fetal breathing movements lasting approximately 2 weeks.[401,402] This phenomenon seems to be related to rupture of membranes *per se*, rather than to infection, hypoxia, or intrauterine growth restriction, even though the precise mechanisms are unknown. Membrane rupture leads to a reduction in intra-amniotic pressure and, thus, favors loss of lung fluid. Teleologically, a reduction in fetal breathing may be a mechanism to protect against lung fluid loss and pulmonary hypoplasia.

Vintzileos et al.[403,404] were the first to document an association between infection and decreased fetal breathing activity in preterm PROM. Subsequently, we confirmed these findings and documented that women with positive amniotic fluid cultures had fewer and shorter episodes of fetal breathing activity than women with negative amniotic fluid cultures.[405] The total time spent breathing differed dramatically between the two groups (Fig. 63.8).

The presence of fetal breathing has a very high negative predictive value (approximately 95%) for MIAC and neonatal sepsis. However, the absence of breathing activity has a limited positive predictive value (approximately 50%) for either of these two outcomes and, thus, it cannot be used as an indication for delivery (Table 63.17). Therefore, the presence of breathing indicates that infection is unlikely.

Why should breathing be reduced in cases of infection? The evidence in support of a role for prostaglandins includes: (1) sepsis is associated with increased plasma concentrations of prostaglandins; (2) prostaglandin administration to fetal lambs reduces breathing activity;[406] and (3) decreased fetal breathing movements in PROM are associated with increased concentrations of prostaglandin E2 in fetal plasma obtained by cordocentesis.[407]

Fetal body movements

Intra-amniotic infection is associated with a dramatic reduction in fetal body movements (Fig. 63.8).[405] The diagnostic indices are displayed in Table 63.17.[408] Decreased fetal motion in the context of infection may be the counterpart of the reduction in motor behavior observed during the course of febrile illnesses in adults and children. We have proposed that IL-1 and TNF-α released in the course of infection may be responsible for this phenomenon (R. Romero, personal communication).

Biophysical profile (BPP)

The BPP has been found to be helpful in the management of patients with PROM.[387,390–393,403,405,409–413] Vintzileos et al.,[403]

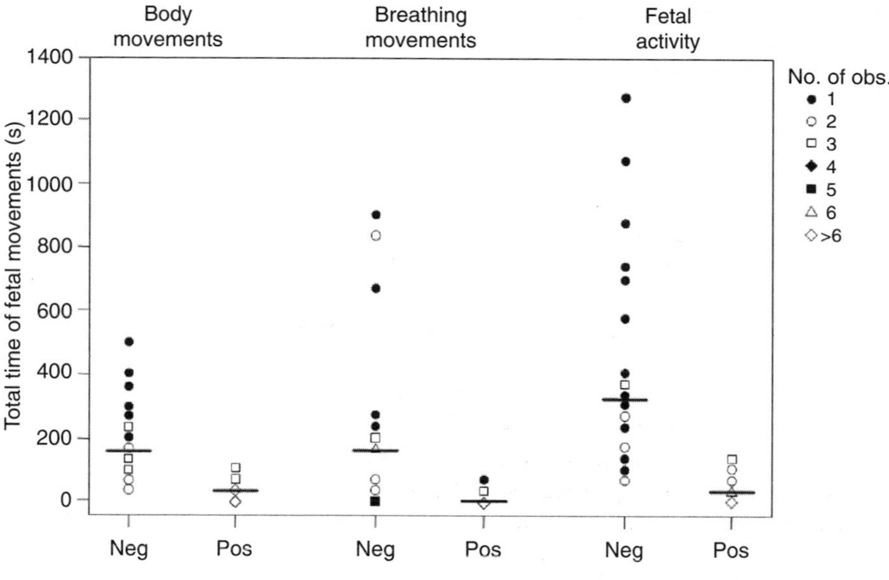

Figure 63.8 The total amount of time (in seconds) of body movements, breathing movements, and fetal activity according to the amniotic fluid culture results. Obs., observations. From ref. 405 with permission from Elsevier.

Table 63.17 Diagnostic indices of fetal breathing movements (less than 30-s duration in 30-min observation period) and fetal body movements (two or fewer body or limb movements in 30 min) in the prediction of infectious outcome.

First author	Diagnostic criteria	Sensitivity	Specificity	Positive predictive value	Negative predictive value	Prevalence (%)
Fetal breathing movements						
Vintzileos[403]	Chorioamnionitis, documented and possible neonatal sepsis	1 (16/16)	0.73 (27/37)	0.61 (16/26)	1 (27/27)	30 (16/53)
Vintzileos[403]	Documented neonatal sepsis	1 (7/7)	0.59 (27/46)	0.27 (7/26)	1 (27/27)	13 (7/53)
Roberts[412]	Positive amniotic fluid culture	0.92 (23/25)	0.49 (19/39)	0.53 (23/43)	0.9 (19/21)	39 (25/64)
Fetal body movements						
Vintzileos[403]	Chorioamnionitis, documented and possible neonatal sepsis	0.5 (8/16)	0.94 (35/37)	0.8 (8/10)	0.81 (35/43)	30 (16/53)
Vintzileos[403]	Documented neonatal sepsis	0.86 (6/7)	0.91 (42/46)	0.60 (6/10)	0.98 (42/43)	13 (7/53)
Roberts[412]	Positive amniotic fluid culture	0.32 (8/25)	0.97 (38/39)	0.89 (8/9)	0.69 (38/55)	39 (25/64)
Gauthier[393]	Positive amniotic fluid culture	0.11 (6/54)	0.98 (56/57)	0.86 (6/7)	0.54 (42/69)	49 (54/111)

using logistic regression analysis, demonstrated that each component of the BPP contains useful information for the prediction of infection-related morbidity (defined as maternal chorioamnionitis, possible neonatal sepsis, and proven neonatal sepsis). In their first study, a modified BPP scoring system that incorporated placental grading (with a maximal score of 12) was used. A BPP score of seven or less was much better than any single component of the BPP in the prediction of infection-related outcome. Placental grading was the only parameter that had no predictive value, hence its exclusion from subsequent studies. The diagnostic indices of a BPP score ≤ 7 (performed 24 h before delivery) were: sensitivity 94%, specificity 97%, positive predictive value 95%, and negative predictive value 97% in a population with a prevalence of infection-related outcome of 30%. This study was observational in nature and, thus, the BPP was not used for patient management.

Subsequently, Vintzileos et al.[414] compared the outcome of pregnancy in patients managed with serial BPPs with two historical control groups: (1) expectant management without BPP or amniocentesis; and (2) management with a single amniocentesis on admission. A BPP score ≤ 7 on two examinations 2 h apart was used as an indication for delivery. An abnormal score required a nonreactive NST and absence of fetal breathing. The results of this study indicated that patients managed with daily BPPs had a lower rate of overall neonatal sepsis (suspected and culture proven) than patients in either control group. This study did not provide the frequency of other

Table 63.18 Relationship between various features of the biophysical profile (BPP) and infectious outcome.

Group	No. of patients	Clinical chorioamnionitis	Neonatal infection	Overall infection
I*	81	4 (4.9%)	3 (3.7%)	6 (7.4%)
II†	13	3 (23%)	9 (69.2%)	9 (69.2%)
III‡	17	9 (52.9%)	15 (88.2%)	16 (94.1%)
		$P = 0.0001$	$P = 0.0001$	$P = 0.0001$

*Fetuses with reactive nonstress test, or fetal breathing movements, or both.

†Fetuses with nonreactive nonstress test, absent fetal breathing movements, normal fetal body movements and tone.

‡Fetuses with nonreactive nonstress test, absent fetal breathing movements, absent fetal body movements and tone.

From ref. 390 with permission from Lippincott Williams & Wilkins.

indices of neonatal morbidity (e.g., RDS, IVH, duration of mechanical ventilation) in the different groups. This issue is important, as 14 patients who were delivered because of a low BPP score showed no evidence of neonatal infection and, thus, could be considered false positives. If intervention was not associated with an increased rate of other neonatal complications, management with serial BPPs would seem a reasonable approach. The investigators found that the BPP had limitations when the interval between the test and delivery was longer than 24 h, and that maternal infection without fetal infection was not correlated with the results of the BPP scoring. Vintzileos and Knuppel[390] subsequently reported on 111 fetuses with preterm PROM followed with daily BPPs, and found that, as more of the biophysical activities became compromised, the higher the incidence of infection-related complications (Table 63.18).

It is noteworthy that, subsequent to this work, three studies[409,410,413] reported an association between the results of the BPP and infection-related outcomes, and three others could not confirm such an association.[411,412] Our explanation for the apparent discrepancy is that studies reporting negative results used the BPP at less frequent testing intervals (48- to 72-h intervals) than the daily testing used in positive reports.

BPP and the results of amniocentesis

Four studies have examined the relationship between components of the BPP scoring and amniotic fluid culture results retrieved by transabdominal amniocentesis.[391,393,405,412] Goldstein et al.[405] made a key observation linking fetal breathing and movements with the likelihood of MIAC: (1) the presence of fetal breathing movements for 30 s or more ruled out intra-amniotic infection; (2) if fetal breathing was absent or lasted less than 30 s and body movements were decreased (lasting less than 50 s), MIAC was detected in all cases; and (3) in intermediate cases (normal fetal body movements but compromised fetal breathing movements), 64% of women had positive amniotic fluid cultures.

Table 63.19 Prediction of positive amniotic fluid cultures: biophysical profile versus total fetal activity.

	Biophysical profile	Total fetal activity
Sensitivity	0.92 (23/25)	0.96 (24/25)
Specificity	0.59 (23/29)*	0.82 (32/39)
Positive predictive value	0.59 (23/29)	0.77 (24/31)
Negative predictive value	0.92 (23/25)	0.97 (32/33)

*$P < 0.05$.

From ref. 412 with permission from John Wiley & Sons Ltd on behalf of the ISUOG.

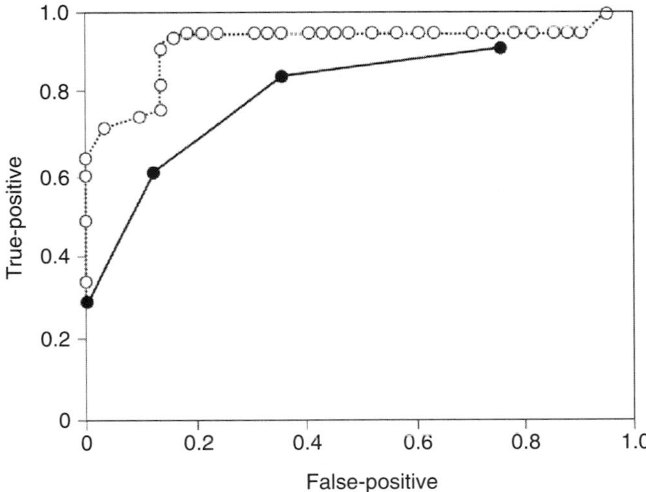

Figure 63.9 Receiver operator characteristic curve for the association between total fetal activity (open circles) and biophysical profile (closed circles) to MIAC. From ref. 412 with permission from John Wiley & Sons Ltd on behalf of the ISUOG.

Roberts et al.[412] compared the diagnostic performance of the BPP with that of total fetal activity (the sum of fetal breathing and body movements in a 30-min period of observation) in the prediction of a positive amniotic fluid culture. Although both methods correlated significantly with the presence of MIAC, the specificity of total fetal activity greater than 10% was significantly better than that of the BPP (Table 63.19; Fig. 63.9). Gauthier et al.[393] reported that the likelihood of a positive amniotic fluid culture was inversely related to the BPP score (Table 63.20). However, 61% (33/54) of patients with positive amniotic fluid cultures had a BPP of eight or more, which may reflect that their fetuses were unaffected.

Devoe et al.[415] examined the ability of the BPP to predict the latency period in 25 women with PROM between 28 and 30 weeks of gestation. The diagnostic indices of the BPP in predicting delivery within 72 h are shown in Table 63.21. In other studies, the sensitivity of the BPP to predict delivery within 72 h varied from 0% to 80%.[392,393,403,405,411] The relationship between a low BPP and the impending onset of labor can be understood in the context that the FIRS (which may be reflected as a low BPP score) is followed by the impending

Table 63.20 Correlation of biophysical score with microbial invasion of the amniotic cavity.

Biophysical profile score	2	4	6	8	10
Negative amniotic fluid culture	0	2 (15%)	3 (27%)	25 (52%)	27 (73%)
Positive amniotic fluid culture	2 (100%)	11 (85%)	8 (73%)	23 (48%)	10 (27%)

%, percentages at each biophysical profile score.

From ref. 393 with permission from Lippincott Williams & Wilkins.

Table 63.21 Diagnostic indices of biophysical profile in predicting delivery within 72 h.[415]

Diagnostic criteria	Sensitivity	Specificity	Positive predictive value	Negative predictive value
Absent fetal breathing movements	0.55	1	1	0.31
Absent fetal body movements	0.25	1	1	0.25
Nonreactive nonstress test	0.2	1	1	0.24

Table 63.22 Diagnostic indices of C-reactive protein.

First author	Cutoff values (mg/dL)	Infectious definition	Prevalence of infection (%)	Sensitivity (%)	Specificity (%)	Positive predictive value (%)	Negative predictive value (%)
Evans[416]	2	Clinical or histologic	69.4	80	100	100	69
Hawrylyshyn[419]	1.25	Histologic	50	88	96	96	89
Farb[417]	2	Clinical	29	56	73	45	80
		Histologic	21	80	68	40	93
Romem[422]	2	Clinical	16.3	86	97	86	97
Ismail[420]	2	Clinical	18	82	55	36	91
		Histologic	63	67	81	90	50
Fisk[418]	2	Histologic	59	50*/92†	81*/73†	79*/73†	53*/92†
Kurki[421]	1.2	Clinical	22.4	94	50	35	97
		Histologic	–	72‡	63‡	48‡	83‡
Kurki[421]	4	Neonatal infection	13	79	43	18	93

*24-h sample to delivery interval.

†12-h sample to delivery interval.

‡Cutoff value 4 mg/dL.

onset of labor in patients with preterm PROM. In summary, there is compelling evidence that a low BPP score is associated with infection-related outcomes.

C-reactive protein

Several studies have examined the value of C-reactive protein (CRP) in monitoring the patient with preterm PROM.[416–422] Most studies indicate a strong relationship between an elevated maternal serum CRP and the presence of histologic chorioamnionitis. Diagnostic indices, cutoff values, and the definition of infection-related morbidity for the different studies are shown in Table 63.22.

In terms of the prediction of a positive amniotic fluid culture, Yoon et al.[423] compared the performance of maternal serum CRP and WBC count with that of the amniotic fluid WBC count in the identification of MIAC, clinical histologic chorioamnionitis, and significant neonatal morbidity. The amniotic fluid WBC count was a better predictor than maternal serum CRP in the identification of MIAC.[423]

DiNaro et al.[424] recently provided evidence indicating that the determination of vaginal fluid CRP can be used in the identification of the fetus with funisitis, the histologic counterpart of FIRS. The rationale for this observation is that CRP in vaginal fluid is thought to be of fetal origin. Thus, an elevation in vaginal CRP concentration is an indicator of a fetal acute-phase response.

Thompson et al.[425] reported a study of fetal serum CRP obtained by cordocentesis in patients with preterm PROM. A fetal CRP of more than 0.8 mg/dL was found in five of six fetuses with positive fetal blood cultures. In contrast, when the CRP concentration was less than 0.6 mg/dL, none of 11 fetuses had positive cultures. These results may extend to the assessment of fetal plasma and umbilical cord cytokines. Some evidence indicates that neonates with an elevated umbilical cord IL-6 (a cytokine that stimulates the production of CRP) are at increased risk for the development of short- and long-term complications such as PVL,[426] cerebral palsy,[258] and BPD.[369]

Management of patients with preterm PROM

The management of patients with preterm PROM depends on the gestational age at the time of membrane rupture (see Fig. 63.10).

Previable PROM (< 24 weeks of gestation)

(see Fig. 63.11)

The major complications of previable PROM are maternal infection, late abortion/preterm labor, low neonatal survival, and a high risk of neurologic handicap.[427,428] Patients are generally offered two options: pregnancy termination or expectant management. The presence of intra-amniotic inflammation/infection in amniotic fluid analysis carries a poor prognosis because of the risk of spontaneous preterm labor as well as fetal morbidity. A more vexing problem is when the preterm PROM occurs in a previable gestation, but delivery occurs when the infant is viable and at very high risk of death and neurologic handicap if survival is achieved. Table 63.23 demonstrates the outcome of patients before viability. Management of these patients requires an in-depth discussion involving the parents, neonatologists, and obstetricians and careful documentation in the medical record. The value of antibiotic or corticosteroid administration in previable PROM has not been established. Leakage of amniotic fluid after second-trimester amniocentesis should be considered as a separate entity from previable PROM. It occurs in 1.2% of patients and is usually transient in nature.[429] The risk of delayed PROM in these cases is no different from that in the general population.[430]

PROM remote from term (24 weeks to 31 weeks and 6 days of gestation) (see Fig. 63.12)

The management goals are: (1) to exclude intra-amniotic infection/inflammation; and (2) to institute expectant management in patients without documented infection/inflammation.

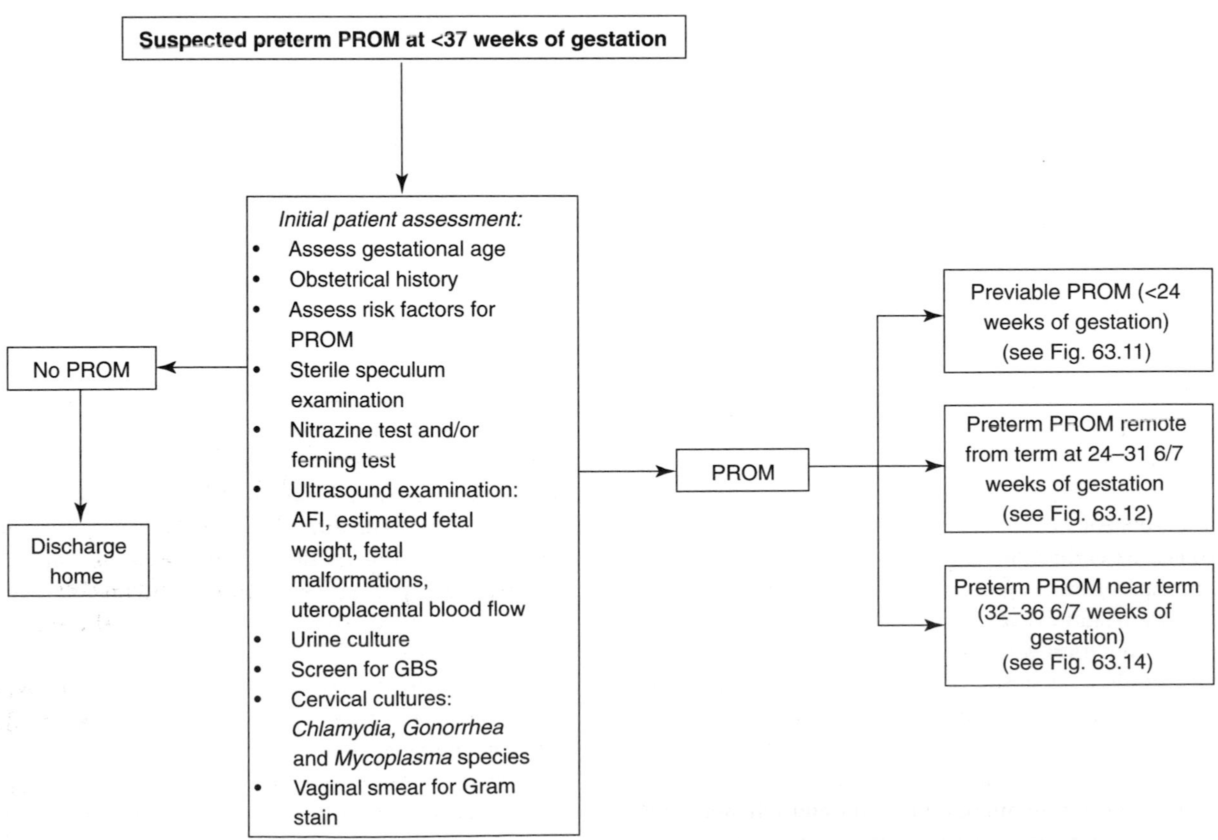

Figure 63.10 Initial assessment of preterm PROM. AFI, amniotic fluid index; GBS, group B *Streptococcus*. Modified from Mercer BM. *Clin Perinatol* 2004;31:765–782[432] with permission from Elsevier.

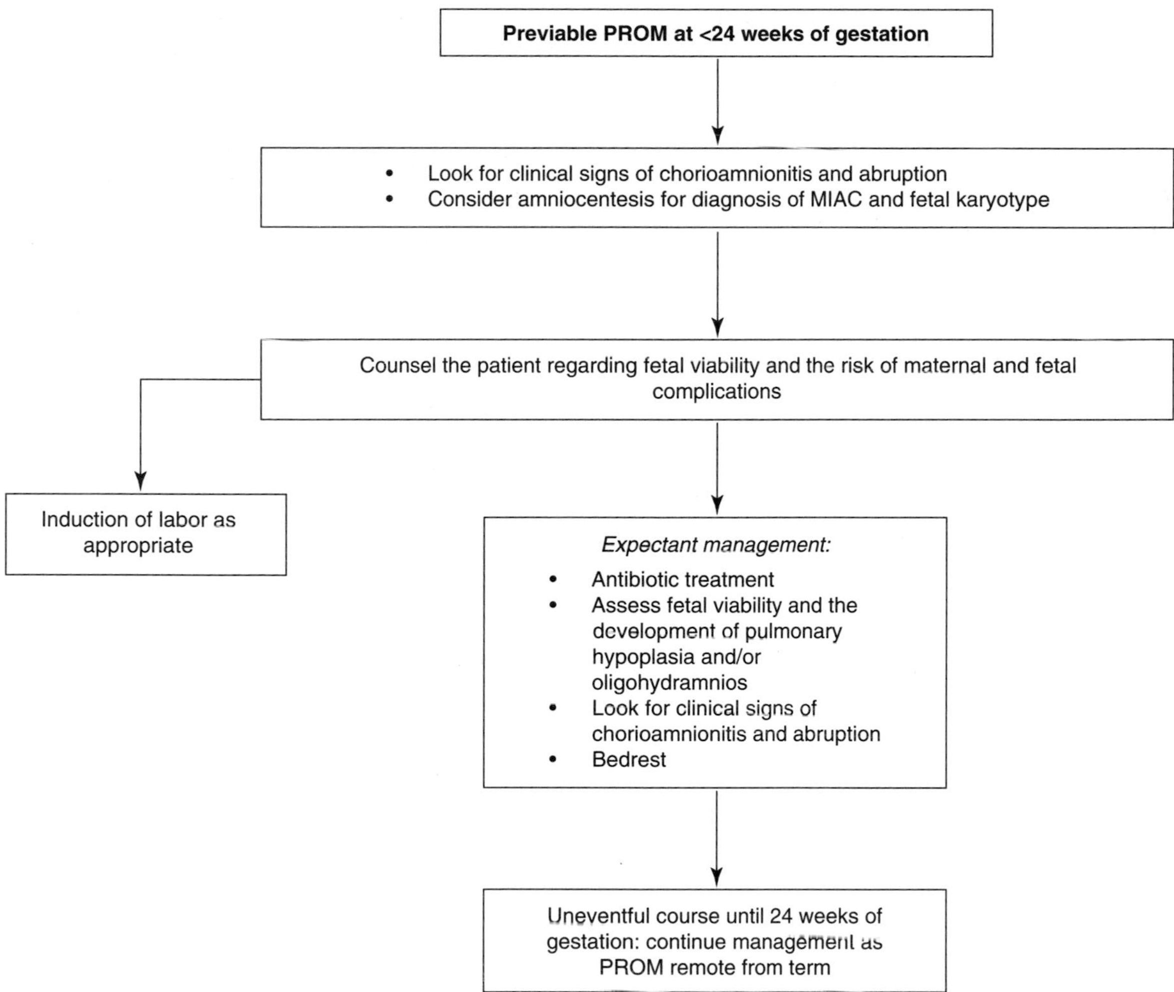

Figure 63.11 Management of previable PROM (before 24 weeks of gestation). MIAC, microbial invasion of the amniotic cavity. Modified from Mercer BM. *Clin Perinatol* 2004;31:765–782[432] with permission from Elsevier.

Intra-amniotic infection/inflammation and its management

The most accurate method for the diagnosis of intra-amniotic infection/inflammation is amniocentesis. Once intra-amniotic infection/inflammation is identified in patients between 24 and 31 completed weeks of gestation, the optimal management is a challenge: the earlier the gestational age, the more difficult the dilemma. In patients who are close to 32 weeks of gestation, delivery would avoid continuous exposure to microbial products and inflammatory agents, and is unlikely to increase neonatal morbidity. These patients are managed in our unit with detailed counseling, antibiotic administration, and delivery. In contrast, in patients close to 24 weeks of gestation, the option of parenteral administration of antibiotics is considered to eradicate intra-amniotic infection and inflammation. Patients are informed that this alternative may prolong pregnancy, eradicate intra-amniotic infection, and reduce the risk of extreme prematurity, but that it requires intensive surveillance and repeat evaluation of the amniotic cavity to ensure eradication of microorganisms and reduced intra-amniotic inflammation (as gauged by the amniotic fluid WBC count). Despite these interventions, the risks of infection and prematurity are not eliminated. Broad coverage is recommended before the results of cultures are available, and this approach should be modified once the specific microorganisms involved are identified. The choice of antibiotics is informed by the results of microbial cultures. Our choice for broad-coverage antibiotics includes azythromycin, clindamycin, and ampicillin. We have also used a combination of ceftriaxone, clindamycin, and erythromycin for 10–14 days.[248] Azythromycin is included because *U. urealyticum* is the most frequent microorganism found in the amniotic cavity.[217]

Antibiotic treatment aimed at the eradication of intra-amniotic infection should not be confused with prophylactic treatment, which is now considered the standard of care for

Table 63.23 Second-trimester premature rupture of the membranes.

Author	Study period	No. of women	Gestational age at PROM (median/mean)	Gestational age at PROM (range)	Latency days (median/mean)	Latency days (range)	Delivered in 1 week (%)	Neonatal survival number (%)	Clinical chorioamnionitis number (%)	Neonatal sepsis number (%)	Normal at 1 year number (%)
Taylor[486]	1979–1982	53	23/22.6	16–25	6.0/16.8	0.5–87	62.3	13/60 (21.6)	22/53 (41)	–	5/8 (62)
*Beydoun[489]	1978–1985	70	23/24.1	20–26	7.5/19.1	2–124	50.7	35/69(50.7)	41/70 (58.6)	4/35 (11.4)	5/17 (29.4)
Moretti[487]	1981–1987	118	24/23.1	16–26	4.2/13	1–152	66.9	34/124 (27.4)	46/118 (39)	20/68 (29.4)	–
Bengston[490]	1982–1985	59	24/23.2	15–26	9/21.5	0.5–161	49.2	31/63 (49.2)	27/59 (46)	7/22 (31.8)	–
Major[488]	1984–1988	70	24/23.7	19–25	–/12	1–60	62.9	45/71 (63.3)	30/70 (43)	12/70 (17)	31/45 (68)
*Hibbard[491]	1986–1989	44	–/23.9	17–26	6/13.1	1–68	40.9	26/48 (54.2)	34/44 (77)	16/43 (41)	–
Morales[492]	1981–1991	97	23/–	17–25	10.5/–	2–126	–	39/97 (40.2)	24/97 (25)	3/97 (4)	19/30 (63)
Fortunato[493]	1987–1991	24	–/25.3	15.5–27	–/21.6	1.4–75.4	21	19/24 (79.2)	2/24 (8)‡	3/24 (12.5)	–
†David[495]	1985–1989	71	–/23	17–25	–/20	0.5–77	40.8	22/71 (31)	28/71 (39.4)	12/52 (23.1)	5/8 (62.5)
Rib[494]	1983–1988	41	–/23.6	19–26	4.2/10.6	1–102	75§	21/45 (47.0)	29/41 (70.7)	10/45 (22.2)	7/18 (38.8)

*Excluded patients delivering in first 24 h.

†Excluded patients delivered < 20 weeks.

‡Histologic chorioamnionitis occurred in 54% in Fortunato et al.

§Two weeks after admission.

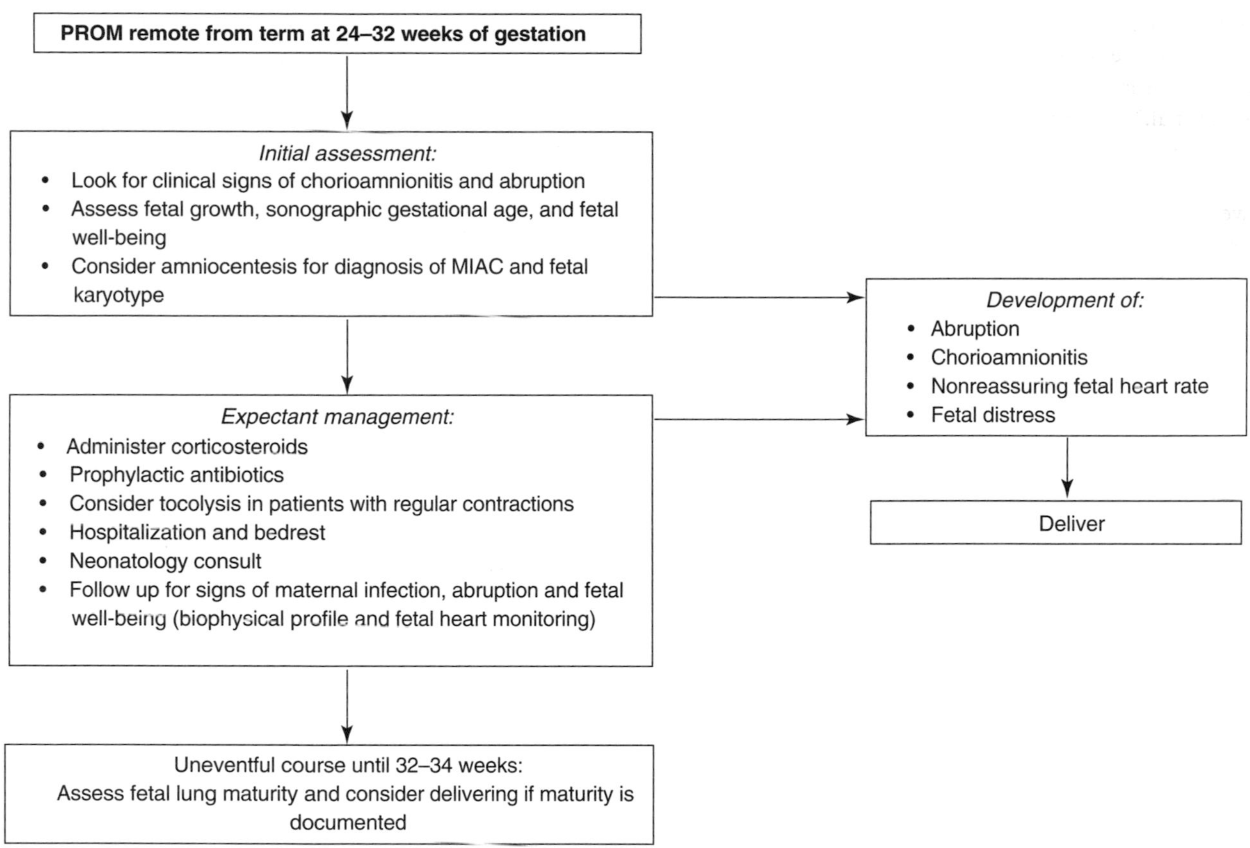

Figure 63.12 Management of PROM remote from term (between 24 weeks and 31 weeks and 6 days of gestation). MIAC, microbial invasion of the amniotic cavity. Modified from Mercer BM. *Clin Perinatol* 2004;31:765–782[432] with permission from Elsevier.

patients with preterm PROM, regardless of whether the inflammatory/infection state of the amniotic fluid is known. Thus, patients in this gestational age range, without evidence of infection and inflammation, are given prophylactic treatment with antibiotics (ampicillin and erythromycin).

In summary, the management of PROM between 24 and 31 completed weeks comprises: (1) maternal and fetal inpatient surveillance in a tertiary medical center; (2) administration of corticosteroids to accelerate fetal lung maturity;[431] and (3) antibiotic administration, which may be therapeutic or prophylactic.[432,433]

"Prophylactic" antibiotic administration

Antibiotic administration has now become the standard of care in patients with preterm PROM. This practice is based upon the results of several randomized clinical trials, in which antibiotic administration was associated with prolongation of pregnancy, a reduced rate of maternal chorioamnionitis,[434] and a reduced frequency of neonatal morbidity, measured as "composite neonatal outcome."[435] This approach has often been referred to as "prophylactic" antibiotic administration. However, this may be a misnomer. One-third of women with preterm PROM have a positive amniotic fluid culture on admission.[120] Furthermore, the frequency of MIAC increases as the patients are being observed in the antepartum ward to the point that, at the time of the onset of labor, 75% of patients will have a positive amniotic fluid culture for microorganisms.[121] These studies were conducted before the administration of prophylactic antibiotics and demonstrate that microorganisms are present at admission, and also that secondary infection of the amniotic cavity occurs during expectant management. It would be inaccurate to refer to "prophylactic" administration as therapy instituted with patients who have a proven infection (one-third of all patients). Antimicrobial therapy may prolong pregnancy by controlling microbial proliferation of an existing infection and preventing secondary infection/inflammation. However, antibiotic administration is not uniformly efficacious in eradicating microbially proven intra-amniotic infection.[248]

Several investigators have conducted randomized clinical trials to assess the potential benefits of prophylactic antibiotic administration in patients with preterm PROM.[435–448]

Mercer et al.[449] reported a randomized clinical trial in which patients were allocated to receive intravenous ampicillin (2 g every 6 h) and erythromycin (250 mg every 6 h for 48 h, followed by oral amoxicillin and erythromycin base (every 8 h for 5 days) versus placebos. Recruitment was restricted to patients with a gestational age ranging between 24 and 32 weeks. GBS carriers were identified and treated, and tocolysis and steroids were not administered after randomization. The primary outcome of the trial was a composite variable that included any of the following: fetal or infant death, RDS, severe IVH, stage II or III of necrotizing enterocolitis (NEC), or sepsis within 72 h of birth.[449] Antibiotic administration was associated with prolongation of pregnancy and a significant reduction in the rate of RDS (RR 0.83, 95% CI 0.69–0.99), NEC (RR 0.4, 95% CI 0.17–0.95), clinical chorioamnionitis, and the composite primary outcome, which is an index of fetal/infant morbidity and mortality (RR 0.84, 95% CI 0.71–0.99). These differences were not demonstrated in GBS carriers, an observation attributable to antibiotic administration to patients allocated to the placebo group for this clinical indication, and thus obscuring the potential effects of antibiotic administration.[449]

In the ORACLE study,[435] 4826 women with preterm PROM were randomly assigned to: (1) erythromycin; (2) co-amoxiclav (amoxicillin and clavulanic acid); (3) erythromycin and co-amoxiclav; and (4) placebo. The study included patients before 36 weeks and 6 days from 161 medical centers. Tocolysis and corticosteroid administration were left to the discretion of the attending physician. The primary outcome measure was a composite variable, which included neonatal death, chronic lung disease, or major cerebral abnormality before discharge from the hospital.

Among neonates of patients with singleton gestations allocated to erythromycin only, fewer had the primary composite outcome than those in the placebo group [11.2% (125/1111) versus 14.4% (166/1149), $P = 0.02$]. Erythromycin treatment alone significantly reduced the proportion of patients delivering within 48 h in comparison with the placebo group. The combination of erythromycin with co-amoxiclav significantly reduced the proportion of patients delivering within 1 week of admission. Similarly, co-amoxiclav administration alone, or in combination with erythromycin, significantly reduced the proportion of patients delivering within 48 h and within 7 days from admission, compared with the placebo group.[435]

The neonatal effects of erythromycin treatment included a reduction in the need for exogenous surfactant, in neonates needing 21% O_2 administration for 48 h after delivery, as well as a reduction in positive neonatal blood cultures.[435] Co-amoxiclav had a similar effect on the proportion of neonates needing 21% O_2 administration for 48 h after delivery. Of note, the rate of suspected and proven NEC was significantly higher in the group of neonates whose mothers were treated with co-amoxiclav as a single or combined therapy. The authors attribute their findings to the wide and nonspecific effect of this broad-spectrum antibiotic, which may change the flora of premature neonates and induce the growth of pathologic bacteria that induce NEC.[435]

Lovett et al.[450] did not demonstrate an association between prophylactic antibiotic treatment of patients with preterm PROM with co-amoxiclav and an increased incidence of NEC in comparison with placebo. The studies differ in the antibiotic regimen, as well as in the gestational age at inclusion and the number of patients. Therefore, comparison of the studies is difficult. The recommendation of the investigators in the ORACLE I trial was to use erythromycin and avoid using co-amoxiclav in patients with preterm PROM.[435] Recently, a systematic review by Kenyon et al.[451,452] confirmed these results.

According to Kenyon et al.,[452] the number of patients needed to treat to prevent one adverse outcome remains high [chorioamnionitis: 10 (95% CI 7–34); delivery within 48 h: 9 (95% CI 6–20); delivery within 7 days: 7 (95% CI 5–15); neonatal infection: 17 (95% CI 12–50); and abnormal cerebral ultrasonography before discharge: 69 (95% CI 35–1842)]. It is possible that the wide confidence intervals reflect the range of gestational ages of patients included in the systematic review.

Can antibiotic treatment of women with documented MIAC alter the natural history of preterm PROM?

The traditional view has been that clinical chorioamnionitis should be managed by immediate delivery, and this view has been extended to the management of MIAC.[453] There is evidence that both these conditions can be treated *in utero* without interruption of pregnancy. Ogita and colleagues[454] first reported the successful treatment of established chorioamnionitis with antibiotic treatment via a transcervical catheter. Subsequently, we reported that giving antibiotics to a mother with preterm PROM at 29 weeks and an amniotic fluid culture positive for *Bacteroides bivius*, *Veillonella parvula*, and *Peptococcus* without clinical signs of chorioamnionitis resulted in eradication of MIAC.[455] In a second case, we were successful in eradicating *U. urealyticum* from the amniotic cavity with antibiotic treatment.[456]

The effects of antibiotics on the natural history of MIAC in patients with preterm PROM has been reported by Gomez et al.[248] Patients who underwent amniocentesis upon admission and those without evidence of intra-amniotic inflammation or MIAC were treated with ampicillin and erythromycin for 7 days. In contrast, patients with intra-amniotic inflammation or MIAC were treated with ceftriaxone, clindamycin, and erythromycin for 10–14 days. Patients who remained undelivered after the conclusion of the course of antibiotics underwent a second amniocentesis. Six of seven patients who had MIAC at the time of the first amniocentesis still had positive amniotic fluid cultures for microorganisms after a full course of antibiotic treatment. Of the 18 patients with intra-amniotic inflammation, most (15/18) still showed evidence of an elevated WBC count in amniotic fluid after antibiotic administration. Therefore, antibiotic administration did not eradicate MIAC or intra-amniotic inflammation. Moreover, among patients with no evidence of intra-amniotic inflammation, 32% (9/28) developed inflammation despite therapy and, among those without MIAC, 55% (5/9) developed a positive amniotic fluid culture.[248] These data raise important questions about the effect of antibiotics and the nature of the invading microorganisms in preterm PROM. Long-term follow-up studies of infants enrolled in the randomized clinical trials are urgently needed because antibiotic treatment of intrauterine infection in animals has been associated with neurologic lesions similar to PVL. Even though the ORACLE I trial observed that the number of neurosonographic lesions was lower in patients who received treatment with erythromycin, it remains to be proven whether the rate of long-term handicap will be lower in these infants.

Should corticosteroids be administrated to patients with preterm PROM remote from term?

A systematic review included 13 randomized clinical trials and demonstrated a reduction in the incidence of RDS, IVH, and NEC (RR 0.56, 95% CI 0.46–0.70; RR 0.47, 95% CI 0.31–0.70; RR 0.21, 95% CI 0.05–0.82 respectively).[457] A nonsignificant trend of reduced neonatal mortality was observed. Moreover, no increase in neonatal and fetal infection was observed.[457] Steroid treatment was associated with a modest, yet significant, increase in the risk of puerperal endometritis (RR 2.42, 95% CI 1.38–4.24), but no significant increase in neonatal sepsis. Similar findings were reported by Crowley[458,459] in an earlier meta-analysis, which included fewer trials.

Clinical investigators have compared expectant management with steroid administration for 48 h followed by delivery. However, induction of delivery immediately after steroid administration is associated with an increased risk of RDS and, therefore, is best avoided.[459]

The 1994 National Institutes of Health Consensus Conference recommended the use of corticosteroids in pregnancies complicated by preterm PROM with expected delivery between 24 and 30–32 weeks of gestation.[431] This recommendation was based largely on data suggesting that the incidence of IVH was lower in neonates exposed to corticosteroids.[431] The modest increased risk of puerperal infection is considered to be easy to manage. A meta-analysis comparing the outcome of treatment with antibiotics and steroids versus antibiotics without steroids found that steroid administration diminished the beneficial effects of antibiotics in reducing the rate of chorioamnionitis, endometritis, neonatal sepsis, and IVH.[460] It seems that this issue requires further study, particularly when MIAC has been demonstrated by amniocentesis. Steroids may compromise the fetal host response to microbial products and potentially increase the risk of adverse outcome.

How many courses of corticosteroids should be administered?

Repeated courses of corticosteroids have been used to enhance their effects. However, recent data, based upon studies in humans and animals, have raised questions about the safety of repeated corticosteroid administration. Guinn et al.[461] performed a double-blind, randomized, controlled trial, in which women at risk of preterm delivery received one course of betamethasone or dexamethasone at admission, and were randomly allocated for subsequent weekly courses of either betamethasone (n = 256) or placebo (n = 246) until 34 weeks of gestation or delivery. There were no significant differences in the frequency of composite neonatal morbidity (severe RDS, BVD, severe IVH, PVL, proven sepsis, NEC, or perinatal death) between the study groups [weekly course 22.5% (56/256) versus single course 28% (66/246), $P = 0.16$]. However, when the analysis was stratified by gestational age, patients who delivered between 24 and 27 weeks and received a single course had a higher rate of composite neonatal morbidity and severe RDS than those in the weekly course group. An important limitation of this study is that the authors did not control for the use of surfactant, which was more frequent in the single course group [single course 24% (59/246) versus the weekly course 15.6% (40/256), $P = 0.01$].[461]

In animal experiments, multiple courses of corticosteroids have been associated with low birthweight in term and preterm sheep, as well as small head diameters in term sheep.[462] Among human neonates born between 27 and 29 weeks of gestation, repeated courses of betamethasone were associated with a smaller neonatal head circumference than those exposed to a single course (multiple courses 25.5 ± 1.6 cm versus single course 26.5 ± 1.4 cm, $P = 0.02$).[463] Similarly, French et al.[464] reported the results of a cohort study that included 477 singleton infants born at less than 33 weeks of gestation. The authors performed a multivariate analysis, which indicated that multiple corticosteroid courses were associated with a significant reduction in birthweight ($P = 0.01$) and head circumference ($P = 0.002$).[464]

Tocolysis

Tocolysis has been employed to attempt to delay delivery and reduce perinatal complications in preterm PROM. Seven randomized clinical trials have studied the effect of tocolysis on pregnancy prolongation and perinatal outcome. Two trials addressed the issue of prophylactic administration of oral ritodrine to patients not in labor,[465,466] while four have examined the effectiveness of intravenous tocolysis in patients with uterine contractions,[467–470] and one has compared short-term (24 h) with long-term tocolysis.[467]

Levy and Warsof[466] randomized 42 women with preterm PROM to receive oral ritodrine (10 mg orally every 4 h) versus no medication or placebo. Drugs were given until the onset of labor. A latency period of more than 7 days was noted more frequently in patients receiving ritodrine than in the control subjects [47% (10/21) versus 14.2% (3/21), $P = 0.04$]. The only perinatal death occurred in the control group. No differences in perinatal morbidity or mortality were documented between groups.

Dunlop and associates[465] randomized 48 women to receive oral ritodrine versus no tocolysis and then subrandomized each group to receive prophylactic antibiotics (cephalexin) versus no antibiotics. The result was a four-limb randomization with 12 patients per group. Steroids were given to all patients. No difference in outcome (perinatal mortality and RDS) was observed between patients receiving ritodrine versus no tocolysis. Therefore, the evidence is inconclusive as to the usefulness of oral tocolysis.

Of the four randomized trials of intravenous tocolysis, only one used a double-blind placebo design.[467] The other three compared tocolysis with bedrest.[468–470] Overall, no change in maternal or neonatal morbidity and mortality was demonstrated between the study group and the control group. Tocolysis, however, resulted in some degree of pregnancy prolongation in three of the trials.[467,469,470]

In the trial by Christensen and coworkers,[467] ritodrine administration was associated with a significant decrease in the proportion of women delivering within 24h after membrane rupture [ritodrine 0% (0/24) versus placebo 37.5% (6/16), $P < 0.05$]. However, no difference in pregnancy prolongation after 24h was observed between the treatment group and the control group. In the study by Weiner and colleagues,[470] the duration of pregnancy was greater in patients receiving tocolysis than in those allocated to bedrest [105h (SD 157h)]. Post-hoc analysis indicated that tocolysis administration resulted in significant pregnancy prolongation for patients with gestational ages of less than 28 weeks at the time of membrane rupture (bedrest 53.4h versus tocolysis 232.8h, $P = 0.05$). This was not associated with a demonstrable reduction in perinatal morbidity or mortality. No difference in pregnancy prolongation was noted in patients with a gestational age greater than 28 weeks. The authors concluded that there was no justification for tocolysis after 28 weeks of gestation. An unresolved issue is whether the prolongation observed in patients with gestational ages of less than 28 weeks (mean prolongation 5 days) could have some beneficial effect. Steroids were not used in this trial.

Garite and associates[468] randomized 79 women with a gestational age of 25–30 weeks to receive either intravenous tocolysis with ritodrine (followed by oral therapy) or expectant management. Steroids were not administered. No difference in pregnancy prolongation or perinatal morbidity and mortality was observed between the two groups. It should be noted that 16 of 39 patients randomized to the tocolytic limb did not receive the treatment.

Matsuda et al.[469] conducted a trial of 81 women with preterm PROM who were allocated to either intravenous antibiotics and tocolysis ($n = 39$: ritodrine and $MgSO_4$ if ritodrine alone failed) and bedrest ($n = 42$). Patients with clinical chorioamnionitis, positive amniotic fluid Gram stain, and fetal distress on heart rate monitoring were excluded. Steroids were not used. Patients who received tocolysis and antibiotics had a longer latency period than those in the control group (longer than 48h 87% versus 50%; and longer than 7 days, 39% versus 12%). No differences in the rate of clinical chorioamnionitis or proven neonatal sepsis (13% versus 12%) were noted. However, suspected neonatal sepsis was significantly higher in the women receiving tocolysis and antibiotics (39% versus 17%). Given that antibiotic administration results in prolongation of the latency period, the value of tocolysis cannot be ascertained.

A randomized trial conducted over a 7-year period in 240 patients with PROM (26 and 35 weeks of gestation) allocated women to short-term tocolysis (24h i.v.) or long-term tocolysis (24h i.v. followed by oral therapy until delivery).[471] Women were excluded if the Bishop score was 5 or more or if tocolysis failed in the first 24h. No difference was found in the duration of the latency period between the two groups. Chorioamnionitis (RR 2.47, 95% CI 1.42–4.66) and postpartum endometritis (RR 1.74, 95% CI 1.10–2.75) were more common in those receiving long-term tocolysis; no differences in neonatal outcome were noted.

Because three of the randomized clinical trials of intravenous tocolysis suggest that treatment results in some prolongation of pregnancy, it is relevant to determine whether enough time could be gained to complete steroid administration and reduce the incidence of RDS.[467,469,470] Meta-analysis of the four trials indicates that tocolysis does result in prolongation of pregnancy of more than 48h. However, because no study has shown an improvement in maternal or neonatal outcomes, there is no evidence to support the use of intravenous tocolysis in women with PROM.

Should a cervical cerclage be removed in a patient who presents with preterm PROM?

Cerclage removal has been advocated to reduce the risk of infection-related complications,[472] while leaving the cerclage in place has been recommended to prolong pregnancy.

Yeast and Garite[473] reported the results of a case–control study in which the outcome of patients with a cervical cerclage removed after preterm PROM was compared with that of patients with PROM of a similar gestational age. There was no difference in the incidence of chorioamnionitis or other infectious complications and neonatal outcome between the two groups. The interval between PROM and delivery was not significantly different between patients with and without cerclage. Blickstein and associates[474] reported similar findings after comparing the outcome of 32 patients with cerclage and 76 without cerclage. In contrast, Goldman and colleagues[475] compared the outcome of 46 women with preterm PROM in whom the cerclage was not removed with that of 46 women with preterm PROM without cerclage. Patients with a cerclage had a significantly shorter PROM-to-delivery interval and lower gestational age at delivery than patients without the cerclage. However, the rates of chorioamnionitis, other infection-related complications, and neonatal outcome were not different between the two groups. Ludmir et al.[476] evaluated the role of immediate cerclage removal in preterm PROM in 30 women. In 20 women, the cerclage was removed immediately after the diagnosis of ruptured membranes was made, while in 10 women, the cerclage was retained after the membranes ruptured. Thirty-three patients with preterm PROM without cerclage served as control subjects. A greater proportion of women with a cerclage left in place delivered after 48 h [90% (9/10) versus 50% (10/20) respectively]. However, perinatal mortality was significantly higher in infants born to women in whom cerclage was retained in comparison with immediate removal or the control group [70% (7/10) versus 10% (2/20) versus 18% (6/33) respectively]. Seventy-one percent of the neonatal morbidity was attributable to sepsis. The authors did not use broad-spectrum antibiotic treatment, which may explain this observation.[476]

McElrath et al.[477] reported a randomized clinical trial conducted over 12 years comparing removal (n = 288) versus nonremoval (n = 114) of cerclage in patients with preterm PROM. All patients were treated with antibiotics and corticosteroids. Patients with retained cerclage had a lower gestational age at membrane rupture and delivered earlier than patients in whom cerclage was removed. However, there was no difference in the latency period between the groups. Neonatal mortality was higher among patients in whom the cerclage was kept. This difference became nonsignificant when the analysis was stratified into three gestational age groups (< 28, 28–30, and > 30 weeks). There were no significant differences in the rate of RDS, IVH, and neonatal sepsis between the study groups.[477]

In summary, patients with preterm PROM and a cerclage could be managed by leaving the cerclage in place and maintaining close surveillance to detect maternal and/or fetal infection.

Home care versus hospital care

Technical Bulletin no. 15 of the American College of Obstetricians and Gynecologists suggested that, "management in hospital or in selected patients at home with careful observation is feasible" in preterm PROM.[478] The potential disadvantages of home care include the risk of delivering a preterm infant outside a tertiary center and the implicit delay in obstetric intervention if fetal distress or infection occurs. The advantages of home care include decreased costs and psychological benefits to the patient.

Two studies have compared home care with hospital care. The first, a small, randomized trial of women with PROM at less than 37 weeks of gestation, had strict criteria for home care.[479] Only patients undelivered after 72 h (60% delivered in less than 72 h), in cephalic presentation, with negative amniotic fluid culture (by amniocentesis), cervical dilation of less than 4 cm on speculum examination, and at least one amniotic fluid pocket of more than 1 cm (22% had oligohydramnios) were eligible for participation. Follow-up included biweekly NST, weekly ultrasound examination, and corticosteroid administration. Fifty-five patients were randomized, 27 to home care and 28 to remain in hospital. There was no difference in the latency period, gestational age at delivery, chorioamnionitis [11.1% (3/27) versus 14.3% (4/28)], neonatal morbidity [3.7% (1/27) versus 7.1% (2/28)], RDS [3.7% (1/27) versus 7.1% (2/28)], or neonatal pneumonia [18.5% (5/27) versus 10.7% (3/28)].[479]

The second study of home care was a retrospective study of patients with preterm PROM between 20 and 30 weeks of gestation, in which 19 of 21 women undelivered after 7 days were discharged home.[480] All patients had "adequate or slightly diminished amniotic fluid volume." Eleven of 19 women delivered at term. No neonatal deaths occurred, and there was one case of maternal and neonatal sepsis in a woman managed at home [she was infected with human immunodeficiency virus (HIV)]. One case of neonatal sepsis occurred in an infant born to a woman who was managed in hospital and delivered preterm.

The data available are insufficient to recommend management of preterm PROM outside tertiary care centers. We believe that fetuses with preterm PROM require careful surveillance, which is rarely available outside a hospital environment.

When to induce?

Expectant management of patients presenting with preterm PROM remote from term is the standard of care today.[20,432,433] This management significantly reduces the neonatal complications related to prematurity;[20,432,433] however, the longer the latency period, the higher the risk of chorioamnionitis and abruption.[385,481–483]

Cox and Leveno[484] performed a prospective study comparing induction versus expectant management of patients presenting with preterm PROM between 30 and 34 weeks. There were no significant differences in neonatal morbidity. However, chorioamnionitis was significantly higher in the expectant management group [2% (1/61) versus 15% (10/68), P = 0.009]. Of note, 74% (50/68) of the expectant management group delivered within 72 h.

The timing of delivery is a determinant of the presence of major, but not minor, composite neonatal morbidity. Indeed, major composite neonatal complications (RDS, IVH, intubation, BPD, seizure, NEC, bowel perforation, retinopathy of prematurity, meningitis, pneumonia, primary pulmonary hypertension, and patent ductus arteriosus) decrease substantially after 32 weeks of gestation.[485] In contrast, minor composite neonatal outcomes (hyperbilirubinemia, transient tachypnea of the newborn, hyper- or hypoglycemia, and hyper- or hyponatremia) decrease only after 34 weeks of gestation (Fig. 63.13). Mercer et al.[386] demonstrated that, in patients with preterm PROM, delivery after 32 weeks of gestation was not associated with a significant increase in neonatal morbidity. The development of chorioamnionitis, placental abruption, or a nonreassuring fetal heart rate tracing often

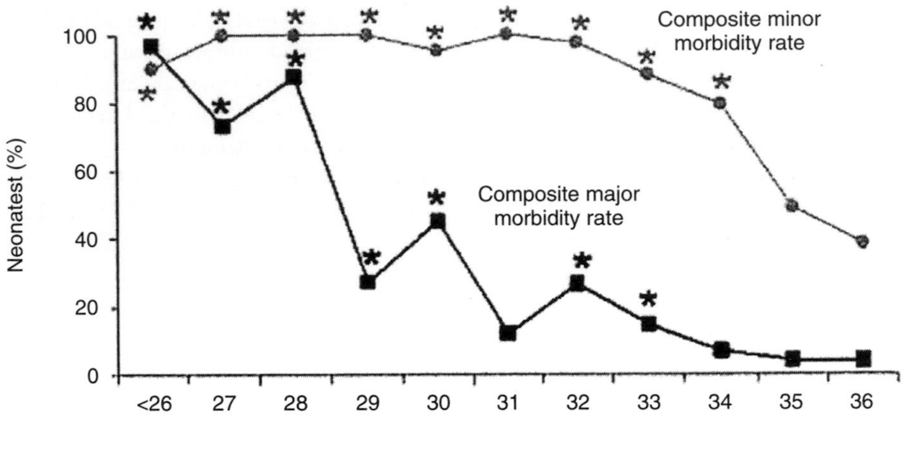

Figure 63.13 Composite major (solid line, square marks) and minor (solid line, circle marks) neonatal morbidity rates for infants born after preterm premature rupture of membranes according to gestational age of delivery. Composite neonatal major morbidity was defined as the presence of any of the following: intraventricular hemorrhage, respiratory distress syndrome, intubation, bronchopulmonary dysplasia, sepsis, seizure, necrotizing enterocolitis, bowel perforation, meningitis, pneumonia or primary pulmonary hypertension, patent ductus arteriosus, or retinopathy of prematurity. Composite neonatal minor morbidity was defined as the presence of any of the following: hyperbilirubinemia, transient tachypnea of the newborn, or metabolic disturbances (hyper- or hypoglycemia or hyper- or hyponatremia). Outcome data for each gestational age group were compared with the respective outcome of a reference group of women with preterm premature rupture of membranes who delivered at 36 weeks to 36 weeks and 6 days of gestation. $^*P < 0.05$. From ref. 485 with permission.

requires induction of labor and delivery, regardless of gestational age.

What are the complications associated with expectant management?

This question has been addressed by many studies, and is summarized in Table 63.23.[486–495] Fetal and neonatal complications include pulmonary hypoplasia, oligohydramnios sequence, RDS, IVH, neonatal sepsis, and NEC. Perinatal survival rates by gestational age in patients with early preterm PROM are displayed in Tables 63.23 and 63.24. The rate of stillbirth reached 15–26% in previable PROM; overall, there were 111 stillbirths and 237 neonatal deaths[496] (these figures exclude the study by Rib et al.,[494] in which no distinction was made between stillbirths and neonatal deaths). Intrauterine fetal deaths were not systematically reported in all studies.

The main maternal complications of expectant management of preterm PROM are chorioamnionitis (39%), endometritis (14%), placental abruption (3%), and postpartum hemorrhage due to retained placenta that requires curettage (12%).[489] No relationship between the duration of membrane rupture and chorioamnionitis has been noted. However, cases of septicemia requiring a hysterectomy, septic shock, and maternal death were reported.[486–488,490]

Expectant management prolonged pregnancy by more than 1 week in 49.8% (254/510),[486–491,493,495] more than 2 weeks in 28% (114/407),[486,488,489,493–495] and more than 1 month in 19.2% of cases (71/370).[486,487,489,490,495] An inverse relationship

Table 63.24 Survival by gestational age in second-trimester premature rupture of membranes.

First author	Gestational age in weeks	Survival number (%)
Moretti[487]	< 20	2/16 (12)
	20–22	2/27 (7.4)
	23–24	9/35 (25)
	25–26	27/46 (58.6)
Major[488]	19–21	3/6 (50)
	21–22	10/15 (66.7)
	23–24	21/25 (84)
	25–26	21/25 (84)
Hibbard[491]	< 24	7/18 (38.9)
	24–26	19/30 (63.3)
Morales[492]	< 20	1/15 (67)
	20–22	7/30 (23.3)
	23–24	31/52 (59.6)
David[495]	< 20	1/6 (16.7)
	20–22	4/21 (19)
	23–25	19/43 (44.2)
Rib[494]	19–22	0/8 (0)
	22–23	9/20 (45)
	24–26	12/17 (70.6)

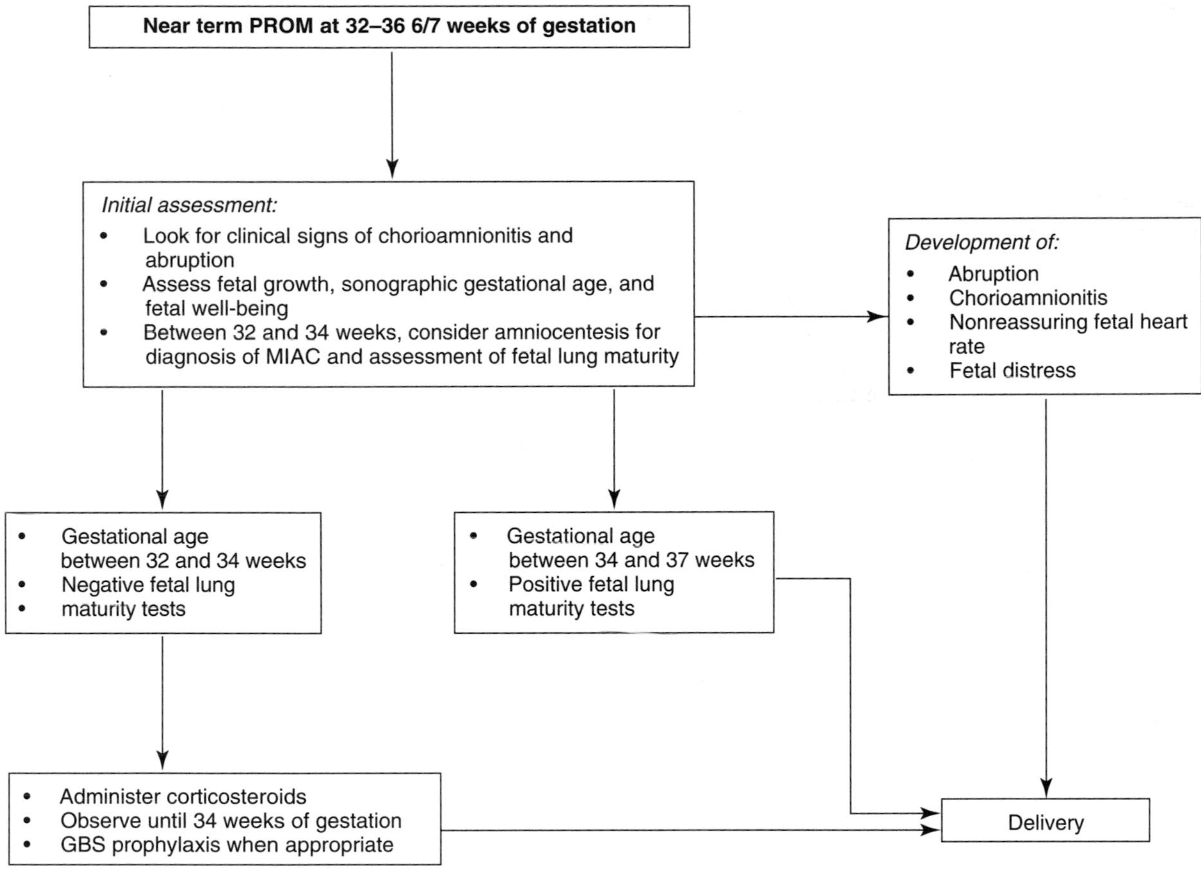

Figure 63.14 Management of near term PROM (between 32 and 37 weeks of gestation). MIAC, microbial invasion of the amniotic cavity; GBS, group B *Streptococcus*. Modified from Mercer BM. *Clin Perinatol* 2004;31:765–782[432] with permission from Elsevier.

between gestational age at preterm PROM and the latency period was noted in four studies.[486,490–492]

PROM near term (32–36 6/7 weeks of gestation) (see Fig. 63.14)

Mercer et al.[386] demonstrated no differences in the maternal and neonatal outcomes of expectant management and induction of labor. However, there was a trend toward a higher incidence of maternal chorioamnionitis in the expectant management group.[386] Cox and Leveno[484] reported a higher incidence of maternal chorioamnionitis. The conventional view is to perform amniocentesis for fetal lung maturity between 32 and 34 weeks and, if the result is positive, to proceed with induction of labor in order to reduce maternal morbidity.[432,484,497] In cases with negative fetal lung maturity, the management is not clear. Some physicians will choose expectant management until 34 weeks, while others will administer corticosteroids and induce labor 48 h later.[498] There are not sufficient data in the literature to support either course of action.

In a survey that was conducted in the USA during 2003 among members of the Society of Maternal Fetal Medicine, 42% will induce labor in patients presenting with premature PROM and positive lung maturity at 32 weeks.[498] In cases with unknown fetal lung maturity, 58% will postpone delivery to 34 weeks of gestation.[498] In summary, patients between 32 and 34 weeks need assessment of lung maturity and, if positive, the patients should be offered induction of labor. In cases without fetal lung maturity, there are not sufficient data as to the optimal management approach. Mercer[12] proposed that women with PROM after 34 weeks should be delivered.

The role of amnioinfusion in preterm PROM

Oligohydramnios is a risk factor for the development of abnormal fetal heart rate patterns during labor.[499] Experimental evidence obtained in rhesus monkeys indicates that loss of amniotic fluid is associated with the appearance of variable fetal heart rate decelerations that disappear after fluid volume is replaced.[500] A similar phenomenon has been observed in women with rupture of membranes. Moberg and coworkers[501] reported that patients with preterm PROM had a higher incidence of Cesarean delivery for fetal distress than patients with preterm labor and intact membranes [7.9% (21/267) versus 1.5% (2/130) respectively, $P < 0.05$]. Seventy-six percent of patients who underwent Cesarean delivery for fetal distress in the PROM group had fetal heart rate patterns consistent with umbilical cord compression. Miyazaki and Taylor[502] were the first to report a clinical trial in which saline amnioinfusion was used in 42 patients in labor with five or more consecutive repetitive variable decelerations or prolonged decelerations (< 100 b.p.m. for at least 3 min) that did not respond to changes in maternal position and oxygen therapy. Amnioinfusion provided relief from repetitive variable decelerations in 67% (19/28) of cases and of prolonged decelerations in 85.7% (12/14).

Subsequently, Miyazaki and Nevarez[503] compared amnioinfusion with standard management of variable decelerations in 96 patients. Amnioinfusion was associated with a significant reduction in the severity and occurrence of variable decelerations and prolonged decelerations (amnioinfusion 51% versus non-infusion group 4.2%, $P < 0.01$). This effect was more dramatic in nulliparous patients. A significant reduction in the incidence of Cesarean delivery for fetal distress was noted in nulliparous, but not in multiparous, patients.

Nageotte and associates[504] compared prophylactic amnioinfusion versus no infusion in a randomized clinical trial of 61 women in preterm PROM in early labor. Patients who received an amnioinfusion had significantly lower incidence of severe decelerations during both the first and the second stage of labor. The incidence of Cesarean delivery for fetal distress was also lower in patients receiving amnioinfusion than in the control group [3% (1/29) versus 22% (7/32), $P = 0.06$]. No umbilical cord pH data were reported.

A meta-analysis of randomized clinical trials using transcervical amnioinfusion has demonstrated that this procedure is associated with a significant reduction in the rate of Cesarean delivery (OR 0.48, 95% CI 0.30–0.77), variable decelerations, 1- and 5-min Apgar score of less than 7, umbilical artery pH of less than 7.20, and meconium aspiration syndrome. The reduction in Cesarean delivery may also lead to a decrease in endometritis.[505] Potential complications of intrapartum amnioinfusion include uterine overdistention, elevated intrauterine pressure, and amniotic fluid embolism.[506] In conclusion, the balance of the evidence supports the use of transcervical amnioinfusion in preterm PROM when there are fetal heart rate abnormalities. However, a recent randomized controlled trial (RCT) in patients admitted at ≥ 36 weeks with thick meconium staining of the amniotic fluid failed to demonstrate a beneficial effect of transcervical amnioinfusion.[507]

The value of transabdominal infusion in the management of PROM remote from term was assessed recently in a RCT in which women with PROM between 24 weeks and 32 weeks and 6 days were allocated to transabdominal amnioinfusion ($n = 17$) or expectant management ($n = 17$). Women in the amnioinfusion group received weekly serial amnioinfusion of isotonic sodium chloride if the AFI was below the fifth percentile and/or a median pocket of amniotic fluid was < 2 cm. The mean volume infused was 250 mL. The transabdominal amnioinfusion was associated with a lower risk of delivery within 7 days (RR 0.18, 95% CI 0.04–0.69).[508]

Another use of amnioinfusion is to improve fetal visualization in cases of severe oligohydramnios. Amnioinfusion was first used by Gembruch and Hansmann[509] to improve sonographic imaging in cases of midtrimester oligohydramnios. Fisk et al.[307] reported improved fetal visualization after expansion of the amniotic volume in a significant number of cases (amnioinfusion was successful in 58/61 cases, enabling sonographic visualization of fetal anatomy in 51 cases). There was one inadvertent aspiration of fetal blood at 34 weeks of gestation followed by profound bradycardia necessitating delivery. The neonate died from pulmonary hypoplasia. Four other fetal losses may have been procedure related.

Prelabor rupture of the membranes at term

The management of patients with PROM at term includes: (1) exclusion of cord prolapse; (2) detection of infection; and (3) evaluation of fetal well-being. If any evidence exists of fetal compromise or infection, induction of labor or delivery is the management of choice. For other patients, the relevant management issues include deciding between (1) induction or expectant management and (2) when and how induction should be undertaken.[510–533]

The natural history of term PROM is that 90% of women will be in spontaneous labor within 24 h.[533] Nulliparous women have a longer latency period than multiparous women.[516,523,528] Patients with an unfavorable cervix at presentation and those who are not in labor within 6 h of rupture of membranes generally do not initiate labor spontaneously within 24 h and represent a management dilemma.[532]

The largest clinical trial in term PROM[517] included 5041 patients who were randomly allocated to four groups: (1) immediate induction with oxytocin; (2) expectant management followed by induction with oxytocin after 4 days; (3) induction of labor with vaginal prostaglandin E_2 (1–2 mg, followed by i.v. oxytocin; if not in labor in 4 h, a second dose of prostaglandin E_2); and (4) expectant management followed by induction of labor with prostaglandin E_2, if labor had not begun within 4 days. The primary outcome of the trial was probable neonatal infection (clinical and laboratory signs). Secondary outcomes were the need for Cesarean delivery and women's evaluation of their treatment. The results showed no difference in neonatal infection and Cesarean delivery rate between the induction groups (oxytocin versus prostaglandin E_2). However, the incidence of chorioamnionitis was lower in patients allocated to induction of labor. Women's satisfaction with their obstetric care was higher for those allocated to induction of labor.

Table 63.25 Pooled odds ratios (ORs) and confidence intervals (CIs) for three treatment policies of term prelabor rupture of the membranes and outcome variables of interest. From ref. 524 with permission from Lippincott Williams & Wilkins.

	Chorioamnionitis		Endometritis		Cesarean delivery		Neonatal infection	
	OR	CI	OR	CI	OR	CI	OR	CI
Oxytocin vs. conservative	0.91	0.51–1.62	0.78	0.50–1.21	1.24	0.89–1.73	0.73	0.47–1.13
Prostaglandins vs. conservative	0.68	0.51–0.91	0.81	0.53–1.23	0.95	0.76–1.20	1.06	0.67–1.66
Prostaglandins vs. oxytocin	1.55	1.09–2.21	0.78	0.23–2.63	0.67	0.34–1.29	1.50	0.91–2.45

Mozurkewich and Wolf,[524] in their meta-analysis of 23 studies including 7493 women, demonstrated that induction of labor is superior to expectant management. The meta-analysis compared three policies: (1) immediate induction with oxytocin; (2) induction of labor with vaginal or endocervical prostaglandin E_2 gel suppositories or tablets; and (3) expectant management that has sometimes included delayed induction with oxytocin. The frequency of chorioamnionitis and endometritis was significantly lower in patients undergoing immediate induction of labor with oxytocin than in those managed expectantly (OR 0.67, 95% CI 0.52–0.85 and OR 0.71, 95% CI 0.51–0.99 respectively). The rate of chorioamnionitis was significantly higher in patients who received vaginal prostaglandins than in those induced with immediate administration of oxytocin, but lower than that of patients in the expectant management group (OR 1.55, 95% CI 1.09–2.21 and OR 0.68, 95% CI 0.51–0.91 respectively). The rates of Cesarean delivery and neonatal infection were not different among the three management schemes (Table 63.25). Based on these data, we endorse a policy of immediate induction of labor in patients with term PROM. Antibiotic administration is justified before Cesarean delivery for obstetric indications or for carriers of GBS.

Tan and Hannah[534] performed a meta-analysis of 18 trials comparing induction of labor with oxytocin versus expectant management in patients with PROM at or near term. Induction of labor with oxytocin was associated with a lower risk of chorioamnionitis (OR 0.63, 95% CI 0.51–0.78), endometritis (OR 0.72, 95% CI 0.52–0.99), and neonatal infection (OR 0.64, 95% CI 0.44–0.93). Cesarean delivery rates were not statistically different. Oxytocin was associated with a more frequent use of pain medication and internal fetal heart rate monitoring. Another meta-analysis of 15 RCTs by Lin et al.[535] included: (1) six studies ($n = 453$) of misoprostol versus placebo or expectant management; and (2) nine studies ($n = 1130$) of misoprostol versus oxytocin for labor induction with term PROM. Surprisingly, there were no significant differences in the frequency of chorioamnionitis, neonatal sepsis, or Cesarean delivery among the study groups. Similarly, a recent systematic review of induction of labor versus expectant management for term PROM by Dare et al.[536] did not find differences in the rate of Cesarean deliveries and neonatal infection. However, the frequency of chorioamnionitis and endometritis was higher in the expectant management group.[536]

Expectant management at home of patients with PROM at term is not recommended. This recommendation is based upon the report by Hanna et al.[537] that home care was associated with an increased risk of neonatal infections (OR 1.97, 95% CI 1.00–3.90) and Cesarean delivery in patients not colonized with GBS (OR 1.48, 95% CI 1.03–2.14).

Novel treatment techniques

Attempts have been made to seal the site of rupture (mostly in iatrogenic cases). These techniques are at the current time in developing stages. However, a description is included because patients or their physician may inquire about these techniques.

Fibrin glue

Fibrin glue is a mixture of fibrinogen, thrombin, and cell fibrin that is injected under ultrasound guidance onto the site of rupture. Genz[538] treated 19 patients, with a success rate of 60%. However, Kurz and Hick[539] (using the same procedure) reported a small series in which there were no successes.

Baumgarten and Moser[540] used an intracervical approach to apply the sealant, following a cervical cerclage in 26 women, with a success rate of 65% (success was defined as the percentage of surviving infants). Pregnancy was prolonged for more than 28 days in six women, and no cases of chorioamnionitis were documented. Uchide et al.[541] reported a case of intracervical fibrin glue instillation and cervical cerclage in which the pregnancy lasted from 24 weeks (time of rupture) to 31 weeks of gestation. Catalano and Zardini[542] reported five cases in which intracervical instillation of fibrin glue resulted in successful pregnancy prolongation. Similar results were found by Sciscione et al.[543] in 12 patients (13 fetuses) with previable PROM using fibrin sealants. All patients had an increase in the AFI and diminution of leakage. The fetal survival rate was 53.8%.

Amniopatch

This approach consists of transabdominally injecting platelets and cryoprecipitate to seal the membranes. The basis for this approach is that the amnion is avascular and, therefore, unable to initiate platelet activation, fibrin deposition, and other events required for wound healing in vascular tissues. The procedure consists of administering platelets (0.5 units) followed by cryoprecipitate (a source of fibrinogen). Quintero et al.[544] pioneered this approach in 1996 and subsequently reported the experience in 28 cases.[545] A key observation is that this approach is successful when applied to rupture of membranes occurring after procedures such as fetoscopy. The rate of successful sealing of the membranes is 64% (18/28). Among the successful cases, one patient had a miscarriage, one patient terminated the pregnancy due to a chromosomal abnormality, and one neonate died of meningitis 2 weeks after discharge from the neonatal intensive care unit. Of the 10 unsuccessful cases, three neonates were alive and well. Some cases resulted in fetal death ($n = 3$), voluntary termination of pregnancy ($n = 2$), and miscarriage ($n = 2$). This option can be offered to patients who have membrane rupture after amniocentesis, skin biopsies, fetal shunts, and diagnostic operative fetoscopy. Precise knowledge of the site of rupture is unnecessary. The hemostatic material does not need to be injected into the site of rupture, and appears to find its way to the defect and seals it. The possibility of fetal death must be explained to patients. This phenomenon has been attributed to the possible effect of vasoactive agents released during the course of platelet activation.

Physical barrier to stop leakage

A group from Lithuania evaluated 16 women between 22 and 32 weeks of gestation with PROM in whom a "cervical cup" was inserted to stop leakage.[546] Outcomes were compared with 19 women with preterm PROM. The average AFI in the women having the adapter almost doubled, whereas the AFI did not change in control subjects. No infections occurred in mothers or infants in either group. The aim of increasing the amniotic fluid volume was to enable easier amniocentesis.

O'Brien et al.[547] had implemented a treatment protocol for patients presenting with previable PROM including amnioinfusion, cervical cerclage, and administration of gelatine sponge into the amniotic cavity. Eight of 15 fetuses (53%) reached viability, two of whom were intrauterine fetal demise, and six were discharged home alive. However, three fetuses had talipes equivarus and bilateral hip dysplasia, while two fetuses had torticolis. This might be an effective, although aggressive, mode of treatment, but further studies are needed to investigate the origin of the higher rate of musculoskeletal disorders. A surgical approach to sealing the membranes in patients with spontaneous rupture and no evidence of infection and inflammation is being explored. The procedure relies on the placement of a graft with laser welding. This has been attempted in animals, but the procedure is still experimental in humans.[545,548]

Acknowledgments

This work was conducted by members of the Perinatology Research Branch of the National Institute of Child Health and Human Development (NICHD) of the National Institutes of Health (NIH) and funded by the Intramural Program of NICHD/NIH.

This chapter was published in previous editions of this book. The current version has been substantially changed. The authors wish to acknowledge the contribution of authors of previous chapters. In particular, the current authors and the editors gratefully acknowledge the intellectual contributions of Dr Neil Athayde, Dr Eli Maymon, and Dr Percy Pacora.

Key points

1 Term PROM occurs in approximately 10% of patients, while the frequency of preterm PROM is 2–3.5%.

2 The "zone of altered morphology" (ZAM) is an anatomical structure that includes amnion and chorion (of fetal origin) and portions of decidua (of maternal origin) apposed to the cervix, which undergoes morphologic changes before the onset of labor.

3 It has been proposed from biophysical studies of chorioamniotic membranes of patients with PROM that the membranes have focal areas of weakness rather than a generalized weakening.

4 Evidence supports the role of matrix metalloproteinases (MMPs), proteases that can degrade several components of the chorioamniotic membranes, in both preterm and term PROM.

5 Preterm PROM is associated with positive amniotic fluid cultures in approximately 30% of cases, while 75% of patients have microbial invasion of the amniotic cavity (MIAC) when amniocenteses are performed at the time of onset of labor.

6 The most important risk factor for preterm PROM is a previous preterm delivery.

7 Vaginal bleeding, a short cervix (≤ 25 mm), a history of previous spontaneous preterm delivery (with intact or ruptured membranes), and smoking are risk factors for preterm PROM in the index pregnancy.

8 The risk of PROM in a subsequent pregnancy is 4% if the patient's first pregnancy went to term and was

not complicated by PROM, while the recurrence rates are 21% for preterm PROM and 26% for term PROM.

9 The main consequences of preterm PROM are: (1) spontaneous onset of labor leading to prematurity; (2) infection; (3) abruptio placentae; (4) fetal death; and (5) the oligohydramnios sequence.

10 The prevalence of positive amniotic fluid cultures in women with preterm PROM is 32.4%, whereas in term PROM, the prevalence is 34.3%.

11 In preterm PROM, genital mycoplasmas (*Ureaplasma urealyticum* and *Mycoplasma hominis*) are the most frequent isolates from the amniotic fluid, followed by *Streptococcus agalactiae*, *Fusobacterium* species, and *Gardnerella vaginalis*.

12 The frequency of positive fetal blood culture is about 10% among patients with preterm PROM.

13 The risk of pulmonary hypoplasia when PROM occurs at 19 weeks has been found to be 50%, yet it was only 10% when the membranes ruptured at 25 weeks.

14 The accuracy of ferning in the diagnosis of PROM is 95%.

15 Fetal lung maturity studies can be performed on amniotic fluid obtained from the vagina. A mature lecithin/sphingomyelin (L/S) ratio or the presence of phosphatidylglycerol (PG) in these samples is associated with a very low risk of respiratory distress syndrome (RDS).

16 The diagnostic indices of a BPP score ≤ 7 (performed 24 h before delivery) for the prediction of infection-related morbidity (defined as maternal chorioamnionitis, possible neonatal sepsis, and proven neonatal sepsis) were: sensitivity 94%, specificity 97%, positive predictive value 95%, and negative predictive value 97%, in a population with a prevalence of infection-related outcome of 30%.

17 The natural history of term PROM is that 90% of women will be in spontaneous labor within 24 h.

18 Expectant management at home of patients with PROM at term was associated with an increased risk of neonatal infections and Cesarean delivery in patients not colonized with group B *Streptococcus* (GBS).

19 In patients with preterm PROM, delivery after 32 weeks of gestation is not associated with a significant increase in neonatal morbidity.

20 Patients with preterm PROM and a cerclage could be managed by leaving the cerclage in place and maintaining close surveillance to detect maternal and/or fetal infection.

References

1 Keirse MJ, Ohlsson A, Treffers PE, Kanhani HHH. Prelabour rupture of the membranes preterm. In: Chalmers I, Enkin M, Keirse MJ, eds. *Effective care in pregnancy and childbirth*. Oxford: Oxford University Press; 1989:666.

2 Johnson JW, Daikoku NH, Niebyl JR, et al. Premature rupture of the membranes and prolonged latency. *Obstet Gynecol* 1981;57:547–556.

3 Hauth JC, Cunningham FG, Whalley PJ. Early labor initiation with oral PGE2 after premature rupture of the membranes at term. *Obstet Gynecol* 1977;49:523–526.

4 Lange AP, Secher NJ, Nielsen FH, Pedersen GT. Stimulation of labor in cases of premature rupture of the membranes at or near term. A consecutive randomized study of prostaglandin E2-tablets and intravenous oxytocin. *Acta Obstet Gynecol Scand* 1981;60:207–210.

5 Lebherz TB, Hellman LP, Madding R, et al. Double-blind study of premature rupture of the membranes. a report of 1,896 cases. *Am J Obstet Gynecol* 1963;87:218–225.

6 Magos AL, Noble MC, Wong TY, Rodeck CH. Controlled study comparing vaginal prostaglandin E2 pessaries with intravenous oxytocin for the stimulation of labour after spontaneous rupture of the membranes. *Br J Obstet Gynaecol* 1983;90:726–731.

7 Tamsen L, Lyrenas S, Cnattingius S. Premature rupture of the membranes – intervention or not. *Gynecol Obstet Invest* 1990;29:128–131.

8 van der WD, Venter PF. Management of term pregnancy with premature rupture of the membranes and unfavourable cervix. *S Afr Med J* 1989;75:54–56.

9 Westergaard JG, Lange AP, Pedersen GT, Secher NJ. Use of oral oxytocins for stimulation of labor in cases of premature rupture of the membranes at term. A randomized comparative study of prostaglandin E2 tablets and demoxytocin resoriblets. *Acta Obstet Gynecol Scand* 1983;62:111–116.

10 Knudsen FU, Steinrud J. Septicaemia of the newborn, associated with ruptured foetal membranes, discoloured amniotic fluid or maternal fever. *Acta Paediatr Scand* 1976;65:725–731.

11 Verber IG, Pearce JM, New LC, et al. Prolonged rupture of the fetal membranes and neonatal outcome. *J Perinat Med* 1989;17:469–476.

12 Mercer BM. Preterm premature rupture of the membranes. *Obstet Gynecol* 2003;101:178–193.

13 Christensen KK, Christensen P, Ingemarsson I, et al. A study of complications in preterm deliveries after prolonged premature rupture of the membranes. *Obstet Gynecol* 1976;48:670–677.

14 Daikoku NH, Kaltreider DF, Khouzami VA, et al. Premature rupture of membranes and spontaneous preterm labor: maternal endometritis risks. *Obstet Gynecol* 1982;59:13–20.

15 Fayez JA, Hasan AA, Jonas HS, Miller GL. Management of premature rupture of the membranes. *Obstet Gynecol* 1978;52: 17–21.

16 Gunn GC, Mishell DR, Jr, Morton DG. Premature rupture of the fetal membranes. A review. *Am J Obstet Gynecol* 1970;106: 469–483.

17 Sachs M, Baker TH. Spontaneous premature rupture of the membranes. *Am J Obstet Gynecol* 1967;97:888.

18 Gibbs RS, Blanco JD. Premature rupture of the membranes. *Obstet Gynecol* 1982;60:671–679.

19 Shubert PJ, Diss E, Iams JD. Etiology of preterm premature rupture of membranes. *Obstet Gynecol Clin North Am* 1992;19: 251–263.

20 Mercer BM. Preterm premature rupture of the membranes: current approaches to evaluation and management. *Obstet Gynecol Clin North Am* 2005;32:411–428.
21 Schwarcz R, Belizan JM, Nieto F, et al. Third progress report on the Latin American collaborative study on the effects of late rupture of membranes on labor and the neonate, submitted to the Director of the Pan-American Health Organization (PAHO/WHO) and the participating groups. Montevideo: Latin American Center of Perinatology and Human Development, 1974.
22 Quintero RA, Morales WJ, Kalter CS, et al. Transabdominal intra-amniotic endoscopic assessment of previable premature rupture of membranes. *Am J Obstet Gynecol* 1998;179:71–76.
23 Bell SC, McParland PC. Fetal membrane rupture. In: Critchley H, Bennett P, Thornton S, eds. *Preterm birth*. London: RCOG Press; 2004:195–212.
24 Bourne GL. The microscopic anatomy of the human amnion and chorion. *Am J Obstet Gynecol* 1960;79:1070–1073.
25 Benirschke K, Kaufmann P. Anatomy and pathology of the placental membranes. In: Benirschke K, Kaufman P (eds) *Pathology of the human placenta*, 3rd edn. New York: Springer-Verlag; 1995:268.
26 Danforth DN, Hull RW. The microscopic anatomy of the fetal membranes with particular reference to the detailed structure of the amnion. *Am J Obstet Gynecol* 1958;75:536.
27 Luckett WP. Amniogenesis in the early human and rhesus monkey embryos. *Anat Rec* 1973;175:375.
28 Malak TM, Bell SC. Structural characteristics of term human fetal membranes: a novel zone of extreme morphological alteration within the rupture site. *Br J Obstet Gynaecol* 1994;101: 375–386.
29 McParland PC, Taylor DJ, Bell SC. Mapping of zones of altered morphology and chorionic connective tissue cellular phenotype in human fetal membranes (amniochorion and decidua) overlying the lower uterine pole and cervix before labor at term. *Am J Obstet Gynecol* 2003;189:1481–1488.
30 McParland PC, Taylor DJ, Bell SC. Myofibroblast differentiation in the connective tissues of the amnion and chorion of term human fetal membranes – implications for fetal membrane rupture and labour. *Placenta* 2000;21:44–53.
31 McParland PC, Pringle JH, Bell SC. Tenascin and the fetal membrane wound hypothesis – programming for fetal membrane rupture? *Br J Obstet Gynaecol* 1998;105:1223–1224.
32 McParland PC, Bell SC, Pringle JH, Taylor DJ. Regional and cellular localization of osteonectin/SPARC expression in connective tissue and cytotrophoblastic layers of human fetal membranes at term. *Mol Hum Reprod* 2001;7:463–474.
33 Bell SC, Malak TM. Structural and cellular biology of the fetal membranes. In: Elder M, Romero R, Lamont R, eds. *Preterm labor*. New York: Churchill Livingstone; 1997:401–428.
34 Malak TM, Mullholland G, Bell SC. Structural characteristics and fibronectin synthesis by the intact term fetal membranes covering the cervix. *Br J Obstet Gynaecol* 1993;100:775.
35 Poppel J. Ueber die Resistenz der Eihaute, ein Beitrag zur Mechanik der Geburt. *Monatsschr Geburtsk* 1863;6:163.
36 Duncan JN. On a lower limit to the power exerted in the function of parturition. *Proc R Soc Edin* 1869;6:163.
37 Millar LK, Stollberg J, DeBuque L, Bryant-Greenwood G. Fetal membrane distention: determination of the intrauterine surface area and distention of the fetal membranes preterm and at term. *Am J Obstet Gynecol* 2000;182:128–134.
38 Parry S, Strauss JF, III. Premature rupture of the fetal membranes. *N Engl J Med* 1998;338:663–670.
39 Lavery JP, Miller CE, Knight RD. The effect of labor on the rheologic response of chorioamniotic membranes. *Obstet Gynecol* 1982;60:87–92.
40 Al Zaid NS, Bou-Resli MN, Goldspink G. Bursting pressure and collagen content of fetal membranes and their relation to premature rupture of the membranes. *Br J Obstet Gynaecol* 1980;87:227–229.
41 Artal R, Sokol RJ, Neuman M, et al. The mechanical properties of prematurely and non-prematurely ruptured membranes. Methods and preliminary results. *Am J Obstet Gynecol* 1976; 125:655–659.
42 Danforth DN, Mcelin TW, States MN. Studies on fetal membranes. I. Bursting tension. *Am J Obstet Gynecol* 1953;65:480–490.
43 Maclachlan TB. A method for the investigation of the strength of the fetal membranes. *Am J Obstet Gynecol* 1965;91:309–313.
44 Meudt R, Meudt E. Rupture of the fetal membranes. An experimental, clinical, and histologic study. *Am J Obstet Gynecol* 1967;99:562–568.
45 Polishuk WZ, Kohane S, Hadar A. Fetal weight and membrane tensile strength. *Am J Obstet Gynecol* 1964;88:247–250.
46 Parry-Jones E, Priya S. A study of the elasticity and tension of fetal membranes and of the relation of the area of the gestational sac to the area of the uterine cavity. *Br J Obstet Gynaecol* 1976;83:205–212.
47 Lavery JP, Miller CE. The viscoelastic nature of chorioamniotic membranes. *Obstet Gynecol* 1977;50:467–472.
48 Lavery JP, Miller CE. Deformation and creep in the human chorioamniotic sac. *Am J Obstet Gynecol* 1979;134:366–375.
49 Bou-Resli MN, Al Zaid NS, Ibrahim ME. Full-term and prematurely ruptured fetal membranes. An ultrastructural study. *Cell Tissue Res* 1981;220:263–278.
50 Ibrahim ME, Bou-Resli MN, Al Zaid NS, Bishay LF. Intact fetal membranes. Morphological predisposal to rupture. *Acta Obstet Gynecol Scand* 1983;62:481–485.
51 Skinner SJ, Campos GA, Liggins GC. Collagen content of human amniotic membranes: effect of gestation length and premature rupture. *Obstet Gynecol* 1981;57:487–489.
52 Kanayama N, Terao T, Kawashima Y, et al. Collagen types in normal and prematurely ruptured amniotic membranes. *Am J Obstet Gynecol* 1985;153:899–903.
53 Evaldson GR, Larsson B, Jiborn H. Is the collagen content reduced when the fetal membranes rupture? A clinical study of term and prematurely ruptured membranes. *Gynecol Obstet Invest* 1987;24:92–94.
54 Vadillo-Ortega F, Gonzalez-Avila G, Karchmer S, et al. Collagen metabolism in premature rupture of amniotic membranes. *Obstet Gynecol* 1990;75:84–88.
55 MacDermott RI, Landon CR. The hydroxyproline content of amnion and prelabour rupture of the membranes. *Eur J Obstet Gynecol Reprod Biol* 2000;92:217–221.
56 Kanayama N, Kamijo H, Terao T, et al. The relationship between trypsin activity in amniotic fluid and premature rupture of membranes. *Am J Obstet Gynecol* 1986;155:1043–1048.
57 Vadillo-Ortega F, Hernandez A, Gonzalez-Avila G, et al. Increased matrix metalloproteinase activity and reduced tissue inhibitor of metalloproteinases-1 levels in amniotic fluids from pregnancies complicated by premature rupture of membranes. *Am J Obstet Gynecol* 1996;174:1371–1376.
58 Lei H, Vadillo-Ortega F, Paavola LG, Strauss JF, III. 92-kDa gelatinase (matrix metalloproteinase-9) is induced in rat amnion immediately prior to parturition. *Biol Reprod* 1995;53:339–344.

59 Rajabi MR, Dean DD, Woessner JF, Jr. Changes in active and latent collagenase in human placenta around the time of parturition. *Am J Obstet Gynecol* 1990;163:499–505.
60 Bryant-Greenwood GD, Yamamoto SY. Control of peripartal collagenolysis in the human chorion-decidua. *Am J Obstet Gynecol* 1995;172:63–70.
61 Artal R, Burgeson RE, Hobel CJ, Hollister D. An in vitro model for the study of enzymatically mediated biomechanical changes in the chorioamniotic membranes. *Am J Obstet Gynecol* 1979;133:656–659.
62 Rajabi M, Dean DD, Woessner JF, Jr. High levels of serum collagenase in premature labor – a potential biochemical marker. *Obstet Gynecol* 1987;69:179–186.
63 Draper D, McGregor J, Hall J, et al. Elevated protease activities in human amnion and chorion correlate with preterm premature rupture of membranes. *Am J Obstet Gynecol* 1995;173:1506–1512.
64 Vadillo-Ortega F, Gonzalez-Avila G, Furth EE, et al. 92-kd type IV collagenase (matrix metalloproteinase-9) activity in human amniochorion increases with labor. *Am J Pathol* 1995;146: 148–156.
65 O'Brien WF, Knuppel RA, Morales WJ, et al. Amniotic fluid alpha 1-antitrypsin concentration in premature rupture of the membranes. *Am J Obstet Gynecol* 1990;162:756–759.
66 Burgos H, Hsi BL, Yeh CJ, Faulk WP. Plasminogen binding by human amniochorion. A possible factor in premature rupture of membranes. *Am J Obstet Gynecol* 1982;143:958–963.
67 Jenkins DM, O'Neill M, Mattar M, et al. Degenerative changes and detection of plasminogen in fetal membranes that rupture prematurely. *Br J Obstet Gynaecol* 1983;90:841–846.
68 Milwidsky A, Hurwitz A, Eckstein L, et al. Proteolytic enzymes in human fetal membranes and amniotic fluid. A comparison of normal and premature ruptured membranes. *Enzyme* 1985;33: 188–196.
69 McGregor JA, Lawellin D, Franco-Buff A, et al. Protease production by microorganisms associated with reproductive tract infection. *Am J Obstet Gynecol* 1986;154:109–114.
70 McGregor JA, French JI, Lawellin D, et al. Bacterial protease-induced reduction of chorioamniotic membrane strength and elasticity. *Obstet Gynecol* 1987;69:167–174.
71 Sbarra AJ, Selvaraj RJ, Cetrulo CL, et al. Infection and phagocytosis as possible mechanisms of rupture in premature rupture of the membranes. *Am J Obstet Gynecol* 1985;153:38–43.
72 Schoonmaker JN, Lawellin DW, Lunt B, McGregor JA. Bacteria and inflammatory cells reduce chorioamniotic membrane integrity and tensile strength. *Obstet Gynecol* 1989;74:590–596.
73 Helmig R, Uldbjerg N, Ohlsson K. Secretory leukocyte protease inhibitor in the cervical mucus and in the fetal membranes. *Eur J Obstet Gynecol Reprod Biol* 1995;59:95–101.
74 Sbarra AJ, Thomas GB, Cetrulo CL, et al. Effect of bacterial growth on the bursting pressure of fetal membranes in vitro. *Obstet Gynecol* 1987;70:107–110.
75 McGregor JA, Schoonmaker JN, Lunt BD, Lawellin DW. Antibiotic inhibition of bacterially induced fetal membrane weakening. *Obstet Gynecol* 1990;76:124–128.
76 Woessner JF, Jr. Matrix metalloproteinases and their inhibitors in connective tissue remodelling. *FASEB J* 1991;5:2145.
77 Romero R, Ray DA, Sepulveda W, et al. Evidence of active forms of 72 kDa and 92 kDa type IV collagenases in human parturition. 39th Annual Meeting of the Society for Gynecologic Investigation, San Antonio, 1992.
78 Fortunato SJ, Menon R, Lombardi S. Induction of MMP-9 and normal presence of MMP-2, TIMP-1 and 2 in human fetal membranes. 17th Annual Meeting of the Society of Perinatal Obstetricians, Anaheim. *Am J Obstet Gynecol* 1997;176:1.
79 Parks WC, Mecham RP. *Matrix metalloproteinases*. San Diego, CA: Academic Press, 1998.
80 Fortunato S, Menon R, Swan K, Baricos W. Presence of extracellular matrix degrading enzymes and tissue inhibitor of metalloproteinases (TIMP-1) in human fetal membranes. *Am J Obstet Gynecol* 1995;172:518.
81 Romero R, Gomez R. Helming R, et al. Amniotic fluid elastase and secretory leukocyte protease natural inhibitor during labor, rupture of membranes and intrauterine infection. *Scientific Abstr* 1994;183:O193.
82 Fortunato SJ, Menon R, Swan K, Baricos W. Expression of matrix degrading enzymes and tissue inhibitors of metalloproteinases (TIMP) in human fetal membranes. 15th Annual Meeting of the Society of Perinatal Obstetricians, Atlanta. *Am J Obstet Gynecol* 1995;170.
83 Fortunato SJ, LaFleur B, Menon R. Collagenase-3 (MMP-13) in fetal membranes and amniotic fluid during pregnancy. *Am J Reprod Immunol* 2003;49:120–125.
84 Maymon E, Romero R, Pacora P, et al. Evidence for the participation of interstitial collagenase (matrix metalloproteinase 1) in preterm premature rupture of membranes. *Am J Obstet Gynecol* 2000;183:914–920.
85 Maymon E, Romero R, Pacora P, et al. Human neutrophil collagenase (matrix metalloproteinase 8) in parturition, premature rupture of the membranes, and intrauterine infection. *Am J Obstet Gynecol* 2000;183:94–99.
86 Maymon E, Romero R, Pacora P, et al. Evidence of in vivo differential bioavailability of the active forms of matrix metalloproteinases 9 and 2 in parturition, spontaneous rupture of membranes, and intra-amniotic infection. *Am J Obstet Gynecol* 2000;183:887–894.
87 Maymon E, Romero R, Pacora P, et al. Matrilysin (matrix metalloproteinase 7) in parturition, premature rupture of membranes, and intrauterine infection. *Am J Obstet Gynecol* 2000;182:1545–1553.
88 Maymon E, Romero R, Pacora P, et al. A role for the 72 kDa gelatinase (MMP-2) and its inhibitor (TIMP-2) in human parturition, premature rupture of membranes and intra-amniotic infection. *J Perinat Med* 2001;29:308–316.
89 Fortunato SJ, Menon R, Lombardi SJ. MMP/TIMP imbalance in amniotic fluid during PROM: an indirect support for endogenous pathway to membrane rupture. *J Perinat Med* 1999;27:362–368.
90 Fortunato SJ, Menon R, Ahmed NU, et al. Amniotic fluid concentrations of collagenase-1 and collagenase-3 are increased in polyhydramnios. *J Perinat Med* 2004;32:122–125.
91 Biggio JR, Jr, Ramsey PS, Cliver SP, et al. Midtrimester amniotic fluid matrix metalloproteinase-8 (MMP-8) levels above the 90th percentile are a marker for subsequent preterm premature rupture of membranes. *Am J Obstet Gynecol* 2005;192:109–113.
92 Morris SM, Stone PJ. Immunocytochemical study of the degradation of elastic fibers in a living extracellular matrix. *J Histochem Cytochem* 1995;43:1145–1153.
93 McDonald JA, Kelley DG. Degradation of fibronectin by human leukocyte elastase. Release of biologically active fragments. *J Biol Chem* 1980;255:8848–8858.
94 Steadman R, Irwin MH, St John PL, et al. Laminin cleavage by activated human neutrophils yields proteolytic fragments with selective migratory properties. *J Leukoc Biol* 1993;53:354–365.

95 Gadek JE, Fells GA, Wright DG, Crystal RG. Human neutrophil elastase functions as a type III collagen "collagenase". *Biochem Biophys Res Commun* 1980;95:1815–1822.

96 Mainardi CL, Hasty DL, Seyer JM, Kang AH. Specific cleavage of human type III collagen by human polymorphonuclear leukocyte elastase. *J Biol Chem* 1980;255:12006–12010.

97 Bergenfeldt M, Axelsson L, Ohlsson K. Release of neutrophil proteinase 4(3) and leukocyte elastase during phagocytosis and their interaction with proteinase inhibitors. *Scand J Clin Lab Invest* 1992;52:823–829.

98 Helmig BR, Romero R, Espinoza J, et al. Neutrophil elastase and secretory leukocyte protease inhibitor in prelabor rupture of membranes, parturition and intra-amniotic infection. *J Matern Fetal Neonatal Med* 2002;12:237–246.

99 Tromp G, Kuivaniemi H, Romero R, et al. Genome-wide expression profiling of fetal membranes reveals a deficient expression of proteinase inhibitor 3 in premature rupture of membranes. *Am J Obstet Gynecol* 2004;191:1331–1338.

100 Romero R, Chaiworapongsa T, Espinoza J, et al. Fetal plasma MMP-9 concentrations are elevated in preterm premature rupture of the membranes. *Am J Obstet Gynecol* 2002;187: 1125–1130.

101 Ognjanovic S, Ku TL, Bryant-Greenwood GD. Pre-B-cell colony-enhancing factor is a secreted cytokine-like protein from the human amniotic epithelium. *Am J Obstet Gynecol* 2005;193: 273–282.

102 Nemeth E, Millar LK, Bryant-Greenwood G. Fetal membrane distention: II. Differentially expressed genes regulated by acute distention in vitro. *Am J Obstet Gynecol* 2000;182:60–67.

103 Nemeth E, Tashima LS, Yu Z, Bryant-Greenwood GD. Fetal membrane distention: I. Differentially expressed genes regulated by acute distention in amniotic epithelial (WISH) cells. *Am J Obstet Gynecol* 2000;182:50–59.

104 Jia SH, Li Y, Parodo J, et al. Pre-B cell colony-enhancing factor inhibits neutrophil apoptosis in experimental inflammation and clinical sepsis. *J Clin Invest* 2004;113:1318–1327.

105 Kettritz R, Gaido ML, Haller H, et al. Interleukin-8 delays spontaneous and tumor necrosis factor-alpha-mediated apoptosis of human neutrophils. *Kidney Int* 1998;53:84–91.

106 Romero R. Prenatal medicine: the child is the father of the man. *Prenatal Neonatal Med* 1996;1:8–11.

107 Romero R, Espinoza J, Mazor M, Chaiworapongsa T. The preterm parturition syndrome. In: Critchley H, Bennett P, Thornton S, eds. *Preterm birth*. London: RCOG Press; 2004:28–60.

108 Mercer BM, Goldenberg RL, Meis PJ, et al. The Preterm Prediction Study: prediction of preterm premature rupture of membranes through clinical findings and ancillary testing. The National Institute of Child Health and Human Development Maternal–Fetal Medicine Units Network. *Am J Obstet Gynecol* 2000;183:738–745.

109 Weiss JL, Malone FD, Vidaver J, et al. Threatened abortion: a risk factor for poor pregnancy outcome, a population-based screening study. *Am J Obstet Gynecol* 2004;190:745–750.

110 Yang J, Hartmann KE, Savitz DA, et al. Vaginal bleeding during pregnancy and preterm birth. *Am J Epidemiol* 2004;160:118–125.

111 Carroll SG, Papaioannou S, Ntumazah IL, et al. Lower genital tract swabs in the prediction of intrauterine infection in preterm prelabour rupture of the membranes. *Br J Obstet Gynaecol* 1996;103:54–59.

112 Fujimoto T, Parry S, Urbanek M, et al. A single nucleotide polymorphism in the matrix metalloproteinase-1 (MMP-1) promoter influences amnion cell MMP-1 expression and risk for preterm premature rupture of the fetal membranes. *J Biol Chem* 2002;277:6296–6302.

113 Ferrand PE, Parry S, Sammel M, et al. A polymorphism in the matrix metalloproteinase-9 promoter is associated with increased risk of preterm premature rupture of membranes in African Americans. *Mol Hum Reprod* 2002;8:494–501.

114 Wang H, Parry S, Macones G, et al. Functionally significant SNP MMP8 promoter haplotypes and preterm premature rupture of membranes (PPROM). *Hum Mol Genet* 2004;13: 2659–2669.

115 Kurki T, Sivonen A, Renkonen OV, et al. Bacterial vaginosis in early pregnancy and pregnancy outcome. *Obstet Gynecol* 1992;80:173–177.

116 Simhan HN, Caritis SN, Krohn MA, Hillier SL. The vaginal inflammatory milieu and the risk of early premature preterm rupture of membranes. *Am J Obstet Gynecol* 2005;192:213–218.

117 Roberts AK, Monzon-Bordonaba F, Van Deerlin PG, et al. Association of polymorphism within the promoter of the tumor necrosis factor alpha gene with increased risk of preterm premature rupture of the fetal membranes. *Am J Obstet Gynecol* 1999;180:1297–1302.

118 Macones GA, Parry S, Elkousy M, et al. A polymorphism in the promoter region of TNF and bacterial vaginosis: preliminary evidence of gene–environment interaction in the etiology of spontaneous preterm birth. *Am J Obstet Gynecol* 2004;190: 1504–1508.

119 Estrada-Gutierrez G, Zaga V, Gonzalez-Jimenez MA, et al. Initial characterization of the microenvironment that regulates connective tissue degradation in amniochorion during normal human labor. *Matrix Biol* 2005;24:306–312.

120 Goncalves LF, Chaiworapongsa T, Romero R. Intrauterine infection and prematurity. *Ment Retard Dev Disabil Res Rev* 2002;8:3–13.

121 Romero R, Quintero R, Oyarzun E, et al. Intraamniotic infection and the onset of labor in preterm premature rupture of the membranes. *Am J Obstet Gynecol* 1988;159:661–666.

122 Cassell GH, Davis RO, Waites KB, et al. Isolation of *Mycoplasma hominis* and *Ureaplasma urealyticum* from amniotic fluid at 16–20 weeks of gestation: potential effect on outcome of pregnancy. *Sex Transm Dis* 1983;10:294–302.

123 Horowitz S, Mazor M, Romero R, et al. Infection of the amniotic cavity with *Ureaplasma urealyticum* in the midtrimester of pregnancy. *J Reprod Med* 1995;40:375–379.

124 Gray DJ, Robinson HB, Malone J, Thomson RB, Jr. Adverse outcome in pregnancy following amniotic fluid isolation of *Ureaplasma urealyticum*. *Prenat Diagn* 1992;12:111–117.

125 Yoon BH, Oh SY, Romero R, et al. An elevated amniotic fluid matrix metalloproteinase-8 level at the time of mid-trimester genetic amniocentesis is a risk factor for spontaneous preterm delivery. *Am J Obstet Gynecol* 2001;185:1162–1167.

126 Arias F, Rodriquez L, Rayne SC, Kraus FT. Maternal placental vasculopathy and infection: two distinct subgroups among patients with preterm labor and preterm ruptured membranes. *Am J Obstet Gynecol* 1993;168:585–591.

127 Arias F, Victoria A, Cho K, Kraus F. Placental histology and clinical characteristics of patients with preterm premature rupture of membranes. *Obstet Gynecol* 1997;89:265–271.

128 Kim YM, Chaiworapongsa T, Gomez R, et al. Failure of physiologic transformation of the spiral arteries in the placental bed in preterm premature rupture of membranes. *Am J Obstet Gynecol* 2002;187:1137–1142.

129 Gomez R, Romero R, Nien JK, et al. Idiopathic vaginal bleeding during pregnancy as the only clinical manifestation of intrauterine infection. *J Matern Fetal Neonatal Med* 2005;18:31–37.
130 Mackenzie AP, Schatz F, Krikun G, et al. Mechanisms of abruption-induced premature rupture of the fetal membranes: Thrombin enhanced decidual matrix metalloproteinase-3 (stromelysin-1) expression. *Am J Obstet Gynecol* 2004;191: 1996–2001.
131 Rosen T, Schatz F, Kuczynski E, et al. Thrombin-enhanced matrix metalloproteinase-1 expression: a mechanism linking placental abruption with premature rupture of the membranes. *J Matern Fetal Neonatal Med* 2002;11:11–17.
132 Stephenson CD, Lockwood CJ, Ma Y, Guller S. Thrombin-dependent regulation of matrix metalloproteinase (MMP)-9 levels in human fetal membranes. *J Matern Fetal Neonatal Med* 2005;18:17–22.
133 Curry TE, Jr, Osteen KG. The matrix metalloproteinase system: changes, regulation, and impact throughout the ovarian and uterine reproductive cycle. *Endocr Rev* 2003;24:428–465.
134 Darby MJ, Caritis SN, Shen-Schwarz S. Placental abruption in the preterm gestation: an association with chorioamnionitis. *Obstet Gynecol* 1989;74:88–92.
135 Naeye RL. Factors that predispose to premature rupture of the fetal membranes. *Obstet Gynecol* 1982;60:93–98.
136 Evaldson G, Lagrelius A, Winiarski J. Premature rupture of the membranes. *Acta Obstet Gynecol Scand* 1980;59:385–393.
137 Buchmayer SM, Sparen P, Cnattingius S. Previous pregnancy loss: risks related to severity of preterm delivery. *Am J Obstet Gynecol* 2004;191:1225–1231.
138 Hassan S, Romero R, Hendler I, et al. A sonographic short cervix as the only clinical manifestation of intra-amniotic infection. *J Perinat Med* 2006;34:13–19.
139 Rizzo G, Capponi A, Vlachopoulou A, et al. Ultrasonographic assessment of the uterine cervix and interleukin-8 concentrations in cervical secretions predict intrauterine infection in patients with preterm labor and intact membranes. *Ultrasound Obstet Gynecol* 1998;12:86–92.
140 Hein M, Helmig RB, Schonheyder HC, et al. An in vitro study of antibacterial properties of the cervical mucus plug in pregnancy. *Am J Obstet Gynecol* 2001;185:586–592.
141 Hein M, Valore EV, Helmig RB, et al. Antimicrobial factors in the cervical mucus plug. *Am J Obstet Gynecol* 2002;187:137–144.
142 Svinarich DM, Wolf NA, Gomez R, et al. Detection of human defensin 5 in reproductive tissues. *Am J Obstet Gynecol* 1997;176:470–475.
143 Lind J, Wallenburg HC. Pregnancy and the Ehlers–Danlos syndrome: a retrospective study in a Dutch population. *Acta Obstet Gynecol Scand* 2002;81:293–300.
144 Peterkofsky B. Ascorbate requirement for hydroxylation and secretion of procollagen: relationship to inhibition of collagen synthesis in scurvy. *Am J Clin Nutr* 1991;54:1135S–1140S.
145 Casanueva E, Avila-Rosas H, Polo E, et al. Vitamin C status, cervico-vaginal infection and premature rupture of amniotic membranes. *Arch Med Res* 1995;26(Spec. no.):S149–S152.
146 Barrett BM, Sowell A, Gunter E, Wang M. Potential role of ascorbic acid and beta-carotene in the prevention of preterm rupture of fetal membranes. *Int J Vitam Nutr Res* 1994;64: 192–197.
147 Harger JH, Hsing AW, Tuomala RE, et al. Risk factors for preterm premature rupture of fetal membranes: a multicenter case–control study. *Am J Obstet Gynecol* 1990;163:130–137.
148 Spinillo A, Nicola S, Piazzi G, et al. Epidemiological correlates of preterm premature rupture of membranes. *Int J Gynaecol Obstet* 1994;47:7–15.
149 Ladfors L, Mattsson LA, Eriksson M, Milsom I. Prevalence and risk factors for prelabor rupture of the membranes (PROM) at or near-term in an urban Swedish population. *J Perinat Med* 2000;28:491–496.
150 Asrat T, Lewis DF, Garite TJ, et al. Rate of recurrence of preterm premature rupture of membranes in consecutive pregnancies. *Am J Obstet Gynecol* 1991;165:1111–1115.
151 Ekwo EE, Gosselink CA, Moawad A. Unfavorable outcome in penultimate pregnancy and premature rupture of membranes in successive pregnancy. *Obstet Gynecol* 1992;80:166–172.
152 Ekwo EE, Gosselink CA, Moawad A. Previous pregnancy outcomes and subsequent risk of preterm rupture of amniotic sac membranes. *Br J Obstet Gynaecol* 1993;100:536–541.
153 Eggers TR, Doyle LW, Pepperell RJ. Premature rupture of the membranes. *Med J Aust* 1979;1:209–213.
154 Townsend L, Aickin DR, Fraillon JM. Spontaneous premature rupture of the membranes. *Aust NZ J Obstet Gynaecol* 1966;6:226–235.
155 Meyer MB, Tonascia JA. Maternal smoking, pregnancy complications, and perinatal mortality. *Am J Obstet Gynecol* 1977;128: 494–502.
156 Williams MA, Mittendorf R, Stubblefield PG, et al. Cigarettes, coffee, and preterm premature rupture of the membranes. *Am J Epidemiol* 1992;135:895–903.
157 Hadley CB, Main DM, Gabbe SG. Risk factors for preterm premature rupture of the fetal membranes. *Am J Perinatol* 1990;7:374–379.
158 Adams MM, Read JA, Rawlings JS, et al. Preterm delivery among black and white enlisted women in the United States Army. *Obstet Gynecol* 1993;81:65–71.
159 Schieve LA, Handler A. Preterm delivery and perinatal death among black and white infants in a Chicago-area perinatal registry. *Obstet Gynecol* 1996;88:356–363.
160 Meis PJ, Ernest JM, Moore ML. Causes of low birth weight births in public and private patients. *Am J Obstet Gynecol* 1987;156:1165–1168.
161 Odibo AO, Talucci M, Berghella V. Prediction of preterm premature rupture of membranes by transvaginal ultrasound: features and risk factors in a high-risk population. *Ultrasound Obstet Gynecol* 2002;20:245–251.
162 Fortunato SJ, Lombardi SJ, Menon R. Racial disparity in membrane response to infectious stimuli: a possible explanation for observed differences in the incidence of prematurity. Community Award Paper. *Am J Obstet Gynecol* 2004;190:1557–1562.
163 Friel L, Kuivaniemi H, Gomez R, et al. Genetic predisposition for preterm PROM: results of a large candidate-gene association study of mothers and their offspring. *Am J Obstet Gynecol* 2005;193(6):S17.
164 Naeye RL, Peters EC. Causes and consequences of premature rupture of fetal membranes. *Lancet* 1980;1:192–194.
165 Mills JL, Harlap S, Harley EE. Should coitus late in pregnancy be discouraged? *Lancet* 1981;2:136–138.
166 Perkins RP. Sexual behavior and response in relation to complications of pregnancy. *Am J Obstet Gynecol* 1979;134:498–505.
167 Rayburn WF, Wilson EA. Coital activity and premature delivery. *Am J Obstet Gynecol* 1980;137:972–974.
168 Ekwo EE, Gosselink CA, Woolson R, et al. Coitus late in pregnancy: risk of preterm rupture of amniotic sac membranes. *Am J Obstet Gynecol* 1993;168:22–31.

169 Casanueva E, Ripoll C, Tolentino M, et al. Vitamin C supplementation to prevent premature rupture of the chorioamniotic membranes: a randomized trial. *Am J Clin Nutr* 2005;81:859–863.
170 Wideman GL, Baird GH, Bolding OT. Ascorbic acid deficiency and premature rupture of fetal membranes. *Am J Obstet Gynecol* 1964;88:592–595.
171 Vadillo OF, Pfeffer BF, Bermejo Martinez ML, et al. [Dietetic factors and premature rupture of fetal membranes. Effect of vitamin C on collagen degradation in the chorioamnion]. *Ginecol Obstet Mex* 1995;63:158–162.
172 Stuart EL, Evans GS, Lin YS, Powers HJ. Reduced collagen and ascorbic acid concentrations and increased proteolytic susceptibility with prelabor fetal membrane rupture in women. *Biol Reprod* 2005;72:230–235.
173 Artal R, Burgeson R, Fernandez FJ, Hobel CJ. Fetal and maternal copper levels in patients at term with and without premature rupture of membranes. *Obstet Gynecol* 1979;53:608–610.
174 Kiilholma P, Gronroos M, Erkkola R, et al. The role of calcium, copper, iron and zinc in preterm delivery and premature rupture of fetal membranes. *Gynecol Obstet Invest* 1984;17:194–201.
175 Sikorski R, Juszkiewicz T, Paszkowski T. Zinc status in women with premature rupture of membranes at term. *Obstet Gynecol* 1990;76:675–677.
176 Sibai BM, Villar MA, Bray E. Magnesium supplementation during pregnancy: a double-blind randomized controlled clinical trial. *Am J Obstet Gynecol* 1989;161:115–119.
177 Villar J, Repke JT. Calcium supplementation during pregnancy may reduce preterm delivery in high-risk populations. *Am J Obstet Gynecol* 1990;163:1124–1131.
178 Simpson J, Palomaki G, Mincr B, et al. Association between adverse perinatal outcomes and serially obtained second and third trimester MSAFP measurements. *Am J Obstet Gynecol* 1995;173:1742.
179 O'Brien WF, Sternlight D, Torres C, et al. The value of early third-trimester maternal serum alpha-fetoprotein determination. *Prenat Diagn* 1990;10:183–188.
180 Waller DK, Lustig LS, Cunningham GC, et al. Second-trimester maternal serum alpha-fetoprotein levels and the risk of subsequent fetal death. *N Engl J Med* 1991;325:6–10.
181 Harlap S, Davies AM. Late sequelae of induced abortion: complications and outcome of pregnancy and labor. *Am J Epidemiol* 1975;102:217–224.
182 Sagot P, Caroit Y, Winer N, et al. Obstetrical prognosis for carbon dioxide laser conisation of the uterine cervix. *Eur J Obstet Gynecol Reprod Biol* 1995;58:53–58.
183 Samson SL, Bentley JR, Fahey TJ, et al. The effect of loop electrosurgical excision procedure on future pregnancy outcome. *Obstet Gynecol* 2005;105:325–332.
184 Lenihan JP, Jr. Relationship of antepartum pelvic examinations to premature rupture of the membranes. *Obstet Gynecol* 1984;63:33–37.
185 McDuffie RS, Jr, Nelson GE, Osborn CL, et al. Effect of routine weekly cervical examinations at term on premature rupture of the membranes: a randomized controlled trial. *Obstet Gynecol* 1992;79:219–322.
186 Main DM, Gabbe SG, Richardson D, Strong S. Can preterm deliveries be prevented? *Am J Obstet Gynecol* 1985;151:892–898.
187 Main DM, Richardson DK, Hadley CB, Gabbe SG. Controlled trial of a Preterm Labor Detection program: efficacy and costs. *Obstet Gynecol* 1989;74:873–877.
188 Holbrook R, Falcon J, Hemass M, et al. Evaluation of the weekly cervical examination in a preterm birth prevention program. *Am J Perinatol* 1987;4:240.
189 Romero R, Mazor M, Oyarzun E, et al. Is genital colonization with *Mycoplasma hominis* or *Ureaplasma urealyticum* associated with prematurity/low birth weight? *Obstet Gynecol* 1989;73: 532–536.
190 Hillier SL, Nugent RP, Eschenbach DA, et al. Association between bacterial vaginosis and preterm delivery of a low-birth-weight infant. The Vaginal Infections and Prematurity Study Group. *N Engl J Med* 1995;333:1737–1742.
191 Romero R, Chaiworapongsa T, Kuivaniemi H, Tromp G. Bacterial vaginosis, the inflammatory response and the risk of preterm birth: a role for genetic epidemiology in the prevention of preterm birth. *Am J Obstet Gynecol* 2004;190:1509–1519.
192 Carey JC, Klebanoff MA, Hauth JC, et al. Metronidazole to prevent preterm delivery in pregnant women with asymptomatic bacterial vaginosis. National Institute of Child Health and Human Development Network of Maternal–Fetal Medicine Units. *N Engl J Med* 2000;342:534–540.
193 McDonald H, Brocklehurst P, Parsons J. Antibiotics for treating bacterial vaginosis in pregnancy. *Cochrane Database Syst Rev* 2005;CD000262.
194 Regan JA, Chao S, James LS. Premature rupture of membranes, preterm delivery, and group B streptococcal colonization of mothers. *Am J Obstet Gynecol* 1981;141:184–186.
195 Matorras R, Garcia PA, Omenaca F, et al. Group B streptococcus and premature rupture of membranes and preterm delivery. *Gynecol Obstet Invest* 1989;27:14–18.
196 Alger LS, Lovchik JC, Hebel JR, et al. The association of *Chlamydia trachomatis*, *Neisseria gonorrhoeae*, and group B streptococci with preterm rupture of the membranes and pregnancy outcome. *Am J Obstet Gynecol* 1988;159:397–404.
197 Newton ER, Clark M. Group B streptococcus and preterm rupture of membranes. *Obstet Gynecol* 1988;71:198–202.
198 Towers CV, Lewis DF, Asrat T, et al. The effect of colonization with group B streptococci on the latency phase of patients with preterm premature rupture of membranes. *Am J Obstet Gynecol* 1993;169:1139–1143.
199 Maxwell GL, Watson WJ. Preterm premature rupture of membranes: results of expectant management in patients with cervical cultures positive for group B streptococcus or *Neisseria gonorrhoeae*. *Am J Obstet Gynecol* 1992;166:945–949.
200 Regan JA, Klebanoff MA, Nugent RP, et al. Colonization with group B streptococci in pregnancy and adverse outcome. VIP Study Group. *Am J Obstet Gynecol* 1996;174:1354–1360.
201 Harrison HR, Alexander ER, Weinstein L, et al. Cervical *Chlamydia trachomatis* and mycoplasmal infections in pregnancy. Epidemiology and outcomes. *JAMA* 1983;250:1721–1727.
202 Sweet RL, Landers DV, Walker C, Schachter J. *Chlamydia trachomatis* infection and pregnancy outcome. *Am J Obstet Gynecol* 1987;156:824–833.
203 Amstey MS, Steadman KT. Asymptomatic gonorrhea and pregnancy. *J Am Vener Dis Assoc* 1976;3:14–16.
204 Handsfield HH, Hodson WA, Holmes KK. Neonatal gonococcal infection. I. Orogastric contamination with *Neisseria gonorrhoeae*. *JAMA* 1973;225:697–701.
205 Edwards LE, Barrada MI, Hamann AA, Hakanson EY. Gonorrhea in pregnancy. *Am J Obstet Gynecol* 1978;132:637–641.
206 Minkoff H, Grunebaum AN, Schwarz RH, et al. Risk factors for prematurity and premature rupture of membranes: a prospective

study of the vaginal flora in pregnancy. *Am J Obstet Gynecol* 1984;150:965–972.
207 Klebanoff MA, Carey JC, Hauth JC, et al. Failure of metronidazole to prevent preterm delivery among pregnant women with asymptomatic *Trichomonas vaginalis* infection. *N Engl J Med* 2001;345:487–493.
208 Carey JC, Klebanoff MA. Is a change in the vaginal flora associated with an increased risk of preterm birth? *Am J Obstet Gynecol* 2005;192:1341–1346.
209 Barabas AP. Ehlers–Danlos syndrome associated with prematurity and premature rupture of fetal membranes; possible increase in incidence. *Br Med J* 1966;2:682–684.
210 Yanagihara T, Ueta M, Hanaoka U, et al. Late second-trimester nonstress test characteristics in preterm delivery before 32 weeks of gestation. *Gynecol Obstet Invest* 2001;51:32–35.
211 Cox SM, Williams ML, Leveno KJ. The natural history of preterm ruptured membranes: what to expect of expectant management. *Obstet Gynecol* 1988;71:558–562.
212 Wilson JC, Levy DL, Wilds PL. Premature rupture of membranes prior to term: consequences of nonintervention. *Obstet Gynecol* 1982;60:601–606.
213 Nelson LH, Anderson RL, O'Shea TM, Swain M. Expectant management of preterm premature rupture of the membranes. *Am J Obstet Gynecol* 1994;171:350–356.
214 Ananth CV, Oyelese Y, Srinivas N, et al. Preterm premature rupture of membranes, intrauterine infection, and oligohydramnios: risk factors for placental abruption. *Obstet Gynecol* 2004;104:71–77.
215 Barfield WD, Tomashek KM, Flowers LM, Iyasu S. Contribution of late fetal deaths to US perinatal mortality rates, 1995–1998. *Semin Perinatol* 2002;26:17–24.
216 Russell KP, Anderson GV. The aggressive management of ruptured membranes. *Am J Obstet Gynecol* 1962;83:930–937.
217 Romero R, Sirtori M, Oyarzun E, et al. Infection and labor. V. Prevalence, microbiology, and clinical significance of intraamniotic infection in women with preterm labor and intact membranes. *Am J Obstet Gynecol* 1989;161:817–824.
218 Romero R, Mazor M, Morretti R, et al. Infection and labor VII. Microbial invasion of the amniotic cavity in spontaneous rupture of membranes at term. *Am J Obstet Gynecol* 1992;166: 129.
219 Yoon BH, Romero R, Kim M, et al. Clinical implications of detection of *Ureaplasma urealyticum* in the amniotic cavity with the polymerase chain reaction. *Am J Obstet Gynecol* 2000;183: 1130–1137.
220 Vintzileos AM, Campbell WA, Nochimson DJ, et al. Qualitative amniotic fluid volume versus amniocentesis in predicting infection in preterm premature rupture of the membranes. *Obstet Gynecol* 1986;67:579–583.
221 Gonik B, Bottoms SF, Cotton DB. Amniotic fluid volume as a risk factor in preterm premature rupture of the membranes. *Obstet Gynecol* 1985;65:456–459.
222 Park JS, Yoon BH, Romero R, et al. The relationship between oligohydramnios and the onset of preterm labor in preterm premature rupture of membranes. *Am J Obstet Gynecol* 2001;184: 459–462.
223 Akinbi HT, Narendran V, Pass AK, et al. Host defense proteins in vernix caseosa and amniotic fluid. *Am J Obstet Gynecol* 2004;191:2090–2096.
224 Espinoza J, Chaiworapongsa T, Romero R, et al. Antimicrobial peptides in amniotic fluid: defensins, calprotectin and bacterial/permeability-increasing protein in patients with microbial invasion of the amniotic cavity, intra-amniotic inflammation, preterm labor and premature rupture of membranes. *J Matern Fetal Neonatal Med* 2003;13:2–21.
225 Otsuki K, Yoda A, Toma Y, et al. Lactoferrin and interleukin-6 interaction in amniotic infection. *Adv Exp Med Biol* 1998;443:267–271.
226 Sachs BP, Stern CM. Activity and characterization of a low molecular fraction present in human amniotic fluid with broad spectrum antibacterial activity. *Br J Obstet Gynaecol* 1979;86: 81–86.
227 Soto E, Espinoza J, Kusanovic, JP, et al. A natural anti-microbial agent present in normal amniotic fluid participates in the host response to intra-amniotic infection. *Am J Obstet Gynecol* 2005;193(6):S169.
228 Averbuch B, Mazor M, Shoham-Vardi I, et al. Intra-uterine infection in women with preterm premature rupture of membranes: maternal and neonatal characteristics. *Eur J Obstet Gynecol Reprod Biol* 1995;62:25–29.
229 Cotton DB, Hill LM, Strassner HT, et al. Use of amniocentesis in preterm gestation with ruptured membranes. *Obstet Gynecol* 1984;63:38–43.
230 Coultrip LL, Grossman JH. Evaluation of rapid diagnostic tests in the detection of microbial invasion of the amniotic cavity. *Am J Obstet Gynecol* 1992;167:1231–1242.
231 Garite TJ, Freeman RK, Linzey EM, Braly P. The use of amniocentesis in patients with premature rupture of membranes. *Obstet Gynecol* 1979;54:226–230.
232 Zlatnik FJ, Cruikshank DP, Petzold CR, Galask RP. Amniocentesis in the identification of inapparent infection in preterm patients with premature rupture of the membranes. *J Reprod Med* 1984;29:656–660.
233 Broekhuizen FF, Gilman M, Hamilton PR. Amniocentesis for gram stain and culture in preterm premature rupture of the membranes. *Obstet Gynecol* 1985;66:316–321.
234 Dudley J, Malcolm G, Ellwood D. Amniocentesis in the management of preterm premature rupture of the membranes. *Aust NZ J Obstet Gynaecol* 1991;31:331–336.
235 Feinstein SJ, Vintzileos AM, Lodeiro JG, et al. Amniocentesis with premature rupture of membranes. *Obstet Gynecol* 1986;68: 147–152.
236 Font GE, Gauthier DW, Meyer WJ, et al. Catalase activity as a predictor of amniotic fluid culture results in preterm labor or premature rupture of membranes. *Obstet Gynecol* 1995;85:656–658.
237 Garite TJ, Freeman RK. Chorioamnionitis in the preterm gestation. *Obstet Gynecol* 1982;59:539–545.
238 Gauthier DW, Meyer WJ, Bieniarz A. Correlation of amniotic fluid glucose concentration and intraamniotic infection in patients with preterm labor or premature rupture of membranes. *Am J Obstet Gynecol* 1991;165:1105–1110.
239 Gauthier DW, Meyer WJ. Comparison of gram stain, leukocyte esterase activity, and amniotic fluid glucose concentration in predicting amniotic fluid culture results in preterm premature rupture of membranes. *Am J Obstet Gynecol* 1992;167:1092–1095.
240 Hazan Y, Mazor M, Horowitz S, et al. The diagnostic value of amniotic fluid Gram stain examination and limulus amebocyte lysate assay in patients with preterm birth. *Acta Obstet Gynecol Scand* 1995;74:275–280.
241 Romero R, Yoon BH, Mazor M, et al. A comparative study of the diagnostic performance of amniotic fluid glucose, white blood cell count, interleukin-6, and gram stain in the detection of microbial invasion in patients with preterm premature rupture of membranes. *Am J Obstet Gynecol* 1993;169:839–851.

242 Ablow RC, Driscoll SG, Effmann EL, et al. A comparison of early-onset group B steptococcal neonatal infection and the respiratory-distress syndrome of the newborn. *N Engl J Med* 1976;294:65–70.

243 Jacobs J, Edwards D, Gluck L. Early-onset sepsis and pneumonia observed as respiratory distress syndrome: assessment of lung maturity. *Am J Dis Child* 1980;134:766–768.

244 Modanlou HD, Bosu SK, Weller MH. Early onset group B streptococcus neonatal septicemia and respiratory distress syndrome: characteristic features of assisted ventilation in the first 24 hours of life. *Crit Care Med* 1980;8:716–720.

245 Romero R, Yoon BH, Goncalves LF, et al. The clinical significance of microbial invasion of the amniotic cavity with mycoplasmas in patients with preterm PROM. Fortieth Annual Meeting of the Society for Gynecologic Investigation, March 31–April 3. *Scientific Abstr* 1993;70:S4.

246 Gauthier DW, Meyer WJ, Bieniarz A. Expectant management of premature rupture of membranes with amniotic fluid cultures positive for *Ureaplasma urealyticum* alone. *Am J Obstet Gynecol* 1994;170:587–590.

247 Horowitz S, Mazor M, Horowitz J, et al. Antibodies to *Ureaplasma urealyticum* in women with intraamniotic infection and adverse pregnancy outcome. *Acta Obstet Gynecol Scand* 1995;74:132–136.

248 Gomez R, Nien JK, Sepulveda G, et al. Antibiotic treatment of patients with preterm PROM does not eradicate intra-amniotic infection or prevent the development of intra-amniotic inflammation. *Am J Obstet Gynecol* 2001;185(6):S142.

249 Carroll SG, Ville Y, Greenough A, et al. Preterm prelabour amniorrhexis: intrauterine infection and interval between membrane rupture and delivery. *Arch Dis Child Fetal Neonatal Ed* 1995;72:F43–F46.

250 Gomez R, Romero R, Ghezzi F, et al. The fetal inflammatory response syndrome. *Am J Obstet Gynecol* 1998;179:194–202.

251 Romero R, Gomez R, Ghezzi F, et al. A fetal systemic inflammatory response is followed by the spontaneous onset of preterm parturition. *Am J Obstet Gynecol* 1998;179:186–193.

252 Romero R, Athayde N, Gomez R, et al. The fetal inflammatory response syndrome is characterized by the outpouring of a potent extracellular matrix degrading enzyme into the fetal circulation. *Am J Obstet Gynecol* 1998;178:S3.

253 Berry SM, Romero R, Gomez R, et al. Premature parturition is characterized by in utero activation of the fetal immune system. *Am J Obstet Gynecol* 1995;173:1315–1320.

254 Berry SM, Gomez R, Athayde N, et al. The role of granulocyte colony stimulating factor in the neutrophilia observed in the fetal inflammatory response syndrome. *Am J Obstet Gynecol* 1998;178:S202.

255 Gomez R, Berry S, Yoon BH, et al. The hematologic profile of the fetus with systemic inflammatory response syndrome. *Am J Obstet Gynecol* 1998;178:S202.

256 Yoon BH, Romero R, Jun JK, et al. An increase in fetal plasma cortisol but not dehydroepiandrosterone sulfate is followed by the onset of preterm labor in patients with preterm premature rupture of the membranes. *Am J Obstet Gynecol* 1998;179: 1107–1114.

257 Romero R, Espinoza J, Goncalves LF, et al. Fetal cardiac dysfunction in preterm premature rupture of membranes. *J Matern Fetal Neonatal Med* 2004;16:146–157.

258 Yoon BH, Jun JK, Romero R, et al. Amniotic fluid inflammatory cytokines (interleukin-6, interleukin-1beta, and tumor necrosis factor-alpha), neonatal brain white matter lesions, and cerebral palsy. *Am J Obstet Gynecol* 1997;177:19–26.

259 Yoon BH, Romero R, Park JS, et al. Fetal exposure to an intra-amniotic inflammation and the development of cerebral palsy at the age of three years. *Am J Obstet Gynecol* 2000;182:675–681.

260 Yoon BH, Romero R, Jun JK, et al. Amniotic fluid cytokines (interleukin-6, tumor necrosis factor-alpha, interleukin-1 beta, and interleukin-8) and the risk for the development of bronchopulmonary dysplasia. *Am J Obstet Gynecol* 1997;177: 825–830.

261 Yoon BH, Romero R, Kim KS, et al. A systemic fetal inflammatory response and the development of bronchopulmonary dysplasia. *Am J Obstet Gynecol* 1999;181:773–779.

262 Kim YM, Kim GJ, Kim MR, et al. Skin: an active component of the fetal innate immune system. *Am J Obstet Gynecol* 2003;189(6):S74.

263 Pacora P, Chaiworapongsa T, Maymon E, et al. Funisitis and chorionic vasculitis: the histological counterpart of the fetal inflammatory response syndrome. *J Matern Fetal Neonatal Med* 2002;11:18–25.

264 D'Alquen D, Kramer BW, Seidenspinner S, et al. Activation of umbilical cord endothelial cells and fetal inflammatory response in preterm infants with chorioamnionitis and funisitis. *Pediatr Res* 2005;57:263–269.

265 Yoon BH, Romero R, Park JS, et al. The relationship among inflammatory lesions of the umbilical cord (funisitis), umbilical cord plasma interleukin 6 concentration, amniotic fluid infection, and neonatal sepsis. *Am J Obstet Gynecol* 2000;183:1124–1129.

266 Wu YW, Colford JM, Jr. Chorioamnionitis as a risk factor for cerebral palsy: a meta-analysis. *JAMA* 2000;284:1417–1424.

267 Leviton A, Paneth N, Reuss ML, et al. Maternal infection, fetal inflammatory response, and brain damage in very low birth weight infants. Developmental Epidemiology Network Investigators. *Pediatr Res* 1999;46:566–575.

268 Cornette L. Fetal and neonatal inflammatory response and adverse outcome. *Semin Fetal Neonatal Med* 2004;9:459–470.

269 Pankuch GA, Appelbaum PC, Lorenz RP, et al. Placental microbiology and histology and the pathogenesis of chorioamnionitis. *Obstet Gynecol* 1984;64:802–806.

270 Romero R, Salafia CA, Athanassiadis AP, et al. The relationship between acute inflammatory lesions of the preterm placenta and amniotic fluid microbiology. *Am J Obstet Gynecol* 1992;166: 1382.

271 Ananth CV, Savitz DA, Williams MA. Placental abruption and its association with hypertension and prolonged rupture of membranes: a methodologic review and meta-analysis. *Obstet Gynecol* 1996;88:309–318.

272 Ananth CV, Smulian JC, Demissie K, et al. Placental abruption among singleton and twin births in the United States: risk factor profiles. *Am J Epidemiol* 2001;153:771–778.

273 Nelson DM, Stempel LE, Zuspan FP. Association of prolonged, preterm premature rupture of the membranes and abruptio placentae. *J Reprod Med* 1986;31:249–253.

274 Vintzileos AM, Campbell WA, Nochimson DJ, Weinbaum PJ. Preterm premature rupture of the membranes: a risk factor for the development of abruptio placentae. *Am J Obstet Gynecol* 1987;156:1235–1238.

275 Gonen R, Hannah ME, Milligan JE. Does prolonged preterm premature rupture of the membranes predispose to abruptio placentae? *Obstet Gynecol* 1989;74:347–350.

276 Major CA, de Veciana M, Lewis DF, Morgan MA. Preterm premature rupture of membranes and abruptio placentae: is there an association between these pregnancy complications? *Am J Obstet Gynecol* 1995;172:672–676.

277 Naeye RL. Coitus and antepartum haemorrhage. *Br J Obstet Gynaecol* 1981;88:765–770.
278 Lockwood CJ, Toti P, Arcuri F, et al. Mechanisms of abruption-induced premature rupture of the fetal membranes: thrombin-enhanced interleukin-8 expression in term decidua. *Am J Pathol* 2005;167:1443–1449.
279 Lauria MR, Gonik B, Romero R. Pulmonary hypoplasia: pathogenesis, diagnosis, and antenatal prediction. *Obstet Gynecol* 1995;86:466–475.
280 Rotschild A, Ling EW, Puterman ML, Farquharson D. Neonatal outcome after prolonged preterm rupture of the membranes. *Am J Obstet Gynecol* 1990;162:46–52.
281 Vergani P, Ghidini A, Locatelli A, et al. Risk factors for pulmonary hypoplasia in second-trimester premature rupture of membranes. *Am J Obstet Gynecol* 1994;170:1359–1364.
282 Moessinger AC, Collins MH, Blanc WA, et al. Oligohydramnios-induced lung hypoplasia: the influence of timing and duration in gestation. *Pediatr Res* 1986;20:951–954.
283 Winn HN, Chen M, Amon E, et al. Neonatal pulmonary hypoplasia and perinatal mortality in patients with midtrimester rupture of amniotic membranes – a critical analysis. *Am J Obstet Gynecol* 2000;182:1638–1644.
284 Johnson A, Callan NA, Bhutani VK, et al. Ultrasonic ratio of fetal thoracic to abdominal circumference: an association with fetal pulmonary hypoplasia. *Am J Obstet Gynecol* 1987;157: 764–769.
285 Nimrod C, Varela-Gittings F, Machin G, et al. The effect of very prolonged membrane rupture on fetal development. *Am J Obstet Gynecol* 1984;148:540–543.
286 Thibeault DW, Beatty EC, Jr, Hall RT, et al. Neonatal pulmonary hypoplasia with premature rupture of fetal membranes and oligohydramnios. *J Pediatr* 1985;107:273–277.
287 Blott M, Greenough A, Nicolaides KH, et al. Fetal breathing movements as predictor of favourable pregnancy outcome after oligohydramnios due to membrane rupture in second trimester. *Lancet* 1987;2:129–131.
288 Moessinger AC, Fox HE, Higgins A, et al. Fetal breathing movements are not a reliable predictor of continued lung development in pregnancies complicated by oligohydramnios. *Lancet* 1987;2:1297–1300.
289 Harding R, Sigger JN, Wickham PJ, Bocking AD. The regulation of flow of pulmonary fluid in fetal sheep. *Respir Physiol* 1984;57:47–59.
290 Badalian SS, Chao CR, Fox HE, Timor-Tritsch IE. Fetal breathing-related nasal fluid flow velocity in uncomplicated pregnancies. *Am J Obstet Gynecol* 1993;169:563–567.
291 Adzick NS, Harrison MR, Glick PL, et al. Experimental pulmonary hypoplasia and oligohydramnios: relative contributions of lung fluid and fetal breathing movements. *J Pediatr Surg* 1984;19:658–665.
292 Alcorn D, Adamson TM, Lambert TF, et al. Morphological effects of chronic tracheal ligation and drainage in the fetal lamb lung. *J Anat* 1977;123:649–660.
293 Fewell JE, Hislop AA, Kitterman JA, Johnson P. Effect of tracheostomy on lung development in fetal lambs. *J Appl Physiol* 1983;55:1103–1108.
294 Wigglesworth JS, Desai R, Hislop AA. Fetal lung growth in congenital laryngeal atresia. *Pediatr Pathol* 1987;7:515–525.
295 Nicolini U, Fisk NM, Rodeck CH, et al. Low amniotic pressure in oligohydramnios – is this the cause of pulmonary hypoplasia? *Am J Obstet Gynecol* 1989;161:1098–1101.
296 Nimrod C, Davies D, Iwanicki S, et al. Ultrasound prediction of pulmonary hypoplasia. *Obstet Gynecol* 1986;68:495–498.
297 Songster GS, Gray DL, Crane JP. Prenatal prediction of lethal pulmonary hypoplasia using ultrasonic fetal chest circumference. *Obstet Gynecol* 1989;73:261–266.
298 Fong K, Ohlsson A, Zalev A. Fetal thoracic circumference: a prospective cross-sectional study with real-time ultrasound. *Am J Obstet Gynecol* 1988;158:1154–1160.
299 D'Alton M, Mercer B, Riddick E, Dudley D. Serial thoracic versus abdominal circumference ratios for the prediction of pulmonary hypoplasia in premature rupture of the membranes remote from term. *Am J Obstet Gynecol* 1992;166:658–663.
300 Ohlsson A, Fong K, Rose T, et al. Prenatal ultrasonic prediction of autopsy-proven pulmonary hypoplasia. *Am J Perinatol* 1992;9:334–337.
301 Roberts AB, Mitchell JM. Direct ultrasonographic measurement of fetal lung length in normal pregnancies and pregnancies complicated by prolonged rupture of membranes. *Am J Obstet Gynecol* 1990;163:1560–1566.
302 Fox HE, Badalian SS, Timor-Tritsch IE, et al. Fetal upper respiratory tract function in cases of antenatally diagnosed congenital diaphragmatic hernia: preliminary observations. *Ultrasound Obstet Gynecol* 1993;3:164–167.
303 van Eyck J, van der MK, Wladimiroff JW. Ductus arteriosus flow velocity modulation by fetal breathing movements as a measure of fetal lung development. *Am J Obstet Gynecol* 1990;163: 558–566.
304 Laudy JA, Tibboel D, Robben SG, et al. Prenatal prediction of pulmonary hypoplasia: clinical, biometric, and Doppler velocity correlates. *Pediatrics* 2002;109:250–258.
305 Vintzileos AM, Campbell WA, Rodis JF, et al. Comparison of six different ultrasonographic methods for predicting lethal fetal pulmonary hypoplasia. *Am J Obstet Gynecol* 1989;161:606–612.
306 Heling KS, Tennstedt C, Chaoui R, et al. Reliability of prenatal sonographic lung biometry in the diagnosis of pulmonary hypoplasia. *Prenat Diagn* 2001;21:649–657.
307 Fisk NM, Ronderos-Dumit D, Soliani A, et al. Diagnostic and therapeutic transabdominal amnioinfusion in oligohydramnios. *Obstet Gynecol* 1991;78:270–278.
308 Nakayama DK, Glick PL, Harrison MR, et al. Experimental pulmonary hypoplasia due to oligohydramnios and its reversal by relieving thoracic compression. *J Pediatr Surg* 1983;18:347–353.
309 Potter E. Bilateral renal agenesis. *J Pediatr* 1946;29:68.
310 Porter HJ. Pulmonary hypoplasia – size is not everything. *Virchows Arch* 1998;432.
311 Wenstrom KD. Pulmonary hypoplasia and deformations related to premature rupture of membranes. *Obstet Gynecol Clin North Am* 1992;19:397–408.
312 Tamura RK, Sabbagha RE, Depp R, et al. Diminished growth in fetuses born preterm after spontaneous labor or rupture of membranes. *Am J Obstet Gynecol* 1984;148:1105–1110.
313 Bukowski R, Gahn D, Denning J, Saade G. Impairment of growth in fetuses destined to deliver preterm. *Am J Obstet Gynecol* 2001;185:463–467.
314 Spinillo A, Montanari L, Sanpaolo P, et al. Fetal growth and infant neurodevelopmental outcome after preterm premature rupture of membranes. *Obstet Gynecol* 2004;103:1286–1293.
315 Blackwell S, Romero R, Chaiworapongsa T, et al. Maternal and fetal inflammatory responses in unexplained fetal death. *J Matern Fetal Neonatal Med* 2003;14:151–157.
316 Gerber S, Vardhana S, Meagher-Villemure K, et al. Association between fetal interleukin-1 receptor antagonist gene polymorphism and unexplained fetal death. *Am J Obstet Gynecol* 2005;193:1472–1477.

317 Reece EA, Chervenak FA, Moya FR, Hobbins JC. Amniotic fluid arborization: effect of blood, meconium, and pH alterations. *Obstet Gynecol* 1984;64:248–250.
318 Friedman ML, Mcelin TW. Diagnosis of ruptured fetal membranes. Clinical study and review of the literature. *Am J Obstet Gynecol* 1969;104:544–550.
319 Lodeiro JG, Hsieh KA, Byers JH, Feinstein SJ. The fingerprint, a false-positive fern test. *Obstet Gynecol* 1989;73:873–874.
320 McGregor JA, Johnson S. "Fig leaf" ferning and positive nitrazine testing: semen as a cause of misdiagnosis of premature rupture of membranes. *Am J Obstet Gynecol* 1985;151:1142–1143.
321 Brookes C, Shand K, Jones WR. A reevaluation of the ferning test to detect ruptured membranes. *Aust NZ J Obstet Gynaecol* 1986;26:260–264.
322 Rosemond RL, Lombardi SJ, Boehm FH. Ferning of amniotic fluid contaminated with blood. *Obstet Gynecol* 1990;75:338–340.
323 Bennett SL, Cullen JB, Sherer DM, Woods JR, Jr. The ferning and nitrazine tests of amniotic fluid between 12 and 41 weeks gestation. *Am J Perinatol* 1993;10:101–104.
324 Adoni A, Ben Chetrit A, Zacut D, et al. Prolongation of the latent period in patients with premature rupture of the membranes by avoiding digital examination. *Int J Gynaecol Obstet* 1990;32:19–21.
325 Lewis DF, Major CA, Towers CV, et al. Effects of digital vaginal examinations on latency period in preterm premature rupture of membranes. *Obstet Gynecol* 1992;80:630–634.
326 Schutte MF, Treffers PE, Kloosterman GJ, Soepatmi S. Management of premature rupture of membranes: the risk of vaginal examination to the infant. *Am J Obstet Gynecol* 1983;146:395–400.
327 Sukcharoen N, Vasuratna A. Effects of digital cervical examinations on duration of latency period, maternal and neonatal outcome in preterm premature rupture of membranes. *J Med Assoc Thai* 1993;76:203–209.
328 Munson LA, Graham A, Koos BJ, Valenzuela GJ. Is there a need for digital examination in patients with spontaneous rupture of the membranes? *Am J Obstet Gynecol* 1985;153:562–563.
329 Brown CL, Ludwiczak MH, Blanco JD, Hirsch CE. Cervical dilation: accuracy of visual and digital examinations. *Obstet Gynecol* 1993;81:215–216.
330 Morgan MA, de Veciana M, Rumney PJ, Schlinke S. Cervical assessment: visual or digital? *J Perinatol* 1996;16:103–106.
331 Smith RP. A technique for the detection of rupture of the membranes. A review and preliminary report. *Obstet Gynecol* 1976;48:172–176.
332 Gahl W, Kazina TR, Furmann D, et al. Diamine oxidase in the diagnosis of ruptured fetal membranes. *Am J Obstet Gynecol* 1969;104:544.
333 Huber JF, Bischof P, Extermann P, et al. Are vaginal fluid concentrations of prolactin, alpha-fetoprotein and human placental lactogen useful for diagnosing ruptured membranes? *Br J Obstet Gynaecol* 1983;90:1183–1185.
334 Koninckx PR, Trappeniers H, Van Assche FA. Prolactin concentration in vaginal fluid: a new method for diagnosing ruptured membranes. *Br J Obstet Gynaecol* 1981;88:607–610.
335 Phocas I, Sarandakou A, Kontoravdis A, et al. Vaginal fluid prolactin: a reliable marker for the diagnosis of prematurely ruptured membranes. Comparison with vaginal fluid alpha-fetoprotein and placental lactogen. *Eur J Obstet Gynecol Reprod Biol* 1989;31:133–141.
336 Gaucherand P, Guibaud S, Rudigoz RC, Wong A. Diagnosis of premature rupture of the membranes by the identification of alpha-feto-protein in vaginal secretions. *Acta Obstet Gynecol Scand* 1994;73:456–459.
337 Kishida T, Hirao A, Matsuura T, et al. Diagnosis of premature rupture of membranes with an improved alpha-fetoprotein monoclonal antibody kit. *Clin Chem* 1995;41:1500–1503.
338 Kishida T, Yamada H, Negishi H, et al. Diagnosis of preterm premature rupture of the membranes using a newly developed AFP monoclonal antibody test kit. *Eur J Obstet Gynecol Reprod Biol* 1995;58:67–72.
339 Lockwood CJ, Wein R, Chien D, et al. Fetal membrane rupture is associated with the presence of insulin-like growth factor-binding protein-1 in vaginal secretions. *Am J Obstet Gynecol* 1994;171:146–150.
340 Buyukbayrak EE, Turan C, Unal O, et al. Diagnostic power of the vaginal washing-fluid prolactin assay as an alternative method for the diagnosis of premature rupture of membranes. *J Matern Fetal Neonatal Med* 2004;15:120–125.
341 Esim E, Turan C, Unal O, et al. Diagnosis of premature rupture of membranes by identification of beta-HCG in vaginal washing fluid. *Eur J Obstet Gynecol Reprod Biol* 2003;107:37–40.
342 Erdemoglu E, Mungan T. Significance of detecting insulin-like growth factor binding protein-1 in cervicovaginal secretions: comparison with nitrazine test and amniotic fluid volume assessment. *Acta Obstet Gynecol Scand* 2004;83:622–626.
343 Anai T, Tanaka Y, Hirota Y, Miyakawa I. Vaginal fluid hCG levels for detecting premature rupture of membranes. *Obstet Gynecol* 1997;89:261–264.
344 Kishida T, Yamada H, Negishi H, et al. Diagnosis of premature rupture of the membranes in preterm patients, using an improved AFP kit: comparison with ROM-check and/or nitrazine test. *Eur J Obstet Gynecol Reprod Biol* 1996;69:77–82.
345 Atterbury JL, Groome LJ, Hoff C. Methods used to diagnose premature rupture of membranes: a national survey of 812 obstetric nurses. *Obstet Gynecol* 1998;92:384–389.
346 Lockwood CJ, Senyei AE, Dische MR, et al. Fetal fibronectin in cervical and vaginal secretions as a predictor of preterm delivery. *N Engl J Med* 1991;325:669–674.
347 Eriksen NL, Parisi VM, Daoust S, et al. Fetal fibronectin: a method for detecting the presence of amniotic fluid. *Obstet Gynecol* 1992;80:451–454.
348 Goldenberg RL, Mercer BM, Meis PJ, et al. The preterm prediction study: fetal fibronectin testing and spontaneous preterm birth. NICHD Maternal Fetal Medicine Units Network. *Obstet Gynecol* 1996;87:643–648.
349 Greenhagen JB, Van Wagoner J, Dudley D, et al. Value of fetal fibronectin as a predictor of preterm delivery for a low-risk population. *Am J Obstet Gynecol* 1996;175:1054–1056.
350 Irion O, Matute S, Bischof P, Beguin F. Cervical oncofetal fibronectin in patients with false labor as a predictor of preterm delivery. *Am J Obstet Gynecol* 1996;394:384.
351 Leeson SC, Maresh MJ, Martindale EA, et al. Detection of fetal fibronectin as a predictor of preterm delivery in high risk asymptomatic pregnancies. *Br J Obstet Gynaecol* 1996;103:48–53.
352 Malak TM, Sizmur F, Bell SC, Taylor DJ. Fetal fibronectin in cervicovaginal secretions as a predictor of preterm birth. *Br J Obstet Gynaecol* 1996;103:648–653.
353 Morrison JC, Allbert JR, McLaughlin BN, et al. Oncofetal fibronectin in patients with false labor as a predictor of preterm delivery. *Am J Obstet Gynecol* 1993;168:538–542.

354 Nageotte MP, Casal D, Senyei AE. Fetal fibronectin in patients at increased risk for premature birth. *Am J Obstet Gynecol* 1994;170:20–25.

355 Rizzo G, Capponi A, Arduini D, et al. The value of fetal fibronectin in cervical and vaginal secretions and of ultrasonographic examination of the uterine cervix in predicting premature delivery for patients with preterm labor and intact membranes. *Am J Obstet Gynecol* 1996;175:1146–1151.

356 Atlay RD, Sutherst JR. Premature rupture of the fetal membranes confirmed by intra-amniotic injection of dye (Evans blue T-1824). *Am J Obstet Gynecol* 1970;108:993–994.

357 Diaz-Garzon J. Indigocarmine test of preterm rupture of membranes. *Rev Columb Obstet Gynecol* 1969;20:373.

358 Fujimoto S, Kishida T, Sagawa T, et al. Clinical usefulness of the dye-injection method for diagnosing premature rupture of the membranes in equivocal cases. *J Obstet Gynaecol* 1995;21:215–220.

359 Meyer BA, Gonik B, Creasy RK. Evaluation of phenazopyridine hydrochloride as a tool in the diagnosis of premature rupture of the membranes. *Am J Perinatol* 1991;8:297–299.

360 Cowett RM, Hakanson DO, Kocon RW, Oh W. Untoward neonatal effect of intraamniotic administration of methylene blue. *Obstet Gynecol* 1976;48:74S–75S.

361 McEnerney J, McEnerney L. Unfavourable neonatal outcomes after intraamniotic injection of methylene blue. *Obstet Gynecol* 1983;1983:351.

362 Troche BI. Methylene blue baby. *N Engl J Med* 1989;320:1756–1757.

363 Divon MY, Chamberlain PF, Sipos L, Platt LD. Underestimation of fetal weight in premature rupture of membranes. *J Ultrasound Med* 1984;3:529–531.

364 Ben Haroush A, Yogev Y, Bar J, et al. Accuracy of sonographically estimated fetal weight in 840 women with different pregnancy complications prior to induction of labor. *Ultrasound Obstet Gynecol* 2004;23:172–176.

365 Edwards A, Goff J, Baker L. Accuracy and modifying factors of the sonographic estimation of fetal weight in a high-risk population. *Aust NZ J Obstet Gynaecol* 2001;41:187–190.

366 Romero R, Goncalves LF, Ghezzi F, et al. Amniocenteses. In: Fleischer AC, Manning FA, Jeanty P, Romero R, eds. *Sonography in obstetrics and gynecology: principles and practice*. Stamford, CT: Appleton & Lange, 1996.

367 Cotton DB, Gonik B, Bottoms SF. Conservative versus aggressive management of preterm rupture of membranes. A randomized trial of amniocentesis. *Am J Perinatol* 1984;1:322–324.

368 Shim SS, Romero R, Hong JS, et al. Clinical significance of intra-amniotic inflammation in patients with preterm premature rupture of membranes. *Am J Obstet Gynecol* 2004;191:1339–1345.

369 Yoon BH, Romero R, Kim CJ, et al. Amniotic fluid interleukin-6: a sensitive test for antenatal diagnosis of acute inflammatory lesions of preterm placenta and prediction of perinatal morbidity. *Am J Obstet Gynecol* 1995;172:960–970.

370 Jalava J, Mantymaa ML, Ekblad U, et al. Bacterial 16S rDNA polymerase chain reaction in the detection of intra-amniotic infection. *Br J Obstet Gynaecol* 1996;103:664–669.

371 Romero R, Gomez R, Nien JK, et al. Metabolomics in premature labor: a novel approach to identify patients at risk for preterm delivery. *Am J Obstet Gynecol* 2004;191(6):S2.

372 Yeast JD, Garite TJ, Dorchester W. The risks of amniocentesis in the management of premature rupture of the membranes. *Am J Obstet Gynecol* 1984;149:505–508.

373 Shaver DC, Spinnato JA, Whybrew D, et al. Comparison of phospholipids in vaginal and amniocentesis specimens of patients with premature rupture of membranes. *Am J Obstet Gynecol* 1987;156:454–457.

374 Stedman CM, Crawford S, Staten E, Cherny WB. Management of preterm premature rupture of membranes: assessing amniotic fluid in the vagina for phosphatidylglycerol. *Am J Obstet Gynecol* 1981;140:34–38.

375 Brame RG, MacKenna J. Vaginal pool phospholipids in the management of premature rupture of membranes. *Am J Obstet Gynecol* 1983;145:992–1000.

376 Golde SH. Use of obstetric perineal pads in collection of amniotic fluid in patients with rupture of the membranes. *Am J Obstet Gynecol* 1983;146:710–712.

377 Estol PC, Poseiro JJ, Schwarcz R. Phosphatidylglycerol determination in the amniotic fluid from a pad placed over the vulva: a method for diagnosis of fetal lung maturity in cases of premature ruptured membranes. *J Perinat Med* 1992;20:65–71.

378 Lewis DF, Towers CV, Major CA, et al. Use of Amniostat-FLM in detecting the presence of phosphatidylglycerol in vaginal pool samples in preterm premature rupture of membranes. *Am J Obstet Gynecol* 1993;169:573–576.

379 Gluck L, Kulovich MV, Borer RC, Jr, Keidel WN. The interpretation and significance of the lecithin-sphingomyclin ratio in amniotic fluid. *Am J Obstet Gynecol* 1974;120:142–155.

380 Schumacher RE, Parisi VM, Steady HM, Tsao FH. Bacteria causing false positive test for phosphatidylglycerol in amniotic fluid. *Am J Obstet Gynecol* 1985;151:1067–1068.

381 Dombroski RA, MacKenna J, Brame RG. Comparison of amniotic fluid lung maturity profiles in paired vaginal and amniocentesis specimens. *Am J Obstet Gynecol* 1981;140:461–464.

382 Goldstein AS, Mangurten HH, Libretti JV, Berman AM. Lecithin/sphingomyelin ratio in amniotic fluid obtained vaginally. *Am J Obstet Gynecol* 1980;138:232–233.

383 Sbarra AJ, Blake G, Cetrulo CL, et al. The effect of cervical/vaginal secretions on measurements of lecithin/sphingomyelin ratio and optical density at 650 nm. *Am J Obstet Gynecol* 1981;139:214–216.

384 Phillippe M, Acker D, Torday J, et al. The effects of vaginal contamination on two pulmonary phospholipid assays. *J Reprod Med* 1982;27:283–286.

385 Spinnato JA, Shaver DC, Bray EM, Lipshitz J. Preterm premature rupture of the membranes with fetal pulmonary maturity present: a prospective study. *Obstet Gynecol* 1987;69:196–201.

386 Mercer BM, Crocker LG, Boe NM, Sibai BM. Induction versus expectant management in premature rupture of the membranes with mature amniotic fluid at 32 to 36 weeks: a randomized trial. *Am J Obstet Gynecol* 1993;169:775–782.

387 Vintzileos AM, Feinstein SJ, Lodeiro JG, et al. Fetal biophysical profile and the effect of premature rupture of the membranes. *Obstet Gynecol* 1986;67:818–823.

388 Vintzileos AM, Campbell WA, Nochimson DJ, Weinbaum PJ. The use of the nonstress test in patients with premature rupture of the membranes. *Am J Obstet Gynecol* 1986;155:149–153.

389 Zeevi D, Sadovsky E, Younis J, et al. Antepartum fetal heart rate characteristics in cases of premature rupture of membranes. *Am J Perinatol* 1988;5:260–263.

390 Vintzileos AM, Knuppel RA. Fetal biophysical assessment in premature rupture of the membranes. *Clin Obstet Gynecol* 1995;38:45–58.

391 Carroll SG, Papaioannou S, Nicolaides KH. Assessment of fetal activity and amniotic fluid volume in the prediction of

intrauterine infection in preterm prelabor amniorrhexis. *Am J Obstet Gynecol* 1995;172:1427–1435.

392 Del Valle GO, Joffe GM, Izquierdo LA, et al. The biophysical profile and the nonstress test: poor predictors of chorioamnionitis and fetal infection in prolonged preterm premature rupture of membranes. *Obstet Gynecol* 1992;80:106–110.

393 Gauthier DW, Meyer WJ, Bieniarz A. Biophysical profile as a predictor of amniotic fluid culture results. *Obstet Gynecol* 1992;80:102–105.

394 Jackson DN, Lewis DF, Nageotte MP, Towers CV. Daily amniotic fluid index study in the management of preterm prolonged ruptured membranes: a prospective study. SPO Abstract 655. *Am J Obstet Gynecol* 1991;164:423.

395 Vintzileos AM, Campbell WA, Nochimson DJ, Weinbaum PJ. Degree of oligohydramnios and pregnancy outcome in patients with premature rupture of the membranes. *Obstet Gynecol* 1985;66:162–167.

396 Hadi HA, Hodson CA, Strickland D. Premature rupture of the membranes between 20 and 25 weeks' gestation: role of amniotic fluid volume in perinatal outcome. *Am J Obstet Gynecol* 1994;170:1139–1144.

397 Lao TT, Cheung VY. Expectant management of preterm prelabour rupture of membranes – the significance of oligohydramnios at presentation. *Eur J Obstet Gynecol Reprod Biol* 1993;48:87–91.

398 Scane TM, Hawkins DF. Antibacterial activity in human amniotic fluid: dependence on divalent cations. *Br J Obstet Gynaecol* 1986;93:577–581.

399 Yoon BH, Kim YA, Romero R, et al. Association of oligohydramnios in women with preterm premature rupture of membranes with an inflammatory response in fetal, amniotic, and maternal compartments. *Am J Obstet Gynecol* 1999;181:784–788.

400 Smith CV, Greenspoon J, Phelan JP, Platt LD. Clinical utility of the nonstress test in the conservative management of women with preterm spontaneous premature rupture of the membranes. *J Reprod Med* 1987;32:1–4.

401 Kivikoski AI, Amon E, Vaalamo PO, et al. Effect of third-trimester premature rupture of membranes on fetal breathing movements: a prospective case–control study. *Am J Obstet Gynecol* 1988;159:1474–1477.

402 Roberts AB, Goldstein I, Romero R, Hobbins JC. Fetal breathing movements after preterm premature rupture of membranes. *Am J Obstet Gynecol* 1991;164:821–825.

403 Vintzileos AM, Campbell WA, Nochimson DJ, et al. The fetal biophysical profile in patients with premature rupture of the membranes – an early predictor of fetal infection. *Am J Obstet Gynecol* 1985;152:510–516.

404 Vintzileos AM, Campbell WA, Nochimson DJ, Weinbaum PJ. Fetal breathing as a predictor of infection in premature rupture of the membranes. *Obstet Gynecol* 1986;67:813–817.

405 Goldstein I, Romero R, Merrill S, et al. Fetal body and breathing movements as predictors of intraamniotic infection in preterm premature rupture of membranes. *Am J Obstet Gynecol* 1988;159:363–368.

406 Kitterman JA, Liggins GC, Clements JA, Tooley WH. Stimulation of breathing movements in fetal sheep by inhibitors of prostaglandin synthesis. *J Dev Physiol* 1979;1:453–466.

407 Thompson PJ, Greenough A, Nicolaides KH. Fetal breathing movements and prostaglandin levels in pregnancies complicated by premature rupture of the membranes. *J Perinat Med* 1992;20:209–213.

408 Manning FA, Morrison I, Lange IR, et al. Fetal assessment based on fetal biophysical profile scoring: experience in 12,620 referred high-risk pregnancies. I. Perinatal mortality by frequency and etiology. *Am J Obstet Gynecol* 1985;151:343–350.

409 Fleming AD, Salafia CM, Vintzileos AM, et al. The relationships among umbilical artery velocimetry, fetal biophysical profile, and placental inflammation in preterm premature rupture of the membranes. *Am J Obstet Gynecol* 1991;164:38–41.

410 Mercer B, Moretti M, Shaver D. Intensive antenatal testing for women with prolonged preterm premature rupture of the membranes. Abstract 420. Presented at 11th Annual Meeting of the Society of Perinatal Obstetricians, San Francisco, 1991.

411 Miller JM, Jr, Kho MS, Brown HL, Gabert HA. Clinical chorioamnionitis is not predicted by an ultrasonic biophysical profile in patients with premature rupture of membranes. *Obstet Gynecol* 1990;76:1051–1054.

412 Roberts AB, Goldstein I, Romero R, Hobbins JC. Comparison of total fetal activity measurement with the biophysical profile in predicting intra-amniotic infection in preterm premature rupture of membranes. *Ultrasound Obstet Gynecol* 1991;1:36–39.

413 Roussis P, Rosemond RL, Glass C, Boehm FH. Preterm premature rupture of membranes: detection of infection. *Am J Obstet Gynecol* 1991;165:1099–1104.

414 Vintzileos AM, Bors-Koefoed R, Pelegano JF, et al. The use of fetal biophysical profile improves pregnancy outcome in premature rupture of the membranes. *Am J Obstet Gynecol* 1987;157:236–240.

415 Devoe LD, Youssef AE, Croom CS, Watson J. Can fetal biophysical observations anticipate outcome in preterm labor or preterm rupture of membranes? *Obstet Gynecol* 1994;84:432–438.

416 Evans MI, Hajj SN, Devoe LD, et al. C-reactive protein as a predictor of infectious morbidity with premature rupture of membranes. *Am J Obstet Gynecol* 1980;138:648–652.

417 Farb HF, Arnesen M, Geistler P, Knox GE. C-reactive protein with premature rupture of membranes and premature labor. *Obstet Gynecol* 1983;62:49–51.

418 Fisk NM, Fysh J, Child AG, et al. Is C-reactive protein really useful in preterm premature rupture of the membranes? *Br J Obstet Gynaecol* 1987;94:1159–1164.

419 Hawrylyshyn P, Bernstein P, Milligan JE, et al. Premature rupture of membranes: the role of C-reactive protein in the prediction of chorioamnionitis. *Am J Obstet Gynecol* 1983;147:240–246.

420 Ismail MA, Zinaman MJ, Lowensohn RI, Moawad AH. The significance of C-reactive protein levels in women with premature rupture of membranes. *Am J Obstet Gynecol* 1985;151:541–544.

421 Kurki T, Teramo K, Ylikorkala O, Paavonen J. C-reactive protein in preterm premature rupture of the membranes. *Arch Gynecol Obstet* 1990;247:31–37.

422 Romem Y, Artal R. C-reactive protein as a predictor for chorioamnionitis in cases of premature rupture of the membranes. *Am J Obstet Gynecol* 1984;150:546–550.

423 Yoon BH, Jun JK, Park KH, et al. Serum C-reactive protein, white blood cell count, and amniotic fluid white blood cell count in women with preterm premature rupture of membranes. *Obstet Gynecol* 1996;88:1034–1040.

424 DiNaro E, Ghezzi F, Raio L, et al. C-reactive protein in vaginal fluid of patients with preterm premature rupture of membranes. *Acta Obstet Gynecol Scand* 2003;82:1072–1079.

425 Thompson PJ, Greenough A, Davies E, Nicolaides KH. Fetal C-reactive protein. *Early Hum Dev* 1993;32:81–85.

426 Yoon BH, Romero R, Yang SH, et al. Interleukin-6 concentrations in umbilical cord plasma are elevated in neonates with white matter lesions associated with periventricular leukomalacia. *Am J Obstet Gynecol* 1996;174:1433–1440.
427 Fanaroff AA, Hack M. Periventricular leukomalacia – prospects for prevention. *N Engl J Med* 1999;341:1229–1231.
428 Hack M, Fanaroff AA. Outcomes of extremely immature infants – a perinatal dilemma. *N Engl J Med* 1993;329:1649–1650.
429 Gold RB, Goyert GL, Schwartz DB, et al. Conservative management of second-trimester post-amniocentesis fluid leakage. *Obstet Gynecol* 1989;74:745–747.
430 Hanson FW, Tennant FR, Zorn EM, Samuels S. Analysis of 2136 genetic amniocenteses: experience of a single physician. *Am J Obstet Gynecol* 1985;152:436–443.
431 NIH Consensus Development Panel on the Effect of Corticosteroids for Fetal Maturation on Perinatal Outcomes. Effect of corticosteroids for fetal maturation on perinatal outcomes. *JAMA* 1995;273:413–418.
432 Mercer BM. Preterm premature rupture of the membranes: diagnosis and management. *Clin Perinatol* 2004;31:765–782, vi.
433 Simhan HN, Canavan TP. Preterm premature rupture of membranes: diagnosis, evaluation and management strategies. *Br J Obstet Gynaecol* 2005;112(Suppl. 1):32–37.
434 Mercer BM, Arheart KL. Antimicrobial therapy in expectant management of preterm premature rupture of the membranes. *Lancet* 1995;346:1271–1279.
435 Kenyon SL, Taylor DJ, Tarnow-Mordi W. Broad-spectrum antibiotics for preterm, prelabour rupture of fetal membranes: the ORACLE I randomised trial. ORACLE Collaborative Group. *Lancet* 2001;357:979–988.
436 Amon E, Lewis SV, Sibai BM, et al. Ampicillin prophylaxis in preterm premature rupture of the membranes: a prospective randomized study. *Am J Obstet Gynecol* 1988;159:539–543.
437 Morales WJ, Angel JL, O'Brien WF, Knuppel RA. Use of ampicillin and corticosteroids in premature rupture of membranes: a randomized study. *Obstet Gynecol* 1989;73:721–726.
438 Johnston MM, Sanchez-Ramos L, Vaughn AJ, et al. Antibiotic therapy in preterm premature rupture of membranes: a randomized, prospective, double-blind trial. *Am J Obstet Gynecol* 1990;163:743–747.
439 Christmas JT, Cox SM, Andrews W, et al. Expectant management of preterm ruptured membranes: effects of antimicrobial therapy. *Obstet Gynecol* 1992;80:759–762.
440 McGregor JA, French JI, Seo K. Antimicrobial therapy in preterm premature rupture of membranes: results of a prospective, double-blind, placebo-controlled trial of erythromycin. *Am J Obstet Gynecol* 1991;165:632–640.
441 Kurki T, Hallman M, Zilliacus R, et al. Premature rupture of the membranes: effect of penicillin prophylaxis and long-term outcome of the children. *Am J Perinatol* 1992;9:11–16.
442 McCaul JF, Perry KG, Jr, Moore JL, Jr, et al. Adjunctive antibiotic treatment of women with preterm rupture of membranes or preterm labor. *Int J Gynaecol Obstet* 1992;38:19–24.
443 Mercer BM, Moretti ML, Prevost RR, Sibai BM. Erythromycin therapy in preterm premature rupture of the membranes: a prospective, randomized trial of 220 patients. *Am J Obstet Gynecol* 1992;166:794–802.
444 Owen J, Groome LJ, Hauth JC. Randomized trial of prophylactic antibiotic therapy after preterm amnion rupture. *Am J Obstet Gynecol* 1993;169:976–981.
445 Blanco JD, Iams J, Artal R, et al. Multicentre double-blind prospective randomized trial of ceftrizoxime versus placebo in women with preterm premature rupture of the membranes. *Am J Obstet Gynecol* 1993;168:378.
446 Lockwood CJ, Costigan K, Ghidini A, et al. Double-blind, placebo-controlled trial of piperacillin prophylaxis in preterm membrane rupture. *Am J Obstet Gynecol* 1993;169:970–976.
447 Ernest JM, Givner LB. A prospective, randomized, placebo-controlled trial of penicillin in preterm premature rupture of membranes. *Am J Obstet Gynecol* 1994;170:516–521.
448 Mercer B, Miodovnik M, Thurnau G, et al. A multi centre randomized masked trial of antibiotics vs placebo therapy after preterm premature rupture of the membranes (Abstract no. 6). *Am J Obstet Gynecol* 1996;174:304.
449 Mercer BM, Miodovnik M, Thurnau GR, et al. Antibiotic therapy for reduction of infant morbidity after preterm premature rupture of the membranes. A randomized controlled trial. National Institute of Child Health and Human Development Maternal–Fetal Medicine Units Network. *JAMA* 1997;278:989–995.
450 Lovett SM, Weiss JD, Diogo MJ, et al. A prospective, double-blind, randomized, controlled clinical trial of ampicillin-sulbactam for preterm premature rupture of membranes in women receiving antenatal corticosteroid therapy. *Am J Obstet Gynecol* 1997;176:1030–1038.
451 Kenyon S, Boulvain M, Neilson J. A systematic review of antibiotics for preterm rupture of membranes in pregnancy (PROM). 1st SGI International Summit: Preterm Birth; 2005:116.
452 Kenyon S, Boulvain M, Neilson J. Antibiotics for preterm rupture of the membranes: a systematic review. *Obstet Gynecol* 2004;104:1051–1057.
453 Brelje MC, Kaltreider DF. The use of vaginal antibiotics in premature rupture of the membranes. *Am J Obstet Gynecol* 1966;94:889.
454 Ogita S, Imanaka M, Matsumoto M, Hatanaka K. Premature rupture of the membranes managed with a new cervical catheter. *Lancet* 1984;1:1330–1331.
455 Romero R, Scioscia AL, Edberg SC, Hobbins JC. Use of parenteral antibiotic therapy to eradicate bacterial colonization of amniotic fluid in premature rupture of membranes. *Obstet Gynecol* 1986;67:15S–17S.
456 Romero R, Hagay Z, Nores J, et al. Eradication of *Ureaplasma urealyticum* from the amniotic fluid with transplacental antibiotic treatment. *Am J Obstet Gynecol* 1992;166:618–620.
457 Harding JE, Pang J, Knight DB, Liggins GC. Do antenatal corticosteroids help in the setting of preterm rupture of membranes? *Am J Obstet Gynecol* 2001;184:131–139.
458 Crowley P. Corticosteroids after prelabour rupture of membranes (revised May 5, 1994). In: Keirse MJ, Renfre MJ, Neilson JP, Crowther C, eds. *Pregnancy and childbirth module*. The Cochrane Pregnancy and Childbirth Database. The Cochrane Collaboration, Issue 2 (available from BMJ Publishing Group, London). Oxford, UK, 1995.
459 Crowley P. Corticosteroids + induction of labour after PROM preterm (revised April 22, 1993). In: Keirse MJ, Renfre MJ, Neilson JP, Crowther C, eds. *Pregnancy and childbirth module*. The Cochrane Pregnancy and Childbirth Database. The Cochrane Collaboration, Issue 2 (available from BMJ Publishing Group, London). Oxford, UK, 1995.
460 Leitich H, Egarter C, Reisenberger K, et al. Concomitant use of glucocorticoids: a comparison of two metaanalyses on antibiotic treatment in preterm premature rupture of membranes. *Am J Obstet Gynecol* 1998;178:899–908.
461 Guinn DA, Atkinson MW, Sullivan L, et al. Single vs weekly courses of antenatal corticosteroids for women at risk of preterm

delivery: a randomized controlled trial. *JAMA* 2001;286:1581–1587.

462 Jobe AH, Wada N, Berry LM, et al. Single and repetitive maternal glucocorticoid exposures reduce fetal growth in sheep. *Am J Obstet Gynecol* 1998;178:880–885.

463 Dirnberger DR, Yoder BA, Gordon MC. Single versus repeated-course antenatal corticosteroids: outcomes in singleton and multiple-gestation pregnancies. *Am J Perinatol* 2001;18:267.

464 French NP, Hagan R, Evans SF, et al. Repeated antenatal corticosteroids: size at birth and subsequent development. *Am J Obstet Gynecol* 1999;180:114–121.

465 Dunlop PD, Crowley PA, Lamont RF, Hawkins DF. Preterm ruptured membranes, no contractions. *J Obstet Gynecol* 1986;7:92.

466 Levy DL, Warsof SL. Oral ritodrine and preterm premature rupture of membranes. *Obstet Gynecol* 1985;66:621–623.

467 Christensen KK, Ingemarsson I, Leideman T, et al. Effect of ritodrine on labor after premature rupture of the membranes. *Obstet Gynecol* 1980;55:187–190.

468 Garite TJ, Keegan KA, Freeman RK, Nageotte MP. A randomized trial of ritodrine tocolysis versus expectant management in patients with premature rupture of membranes at 25 to 30 weeks of gestation. *Am J Obstet Gynecol* 1987;157:388–393.

469 Matsuda Y, Ikenoue T, Hokanishi H. Premature rupture of the membranes – aggressive versus conservative approach: effect of tocolytic and antibiotic therapy. *Gynecol Obstet Invest* 1993;36:102–107.

470 Weiner CP, Renk K, Klugman M. The therapeutic efficacy and cost-effectiveness of aggressive tocolysis for premature labor associated with premature rupture of the membranes. *Am J Obstet Gynecol* 1988;159:216–222.

471 Decavalas G, Mastrogiannis D, Papadopoulos V, Tzingounis V. Short-term versus long-term prophylactic tocolysis in patients with preterm premature rupture of membranes. *Eur J Obstet Gynecol Reprod Biol* 1995;59:143–147.

472 Harger JH. Comparison of success and morbidity in cervical cerclage procedures. *Obstet Gynecol* 1980;56:543–548.

473 Yeast JD, Garite TR. The role of cervical cerclage in the management of preterm premature rupture of the membranes. *Am J Obstet Gynecol* 1988;158:106–110.

474 Blickstein I, Katz Z, Lancet M, Molgilner BM. The outcome of pregnancies complicated by preterm rupture of the membranes with and without cerclage. *Int J Gynaecol Obstet* 1989;28:237–242.

475 Goldman JM, Greene MF, Tuomala R, et al. Outcome of expectant management in preterm premature rupture of membranes with cervical cerclage in place. Abstract 139. Presented at the Tenth Annual Meeting of the Society of Perinatal Obstetricians, Houston, Texas, 1990.

476 Ludmir J, Bader T, Chen L, et al. Poor perinatal outcome associated with retained cerclage in patients with premature rupture of membranes. *Obstet Gynecol* 1994;84:823–826.

477 McElrath TF, Norwitz ER, Lieberman ES, Heffner LJ. Perinatal outcome after preterm premature rupture of membranes with in situ cervical cerclage. *Am J Obstet Gynecol* 2002;187:1147–1152.

478 ACOG Technical Bulletin No. 15. *Premature rupture of the membranes*. Washington, DC: ACOG, 1988.

479 Carlan SJ, O'Brien WF, Parsons MT, Lense JJ. Preterm premature rupture of membranes: a randomized study of home versus hospital management. *Obstet Gynecol* 1993;81:61–64.

480 Philipson EH, Hoffman DS, Hansen GO, Ingardia CJ. Preterm premature rupture of membranes: experience with latent periods in excess of seven days. *Am J Perinatol* 1994;11:416–419.

481 Curet LB, Rao AV, Zachman RD, et al. Association between ruptured membranes, tocolytic therapy, and respiratory distress syndrome. *Am J Obstet Gynecol* 1984;148:263–268.

482 Ustun C, Kokcu A, Cil E, Kandemir B. Relationship between endomyometritis and the duration of premature membrane rupture. *J Matern Fetal Med* 1998;7:243–246.

483 McElrath TF, Allred EN, Leviton A. Prolonged latency after preterm premature rupture of membranes: an evaluation of histologic condition and intracranial ultrasonic abnormality in the neonate born at < 28 weeks of gestation. *Am J Obstet Gynecol* 2003;189:794–798.

484 Cox SM, Leveno KJ. Intentional delivery versus expectant management with preterm ruptured membranes at 30–34 weeks' gestation. *Obstet Gynecol* 1995;86:875–879.

485 Lieman JM, Brumfield CG, Carlo W, Ramsey PS. Preterm premature rupture of membranes: is there an optimal gestational age for delivery? *Obstet Gynecol* 2005;105:12–17.

486 Taylor J, Garite TJ. Premature rupture of membranes before fetal viability. *Obstet Gynecol* 1984;64:615–620.

487 Moretti M, Sibai BM. Maternal and perinatal outcome of expectant management of premature rupture of membranes in the midtrimester. *Am J Obstet Gynecol* 1988;159:390–396.

488 Major CA, Kitzmiller JL. Perinatal survival with expectant management of midtrimester rupture of membranes. *Am J Obstet Gynecol* 1990;163:838–844.

489 Beydoun SN, Yasin SY. Premature rupture of the membranes before 28 weeks: conservative management. *Am J Obstet Gynecol* 1986;155:471–479.

490 Bengtson JM, VanMarter LJ, Barss VA, et al. Pregnancy outcome after premature rupture of the membranes at or before 26 weeks' gestation. *Obstet Gynecol* 1989;73:921–927.

491 Hibbard JU, Hibbard MC, Ismail M, Arendt E. Pregnancy outcome after expectant management of premature rupture of the membranes in the second trimester. *J Reprod Med* 1993;38:945–951.

492 Morales WJ, Talley T. Premature rupture of membranes at < 25 weeks: a management dilemma. *Am J Obstet Gynecol* 1993;168: 503–507.

493 Fortunato SJ, Welt SI, Eggleston MK, Jr, Bryant EC. Active expectant management in very early gestations complicated by premature rupture of the fetal membranes. *J Reprod Med* 1994;39:13–16.

494 Rib DM, Sherer DM, Woods JR, Jr. Maternal and neonatal outcome associated with prolonged premature rupture of membranes below 26 weeks' gestation. *Am J Perinatol* 1993;10: 369–373.

495 David J, Permezel M. Pregnancy outcomes following preterm premature rupture of the membranes at less than 26 weeks' gestation. *Aust NZ J Obstet Gynaecol* 1992;32:120.

496 Mercer BM. Management of premature rupture of membranes before 26 weeks' gestation. *Obstet Gynecol Clin North Am* 1992;19:339–351.

497 ACOG Practice Bulletin. *Clinical management guidelines for obstetrician–gynecologists*, No. 1. Washington, DC: ACOG; 1998:586.

498 Healy AJ, Veille JC, Sciscione A, et al. The timing of elective delivery in preterm premature rupture of the membranes: a survey of members of the Society of Maternal–Fetal Medicine. *Am J Obstet Gynecol* 2004;190:1479–1481.

499 Strong TH, Jr. Amnioinfusion with preterm, premature rupture of membranes. *Clin Perinatol* 1992;19:399–409.

500 Gabbe SG, Ettinger BB, Freeman RK, Martin CB. Umbilical cord compression associated with amniotomy: laboratory observations. *Am J Obstet Gynecol* 1976;126:353–355.
501 Moberg LJ, Garite TJ, Freeman RK. Fetal heart rate patterns and fetal distress in patients with preterm premature rupture of membranes. *Obstet Gynecol* 1984;64:60–64.
502 Miyazaki FS, Taylor NA. Saline amnioinfusion for relief of variable or prolonged decelerations. A preliminary report. *Am J Obstet Gynecol* 1983;146:670–678.
503 Miyazaki FS, Nevarez F. Saline amnioinfusion for relief of repetitive variable decelerations: a prospective randomized study. *Am J Obstet Gynecol* 1985;153:301–306.
504 Nageotte MP, Freeman RK, Garite TJ, Dorchester W. Prophylactic intrapartum amnioinfusion in patients with preterm premature rupture of membranes. *Am J Obstet Gynecol* 1985; 153:557–562.
505 Hofmeyr GJ. Amnioinfusion: a question of benefits and risks. *Br J Obstet Gynaecol* 1992;99:449–451.
506 Wenstrom KD, Andrews WW, Maher JE. Prevalence and complications associated with amnioinfusion. *Am J Obstet Gynecol* 1994;170:341.
507 Fraser WD, Hofmeyr J, Lede R, et al. Amnioinfusion for the prevention of the meconium aspiration syndrome. *N Engl J Med* 2005;353:909–917.
508 Tranquilli AL, Giannubilo SR, Bezzeccheri V, Scagnoli C. Transabdominal amnioinfusion in preterm premature rupture of membranes: a randomised controlled trial. *Br J Obstet Gynaecol* 2005;112:759–763.
509 Gembruch U, Hansmann M. Artificial instillation of amniotic fluid as a new technique for the diagnostic evaluation of cases of oligohydramnios. *Prenat Diagn* 1988;8:33–45.
510 Chua S, Arulkumaran S, Yap C, et al. Premature rupture of membranes in nulliparas at term with unfavorable cervices: a double-blind randomized trial of prostaglandin and placebo. *Obstet Gynecol* 1995;86:550–554.
511 Chung T, Rogers MS, Gordon H, Chang A. Prelabour rupture of the membranes at term and unfavourable cervix; a randomized placebo-controlled trial on early intervention with intravaginal prostaglandin E2 gel. *Aust NZ J Obstet Gynaecol* 1992;32:25–27.
512 Duff P, Huff RW, Gibbs RS. Management of premature rupture of membranes and unfavorable cervix in term pregnancy. *Obstet Gynecol* 1984;63:697–702.
513 Ekman-Ordeberg G, Uldbjerg N, Ulmsten U. Comparison of intravenous oxytocin and vaginal prostaglandin E2 gel in women with unripe cervixes and premature rupture of the membranes. *Obstet Gynecol* 1985;66:307–310.
514 Gonen R, Samberg I, Degani S. Intracervical prostaglandin E2 for induction of labor in patients with premature rupture of membranes and an unripe cervix. *Am J Perinatol* 1994;11: 436–438.
515 Grant JM, Serle E, Mahmood T, et al. Management of prelabour rupture of the membranes in term primigravidae: report of a randomized prospective trial. *Br J Obstet Gynaecol* 1992;99:557–562.
516 Hagskog K, Nisell H, Sarman I, Westgren M. Conservative ambulatory management of prelabor rupture of the membranes at term in nulliparous women. *Acta Obstet Gynecol Scand* 1994;73:765–769.
517 Hannah ME, Ohlsson A, Farine D, et al. Induction of labor compared with expectant management for prelabor rupture of the membranes at term. TERMPROM Study Group. *N Engl J Med* 1996;334:1005–1010.
518 Hjertberg R, Hammarstrom M, Moberger B, et al. Premature rupture of the membranes (PROM) at term in nulliparous women with a ripe cervix. A randomized trial of 12 or 24 hours of expectant management. *Acta Obstet Gynecol Scand* 1996;75:48–53.
519 Ladfors L, Mattsson LA, Eriksson M, Fall O. A randomised trial of two expectant managements of prelabour rupture of the membranes at 34 to 42 weeks. *Br J Obstet Gynaecol* 1996;103:755–762.
520 Mahmood TA, Dick MJ, Smith NC, Templeton AA. Role of prostaglandin in the management of prelabour rupture of the membranes at term. *Br J Obstet Gynaecol* 1992;99:112–117.
521 Mahmood TA, Dick MJ. A randomized trial of management of pre-labor rupture of membranes at term in multiparous women using vaginal prostaglandin gel. *Obstet Gynecol* 1995;85:71–74.
522 Malik N, Gittens L, Gonzalez D, et al. Clinical amnionitis and endometritis in patients with premature rupture of membranes: endocervical prostaglandin E2 gel versus oxytocin for induction of labor. *Obstet Gynecol* 1996;88:540–543.
523 Morales WJ, Lazar AJ. Expectant management of rupture of membranes at term. *South Med J* 1986;79:955–958.
524 Mozurkewich E, Wolf F. Premature rupture of membranes at term: a meta-analysis of three management schemes. *Obstet Gynecol* 1997;89:1035–1043.
525 Natale R, Milne JK, Campbell MK, et al Management of premature rupture of membranes at term: randomized trial. *Am J Obstet Gynecol* 1994;171:936–939.
526 Ngai SW, To WK, Lao T, Ho PC. Cervical priming with oral misoprostol in pre-labor rupture of membranes at term. *Obstet Gynecol* 1996;87:923–926.
527 Ray DA, Garite TJ. Prostaglandin E2 for induction of labor in patients with premature rupture of membranes at term. *Am J Obstet Gynecol* 1992;166:836–843.
528 Rydhstrom H, Ingemarsson I. No benefit from conservative management in nulliparous women with premature rupture of the membranes (PROM) at term. A randomized study. *Acta Obstet Gynecol Scand* 1991;70:543–547.
529 Rymer J, Parker A. A comparison of Syntocinon infusion with prostaglandin vaginal pessaries when spontaneous rupture of the membranes occurs without labour after 34 weeks gestation. *Aust NZ J Obstet Gynaecol* 1992;32:22–24.
530 Shalev E, Schantz A, Wahlin A, et al. Management of prelabor rupture of membranes at term. A randomized study. *Acta Obstet Gynecol Scand* 1993;72:627.
531 Shalev E, Peleg D, Eliyahu S, Nahum Z. Comparison of 12- and 72-hour expectant management of premature rupture of membranes in term pregnancies. *Obstet Gynecol* 1995;85:766–768.
532 Wagner MV, Chin VP, Peters CJ, et al. A comparison of early and delayed induction of labor with spontaneous rupture of membranes at term. *Obstet Gynecol* 1989;74:93–97.
533 Zlatnik FJ. Management of premature rupture of membranes at term. *Obstet Gynecol Clin North Am* 1992;19:353–364.
534 Tan BP, Hannah ME. Oxytocin for prelabour rupture of membranes at or near term. *Cochrane Database Syst Rev* 2000;CD000157.
535 Lin MG, Nuthalapaty FS, Carver AR, et al. Misoprostol for labor induction in women with term premature rupture of membranes: a meta-analysis. *Obstet Gynecol* 2005;106:593–601.
536 Dare MR, Middleton P, Crowther CA, et al. Planned early birth versus expectant management (waiting) for prelabour rupture of membranes at term (37 weeks or more). *Cochrane Database Syst Rev* 2006;1:CD005302.
537 Hannah ME, Hodnett ED, Willan A, et al. Prelabor rupture of

the membranes at term: expectant management at home or in hospital? The TermPROM Study Group. *Obstet Gynecol* 2000;96:533–538.

538 Genz HJ. [Treatment of premature rupture of the fetal membranes by means of fibrin adhesion]. *Med Welt* 1979;30:1557–1559.

539 Kurz C, Hick A. Fibrin sealing: an advanced therapy in dealing with premature rupture of membranes. *J Perinat Med* 1982;66.

540 Baumgarten K, Moser S. The technique of fibrin adhesion for premature rupture of the membranes during pregnancy. *J Perinat Med* 1986;14:43–49.

541 Uchide K, Terada S, Hamasaki H, et al. Intracervical fibrin instillation as an adjuvant to treatment for second trimester rupture of membranes. *Arch Gynecol Obstet* 1994;255:95–98.

542 Catalano A, Zardini E. [Premature rupture of the membranes. Spontaneous course of the event and the therapeutic approach with a human fibrin glue]. *Minerva Ginecol* 1994;46:675–680.

543 Sciscione AC, Manley JS, Pollock M, et al. Intracervical fibrin sealants: a potential treatment for early preterm premature rupture of the membranes. *Am J Obstet Gynecol* 2001;184: 368–373.

544 Quintero RA, Romero R, Dzieczkowski J, et al. Sealing of ruptured amniotic membranes with intra-amniotic platelet-cryoprecipitate plug. *Lancet* 1996;347:1117.

545 Quintero RA. Treatment of previable premature ruptured membranes. *Clin Perinatol* 2003;30:573–589.

546 Vaitkiene D, Bergstrom S. Management of amniocentesis in women with oligohydramnios due to membrane rupture: evaluation of a cervical adapter. *Gynecol Obstet Invest* 1995;40:28–31.

547 O'Brien JM, Barton JR, Milligan DA. An aggressive interventional protocol for early midtrimester premature rupture of the membranes using gelatin sponge for cervical plugging. *Am J Obstet Gynecol* 2002;187:1143–1146.

548 Quintero RA. New horizons in the treatment of preterm premature rupture of membranes. *Clin Perinatol* 2001;28:861–875.

549 Ferrand PE, Fujimoto T, Chennathukuzhi V, et al. The CARD15 2936insC mutation and TLR4 896 A→G polymorphism in African Americans and risk of preterm premature rupture of membranes (PPROM). *Mol Hum Reprod* 2002;8:1031–1034.

550 Kalish RB, Vardhana S, Gupta M, et al. Interleukin-1 receptor antagonist gene polymorphism and multifetal pregnancy outcome. *Am J Obstet Gynecol* 2003;189:911–914.

551 Kalish RB, Vardhana S, Gupta M, et al. Polymorphisms in the tumor necrosis factor-alpha gene at position –308 and the inducible 70 kd heat shock protein gene at position +1267 in multifetal pregnancies and preterm premature rupture of fetal membranes. *Am J Obstet Gynecol* 2004;191:1368–1374.

552 Kalish RB, Nguyen DP, Vardhana S, et al. A single nucleotide A→G polymorphism at position –670 in the Fas gene promoter: relationship to preterm premature rupture of fetal membranes in multifetal pregnancies. *Am J Obstet Gynecol* 2005;192:208–212.

553 Annells MF, Hart PH, Mullighan CG, et al. Interleukins-1, -4, -6, -10, tumor necrosis factor, transforming growth factor-beta, FAS, and mannose-binding protein C gene polymorphisms in Australian women: risk of preterm birth. *Am J Obstet Gynecol* 2004;191:2056–2067.

554 Fuks A, Parton LA, Polavarapu S, et al. Polymorphism of Fas and Fas ligand in preterm premature rupture of membranes in singleton pregnancies. *Am J Obstet Gynecol* 2005;193:1132–1136.

555 Hussey MJ, Levy ES, Pombar X, et al. Evaluating rapid diagnostic tests of intra-amniotic infection: Gram stain, amniotic fluid glucose level, and amniotic fluid to serum glucose level ratio. *Am J Obstet Gynecol* 1998;179:650–656.

556 Maymon E, Romero R, Chaiworapongsa T, et al. Value of amniotic fluid neutrophil collagenase concentrations in preterm premature rupture of membranes. *Am J Obstet Gynecol* 2001;185: 1143–1148.

557 Romero R, Ghidini A, Bahado-Singh R. Premature rupture of the membranes. In: Reece E, Hobbins J, Mahoney M, Petrie R, eds. *Medicine of the fetus and mother*. Philadelphia: Lippincott; 1992:1430–1468.

558 Goldstein I, Copel J, Hobbins J. Fetal behavior in preterm premature rupture of the membranes. *Clin Perinatol* 1989;16:735.

559 Asrat T, Nageote M, Garite T, et al. Gram stain results from amniocentesis in patients with preterm premature rupture of the membranes. *Am J Obstet Gynecol* 1991;163:887.

560 Romero R, Gomez R, Galasso M, et al. Is oligohydramnios a risk factor for infection in term premature rupture of membranes? *Ultrasound Obstet Gynecol* 1994;4:95–100.

64 Prolonged pregnancy

Curtis L. Lowery and Paul Wendel

Prolonged pregnancy may be defined as any pregnancy that continues past 294 days.[1,2] It is well established that the prolonged pregnancy is associated with increased maternal and fetal morbidity and mortality.[3–5] Postdatism implies that the pregnancy has endured longer than the estimated due date of 40 weeks. The postmature syndrome is associated with intrauterine growth restriction and occurs when there is placental insufficiency often caused by an aging placenta.[6–8] The most common cause of the prolonged pregnancy is inaccurate dating. Ultrasound has proved effective in reducing the number of inappropriate inductions.[9,10] Anencephaly and adrenal hypoplasia have been associated with prolonged pregnancy, and both share a common feature of pituitary insufficiency, and show an absence of the usually high estrogen levels that characterize normal pregnancy.[11,12] Despite improvements in pregnancy dating, the prolonged pregnancy continues to present a significant problem for healthcare providers.

Definitions

Multiple terms including postterm, prolonged, postdates, and postmature have been used to describe pregnancies exceeding their due date. The lack of standardized definitions has made comparison between studies on the prolonged pregnancy extremely difficult. Postterm or prolonged pregnancy should be the preferred terminology for the pregnancy extended beyond 42 weeks. Postmaturity is a neonatal diagnosis and should be used to describe the infant with recognizable clinical features associated with postmaturity, including peeling, parchment-like skin, and meconium staining of skin, membranes, and the umbilical cord. In addition, these infants may also have overgrown nails, well-developed creases on the palms and soles, abundance of scalp hair, little vernix or lanugo hair, scaphoid abdomen, and minimal subcutaneous fat.[13,14] Like most medical conditions, the syndrome exhibits a continuum that varies from mild placental insufficiency to a more severe medical problem with significant growth restriction and a greater probability of associated hypoxia.

Incidence

Around 20% of women cannot remember their last menstrual period and, when there is late entry to prenatal care, there is often confusion regarding the dating of the pregnancy.[15] The incidence of prolonged pregnancy varies from 3% to as high as 14%, depending on whether first-trimester ultrasound dating or last menstrual period dating has been used to determine the estimated date of delivery.[10,16] Women with one previous prolonged pregnancy have a 30% chance of a recurrent prolonged pregnancy.[17] In centers in which patients are seen early in pregnancy and have ultrasounds in the first trimester, the incidence of the prolonged pregnancy has been reduced by half to two-thirds.[10,16] Perinatal mortality has been noted to increase in pregnancies with unknown dates.[18] It is possible that some of these deaths are due to a failure to diagnose the prolonged pregnancy. It is also important to remember, when managed conservatively, 40–50% of women will deliver within 4–5 days of the 42nd week.[19]

Maternal and fetal risks

Maternal risks

The maternal risks from the prolonged pregnancy are associated with the increased need for operative delivery in both spontaneous and induced labor. Controversy remains as to whether spontaneous labor has a lower incidence of operative delivery than those patients who require induction.[20,21] There may also be an increase in fetal macrosomia and uteroplacental insufficiency, which predisposes the patient to an increased incidence of operative delivery. Conservative therapy and awaiting labor may not avoid the need for operative interventions resulting from these problems.[22,23] The National Institute of Child Health and Human Development Network of Maternal–Fetal Medicine Units reported that induction of labor in pregnancies ≥ 41 weeks was not associated with a significant increase in Cesarean delivery rates

Table 64.1 Summary odds ratios for Cesarean section in randomized trials of elective induction versus expectant management.*

Group	Odds ratio	95% confidence interval
By gestational age:		
< 41 weeks	0.6	0.35–1.03
> 41 weeks	0.87	0.77–0.99
By parity:		
Primigravid	0.75	0.64–0.88
Multigravid		
Bishop score < 6	1.02	0.75–1.38
By overall Cesarean section rate:		
< 10%	0.89	0.58–1.39
> 10%	0.87	0.77–1.00
By class of induction agent:		
Oxytocin	0.85	0.74–0.98
Prostaglandins	0.84	0.65–1.08

Data from Crowley (2000);[9] odds ratios < 1 indicate that the Cesarean section rate was lower in the elective induction group.

compared with awaiting spontaneous labor. In this study, 440 patients with uncomplicated pregnancies at 41 weeks' gestation were randomized to either immediate induction of labor ($n = 265$) or expectant management ($n = 175$). The Cesarean delivery rate was not significantly different in the expectant (18%), prostaglandin E_2 gel (23%), or placebo gel (18%) groups.[24]

In the Canadian Multicenter study involving 3407 women at > 42 weeks' gestation, there was a statistically significant lower Cesarean section rate in the induction group of 21.2% compared with the conservatively managed group with a Cesarean section rate of 24.5%.[25] The higher Cesarean section rate was felt to be the result of a greater incidence of fetal distress in the conservatively managed group. A later cost estimate of this trial showed that induction of labor was associated with a significantly lower cost (US$2502 versus US$2684).[26] In Table 64.1, data from the Cochrane database are summarized, and it would appear from these studies that the prolonged pregnancy is associated with an increased need for operative vaginal delivery, induction of labor, and Cesarean section. The study shows that inductions prior to 42 weeks may reduce the need for Cesarean sections.

Fetal and neonatal risks

Multiple studies have demonstrated an increased risk of perinatal mortality after 42 weeks.[6,16,27–42] Perinatal mortality reaches its nadir at 39–40 weeks and then increases as pregnancy exceeds 41 weeks.[43] These deaths occur during the antepartum, intrapartum, and neonatal period as the result of events related to either uteroplacental insufficiency or through the development of fetal macrosomia and commonly associated birth trauma. During the antepartum period, the fetus may suffer hypoxic ischemic insults that can result in either stillbirth or intrauterine growth restriction and the development of the postmature syndrome.

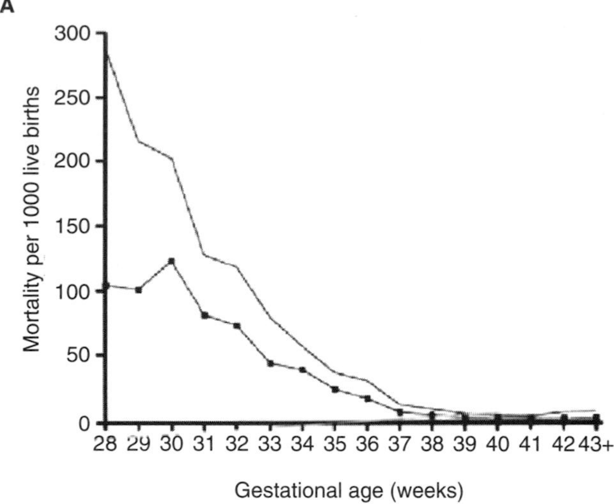

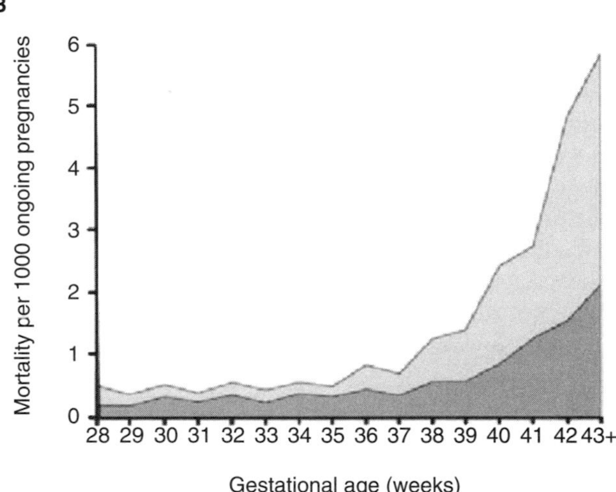

Figure 64.1 (A) The rates of stillbirth (-■-) and infant mortality (—) for each week of gestation from 28 to 43+ weeks expressed per 1000 live births. (B) The rates of stillbirth (dark gray) and infant mortality (light gray) in the same population of 171 527 singleton births expressed as a function of 1000 ongoing (undelivered) pregnancies. Data from Hilder et al.[44] (with permission of Blackwell Science Ltd).

Traditional reports of stillbirth rates have commonly used, as the denominator, the number of deaths per 1000 newborns. This estimate fails to provide a realistic risk assessment, which is the number of deaths per continuing pregnancies. Stillbirth rates should be reported based on a denominator that will provide the most appropriate statement of risk. Studies have shown that pregnancies that continue beyond 42 weeks have an increased risk of stillbirth (see Fig. 64.1A) but, when the risk of stillbirth is expressed as a function of ongoing

Table 64.2 Observed relationship between gestational age and stillbirth risk.

Study	Location	Dates	*n*	Stillbirth risk per 1000													
				Denominator: 1000 deliveries in specified gestational week							Denominator: 1000 continuing pregnancies						
				37	38	39	40	41	42	43	37	38	39	40	41	42	43
Yudkin et al. (1987)	Oxford	1978–1985	40 888	2.14		0.43		1.24			0.42		0.29		1.24		
Hilder et al. (1998)	London	1989–1991	171 527	6.2	3.8	2.2	1.5	1.7	1.9	2.1	0.35	0.56	0.57	0.86	1.27	1.55	2.12
Cotzias et al. (1999)	London	1989–1991	171 527	–	–	–	–	–	–	–	1.55	1.37	1.19	1.08	1.21	1.30	1.58
Smith (2001)	Scotland	1985–1996	700 878	–	–	–	–	–	–	–	0.4	0.4	0.5	0.9	1.2	1.9	6.3

From ref. 58.

pregnancies (stillbirth divided by total births), the mortality rate is even greater. In a retrospective study by Hilder et al.[44] of 177 527 singleton births (1989–1991), the rate of stillbirths increases sixfold from 0.35 per 1000 ongoing pregnancies at 37 weeks to 2.12 per 1000 ongoing pregnancies at 43 weeks (see Fig. 64.1B). This difference was even more striking when the infant mortality statistics were included, showing an eight-fold increased risk of pregnancy loss (stillbirth plus death within the first year of life) from 0.7 per 1000 ongoing pregnancies at 37 weeks to 5.8 per 1000 pregnancies at 43 weeks' gestation (Table 64.2).

The literature has been inconsistent in reporting the frequency and type of antenatal surveillance of the prolonged pregnancy.[2] No single method of fetal assessment has proved superior in either sensitivity or specificity of fetal evaluation in the prolonged pregnancy, and there have been no randomized, controlled trials in which surveillance was compared with no surveillance. The Agency for Healthcare Research and Quality (AHRQ) published an evidence-based report/technology assessment on the management of the prolonged pregnancy.[45,46] A detailed description of the tests used to evaluate the prolonged pregnancy is undertaken in the chapter entitled "Normal and abnormal placentation." This group estimated that, if the perinatal mortality rate was 1.2 per 1000 births at 41 weeks, a randomized file would need over 40 000 women in each arm to determine a twofold difference in the risk of stillbirth between two competing methods of surveillance. As with most tests, there is a tradeoff between specificity and sensitivity. Tests that are more sensitive are usually less specific. As it has been well established that the probability of adverse fetal outcome increases with increasing gestational age, then antepartum tests with high negative predictive values are needed. Data reported by Bochner et al.[47] are consistent with this concept and showed positive predictive values for adverse outcomes were better when testing began at 42 weeks (21.1% versus 11.9% at 41 weeks), but negative predictive values were worse (98.5% at 42 weeks versus 99.1% at 41 weeks). Assuming that induction of labor does not carry increased perinatal risk, planned induction of labor at any gestational age should always result in fewer adverse perinatal outcomes than continuing pregnancies with testing strategies.

A fetal mortality rate of 1.12 per 1000 was reported in a review of 8038 consecutive postterm pregnancies with twice-weekly antepartum fetal surveillance protocols using nonstress tests, fluid indices, and biophysical profiles as needed.[9,48] As noted above, most prolonged pregnancies occur as a result of poor dating and are often not in fact prolonged. Combined with improved antepartum fetal surveillance, it will be difficult to show that induction of labor at 41 weeks as opposed to 42 weeks will significantly improve mortality rates.

Most of the excessive perinatal mortality associated with a prolonged pregnancy occurs in the intrapartum and neonatal periods.[49] Intrapartum asphyxia and meconium aspiration were implicated in 25% of the deaths. Also, 5.4 per 1000 postterm infants compared with 0.9 per 1000 term infants exhibited early neonatal seizures. Meconium aspiration syndrome is significantly increased in these patients.[29,50–54]

Fetal macrosomia

It is important to remember that the most common complication of the prolonged pregnancy is fetal macrosomia. Macrosomia has been defined as newborn birthweights of either 4000 g or 4500 g. Macrosomia can result in dystocia and associated brachioplexus injuries and fractures. In a study by Pollack et al.,[55] 21% of the pregnancies beyond 41 weeks had infants weighing more than 4000 g, and 4% of these fetuses weighed more than 4500 g. Labor induction, Cesarean delivery, fetal macrosomia, and shoulder dystocia are also significantly increased.[51] The clinical significance of birthweights between 4000 and 4500 g is unclear, but it has been well established that shoulder dystocia is greatest for infants weighing > 4500 g.[53,56,57]

As both mother and fetus are at risk from macrosomia, attempts have been made to determine fetal weights in prolonged pregnancies. Table 64.3 reports on test performance characteristics for studies outlining the association between estimated fetal weights and macrosomia, as compiled by

Table 64.3 Accuracy of antenatal fetal weight estimation for predicting macrosomia.

Study	Screening test threshold	Rate of abnormal tests	Outcome threshold	Rate of outcome event	Sensitivity	Specificity	Positive predictive value	Negative predictive value
Chauhan et al. (1995)	> 4000 g	0.21	> 4000 g	0.26	0.61	0.92	0.73	0.87
O'Reilly-Green and Divon (1997)	> 3710 g	0.42	> 4000 g	0.24	0.85	0.72	0.49	0.94
Chervenak et al. (1989)	> 4000 g	0.22	> 4000 g	0.26	0.60	0.91	0.69	0.87
Pollack et al. (1992)	> 4000 g	0.20	> 4000 g	0.23	0.56	0.91	0.65	0.88
Jazayeri et al. (1999)	Abdominal circumference > 34 cm	0.48	> 4000 g	0.50	0.89	0.93	0.93	0.90
Gilby et al. (2000)	Abdominal circumference > 38 cm	0.05	> 4500 g	0.03	0.54	0.97	0.37	0.98
O'Reilly-Green and Divon (1997)	> 4500 g	0.02	> 4500 g	0.04	0.22	0.99	0.44	0.97
O'Reilly-Green and Divon (1997)	> 4191 g	0.11	> 4500 g	0.04	0.83	0.92	0.30	0.99
Pollack et al. (1992)	> 4500 g	0.02	> 4500 g	0.04	0.14	0.99	0.33	0.96
Gilby et al. (2000)	Abdominal circumference > 34 cm	0.38	> 4500 g	0.03	0.99	0.65	0.09	1.00

Myers et al.[58] for the AHRQ publication *Management of prolonged pregnancy: evidence report/technology assessment no. 53*. Chauhan et al.[59] compared estimates of fetal weight by clinicians using Leopold maneuvers in early labor with ultrasound measures with the actual newborn birthweights (see Table 64.3). In this study, the clinical estimates were significantly better at estimating within 10% of actual weight than ultrasound calculations (clinical 65.4% versus sonographic 42.8%; $P < 0.005$). Chervenak et al.[60] calculated fetal weights in 317 women followed conservatively for the management of prolonged pregnancy. In this study, 24% of women had infants born weighing more than 4000 g and, of this group, 22% versus 10% of the control subjects ($P < 0.01$) had Cesarean sections for protracted disorders. The sensitivity of ultrasound for predicting birthweight > 4000 g was 61%, specificity 91%, positive predictive value 70%, and predictive value 87%. In Table 64.3, we see the effects of test threshold on outcome prediction.

Gilby et al.[61] compared fetal abdominal circumference measurements of 34–38 cm and prediction of birthweight > 4000 g. At 34 cm, 38% of the population was selected; however, when 38 cm was used, only 5% of the population met this threshold. At the 34-cm threshold, the sensitivity was 99%, while at 38 cm, the sensitivity was only 54%. The specificity was much lower at 65% for the less stringent 34-cm value, whereas the 38-cm measurement gave a specificity of 97%. The positive predictive values yielded 9% and 37% respectively. Similar results were obtained from the 1997 O'Reilly-Green and Divon[62] study when comparing ultrasound weight calculated thresholds (4191–4500 g). From these comparisons, we can determine that stringent thresholds for the diagnosis of macrosomia yield poor sensitivities but improved specificities and positive predictive values. The obvious question is where the threshold for intervention should be set. In 1996, Rouse et al.[63] performed a cost analysis finding that, if Cesarean sections are performed on all pregnancies with estimated fetal weights of 4500 g, 3695 Cesarean sections at a cost of US$8 million would be performed to prevent one permanent brachioplexus injury. There are limited data to support whether induction of labor in patients with estimated fetal weights between 4000 and 4500 g reduces newborn or maternal morbidity. Methods for prediction of birthweights more than 4500 g in the routine prolonged pregnancy are imprecise. There is no evidence that ultrasound-guided clinical decision-making can accurately identify macrosomia and whether the use of this modality can change clinical outcomes.

Management

While there is no clear consensus as to the most clinically correct method for the management of the prolonged pregnancy in recent times, most physicians now plan inductions at 41 or 42 weeks. While there is an increased incidence of stillbirth with increasing gestational age, this incidence does not become significant until 42 weeks, and most studies have shown no clear benefit from the induction of labor versus conservative management with aggressive fetal assessment. The two big questions to be answered are whether induction of labor before 42 weeks increases the incidence of Cesarean section and does this approach result in a greater cost than conservative therapy? The absolute goal for the management of the prolonged pregnancy is to reduce newborn morbidity and prevent all stillbirths, while at the same time keeping the Cesarean section and operative vaginal delivery rates as low as possible.

Pregnancy dating

The most important way to minimize the incorrect diagnosis of postterm pregnancy is to establish accurate pregnancy dating as early as possible. With accurate dating, making decisions regarding induction or conservative management can be improved based upon more objective information. The estimated delivery date (EDD), as calculated from the last menstrual period (LMP), can be used reliably in women with regular normal menstrual cycles, especially when these women are seen early in the pregnancy and a detailed history is obtained during their first visits. It is important to remember that many women cannot accurately recall their LMP, particularly when they start prenatal care late in their pregnancies. In women for whom there is uncertainty regarding their pregnancy dating, an ultrasound in the first or second trimesters should be obtained. The crown–rump length can determine gestational age to within 5 days.[10,64] Most clinicians accept the variation in ultrasonography generally as ± 7 days up to 20 weeks of gestation, ± 14 days between 20 and 30 weeks of gestation, and ± 21 days beyond 30 weeks of gestation. The use of ultrasound dating in these situations has significantly reduced the false diagnosis of prolonged pregnancy.[16,64,65]

When the ultrasound measurements differ from the LMP by more than these ranges, ultrasound estimates of EDD should be used. Serial measurements of symphysis fundal height may be useful in identifying the occasional case of growth restriction or macrosomia; however, these measurements are of no value in establishing gestational age. Again, ultrasound measurements should be obtained when there are variations in the fundal height before clinical interventions are undertaken.

Induction versus expectant management

Physicians concerned about adverse events in patients beyond 40 weeks' gestation lean toward induction of labor. A stillbirth occurring during this period is often viewed as preventable among patients and physicians alike, who often believe that induction of labor may have avoided this untoward event. In the NIH-sponsored Maternal–Fetal Medicine Network trial, induction of labor at 41 weeks was compared with expectant management. The expectant management group's surveillance consisted of nonstress testing and amniotic fluid assessment. There were 265 patients in the induction group and 175 patients in the expectant management group. The rate of Cesarean section was similar between the two groups, with no difference in perinatal deaths.[24]

In the Canadian Multicenter postterm pregnancy trial by Hannah et al.,[25] singleton pregnancies at 41 weeks or more were assigned to induction or antepartum monitoring. Patients in the monitored group were asked to perform kick counts each day, while receiving nonstress testing three times a week and amniotic fluid assessment two to three times per week. The monitored patients were delivered at 44 weeks or the time at which there were maternal or fetal indications. In this study, which was performed in 22 hospitals over a period of 5 years, perinatal morbidity and mortality were not statistically significant between groups, whereas Cesarean section rates were significantly lower in the induction of labor group.

In a study at Parkland Hospital performed by Alexander et al.,[66] a retrospective analysis assessed 56317 pregnancies delivered with gestational ages > 40 weeks. These patients were separated into three groups as determined by the gestational age at delivery, making 29136 at 40 weeks, 16386 at 41 weeks, and 10795 at 42 weeks. Patients with hypertension, prior Cesarean, diabetes, fetal malformations, breech presentation, and placenta previa were excluded. Labor complications including need for oxytocin, prolonged second stage of labor, overall length of labor, need for forceps delivery, and Cesarean section all increase with increasing gestational age. Neonatal outcomes were similar across all three groups. This study concluded that routine induction at 41 weeks would likely increase the need for operative obstetrics without changing neonatal outcome.

In a systematic review with meta-analysis, Sanchez-Ramos et al.[67] reviewed computerized databases, references and published studies, and textbook chapters in all languages to identify randomized, controlled trials evaluating induction and expected management of labor for postterm pregnancies. The primary outcome assessments were Cesarean delivery rates and perinatal mortality. Sixteen studies met the inclusion criteria, and women allocated to induction management compared with those who underwent expectant management had lower Cesarean section rates (20.0% versus 22.1%) [odds ratio (OR) 0.88; 95% confidence interval (CI) 0.78–0.99]. Perinatal mortality rates did not differ significantly between the groups; however, a sample size of 16 000 patients would be required for a power of 80% to detect a 50% reduction in perinatal mortality. This review concluded that a policy of labor induction at 41 weeks' gestation for uncomplicated singleton pregnancies would reduce Cesarean section delivery rates without compromising perinatal outcomes.

Similarly, a meta-analysis of 19 controlled trials for prolonged pregnancy at or beyond 290 days compared induction with intention to await spontaneous labor.[47] Conservative management was associated with a higher Cesarean section rate, 20.6% compared with 19.5%. The OR for perinatal mortality was 0.18 in favor of induction (95% CI 0.04–0.80).[46]

Induction of labor

The Bishop score was first reported in 1964 and has been used since that time as a tool to predict the success of induction.[68]

Table 64.4 Components of the Bishop score.

Examination findings	Score			
	0	1	2	3
Dilatation (cm)	Closed	1–2	3–4	> 5
Effacement (%)	0–30	40–50	60–70	> 80
Station	−3	−2	−1 or 0	+1, +2
Consistency	Firm	Medium	Soft	–
Position of cervix	Posterior	Midposition	Anterior	–

The Bishop score is based on five components: cervical dilation, cervical effacement, cervical consistency, cervical position, and the fetal station (see Table 64.4). From Bishop's original work, when the score was > 9, 100% of the cases were successfully induced.[69] Studies to date have provided only limited information that Bishop's scoring predicts the success of induction.[70] Hendrix et al.[71] evaluated Bishop score in women to determine its ability to predict the success of induction. This group concluded that the Bishop score was of limited value in predicting successful induction as there was no significant difference in the Bishop score between 253 women who delivered vaginally and 38 women who required Cesarean section. Several groups have reported that the Bishop score suffers from significant intraobserver variability, which may explain the poor predictive value of the test.[72] Given the intraobserver variability, the demonstrated poor predictive power, and the demonstrated success rates of induction protocols, Bishop scoring in the prolonged pregnancy should have limited applications.

Induction protocols

Based on current evidence, induction of labor at 41 weeks should be effective in reducing mortality. Many different approaches to cervical ripening and induction of labor have been reported. At present, there is no universally agreed upon method for the induction of labor. Recently, there has been a report of a randomized, controlled trial of castor oil for the promotion of labor. In this study, 52 women given 60 mg of castor oil were compared with 48 women with no treatment. In the castor oil group, 57.7% of the subjects went into labor within 24 h, but only 4.2% of the control patients experienced labor ($P < 0.001$).[73] Cesarean section rates were 19.2% in the castor oil group and 8.3% in the nontreatment group ($P = 0.20$). The most recent Cochrane review and AHRQ-evidenced reports on the management of prolonged pregnancy both felt that this was a significant finding.[45]

Sweeping or stripping of the membranes is a simple procedure performed during pelvic examination in which a finger placed in the cervix is swept in a circular fashion detaching the amniotic membranes from the cervical tissues. This procedure is felt to initiate labor due to the local release of prostaglandins when the membranes are detached. Most studies have shown that sweeping of the membranes can initiate labor in the term patient.[74–81] These studies have failed to show an increase in any adverse outcomes including infections or bleeding. Sweeping or stripping of the membranes appears to be a safe and effective method to aid in the induction of labor. As it is impossible to predict which patients will not be delivered at 41 weeks, a policy of stripping of membranes between 38 and 40 weeks does not seem justified. In those patients at 40 weeks or more with good pregnancy dating, consideration should be given to membrane stripping.

There have been a large number of trials that have evaluated the effects of inducing agents in the promotion of labor. Variations in patient populations and the relatively low number of women studied in each of these trials make it exceedingly difficult to arrive at definitive statements about the benefits and risks of these agents for use in the prolonged pregnancy. As a general rule, the more effective these agents are in initiating labor and shortening induction to delivery times, the more likely are these agents to produce uterine hyperstimulation and the subsequent associated fetal distress.[45] Prostaglandin E_2 (PGE_2) appears to be more effective than oxytocin, and misoprostol is more effective than PGE_2. Sweeping of the amniotic membranes may decrease the need for inducing agents.

Summary

Prolonged pregnancy is the preferred term to be used when pregnancies continue past 294 days. The incidence of prolonged pregnancy varies from 3% to 14%, and the most common cause of the prolonged pregnancy is inaccurate pregnancy dating. Approximately 20% of women cannot remember their last menstrual period. Studies have shown that, when women obtain prenatal care in the first trimester and have ultrasound performed when pregnancy dating is in question, the incidence of prolonged pregnancy is reduced by at least 50%. The postmature syndrome is a neonatal diagnosis made when newborns exhibit peeling, parchment-like skin, meconium staining of the skin, overgrown nails, abundant scalp hair, and minimal subcutaneous fat. This condition is likely the result of uteroplacental insufficiency and is associated with a greater probability of associated hypoxia. Maternal risks from the prolonged pregnancy are associated with an increased need for induction of labor, operative vaginal delivery, and increased need for Cesarean sections. Induction of labor at or beyond 41 weeks does not increase the incidence of Cesarean section and may be associated with a decrease in stillbirth rates and perinatal morbidity and mortality. As the incidence of stillbirth is low prior to 42 weeks, antepartum testing in the low-risk patient is probably not indicated prior to this time. Cervical ripening may reduce induction to delivery times, but may also increase uterine hypertonicity and fetal distress. Every attempt should be made to obtain accurate pregnancy dating as early as possible. Induction of labor at 41 weeks does not increase Cesarean section rates or pregnancy cost and may reduce the incidence of stillbirth and newborn morbidity and mortality.

Key points

1 Prolonged pregnancy may be defined as any pregnancy that continues past 294 days.

2 Prolonged pregnancy is associated with increased maternal and fetal morbidity and mortality.[4–6]

3 The most common cause of the prolonged pregnancy is inaccurate dating.

4 Postterm or prolonged pregnancy should be the preferred terminology for the pregnancy extending beyond 42 weeks.

5 Postmaturity is a neonatal diagnosis and should be used to describe the infant with recognizable clinical features associated with postmaturity including peeling, parchment-like skin, and meconium staining of skin, membranes, and the umbilical cord, with a possible incidence of overgrown nails, well-developed creases on the palms and soles, abundance of scalp hair, little vernix or lanugo hair, scaphoid abdomen, and minimal subcutaneous fat.[14,15]

6 Around 20% of women cannot remember their last menstrual period and, when there is late entry to prenatal care, there is often confusion regarding the dating of the pregnancy.[16]

7 The maternal risks from the prolonged pregnancy are associated with the increased need for operative delivery in both spontaneous and induced labor.

8 Induction of labor at 41 weeks does not increase Cesarean section rates or pregnancy cost and may reduce the incidence of stillbirth and newborn morbidity and mortality.

9 Multiple studies have demonstrated an increased risk of perinatal mortality after 42 weeks.[7,17,28–43]

10 Perinatal mortality reaches its nadir at 39–40 weeks and then increases as pregnancy exceeds 41 weeks.[44]

11 Studies have shown that pregnancies that continue beyond 42 weeks have an increased risk of stillbirth, but when the risk of stillbirth is expressed as a function of ongoing pregnancies (stillbirth divided by total births), the mortality rate is even greater.

12 Assuming that induction of labor does not carry increased perinatal risk, planned induction of labor at any gestational age should always result in fewer adverse perinatal outcomes and testing strategies.

13 Most of the excessive perinatal mortality associated with a prolonged pregnancy occurs in the intrapartum and neonatal periods.[50]

14 Conditions associated with prolonged pregnancy include intrapartum asphyxia, meconium aspiration, neonatal seizures,[50] fetal macrosomia resulting in dystocia and associated brachioplexus injuries and fractures, anencephaly, and adrenal hypoplasia with pituitary insufficiency.[12,13]

15 Given the intraobserver variability, the demonstrated poor predictive power, and the demonstrated success rates of induction protocols, Bishop scoring in the prolonged pregnancy should have limited applications.

16 The most important way to minimize the incorrect diagnosis of postterm pregnancy is to establish accurate pregnancy dating as early as possible.

17 In women for whom there is uncertainty regarding their pregnancy dating, an ultrasound in the first or second trimesters should be obtained.

18 The crown–rump length can determine gestational age to within 5 days.[10,66]

19 When the ultrasound measurements differ from the last menstrual period by more than the ranges shown, then ultrasound estimates of EDD should be used: up to 20 weeks' gestation, ± 7 days; between 20 and 30 weeks' gestation, ± 14 days; beyond 30 weeks' gestation, ± 21 days.

20 Induction of labor at or beyond 41 weeks does not increase the incidence of Cesarean section and may be associated with a decrease in stillbirth rates and perinatal morbidity and mortality.

References

1 Schmid S, Hendry M. [Prolonged pregnancy. Risks in pregnancy duration over 294 days and obstetric consequences.] *Gynakol Rundsch* 1991;31(3):144–152.

2 American College of Obstetricians and Gynecologists (ACOG). Management of postterm pregnancy. *ACOG Practice Patterns* 1997;6.

3 Bergsjo P, Huang GD, Yu SQ, et al. Comparison of induced versus non-induced labor in post-term pregnancy. A randomized prospective study. *Acta Obstet Gynecol Scand* 1989;68(8):683–687.

4 Cucco C, Osborne MA, Cibils LA. Maternal–fetal outcomes in prolonged pregnancy. *Am J Obstet Gynecol* 1989;161(4):916–920.

5 Maly Z, Grosmanova A, Pulkrabkova S, Gogela J. [Effect of birth weight on neonatal and maternal morbidity in expectant management of post-term pregnancy.] *Ceska Gynekol* 2002;67(Suppl. 1):20–22.

6 Bach HG. [Postmaturity syndrome, prolonged pregnancy and perinatal mortality.] *Gynaecologia* 1960;150:197–204.

7 Field TM, Dabiri C, Hallock N, Shuman HH. Developmental effects of prolonged pregnancy and the postmaturity syndrome. *J Pediatr* 1977;90(5):836–839.
8 Vorherr H. Placental insufficiency and postmaturity. *Eur J Obstet Gynecol Reprod Biol* 1975;5(1–2):109–122.
9 Crowley P. Interventions for preventing or improving the outcome of delivery at or beyond term. *Cochrane Database Syst Rev* 2000;2:CD000170.
10 Gardosi J, Geirsson RT. Routine ultrasound is the method of choice for dating pregnancy. *Br J Obstet Gynaecol* 1998;105(9): 933–936.
11 O'Donohoe NV, Holland PD. Familial congenital adrenal hypoplasia. *Arch Dis Child* 1968;43(232):717–723.
12 Roberts G, Cawdery JE. Congenital adrenal hypoplasia. *J Obstet Gynaecol Br Commonw* 1970;77(7):654–656.
13 Clifford SH. Postmaturity with placental dysfunction: clinical syndrome and pathologic findings. *J Pediatr* 2005;44:1–13.
14 Culikova V, Culik J, Topolsky L. [Amnioscopy, Clifford's syndrome and serologic conflict.] *Cesk Gynekol* 1974;39(1):34–35.
15 Hall MH, Carr-Hill RA. The extent and antecedents of uncertain gestation. *Br J Obstet Gynaecol* 1980;92:445–451.
16 Hogberg U, Larsson N. Early dating by ultrasound and perinatal outcome. A cohort study. *Acta Obstet Gynecol Scand* 1997; 76(10):907–912.
17 Bakketeig L, Bergsjo P. Postterm pregnancy: magnitude of the problem. *Effect Care Pregnancy Childbirth* 1989;I:765–775.
18 Dewhurst CJ, Beazley JM, Campbell S. Assessment of fetal maturity and dysmaturity. *Am J Obstet Gynecol* 1972;113(2):141–149.
19 Ingemarsson I, Heden L. Cervical score and onset of spontaneous labor in prolonged pregnancy dated by second-trimester ultrasonic scan. *Obstet Gynecol* 1989;74(1):102–105.
20 Cardozo L, Fysh J, Pearce JM. Prolonged pregnancy: the management debate. *Br Med J (Clin Res Ed)* 1986;293(6554): 1059–1063.
21 Gibb DM, Cardozo LD, Studd JW, Cooper DJ. Prolonged pregnancy: is induction of labour indicated? A prospective study. *Br J Obstet Gynaecol* 1982;89(4):292–295.
22 Dyson DC. Fetal surveillance vs. labor induction at 42 weeks in postterm gestation. *J Reprod Med* 1988;33(3):262–270.
23 Dyson DC, Miller PD, Armstrong MA. Management of prolonged pregnancy: induction of labor versus antepartum fetal testing. *Am J Obstet Gynecol* 1987;156(4):928–934.
24 The National Institute of Child Health and Human Development Network of Maternal–Fetal Medicine Units. A clinical trial of induction of labor versus expectant management in postterm pregnancy. *Am J Obstet Gynecol* 1994;170(3):716–723.
25 Hannah ME, Hannah WJ, Hellmann J, et al. Induction of labor as compared with serial antenatal monitoring in post-term pregnancy. A randomized controlled trial. The Canadian Multicenter Post-term Pregnancy Trial Group. *N Engl J Med* 1992;326(24): 1587–1592.
26 Goeree R, Hannah M, Hewson S. Cost-effectiveness of induction of labour versus serial antenatal monitoring in the Canadian Multicentre Postterm Pregnancy Trial. *Can Med Assoc J* 1995;152(9): 1445–1450.
27 Backer JE. [Perinatal mortality in relation to duration of pregnancy and weight of infant at birth.] *Tidsskr Nor Laegeforen* 1968;88(22):2106–2111.
28 Bastian H, Keirse MJ, Lancaster PA. Perinatal death associated with planned home birth in Australia: population based study (see comment). *Br Med J* 1998;317(7155):384–388.
29 Eden RD, Seifert LS, Winegar A, Spellacy WN. Postdate pregnancies: a review of 46 perinatal deaths. *Am J Perinatol* 1987;4(4):284–287.
30 Anderson GG. Postmaturity: a review. *Obstet Gynecol Surv* 1972;27:65–73.
31 Harper RG, Sokal MM, Sokal S, et al. The high-risk perinatal registry. A systematic approach for reducing perinatal mortality. *Obstet Gynecol* 1977;50(3):264–268.
32 Iffy L, Apuzzio JJ, Mitra S, et al. Rates of cesarean section and perinatal outcome. Perinatal mortality. *Acta Obstet Gynecol Scand* 1994;73(3):225–230.
33 Kallen K. Increased risk of perinatal/neonatal death in infants who were smaller than expected at ultrasound fetometry in early pregnancy. *Ultrasound Obstet Gynecol* 2004;24(1):30–34.
34 Kolonja S. [Possible effect of prolonged pregnancy on perinatal fetal mortality.] *Riv Ostet Ginecol Prat* 1957;39(7):583–587.
35 Kolonja S. [Does prolonged pregnancy really increase perinatal mortality.] *Wien Med Wochenschr* 1957;107(48):989.
36 Kumari S, Jain S, Pruthi PK, et al. Perinatal risks in postdated pregnancy. *Indian Pediatr* 1984;21(1):21–27.
37 Lattanzi WE. Perinatal morbidity and mortality committee. Case history and commentary. *Conn Med* 1974;38(5):251–252.
38 Naeye RL. Causes of perinatal mortality excess in prolonged gestations. *Am J Epidemiol* 1978;108(5):429–433.
39 Onah HE. Effect of prolongation of pregnancy on perinatal mortality. *Int J Gynaecol Obstet* 2003;80(3):255–261.
40 Papiernik E, Alexander GR, Paneth N. Racial differences in pregnancy duration and its implications for perinatal care. *Med Hypotheses* 1990;33(3):181–186.
41 Stamm O, Mattern L. [V. Perinatal mortality in prolonged pregnancy.] *Bull Fed Soc Gynecol Obstet Lang Fr* 1957;9(1, bis):133–142.
42 Stubblefield PG, Berek JS. Perinatal mortality in term and postterm births. *Obstet Gynecol* 1980;56(6):676–682.
43 Cnattingius S, Taube A. Stillbirths and rate of neonatal deaths in 76,761 postterm pregnancies in Sweden, 1982–1991; a register study. *Acta Obstet Gynecol Scand* 1998;77(5):582–583.
44 Hilder L, Costeloe K, Thilaganathan B. Prolonged pregnancy: evaluating gestation-specific risks of fetal and infant mortality. *Br J Obstet Gynaecol* 1998;105(2):169–173.
45 Agency for Healthcare Research and Quality. *Management of prolonged pregnancy (summary)*. US Department of Health and Human Services Public Health Service 2005, No. 53. Available at: URL: www.AHRQ.gov.
46 Crowley P. Interventions for preventing or improving the outcome of delivery at or beyond term. *The Cochrane Library* 2004;Issue 2.
47 Bochner CJ, Williams J, III, Castro L, et al. The efficacy of starting postterm antenatal testing at 41 weeks as compared with 42 weeks of gestational age. *Am J Obstet Gynecol* 1988;159(3):550–554.
48 Grubb DK, Rabello YA, Paul RH. Post-term pregnancy: fetal death rate with antepartum surveillance (see comment). *Obstet Gynecol* 1992;79(6):1024–1026.
49 Curtis PD, Matthews TG, Clarke TA, et al. Neonatal seizures: the Dublin Collaborative Study. *Arch Dis Child* 1988;63(9):1065–1068.
50 Eden RD, Seifert LS, Winegar A, Spellacy WN. Perinatal characteristics of uncomplicated postdate pregnancies. *Obstet Gynecol* 1987;69(3 Pt 1):296–299.
51 Mannino F. Neonatal complications of postterm gestation. *J Reprod Med* 1988;33(3):271–276.
52 Saunders K. Should we worry about meconium? A controlled study of neonatal outcome. *Trop Doct* 2002;32(1):7–10.

53 Yeh SY, Bruce SL, Thornton YS. Intrapartum monitoring and management of the postdate fetus. *Clin Perinatol* 1982;9(2):381–386.

54 Yoder BA, Kirsch EA, Barth WH, Gordon MC. Changing obstetric practices associated with decreasing incidence of meconium aspiration syndrome. *Obstet Gynecol* 2002;99(5 Pt 1):731–739.

55 Pollack RN, Hauer-Pollack G, Divon MY. Macrosomia in postdates pregnancies: the accuracy of routine ultrasonographic screening. *Am J Obstet Gynecol* 1992;167(1):7–11.

56 Acker DB, Sachs BP, Friedman EA. Risk factors for shoulder dystocia. *Obstet Gynecol* 1985;66(6):762–768.

57 Spellacy WN, Miller S, Winegar A, Peterson PQ. Macrosomia – maternal characteristics and infant complications. *Obstet Gynecol* 1985;66(2):158–161.

58 Myers ER, Blumrick R, Christian AL, et al. *Management of prolonged pregnancy*. Evidence Report/Technology Assessment No. 53 (Prepared by Duke Evidence-based Practice Center, Durham, NC, under Contract No. 290-97-0014). AHRQ Publication No. 02-E018. Rockville, MD: Agency for Healthcare Research and Quality, 2002.

59 Chauhan SP, Sullivan CA, Lutton TC, et al. Parous patients' estimate of birth weight in postterm pregnancy. *J Perinatol* 1995;15(3):192–194.

60 Chervenak JL, Divon MY, Hirsch J, et al. Macrosomia in the postdate pregnancy: is routine ultrasonographic screening indicated? *Am J Obstet Gynecol* 1989;161(3):753–756.

61 Gilby JR, Williams MC, Spellacy WN. Fetal abdominal circumference measurements of 35 and 38 cm as predictors of macrosomia. A risk factor for shoulder dystocia (see comment). *J Reprod Med* 2000;45(11):936–938.

62 O'Reilly-Green CP, Divon MY. Receiver operating characteristic curves of sonographic estimated fetal weight for prediction of macrosomia in prolonged pregnancies. *Ultrasound Obstet Gynecol* 1997;9(6):403–408.

63 Rouse DJ, Owen J, Goldenberg RL, Cliver SP. The effectiveness and costs of elective cesarean delivery for fetal macrosomia diagnosed by ultrasound. *JAMA* 1996;276(18):1480–1486.

64 Mongelli M, Yuxin NG, Biswas A, Chew S. Accuracy of ultrasound dating formulae in the late second-trimester in pregnancies conceived with in-vitro fertilization. *Acta Radiol* 2003;44(4):452–455.

65 Savitz DA, Terry JW, Jr, Dole N, et al. Comparison of pregnancy dating by last menstrual period, ultrasound scanning, and their combination. *Am J Obstet Gynecol* 2002;187(6):1660–1666.

66 Alexander JM, McIntire DD, Leveno KJ. Forty weeks and beyond: pregnancy outcomes by week of gestation. *Obstet Gynecol* 2000;96(2):291–294.

67 Sanchez-Ramos L, Olivier F, Delke I, Kaunitz AM. Labor induction versus expectant management for postterm pregnancies: a systematic review with meta-analysis. *Obstet Gynecol* 2003;101(6):1312–1318.

68 Semczuk M, Lopucka M. Evaluation of cervix condition according to Bishop score in post term pregnancy. *Ann Univ Mariae Curie Sklodowska [Med]* 1986;41:125–131.

69 Bishop EH. Pelvic scoring for elective induction. *Obstet Gynecol* 1964;24:266–268.

70 Harris BA, Jr, Huddleston JF, Sutliff G, Perlis HW. The unfavorable cervix in prolonged pregnancy. *Obstet Gynecol* 1983;62(2):171–174.

71 Hendrix NW, Chauhan SP, Morrison JC, et al. Bishop score: a poor diagnostic test to predict failed induction versus vaginal delivery. *South Med J* 1998;91(3):248–252.

72 Goldberg J, Newman RB, Rust PF. Interobserver reliability of digital and endovaginal ultrasonographic cervical length measurements. *Am J Obstet Gynecol* 1997;177(4):853–858.

73 Garry D, Figueroa R, Guillaume J, Cucco V. Use of castor oil in pregnancies at term. *Alternative Ther Health Med* 2000;6(1):77–79.

74 Boulvain M, Fraser WD, Marcoux S, et al. Does sweeping of the membranes reduce the need for formal induction of labour? A randomised controlled trial. *Br J Obstet Gynaecol* 1998;105(1):34–40.

75 Boulvain M, Irion O, Marcoux S, Fraser W. Sweeping of the membranes to prevent post-term pregnancy and to induce labour: a systematic review. *Br J Obstet Gynaecol* 1999;106(5):481–485.

76 Cammu H, Haitsma V. Sweeping of the membranes at 39 weeks in nulliparous women: a randomised controlled trial. *Br J Obstet Gynaecol* 1998;105(1):41–44.

77 Crane J, Bennett K, Young D, et al. The effectiveness of sweeping membranes at term: a randomized trial. *Obstet Gynecol* 1997;89(4):586–590.

78 el Torkey M, Grant JM. Sweeping of the membranes is an effective method of induction of labour in prolonged pregnancy: a report of a randomized trial. *Br J Obstet Gynaecol* 1992;99(6):455–458.

79 Grant JM. Sweeping of the membranes in prolonged pregnancy. *Br J Obstet Gynaecol* 1993;100(10):889–890.

80 Salamalekis E, Vitoratos N, Kassanos D, et al. Sweeping of the membranes versus uterine stimulation by oxytocin in nulliparous women. A randomized controlled trial. *Gynecol Obstet Invest* 2000;49(4):240–243.

81 Weerasekera DS. Sweeping of the membranes is an effective method of induction of labour in prolonged pregnancy: a report of a randomised trial. *Br J Obstet Gynaecol* 1993;100(2):193–194.

65 Anesthesia in the high-risk patient

Danny Wilkerson and Richard B. Clark

Normal parturients require special anesthetic considerations because of the physiological changes of pregnancy. Patients in high-risk categories have concomitant disease states that increase their risk of morbidity or mortality. Understanding and evaluating these comorbidities allow for the maximum provision of safe anesthesia in labor and spontaneous vaginal delivery or Cesarean section. The goal of maintaining fetal well-being, maternal cardiovascular stability, and uteroplacental blood flow must remain paramount. There are many high-risk categories but this chapter will focus on the topics below; recommendations and special considerations for these commonly encountered high-risk conditions are given.

Obesity

Obesity can be defined as a body mass index of ≥ 30 (BMI; equal to weight in pounds divided by height in inches squared × 703, or weight in kilograms divided by height in meters squared). Extreme or morbid obesity is defined as a BMI ≥ 40 (see Table 65.1).[1] Obesity is associated with increased morbidity and mortality and with certain disease states including diabetes mellitus, coronary artery disease, and hypertension.[2] It is also associated with profound physiological changes, such as an increase in oxygen consumption, carbon dioxide production, and alveolar ventilation. An increase in abdominal mass forces the diaphragm cephalad, accentuating the decrease in functional residual capacity (FRC) and expiratory reserve volume (ERV; Fig. 65.1).

In obesity, the work of breathing is increased. The increase in adipose tissue over the chest wall together with poor lung compliance resembles a restrictive lung disease. The lithotomy, supine, and Trendelenburg positions accentuate the reduction in lung volume. This, together with the decrease in FRC and ERV, may lead to ventilation/perfusion mismatch, hypoxemia, and postoperative atelectasis.

The pickwickian syndrome (obesity–hypoventilation syndrome) may occur in pregnancy and is characterized by somnolence, hypercarbia, right-sided heart failure, and chronic hypoxemia.[3] It may be associated with obstructive sleep apnea and so difficult airway management should be anticipated. Obesity is also associated with an increase in gastric volume, poor gastric emptying, and hyperacidity as well as an increased risk of aspiration.[4]

Intravenous narcotics in the laboring obese patient should be used cautiously because of the risk of respiratory compromise. Continuous lumbar epidural anesthesia is the preferred regional anesthetic technique for pain relief during labor although some practitioners use combined spinal epidural (CSE) or single-shot spinal techniques. All three may be technically difficult in the morbidly obese patient.

In obesity, anesthesia for Cesarean section and labor must include a thorough evaluation of the airway. A difficult intubation must be anticipated and planned for. Regional anesthesia is preferred to general anesthesia; if general anesthesia is selected, a rapid sequence induction with endotracheal intubation must be performed. Patients should receive an H2 antagonist and a nonparticulate antacid preoperatively. Extubation should be performed when the patient is awake with airway reflexes intact.

For Cesarean section, it is appropriate to use regional anesthesia to achieve a T4–T6 spinal level; spinal epidural, CSE, or epidural techniques can be used. Some practitioners advocate a continuous spinal technique if an inadvertent dural puncture occurs during attempted epidural placement.[5] Left uterine displacement (LUD) and supplemental oxygen by mask are standard.

Hypertensive disorders in pregnancy

Hypertensive disorders in pregnancy include gestational hypertension, preeclampsia, eclampsia, preeclampsia superimposed on chronic hypertension, and chronic hypertension. The first three disorders were previously known as pregnancy-induced hypertension (PIH)[6] (see Table 65.2). Most of these disorders result in hypertension, proteinuria, and edema, and may cause seizures. Hypertension of 140/90 mmHg or more is termed mild preeclampsia, whereas a pressure of 160/110 mmHg results in severe preeclampsia. These conditions are associated with a decreased blood volume and there are many implications for the anesthesiologist.[7] The remainder of this discussion will focus on preeclampsia. The circulation in preeclampsia can be characterized as hyperdynamic (see Table 65.3).

The standard treatment for preeclampsia is magnesium sulfate. A 4-g bolus is given intravenously, followed by 2 g/h intravenously. The therapeutic blood levels are 4.0–6.0 mequiv./L. Although magnesium is not specific for preeclampsia, it has been found to be very effective. Magnesium sulfate has a peripheral and a central action, and is used primarily to treat or prevent seizures. Antihypertensives such as hydralazine, labetalol, and methyldopa are utilized to control blood pressure. The HELLP syndrome [a group of symptoms that occur in pregnant women who have (H) hemolytic anemia, (EL) elevated liver enzymes, and (LP) low platelet count] may develop. Monitoring of the central circulation (central venous pressure) or use of a pulmonary artery catheter may be indicated.

Anesthesia for labor and delivery in the preeclamptic patient is necessary and desirable; we believe that lumbar epidural anesthesia is the preferred method. Blood volume is reduced in preeclampsia and, therefore, before the block is given, infusion of a balanced salt solution begins, with the aim of administering at least 500 cm^3. A further infusion may be given if hypotension occurs after the block takes effect. If a clotting disorder is present, spinal or epidural anesthesia may be contraindicated because of the risk of an epidural hematoma. Obtaining a prothrombin time, partial thromboplastin time (PTT), and platelet count is standard practice in the severely preeclamptic woman. If there are obvious signs such as bruising or bleeding at the intravenous site, or into the Foley catheter, an epidural should be avoided. A dramatic drop in the platelet count over a 2–3 h period indicates a worsening of the preeclampsia and cautious clinical judgment should be used when deciding whether to place an epidural catheter. Thromboelastography (TEG) may also be helpful.[8] In a retrospective survey of Cesarean delivery in severely preeclamptic patients, Hood and Curry[9] found no difference in hemodynamic effects between those receiving spinal anesthesia and those receiving epidural anesthesia.

Preeclamptic patients may require a Cesarean section for delivery and we believe that regional anesthesia is preferable. For many years, there was a prejudice against regional anesthesia because of the fear of profound hypotension. With the recognition that there is a decrease in blood volume in preeclampsia and the use of liberal amounts of balanced salt solution (1000 cm^3), hypotension is much less of a problem. The significant work of Wallace and colleagues[10] has shown that spinal, epidural, or general anesthesia can all be used successfully for Cesarean section in preeclamptic patients. General anesthesia is less desirable than regional but may be necessary if regional anesthesia is not possible; for example clotting defects may contraindicate regional anesthesia. General anesthesia carries with it the risks of regurgitation and aspiration, and also severe hypertension on endotracheal intubation and surgical incision. Antihypertensives should be given before and after induction if necessary. The anesthetic technique consists of induction with thiopental, followed by administration of succinylcholine, intubation, and maintenance with 50% nitrous oxide/oxygen, and 0.5% isoflurane. A narcotic is given intravenously to the mother after delivery. Nondepolarizing neuromuscular blocking agents may be needed for abdominal relaxation. The anesthesiologist must be aware of the synergistic action of muscle relaxants and magnesium. Extubation should take place with the patient awake and with airway reflexes intact.

Prematurity

The premature infant is generally considered to have a gestational age of 20–37 weeks and a weight of less than 2500 g.[11] However, some small for gestational age infants with a low birthweight are born near term. A more appropriate definition is therefore preterm infant. About 7–8% of deliveries in the USA are preterm.

It would seem inherently obvious that these small, fragile infants should not be subjected to the effects of maternally administered depressants such as narcotics and tranquilizers. Very little information has been published on this subject, although one older study[12] found no differences in the Apgar scores of infants when meperidine was used during labor.[12] It is recommended, however, that these drugs be kept to a minimum during labor.[13]

Mothers in preterm labor are often treated with drugs that inhibit labor. Ritodrine was popular for several years but has been associated with pulmonary edema. Magnesium sulfate is now frequently used for the treatment of preterm labor. The anesthesiologist must be aware of the effect that this therapy has on the motor end plate and that it can also alter the response of vasopressor agents.

Preterm infants should not be subjected to the hazards of precipitous delivery as this can cause cerebral trauma. Because of this, and to minimize the use of depressant drugs, lumbar epidural anesthesia is considered to be the best option for vaginal delivery.[13] Spinal or epidural anesthesia is preferred for abdominal delivery, so that neonatal depression can be minimized.

Cardiac disease

About 1% of all pregnancies are complicated by heart disease, and 60–80% of these complications are caused by congenital heart disease.[14] The remainder of cases are mostly valvular, caused by rheumatic heart disease. The New York Heart Association (NYHA) has provided a simple way of classifying the

Table 65.1 Body mass index.

	Normal						Overweight					Obese					
BMI	19	20	21	22	23	24	25	26	27	28	29	30	31	32	33	34	35
Height (inches)	Body weight (pounds)																
58	91	96	100	105	110	115	119	124	129	134	138	143	148	153	158	162	167
59	94	99	104	109	114	119	124	128	133	138	143	148	153	158	163	168	173
60	97	102	107	112	118	123	128	133	138	143	148	153	158	163	168	174	179
61	100	106	111	116	122	127	132	137	143	148	153	158	164	169	174	180	185
62	104	109	115	120	126	131	136	142	147	153	158	164	169	175	180	186	191
63	107	113	118	124	130	135	141	146	152	158	163	169	175	180	186	191	197
64	110	116	122	128	134	140	145	151	157	163	169	174	180	186	192	197	204
65	114	120	126	132	138	144	150	156	162	168	174	180	186	192	198	204	210
66	118	124	130	136	142	148	155	161	167	173	179	186	192	198	204	210	216
67	121	127	134	140	146	153	159	166	172	178	185	191	198	204	211	217	223
68	125	131	138	144	151	158	164	171	177	184	190	197	203	210	216	223	230
69	128	135	142	149	155	162	169	176	182	189	196	203	209	216	223	230	236
70	132	139	146	153	160	167	174	181	188	195	202	209	216	222	229	236	243
71	136	143	150	157	165	172	179	186	193	200	208	215	222	229	236	243	250
72	140	147	154	162	169	177	184	191	199	206	213	221	228	235	242	250	258
73	144	151	159	166	174	182	189	197	204	212	219	227	235	242	250	257	265
74	148	155	163	171	179	186	194	202	210	218	225	233	241	249	256	264	272
75	152	160	168	176	184	192	200	208	216	224	232	240	248	256	264	272	279
76	156	164	172	180	189	197	205	213	221	230	238	246	254	263	271	279	287

Table reprinted from National Heart Lung and Blood Institute. World Wide Web URL: http://www.nhlbi.nih.gov.

To use the table, find the appropriate height in the left-hand column labeled "height." Move across to the given weight (in pounds). The number at the top of the column is the BMI for that height and weight.

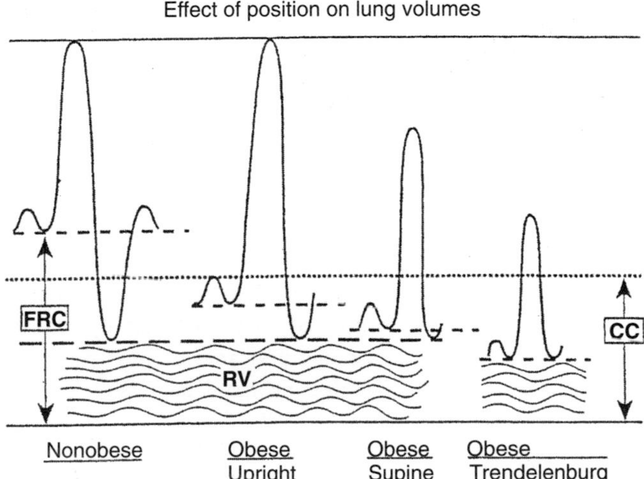

Figure 65.1 Changes in lung mechanics in obese and nonobese patients. In obesity, functional residual capacity (FRC) decreases at the expense of expiratory reserve volume (ERV). Closing capacity (CC) remains normal. From Vaughan RW. Pulmonary and cardiovascular derangements in the obese patient. In: Brown BR, ed. *Anesthesia and the obese patient*. Philadelphia, PA: FA Davis; 1982:26, with permission.

Table 65.2 Diagnosis of hypertensive disorders complicating pregnancy.

Hypertensive disorder	Characteristics
Gestational hypertension	Blood pressure ≥ 140/90 mmHg for first time during pregnancy No proteinuria
Preeclampsia	Blood pressure ≥ 140/90 mmHg after 30 weeks' gestation Proteinuria ≥ 300 mg/24 h or ≥ 1+ on dipstick reading
Eclampsia with preeclampsia	Seizures that cannot be attributed to other causes in a woman
Preeclampsia superimposed on chronic hypertension	New onset proteinuria ≥ 300 mg/24 h
Chronic hypertension	Blood pressure ≥ 140/90 mmHg before pregnancy or diagnosed before 20 weeks' gestation

Adapted from ref. 6, with permission.

				Extreme obesity														
36	37	38	39	40	41	42	43	44	45	46	47	48	49	50	51	52	53	54
172	177	181	186	191	196	201	205	210	215	220	224	229	234	239	244	248	253	358
178	183	188	193	198	203	208	212	217	222	227	232	237	242	247	252	257	262	267
184	189	194	199	204	209	215	220	225	230	235	240	245	250	255	261	266	271	276
190	195	201	206	211	217	222	227	232	238	243	248	254	259	264	269	275	280	285
196	202	207	213	218	224	229	235	240	246	251	256	262	267	273	278	284	289	295
203	208	214	220	225	231	237	242	248	254	259	265	270	278	282	287	293	299	304
209	215	221	227	232	238	244	250	256	262	267	273	279	285	291	296	302	308	314
216	222	228	234	240	246	252	258	264	270	276	282	288	294	300	306	312	318	324
223	229	235	241	247	253	260	266	272	278	264	291	297	303	309	315	322	328	334
230	236	242	249	255	261	268	274	280	287	293	299	306	312	319	325	331	338	344
236	243	249	256	262	269	276	282	289	295	302	308	315	322	328	335	341	348	354
243	250	257	263	270	277	284	291	297	304	311	318	324	331	338	345	351	358	365
250	257	264	271	278	285	292	299	306	313	320	327	334	341	348	355	362	369	376
257	265	272	279	286	293	301	308	315	322	329	338	343	351	358	365	372	379	386
265	272	279	287	294	302	309	316	324	331	338	346	353	361	368	375	383	390	397
272	280	288	295	302	310	318	325	333	340	348	355	363	371	378	386	393	401	408
280	287	295	303	311	319	326	334	342	350	358	365	373	381	389	396	404	412	420
287	295	303	311	319	327	335	343	351	359	367	375	383	391	399	407	415	423	431
295	304	312	320	328	336	344	353	361	369	377	385	394	402	410	418	426	435	443

Table 65.3 Cardiovascular parameters of normal nonpregnant, normal pregnant, and severely preeclamptic women.

Cardiovascular parameter	Normal nonpregnancy	Normal pregnancy	Severe preeclampsia	Severe preeclampsia with pulmonary edema
Mean arterial pressure (mmHg)	86.4	90.3	130	136
Central venous pressure (mmHg)	3.7	3.6	4.8	11.0
Pulmonary capillary wedge pressure (mmHg)	6.3	7.5	8.3	18.0
Cardiac output (L/min)	4.3	6.2	8.4	10.5
Systemic vascular resistance (dynes)	1530	1210	1226	964

Adapted from Hughes SC, Levinson G, Rosen MA, eds. *Shnider and Levinson's anesthesia for obstetrics*, 4th edn. Philadelphia, PA: Lippincott Williams & Wilkins 2002:300, with permission.

extent of heart failure. Class I and II patients have a maternal mortality rate of 1% or less, whereas class III or IV patients have a maternal mortality rate of 5–15% and a perinatal mortality rate of 20–30%.[15] Most deaths from cardiac disease in pregnancy are parturients with right-to-left shunts or stenotic heart disease.

Left-to-right shunts occur with congenital lesions such as patent ductus arteriosus (PDA), ventricular septal defect (VSD), and atrial septal defect (ASD). These patients usually tolerate pregnancy well. Early epidural placement with a slow onset of anesthesia is preferred, using saline for loss of resistance (LOR) instead of air, to prevent paradoxical air emboli. Epidural analgesia prevents maternal increases in systemic vascular resistance (SVR) and catecholamine levels. Increases in SVR may lead to pulmonary hypertension. Hypercarbia and acidosis may lead to an increase in pulmonary vascular resistance and should be avoided.

Eisenmenger syndrome is caused by a left-to-right shunt which results in an increase in pulmonary artery pressure if left untreated. This fixed, high pressure can change the

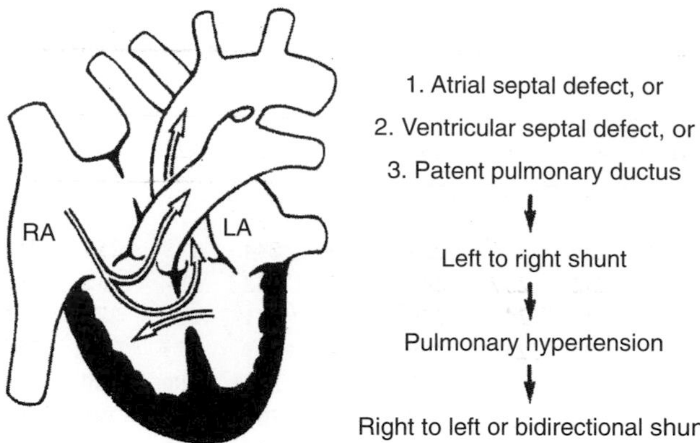

Figure 65.2 Pathophysiology of Eisenmenger syndrome. RA, right atrium; LA, left atrium. Reprinted from Hughes SC, Levinson G, Rosen MA, eds. *Shnider and Levinson's anesthesia for obstetrics*, 4th edn. Philadelphia, PA: Lippincott Williams & Wilkins; 2002:469, with permission.

Table 65.4 Eisenmenger syndrome: anesthetic considerations.

Avoid decreases in systemic vascular resistance
Avoid decreases in venous return
Avoid increases in pulmonary vascular resistance (e.g., hypercarbia, acidosis, hypoxia)

Reprinted from Hughes SC, Levinson G, Rosen MA, eds. *Shnider and Levinson's anesthesia for obstetrics*, 4th edn. Philadelphia, PA: Lippincott Williams & Wilkins; 2002:469, with permission.

primary left-to-right shunt into a right-to-left shunt (Fig. 65.2), leading to hypoxemia and right ventricular failure.[16] Labor analgesia can be accomplished with a lumbar epidural, intrathecal opioids, or a pudendal block early in the second stage of labor. Care must be taken to avoid pain, hypoxemia, hypercarbia, and acidosis, which will increase pulmonary vascular resistance and increase the right-to-left shunt (Table 65.4). Maintenance of intravascular volume, venous return, and an adequate SVR is essential. For anticoagulated parturients in which regional anesthesia is contraindicated, a patient-controlled anesthesia (PCA) with remifentanil may be a good option.[17]

Primary pulmonary hypertension may be treated with supplemental oxygen, inhaled nitric oxide, nitroglycerin, prostaglandins, or calcium channel blockers. Single-shot spinal anesthesia should be avoided; slow induction of continuous epidural anesthesia is preferred. Increases in pulmonary artery pressures caused by general anesthesia for Cesarean section can be minimized using a narcotic-based induction and maintenance technique. The use of pulmonary artery catheters is controversial.

The most common cyanotic heart lesion is tetralogy of Fallot. This consists of VSD, overriding aorta, right ventricular outflow tract obstruction, and right ventricular hypertrophy. Care should be taken to avoid a decrease in SVR, as with single-shot spinal anesthesia, which may cause shunt increase and a worsening hypoxemia. Labor and delivery analgesia is best managed with systemic medications and a pudendal block.[18] Spinal opioids can offer a good alternative, and epidural can be used with caution.[18] The goal is to avoid a decrease in SVR, and to maintain a sufficient venous return and adequate intravascular volume. Hypotension, straining, or coughing is best avoided. General anesthesia is usually well tolerated but hypotension and "bucking" should be avoided.[19,20] It is advisable to maintain a normal or slightly increased SVR.[21]

Most mild to moderately symptomatic pregnant patients with valvular disease tolerate epidural anesthesia for labor and it is recommended as it eliminates pain and tachycardia. Patients with severe symptomatic aortic stenosis may not tolerate even mild hypotension or tachycardia. During the first stage of labor, intrathecal narcotics have been used, followed by a pudendal block in the second stage. Myocardial depression with halogenated agents during general anesthesia should be avoided. Maintenance of sinus rhythm, adequate SVR, and intravascular volume and venous returns are a must.

Peripartum cardiomyopathy is characterized by biventricular hypokinesis, low cardiac output, and elevated filling pressures. Its onset is often insidious and its etiology is unknown. The maternal mortality rate is high. Management is supportive with treatment of symptomatic heart failure. Vaginal delivery or Cesarean section may be facilitated by epidural anesthesia,[21] unless the patient has a contraindication to regional anesthesia. General anesthesia for Cesarean section may result in profound myocardial depression.[22] Echocardiography and invasive pressure monitoring can prove invaluable. The use of a continuous spinal anesthetic for Cesarean section in a patient with severe recurrent peripartum cardiomyopathy has been reported.[23]

Neurological disease

Multiple sclerosis

Multiple sclerosis is a demyelinating disease of the central nervous system. It is a progressive disease with intermittent exacerbations and remissions. The etiology is unknown and treatment includes symptomatic care and physical therapy. There is a tendency for remission during pregnancy; however, in the 3- to 6-month period after delivery there may be an increase in exacerbations of symptoms.[24]

The data currently available do not contraindicate regional anesthesia for labor, delivery, or Cesarean section. There is a high incidence of postpartum relapse, regardless of the type of anesthesia delivered. A dilute solution of local anesthetic, with or without opioid, may be used safely for labor analgesia.[25] Conditions known to exacerbate multiple sclerosis, such as stress, infection, and hyperpyrexia, should be avoided.[26]

Myasthenia gravis

Myasthenia gravis is characterized by episodes of muscle weakness, which is made worse by activity. It is an autoimmune disorder; antiacetylcholine receptor antibodies are produced which destroy acetylcholine receptors and produce an antibody-induced blockade of any remaining receptors.[27] This affects muscles of respiration, laryngeal muscles, and facial and ocular muscles. The disease does not affect cardiac or smooth muscle contraction; however, an electrocardiogram (ECG) should be obtained because there have been reports of focal myocardial necrosis in patients with myasthenia gravis.[28] The degree of bulbar involvement and respiratory compromise should be thoroughly evaluated. The course of the disease varies during pregnancy. Anticholinesterases, which increase the amount of acetylcholine available, are the first line of treatment. Corticosteroids, plasmapheresis (decreases antibody levels), and thymectomy have been used in the treatment of myasthenia gravis.

Myasthenia gravis does not affect the first stage of labor; however, a vacuum-assisted or forceps delivery is often required for the second stage. Cesarean section should be reserved for obstetric indications. Drugs that can potentiate muscle weakness, for example magnesium sulfate, should be avoided.

For labor, epidural analgesia is the preferred method of pain relief.[29] Parenteral opioids should be used cautiously to avoid further respiratory compromise. Plasma cholinesterase activity is decreased, which may prolong the half-life of ester local anesthetics if used for epidural analgesia. If the CSE technique is used, the increased risk of respiratory depression from intrathecal opioids must be considered.

For Cesarean delivery, regional anesthesia is preferred.[30] The small amount of local anesthesia used for spinal anesthesia allows either amide or ester local anesthetic agents to be used safely. General anesthesia may be preferred in patients with significant respiratory compromise, in order to secure the airway and avoid any further respiratory compromise that could be produced with regional anesthesia.[31] Propofol, ketamine, and thiopental may be used for induction, with rapid sequence induction being used; however, succinylcholine may not be metabolized as rapidly. Myasthenia gravis patients are extremely sensitive to nondepolarizing muscle relaxants, which should be used cautiously, if at all. Postoperative ventilation may be required, especially in patients with severe bulbar involvement. Neuromuscular blockade should be monitored with a nerve stimulator. It must be remembered that volatile agents potentiate muscle relaxants. Because symptoms of myasthenia gravis may worsen postoperatively, the myasthenia gravis patient should be monitored in an acute care area.

Substance abuse

Many pregnant patients use both legal and illegal drugs that can have dire consequences on both mother and fetus. The following discussion will focus on the commonly used illicit drugs.

Opioids

Opioids can be smoked, inhaled, or injected intravenously or intramuscularly. Heroin appears to be the most common opioid abused during pregnancy although fentanyl, meperidine, morphine, and methadone are also abused; polysubstance abuse is also common.[32] Opioid exposure during pregnancy is associated with preterm labor, chorioamnionitis, intrauterine growth restriction (IUGR), and placental abruption. Neonates of opioid addicts can exhibit narcotic withdrawal, hyperthermia, seizures, and an increased risk of sudden infant death syndrome (SIDS). Other maternal complications include thrombophlebitis, HIV, AIDS, hepatitis, and endocarditis.[33]

The administration of anesthesia can be complicated by limited intravenous access and the need for emergency Cesarean section because of fetal distress. The patient may present in opioid withdrawal, acutely opioid intoxicated, or even in opioid overdose. If the newborn of an opioid addict presents with respiratory depression then the infant should be given ventilation assistance, but naloxone should not be administered as this may precipitate acute withdrawal syndrome. Regional anesthetic techniques are preferred unless there is a contraindication;[32] however, HIV is not a contraindication for regional anesthesia.[34] Intravenous drug abusers are prone to an increased incidence of epidural abscesses, therefore a neurological assessment should be carried out before regional anesthesia is administered. The addict's daily narcotic dose should be met, and opioid agonist–antagonists should be avoided. General anesthesia can be provided with the typical induction agents. Cross-tolerance is not a problem during maintenance provided the patient's physiological opioid requirements are met.

Cocaine

Cocaine is a local anesthetic of the ester group. Its potent sympathomimetic effects (hypertension, vasoconstriction, myocardial effects) result primarily from inhibition of reuptake of norepinephrine at nerve terminals.[35] Cocaine can cause complications such as placental abruption, fetal demise *in utero*, premature labor and delivery, fetal distress (leading to emergency Cesarean section), uterine rupture, uteroplacental insufficiency, and spontaneous abortion. Maternal hypertension, seizures, and hyperreflexia, as a result of acute cocaine intoxication, may be confused with preeclampsia/eclampsia. Smoking "crack" cocaine can lead to significant pulmonary problems.

Anesthetic considerations revolve around the acutely intoxicated patient with catecholamine excess, or the chronically catecholamine-depleted addict. Early placement of labor epidural will decrease maternal pain, lower catecholamine levels, and potentially minimize increases in uterine vascular resistance (potentially benefiting a compromised fetus). Hypertension may be treated with hydralazine, labetalol, or nitroglycerin.[36] Small doses of benzodiazepine may prove helpful. Seizures in the acutely intoxicated patient may be treated with thiopental and airway protection, oxygenation, and ventilation. Hypotension may be increased in cocaine abusers who are volume depleted. Ephedrine may be ineffective in the catecholamine-depleted cocaine abuser; hypotension that is refractory to ephedrine can be treated with incremental doses of phenylephrine.

For Cesarean section, the epidural level can be raised slowly to achieve a T4 level. Spinal anesthesia can be administered provided that adequate hydration and LUD are used, and vasopressors are immediately available. General anesthesia for Cesarean section in cases of fetal distress can be complicated by maternal tachycardia, hypertension, arrhythmias, and myocardial ischemia, and the anesthesiologist should be prepared to treat these complications. Nitroprusside may be needed if there is a hypertensive crisis.

Key points

1. Patients in high-risk categories have concomitant disease states that increase the risk of morbidity or mortality.
2. Obesity is associated with increased morbidity and mortality, and with disease states, including diabetes mellitus, coronary artery disease, and hypertension.
3. Obesity increases oxygen consumption, carbon dioxide production, and alveolar ventilation, and decreases functional residual capacity and expiratory reserve volume.
4. In the obese patient, regional anesthesia is preferred for labor and delivery, including Cesarean section.
5. General anesthesia in the obese parturient requires a thorough airway examination and an anticipation of a difficult intubation.
6. Hypertensive disorders in pregnancy include gestational hypertension, preeclampsia, eclampsia, chronic hypertension, and preeclampsia superimposed on chronic hypertension.
7. Wallace and colleagues[10] have shown that spinal, epidural, and general anesthesia can all be used successfully for Cesarean section in preeclamptic patients.
8. Delivery of the premature infant is best accomplished with lumbar epidural anesthesia for vaginal delivery, and spinal or epidural anesthesia for Cesarean section.
9. Patients with left-to-right cardiac shunts usually tolerate pregnancy well.
10. The most common cyanotic heart lesion is tetralogy of Fallot.
11. Peripartum cardiomyopathy is characterized by biventricular hypokinesis, low cardiac output, and elevated filling pressures.
12. Data available at present do not contraindicate regional anesthesia for labor, delivery, or Cesarean section in patients with multiple sclerosis and myasthenia gravis.
13. For patients with myasthenia gravis, epidural analgesia is the preferred method of pain relief during labor.
14. Patients with myasthenia gravis are extremely sensitive to nondepolarizing muscle relaxants, and these should be used cautiously, if at all.
15. Heroin appears to be the most common opioid abused during pregnancy.
16. Opioid exposure during pregnancy is associated with preterm labor, placental abruption, intrauterine growth restriction, and chorioamnionitis.
17. HIV is not a contraindication for regional anesthesia.
18. The addict's daily narcotic dose should be met.
19. Cocaine use during pregnancy can cause complications such as placenta abruption, fetal demise *in utero*, spontaneous abortions, uterine rupture, premature labor and delivery, uteroplacental insufficiency, and fetal distress.
20. Ephedrine may be ineffective in the catecholamine-depleted cocaine abuser.

References

1 Adams JP, Murphy PG. Obesity in anesthesia and intensive care. *Br J Anaesth* 2000;85:91–108.

2 Kumari AS. Pregnancy outcome in women with morbid obesity. *Int J Gynecol Obstet* 2001;73:101–107.

3 Loadsman JA, Hillman DR. Anaesthesia and sleep apnea. *Br J Anaesth* 2001;86:254–266.

4 Ng A, Smith G. Gastroesophageal reflux and aspiration of gastric contents in anesthetic practice. *Anesth Analg* 2001;93:496–513.

5 Reyes M, Pan PH. Very low dose spinal anesthesia for cesarean section in a morbidly obese preeclamptic patient and its potential implications. *Int J Obstet Anesth* 2004;13:99–102.

6 Cunningham F, Gant N, Leveno K, et al., eds. *Williams obstetrics*, 21st edn. New York: McGraw-Hill; 2001:568.

7 Hughes S, Levinson G, Rosen M, eds. *Shnider and Levinson's*

anesthesia for obstetrics, 4th edn. Philadelphia, PA: Lippincott Williams & Wilkins; 2002:297.
8 Chestnut D. *Obstetric anesthesia principles and practice*, 3rd edn. Philadelphia, PA: Elsevier Mosby; 2004:770.
9 Hood DD, Curry R. Spinal versus epidural anesthesia for cesarean section in severely preeclamptic patients: a retrospective survey. *Anesthesiology* 1999;90:1276–1292.
10 Wallace DH, Leveno KJ, Cunninghan FG. Randomized comparison of general and regional anesthesia for cesarean delivery in pregnancy complicated by severe preeclampsia. *Obstet Gynecol* 1995;86:193–199.
11 Chestnut D. *Obstetric anesthesia principles and practice*, 3rd edn. Philadelphia, PA: Elsevier Mosby; 2004:605.
12 Kaltreider DF. Premature labor and meperidine analgesia. *Am J Obstet Gynecol* 1967;99:989–993.
13 Santos AC, Finster M. Anesthesia in the high-risk patient. In: Reece EA, Hobbins JC, eds. *Medicine of the fetus and mother*, 2nd edn. Philadelphia, PA: Lippincott-Raven, 1999.
14 Siu SC, Colman JM. Heart disease and pregnancy. *Heart* (British Cardiac Society) 2001;85:710–715.
15 Harnett M, Mushlin PS, Camann WR. Cardiovascular disease. In: Chestnut D, ed. *Obstetric anesthesia principles and practice*, 3rd edn. Philadelphia, PA: Elsevier Mosby; 2004:707–733.
16 Gambling DR, Douglas MJ. *Obstetric anesthesia and uncommon disorders*. Philadelphia: WB Saunders Co.; 1998:7.
17 Owen MD, Poss MJ, Dean LS, et al. Prolonged intravenous remifentanil infusion for labor analgesia. *Anesth Analg* 2002; 94:918–919.
18 Kuczkowski KM. Labor analgesia for the parturient with cardiac disease. What does an obstetrician need to know? *Acta Obstet Gynecol Scand* 2004;83:223–233
19 Spinnato JA, Kraynack BJ, Cooper MW. Eisenmenger's syndrome in pregnancy: epidural analgesia for elective cesarean section. *N Engl J Med* 1981;304:1215–1217.
20 Ghai B, Mohan V, Khetarpal M, et al. Epidural anesthesia for cesarean section in a patient with Eisenmenger's syndrome. *Int J Obstet Anesth* 2002;11:44–47.
21 Mangano DT. Anesthesia for the pregnant cardiac patient. In: Hughes SC, Levinson G, Rosen MA, eds. *Shnider and Levinson's anesthesia for obstetrics*, 4th edn. Philadelphia, PA: Lippincott Williams & Wilkins, 2002.
22 Breen TW, Janzen JA. Pulmonary hypertension and cardiomyopathy: anaesthetic management for caesarean section. *Can J Anaesth* 1991;38:895–899.
23 Velickovic IA, Leicht CH. Continuous spinal anesthesia for cesarean section in a parturient with severe recurrent peripartum cardiomyopathy. *Int J Obstet Anesth* 2004;13:40–43.
24 Confavreux C, Hutchinson M, Hours MM, et al. Rate of pregnancy-related relapse in multiple sclerosis. *N Engl J Med* 1998;339:285–291.
25 Ferrero S, Pretta S, Ragni N. Multiple sclerosis: management issues during pregnancy. *Eur J Obstet Gynecol* 2004;115:3–9.
26 Bader AM. Neurologic and neuromuscular disease. In: Chestnut D, ed. *Obstetric anesthesia practice and principles*, 3rd edn. Philadelphia, PA: Elsevier Mosby; 2004:873.
27 Richman DP, Agius MA. Acquired myasthenia gravis: immunology. *Neurol Clin* 1994;12:273–284.
28 Baraka A. Anesthesia and myasthenia gravis. *Can J Anaesth* 1992;39:476.
29 Rolbin WH, Levinson G, Shnider SM, et al. Anesthetic consideration for myasthenia gravis and pregnancy. *Anesth Analg* 1978;57:441–447.
30 Saito Y, Sakura S, Takatori T, et al. Epidural anesthesia in a patient with myasthenia gravis. *Acta Anaesth Scand* 1993;37:513–515.
31 Gambling DR, Douglas MJ. *Obstetric anesthesia and uncommon disorders*. Philadelphia: WM Saunders Co.; 1998:435.
32 Kuczkowski KM. The cocaine abusing parturient; a review of anesthetic considerations. *Can J Anaesth* 2004;51:145–154.
33 Kuczkowski KM. Anesthetic implications of drug abuse in pregnancy. *J Clin Anesth* 2003;15:382–394.
34 Hughes S, Dailey PA. Human immunodeficiency virus in the delivery suite. In: Hughes S, Levinson G, Rosen M, eds. *Shnider and Levinson's anesthesia for obstetrics*, 4th edn. Philadelphia, PA: Lippincott Williams & Wilkins; 2002:591.
35 Berde CB, Strichartz GR. Local anesthetics. In: Miller RD, ed. *Anesthesia*, 5th edn. Philadelphia, PA: Churchill Livingstone; 2000:513.
36 Hughes SC, Kessin C. Anesthesia and the drug-addicted mother; In: Hughes S, Levinson G, Rosen M, eds. *Shnider and Levinson's anesthesia for obstetrics*, 4th edn. Philadelphia, PA: Lippincott Williams & Wilkins; 2002: 607.

Further reading

Birnbach DJ. *Ostheimer's manual of obstetric anesthesia*, 3rd edn. New York: Churchill Livingstone, 2000.
Chestnut DH. *Obstetric anesthesia principles and practice*, 3rd edn. Philadelphia, PA: Elsevier Mosby, 2004.
Datta S. *The obstetric anesthesia handbook*, 3rd edn. New York: Hanley & Belfus, 2000.
Datta S. *Anesthetic and obstetric management of high-risk pregnancy*, 3rd edn. New York: Springer-Verlag, 2004.
Gambling DR, Douglas MJ. *Obstetric anesthesia and uncommon disorders*. Philadelphia: WB Saunders Co., 1998.
Hughes SC, Levinson G, Rosen MA, eds. *Shnider and Levinson's anesthesia for obstetrics* Philadelphia, PA: Lippincott, Williams & Wilkins, 2002.
Miller RD, ed. *Anesthesia*, 5th edn. Philadelphia, PA: Churchill Livingstone, 2000.
Stoelting RE, Dierdorf SF. *Anesthesia and co-existing disease*, 4th edn. Philadelphia: Churchill Livingstone, 2002.
Tsen LC. The Gerald W Ostheimer "What's new in obstetric anesthesia" lecture. *Anesthesiology* 2005;102.672–679.

Puerperium and lactation: physiology of the reproductive system

Judy M. Hopkinson, Pamela D. Berens, and E. Albert Reece

The puerperium is typically described as the postpartum period approximately 6–8 weeks after delivery, during which time many physiologic changes of pregnancy will revert to their prepartum state.

Reproductive system

Involution of the uterus is most dramatic on the first day after delivery. From a uterine weight of about 1100 g at term, by 24 h postpartum, the uterine fundus is typically palpable near the umbilicus. Two weeks postpartum, the uterus is no longer palpated on abdominal examination and, at 6 weeks, it will return to a weight of less than 100 g, although commonly heavier than the prepregnancy weight. Ultrasound evaluation of the postpartum uterus suggests a slight increase in puerperal uterine size in women delivered via Cesarean, although little difference in involution is noted between breastfeeding and formula-feeding mothers.[1,2] Some studies suggest an increased uterine size during the puerperium in multiparous women, although others do not support this finding.[3,4] Fluid and debris may be noted in the uterine cavity of asymptomatic women in the midpuerperium.[5]

Initially, postpartum women experience a discharge of decidua and blood known as lochia rubra. This becomes more watery and pale, referred to as lochia serosa and, finally, the more yellow to whitish lochia alba. Total lochial volume is estimated at 200–500 mL.[6] The mean duration of lochia is 33 days with 15% of women continuing to experience lochial discharge at 6 weeks postpartum.[7] The duration of lochia does not appear to be well correlated with lactational status.

Painful postpartum uterine contractions are commonly referred to as "afterpains." This appears to be more problematic in multiparous women.[8] Breastfeeding mothers frequently note an association of afterpains with nursing episodes due to oxytocin release. Holdcroft et al.[9] noted that 96% of women reported pains during breastfeeding, with the intensity of these pains being significantly associated with parity. Mean duration and number of contractions were also related to parity. Nonsteroidal anti-inflammatory agents such as ibuprofen may be used for analgesia.

Cervix and vagina

Immediately after vaginal delivery, the cervix has a loose, pliable tone, and may have several small excoriations. Over the first week postpartum, the cervix assumes a more typical gross appearance, although it may remain slightly dilated for the first few days. Persistent heavy bleeding and a continued open cervical os should alert the physician to the possibility of retained placental fragments. Cervical dysplasia may regress in the postpartum period. Kaplan et al.[10] studied 157 women with antepartum cervical squamous intraepithelial neoplasia and their subsequent postpartum course. Sixty-two percent of patients with low-grade antepartum dysplasia had regression, while only 6% experienced disease progression, although 60% developed recurrent disease within 5 years. All 28 cases of antepartum high-grade dysplasia in this study persisted postpartum.

The typical rugated appearance of the vagina is temporarily lost, with it appearing more edematous, vascular, and smooth after delivery. Rugae typically reappear about 3 weeks postpartum as these changes resolve. The vagina may initially appear relatively estrogen deficient in postpartum lactating women or women using progesterone-only contraception. A vaginal lubricant may be beneficial if dyspareunia occurs.

Hormonal regulation

Resumption of ovulation and subsequent menses differs greatly in breastfeeding compared with nonbreastfeeding mothers. Nonlactating mothers experience ovulation on average 45 days after delivery with return of menses in many by 7–9 weeks postpartum. Lactating mothers experience a delayed and much more variable return to both ovulation and menstruation, which may relate to specific breastfeeding practices.[11,12] Lactational amenorrhea is useful in predicting the return of fertility in nursing women. During the first 6 months after delivery, women who are amenorrheic and breastfeeding frequently (≥ 8 times/24 h) without giving supplements have a less than 2% risk of pregnancy.[13–19]

The control of fertility generated by lactation is incompletely understood. Current theory suggests a prolactin-mediated dysfunction of the gonadotropin-releasing hormone (GnRH) pulse generator in the hypothalamus as the underlying cause of lactation-related reduction in fertility.[20]

Urinary system

The urinary system and pelvic floor are altered by pregnancy and the birthing process. Intravenous fluids and oxytocin (which is antidiuretic during infusion) may increase postpartum diuresis. Conduction anesthetics may also disrupt neural bladder control. Urinary retention with overdistention, urinary tract infection, and stress urinary incontinence are common transient problems. Dilation of the ureters may persist for 3 months or more postpartum.[21,22]

Lactation

Exclusive breastfeeding during approximately the first 6 months of life with continued breastfeeding through at least the second half of infancy is associated with reduced risk of adverse outcomes in mother and infant[23] (Table 66.1). Environmental factors have a marked influence on breastfeeding success. Obstetric practices must be evaluated for their potential impact on lactation performance.

Mammary development

Figure 66.1 illustrates the general anatomic structures of the developed human breast. Recently, ultrasound imaging of the lactating breast has raised questions regarding the permanent existence of lactiferous sinuses.[24] During pregnancy, lobuloalveolar growth increases dramatically. Terminal end buds differentiate into alveoli composed of a single layer of milk-secreting epithelial cells surrounding a central lumen. Alveoli are surrounded by myoepithelial cells and capillaries. The lumen of the alveoli empty into intralobular ducts, which coalesce to form a central duct in each lobe exiting through one of 5–9 ductal orifices.

Onset of milk production and early lactation failure

By 16 weeks' gestation, the breast is fully competent to produce milk. This is prevented by the high level of circulating progesterone, which blocks prolactin activation of alfa-lactalbumin formation. Onset of copious milk production (lactogenesis stage II or LS-II) begins after delivery of the placenta and subsequent fall in progesterone.[25] The mean time for LS-II is 50–73 h postpartum.[26] LS-II occurs later following stressful deliveries[27] and in primiparious,[28], obese,[29–31] and diabetic[26] women. Delayed onset of LS-II is a risk factor for premature weaning, and these dyads should be monitored closely.

Tissue swelling and edema are common during LS-II, but the experience of painful engorgement varies. Analgesics are appropriate treatment for pain. Skilled assistance may be needed to achieve effective latch and efficient milk removal.

Table 66.1 Associations between breastfeeding and risk of adverse outcomes.

	Infant risk		
Adverse outcome	During breastfeeding	After weaning	Maternal risk
Gastrointestinal and respiratory illnesses	Decreased[127]	Decreased if exclusively BF for >3 months[127,128]	
Celiac disease	Decreased[129]	Delayed onset/possibly reduced severity[129]	
Wheezing	Decreased[130]	Decreased[130]	
Urinary infections	Decreased[127]		
Diabetes		Decreased[131,132]	Decreased[133]
Leukemia		Decreased[134,135]	
Atopic dermatitis	Decreased		
Obesity		Decreased[136,137]	
Chron's disease		Decreased[129]	
Rheumatoid arthritis		Decreased[138]	Decreased[139]
Breast cancer			Decreased[140]
Ovarian cancer			Decreased[141]
Bone density			Temporary decrease followed by increase over baseline with resumption of menses[142,143]
Visual acuity	Increased[127]		
Cognition/psychomotor performance		Increased[144,145]	

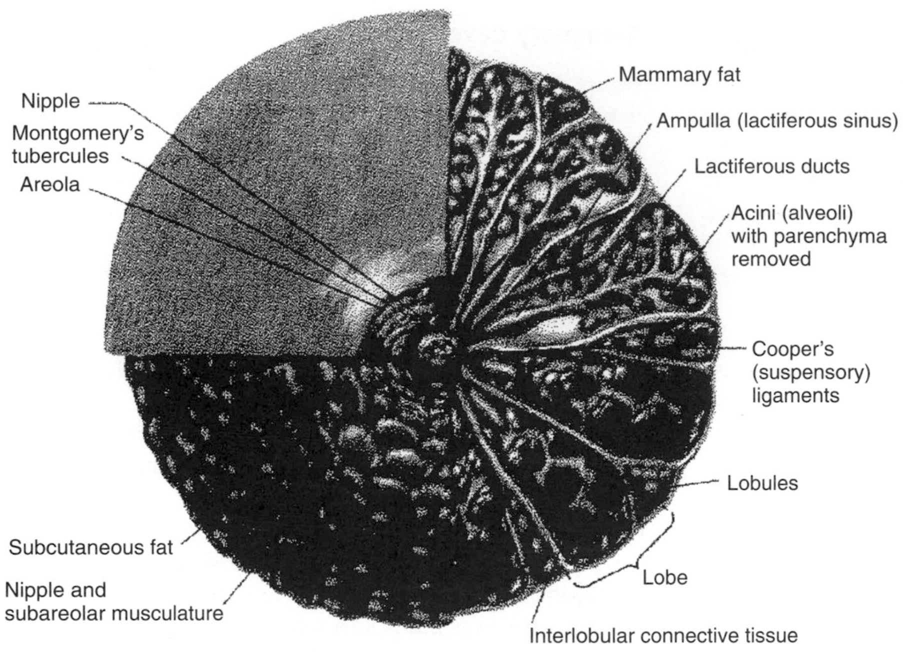

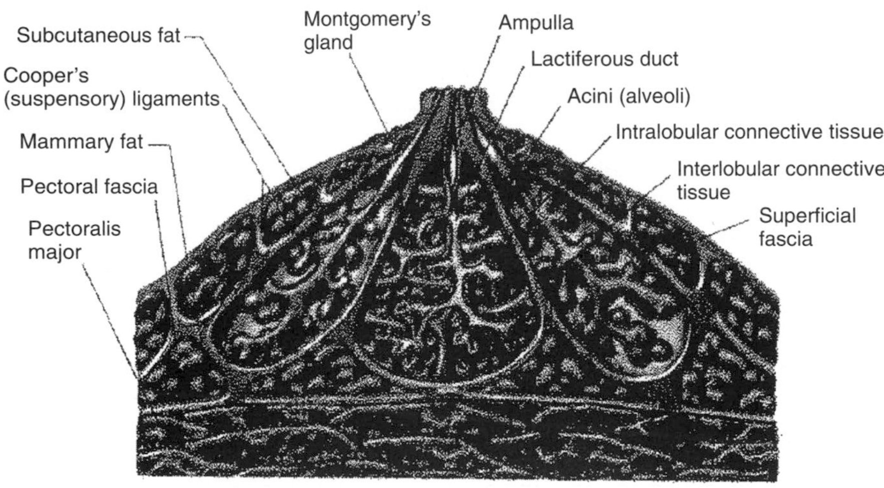

Figure 66.1 Anatomy of the human breast. (Copyright 1980 CIBA-GEIGY Corporation. Reproduced with permission from the Clinical Symposia by Frank H. Netter, MD. All rights reserved.)

Early lactation failure or partial inhibition of milk production can result from primary glandular insufficiency, retained placenta,[25] and severe postpartum hemorrhage resulting in ischemic pituitary necrosis and Sheehan's syndrome.[32]

Regulation of milk volume

Following LS-II, milk production increases to a mean of 750 mL/day by 4 weeks after delivery and remains there throughout exclusive breastfeeding.[33] For individual women, milk volume increases or decreases in response to alterations in mammary stimulation and the degree of breast emptying.

Prolactin is the primary endocrine regulator of milk production. Baseline levels vary with physiological state. Prolactin increases from 8–14 ng/mL prepregnancy to 200–500 ng/mL at term, and declines to 30–40 ng/mL between 180 and 360 days of lactation. Suckling causes a sharp rise in prolactin levels at all stages of lactation through at least the second year.[34–37] Suckling triggers a prolactin rise, which peaks at 30 min and returns to baseline after 2.5–3.0 h. Relationships between milk production and prolactin levels are not straightforward. This may reflect numerical or functional differences in prolactin receptors.

Pituitary release of oxytocin is triggered by suckling, auditory, olfactory, or emotional cues.[38] Unlike prolactin, oxytocin can be released through a conditioned reflex. Milk ejection results from oxytocin-induced contraction of myoepithelial cells surrounding the alveoli. Lactiferous ducts then increase in diameter facilitating milk flow.[24]

Weaning and involution of the mammary gland

Involution of the mammary gland is triggered by prolonged milk stasis and termination of suckling. Peaker and Wilde[39] detected a feedback inhibitor of lactation (termed FIL), which accumulates during milk stasis and blocks the secretion of milk constituents. Locally produced serotonin has been identified as a possible candidate for FIL,[40] although additional milk proteins may be involved.

Composition of human milk

Human milk is a complex, highly structured fluid containing a wide variety of nutrients and other bioactive factors, which impact infant growth, development, and immune function. Its composition is dynamic, varying with duration of lactation, degree of breast emptying, during a nursing, with the mother's diet, with maternal antigen response, maternal genotype, and other particulars. Changes over the course of lactation appear to match the changing needs of the growing infant.[41] Human milk components are multifunctional, serving not only as nutrients but also in a variety of ways that promote infant health and development. Proteins, for example, are a source of peptides, amino acids, and nitrogen, but are also involved in the development of the immune response (immunoglobulins), nonimmunologic defense (lactoferrin, lysozyme), growth stimulation (neural growth factor), and other functions. Carbohydrates provide nutritional support (lactose) and prevent bacterial adhesion to mucosal surfaces (oligosaccharides).[42–46] Human milk oligosaccharides (HMOs) are dietary fibers that pass through the digestive tract largely intact,[47] acting as prebiotics and presumably promoting gastric motility. Concentrations of HMOs vary over time[48–52] and this, along with variations in the type of oligosaccharides present, may be genetically determined.[44,48,49,53,54]

Colostrum, the initial milk produced in the first 3–7 days postpartum, is uniquely suited for the neonate. It contains a threefold higher protein concentration than mature milk, higher concentrations of immunoglobulins, leukocytes, and other immunologically active proteins, and lower concentrations of lactose, energy, and fat than more mature milk.[55] Throughout lactation, the specificity of secretory immunoglobulin A (SIgA) in milk depends on the mother's antigen exposure and response. In this sense, human milk is location specific. Infants themselves can control the nutrient content of received milk by varying the degree of breast emptying. Fat content (and calorie density) increases with the degree of breast emptying, progressing from low-fat "foremilk" to high-fat "hindmilk" during the course of a feed. The influence of maternal diet is more pronounced among malnourished women and relatively minor among those with normal body nutrient stores. The role of maternal genotype in milk composition – particularly oligosaccharide and cytokine content – is the subject of current research.[54,56]

Maternal diet and milk composition

In well-nourished women, normal dietary fluctuations influence the flavor and odor of milk, which influences infant dietary preferences.[57] In general, the nutrient content of milk is more responsive to maternal diet during lactation in malnourished than in well-nourished women.[58] Women can and do produce adequate and abundant milk on inadequate diets.[34] Complicated "rules" about diet during lactation that fail to consider the mother's nutrient stores and dietary preferences can undermine maternal resolve to breastfeed.[59]

Two nutrients may not be supplied in adequate amounts in milk from normal, well-nourished women: vitamin K[60] and vitamin D.[61] Routine intramuscular injection of vitamin K1 at birth provides all the vitamin K needed. The American Academy of Pediatrics recommends daily supplementation with 200 IU of vitamin D to all infants unless they consume at least 500 mL/day vitamin D-fortified formula or milk.[62]

Other nutritional deficiencies may be observed in breastfed infants of severely malnourished or diet-restricted mothers, including deficiencies in vitamin B12, folic acid, ascorbic acid, iodine, zinc, and carnitine.[63–65] Without supplements, strict vegans will eventually develop B12 deficiencies and produce milk deficient in B12.[66,67] Infants may become symptomatic before the mother.[67] Although infant symptoms can be partially reversed with B12 shots, neurologic deficits can be irreversible. Vegetarians should consume B12 supplements, particularly during pregnancy and lactation. Other circumstances that may lead to B12-deficient breast milk are: (1) severe maternal malnutrition – particularly if accompanied by intestinal parasites and resulting nutrient malabsorption;[68,69] (2) gastric bypass surgery or partial gastrectomy.[70,71] In these cases, maternal oral supplementation may not be sufficient, and intravenous vitamin B12 may be required.[70]

Maternal fat intake affects the relative concentration of milk fatty acids without appreciably altering total fat content. For example, while all human milk contains docosahexanoic acid (DHA), 10-fold elevations can result from increased maternal dietary intake. DHA is critical for neurologic development. In a supplementation study, children's mental processing scores at age 4 years correlated with maternal intake of DHA and eicosapentanoic acid during pregnancy.[72] Supplementation during lactation alone has not been found to improve mental functioning,[73] but may improve psychomotor functioning.[74] Conversely, milk cholesterol levels do not respond to maternal diet, and are elevated in mothers with familial hypercholesterolemia.[75]

Milk ascorbic acid (AA) content can be low if maternal intakes are low, and low (but not average or high) milk AA can be doubled or tripled by increasing maternal dietary intake.[76] Similarly, maternal dietary intake normally influences milk iodine content only when maternal status is inadequate[77] or iodine intake is extremely elevated.[78] Milk iodine is reduced in healthy mothers who smoke cigarettes,[79] and is inversely related to milk perchlorate levels (an environmental contaminant).[80]

Contaminants in human milk

Environmental contaminants are ubiquitous. An extensive review of research on contamination of human milk was published by LaKind et al. in 2004.[81] In spite of the ubiquitous presence of contaminants in human milk, breastfed infants are healthier than infants who are not breastfed. Much work remains to be done to identify circumstances in which the adverse effects of milk contaminants may outweigh the adverse effects of failure to provide human milk.

Exercise and calorie restriction diets during lactation

While postpartum women lose an average of 0.5–1.0 kg/month after postpartum diuresis,[82,83] individual weight loss varies. The myth that breastfeeding assures postpartum weight loss is prevalent, and prenatal education regarding the realities of postpartum weight management is advisable. In the US, each pregnancy increases the risk of becoming overweight by 60% and the risk of obesity by 110%.[84] Failure to return to prepregnancy weight by 6 months postpartum increases the risk of obesity a decade later.[85] In spite of the estimated 650 kcal/day required to support full lactation, breastfeeding has little impact on short-term postpartum weight loss in societies where food is abundant.[86] Energy required for lactation is derived from increased intake in preference to body fat mobilization.[87]

Obese women have lower breastfeeding initiation rates[30,88–90] and shorter breastfeeding durations than women of normal weight. Breastfeeding women who desire to initiate or increase weight loss may be advised to begin moderate calorie restriction (500 kcal/day) and regular exercise after breastfeeding is well established. Severe calorie restriction may be associated with decreased milk production.[91] Early warning signs include infant loss of appetite, irritability, or restlessness, and maternal fatigue. In all cases, dyads should be closely monitored for signs of compromised milk production.

Exercise has no apparent impact on milk composition, excluding a temporary rise in lactate after prolonged, heavy exercise.[92] Mineral content of milk did not change in response to exercise in a randomized crossover trial comparing the phosphorus, calcium, magnesium, sodium, and potassium content of milk from women at rest with milk from the same women at 10, 30, and 60 min after maximal graded exercise.[93] Similarly, in well-nourished women, maternal dietary intake has relatively little impact on milk mineral content.[77,94] Larson-Meyer[92] published an excellent review on the effect of exercise on postpartum women and their offspring. Women should be advised to consume a balanced diet during calorie restriction to protect their health.

Prenatal and perinatal practices and conditions that affect breastfeeding

Breastfeeding should be recommended at the initial prenatal examination. Further education can be offered during prenatal care for women planning to breastfeed and those initially inclined to formula feed. Women with specific concerns such as breast implants, prior breast surgery, inverted nipples, time constraints, or lack of confidence should be educated regarding their particular situation. Prior breast reduction or other surgery involving a periareolar incision should prompt counseling regarding the importance of communicating that information to the pediatrician and the need to monitor infant growth. Multiparous women should be questioned regarding their prior breastfeeding experiences, and any concerns should be addressed.

Cigarettes

Smoking cessation is strongly encouraged during pregnancy. Parents who continue to smoke should do so in an environment that is away from the newborn. Nicotine and its metabolite cotinine are present in human milk. Urinary cotinine levels in breastfed infants of smoking mothers have been reported to be 10-fold higher than those of formula-fed infants.[95] Importantly, however, neurologic deficits associated with maternal cigarette smoking in formula-fed infants were not observed in a comparison group of infants breastfed for > 3 weeks.[96]

Caffeine

Peak caffeine levels in breast milk are reached about 1 h after ingestion and are typically about 1% of the maternal dose.[97] Thus, infants should receive only a very small percentage of the maternal dose. However, clearance of caffeine in the infant is slower than in the adult.[98] Rare concerns with irritability and insomnia have been reported, but would be unlikely with occasional and moderate consumption.

Alcohol

Alcohol consumption should be avoided during pregnancy. Excessive consumption of alcohol should be avoided by new parents regardless of the planned infant feeding method because of the implications for parenting skills. Research has suggested that the consumption of ethanol has a potentially deleterious effect on the quantity of breast milk consumed by the baby. Milk transfer decreased during breastfeeding for 4 h after maternal alcohol consumption and then increased 8–16 h after consumption ceased.[99] These studies do not support the folklore that small amounts of alcohol improve lactation.

In general, after consumption of a relatively small amount of alcohol and the passage of sufficient time so that the mother no longer feels the effects of the alcohol, breastfeeding can resume. Using a nomogram published by Ho et al.,[100] a 140-pound lactating woman would require 2 h and 19 min after consuming one drink to achieve a zero level of milk alcohol.

Substances of abuse

Substances of abuse are contraindicated during pregnancy and lactation. The exception is methadone supplied within the context of a successful maintenance program. Mothers on methadone should be monitored carefully and the infant

Table 66.2 Contraindications for breastfeeding.

Condition	Contraindication
Substances of abuse (except methadone maintenance program and free of other drugs)	Absolute
Alcohol abuse	Absolute
Chemotherapeutic agents	Absolute or relative (depending on prior fetal exposure, duration of agent, and particular agent involved)
Maternal HIV	Absolute in US Relative in non-US regions with insufficient access to formula or clean water
Maternal HSV infection of nipple	Temporary cessation from involved nipple/areola until lesions resolved
Active untreated maternal tuberculosis	Temporary until after treatment established
Radioactive ^{131}I therapy	Absolute due to long half-life and potential to concentrate in thyroid and breast
Infant galactosemia	Absolute

observed for methadone withdrawal after delivery regardless of feeding method. Breast milk exposure may mitigate neonatal abstinence syndrome, but is not sufficient to prevent withdrawal.[101] Mothers engaging in continued substance abuse postpartum should be provided with support services for drug dependency treatment and counseled not to breastfeed. A study of breast milk from 11 mothers who admitted using drugs during pregnancy detected cocaine in six of the specimens.[102] It is suspected that cocaine has a high milk to plasma ratio. Serious adverse effects have been reported. Similarly, marijuana has a high milk to plasma ratio, suggesting that it is concentrated in breast milk.[103]

Medication use

Advice regarding the use of a medication during breastfeeding should reflect not only the efficacy of the drug in treating the mother's condition but also the impact of the drug on lactation and the breastfed infant. Few studies examine drug use during lactation, and specialized references are required to formulate appropriate advice. Those drugs that have been shown to be safe for use during breastfeeding and/or those used in pediatric populations are generally preferred. Thus, the drug of choice for a particular condition may well differ depending on whether or not the mother is breastfeeding. The healthcare provider should review available information with the parents and discuss their individual situation. The age, weight, and health of the child, in addition to the amount of breast milk in the diet and any medications the child is taking, should be considered when choosing which medication is the best choice. Many characteristics of medications influence their potential to pass into breast milk and then reach and affect the breastfed child. These include the molecular weight, half-life, pH, protein binding, lipid solubility, oral bioavailability, and acid stability.

Maternal health problems

Table 66.2 lists circumstances in which breastfeeding is contraindicated. Table 66.3 lists concerns regarding breastfeeding by women with specific diseases.

Thyroid disease

Postpartum thyroid dysfunction is common and, occasionally, lactation difficulties in the previously successfully breastfeeding mother could be a presenting symptom of thyroid dysfunction. Breastfeeding can be continued during many treatments for either hypothyroidism or hyperthyroidism. Radioactive ablation of the thyroid with ^{131}I is not recommended during breastfeeding

Diabetes mellitus

The gestational diabetic will not need further therapy after delivery, although her infant is still at risk of neonatal hypoglycemia, and infant glucose monitoring is warranted within 30 min of birth. Some gestational diabetics have previously undiagnosed diabetes. Therefore, it is recommended that gestational diabetics undergo glucose testing at the postpartum visit. Insulin can be continued safely during lactation. Metformin has been studied in a small number of breastfeeding women.[104] No adverse reactions were noted in the infants. Owing to the concern over lactic acidosis, use in either a mother or an infant with renal dysfunction may not be advisable.

Cystic fibrosis (CF)

Recent studies have shown that electrolyte concentrations in the breast milk of women with CF are within normal limits as the mammary gland does not reabsorb sodium in excess of water.[105–107] Preliminary information indicates that women with CF can breastfeed while receiving close monitoring of their disease.

Maternal phenylketonuria (PKU)

Limited data indicate that a mother with PKU under strict dietary control should be allowed to breastfeed. Although milk phenylalanine concentrations are dramatically elevated,[108] successful management of PKU and breastfeeding have been described with complementary low phenylalanine infant formula in women using strict dietary control.[109]

Table 66.3 Maternal disease and breastfeeding considerations.

Infection	Route of transmission	Breastfeeding considerations
HIV	Blood and body fluids	Contraindicated in US and regions where safe alternatives to breast milk are available
Hepatitis A	Fecal and oral	Continued breastfeeding: encourage good hygiene
Hepatitis B	Blood and body fluids	Continued breastfeeding: infant to receive hepatitis B immunoglobulin (HBIG) within 12 h of birth and hepatitis B vaccination
Hepatitis C	Blood and body fluids	Continued breastfeeding: no difference in transmission rate (~4%) in breastfed versus formula-fed infants. Some experts recommend temporary interruption of breastfeeding when bleeding nipples are present
Cytomegalovirus	Respiratory	Continued breastfeeding of healthy term infant Breastfeeding of premature infant during infection deserves individual consideration
Herpes simplex virus	Direct contact	Continued breastfeeding unless lesions on nipple/areola (see above). Cover lesions in potential contact with infant, good hygiene
Varicella virus	Respiratory, direct contact	Maternal primary infection: infant varicella immune globulin (VZIG) and possible vaccination depending on infant age Maternal shingles: continued breastfeeding, cover lesions in potential contact with infant and encourage good hygiene. Consider VZIG

Human immunodeficiency virus (HIV)

The current estimate of the prevalence of HIV in pregnant US women is 1–2 per 1000. Without treatment, the transmission rate from mother to child related to pregnancy and delivery is approximately 25%. Antiretroviral therapy with zidovudine during pregnancy and labor with infant treatment during the first 6 weeks postpartum and not breastfeeding reduces the risk of transmission to approximately 6–8%. Women with an unknown HIV status prior to labor account for 40% of mother to child transmission of HIV in the US. Optimal treatment in labor with the use of intrapartum zidovudine or initiating infant therapy by 48 h of life significantly reduces the risk of transmission. The recommendation to avoid breastfeeding should also be provided in this situation. For women with unknown HIV status upon entry to the labor suite, rapid HIV testing could allow for treatment and recommendations that could significantly improve outcome.

Support strategy for mother and infant

Intrapartum influences

During an uncomplicated pregnancy and delivery, the infant can be given to the mother at delivery, and breastfeeding initiation should be encouraged within the first hour after birth. Labor companionship and support have been associated with improved breastfeeding initiation and continuation rates.[110–112] Avoidance of unnecessary interventions is recommended. Having staff trained in lactation support can mitigate potential obstacles to breastfeeding that may present with complicated pregnancies and/or medical interventions associated with delivery.

Labor induction and delivery method

Studies evaluating the influence of labor induction on breastfeeding success reach varying conclusions and may be confounded by maternal confidence or intentionality. In a study by Out et al.,[113] women undergoing medically indicated labor induction were more likely to continue their antepartum intention to breastfeed than women in the "elective" induction group. Similarly, emergent Cesarean delivery appears to be a more significant obstacle to breastfeeding success than non-emergent Cesarean delivery.[114,115] Delayed onset of lactation in mothers undergoing Cesarean delivery has also been reported.[116] Grajeda and Perez-Escamilla[117] found that primiparous vaginally delivered women experienced onset of lactation at day 2.9 on average as opposed to day 3.4 for those undergoing emergent Cesarean delivery. No difference was noted related to mode of delivery in multiparas.

Regional anesthesia appears to be associated with improved lactation performance compared with general anesthesia.[118,119] Patient-controlled analgesia with morphine or continuous extradural anesthesia in the initial postoperative period is preferred over the use of meperidine because of the association of meperidine with an adverse effect on infant suckling behavior.[120]

Maternal–infant contact

The vigorous term infant with clear amniotic fluid may be placed on the maternal abdomen at delivery. The family may participate in cutting the cord if the situation is deemed appropriate. The infant can then be dried, stimulated, and placed skin to skin with the mother with warm blankets placed over the dyad to maintain the infant's temperature. Infant interventions such as vitamin K injection, the application of

Table 66.4 Breastfeeding information for new parents.

1 Normal milk production is quite low until after the onset of lactogenesis stage II between the first and fifth days postpartum
2 Most infants nurse 8–14 times/day in the first 1–2 weeks. This decreases to 7–10 times/day by 4 weeks
3 Each infant's "demand" breastfeeding frequency reflects his own developmental status and nursing skill as well as the mother's milk flow
4 After the third day of life, exclusively breastfed infants usually soak six or more diapers and have three or more stools of 1 tablespoon or greater/day
5 Infant stools normally change from dark (green or brown) to mustard yellow by the fifth day. This happens after the mother's milk "comes in" and the baby begins to receive larger volumes of milk, which clears the meconium from the gastrointestinal tract
6 Healthcare provider should be notified promptly if urine or stool patterns deviate from norms indicated in items 4 and 5 or if parents are concerned about adequacy of infant intake or maternal milk production

ophthalmic ointment, newborn screening, and measurements may be obtained later. The mother can be encouraged to breastfeed soon after delivery, ideally within the first hour after birth. A Cochrane review evaluating 17 studies found a significant positive impact of skin to skin contact on the maintenance of infant body temperature, infant glucose levels, and continued breastfeeding at 1 and 3 months.[121]

Unless medically indicated, newborn interventions should be delayed until after the first hour of life. In an ideal situation, these procedures can be performed in the room of the new family. The family should be encouraged to room in with the infant and breastfeed on demand. Rooming in will facilitate the acquisition of parental roles and the development of nonverbal parent–infant communication skills, such as recognition of infant hunger and satiety cues required for successful breastfeeding.

Latch and milk transfer during feeding should be assessed by trained personnel within 8 h prior to hospital discharge. Predischarge teaching should include the elements listed in Table 66.4. Parents should be advised to report promptly deviations from normal urine and stool patterns or concerns about low milk production to the healthcare provider. Breastfed infants discharged 1–2 days after delivery should return to their healthcare provider in the first few days after discharge to assure that the mother's milk has come in, infant weight loss has ceased, and jaundice and dehydration are not significant.

Common problems in postpartum care

Mastitis

Mastitis occurs in approximately 9.5% of breastfeeding women during the first 12 weeks postpartum.[122] Risk factors include unrelieved engorgement or plugged ducts, past history of mastitis, and nipple trauma which provides a portal of entry for the offending organisms. *Staphylococcus aureus* is the most common organism cultured from the mastitic breast.

Signs and symptoms of mastitis include an erythematous, tender breast, fever, and flu-like symptoms such as myalgia, nausea, and headache. A localized tender knot in the breast in the absence of symptoms of infection suggests a plugged duct, which can be managed with frequent nursing and warm compresses. Persistent breast masses should be pursued regardless of lactation status. More diffuse firmness in both breasts in the initial week postpartum is suggestive of engorgement and is usually associated with normal or low-grade fever. The presence of a fluctuant palpable and tender mass in the mastitic breast is suggestive of a breast abscess.

Mastitis is treated with a penicillinase-resistant antibiotic such as Dicloxicillin or a cephalosporin for 10–14 days. If symptoms do not improve after 24–48 h of therapy, milk should be cultured for resistant organisms, and the breast should be re-examined for possible abscess. Nonsteroidal anti-inflammatory agents such as ibuprofen are useful in pain control. In addition to antibiotic therapy, breastfeeding should be assessed, and factors that predisposed to the infection should be addressed, such as latch difficulties leading to nipple trauma. Otherwise, the mother may be more likely to experience a recurrent episode of infection. Breastfeeding the healthy, term infant during treatment of mastitis should be continued, and excellent drainage of the infected breast is important in recovery. Abrupt weaning during mastitis increases the risk of abscess.

The risk of breast abscess is 0.4% for breastfeeding women generally, and 3% for those with mastitis.[123] Management of breast abscesses requires the use of antibiotics with the addition of drainage of the abscess collection. Prior management using open incision and drainage is being replaced by repeat ultrasound-guided aspirations of the abscess either with or without the placement of a drainage catheter.[124–126]

Contraception

If the patient is using lactational amenorrhea as a means of contraception, provision should be made for easy access to additional contraception at 6 months, or sooner if the need arises. Nonhormonal contraceptive options do not affect breast milk composition or quantity. If a hormonal contraceptive is chosen, a progesterone-only alternative has less potential impact on milk supply. In breastfeeding mothers, estrogen-containing contraceptive options have the theoretical concern of adversely affecting milk supply. If a breastfeeding mother is inclined to pursue an estrogen-containing option, the lower estrogen dosage appears prudent. The mother should be counseled regarding the potential for an adverse effect on milk supply, and the contraceptive should be initiated as late after established lactation as possible.

Low milk production

If a mother expresses concern about low milk production in the early postpartum period, the infant should be evaluated and the mother assessed for possible causes of failed LS-II (see Onset of milk production and early lactation failure). If infant status is normal and the child is exclusively breastfed, maternal concerns likely reflect misinterpretation of infant behavior. If the infant is not thriving or is receiving formula supplements, it suggests that maternal milk volume is low. Medications and over-the-counter drugs should be reviewed for potential impact on milk production. If no medical or pharmacologic cause is apparent, milk volume usually increases in response to increased frequency of breast stimulation (nursing or pumping) and/or the increased degree of breast emptying (improved infant latch or breast massage during nursing). Referral to a certified lactation consultant is appropriate for both perceived and confirmed low milk production.

Key points

1. In controlled studies, lack of breastfeeding and/or earlier introduction of supplements and weaning are associated with increased risk of a variety of adverse outcomes in mothers and infants (see Table 66.1).
2. Onset of copious milk production (stage II lactogenesis) begins after delivery of the placenta in response to the subsequent fall in circulating progesterone. Delay of lactogenesis stage II beyond day 5 postpartum should prompt evaluation.
3. Failed lactogenesis can result from primary glandular insufficiency, retained placenta, or severe postpartum hemorrhage resulting in ischemic pituitary necrosis and Sheehan's syndrome.
4. When engorgement becomes severe, analgesics are appropriate treatment for pain, and immediate skilled assistance may be needed to achieve effective latch on and efficient milk removal.
5. In established lactation, milk volume averages 750 mL/day and increases or declines in response to alterations in mammary stimulation and the degree of breast emptying.
6. The nutrient content of human milk is conveyed to the infant within, and does not exist apart from, a redundant milieu of anti-infective, growth-stimulating, and anti-inflammatory agents.
7. Strict vegetarians should consume vitamin B12 supplements during pregnancy and lactation for their own health and to prevent vitamin B12 deficiencies in their infants.
8. In spite of the ubiquitous presence of environmental contaminants in human milk, breastfed infants are healthier than infants who are not breastfed.
9. Breastfeeding women who desire to lose weight may be advised to initiate moderate caloric restriction (500 kcal/day below maintenance levels), consume a balanced diet, and undertake regular exercise after breastfeeding is well established.
10. During the first 6 months postpartum, women who are amenorrheic and breastfeeding frequently (≥ 8 times/24 h) without giving supplements have a less than 2% risk of pregnancy.
11. Women with specific breastfeeding-related concerns, such as breast implants, prior breast surgery, inverted nipples, time constraints, or lack of confidence, should be educated regarding their particular situation.
12. Advice regarding medication use during breastfeeding should be formulated only after reviewing information on that medication, exploring alternative treatments, and discussing that individual situation with the parents. The age, weight, and health of the child, in addition to the amount of breast milk in the diet and medications the child is taking, should all be considered when prescribing medication for breastfeeding women.
13. Maternal contraindications to breastfeeding are rare and include continued use of substances of abuse, rare chemotherapeutic and other medications, and maternal HIV infection. Temporary interruption is warranted with maternal herpes simplex virus (HSV) involving the nipple and untreated maternal tuberculosis.
14. Having staff trained in lactation support can help to minimize the impact of potential obstacles to breastfeeding, which may present with medically complicated pregnancies and/or medical interventions associated with delivery.
15. During an uncomplicated pregnancy and delivery, the infant can be placed skin to skin with the mother at delivery with warm blankets covering them, and breastfeeding initiation should be encouraged within the first hour after birth.
16. In the initial postCesarean period, patient-controlled analgesia with morphine or continuous extradural anesthesia is preferred over the use of meperidine because of the association of meperidine with poor infant suckling behavior in the early postpartum period.
17. New parents should be specifically and carefully advised of the ranges of normal for volume of colostrum, time of onset of copious milk production, frequencies of infant feeding, stooling, and urination, and the timing of meconium passage, with clear instructions to contact the care provider should the infant deviate from expected norms (Table 66.4).

18 Breastfed infants discharged 1–2 days after delivery should return to their healthcare provider in the first few days after discharge to assure that the mother's milk has come in, infant weight loss has ceased, and jaundice and dehydration are not significant.

19 Evaluation of persistent breast masses should be pursued regardless of lactation status.

20 Breastfeeding the healthy, term infant should be continued during treatment of mastitis with antibiotics; excellent drainage of the infected breast is important in maternal recovery.

References

1 Negishi H, Kishida T, Yamada H, et al. Changes in uterine size after vaginal delivery and cesarean section determined by vaginal sonography in the puerperium. *Arch Gynecol Obstet* 1999; 263(1–2):13–16.
2 Shalev J, Royburt M, Fite G, et al. Sonographic evaluation of the puerperal uterus: correlation with manual examination. *Gynecol Obstet Invest* 2002;53(1):38–41.
3 Olayemi O, Omigbodun AA, Obajimi MO, et al. Ultrasound assessment of the effect of parity on postpartum uterine involution. *J Obstet Gynaecol* 2002;22(4):381–384.
4 Mulic-Lutvica A, Bekuretsion M, Bakos O, Axelsson O. Ultrasonic evaluation of the uterus and uterine cavity after normal, vaginal delivery. *Ultrasound Obstet Gynecol* 2001;18(5):491–498.
5 Al-Bdour AN, Akasheh HF, Al-Husban NA. Ultrasonography of the uterus after normal vaginal delivery. *Saudi Med J* 2004; 25(1):41–44.
6 Sherman D, Lurie S, Frenkel E, et al. Characteristics of normal lochia. *Am J Perinatol* 1999;16(8):399–402.
7 Oppenheimer LW, Sherriff EA, Goodman JD, et al. The duration of lochia. *Br J Obstet Gynaecol* 1986;93(7):754–757.
8 Murray A, Holdcroft A. Incidence and intensity of postpartum lower abdominal pain. *Br Med J* 1989;298(6688):1619.
9 Holdcroft A, Snidvongs S, Cason A, et al. Pain and uterine contractions during breast feeding in the immediate post-partum period increase with parity. *Pain* 2003;104(3):589–596.
10 Kaplan KJ, Dainty LA, Dolinsky B, et al. Prognosis and recurrence risk for patients with cervical squamous intraepithelial lesions diagnosed during pregnancy. *Cancer* 2004;102(4): 228–232.
11 Howie PW, McNeilly AS. Breast-feeding and postpartum ovulation. *IPPF Med Bull* 1982;16(2):1–3.
12 Rogers IS. Lactation and fertility. *Early Hum Dev* 1997; 49(Suppl.):S185–190.
13 Lactation amenorrhea: experts recommend full breastfeeding as a child spacing method. *Network* 1988;10(2):12.
14 Short RV, Lewis PR, Renfree MB, Shaw G. Contraceptive effects of extended lactational amenorrhoea: beyond the Bellagio Consensus. *Lancet* 1991;337(8743):715–717.
15 Kennedy KI, Visness CM. Contraceptive efficacy of lactational amenorrhoea. *Lancet* 1992;339(8787):227–230.
16 Perez A, Labbok MH, Queenan JT. Clinical study of the lactational amenorrhoea method for family planning. *Lancet* 1992;339(8799):968–970.
17 Gross BA. Is the lactational amenorrhea method a part of natural family planning? Biology and policy. *Am J Obstet Gynecol* 1991;165(6 Pt 2):2014–2019.
18 World Health Organization Task Force on Methods for the Natural Regulation of Fertility. The World Health Organization multinational study of breast-feeding and lactational amenorrhea. III. Pregnancy during breast-feeding. *Fertil Steril* 1999;72(3):431–440.
19 Labbok MH, Hight-Laukaran V, Peterson AE, et al. Multicenter study of the Lactational Amenorrhea Method (LAM): I. Efficacy, duration, and implications for clinical application. *Contraception* 1997;55(6):327–336.
20 McNeilly AS. Lactational control of reproduction. *Reprod Fertil Dev* 2001;13(7–8):583–590.
21 Bailey RR, Rolleston GL. Kidney length and ureteric dilatation in the puerperium. *J Obstet Gynaecol Br Commonw* 1971;78(1): 55–61.
22 Beydoun SN. Morphologic changes in the renal tract in pregnancy. *Clin Obstet Gynecol* 1985;28(2):249–256.
23 Gartner LM, Morton J, Lawrence RA, et al. Breastfeeding and the use of human milk. *Pediatrics* 2005;115(2):496–506.
24 Ramsay DT, Kent JC, Owens RA, Hartmann PE. Ultrasound imaging of milk ejection in the breast of lactating women. *Pediatrics* 2004;113(2):361.
25 Neifert MR, McDonough SL, Neville MC. Failure of lactogenesis associated with placental retention. *Am J Obstet Gynecol* 1981;140(4):477–478.
26 Perez-Escamilla R, Chapman DJ. Validity and public health implications of maternal perception of the onset of lactation: an international analytical overview. *J Nutr* 2001;131(11):3021S–3024S.
27 Dewey KG. Maternal and fetal stress are associated with impaired lactogenesis in humans. *J Nutr* 2001;131(11):3012S–3015S.
28 Hilson JA, Rasmussen KM, Kjolhede CL. High prepregnant body mass index is associated with poor lactation outcomes among white, rural women independent of psychosocial and demographic correlates. *J Hum Lact* 2004;20(1):18.
29 Rasmussen KM, Kjolhede CL. Prepregnant overweight and obesity diminish the prolactin response to suckling in the first week postpartum. *Pediatrics* 2004;113(5):e465–471
30 Donath SM, Amir LH. Does maternal obesity adversely affect breastfeeding initiation and duration? *Breastfeed Rev* 2000;8(3): 29–33.
31 Hilson JA, Rasmussen KM, Kjolhede CL. Maternal obesity and breast-feeding success in a rural population of white women. *Am J Clin Nutr* 1997;66(6):1371–1378.
32 Kelestimur F. Sheehan's syndrome. *Pituitary* 2003;6(4):181–188.
33 Butte NF, Garza C, Smith EO, Nichols BL. Human milk intake and growth in exclusively breast-fed infants. *J Pediatr* 1984;104(2):187–195.
34 Lawrence RA, Lawrence R. *Breastfeeding: a guide for the medical profession*, 6th edn. St. Louis, MO: Mosby (Elsevier Inc.); 2005:318.
35 Diaz S. Determinants of lactational amenorrhea. *Int J Gynecol Obstet* 1989;1(Suppl.):83–89.
36 Freeman ME, Kanyicska B, Lerant A, Nagy G. Prolactin: structure, function, and regulation of secretion. *Physiol Rev* 2000;80(4):1523–1631.

37 Stern JM, Reichlin S. Prolactin circadian rhythm persists throughout lactation in women. *Neuroendocrinology* 1990;51(1):31–37.
38 Newton M, Newton NR. The let-down reflex in human lactation. *J Pediatr* 1948;33:698.
39 Peaker M, Wilde CJ. Feedback control of milk secretion from milk. *J Mammary Gland Biol Neoplasia* 1996;1(3):307–315.
40 Matsuda M, Imaoka T, Vomachka AJ, et al. Serotonin regulates mammary gland development via an autocrine–paracrine loop. *Dev Cell* 2004;6(2):193–203.
41 Kunz C, Rodriguez-Palmero M, Koletzko B, Jensen R. Nutritional and biochemical properties of human milk, Part I: General aspects, proteins, and carbohydrates. *Clin Perinatol* 1999;26(2):307.
42 Morrow AL, Ruiz-Palacios GM, Jiang X, Newburg DS. Human-milk glycans that inhibit pathogen binding protect breast-feeding infants against infectious diarrhea. *J Nutr* 2005;135(5):1304.
43 Morrow AL, Ruiz-Palacios GM, Altaye M, et al. Human milk oligosaccharide blood group epitopes and innate immune protection against campylobacter and calicivirus diarrhea in breastfed infants. *Adv Exp Med Biol* 2004;554:443.
44 Morrow AL, Ruiz-Palacios GM, Altaye M, et al. Human milk oligosaccharides are associated with protection against diarrhea in breast-fed infants. *J Pediatr* 2004;145(3):297.
45 Clemens K, Silvia R. Physiology of oligosaccharides in lactating women and breast fed infants. *Adv Exp Med Biol* 2000;478:241.
46 Newburg DS. Human milk glycoconjugates that inhibit pathogens. *Curr Med Chem* 1999;6(2):117.
47 Gnoth MJ, Kunz C, Kinne-Saffran E, Rudloff S. Human milk oligosaccharides are minimally digested in vitro. *J Nutr* 2000;130(12):3014.
48 Chaturvedi P, Warren CD, Buescher CR, et al. Survival of human milk oligosaccharides in the intestine of infants. *Adv Exp Med Biol* 2001;501:315.
49 Erney RM, Malone WT, Skelding MB, et al. Variability of human milk neutral oligosaccharides in a diverse population. *J Pediatr Gastroenterol Nutr* 2000;30(2):181.
50 Landberg E, Huang Y, Stromqvist M, et al. Changes in glycosylation of human bile-salt-stimulated lipase during lactation. *Arch Biochem Biophys* 2000;377(2):246.
51 Coppa GV, Pierani P, Zampini L, et al. Oligosaccharides in human milk during different phases of lactation. *Acta Paediatr Suppl* 1999;88(430):89.
52 Miller JB, Bull S, Miller J, McVeagh P. The oligosaccharide composition of human milk: temporal and individual variations in monosaccharide components. *J Pediatr Gastroenterol Nutr* 1994;19(4):371.
53 Sumiyoshi W, Urashima T, Nakamura T, et al. Determination of each neutral oligosaccharide in the milk of Japanese women during the course of lactation. *Br J Nutr* 2003;89(1):61.
54 Newburg DS, Ruiz-Palacios GM, Altaye M, et al. Innate protection conferred by fucosylated oligosaccharides of human milk against diarrhea in breastfed infants. *Glycobiology* 2004;14(3):253.
55 Garza C, Hopkinson J. Physiology of lactation. In: Tsang RC, Nichols BL, eds. *Nutrition during infancy*. Philadelphia: Hanley & Belfus; 1988:20.
56 Fituch CC, Palkowetz KH, Goldman AS, Schanler RJ. Concentrations of IL-10 in preterm human milk and in milk from mothers of infants with necrotizing enterocolitis. *Acta Paediatr* 2004;93(11):1496–1500.
57 Mennella JA, Beauchamp GK. Experience with a flavor in mother's milk modifies the infant's acceptance of flavored cereal. *Dev Psychopathol* 1999;35(3):197–203.
58 Allen LH. Multiple micronutrients in pregnancy and lactation: an overview. *Am J Clin Nutr* 2005;81(5):1206S.
59 Lawrence RA, Lawrence R. *Breastfeeding: a guide for the medical profession*, 6th edn. St. Louis, MO: Mosby (Elsevier Inc.); 2005:317.
60 Canfield LM, Hopkinson JM, Lima AF, et al. Vitamin K in colostrum and mature human milk over the lactation period – a cross-sectional study. *Am J Clin Nutr* 1991;53(3):730–735.
61 Lammi-Keefe CJ. Vitamins D and E in human milk. In: Jensen RG, ed. *Handbook of milk composition (food science and technology international)*. San Diego, CA: Academic Press (Division of Harcourt Brace & Co.); 1995:706–717.
62 Gartner LM, Greer FR. Prevention of rickets and vitamin D deficiency: new guidelines for vitamin D intake. *Pediatrics* 2003;111(4 Pt 1):908–910.
63 Zmora E, Gorodischer R, Bar-Ziv J. Multiple nutritional deficiencies in infants from a strict vegetarian community. *Am J Dis Child* 1979;133(2):141–144.
64 Kanaka C, Schutz B, Zuppinger KA. Risks of alternative nutrition in infancy: a case report of severe iodine and carnitine deficiency. *Eur J Pediatr* 1992;151(10):786–788.
65 Hey E. Vitamin K – what, why, and when. *Arch Dis Child Fetal Neonatal Ed* 2003;88(2):F80–83.
66 Specker BL, Black A, Allen L, Morrow F. Vitamin B-12: low milk concentrations are related to low serum concentrations in vegetarian women and to methylmalonic aciduria in their infants. *Am J Clin Nutr* 1990;52(6):1073–1076.
67 Hamosh M, Dewey KG, Garza C, et al. Infant outcomes. In: *Nutrition during lactation*, 1st edn. Washington, DC: National Academy Press; 1991:153–196.
68 Casterline JE, Allen LH, Ruel MT. Vitamin B-12 deficiency is very prevalent in lactating Guatemalan women and their infants at three months postpartum. *J Nutr* 1997;127(10):1966–1972.
69 Allen LH, Rosado JL, Casterline JE, et al. Vitamin B-12 deficiency and malabsorption are highly prevalent in rural Mexican communities. *Am J Clin Nutr* 1995;62(5):1013–1019.
70 Grange DK, Finlay JL. Nutritional vitamin B12 deficiency in a breastfed infant following maternal gastric bypass. *Pediatr Hematol Oncol* 1994;11(3):311.
71 Wardinsky TD, Montes RG, Friederich RL, et al. Vitamin B12 deficiency associated with low breast-milk vitamin B12 concentration in an infant following maternal gastric bypass surgery. *Arch Pediatr Adolesc Med* 1995;149(11):1281–1284.
72 Helland IB, Smith L, Saarem K, et al. Maternal supplementation with very-long chain n-3 fatty acids during pregnancy and lactation augments children's IQ at 4 years of age. *Pediatrics* 2003;111(1):e39–44.
73 Lauritzen L, Jorgensen MH, Olsen SF, et al. Maternal fish oil supplementation in lactation: effect on developmental outcome in breast-fed infants. *Reprod Nutr Dev* 2005;45(5):535–547.
74 Jensen CL, Voigt RG, Prager TC, et al. Effects of maternal docosahexaenoic acid intake on visual function and neurodevelopment in breastfed term infants. *Am J Clin Nutr* 2005;82(1):125–132.
75 Picciano MF. Human milk: nutritional aspects of a dynamic food. *Biol Neonate* 1998;74(2):84–93.
76 Daneel-Otterbech S, Davidsson L, Hurrell R. Ascorbic acid supplementation and regular consumption of fresh orange juice increase the ascorbic acid content of human milk: studies in

European and African lactating women. *Am J Clin Nutr* 2005;81(5):1088–1093.

77 Chierici R, Saccomandi D, Vigi V. Dietary supplements for the lactating mother: influence on the trace element content of milk. *Acta Paediatr Suppl* 1999;88(430):7–13.

78 Moon S, Kim J. Iodine content of human milk and dietary iodine intake of Korean lactating mothers. *Int J Food Sci Nutr* 1999;50(3):165–171.

79 Laurberg P, Nohr SB, Pedersen KM, Fuglsang E. Iodine nutrition in breast-fed infants is impaired by maternal smoking. *J Clin Endocrinol Metab* 2004;89(1):181–187.

80 Kirk AB, Martinelango PK, Tian K, et al. Perchlorate and iodide in dairy and breast milk. *Environ Sci Technol* 2005;39(7): 2011–2017.

81 LaKind JS, Amina Wilkins A, Berlin CM, Jr. Environmental chemicals in human milk: a review of levels, infant exposures and health, and guidance for future research. *Toxicol Appl Pharmacol* 2004;198(2):184–208.

82 Prentice AM, Prentice A. Energy costs of lactation. *Annu Rev Nutr* 1988;8:63–79.

83 Butte NF, Hopkinson JM. Body composition changes during lactation are highly variable among women. *J Nutr* 1998;128(2 Suppl.):381S–385S.

84 Keppel KG, Taffel SM. Pregnancy-related weight gain and retention: implications of the 1990 Institute of Medicine guidelines. *Am J Public Health* 1993;83(8):1100–1103.

85 Rooney BL, Schauberger CW. Excess pregnancy weight gain and long-term obesity: one decade later. *Obstet Gynecol* 2005; 100(2):245–252.

86 Fraser AB, Grimes DA. Effect of lactation on maternal body weight: a systematic review. *Obstet Gynecol Surv* 2003;58(4):265–269.

87 Butte NF, Wong WW, Hopkinson JM. Energy requirements of lactating women derived from doubly labeled water and milk energy output. *J Nutr* 2001;131(1):53–58.

88 Baker JL, Michaelsen KF, Rasmussen KM, Sorensen TI. Maternal prepregnant body mass index, duration of breastfeeding, and timing of complementary food introduction are associated with infant weight gain. *Am J Clin Nutr* 2004;80(6):1579–1588.

89 Kugyelka JG, Rasmussen KM, Frongillo EA. Maternal obesity is negatively associated with breastfeeding success among Hispanic but not Black women. *J Nutr* 2004;134(7):1746–1753.

90 Li R, Jewell S, Grummer-Strawn L. Maternal obesity and breastfeeding practices. *Am J Clin Nutr* 2003;77(4):931–936.

91 Dusdieker LB, Hemingway DL, Stumbo PJ. Is milk production impaired by dieting during lactation? *Am J Clin Nutr* 1994;59(4):833–840.

92 Larson-Meyer DE. Effect of postpartum exercise on mothers and their offspring: a review of the literature. *Obes Res* 2002; 10(8):841–853.

93 Fly AD, Uhlin KL, Wallace JP. Major mineral concentrations in human milk do not change after maximal exercise testing. *Am J Clin Nutr* 1998;68(2):345–349.

94 Prentice A. Micronutrients and the bone mineral content of the mother, fetus and newborn. *J Nutr* 2003;133(5 Suppl. 2):1693S–1699S.

95 Mascola MA, Van Vunakis H, Tager IB, et al. Exposure of young infants to environmental tobacco smoke: breast-feeding among smoking mothers. *Am J Public Health* 1998;88(6):893–896.

96 Batstra L, Neeleman J, Hadders-Algra M. Can breast feeding modify the adverse effects of smoking during pregnancy on the child's cognitive development? *J Epidemiol Commun Health* 2003;57(6):403–404.

97 Berlin CM, Jr, Denson HM, Daniel CH, Ward RM. Disposition of dietary caffeine in milk, saliva, and plasma of lactating women. *Pediatrics* 1984;73(1):59–63.

98 Le Guennec JC, Billon B. Delay in caffeine elimination in breast-fed infants. *Pediatrics* 1987;79:264–268.

99 Mennella JA. Regulation of milk intake after exposure to alcohol in mothers' milk. *Alcohol Clin Exp Res* 2001;25(4):590–593.

100 Ho E, Collantes A, Kapur BM, et al. Alcohol and breast feeding: calculation of time to zero level in milk. *Biol Neonate* 2001;80(3):219–222.

101 Jansson LM, Velez M, Harrow C. Methadone maintenance and lactation: a review of the literature and current management guidelines. *J Hum Lact* 2004;20(1):62–71.

102 Winecker RE, Goldberger BA, Tebbett IR, et al. Detection of cocaine and its metabolites in breast milk. *J Forensic Sci* 2001;46(5):1221–1223.

103 Hale TW. *Medications and mother's milk: a manual of lactational pharmacology*, 11th edn. Amarillo, TX: Pharmasoft Publishing; 2004:937.

104 Hale TW, Kristensen JH, Hackett LP, et al. Transfer of metformin into human milk. *Diabetologia* 2002;45(11):1509–1514.

105 Shiffman ML, Seale TW, Flux M, et al. Breast-milk composition in women with cystic fibrosis: report of two cases and a review of the literature. *Am J Clin Nutr* 1989;49(4):612–617.

106 Alpert SE, Cormier AD. Normal electrolyte and protein content in milk from mothers with cystic fibrosis: an explanation for the initial report of elevated milk sodium concentration. *J Pediatr* 1983;102(1):77–80.

107 Stead RJ, Brueton MJ, Hodson ME, Batten JC. Should mothers with cystic fibrosis breast feed? *Arch Dis Child* 1987;62(4): 433.

108 Bradburn NC, Wappner RS, Lemons JA, et al. Lactation and phenylketonuria. *Am J Perinatol* 1985;2(2):138–141.

109 Purnell H. Phenylketonuria and maternal phenylketonuria. *Breastfeed Rev* 2001;9(2):19–21.

110 Scott JA, Binns CW. Factors associated with the initiation and duration of breastfeeding: a review of the literature. *Breastfeed Rev* 1999;7(1):5–16.

111 Hofmeyr GJ, Nikodem VC, Wolman WL, et al. Companionship to modify the clinical birth environment: effects on progress and perceptions of labour, and breastfeeding. *Br J Obstet Gynaecol* 1991;98(8):756–764.

112 Langer A, Campero L, Garcia C, Reynoso S. Effects of psychosocial support during labour and childbirth on breastfeeding, medical interventions, and mothers' wellbeing in a Mexican public hospital: a randomised clinical trial. *Br J Obstet Gynaecol* 1998;105(10):1056.

113 Out JJ, Vierhout ME, Wallenburg HC. Breast-feeding following spontaneous and induced labour. *Eur J Obstet Gynecol Reprod Biol* 1988;29(4):275–279.

114 Victora CG, Huttly SR, Barros FC, Vaughan JP. Caesarean section and duration of breast feeding among Brazilians. *Arch Dis Child* 1990;65(6):632–634.

115 Mathur GP, Pandey PK, Mathur S, et al. Breastfeeding in babies delivered by cesarean section. *Indian Pediatr* 1993;30(11): 1285–1290.

116 Dewey KG, Nommsen-Rivers LA, Heinig MJ, Cohen RJ. Risk factors for suboptimal infant breastfeeding behavior, delayed onset of lactation, and excess neonatal weight loss. *Pediatrics* 2003;112(3 Pt 1):607–619.

117 Grajeda R, Perez-Escamilla R. Stress during labor and delivery is associated with delayed onset of lactation among urban Guatemalan women. *J Nutr* 2002;132(10):3055–3060.

118 Albani A, Addamo P, Renghi A, et al. [The effect on breastfeeding rate of regional anesthesia technique for cesarean and vaginal childbirth.] *Minerva Anestesiol* 1999;65(9):625–630.

119 Lie B, Juul J. Effect of epidural vs. general anesthesia on breastfeeding. *Acta Obstet Gynecol Scand* 1988;67(3):207–209.

120 Wittels B, Glosten B, Faure EA, et al. Postcesarean analgesia with both epidural morphine and intravenous patient-controlled analgesia: neurobehavioral outcomes among nursing neonates. *Anesth Analg* 1997;85(3):600–606.

121 Anderson A. Breastfeeding: societal encouragement needed. *J Hum Nutr Diet* 2003;16(4):217–218.

122 Foxman B, D'Arcy H, Gillespie B, et al. Lactation mastitis: occurrence and medical management among 946 breastfeeding women in the United States. *Am J Epidemiol* 2002;155(2):103–114.

123 Amir LH, Lumley J, Garland SM. A failed RCT to determine if antibiotics prevent mastitis: cracked nipples colonized with *Staphylococcus aureus*: a randomized treatment trial [ISRCTN65289389]. *BMC Pregnancy Childbirth* 2004;4(1):19.

124 Dixon JM. Repeated aspiration of breast abscesses in lactating women. *Br Med J* 1988;297(6662):1517–1518.

125 Christensen AF, Al-Suliman N, Nielsen KR, et al. Ultrasound-guided drainage of breast abscesses: results in 151 patients. *Br J Radiol* 2005;78(927):186–188.

126 Ulitzsch D, Nyman MK, Carlson RA. Breast abscess in lactating women: US-guided treatment. *Radiology* 2004;232(3):904–909.

127 Gartner LM, Morton J, Lawrence RA, et al. Breastfeeding and the use of human milk. *Pediatrics* 2005;115:496–506.

128 Wright AL, Bauer M, Naylor A, et al. Increasing breastfeeding rates to reduce infant illness at the community level. *Pediatrics* 1998;101:837–844.

129 Akobeng AK, Ramanan AV, Buchan I, Heller RF. Effect of breastfeeding on risk of coeliac disease: A systematic review and meta-analysis of observational studies. *Arch Dis Child* 2005;91:39–43.

130 Oddy WH, Halonen M, Martinez FD, et al. TGF-beta in human milk is associated with wheeze in infancy. *J Allergy Clin Immunol* 2003;112:723–728.

131 Taylor JS, Kacmar JE, Nothnagle M, Lawrence RA. A systematic review of the literature associating breastfeeding with type 2 diabetes and gestational diabetes. *J Am Coll Nutr* 2005;24: 320–326.

132 Rodekamp E, Harder T, Kohlhoff R, et al. Long-term impact of breast-feeding on body weight and glucose tolerance in children of diabetic mothers: role of the late neonatal period and early infancy. *Diabetes Care* 2005;28:1457–1462.

133 Stuebe AM, Rich-Edwards JW, Willett WC, et al. Duration of lactation and incidence of type 2 diabetes. *JAMA* 2005;294: 2601–2610.

134 Kwan ML, Buffler PA, Abrams B, Kiley VA. Breastfeeding and the risk of childhood leukemia: a meta-analysis. *Public Health Rep* 2004;119:521–535.

135 Martin RM, Gunnell D, Owen CG, Smith GD. Breast-feeding and childhood cancer: A systematic review with metaanalysis. *Int J Cancer* 2005;117:1020–1031.

136 Arenz S, Ruckerl R, Koletzko B, von KR. Breast-feeding and childhood obesity – a systematic review. *Int J Obes Relat Metab Disord* 2004;28:1247–1256.

137 Owen CG, Martin RM, Whincup PH, et al. Effect of infant feeding on the risk of obesity across the life course: a quantitative review of published evidence. *Pediatrics* 2005;115:1367–1377.

138 Jacobsson LT, Jacobsson ME, Askling J, Knowler WC. Perinatal characteristics and risk of rheumatoid arthritis. *Br Med J* 2003;326:1068–1069.

139 Karlson EW, Mandl LA, Hankinson SE, Grodstein F. Do breast-feeding and other reproductive factors influence future risk of rheumatoid arthritis? Results from the Nurses' Health Study. *Arthritis Rheum* 2004;50:3458–3467.

140 Martin RM, Middleton N, Gunnell D, et al. Breast-feeding and cancer: the Boyd Orr cohort and a systematic review with meta-analysis. *J Natl Cancer Inst* 2005;97:1446–1457.

141 Ness RB, Grisso JA, Cottreau C, et al. Factors related to inflammation of the ovarian epithelium and risk of ovarian cancer. *Epidemiology* 2000;11:111–117.

142 Chantry CJ, Auinger P, Byrd RS. Lactation among adolescent mothers and subsequent bone mineral density. *Arch Pediatr Adolesc Med* 2004;158:650–656.

143 Hopkinson JM, Butte NF, Ellis K, Smith EO. Lactation delays postpartum bone mineral accretion and temporarily alters its regional distribution in women. *J Nutr* 2000;130:777–783.

144 Drane DL, Logemann JA. A critical evaluation of the evidence on the association between type of infant feeding and cognitive development. *Paediatr Perinat Epidemiol* 2000;14:349–356.

145 Mortensen EL, Michaelsen KF, Sanders SA, Reinisch JM. The association between duration of breastfeeding and adult intelligence. *JAMA* 2002;287:2365–2371.

Part XIII

The Newborn Infant

67 Premature birth and neurological complications

Alan Hill

Prematurity is a major risk factor for neonatal brain injury. Recent statistics indicate that the rate of premature delivery has increased during recent decades such that very low birth-weight (VLBW) infants now comprise approximately 1.5% of live births and more than 85% of such infants survive. However, enthusiasm over the improved survival of VLBW infants is tempered by concern regarding the high risk of neurological morbidity in survivors, e.g., approximately 5–15% develop cerebral palsy and an additional 25–50% have developmental disabilities affecting cognitive function, behavior, and school performance.[1–3] In addition, survivors have an increased incidence of non-neurological problems (e.g., congenital anomalies, respiratory infections, and sudden infant death syndrome).

In this chapter, discussion is limited to a review of the major types of cerebral injury that occur in premature infants, e.g., germinal matrix–intraventricular hemorrhage (GMH–IVH) and its complications of periventricular hemorrhagic infarction (PVI) and posthemorrhagic hydrocephalus (PHH), hypoxic–ischemic injury, and common metabolic disturbances. Although hemorrhagic and hypoxic–ischemic injury are discussed separately, there is a close relationship between these two major categories of premature brain injury.

Anatomic and physiological features of the premature brain

The specific patterns of brain injury observed in the premature newborn are related to unique anatomic and physiological features of the immature brain as follows.

Vascular supply of the premature brain

Subependymal germinal matrix

The subependymal germinal matrix is a richly vascularized site of active cellular proliferation located immediately ventrolateral to the lateral ventricles in the premature brain (Fig. 67.1). It is a source of neuronal precursors between 10 and 20 weeks of gestation, followed by production of glioblasts during the third trimester. These latter elements subsequently differentiate into oligodendroglia and astrocytes. The size of the germinal matrix decreases progressively during gestation until it has virtually disappeared by term. The immature, fragile, endothelium-lined vessels have a propensity to rupture, causing a GMH, which may then break through the adjacent wall of the lateral ventricles to produce IVH.[1,3]

Arterial blood supply

The arterial supply of the premature brain is a major determinant of the unique patterns of hypoxic–ischemic injury. Thus, injury occurs predominantly in the relatively avascular periventricular white matter in the border zones (watershed areas) between the long penetrating branches of the middle and posterior cerebral arteries, in the posterior white matter around the trigone of the lateral ventricles, and in the border zones between long penetrators of the middle and anterior cerebral arteries in the frontal periventricular white matter around the foramen of Monro. The cerebral cortex is relatively resistant to hypoxic–ischemic insult because of the rich, interarterial anastomoses of meningeal vessels during early development of the arterial system.[1,4]

Venous drainage

Whereas arterial blood supply plays a major role in the genesis of hypoxic–ischemic injury, the distinctive deep venous drainage of the premature brain may render particular sites (e.g., the subependymal germinal matrix) vulnerable to hemorrhage. Thus, there is a sharp reversal in the direction of venous flow at the confluence of the choroidal, thalamostriate, and medullary veins where they form the terminal and internal cerebral veins, which predisposes to venous stasis. This, in turn, may cause an increase in intravascular pressure proximally and capillary rupture, especially in situations associated with elevations in venous pressure (e.g., labor, delivery, and asphyxia).[1,3,5,6]

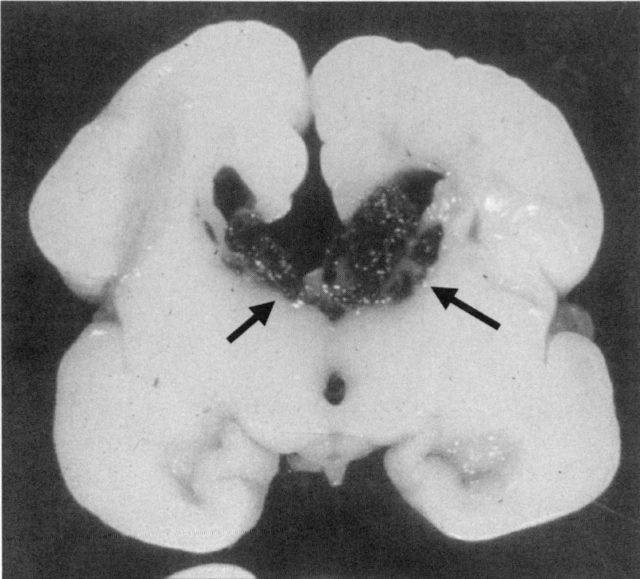

Figure 67.1 Coronal section of pathological specimen of brain of premature infant: note paucity of gyri, bilateral germinal matrix hemorrhage (arrows), and intraventricular hemorrhage.

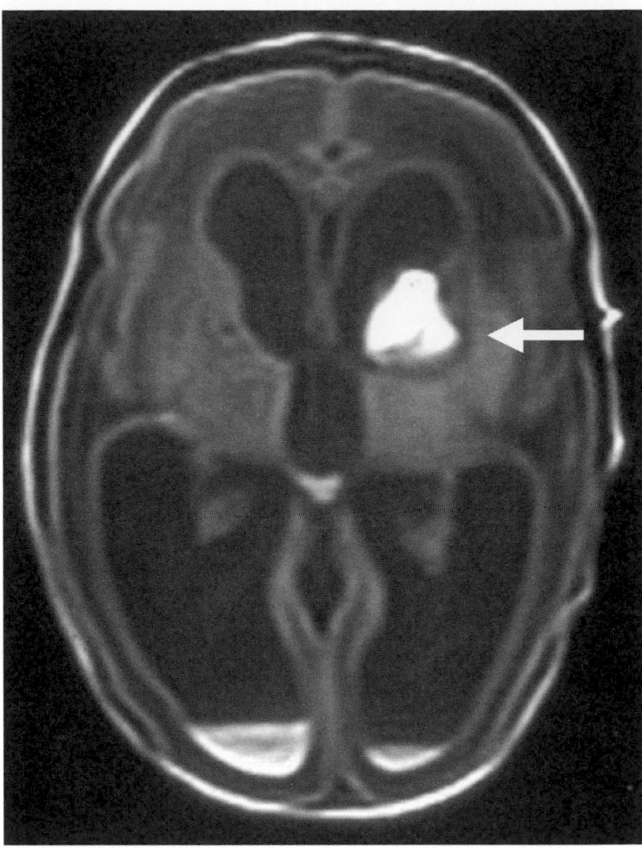

Figure 67.2 Periventricular leukomalacia on T1-weighted MRI of premature infant at age 3 days: note germinal matrix hemorrhage on left (arrow) and layered hemorrhage in third ventricle and occipital horns of lateral ventricles.

Cerebrovascular autoregulation

Cerebrovascular autoregulation is the homeostatic mechanism that maintains constant cerebral perfusion over a wide range of systemic arterial pressures. This mechanism appears to be incompletely developed in a subset of premature newborns, resulting in a "pressure-passive" relationship between systemic blood pressure and cerebral perfusion and increased risk of ischemic and hemorrhagic brain injury.[1,3,7]

Composition of cerebral tissue

The relatively close packing of cortical neurons and lack of Nissl substance in the premature brain makes it difficult to detect cortical neuronal necrosis after hypoxic–ischemic insult. Furthermore, the normally high water content in the premature brain makes it unlikely that cerebral edema plays a major role in the pathogenesis of hypoxic–ischemic injury. The propensity for cystic cavitation of periventricular lesions relates to this relatively high water content, together with the paucity of myelin and poor astroglial response of the premature brain.[1,4] In addition, advances in cellular neurobiology provide increasing evidence that white matter injury in the premature newborn arises, in part, because of a unique developmental vulnerability of oligodendrocyte precursor cells. Cell death and necrosis appear to occur via apoptosis.[1,4,8,9] This raises the possibility that apoptotic cell death and white matter injury may be preventable by using free radical scavengers.[10]

Major types of cerebral injury in the premature newborn

Germinal matrix–intraventricular hemorrhage (GMH–IVH)

As discussed previously, GMH–IVH originates from spread of GMH into the ventricular system (Figs 67.1 and 67.2). The incidence of GMH–IVH has declined in recent decades to less than 20%.[3] However, because the incidence of GMH–IVH correlates closely with the degree of prematurity, the improved survival of extremely premature infants suggests that GMH–IVH will remain a significant problem. GMH–IVH occurs during the first 24 h of life in approximately 50% of cases and before 3 days of age in 90%.[1]

Pathogenesis

The pathogenesis of GMH–IVH is multifactorial and includes a combination of intravascular, vascular, and extravascular factors that are summarized in Table 67.1.

Diagnosis and clinical features

All premature newborns are at risk of GMH–IVH, particularly those who require mechanical ventilation and/or sustain hypoxic–ischemic insult or other major systemic complications (e.g., sepsis, pneumothorax). In infants with severe GMH–IVH, hemorrhage may be suspected on the basis of clinical features (e.g., abnormal neurological signs, decreasing hematocrit, hypotension, bulging fontanelle, and metabolic acidosis). However, GMH–IVH can be diagnosed on the basis of clinical criteria alone in only 50% of cases.[1] Definitive diagnosis requires confirmation by neuroimaging, usually by cranial ultrasonography (Fig. 67.3). Because extension of GMH–IVH may occur during the first week, routine screening by ultrasonography between 7 and 14 days of age is often performed in all infants < 30 weeks' gestation in order to demonstrate the maximal extent of hemorrhage. Subsequently, serial ultrasound scanning and close clinical surveillance may be necessary for the identification of potential complications, e.g., during subsequent months.[11]

Table 67.1 Pathogenetic factors for intraventricular hemorrhage.

Disturbed cerebrovascular autoregulation
Altered cerebral blood flow (increase or decrease, fluctuating pattern)
Increased cerebral venous pressure
Disturbance of coagulation
Fragility and poor mechanical support of germinal matrix vasculature
Increased fibrinolytic activity within germinal matrix
Decreased extravascular tissue pressure

Complications of germinal matrix–intraventricular hemorrhage

Posthemorrhagic hydrocephalus (PHH)

Progressive ventricular dilation has been reported to develop in approximately 35% of premature infants with GMH–IVH. Progressive hydrocephalus with increased intracranial pressure may develop rapidly after major GMH–IVH, either related to a large volume of intraventricular blood or because of obstruction or impaired reabsorption of cerebrospinal fluid. More commonly, progressive ventriculomegaly develops gradually, over several weeks, related principally to obliterative arachnoiditis in the posterior fossa that obstructs the flow of cerebrospinal fluid. Such ventricular dilation may resolve or arrest spontaneously in approximately 65% of cases, usually within 4 weeks of onset. In the remainder, intervention is usually required by temporizing measures to drain cerebrospinal fluid (e.g., serial lumbar punctures, external ventriculostomy, placement of a subcutaneous reservoir, subgaleal shunt) or, rarely, pharmacological interventions with medications to decrease cerebrospinal fluid production (e.g., acetazolamide). In instances in which progressive ventricular dilation continues, placement of a permanent ventriculoperitoneal shunt may be required.[1] When planning intervention, it is critical to distinguish between progressive hydrocephalus with increased intracranial pressure and ventriculomegaly related principally to cerebral atrophy, which is associated with normal intracranial pressure. In many instances, the two processes may coexist.[3,12] Recent data after 1994 suggest that the natural history of posthemorrhagic ventriculomegaly may be evolving, in that the overall incidence has decreased to

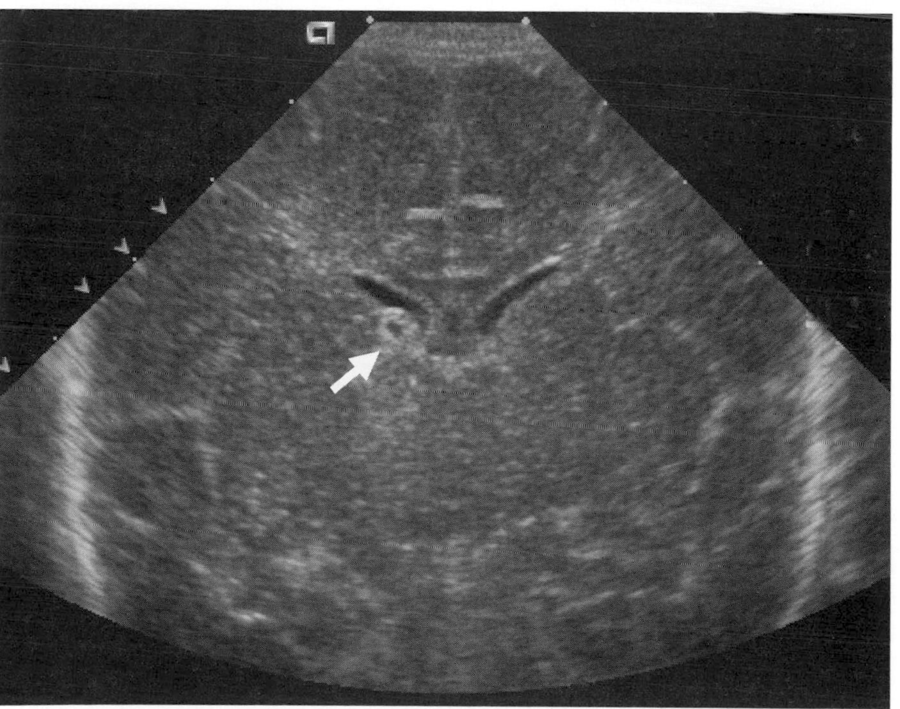

Figure 67.3 Coronal cranial ultrasound at age 7 days: note resolving germinal matrix hemorrhage on right (arrow).

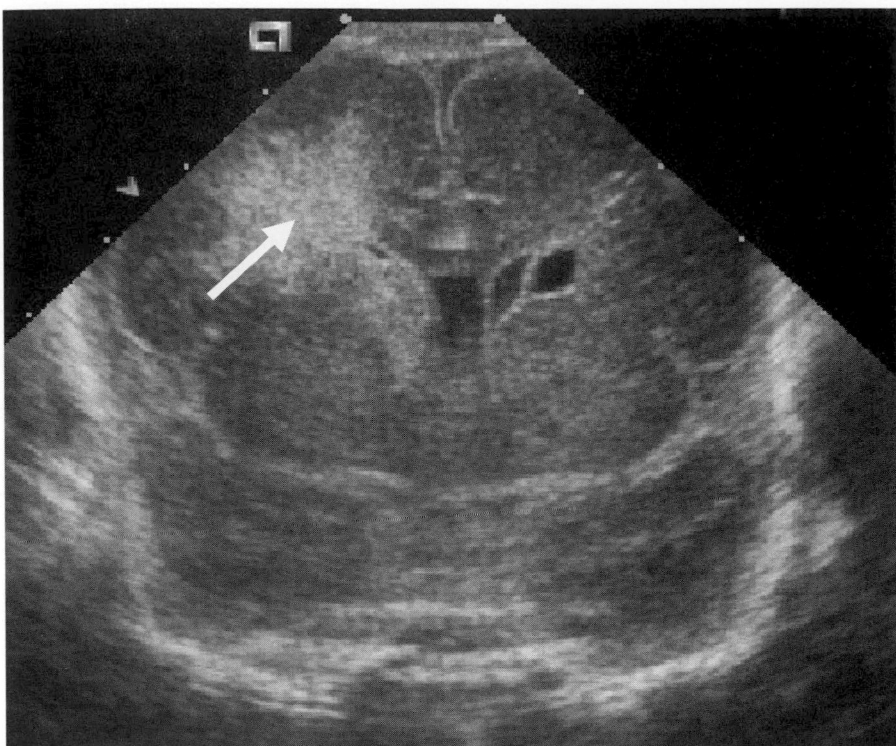

Figure 67.4 Coronal cranial ultrasound: note periventricular hemorrhage infarction (PVI) on right (arrow).

approximately 25% of infants with GMH–IVH. However, in this cohort, ventriculomegaly arrested or resolved spontaneously in only 33%.[13]

Periventricular hemorrhagic infarction (PVI)

Hemorrhagic necrosis in the periventricular white matter (PVI) is observed in approximately 15% of infants with IVH, most commonly in association with large GMH (Fig. 67.4). These parenchymal lesions may be extensive and are either unilateral or strikingly asymmetric, often with a fan-shaped appearance.[1,14] Neuropathological and radiological studies have demonstrated that PVI is not simply an extension of GMH–IVH, but rather represents venous infarction from obstruction of flow in the terminal vein in the subependymal region by an ipsilateral large GMH or GMH–IVH.[15] Thus, this lesion is distinct from secondary hemorrhage into areas of periventricular leukomalacia (PVL), which is bilateral (discussed later). However, distinction between the two lesions is often difficult, and both lesions frequently coexist.[16]

Hypoxic–ischemic cerebral injury

Complications of intrapartum hypoxic–ischemic insult associated with preterm delivery, together with a high incidence of postnatal cardiorespiratory problems (e.g., respiratory distress syndrome, patent ductus arteriosus, apnea of prematurity), render the premature infant at high risk of hypoxic–ischemic cerebral injury. The specific neuropathological patterns relate principally to the stage of maturation of the immature brain (Table 67.2).

Table 67.2 Major patterns of hypoxic–ischemic cerebral injury in the premature newborn.

Pattern	Major anatomic location
Selective neuronal necrosis	Diencephalon, thalamus, brainstem
Periventricular leukomalacia	Periventricular white matter, particularly in peritrigonal region (bilateral)
Focal/multifocal necrosis	Cortex and white matter
Periventricular hemorrhagic infarction	Periventricular white matter, unilateral or asymmetric

Selective neuronal necrosis

During the third trimester, neurons in the thalamus, hypothalamus, and brainstem appear to be particularly vulnerable to hypoxic–ischemic insult.[17,18] In one neuropathological series, pontine neuronal necrosis was documented in 46% of premature infants with IVH, all of whom had died of respiratory failure.[19]

Periventricular leukomalacia (PVL)

As discussed previously, ischemic injury in the premature brain principally involves the periventricular watershed zones of arterial supply in white matter. In addition, there is often more diffuse white matter injury related to diffuse loss of early differentiating oligodendroglia.[1,4] Considerable advances have been made in the understanding of the pathogenesis of PVL.[4,20] Thus, in addition to the role of vascular anatomic factors in the periventricular region and the pressure-passive cerebral circulation observed in some unstable premature newborns (discussed previously), there appears to be an intrinsic vulnerability of early, differentiating oligodendrocyte precursors to attack by free radicals, leading to apoptotic cell death.[4,8,9] In addition, there is mounting evidence of direct injury to white matter from inflammatory mediators (e.g., endotoxins, cytokines). The possible role of inflammatory factors has been suggested by epidemiological studies and studies of placental pathology, which suggest an increased incidence of PVL in preterm infants of mothers with chorioamnionitis.[20–23]

Neuropathological studies reveal a spectrum of severity of PVL ranging from minor reduction in the quantity of myelin and gliosis to extensive encephalomalacia. Neuropathological studies have also emphasized the frequent association between PVL and GMH–IVH in as many as 75% of infants.[19]

The diagnosis of PVL during the neonatal period cannot be based reliably on clinical criteria and must be established by detection of abnormalities on serial neuroimaging. Cranial ultrasonography may demonstrate transient increased echogenicity in periventricular white matter during the first days of life, followed by the development of echolucent cysts in these regions after several weeks in severe cases and ventricular dilation after several months[1,24,25] (Fig. 67.5). However, correlative neuropathological studies have demonstrated the relatively poor sensitivity of ultrasonography for detection of PVL (approximately 70% of mild cases are not diagnosed consistently).[26] More recently, studies with magnetic resonance imaging (MRI), especially diffusion-weighted studies, may identify less severe white matter lesions.[17,27]

The clinical features of PVL in the premature newborn are variable, and detailed neurological examination may be difficult in the presence of complex life support apparatus. The principal long-term neurological sequela of PVL is motor handicap (e.g., spastic diplegia or quadriplegia). Injury to optic radiation may result in visual impairment, and more diffuse white matter injury may result in behavioral disturbances and intellectual deficits.[1] The possible role of PVL in causing abnormal cerebral cortical neuronal organization and significant intellectual deficits, because of either injury to subplate neurons or late migrating astrocytes, awaits further clarification.[28]

In older children with cerebral palsy who were born prematurely, the clinical suspicion of PVL as the cause can be confirmed by documentation of characteristic abnormalities on brain imaging [computed tomography (CT) or MRI]. Abnormalities on CT scans performed after 6 months of age include ventriculomegaly with irregular ventricular walls and reduction in the quantity of periventricular white matter, particularly in the peritrigonal region, and prominent sylvian fissures

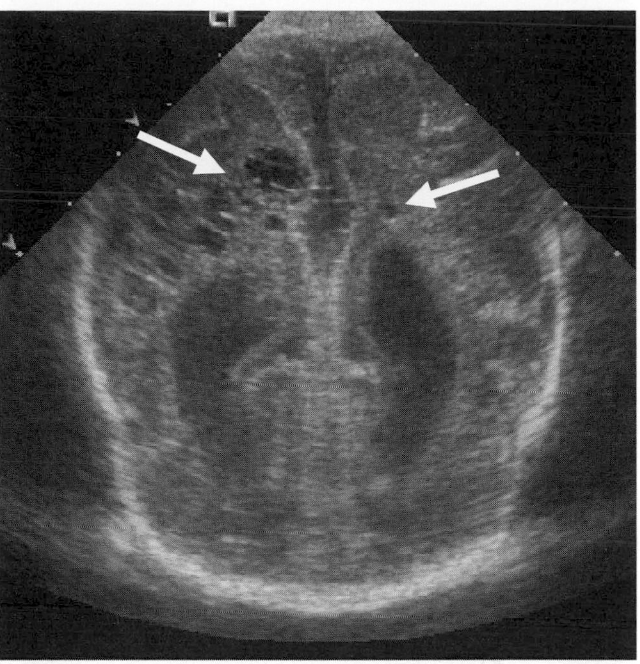

Figure 67.5 Coronal cranial ultrasound at age 5 weeks: note cystic periventricular leukomalacia (arrows) more prominent on the right.

(Fig. 67.6).[29] Similar abnormalities may be recognized with greater definition by MRI (Fig. 67.7).[30]

Focal–multifocal brain necrosis

Focal ischemic cerebral lesions associated with arterial occlusion occur uncommonly in premature infants. In one large series, none was observed in infants who were less than 28 weeks of gestational age. Five percent of all cases of infarction occurred in infants between 28 and 32 weeks, and 10% occurred in infants between 32 and 37 weeks of gestation. Multiple small scattered infarcts, related to occlusion of small vessels, are more common in this age group than in term infants.[31] Focal cerebral necrosis in the premature brain frequently results in cavitation, with the formation of porencephalic cysts or multicystic encephalomalacia. Neurological sequelae (e.g., cerebral palsy, mental retardation, and seizures) are variable and correlate with the anatomic location and the extent of cerebral injury.[1]

Bilirubin encephalopathy

Unconjugated hyperbilirubinemia in the newborn may result in kernicterus, which involves localized staining of basal ganglia and brainstem nuclei associated with microscopic neuronal destruction. Despite the extensive literature on bilirubin metabolism, its central nervous system toxicity remains poorly understood.

Bilirubin staining of the brain has been documented in premature newborns even at relatively low bilirubin levels, often in regions of the brain injured by other insults (e.g., PVL). In

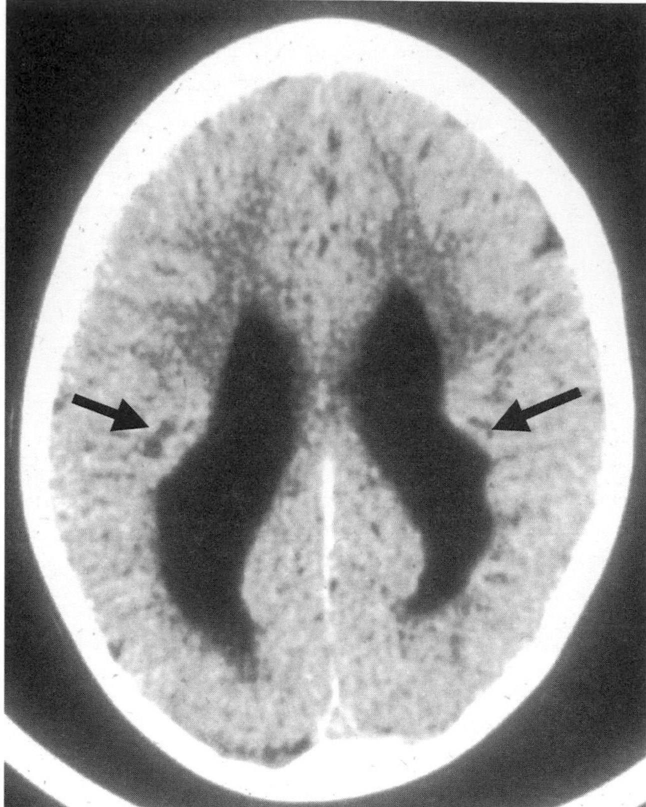

Figure 67.6 Periventricular leukomalacia on axial CT scan at age 2 years: note dilated lateral ventricles with irregular ependymal border, paucity of white matter, and deep sulci (arrows).

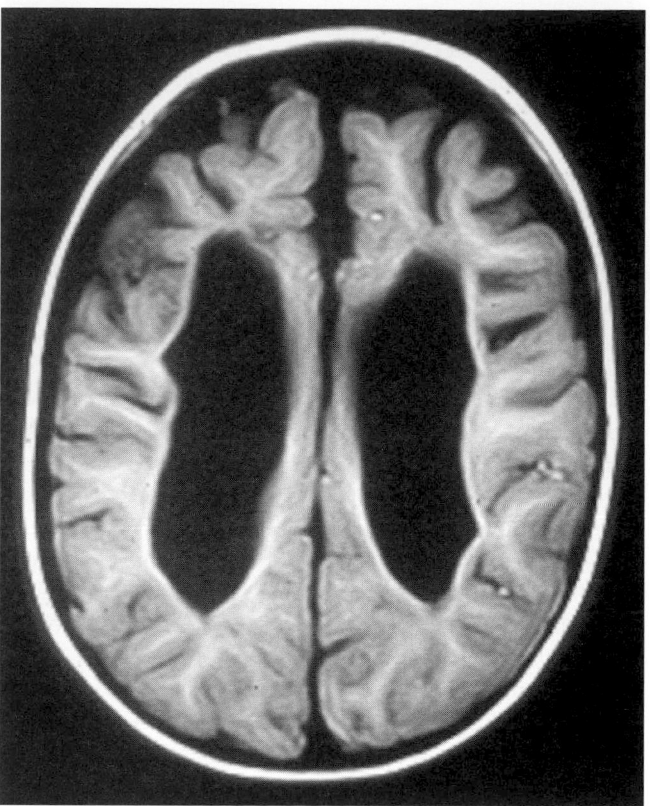

Figure 67.7 Periventricular leukomalacia on T1-weighted MRI at age 3 years: note ventriculomegaly with irregular ependymal border, almost complete loss of white matter, and deep sulci abutting ependyma.

addition, bilirubin staining without structural neuronal injury has been documented in premature infants with moderate hyperbilirubinemia.[1,32] Interestingly, sick premature newborns do not generally demonstrate the classic neonatal neurological encephalopathy or later kernicterus. Furthermore, there is no proven definite relationship between moderate hyperbilirubinemia and neurological outcome in premature newborns. Because extrapyramidal movement abnormalities are less common in infants born prematurely, the possibility exists that the maturational stage of the brain at the time of insult may be critical in determining neurological sequelae, as is the case in hypoxic–ischemic cerebral injury. To date, there is some evidence that hearing loss may be the major manifestation of bilirubin neurotoxicity in the premature newborn.[1,32,33]

Hypoglycemic brain injury

Transient hypoglycemia occurs commonly in the stressed premature newborn, often in association with hypoxic–ischemic cerebral injury. At present, many issues remain unresolved, including the threshold and duration of significant hypoglycemia, as well as the suspected additive and potentiating effects of hypoglycemia in the context of other types of insult.[34,35] Furthermore, there may be an important role for glucose in the regulation of cerebral blood flow, in that moderate hypoglycemia has been shown to be associated with a two- to threefold increase in cerebral blood flow.[36] The clinical significance of this observation remains to be determined, e.g., its role in an increased risk of GMH–IVH. Severe hypoglycemia has become a relatively rare problem in most neonatal units because of routine frequent monitoring of blood glucose levels and early intravenous glucose supplementation.

Prevention and management of hemorrhagic and hypoxic–ischemic brain injury

Although hypoxic–ischemic cerebral injury and GMH–IVH have distinct pathogenetic mechanisms, in many instances, similar strategies for intervention are used to decrease both types of injury. For practical purposes, major approaches to management are discussed in terms of the timing of intervention, i.e., antepartum, intrapartum, or postpartum (Table 67.3).

Table 67.3 Prevention and management of cerebral injury.

Antepartum intervention
Prevention of premature delivery
Intrauterine transport
Pharmacological interventions: corticosteroids, others (?)
Intrapartum interventions
Avoidance of prolonged labor (?)
Delivery by Cesarean section (?)
Postnatal interventions
Adequate ventilation
Prevention and correction of hemodynamic disturbances
Correction of coagulation abnormalities
Pharmacological interventions (?): indomethacin

Antepartum interventions

Prevention of premature delivery

Although the prevention of premature delivery receives ongoing major attention, current public education programs and medical interventional strategies appear to be losing ground, in that the incidence of premature delivery has actually increased during the last two decades.[1–3] Major strategies for such prevention are discussed in detail elsewhere in this book.

One approach to the prevention of preterm delivery that is particularly appealing involves the treatment of women with bacterial vaginosis with antimicrobial agents, which may also decrease premature rupture of membranes and chorioamnionitis, which, in turn, are associated with adverse neonatal outcome including GMH–IVH and PVL.[37]

Intrauterine transportation

If premature delivery is unavoidable, concerted effort should be directed toward transfer of the mother to a high-risk perinatal center before delivery to ensure the optimal condition of the infant at birth as well as the availability of state-of-the-art neonatal management to minimize postnatal complications.

Prenatal pharmacological interventions

Prenatal pharmacological interventions for the prevention of premature delivery and, hence, possibly GMH–IVH and its complications are under investigation.

Antenatal tocolytic therapy

Attempts to stop premature labor by aggressive tocolytic therapy have been disappointing,[38] and there is concern that tocolytic agents may affect fetal systemic hemodynamics and cerebral perfusion, thereby increasing the risk of GMH–IVH and PVL.

Antenatal corticosteroids

Antenatal corticosteroids, administered primarily to induce fetal lung maturation, thereby reducing the risk of respiratory distress syndrome, also have the additional beneficial effects of stabilizing cell membranes in other organs, including vessels of the germinal matrix.[39] Numerous controlled trials indicate that antenatal corticosteroids reduce mortality as well as the overall incidence and severity of IVH. Furthermore, even an incomplete course of antenatal corticosteroid treatment is beneficial in that regard.[40] Clearly, there is convincing evidence to suggest that prompt treatment with antenatal corticosteroids may be indicated for most women who are at imminent risk of preterm delivery.

Other medications

Although earlier studies suggested that antenatal phenobarbital and vitamin K may be associated with a reduction in GMH–IVH, recent comprehensive reviews of the combined data from all clinical trials for the Cochrane Database failed to demonstrate a benefit from either medication. Further well-designed clinical trials are required to determine the usefulness of these medications.[41,42]

Intrapartum management

Because approximately 50% of cases of GMH–IVH occur within the first 24 h of life, careful consideration must be given to the role of intrapartum factors in the pathogenesis of GMH–IVH. Mechanical forces on the compliant skull of the premature infant during uterine contractions and vaginal delivery may result in considerable perturbations of fetal cerebral hemodynamics. Despite earlier conflicting data about the role of labor and mode of delivery as a risk factor for IVH, the data suggest that prolonged labor and vaginal delivery may increase the risk of IVH in very low birthweight infants.[43,44] Clearly, further investigations are needed to clarify the role of specific obstetric factors.

Postnatal interventions

Adequate ventilation of the newborn

Immediate provision of adequate ventilation to prevent ongoing hypoxemia and hypercarbia is of major importance in the management of the premature newborn. Major advances in the management of respiratory distress syndrome have occurred in recent years. Contrary to initial expectations, the reported prevalence of IVH in surfactant-treated infants is higher than in control subjects, related perhaps to fluctuations in cerebral hemodynamics associated with the rapid changes in the lung mechanics of surfactant-treated infants.[45] The risk of IVH or PVL associated with newer methods of ventilation (e.g., high-frequency oscillatory ventilation and nitric oxide therapy) have not been clarified to date.[12]

Prevention and correction of hemodynamic disturbances

Rapid fluctuations in systemic hemodynamics may result in significant perturbations of cerebral perfusion, especially in the context of impaired cerebrovascular autoregulation in the immature brain. Avoidance of prolonged labor and vaginal (especially breech) delivery may be significant in this regard.[43,44] Systemic hemodynamic disturbances have been documented during management in the intensive care setting, e.g., routine monitoring, handling, tracheal suctioning. The use of muscle paralysis with pancuronium appears to be particularly effective in preventing pneumothorax, as well as abrupt fluctuations in cerebral blood flow associated with tracheal suctioning and other routine handling procedures. Thus, comprehensive analysis of data for the Cochrane Database demonstrated significant reduction in GMH–IVH after neuromuscular paralysis.[46] However, because long-term pulmonary and neurological effects are uncertain, routine pancuronium is not recommended for ventilated newborns.

Correction of coagulation abnormalities

Although abnormal coagulation is a risk factor for the development of GMH–IVH, review of combined data from randomized trials has failed to support the routine use of fresh frozen plasma, albumin, or blood substitutes, in that there was no reduction in severe GMH–IVH, mortality, or cerebral palsy.[47]

Pharmacological interventions

Prophylactic indomethacin, used to treat symptomatic ductus arteriosus, is associated with a reduction in severe GMH–IVH and no apparent long-term adverse effects.[48]

Neurological outcome in the premature newborn

The long-term neurological outcome of the premature newborn is determined principally by the extent of parenchymal hypoxic–ischemic injury and the occurrence of complications of GMH–IVH (e.g., PHH and PVI), rather than the occurrence of GMH–IVH itself. The significance of metabolic derangements (e.g., moderate hyperbilirubinemia, asymptomatic hypoglycemia) is less well established. The major factors that may assist in the prediction of neurological outcome are listed in Table 67.4.

Table 67.4 Useful factors for predicting neurological outcome.

Neurological examination (seizures, abnormalities that persist to 40 weeks' postconceptional age)
Location and extent of periventricular ischemic/hemorrhagic lesions documented by cranial ultrasonography or computed tomography
Posthemorrhagic hydrocephalus (associated with cerebral atrophy, surgical drainage required)
? Other metabolic disturbances (e.g., hyperbilirubinemia, hypoglycemia)

The neurological examination of the premature infant is often limited by the presence of complex life support apparatus. Nevertheless, certain clinical features (e.g., occurrence of seizures) correlate closely with poor neurological outcome.[49] Clinically recognizable seizure activity occurs uncommonly in the premature newborn because the immaturity of cortical interconnections tends to impede the propagation of abnormal electrical discharges. Electroencephalography may assist in the more accurate documentation of seizures. Serial neurological examinations are also invaluable for accurate prediction of outcome.[50]

In addition to clinical examination, detailed assessment of the precise location and extent of cerebral injury by neuroimaging is of major predictive value. Thus, follow-up studies of VLBW infants report severe neurological abnormalities in those with major cranial ultrasonographic abnormalities. However, occasionally, if there is only minor parenchymal involvement or if injury is localized to a relatively clinically silent region of the brain, especially the frontal or occipital regions, the eventual handicap may be surprisingly mild.[1]

Several studies have a high incidence of major neurological sequelae in infants with PHH, especially in those who require a ventriculoperitoneal shunt. Although poor outcome is related to concomitant parenchymal injury and in part to shunt-related complications (e.g., infection, shunt obstruction), there is increasing evidence that progressive PHH itself may be detrimental.[51,52] The occurrence of major sequelae in children born prematurely who had abnormal neuroimaging is not surprising. More concerning is the mounting evidence of neurodevelopmental abnormalities in children who had normal neonatal cranial ultrasound scans.[53]

Key points

1 Premature delivery occurs in approximately 1.5% of live births, and more than 85% of very low birthweight infants (birthweight < 1500 g) survive.

2 The topography of hemorrhagic and hypoxic–ischemic brain injury in premature newborns relates to unique anatomic and physiological features of the immature brain.

3 Diagnosis of the various types of hemorrhagic and hypoxic–ischemic premature brain injury in the newborn period can be made on the basis of clinical

features alone in only a minority of cases. Accurate diagnosis usually requires confirmation by neuroimaging, usually cranial ultrasonography. Routine screening by ultrasonography is recommended in premature newborns of < 30 weeks' gestation between 7 and 14 days of age and should be repeated at term.

4 Germinal matrix–intraventricular hemorrhage (GMH–IVH) originates from hemorrhage from fragile vessels in the subependymal germinal matrix, which then ruptures through the wall of the lateral ventricles to cause IVH.

5 The incidence of GMH–IVH in premature newborns has declined to less than 20%, and long-term sequelae are usually related more to its major complications (posthemorrhagic hydrocephalus and periventricular hemorrhagic infarction) and to parenchymal ischemic injury than to GMH–IVH itself.

6 Progressive posthemorrhagic hydrocephalus (PHH), related to obstruction of cerebrospinal fluid by obliterative arachnoiditis in the posterior fossa, usually develops gradually over weeks and may arrest or resolve spontaneously in 35–65% of cases. Such PHH with increased intracranial pressure must be distinguished from ventriculomegaly related to cerebral atrophy. This distinction may be difficult, and both causes of ventricular enlargement may coexist.

7 Periventricular hemorrhagic infarction (PVI) occurs as a result of hemorrhagic venous infarction from obstruction of the terminal vein by ipsilateral large GMH. It may be visualized on cranial ultrasonography as a unilateral, fan-shaped lesion with ipsilateral large GMH.

8 Periventricular leukomalacia (PVL) is the major pattern of hypoxic–ischemic brain injury in premature newborns, which results in long-term sequelae of spastic diplegia and often visual impairment.

9 Periventricular leukomalacia may be distinguished from periventricular hemorrhage infarction on cranial ultrasonography, in that it appears as bilateral, increased echoes in periventricular white matter in the first days of life, whereas PVI is mostly unilateral.

10 Approximately 70% of mild cases of PVL may remain undetectable by cranial ultrasonography. MRI, especially diffusion-weighted studies, may identify less severe white matter injury.

11 The pathogenesis of PVL relates to hypoxic–ischemic insult affecting watershed zones of arterial supply in periventricular white matter in the immature brain. Impaired cerebrovascular autoregulation, intrinsic vulnerability of oligodendrocyte precursors to free radical attack, and direct white mater injury from inflammatory mediators, e.g., cytokines, endotoxins, are considered to be major pathogenetic factors.

12 PVL may be followed by reduced volume of cortical gray matter at term, as documented on MRI studies. This may account for later cognitive dysfunction.

13 Central nervous system toxicity of unconjugated hyperbilirubinemia remains poorly understood in premature newborns, in that they often do not demonstrate neonatal encephalopathy or classic features of kernicterus.

14 Hearing loss may be the major manifestation of bilirubin neurotoxicity in infants born prematurely.

15 The threshold and duration of significant hypoglycemia that results in cerebral injury as well as its suspected synergistic effect with hypoxia–ischemia remain unresolved. Moderate hypoglycemia is associated with a two- to threefold increase in cerebral blood flow.

16 Antenatal corticosteroids reduce mortality as well as the overall incidence and severity of GMH–IVH, perhaps by reducing the risk of hemodynamic disturbances from respiratory distress syndrome and by stabilization of vessels in the germinal matrix.

17 Prolonged labor and vaginal delivery appear to increase the risk of GMH–IVH in very low birthweight infants.

18 Neuromuscular paralysis with pancuronium in premature newborns who require mechanical ventilation is associated with significant reduction in GMH–IVH.

19 Long-term neurological sequelae in infants born prematurely correlate closely with the abnormal neurological examination at term and the extent of abnormalities on neuroimaging, especially MRI.

20 Approximately 5–15% of infants born prematurely develop cerebral palsy, and an additional 25–50% develop cognitive and behavioral difficulties.

References

1 Volpe JJ. *Neurology of the newborn.* Philadelphia, PA: W.B. Saunders, 2001.

2 McIntire DD, Bloom SL, Casey BM, et al. Birth weight in relation to morbidity and mortality among newborn infants. *N Engl J Med* 1999;340:1234.

3 Roland EH, Hill A. Germinal matrix-intraventricular hemorrhage in the premature newborn: management and outcome. *Neurol Clin North Am* 2003; 21:833.

4 Volpe JJ. Neurobiology of periventricular leukomalacia in the premature infant. *Pediatr Res* 2001;50:553.

5 Ghazi-Birry HS, Brown WR, Moody DM, et al. Human germinal matrix: venous origin and vascular characteristics. *Am J Neuroradiol* 1997;18:219.

6 Shalak L, Perlman JM. Hemorrhagic–ischemic cerebral injury in the preterm infant – current concepts. *Clin Perinatol* 2002;29: 745.

7 Tsuji M, Soul JP, du Plessis A, et al. Cerebral intravascular oxygenation correlates with mean arterial pressure in coitically ill premature infants. *Pediatrics* 2000;106:625.

8 Back SA, Luo NL, Borenstein NS, et al. Late oligodendrocyte progenitors coincide with the developmental window of vulnerability for human perinatal white matter injury. *J Neurosci* 2001;21:1302.
9 Ferreiro DM. Neonatal brain injury. *N Engl J Med* 2004;351:1985.
10 Ferreiro DM. Timing is everything – delaying therapy for delayed cell death. *Dev Neurosci* 2002;24:349.
11 Ment LR, Boda HS, Barnes P, et al. Practice parameter: neuroimaging of the neonate: report of the quality standards subcommittee of the American Academy of Neurology and the Practice Committee of the Child Neurology Society. *Neurology* 2002;57:1726.
12 du Plessis AJ. Posthemorrhagic hydrocephalus and brain injury in the preterm infant: dilemmas in diagnosis and management. *Semin Pediatr Neurol* 1998;5:161.
13 Murphy BP, Inder TE, Rooks V, et al. Posthemorrhagic ventricular dilatation in the premature infant: natural history and predictors of outcome. *Arch Dis Child Fetal Neonatal Ed* 2002;87:F37.
14 Counsell SJ, Maalouf EF, Rutherford MA, et al. Periventricular hemorrhagic infarct in a preterm neonate. *Eur J Pediatr Neurol* 1999;3:25.
15 Taylor GA. Effect of germinal matrix hemorrhage on terminal vein position and patency. *Pediatr Radiol* 1995;25:537.
16 De Vries LS, Roelants-van Rijn AM, Rademaker KJ, et al. Unilateral parenchymal hemorrhagic infarction in the preterm infant. *Eur J Pediatr Neurol* 2001;5:139.
17 Madouf EF, Duggan PJ, Counsell SJ, et al. Comparison of findings on cranial ultrasound and magnetic resonance imaging in preterm infants. *Pediatrics* 2001;107:719.
18 Inder TE, Warfield SK, Wang H, et al. Abnormal cerebral structure is present at term in premature infants. *Pediatrics* 2005;115:286.
19 Armstrong DL, Sauls CD, Goddard-Finegold J. Neuropathologic findings in short-term survivors of intraventricular hemorrhage. *Am J Dis Child* 1987;141:617–621.
20 du Plessis AJ, Volpe JJ. Perinatal brain injury in the preterm and term newborn. *Curr Opin Neurol* 2002;15:151.
21 Wu YW. Systematic review of chorioamnionitis and cerebral palsy. *Ment Retard Dev Disabil Res Rev* 2002;8:25.
22 Willoughby RE, Jr, Nelson KB. Chorioamnionitis and brain injury. *Clin Perinatol* 2002;29:603.
23 Nelson KB, Grether JK, Dambrosia JM, et al. Neonatal cytokines and cerebral palsy in very preterm infants. *Pediatr Res* 2003;53:60.
24 Groenendahl F, de Vries LS. Cranial ultrasound detection of white matter echolucencies. *Pediatr Res* 2001;50:772.
25 Childs AM, Corrette L, Remenghi LA, et al. Magnetic resonance and cranial ultrasound characteristics of periventricular white matter abnormalities in newborn infants. *Clin Radiol* 2001;56:647.
26 Ment LM, Schneider AC, Ainley MA, Allan WC. Adaptive mechanisms of developing brain. The neuroradiologic assessment of the preterm infant. *Clin Perinatol* 2000;27:303.
27 Inder TE, Anderson NJ, Spencer C, et al. White matter injury in the premature infant: a comparison between serial cranial sonographic and MR findings at term. *Am J Neuroradiol* 2003;24:805.
28 Inder TE, Huppi PS, Warfield S, et al. Periventricular white matter injury in the premature infant is followed by reduced cerebral cortical gray matter volume at term. *Am Neurol* 1999;46:755.
29 Flodmark O, Roland EH, Hill A, Whitfield MF, Periventricular leukomalacia: radiologic diagnosis. *Radiology* 1986;162:119.
30 Roelants-van Rijn, Groenendahl F, Beek FS, et al. Parenchymal brain injury in the preterm infant: comparison of cranial ultrasound, MRI and neurodevelopmental outcome. *Neuropediatrics* 2001;32:80.
31 Barmada MA, Moosy J, Shumann RM. Cerebral infarcts with arterial occlusion in neonates. *Ann Neurol* 1979;6:495.
32 Watchko JF, Meisels MJ. Jaundice in low birth weight infants: pathobiology and outcome. *Arch Dis Child Fetal Neonatal Ed* 2003;88:F455.
33 Oh W, Tyson JE, Fanaroff AA, et al. Association between peak serum bilirubin and neurodevelopmental outcome in extremely low birth weight infants. *Pediatrics* 2003;112:773.
34 Hawden JM. Hypoglycemia and the neonatal brain. *Eur J Pediatr* 1999;158:59.
35 Kalhan S, Peter-Wohl S. Hypoglycemia: what is it for the neonate? *Am J Perinatol* 2000;17:11.
36 Pryds O, Christensen NJ, Friis HB. Increased cerebral blood flow and plasma epinephrine in hypoglycemic, preterm neonates. *Pediatrics* 1990;85:172.
37 Goncalve LF, Chaiwaraponga T, Romaro R. Intrauterine infection and prematurity. *Ment Retard Dev Dis Res Rev* 2002;8:3.
38 Weibtraub Z, Solovechick M, Reichman B, et al. Effect of maternal tocolysis on the incidence of severe periventricular/intraventricular hemorrhage in very low birthweight infants. *Arch Dis Child Fetal Neonatal Ed* 2001;85:F13.
39 Ment LR, Oh W, Ehrenkranz Z, et al. Antenatal steroids delivery mode and intraventricular hemorrhage in preterm infants. *Am J Obstet Gynecol* 1995;172:795.
40 Harding JE, Pang J, Knight DB, et al. Do antenatal corticosteroids help in the setting of preterm rupture of membranes. *Am J Obstet Gynecol* 2001;184:131.
41 Crowther CA, Henderson-Smart DJ. Phenobarbital prior to preterm birth for preventing neonatal periventricular hemorrhage. *Cochrane Database Syst Rev* 2001;2:CD000164.
42 Crowther CA, Henderson-Smart DJ. Vitamin K prior to preterm birth for preventing neonatal periventricular hemorrhage. *Cochrane Database Syst Rev* 2001;1:CD00029.
43 Leviton A, Fenton F, Kubon KC, et al. Labor and delivery characteristics and the risk of germinal matrix hemorrhage in low birthweight infants. *J Child Neurol* 1991;6:35.
44 Shaver DC, Bada HS, Korones SB, et al. Early and late intraventricular hemorrhage – the role of obstetric factors. *Obstet Gynecol* 1992;80:831.
45 Soll RF, Morley CJ. Prophylactic versus selective use of surfactant in preventive morbidity and mortality in preterm infants. *Cochrane Database Syst Rev* 2001;2:CD000510.
46 Cools F, Offinga M. Neuromuscular paralysis for newborn infants receiving mechanical ventilation. *Cochrane Database Syst Rev* 2000;4:CD002773.
47 Osborn DA, Evans N. Early volume expansion for prevention of morbidity and mortality in very preterm infants. *Cochrane Database Syst Rev* 2001;4:CD002055.
48 Fowlie PW, Davis PG. Prophylactic intravenous indomethacin for preventing mortality and morbidity in preterm infants. *Cochrane Database Syst Rev* 2002;3:CD000174.
49 Ames PN, Bandir J, Townsend J, et al. Epilepsy in very preterm infants: neonatal cranial ultrasound reveals a high risk subcategory. *Dev Med Child Neurol* 1998;40:724.
50 Dubowitz LMS, Dubowitz V, Palmer PG, et al. Correlation of neurologic assessment in the preterm infant with outcome at one year. *J Pediatr* 1984;105:452.

51 Resch B, Gedermann A, Maurer U, et al. Neurodevelopmental outcome of hydrocephalus following intra/periventricular hemorrhage in preterm infants: short and longterm results. *Childs Neurol Syst* 1996;12:27.
52 Ventriculomegaly Trial Group. Randomized trial of early tapping in neonatal posthemorrhagic ventricular dilatation: results at 30 months. *Arch Dis Child* 1994;70:129.
53 Torrioli MG, Fisone MF, Bonvini L, et al. Perceptual-motor, visual and cognitive ability in very low birthweight preschool children without neonatal ultrasound abnormalities. *Brain Dev* 2000;22: 163.

68 Common problems of the newborn

Fernando R. Moya and Matthew Laughon

Neonatal adaptation to extrauterine life

At birth, the infant must adapt quickly to the more demanding extrauterine environment, in which he or she must take control of vital functions such as gas exchange and body temperature regulation. In preparation for birth, many adaptations are initiated *in utero*, particularly with the onset of labor. Many of the problems that newborns exhibit over the first several days after birth arise from difficulties with this transition.

Circulatory adaptation

The fetal circulation is characterized by a low systemic resistance and a high pulmonary vasomotor tone. *In utero*, the placenta serves as the organ for gas exchange. The distribution of the cardiac output is markedly different between the fetus and the adult. Approximately 30–40% of the fetal cardiac output is conveyed through both umbilical arteries to the placenta. This systemic blood has a $P\text{O}_2$ of approximately 25–30 mmHg and a $P\text{CO}_2$ of 40–45 mmHg. There is a small, but progressive, decrease in umbilical arterial $P\text{O}_2$ with advancing gestational age. However, because this is paralleled by an increase in fetal hemoglobin, the oxygen content of the blood remains constant.[1] After circulation through the placenta, the umbilical venous $P\text{O}_2$ rises to 35–55 mmHg, whereas the $P\text{CO}_2$ drops to 35–40 mmHg. This more oxygenated blood returns to the right atrium via the umbilical vein and the inferior vena cava. The stream from the inferior vena cava is directed preferentially across the foramen ovale to the left atrium, left ventricle, and ascending aorta, thereby perfusing primarily the head and neck vessels as well as the coronary arteries. A smaller fraction of the inferior vena cava return mixes with the superior vena cava flow and passes into the right ventricle and pulmonary artery. During fetal life, the pulmonary vascular resistance is high and opposes pulmonary blood flow. Less than 10% of the fetal cardiac output goes through the lungs and, on returning through the pulmonary veins, mixes with more oxygenated blood in the left atrium. Most of the pulmonary artery blood flow crosses into the descending aorta through the ductus arteriosus (DA). The high pulmonary vascular resistance is secondary to the low fetal $P\text{O}_2$, underventilation of the fluid-filled fetal lungs, and the predominance of prostaglandins promoting increased pulmonary vasomotor tone.[2]

At birth, several events determine a rapid change in the circulatory pattern, ultimately separating the pulmonary and systemic circuits. With the clamping of the cord, systemic vascular resistance increases. The initiation of lung expansion increases the alveolar oxygen concentration and the $P\text{O}_2$ of the blood perfusing the lungs. This increase in oxygenation as well as local production of endogenous vasodilators, such as nitric oxide (NO) and prostacyclin, result in an increase in pulmonary blood flow. The increased venous return to the left atrium via pulmonary veins and the increase in systemic vascular resistance elevate left atrial pressure above that of the right atrium. This causes a functional closure of the foramen ovale. Anatomic closure of this structure usually happens in the weeks following birth, but it may remain open for life. The increased pressures on the systemic circuit, along with the decrease in pulmonary artery pressure, reverse the ductal flow to a predominantly left-to-right shunt. Ductal closure results from constriction of its spiral musculature in response to a higher $P\text{O}_2$ and predominant stimulation of constrictor prostaglandins. The decreasing radius of the DA compromises the nourishment of its endothelium, which ultimately necroses, obliterating its lumen. Permanent anatomic ductal closure may occur up to several weeks after birth. When the DA remains patent, the sustained left-to-right shunt can lead to substantial pulmonary overflow and pulmonary edema. The ability of the DA to respond to oxygen and prostaglandins may be markedly reduced in very immature neonates; hence the higher incidence of symptomatic DA at lower gestational ages. Hypoxemia, the lack of lung expansion, and acidosis at birth are both causes of a persistently elevated pulmonary vascular resistance that can interfere with the transition of the circulation from the fetal to the adult pattern.

Lung expansion and initiation of breathing

The human fetus initiates respiratory movements late in the first trimester of gestation. Subsequently, these movements become stronger and more organized and, near term, there is a pattern of regular breathing at rates similar to those found after birth. Just before the initiation of labor, fetal breathing decreases from 75–85% to only about 15–30% of the time. In preparation for birth, the fetal lungs undergo several changes. The biochemical maturation of the lung in terms of surfactant production is discussed elsewhere in this textbook. *In utero*, the fetal lungs are filled with a fluid rich in chloride (> 150 mEq/L) and relatively free of protein (< 0.3 mg/mL). The volume of fluid that occupies the alveolar spaces and airways is similar to the functional residual capacity (FRC) during the neonatal period, namely 30–35 mL/kg body weight.[3] Fetal lung fluid is produced at an hourly rate of 4–6 mL/kg body weight. Before delivery, production of fetal lung fluid decreases and active reabsorption begins. This is secondary to hormonal changes that occur with the onset of labor, such as increases in circulating catecholamines and elevations in arginine vasopressin.[4] At birth, a small proportion of the lung fluid that occupies the airways is squeezed out of the trachea during passage through the birth canal. The majority of the lung fluid is reabsorbed from the alveolar spaces into the pulmonary circulation, which increases with lung expansion in a process involving several ion transporters such as Na-K ATPase and epithelial sodium channels (ENaC).[5] Approximately 10–15% of this fluid is reabsorbed into the pulmonary lymphatics. The clearance of lung fluid continues for several hours after birth.

To expand the lungs at birth, the infant must generate a large transpulmonary pressure and overcome the resistance of the fluid-filled airways.[3] Initial respiratory efforts can generate transpulmonary pressures of 80–90 cmH_2O. This may explain why the spontaneous occurrence of pneumothorax in healthy newborns is not uncommon. The FRC is rapidly established with the first several breaths; however, this may continue to expand to a lesser degree several hours after birth. Infants born by elective Cesarean section have smaller lung volumes than those observed in vaginally delivered newborns.[6] This difference may persist for up to 48 h after birth. Infants born by Cesarean section with preceding labor constitute an intermediate group. Very immature neonates may have difficulties establishing an adequate FRC with the first few breaths, particularly if they lack adequate amounts of surfactant. The synthesis and metabolism of pulmonary surfactant are discussed in Chapter 6.

Thermoregulation

In utero, the heat generated by the fetus is dissipated by the placenta. Because of the higher metabolic rate of the fetus, its temperature is at or slightly above the maternal core temperature. When there is maternal fever or placental insufficiency, the ability of the fetus to transfer heat to the mother can be impaired, and the infant may be born with an elevated body temperature.

Heat is exchanged by conduction, convection, evaporation, and radiation. The relative importance of any of these forms of heat exchange varies, depending on the clinical situation. For instance, at birth, the infant is delivered from a fluid, warm environment to cooler and dry surroundings. Hence, evaporation is the main source of heat loss right after delivery.[7] Unless the infant is dried soon after birth, preferably with warm towels or blankets, rapid cooling will occur. If the term infant is not in need of resuscitation or assistance in transition (suctioning of meconium, poor respiratory effort), close contact with the mother's skin may serve to decrease the surface area for evaporation and to gain heat through conduction from the mother. This beneficial effect in temperature control is in addition to the immeasurable gains that result from early mother–infant bonding.

The newborn infant is at a significant disadvantage in terms of temperature control because of a relatively large surface area, poor thermal insulation from the environment, decreased ability to generate heat through physical activity (shivering thermogenesis), and, especially, no ability to adjust his or her own protection (clothing) from the thermal stress of the environment. Preterm and growth-retarded infants are at an even higher risk of heat loss and hypothermia. Small preterm infants have an incomplete development of the stratum corneum of the skin and poor keratinization. The smaller the infant, preterm or growth retarded, the fewer subcutaneous fat stores it has, which act as insulation from the environment.

For body temperature to remain constant, heat must be generated at the same rate at which it is lost. Neonates have difficulties not only with heat loss, but also with heat production. Most heat production in the newborn is chemically derived from the breakdown of high-energy triglycerides (nonshivering thermogenesis) stored preferentially in brown fat.[7] This is distributed in the subscapular areas, around the great vessels of the neck and thorax, and around the adrenal glands. Brown fat has numerous capillaries and sympathetic nerve endings. In response to catecholamine stimulation, heat generated through triglyceride breakdown is transferred into the circulation for distribution throughout the body. When the availability of brown fat and substrates is decreased (preterm or growth-retarded infant) or this mechanism is impaired (hypoxia, drugs), heat production is markedly decreased and hypothermia may ensue. The consequences of hypothermia are hypoglycemia, metabolic acidosis, lethargy, and increased oxygen requirements. Also, hypothermia has been associated with a higher mortality at all gestational ages.

After delivery and drying, the newborn should be cared for in a "neutral thermal environment." This refers to that environmental temperature at which the energy expenditure and oxygen consumption for heat production and maintenance of a normal body temperature is the lowest. The neutral thermal environment varies inversely with gestational age and postnatal age.[8]

Asphyxia and neonatal resuscitation

During the transition period from fetal life to extrauterine existence, asphyxia, now more commonly known as either neonatal or perinatal depression, is one of many adverse events that may affect the ability of the neonate to survive or to develop to its fullest potential. Although there is disagreement on the definition of asphyxia or neonatal/perinatal depression,[9,10] the term generally refers to "a condition of impaired blood gas exchange leading, if it persists, to progressive hypoxemia and hypercapnia."[11] Most of the disagreements in its diagnosis arise from attempting to define asphyxia objectively based on Apgar score, fetal heart rate alterations, umbilical cord blood gases, the presence of neurologic abnormalities during the neonatal period, or a combinations of these and other factors. With this approach, asphyxia can be diagnosed reliably only in severely depressed infants. Asphyxia occurs in 2–9 per 1000 births; however, a recent epidemiologic report demonstrates a 90% decrease in the diagnosis of asphyxia from 1991 to 2000.[12]

Mechanisms that result in acute fetal asphyxia usually interfere with the ability of the placenta to exchange oxygen and carbon dioxide. When poor perfusion of the uteroplacental circulation (e.g., maternal hypotension) or separation of the placenta from its insertion (e.g., in abruptio placentae) occurs, the primary consequence is fetal hypoxemia; superimposed ischemia may take place. When the umbilical circulation is compromised (e.g., cord prolapse), the primary consequence is fetal hypercarbia. The severity and rate of progression of asphyxia are highly variable. Asphyxiated infants redistribute cardiac output to the brain, myocardium, and adrenal glands at the expense of blood flow to less vital areas such as the gut, kidneys, muscle, and skin. In addition, the resulting hypoxemia and acidosis may compromise myocardial function to a point at which cardiac output drops. This compromises further oxygen delivery to the tissues.

The best approach to the management of asphyxia is prevention and anticipation. Although asphyxia occurs primarily in high-risk pregnancies, a sizeable proportion of asphyxiated neonates still present without warning. For this reason, personnel skilled in initiating resuscitation must be present at all deliveries.[13] At birth, an initial assessment of the infant is made. If the infant appears depressed, then the initial steps of resuscitation include: providing warmth; positioning the infant to open the airway and clearing it as necessary; drying, stimulating, and repositioning; plus giving oxygen as necessary. If there is a history of meconium in the amniotic fluid, management may include endotracheal intubation and suctioning, although this is now reserved primarily for nonvigorous infants[14] (see section on Meconium aspiration syndrome). Moreover, the efficacy of attempting perineal suctioning in the presence of meconium-stained amniotic fluid has been questioned.[15] Subsequent actions are focused on establishing adequate respirations and circulation, and evaluating the neonate.[16]

The Apgar score is a useful method to assess the neonate during the early period of transition, as well as to evaluate the response to interventions such as resuscitation (Table 68.1). Respirations, heart rate, and color are more useful in assessing neonatal status and need for intervention than the other components of the Apgar score. Thus, appropriate interventions should not be delayed until the 1-min Apgar score is obtained. A repeat Apgar score must be obtained at 5 min after birth in all infants and every 5 min thereafter up to 20 min of age or until the neonate achieves two consecutive scores above 7 if he/she was depressed at birth. The Apgar score is influenced by gestational age.[17] After performing the initial resuscitative steps, infants who are vigorous, are breathing spontaneously, and have a heart rate above 100 need to be observed closely. Blow-by oxygen must be supplied to those who remain cyanotic despite adequate respirations and heart rate. If the infant is apneic, has inadequate respirations, or has a heart rate below 100, current guidelines recommend initiating positive pressure ventilation with 100% oxygen.[13,16] However, there is increasing evidence that resuscitation with room air is as effective as 100% oxygen and may result in less mortality in near-term or term infants.[18,19] Thus, if resuscitation is initiated with less than 100% oxygen, supplemental oxygen up to 100% should be administered if there is no appreciable improvement within 90 s following birth.[16] A good response is primarily indicated by rapid increases in heart rate, although improvements in color and initiation of spontaneous respiratory efforts are also indicators of a positive response. Persistent or prolonged apnea may be a sign of asphyxia or depression by narcotics. Nalox-

Table 68.1 The Apgar score.

Sign	0	1	2
Heart rate	Absent	< 100 b.p.m.	> 100 b.p.m.
Respirations	Absent	Weak cry; hypoventilation	Good, strong cry
Muscle tone	Flaccid	Some flexion	Active motion
Reflex irritability	No response	Grimace	Cough or sneeze
Color	Blue or pale	Body pink; extremities blue	Completely pink

Table 68.2 Medications for delivery room resuscitation.

Drug	Indication	Dose	Route
Epinephrine	Asystole or heart rate of < 60 despite positive pressure ventilation with 100% oxygen and chest compressions	0.01–0.03 mg/kg or 0.1–0.3 mL/kg of 1 : 10 000 solution up to	i.v.
		0.1 mg/kg or 0.3–1 mL/kg of 1 : 10 000 solution	i.t.
Sodium bicarbonate	Metabolic acidosis	2 mEq/kg The use of 4.2% solution is recommended	i.v.
Naloxone (Narcan)	Respiratory depression and maternal exposure to narcotics in previous 4 h	0.1 mg/kg The use of 0.4 mg/mL or1.0 mg/mL solutions is recommended	i.v., i.t., s.c., i.m.
Volume expander: normal saline, whole blood	Evidence of hypovolemia	10 mL/kg	i.v.

i.m., intramuscular; i.t., intracheal; i.v., intravenous; s.c., subcutaneous.

one (Narcan) can be given in neonates with poor or absent respiratory efforts exposed to maternally administered narcotics within 4 h of delivery.

When the heart rate is less than 60 beats per minute (b.p.m.) and there is no rapid response to positive pressure ventilation, chest compressions must be initiated to maintain an acceptable cardiac output. After 30 s without improvement, epinephrine should be administered. At this time, endotracheal intubation must be performed if it has not been done previously. The main indications for endotracheal intubation are persistent apnea, need for positive pressure ventilation for several minutes, and lack of response to resuscitative maneuvers.[16]

The medications needed for delivery room resuscitation are listed in Table 68.2. Administration of epinephrine, preferably intravenously, usually results in a rapid increase in heart rate and cardiac output. The dose may be repeated after 5 min if there is no response. Reasons for poor response to epinephrine are significant acidosis and hypovolemia. If acidosis is suspected, an effort should be made to obtain arterial blood gases. Current guidelines acknowledge that correction of metabolic acidosis with sodium bicarbonate is controversial.[16] Hypovolemia should be suspected when there is a poor response to resuscitation and evidence of poor perfusion, especially if there is a history of abruption, tight nuchal cord, or bleeding. Ideally, group O Rh-negative whole blood should be used when bleeding and acute anemia are suspected. However, crystalline solutions such as normal saline and lactated Ringer's are more readily available and are usually effective.

Infants who suffer any degree of perinatal depression must be observed closely during the first 24–48 h after birth. Vital signs, neurologic findings, and functioning of other systems must be assessed periodically. Multiorgan dysfunction involving the kidneys, liver, and heart is common among neonates with severe perinatal depression.[20,21] Finally, it is very difficult to correlate asphyxia, using any definition, with long-term neurodevelopmental outcome.[22–24] Recent clinical trials have suggested that institution of hypothermia may be of some benefit in reducing the likelihood of a poor outcome among term and near-term neonates born with significant depression and signs of hypoxic–ischemic encephalopathy.[25,26]

Respiratory problems

Signs of respiratory distress, such as tachypnea, retractions, nasal flaring, end-expiratory grunting, and cyanosis, may be the result of many diseases, some of which involve systems other than the respiratory system (Table 68.3). An adequate history and thorough physical examination may be sufficient to suspect or diagnose the etiology of the respiratory distress. Nevertheless, part of the workup of any neonate with signs of respiratory distress generally includes obtaining a chest radiograph and determining arterial blood gases, even if there is no need for supplemental oxygen.

Respiratory distress syndrome

Respiratory distress syndrome (RDS) due to surfactant deficiency and lung immaturity is one of the most common causes of respiratory difficulty in the neonatal period. Acute and chronic complications resulting from RDS or its treatment remain as frequent causes of morbidity and mortality in neonatal intensive care units.[27] The most important risk factor for the development of RDS is preterm birth. The incidence of RDS varies inversely with gestational age and can be as high as 60–70% among infants less than 28–29 weeks of gestation. Conversely, RDS is seldom seen beyond 38 weeks of gestation. Additional risk factors are male sex, Cesarean section delivery, perinatal asphyxia, second twin pregnancy, and maternal diabetes. Preterm delivery is associated with variable degrees of immaturity of surfactant metabolism. Infants who develop RDS have lower amounts of surfactant phospholipids and

Table 68.3 Common causes of respiratory distress in the newborn.

I. Respiratory disorders:
  A. Pulmonary diseases
    Respiratory distress syndrome
    Meconium aspiration syndrome
    Transient tachypnea
    Pneumonia
    Pneumothorax and other air leaks
    Developmental anomalies (congenital lobar emphysema, chylothorax, pulmonary hypoplasia)
  B. Airway obstruction
    Choanal atresia
    Pierre Robin syndrome
  C. Rib cage abnormalities
    Asphyxiating thoracic dystrophy
  D. Diaphragmatic disorders
    Diaphragmatic hernia
    Phrenic nerve injury

II. Extrarespiratory disorders:
  A. Congenital heart disease
  B. Acid–base abnormalities (inherited disorders of metabolism, other causes of metabolic acidosis)
  C. Central nervous system disorders (cerebral edema, hemorrhage, infection)

proteins in the airway than control subjects.[28,29] This deficiency may be the result of abnormalities of surfactant synthesis, secretion, reutilization, or combinations of these factors. Among very immature neonates, there is also substantial structural lung immaturity. The relative importance of this aspect has become more apparent with surfactant replacement therapy. Alterations in lung mechanics that persist after surfactant administration are primarily a reflection of the anatomic immaturity of the preterm lung. Both surfactant deficiency and structural lung immaturity lead to decreased pulmonary compliance and atelectasis. Hypoxemia develops as a consequence of the resulting right-to-left intrapulmonary shunting. Hypercarbia may also occur due to hypoventilation of the lungs. Lack of ductal closure is a common finding among small infants with RDS. This may provide the route for left-to-right shunting and, potentially, pulmonary edema. Leakage of pulmonary capillaries due to hyperemia, hypoxic injury to the alveolar and capillary walls, and volutrauma (overstretching of lung tissue) gives access to plasma proteins into the alveolar sacs. Several of these proteins can inhibit surfactant function.[30,31] Thus, capillary leakage may play an important role in the pathogenesis of RDS by inactivation of secreted surfactant.

The clinical signs of RDS are tachypnea, nasal flaring, grunting, retractions, and cyanosis in room air. Decreased air entry is found on auscultation. Because these signs are common to other diseases such as pneumonia and heart disease, the diagnosis of RDS is based not only on clinical assessment, but also on the presence of radiographic findings, such as a diffuse reticulogranular pattern, poor lung expansion, and air bronchograms. Because this radiographic pattern is also observed with group B streptococcal pneumonia, exclusion of the possibility of infection is necessary.[32] Typically, in neonates not treated with exogenous surfactant, the severity of RDS increases up to 48–72 h, followed by a gradual improvement. This phase is often preceded by or occurs in association with a marked diuresis. The clinical course of RDS is substantially modified by the administration of exogenous surfactant; however, the timing of diuresis is not influenced by this therapy.[33,34]

The management of infants with RDS involves general measures such as maintenance of vital signs and thermoregulation, fluid and electrolyte management, nutritional support, and correction of hematologic or acid–base abnormalities. Specific measures consist of oxygen therapy and the use of positive airway pressure, either continuously (CPAP) or by assisted ventilation.[35] The goals of this therapy are to maintain acceptable arterial blood gases with as little support as possible, in order to minimize the likelihood of volutrauma and oxygen toxicity. Because neonates have mostly fetal hemoglobin, an arterial $P\text{O}_2$ between 50 and 70 mmHg is sufficient to saturate 90–95% of the hemoglobin. Higher values are not needed and can be deleterious. In fact, it is also possible that arterial $P\text{O}_2$ values slightly below 50 mmHg (saturation readings generally between 85% and 90%) may be as safe in the early neonatal period. Infants receiving oxygen or any form of ventilator assistance must be monitored closely with pulse oximetry and intermittent blood gas analysis. Also, $P\text{CO}_2$ values of less than 40–45 mmHg should be avoided because they have been associated with a higher risk of developing bronchopulmonary dysplasia.[36] The role of high-frequency ventilation in the management of infants with RDS remains controversial and is generally reserved for specific instances such as the presence of severe air leaks and pulmonary interstitial emphysema.[37]

Administration of exogenous surfactant has become the standard of therapy for infants with RDS who are intubated.[33,38,39] Several types of exogenous surfactant are available for use in neonates. Currently available surfactant preparations consist of either synthetic mixtures of phospholipids or extracts of animal lung surfactant; the latter are currently the most used type (Table 68.4). Animal-derived lung surfactants contain specific surfactant proteins, which are important for the function of surfactant. Their animal origin is of some concern; however, to date, no major significant immune reaction to these proteins has been demonstrated.[40,41] Clinical trials of newer generation surfactants that contain synthetic peptides that mimic the action of surfactant proteins have shown substantial efficacy and may become widely used in the future.[42,43] Administration of surfactant can be performed at birth (prophylactic) or after RDS has already been diagnosed (rescue/treatment). With the prophylactic approach, many infants are intubated and may be given surfactant unnecessarily. However, this approach has been shown

Table 68.4 Composition of exogenous surfactants.

Surfactant	Source	Contents	Initial dose (mL/kg)
Exosurf	Synthetic	DPPC, hexadecanol, tyloxapol	5
Survanta	Minced cow lung with synthetic lipids added	Phospholipids, SP-B, SP-C	4
Infasurf	Calf lung lavage	Phospholipids, SP-B, SP-C	3
Curosurf	Pig lung	Phospholipids, SP-B, SP-C	2.5
Surfaxin	Synthetic, new generation	DPPC, PG, synthetic SP-B-like peptide	5.8

DPPC, dipalmitoyl-phosphatidylcholine; SP, surfactant proteins; PG, phosphatidylglycerol.

to result in improved survival in very immature infants in systematic reviews of the subject.[44] Soon after intratracheal administration of a dose of surfactant, rapid improvements in oxygenation and lung compliance are observed, especially with preparations containing surfactant proteins or a synthetic mimic of them. Accordingly, ventilatory support can be decreased rapidly. Nonetheless, these effects can be transient, and repeat doses of surfactant may be necessary. Administration of surfactant, whether as prophylaxis or as rescue therapy, results in substantial decreases in neonatal mortality and a markedly lower incidence of air leaks such as pneumothorax, pneumomediastinum, and pulmonary interstitial emphysema. The occurrence of complications such as intraventricular hemorrhage and bronchopulmonary dysplasia (BPD), however, has not decreased consistently with surfactant replacement therapy.[38,39]

Despite widespread availability of surfactant replacement, RDS and other complications of prematurity continue to be responsible for a substantial proportion of deaths and morbidity among preterm infants. Thus, all efforts directed toward prevention of preterm delivery need to be continued and strengthened. In addition, attempts to accelerate fetal maturation with antenatal corticosteroids must be undertaken whenever feasible.[45] Despite multiple animal studies and promising preliminary clinical data, the addition of thyrotropin-releasing hormone to prenatal corticosteroid therapy has not been shown to be more effective than corticosteroids alone to prevent RDS in the era of widespread surfactant use.[46] Currently available data strongly suggest that prenatal administration of corticosteroids followed by postnatal surfactant replacement for those infants who develop RDS is the best possible approach to the prevention and treatment of RDS and its complications.[47]

Bronchopulmonary dysplasia

Most neonates with RDS recover completely from their lung disease within the first week after birth. Some, however, develop a form of chronic respiratory disease called BPD. The diagnosis of BPD is based on the presence of tachypnea, retractions, and supplemental oxygen requirement at 28 days after birth. However, a more stringent diagnostic criterion for BPD of need for oxygen therapy at 36 weeks adjusted gestational age has been recommended because it has been shown to be a more specific predictor of long-term pulmonary morbidity in very low-birthweight infants.[48,49] Associated chest radiographic findings in infants with BPD include interstitial fibrosis, cystic changes, hyperinflation, and segmental atelectasis. The term chronic lung disease of prematurity (CLD) defined on the basis of clinical criteria (oxygen requirement) only, at either 28 days of age or 36 weeks adjusted gestational age, has also been used to describe infants with prolonged needs for supplemental oxygen due to lung disease. As neonatal intensive care has become more sophisticated over the past three decades, the survival of very low-birthweight infants has increased dramatically, and BPD is now seen in very small infants who did not have RDS or pneumonia in the first week after birth.[50] This "new BPD" seems to be more the consequence of chronic inflammation, deleterious effects of cytokines and other mediators, and an arrest of the process of normal lung development.[51] The incidence of BPD or CLD varies according to the definition used and the population studied, but is clearly inversely proportional to gestational age. In a retrospective study of 1625 infants with birthweights between 700 and 1500 g treated in eight major medical centers in the United States, the incidence of CLD, defined as an oxygen requirement at 28 days of age, ranged from 6% to 33% in the different medical centers.[52] Within the entire study population, lower birthweight, white race, and male sex were identified as risk factors for the development of CLD.

The pathogenesis of BPD is multifactorial.[50–52] Oxygen toxicity and volutrauma have frequently been implicated in the pathogenesis of BPD, but it is very difficult to isolate these factors from the pulmonary immaturity and acute lung injury for which these treatment modalities are used. Pulmonary air leaks, pulmonary edema, patent DA, acquired pneumonia, and poor nutrition are also risk factors for the development of BPD. More recently, it has been reported that various cytokines may play a major role in the pathogenesis of BPD. Moreover, the detrimental effect of these mediators may, in fact, start *in utero*.[53,54] Pulmonary hypertension and cor pulmonale can be observed in more advanced forms of BPD. Infants with BPD also have an increased susceptibility to severe bacterial and viral infections.

Management of infants with BPD is directed at treating symptoms, optimizing lung growth and healing, supporting general growth and development, and preventing complications.[55,56] Treatment strategies include chronic administration of oxygen to attempt to prevent cor pulmonale, aggressive nutritional support, fluid restriction, use of chronic diuretics, bronchodilators, and environmental measures to minimize the risk of respiratory infection. However, the use of many of these interventions is not supported by well-controlled clinical trials.[57,58] Nonetheless, they are widely used in neonatal intensive care units. Treatment with postnatal corticosteroids has been shown to be of short-term benefit primarily for ventilator-dependent infants with BPD. However, there is increasing evidence of serious adverse neurodevelopmental risks associated with prolonged postnatal corticosteroid therapy.[59,60] Thus, their use should be extremely limited and should include thorough parental disclosure of the potential side-effects of their use.

The mortality for infants with BPD has decreased over the past decades, but morbidity remains high. Most deaths in infants with BPD are a consequence of cor pulmonale or respiratory infections. In survivors, pulmonary function improves over the first several years of age, although some evidence of increased airway reactivity persists into early adulthood. The association between BPD and long-term neurodevelopmental abnormalities remains a major concern.[49] With carefully monitored long-term oxygen therapy to reduce the risk of cor pulmonale and aggressive management of nutrition and respiratory infections, the prognosis for infants with BPD may continue to improve.

Meconium aspiration syndrome

Meconium is composed of desquamated cells from the skin and gastrointestinal tract, lanugo, amniotic fluid, and various intestinal secretions, including bile. Whereas meconium is present in the intestine of immature fetuses, it is rarely found in amniotic fluid before 34 weeks of gestation. Beyond this period, meconium can be detected in 10–18% of all deliveries.[15,61] *In utero* passage of meconium can be a sign of maturation, or it may be triggered by fetal hypoxemia and acidosis. However, there is a poor correlation between meconium staining of the amniotic fluid and umbilical cord acid–base status.[61] Of all infants delivered through meconium-stained amniotic fluid, between 1% and 9% may develop meconium aspiration syndrome (MAS).[14,15] Many of these cases have delivered through thick meconium.[62,63]

The presence of meconium in the airway may interfere with the initiation of breathing and may be a cause of difficult resuscitation. In MAS, overall airway resistance is increased, although the airway obstruction is not homogeneous throughout the lungs. Segments of the lungs exhibit alveolar overdistention and air trapping, whereas in others, alveolar collapse predominates. Air leaks (pneumothorax, pneumomediastinum) may frequently be seen among infants with MAS, particularly those who require mechanical ventilation.[14,15] These alterations lead to variable degrees of ventilation–perfusion abnormalities and intrapulmonary shunting with resulting hypoxemia.[64,65] Infants with severe MAS also develop respiratory acidosis. Hypoxemia and acidosis can increase pulmonary vascular resistance and cause right-to-left shunting through the DA, foramen ovale, or both, a condition known as persistent pulmonary hypertension of the newborn (PPHN). This condition may worsen the oxygenation status of the infant. The presence of meconium in the amniotic fluid is a known risk factor for the development of PPHN.[65] Some infants who have fatal MAS and PPHN have been shown to have excessive development of the muscle layer around the small intra-acinar arterioles of the lung, which predisposes them to PPHN. It has been suggested that these changes result from a chronic and often subclinical hypoxemia *in utero* or subclinical infection.[66,67] Additional factors that play a role in the pathogenesis of MAS are the chemical pneumonitis induced by the free fatty acids in meconium.[68]

Infants with MAS manifest tachypnea and variable degrees of nasal flaring, retractions, and cyanosis in room air; grunting is less common. The chest appears to be hyperexpanded, and aeration may be decreased on auscultation. Meconium staining of the skin is not uniformly present. Usually, these infants are appropriately grown. However, they may have a low ponderal index, because of recent intrauterine weight loss, or other signs may be present. Radiographic examination reveals hyperexpansion of the lungs, asymmetric areas of atelectasis, and areas that may be completely spared. Pneumothorax and pneumomediastinum are frequent findings.

The management of infants with MAS must begin before delivery. Careful surveillance of fetal well-being is important, particularly if meconium is found in the amniotic fluid. Delivery with intact fetal membranes can obscure the detection of meconium. Detection of meconium in the amniotic fluid mandates the need for the presence of a team skilled in neonatal intubation and resuscitation at delivery.[16] Use of a DeLee catheter to suction the nose and pharynx as soon as the head is delivered and while it is still on the perineum has not been shown to reduce the risk of MAS.[15] Not all infants with meconium-stained amniotic fluid need to be intubated after birth for the purpose of suctioning. The best approach for term infants who have already initiated vigorous respiratory efforts is probably just observation, regardless of the characteristics of the meconium.[14] Efforts to intubate these neonates may be more harmful than helpful. Direct visualization of the larynx and tracheal suctioning is now reserved primarily for infants in need of resuscitation. Thorough endotracheal suctioning will not prevent all cases of MAS.[69] Furthermore, the use of amnioinfusion also does not prevent MAS.[70] Subsequent management depends on whether the infant develops clinical signs of MAS. Adequate oxygenation, correction of metabolic acidosis, and support of the circulation are critical to minimize the stimuli for pulmonary vasoconstriction. The routine use of antibiotics in infants with MAS remains controversial.[71] Controlled clinical trials have shown improvements in oxygenation and a lower need for extracorporeal membrane oxygenation (ECMO) with bolus administration of exogenous surfactant to infants with severe MAS, although this practice remains controversial.[72,73] A new approach using lavage with surfactant may also prove to be of use in established MAS.[74]

The mortality of infants with MAS used to be as high as 40%, but it has declined dramatically with improvements in care and the availability of ECMO. Most MAS deaths result from PPHN or the consequences of asphyxia. Up to one-third of survivors of MAS may exhibit pulmonary function abnormalities later in childhood, such as airway obstruction and exercise-induced bronchospasm.[75,76] Meconium contamination of the middle ear at birth may also increase the risk of otitis media in these infants.[77] The long-term neurologic outcome of infants with MAS can be quite variable and is influenced by the presence or absence of signs of perinatal asphyxia.

Persistent pulmonary hypertension of the newborn

Although right-to-left shunting through the foramen ovale and DA is necessary for fetal survival, persistence of this pattern of circulation results in marked hypoxemia in extrauterine life. Hypercarbia, however, is not a consequence of PPHN. Under normal circumstances, the high fetal pulmonary vascular resistance progressively decreases after birth. Endogenous production of nitrous oxide (NO) seems to play a pivotal role in this process.[78] With hypoxemia and acidosis, pulmonary vascular resistance will remain high, or it may increase if it had already decreased. Experiments in animal models of PPHN suggest that a lower expression of the enzyme responsible for endogenous NO production, NO synthase, may account for the predisposition to develop PPHN in diseases such as congenital diaphragmatic hernia.[79] Pulmonary vasoconstriction can also be induced by mediators such as thromboxane A_2 and leukotrienes.[80] These mediators may play a role in PPHN associated with group B streptococcal infections.

Using an anatomic approach, infants with PPHN can be divided into a group with normal pulmonary vasculature who develop PPHN because of a transient maladaption (acute asphyxia, pneumonia), another group in which there is underdevelopment of the pulmonary vasculature (pulmonary hypoplasia), and a last group of infants in whom the number of pulmonary vessels is normal, but in whom development of the muscle layer around the intra-acinar arteries is excessive.[81] In the last two groups, the pulmonary vascular abnormalities probably develop days or weeks before birth. Clinically, PPHN has also been classified as primary (i.e., without associated disorders) or secondary to respiratory or other diseases (Table 68.5). A recent study has associated maternal exposure to selective serotonin reuptake inhibitors with a higher likelihood of PPHN.[82] The diagnosis of PPHN should be suspected when there is a high alveolar to arterial difference of oxygen, even if there is no hypoxemia ($Po_2 < 50$ mmHg). The presence of right-to-left ductal shunting is established clinically by comparing preductal and postductal arterial blood gases or by showing a lower hemoglobin (Hb) saturation in areas perfused by postductal blood with simultaneous preductal readings.

Table 68.5 Diseases commonly associated with persistent pulmonary hypertension of the newborn.

Perinatal asphyxia
Meconium aspiration syndrome
Pneumonia
Respiratory distress syndrome
Polycythemia
Diaphragmatic hernia
Pulmonary hypoplasia
Maternal salicylate use during pregnancy
Maternal selective serotonin reuptake inhibitor use during pregnancy

The absence of ductal shunting does not rule out PPHN as this could be occurring at the level of the foramen ovale. The diagnosis must be done by echocardiography, which also serves to discount the possibility of congenital heart disease and assess myocardial contractility.

The treatment of infants with PPHN is controversial.[83] In general, therapy is focused on supporting the systemic circulation by fluid administration and the use of pressor agents, and a series of measures to overcome hypoxemia and acidosis in order to decrease the elevated pulmonary vascular resistance. These have included hyperventilation, alkalization with sodium bicarbonate, and administration of a variety of other medications seeking to dilate the pulmonary vasculature (tolazoline, chlorpromazine, nitroprusside, prostaglandins, nifedipine, amrinone) and provide sedation and muscle paralysis (fentanyl, pancuronium). However, there few if any controlled trials to support the use of most of these therapies.[83] A more conservative approach to avoiding the volutrauma resulting from attempts to hyperventilate has been suggested.[84] With a conservative approach, survival rates of 80–90% have been reported in PPHN.[85] High-frequency ventilation and ECMO are additional therapies used to treat infants with PPHN.[86,87] Several controlled clinical trials have shown that the use of inhaled NO therapy improves oxygenation and can reduce the need for ECMO among term infants with PPHN.[88,89]

Neurologic abnormalities and hearing loss have been reported in up to 50% of survivors of PPHN.[90,91] However, severe neurodevelopmental impairment is uncommon. It is not well known whether these abnormalities result from hypoxia, associated conditions (hypoglycemia, asphyxia), therapeutic interventions, or combinations of these factors.[92]

Transient tachypnea of the newborn

The pathogenesis of transient tachypnea of the newborn (TTN) is related primarily to lung fluid reabsorption. This respiratory disease is seen mostly in term or near-term infants but may also affect premature infants.[93] With the onset of labor, lung fluid production decreases, and its absorption increases under the influence of catecholamines, vasopressin, and corticosteroids.

Labor markedly influences pulmonary epithelial ion transport so that term infants born by Cesarean section without labor exhibit a delay in the transition from chloride secretion to sodium absorption. Infants with TTN demonstrate a similar abnormality.[94] Thus, delivery by Cesarean section without labor constitutes a risk factor for TTN.[95] Some infants who develop TTN have also been shown to have borderline lung maturity on prenatal amniotic fluid analysis.[96] Additional risk factors are maternal diabetes, prolonged labor, male sex, macrosomia, and asphyxia.[97] This last complication not only interferes with lung fluid reabsorption, but may also lead to a variable degree of left or combined ventricular failure.[98,99]

The manifestations of TTN are tachypnea, retractions, grunting, and hyperexpansion of the thorax. These signs are usually manifest by 6–8 h after birth. Onset of respiratory symptoms beyond 24–48 h after birth is usually not due to TTN; hence, other explanations should be sought. The radiologic features of TTN are mild hyperinflation, increased interstitial and vascular markings (primarily around the hilar areas), fluid in the horizontal fissure, and, at times, mild cardiomegaly. Small pleural effusions, mostly on the right side, can be present. A pleural effusion, revealed by radiographic examination where none existed earlier, is more suggestive of infection than of TTN. The presence of radiographic abnormalities indicative of delayed clearance of lung fluid is not necessarily associated with clinical manifestations, especially on radiography performed soon after delivery. There can be variable degrees of hypoxemia and respiratory acidosis. Treatment consists primarily of supportive therapy and administration of supplemental oxygen. Oxygen requirements are variable and can be very high. In addition, some infants may require the use of CPAP or mechanical ventilation for significant respiratory distress or blood gas derangements. The association of TTN with PPHN has also been reported.[99] The signs of TTN usually last less than 72 h, and pulmonary sequelae are rare.

Hematologic problems

Fetal erythropoiesis occurs primarily in the liver and bone marrow and, to a lesser extent, in the spleen. Extramedullary erythropoiesis may persist for up to 1–2 weeks after delivery. During the second trimester and early third trimester, over 90% of the hemoglobin of the fetus is HbF, which binds oxygen more avidly than HbA. The *p*50 and *p*90 (i.e., the partial pressure of oxygen at which 50% and 90%, respectively, of the Hb is saturated) are considerably lower in HbF than in HbA. The synthesis of HbA increases as the fetus approaches term, resulting in an increase in total body hemoglobin mass and a decrease in the proportion of HbF to 50–85% of the total.[100] After birth, there is a gradual decline in circulating HbF levels to about 10–15% at 3–4 months of age, and less than 2% by 2 years of age. In certain disorders of HbA synthesis (sickle cell anemia, thalassemia major), the rate of decline of HbF is much slower. The fetal red blood cell has a survival of only 80–90 days.

The normal hematologic values for term infants are seen in Table 68.6. Abnormalities in the white blood cell (WBC) count, such as leukopenia (< 5000/mL), marked leukocytosis (> 30 000/mm^3), and an increase in the immature–mature neutrophil ratio (> 0.2–0.3) are suggestive of neonatal infection.[101,102] The platelet count is similar in both preterm and term infants. Although an occasional healthy newborn will have less than 150 000 platelets/mL, counts below this level should be considered suspicious; a number below 100 000/mL is definitely abnormal.

Under normal circumstances, the level of Hb in cord blood is influenced by gestational age and placental transfusion. The increase in Hb with advancing gestation is associated with a mild but significant decrease in umbilical venous Po_2, ensuring constant oxygen content of the fetal umbilical venous blood throughout gestation. The pool of blood shared by the fetus and the placenta may be preferentially transfused to either of them at the time of delivery. If there is delayed cord clamping, the infant is held lower than the placenta, or if there is a hypoxia-induced increase in placental vascular resistance, the blood volume of the infant may be increased by up to 60%.[103,104] Conversely, positioning the infant above the placenta or rapid cord clamping may partially deprive the neonate of the placental transfusion. This mechanism may explain the lower cord blood Hb levels observed in neonates born by Cesarean section.

Table 68.6 Normal hematologic values for term newborns.*

Age	Hb (g/dL)	Hct (%)	Reticulocytes (%)	WBC (× 10^3/mL)	Platelets (× 10^3/mL)
Cord	16.5 ± 3.0	51 ± 9	3–10	18 ± 9	300 ± 150
1–3 days	18.5 ± 4.0	56 ± 9	3–7	15 ± 9†	300 ± 150
1 week	17.5 ± 4.0	54 ± 12	< 2–3	12 ± 5	300 ± 150
1 month	14.0 ± 4.0	43 ± 12	–	–	300 ± 150

Hb, hemoglobin, Hct, hematocrit; WBC, white blood cell.

*All values are approximate mean ± 2 standard deviations; from Oski FA, Naiman JL, eds. *Hematologic problems in the newborn*, 3rd edn. Philadelphia: W.B. Saunders, 1982; and Avery GB, ed. *Neonatology*, 3rd edn. Philadelphia, PA: J.B. Lippincott, 1987.

†Values increase 12–24 h after birth.

Table 68.7 Common causes of anemia in the newborn.

Hemorrhage	Hemolysis	Decreased RBC production
External	*Immune*	Diamond–Blackfan syndrome
Placenta abruptio	ABO	Transcobalamin II deficiency
Placenta previa	Rh	Congenital leukemia
Tumors	Minor groups	
Cord	Maternal autoimmune	
Nuchal cord	Drug-induced	
Velamentous insertion		
Fetoplacental	*Nonimmune*	
Fetomaternal	Infection	
Twin–twin transfusion	RBC membrane defects	
	Glucose-6-phosphate dehydrogenase deficiency	
Internal		
Cephalhematoma	Pyruvate kinase deficiency	
Intracranial	Hemoglobinopathies	
Ruptured liver, spleen		
Adrenal		
Retroperitoneal		
Iatrogenic		

RBC, red blood cell.

Table 68.8 Differential diagnosis of anemia in the newborn: clinical and laboratory findings.

	Hemorrhage			
	Acute	Chronic	Hemolysis	Decreased RBC production
Clinical				
Pallor	(−) to +++	+ to +++	+ to +++	+ to +++
Hepatosplenomegaly	(−)	(−) to +++	++ to +++	(−)
Early jaundice	(−)	(−)	++ to +++	(−)
Hypovolemia	+ to +++	(−)	(−)	(−)
Laboratory				
Cord hemoglobin	Nl or ↓	↓ to ↓↓↓	↓ to ↓↓↓	↓ to ↓↓↓
Bilirubin (cord or day 1)	Nl	Nl	↑ to ↑↑↑	Nl
Direct Coombs' test	(−)	(−)	(−) to +++	(−)
Reticulocytes	Nl to ↑↑↑	↑ to ↑↑↑	↑ to ↑↑↑	Low

↓, mild decrease; ↑, mild increase; ↓↓↓, marked decrease; ↑↑↑, marked increase; (−), absent; +, mild; +++, severe; Nl, normal; RBC, red blood cell.

Anemia

Anemia, defined as a Hb < 13 g/dL in term infants, can be the result of hemorrhage, hemolysis, or decreased red cell production (Table 68.7). It is uncommon to see anemia secondary to combinations of these factors. Clinical and laboratory findings that are helpful in establishing the differential diagnosis of anemia in the newborn are listed in Table 68.8.

Anemia secondary to hemorrhage

Anemia secondary to hemorrhage is a frequent etiology of anemia presenting at birth or soon thereafter. Acute blood loss presents as signs of hypovolemia including lethargy, poor capillary refill, tachycardia, weak pulses, hypotension, or pallor. Significant blood loss may render an infant unresponsive to the usual resuscitative maneuvers until the intravascular volume depletion is restored. Chronic blood loss over a period of days or weeks permits substantial hemodynamic compensation, so that the main presenting sign is pallor.[105] If the hemorrhage is external, there is no additional bilirubin load to the liver once the postnatal breakdown of Hb begins. This is in contrast to internal hemorrhages (e.g., cephalhematoma) that contribute to elevations in the serum bilirubin and jaundice beyond the first 24–48 h after birth.

External bleeding may be apparent by history (vaginal bleeding in the mother in placenta previa) or physical examination (ruptured umbilical cord). Twin-to-twin transfusion is a type of external hemorrhage that is seen primarily in monochorionic twins. The donor twin becomes anemic while the recipient's Hb is increased. Abnormalities of the umbilical cord, such as varices, aneurysm, or velamentous insertion, make it more prone to rupturing; however, a normal umbilical cord may also rupture when stretched excessively, such as in a precipitous delivery, or when attempting to reduce a very tight nuchal cord. Fetal blood loss may occur with an intact tight nuchal cord as the umbilical vein is compressed before the arteries, which continue to direct blood to the placenta.

Substantial bleeding may be occult and thus more difficult to diagnose (fetal–maternal hemorrhage or FMH). FMH is more likely to happen when there are abnormalities of the placenta or instrumentation such as amniocentesis, Cesarean section, or external version. Placental abnormalities such as abruptio placentae, placenta previa, choriocarcinoma, and chorioangioma have been associated with severe FMH.[106] The diagnosis is confirmed by demonstration of fetal erythrocytes in the maternal circulation by Kleihauer–Betke staining or other techniques such as determination of fetal hemoglobin by flow cytometry. The amount of red blood cells lost into the mother can be approximated using several formulas, as reviewed recently by Giacoia.[107]

Anemia secondary to hemolysis

Hemolytic anemias usually manifest with pallor and early onset of jaundice, but without signs of hypovolemia. The etiology of hemolysis may be quite variable. ABO or Rh incompatibility and infection are the most common causes of hemolytic anemia in the newborn. Clinical and laboratory findings useful in differentiating hemolysis from other causes of anemia are listed in Table 68.8. ABO hemolytic disease has a wide spectrum from immune hemolysis only, demonstrated by a decreased RBC survival, to severe anemia and, rarely, hydrops fetalis.[108] It usually affects firstborn infants. The diagnosis should be suspected in any newborn with early onset of jaundice with or without significant anemia. Generally, the mother is type O and the infant either type A or type B. The direct Coombs' test can be positive; however, it is often negative because of a low antibody titer and because A or B antigens are more sparsely located in the fetal red blood cells (RBCs). The hemolysis is less aggressive than in Rh isoimmunization.

In contrast, Rh isoimmunization frequently results in more significant degrees of anemia and hyperbilirubinemia.[109] The severity of the hemolysis increases with subsequent pregnancies with Rh-positive fetuses. At birth, affected infants are generally anemic and develop rapidly rising indirect bilirubin levels (> 0.4–0.5 mg/h). Hepatosplenomegaly is more common than in ABO hemolytic disease. A positive direct Coombs' test is the rule. The blood smear reveals numerous reticulocytes and nucleated RBCs, but rare spherocytes. In cases with severe hemolysis, thrombocytopenia is often found.

Other causes of immune hemolysis should be suspected in the presence of a positive direct Coombs' test but compatible ABO and Rh types between mother and infant. Minor group sensitization is occasionally a cause of immune hemolysis.[110] The maternal history may be suggestive of an autoimmune disorder or of the use of medications capable of inducing an immune hemolytic anemia. In these cases, the maternal direct Coombs' test can be positive.

Viral or bacterial infections are the most common cause of nonimmune hemolysis. These infants usually exhibit signs such as hepatosplenomegaly, petechiae, cutaneous rash, growth retardation, and chorioretinitis. Laboratory findings include thrombocytopenia, leukopenia, evidence of disseminated intravascular coagulation, and increases in direct bilirubin. Abnormalities of the RBC membrane, enzymes, or hemoglobin are uncommon causes of hemolytic anemia in the newborn. Their presence should be suspected with a positive family history, evidence of hemolysis with negative direct Coombs' test, and suggestive findings on a blood smear. The diagnosis is made by identifying the specific defect.

Decreased RBC production

Neonatal anemia due to decreased RBC production is very uncommon. It should be suspected in the presence of anemia with a low reticulocyte count (< 2%) not explained by other obvious causes. Isolated hypoplastic anemia is suggestive of the Diamond–Blackfan syndrome, which also features physical anomalies (cleft palate, abnormal thumbs, ocular defects, short or webbed neck) in 30% of cases. Involvement of WBC and platelet precursors is found in transcobalamin II deficiency and congenital leukemia.

Polycythemia

Polycythemia is defined as a spun peripheral venous hematocrit (Hct) of more than 65%. The site and time of sampling are critical to make the diagnosis.[111] The venous Hct peaks at 2 h after birth and then declines;[112] capillary samples are 5–10% higher than simultaneously obtained venous samples. The incidence of polycythemia varies from 1.4% to 1.8% at sea level and is higher at higher altitudes, in small for gestational age (SGA) and large for gestational age infants, and in term and postterm newborns compared with preterm infants.[113,114] The most common signs and symptoms associated with polycythemia are plethora, lethargy, tachypnea, feeding difficulties, hypotonia, and jitteriness. These signs are also common to other neonatal diseases and are not pathognomonic of polycythemia. Many neonates with venous Hct above 65% are asymptomatic; the majority of those exhibiting symptoms are hyperviscous.[111,115] However, viscosity measurements are not widely available, and it is uncertain what actually represents hyperviscous values.[111,116] The symptomatology in these infants may be secondary to sluggish tissue

Table 68.9 Etiology of neonatal polycythemia.

Increased erythropoiesis	Transfusion
Intrauterine hypoxia:	Delayed cord clamping
Small for gestational age	Intentional
Postmaturity	Unassisted delivery
Toxemia	Twin–twin transfusion
Hyperinsulinemia:	Monochorionic placenta
Maternal diabetes	Maternal–fetal transfusion
Beta-cell hyperplasia	
Beckwith–Wiedemann syndrome	
Chromosomal abnormalities:	
Trisomy 21	
Trisomy 13	
Trisomy 18	
Congenital adrenal hyperplasia	
Thyrotoxicosis	

blood flow and to associated problems, such as hypoglycemia, hypocalcemia, or asphyxia.

Polycythemia may result from either a chronic increase in the RBC mass or an acute expansion of the circulating blood volume with subsequent increases in Hct when transudation to the interstitial compartment occurs (Table 68.9). *In utero*, hypoxia stimulates erythropoietin production, which in turn promotes erythropoiesis (SGA, postmaturity). These infants are generally not hypervolemic and can have elevated reticulocyte counts.[117] Conversely, infants with polycythemia due to transfusion may be hypervolemic.

Although there are no generally accepted criteria for the treatment of polycythemia, most centers will intervene in all infants with central venous Hct above 70% or those with Hct above 65% if they are symptomatic.[118] Treatment consists of a partial exchange transfusion to lower the Hct to a range at which blood viscosity will also be much lower. The formula used to calculate the volume to exchange is: volume (mL) = blood volume × (observed Hct–desired Hct)/observed Hct, where blood volume is 80–100 mL/kg body weight. The use of normal saline or lactated Ringer's for the isovolemic exchange effectively lowers viscosity, although albumin can also be used.[118,119] However, the long-term benefits of partial exchange transfusion have not been clearly demonstrated. The long-term outcome of these infants depends on the etiology of the problem, and the presence of associated conditions that may also have an effect on neurologic development (hypoglycemia, asphyxia, infection). Regardless of treatment, infants with polycythemia and hyperviscosity are at increased risk of neurologic deficits and developmental delay.[115,120]

Hyperbilirubinemia

Although all newborns will have elevated levels of serum bilirubin compared with adult standards, not all will have a serum

Table 68.10 Physiologic and pathologic jaundice.

	Physiologic	Pathologic
Time of onset	> 24 h	< 24 h or > 1 week
Peak bilirubin level	8–12 mg/dL	> 12 mg/dL (term) > 12 mg/dL (preterm) > 5 mg/dL/day
Timing of peak	3–4 days	> 1 week (term) > 2 weeks (preterm)

level exceeding 4 mg/dL and become visibly jaundiced.[121] The toxicity of bilirubin results from its binding to key proteins in the cell and mitochondria, leading to the uncoupling of oxidative phosphorylation and resultant lack of internal energy for cellular metabolism, although other mechanisms are also involved.[122] This is most crucial in tissues of high metabolic rate and with little capability of regeneration (e.g., the brain).

Between 75% and 90% of bilirubin is derived from the breakdown of hemoglobin from either aged RBCs or ineffective erythropoiesis.[123] Bilirubin is bound to albumin in the bloodstream and transported to the liver. There, it is conjugated by glucuronyl transferase and excreted through the bile into the intestinal tract. After the first week after birth, intestinal bacteria convert the conjugated bilirubin to stercobilin, excreted in the stool, and to urobilinogen, a water-soluble colorless pigment that is excreted into the urine.

Table 68.10 outlines the primary definitions of physiologic and pathologic jaundice. Pathologic jaundice most commonly results from excess RBC mass as in polycythemia, or excess RBC destruction. Examples of excess destruction include hemolysis (as in hemolytic disease of the newborn), RBC defects (e.g., spherocytosis), and internal hemorrhages (e.g., cephalhematoma). Several factors, such as acidosis, hypoxia, hypothermia, and medications, reduce binding of bilirubin to albumin and may interfere with its transport to the liver.[123] Decreased conjugation of bilirubin is seen in neonatal hypoglycemia and hypothyroidism. Decreased excretion occurs with certain infections (e.g., transplacental infections, bacterial sepsis, urinary tract infections), genetic enzymatic defects (e.g., Dubin–Johnson), biliary atresia, cystic fibrosis, galactosemia, and with prolonged use of parenteral nutrition.

All term infants should be examined periodically for the presence of jaundice.[124] Recently, a risk index or score has been developed to predict which infants will develop a serum bilirubin > 25 g/dL.[125] Some authors advocate a system-based approach to prevent kernicterus by performing universal screening and plotting the results on an hour-specific nomogram to guide follow-up (Fig. 68.1).[126,127] Regardless, the jaundiced infant should be carefully evaluated prior to institution of therapy. A complete blood count (CBC) should be performed looking to ascertain red cell number and morphology. A high reticulocyte count indicates rapid RBC turnover. If the direct fraction of bilirubin is elevated, transplacental viral and

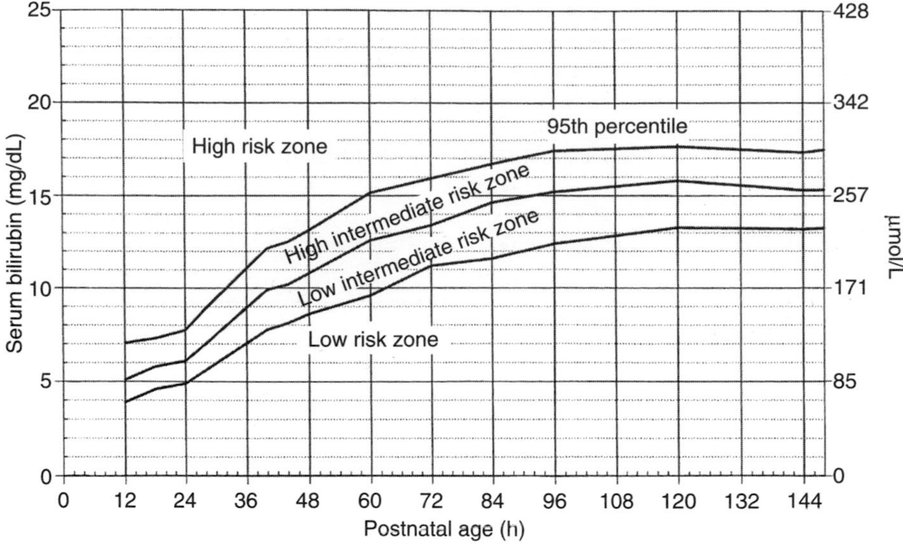

Figure 68.1 Nomogram for designation of risk in well newborns based on the hour-specific serum bilirubin values. From Bhutani VK, Johnson LH, Keren R. Diagnosis and management of hyperbilirubinemia in the term neonate: for a safer first week. *Pediatr Clin North Am* 2004;51:843–861.

parasitic infections should be considered. Blood type determination should be performed on the mother and infant, looking for incompatibility, primarily within the ABO and Rh blood group systems. The presence of an antibody should be sought by performing a Coombs' test. If no etiology is ascertained, a urinalysis and urine culture (urinary tract infection), and possibly a urine-reducing substance test (galactosemia) and a serum T_4 (hypothyroidism) should be performed, even though these etiologies usually present with jaundice either after feedings (lactose) have been introduced or beyond the first several days respectively.[124]

The goal of treatment is to reduce bilirubin encephalopathy, which is the toxicity of an elevated serum bilirubin; this is commonly called kernicterus. However, the term kernicterus refers specifically to bilirubin staining of the basal ganglia, which may be a perimortem or postmortem event.[128] No "toxic" level of bilirubin has been adequately defined.[129] Historically, a level of > 20 mg/dL has been associated with an increased risk of central nervous system pathology among term or near-term neonates. However, the basis for this assumption continues to be questioned.[130] The primary therapies for hyperbilirubinemia have been exchange transfusion and phototherapy. Exchange transfusion has many complications including thrombosis, cardiac arrhythmias, electrolyte disturbances, problems of coagulation, and a potential for infection from the invasive procedure and from the donor blood. The historical mortality is approximately 1%, with morbidity as high as 30–79%, although the majority of adverse events associated with exchange transfusion are laboratory abnormalities and are asymptomatic and treatable.[131,132] Phototherapy is the mainstay of therapy for hyperbilirubinemia. Phototherapy causes photoisomerization of bilirubin molecules into structural isomers that are excreted through the liver and urine.[133] Although phototherapy helps to slow the rate of rise of bilirubin, once it is discontinued, there tends to be a 1–2 mg/dL rebound in the next 12–24 h.

Table 68.11 Adverse effects of phototherapy.

Metabolic
Increased insensible water loss
Overheating
Hypocalcemia (white phototherapy)
Decreased riboflavin (blue phototherapy)
Gastrointestinal
Loose, watery stools
Lactase deficiency
Skin
Bronzing
Rashes
Dark-skinned infants pigment faster
Other
? Retinal degeneration
? DNA damage
Electrical shock

Phototherapy has numerous side-effects, which are listed in Table 68.11.[131,133]

Despite the rising tide of technology in medicine, there is much we presently do not know about the long-range and more subtle types of developmental influences of bilirubin.[129] Hyperbilirubinemia affects each child on an individual basis, and clinicians must be aware of the possible ramifications that even moderate levels of jaundice may contribute in very subtle ways to developmental disability.

Metabolic problems

Hypoglycemia

At the time of delivery, blood or plasma glucose in the fetus is approximately 80–90% of the maternal concentration. SGA fetuses may have below normal blood glucose values. This has been attributed primarily to reduced supply across the placenta.[134] With cord clamping, the neonate is separated from the steady supply of maternal glucose and must resort primarily to mobilization of glycogen stores or an exogenous supply of glucose (feeding, parenteral) to remain normoglycemic. Maintenance of an adequate circulating glucose concentration is critical because it is the principal nutrient used by the neonatal brain, although use of ketone bodies may also provide energy to the brain of the neonate. Gluconeogenesis, mainly through alanine, also contributes to glucose homeostasis after birth.[135] The processes of glycogen breakdown and gluconeogenesis are influenced by hormones such as glucagon, growth hormone, and cortisol, all of which increase markedly after birth. Epinephrine is not an important regulator of glucose metabolism at birth; however, its concentration increases with hypoglycemia. Glucose homeostasis depends not only on its availability, but also on its rate of use. Imbalances between glucose availability and the rate at which it is removed from the circulation result in either hypoglycemia or hyperglycemia.

The cord blood glucose concentration is influenced by the maternal concentration of glucose during labor and delivery.[136] Maternal hydration with glucose-containing solutions prior to Cesarean section or during oxytocin induction can result in maternal and fetal hyperglycemia and fetal hyperinsulinemia. This relative insulin excess may precipitate a more rapid or profound decrease in postnatal glucose concentrations.[137,138] An exaggeration of this mechanism is responsible for the early onset of hypoglycemia in the infants of diabetic mothers.

In normal term neonates delivered vaginally to healthy mothers, there is a rapid fall in plasma glucose to 56 ± 19 mg/dL (mean ± standard deviation) at 1 h and 70 ± 13 mg/dL at 3 h after birth. Then, plasma glucose values remain fairly stable for the first week after birth.[139,140] Normal glucose values in preterm infants are slightly less than those in term infants. Although the definition of hypoglycemia remains controversial, adoption of pragmatic threshold blood glucose concentrations when clinical intervention should be considered has been recommended, particularly in the presence of neurological signs suggestive of hypoglycemia.[141–143] Attention must be paid to whether the values represent plasma or whole blood glucose, as the former are usually between 10% and 15% higher. The common use of rapid reagent strips is acceptable for screening and follow-up of blood glucose levels well within the normal range. However, low values must be confirmed by laboratory determination of true glucose concentrations.[144,145] The presence of a high Hct level may interfere with blood glucose determinations using reagent strips.[146]

The causes of neonatal hypoglycemia are listed in Table 68.12. An altered endogenous glucose production secondary to lack of glycogen storage is the main reason for the common occurrence of hypoglycemia in preterm and SGA infants. Both these groups are also at risk of complications that may increase peripheral glucose use, such as hypoxia, cold stress,

Table 68.12 Common causes of neonatal hypoglycemia.

I. Altered glucose production:
- A. Lack of glycogen stores
    - Prematurity
    - Small for gestational age
- B. Failure of glucose mobilization
    - Endocrine disorders
        - Panhypopituitarism
        - Cortisol deficiency
        - Glucagon deficiency
    - Metabolic disorders
        - Galactosemia
        - Glycogen storage disease, type 1
        - Hereditary fructose intolerance
        - Tyrosinemia

II. Excess glucose utilization:
- A. Hyperinsulinism
    - Infant of diabetic mother
    - Excess glucose administration during labor/delivery
    - Erythroblastosis fetalis
    - Beckwith–Wiedemann syndrome
    - Beta-cell hyperplasia/nesidioblastosis
    - Malposition of umbilical arterial catheter (T11–L1)
    - Leucine sensitivity
    - Maternal drugs (thiazides, beta-adrenergic tocolytics)
- B. Increased peripheral demands
    - Hypoxia
    - Cold stress
    - Infection
    - Polycythemia/hyperviscosity

and infection. Hypoglycemia may also result from endocrine or metabolic disorders that lead to decreased hepatic glucose output. As a group, these disorders are uncommon; however, hypoglycemia is sometimes the presenting manifestation. Infants with panhypopituitarism are of normal weight and length at birth, but the finding of hypoplastic genitalia in male infants (small phallus and scrotum, undescended testis) may suggest this diagnosis. Hepatomegaly, jaundice, and metabolic acidosis are all findings suggestive of a metabolic disorder.

Hypoglycemia due to an insulin excess is most often a result of maternal diabetes. Excessive maternal glucose administration during labor and delivery may produce a transient neonatal hyperinsulinemia and rapid fall in glucose. However, persistently low glucose values should be interpreted as secondary to other causes of hypoglycemia. Infants of diabetic mothers can be large for gestational age, mostly on the basis of weight, but have a head circumference within normal limits. They may exhibit mild degrees of organomegaly and signs of plethora. They are also at high risk of having other metabolic abnormalities (hypocalcemia, hypomagnesemia), respiratory distress, and congenital anomalies most commonly involving the central nervous and cardiovascular systems. Infants of diabetic mothers may develop hypoglycemia soon after birth, and they often remain asymptomatic despite very low glucose values. Organomegaly and other anomalies (e.g., macroglossia, omphalocele, hemihypertrophy, and abnormal ear lobe grooves) are suggestive of Beckwith–Wiedemann syndrome. Hyperplasia of islet cells has been demonstrated in infants with this syndrome and in those with erythroblastosis fetalis. In erythroblastosis fetalis, it has been postulated that the massive hemolysis results in the release of glutathione and inhibition of circulating insulin, with compensatory islet cell hyperplasia. Hypoglycemia secondary to any form of beta-cell hyperplasia may be severe and can persist for several weeks to months. Increased peripheral use of glucose can be seen with hypoxia, cold stress, infection, and polycythemia, despite the presence of adequate glycogen storage and normal insulin levels.

The management of hypoglycemia begins with recognition of the factors that place the neonate at high risk of this condition, so that early glucose screening can be instituted. Attempts to avoid maternal hyperglycemia during labor and delivery must be stressed. The treatment of neonatal hypoglycemia depends on its severity and the availability of the enteral route. In infants with borderline low values detected by reagent strip and no contraindication for feedings, a confirmatory blood or plasma glucose test must be made followed by feeding of 5% dextrose or formula. The latter provides other nutritional sources for energy and gluconeogenesis besides carbohydrates. If correction to euglycemic levels is observed with this intervention, feedings should be advanced as tolerated, and close monitoring of glucose must be continued for at least 24–48 h. Failure to correct glucose levels with this approach or an inability to use the enteral route are indications for parenteral glucose administration. Correction of very low glucose values (< 20–25 mg/dL) is best accomplished by intravenous administration of a minibolus of 200 mg/kg of glucose followed by a constant glucose infusion of 6–8 mg/kg/min.[147] The use of boluses of 25–50% dextrose can result in significant hyperglycemia and rebound hypoglycemia, and should therefore be avoided. A peripheral vein is the preferred route for parenteral glucose administration. The umbilical vein can be used for short-term glucose infusion; however, concerns about infection make it a less desirable route for long-term use. Glucose administration through umbilical arterial catheters placed between T11 and L1 can result in high rates of glucose delivered to the pancreatic vessels and reactive hyperinsulinemia, which resolves after withdrawal of the catheter tip to a lower position. The rate of glucose infusion should be adjusted to maintain normoglycemia. Feedings should be given concomitantly with parenteral glucose whenever possible, unless they constitute the etiology of the hypoglycemia (i.e., galactosemia, tyrosinemia). A high glucose requirement to maintain normoglycemia is suggestive of hyperinsulinism and excess glucose use. If rates in excess of 12–15 mg/kg/min glucose are required, additional therapy is indicated. Corticosteroids (hydrocortisone, 5 mg/kg/day, or prednisone, 2 mg/kg/day), glucagon (300 μg/kg), diazoxide (10–15 mg/kg/day), and epinephrine have been used for the control of hypoglycemia. Corticosteroids act primarily by enhancing gluconeogenesis, whereas glucagon and epinephrine increase glycogen breakdown. Epinephrine also has a powerful anti-insulin effect. Diazoxide suppresses pancreatic insulin secretion. Also, the hormone somatostatin has been used for control of hypoglycemia when hyperinsulinism is suspected.[141]

The prognosis for infants with neonatal hypoglycemia depends on its etiology, the presence of clinical signs and associated conditions, and the duration of hypoglycemia. Neonates with significant seizures secondary to hypoglycemia have a risk of up to 50% of an abnormal neurologic outcome.[142] Abnormal neurologic features observed after neonatal hypoglycemia include low IQ score, seizure disorder, and motor deficits (spasticity, ataxia). These features are the neuropathologic reflection of cortical damage due to the lack of glucose.[148,149] A still unresolved issue is whether marginal or transient hypoglycemia can lead to or worsen damage. Data from a study in preterm neonates suggested that, contrary to general belief, moderate degrees of hypoglycemia can have a significant effect on long-term neurodevelopmental performance.[150] Whether the same is true for term and postterm neonates is not known. However, until the safety of moderate and usually asymptomatic hypoglycemia is demonstrated, neonates with borderline or mildly decreased glucose levels should be properly identified and treated expeditiously.

Hypocalcemia

During the second half of pregnancy, there is rapid fetal accretion of calcium at rates of 110–150 mg/kg/day. Fetal accretion of phosphorus and magnesium is also high. The concentrations of these minerals are higher in cord blood than in the maternal circulation.[151] The cord blood levels of hormones involved in calcium homeostasis are also different from the mother and reflect attempts by the fetus to maximize bone mineralization (Table 68.13). A steady decrease in serum

Table 68.13 Approximate mineral and hormonal levels in maternal and cord blood.

	Maternal	Cord
Minerals (mg/dL)		
Ca	9.2 ± 0.3	10.4 ± 0.5*
iCa	4.5 ± 0.2	5.6 ± 0.3*
P	4.3 ± 1.6	5.8 ± 1.2*
Mg	1.8 ± 0.1	2.0 ± 0.1*
Hormones (% of maternal level)		
Calcitonin	–	180%
Parathormone	–	80–100%
25-OH vitamin D	–	80
1-25 $(OH)_2$ vitamin D	–	30–40%

*Significantly different from the maternal value.

calcium and ionized calcium (iCa) is observed after birth, reaching a nadir at approximately 24 h of age and remaining low for 48–72 h.[152] This decrease in circulating calcium is due to interruption of the transplacental supply and the predominance of hypocalcemic hormones such as calcitonin and glucagon. Both these hormones increase after birth in normal term neonates, and even further elevations are seen with neonatal asphyxia.[153,154] Unlike small preterm infants, term neonates are able to increase parathyroid hormone (PTH) levels in response to decreasing calcium concentrations.[155] The postnatal decrease in serum calcium is also prompted by the transient endogenous phosphorous load secondary to tissue breakdown, which cannot be excreted rapidly by the kidneys.

Neonatal hypocalcemia has been defined as a serum calcium level of < 7–8 mg/dL.[156] In a large proportion of sick preterm infants, serum calcium levels fall to < 7 mg/dL. Because the physiologically important fraction is the iCa, and its concentration cannot be reliably predicted from total calcium determinations, direct measurement of iCa with new electrodes suitable for this purpose has been advocated.[152] Hypocalcemia has been classified as early, which occurs in the first few days after birth, and late, which presents after day 4 or 5. At term, early neonatal hypocalcemia is most commonly seen in asphyxiated neonates and infants of diabetic mothers. In asphyxia, the pathogenesis of hypocalcemia is related to the large phosphorus load secondary to tissue damage and to exaggerated increases in calcitonin and glucagon. In these infants, hypocalcemia may occur despite increased levels of PTH.[154] In contrast, infants of diabetic mothers can show a decrease in PTH secretion during the first days after birth.[157] This has been attributed to fetal and neonatal magnesium deficiency secondary to the chronic maternal loss of magnesium seen with diabetes. Secretion of PTH depends on magnesium concentrations. Other infants at risk of hypocalcemia are those subjected to rapid changes in serum pH, either by correction of acidosis or by hyperventilation, and those who undergo exchange transfusions with blood containing citrate and phosphate as anticoagulants or buffers, which can bind calcium.[158] Late neonatal hypocalcemia may be secondary to a variety of disorders. Abnormalities of calcium and magnesium absorption may present at this time. These may be due to primary intestinal abnormalities or deficiencies in vitamin D metabolism. Ingestion of large phosphorus loads (e.g., from cow's milk) or deficient renal excretion (renal failure) may cause hyperphosphatemia and secondary hypocalcemia. Parathyroid disorders may also present at this time. Primary hypoparathyroidism is seen in DiGeorge's syndrome, which also features abnormal facies, cardiac anomalies (usually conotruncal or of the aortic arch), and defects in T-cell function because of thymic hypoplasia. Maternal PTH excess usually results in transient suppression of neonatal parathyroid function.[159] Protracted hypocalcemia with varying degrees of hyperphosphatemia is suggestive of this diagnosis even in the absence of a positive maternal history.

Neonatal hypocalcemia is often asymptomatic. The signs suggestive of hypocalcemia are primarily jitteriness and irritability, although apnea or seizures can sometimes occur. However, they are not specific and can also be elicited by hypoglycemia, hypomagnesemia, narcotic withdrawal, neurologic disorders, or infection. Chvostek's and Trousseau's signs are uncommon. Heart failure has also been described with severe hypocalcemia.[160] Signs of hypocalcemia are generally seen only when the iCa falls to very low levels. Disappearance of the symptomatology with calcium treatment supports the diagnosis of hypocalcemia. Serial determinations of serum calcium should be performed in neonates at high risk of hypocalcemia and those with suggestive signs. Although iCa measurements are ideal for diagnosing hypocalcemia, they may not be widely available. Persistently low serum calcium values constitute an indication for magnesium and phosphorous determinations. Total protein and albumin measurements are also useful because hypoproteinemia is associated with low serum calcium values; however, in these cases, the iCa is normal. Although the QT interval of the electrocardiogram may be prolonged in hypocalcemia, it is generally not useful in the nursery.[161] Chest radiography and echocardiography are useful when DiGeorge's syndrome is suspected. Despite the thymic hypoplasia of these infants, their lymphocyte count may be normal soon after birth.

Treatment of hypocalcemia is reserved primarily for symptomatic infants. The therapy consists of intravenous administration of 10% calcium gluconate (9.4 mg of elemental calcium/mL) in doses of 100–200 mg/kg, followed by a continuous infusion of approximately 400–800 mg/kg/day. Intravenous calcium gluconate must be administered slowly and with cardiac monitoring because of the possibility of bradycardia. Bolus infusion of calcium gluconate results in marked and transient elevations in serum calcium and iCa. The patency of the vein must be ascertained because extravasation of calcium salts results in skin necrosis. Whether asymptomatic neonates with low serum calcium (< 7 mg/dL), particularly preterm neonates, should be treated is controversial because serum calcium usually returns to normal values spontaneously after the first 3–4 days after birth. Furthermore, controlled studies to evaluate the treatment of hypocalcemia conducted in sick preterm infants with serum calcium levels of < 6–7 mg/dL have failed to show any significant benefit of parenteral calcium administration.[162,163] These findings suggest that, for a majority of newborns, hypocalcemia primarily represents a biochemical abnormality that only merits treatment in a few of them. If serum calcium remains low beyond 4–5 days after birth, or it is refractory to the usual therapy, further evaluation is necessary. Oral calcium gluconate or vitamin D analogs have been used with very limited success to treat or prevent neonatal hypocalcemia. However, the majority of infants with low serum calcium levels either are too sick to be fed or develop hypocalcemia before feedings are initiated or advanced to substantial volumes. The therapy also depends on the etiology of hypocalcemia (e.g., use of low-phosphorous formula for hypocalcemia secondary to hyperphosphatemia, administration of vitamin D for its deficiency, or hypoparathyroidism).

The long-term outcome of neonates with hypocalcemia depends primarily on the associated problems (asphyxia, DiGeorge's syndrome) rather than on the presence of symptoms or serum calcium values. If seizures due to late-onset hypocalcemia are recognized and treated appropriately, the prognosis is almost invariably normal.[164]

Hypomagnesemia and hypermagnesemia

Fetal serum magnesium as well as magnesium accretion increase during the third trimester of pregnancy. Preterm infants have slightly higher serum magnesium than those born at term, probably as a reflection of lower renal excretion. Magnesium and calcium homeostasis is related primarily through PTH and the exchange of these ions in bone. Acute changes in serum magnesium concentrations are inversely related to PTH secretion, but not to calcitonin secretion.[165,166] However, a chronic magnesium deficiency with depletion of tissue stores reduces PTH secretion. This mechanism may be largely responsible for the hypomagnesemia and hypocalcemia of infants of diabetic mothers.[167,168] Magnesium is actively transported across the placenta and, after therapeutic use of magnesium salts in the mother, fetal serum magnesium also increases to approximately 80–90% of the maternal concentration.[169] Under normal circumstances, there is a slow and small increase in serum magnesium after birth.[170] Retrospective evidence had associated prenatal exposure to magnesium sulfate with lower rates of cerebral palsy and intracranial hemorrhage. However, a recent systematic review does not suggest a major role for antenatal administration of magnesium as a useful neuroprotective intervention.[171]

Neonatal hypomagnesemia is defined as a serum magnesium level of < 1.6 mg/dL.[170] It has been described in 9–38% of infants of diabetic mothers and in SGA infants.[172,173] Low serum magnesium has been reported in up to 30% of infants with polycythemia; however, a good correlation between Hct and serum magnesium does not exist. Whether birth asphyxia is, *per se*, a risk factor for hypomagnesemia is controversial. Hypocalcemia often coexists in neonates with hypomagnesemia. Hypoparathyroidism, hyperphosphatemia, and exchange transfusions with citrated blood also constitute risk factors for hypomagnesemia.[158] Deficient magnesium absorption leading to low serum magnesium levels has been described as a primary disorder and is also seen in infants with short gut.

The signs of hypomagnesemia are similar to those of hypocalcemia. Signs of hyperexcitability soon after birth often present despite normal serum iCa and glucose.[173] The treatment of hypomagnesemia consists of administration of magnesium sulfate 50% (50 mg of elemental magnesium/mL) in doses of 0.05–0.25 mL/kg intravenously. Oral supplementation using the same dose can be used in neonates without severe signs such as seizures. Only careful follow-up of serum magnesium is indicated in asymptomatic infants with normocalcemia but low serum magnesium levels because hypomagnesaemia, with few exceptions, is usually transient.

The upper range of serum magnesium in infancy has been reported as 2.8 mg/dL. However, studies have shown that normal term infants usually have serum magnesium below 2.4 mg/dL.[170] Thus, neonatal hypomagnesemia at term is best defined as serum magnesium above 2.5 mg/dL in the first few days after birth. The pathogenesis of neonatal hypermagnesemia is almost invariably the use of magnesium salts in the mother. The adverse neuromuscular effects of magnesium excess derive mostly from its interference with the acetylcholine release at the neuromuscular junction. Clinically, this translates primarily as muscle weakness and lethargy. These signs may interfere with gestational age assessment using neurologic signs.[174] There is no good correlation between serum magnesium and presence of signs of hypermagnesemia. Delayed passage of stools, abdominal distention, and even meconium plug syndrome have also been described in preterm neonates of hypertensive mothers with hypermagnesemia.[174,175] Term infants with serum magnesium below 4 mg/dL are usually asymptomatic or exhibit mild hypotonia. Respiratory depression and apnea may occur with higher levels, particularly in preterm infants.[176] However, asphyxia is uncommon among term infants born to mothers exposed to the usual doses of magnesium sulfate. Although hypermagnesemia suppresses PTH secretion, a decrease in serum calcium following magnesium sulfate therapy has been observed primarily in the mothers and not in their offspring. Despite the suppression of PTH in the infant, serum calcium remains stable or may even increase as a result of an enhanced exchange of magnesium in the bone surface. The treatment of hypermagnesemia consists of support of the cardiorespiratory and renal function as serum magnesium decreases quickly in 48–72 h to levels not usually associated with symptoms. More aggressive therapy, such as exchange transfusion, is not indicated unless there are signs of cardiovascular collapse and renal failure. In these rare cases, the potential benefits of an exchange transfusion must clearly outweigh those of supportive therapy to justify the use of exchange transfusion.

Sepsis/infection

Sepsis, the common term for any viral, bacterial, or parasitic systemic infection of the newborn, is seen in approximately 32 000 full-term births each year in the United States.[177] The two primary modes of infection in the neonatal period are transplacental infection of the fetus and ascending infection in the perinatal period.[178] The term TORCH was popularized in the mid-1970s to denote the transplacental infections of toxoplasmosis (TO), rubella (R), cytomegalovirus (C), and herpes (H). This acronym is easy to remember but, unfortunately, has diverted the focus from the likelihood and evaluation of specific transplacental infections including those mentioned above and a variety of other organisms.[178,179] The neonatal problems observed with infections caused by agents in this group are reviewed in detail in Part V. Infections may have profound effects on development early in the pregnancy, altering the growth of the fetus; in later pregnancy and after birth, they may disrupt the normal formation and function of tissues and organs.

Signs and symptoms of infection may resemble or be disguised by other illnesses of the newborn.[180] Common signs of infection are poor temperature control and apnea; fever is very uncommon in the newborn. Other signs include respiratory distress, poor perfusion, lethargy or irritability, poor feeding tolerance, and hypoglycemia. Irritability may arise from inflammation of the membranes surrounding the brain, but is seen more often with birth asphyxia, drug withdrawal, or central nervous system hemorrhage. Similarly, rather than identifying an infected newborn, hypoglycemia is seen more commonly in the growth-retarded or large for gestational age infant. Physical findings suggesting infection include skin lesions, petechiae, and organomegaly. However, these are generally uncommon.

Neonatal sepsis has been divided into "early onset infections," which usually present at birth or during the first 48–72 h after delivery, and "late onset infections," which appear beyond this period. The most common organisms causing either early or late onset bacterial or fungal sepsis in the neonatal period are listed in Table 68.14. The incidence of group B streptococcal (GBS) infection has fallen dramatically (to less than 1 per 1000 live births) over the past 10 years, primarily because of intrapartum antibiotic prophylaxis.[177] This is usually an ascending infection, and the newborn, although colonized at birth, may not be symptomatic for several days. Infections with Gram-negative bacteria are even less common than GBS infection.[181] It has been suggested recently that the widespread use of antibiotic prophylaxis to prevent GBS disease with drugs such as ampicillin has led to an increase in the rate of significant neonatal infections by Gram-negative bacteria.[182] Nosocomial infections usually manifest beyond 5–7 days after birth and are more common among very premature infants.[183] They are caused most frequently by coagulase-negative *Staphylococcus* species, although other Gram-positive and Gram-negative organisms are detected not infrequently. *Candida* species are most common among extremely low-birthweight infants and generally carry a poor long-term outcome.[184]

The treatment of the neonate with a bacterial or fungal infection is relatively simple. If infection is suspected, cultures of blood, spinal fluid, and urine should be taken. Initially, the choice of antibiotics depends on the suspected organisms. Once culture results are available, they can be adjusted to the specific organisms. Viral and protozoan infections are difficult to treat. The antibiotics available to treat them are generally toxic and have very limited application.

Table 68.14 Common organisms causing sepsis during the neonatal period.

Early-onset sepsis
Group B streptococcus
Escherichia coli
Klebsiella pneumoniae
Listeria monocytogenes
Staphylococcus aureus
Late-onset sepsis
Staphylococcus coagulase negative
Escherichia coli
Enterococcus fecalis
Klebsiella pneumoniae
Staphylococcus aureus
Candida species

Necrotizing enterocolitis

Necrotizing enterocolitis (NEC) is a multifactorial disease.[185] It is the most commonly acquired serious gastrointestinal disease in the neonatal intensive care unit. It affects predominantly premature infants of less than 34 weeks' gestation, with an incidence of 5–15%. It has a wide spectrum of clinical manifestations and may occur in both endemic and epidemic forms. Numerous epidemiologic studies have revealed primarily two associations with NEC: prematurity, with an increased risk of NEC with decreasing gestational age; and feeding, especially with formula.[186,187] Although intestinal ischemia has been suggested as an etiology, only a small proportion of the reported cases of neonatal NEC can be linked to a known ischemic insult.

Studies in animal models have suggested that NEC begins when undigested carbohydrate and other substrates become available to the intestinal flora.[188] Organic acids produced by carbohydrate fermentation lower the luminal pH. There is an alteration in the mucosal tight junctions, allowing luminal proteins to be exposed to the mast cell. This initiates an inflammatory response that may ultimately lead to bowel necrosis. Also, several proinflammatory mediators have been implicated in the pathogenesis of NEC. For instance, elevated levels of platelet-activating factor (PAF) and decreased activity of the enzyme that inactivates this mediator, PAF-acetylhydrolase, have been described in preterm neonates with NEC.[189] Also, it has been shown that human milk, particularly that of mothers delivering preterm, contains this enzyme.[190] Elevated circulating levels of tumor necrosis factor have also been reported among infants with NEC.[189] Proinflammatory cytokines such as interleukin (IL)-6 and anti-inflammatory cytokines such as IL-8 are also increased during NEC.[191,192] However, direct causality attributable to these mediators has not been demonstrated conclusively.

Generally, there are two types of NEC. The first, which accounts for approximately 10% or less of infants with NEC, is found within the first week of life in critically ill neonates who have not been fed enterally. They usually have multiple organ involvement, including renal dysfunction, central nervous system hemorrhage, and tricuspid regurgitation, along with intestinal injury, which may be distributed anywhere within the gastrointestinal tract. Bacteria are not commonly involved because the intestine is only in the first stages of colonization. The cause of this variety is probably intestinal hypoxia associated with birth asphyxia or polycythemia leading to ischemia–reperfusion injury, although the use of exchange transfusions has also been associated with the development of NEC among polycythemic infants.[193] This mechanism has also been implicated in those cases of NEC seen among infants with congenital heart disease.[194] The latter presentation of NEC is generally seen in the healthier growing preterm infant who is being fed enterally. In this situation, the intestine is colonized with bacteria, and the disease is often localized primarily to the terminal ileum and proximal colon, although nearly all areas of the gastrointestinal tract can be involved. Occasionally, NEC affects the entire length of the intestinal tract.

The symptoms of NEC include bloody stools, decreased number of stools, abdominal distention, gastric residuals, along with variable signs of systemic involvement such as lethargy, poor perfusion, and metabolic acidosis. Abdominal radiography may reveal pneumatosis intestinalis, air in the hepatic vascular tree, and/or bowel wall edema. Uncommonly, free air in the peritoneal cavity, due to bowel perforation, is the presenting sign. Classification of the stages of NEC using the criteria proposed by Bell et al.[195] is useful to define its severity and potential prognosis (Table 68.15). However, only stages II and III of NEC from this classification are considered "proven" NEC, whereas the presentation of stage I NEC is frequently seen with sepsis (without NEC), feeding intolerance, and other etiologies.

The therapy for NEC has remained relativity unchanged for the last 20 years. Feedings should be stopped and the infant placed on intravenous fluids, while attempts are made to decompress the bowel with the use of low intermittent suction. Broad-spectrum antibiotics should be started after appropriate cultures have been taken, along with general supportive care, including correction of metabolic acidosis. Only about 30–50% of cases of NEC are associated with positive blood culture results, usually for Gram-negative bacteria in the most severe cases.[187] Should the disease progress to the point of intestinal perforation, the necrotic portion of the intestine is removed surgically, usually leaving an intestinal ostomy. Bowel perforation is the main indication for surgical intervention in infants with NEC, although a lack of clinical improvement with medical therapy, the persistence of a fixed loop of bowel on abdominal radiography (suggestive of bowel necrosis), and signs of intestinal obstruction are often the reason for surgical involvement. Feedings may be resumed after several weeks of bowel recovery. The mortality still ranges from 30% to 50% for the most severe forms of NEC, even with aggressive medical and surgical management.[187]

Predictors of outcome, for both the intestine and the neonate, relate to the extent and severity of intestinal inflammation and the presence of severe systemic involvement. Neutropenia and thrombocytopenia suggest active consumption in the intestinal and systemic inflammatory process. Those infants who have severe metabolic acidosis refractory to therapy, hypotension, shock, and disseminated intravascular coagulation have the poorest prognosis. Even if the infant survives, he or she will usually have a prolonged hospital course.[196] Long-term complications in infants who recover include strictures, enterocolonic fistulas, malabsorption, and postsurgical short bowel syndrome.[197] There may also be complications of parenteral nutrition, such as infection and cholestasis. Moreover, recent evidence suggests that infants

Table 68.15 Bell's staging for necrotizing enterocolitis (NEC).

Stage I Suspect	Stage II Definite	Stage III Advanced
Any one or more historical factors producing perinatal stress	Any one or more historical factors	Any one or more historical factors
Systemic manifestations – temperature instability, lethargy, apnea, bradycardia	Signs and symptoms as in Stage 1 plus persistent occult or gross gastrointestinal bleeding; marked abdominal distention	Signs and symptoms as in Stage II plus deterioration of vital signs, evidence of septic shock, or marked gastrointestinal hemorrhage
Gastrointestinal manifestations – poor feeding, increasing pregavage residuals, emesis (may be bilious or test positive for occult blood, which may be present in stool with no fissure)	Abdominal radiographs show significant intestinal distention with ileus; small bowel separation (edema in bowel wall or peritoneal fluid), unchanging or persistent "rigid" bowel loops, pneumatosis intestinalis, portal vein gas	Abdominal radiographs may show pneumoperitoneum in addition to signs listed for Stage II
Exclude other disorders via bacterial cultures, electrolyte analysis, maternal drug history, coagulation studies, and contrast studies		

with severe NEC are also at very high risk of poor long-term neurologic outcome.[198]

Retinopathy of prematurity

Retinopathy of prematurity (ROP), formerly called retrolental fibroplasia, is a vasoproliferative retinopathy that occurs almost exclusively in preterm infants. Normal vascularization of the retina begins at the optic disk and advances peripherally between 16 and 44 weeks' gestation. After preterm birth, there may be a cessation of normal vascular growth followed by a period of neovascularization. When this vascular regrowth proliferates out of the plane of the retina and into the vitreous, partial or total retinal detachment can result. The factors that control these processes are currently not well understood.[199] ROP is most common in extremely low-birthweight infants. After adjusting for birthweight and gestational age, black infants are less susceptible to ROP than white infants. Additional factors that have been implicated in its pathogenesis by either association or anecdotal evidence include hypercarbia, multiple transfusions, severe apnea and bradycardia, acidosis, and RDS. In general, infants who are sicker and more unstable seem to be at higher risk. Hyperoxia has long been implicated as a cause of ROP. Current evidence suggests that hyperoxia alone is neither a necessary nor a sufficient cause of ROP.[200] Recent speculations that exposure to a bright environmental light might contribute to ROP were not supported by clinical trials of light reduction.[201]

An international classification has been developed for ROP, which allows for assessment of its severity and consistent reporting (Table 68.16).[202] Approximately 90% of cases of ROP regress spontaneously. The remaining 10% of cases progress to severe ROP. Based on data from the Cryotherapy Study conducted in the mid-1980s on 4099 infants with birthweights of less than 1251 g, 66% of surviving infants weighing less than 1251 g developed ROP.[203] Approximately 6% of the infants in this study developed severe (threshold) ROP. In infants weighing less than 751 g, 90% developed ROP and 16% developed threshold ROP. It is unclear whether the increased use of surfactant or corticosteroids has changed the incidence of ROP over the past decade. Laser surgery is now the treatment of choice for threshold or severe ROP. The risk of blindness with threshold ROP has been reduced substantially with laser or cryotherapy treatment.[203,204] Once retinal detachment has occurred, there is little likelihood of restoring vision. Even in infants with mild or regressed ROP, the incidence of myopia, strabismus, and amblyopia is more common than in infants without ROP.[205]

Overall mortality and morbidity of the preterm infant

Over the past 15 years, the survival of preterm infants has been increasing at the lowest end of gestational age, that is around 23–26 weeks (Fig. 68.2).[206] However, clinicians generally underestimate the chances of survival and overestimate the chances of serious morbidity.[207] This may lead clinicians to restrict potentially beneficial or life-saving therapies.[208]

In preterm infants, decreasing birthweight and gestational age are the most important determinants of mortality and morbidity (Table 68.17).[209] At a given birthweight, infants who are more mature have a lower mortality. Similarly, at a given gestational age, infants with higher birthweight have a lower mortality. For reasons that are not fully understood, even after adjustment for birthweight and gestational age, black and female infants have a lower mortality than white and male infants respectively.[209] Higher national neonatal mortality for black infants, compared with white infants, is largely due to the higher proportion of black infants born prematurely and/or with low birthweight.

Acute morbidities increase with decreasing birthweight as shown in Table 68.18. There is also substantial variability

Table 68.16 International classification for ROP.*

Zones	Zone 1 From the center of the optic nerve to twice the distance from the optic nerve to the macula in a circle Zone 2 Circle surrounding the zone 1 circle with the nasal ora serrata as its nasal border Zone 3 Crescent of the circle of zone 2 that did not encompass temporally
Stages	Stage 0 Immature retinal vasculature Stage I Mildly abnormal blood vessel growth. A line is present between the vascular and avascular region Stage II Moderately abnormal blood vessel growth. A ridge is present between the vascular and avascular region Stage III Severely abnormal blood vessels growing toward the center of the eye on or over the ridge Stage IV Partially detached retina Stage V Completely detached retina
Plus disease	Dilation and tortuosity of the peripheral retinal vessels, part of the subclassification given to the above stages

*International Committee for the Classification of Retinopathy of Prematurity. The International Classification of Retinopathy of Prematurity revisited. *Arch Ophthalmol* 2005;123:991–999.

Table 68.17 Mortality by gestational age and birthweight, 1995–1997.

Mortality (%)							
Gestation (weeks)	22–23	24–25	26–27	28–29	30–31	32–33	Total
Total	63.7	27.0	12.0	5.0	2.2	1.0	
Weight (g)							
1750–1999				1.8	1.5	1.2	1.4
1500–1749			4.5	2.7	2.0	1.1	2.2
1250–1499		3.7	3.4	2.7	2.1	2.0	2.8
1000–1249	12.8	7.9	5.3	3.5	3.2	4.5	4.5
750–999	17.4	14.0	8.5	6.6	5.8		10.2
500–749	61.5	31.9	23.7	19.6	23.3		40.0
250–499	87.3	70.5	62.7				84.2

Adapted from Alexander GR, Kogan M, Bader D, et al. US birth weight/gestational age-specific neonatal mortality: 1995–1997 rates for whites, hispanics, and blacks. *Pediatrics* 2003;111:c61–66.

Table 68.18 Common morbidities of infants 501–1500 g as reported by centers of the Vermont Oxford Network in 2004.

	Birthweight (g)				
	501–1500	501–750	751–1000	1001–1250	1251–1500
Respiratory					
RDS	74 (65, 85)	94 (91, 100)	87 (82, 100)	72 (63, 88)	54 (40, 71)
Pneumothorax	5 (2, 6)	10 (0, 14)	6 (0, 10)	3 (0, 5)	3 (0, 4)
Chronic lung disease					
Oxygen at:					
28 days	53 (41, 61)	92 (88, 100)	74 (63, 88)	43 (28, 57)	22 (9, 30)
36 weeks	36 (21, 45)	70 (50, 92)	49 (25, 65)	27 (8, 38)	15 (0, 22)
Symptomatic PDA	37 (26, 45)	57 (40, 71)	51 (33, 65)	33 (20, 44)	19 (8, 25)
NEC	6 (2, 8)	10 (0, 16)	8 (0, 11)	5 (0, 7)	3 (0, 4)
GI perforation	2 (0, 3)	5 (0, 8)	3 (0, 5)	1 (0, 0)	1 (0, 0)
Intraventricular hemorrhage (IVH)	26 (18, 33)	46 (30, 59)	32 (19, 43)	21 (10, 28)	16 (6, 21)
Ultrasound grade					
0	74 (67, 82)	54 (41, 70)	68 (57, 81)	79 (72, 90)	84 (79, 94)
1	11 (5, 15)	12 (0, 18)	12 (0, 18)	11 (0, 15)	10 (0, 14)
2	6 (2, 8)	11 (0, 15)	7 (0, 11)	5 (0, 7)	3 (0, 5)
3	4 (1, 6)	9 (0, 14)	6 (0, 9)	3 (0, 5)	2 (0, 2)
4	5 (2, 7)	14 (0, 21)	7 (0, 11)	2 (0, 3)	1 (0, 0)
Cystic PVL	3 (0, 5)	5 (0, 7)	4 (0, 6)	3 (0, 5)	2 (0, 3)
Retinopathy of prematurity					
ROP (any)	41 (26, 51)	79 (67, 100)	56 (38, 73)	28 (11, 41)	13 (0, 20)
ROP stage					
0	59 (49, 74)	21 (0, 33)	44 (27, 62)	72 (59, 89)	87 (80, 100)
1	18 (8, 23)	19 (0, 28)	24 (8, 33)	18 (0, 25)	10 (0, 14)
2	13 (5, 18)	28 (6, 40)	19 (4, 29)	8 (0, 11)	3 (0, 0)
3	9 (4, 13)	29 (10, 42)	12 (0, 17)	3 (0, 3)	1 (0, 0)
4	1 (0, 0)	2 (0, 0)	1 (0, 0)	0 (0, 0)	0 (0, 0)

Numbers are percentiles (Network Quartiles).

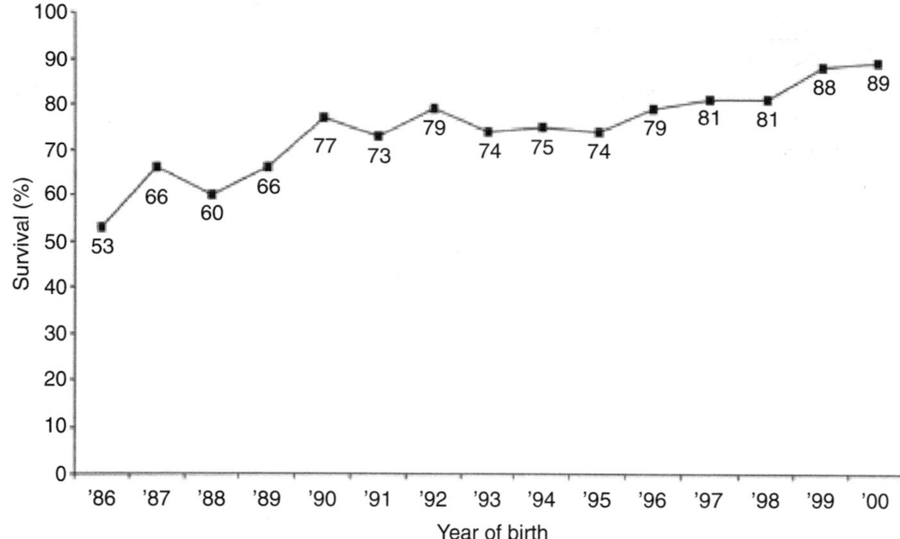

Figure 68.2 Survival by year from 1986 to 2000 for patients with gestational ages of 23–26 weeks. From Hoekstra RE, Ferrera TB, Couser RJ, et al. Survival and long-term neurodevelopmental outcome of extremely premature infants born at 23–26 weeks' gestational age at a tertiary center. *Pediatrics* 2004;113:e1–6.

between centers in the frequency of these complications. The long-term morbidities associated with preterm birth include cerebral palsy, neurodevelopmental delay, chronic lung disease, short bowel syndrome, poor growth, and visual and hearing deficits.

Newborn intensive care is very expensive. The cost is roughly proportional to the length of hospital stay, which is inversely proportional to gestational age.[210] For these reasons, the costs of neonatal care have been increasing for extremely low-birthweight infants. Although these costs are quite high, the cost per life-year gained is quite favorable when compared with adult medical interventions.[211]

Key points

1 The best approach to the management of asphyxia is prevention and anticipation. Although asphyxia occurs primarily in high-risk pregnancies, a sizeable proportion of asphyxiated neonates still present without warning. For this reason, personnel skilled in initiating resuscitation must be present at all deliveries.

2 A good response to neonatal resuscitation is primarily indicated by rapid increases in heart rate, although improvements in color and initiation of spontaneous respiratory efforts are also indicators of a positive response.

3 The most important risk factor for the development of respiratory distress syndrome (RDS) is preterm birth. The incidence of RDS varies inversely with gestational age and can be as high as 60–70% among infants less than 28–29 weeks of gestation. Conversely, RDS is seldom seen beyond 38 weeks of gestation.

4 Administration of exogenous surfactant has become the standard of therapy for infants with RDS who are intubated. Whether used as prophylaxis or rescue therapy, it results in decreases in neonatal mortality and air leaks. However, the occurrence of complications such as intraventricular hemorrhage and bronchopulmonary dysplasia (BPD) is not decreased with surfactant therapy.

5 The incidence of BPD is inversely proportional to gestational age. As the survival of very low-birthweight infants has increased, a "new BPD" is now seen in very small infants who did not have RDS or pneumonia in the first week after birth. This seems to be more the consequence of chronic inflammation, deleterious effects of cytokines and other mediators, and an arrest of the process of normal lung development.

6 The best approach for term infants born through meconium-stained amniotic fluid who have initiated vigorous respiratory efforts is probably just observation, regardless of the characteristics of the meconium. Direct visualization of the larynx and tracheal suctioning are now reserved primarily for infants in need of resuscitation. Thorough endotracheal suctioning will not prevent all cases of meconium aspiration syndrome (MAS).

7 Delivery by Cesarean section without labor constitutes a risk factor for transient tachypnea of the newborn (TTN). Some infants who develop TTN have also been shown to have borderline lung maturity on prenatal amniotic fluid analysis. Additional risk factors are maternal diabetes, prolonged labor, male sex, macrosomia, and asphyxia.

8 Anemia, defined as a Hb below 13 g/dL in term infants, can be the result of hemorrhage, hemolysis, or decreased red cell production. It is uncommon to see anemia secondary to combinations of these factors.

9 Anemia secondary to acute hemorrhage presents with signs of hypovolemia including lethargy, poor capillary refill, tachycardia, weak pulses, hypotension, or pallor. Chronic blood loss over a period of days or weeks permits substantial hemodynamic compensation, so that the main presenting sign is pallor.

10 Hemolytic anemias usually manifest with pallor and early onset of jaundice, but without signs of hypovolemia. ABO or Rh incompatibility and infection are the most common causes of hemolytic anemia in the newborn.

11 Rh isoimmunization frequently results in more significant degrees of anemia and hyperbilirubinemia than ABO incompatibility. The severity of the hemolysis increases with subsequent pregnancies of Rh-positive fetuses.

12 Although there are no generally accepted criteria for the treatment of polycythemia, most centers will intervene on all infants with central venous hematocrit (Hct) above 70% or those with Hct above 65% if they are symptomatic. Treatment consists of a partial exchange transfusion to lower the Hct to a range at which blood viscosity will also be much lower, usually around 50–55%. However, the long-term benefits of partial exchange transfusion have not been clearly demonstrated.

13 All newborns should be examined periodically for the presence of jaundice. The jaundiced infant should be carefully evaluated prior to the institution of therapy.

14 Although the definition of hypoglycemia remains controversial, adoption of pragmatic threshold blood glucose concentrations when clinical intervention should be considered is recommended, particularly in the presence of neurological signs suggestive of hypoglycemia.

15 Correction of very low glucose values (< 20–25 mg/dL) is best accomplished by intravenous administration of a minibolus of 200 mg/kg of glucose followed by a constant glucose infusion of 6–8 mg/kg/min. The use of boluses of 25–50% dextrose can result in significant hyperglycemia and rebound hypoglycemia, and should therefore be avoided.

16 Neonatal hypocalcemia is often asymptomatic. The signs suggestive of hypocalcemia are primarily jitteriness and irritability, although apnea or seizures can sometimes occur. However, they are not specific and can also be elicited by hypoglycemia, hypomagnesemia, narcotic withdrawal, neurologic disorders, or infection.

17 Signs and symptoms of infection may resemble or be disguised by other illnesses of the newborn. Common signs of infection are poor temperature control and apnea; fever is very uncommon in the newborn. Other signs include respiratory distress, poor perfusion, lethargy or irritability, poor feeding tolerance, and hypoglycemia.

18 Necrotizing enterocolitis (NEC) is the most commonly acquired serious gastrointestinal disease in the neonatal intensive care unit. It affects predominantly premature infants of less than 34 weeks' gestation, with an incidence of 5–15%.

19 Hyperoxia has long been implicated as a cause of retinopathy of prematurity (ROP). Current evidence suggests that hyperoxia alone is neither a necessary nor a sufficient cause of ROP. Additional factors that have been implicated in its pathogenesis by either association or anecdotal evidence include hypercarbia, multiple transfusions, severe apnea and bradycardia, acidosis, infection, and RDS.

20 In preterm infants, decreasing birthweight and gestational age are the most important determinants of mortality and morbidity. At a given birthweight, infants who are more mature have a lower mortality. Similarly, at a given gestational age, infants with higher birthweight have a lower mortality. Acute morbidities increase with decreasing birthweight.

References

1 Soothill P, Nicolaides KH, Rodeck CH, Campbell S. Effect of gestational age on fetal and intervillous blood gas and acid–base values in human pregnancy. *Fetal Ther* 1986;13:168.

2 Alvaro RE, Rigatto H. Cardiorespiratory adjustments at birth. In: MacDonald MG, Seshia MMK, Mullet MD, eds. *Avery's neonatology: Pathophysiology and management of the newborn*, 6th edn. Philadelphia: Lippincott, Williams and Wilkins; 2005: 284–303.

3 Milner AD, Vyas H. Lung expansion at birth. *J Pediatr* 1982;101:879.

4 Bland R. Edema formation in the newborn lung. *Clin Perinatol* 1982;9:593.

5 Barker PM, Southern KW. Regulation of liquid secretion and absorption by the fetal and neonatal lung. In: Polin R, Fox W, Abman S, eds. *Fetal and neonatal physiology*, 3rd edn. Philadelphia: Elsevier; 2004:822.

6 Milner AD, Saunders RA, Hoplain IE. Effects of delivery by caesarean section on lung mechanics and lung volume in the human neonate. *Arch Dis Child* 1978;53:545.

7 Sahni R, Schulze K. Temperature control in newborn infants. In: Polin R, Fox W, Abman S, eds. *Fetal and neonatal physiology*, 3rd edn. Philadelphia: Elsevier ;2004:548.

8 Hey E, Katz G. The optimum thermal environment for naked babies. *Arch Dis Child* 1970;45:328.

9 Gilstrap LC, 3rd, Leveno KJ, Burris J, et al. Diagnosis of birth asphyxia on the basis of fetal pH, Apgar score, and newborn cerebral dysfunction. *Am J Obstet Gynecol* 1989;161:825–830.
10 Use and abuse of the Apgar score. Committee on Fetus and Newborn, American Academy of Pediatrics, and Committee on Obstetric Practice, American College of Obstetricians and Gynecologists. *Pediatrics* 1996;98:141–142.
11 Bax M, Nelson KB. Birth asphyxia: a statement. World Federation of Neurology Group. *Dev Med Child Neurol* 1993;35:1022–1024.
12 Wu YW, Backstrand KH, Zhao S, et al. Declining diagnosis of birth asphyxia in California: 1991–2000. *Pediatrics* 2004;114: 1584–1590.
13 Niermeyer S, Kattwinkel J, Van Reempts P, et al. International Guidelines for Neonatal Resuscitation: an excerpt from the Guidelines 2000 for Cardiopulmonary Resuscitation and Emergency Cardiovascular Care: International Consensus on Science. Contributors and Reviewers for the Neonatal Resuscitation Guidelines. *Pediatrics* 2000;106:E29.
14 Wiswell TE, Gannonn CM, Jacob J, et al. Delivery room management of the apparently vigorous meconium-stained neonate: results of the multicenter, international collaborative trial. *Pediatrics* 2000;105:1–5.
15 Vain NE, Szyld EG, Prudent LM, et al. Oropharyngeal and nasopharyngeal suctioning of meconium-stained neonates before delivery of their shoulders: multicentre, randomized trial. *Lancet* 2004;364:597–602.
16 Neonatal Resuscitation Guidelines. *Circulation* 2005;112(Suppl. I):IV-188–IV-195.
17 Catlin EA, Carpenter MW, Braun BS, et al. The Apgar score revisited: influence of gestational age. *J Pediatr* 1986;109: 865.
18 Davis PG, Tan A, O'Donnell CP, Schulze A. Resuscitation of newborn infants with 100% oxygen or air: a systematic review and meta-analysis. *Lancet* 2004;364:1329–1333.
19 Saugstad OD, Ramji S, Vento M. Resuscitation of depressed newborn infants with ambient air or pure oxygen: a meta-analysis. *Biol Neonate* 2004;87:27–34.
20 Perlman JM. Systemic abnormalities in term infants following perinatal asphyxia. Relevance to long-term neurologic outcome. *Clin Perinatol* 1989;16:475.
21 Shah P, Riphagen S, Beyene J, Perlman M. Multiorgan dysfunction in infants with post-asphyxial hypoxic-ischaemic encephalopathy. *Arch Dis Child Fetal Neonatal Ed* 2004;89: F152–155.
22 Paneth N, Stark R. Cerebral palsy and mental retardation in relation to indicators of perinatal asphyxia. *Am J Obstet Gynecol* 1983;147:960.
23 Blair E, Stanley FJ. Intrapartum asphyxia: a rare cause of cerebral palsy. *J Pediatr* 1988;112:515.
24 Grant A, O'Brien N, Joy MT, et al. Cerebral palsy among children born during the Dublin randomized trial of intrapartum monitoring. *Lancet* 1989;2:1233.
25 Gluckman PD, Wyatt JS, Azzopardi D, et al. Selective head cooling with mild systemic hypothermia after neonatal encephalopathy: multicentre randomised trial. *Lancet* 2005;365:663–670.
26 Shankaran S, Laptook AR, Ehrenkranz RA, et al. Whole-body hypothermia for neonates with hypoxic-ischemic encephalopathy. *N Engl J Med* 2005;353:1574–11584.
27 Wegman ME. Annual summary of vital statistics – 1993. *Pediatrics* 1994;94:792–803.
28 Ikegami M, Jacobs H, Jobe A. Surfactant function in respiratory distress syndrome. *J Pediatr* 1983;102:443.
29 Moya F, Montes H, Thomas V, et al. Surfactant protein A and disaturated phosphatidylcholine in tracheal fluid from infants with respiratory distress syndrome. *Am J Resp Crit Care Med* 1994;150:1672–1677.
30 Ikegami M, Rebello CM, Jobe AH. Surfactant inhibition by plasma: gestational age and surfactant treatment effects in preterm lambs. *J Appl Physiol* 1996;81:2517–2522.
31 Ikegami M, Jobe AH. Surfactant metabolism. *Semin Perinatol* 1993;17:233–240.
32 Ablow RC, Gross I, Effmann EI, et al. The radiographic features of early onset group B streptococcal neonatal sepsis. *Radiology* 1977;124:771.
33 Suresh GK, Soll RF. Overview of surfactant replacement trials. *J Perinatol* 2005;25(Suppl. 2):S40–44.
34 Bhat R, John E, Diaz-Blanco J, et al. Surfactant therapy and spontaneous diuresis. *J Pediatr* 1989;114:443.
35 Donn SM, Sinha SK. Respiratory distress syndrome. In: Sinha SK, Donn SM, eds. *Manual of neonatal respiratory care*. Armonk, NY: Futura Publishing Co.; 2000:260–265.
36 Garland JS, Buck RK, Allred EN, Leviton A. Hypocarbia before surfactant therapy appears to increase bronchopulmonary dysplasia risk in infants with respiratory distress syndrome. *Arch Pediatr Adolesc Med* 1995;149:617–622.
37 Plavka R, Keszler M. Interaction between surfactant and ventilatory support in newborns with primary surfactant deficiency. *Biol Neonate* 2003;84:89–95.
38 Soll RF. Synthetic surfactant for respiratory distress syndrome in preterm infants. *Cochrane Database Syst Rev* 2000;2: CD001149.
39 Soll RF, Blanco F. Natural surfactant extract versus synthetic surfactant for neonatal respiratory distress syndrome. *Cochrane Database Syst Rev* 2001;2:CD000144.
40 Merritt TA, Strayer DS, Hallman M, et al. Immunologic consequences of exogenous surfactant administration. *Semin Perinatol* 1988;12:221–230.
41 Hamvas A, Nogee LM, Mallory GB, Jr, et al. Lung transplantation for treatment of infants with surfactant protein B deficiency. *J Pediatr* 1997;130:231–239.
42 Moya FR, Gadzinowski J, Bancalari E, et al. A multicenter, randomized, masked, comparison trial of lucinactant, colfosceril palmitate, and beractant for the prevention of respiratory distress syndrome among very preterm infants. *Pediatrics* 2005;115: 1018–1029.
43 Sinha SK, Lacaze-Masmonteil T, Valls i Soler A, et al. A multicenter, randomized, controlled trial of lucinactant versus poractant alfa among very premature infants at high risk for respiratory distress syndrome. *Pediatrics* 2005;115:1030–1038.
44 Soll RF, Morley CJ. Prophylactic versus selective use of surfactant in preventing morbidity and mortality in preterm infants. *Cochrane Database Syst Rev* 2001;2:CD000510.
45 Crowley P. Antenatal corticosteroids – current thinking. *Br J Obstet Gynaecol* 2003;110(Suppl. 20):77–78.
46 Gross I, Moya FR. Is there a role for antenatal TRH therapy for the prevention of neonatal lung disease? *Semin Perinatol* 2001;25:406–416.
47 Jobe AH, Mitchell BR, Gunkel JH. Beneficial effects of the combined use of prenatal corticosteroids and postnatal surfactant on preterm infants. *Am J Obstet Gynecol* 1993;168:508–513.
48 Jobe AH, Bancalari E. Bronchopulmonary dysplasia. *Am J Respir Crit Care Med* 2001;163:1723–1729.

Index

Page numbers in *italics* and **bold** represent figures and tables respectively